The American Psychiatric Publishing
Textbook of
NEUROPSYCHIATRY AND
BEHAVIORAL NEUROSCIENCES

Fifth Edition

The American Psychiatric Publishing Textbook of

NEUROPSYCHIATRY AND BEHAVIORAL NEUROSCIENCES

Fifth Edition

Edited by

STUART C. YUDOFSKY, M.D.

ROBERT E. HALES, M.D., M.B.A.

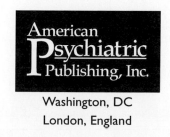

American Psychiatric Publishing, Inc.

Washington, DC
London, England

Manufactured in the United States of America on acid-free paper
11   10   09   08   07   5   4   3   2   1
Fifth Edition

Typeset in Adobe's Revival and Gill Sans.

American Psychiatric Publishing, Inc.
1000 Wilson Boulevard
Arlington, VA 22209-3901
www.appi.org

Library of Congress Cataloging-in-Publication Data
The American Psychiatric Publishing textbook of neuropsychiatry and behavioral neurosciences / edited by Stuart C. Yudofsky, Robert E. Hales. — 5th ed.
   p. ; cm.
   Rev. ed. of The American Psychiatric Press textbook of neuropsychiatry and clinical neurosciences. 4th ed. c2002.
   Includes bibliographical references and index.
   ISBN 978-1-58562-239-9 (hardcover : alk. paper)
   1. Neuropsychiatry. I. Yudofsky, Stuart C. II. Hales, Robert E. III. American Psychiatric Publishing. IV. American Psychiatric Press textbook of neuropsychiatry and clinical neurosciences. V. Title: Textbook of neuropsychiatry and behavioral neurosciences. VI. Title: Neuropsychiatry and behavioral neurosciences.
   [DNLM: 1. Delirium, Dementia, Amnestic, Cognitive Disorders. 2. Nervous System Diseases. 3. Neuropsychology. WM 140 A51277 2008]
   RC341.A44 2008
   616.8—dc22

                                                                                            2007007102

British Library Cataloguing in Publication Data
A CIP record is available from the British Library.

To the women in our lives,

With love...

Beth, Elissa, Lynn, and Emily Yudofsky

Dianne and Julia Hales

Through two decades and five editions of the Textbook,

We are still happily married,

And our daughters still speak with us.

CONTENTS

PART I
BASIC PRINCIPLES OF
NEUROSCIENCE

PART II
NEUROPSYCHIATRIC ASSESSMENT

PART III
NEUROPSYCHIATRIC SYMPTOMATOLOGIES

PART IV
NEUROPSYCHIATRIC
DISORDERS

PART V
NEUROPSYCHIATRIC
TREATMENTS

CONTRIBUTORS

Oyetunde O. Alagbe, M.D.
Postdoctoral Fellow, Department of Psychiatry and Behavioral Sciences, Emory University School of Medicine, Atlanta, Georgia

Susan L. Andersen, Ph.D.
Associate Professor, Department of Psychiatry, Harvard Medical School, Laboratory of Developmental Psychopharmacology and Developmental Biopsychiatry Research Program, McLean Hospital, Belmont, Massachusetts

Theodore J. Anfinson, M.D.
Associate Professor, Department of Psychiatry and Behavioral Sciences, Emory University School of Medicine, Atlanta, Georgia

Liana G. Apostolova, M.D.
Assistant Professor, Department of Neurology, David Geffen School of Medicine, University of California at Los Angeles, Los Angeles, California

Heather A. Berlin, Ph.D., M.P.H.
Postdoctoral Fellow, Department of Psychiatry, Mount Sinai School of Medicine, New York, New York

Rashmi Bhandari, Ph.D.
Clinical Assistant Professor of Anesthesia, Stanford University School of Medicine, Stanford, California

Elizabeth B. Boswell, M.D.
Private practice of psychiatry, Atlanta, Georgia

Nash N. Boutros, M.D.
Professor of Psychiatry and Neurology, Wayne State University School of Medicine, Detroit, Michigan

William G. Brose, M.D.
Adjunct Clinical Professor of Anesthesia, Stanford University School of Medicine, Stanford, California

Michael J. Burke, M.D., Ph.D.
Associate Professor, Department of Psychiatry and Behavioral Health Sciences, Director, Medical Student Education, and Director, Inpatient Psychiatry Services, University of Kansas School of Medicine, Wichita, Kansas

David Glenn Clark, M.D.
Assistant Professor of Neurology, University of Alabama School of Medicine, Birmingham, Alabama

Ronald A. Cohen, Ph.D.
Professor, Department of Psychiatry and Human Behavior, Brown University, and Director of Neuropsychology, Centers for Behavioral Medicine, the Miriam Hospital, Providence, Rhode Island

Cheryl Corcoran, M.D., M.S.P.H.
Assistant Professor of Clinical Psychiatry, Department of Psychiatry, Columbia University College of Physicians and Surgeons, New York, New York

Monica Kelly Cowles, M.D., M.S.
Psychiatry Resident, Department of Psychiatry and Behavioral Sciences, Emory University School of Medicine, Atlanta, Georgia

Jeffrey L. Cummings, M.D.
Augustus S. Rose Professor, Departments of Neurology, Psychiatry, and Biobehavioral Neurosciences, David Geffen School of Medicine, University of California at Los Angeles, Los Angeles, California

Shreenath V. Doctor, M.D., Ph.D.
Private practice of neuropsychiatry, Bellaire, Texas

Dwight L. Evans, M.D.
Ruth Meltzer Professor and Chairman of Psychiatry, Professor of Medicine, Professor of Neuroscience, University of Pennsylvania School of Medicine, Philadelphia, Pennsylvania

Francisco Fernandez, M.D.
Professor and Chair, Department of Psychiatry and Behavioral Medicine, University of South Florida, Tampa, Florida

Ronald E. Fisher, M.D., Ph.D.
Assistant Professor, Departments of Radiology and Neuroscience, Baylor College of Medicine, Houston, Texas; Director of Nuclear Medicine, The Methodist Hospital, Houston, Texas

David V. Forrest, M.D.
Clinical Professor of Psychiatry, Consultation-Liaison Psychiatrist in Neurology, and Faculty, Psychoanalytic Center, Columbia University College of Physicians and Surgeons, New York, New York

Michael D. Franzen, Ph.D.
Associate Professor of Psychiatry, Drexel University College of Medicine, Allegheny General Hospital, Pittsburgh, Pennsylvania

Raymond Gaeta, M.D.
Associate Professor of Anesthesia, Stanford University School of Medicine, Stanford, California

Silvana Galderisi, M.D.
Professor of Psychiatry, University of Naples SUN, Naples, Italy

Subroto Ghose, M.D., Ph.D.
Assistant Professor of Psychiatry, University of Texas Southwestern Medical Center, Dallas, Texas

Kenneth L. Goetz, M.D.
Associate Professor, Department of Psychiatry, Drexel University School of Medicine, Pittsbugh, Pennsylvania

Brenda Golianu, M.D.
Assistant Professor of Anesthesia (Pediatric Anesthesia), Stanford University School of Medicine, Stanford, California

Robert E. Hales, M.D., M.B.A.
Joe P. Tupin Professor and Chair, Department of Psychiatry and Behavioral Sciences, University of California–Davis School of Medicine, Sacramento, California; Medical Director, Sacramento County Mental Health Services, Sacramento, California; Editor-in-Chief, American Psychiatric Publishing, Inc., Arlington, Virginia

Steven P. Hamilton, M.D., Ph.D.
Associate Professor, Department of Psychiatry, University of California–San Francisco, San Francisco, California

Brian T. Harel, Ph.D.
Postdoctoral Resident, Department of Neurology, University of Iowa Hospitals and Clinics, Iowa City, Iowa

Max Hirshkowitz, Ph.D.
Associate Professor, Department of Psychiatry and Department of Medicine, Baylor College of Medicine; Michael E. DeBakey VAMC Sleep Disorders and Research Center, Houston, Texas

Eric Hollander, M.D.
Professor of Psychiatry; Director, Seaver and New York Autism Center of Excellence; Director, Clinical Psychopharmacology; and Director, Compulsive, Impulsive and Anxiety Disorders Program, Department of Psychiatry, Mount Sinai School of Medicine, New York, New York

Paul E. Holtzheimer III, M.D.
Assistant Professor, Department of Psychiatry and Behavioral Sciences, Emory University School of Medicine, Atlanta, Georgia

W. Dale Horst, Ph.D.
Director Emeritus, Psychiatric Research Institute, and Research Professor, Department of Psychiatry and Behavioral Health Sciences, University of Kansas School of Medicine, Wichita, Kansas

Diane B. Howieson, Ph.D.
Associate Professor of Neurology and Psychiatry, Oregon Health and Science University, Portland, Oregon

Robin A. Hurley, M.D., FANPA
Associate Professor, Departments of Psychiatry and Radiology, Wake Forest University School of Medicine, Winston-Salem, North Carolina; Clinical Associate Professor, Department of Psychiatry, Baylor College of Medicine, Houston, Texas; Acting Chief of Staff and Associate Chief of Staff for Mental Health, W.G. "Bill" Hefner VAMC, Salisbury, North Carolina; Co-Director for Education, Mid Atlantic MIRECC, Salisbury, North Carolina

Dennis Kim, M.D.
Instructor, Department of Psychiatry, Harvard Medical School, Developmental Biopsychiatry Research Program, McLean Hospital, Belmont, Massachusetts

H. Florence Kim, M.D.
Assistant Professor, Menninger Department of Psychiatry and Behavioral Sciences, Baylor College of Medicine, and Medical Director, Diagnostic Assessment Unit, The Menninger Clinic, Houston, Texas

Alan J. Lerner, M.D.
Associate Professor of Neurology, Case Western Reserve University, and Director, Memory and Cognition Center, Neurological Institute, University Hospitals Case Medical Center, Cleveland, Ohio

Muriel D. Lezak, Ph.D.
Professor Emerita, Neurology, Oregon Health and Science University, Portland, Oregon

Mark R. Lovell, Ph.D.
Assistant Professor, Department of Orthopedic Surgery, University of Pittsburgh School of Medicine, and Director, Sports Medicine Concussion Program, UPMC Center for Sports Medicine, Pittsburgh, Pennsylvania

Dolores Malaspina, M.D., M.S.P.H.
Professor and Chairman, Department of Psychiatry, New York University Medical Center, New York, New York

Helen S. Mayberg, M.D.
Professor, Department of Psychiatry and Behavioral Sciences, Department of Neurology, Emory University School of Medicine, Atlanta, Georgia

A. Kimberley McAllister, Ph.D.
Associate Professor of Neuroscience, Center for Neuroscience, University of California–Davis, Davis, California

David J. Meagher, M.D., M.R.C.Psych.
Consultant Psychiatrist and Director of Clinical Research, Department of Psychiatry, Midwestern Regional Hospital, Dooradoyle, Limerick, Ireland

Mario F. Mendez, M.D., Ph.D.
Professor of Neurology and of Psychiatry and Biobehavioral Sciences, David Geffen School of Medicine, University of California at Los Angeles, Los Angeles, California

Andrew H. Miller, M.D.
William P. Timmie Professor of Psychiatry and Behavioral Sciences and Director, Psychiatric Oncology/Winship Cancer Institute, Emory University School of Medicine, Atlanta, Georgia

Carryl P. Navalta, Ph.D.
Instructor, Department of Psychiatry, Harvard Medical School, Developmental Biopsychiatry Research Program and Child Outpatient Program, McLean Hospital, Belmont, Massachusetts

Charles B. Nemeroff, M.D., Ph.D.
Reunette W. Harris Professor and Chairman, Department of Psychiatry and Behavioral Sciences, Emory University School of Medicine, Atlanta, Georgia

Eric J. Nestler, M.D., Ph.D.
Professor and Chair, Department of Psychiatry and Center for Basic Neuroscience, University of Texas Southwestern Medical Center, Dallas, Texas

Stephen C. Noctor, Ph.D.
Research Scientist, Institute for Regenerative Medicine, Department of Neurology, University of California–San Francisco, San Francisco, California

Fred Ovsiew, M.D., FANPA
Professor of Psychiatry, University of Chicago; Chief, Clinical Neuropsychiatry Service; and Medical Director, Adult Inpatient Psychiatry, University of Chicago Hospitals, Chicago, Illinois. Diplomate in Behavioral Neurology and Neuropsychiatry.

Ann Polcari, Ph.D., R.N.
Instructor, Department of Psychiatry, Harvard Medical School, Developmental Biopsychiatry Research Program, McLean Hospital, Belmont, Massachusetts

Trevor R.P. Price, M.D.
Private practice of psychiatry, Bryn Mawr, Pennsylvania

Scott L. Rauch, M.D.
Professor of Psychiatry, Harvard Medical School, Boston, Massachusetts; Chair, Partners Psychiatry and Mental Health, and President and Psychiatrist-in-Chief, McLean Hospital, Belmont, Massachusetts

Stephen Rayport, M.D., Ph.D.
Associate Professor of Clinical Neuroscience, Department of Psychiatry, Columbia University College of Physicians and Surgeons, New York, New York

David Riley, M.D.
Professor of Neurology, Case Western Reserve University, and Director, Movement Disorders Center, Neurological Institute, University Hospitals Case Medical Center, Cleveland, Ohio

Robert G. Robinson, M.D.
Paul W. Penningroth Chair, Professor and Head, Department of Psychiatry, University of Iowa College of Medicine, Iowa City, Iowa

Peter P. Roy-Byrne, M.D.
Professor and Vice-Chair, Department of Psychiatry and Behavioral Sciences, University of Washington, Seattle, Washington

Harold A. Sackeim, Ph.D.
Professor of Clinical Psychology in Psychiatry and Radiology, Columbia University College of Physicians and Surgeons; Chief, Department of Biological Psychiatry, New York State Psychiatric Institute, New York, New York

Stephen Salloway, M.D.
Professor, Departments of Clinical Neurosciences and Psychiatry, Brown Medical School, and Director of Neurology and the Memory and Aging Program, Butler Hospital, Providence, Rhode Island

Scott Schobel, M.D.
Postdoctoral Clinical Fellow, Department of Psychiatry, Columbia University College of Physicians and Surgeons, New York, New York

David W. Self, Ph.D.
Associate Professor, Department of Psychiatry and Center for Basic Neuroscience, University of Texas Southwestern Medical Center, Dallas, Texas

Mujeeb U. Shad, M.D.
Assistant Professor of Psychiatry, University of Texas Southwestern Medical Center, Dallas, Texas

Amir Sharafkhaneh, M.D.
Assistant Professor, Department of Medicine, Baylor College of Medicine, and Medical Director, Michael E. DeBakey VAMC Sleep Disorders and Research Center, Houston, Texas

Richard J. Shaw, M.B., B.S.
Associate Professor of Psychiatry and Behavioral Sciences (Child and Adolescent Psychiatry), Stanford University School of Medicine, Stanford, California

Jonathan M. Silver, M.D.
Clinical Professor of Psychiatry, New York University School of Medicine, New York, New York

Mark Snowden, M.D., M.P.H.
Associate Professor, Department of Psychiatry and Behavioral Sciences, University of Washington, Seattle, Washington

Solomon H. Snyder, M.D.
University Distinguished Service Professor of Neuroscience, Pharmacology, and Psychiatry and Director, Department of Neuroscience, Johns Hopkins University School of Medicine, Baltimore, Maryland

David Spiegel, M.D.
Jack, Samuel and Lulu Willson Professor in Medicine, Department of Psychiatry and Behavioral Sciences, Stanford University School of Medicine, Stanford, California

Sergio E. Starkstein, M.D., Ph.D.
Professor of Psychiatry and Clinical Neurosciences, University of Western Australia, Fremantle, Australia

Dan J. Stein, M.D., Ph.D.
Professor, Department of Psychiatry, University of Cape Town, Groote Schuur Hospital, Cape Town, South Africa; Mount Sinai School of Medicine, New York, New York

Yaakov Stern, Ph.D.
Professor of Clinical Neuropsychology in Departments of Neurology, Psychiatry, and the Sergievsky Center, Columbia University College of Physicians and Surgeons; Director of Neuropsychology, Memory Disorders Clinic, Department of Biological Psychiatry, New York State Psychiatric Institute, New York, New York

Lawrence H. Sweet, Ph.D.
Assistant Professor, Psychiatry and Human Behavior, Brown Medical School, and Research Psychologist, Butler Hospital, Providence, Rhode Island

Katherine H. Taber, Ph.D., FANPA
Research Professor, Division of Biomedical Sciences, Virginia College of Osteopathic Medicine, Blacksburg, Virginia; Adjunct Associate Professor, Department of Physical Medicine and Rehabilitation, Baylor College of Medicine, Houston, Texas; Assistant Co-Director for Education, Mid Atlantic MIRECC, Salisbury, North Carolina; Research Scientist, W.G. "Bill" Hefner VAMC, Salisbury, North Carolina

Carol A. Tamminga, M.D.
Professor and Vice Chair of Clinical Research, Department of Psychiatry, University of Texas Southwestern Medical Center, Dallas, Texas

Jun Tan, M.D., Ph.D.
Associate Professor, Department of Psychiatry and Behavioral Medicine, University of South Florida, Tampa, Florida

Martin H. Teicher, M.D., Ph.D.
Associate Professor, Department of Psychiatry, Harvard Medical School, Developmental Biopsychiatry Research Program and Laboratory of Developmental Psychopharmacology, McLean Hospital, Belmont, Massachusetts

Robert W. Thatcher, Ph.D.
Professor, Department of Neurology, University of South Florida, and Director, NeuroImaging Laboratory, Bay Pines VAMC, Bay Pines, Florida

Akemi Tomoda, M.D., Ph.D.
Associate Professor, Department of Child Developmental Sociology, Kumamoto University Hospital, Kumamoto, Japan

Daniel Tranel, Ph.D.
Professor of Neurology and Psychology, Division of Behavioral Neurology and Cognitive Neuroscience, Department of Neurology, University of Iowa College of Medicine, Iowa City, Iowa

Paula T. Trzepacz, M.D.
Medical Fellow, II, Neurosciences Research, Eli Lilly and Company, Indianapolis, Indiana; Clinical Professor of Psychiatry, University of Mississippi Medical School, Jackson, Mississippi; Adjunct Professor of Psychiatry, Tufts University School of Medicine, Boston, Massachusetts; Clinical Professor of Psychiatry, Indiana University School of Medicine, Indianapolis, Indiana

Gary J. Tucker, M.D. (deceased)
Department of Psychiatry and Behavioral Sciences, University of Washington, Seattle, Washington

W. Martin Usrey, Ph.D.
Associate Professor of Neurology, Center for Neuroscience, University of California–Davis, Davis, California

Stuart C. Yudofsky, M.D.
D.C. and Irene Ellwood Professor and Chairman, Menninger Department of Psychiatry and Behavioral Sciences, Baylor College of Medicine; Chairman, Department of Psychiatry, The Methodist Hospital, Houston, Texas

DISCLOSURE OF INTERESTS

The contributors have declared all forms of support received within the 12 months prior to manuscript submittal that may represent a competing interest in relation to their work published in this volume, as follows:

Theodore J. Anfinson, M.D. *Speakers' Bureau:* Bristol-Myers Squibb, GlaxoSmithKline, Janssen, Pfizer.

Jeffrey L. Cummings, M.D. *Grants/Research Support:* Janssen. *Consultant:* Avanir, Eisai, Eli Lilly, EnVivo, Forest, Janssen, Lundbeck, Merz, Myriad, Neurochem, Novartis, Ono, Pfizer, Sanofi-Aventis, Sepracor, Takeda. *Speakers' Bureau:* Eisai, Forest, Janssen, Lundbeck, Merz, Novartis, Pfizer. *Honoraria:* Avanir, Eisai, Janssen, Forest, Lundbeck, Merz, Myriad, Neurochem, Novartis, Ono, Pfizer, Sanofi-Aventis, Sepracor, Takeda. *Board Member:* EnVivo, Myriad, Pfizer.

Dwight L. Evans, M.D. *Grants/Research Support:* National Institute of Mental Health (NIMH). *Consultant:* Abbott, AstraZeneca, Bristol-Myers Squibb/Otsuka, Cephalon, Eli Lilly, Forest, Janssen/Johnson & Johnson, Neuronetics, Pamlab, LLC, Wyeth-Ayerst.

Francisco Fernandez, M.D. *Grants/Research Support:* Cyberonics. *Speakers' Bureau:* Wyeth-Ayerst.

Robert E. Hales, M.D., M.B.A. Symposium chair, American Psychiatric Association Annual Meeting CME program supported by Bristol-Myers Squibb. Teleconference program on poster presentation involving aripiprazole, supported by Bristol-Myers Squibb.

Max Hirshkowitz, Ph.D. *Grants/Research Support:* Sleep center has federally funded research protocols and foundation support. *Consultant:* Cephalon, Takeda, Sanofi-Synthelabo. *Contracts:* Sleep center has contracts with Cephalon, GlaxoSmithKline, Merck, NBI, ResMed, Respironics, Sanofi-Aventis, Sepracor, Takeda. *Speakers' Bureau:* Cephalon, Sanofi, Takeda. *Other:* Sleep center has received free use of equipment for test purposes from Fisher-Paykel, Itamar, Nasal Aire, Puritan Bennett, ResMed, Respironics, Sunrise.

Eric Hollander, M.D. *Grants/Research Support:* National Institute on Drug Abuse (NIDA), NIMH, National Institute on Neurological Disorders and Stroke (NINDS), U.S. Food and Drug Administration Office of Orphan Products Development (OPD-FDA), Abbott, Ortho-McNeil, Somaxon.

Paul E. Holtzheimer III, M.D. *Grants/Research Support/Honoraria:* Abbott, American Psychiatric Association, American Federation for Aging Research, Cyberonics, GlaxoSmithKline, National Center for Research Resources, National Institutes of Health Loan Repayment Program, Neuronetics.

Alan J. Lerner, M.D. *Speakers' Bureau:* Forest, Novartis, Pfizer.

Helen S. Mayberg, M.D. *Grants/Research Support:* Canadian Institutes of Health Research, NIMH, National Alliance for Research on Schizophrenia and Depression (NARSAD). *Consultant:* Advanced Neuromodulation Systems, AstraZeneca, Cyberonics, Eli Lilly, GlaxoSmithKline, Novartis. *Other:* Patent application filed for deep brain stimulation for treatment-resistant depression.

David J. Meagher, M.D., MRCPsych *Grants/Research Support:* Unrestricted educational grant, AstraZeneca.

Andrew H. Miller, M.D. *Grants/Research Support:* NIMH, National Heart, Lung and Blood Institute (NHLBI), GlaxoSmithKline, Janssen, Schering-Plough. *Consultant:* Centecor, Schering-Plough.

Charles B. Nemeroff, M.D., Ph.D. *Grants/Research Support:* NARSAD, NIMH, American Foundation for Suicide Prevention (AFSP), AstraZeneca, Bristol-Myers Squibb, Forest, Janssen, Pfizer, Wyeth-Ayerst. *Consultant:* Abbott, Acadia, Bristol-Myers Squibb, Corcept, Cypress Biosciences, Cyberonics, Lilly, Entrepreneur's Fund, Forest, GlaxoSmithKline, i3 DLN, Janssen, Lundbeck, Otsuka, Pfizer, Quintiles, UCB Pharma, Wyeth-Ayerst. *Speakers' Bureau:* Abbott, GlaxoSmithKline, Janssen, Pfizer. *Board of Directors:* AFSP, American Psychiatric Institute for Research and Education (APIRE), George West Mental Health Foundation, Novell Pharma, National Foundation for Mental Health. *Stockholder:* Acadia, Corcept, Cypress Biosciences, NovaDel. *Equity:* BMC-JR LLC, CeNeRx, Reevax. *Patents:* Method and devices for transdermal delivery of lithium (US 6,375,990 B1); method to estimate serotonin and norepinephrine transporter occupancy after drug treatment using patient or animal serum (provisional filing, April 2001).

Eric J. Nestler, M.D., Ph.D. *Scientific Advisory Board:* Eli Lilly (chair), Helicon, Intra-Cellular Therapies, Neurogen, Neurologix, Neuro-Molecular, Predix Pharmaceuticals, Psychogenics (founder and chair), RxGen.

Scott L. Rauch, M.D. *Grants/Research Support:* Cephalon, Cyberonics, Medtronic Inc, Northstar. *Fellowship Support:* Pfizer. *Consultant:* Cyberonics, Novartis.

David Riley, M.D. *Honoraria:* Boehringer Ingelheim, GlaxoSmithKline.

Peter P. Roy-Byrne, M.D. *Grants/Research Support:* Forest, GlaxoSmithKline, Pfizer. *Consultant/Advisor:* Alza, Cephalon, GlaxoSmithKline, Eli Lilly, Forest, Janssen, Jazz, Pfizer, Pharmacia, Roche, Wyeth-Ayerst. *Speaker's Honoraria:* Forest, GlaxoSmithKline, Novartis, Pfizer, Pharmacia, Wyeth-Ayerst.

Harold A. Sackeim, Ph.D. *Consultant:* Cyberonics, MECTA Lab Corp., Neuronetics, NeuroPace, Pfizer.

Amir Sharafkhaneh, M.D. *Consultant:* Avanir Pharmaceuticals, Hamilton Pharmaceuticals. *Speakers' Bureau:* Forest, Pfizer.

Jonathan M. Silver, M.D. *Consultant:* Novartis. *Speaker:* Avanir.

Mark Snowden, M.D., M.P.H. *Speakers' Bureau:* Pfizer.

Dan J. Stein, M.D., Ph.D. *Grants/Research Support or Consultancy Honoraria:* AstraZeneca, Eli Lilly, GlaxoSmithKline, Lundbeck, Orion, Pfizer, Pharmacia, Roche, Servier, Solvay, Sumitomo, Wyeth-Ayerst.

Carol A. Tamminga, M.D. *Grants/Research Support:* Bristol-Myers Squibb for Physicians Postgraduate Press monograph. *Speaker:* AstraZeneca (once). *Consultant, ad hoc:* Abbott, ARYx Therapeutics, Becker Pharma, Organon, Patterson, Balknap, Webb & Tyler for Johnson & Johnson (once), Saegis, Sumitomo. *Consultant, Drug Development:* Nupathe. *Advisory Board, Drug Development:* Acadia, Avera, Intracellular Therapies, Neurogen.

Martin H. Teicher, M.D., Ph.D. *Grants/Research Support:* NIDA, NIMH, NARSAD, Kodak Inc., Simches family. *Sponsored Research:* Federally sponsored research on a nonpharmacological treatment for ADHD developed by Ambulatory Monitoring, Inc. *Patents:* M.H.T. largely developed the M-MAT technology used in this report for assessing activity and attention disturbances in ADHD and is the holder of six patents relating to assessment of ADHD involving this technology or T2 relaxometry. M-MAT is owned by McLean Hospital and has been licensed to BioBehavioral Diagnostics, Inc, for commercial development, with the potential for M.H.T. to profit in accordance with conflict of interest policies established by Harvard Medical School. M.H.T. also holds four patents on the use of pharmaceutical agents, including *l-threo* methylphenidate for treatment of depression, and for the delivery of methylphenidate, along with a second central nervous system stimulant, for treatment of ADHD. *Other:* M.H.T. has not signed any agreement that would prevent a) publishing both positive and negative results, b) collaborating with other investigators to pool data across sites, or c) publishing without the approval of the sponsor.

Robert W. Thatcher, Ph.D. R.W.T. is an officer in and is affiliated with Applied Neuroscience, Inc, but received no financial or other support from that firm while writing or contributing to this chapter.

Paula T. Trzepacz, M.D. Dr. Trzepacz is a full-time salaried employee of and shareholder in Eli Lilly and Company.

Stuart C. Yudofsky, M.D. Co-chairman, Psychopharmacology Update Breakfast Symposium, sponsored by Bristol-Myers Squibb, at the American Psychiatric Association Annual Meeting. Vice President, Diamond Healthcare Corporation, a private company that specializes in providing inpatient psychiatric, alcoholism, and substance use disorders treatment services.

The following contributors stated that they had no competing interests during the year preceding manuscript submittal: Oyetunde O. Alagbe, M.D.; Susan L. Andersen, Ph.D.; Liana G. Apostolova, M.D.; Heather A. Berlin, Ph.D., M.P.H.; Rashmi Bhandari, Ph.D.; Elizabeth B. Boswell, M.D.; Nash N. Boutros, M.D.; William G. Brose, M.D.; Michael J. Burke, M.D., Ph.D.; David Glenn Clark, M.D.; Ronald A. Cohen, Ph.D.; Cheryl Corcoran, M.D., M.S.P.H.; Monica Kelly Cowles, M.D., M.S.; Shreenath V. Doctor, M.D., Ph.D.; Ronald E. Fisher, M.D., Ph.D.; David V. Forrest, M.D.; Michael D. Franzen, Ph.D.; Raymond Gaeta, M.D.; Silvana Galderisi, M.D.; Subroto Ghose, M.D., Ph.D.; Kenneth L. Goetz, M.D.; Brenda Golianu, M.D.; Steven P. Hamilton, M.D., Ph.D.; Brian T. Harel, Ph.D.; W. Dale Horst, Ph.D.; Diane B. Howieson, Ph.D.; Robin A. Hurley, M.D.; Dennis Kim, M.D.; H. Florence Kim, M.D.; Muriel D. Lezak, Ph.D.; Mark R. Lovell, Ph.D.; Dolores Malaspina, M.D., M.S.P.H.; A. Kimberley McAllister, Ph.D.; Mario F. Mendez, M.D., Ph.D.; Carryl P. Navalta, Ph.D.; Stephen C. Noctor, Ph.D.; Fred Ovsiew, M.D.; Ann Polcari, Ph.D., R.N.; Trevor R. P. Price, M.D.; Stephen Rayport, M.D., Ph.D.; Robert G. Robinson, M.D.; Stephen Salloway, M.D.; Scott Schobel, M.D.; David W. Self, Ph.D.; Mujeeb U. Shad, M.D.; Richard J. Shaw, M.B., B.S.; David Spiegel, M.D.; Sergio E. Starkstein, M.D., Ph.D.; Yaakov Stern, Ph.D.; Lawrence H. Sweet, Ph.D.; Katherine H. Taber, Ph.D.; Jun Tan, M.D., Ph.D.; Akemi Tomoda, M.D., Ph.D.; Daniel Tranel, Ph.D.; W. Martin Usrey, Ph.D.

PREFACE

The roots of the fifth edition of *The American Psychiatric Publishing Textbook of Neuropsychiatry and Behavioral Neurosciences* extend back almost a quarter of a century, to the mid-1980s. At that time in American medicine, "neuropsychiatry" was mostly a historical term that referred primarily to a remarkable era of European psychiatry and neurology that extended from about 1830 to 1900. There were very few psychiatrists in America who identified themselves as being subspecialists in neuropsychiatry, and little original research had been published in this realm in prominent psychiatric or neurological journals.

In 1983, one of us, Robert E. Hales, M.D., was Chairperson of the Scientific Program Committee of the American Psychiatric Association and was responsible for editing the annual Psychiatry Update Series of the American Psychiatric Association. Dr. Hales asked the other of us, Stuart C. Yudofsky, M.D., to edit a section on neuropsychiatry for the fourth volume of the American Psychiatric Association's *Annual Review* series. At that time, Dr. Yudofsky was an Assistant Professor of Psychiatry at Columbia College of Physicians and Surgeons and the chief of an inpatient neuropsychiatry service that was located in the Neurological Institute of Columbia Presbyterian Medical Center. Dr. Hales, a West Point graduate, was also an Assistant Professor and Staff Psychiatrist at Uniformed Services University of Health Sciences in Bethesda, Maryland. By virtue of our clinical assignments—Dr. Hales in a military hospital and Dr. Yudofsky directing an inpatient neuropsychiatric unit in a neurological hospital—we both had treated many patients with psychiatric symptoms associated with traumatic brain injuries and other central nervous system disorders.

The section on Neuropsychiatry for the 1985 *Psychiatry Update: American Psychiatric Association Annual Review* comprised the following chapters and authors (Yudofsky 1985): The Neuropsychiatric Evaluation, by Michael A. Taylor, M.D., Frederick Sierles, M.D., and Richard Abrams, M.D.; Psychiatric Aspects of Brain Injury: Trauma, Stroke, and Tumor, by Stuart C. Yudofsky, M.D., and Jonathan M. Silver, M.D.; Psychiatric Aspects of Movement Disorders and Demyelinating Diseases, by Dilip V. Jeste, M.D., Jack A. Grebb, M.D., and Richard J. Wyatt, M.D.; Interictal Behavioral Changes in Patients with Temporal Lobe Epilepsy, by David Bear, M.D., Roy Freeman, M.D., David Schiff, B.A., and Mark Greenberg, Ph.D.; Dementia Syndrome, by Stephen L. Read, M.D., Gary W. Small, M.D., and Lissy F. Jarvik, M.D., Ph.D.; Substance-Induced Organic Mental Disorders, by Mark S. Gold, M.D., Todd Wilk Estroff, M.D., and A.L.C. Pottash, M.D.; and Future Interfaces Between Psychiatry and Neurology, by Robert M. Post, M.D. Many of these authors became pioneers and leaders in the reemergence of neuropsychiatry that has occurred over the ensuing quarter of a century.

To our surprise and delight, Volume 4 of *Psychiatry Update: The American Psychiatric Association Annual Review* proved to set sales records for the *Annual Review* series, with highly positive reviews and enthusiastic readership responses for the section on neuropsychiatry. This reaction by readers, combined with our ongoing teaching experiences with medical students and psychiatry residents, prompted us to consider writing a different type of neuropsychiatry textbook from that which had heretofore been available:

> We became convinced that the data base, complexity, and relevance of the field have expanded to the point that a new format, utilizing many individual investigators and clinicians with specialized knowledge of critical areas of neuropsychiatry, would have value and usefulness. (Hales and Yudofsky 1987)

Over many decades prior to the first edition of *The American Psychiatric Textbook of Neuropsychiatry*, the standard textbook in neuropsychiatry and behavioral neurology was a singled-authored book by British neuropsychiatrist William Alwyn Lishman entitled *Organic Psychiatry: The Psychological Consequences of Cerebral Disorder*, which in 1987 was in its second edition. European neuropsychiatry can trace its academic origins to the middle of the nineteenth century. During that period, neurology and psychiatry were unified under great academic leaders such as

Wilhelm Griesinger, M.D., who was chairman of a conjoined Department of Neurology and Psychiatry at the University of Berlin (Yudofsky 1995). Although widely recognized as the founder of neuropsychiatry, Griesinger is also acknowledged by some historians as "the first genuine psychiatrist" (Roback 1961). It is worth noting that the conceptual confluence of these two specialties under the leadership of Griesinger had a direct influence on some extraordinarily inventive and productive neuropsychiatrists, including Alois Alzheimer, Arnold Pick, Theodor Meynert, Sigmund Freud, Emil Kraepelin, and Adolf Meyer (Sulloway 1979).

In the Preface to the fourth edition of the *Textbook of Neuropsychiatry and Clinical Neurosciences*, we wrote that since the conception of the Textbook, we were mindful of the seminal European origins of neuropsychiatry, and at the same time especially concerned that our new textbook would be easy to utilize both in clinical settings by American medical practitioners and in academic settings by American students and residents:

> We also set forth what we considered to be the "new turf" of the Textbook: if the previous, grand European texts could be considered an elegant Rolls Royce, we wished to offer a book that could be likened to a hardworking, dependable American Jeep. (Yudofsky and Hales 2002)

We believe that in the fifth edition we have adhered to our original goals. Nonetheless, the Textbook has continuously evolved over each of its editions. Permit us to trace its development in the context of the growth of neuroscience discovery and the advancement of clinical neuropsychiatry over the past two decades.

The second edition of the Textbook, which was published in 1992, was expanded by 32%, from 25 chapters to 33—along with a 60% increase in pages, from 490 to 839. The Textbook's third edition, published in 1997, exactly one decade after the first edition, was again enlarged, this time by four additional chapters and another 285 pages. Most of these increases related to the dramatic strides made in basic neuroscience. In the second and third editions of the textbook, a new section was added that was entitled Basic Principles of Neuroscience. The new section included the chapters Cellular and Molecular Biology of the Neuron; Human Electrophysiology: Cellular Mechanisms and Control of Wakefulness and Sleep; Intracellular and Intercellular Principles of the Pharmacotherapy of Patients with Neuropsychiatric Disorders (third edition), and Functional Neuroanatomy: Neuropsychological Correlates of Cortical and Subcortical Damage. We had thus revised and expanded the second and third editions of the *Textbook of Neuropsychiatry* to

reflect many of the research advances—both clinical and in basic science—that had taken place over the 1990s, which had been termed "The Decade of the Brain."

By the time the third edition was published in 1997, many changes had occurred both in psychiatry and in the status of neuropsychiatry in America. In 1988, American Psychiatric Press, Inc. (APPI) inaugurated the publication of *The Journal of Neuropsychiatry and Clinical Neurosciences* (the *Journal*), with one of us (Dr. Yudofsky) as Editor, and the other (Dr. Hales) as Deputy Editor. Sol Snyder, M.D., Eric Kandel, M.D., Lewis L. Judd, M.D., and the late Gary J. Tucker, M.D., agreed to serve as Consulting Editors. We express especial gratitude to each of these gifted leaders for their contributions to neuropsychiatry and the *Journal* and particularly to Dr. Snyder for the brilliant Introduction to this edition of the Textbook. Dr. Snyder, a psychiatrist, is one of the world's leading researchers in basic neuroscience, and we were fortunate that he, with Brian L. Largent, Ph.D., also contributed an original research article to the inaugural issue of *The Journal of Neuropsychiatry and Clinical Neurosciences* entitled "Receptor Mechanisms in Antipsychotic Drug Action: Focus on Sigma Receptors" (Snyder 1989).

Also in 1988, the American Neuropsychiatric Association (the Association) was founded, and this organization attracted psychiatrists, neurologists, and psychologists whose primary identities were in neuropsychiatry, behavioral neurology, and neuropsychology. In 1991, the *Journal* became the official journal of the Association. Many of the editors of and contributors to the *Journal*, as well as officers and members of the Association, became chapter authors for the third, fourth, and fifth editions of the Textbook. Gradually, the focus and clinical philosophies related to neuropsychiatry, as articulated and manifested in the Association, the Textbook, and the *Journal* became mainstream psychiatry.

One example of this influence was the appointment of Nancy C. Andreasen, M.D., Ph.D., as Editor-in-Chief of the *American Journal of Psychiatry*, the official journal of the American Psychiatric Association. Dr. Andreasen, an Associate Editor of and regular contributor to *The Journal of Neuropsychiatry and Clinical Neurosciences* since its inception, has many research interests in neuropsychiatry, including the study of the brains of living patients with schizophrenia through functional brain imaging. The content of the *American Journal of Psychiatry* progressively included key articles on clinical neuroscience and neuropsychiatry over the years that Dr. Andreasen was Editor-in-Chief, and this focus both reflected and influenced the emphasis of the field of psychiatry.

The Textbook was again expanded significantly in its fourth edition, published in 2002, largely reflecting the continuing influence of neuroscience discovery on neuropsychiatry and behavioral neurology. Highlighting this expansion, we wrote in the Preface to the fourth edition:

> For the Fourth Edition, we have labored to maintain the original goals of the Textbook. Additionally, in light of the great advances in the basic and clinical sciences that comprise the scholarly underpinnings and foundations, the focus on the neurosciences has been expanded in this edition. Great strides have been made over the past decade in the clinical neurosciences, which include, but are not limited to, structural and functional brain imaging, electrophysiology and electrodiagnosis, cell and molecular biology, genetics, and neuropsychopharmacology. Reflecting this intensification, the title of the Textbook has been changed and now includes Clinical Neurosciences. (Yudofsky 2002)

One example of this expansion was Dr. Dolores Malaspina and colleagues' chapter on epidemiologic and genetic aspects of neuropsychiatric disorders. This chapter increased by 60%. The total number of pages in the fourth edition again increased from the previous edition, this time by 261 pages, for a total of 1,375 pages.

One of the most obvious of the many changes in the fifth edition of the Textbook is its change in title. The title has been altered from *The American Psychiatric Publishing Textbook of Neuropsychiatry and Clinical Neurosciences* to *The American Psychiatric Publishing Textbook of Neuropsychiatry and Behavioral Neurosciences*. We decided to change "Clinical" to "Behavioral" for several reasons. First, "clinical neurosciences" is now used to encompass a broad range of medical disciplines, including ophthalmology, otolaryngology, and even anesthesiology. The term "behavioral neurosciences" has recently gained favor and some consensus as the basic science domain of neuropsychiatry and behavioral neurology. Second, many of the readers of the Textbook are neurologists who subspecialize in behavioral neurology. Quite a few behavioral neurologists have suggested that we change the title to be more appealing to their ranks, their students, and their residents. Finally, subspecialty certification as advanced by the American Neuropsychiatric Association now includes both neuropsychiatry (for psychiatrists) and behavioral neurology (for neurologists).

Since the publication of the first edition, we have maintained close contact with our readership and have encouraged their input, criticisms, and suggestions. Increasingly, our readers—especially medical students and residents—have been expressing concern about the ever-expanding size (and cost) of the book. We realized that if this trend continued the Textbook would require two volumes, and perhaps lose sight of its primary mission as stated in the previous prefaces:

> We strove to craft a comprehensive text that would be also clinically relevant and practical to use by medical students, residents of a broad range of medical specialties psychiatrists, neurologists, psychologists and neuropsychologists, and a broad range of professionals who work in a wide range of clinical settings. Thus, it was our intention that the Textbook would be useful to students and clinicians who treat patients in the general hospital setting, in physical medicine/rehabilitation hospitals, in psychiatric institutes and community mental health centers, in alcohol and chemical dependency programs, and in outpatient services and doctors' offices. (Yudofsky 2002)

In summary, with some surprise, we realized that although we had not replicated Professor Lishman's English Rolls Royce, we were well on the way to transforming the Textbook from the practical Jeep originally envisioned into an enormous American Hummer. Practicality and utility had to be reconsidered. Therefore, after much painful decision-making, we have somewhat reduced rather than expanded the size of the fifth edition of the Textbook. Six chapters were removed, including the chapter on Human Electrophysiology and Basic Sleep Mechanisms, some of which was consolidated into the chapter on Neuropsychiatric Aspects of Sleep and Sleep Disorders. Notwithstanding these reductions, several key chapters were not cut, and some even increased in length. Among the latter are Cellular and Molecular Biology of the Neuron; Clinical and Functional Imaging in Neuropsychiatry; and Neuropsychiatric Aspects of Delirium. The chapter on delirium, in fact, was expanded by almost 30 pages, which reflects the aging of the most susceptible populations, the lethality, and the potential reversibility of this condition.

Consistent with the fields of neuropsychiatry and behavioral neurosciences over the past two decades, the Textbook has been a living and evolving entity since it was first published. It is our abiding hope that our efforts and those of our dedicated chapter authors and the extraordinary staff of APPI will be reified in a useful book for professionals who care deeply about understanding and helping the many people among us who suffer from neuropsychiatric disorders.

Stuart C. Yudofsky, M.D.
Robert E. Hales, M.D., M.B.A.

REFERENCES

Hales RE, Yudofsky, SC: Preface. The American Psychiatric Press Textbook of Neuropsychiatry. Edited by Hales RE, Yudofsky, SC. Washington, DC, American Psychiatric Press, 1987, pp xv–xvi

Lishman WA: Organic Psychiatry: The Psychological Consequences of Cerebral Disorder, 2nd Edition. Oxford, UK, Blackwell Scientific, 1987

Roback AA: History of Psychology and Psychiatry. New York, Philosophical Library, 1961

Snyder SH, Largent BL: Receptor mechanisms in antipsychotic drug action: focus on sigma receptors. J Neuropsychiatry Clin Neurosci 1:7–15, 1989

Sulloway FJ: Freud, Biologist of the Mind: Beyond the Psychoanalytic Legend. New York, Basic Books, 1979

Yudofsky SC: Neuropsychiatry, in Psychiatry Update: American Psychiatric Association Annual Review, Vol 4. Edited by Hales RE, Frances, AJ. Washington, DC, American Psychiatric Press, 1985, pp 101–255

Yudofsky SC: Images in psychiatry: Wilhelm Griesinger, M.D., 1817–1868. Am J Psychiatry 152:1203, 1995

Yudofsky SC, Hales RE: Preface. The American Psychiatric Publishing Textbook of Neuropsychiatry and Clinical Neurosciences, 4th Edition. Edited by Yudofsky, SC, Hales RE. Washington, DC, American Psychiatric Publishing, 2002, p xix

ABOUT THE COVER IMAGE

This image was created by Elisabeth Wilde, Ph.D. (Department of Physical Medicine and Rehabilitation, Baylor College of Medicine, Houston, Texas), with the assistance of Jill V. Hunter, M.D. (Texas Children's Hospital, Houston), Zili Chu, Ph.D. (Texas Children's Hospital, Houston), Marco Ramos, B.S. (Baylor College of Medicine), and Jon Chis, M.S. (Phillips Medical Systems). The image portrays fibers emanating from the corpus callosum of a healthy individual, using diffusion tensor imaging (DTI) with fiber tractography generated by utilizing a 30-direction protocol on a 3-tesla Philips magnet (Philips; Best, The Netherlands). Philips PRIDE software was employed to generate the tractographic image. Consistent with convention, red color indicates fibers coursing in a left-right orientation; green, an anterior-posterior direction; and blue, an inferior-superior direction. Though currently considered a research tool, DTI is rapidly evolving and is likely to gain widespread clinical application in the coming years. Because of its sensitivity to alteration in white matter microstructure, DTI has shown remarkable promise in diagnosis, observation of the natural history of disease/recovery, and evaluation of treatment and intervention in several psychiatric and neurological disorders that affect white matter. Several studies have suggested that DTI is capable of detecting clinically relevant changes that may not be as evident using conventional structural imaging sequences.

ACKNOWLEDGMENTS

This book would not have been possible without the generous help and hard work of many people. First, we wish to thank again Solomon H. Snyder, M.D., for his extraordinary and gracious Introduction and our chapter authors who have crafted contributions that are up to date, relevant, and enjoyable to read. We believe we have succeeded in recruiting chapter authors who are not only leaders in their respective fields, but also are excellent at organizing and presenting their material.

Second, we thank the officers and members of the American Neuropsychiatric Association. As are we, many of our authors are members of this association that provides inspiration, leadership, and services through its many educational and public service activities. Since the publication of the Textbook's fourth edition, the Association has helped to spur recognized subspecialty certification in neuropsychiatry and behavioral neurology through its fellowship guidelines and examination programs. Almost every chapter author has been a peer reviewer for, and author of, original research articles in *The Journal of Neuropsychiatry and Clinical Neurosciences*. We believe that the *Journal*, now flourishing in its twentieth year, is a fine complement to this textbook, in that the scientific and clinical information presented here will be systematically updated and expanded by articles that appear in the *Journal*. We encourage readers to consider joining the American Neuropsychiatric Association. For information on membership, please consult the association's Web site at www.neuropsychiatry.com. For subscription information for the *Journal*, please consult the Web site of American Psychiatric Publishing, Inc. (APPI) at www.appi.org.

Since its inception almost a quarter of a century ago, Ronald E. McMillen, Chief Executive Officer of APPI, has participated actively in, or contributed substantively to, each publishing element of each edition of this textbook. We cherish and value our long and productive partnership—and friendship—with Ron. We have also had many prior rewarding collaborations with Roxanne Rhodes, APPI Project Editor for this edition of the textbook. Roxanne is creative, thoughtful, and diligent and understands the value of collegial enterprise and teamwork; she remains on top of all the seemingly endless details required to put together a textbook of this size and complexity, and manages to do so with a positive attitude and a cheerful temperament. Additionally, we express our heartfelt deep appreciation to Lynn Sanders, assistant to Dr. Yudofsky at the Menninger Department of Psychiatry of Baylor College of Medicine. Truly gifted with organizational details and with information technology, Lynn has labored on a daily basis to help coordinate this entire project from its inception. As the friendly but persistent liaison among the authors, APPI staff, and us, she has left no detail overlooked and no question unaddressed.

Since the last edition of the Textbook, the field of neuropsychiatry has lost a great and productive pioneer, and we have lost a close friend. Gary J. Tucker, M.D., has been the author of the chapter on Neuropsychiatric Aspects of Seizure Disorders for the last three editions of the Textbook, as well as having served on its Editorial Board for the third and fourth editions. A beloved mentor, Gary has helped the two of us in incalculable ways in our careers and publishing projects. We are pleased that we were able to dedicate the fourth edition of the Textbook in his honor, while he was still alive. On behalf of the editors, authors and readers of the Textbook, we both wish to express our condolences to his lovely wife, Sharon, and his children, Adam and Clair.

Finally, we thank the many people who purchased the previous four editions of the Textbook. We are grateful for the many e-mails, letters, calls, and face-to-face communications from psychiatrists, neurologists, neuropsychologists, and other professionals and trainees about their experiences with the previous editions. They offered many suggestions and told us what they found helpful and useful about the book in their practices, teaching duties, certification and recertification examinations, and personal edifications. They have informed us about what they believed should have been included, or should have been omitted, in past editions. We have listened and have tried to respond accordingly.

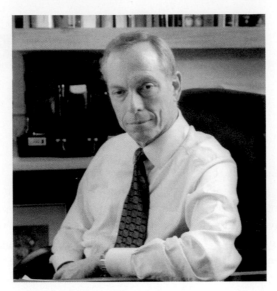

SOLOMON H. SNYDER, M.D.

Solomon H. Snyder was born in Washington, D.C., in December 1938. Dr. Snyder received his undergraduate and medical training at Georgetown University (M.D. 1962); Research Associate training with Julius Axelrod at the National Institutes of Health (1963–1965); and psychiatric training at the Johns Hopkins Hospital (1965–1968). In 1966 he joined the faculty of the Johns Hopkins University School of Medicine (Assistant Professor of Pharmacology, 1966–1968; Associate Professor, Pharmacology/Psychiatry, 1968–1970; Professor, 1970). In 1980 he established the Department of Neuroscience and served as Director (1980–2006). He is presently Distinguished Service Professor of Neuroscience, Pharmacology, and Psychiatry.

Dr. Snyder is the recipient of numerous professional honors, including the Albert Lasker Award for Basic Biomedical Research (1978); the National Medal of Science (2005); the Albany Medical Center Prize (2007); Honorary Doctor of Science degrees from Northwestern University (1981), Georgetown University (1986), Ben-Gurion University (1990), Albany Medical College (1998), Technion University of Israel (2002), Mount Sinai Medical School (2004), and the University of Maryland (2006); the Wolf Foundation Prize in Medicine (1983); the Dickson Prize of the University of Pittsburgh (1983); the Bower Award of the Franklin Institute (1991); the Bristol-Myers Squibb Award for Distinguished Achievement in Neuroscience Research (1996); and the Gerard Prize of the Society for Neuroscience (2000). He is a member of the United States National Academy of Sciences and a Fellow of the American Academy of Arts and Sciences and the American Philosophical Society. He is the author of more than 1,000 journal articles and several books, including *Uses of Marijuana* (1971), *Madness and the Brain* (1974), *The Troubled Mind* (1976), *Biological Aspects of Abnormal Behavior* (1980), *Drugs and the Brain* (1986), and *Brainstorming* (1989).

Many advances in molecular neuroscience have followed from Dr. Snyder's identification of receptors for neurotransmitters and drugs and elucidation of the actions of psychotropic agents. He pioneered the labeling of receptors by reversible ligand binding in the identification of opiate receptors and extended this technique to all the major neurotransmitter receptors in the brain. In characterizing each new group of receptors, he also elucidated actions of major neuroactive drugs. The isolation and subsequent cloning of receptor proteins stems from the ability to label, and thus monitor, receptors by these ligand binding techniques. The application of Dr. Snyder's techniques has enhanced the development of new agents in the pharmaceutical industry by enabling rapid screening of large numbers of candidate drugs. Dr. Snyder applied receptor techniques to elucidate intracellular messenger systems including isolation of inositol 1,4,5,-trisphosphate receptors and elucidation of inositol pyrophosphates as phosphorylating agents. He has established gases as a new class of neurotransmitters, beginning with his demonstrating the role of nitric oxide in mediating glutamate synaptic transmission and neurotoxicity. His isolation and molecular cloning of nitric oxide synthase led to major insights into the neurotransmitter functions of nitric oxide throughout the body. Subsequently, he established carbon monoxide as another gaseous transmitter and D-serine as a glial-derived endogenous ligand of glutamate-NMDA receptors. He has discovered novel mechanisms of cell death involving a nitric oxide-glyceraldehyde-3-phosphate dehydrogenase-Siah pathway as well as an IP_3-cytochrome C-calcium cascade.

Part I

Basic Principles of Neuroscience

CELLULAR AND MOLECULAR BIOLOGY OF THE NEURON

A. Kimberley McAllister, Ph.D.
W. Martin Usrey, Ph.D.
Stephen C. Noctor, Ph.D.
Stephen Rayport, M.D., Ph.D.

Neuropsychiatric disorders are due to disordered functioning of neurons and, in particular, their synapses. Many neuropsychiatric disorders arise from aberrations in neurodevelopmental mechanisms. In the initial stages of brain development, cell-cell interactions are the dominant force in the assembly of the brain (Wichterle et al. 2002). As circuits form, individual neurons and connections are pruned on an activity-dependent basis, driven by intrinsic activity and competition for trophic factors. Neurogenesis does not stop with maturation but in fact continues in some brain regions and appears to be required for mood regulation (Santarelli et al. 2003; Warner-Schmidt and Duman 2006). With further maturation, experience becomes the dominant force in shaping neuronal connections and regulating their efficacy. In the mature brain, these neurodevelopmental mechanisms are harnessed in muted form and mediate most plastic processes (Black 1995; Kandel and O'Dell 1992). Neuropsychiatric disorders arising from problems in early brain development are more likely to be intrinsically or genetically based, whereas those arising during later stages are more likely to be experience based (Toga and Thompson 2005). In senescence, neurodegenerative processes may unravel neural circuits by aberrantly engaging neurodevelopmental mechanisms (Luo and O'Leary 2005).

Experience is so pivotal in fine-tuning neural connectivity that aberrant experience—particularly during critical periods in development—may give rise to or exacerbate neuropsychiatric disorders. For example, monocular occlusion or strabismus in young animals results in permanent pathologic connectivity of the visual system (Hubel et al. 1977). In humans, failure to achieve conjugate gaze in childhood results in permanent visual loss. In mice, early blockade of the serotonin transporter with fluoxetine engenders an anxious phenotype when the mice grow up (Ansorge et al. 2004). In humans, early life stress engenders greater vulnerability to depression in adult life (Caspi et al. 2003). Similar but subtler changes occur in adulthood during learning. From work on the simple nervous systems of organisms such as the marine snail *Aplysia* (Kandel 2001b), it is known that changes in synaptic connections encode memories. Here, too, abnormal experiences may permanently alter patterns of neuronal connectivity. In the human brain, imaging studies have begun to reveal changes in regional brain activity that occur after learning and that are suggestive of changes in the strength of neuronal connections (Maguire et al. 2000; Pantev et al. 1998; Sadato et al. 1996). Some functional neuropsychiatric disorders have now been shown to have a direct impact on brain structure; for example, posttraumatic stress disorder has been associated with alterations in hippocampal size (Kitayama et al. 2005).

In this chapter, we focus first on the cellular function of neurons and then on how they develop. The accelerating pace of recent advances begins now to offer a glimmer of how therapeutic interventions to correct aberrant neuronal growth and differentiation during development and maturation, or later to normalize neuronal signaling, may translate into revolutionary treatments for neuropsychiatric disorders.

CELLULAR FUNCTION OF NEURONS

Individual neurons in the brain receive signals from thousands of neurons and, in turn, send information to thousands of others. Whereas activity in peripheral sensory neurons may represent particular bits of information, activity of networks of neurons in the central nervous system (CNS) represents integrated sensory and associational information. CNS neurons may be seen as part of dynamic cellular ensembles that shift their participation from one network to another as information is used in varied tasks. The sophistication of these networks depends on both the properties of the neurons themselves and the patterns and strength of their connections.

CELLULAR COMPOSITION OF THE BRAIN

Brain cells comprise two principal types: *neurons* and *glia*. Neurons are the substrate for most information processing, whereas glia are classically believed to play a supporting role. Neurons are highly differentiated cells that show considerable heterogeneity in shape and size; in fact, there are more types of neurons than types of cells in any other part of the body. Some are among the largest cells in the body, as in the case of the upper motor neurons that project to the lumbar spinal cord and have axons that are a meter or more in length; others are among the smallest cells in the body, as in the case of the granule cells of the cerebellum. Neurons are quite numerous, and they interconnect via synapses that are still more numerous. The human brain contains 10^{12}–10^{13} neurons. Each neuron forms an average of 10^3 connections, which is a minimal estimate, so the brain has on the order of 10^{15}–10^{16} synapses. In childhood and continuing throughout the life span to a more limited extent, the numbers of neurons and synapses show dramatic changes. During early development, neurogenesis can occur at a rate of up to 250,000 neurons per minute. In childhood, there is considerable refinement in neural circuits, associated with programmed cell death, or apoptosis, and a reduction in the number of synapses. In adulthood, neurogenesis continues, but in a very limited way. In later life, neurodegenerative disorders produce losses in the number of neurons and synapses.

Glial cells can be divided into three classes: 1) astrocytes, 2) oligodendrocytes, and 3) microglia. *Astrocytes* have three traditional functions: they provide the scaffolding of the brain, form the blood-brain barrier, and guide neuronal migration during development. Evidence is accumulating, however, that astroglial cells are more dynamic than previously suspected and are capable of cell-cell signaling over long distances (Dani et al. 1992; Fellin and Carmignoto 2004; Murphy et al. 1993). Moreover, they can influence neuronal activity, enhance neuronal connectivity, and play critical roles in regulating neuronal excitability during normal processes as well as in disease states (Araque et al. 1999; Mennerick and Zorumski 1994; Nedergaard 1994; Pfrieger and Barres 1997). And, they are neural progenitor cells (Noctor et al. 2002). *Oligodendrocytes* produce the myelin sheath that speeds conduction of the action potential along axons. In patients with multiple sclerosis, which results from an immune attack on the principal protein of the myelin sheath, myelin basic protein, there is a failure in action potential conduction (Graham and Lantos 2002). *Microglia* are the macrophages of the brain: quiescent until activated by brain injury.

NEURONAL SHAPE

Neurons share a common organization dictated by their function, which is to receive, process, and transmit information. The great Spanish neuroanatomist Santiago Ramón y Cajal called this *dynamic polarization* (Ramón y Cajal 1894). Although neurons show a wide diversity of sizes and shapes, they generally have four well-defined regions (Figure 1–1): 1) dendrites, 2) cell body, 3) axon, and 4) synaptic specializations. Each region has distinct functions. *Dendrites* receive signals from other neurons, process and modify this information, and then convey these signals to the cell body. As in all cells, the *cell body* contains the genetic information resident in the nucleus that codes for the fabrication of the necessary elements of cellular function, as well as sites for their manufacture, processing, and transport. The *axon* makes highly specific connections and conveys information over long distances to its terminals. Finally, *synaptic specializations* comprise the active zone and synaptic terminal on the presynaptic axon and the postsynaptic density on the postsynaptic dendrite.

A neuron's shape is determined by the cytoskeleton. The cytoskeleton is composed primarily of three filamen-

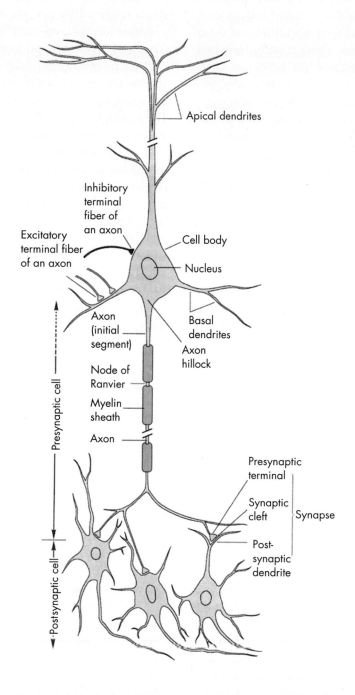

FIGURE I–I.   Functional organization of the neuron. Neurons have distinct cellular regions subserving the input, integration, conduction, and output of information: the dendrites, cell body, axon, and synaptic specializations, respectively. Excitatory and inhibitory neurotransmitters released by other neurons induce depolarizing or hyperpolarizing current flow in dendrites. These currents converge in the cell body, and if the resulting polarization is sufficient to bring the initial segment of the axon to threshold, an action potential is initiated. The action potential travels down the axon, speeded by myelination, to reach the synaptic terminals. Axon terminals form synapses with other neurons or effector cells, renewing the cycle of information flow in postsynaptic cells. As in all cells, the cell body (or perikaryon) is also the repository of the neuron's genetic information (in the nucleus) and the principal site of macromolecular synthesis.

Source.   Reprinted from Kandel ER: "Nerve Cells and Behavior," in *Principles of Neural Science, 4th Edition.* Edited by Kandel ER, Schwartz JH, Jessell TM. New York, McGraw-Hill, 2000, pp. 19–35. Copyright 2000, The McGraw-Hill Companies, Inc. Used with permission.

tous components: 1) microtubules, 2) neurofilaments, and 3) actin (Pigino et al. 2006). *Microtubules* are composed of tubulin subunits and form a scaffold that determines the shape of the neuron. These tubules form bundles that extend throughout the major processes of the neuron and are stabilized by microtubule-associated proteins, called MAPs. *Neurofilaments* are the most abundant cytoskeletal components of the axon and are much more stable than microtubules. These neurofilaments are constituents of neurofibrillary tangles, characteristic of Alzheimer's disease. Finally, *actin* filaments form a dense network concentrated just under the cell membrane. Together with a large number of actin-binding proteins, this network facilitates cell motility and formation of synaptic specializations and allows for plasticity of axonal and dendritic structure (Dillon and Goda 2005). In addition to its important structural role, the cytoskeleton is essential for intracellular trafficking of proteins and organelles and facilitates the selective transport of axonal and dendritic proteins (Burack et al. 2000; Kamal and Goldstein 2002). Thus, cytoskeletal defects are likely to cause devastating neuronal damage—impairing axonal and dendritic transport and cell signaling, and eventually causing cell death (Hirokawa and Takemura 2003). Many neurodegenerative disorders are associated with defects in the trafficking of molecules or synaptic function (Cummings 2003).

NEURONAL EXCITABILITY

Neurons are capable of transmitting information because they are electrically and chemically excitable. This excitability is conferred by a number of classes of ion channels that are selectively permeable to specific ions and that are regulated by voltage (voltage-gated channels), neurotransmitter binding (ligand-gated channels), or by pressure or stretch (mechanically gated channels) (reviewed in Hille 2001). In general, neuronal ion channels conduct ions across the plasma membrane at extremely rapid rates—100 million ions may pass through a single channel in a second. This large flow of current causes rapid changes in membrane potential and is the basis for the action potential, the substrate for information transfer *within* neurons, and for fast synaptic responses, the substrate for information transfer *between* neurons. Ligand-gated channels are often targets for psychiatric drugs, anesthetics, and neurotoxins. As expected, diseases caused by defects in ion channels are diverse and devastating. For example, in myasthenia gravis the immune system mounts an attack on nicotinic acetylcholine receptors; in hyperkalemic periodic paralysis, muscle stiffness and weakness following exercise result from a point mutation in voltage-gated

Na^+ channels; and in episodic ataxia, the generalized ataxia triggered by periods of stress results from point mutation in a delayed-rectifier voltage-gated K^+ channel (reviewed in Koester and Siegelbaum 2000).

Neurotransmitters released by one neuron at synapses activate receptors (ligand-gated channels) on dendrites of other neurons and induce ion flux across the membrane. The resulting electrical signals spread passively over some distance, often reaching the cell body in this way. In addition to passive conductances, localized regenerative mechanisms similar to those that give rise to the action potential (discussed later in this section) amplify dendritic input signals, boosting them so that they can reach the cell body (Eilers and Konnerth 1997; Magee and Carruth 1999; Yuste and Tank 1996). In the cell body, these synaptic inputs combine and, if sufficient, depolarize the initial segment of the axon, or axon hillock, which is the part of the axon closest to the cell body that has the lowest threshold for activation. When a threshold level of depolarization is reached, the action potential is initiated. The action potential, or spike, is an electrical wave that propagates down the axon. In the axon terminals, this wave triggers an influx of calcium (Ca^{2+}), which leads to exocytosis of neurotransmitters from synaptic vesicles at specialized sites called active zones. The released neurotransmitter reaches and activates closely apposed receptors in the postsynaptic density on the postsynaptic cell's dendrites. Ultimately, this information flow reaches effector cells, principally motor fibers that mediate movement and thus generate behavior. Action potentials also back-propagate into dendrites (Johnston et al. 2003), which contributes to the crucial postsynaptic depolarization necessary for long-term potentiation (LTP).

The ability of neurons to generate an action potential derives from the presence of strong ionic gradients across the membrane; sodium (Na^+) and chloride (Cl^-) are highly concentrated outside the membrane, while potassium (K^+) is highly concentrated inside. These gradients are generated by the continuous action of membrane pumps energized by the hydrolysis of adenosine triphosphate (ATP). Also in the membrane are voltage-gated ion channels that regulate the flow of Na^+, K^+, and Ca^{2+} ions across the membrane. At rest, K^+ and Cl^- channels are open so that K^+ and Cl^- gradients determine the membrane potential, causing the cell to be negative inside by about –50 mV to –75 mV. However, if the membrane is depolarized past the threshold potential for generating an action potential, voltage-gated Na^+ channels open rapidly. Because inflow of Na^+ depolarizes the membrane, this confers a regenerative property—once a threshold potential is reached, increased Na^+ influx leads to further depolarization, which opens more Na^+ channels, further enhancing Na$^+$ influx, and so on. Thus, once threshold is reached, the membrane potential switches to +50 mV very rapidly. The membrane potential stays depolarized for only about a millisecond, because Na$^+$ channels then show a time-dependent inactivation (Figure 1–2). Simultaneously, voltage-dependent K$^+$ channels, which are also activated by depolarization but more slowly, increase their permeability. Because K$^+$ flows along its concentration gradient out of the cell, this, together with reduction in Na$^+$ current, leads to the repolarization of the membrane. Thus, the membrane potential peaks at a depolarized level determined by the Na$^+$ gradient and then rapidly returns to the resting potential, determined by the K$^+$ gradient. Once the membrane is repolarized, Na$^+$ inactivation wears off (the time this takes accounts for the refractory period of the neuron, a brief period when the threshold for firing an action potential is elevated), and the cell can fire again.

The regenerative property of the action potential not only serves to amplify threshold potentials (its principal function in dendrites) but also confers long-distance signaling capabilities in the axon (Figure 1–3). When the membrane potential peaks under the control of the increase in Na$^+$ permeability, adjacent regions of the axon become sufficiently depolarized that they, in turn, are brought to threshold and generate an action potential. As successive axonal segments are depolarized, the action potential conducts at great speed down the axon. This is further enhanced by myelination, which increases the rate of conduction several fold by restricting the current flow required for action potential generation to the gaps between myelin segments, the nodes of Ranvier (see Figure 1–3). Because of its all-or-none characteristics and ability to conduct over long distances, the action potential provides a high-quality digital signaling mechanism in neurons.

Although the information that a neuron integrates comes from synaptic input, how the neuron processes that information depends on its intrinsic properties (Llinás 1988; London and Häusser 2005). Many CNS neurons have the ability to generate their own patterns of activity in the absence of synaptic input, firing either at a regular rate (pacemaker firing) or in clusters of spikes (burst firing) (McCormick and Bal 1997). This endogenous activity is driven by specialized ion channels with their own voltage and time dependence that periodically bring the initial segment of the axon to threshold. These channels can be modulated by the membrane potential of the cell or by second-messenger systems. Depending on the activation of these specialized channels, neurons may profoundly change how they respond to a given synaptic input. For example, a thalamic neuron fires as a pacemaker when stimulated from slightly depolarized levels, whereas it fires in bursts of action potentials when stimulated from hyperpolarized levels

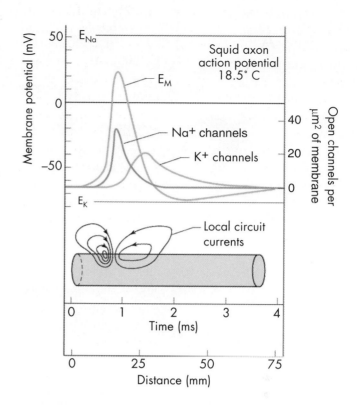

FIGURE 1–2. Opening of ion channels gives rise to the action potential. The upper traces show the two principal currents shaping the action potential, sodium (Na$^+$) and potassium (K$^+$) currents. Once a neuron reaches threshold for firing an action potential, voltage-activated Na$^+$ channels open, giving rise to a rapid inward Na$^+$ current and to the rapid rising phase of the action potential (*green trace*; membrane potential, E$_M$). Once the membrane is depolarized, Na$^+$ channels rapidly inactivate, reducing the Na$^+$ current (*purple trace*) and thereby contributing to the falling phase of the action potential. Then, outward K$^+$ current (*yellow trace*) activates, driving the falling phase of the action potential. K$^+$ channels are slow to open but stay open for much longer than Na$^+$ channels, pulling the E$_M$ back to the resting level. Abbreviations: E$_{Na}$ and E$_K$=the reversal potentials for Na$^+$ and K$^+$, respectively, to which the opening of channels drives the membrane potential (E$_M$). The lower schematic shows the local circuit currents that underlie the propagation of the action potential. The intense loop on the left spreads the depolarization to the right into unexcited membrane, which then renews the cycle, depolarizing the next segment and thereby propagating the action potential.

Source. Reprinted from Hille B, Catterall WA: "Electrical Excitability and Ion Channels," in *Basic Neurochemistry: Molecular, Cellular and Medical Aspects, 7th Edition.* Edited by Siegel GJ, Albers RW, Brady S, Price DL. Burlington, MA, Elsevier Academic, 2006, pp. 95–109. Copyright 2006. Used with permission from Elsevier.

(Llinás and Jahnsen 1982; Sherman 2001) (Figure 1–4). Changes in second-messenger levels may also profoundly

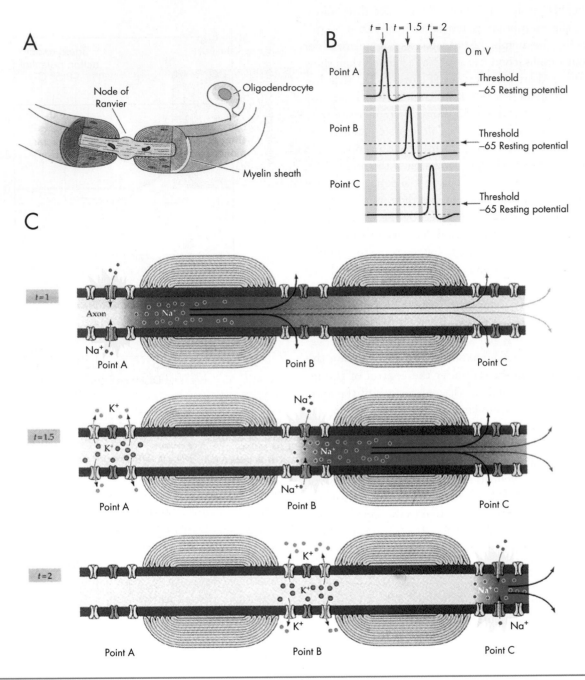

FIGURE 1–3. Action potential conduction in myelinated axon. *Panel A.* Schematic of a myelinated axon. Oligodendrocytes produce the insulating myelin sheath that surrounds the axon in segments. Myelination restricts current flow to the gaps between myelin segments, the nodes of Ranvier, where Na⁺ channels are concentrated. The result is a dramatic enhancement of the conduction velocity of the action potential. *Panel B.* Because sodium channels are activated by membrane depolarization and also cause depolarization, they have regenerative properties. This underlies the "all-or-nothing" properties of the action potential and also explains its rapid spread down the axon. The action potential is an electrical wave; as each node of Ranvier is depolarized, it in turn depolarizes the subsequent node. *Panel C.* The Na⁺ current underlying the action potential is shown in three successive images at 0.5-millisecond intervals and corresponds to the current traces in Panel B. As the action potential (*red shading*) travels to the right, Na⁺ channels go from closed to open to inactivated to closed. In this way, an action potential initiated at the initial segment of the axon conducts reliably to the axon terminals. Because Na⁺ channels temporarily inactivate after depolarization, there is a brief refractory period following the action potential that blocks backward spread of the action potential and thus ensures reliable forward conduction.

Source. Reprinted from Purves D, Augustine GJ, Fitzpatrick D, et al. (eds): *Neuroscience, 3rd Edition.* Sunderland, MA, Sinauer Associates, 2004, p. 64. Used with permission.

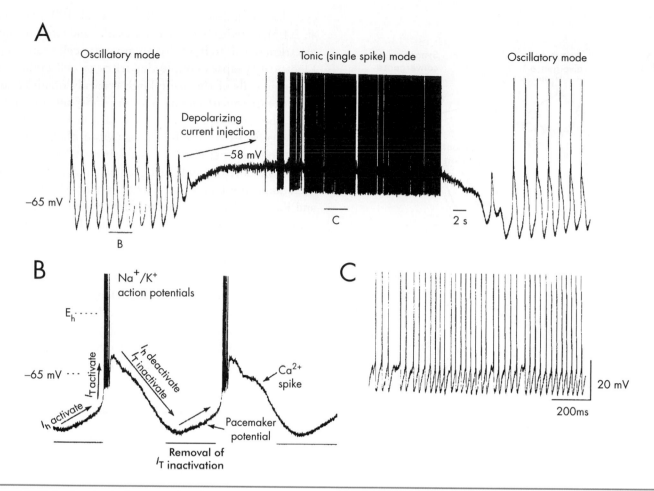

A

Oscillatory mode   Tonic (single spike) mode   Oscillatory mode

Depolarizing
current injection

−58 mV

−65 mV

C

2 s

B

B

Na$^+$/K$^+$
action potentials

E$_h$

−65 mV

I_T activate

I_h activate

I_h deactivate
I_T inactivate

Ca^{2+}
spike

Pacemaker
potential

Removal of
I_T inactivation

C

20 mV

200ms

FIGURE 1–4. Intrinsic properties determine neuronal responses. Many CNS neurons respond differently to the same inputs, depending on their level of depolarization. *Panel A.* Thalamic neurons spontaneously generate bursts of action potentials, resulting from interactions between an inward pacemaker current and a Ca^{2+} current. Depolarization of these neurons changes their firing to a tonic mode. *Panel B.* Action potential bursts at higher time resolution from trace in Panel A. *Panel C.* Higher time resolution of currents in the tonic mode from Panel A. I_h and I_T = the currents through a hyperpolarization-activated channel and a T-type calcium channel, respectively.

Source.   Reprinted from McCormick DA: "Membrane Potential and Action Potential," in *Fundamental Neuroscience, 2nd Edition.* Edited by Squire LR, Roberts JL, Spitzer NC, Zigmond MZ, McConnell SK, Bloom FE. San Diego, CA, Academic Press, 2003, pp. 139–161. Copyright Elsevier 2004. Used with permission.

affect the activity or response properties of neurons, lending still a greater repertoire to the functioning of individual neurons. Thus, synaptic inputs may not only evoke a response in a postsynaptic neuron, but may also shape intrinsic firing patterns, cause a cell to shift from one mode of activity to another, or modulate responses to other synaptic inputs.

SIGNALING BETWEEN NEURONS

Neurons communicate with one another at specialized sites of close membrane apposition called *synapses*. The prototypic axodendritic synapse connects a presynaptic axon terminal with a postsynaptic dendrite. This arrangement is typical for projection neurons that convey informa-

tion from one region of the brain to another. In contrast, local circuit interneurons interact with neighboring neurons. While interneurons may make axodendritic and axosomatic connections, they can also form several other kinds of synaptic contacts that greatly increase their functional sophistication (Figure 1–5). In some cases, dendrites may synapse with dendrites (*dendrodendritic* connections) or cell bodies with cell bodies (*somasomatic* connections), forming local neural circuits that convey information without action potential firing. Axons may synapse onto the axon terminals of other axons (*axoaxonic* connections) and modulate transmitter release by presynaptic inhibition or facilitation. Some neurons may function as both interneurons and projection neurons, the most prominent example

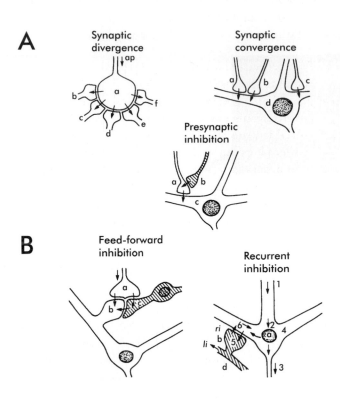

FIGURE 1–5. Modes of interneuronal communication. *Panel A.* Different connection patterns dictate how information flows between neurons. In synaptic divergence, one neuron (a) may disseminate information to several postsynaptic cells (b–f) simultaneously (information flow is shown by *arrows*). Alternatively, in the case of synaptic convergence, a single neuron (d) may receive input from an array of presynaptic neurons (a–c). In presynaptic inhibition, one neuron (b) can modulate information flowing between two other neurons (from a to c) by influencing neurotransmitter release from the presynaptic neuron's terminals; this can be inhibitory (as shown) or facilitatory. *Panel B.* Neurons may modulate their own actions. In feed-forward inhibition, the presynaptic cell (a) may directly activate a postsynaptic cell (b) and at the same time modulate its effects via activation of an inhibitory cell (c), which in turn inhibits the cell (b). In recurrent inhibition, a presynaptic cell (a) activates an inhibitory cell (b) that synapses back onto the presynaptic cell (a), limiting the duration of its activity. ap=action potential; li=lateral inhibition; ri=recurrent inhibition.

Source. Adapted from Shepherd GM, Koch C: "Introduction to Synaptic Circuits," in *The Synaptic Organization of the Brain, 3rd Edition.* Edited by Shepherd GM. New York, Oxford University Press, 1990, pp. 3–31.

being the medium spiny γ-aminobutyric acid (GABA) neurons of the striatum, which comprise about 95% of the neurons in the region (Smith and Bolam 1990).

A minority of local connections are mediated by electrical synapses that do not require chemical neurotransmitters at all. Electrical synapses are formed by multisubunit channels, called *gap junctions*, that link the

cytoplasm of adjacent cells (Bennett et al. 1991; Sohl et al. 2005), allowing both small molecules and ions carrying electrical signals to flow directly from one cell to another. Electrical synapses couple dendrites or cell bodies of adjoining cells of the same kind, typically dendrite-to-dendrite or soma-to-soma. During embryonic development, the ability to pass small molecules, including second messengers, between cells is important for the generation of morphogenic gradients (Dealy et al. 1994). During early brain development, such gradients regulate cell proliferation and establish patterns of connectivity (Kandler and Katz 1995). In the mature brain, electrical synapses act to synchronize the electrical activity of groups of neurons and mediate high-frequency transmission of signals (Bennett 1977; Brivanlou et al. 1998; Tamas et al. 2000). Glial cells are also connected by gap junctions, which link these cells into large syncytia, providing avenues for intercellular propagation of chemical signals mediated by small molecules and ions, such as Ca^{2+}. The importance of gap junctions for glial cell function is underscored by the fact that the X-linked form of Charcot-Marie-Tooth disease results from a single mutation in a connexin gene required for formation of gap junctions between Schwann cells (reviewed in Schenone and Mancardi 1999).

Most CNS synaptic connections are mediated by chemical neurotransmitters. Although chemical synapses are slower than electrical ones, they allow for signal amplification, may be inhibitory as well as excitatory, are susceptible to a wide range of modulation, and can modulate the activities of other cells through the release of transmitters activating second-messenger cascades. There are primarily two classes of neurotransmitters in the nervous system: 1) small molecule transmitters and 2) neuropeptides. In general, *small molecule transmitters* mediate fast synaptic transmission; are stored in small, clear synaptic vesicles; and include glutamate, GABA, glycine, acetylcholine, serotonin, dopamine, norepinephrine, epinephrine, and histamine. The cellular and molecular mechanisms of release of these synaptic vesicles are described in the remainder of this section. In contrast, the *neuropeptides* are a very large family of neurotransmitters that modulate synaptic transmission, are stored in large dense-core vesicles, and include somatostatin, the hypothalamic-releasing hormones, endorphins, enkephalins, and the opioids. Interestingly, small molecule transmitters and neuropeptides are often released from the same neuron and can act together on the same target (Hökfelt 1991).

Small neurotransmitter molecules are stored in small, clear, membrane-bound granules called *synaptic vesicles* (Figure 1–6). Each synaptic vesicle contains several thousand neurotransmitter molecules. When an action potential invades the presynaptic region, the depolarization ac-

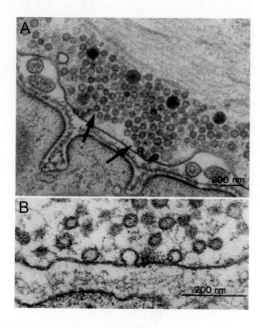

FIGURE 1–6. Synaptic ultrastructure. Neuromuscular junctions from frog sartorius muscle were flash-frozen milliseconds after high potassium treatment to increase synaptic transmission. *Panel A.* Synaptic vesicles are clustered at two active zones (*arrows*), which are sites where vesicles fuse with the plasma membrane to release their neurotransmitter. *Panel B.* At higher magnification, and after stimulation, omega profiles of vesicles in the process of releasing their neurotransmitter are visible.

Source. Reprinted from Schwarz TL: "Release of Neurotransmitters," in *Fundamental Neuroscience, 2nd Edition.* Edited by Squire LR, Roberts JL, Spitzer NC, Zigmond MZ, McConnell SK, Bloom FE. San Diego, CA, Academic Press, 2003, pp. 197–224; original source Heuser JE: "Synaptic Vesicle Endocytosis Revealed in Quick-Frozen Frog Neuromuscular Junctions Treated With 4 Aminopyridine and Given a Single Electrical Shock." *Society for Neuroscience Symposia* 1977; 2:215–239. Copyright 1977.

tivates voltage-dependent Ca^{2+} channels and triggers transmitter release (Figure 1–7). The subsequent Ca^{2+} influx raises the local Ca^{2+} concentration near the active zone, promoting synaptic vesicle fusion and neurotransmitter release via *exocytosis*. Neurotransmitter then diffuses a short distance across the synaptic cleft and binds to postsynaptic receptors. The dynamics and modulation of synaptic transmission are fundamental to alterations in synaptic connections that underlie both normal and pathologic learning and memory. Recently, the molecular machinery (Figure 1–8) involved in synaptic transmission has been increasingly clarified (Sudhof 2004). Interestingly, several potent neurotoxins act directly on this machinery. Current theory is that synaptic transmission comprises a large number of consecutive steps that occur both pre- and

postsynaptically. Within the general events described in Figure 1–7, synaptic vesicles undergo a six-step cycle:

1. Vesicles dock at active zones before exocytotic release.
2. Priming occurs, whereby vesicles become ready to respond to increases in intracellular Ca^{2+}. (The potent neurotoxins botulinum and tetanus toxin block synaptic transmission by proteolysis of key molecules involved in priming.)
3. Triggered by an influx in Ca^{2+}, fusion/exocytosis then occurs in less than a millisecond, releasing the neurotransmitter into the synaptic cleft.
4. Endocytosis recovers the synaptic vesicle membrane.
5. Synaptic vesicles are refilled with neurotransmitter, driven by an acidic intravesicular gradient.
6. The filled synaptic vesicles are transported back to the active zone to complete the cycle.

Neurotransmitter activity is typically limited in duration by several mechanisms that rapidly remove released neurotransmitter from the synapse. First, simple diffusion out of the synaptic cleft limits the duration of action of all neurotransmitters. Second, neurotransmitters may be enzymatically degraded; for example, acetylcholine is hydrolyzed by acetylcholinesterase bound to the postsynaptic membrane adjacent to the receptors. Finally, although the monoamine and amino acid neurotransmitters are also metabolized, they are principally removed from the synaptic cleft by rapid reuptake mechanisms, whereby they are repackaged in synaptic vesicles or metabolized (Masson et al. 1999).

The monoamine neurotransmitter transporters (Figure 1–9), which mediate this rapid reuptake process, are the sites of action of a number of drugs and neurotoxins (Gainetdinov and Caron 2003). Prominent among these are the tricyclic antidepressants, selective serotonin reuptake inhibitors (SSRIs), the psychostimulants, and the neurotoxin 1-methyl-4-phenyl-1,2,3,4-tetrahydropyridine (MPTP). The tricyclics block serotonin and norepinephrine reuptake, while the SSRIs, as their name suggests, block serotonin reuptake. Other newer antidepressants block feedback inhibition of release, thereby increasing synaptic serotonin levels. Cocaine prevents dopamine and serotonin reuptake, whereas amphetamine both slows reuptake of dopamine and serotonin and induces dopamine release (Ramamoorthy and Blakely 1999; Sulzer et al. 2005). Molecular studies have also suggested that cocaine binding and dopamine reuptake occur at separate sites on the transporter, suggesting the possibility that cocaine action could be successfully blocked without impeding normal reuptake (Lin et al. 2000). Mice lacking the dopamine transporter (DAT) show a profound persistence of synaptic dopamine, so

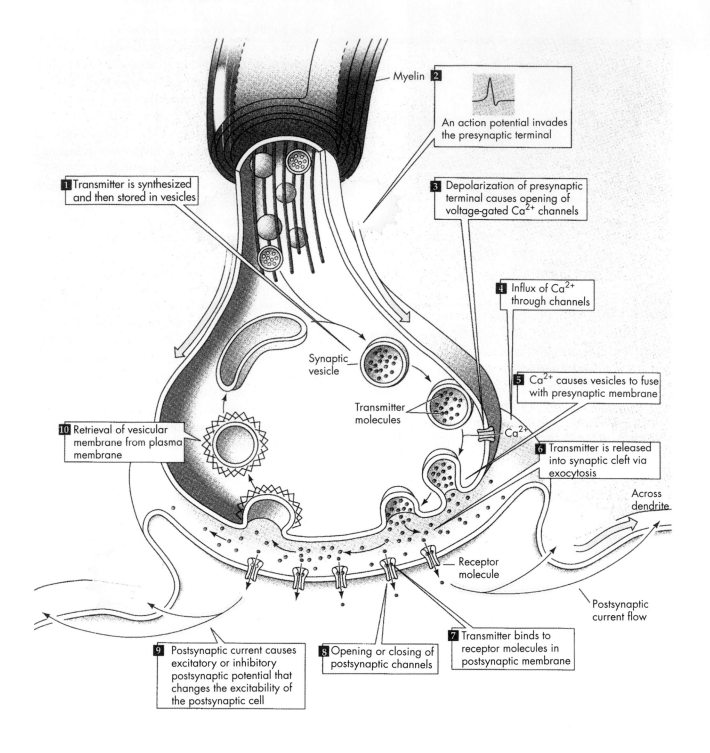

FIGURE 1–7.   Steps in synaptic transmission at a chemical synapse. Essential steps in the process of synaptic transmission are numbered.

Source.   Reprinted from Purves D, Augustine GJ, Fitzpatrick D, et al. (eds): *Neuroscience, 3rd Edition.* Sunderland, MA, Sinauer Associates, 2004, p 97. Used with permission.

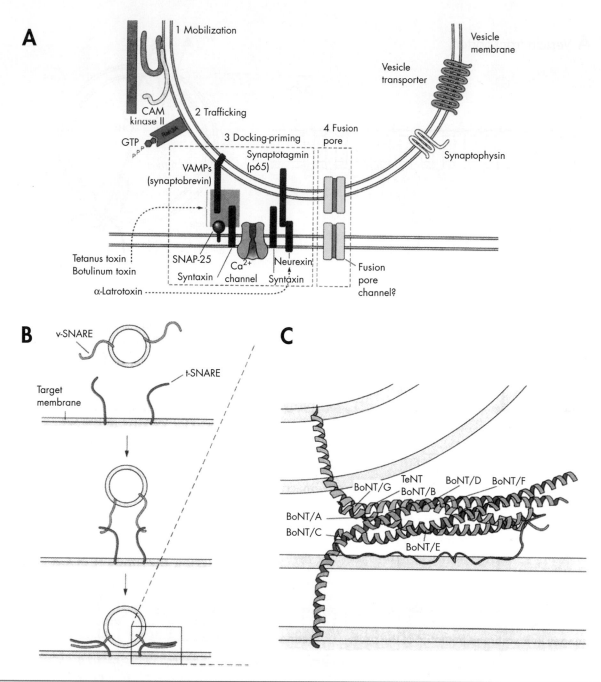

FIGURE 1–8. Molecular events in synaptic vesicle docking and fusion. A coordinated set of proteins is involved in the positioning of vesicles at the presynaptic membrane and in controlling release by membrane fusion. *Panel A.* Many of the synaptic vesicle proteins that have recently been cloned are integral to this process. Some of these proteins interact with the cytoskeleton to position the vesicles at the terminal, while other proteins are integral to the fusion process. In addition, several of these synaptic vesicle proteins are targets for neurotoxins that function by influencing neurotransmitter release. *Panel B.* The current theory for how synaptic vesicles fuse with the membrane and release neurotransmitter is called the SNARE hypothesis. Both the synaptic vesicles and the plasma membrane express specific proteins that mediate docking and fusion: v-SNAREs (synaptic vesicles) and t-SNAREs (plasma membrane). Vesicles are brought close to the membrane through interactions between VAMP (synaptobrevin), syntaxin, and SNAP-25. *N*-ethylmaleimide-sensitive fusion protein (NSF) then binds to the complex to facilitate fusion. Calcium influx is required to stimulate fusion, but the precise binding partner for calcium and the exact events leading to fusion remain obscure. *Panel C.* The crystal structure of the fusion complex, as shown here, is consistent with the SNARE hypothesis. BoNT=botulinum; TeNT=tetanus toxin.

Source. Adapted from Kandel ER, Siegelbaum SA: "Transmitter Release," in *Principles of Neural Science, 4th Edition.* Edited by Kandel ER, Schwartz JH, Jessell TM. New York, McGraw-Hill, 2000, pp. 253–279. Copyright 2000, The McGraw-Hill Companies, Inc. Used with permission.

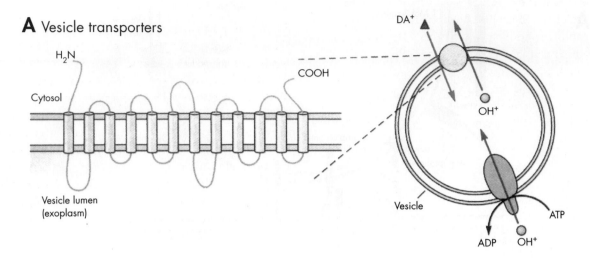

A Vesicle transporters

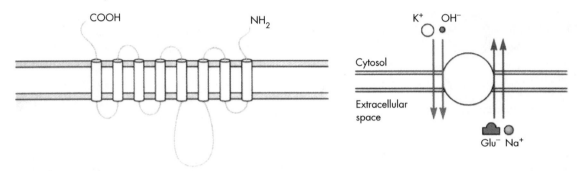

B Glutamate uptake

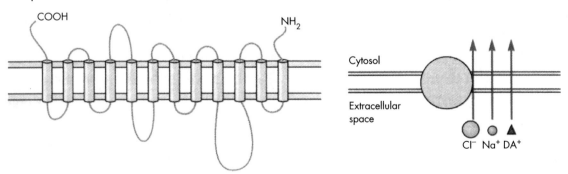

C Uptake of other transmitters

FIGURE 1–9. Neurotransmitter transporters. Synaptic transmission in the CNS is terminated for the most part by reuptake of neurotransmitter by specific transporters with shared molecular motifs. These transporters carry neurotransmitters across membranes against concentration gradients, and thus require metabolic energy. Most often, this energy is provided by cotransport of an ion down its concentration gradient. *Panel A.* One family of transporters in synaptic vesicles serves to load neurotransmitter or transmitter precursors into synaptic vesicles. *Panel B.* A second family of transporters in the plasma membrane with eight transmembrane domains handles amino acid neurotransmitters, such as glutamate and GABA. *Panel C.* A third family of transporters in the plasma membrane with twelve transmembrane domains handles the monoamines dopamine, norepinephrine, and serotonin.

Source.   Reprinted from Schwartz JH: "Neurotransmitters," in *Principles of Neural Science, 4th Edition.* Edited by Kandel ER, Schwartz JH, Jessell TM. New York, McGraw-Hill, 2000, pp. 280–297. Copyright 2000, The McGraw-Hill Companies, Inc. Used with permission.

they appear as if they are permanently on psychostimulants (Giros et al. 1996); psychostimulants have no effect on these animals, confirming that the dopamine transporter is critical to the action of these drugs. MPTP is taken up by the dopamine transporter selectively; once in dopamine neurons, it increases oxidative stress, leading to the demise of the neurons and behaviorally to parkinsonism (Pifl et al. 1996).

RAPID POSTSYNAPTIC RESPONSES

The action of a neurotransmitter depends on the properties of the postsynaptic receptors to which it binds. Postsynaptic receptors activated by neurotransmitter fall into two classes: 1) ionotropic and 2) metabotropic (discussed in the following section). Ionotropic receptors are directly linked to an ion channel; these receptors undergo a conformational change upon neurotransmitter binding that opens the channel. This results in either depolarization, giving rise to an excitatory postsynaptic potential, or hyperpolarization, giving rise to an inhibitory postsynaptic potential. The neuromuscular junction is the prototypic excitatory synapse; simultaneous binding of two acetylcholine molecules opens a channel in the receptor that is permeable to both Na^+ and K^+ (Karlin and Akabas 1995). This results in a strong depolarization of the postsynaptic membrane mediated by Na^+ influx (and moderated by K^+ efflux), leading to an action potential in the motor fiber that evokes contraction. Ligand-gated channels are found at synapses such as the neuromuscular junction, where rapid and reliable activation of the postsynaptic cell is required. At the neuromuscular junction, the postsynaptic response is sufficiently strong so that there is a one-to-one translation of motor neuron spikes into muscle fiber spikes, thus ensuring reliable muscle contraction.

Unlike the neuromuscular junction, CNS neurons function in dynamic networks (Vogels et al. 2005) so that generally no individual cell has so strong a synaptic connection with another cell that it alone brings it to threshold. Rather, groups of neurons—active in concert—converge on a postsynaptic neuron to generate multiple postsynaptic potentials. These potentials may summate within regions of the postsynaptic neuron (*spatial summation*) if they occur sufficiently close together in time to cause the postsynaptic neuron to fire. As a rule, fast ligand-gated channels mediate the flow of information representing patterns of sensory input and associations between sensory modalities, underlying central representations that ultimately give rise to motor outputs. In the CNS, glutamate receptors mediate most fast excitatory transmission; GABA and glycine are the most common inhibitory neurotransmitters.

GLUTAMATE RECEPTORS

Excitatory postsynaptic potentials are mediated by two classes of ionotropic glutamate receptors: N-methyl-D-aspartate (NMDA) receptors and non-NMDA, or α-amino-3-hydroxy-5-methylisoxazole-4-propionic acid (AMPA), receptors (Hassel and Dingledine 2006). Ionotropic glutamate receptors are multimeric proteins, usually composed of four subunits. NMDA receptors are formed from combinations of NR1 and NR2 subunits; the NR1 subunit is universally expressed in neurons, whereas the NR2, which comes in several subtypes, is heterogeneously expressed both during development and among different neurons, giving rise to different response properties (Schoepfer et al. 1994). NMDA receptors depolarize cells by opening channels that principally allow Ca^{2+} to enter the cell. The most striking property of NMDA receptors is that the ion channel is usually blocked by Mg^{2+} at membrane potentials more negative than about –40 mV (MacDermott et al. 1986; Nowak et al. 1984). As a result, at the resting potential of most neurons, the NMDA receptor channel is occluded. For current to flow through NMDA channels, glutamate must bind to the receptor and the membrane must be depolarized simultaneously to displace the Mg^{2+}. This dual requirement underlies the unique role of NMDA receptors in processes as varied as synaptogenesis, learning and memory, and even cell death. NMDA receptors are also likely to be critical for proper mental functioning. NMDA receptor hypofunction has been implicated as a pathogenic mechanism in schizophrenia (Coyle 2006), and transgenic mice with reduced NMDA receptor expression display aberrations in behavior similar to those seen in patients with schizophrenia (Gainetdinov et al. 2001).

The non-NMDA glutamate receptors are further divided into AMPA receptors and kainate receptors on the basis of their affinities for these glutamate analogs. AMPA receptors are formed from combinations of subunits GluR1 to GluR4, and kainate receptors are formed from combinations of GluR5 to GluR7 plus KA1 and KA2. The complexity in the types of possible glutamate receptors is further increased by the existence of flip and flop conformations of GluR1 to GluR4 subunits and posttranslational editing of glutamate receptor mRNA. Non-NMDA receptors generally gate channels that allow Na^+ but not Ca^{2+} to cross the membrane. The GluR2 subunit of the AMPA receptor channel is responsible for blocking Ca^{2+} passage. Neurons that express such Ca^{2+}-permeable AMPA receptors may be particularly vulnerable to excitotoxic cell death in disease states such as amyotrophic lateral sclerosis (Van Den Bosch et al. 2006). Ca^{2+}-permeable AMPA receptors mediate non-NMDA-dependent long-term potentiation, which has been implicated in anxiety states (Mahanty and Sah 1998).

GABA RECEPTORS

Inhibitory postsynaptic potentials in the brain are mediated primarily by GABA receptors (Olsen and Betz 2006). Several classes of GABA receptors have been identified. $GABA_A$ receptors are ionotropic receptors that form Cl^--selective channels and mediate fast synaptic inhibition in the brain. $GABA_B$ receptors are metabotropic receptors that tend to be slower acting and play a modulatory role; they are often found on presynaptic terminals, where they inhibit transmitter release. $GABA_A$ receptors are members of the nicotinic acetylcholine receptor superfamily. The $GABA_A$ receptor-channel complex is composed of a mixture of five subunits from α, β, γ, and ρ families. This gives rise to receptors with varying properties, depending on the specific receptor subunit composition. Because most of the subunit families have multiple subtypes, some of which can undergo RNA splicing, there is the potential for an extraordinary diversity of $GABA_A$ receptor function. During early development, intracellular chloride levels are high, so $GABA_A$ receptors in fact mediate excitation (H. Lee et al. 2005). Recent studies indicate that at some synapses, in particular those projecting onto the initial segments of cortical pyramidal neurons, GABA may continue to be depolarizing in adulthood (Szabadics et al. 2006).

The mRNA sequences for individual or multiple receptor subunits can be injected into oocytes or cultured mammalian cells, and the properties of the subsequently expressed receptor subunit combinations elucidated. This approach has shown how the properties of a particular $GABA_A$ receptor depend on the subunit composition as well as on interactions among the subunits. Site-directed mutagenesis has been applied to localize binding sites of specific ligands on receptor subunits. Benzodiazepines bind to a recognition site formed by the α and γ subunits. The α_1 subunits mediate the sedating effects of benzodiazepines and are targeted selectively by the newer-generation soporifics such as zolpidem, while the α_2 subunits mediate the anxiolytic effects. The clinical actions of benzodiazepines, along with two other classes of CNS-depressant drugs, barbiturates and anesthetic steroids, as well as ethanol seem to be related to their ability to bind to $GABA_A$ receptors and to enhance $GABA_A$ receptor currents (Yamakura et al. 2001). Individual $GABA_A$ channels do not open continuously in the presence of GABA but rather flicker open and closed, often in bursts. Benzodiazepines increase GABA current by increasing the frequency of channel openings without altering open time or conductance. Barbiturates prolong the channel open time without altering opening fre-

quency or conductance. Steroids such as androsterone and pregnenolone increase the open time and the frequency of bursts. Despite the different mechanisms of action, each drug enhances GABAergic transmission, accounting for their shared properties as anticonvulsants. In fact, they may directly counteract a GABA deficit due to a reduction in GABA transporter numbers in epileptogenic cortex that may be etiological in epilepsy (During et al. 1995).

METABOTROPIC RECEPTORS

Longer-term modulatory effects are generally mediated by metabotropic receptors (Greengard 2001). These non-channel-linked receptors regulate cell function via activation of G proteins that couple to second-messenger cascades. Although other non-channel-linked receptors may also be catalytic, in the CNS only G protein–linked receptors are found. In fact, the majority of neurotransmitters and neuromodulators exert their effects through binding to G protein receptors. G protein–linked receptors are so named because they couple to intracellular guanosine triphosphate (GTP)-binding regulatory proteins. G proteins are formed from a complex of three membrane-bound proteins ($G\alpha_{\beta\gamma}$); when the receptor is activated, the α subunit (G_α) binds GTP and dissociates from a complex of the β and γ subunits ($G_{\beta\gamma}$). Both G_α and $G_{\beta\gamma}$ may go on to trigger subsequent events. Activated G proteins have a life span of seconds to minutes; G_α auto-inactivates by hydrolyzing its bound GTP, after which it reaggregates with $G_{\beta\gamma}$, returning to the resting state. Continued transmitter binding to the receptor may reinitiate the cycle.

G proteins are the first link in signaling cascades that either directly activate protein kinases—enzymes that phosphorylate cellular proteins (Walaas and Greengard 1991)—or raise intracellular Ca^{2+} and indirectly activate kinases (Figure 1–10) (Ghosh and Greenberg 1995). Proteins undergo conformational changes when they are phosphorylated that may lead to either their activation or inactivation. Proteins affected may include membrane channels, cytoskeletal elements, and transcriptional regulators of gene expression. In this way, modulatory actions mediated by second messengers control most cellular processes. The potential for amplification, combined with divergence and convergence of signals, provides the requisite mechanisms for enduring changes in neuronal function, especially for mechanisms essential for learning and memory and for development. The three major second-messenger cascades involving G proteins and their interaction with Ca^{2+} are schematized in Figure 1–10.

As these G protein coupled receptors are the targets of many therapeutic and abused drugs, understanding their

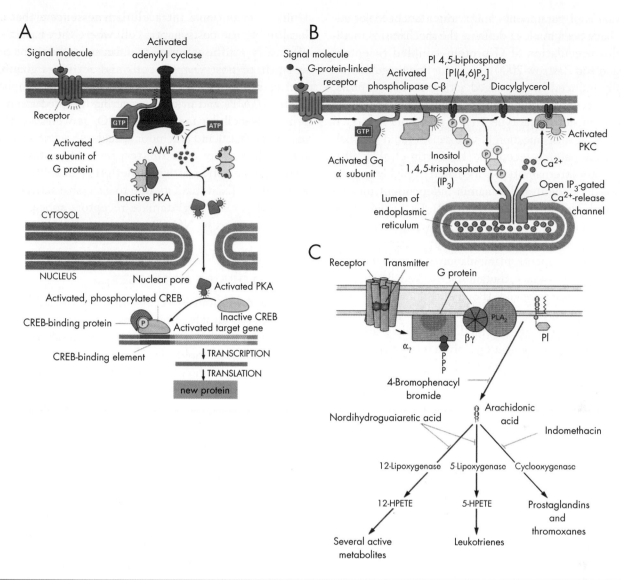

FIGURE I–10. Major intracellular signaling pathways in neurons. Ligand binding to receptors activates three major signaling pathways via G proteins. *Panel A.* In the cyclic adenosine monophosphate (cAMP) system, a G protein link couples ligand binding to activation of adenylyl cyclase. This in turn generates cAMP, which binds to the regulatory units (R) of cAMP-dependent protein kinase, releasing the catalytic subunits (activated PKA). After being phosphorylated (activated, phosphorylated CREB), CREB binds to cAMP response elements (CREB-binding element) to regulate gene expression. *Panel B.* In the inositol phospholipid system, G proteins activate phospholipase C, which hydrolyzes membrane phospholipids to produce two second messengers, diacylglycerol and inositol triphosphate (IP_3). IP_3 triggers the release of Ca^{2+} from the endoplasmic reticulum. Ca^{2+}, in turn, triggers the translocation of protein kinase C (PKC) to the cell membrane, where it is activated by diacylglycerol. Because it becomes membrane bound with activation, PKC may be especially important in the modulation of membrane channels. Ca^{2+} released from intracellular stores may act similarly to Ca^{2+} that enters from outside the cell (not shown), allowing temporal coincidence through activation of voltage-dependent Ca^{2+} channels. *Panel C.* In the arachidonic acid system, G proteins may couple to phospholipase A_2 (PLA_2), forming arachidonic acid by hydrolysis of membrane phospholipids. Arachidonic acid is either a second messenger in its own right or a precursor of the lipoxygenase pathway giving rise to a family of membrane-permeant second messengers. The cyclooxygenase pathway is principally important outside the brain in prostaglandin production. HPETE=hydroperoxyeicosatetraenoic acid; PI=phosphatidylinositol.

Source. Panels A and B copyright 2002 from *Molecular Biology of the Cell,* by Alberts B, Johnson A, Lewis J, Raff M, Roberts K, Walter P. New York, Garland Science, 2002. Reproduced by permission of Garland Science/Taylor & Francis LLC.
Panel C reprinted from Siegelbaum SA, Schwartz JH, Kandel ER: "Modulation of Synaptic Transmission: Second Messengers," in *Principles of Neural Science, 4th Edition.* Edited by Kandel ER, Schwartz JH, Jessell TM. New York, McGraw-Hill, 2000, pp. 229–252. Copyright 2000 The McGraw-Hill Companies, Inc. Used with permission.

regulation is of paramount clinical importance. Major advances have been made in defining the mechanisms mediating downregulation of G protein–coupled receptors (Tsao and von Zastrow 2000). Receptor downregulation is generally induced by prolonged activation of receptors, leading to receptor internalization. For example, prolonged activation of dopamine type 1 (D_1) receptors in striatal neurons by agonist injection in vivo causes rapid internalization of dopamine receptors (Dumartin et al. 1998). This receptor internalization is mediated by highly specific dynamin-dependent and dynamin-independent mechanisms (Vickery and von Zastrow 1999). Determining the mechanisms of G protein receptor downregulation may identify targets for development of new classes of drugs useful for the therapeutic manipulation of G protein receptor signaling. For instance, mutant mice lacking β-arrestin 2 show no tolerance to opioids (Bohn et al. 1999).

The slower actions of metabotropic receptors are responsible for altering neuronal excitability and the strength of synaptic connections, often reinforcing neural pathways involved in learning (Bailey and Kandel 2004). Activation of these receptors generally does not change the membrane potential at all. Rather, receptor binding activates second-messenger cascades that can dramatically alter the response properties of other receptors. Most profoundly, second messengers may translocate to the nucleus, where they may control gene expression, exerting longer-term changes in cell function via the activation of genes in a temporal sequence (Girault and Greengard 2004). Many long-term adaptations, such as those induced by psychotropic agents, appear to be mediated by adaptations in metabotropic receptor signaling. For instance, the antidepressant effects of SSRIs are not due to the immediate surge in serotonin associated with the blockade of the serotonin reuptake transporter (SERT), but rather to longer-term adaptations in signaling mediated by $5HT_{1A}$ and $5HT_{2A}$ serotonin receptors (Blier and Abbott 2001). Dopaminergic actions in cortex, implicated in the modulation of working memory (Goldman-Rakic et al. 2000), result in long-term adaptations in cortical signaling (Seamans and Yang 2004).

GASES AS TRANSCELLULAR MODULATORS

Surprisingly, nitric oxide (NO), a gas, has been shown to mediate interneuronal signaling, functioning as a second messenger with neurotransmitter properties (Brenman and Bredt 1997; Schulman 1997). NO is extremely short lived and is rapidly synthesized on demand from arginine by the enzyme nitric oxide synthase (NOS). NOS is activated by increases in intracellular Ca^{2+} concentration.

Unlike conventional intracellular messengers that are localized to the postsynaptic cell, where they have their effects, NO diffuses across membranes to adjacent presynaptic or postsynaptic cells and activates guanylyl cyclase, raising levels of cyclic guanosine 3′,5′-monophosphate (cGMP) and in turn triggering the production of other intracellular messengers. NO, as well as carbon monoxide (CO) and arachidonic acid, other transcellular modulators, may coordinate pre- and postsynaptic changes in synaptic plasticity (Meffert et al. 1996; O'Dell et al. 1994). Excitotoxicity due to excessive activation of the NMDA class of glutamate receptors appears to be mediated in part by NO (Dawson et al. 1994).

ORGANIZATION OF POSTSYNAPTIC RECEPTORS AT SYNAPSES

Most neurotransmitter receptors are clustered at postsynaptic sites closely apposed to the presynaptic terminal. Several laboratories have made remarkable progress in identifying the molecular components of the postsynaptic scaffold that holds synaptic receptors in place (Figure 1–11) (Lee and Sheng 2000; O'Brien et al. 1998). One of the most abundant proteins in the postsynaptic density is PSD-95 (a postsynaptic density protein of 95 kd). PSD-95 is a cytoplasmic protein that contains three domains important for protein binding, called *PDZ domains* (named after the initials of the first three proteins found to share a common sequence of 80–90 amino acids important for their stabilization at the postsynaptic membrane). These domains of PSD-95 bind to the NMDA receptor, to the Shaker K^+ channel, and to cell adhesion proteins called *neuroligins*. In contrast, AMPA receptors bind a distinct PDZ domain protein called GRIP, and metabotropic glutamate receptors interact with HOMER. These PDZ proteins are believed to cluster neurotransmitter receptors and other important components of the synapse at the postsynaptic density and to mediate rapid insertion or removal of receptors from the synapse, as may occur during synaptic plasticity (Kennedy and Ehlers 2006).

SYNAPTIC MODULATION IN LEARNING AND MEMORY

Learning and memory require both short- and long-term changes at synapses. In addition to rapid signals, neurotransmitters activate second messenger systems that profoundly increase the range of responses a neuron shows to synaptic input. Second messengers activate kinases that both amplify and prolong signals by phosphorylating other proteins. Phosphorylated proteins remain

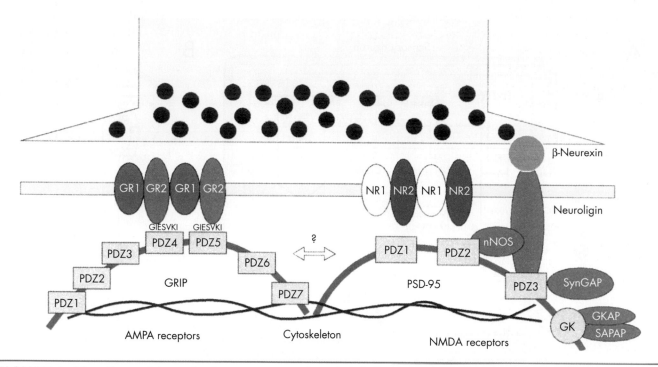

FIGURE 1–11. Some of the molecular components of a typical CNS glutamatergic synapse. α-Amino-3-hydroxy-5-methyl-isoxazole-4-propionic acid (AMPA) receptor subunits are tethered to GRIP through PDZ domain interactions, and the *N*-methyl-D-aspartate (NMDA) receptor subunits are bound to PSD-95. Both GRIP and PSD-95 also interact with the cytoskeleton, providing a protein scaffold for glutamate receptors in the postsynaptic density. This scaffold may regulate the dynamic, activity-dependent insertion or removal of glutamate receptors from CNS synapses. GIESVKI=the amino acids critical for binding GR2 to PDZ4 and PDZ5; nNOS=neuronal nitric oxide synthase.

Source. Reprinted from O'Brien RJ, Lau LF, Huganir RL: "Molecular Mechanisms of Glutamate Receptor Clustering at Excitatory Synapses." *Current Opinion in Neurobiology* 8:364–369, 1998. Copyright 1998. Used with permission from Elsevier.

active—often for a much longer period than agonist remains bound to receptor—until they are dephosphorylated by protein phosphatases. Because second messengers trigger numerous cellular functions, activation of a single receptor may trigger a coordinated cellular response involving several systems. This may include activity-dependent modulation of genomic transcription, leading to enduring changes in cellular function.

SENSITIZATION IN *APLYSIA*

Investigations using the marine mollusk *Aplysia californica* have been fundamental to current understanding of the cellular mechanisms of learning and memory (Hawkins et al. 2006; Kandel 2001a). Because its nervous system is composed of relatively few neurons and these neurons are identifiable from animal to animal, changes in *Aplysia* behavior can be traced to alterations in individual synaptic connections. *Aplysia* exhibits a simple defensive behavior, the gill-withdrawal reflex, that shows several elementary forms of learning. Mild stimulation to the siphon skin overlying the gill leads to its reflex withdrawal. If a shock is

delivered to the tail, the reflex shows sensitization; subsequent siphon stimulation elicits a more brisk reflex. If siphon stimulation is paired with tail shock, the animal shows associative learning manifested in an increased reflex response to the mild siphon stimulation. In effect, *Aplysia* learns that mild siphon stimulation predicts tail shock.

Sensitizing stimuli to the tail activate serotonergic facilitator neurons that synapse on sensory neuron terminals. The serotonin released produces presynaptic facilitation by activating adenylyl cyclase via a G protein link; cyclic adenosine monophosphate (cAMP) binds to the regulatory subunits of cAMP-dependent protein kinase (PKA), releasing the catalytic subunits, which phosphorylate a class of voltage-dependent K^+ channels (S-K^+ channels) and inactivate them. Because less K^+ current is evoked, the membrane remains depolarized a bit longer with a given action potential, there is more Ca^{2+} influx, and thus more transmitter release. Associative learning appears to be due to facilitator neuron activation closely following sensory neuron activation. The spike-triggered Ca^{2+} influx in the sensory neuron terminal and serotonin-activated second-messenger systems, when activated

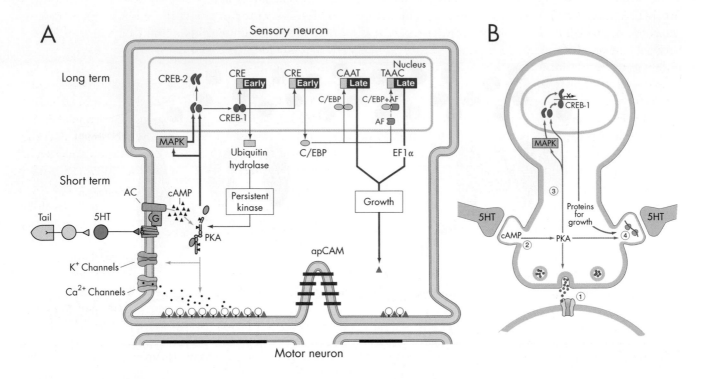

FIGURE 1–12.   Molecular mechanisms of short-term and long-term memory storage. *Panel A.* Schematic shows a single synaptic connection between a sensory and motor neuron in the neural circuit mediating defensive gill-withdrawal reflex in the marine snail *Aplysia californica.* Serotonin (5HT) triggers an increase in synaptic strength, which underlies the animal's heightened reflex withdrawal response when stressed. In short-term sensitization (lasting on the order of an hour), one electric shock to the tail activates serotonin interneurons (*blue*), activating serotonin receptors (also in *blue*) that activate protein kinase A (PKA), which phosphorylates existing proteins, leading to a short-term enhancement of synaptic transmission. With repeated stress, persistent elevation of cyclic adenosine monophosphate (cAMP) levels engages nuclear regulatory pathways. PKA in turn activates another kinase (MAPK), and together they phosphorylate CREB-2, releasing active CREB-1. CREB-1 then activates directly and indirectly a series of genes in temporal sequence, locking in the activation of PKA via ubiquitin hydrolase and encoding proteins necessary for synaptic growth. One example is *Aplysia* cell-adhesion molecule (apCAM), a molecule important in synaptic development, which plays a similar role in the further growth of synaptic connections with learning. *Panel B.* The signaling mechanisms involved in sensitization are summarized in broader strokes in this schematic: 1) sensory neurons activate motor neurons via exocytic release of the excitatory transmitter glutamate; 2) stress stimuli activate protein kinase, which both enhances transmitter release locally and 3) translocates to the nucleus to orchestrate long-term changes. The proteins for growth are utilized at synapses marked by serotonin stimulation, leading to long-term strengthening of stressed synapses.

Source.   Reprinted from Kandel ER: "The Molecular Biology of Memory Storage: A Dialogue Between Genes and Synapses." *Science* 294:1030–1038, 2001, with permission from AAAS and the Nobel Foundation. Copyright Nobel Foundation 2000.

together, produce enhanced protein kinase C (PKC) activity. This is termed *activity-dependent enhancement of presynaptic facilitation,* and it provides the coincidence detection inherent in associative learning (Figure 1–12A, *Short Term*). In all of these short-term forms of learning, the mechanisms involve covalent modification of existing proteins, principally by phosphorylation.

In contrast, long-term memory requires changes in gene transcription. The same mechanisms that mediate short-term sensitization initiate long-term memory formation. In long-term as in short-term sensitization, the

memory is encoded by a strengthening of sensorimotor synapses. There is increased transmitter release, and S-K⁺ channels are closed, leading to increased Ca²⁺ influx. Synaptic vesicles are trafficked to release sites, accounting for about a third of the increment in synaptic strength, with the balance mediated by growth of new varicosities (Kim et al. 2003). With such structural changes, there is an absolute requirement for gene transcription and the synthesis of new proteins. cAMP affects gene transcription by binding to the cAMP response element–binding protein (CREB), which then binds to regulatory cAMP-response element sites to activate gene transcription (Figure 1–12A, *Long term*). CREB in turn induces ubiquitin transcription, which leads to the cleavage of the regulatory subunit of cAMP-dependent protein kinase and an enduring upregulation of the kinase. Ultimately, the changes triggered by repeated sensory input, activation of facilitatory interneurons, serotonin application, or cAMP injection lead to enduring structural changes involving the growth of new processes and increased numbers and size of synapses. These morphological changes are mediated in part by cell adhesion molecules, akin to ones that play crucial roles in the assembly of the nervous system. Changes in gene expression lead to protein synthesis at the cellular but not synaptic level, raising the question as to how specific connections are strengthened selectively. Once sensitization has been initiated by repeated serotonin application, subsequent serotonin stimulation at the level of single synapses appears to mark the synapses for growth (Figure 1–12B). Additionally, neurons appear to be capable of limited local protein synthesis at synapses, providing further means for synapse-specific plasticity (Brittis et al. 2002). Thus, short-term changes in synaptic strength translate into enduring structural changes through interactions among second-messenger systems orchestrating gene transcription.

LONG-TERM POTENTIATION

Since the pioneering observations more than 50 years ago on patient H.M., who following bilateral hippocampal resection was no longer able to encode memories, studies of memory have focused on the circuitry of the hippocampus (Lynch 2004). This focus was further strengthened, more than 30 years ago, by the discovery that brief high-frequency stimulation of hippocampal pathways leads to long-term potentiation of the synaptic connections (Bliss and Lomo 1973). In intact animals, LTP may last for days to weeks, and so has come to be seen as the crucial synaptic process underlying memory formation. In the hippocampus, each of the three major synaptic circuits shows LTP, with distinct but shared mechanisms. At the most studied synapse, the Schaffer collateral synapse made by the projections of CA3 onto CA1 pyramidal neurons (Figure 1–13), LTP is initiated by Ca^{2+} influx into the postsynaptic neuron via NMDA receptors. Although glutamate released by CA3 neurons acts on NMDA and AMPA receptors, only high-frequency firing activates sufficient numbers of AMPA receptors to depolarize the postsynaptic membrane, relieve the voltage-dependent Mg^{2+} block of the NMDA receptor, and allow Ca^{2+} influx, initiating LTP (Blitzer et al. 2005). Because NMDA receptor activation requires both binding of

neurotransmitter and postsynaptic depolarization, the NMDA receptor provides the molecular coincidence detector originally postulated by Donald Hebb (1949), who predicted that alterations in synaptic strength would involve coordinated pre- and postsynaptic activity.

The influx of Ca^{2+} into the postsynaptic CA3 neuron activates Ca^{2+}/calmodulin-dependent protein kinase II (CaMKII), which mediates the phosphorylation of AMPA receptors, increasing their sensitivity (Lisman et al. 2002). CaMKII is capable of autophosphorylation and locks itself in an active catalytic state. This provides a molecular basis for early LTP. Ca^{2+} also activates calcineurin (PP2b), a phosphatase, which modulates PP1, which in turn can dephosphorylate CaMKII and block LTP. Calcineurin's action is modulated by cAMP, which acting through PKA blocks PP1 activity (Blitzer et al. 1998). This pathway, which is activated by catecholamines and Ca^{2+}, serves a gating function. Dopamine acting via D_1 receptors is required for late LTP (Huang and Kandel 1995). Switching off calcineurin in adult mice enhances LTP in the hippocampus and spatial learning (Malleret et al. 2001), arguing further for the significance of LTP for memory. Interestingly, however, mice with genetic deletion of calcineurin in the forebrain show working memory deficits reminiscent of those seen in schizophrenia (Miyakawa et al. 2003).

LTP is composed of at least two phases: early and late LTP. Early LTP lasts for the first 3 hours after induction and does not require protein synthesis. In contrast, late LTP lasts for several hours and requires both gene transcription and protein translation. As is true for long-term synaptic enhancement in *Aplysia*, late LTP involves activation of CamKII, production of cAMP, and activation of gene transcription through a CREB-dependent process. LTP can also stimulate the growth of new synaptic connections. Such changes are likely to underlie the more permanent synaptic alterations necessary for learning and memory (Bailey and Kandel 2004). In early LTP, synaptic strengthening occurs postsynaptically via increased sensitivity of existing AMPA receptors. As memory is encoded in late LTP, AMPA receptors are inserted in functionally silent synapses, and altogether new postsynaptic structures develop (Lisman et al. 2002) (Figure 1–14). In particular, *silent* synapses—synapses that contain only NMDA receptors before induction of LTP—may be activated by activity-dependent insertion of new AMPA receptors. Increases in AMPA-receptor function at previously silent synapses after LTP-inducing stimuli have been visualized directly by following the trafficking of AMPA receptors tagged with green fluorescent protein (GFP) (Shi et al. 1999). Relatively subtle changes in AMPA receptor trafficking are crucial, as has been shown in the amygdala for fear conditioning (Rumpel et al. 2005).

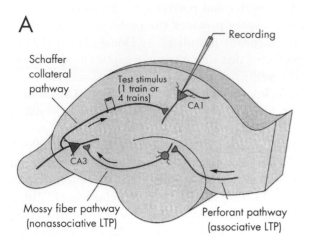

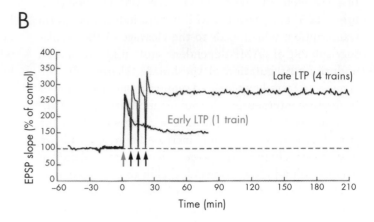

FIGURE 1–13.   Long-term potentiation (LTP) in the hippocampus. *Panel A.* A brain slice preparation from the rodent hippocampus is shown with the postsynaptic recording electrode in a CA1 pyramidal cell and a presynaptic stimulating electrode (coil) on the Schaffer collateral pathway axon of a CA3 pyramidal cell. *Panel B.* Stimulating the Schaffer collateral pathway at low frequency (once a minute) causes the CA3 axon terminals to release glutamate, which evokes a stable excitatory response (measured as the rising slope of the excitatory postsynaptic potential, EPSP; the control response is normalized to 100%). A single tetanus (*blue arrow*, 100 stimuli in 1 second) evokes early LTP, which is weak and lasts on the order of an hour. In contrast, with four tetani (*blue and black arrows*), the postsynaptic response is dramatically increased. Late LTP lasts for over 24 hours, as would be required for a synaptic mechanism encoding long-term memory.

Source.   Adapted from Kandel ER: "Cellular Mechanisms of Learning and the Biological Basis of Individuality," in *Principles of Neural Science, 4th Edition.* Edited by Kandel ER, Schwartz JH, Jessell TM. New York, McGraw-Hill, 2000, pp. 1247–1279. Copyright 2000, The McGraw-Hill Companies, Inc. Used with permission.

Whereas the *induction* of LTP is postsynaptic and depends on Ca^{2+} and the activation of CaMKII, the *expression* of LTP involves coordinated pre- and postsynaptic changes. Such an LTP-dependent increase in synaptic transmission has been visualized using antibody uptake (Malgaroli et al. 1995) and demonstrated in recordings from single synapses that have shown that the expression of LTP is associated with an increase in the numbers of synaptic vesicles released (Bolshakov et al. 1997). The question then arises, how do postsynaptic events triggered by NMDA receptor activation lead to changes in presynaptic neurotransmitter release? A retrograde second messenger that could diffuse across the synapse and act on the presynaptic terminal seems to be required. Several experiments indicate that NO or CO can convey such a retrograde signal, diffusing from postsynaptic to nearby presynaptic sites, and activate guanylyl cyclase to induce an elevation in cGMP in the presynaptic terminal (Wang et al. 2005). Neurotrophins may also act as retrograde signals in LTP (McAllister et al. 1999).

How is the strengthening of synapses by LTP kept in check? Hippocampal synapses also show long-term depression (LTD), which involves a similar array of mecha-

nisms activated by low-frequency synaptic activation (Anwyl 2006). LTD may be mediated by a decrease in neurotransmitter release and/or a decrease in postsynaptic responsiveness due to lowered numbers or sensitivity of glutamate receptors. Thus, through a dynamic balance between LTP and LTD, memories of irrelevant information may be eliminated and lasting memories fine-tuned. The regulation of synaptic strength appears to be controlled in the hippocampus by the predominant theta rhythm. Stimulation at the theta frequency produces LTP, whereas stimulation that is slower or specifically associated with the troughs of the rhythm produces LTD (Huerta and Lisman 1996). Possibly alterations in brain rhythms, implicated in several neuropsychiatric disorders (Behrendt and Young 2004; Spencer et al. 2004), act in part via modulation of synaptic plasticity.

DEVELOPMENT OF NEURONS

BIRTH AND MIGRATION

The human nervous system is the most complex organ system in vertebrates and contains a greater variety of cell types

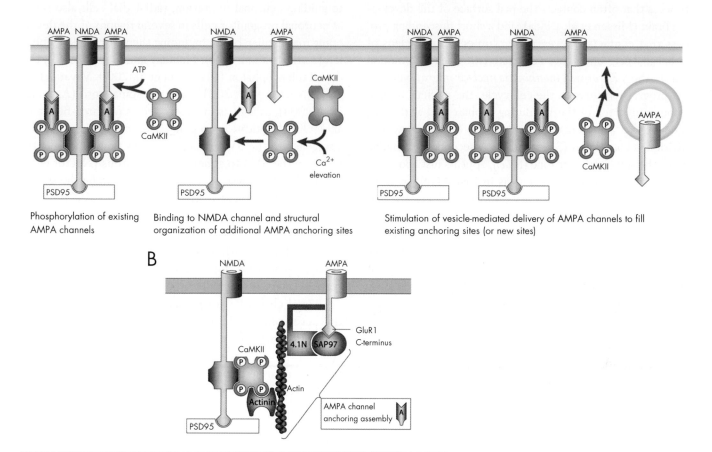

FIGURE 1–14. Molecular basis for long-term potentiation in the postsynaptic membrane of a CA1 pyramidal neuron. *Panel A.* With sufficient stimulation (or coincident postsynaptic depolarization), *N*-methyl-D-aspartate (NMDA)–type glutamate receptors are activated and Ca²⁺ fluxes into the cell. Ca²⁺ activates calcium/calmodulin-dependent protein kinase II (CaMKII), which increases the responsiveness of α-amino-3-hydroxy-5-methylisoxazole-4-propionic acid (AMPA)–type glutamate receptors. CaMKII can phosphorylate itself, locking it in the active mode. With continued activity, CaMKII organizes the further insertion of AMPA receptors into the postsynaptic membrane. *Panel B.* AMPA receptor recruitment to the postsynaptic membrane is mediated by the contractile protein actin. Actin is a ubiquitous contractile protein, the same protein involved peripherally in muscle contraction. CaMKII thus plays a pivotal role at all steps in the enhancement of synaptic transmission with long-term potentiation.

Source. Lisman J, Schulman H, Cline H: "The Molecular Basis of CaMKII Function in Synaptic and Behavioural Memory." *Nature Reviews Neuroscience* 3:175–190, 2002. Copyright 2002. Reprinted by permission from Macmillan Publishers Ltd.

than is found in any other organ. Remarkably, the diversity of cell types that regulate every aspect of our lives is accomplished during a brief span of development encompassing just 3–4 months in humans. It is therefore not surprising that this critical period of gestation is sensitive to interference through environmental factors and pathogens, as well as genetic mutations. For example, extrinsic factors such as alcohol exposure have been shown to decrease neuronal production, and in severe cases to produce microcephaly and mental retardation (M.W. Miller 1989). In addition, mutations in the doublecortin gene have been shown to dramatically interfere with neocortical development, resulting

in epilepsy and in severe cortical malformations such as lissencephaly (des Portes et al. 1998; Gleeson et al. 1998).

The principal cell types in the brain, neurons and glia, are generated in two proliferative zones that line the ventricular system during development, after which they migrate into the overlying cortical mantle. Each proliferative zone is comprised of a different class of progenitor cells. The ventricular zone (VZ), which is adjacent to the ventricular lumen during CNS development, consists primarily of pseudostratified columnar epithelial cells (Boulder Committee 1970). These cells were first characterized in the late nineteenth century and have gone by various names but are now called *radial glial cells* (Rakic 1971). Radial glia are bipolar cells with a soma located in the VZ, a long, thin ascending process that often contacts the pial surface of the developing brain (Misson et al. 1988a), and a short descending process that contacts the ventricular lumen. The nucleus of radial glial cells undergoes a characteristic to and fro motion within the VZ, termed *interkinetic nuclear migration*. During progression through the cell cycle, the nucleus is positioned at the top of the VZ during S-phase and at the surface of the ventricular lumen during M-phase, where division is completed (Sauer 1935). A second proliferative zone, the subventricular zone (SVZ), appears just above the VZ at the onset of neurogenesis in many CNS regions (Boulder Committee 1970). SVZ progenitor cells are generated by VZ precursor cells but have distinguishing features. SVZ cells are multipolar, they do not maintain contact with the pial and ventricular surfaces as do radial glial cells, they do not undergo interkinetic nuclear migration as they proceed through the cell cycle, and they divide away from the ventricular lumen (Takahashi et al. 1995).

IDENTIFICATION OF NEURONAL PROGENITOR CELLS

Early studies of nervous system development described mitotic cells adjacent to the ventricle that were assumed to be neuronal progenitor cells (Ramón y Cajal 1911). Nevertheless, the exact identity of the neural progenitor cells remained elusive until recent advances in molecular biology provided new tools with which to study nervous system development. Replication-incompetent retroviruses carrying reporter genes (Sanes et al. 1986) and the delivery of plasmid DNA to progenitor cells through electroporation to modify gene expression (Saito and Nakatsuji 2001) are now common tools in many laboratories. These techniques can deliver genes and fluorescent reporter proteins, such as GFP. Fluorescent reporter proteins have proven invaluable for detailed characterization of targeted cells in living tissue. Thus, it has become possible to study the expression of mRNA and protein, as well as the physiological properties of the labeled cells. Furthermore, it is now possible to study the behaviors of labeled precursor cells through time-lapse imaging in cultured tissue.

Retroviral lineage studies performed in the 1980s and 1990s reported clones containing either neuronal or glial cells, but rarely both (Luskin et al. 1988; Walsh and Cepko 1990). Although radial glial cells divide during neurogenesis (Misson et al. 1988b), they were thought to serve primarily as migratory guides for immature neurons (Rakic 1971). Thus, it was commonly thought that distinct classes of progenitor cells generate neuronal and glial cells. However, new studies have shown that neuronal

and glial cell lineages are not as divergent as previously thought. Indeed, it has now been shown that in addition to guiding neuronal migration, radial glial cells also serve as neuronal progenitor cells in several regions of the developing mammalian brain, including the ventral telencephalon (Anthony et al. 2004; Halliday and Cepko 1992), the dorsal telencephalon (Malatesta et al. 2000; Miyata et al. 2001; Noctor et al. 2001), and the spinal cord (Anthony et al. 2004), as well as in other species (Alvarez-Buylla et al. 1990). In addition to generating neurons, radial glia also generate the SVZ progenitor cells that subsequently divide in the SVZ to generate two neurons (Noctor et al. 2004). The SVZ was previously thought to be the site of gliogenesis, but recent evidence shows that SVZ progenitor cells provide a major contribution to neurogenesis (Haubensak et al. 2004; Kriegstein and Noctor 2004; Letinic et al. 2002; Miyata et al. 2004; Tarabykin et al. 2001), particularly during the genesis of the upper neocortical layers as originally proposed by Smart (1973).

Radial glial cells are present along the entire axis of the developing CNS (Ramón y Cajal 1911), raising the possibility that they might be universal neural progenitor cells. However, evidence suggests that while cerebellar Purkinje neurons are generated by radial glial cells in the VZ (Miale and Sidman 1961), cerebellar granule cells are generated by a distinct class of neural progenitor cells that reside in the external granular layer (EGL) of the developing cerebellum (Kamei et al. 1998; Miale and Sidman 1961). Nevertheless, EGL progenitors in the cerebellum may be homologous to SVZ progenitors in the neocortex. Thus, the lineage relationship between EGL precursors and radial glial cells in the developing cerebellum should be worked out in future research.

When neurogenesis is complete, radial glial cells migrate away from the proliferative zones into the cortical mantle and transform into mature astrocytes in several brain regions (Schmechel and Rakic 1979). Individual radial glial cells have been shown to generate neurons before transforming into astrocytes (Noctor et al. 2004). Astrocytes remain capable of division in the postnatal brain and, interestingly, have been shown to generate neurons in specific regions of the adult brain such as the hippocampus (Doetsch et al. 1999; Seri et al. 2001). It not yet known if adult neurogenic astrocytes are descended from embryonic radial glial cells, but it is likely that a specific astroglial lineage may serve as neuronal progenitor cells throughout life. Identification and characterization of these important progenitor cells has fundamentally altered our understanding of developmental processes in the brain. More importantly, this research has identified a potential source of cells for replacement strategies in the treatment of neurodegenerative disorders.

REGULATION OF PROLIFERATION

A number of factors, including neurotransmitter substances, growth factors, and even hormones, are present in proliferative regions of the brain and are known to regulate cell division in the developing and adult brain. For example, it has been shown that the classical neurotransmitters GABA and glutamate differentially regulate proliferation in the ventricular and subventricular zones during neocortical development (Haydar et al. 2000; LoTurco et al. 1995). Proliferative VZ radial glial cells are coupled to one another through connexin gap junction channels (LoTurco and Kriegstein 1991). New evidence indicates that waves of Ca^{2+} activity in radial glial cells are transmitted through connexin channels (gap junctions) and may be instrumental in regulating the proliferation of radial glial cells and thereby neurogenesis (Weissman et al. 2004). Finally, proteins such as β-catenin, a structural component of the adherens junctions that form between progenitor cells in the VZ, have been shown to promote proliferation versus differentiation of progenitor cells during cortical development (Chenn and Walsh 2002). These varied factors thus work in conjunction to regulate the proliferative behavior of progenitor cells during specific stages of brain development.

DETERMINATION OF CELL FATE

The determination of cell fate occurs at regional, local, and cellular levels. The expression of different transcription factors along the rostrocaudal axis of the developing nervous system reveals one mechanism by which cortical cells acquire specific identities (Schuurmans and Guillemot 2002). Although all radial glial cells share characteristic morphological features, they nonetheless constitute a heterogeneous population based on protein expression patterns (Kriegstein and Gotz 2003). This may explain how different regions of the developing telencephalon generate different classes of cortical cells. For example, excitatory pyramidal cells and astrocytes are generated by Pax6-expressing cells in the dorsal telencephalon, while inhibitory interneurons are generated by Dlx-1/2-expressing cells in the ganglionic eminences of the embryonic ventral telencephalon (Anderson et al. 1997). The expression of transcription factors such as Dlx-1/2 is likely an early step in the commitment of telencephalic cells to a specific fate. The expression of these factors may even correlate with the phenotype of specific neuronal subtypes. Indeed, new evidence indicates that subregions of the ganglionic eminences express different transcription factors and give rise to interneuron subtypes (Nery et al. 2002). Local environmental factors also play a role in determining the fate of neurons in the developing cortex. Transplantation studies demonstrate that the laminar fate of cortical neurons can be altered when transplantation of cortical precursor cells occurs during specific phases of the cell cycle (McConnell and Kaznowski 1991). Furthermore, expression of transcription factors is crucial for the normal differentiation of cortical neurons. For example, the absence of the transcription factor Foxg1 during cortical neurogenesis induces deep-layer cortical neurons to adopt the phenotype of Cajal-Retzius neurons that are normally found in the superficial layer 1 of the neocortex (Hanashima et al. 2004).

The generation of sufficient numbers of the diverse cell types in the nervous system is accomplished through two basic types of progenitor cell divisions: symmetric and asymmetric (Gotz and Huttner 2005). Symmetric divisions generate two daughter cells that are similar, whereas asymmetric divisions generate two daughter cells that differ from one another. Recent evidence indicates that these types of divisions might occur in different proliferative zones—asymmetric divisions occur more frequently at the surface of the ventricular lumen, while symmetric divisions occur more frequently in the SVZ (Noctor et al. 2004).

Radial glial cells divide asymmetrically at the ventricular lumen to generate either a single neuron or an SVZ progenitor that will subsequently generate two neurons. Therefore, each radial glial cell division can generate either one neuron directly or two neurons indirectly (Figure 1–15). Determination of daughter cell fate after radial glial divisions, for either neuronal or SVZ progenitors, thus affects the total number of neurons generated at a given time. A shift toward neuronal fate would decrease the total numbers of neurons being generated, whereas a shift toward SVZ progenitor fate for the radial glial daughter cells would double the neuronal output at a given time. Regulation of daughter cell fate during neurogenesis may thus affect the neuronal density for a given neocortical layer or structure. Invertebrate studies have revealed a number of important fate-determining molecules that are differentially segregated to nascent daughter cells during progenitor cell divisions. Some of these molecules, such as Notch and Numb, are also expressed in mammalian proliferative zones, and research into their role in determining daughter cell fate continues (Pearson and Doe 2004).

MIGRATION

Neurons in the adult brain are organized into complex, intricately interconnected groups of nuclei and laminae. One of the remarkable aspects of brain development is that neurons are not born in their final locations. Instead, neurons are generated in proliferative zones surrounding the ventricular lumen and then must migrate substantial distances, up

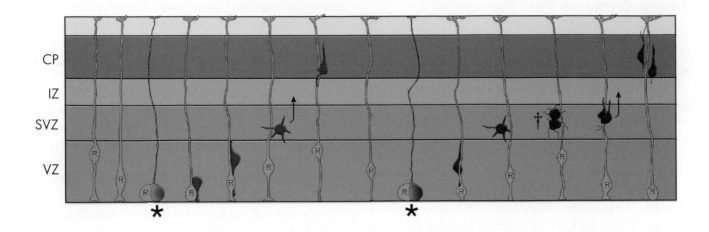

FIGURE 1–15.   Scheme depicting key events in the generation of cortical neurons during embryogenesis. Radial glial cells (R, shown in *green*) undergo interkinetic nuclear migration and divide asymmetrically at the ventricular surface (*) to self-renew and to generate neurons either directly (*red cell*) or indirectly through the generation of an intermediate progenitor cell (*blue*). Intermediate progenitor cells subsequently undergo terminal symmetric division in the subventricular zone (SVZ, †) to generate two neurons.   CP=cortical plate; IZ=intermediate zone; SVZ=subventricular zone; VZ=ventricular zone.

to 7,000 μm or longer, to reach their destination. Despite the complexity of the task, this feat is achieved with such regularity and precision that there is little variation in the architectonic pattern of brain structures from one person to the next, and even between species. In the developing neocortex, cortical neurons are generated in an inside-out sequence such that the deepest layers of the cerebral cortex form first, and subsequent waves of migrating neurons traverse the established layers as they migrate into the cortical mantle. Thus, as development proceeds, neurons must migrate progressively longer distances and through increasing numbers of cortical cells. Migration relies on cell-cell adhesion ligand molecules that signal between the radial glial fibers and migrating neurons (Hatten 1990). Neuronal migration is also regulated by a number of extracellular signaling molecules, such as neurotransmitter substances acting through the NMDA receptor (Komuro and Rakic 1993) and reelin protein acting through its constituent receptor molecules (Tissir and Goffinet 2003).

Recent experiments employing time-lapse imaging of fluorescently labeled cells in cultured brain tissue have revealed that the patterns of neuronal migration in the neocortex are more complex than originally thought. Neurons undergo several distinct stages of migration that can be identified based on the morphology and position of the neurons. After being generated, the cortical neurons leave the ventricular surface and rapidly ascend to the SVZ, where they acquire a multipolar morphology and remain stationary for one day or longer. After sojourning in the SVZ (Bayer and Altman 1991), many cortical neurons make a retrograde movement back toward the ventricular lumen

before reversing orientation toward the cortical plate and commencing radial migration (Noctor et al. 2004) (Figure 1–16). Similar ventricule-directed movements have been reported for GABAergic interneurons during their migration into the dorsal cortex (Nadarajah and Parnavelas 2002). The similarity in the ventricle-directed movements of these distinct cell types indicates that excitatory and inhibitory neurons are capable of responding to similar cues during their cortical migrations, and it hints at a potential source of important migration-guidance molecules located near the ventricular lumen of the developing brain.

Different forms of migration have been identified in other regions of the developing brain, such as the tangential migration of interneurons from the ganglionic eminences of the ventral telencephalon into the dorsal telencephalon. Interneurons do not appear to migrate along radial glial fibers during their journey from the ventral into the dorsal telencephalon. But it has yet to be determined whether they rely on cellular guides, such as developing axonal pathways in the intermediate zone of the developing cortex, or rather are guided solely along gradients of chemoattractive and repulsive factors (Marin and Rubenstein 2003). The picture is further complicated because interneurons migrate along several different complex pathways en route to their destination in the dorsal cortex (Kriegstein and Noctor 2004). The significance of these divergent pathways has yet to be determined, but it is possible that specific interneuron subtypes respond to different migration cues and thus adopt different routes of migration. Yet another form of migration, termed *chain migration*, has been identified for olfactory bulb interneurons as they migrate from their

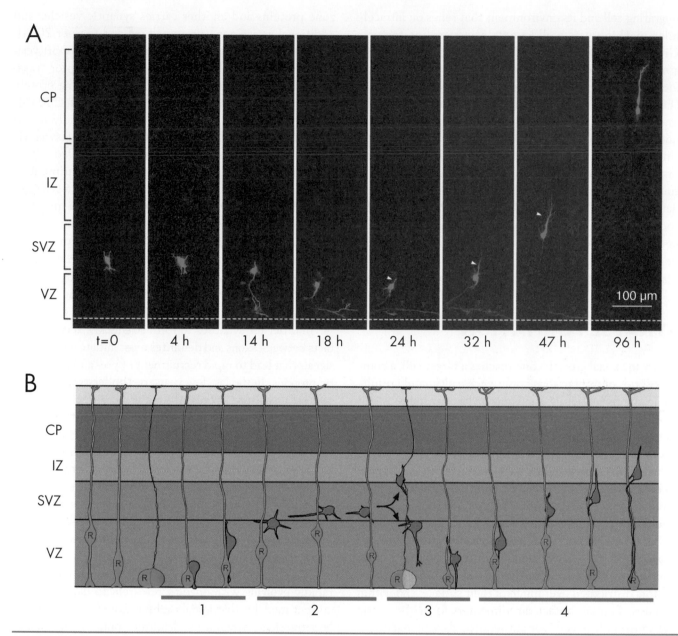

FIGURE 1–16. During development, neocortical neurons exhibit four distinct phases in migration. *Panel A.* A time-lapse sequence of a retrovirally labeled neuron expressing the reporter protein green fluorescent protein (GFP) undergoing migration from the proliferative zone to the cortical plate in a cultured brain slice. The sequence begins when the neuron is in the second phase, which consists of migratory arrest for 24 hours or more (shown here at the end of phase two, t=0 h), followed by a third phase of retrograde migration toward the ventricle (t=14–18 h) and a final phase of polarity reversal and migration toward the cortical plate (CP) (t=24–96 h). Before initiating the final phase of radial migration, the neuron develops a leading process oriented toward the CP (*white arrowhead*). After 96 hours in culture, the migrating neuron had reached its destination at the top of the cortical plate. These neurons often leave a trailing axon in the ventricular zone (VZ, *red arrowheads*). *Panel B.* Schematic depicting a neuron (shown in *dark green*) undergoing the four phases of migration: 1) After being generated by its mother radial glial cell (R, shown in *light green*), the neuron commences initial radial migration, 2) migratory arrest in the SVZ, 3) retrograde migration, and 4) secondary radial migration. IZ=intermediate zone; SVZ=subventricular zone; VZ=ventricular zone.

birthplace in the cortical SVZ along the rostral migratory stream into the olfactory bulb (Lois et al. 1996).

Despite differences in the identified forms of migration, each appears to rely on a shared set of intracellular molecules that are involved in the extension of leading processes and the transportation of cellular structures such as the nucleus (Feng and Walsh 2001). Neuronal migration is thus a complex interplay between the migrating cell and its environment that relies on intracellular machinery as well as extrinsic signaling factors. Given the complexity of this task it is not surprising that a number of nervous system malformations have been identified that result from defects in neuronal migration (Feng and Walsh 2001). These range from severe brain malformations such as lissencephaly to periventricular nodular heterotopia to more moderate cases involving small ectopic clusters of neurons. In each case, varying proportions of neurons fail to migrate to their proper destinations. Afflicted individuals present with mental retardation in severe cases. Mild malformations are often associated with epilepsy. The lifelong impact of these neurological disorders on affected individuals and families cannot be overstated and necessitates our further search for the root causes of these conditions.

SYNAPSE FORMATION

When an axonal growth cone reaches a target cell, a complex series of interactions commences, ultimately resulting in the formation of a synapse. Although there is still much to be learned about the formation of synapses in the CNS, the basic process of synaptogenesis at the neuromuscular junction (the synapse between a motor neuron and a muscle cell) has been well described (Figure 1–17). Both the motor neuron and the muscle cell have the necessary molecular machinery prefabricated before synapse formation (Sanes and Lichtman 1999). The motor neuron growth cone functions like a protosynapse, showing activity-dependent neurotransmitter release. Non-innervated postsynaptic cells have transmitter receptors distributed over much of their surface, and within minutes of initial contact, a rudimentary form of synaptic transmission begins. Over subsequent days, connections become stronger and stabilize as the growth cone matures into a presynaptic terminal, gathering the cellular elements necessary for focused release of neurotransmitter at active zones. In parallel, the postsynaptic cell concentrates receptors at the site of contact, removing them from other regions, and over the course of days it develops postsynaptic specializations.

Although there are many differences between the neuromuscular junction (NMJ) and CNS synapses, the general principles of synapse formation appear to be conserved. As at the NMJ, presynaptic and postsynaptic proteins are present in axons and dendrites, respectively, of CNS neurons prior to synapse formation. Presynaptic proteins are transported in at least two separate multiprotein-containing transport vesicles that are mobile before synapse formation—one carries a subset of active zone proteins and another carries synaptic vesicles and additional active zone proteins (Ziv and Garner 2004). Postsynaptic proteins are also trafficked in transport vesicles prior to synapse formation; NMDA receptor transport vesicles also contain SAP102, a scaffolding protein found at young synapses (Washbourne et al. 2004b). These mobile transport vesicles accumulate rapidly at new sites of contact between presynaptic and postsynaptic CNS neurons. Axo-dendritic contact is followed within minutes by the rapid and simultaneous recruitment of synaptic vesicles and NMDA receptors to new synapses (Washbourne et al. 2002). This early recruitment of NMDA receptors, but not AMPA receptors, to new synapses has been described in multiple systems; the resulting synapses are electrically "silent" until AMPA receptors are inserted (Isaac 2003). In the hours following contact, scaffolding proteins are also recruited to nascent synapses by as yet unknown mechanisms (Kim and Sheng 2004).

In order for synapses to form so quickly, specific contacts between axons and dendrites must initiate intracellular signals that lead to rapid recruitment of pre- and postsynaptic proteins. In the last few years, our understanding of the molecular signals that cause the initial recruitment of synaptic proteins to new sites of axo-dendritic contact has increased dramatically (Scheiffele 2003; Waites et al. 2005). In general, there are three major classes of signals that regulate synapse formation: adhesion molecules, diffusible molecules, and molecules secreted from glial cells. The first class of these synaptogenic molecules are the cell adhesion molecules, which include integrins, neural cell adhesion molecules (NCAMs), nectins, cadherins, neurexin-neuroligin, synaptic cell adhesion molecule (SynCAM), and the ephrins (Washbourne et al. 2004a). Although models are rapidly evolving with ongoing research, to date the most current model is that initial cadherin-based adhesion stabilizes transient, dynamic axodendritic contacts long enough to allow other classes of synaptogenic molecules to interact and activate intracellular cascades that recruit synaptic proteins. After rapid cadherin-based adhesion, trans-synaptic molecules such as neuroligin and SynCAM then lead to simultaneous bidirectional signaling in the axon and dendrite; this kind of signaling could be critical for the rapid and simultaneous recruitment of synaptic transport vesicles and NMDA receptor transport packets to new axodendritic contacts. Recent studies have begun to provide strong evidence that a lack, or abnormal expression, of trans-synaptic adhesion molecules may cause neurodevelopmental disorders. For example, intense interest has recently been focused on the possibility that mutations in one or more of the genes that encode neuroligins—a synaptogenic molecule that mediates both presynaptic and postsynaptic differentiation—cause autism (Chih et al. 2004).

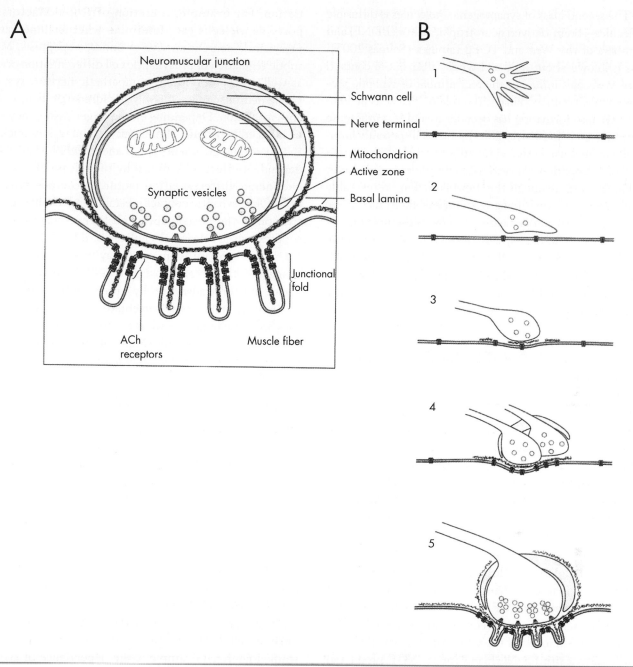

FIGURE 1–17. Synapse formation of the neuromuscular junction (NMJ). *Panel A.* Schematic view of the molecular components of a typical neuromuscular junction. At a mature NMJ, the presynaptic terminal is separated from the postsynaptic muscle cell by the synaptic cleft. Synaptic vesicles filled with acetylcholine (ACh) are clustered at active zones, where they can fuse with the plasma membrane upon depolarization to release their transmitter into the synaptic cleft. Acetylcholine receptors are found postsynaptically, and glial cells called Schwann cells surround the synaptic terminal. *Panel B.* Stages in the formation of the NMJ: 1) An isolated growth cone from a motor neuron is guided to the muscle by axon guidance cues. 2) The first contact is an unspecialized physical contact. 3) However, synaptic vesicles rapidly cluster in the axon terminal, acetylcholine receptors start to cluster under the forming synapse, and a basal lamina is deposited in the synaptic cleft. 4) As development proceeds, multiple motor neurons innervate each muscle. 5) Over time, however, all but one of the axons are eliminated through an activity-dependent process, and the remaining terminal matures.

Source.   Reprinted from Sanes JR, Jessell TM: "The Formation and Regeneration of Synapses," in *Principles of Neural Science, 4th Edition.* Edited by Kandel ER, Schwartz JH, Jessell TM. New York, McGraw-Hill, 2000, pp. 1087–1114. Copyright 2000, The McGraw-Hill Companies, Inc. Used with permission.

The second class of synaptogenic molecules is diffusible molecules—brain-derived neurotrophic factor (BDNF) and members of the Wnt and TGFβ families (Salinas 2005). Less is known about how and when, after initial contact, these molecules influence the recruitment of synaptic proteins to new contacts. Finally, the role of glial cells in regulating synapse formation has been an area of recent intense research (Allen and Barres 2005). Glial cells potently influence synapse formation and function through the secretion of thrombospondins, cholesterol, and tumor necrosis factor alpha. In sum, although this field is making remarkably rapid progress in identifying synaptogenic molecules, there is not yet a clear understanding of how these many molecules interact to initiate synapse formation. Moreover, little is known about the molecular mechanisms of synapse stabilization or elimination in the CNS—processes that are critical for learning and memory and that are likely to give rise to cellular deficits in neurodegenerative disorders.

NEURONAL MATURATION AND SURVIVAL

Maturation of the postsynaptic cell requires de novo protein synthesis, as do learning-dependent, long-term changes in the adult CNS. Immediate-early response genes (IEGs) (Morgan and Curran 1989, 1995) are among the first genes activated by postsynaptic depolarization, stimulated by elevations in Ca^{2+}, cAMP, cGMP, inositol 1,4,5-triphosphate (IP_3), or diacylglycerol (DAG) (Figure 1–10). The prototype of this family of proto-oncogenes is *c-fos*. Transcription of IEGs leads to the synthesis of proteins that modulate or induce transcription of other genes that induce structural changes in the cell. For instance, nerve growth factor (NGF) synthesis may be controlled by *c-fos* transcription; lesions of the sciatic nerve lead to a rapid increase in levels of fos, which binds to the transcription initiation site for NGF and causes NGF production (Hengerer et al. 1990). Long-term sensitization in *Aplysia* (Barzilai et al. 1989), hippocampal LTP (Cole et al. 1989; Wisden et al. 1990), and structural plasticity of dendrites and dendritic spines are also associated with the specific activation of other IEGs such as Arc and CREB (Lyford et al. 1995; Steward and Worley 2002). Current models for synaptic plasticity propose that local activation of IEGs by correlated activity at individual synapses may lead to local protein synthesis specifically at those strengthened synapses. This local protein synthesis has been proposed to play a role in synaptic plasticity and memory consolidation (Steward and Worley 2002).

Interactions between presynaptic and postsynaptic neurons can act to enhance and modulate their differentiation. For example, secretion of trophic factors by postsynaptic cells can determine whether innervating presynaptic neurons survive or undergo apoptosis. More subtle regulation of presynaptic cell differentiation occurs as well. In the developing sympathetic nervous system, young neurons are exclusively noradrenergic before synapse formation. Depending on the target tissue, they may be induced to become cholinergic, retaining only traces of the noradrenergic phenotype (Landis 1990). This target-dependent effect is mediated by the release of a soluble cholinergic-differentiation factor by the postsynaptic cells. Once synaptic contact is established, cholinergic activation of the postsynaptic cell by presynaptic spikes suppresses the release of cholinergic differentiation factor. Thus, synapse formation may trigger far-reaching changes, both pre- and postsynaptically, extending to the choice of neurotransmitter by a presynaptic neuron.

In many areas of the vertebrate nervous system, neurons are initially produced in excess. To survive, neurons must receive an adequate supply of one or more trophic factors produced by their target neurons. Competition for limited supplies of these factors ensures that surviving neurons will be correctly connected and that the number of neurons will be matched to the size of the target. In general, cells deprived of neurotrophic factors undergo apoptosis, a genetically programmed form of cell death characterized by cytoplasmic shrinkage, chromatin condensation, and degradation of DNA into oligonucleosomal fragments (Edwards et al. 1991). Unlike necrosis, this process does not stimulate an inflammatory response. Apoptosis is an active process that requires RNA and protein synthesis (Oppenheim et al. 1991; Scott and Davies 1990). Data are accumulating to support the remarkable hypothesis that apoptosis is the default program for most cells and that widespread cell suicide is prevented only by the continual presence of survival signals that suppress the intrinsic cell death program (Raff et al. 1993). The best-studied neuronal example is the dependence of sympathetic and sensory neurons on NGF, which is produced by the target tissue. Although approximately half of the sympathetic neurons normally undergo apoptosis, exogenously applied NGF prevents most of the cells from dying; in contrast, neutralizing antibodies to NGF produce widespread sympathetic cell death (Raff et al. 1993).

Several families of growth factors and their receptors have been identified (Figure 1–18), including the neurotrophins that bind to members of the Trk family of receptor tyrosine kinases. These include NGF, BDNF, and neurotrophins 3, 4/5, and 6. Another family includes ciliary neurotrophic factor, growth-promoting activity, and leukemia inhibitory factor. Additional neurotrophic factors include basic fibroblast growth factor and glia cell

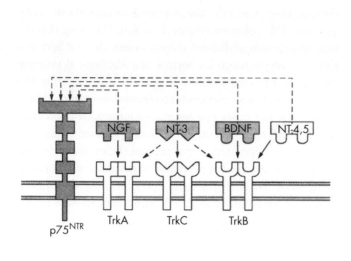

FIGURE 1–18. Neurotrophins exert their effects through binding to two types of receptors: the low-affinity nerve growth factor receptor, also called p75, and high-affinity tyrosine kinase receptors (Trk receptors). Nerve growth factor (NGF) binds primarily to TrkA, and brain-derived neurotrophic factor (BDNF) and neurotrophin-4 (NT-4) bind primarily to TrkB. The specificity of neurotrophin-3 (NT-3) is less precise. Although it mostly binds to TrkC, it can also bind TrkA and TrkB. In addition, all of the neurotrophins bind to p75.

Source. Adapted from Jessell TM, Sanes JR: "The Generation and Survival of Nerve Cells," in *Principles of Neural Science, 4th Edition.* Edited by Kandel ER, Schwartz JH, Jessell TM. New York, McGraw-Hill, 2000, pp. 1041–1062. Copyright 2000, The McGraw-Hill Companies, Inc. Used with permission.

line–derived neurotrophic factor. Transgenic mice with targeted null mutations in neurotrophic genes or their receptors have been produced and have abnormalities in selected populations of neurons (Davies 1994). Neuronal survival factors are not exclusively target-derived. Sources also include innervating neurons, glial cells, and circulating hormones. The ability of trophic factors to promote neuronal survival has been attributed to the phosphatidylinositide 3'-OH kinase/c-Akt kinase cascade acting through at least two components of the intracellular cell death pathway, Bad and caspase-9, and the transcription factor NF-κB (Datta et al. 1999). In addition to their clear roles as survival factors, neurotrophins can also promote cell death through the activation of the p75 receptor, which competes with the Trk receptors for binding to the neurotrophins. Thus, a neuron's decision to live or die is determined by a balance between neurotrophin binding to Trk and p75 receptors (Miller and Kaplan 2001).

The cellular mechanisms of apoptosis appear to involve a complex interplay of several signaling cascades

(Putcha and Johnson 2004; Sastry and Rao 2000). In the worm C. *elegans, ced-3* and *ced-4* are required for apoptosis (Ellis et al. 1991). The gene product of *ced-3* is a cysteine protease and has a mammalian homologue called interleukin-1b converting enzyme (ICE). A large number of cysteine proteases have recently been discovered in many species that play diverse roles in cell death; these proteins are classified as members of the large caspase (for *cysteine-requiring aspartate protease*) family of proteins. Some of the caspases are considered the final effector proteins in the cell death cascade. In contrast to the cell death genes *ced-3* and *ced-4, ced-9* acts to prevent apoptosis in normally surviving C. *elegans* cells. A mutation in *ced-9* leads to widespread apoptosis and death of the embryo (Hengartner et al. 1992). The *ced-9* gene found in worms is homologous to the human oncogene *Bcl-2*, which is overexpressed in human B cell lymphomas (Tsujimoto et al. 1984). The human gene can block cell death in several in vivo and in vitro systems and has been transferred to C. *elegans*, where, remarkably, it can substitute for *ced-9* and prevent apoptosis of C. *elegans* cells. These studies have led to the current "central dogma" of apoptosis: a protein called Egl-1 is induced in cells destined to undergo apoptosis; Egl-1 interacts with Ced-9, displacing the adapter Ced-4, which then activates Ced-3 and causes cell death (Putcha and Johnson 2004). In recent years, results suggest that there may be several apoptotic pathways that depend on cell type and the inducing agent; however, most of these pathways appear to converge at the ICE/caspase step. Although some of the more specific steps in the cell death pathway remain unclear, the basic molecular mechanisms of apoptosis show a remarkable conservation across evolution.

The molecular events that underlie apoptosis in neuronal and nonneuronal cells are likely to include an array of initiators, mediators, and inhibitors, but several common features are emerging. There is evidence that reactive oxygen species can trigger apoptosis in neurons (Greenlund et al. 1995), and *Bcl-2* may prevent apoptosis by suppressing free-radical production (Hockenbery et al. 1990; Kane et al. 1993). This hypothesis has led to attempts to use antioxidants and inhibitors of free-radical production as therapeutic agents in several neurodegenerative diseases, trauma, and stroke. For example, superoxide dismutase (a free-radical scavenger) protects neurons from ischemic injury. Transgenic mice that overexpress superoxide dismutase have smaller infarcts after arterial occlusion (Kinouchi et al. 1991). Mutations in the Cu/Zn superoxide dismutase gene are associated with certain forms of familial amyotrophic lateral sclerosis, suggesting that oxygen radicals may be responsible for motor neuron degeneration in patients with this disease (Rosen et al. 1993).

EXPERIENCE-DEPENDENT SYNAPTIC REFINEMENT

Normal sensory experience is essential to the maturation of neural connections in both the peripheral and central nervous systems. Sensory experience shapes the development of many diverse brain regions during a specific time window during development called the *critical period*. The process of synaptic refinement becomes clinically significant as it continues to be important throughout the life span, providing mechanisms for activity-dependent modification of neuronal structure and connectivity that may be the basis for learning, memory, and forgetting. The integral role of sensory activity in brain development and the ability of experience to alter perception have been most extensively documented in the visual system. In the visual system, overlapping visual input from the two eyes must be combined in an orderly way to maximize acuity and stereopsis (Figure 1–19). In animals with binocular vision, such as humans, cats, and monkeys, visual stimuli from a specific region of visual space activate neurons in the contralateral visual cortex. Neurons in the left hemi-retinas of right and left eyes both convey signals to the left cortex, and similarly, neurons in the right hemi-retinas convey signals to the right cortex (Figure 1–19A). Thus, visual information emanating from the same external source is temporarily separated into right and left eye–specific pathways and then reunited in the same cortical hemisphere.

How is this visual information recombined? The eye-specific segregation of inputs from each retina is maintained in the visual thalamus, or lateral geniculate nucleus (LGN), and in the projection layers of the visual cortex, but then eventually converges in other layers of the primary visual cortex (V1). In geniculate-recipient layers of V1 in the adult, inputs from the two eyes project to separate columns of cells. The ocular dominance columns (OD columns) thus formed are arranged adjacent to each other in alternate stripes dominated by one eye or the other (Figure 1–19) (Hubel and Wiesel 1977). The pattern of stripes formed on the surface of the cortex resembles those of a zebra (Figure 1–19B, D). Output neurons in the OD columns project to other cortical layers, where the visual information derived from inputs to both eyes is recombined and stereopsis clues are extracted. How separate signals from each eye are handled in parallel, recombined, and separated again is representative of a more general pattern in the processing of visual information (Livingstone and Hubel 1988).

Although there are some conflicting reports (Crowley and Katz 2002), most evidence suggests that during development, OD columns arise through activity-dependent processes (Hubel and Wiesel 1977). Initially, geniculate axons carrying information from both eyes overlap. However, as

development proceeds, these axons slowly begin to segregate into OD columns (Figure 1–19B, C). During this period, the pattern of distinct stripes, evenly divided between the two eyes, depends on normal visual activity. If vision in one eye is impaired or there is strabismus, input from the normal or dominant eye comes to control most of the visual cortex, and the other eye becomes functionally blind (Figure 1–19E). In the cortex, the ocular dominance columns of the normal or dominant eye expand at the expense of those of the impaired eye. The columnar segregation of inputs carrying information from each eye is activity dependent (Constantine-Paton et al. 1990; Shatz and Stryker 1988). It depends on discordant inputs from the two retinas; segregation fails if all visual input to the cortex is blocked (with tetrodotoxin) or artificially synchronized in both eyes (by simultaneous electrical stimulation) (Shatz 1990).

Different patterns of electrical activity from each eye, as occur normally, mediate OD segregation. But segregation also requires the activity of postsynaptic cortical cells; infusion of the inhibitory drug muscimol (a GABA$_A$ agonist) causes a reversal of ocular dominance so that, paradoxically, the weak rather than the strong eye gains the larger cortical influence (Reiter and Stryker 1988). Thus, appropriate segregation of cortical inputs requires the coordination of both normal presynaptic activity and postsynaptic responses. Similar activity dependence is also found in retinal axons impinging on LGN cells (Goodman and Shatz 1993). Indeed, activity-dependent segregation of sensory inputs into functional columns appears to be an inherent property of topographic projections in sensory systems. In frogs, which have neither binocular vision nor OD columns, when an extra eye is transplanted into a tadpole, the optic fibers from the third eye compete with the other eye innervating that side of the brain and produce OD columns (Constantine-Paton and Law 1978).

The cellular and molecular mechanisms underlying activity-dependent synaptic refinement are just beginning to be elucidated. Many of these mechanisms are remarkably similar to the cellular mechanisms that underlie learning and memory in the adult brain. In the visual system, geniculate afferents are believed to undergo segregation into OD columns based on a Hebbian learning rule (Hebb 1949), whereby neurons that fire together are selectively strengthened. This rule predicts that neurons that fire synchronously will strengthen their synapses, whereas asynchronous firing will weaken synapses. LTP and LTD are attractive candidates for mediating the process of OD column formation (Bear and Rittenhouse 1999). In addition to activity, other factors may also act to selectively strengthen coincidentally active synapses. One of the most attractive candidates for such a role is the neurotrophin family of growth factors. The neurotro-

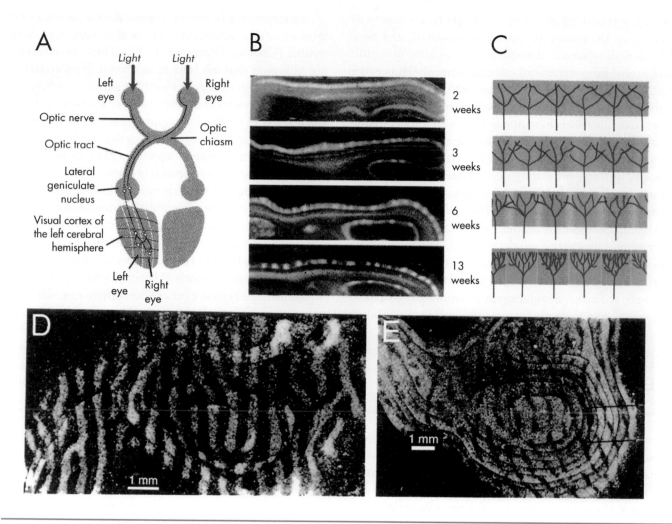

FIGURE 1–19. Ocular dominance columns in visual cortex. *Panel A.* In the human visual pathway, optic fibers from each eye split at the optic chiasm, half going to each side of the brain. In this schematic drawing, fibers conveying visual information from the left sides of each retina are shown projecting to the left lateral geniculate nucleus (LGN). LGN neurons (in different layers) in turn project to ipsilateral visual cortex (principally to layer 4c). In the geniculate-recipient layers of the mature visual cortex, inputs from the eyes segregate into ocular dominance (OD) columns. *Panel B.* Radioactive proline injections into one eye of a two-week-old kitten uniformly label layer 4 in coronal sections of visual cortex, indicating that afferents from that eye are evenly distributed in cortex at this age. However, over the next few weeks, similar injections show a segregation of geniculate afferents into OD columns. *Panel C.* Schematic diagram of the formation of OD columns within layer 4 of cortex during normal development. *Panel D.* One eye of a normal monkey was injected with a radioactive tracer that was transported transsynaptically along the visual pathways. Cortical areas receiving inputs from the injected eye are labeled white, revealing an alternating pattern of evenly spaced stripes (section cut tangentially through layer 4c). *Panel E.* Monocular deprivation alters the development of OD columns. Here the tracer was injected into the nondeprived eye, revealing broader stripes and thus an expansion of the area innervated by the nondeprived eye. Thus, normal experience is a prerequisite to the correct wiring of the cortex.

Source. Panel A reprinted from Kandel ER, Jessell T: "Early Experience and the Fine Tuning of Synaptic Connections," in *Principles of Neural Science.* Edited by Kandel ER, Schwartz JHS, Jessell TM. Stamford, CT, Appleton and Lange, 1991, pp. 945–958. Copyright 1991, The McGraw-Hill Companies, Inc. Used with permission.
Panel B adapted from LeVay S, Stryker MP, Shatz CJ: "Ocular Dominance Columns and Their Development in Layer IV of the Cat's Visual Cortex: A Quantitative Study." *Journal of Comparative Neurology* 179:223–244, 1978. Used with permission.
Panel C reprinted from Purves D, Augustine GJ, Fitzpatrick D, et al. (eds): *Neuroscience.* Sunderland, MA, Sinauer Associates, 1997, p. 427. Used with permission.
Panels D and E reprinted from Hubel DH, Wiesel TN, LeVay S: "Plasticity of Ocular Dominance Columns in Monkey Striate Cortex." *Philosophical Transactions of the Royal Society of London—Series B: Biological Sciences* 278:377–409, 1977. Used with permission.

phins are produced in limiting amounts by cortical neurons, their expression is increased by activity, and they can increase synaptic strength as well as alter dendritic and axonal arborizations of cortical neurons (Huberman and McAllister 2002). Consistent with this hypothesis, either infusion of excess neurotrophins or blockade of the neurotrophins prevents the formation of OD columns (Cabelli et al. 1995, 1997). Thus, the neurotrophins are in a prime position to mediate experience-dependent synaptic refinement during development. Finally, in recent years, a critical role for inhibitory neurons in mediating activity-dependent changes in circuitry has been revealed. Experience-dependent plasticity is deficient in transgenic mice that have decreased GABAergic transmission (Hensch and Fagiolini 2005), and the end of the critical period for activity-dependent plasticity correlates strongly with the development of inhibitory synaptic transmission in multiple systems (Berardi et al. 2003).

NEUROTROPHIC AND NEUROTOXIC ACTIONS OF NEUROTRANSMITTERS

Neurotransmitters themselves may have trophic or toxic roles in the shaping of neurons and their interconnections (Lipton and Kater 1989). Excitatory neurotransmitters such as glutamate trigger Ca^{2+} influx that controls the progress of growth cones. Local intracellular levels of Ca^{2+} act within a narrow window. When levels are low, growth cones are quiescent; when levels rise, growth cones begin to move. Above a certain level, however, further elevations of Ca^{2+} arrest growth and cause retraction or destruction of neuronal processes (al-Mohanna et al. 1992). This can be countered by inhibitory neurotransmitters as well as by provision of neurotrophic factors (Kater et al. 1989; Mattson and Kater 1989).

Higher levels of glutamate produce excitotoxicity, perhaps reflecting the pathologic functioning of these developmental signaling systems (Kater et al. 1989). Alternatively, excitotoxicity may have a normal function in regulating cell numbers and connectivity. Excitotoxicity appears to be mediated acutely by the entry of Na^+ through AMPA channels. This leads to neuronal swelling (resulting in brain edema). Sustained Ca^{2+} entry through NMDA receptor channels causes a delayed mode of excitotoxicity that kills neurons, probably by activation of intracellular proteases and/or generation of free radicals, including NO (Arundine and Tymianski 2003; Choi 1994; Dawson et al. 1994). In addition to mediating Na^+ influx and swelling, AMPA receptors may be coupled to the IP_3/DAG pathway, leading also to increases in intracellular Ca^{2+} and C kinase activation.

Excitotoxicity figures prominently in neuronal loss in strokes, status epilepticus, hypoglycemia, and head trauma (Choi and Rothman 1990). These brain insults are linked in that all lead to neuronal depolarization, which results in excessive electrical activity, evoking excessive increases in glutamate release. In each case, elevated levels of extracellular glutamate are present in experimental models, and their cytopathology can be mimicked by intracerebral injections of excitatory amino acids. The same neurons spared in these disease states are also less affected in the experimental models, probably because they have fewer excitatory amino acid receptors. Injured neurons show increased intracellular levels of Ca^{2+}, and excitatory amino acid antagonists, particularly those blocking NMDA receptors or channels, prevent or dramatically reduce neuronal loss in these conditions.

Similarities between other neuropsychiatric disorders and idiopathic neurodegenerative disorders suggest a pervasive role for excitotoxic mechanisms (Arundine and Tymianski 2003). Intriguingly, a growing body of findings implicates excitotoxic mechanisms in the pathology of Huntington's disease. The neuropathology of Huntington's disease is mimicked by the injection of excitatory amino acids, and the same classes of striatal neurons are spared in both cases (Wexler et al. 1991).

PERSPECTIVES

Brain development is not determined merely by cell-autonomous genetic programs but is instead highly interactive, depending on complex hierarchies of signaling factors operating to progressively restrict cell fate. Once cells have achieved a specific phenotype and have arrived at an appropriate location, competition for survival factors provides another opportunity for environmental influence over developmental outcome. The cellular development of the brain is therefore not strictly lineage dependent, but rather involves a remarkable degree of interactive signaling. In many brain areas, pruning of exuberant synaptic contacts on an activity-dependent basis is yet another example of a mechanism by which experience can refine structural aspects of brain development. One consequence of these developmental mechanisms is that no two outcomes will be exactly the same, even in a case of twins with identical genetic makeup. Another consequence is the potential for pathologic disruption of normal development by physical, chemical, or infectious agents in the fetal or neonatal period.

It is becoming increasingly clear that the adult brain retains a significant degree of plasticity throughout life and that changes in cortical organization can be induced by behaviorally important, temporally coincident sensory inputs (Buonomano and Merzenich 1998). Behavioral training of adult owl monkeys in discrimination of the temporal features of a tactile stimulus can alter the spatial and temporal response properties of cortical neurons. When adult owl monkeys are rewarded for responding to a 30-Hz tactile stimulation of one finger, there is a progressive increase in the area of somatosensory cortex over which neurons respond to the 30-Hz stimulation.

The kinds of changes that take place in the organization of somatosensory cortex also occur in primary auditory cortex. Owl monkeys trained for several weeks to discriminate small differences in the frequency of sequentially presented tones demonstrate progressive improvement in performance with training. At the end of the training period, the amount of cortex responding to behaviorally relevant frequencies is increased. In control studies with equivalent stimulation procedures in which stimuli are unattended, no significant representational changes are recorded. Thus, attended, rewarded behaviors can induce changes in the organization of primary sensory cortex that are correlated with an improvement in perceptual acuity. These experiments begin to suggest ways in which life experiences, including psychotherapy (Etkin et al. 2005), can potentially modify cortical function and alter perception or behavior.

These plastic changes appear to share a common molecular language, first expressed during development involving activity-dependent mechanisms. Neural activity is essential to activity-dependent synaptic refinement, LTP, LTD, and excitotoxicity (Bailey et al. 2000; Brown et al. 1990; Choi and Rothman 1990; Constantine-Paton et al. 1990; Lipton and Kater 1989). The key player is the NMDA receptor, which requires both agonist binding and depolarization for activation. This appears to be the essential requirement for pairing specificity, a mode of synaptic plasticity initially postulated by Hebb (1949), whereby simultaneous activation of presynaptic and postsynaptic elements strengthens connections. Simultaneously, correlation of presynaptic activity with postsynaptic inhibition may selectively weaken connections (Reiter and Stryker 1988). The Ca^{2+} influx mediated by the NMDA receptor may trigger changes in the strength of synapses, in time leading to more permanent structural changes in synapse number. At higher levels, Ca^{2+} may arrest the growth of neurites, cause their retraction, or selectively lesion the susceptible cell.

Many neuropsychiatric disorders no doubt play out in this context. To consider a few examples, most of which have already been mentioned, striatal degeneration in Huntington's disease appears to be due to the overproduction of huntingtin, a synaptic vesicle–associated protein (DiFiglia et al. 1995) that among a multiplicity of actions may trigger NMDA receptor–mediated excitotoxicity (Rego and de Almeida 2005). In Parkinson's disease, a selective loss of dopaminergic neurons in the substantia nigra may be the delayed result of a viral process, lesioning by dopaminergic neurotoxins exemplified by MPTP, or a deficiency in BDNF or glia cell line–derived neurotrophic factor, both of which may be essential for the survival of dopaminergic neurons (Cardoso et al. 2005). In Alzheimer's disease, the loss of cholinergic neurons may result from a deficiency or perhaps aberrant handling of NGF once it is taken up by neurons in the basal forebrain (Pereira et al. 2005). Clearly, elucidation of the cellular and molecular events that occur during normal brain development, maturation, and aging, as well as those that underlie neuropsychiatric disorders, will greatly enhance approaches to their treatment and prevention.

Perhaps the most exciting and revolutionary possible intervention to treat neuropsychiatric diseases is the potential use of stem cells to repair the damaged brain (Lee et al. 2000). Despite tremendous efforts by the neuroscience community during the last century, there are currently no feasible therapies for repairing the damaged adult human brain. Clearly, treatment of many neuropsychiatric diseases would be greatly enhanced if new neurons could be added to a particular damaged brain region and stimulated to differentiate into the appropriate neuronal type and to form appropriate connections. There are currently two approaches to achieving this goal. First, pluripotent stem cells are being used, with increasing success, to repopulate damaged brain regions. For example, adult rats with symptoms similar to Parkinson's disease can regain function after implantation of dopaminergic neurons created in vitro from fetal rat neuronal precursors (Studer et al. 1998). Second, newly discovered intrinsic repair mechanisms in the adult brain are being studied for their therapeutic potential. Neurogenesis has been discovered in several regions of the adult brain, including the dentate gyrus of the hippocampal formation (Fuchs and Gould 2000). These neurons migrate within the brain regions, differentiate, and form functional connections. Moreover, experience, learning, and physical exercise enhance neuronal proliferation in the adult (Fuchs and Gould 2000; Kempermann et al. 2004). The discovery of neurogenesis in the adult brain suggests that the adult brain may have intrinsic mechanisms for repair that could be manipulated to treat neurodegenerative disorders (Kozorovitskiy and Gould 2003; Lie et al. 2004). As the mechanisms of neuropsychiatric disorders are resolved at the cellular and molecular levels, and the tremendous potential of stem cell research is harnessed, it is likely that revolutionary treatments for many neuropsychiatric diseases will be forthcoming.

Highlights for the Clinician

◆ Neuropsychiatric disorders result from disordered functioning of neurons, and in particular their synapses.

◆ Individual neurons in the brain receive synaptic input from thousands of neurons and, in turn, send information to thousands of others.

◆ Learning and memory involve both short-term and long-term changes at synapses; for example, high-frequency stimulation of hippocampal pathways leads to long-term potentiation (LTP).

◆ Neurotransmitters activate second messenger systems that profoundly increase the range of responses a neuron shows to synaptic input, extending to changes in gene transcription.

◆ During development, neurons and glia are generated in proliferative zones lining the ventricular system and then migrate into the overlying cortical mantle.

◆ The determination of cell fate occurs at regional, local, and cellular levels.

◆ Neurotransmitters themselves may have trophic or toxic roles in the shaping of neurons and their interconnections.

◆ Neurons are initially produced in excess; their survival depends on trophic factors produced by their targets.

◆ Normal sensory experience is essential to the maturation of neural connections.

◆ The adult brain retains a significant degree of plasticity; changes in cortical organization can be induced by behaviorally important, temporally coincident sensory input.

◆ In both learning and development, the key molecular coincidence detector is the NMDA receptor, which requires both neurotransmitter binding and depolarization for activation.

◆ Ca^{2+} influx mediated by the NMDA receptor triggers changes in the strength of synapses, in time leading to changes in synapse number.

◆ Ca^{2+} regulates the growth or retraction of neurites, programmed cell death.

◆ The discovery of neurogenesis in the adult brain suggests that the adult brain may have intrinsic mechanisms for repair that could be manipulated to treat neurodegenerative disorders.

RECOMMENDED READINGS

Cummings JL: Toward a molecular neuropsychiatry of neurodegenerative diseases. Ann Neurol 54:147–154, 2003

Graham D, Lantos P: Greenfield's Neuropathology, 7th Edition. London, Arnold, 2002

Kandel ER, Schwartz JH, Jessell TM: Principles of Neural Science, 4th Edition. New York: McGraw-Hill, 2000

Siegel GJ, Albers RW, Brady S, et al: Basic Neurochemistry: Molecular, Cellular and Medical Aspects, 7th Edition. New York, Elsevier, 2006

REFERENCES

al-Mohanna FA, Cave J, Bolsover SR: A narrow window of intracellular calcium concentration is optimal for neurite outgrowth in rat sensory neurones. Brain Res Dev Brain Res 70:287–290, 1992

Allen NJ, Barres BA: Signaling between glia and neurons: focus on synaptic plasticity. Curr Opin Neurobiol 15:542–548, 2005

Alvarez-Buylla A, Kirn JR, Nottebohm F: Birth of projection neurons in adult avian brain may be related to perceptual or motor learning. Science 249:1444–1446, 1990

Anderson SA, Eisenstat DD, Shi L, et al: Interneuron migration from basal forebrain to neocortex: dependence on Dlx genes. Science 278:474–476, 1997

Ansorge MS, Zhou M, Lira A, et al: Early life blockade of the 5-HT transporter alters emotional behavior in adult mice. Science 306:879–881, 2004

Anthony TE, Klein C, Fishell G, et al: Radial glia serve as neuronal progenitors in all regions of the central nervous system. Neuron 41:881–890, 2004

Anwyl R: Induction and expression mechanisms of postsynaptic NMDA receptor-independent homosynaptic long-term depression. Prog Neurobiol 78:17–37, 2006

Araque A, Parpura V, Sanzgiri RP, et al: Tripartite synapses: glia, the unacknowledged partner. Trends Neurosci 22:208–215, 1999

Arundine M, Tymianski M: Molecular mechanisms of calcium-dependent neurodegeneration in excitotoxicity. Cell Calcium 34:325–337, 2003

Bailey C, Kandel E: Synaptic growth and the persistence of long-term memory: a molecular perspective, in The Cognitive Neurosciences, 3rd Edition. Edited by Gazzaniga MS. Cambridge, MA, MIT Press, 2004, pp 647–663

Bailey CH, Giustetto M, Huang YY, et al: Is heterosynaptic modulation essential for stabilizing Hebbian plasticity and memory? Nat Rev Neurosci 1:11–20, 2000

Barzilai A, Kennedy TE, Sweatt JD, et al: 5-HT modulates protein synthesis and the expression of specific proteins during long-term facilitation in *Aplysia* sensory neurons. Neuron 2:1577–1586, 1989

Bayer SA, Altman J: Neocortical Development. New York, Raven, 1991

Bear MF, Rittenhouse CD: Molecular basis for induction of ocular dominance plasticity. J Neurobiol 41:83–91, 1999

Behrendt RP, Young C: Hallucinations in schizophrenia, sensory impairment, and brain disease: a unifying model. Behav Brain Sci 27:771–830, 2004

Bennett MVL: Electrical transmission: a functional analysis and comparison to chemical transmission, in Handbook of Physiology, Vol I: The Nervous System. Bethesda, MD, American Physiological Society, 1977, pp 357–416

Bennett MVL, Barrio LC, Bargiello TA, et al: Gap junctions: new tools, new answers, new questions. Neuron 6:305–320, 1991

Berardi N, Pizzorusso T, Ratto GM, et al: Molecular basis of plasticity in the visual cortex. Trends Neurosci 26:369–378, 2003

Black IB: Trophic interactions and brain plasticity, in The Cognitive Neurosciences. Edited by Gazzaniga MS. Cambridge, MA, MIT Press, 1995, pp 9–17

Blier P, Abbott FV: Putative mechanisms of action of antidepressant drugs in affective and anxiety disorders and pain. J Psychiatry Neurosci 26:37–43, 2001

Bliss TV, Lomo T: Long-lasting potentiation of synaptic transmission in the dentate area of the anaesthetized rabbit following stimulation of the perforant path. J Physiol 232:331–356, 1973

Blitzer RD, Connor JH, Brown GP, et al: Gating of CaMKII by cAMP-regulated protein phosphatase activity during LTP. Science 280:1940–1942, 1998

Blitzer RD, Iyengar R, Landau EM: Postsynaptic signaling networks: cellular cogwheels underlying long-term plasticity. Biol Psychiatry 57:113–119, 2005

Bohn LM, Lefkowitz RJ, Gainetdinov RR, et al: Enhanced morphine analgesia in mice lacking beta-arrestin 2. Science 286:2495–2498, 1999

Bolshakov VY, Golan H, Kandel ER, et al: Recruitment of new sites of synaptic transmission during the cAMP-dependent late phase of LTP at CA3-CA1 synapses in the hippocampus. Neuron 19:635–651, 1997

The Boulder Committee: Embryonic vertebrate central nervous system: revised terminology. Anat Rec 166:257–261, 1970

Brenman JE, Bredt DS: Synaptic signaling by nitric oxide. Curr Opin Neurobiol 7:374–378, 1997

Brittis PA, Lu Q, Flanagan JG: Axonal protein synthesis provides a mechanism for localized regulation at an intermediate target. Cell 110:223–235, 2002

Brivanlou IH, Warland DK, Meister M: Mechanisms of concerted firing among retinal ganglion cells. Neuron 20:527–539, 1998

Brown TH, Kairiss EW, Keenan CL: Hebbian synapses: biophysical mechanisms and algorithms. Annu Rev Neurosci 13:475–511, 1990

Buonomano DV, Merzenich MM: Cortical plasticity: from synapses to maps. Annu Rev Neurosci 21:149–186, 1998

Burack MA, Silverman MA, Banker G: The role of selective transport in neuronal protein sorting. Neuron 26:465–472, 2000

Cabelli RJ, Hohn A, Shatz CJ: Inhibition of ocular dominance column formation by infusion of NT-4/5 or BDNF. Science 267:1662–1666, 1995

Cabelli RJ, Shelton DL, Segal RA, et al: Blockade of endogenous ligands of trkB inhibits formation of ocular dominance columns. Neuron 19:63–76, 1997

Cardoso SM, Moreira PI, Agostinho P, et al: Neurodegenerative pathways in Parkinson's disease: therapeutic strategies. Curr Drug Targets CNS Neurol Disord 4:405–419, 2005

Caspi A, Sugden K, Moffitt TE, et al: Influence of life stress on depression: moderation by a polymorphism in the *5-HTT* gene. Science 301:386–389, 2003

Chenn A, Walsh CA: Regulation of cerebral cortical size by control of cell cycle exit in neural precursors. Science 297:365–369, 2002

Chih B, Afridi SK, Clark L, et al: Disorder-associated mutations lead to functional inactivation of neuroligins. Hum Mol Genet 13:1471–1477, 2004

Choi DW: Calcium and excitotoxic neuronal injury. Ann N Y Acad Sci 747:162–171, 1994

Choi DW, Rothman SM: The role of glutamate neurotoxicity in hypoxic-ischemic neuronal death. Annu Rev Neurosci 13:171–182, 1990

Cole AJ, Saffen DW, Baraban JM, et al: Rapid increase of an immediate early gene messenger RNA in hippocampal neurons by synaptic NMDA receptor activation. Nature 340:474–476, 1989

Constantine-Paton M, Law MI: Eye-specific termination bands in tecta of three-eyed frogs. Science 202:639–641, 1978

Constantine-Paton M, Cline HT, Debski E: Patterned activity, synaptic convergence, and the NMDA receptor in developing visual pathways. Annu Rev Neurosci 13:129–154, 1990

Coyle JT: The neurochemistry of schizophrenia, in Basic Neurochemistry: Molecular, Cellular and Medical Aspects, 7th Edition. Edited by Siegel GJ, Albers RW, Brady S, et al. Burlington, MA, Elsevier Academic, 2006, pp 875–885

Crowley JC, Katz LC: Ocular dominance development revisited. Curr Opin Neurobiol 12:104–109, 2002

Cummings JL: Toward a molecular neuropsychiatry of neurodegenerative diseases. Ann Neurol 54:147–154, 2003

Dani JW, Chernjavsky A, Smith SJ: Neuronal activity triggers calcium waves in hippocampal astrocyte networks. Neuron 8:429–440, 1992

Datta SR, Brunet A, Greenberg ME: Cellular survival: a play in three Akts. Genes Dev 13:2905–2927, 1999

Davies AM: The role of neurotrophins in the developing nervous system. J Neurobiol 25:1334–1348, 1994

Dawson TM, Zhang J, Dawson VL, et al: Nitric oxide: cellular regulation and neuronal injury. Prog Brain Res 103:365–369, 1994

Dealy CN, Beyer EC, Kosher RA: Expression patterns of mRNAs for the gap junction proteins connexin43 and connexin42 suggest their involvement in chick limb morphogenesis and specification of the arterial vasculature. Dev Dyn 199:156–167, 1994

des Portes V, Pinard JM, Billuart P, et al: A novel CNS gene required for neuronal migration and involved in X-linked subcortical laminar heterotopia and lissencephaly syndrome. Cell 92:51–61, 1998

DiFiglia M, Sapp E, Chase K, et al: Huntingtin is a cytoplasmic protein associated with vesicles in human and rat brain neurons. Neuron 14:1075–1081, 1995

Dillon C, Goda Y: The actin cytoskeleton: integrating form and function at the synapse. Annu Rev Neurosci 28:25–55, 2005

Doetsch F, Caille I, Lim DA, et al: Subventricular zone astrocytes are neural stem cells in the adult mammalian brain. Cell 97:703–716, 1999

Dumartin B, Caille I, Gonon F, et al: Internalization of D_1 dopamine receptor in striatal neurons in vivo as evidence of activation by dopamine agonists. J Neurosci 18:1650–1661, 1998

During MJ, Ryder KM, Spencer DD: Hippocampal GABA transporter function in temporal-lobe epilepsy. Nature 376:174–177, 1995

Edwards SN, Buckmaster AE, Tolkovsky AM: The death programme in cultured sympathetic neurones can be suppressed at the posttranslational level by nerve growth factor, cyclic AMP, and depolarization. J Neurochem 57:2140–2143, 1991

Eilers J, Konnerth A: Dendritic signal integration. Curr Opin Neurobiol 7:385–390, 1997

Ellis RE, Yuan JY, Horvitz HR: Mechanisms and functions of cell death. Annu Rev Cell Biol 7:663–698, 1991

Etkin A, Pittenger C, Polan HJ, et al: Toward a neurobiology of psychotherapy: basic science and clinical applications. J Neuropsychiatry Clin Neurosci 17:145–158, 2005

Fellin T, Carmignoto G: Neurone-to-astrocyte signalling in the brain represents a distinct multifunctional unit. J Physiol 559:3–15, 2004

Feng Y, Walsh CA: Protein-protein interactions, cytoskeletal regulation and neuronal migration. Nat Rev Neurosci 2:408–416, 2001

Fuchs E, Gould E: Mini-review: in vivo neurogenesis in the adult brain: regulation and functional implications. Eur J Neurosci 12:2211–2214, 2000

Gainetdinov RR, Caron MG: Monoamine transporters: from genes to behavior. Annu Rev Pharmacol Toxicol 43:261–284, 2003

Gainetdinov RR, Mohn AR, Caron MG: Genetic animal models: focus on schizophrenia. Trends Neurosci 24:527–533, 2001

Ghosh A, Greenberg ME: Calcium signaling in neurons: molecular mechanisms and cellular consequences. Science 268:239–247, 1995

Girault JA, Greengard P: Principles of signal transduction, in Neurobiology of Mental Illness, 2nd Edition. Edited by Charney DS, Nestler EJ. New York, Oxford University Press, 2004, pp 41–65

Giros B, Jaber M, Jones SR, et al: Hyperlocomotion and indifference to cocaine and amphetamine in mice lacking the dopamine transporter. Nature 379:606–612, 1996

Gleeson JG, Allen KM, Fox JW, et al: Doublecortin, a brain-specific gene mutated in human X-linked lissencephaly and double cortex syndrome, encodes a putative signaling protein. Cell 92:63–72, 1998

Goldman-Rakic PS, Muly EC 3rd, Williams GV: D(1) receptors in prefrontal cells and circuits. Brain Res Brain Res Rev 31:295–301, 2000

Goodman CS, Shatz CJ: Developmental mechanisms that generate precise patterns of neuronal connectivity. Cell 72(suppl):77–98, 1993

Gotz M, Huttner WB: The cell biology of neurogenesis. Nat Rev Mol Cell Biol 6:777–788, 2005

Graham D, Lantos P: Greenfield's Neuropathology, 7th Edition. London, Arnold, 2002

Greengard P: The neurobiology of slow synaptic transmission. Science 294:1024–1030, 2001

Greenlund LJ, Deckwerth TL, Johnson E Jr: Superoxide dismutase delays neuronal apoptosis: a role for reactive oxygen species in programmed neuronal death. Neuron 14:303–315, 1995

Halliday AL, Cepko CL: Generation and migration of cells in the developing striatum. Neuron 9:15–26, 1992

Hanashima C, Li SC, Shen L, et al: Foxg1 suppresses early cortical cell fate. Science 303:56–59, 2004

Hassel B, Dingledine R: Glutamate, in Basic Neurochemistry: Molecular, Cellular and Medical Aspects, 7th Edition. Edited by Siegel GJ, Albers RW, Brady S, et al. Burlington, MA, Elsevier Academic, 2006, pp 267–290

Hatten ME: Riding the glial monorail: a common mechanism for glial-guided neuronal migration in different regions of the developing mammalian brain. Trends Neurosci 13:179–184, 1990

Haubensak W, Attardo A, Denk W, et al: Neurons arise in the basal neuroepithelium of the early mammalian telencephalon: a major site of neurogenesis. Proc Natl Acad Sci USA 101:3196–3201, 2004

Hawkins RD, Kandel ER, Bailey CH: Molecular mechanisms of memory storage in Aplysia. Biol Bull 210:174–191, 2006

Haydar TF, Wang F, Schwartz ML, et al: Differential modulation of proliferation in the neocortical ventricular and subventricular zones. J Neurosci 20:5764–5774, 2000

Hebb DO: The Organization of Behavior: A Neuropsychological theory. New York, Wiley, 1949

Hengartner MO, Ellis RE, Horvitz HR: Caenorhabditis elegans gene ced-9 protects cells from programmed cell death. Nature 356:494–499, 1992

Hengerer B, Lindholm D, Heumann R, et al: Lesion-induced increase in nerve growth factor mRNA is mediated by c-fos. Proc Natl Acad Sci USA 87:3899–3903, 1990

Hensch TK, Fagiolini M: Excitatory-inhibitory balance and critical period plasticity in developing visual cortex. Prog Brain Res 147:115–124, 2005

Hille B: Ion Channels of Excitable Membranes, 3rd Edition. Sunderland, MA, Sinauer Associates, 2001

Hirokawa N, Takemura R: Biochemical and molecular characterization of diseases linked to motor proteins. Trends Biochem Sci 28:558–565, 2003

Hockenbery D, Nunez G, Milliman C, et al: Bcl-2 is an inner mitochondrial membrane protein that blocks programmed cell death. Nature 348:334–336, 1990

Hökfelt T: Neuropeptides in perspective: the last ten years. Neuron 7:867–879, 1991

Huang YY, Kandel ER: D1/D5 receptor agonists induce a protein synthesis-dependent late potentiation in the CA1 region of the hippocampus. Proc Natl Acad Sci USA 92:2446–2450, 1995

Hubel DH, Wiesel TN: Ferrier lecture: functional architecture of macaque monkey visual cortex. Proc R Soc Lond B Biol Sci 198:1–59, 1977

Hubel DH, Wiesel TN, LeVay S: Plasticity of ocular dominance columns in monkey striate cortex. Philos Trans R Soc Lond B Biol Sci 278:377–409, 1977

Huberman AD, McAllister AK: Neurotrophins and visual cortical plasticity. Prog Brain Res 138:39–51, 2002

Huerta PT, Lisman JE: Low-frequency stimulation at the troughs of theta-oscillation induces long-term depression of previously potentiated CA1 synapses. J Neurophysiol 75:877–884, 1996

Isaac JT: Postsynaptic silent synapses: evidence and mechanisms. Neuropharmacology 45:450–460, 2003

Johnston D, Christie BR, Frick A, et al: Active dendrites, potassium channels and synaptic plasticity. Philos Trans R Soc Lond B Biol Sci 358:667–674, 2003

Kamal A, Goldstein LS: Principles of cargo attachment to cytoplasmic motor proteins. Curr Opin Cell Biol 14:63–68, 2002

Kamei Y, Inagaki N, Nishizawa M, et al: Visualization of mitotic radial glial lineage cells in the developing rat brain by Cdc2 kinase-phosphorylated vimentin. Glia 23:191–199, 1998

Kandel ER: The molecular biology of memory storage: a dialog between genes and synapses. Biosci Rep 21:565–611, 2001a

Kandel ER: The molecular biology of memory storage: a dialogue between genes and synapses. Science 294:1030–1038, 2001b

Kandel ER, O'Dell TJ: Are adult learning mechanisms also used for development? Science 258:243–245, 1992

Kandler K, Katz LC: Neuronal coupling and uncoupling in the developing nervous system. Curr Opin Neurobiol 5:98–105, 1995

Kane DJ, Sarafian TA, Anton R, et al: Bcl-2 inhibition of neural death: decreased generation of reactive oxygen species. Science 262:1274–1277, 1993

Karlin A, Akabas MH: Toward a structural basis for the function of nicotinic acetylcholine receptors and their cousins. Neuron 15:1231–1244, 1995

Kater SB, Mattson MP, Guthrie PB: Calcium-induced neuronal degeneration: a normal growth cone regulating signal gone awry (?). Ann N Y Acad Sci 568:252–261, 1989

Kempermann G, Wiskott L, Gage FH: Functional significance of adult neurogenesis. Curr Opin Neurobiol 14:186–191, 2004

Kennedy MJ, Ehlers MD: Organelles and trafficking machinery for postsynaptic plasticity. Annu Rev Neurosci 29:325–362, 2006

Kim E, Sheng M: PDZ domain proteins of synapses. Nat Rev Neurosci 5:771–781, 2004

Kim JH, Udo H, Li HL, et al: Presynaptic activation of silent synapses and growth of new synapses contribute to intermediate and long-term facilitation in Aplysia. Neuron 40:151–165, 2003

Kinouchi H, Epstein CJ, Mizui T, et al: Attenuation of focal cerebral ischemic injury in transgenic mice overexpressing CuZn superoxide dismutase. Proc Natl Acad Sci USA 88:11158–11162, 1991

Kitayama N, Vaccarino V, Kutner M, et al: Magnetic resonance imaging (MRI) measurement of hippocampal volume in posttraumatic stress disorder: a meta-analysis. J Affect Disord 88:79–86, 2005

Koester J, Siegelbaum S: Propagated signaling: the action potential, in Principles of Neural Science, 4th Edition. Edited by Kandel ER, Schwartz JH, Jessell TM. New York, McGraw-Hill, 2000, pp 167–169

Komuro H, Rakic P: Modulation of neuronal migration by NMDA receptors. Science 260:95–97, 1993

Kozorovitskiy Y, Gould E: Adult neurogenesis: a mechanism for brain repair? J Clin Exp Neuropsychol 25:721–732, 2003

Kriegstein AR, Gotz M: Radial glia diversity: a matter of cell fate. Glia 43:37–43, 2003

Kriegstein AR, Noctor SC: Patterns of neuronal migration in the embryonic cortex. Trends Neurosci 27:392–399, 2004

Landis SC: Target regulation of neurotransmitter phenotype. Trends Neurosci 13:344–350, 1990

Lee H, Chen CX, Liu YJ, et al: KCC2 expression in immature rat cortical neurons is sufficient to switch the polarity of GABA responses. Eur J Neurosci 21:2593–2599, 2005

Lee SH, Sheng M: Development of neuron-neuron synapses. Curr Opin Neurobiol 10:125–131, 2000

Lee SH, Lumelsky N, Studer L, et al: Efficient generation of midbrain and hindbrain neurons from mouse embryonic stem cells. Nat Biotechnol 18:675–679, 2000

Letinic K, Zoncu R, Rakic P: Origin of GABAergic neurons in the human neocortex. Nature 417:645–649, 2002

Lie DC, Song H, Colamarino SA, et al: Neurogenesis in the adult brain: new strategies for central nervous system diseases. Annu Rev Pharmacol Toxicol 44:399–421, 2004

Lin Z, Wang W, Uhl GR: Dopamine transporter tryptophan mutants highlight candidate dopamine- and cocaine-selective domains. Mol Pharmacol 58:1581–1592, 2000

Lipton SA, Kater SB: Neurotransmitter regulation of neuronal outgrowth, plasticity and survival. Trends Neurosci 12:265–270, 1989

Lisman J, Schulman H, Cline H: The molecular basis of CaMKII function in synaptic and behavioural memory. Nat Rev Neurosci 3:175–190, 2002

Livingstone M, Hubel D: Segregation of form, color, movement, and depth: anatomy, physiology, and perception. Science 240:740–749, 1988

Llinás R: The intrinsic electrophysiological properties of mammalian neurons: insights into central nervous system function. Science 242:1654–1664, 1988

Llinás R, Jahnsen H: Electrophysiology of mammalian thalamic neurones *in vitro*. Nature 297:406–408, 1982

Lois C, Garcia-Verdugo JM, Alvarez-Buylla A: Chain migration of neuronal precursors. Science 271:978–981, 1996

London M, Häusser M: Dendritic computation. Annu Rev Neurosci 28:503–532, 2005

LoTurco JJ, Kriegstein AR: Clusters of coupled neuroblasts in embryonic neocortex. Science 252:563–566, 1991

LoTurco JJ, Owens DF, Heath MJS, et al: GABA and glutamate depolarize cortical progenitor cells and inhibit DNA synthesis. Neuron 15:1287–1298, 1995

Luo L, O'Leary DD: Axon retraction and degeneration in development and disease. Annu Rev Neurosci 28:127–156, 2005

Luskin MB, Pearlman AL, Sanes JR: Cell lineage in the cerebral cortex of the mouse studied in vivo and in vitro with a recombinant retrovirus. Neuron 1:635–647, 1988

Lyford GL, Yamagata K, Kaufmann WE, et al: Arc, a growth factor and activity-regulated gene, encodes a novel cytoskeleton-associated protein that is enriched in neuronal dendrites. Neuron 14:433–445, 1995

Lynch MA: Long-term potentiation and memory. Physiol Rev 84:87–136, 2004

MacDermott AB, Mayer ML, Westbrook GL, et al: NMDA-receptor activation increases cytoplasmic calcium concentration in cultured spinal cord neurones. Nature 321:519–522, 1986

Magee JC, Carruth M: Dendritic voltage-gated ion channels regulate the action potential firing mode of hippocampal CA1 pyramidal neurons. J Neurophysiol 82:1895–1901, 1999

Maguire EA, Gadian DG, Johnsrude IS, et al: Navigation-related structural change in the hippocampi of taxi drivers. Proc Natl Acad Sci USA 97:4398–4403, 2000

Mahanty NK, Sah P: Calcium-permeable AMPA receptors mediate long-term potentiation in interneurons in the amygdala. Nature 394:683–687, 1998

Malatesta P, Hartfuss E, Gotz M: Isolation of radial glial cells by fluorescent-activated cell sorting reveals a neuronal lineage. Development 127:5253–5263, 2000

Malgaroli A, Ting AE, Wendland B, et al: Presynaptic component of long-term potentiation visualized at individual hippocampal synapses. Science 268:1624–1628, 1995

Malleret G, Haditsch U, Genoux D, et al: Inducible and reversible enhancement of learning, memory, and long-term potentiation by genetic inhibition of calcineurin. Cell 104:675–686, 2001

Marin O, Rubenstein JL: Cell migration in the forebrain. Annu Rev Neurosci 26:441–483, 2003

Masson J, Sagn C, Hamon M, et al: Neurotransmitter transporters in the central nervous system. Pharmacol Rev 51:439–464, 1999

Mattson MP, Kater SB: Excitatory and inhibitory neurotransmitters in the generation and degeneration of hippocampal neuroarchitecture. Brain Res 478:337–348, 1989

McAllister AK, Katz LC, Lo DC: Neurotrophins and synaptic plasticity. Annu Rev Neurosci 22:295–318, 1999

McConnell SK, Kaznowski CE: Cell cycle dependence of laminar determination in developing neocortex. Science 254:282–285, 1991

McCormick DA, Bal T: Sleep and arousal: thalamocortical mechanisms. Annu Rev Neurosci 20:185–215, 1997

Meffert MK, Calakos NC, Scheller RH, et al: Nitric oxide modulates synaptic vesicle docking/fusion reactions. Neuron 16:1229–1236, 1996

Mennerick S, Zorumski CF: Glial contributions to excitatory neurotransmission in cultured hippocampal cells. Nature 368:59–62, 1994

Miale IL, Sidman RL: An autoradiographic analysis of histogenesis in the mouse cerebellum. Exp Neurol 4:277–296, 1961

Miller FD, Kaplan DR: Neurotrophin signalling pathways regulating neuronal apoptosis. Cell Mol Life Sci 58:1045–1053, 2001

Miller MW: Effects of prenatal exposure to ethanol on neocortical development, II: cell proliferation in the ventricular and subventricular zones of the rat. J Comp Neurol 287:326–338, 1989

Misson JP, Edwards MA, Yamamoto M, et al: Identification of radial glial cells within the developing murine central nervous system: studies based upon a new immunohistochemical marker. Brain Res Dev Brain Res 44:95–108, 1988a

Misson JP, Edwards MA, Yamamoto M, et al: Mitotic cycling of radial glial cells of the fetal murine cerebral wall: a combined autoradiographic and immunohistochemical study. Brain Res 466:183–190, 1988b

Miyakawa T, Leiter LM, Gerber DJ, et al: Conditional calcineurin knockout mice exhibit multiple abnormal behaviors related to schizophrenia. Proc Natl Acad Sci USA 100:8987–8992, 2003

Miyata T, Kawaguchi A, Okano H, et al: Asymmetric inheritance of radial glial fibers by cortical neurons. Neuron 31:727–741, 2001

Miyata T, Kawaguchi A, Saito K, et al: Asymmetric production of surface-dividing and non-surface-dividing cortical progenitor cells. Development 131:3133–3145, 2004

Morgan JI, Curran T: Stimulus-transcription coupling in neurons: role of cellular immediate-early genes. Trends Neurosci 12:459–462, 1989

Morgan JI, Curran T: Immediate-early genes: ten years on. Trends Neurosci 18:66–67, 1995

Murphy TH, Blatter LA, Wier WG, et al: Rapid communication between neurons and astrocytes in primary cortical cultures. J Neurosci 13:2672–2679, 1993

Nadarajah B, Parnavelas JG: Modes of neuronal migration in the developing cerebral cortex. Nat Rev Neurosci 3:423–432, 2002

Nedergaard M: Direct signaling from astrocytes to neurons in cultures of mammalian brain cells. Science 263:1768–1771, 1994

Nery S, Fishell G, Corbin JG: The caudal ganglionic eminence is a source of distinct cortical and subcortical cell populations. Nat Neurosci 5:1279–1287, 2002

Noctor SC, Flint AC, Weissman TA, et al: Neurons derived from radial glial cells establish radial units in neocortex. Nature 409:714–720, 2001

Noctor SC, Flint AC, Weissman TA, et al: Dividing precursor cells of the embryonic cortical ventricular zone have morphological and molecular characteristics of radial glia. J Neurosci 22:3161–3173, 2002

Noctor SC, Martinez-Cerdeno V, Ivic L, et al: Cortical neurons arise in symmetric and asymmetric division zones and migrate through specific phases. Nat Neurosci 7:136–144, 2004

Nowak L, Bregestovski P, Ascher P, et al: Magnesium gates glutamate-activated channels in mouse central neurones. Nature 307:462–465, 1984

O'Brien RJ, Lau LF, Huganir RL: Molecular mechanisms of glutamate receptor clustering at excitatory synapses. Curr Opin Neurobiol 8:364–369, 1998

O'Dell TJ, Huang PL, Dawson TM, et al: Endothelial NOS and the blockade of LTP by NOS inhibitors in mice lacking neuronal NOS. Science 265:542–546, 1994

Olsen R, Betz H: GABA and glycine, in Basic Neurochemistry: Molecular, Cellular and Medical Aspects, 7th Edition. Edited by Siegel GJ, Albers RW, Brady S, et al. Burlington, MA, Elsevier Academic, 2006, pp 291–301

Oppenheim A, Altuvia S, Kornitzer D, et al: Translation control of gene expression. J Basic Clin Physiol Pharmacol 2:223–231, 1991

Pantev C, Oostenveld R, Engelien A, et al: Increased auditory cortical representation in musicians. Nature 392:811–814, 1998

Pearson BJ, Doe CQ: Specification of temporal identity in the developing nervous system. Annu Rev Cell Dev Biol 20:619–647, 2004

Pereira C, Agostinho P, Moreira PI, et al: Alzheimer's disease-associated neurotoxic mechanisms and neuroprotective strategies. Curr Drug Targets CNS Neurol Disord 4:383–403, 2005

Pfrieger FW, Barres BA: Synaptic efficacy enhanced by glial cells in vitro. Science 277:1684–1687, 1997

Pifl C, Giros B, Caron MG: The dopamine transporter: the cloned target site of parkinsonism-inducing toxins and of drugs of abuse. Adv Neurol 69:235–238, 1996

Pigino G, Kirkpatrick L, Brady S: The cytoskeleton of neurons and glia, in Basic Neurochemistry: Molecular, Cellular and Medical Aspects, 7th Edition. Edited by Siegel GJ, Albers RW, Brady S, et al. Burlington, MA, Elsevier Academic, 2006, pp 123–137

Putcha GV, Johnson EM Jr: Men are but worms: neuronal cell death in C elegans and vertebrates. Cell Death Differ 11:38–48, 2004

Raff MC, Barres BA, Burne JF, et al: Programmed cell death and the control of cell survival: lessons from the nervous system. Science 262:695–700, 1993

Rakic P: Guidance of neurons migrating to the fetal monkey neocortex. Brain Res 33:471–476, 1971

Ramamoorthy S, Blakely RD: Phosphorylation and sequestration of serotonin transporters differentially modulated by psychostimulants. Science 285:763–766, 1999

Ramón y Cajal S: Les nouvelles idées sur la structure du système nerveux chez l'homme et chez les vertébrés [New ideas on the structure of the nervous system in man and in vertebrates]. Paris, C. Reinwald, 1894

Ramón y Cajal S: Histologie du système nerveux de l'homme et des vertébrés [Histology of the nervous system in man and in vertebrates]. Paris, Maloine, 1911

Rego AC, de Almeida LP: Molecular targets and therapeutic strategies in Huntington's disease. Curr Drug Targets CNS Neurol Disord 4:361–381, 2005

Reiter HO, Stryker MP: Neural plasticity without postsynaptic action potentials: less-active inputs become dominant when kitten visual cortical cells are pharmacologically inhibited. Proc Natl Acad Sci USA 85:3623–3627, 1988

Rosen DR, Siddique T, Patterson D, et al: Mutations in Cu/Zn superoxide dismutase gene are associated with familial amyotrophic lateral sclerosis. Nature 362:59–62, 1993

Rumpel S, LeDoux J, Zador A, et al: Postsynaptic receptor trafficking underlying a form of associative learning. Science 308:83–88, 2005

Sadato N, Pascual-Leone A, Grafman J, et al: Activation of the primary visual cortex by Braille reading in blind subjects. Nature 380:526–528, 1996

Saito T, Nakatsuji N: Efficient gene transfer into the embryonic mouse brain using in vivo electroporation. Dev Biol 240:237–246, 2001

Salinas PC: Signaling at the vertebrate synapse: New roles for embryonic morphogens? J Neurobiol 64:435–445, 2005

Sanes JR, Lichtman JW: Development of the vertebrate neuromuscular junction. Annu Rev Neurosci 22:389–442, 1999

Sanes SR, Rubenstein JL, Nicolas JF: Use of a recombinant retrovirus to study post-implantation cell lineage in mouse embryos. EMBO J 5:3133–3142, 1986

Santarelli L, Saxe M, Gross C, et al: Requirement of hippocampal neurogenesis for the behavioral effects of antidepressants. Science 301:805–809, 2003

Sastry PS, Rao KS: Apoptosis and the nervous system. J Neurochem 74:1–20, 2000

Sauer FC: Mitosis in the neural tube. J Comp Neurol 62:377–405, 1935

Scheiffele P: Cell-cell signaling during synapse formation in the CNS. Annu Rev Neurosci 26:488–508, 2003

Schenone A, Mancardi GL: Molecular basis of inherited neuropathies. Curr Opin Neurol 12:603–616, 1999

Schmechel DE, Rakic P: A Golgi study of radial glial cells in developing monkey telencephalon: morphogenesis and transformation into astrocytes. Anat Embryol 156:115–152, 1979

Schoepfer R, Monyer H, Sommer B, et al: Molecular biology of glutamate receptors. Prog Neurobiol 42:353–357, 1994

Schulman H: Nitric oxide: a spatial second messenger. Mol Psychiatry 2:296–299, 1997

Schuurmans C, Guillemot F: Molecular mechanisms underlying cell fate specification in the developing telencephalon. Curr Opin Neurobiol 12:26–34, 2002

Scott SA, Davies AM: Inhibition of protein synthesis prevents cell death in sensory and parasympathetic neurons deprived of neurotrophic factor in vitro. J Neurobiol 21:630–638, 1990

Seamans JK, Yang CR: The principal features and mechanisms of dopamine modulation in the prefrontal cortex. Prog Neurobiol 74:1–58, 2004

Seri B, García-Verdugo JM, McEwen BS, et al: Astrocytes give rise to new neurons in the adult mammalian hippocampus. J Neurosci 21:7153–7160, 2001

Shatz CJ: Impulse activity and the patterning of connections during CNS development. Neuron 5:745–756, 1990

Shatz CJ, Stryker MP: Prenatal tetrodotoxin infusion blocks segregation of retinogeniculate afferents. Science 242:87–89, 1988

Sherman SM: Tonic and burst firing: dual modes of thalamocortical relay. Trends Neurosci 24:122–126, 2001

Shi SH, Hayashi Y, Petralia RS, et al: Rapid spine delivery and redistribution of AMPA receptors after synaptic NMDA receptor activation. Science 284:1811–1816, 1999

Smart IH: Proliferative characteristics of the ependymal layer during the early development of the mouse neocortex: a pilot study based on recording the number, location and plane of cleavage of mitotic figures. J Anat 116:67–91, 1973

Smith AD, Bolam JP: The neural network of the basal ganglia as revealed by the study of synaptic connections of identified neurones. Trends Neurosci 13:259–265, 1990

Sohl G, Maxeiner S, Willecke K: Expression and functions of neuronal gap junctions. Nat Rev Neurosci 6:191–200, 2005

Spencer KM, Nestor PG, Perlmutter R, et al: Neural synchrony indexes disordered perception and cognition in schizophrenia. Proc Natl Acad Sci USA 101:17288–17293, 2004

Steward O, Worley P: Local synthesis of proteins at synaptic sites on dendrites: role in synaptic plasticity and memory consolidation? Neurobiol Learn Mem 78:508–527, 2002

Studer L, Tabar V, McKay RDG: Transplantation of expanded mesencephalic precursors leads to recovery in parkinsonian rats. Nature Neurosci 1:290–295, 1998

Sudhof TC: The synaptic vesicle cycle. Annu Rev Neurosci 27:509–547, 2004

Sulzer D, Sonders MS, Poulsen NW, et al: Mechanisms of neurotransmitter release by amphetamines: a review. Prog Neurobiol 75:406–433, 2005

Szabadics J, Varga C, Molnar G, et al: Excitatory effect of GABAergic axo-axonic cells in cortical microcircuits. Science 311:233–235, 2006

Takahashi T, Nowakowski RS, Caviness VS Jr: Early ontogeny of the secondary proliferative population of the embryonic murine cerebral wall. J Neurosci 15:6058–6068, 1995

Tamas G, Buhl EH, Lorincz A, et al: Proximally targeted GABAergic synapses and gap junctions synchronize cortical interneurons. Nat Neurosci 3:366–371, 2000

Tarabykin V, Stoykova A, Usman N, et al: Cortical upper layer neurons derive from the subventricular zone as indicated by Svet1 gene expression. Development 128:1983–1993, 2001

Tissir F, Goffinet AM: Reelin and brain development. Nat Rev Neurosci 4:496–505, 2003

Toga AW, Thompson PM: Genetics of brain structure and intelligence. Annu Rev Neurosci 28:1–23, 2005

Tsao P, von Zastrow M: Downregulation of G protein-coupled receptors. Curr Opin Neurobiol 10:365–369, 2000

Tsujimoto Y, Yunis J, Onorato-Showe L, et al: Molecular cloning of the chromosomal breakpoint of B-cell lymphomas and leukemias with the t(11;14) chromosome translocation. Science 224:1403–1406, 1984

Van Den Bosch L, Van Damme P, Bogaert E, et al: The role of excitotoxicity in the pathogenesis of amyotrophic lateral sclerosis. Biochim Biophys Acta 2006

Vickery RG, von Zastrow M: Distinct dynamin-dependent and -independent mechanisms target structurally homologous dopamine receptors to different endocytic membranes. J Cell Biol 144:31–43, 1999

Vogels TP, Rajan K, Abbott LF: Neural network dynamics. Annu Rev Neurosci 28:357–376, 2005

Waites CL, Craig AM, Garner CC: Mechanisms of vertebrate synaptogenesis. Annu Rev Neurosci 28:251–274, 2005

Walaas SI, Greengard P: Protein phosphorylation and neuronal function. Pharmacol Rev 43:299–349, 1991

Walsh C, Cepko CL: Cell lineage and cell migration in the developing cerebral cortex. Experientia 46:940–947, 1990

Wang HG, Lu FM, Jin I, et al: Presynaptic and postsynaptic roles of NO, cGK, and RhoA in long-lasting potentiation and aggregation of synaptic proteins. Neuron 45:389–403, 2005

Warner-Schmidt JL, Duman RS: Hippocampal neurogenesis: opposing effects of stress and antidepressant treatment. Hippocampus 16:239–249, 2006

Washbourne P, Bennett JE, McAllister AK: Rapid recruitment of NMDA receptor transport packets to nascent synapses. Nat Neurosci 5:751–759, 2002

Washbourne P, Dityatev A, Scheiffele P, et al: Cell adhesion molecules in synapse formation. J Neurosci 24:9244–9249, 2004a

Washbourne P, Liu XB, Jones EG, et al: Cycling of NMDA receptors during trafficking in neurons before synapse formation. J Neurosci 24:8253–8264, 2004b

Weissman TA, Riquelme PA, Ivic L, et al: Calcium waves propagate through radial glial cells and modulate proliferation in the developing neocortex. Neuron 43:647–661, 2004

Wexler NS, Rose EA, Housman DE: Molecular approaches to hereditary diseases of the nervous system: Huntington's disease as a paradigm. Annu Rev Neurosci 14:503–529, 1991

Wichterle H, Lieberam I, Porter JA, et al: Directed differentiation of embryonic stem cells into motor neurons. Cell 110:385–397, 2002

Wisden W, Errington ML, Williams S, et al: Differential expression of immediate early genes in the hippocampus and spinal cord. Neuron 4:603–614, 1990

Yamakura T, Bertaccini E, Trudell JR, et al: Anesthetics and ion channels: molecular models and sites of action. Annu Rev Pharmacol Toxicol 41:23–51, 2001

Yuste R, Tank DW: Dendritic integration in mammalian neurons, a century after Cajal. Neuron 16:701–716, 1996

Ziv NE, Garner CC: Cellular and molecular mechanisms of presynaptic assembly. Nat Rev Neurosci 5:385–399, 2004

2

FUNCTIONAL NEUROANATOMY

Neuropsychological Correlates of Cortical and Subcortical Damage

Brian T. Harel, Ph.D.
Daniel Tranel, Ph.D.

Nearly a century and a half ago, investigators began to note that damage to discrete brain regions could lead to highly selective deficits in behavior (for a historical review, see Feinberg and Farah 2003). For example, in the 1860s, the surgeon and physical anthropologist Paul Broca (1863, 1865) observed that damage to the anterior part of the left side of the brain led to a deficit in the production of speech while sparing speech comprehension. A complementary observation was reported some 10 years later by the neuropsychiatrist Carl Wernicke (1874), who noted that damage to the posterior part of the left hemisphere led to a disturbance in the comprehension of speech while sparing speech production. These observations eventually led to the notion that humans speak and process language with the left side of the brain. In fact, these early writings became the cornerstones on which the fields of neuropsychology, neuropsychiatry, and cognitive neuroscience were established. Many consistent relations between brain and behavior now have been established, and a wide range of cognitive and behavioral capacities associated with partic-

ular brain regions can be highlighted. In this chapter, we describe various brain-behavior relations, with a focus on the correlations between brain and behavior that are scientifically most consistent and clinically most important.

Much of the work described in this chapter was done with the lesion method approach in humans. In this method, the demonstration of reliable relations between particular cognitive defects and damage to particular neural structures is taken as evidence that those neural structures are related to those cognitive functions in the normal human brain. This level of analysis focuses on neural systems—that is, macroscopic neural structures and their interconnections—and on higher-order cognitive and behavioral capacities such as memory, language, decision making, and moral reasoning. This level of analysis is to be distinguished from other levels of analysis regarding the central nervous system (e.g., single-cell recording, analysis of molecular and cellular mechanisms), which, although very much valid in their own right, do not figure as prominently in current understanding of higher-order brain-behavior

Supported by National Institute of Neurological Disorders and Stroke Grant P01 NS19632.

relations. The lesion method is grounded in the notion that dysfunction in varied neuroanatomical systems in the human brain leads to predictable and reliable cognitive and behavioral manifestations, which may include, depending on the area of neural damage, changes in intellect, memory, language, perception, judgment and decision making, or personality. The method has benefited enormously from recent advances in neuroanatomical analysis, which were fueled by the development of modern neuroimaging techniques—computed tomography (CT) in the 1970s and magnetic resonance (MR) scanning in the early 1980s (H.Damasio 1995, 2005; H. Damasio and Damasio 2003; H. Damasio and Frank 1992; Frank et al. 1997). Dating back to the innovative formulations of Geschwind (1965), there has been a resurgence of interest in the lesion method. The aforementioned increased precision and reliability of neuroimaging definition, together with advances in neuropsychological measurement and cognitive experimentation (Benton 1988, 1994; Lezak et al. 2004; Oliveira-Souza et al. 2004; Tranel 1996), have allowed more powerful analyses of brain-behavior relations and more elaborate theoretical specification (cf. A.R. Damasio 1989a, 1989b; A.R. Damasio and Damasio 1993, 1994; Kosslyn and Koenig 1995). Such advances have enhanced the viability of the lesion method as a technique for scientific inquiry and have helped overcome the limitations of small subject groups and single case studies. Our understanding of brain-behavior relations has reached a level only hinted at in the work of two or three decades past.

In this chapter, several important background assumptions warrant brief comment. Unless otherwise indicated, it is assumed that the human brain under consideration is endowed with conventional hemispheric dominance, whereby speech and language functions are lateralized to the left hemisphere and nonverbal, visuospatial functions are lateralized to the right hemisphere (e.g., Levy 1990). Also, normal acquisition and development of cognitive capacities are assumed; thus, the principles outlined here may not apply to persons with developmental learning disabilities, long-standing psychiatric disease, or inadequate educational opportunity. Finally, as mentioned earlier, many of the findings reviewed here were derived from research focusing on cognitive experimentation in adult humans with focal brain lesions. In general, such lesions are caused by cerebrovascular disease, surgical ablation of nonmalignant cerebral tumors, some viral infections of the central nervous system (especially herpes simplex encephalitis), and traumatic brain injury and degenerative diseases.

Other approaches to the investigation of brain-behavior relations include techniques referred to under the rubric of functional imaging (for excellent reviews of these, see Aguirre 2003; Herscovitch 2004; Price and Friston 2003;

Raichle 1997; Roberts and McGonigle 2004); these techniques have witnessed an explosion in popularity over the past decade and have come to occupy a prominent position in the exploration of brain-behavior relations (for a comprehensive review, see Cabeza and Nyberg 2000; Stephan 2004). Positron emission tomography (PET) involves the measurement of brain cell activity such as glucose metabolism and local blood flow. PET is used to study which brain regions are "active" during particular cognitive tasks, which permits inferences about how certain neural units are related to certain mental functions (Grabowski et al. 1995; McCarthy 1995; Posner et al. 1988; Raichle 1990, 1997; Roland 1993; Silverman and Alavi 2005). Another powerful technique is functional magnetic resonance imaging (fMRI). Similar to PET, fMRI can be used to measure activity levels in various brain regions during cognitive tasks, permitting inferences about how neural units relate to mental activity. Magnetoencephalography (e.g., Poolos 1995; Roberts and McGonigle 2004), event-related potentials (e.g., Deouell et al. 2003; Fabiani et al. 2000; Polich 2004), and transcranial magnetic stimulation (e.g., Deouell et al. 2003; Hallett 2000) are other methods used to investigate brain-behavior relations.

BRAIN-BEHAVIOR RELATIONS

LATERAL SPECIALIZATION: LEFT VERSUS RIGHT

As hinted at in the early observations of Broca and Wernicke, several fundamental differences between the left and the right hemispheres of the human brain constitute some of the most consistent principles of neuropsychology. In the vast majority of adults, the left side of the brain is specialized for language and for processing verbally coded information. This is true of nearly all (about 88%) right-handed individuals (who constitute about 90% of the adult population), the majority (about 75%) of left-handed persons, and 43% of mixed-handed persons (Khedr et al. 2002). This principle applies irrespective of the mode of input. Thus, verbal information apprehended through either the auditory (e.g., speech) or the visual (e.g., written text) channel is processed preferentially by the left hemisphere. The principle also applies to both the input and the output aspects of language—we not only understand language with our left hemisphere but also produce language (spoken and written) with our left hemisphere. Moreover, compelling evidence now indicates that this applies not only to languages that are auditory based but also to languages that are based on visuogestural signals (e.g., American Sign Language) (Bellugi et al. 1989; Hickok et al. 1996;

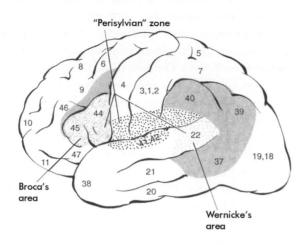

FIGURE 2–1. Lateral view of left hemisphere. The principal language-related regions are highlighted, including Broca's area and Wernicke's area. The "perisylvian" zone includes Broca's and Wernicke's areas and the zone marked with dots. Broca's area is dedicated to speech output, that is, language expression, whereas Wernicke's area is responsible for language comprehension. Other language-related regions highlighted include the supramarginal gyrus (area 40), the angular gyrus (area 39), part of area 37, and the region immediately above and anterior to Broca's area. Not pictured are left-sided subcortical structures (basal ganglia, thalamus) that also participate in speech and language functions.

Source. Reprinted from Tranel D: "Higher Brain Function," in *Neuroscience in Medicine.* Edited by Conn PM. Philadelphia, PA, JB Lippincott, 1995a, pp. 555–580. Used with permission.

Poizner et al. 1987). Figure 2–1 illustrates the typical arrangement of language in the left hemisphere.

The right hemisphere has a very different type of specialization. It processes nonverbal information such as complex visual patterns (e.g., faces) or auditory signals (e.g., music) that are not coded in verbal form. Structures in the right temporal and occipital regions are critical for learning and navigating geographic routes (Barrash et al. 2000a). Although the right hemisphere is more dominant for spatial processing, a closer examination of moderating variables (e.g., gender, type of task) suggests a more complex picture (see Vogel et al. 2003 for details). The right side of the brain is also dedicated to the mapping of "feeling states," that is, patterns of bodily sensations linked to emotions such as anger and fear. A related right hemisphere capacity concerns the perception of our bodies in space, in both intrapersonal and extrapersonal terms. For example, an understanding of where our limbs are in relation to our trunk, and where our body is in relation to the space around us, is under the purview of the right hemisphere. Figure 2–2 depicts some of the fundamental capacities of the right hemisphere.

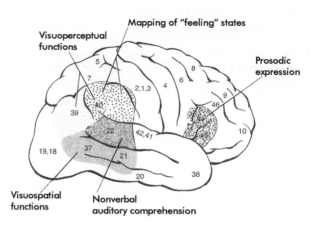

FIGURE 2–2. Lateral view of right hemisphere, depicting several primary regions with a label corresponding to their functional correlates. Many of these functions overlap both psychologically and anatomically, and the areas depicted in the figure should be considered approximate.

Source. Reprinted from Tranel D: "Higher Brain Function," in *Neuroscience in Medicine.* Edited by Conn PM. Philadelphia, PA, JB Lippincott, 1995a, pp. 555–580. Used with permission.

In early conceptualizations of the left and right hemispheres, a prevailing notion was that the left hemisphere was major, or dominant, whereas the right hemisphere was minor, or nondominant. This attitude reflected an emphasis on language in human cognition and behavior. As a highly observable capacity, language received the most scientific and clinical attention and was considered the quintessential and most important human faculty. In fact, for many decades the right hemisphere was believed to contribute little to higher-level cognitive functioning. Because lesions to the right hemisphere typically did not produce language disturbances, it was often concluded that a patient had lost little in the way of higher-order function after right-sided brain injury.

As the field evolved, and it became clear that each hemisphere was dedicated to specific—albeit different—cognitive capacities, the notion of dominance gave way to the idea of specialization. Each hemisphere was "dominant" for certain cognitive functions. Early work had already established the role of the left hemisphere in language. Other studies documented the role of the right hemisphere in visuospatial capacities. Many of the breakthroughs came from studies of split-brain patients, a line of work led by the late psychologist Roger Sperry (1968). To prevent partial seizures from spreading from one side of the brain to the other, patients underwent an operation in which the corpus callosum was cut. The left and right hemispheres were no longer in communication. Careful investigations of these patients found that each

TABLE 2–1. Functional dichotomies of left and right hemispheric dominance

Left	Right
Verbal	Nonverbal
Serial	Parallel
Analytic	Holistic
Controlled	Creative
Logical	Pictorial
Propositional	Appositional
Rational	Intuitive
Social	Physical

Source.   Adapted from Benton 1991.

side of the brain had its own "consciousness," with the left side operating in a verbal mode and the right in a nonverbal mode. Sperry's work and that of others (e.g., Arvanitakis and Graff-Radford 2004; Gazzaniga 1987, 2000; Zaidel et al. 2003; for reviews, see Trevarthen 1990) led to several fundamental distinctions between the cognitive functions for which the left and right hemispheres are specialized (Table 2–1).

LONGITUDINAL SPECIALIZATION: ANTERIOR VERSUS POSTERIOR

Another useful organizational principle for understanding brain-behavior relations is an anterior-posterior distinction. The major demarcation points are the rolandic sulcus, the major fissure separating the frontal lobes from the parietal lobes, and the sylvian fissure, the boundary between the temporal lobes and the frontal and parietal lobes (Figure 2–3).

In general, the posterior regions of the brain are dedicated to sensation and perception. The primary sensory cortices for vision, audition, and somatosensory perception are located in the posterior sectors of the brain in occipital, temporal, and parietal regions, respectively. Thus, apprehension of sensory data from the world outside is mediated by posterior brain structures. Note that the "world outside" is actually two distinct domains: 1) the world that is outside the body and brain and 2) the world that is outside the brain but inside the body. The latter, the soma, comprises the smooth muscle, the viscera, and other bodily structures innervated by the central nervous system.

Anterior brain regions, by contrast, generally comprise effector systems, specialized for the execution of behavior. For example, the primary motor cortices are located immediately anterior to the rolandic sulcus. The motor area for speech, known as Broca's area, is located in the left frontal operculum. The right hemisphere counterpart of Broca's area, in the right frontal operculum, is important for executing stresses and intonations that infuse speech with emotional meaning (prosody). Perhaps most important, a variety of "executive functions" such as judgment, decision making, and the capacity to construct and implement various plans of action are associated with structures in the frontal lobes.

In the following sections, we review a variety of brain-behavior relations. We have used as an organizing principle gross anatomical subdivisions—for example, different lobes of the brain and various sectors within each lobe—and for each, we discuss the most well-established cognitive and behavioral correlates. We hasten to point out, however, that the neuroanatomical arrangement is partly one of efficiency and economy—in several places, we have taken the liberty of including topics because they fit best within the overall context of the discussion and not because they necessarily belong to the anatomical division under consideration (e.g., the basal forebrain is discussed in the section on the frontal lobes; the posterior superior temporal gyrus is discussed as part of the temporoparietal junction).

THE TEMPORAL LOBES

Several major subdivisions can be designated within the temporal lobe: 1) the mesial temporal lobe, including the hippocampus, amygdala, entorhinal and perirhinal cortices, and an additional portion of the anterior parahippocampal gyrus; 2) the remaining nonmesial portion of the temporal lobe, which includes the temporal pole (TP), the inferotemporal (IT) region, and, for purposes of the current discussion, the region of transition between the posterior temporal lobe and the inferior occipital lobe (the occipitotemporal junction); and 3) the posterior portion of the superior temporal gyrus (area 22), which, on the left side, forms the heart of what is traditionally known as Wernicke's area (Figure 2–4). Neuropsychological correlates of the mesial, TP, and IT subdivisions are summarized in the table "Highlights for the Clinician" at the end of this chapter. Correlates of the posterior superior temporal region are considered in the later section "Temporoparietal Junction."

MESIAL TEMPORAL REGION

The mesial temporal lobe comprises the hippocampus, amygdala, entorhinal and perirhinal cortices, and the anterior portion of parahippocampal gyrus not occupied by the entorhinal cortex (see Figure 2–4). Many of these structures play a crucial role in memory.

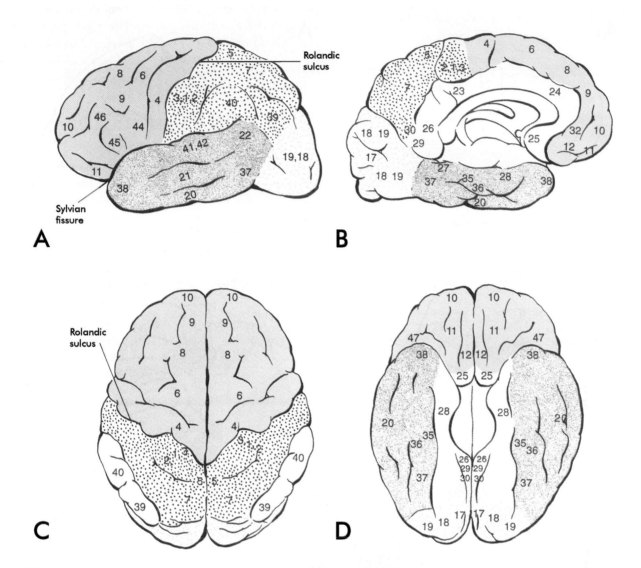

FIGURE 2–3. Lateral (*A*), mesial (*B*), superior (*C*), and inferior (*D*) views of the brain, depicting major demarcation points, including the rolandic sulcus and the sylvian fissure. The four main lobes are shown as follows: frontal=*light blue*; parietal=*dark dots*; occipital=*light dots*; temporal=*blue/gray pattern*. [Only the left hemisphere is depicted in the lateral and mesial views (*A* and *B*), but the mapping would be the same on the right hemisphere.] The unmarked zone—including the cingulate gyrus (areas 24 and 23) and areas 25, 26, 27, and 28—corresponds to a region commonly referred to as the *limbic lobe* (the reader is referred to A.R. Damasio and Van Hoesen 1983 for a more extensive discussion of the anatomy and functional correlates of the limbic lobe). In the superior perspective (*C*), the left hemisphere is on the left, and the right hemisphere is on the right; the sides are reversed in the inferior perspective (*D*).

Source. Reprinted from Tranel D: "Higher Brain Function," in *Neuroscience in Medicine.* Edited by Conn PM. Philadelphia, PA, JB Lippincott, 1995a, pp. 555–580. Used with permission.

Hippocampal Complex

The hippocampus and the adjacent entorhinal and perirhinal cortices can be referred to as the *hippocampal complex*. The components of the hippocampal complex are highly interconnected by means of recurrent neuroanatomical circuits. In turn, the hippocampal complex is extensively interconnected with higher-order association cortices located in the temporal lobe. Those cortices receive signals from the association cortices of all sensory modalities and also receive feedback projections from the hippocampus (Hyman et al. 1988; Lavenex and Amaral 2000; Van Hoesen 1982). Hence structures in the hippocampal complex have access to, and influence over, signals from virtually the entire brain. The system is thus in a position to create integrated records of various aspects of memory experiences, including visual, auditory, and somatosensory information.

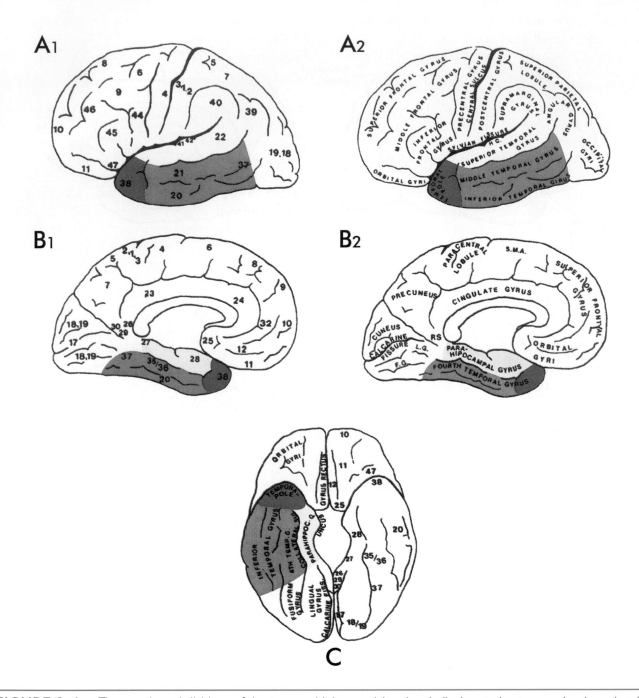

FIGURE 2–4.   Three major subdivisions of the temporal lobe: mesial region (*yellow*), anterior temporal pole region (*red*), and inferotemporal region (*green*). Numbers corresponding to Brodmann's cytoarchitectonic areas are depicted in *Panels A1* and *B1* and the right side (left hemisphere) of *Panel C*, and standard gyrus names are shown in the corresponding *Panels A2* and *B2* and the left side (right hemisphere) of *Panel C*. Lateral (*A1* and *A2*), mesial (*B1* and *B2*), and inferior (*C*) views are represented.

In a general sense, it is reasonable to describe the principal function of the hippocampal complex as the acquisition of new factual knowledge (*declarative memory*). The system is essential for acquiring records of interactions between the organism and the world outside, as well as thought processes such as those engaged in planning. It has been posited that the hippocampal complex is primarily involved in encoding memories in terms of the rela-

tions among objects and events, even when there are no intrinsic qualities that relate them (e.g., names with faces, names with telephone numbers). This allows for multiple means of accessing information, as well as the ability for information to be used in novel situations. This is accomplished through its extensive connections with many higher-order cortical processing areas. As noted earlier, information about the perceptual characteristics of objects and events and the affective and behavioral responses elicited are all sent to the hippocampal complex, which has reciprocal connections with these areas. Thus, these higher-order cortical processing areas are interconnected via the hippocampal complex to form multiple networks. These networks, because of their interconnectedness throughout the cortex, are by their nature relational. The types of relational information range from basic sensory (e.g., relative size or shape) to higher-order relationships (e.g., Cohen and Eichenbaum 1993; Eichenbaum and Cohen 2001). The precise computational operations performed by the hippocampus, however, have not been fully clarified (cf. Kopelman 2002; McClelland et al. 1995; Mishkin 1978; Nadel and Moscovitch 2001; Nadel et al. 2000; Squire 1992; Squire et al. 2004).

There are two hippocampal complexes, one in the left hemisphere and one in the right. Anatomically, the two are roughly equivalent, but major differences are seen in their functional roles. Specifically, the two hippocampal complexes are specialized for different types of material in a manner that parallels the overall functional arrangement of the brain: the left has verbal specialization and the right, nonverbal.

The landmark report by Scoville and Milner (1957) on patient HM, who became severely amnesic after undergoing bilateral mesial temporal lobe resection for control of intractable seizures, established the mesial aspect of the temporal lobes—and the hippocampus in particular—as being unequivocally linked to memory—specifically, to the acquisition of new information (i.e., anterograde memory). More than four decades of research on HM (summarized in Corkin 1984; see also Corkin 2002; Corkin et al. 1997; Gabrieli et al. 1988) and studies in similar patients (e.g., patient EP described in Stefanacci et al. 2000) have confirmed this relation. Patient RB of Zola-Morgan and colleagues (1986), who had pathologically confirmed bilateral lesions limited to the CA1 sector of the hippocampus, is another important example of the marked anterograde amnesia that can occur after circumscribed bilateral hippocampal lesions; this finding was replicated and extended in another study in which postmortem pathological confirmation was available (Rempel-Clower et al. 1996). It has been established that more extensive mesial temporal damage, involving the perirhinal cortex and parahippocampal gyrus in addition to the hippocampal region and entorhinal cortex, tends to produce a proportionate increase in the severity of amnesia (Squire and Zola 1996). Another source of evidence comes from patient Boswell, who had bilateral damage to the entire mesial sector of the temporal lobes (hippocampus, amygdala, entorhinal cortex) and also nonmesial temporal damage (Figure 2–5). In the anterograde compartment,

Boswell's profile is similar to the patterns reported for HM and RB; however, unlike HM and RB, Boswell also had a severe impairment on the retrograde side (A.R. Damasio et al. 1985a, 1989a; Tranel et al. 2000b). Similar to Boswell, EP was found to have severe retrograde amnesia for facts and events, as well as anterograde amnesia (Stefanacci et al. 2000). Studies with functional imaging also have confirmed the role of the mesial temporal lobe in memory (Nyberg et al. 1996; for review, see Rugg 2002).

With respect to the nature of the amnesia associated with hippocampal damage, several relations have been firmly established. First, neuropsychological findings have identified selective impairments in relational memory (e.g., Ryan et al. 2000). This finding has been supported by functional neuroimaging research as well (e.g., Cohen et al. 1999; Giovanello et al. 2004). More recent work has suggested that the hippocampal system specifically mediates long-term relational memory (Ryan and Cohen 2004). Interestingly, this appears to be at odds with recent functional neuroimaging studies that have found activation in the hippocampal system during working memory tasks, as well as long-term memory tasks. However, Ryan and Cohen (2004) posited that these findings reflect the "automatic and obligatory role the hippocampus has in forming long-term memory representations of presented information even when the information need be maintained only over a short delay." Second, a consistent relation is found between the side of the lesion and the type of learning impairment. Specifically, damage to the left hippocampal system produces an amnesic syndrome that affects verbal material (e.g., spoken words, written material) but spares nonverbal material; conversely, damage to the right hippocampal system affects nonverbal material (e.g., complex visual and auditory patterns) but spares verbal material (e.g., Frisk and Milner 1990; Milner 1968, 1972; O'Connor and Verfaellie 2002; M.L. Smith and Milner 1989). For example, after damage to the left hippocampus, a patient may lose the ability to learn new names but remain capable of learning new faces and spatial arrangements (e.g., Tranel 1991a). By contrast, damage to the right hippocampal system frequently impairs the ability to learn new geographic routes (Barrash et al. 2000a).

A third point is that the hippocampal system does not appear to play a role in the learning of perceptuomotor skills and other knowledge that has been referred to as *nondeclarative memory* (e.g., Squire 1992). Patient HM, for example, can learn skills such as mirror drawing and mirror reading (Corkin 1965, 1968; Gabrieli et al. 1993), even though he has no recall of the situation in which the learning of those skills took place. Similar findings have been reported in patient Boswell and other patients with bilateral mesial temporal lobe damage (Tranel et al.

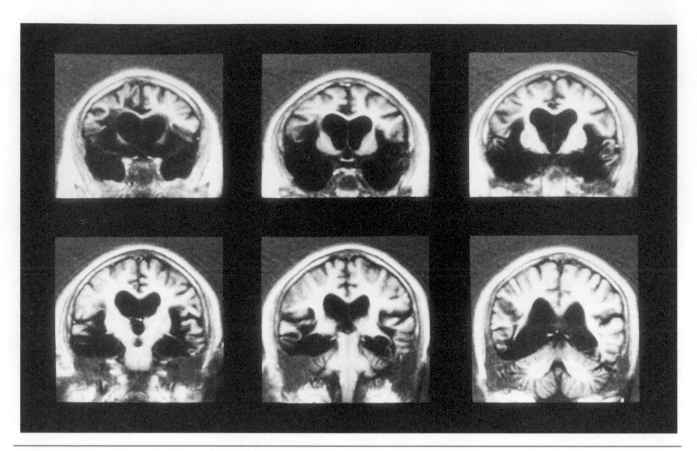

FIGURE 2–5.   T1-weighted magnetic resonance images of patient Boswell, who developed severe global amnesia after having herpes simplex encephalitis. In these coronal sectional images, the left hemisphere is on the right, and the most anterior image is in the upper left corner of the figure. The lesions, which show as black areas, include the anterior temporal regions (amygdala, hippocampus, parahippocampal gyrus, and temporal pole [area 38]) and the anterior portion of the inferior, middle, and superior temporal gyri (areas 20, 21, and anterior 22).

1994b, 2000b). In fact, Boswell not only can acquire perceptuomotor skills such as rotor pursuit and mirror tracing at a normal level but also can retain those skills for many years after the initial learning, even though he cannot recall any shred of knowledge regarding the circumstances of the learning situations. Thus, the role of the hippocampus in memory is principally for acquiring declarative knowledge—that is, facts, faces, names, and other information that can be "declared" and brought into the mind's eye.

Another source of evidence comes from patients with Alzheimer's disease. In the early and middle stages of the disease, patients with Alzheimer's disease develop a marked impairment of anterograde memory, which, as in patients HM and Boswell, spares the learning of nondeclarative information such as new perceptuomotor skills (Eslinger and Damasio 1986; Gabrieli et al. 1993). The neural hallmark in Alzheimer's disease is damage to the hippocampal system (Hyman et al. 1984; Van Hoesen and Damasio 1987; Van Hoesen et al. 1986). The cerebellum and neostriatum, which are intact in the various patients cited earlier, have

been implicated as crucial structures underlying acquisition of motor skills (Eslinger and Damasio 1986; Fiez et al. 1992; Gao et al. 1996; Grafman et al. 1992; Heindel et al. 1993; McCormick and Thompson 1984; Saint-Cyr et al. 1988; Schmahmann 1991; Thompson 1986).

A final comment pertains to the role of the hippocampus in the retrieval of old (sometimes referred to as *remote*) information (retrograde memory). Milner (1972) argued that the hippocampus is not needed for the retrieval of remote memories, and findings in HM and RB, neither of whom had defects in the retrograde compartment, support this contention. Patient Boswell is also consistent with this notion, inasmuch as his severe defects in the retrograde compartment are attributable to his extensive nonmesial, anterior temporal lobe damage (A.R. Damasio et al. 1985a; Tranel et al. 2000b). The weight of the evidence points to the conclusion that the hippocampal system is not the principal repository for old memories. The role of mesial temporal structures in retrograde memory also has been explored in experimental animals (e.g., Horel 1978; Murray 1990; Squire et al. 2004; Zola-Morgan and Squire 1986), as well as with functional imaging (for reviews, see Kopelman 2002; Squire et al. 2004).

Amygdala

The role of the amygdala in memory has been a source of controversy. Studies in nonhuman primates have yielded conflicting results, with some laboratories reporting that the amygdala is critical for normal learning (e.g., Mishkin 1978; Murray 1990; Murray and Mishkin 1985, 1986) and others maintaining that the amygdala does not play a crucial role (e.g., Zola-Morgan et al. 1989). Results in the few human cases available are also equivocal (Lee et al. 1988b; Nahm et al. 1993; Tranel and Hyman 1990).

Recently, however, studies have begun to clarify this issue, and it now appears that the amygdala is important for the acquisition and expression of emotional memory, but perhaps not for neutral memory. Specifically, the amygdala contributes critically to the potentiation of memory traces for emotional stimuli during their acquisition and consolidation into long-term declarative memory (Adolphs et al. 2000, 2005b; Cahill et al. 1995; Phelps et al. 1998). This conclusion is also supported by functional imaging studies (Cahill et al. 1996; Hamann et al. 1999; Richardson et al. 2004). These findings are in accord with other evidence indicating that the amygdala is important for the recognition of emotion, especially fear, in facial expressions (Adolphs 2003; Adolphs et al. 2005a; Young et al. 1995) and in the processing of other information that has emotional significance (Markowitsch et al. 1994). Also, it has been shown that the amygdala is important for classical conditioning of autonomic responses. Bechara et al. (1995) found that a patient with circumscribed bilateral amygdala damage was able to acquire declarative knowledge normally but was impaired in acquiring conditioned autonomic responses; a patient with circumscribed bilateral hippocampal damage (but with intact amygdala) showed the opposite pattern. These findings have led to the idea that the amygdala is important for processing stimuli that communicate emotional significance in social situations; specifically, the amygdala may orchestrate patterns of neural activation in disparate sectors of the brain that would encode both the intrinsic physical features of stimuli (e.g., shape, position in space) and the value that certain stimuli have to the organism, especially emotional significance (Adolphs 2003; Adolphs and Tranel 2000).

Decision making also has been posited to be mediated by the amygdala, which is believed to be part of the neural circuitry subserving emotional and social intelligence (Bar-On et al. 2003). Specifically, it is believed to do this via its ability to associate features of pleasurable or aversive stimuli with the somatic state related to the stimuli (Bechara et al. 2003). This theory has been supported by lesion studies in humans (Lee et al. 1988a, 1998) and by functional neuroimaging studies (LaBar et al. 1998).

ANTERIOR, LATERAL, AND INFERIOR TEMPORAL REGIONS

Retrograde Memory

The anterior and nonmesial sectors of the temporal lobes play important roles in retrograde memory—specifically, the retrieval of knowledge that was acquired before the onset of a brain injury (e.g., Hunkin et al. 1995; for reviews, see Kapur 1993; Kopelman 1992; Markowitsch et al. 1993). In a case reported by Kapur et al. (1994), the patient had damage to anterior, lateral, and ventral temporal structures but not to mesial structures, forming a pattern the authors described as a "mirror-image" lesion to that of HM. The patient's amnesia profile was the inverse of HM's, with severe disruption of retrograde memory and relative sparing of anterograde memory. Other case studies of retrograde amnesia have been reported (e.g., Cermak and O'Connor 1983; De Renzi and Lucchelli 1993; O'Connor et al. 1992; J.M. Reed and Squire 1998; Tulving et al. 1988), and in cases for which anatomical information is available, the findings appear to be consistent with the notion that retrograde memory is related to nonmesial, anterior and lateral temporal regions and not to the hippocampal complex. Recent work in which structural MRI was used (Kopelman et al. 2001) provided further evidence that remote memories rely on nonmesial sectors of the temporal lobes.

We reported a case in which serial neuropsychological assessments and serial structural and functional neuroimaging studies provided further support for the notion that the retrieval of old, factual, concrete knowledge (retrograde memory) and learning of new, factual, concrete knowledge (anterograde memory) depend on distinct systems in the temporal lobe (Jones et al. 1998). A 70-year-old right-handed woman with limbic encephalitis attributed to thymoma was evaluated 4 months after diagnosis. Severe multimodal anterograde and retrograde memory defects were found. A fluorodeoxyglucose (FDG) ^{18}F resting PET scan showed diffuse cortical—but especially right anterolateral—temporal hypometabolism. Two years later, marked resolution of the retrograde memory defect was seen, with persistent anterograde amnesia. A follow-up FDG resting PET scan showed improved metabolism in the anterolateral temporal cortex and in other cortical regions. Metabolism in both mesial temporal regions declined markedly. Striking recovery of retrograde memory occurred in conjunction with the improvement in anterolateral temporal metabolism and despite reduction in mesial temporal metabolism. These findings provide further support for the hypotheses that 1) mesial temporal structures are not the repository of retrograde factual knowledge, and 2) anterolateral temporal lobe structures, especially on the right, may be critical for retrieval of retrograde factual knowledge.

Lexical Retrieval

Structures in the anterior and inferolateral left temporal lobe play a key role in lexical retrieval, or what is commonly known as *naming*. For example, when a familiar person or object is encountered, the word that denotes that person or object is normally recalled. This process occurs virtually automatically, although it may be encumbered by factors such as fatigue, distraction, or aging (Burke et al. 1991). Recent evidence has shown that neural structures in different parts of the left temporal lobe are important for the naming of objects from different conceptual categories.

The neural regions under consideration here include the TP and the IT region (Figure 2–6). These regions are mostly outside the classic language areas in the left hemisphere. Preliminary studies in neurological patients hinted that these regions might have an important role in lexical retrieval (A.R. Damasio et al. 1990a; Goodglass et al. 1986; Graff-Radford et al. 1990a; Hart et al. 1985; Heilman et al. 1972; Semenza and Zettin 1989; Stafiniak et al. 1990; Warrington and McCarthy 1983).

More recent studies have confirmed and extended these observations (e.g., H. Damasio et al. 1996, 2004; Etard et al. 2000; Gorno-Tempini et al. 2000; Grabowski et al. 2000b, 2001, 2003; Sugiura et al. 2001; Tranel et al. 1997b; Tsukiura et al. 2000; Whatmough et al. 2002). Specifically, evidence indicates that the left temporal lobe has separable neural sectors that are relatively specialized for naming entities from different conceptual categories. With regard to concrete entities, naming of unique persons (e.g., John Wayne, Joe Montana) was associated with the left TP; naming of nonunique animals (e.g., skunk, zebra) was associated with the anterior aspect of IT, in a region immediately posterior to the TP; and naming of nonunique tools (e.g., hammer, wrench) was associated with the posterior aspect of IT and an adjacent area in the temporo-occipitoparietal junction (Figure 2–6). It is important to note that lesions in these regions do not typically cause permanent defects in other aspects of language operation; in particular, grammar, syntax, phonetic implementation, and repetition are normal. The defect is confined to lexical access, and the findings have been interpreted as supporting the idea that these neural structures play an intermediary or a mediational role

in lexical retrieval. For example, when the concept of a given tool is evoked (based on the activation of several regions that support pertinent conceptual knowledge and promote its explicit representation in sensorimotor terms), an intermediary region becomes active and promotes (in the appropriate sensorimotor structures) the explicit representation of phonemic knowledge pertaining to the word form that denotes the given tool. When a concept from another category is evoked, such as that of a particular person, a different intermediary region is engaged. The process can operate in reverse to link word form information to conceptual knowledge; for example, hearing the word *buffalo* would activate an intermediary region that would allow us to conjure up the image of a buffalo and other pertinent semantic knowledge that defines our concept of buffalo (for a detailed discussion of this model, see Tranel et al. 1997b).

Neuropsychological correlates of damage to the right anterolateral temporal region remain poorly understood, but several intriguing findings are available thus far. In two cases with this type of lesion, the patients had a selective defect in naming facial expressions (e.g., happiness, fear) (Rapcsak et al. 1989, 1993). The patients did not have difficulty naming other entities, such as objects and actions, and they had no defect in proper naming (e.g., famous faces, buildings). Also, the patients did not have impaired recognition, even with regard to emotional facial expressions not named correctly. For example, the patients could match facial expressions to emotional prosody, and to emotional scenes, at a normal level.

Structures in the right anterolateral temporal region appear to play an important role in the recognition of unique entities (e.g., familiar persons and landmarks). For example, it has been shown that lesions in the right TP produce impairments in the retrieval of conceptual knowledge for familiar persons (Gainotti et al. 2003; Tranel et al. 1997a). This finding has been corroborated by a PET study, which reported activation of this region when subjects were identifying familiar persons and landmarks (Grabowski et al. 2000a). These results are also consistent with the discussion earlier, which emphasized the importance of anterior and lateral aspects of the right temporal lobe in the retrieval of retrograde memories. Together with interconnected right prefrontal cortices, the right anterolateral temporal region is probably of critical importance for the retrieval of unique factual memories (Tranel et al. 2000b). However, the precise role of the right anterolateral temporal region with regard to recognition is unclear in light of more recent research suggesting that recognition defects are not the result of predominantly right hemisphere lesions but rather are more evenly distributed across the two hemispheres (H. Damasio et al. 2004).

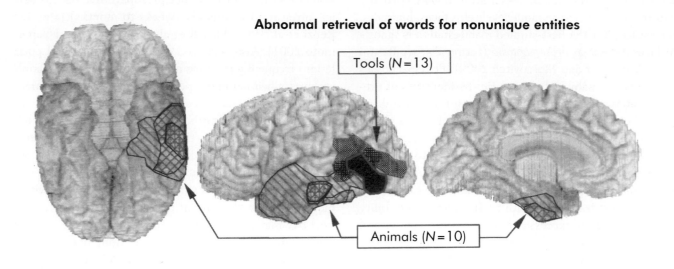

Abnormal retrieval of words for nonunique entities

Tools (N=13)

Animals (N=10)

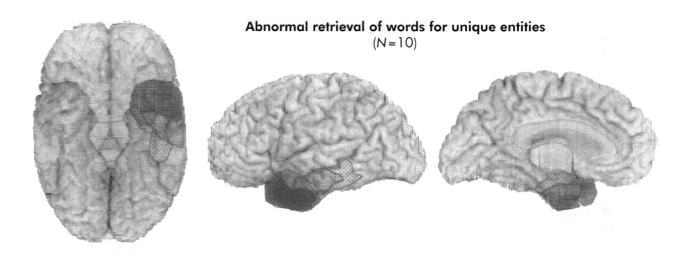

Abnormal retrieval of words for unique entities
(N=10)

FIGURE 2–6. Regions in the left temporal lobe that are important for lexical retrieval, including the left temporal pole (TP) and the inferotemporal (IT) region. Results of analysis based on magnetic resonance (or computed tomographic) scans processed for three-dimensional reconstruction in each subject with Brainvox (H. Damasio and Frank 1992). The top section depicts defective retrieval of words for animals or tools; the bottom section depicts defective retrieval of words for persons. Abnormal retrieval of words for persons correlated with damage clustered in the left TP. Abnormal retrieval of words for animals correlated with damage in the left IT region; maximal overlap occurred in lateral and inferior IT regions. Abnormal retrieval of words for tools correlated with damage in the posterolateral IT region, along with the junction of lateral temporo-occipitoparietal cortices (posterior IT+).

Visual Recognition

Disorders of visual recognition are associated with damage to the posterior part of the IT region, along with the inferior portion of Brodmann areas 18 and 19 in the occipital region, a transition area known as the *occipitotemporal junction*. Lesions to the occipitotemporal junction, especially when they are bilateral, produce unimodal, visually based disorders of recognition. Patients lose the ability to recognize visual stimuli at the level of unique identity. They cannot recognize familiar faces or familiar landmarks. Usually, basic visual perception is largely unaltered, and the presentation thus conforms to the classic notion of associative agnosia—that is, a "normal percept stripped of its meaning" (Teuber 1968). The disturbance can affect any number of visual stimuli that normally require recognition at a unique level (e.g., faces, buildings, landmarks), but the best-studied manifestation is agnosia for faces, known as *prosopagnosia* (for review, see Barton 2003; Kanwisher and Moscovitch 2000). Prosopagnosia's hallmark is an inability to recognize the identities of previously known faces and an inability to learn new ones. The defect can be severe, as patients may lose the ability to recognize faces of family members, close friends, and even themselves in a mirror, but it is confined to the visual channel, and exposure to the voice that belongs to the unrecognized face will elicit prompt and accurate recognition. In most individuals with prosopagnosia, the ability to recognize facial expressions, and to judge gender and estimate age from face information, is well preserved (Bruyer et al. 1983; Davidoff and Landis 1990; Tranel et al. 1988). Also, many patients with prosopagnosia remain capable of recognizing identity based on visual but nonfacial information, such as characteristics of gait or posture (A.R. Damasio et al. 1982b, 1989b, 1990a, 1990b). Some patients with prosopagnosia have impaired perception of texture (Newcombe 1979), and defects in color perception are common (A.R. Damasio et al. 1980; Meadows 1974b). Finally, intriguing evidence shows that many patients with severe prosopagnosia are capable of generating discriminatory autonomic responses to familiar faces, indicating that some preservation of face recognition occurs at a nonconscious level (Bauer 1984; Tranel 2000; Tranel and Damasio 1985; Tranel et al. 1995).

Associative prosopagnosia (Figure 2–7) is nearly always associated with bilateral lesions to the occipitotemporal junction (Benton 1990; A.R. Damasio et al. 1982b, 1990b; Meadows 1974a). Prosopagnosia resulting from unilateral right-sided lesions nearly always has a substantial perceptual component, thus constituting a more apperceptive form of the condition (see subsection "Apperceptive Visual Agnosia" later in this chapter). Unilateral occipitotemporal lesions usually do not cause severe and lasting prosopagnosia, although such lesions may cause significant disturbances in face recognition. On the left, such lesions can produce a partial recognition defect that has been termed *deep prosopagnosia* (A.R. Damasio et al. 1988), in which target faces are misidentified as someone who is very similar to the correct person in terms of gender, age, activity, and so forth (e.g., recognizing Betty Grable as Marilyn Monroe, or recognizing Magic Johnson as Michael Jordan). Right-sided occipitotemporal lesions may cause slow and erratic face recognition, but again, pervasive prosopagnosia is uncommon (A.R. Damasio et al. 1990b). More recent work suggests that right-sided le-

sions are sufficient to produce prosopagnosia, but the deficit often resolves quickly (weeks to months) (e.g., De Renzi et al. 1994; Mesad et al. 2003; Wada and Yamamoto 2001). Also, as noted earlier, right temporal polar lesions frequently produce impaired recognition of familiar faces, albeit not in the pervasive manner that is characteristic of the classic conceptualization of prosopagnosia.

In addition to disturbances of recognition of unique visual stimuli, lesions in the vicinity of the occipitotemporal junction may cause impairments in the visual recognition of nonunique stimuli from various categories, such as animals or tools. For example, when confronted with a picture of a fox, the patient may indicate that it is an animal but may not be able to come up with the specific type. Shown a screwdriver, the patient may respond "some kind of tool; I can't think of which one." This impairment affects recognition at the level of basic objects. In general, the patients can still recognize the superordinate category to which the entity belongs but not the subordinate, basic object level.

An especially intriguing discovery is that an impairment of visual recognition may not affect all types of entities equally but instead may be restricted to one or a few conceptual categories. Several investigators have reported patients who had category-related impairments in visual recognition of entities such as animals, fruits and vegetables, and tools and utensils. For example, patients have been described in whom recognition of animals was impaired but recognition of objects from other categories was normal; conversely, some patients have shown impaired recognition of tools and utensils but normal recognition of animals (for reviews, see Caramazza 2000; Forde and Humphreys 1999; Gainotti 2000; Gainotti et al. 1995; Humphreys and Forde 2001). In a large-scale lesion-based study of this phenomenon, we found a double dissociation relative to recognition profile and lesion site (Tranel et al. 1997a). Specifically, one group of patients had defects in the recognition of animals, but recognition of tools was normal; another group had defective recognition of tools but normal recognition of animals. Defective recognition of animals was associated with lesions in the right mesial occipital/ventral temporal region and also in the left mesial occipital region, whereas defective recognition of tools was associated with lesions in the occipital-temporal-parietal junction in the left hemisphere. These findings, which have been supported by functional imaging studies (for review, see Martin et al. 2000), support the idea that recording and retrieving knowledge for different conceptual categories depends on partially segregated neural systems.

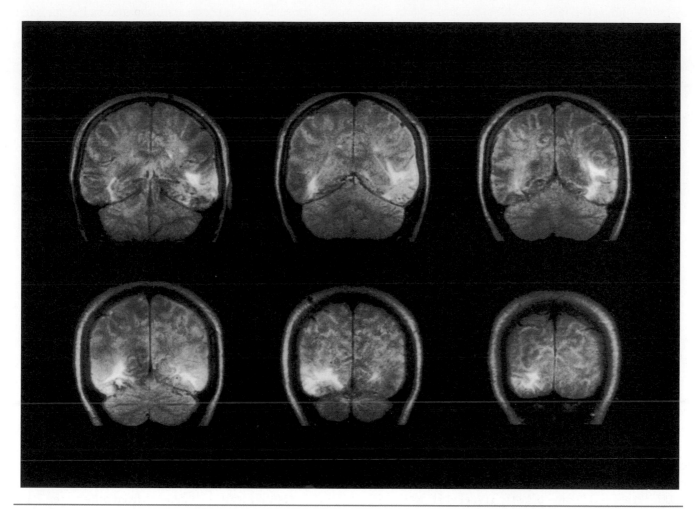

FIGURE 2–7.   T2-weighted magnetic resonance image of a 67-year-old, right-handed woman, which shows bilateral occipito-temporal lesions (showing as white or "bright" signal). In these coronal sections, the left hemisphere is on the right, and the most anterior image is in the upper left corner of the figure. The woman developed severe, permanent prosopagnosia after sustaining these lesions.

THE OCCIPITAL LOBES

The neuroanatomical arrangement of structures in and near the occipital lobes is depicted in Figure 2–8. On the lateral aspect of the hemispheres, the occipital lobes comprise the visual association cortices in Brodmann areas 18 and 19. These areas continue in the mesial aspect. The mesial sector also includes the primary visual cortices (area 17), which are formed by the cortex immediately above and below the calcarine fissure. For purposes of establishing neuropsychological correlates of the occipital lobes, the region can be subdivided in the vertical plane at the level of the calcarine fissure, so that dorsal (superior) and ventral (inferior) components can be designated (Figure 2–8). Neuropsychological correlates of occipital lobe lesions are summarized in the table "Highlights for the Clinician" at the end of the chapter.

DORSAL COMPONENT

The dorsal component of the occipital lobes comprises the primary visual cortex superior to the calcarine fissure (area 17) and the superior portion of the visual association cortices (areas 18 and 19). This region is considered in combination with the anteriorly adjacent parietal areas, including the posterior part of the superior parietal lobule (area 7) and the posterior part of the angular gyrus (area 39). When situated in the primary visual cortex of area 17 and/or its connections, lesions to the dorsal sector of the occipital region lead to a loss of form vision (i.e., blindness) in the inferior visual field contralateral to the lesion, and bilateral lesions of this type will produce an inferior altitudinal hemianopia. An intriguing presentation occurs when the lesions spare the primary visual cortex and involve the association cortices of areas 18 and 19. When such lesions

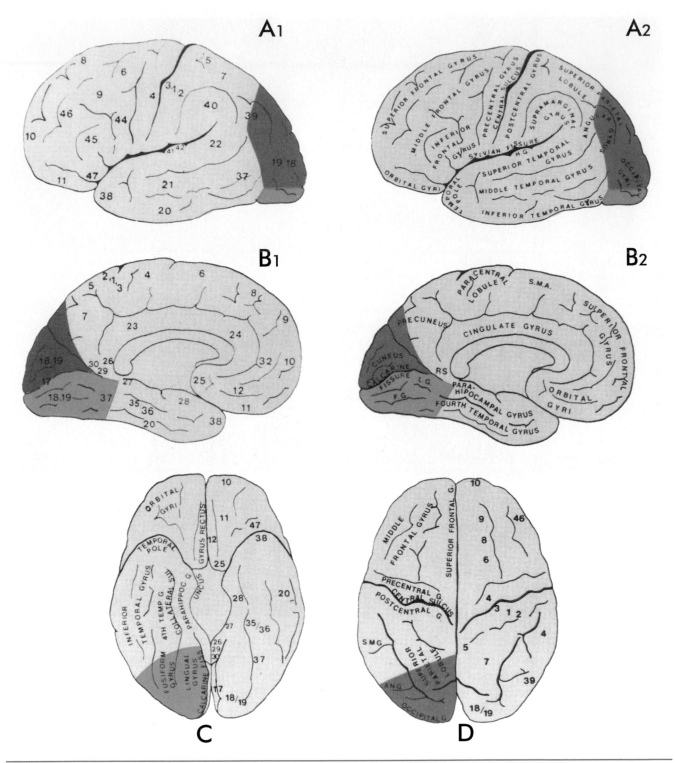

FIGURE 2–8.   Two major subdivisions of the occipital lobe: dorsal (superior) component (*red*) and ventral (inferior) component (*green*). Numbers corresponding to Brodmann's cytoarchitectonic areas are depicted in *Panels A1* and *B1* and the right side (left hemisphere) of *Panels C* and *D*; standard gyrus names are shown on corresponding *Panels A2* and *B2* and the left side (right hemisphere) of *Panels C* and *D*. Lateral (*A1* and *A2*), mesial (*B1* and *B2*), inferior (*C*), and superior (*D*) views are represented.

encroach into the adjacent parietal region comprising areas 39 and 7, patients commonly develop a constellation of defects known as *Balint's syndrome*. An example of a CT

scan of a patient with this type of presentation is shown in Figure 2–9. Balint's syndrome is based on the presence of three components: 1) visual disorientation (also known as

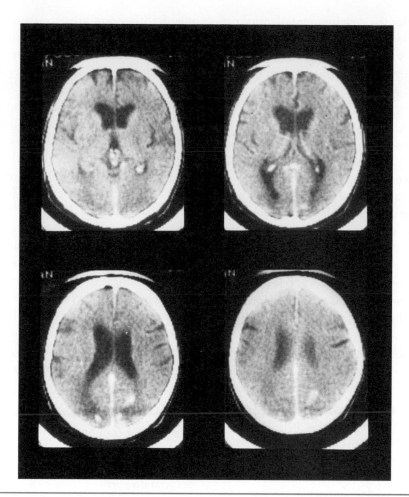

FIGURE 2–9. Contrast-enhanced computed tomographic scan of a 74-year-old right-handed man, showing bilateral lesions (areas of increased density) in the superior occipital region corresponding to the supracalcarine visual association cortices. The man developed a complex visual disturbance (Balint's syndrome) in connection with these lesions.

simultanagnosia), 2) ocular apraxia (also known as *psychic gaze paralysis*), and 3) optic ataxia. The key constituent in the syndrome is visual disorientation, and there is considerable variability in the emphasis that is placed on the other components (A.R. Damasio 1985; Jones and Tranel 2002; Newcombe and Ratcliff 1989; Rizzo 1993; Rizzo and Nawrot 1993; Rizzo and Vecera 2002; Valenza et al. 2004).

Visual Disorientation

Visual disorientation (simultanagnosia) can be conceptualized as an inability to attend to more than a very limited sector of the visual field at any given moment. Patients report that they can see clearly in only a small part of the field, the rest being "out of focus" and in a sort of "fog." The sector of clear vision is unstable and may shift without warning in any direction, so that patients experience a literal "jumping about" of their visual perception. Such patients are incapable of constructing a spatially coherent visual field, and they cannot follow trajectories of stimuli or place stimuli in their proper locations in space. Percep-

tion of motion is often impaired, and such patients fail to notice when objects have moved about in their visual field or fail to recognize the meaning of movements they have otherwise perceived correctly. For example, patients may fail to recognize a familiar gait or stride or fail to understand pantomime (A.R. Damasio et al. 1989b, 1990b). Isolated disturbances of motion detection, however, are quite rare; one of the few such cases was described by Zihl et al. (1983). Patients with visual disorientation can perceive color and shape normally, if the objects are appreciated within a clear sector of the visual field.

Ocular Apraxia

Ocular apraxia (psychic gaze paralysis) is a deficit of visual scanning. It consists of an inability to direct the gaze voluntarily toward a stimulus located in the peripheral vision to bring it into central vision. Thus, patients fail to direct saccades toward stimuli that have appeared in the panorama of their visual fields, or they produce saccades that are inaccurate and miss the target. Ocular apraxia is not necessary for the development of visual disorientation (Newcombe and Ratcliff 1989; Rizzo and Hurtig 1987; Rizzo and Vecera 2002), although it always occurs together with either visual disorientation or optic ataxia (A.R. Damasio et al. 2000).

Optic Ataxia

Optic ataxia is a disturbance of visually guided reaching behavior. Patients are not able to point accurately at a target, under visual guidance. They cannot point precisely to the examiner's fingertip or to items such as a cup or coin. Interestingly, pointing to targets on their own body does not pose a problem because this can be accomplished on the basis of somatosensory information. Also, the patients have no difficulty pointing to sound sources (A.R. Damasio and Benton 1979). Optic ataxia can occur in isolation, particularly when lesions are at the border of the occipital and parietal regions or in the parietal region exclusively.

The full Balint's syndrome is generally associated with bilateral occipitoparietal lesions, although a unilateral lesion, especially on the right, also can produce the syndrome. When lesions are confined to the superior occipital cortices without extension into the parietal region, visual disorientation is likely to occur without associated ocular apraxia or optic ataxia. The defects in motion perception that occur frequently in patients with Balint's syndrome are probably related to damage in the lower parietal and lateral occipital regions. (In fact, there is a growing body of evidence, especially from functional imaging studies, that structures in the vicinity of the temporal-occipital-parietal junction may play an important role in retrieving knowledge about the typical motion patterns of objects [Kourtzi and Kanwisher 2000; Martin et al. 2000; Tootell et al. 1995]). Many patients with Balint's syndrome have an impairment of stereopsis—that is, the process of depth perception from visual information dependent on binocular visual interaction—although complete astereopsis is seen only in the setting of bilateral lesions (Rizzo 1989; Rizzo and Hurtig 1987).

As noted earlier, bilateral damage to the ventral occipitotemporal sector has been linked to prosopagnosia, whereas damage to the dorsal occipitoparietal sector has been linked to simultanagnosia. It was also mentioned that some patients with prosopagnosia produce discriminatory autonomic responses (skin conductance responses) to familiar faces even though the faces are not recognized consciously. Such a finding has never been reported in connection with dysfunction of the dorsal visual system, but we have encountered just such a case (Denburg et al. 2000). LA is a 50-year-old woman diagnosed with a rare visual variant of Alzheimer's disease, with associated Balint's syndrome, including simultanagnosia. MR and PET studies confirmed focal damage to and dysfunction in the occipitoparietal cortices bilaterally. Neuropsychological testing found preservation of anterograde memory, language, and executive functions, in the context of severely defective complex visual skills. Neuro-ophthalmological studies detected normal visual fields and acuity. We conducted an experiment in which the patient's skin conductance responses were measured during presentation of each of 20 neutrally and 20 negatively valenced visual stimuli. The patient consistently showed large-amplitude skin conductance responses to negative stimuli, even though her conscious report indicated that those stimuli were severely misperceived and rated as neutral in valence. In contrast, neutral stimuli that were accurately perceived and rated as neutral in valence evoked significantly smaller skin conductance responses. This case shows nonconscious recognition of affective valence in a patient with simultanagnosia and dorsal visual system dysfunction.

VENTRAL COMPONENT

The ventral component of the occipital lobes comprises the primary visual cortex immediately below the calcarine fissure (area 17) and the inferior portion of the visual association cortices (areas 18 and 19). The latter component corresponds to the lingual and fusiform gyri (see Figure 2–8C). This region is considered together with the posterior part of area 37, that is, the occipitotemporal junction. Damage to primary visual cortex and/or its connections in the inferior bank of the calcarine fissure will produce a form vision defect (blindness) in the contralateral superior visual field. Damage to nearby structures may spare vision for form, either partially or entirely, while producing some other higher-order visual impairments. Several examples are elaborated below, including acquired achromatopsia, apperceptive visual agnosia, and acquired alexia.

Acquired (Central) Achromatopsia

Acquired (central) achromatopsia is a disorder of color perception involving all or part of the visual field, with preservation of form vision, caused by damage to the inferior visual association cortex and/or its subjacent white matter (A.R. Damasio et al. 1980, 2000; Meadows 1974b; Paulson et al. 1994; Rizzo et al. 1993; for review, see Heywood and Kentridge 2003; Tranel 2001). Patients lose color vision in a quadrant, a hemifield, or the entire visual field. The loss may be partial, in which case patients complain that colors appear "washed out" or "dirty," or may be complete, in which case everything is seen in shades of black and white. Perception of form is unaltered, and depth and motion perception are also normal. It is important to note that the disorder is acquired. It is not a hereditary (retinal) disorder of color vision, such as the red-green color blindness that is fairly common in men, hence the designation *central* achromatopsia. Also, the inability to name colors is not part of the disorder. The latter type of patient has, instead, *color anomia*, and it can be shown that this patient is capable of passing color perception tests such as the Ishihara Color Plate Test and the Farnsworth-Munsell 100-Hue Test. Nor is achromatopsia a disturbance of color association (a disorder known as *color agnosia*); patients with achromatopsia can correctly answer prompts such as "the color of grass is _____" or "the color of blood is _____" (for further discussion of these distinctions, see Heywood and Kentridge 2003; Tranel 2001).

The purest form of central achromatopsia is left hemiachromatopsia associated with a unilateral right occipitotemporal lesion, unaccompanied by other neuropsychological defects. A comparable lesion on the left will produce right hemiachromatopsia, but most of those patients will typically also have alexia. An example of a CT scan from the latter type of patient is shown in Figure 2–10. As the case illustrates, an upper-quadrant form vision defect is generally encountered in the colorless hemifield. This is because the occipitotemporal lesion generally disrupts optic radiations or encroaches into primary visual cortex on the inferior bank of the calcarine fissure. Bilateral occipitotemporal lesions may cause full-field achromatopsia, and such patients often will also manifest associative visual agnosia (especially prosopagnosia).

The most precise anatomical studies based on the lesion method have indicated that the middle third of the lingual gyrus is the most common site of damage in patients with central achromatopsia (Rizzo et al. 1993), followed by damage to the white matter immediately behind the posterior tip of the lateral ventricle. In our experience, lesions confined to the fusiform gyrus or to the white matter beneath the ventricle do not produce achromatopsia. Studies that used functional neuroimaging techniques have corroborated and extended the lesion-based work. It has been shown that when subjects are given tasks requiring inspection or searching for colored stimuli, there are areas of activation in the region of the lingual and fusiform gyri, or putative human area V4, essentially the same area implicated by lesion work (Bartels and Zeki 2000; Chao and Martin 1999; Clark et al. 1997; Corbetta et al. 1990; Sakai et al. 1995). The functional imaging and lesion studies are also consistent with

neurophysiology work in animals (Hubel and Livingstone 1987; Livingstone and Hubel 1988; for review, see Zeki 1990) and with studies in which event-related potentials were used (Rosler et al. 1995). The work in nonhuman primates has indicated that separate cellular channels within area 17 are differently dedicated to the processing of color, form, and motion (Hubel and Livingstone 1987; Livingstone and Hubel 1988) and that some visual association cortices have an important specialization for color processing (Van Essen and Maunsell 1983; Zeki 1973).

A disorder closely related to achromatopsia involves defective color imagery; that is, the inability to imagine objects in color. In fact, it has been argued that defective color perception invariably results in defective color imagery (Beauvois and Saillant 1985; Farah 1989, 2003). This conclusion is supported by functional imaging studies, which have shown that imagining and naming the colors associated with various entities activate a region in the fusiform gyrus bilaterally, but more strongly on the left (Martin et al. 1995). Disorders of color recognition (color agnosia) tend to be associated with unilateral left or bilateral lesions to the occipitotemporal junction, although the neural correlates of color agnosia are very poorly understood (Luzzatti and Davidoff 1994; Schnider et al. 1992; Tranel 2001).

Apperceptive Visual Agnosia

Apperceptive agnosia was originally attributed to the disturbed integration of otherwise normally perceived components of a stimulus (Lissauer 1890), and in general, the concept has persisted as a useful designation for recognition defects that have a substantial perceptual component (Bauer and Demery 2003; Riddoch and Humphreys 2003; Tranel and Damasio 1996). Like associative agnosia described earlier, apperceptive agnosia involves the defective recognition of familiar stimuli. Perception and recognition, rather than being discrete processes, operate on a physiological continuum; thus, the distinction between apperceptive and associative agnosia can be somewhat arbitrary. The term *agnosia* should not be applied to patients in whom recognition defects develop in connection with major disturbances of basic perception (Tranel and Damasio 1996).

A common form of apperceptive agnosia occurs in the visual modality in connection with right-sided lesions involving both the inferior and the superior sectors of the posterior visual association cortices. Such a lesion in a patient of this type is illustrated in Figure 2–11. Several authors have described cases of prosopagnosia following this type of lesion (A.R. Damasio et al. 1989b, 1990b; De Renzi 1986; Landis et al. 1986; Michel et al. 1986; Sergent

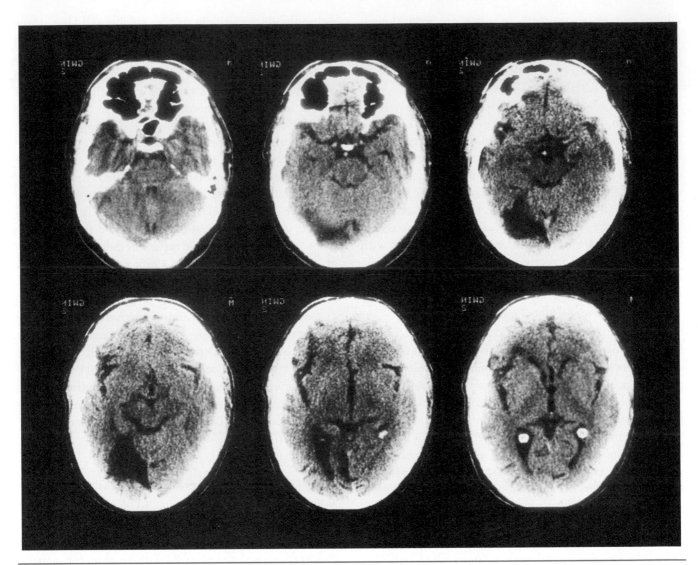

FIGURE 2–10.   Computed tomographic scan of a 67-year-old right-handed man, showing a lesion (area of decreased density) in the left infracalcarine visual association cortices. The man had a right superior quadrantanopia. In the lower right field, form vision was normal, but the patient was unable to see color (achromatopsia). He also had acquired ("pure") alexia.

and Villemure 1989). Patients with apperceptive visual agnosia have difficulty in perceiving all parts of a visual array simultaneously and in generating the image of a whole entity when given a part. When shown a part of a house or a car, for example, the patient will be unable to imagine the whole object to which the part belongs and will fail to recognize the stimulus. A related defect is the inability to assemble parts of a model into a meaningful ensemble. For instance, the patient will be unable to assemble various face parts to form a spatially correct whole. This type of defect has been described in connection with faces and other objects (e.g., A.R. Damasio et al. 1990b). Many such patients also report an inability to image faces (Farah 1989; Kosslyn 1988). Unlike those with associative prosopagnosia, persons with apperceptive agnosia will fail many standard neuropsychological tests of visual perception, such as

matching differently lit photographs of faces and mentally assembling puzzle pieces to form a whole object.

Acquired (Pure) Alexia

Lesions that disconnect both right- and left-sided visual association cortices from the dominant, language-related temporoparietal cortices can produce a complete or partial impairment in reading, a condition known as *acquired (pure) alexia*. Pure alexia can be caused by a single lesion strategically placed in the region behind, beneath, and under the occipital horn of the left lateral ventricle, by damaging pathways from the corpus callosum and from the left visual association cortex (A.R. Damasio and Damasio 1983). Another setting is the combination of a lesion in the corpus callosum, which disconnects right-to-left visual information transfer, and a lesion in the left occipi-

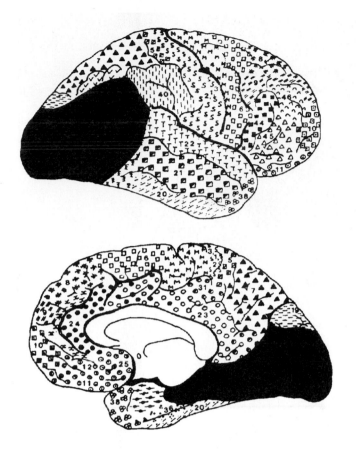

FIGURE 2–11. Depiction of the lesion of a 68-year-old right-handed man who had an infarction that destroyed the right posterior parietal and occipital cortices. Note that the lesion (marked in *black*) includes visual association cortices both above and below the calcarine fissure. The man had apperceptive prosopagnosia.

tal lobe, which disconnects the left visual association cortex from the left language cortex (Benson and Geschwind 1985; Geschwind 1965; Greenblatt 1983). Such lesions are likely to produce right hemianopia, and this sign is a frequent, although not invariable (Greenblatt 1973; Jones and Tranel 2002), accompaniment of pure alexia. Another neuropsychological correlate of pure alexia is color anomia (Davidoff and De Bleser 1994). The "purity" of the condition stems from the fact that patients with these lesions do not develop disturbances in writing or in other aspects of speech and linguistic functioning, separating this type of alexia from the types of reading defects that are common in aphasic patients (Benson et al. 1971). In this sense, pure alexia can be construed as a disturbance of visual pattern recognition. Pure alexia is also known as *alexia without agraphia* or *pure word blindness*.

Patients with pure alexia are unable to read most words and sentences, and in severe cases, even reading of single letters is impaired. The problem is not one of visual acuity. The fact that the patient can see the sentences, words, and letters that cannot be read can be readily confirmed by having the patient copy those stimuli, a task that will be executed normally (Burns 2004; Jones and Tranel 2002; Tranel 1994b). Thus, most patients with pure alexia have normal visual acuity (although a quadrantanopia or hemianopia may be present), and most have normal recognition of nonverbal visual stimuli such as objects and faces.

THE PARIETAL LOBES

On the lateral aspect of the cerebral hemispheres, the parietal lobes comprise a large expanse of cortex bounded by the central sulcus anteriorly, the sylvian fissure inferiorly, and the occipital cortices posteriorly (Figure 2–12). It is important to maintain a clear distinction between the right and the left hemispheres because many cognitive and behavioral correlates of the parietal region are highly lateralized. The parietal lobes are considered together with several anatomically and functionally related neighboring regions. Principal neuropsychological correlates of lesions in these regions are summarized in the table "Highlights for the Clinician."

TEMPOROPARIETAL JUNCTION

In the left hemisphere, an area of cortex formed by the posterior part of the superior temporal gyrus (posterior area 22) constitutes the core of a region known as *Wernicke's area*. The posterior part of the inferior parietal lobule (including parts of the supramarginal and angular gyri) is usually included as part of greater Wernicke's area. This region subserves a set of core speech and language functions whose disruption constitutes the syndrome known as *Wernicke's aphasia* (Caplan 2003; H. Damasio 1998; Tranel and Anderson 1999). Wernicke's aphasia is characterized by fluent, paraphasic speech, impaired repetition, and defective aural comprehension. Patients produce speech without hesitation, and the phrase length and melodic contour of utterances are normal; however, patients make frequent errors in the choice of individual words used to express an idea (paraphasias). Phonemic (also known as *literal*) (e.g., substituting *sephalot* for *elephant*) and semantic (also known as *verbal*) (e.g., substituting *superintendent* for *president*) paraphasias are common. Repetition of sentences is impaired and may be limited to single words. Repetition of digits is usually impaired as well. The comprehension defect can be quite severe and frequently involves both aural and written forms of language. The typical lesion associated with Wernicke's aphasia is depicted in Figure 2–13.

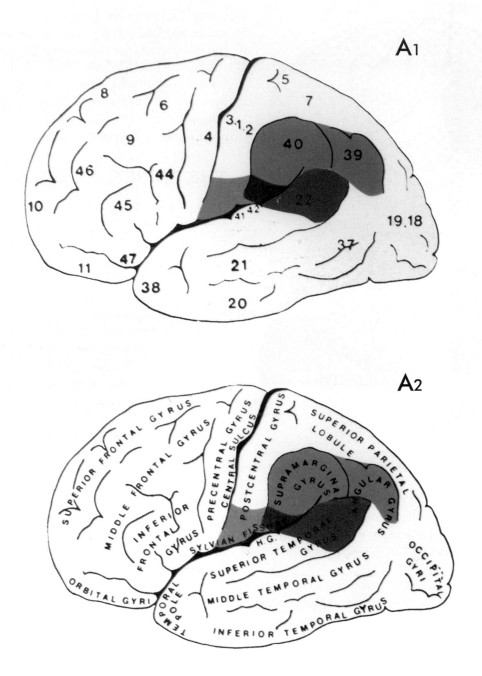

FIGURE 2–12.   Subdivisions of the parietal lobe and nearby regions. The temporoparietal junction, formed by the posterior part of the superior temporal gyrus (area 22), is shown in *red*. The inferior parietal lobule, depicted in *green*, is formed by the angular (area 39) and supramarginal (area 40) gyri. The parietal operculum is formed by the inferior aspect of the postcentral gyrus (shown in *orange*) and a bit of the anteroinferior aspect of the supramarginal gyrus (shown in overlapping *orange* and *green*). Numbers corresponding to Brodmann's cytoarchitectonic areas are depicted in *Panel A1*, and standard gyrus names are shown on the corresponding *Panel A2*. The panels depict a lateral view.

In the right hemisphere, lesions in the region of the temporoparietal junction do not cause disturbances of propositional speech but instead may impair the processing of music and spectral auditory information. A patient of this type was reported by A.R. Damasio et al. (1990d; for a further description of this case, see Tranel 2000). After sustaining a lesion to the right temporoparietal region, the patient developed a severe defect in music recognition. The case was of particular interest because the patient was a trained musician and singer, and the loss of

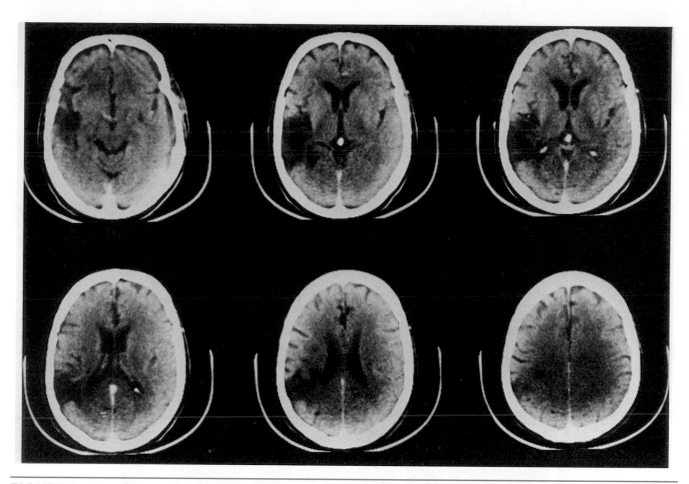

FIGURE 2–13.   Computed tomographic scan of a 56-year-old right-handed man who developed Wernicke's aphasia after sustaining a left middle cerebral artery infarction. The lesion (area of low density) is centered squarely in Wernicke's area, including the posterior superior temporal gyrus (*top row*) and part of the inferior parietal lobule (*bottom row*).

the ability to identify specific singing voices and musical arrangements was especially striking.

Another intriguing neuropsychological correlate of this region is the ability to recognize familiar voices. Van Lancker and her associates reported that lesions to the right parietal cortices disrupt this function, even though auditory acuity is fundamentally unaltered, a condition the authors termed *phonagnosia* (Van Lancker and Kreiman 1988; Van Lancker et al. 1988). More inferior lesions, confined to the temporal cortices, tend to disrupt perception of auditory spectral information (Robin et al. 1990) but may not disrupt voice recognition (Van Lancker et al. 1989).

Bilateral lesions to the posterior part of the superior temporal gyrus lead to the syndrome of auditory agnosia, in which the patient is unable to recognize both speech and nonspeech sounds (Burns 2004; Vignolo 1982; for reviews, see Bauer and Demery 2003; Tranel and Damasio 1996). Almost always caused by stroke, the condition involves the sudden and complete inability to identify the meaning of verbal and nonverbal auditory signals, including spoken words and familiar environmental sounds such as a

telephone ringing or a knock at the door. Full-blown auditory agnosia is rare. In most cases, there is a good deal of perceptual impairment together with a recognition defect, and the term *agnosia* should be applied with qualification.

INFERIOR PARIETAL LOBULE

The inferior parietal lobule comprises the supramarginal and angular gyri. On the left side, lesions to the supramarginal gyrus and the neighboring parietal operculum (the area of cortex formed by the inferiormost portion of the postcentral gyrus) or the underlying white matter, or both, cause a speech and language disturbance known as *conduction aphasia* (e.g., Caplan 2003). An example of a CT scan from such a patient is shown in Figure 2–14. The core feature of this aphasia is a marked defect in verbatim repetition, which is disproportionately severe compared with other speech and language defects. Speech production is fluent but is dominated by phonemic paraphasias. Comprehension is only mildly compromised. Naming is defective and is dominated by phonemic errors, such as substi-

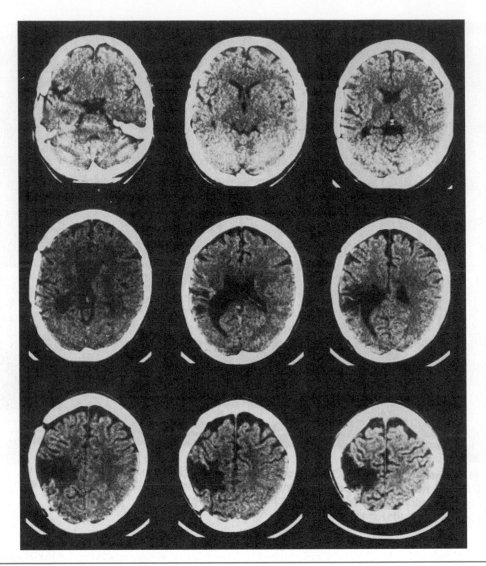

FIGURE 2–14.   Computed tomographic scan of a 35-year-old right-handed woman, showing a lesion (area of low density) in the left supramarginal gyrus (area 40). Note that the lesion spares the primary auditory cortex and the main part of Wernicke's area (posterior area 22). The woman had conduction aphasia.

tution of incorrect phonemes into target naming responses. Reading aloud is impaired, but reading comprehension may be normal. Another distinctive feature of conduction aphasia is that patients cannot write to dictation; however, they can write normally or nearly normally when writing spontaneously or when copying a written example.

Conduction aphasia also has been reported with lesions that damage the primary auditory cortex (areas 41 and 42) and extend into the insular cortex and underlying white matter (H. Damasio and Damasio 1980). Another interesting example is a case described by Hyman and Tranel (1989), in which conduction aphasia occurred together with a complete right hemianesthesia. The lesion in this patient was in the white matter subjacent to the inferior parietal and posterior temporal cortices, with extension into the posterior part of the insula.

Left-sided lesions to the parietal region, especially in the inferior parietal lobule, also have been associated with an acquired disturbance in mathematical abilities, a condition known as *acalculia* (for review, see Denburg and Tranel 2003). Patients lose the ability to perform various calculations—such as adding, subtracting, multiplying, and dividing—and may even be impaired in the simple reading or writing of numbers. A careful review of the literature indicates that the neural correlates of acalculia are not well understood; moreover, the condition is frequently accompanied by disturbances of language (e.g., aphasia) or visuospatial processing that confound its interpretation. Nonetheless, it has been suggested that the left parietal region constitutes the "mathematical brain" in humans, and this idea has attracted a reasonable amount of scientific support (Butterworth 1999).

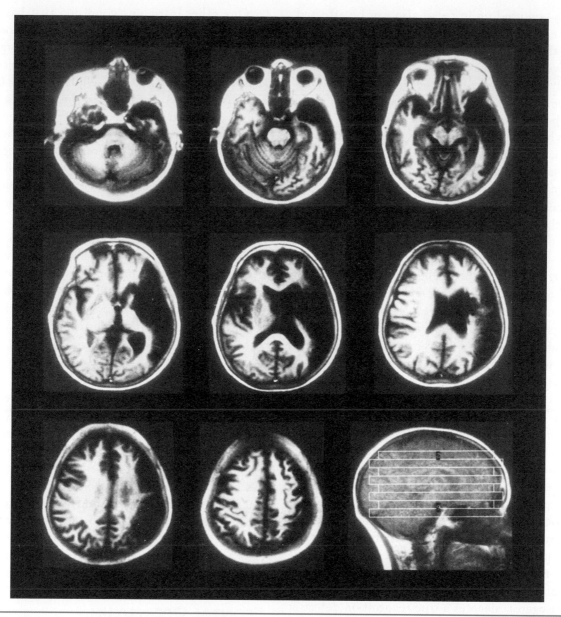

FIGURE 2–15. T1-weighted magnetic resonance images of a 34-year-old right-handed woman, showing a large right middle cerebral artery infarction. The lesion (shown as a *black region*) includes a significant portion of the inferior parietal lobule (areas 39 and 40). The woman had severe left-sided neglect, anosognosia, and visuospatial deficits.

On the right side, the most consistent and striking neuropsychological correlates of lesions to the inferior parietal lobule are neglect and anosognosia. *Neglect*, associated especially with temporoparietal lesions that include areas 39 and 40 as well as the underlying white matter (e.g., Heilman et al. 2003; for review, see Robertson and Marshall 1993; Vallar et al. 2003), refers to a condition whereby the patient fails to attend to stimuli in the contralateral hemispace (spatial neglect). In the visual modality, for example, the patient will not attend to the left hemifield and will fail to report stimuli from that side even when it can be shown that form vision is not impaired (hemianopia). In principle, neglect can occur in re-

lation to any sensory modality, but in practice, the visual and auditory varieties are most common. Some investigators have attributed neglect to an impairment of the attentional mechanisms necessary for normal perception (e.g., Heilman et al. 2003; Vallar et al. 2003; Weintraub and Mesulam 1989). Figure 2–15 shows a typical example of a patient with a large right hemisphere lesion that includes the inferior parietal lobule. The patient had severe neglect, anosognosia, and visuospatial impairments.

Neglect can also involve intrapersonal space. For example, patients may fail to use, or even deny the existence of, the contralateral arm and leg, even when they have no motor impairment (e.g., Tranel 1995b). Representations conjured up in recall also can be affected. When asked to imagine or draw an object, the patient may omit the left half as though it did not exist. Asked to describe well-known scenes from memory, patients may report only the elements from the right side of the representation. The omissions, however, are specific to the patient's perspective, and it can be shown that the patient does have the capacity to access the full array of information. Bisiach and Luzzatti (1978), for example, asked patients to describe a well-known scene from a particular perspective and then rotated the perspective by 180 degrees and asked the patients again to describe the scene. In the first description, patients reported information from only the right side of the scene. In the second condition, the patients again reported information from only the right side of the scene, but because the perspective had been rotated, this was precisely the same information that had been neglected in the first description.

Anosognosia is another frequent correlate of damage to the right inferior parietal lobule (for review, see Adair et al. 2003). However, there is some debate regarding the anatomical localization and lateralization of this phenomenon. For instance, Venneri and Shanks (2004) identified a lesion in the right parietotemporal region in a woman (EN) with persisting anosognosia for hemiplegia and left-sided neglect following a hemorrhagic stroke, whereas others have documented cases of anosognosia following subcortical injuries (see Adair et al. 2003 for details). The term was originally applied to patients who denied that a paretic limb was in fact paretic or that it even belonged to them (Babinski 1914). Denial of sensory loss (e.g., a visual field defect) and cognitive disturbance (e.g., amnesia, dementia, aphasia) also have been included under the concept of anosognosia (Adair et al. 2003; Anderson and Tranel 1989). In a strict sense, anosognosia denotes a true recognition defect in which the patient is unaware of acquired motor, sensory, or cognitive deficits. This can be distinguished from denial of illness, which refers to the adaptive psychological condition that allows patients under severe stress to adapt to the calamitous consequences of disease. Anosognosia can be operationally defined as a significant discrepancy between patients' reporting of their disabilities and the objective evidence regarding their level of functioning. A related term is *anosodiaphoria*, which refers to the condition in which patients appear unconcerned with or minimize the significance of neurological and neuropsychological deficits. It is common for patients to manifest anosognosia early in the course of illness and then for this to evolve gradually into anosodiaphoria. In both conditions, common neuropsychological correlates are defects in visuospatial and visuoconstructional abilities and left hemispatial neglect (Benton 1985; Benton and Tranel 1993).

One other intriguing condition that has been described in connection with lesions to the inferior parietal lobule and nearby posterior/superior temporal cortices on either the right or the left side is tactile object agnosia (Bauer and Demery 2003; Caselli 1991, 1993; C.L. Reed and Caselli 1994). Patients lose the ability to recognize objects presented via the tactile modality, even when basic aspects of somatosensory function are normal or near normal. The condition is different from prosopagnosia in that it involves a disruption of recognition at the basic object level rather than at the level of unique identity (Tranel 1991b). Thus, patients with tactile agnosia cannot recognize stimuli such as keys, pencils, and eating utensils when those items are presented in the somatosensory modality. The condition is far less disabling than a disorder such as prosopagnosia, and many patients with tactile object agnosia will not even complain of a defect. In fact, the impairment may only be demonstrable under careful laboratory testing conditions.

THE FRONTAL LOBES

The frontal lobes constitute about half of the entire cerebral mantle, and this portion of the brain has numerous functional correlates. For reviews of functional correlates of the frontal lobes, the reader is referred to Boller and Spinnler (1994), A.R. Damasio and Anderson (2003), Fuster (1989), Levin et al. (1991), and Stuss and Levine (2002). To consider cognitive and behavioral correlates, it is helpful to divide the frontal lobes into several distinct anatomical sectors (Figure 2–16). The specific neuropsychological correlates of these different sectors are summarized in the table "Highlights for the Clinician."

FRONTAL OPERCULUM

The frontal operculum is formed by areas 44, 45, and 47 (see Figure 2–16). On the left side, the heart of this region (areas 44 and 45) is known as *Broca's area*. The region is dedicated to a set of speech and language functions whose disruption produces a distinctive pattern of aphasia termed *Broca's aphasia*. Patients with Broca's aphasia have nonfluent speech, characterized by short utterances, long response latencies, and flat melodic contour. There is a marked decrease in the density of words per unit time, and the speech production has long gaps in which the patient is struggling unsuccessfully to produce sounds. A severe disturbance of grammar is also characteristic of Broca's aphasia. Paraphasias are common, usually involving omission of phonemes or addition of incorrect phonemes (phonemic paraphasias). In severe cases, speech may be virtually unintelligible. A defect in repeti-

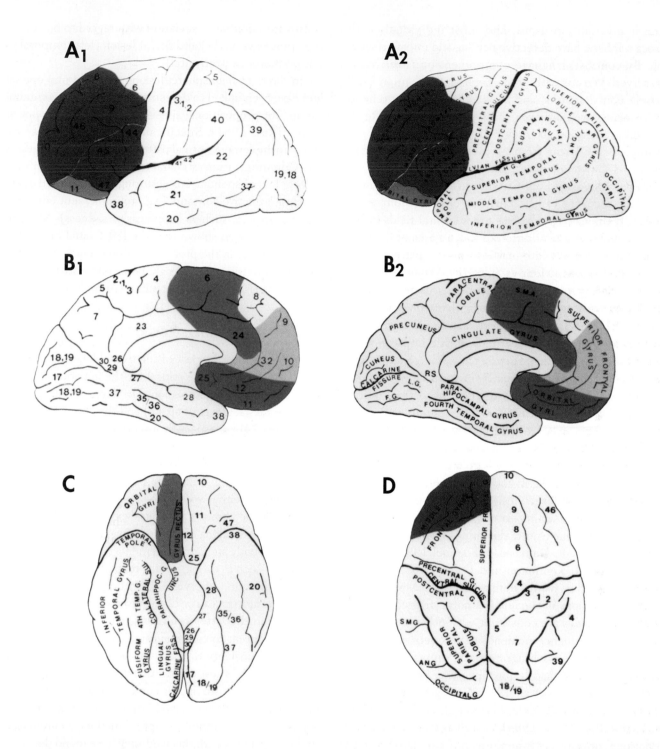

FIGURE 2–16. Major subdivisions of the frontal lobe: the frontal operculum, formed by areas 44, 45, and 47 (*red*); the superior mesial region, formed by the mesial aspect of area 6 and the anterior part of the cingulate gyrus (area 24) (*green*); the inferior mesial region, formed by the orbital cortices (areas 11, 12, and 25) (*orange*) (the basal forebrain is immediately posterior to this region); and the lateral prefrontal region, formed by the lateral aspects of areas 8, 9, 46, and 10 (*purple*). The ventromedial frontal lobe comprises the orbital (*orange*) and the lower mesial (area 32 and the mesial aspect of areas 10 and 9) cortices (*tan*). Numbers corresponding to Brodmann's cytoarchitectonic areas are depicted in *Panels A1* and *B1* and on the right side (left hemisphere) of *Panels C* and *D*, and the standard gyrus names are shown in the corresponding *Panels A2* and *B2* and on the left side (right hemisphere) of *Panels C* and *D*. Lateral (*A1* and *A2*), mesial (*B1* and *B2*), inferior (*C*), and superior (*D*) views are represented.

tion is invariably present, and most individuals with Broca's aphasia have defective naming and impaired writing. By contrast, language comprehension is relatively preserved. Persons with Broca's aphasia can comprehend simple conversations, and they generally comprehend and execute two- and even three-step commands. Reading comprehension also may be relatively preserved. An example of a CT scan from a typical patient with Broca's aphasia is shown in Figure 2–17.

When lesions are confined to Broca's area, speech and language recovery can be fairly extensive (Mohr et al. 1978). If the damage involves other frontal fields in the dorsolateral sector in addition to Broca's area or if it cuts deeper into frontal white matter, a poorer pattern of recovery is observed (Mohr et al. 1978). When lesions involve the lower motor or premotor cortices or the subjacent white matter, aphemia rather than aphasia results (Schiff et al. 1983). Patients develop articulatory defects and hesitant speech, but a true linguistic impairment is not present. Lesions in structures anterior, superior, and deep to Broca's area, but sparing most or all of areas 44 and 45, will commonly produce transcortical motor aphasia (e.g., Rubens 1976), which resembles Broca's aphasia except that no repetition defect is present.

Several studies have detected an intriguing pattern of naming impairment associated with lesions in the premotor or prefrontal region, in and near the left frontal operculum. Patients with such lesions have a disproportionate impairment in the ability to name actions (with verbs) and, by contrast, have normal naming of concrete entities (with nouns) (A.R. Damasio and Tranel 1993; Hillis et al. 2002b, 2004; Kemmerer and Tranel 2003; Tranel et al. 2001). In other words, defective verb retrieval is associated with lesions in the left premotor or prefrontal region. The findings are consistent with other studies that have reported a higher incidence of verb retrieval impairment in patients with agrammatic aphasia, many of whom presumably had lesions involving the left frontal operculum (Daniele et al. 1994; Goodglass et al. 1994; Hillis and Caramazza 1995; Hillis et al. 2002a; Miceli et al. 1988; Miozzo et al. 1994), as well as studies that used functional imaging with nonimpaired participants (e.g., Tranel et al. 2005). An example of a CT scan from a patient with this type of naming pattern is shown in Figure 2–18. The patient had normal retrieval of common and proper nouns (naming of concrete entities) but defective retrieval of verbs (naming of actions). It is intriguing that this is the opposite pattern of that associated with left temporal lobe lesions (see subsection "Lexical Retrieval" earlier in this chapter); those patients have defective retrieval of words for concrete entities (nouns) but normal retrieval of words for actions (verbs). These findings thus constitute a double dissociation with regard to both word type (nouns vs. verbs) and site of lesion (left temporal vs. left premotor or prefrontal).

In the right hemisphere, lesions to the frontal operculum have been linked to defects in paralinguistic communication, but propositional speech and language are not affected (Ross 1981). Specifically, patients may lose the ability to implement normal patterns of prosody and gesturing. Communication is characterized by flat, monotone speech; loss of spontaneous gesturing; and impaired ability to repeat affective contours (e.g., to implement emotional tones in speech, such as happiness or sadness). More recently, it has been shown that the left frontal operculum also plays a role in the processing of emotional prosody, although not to the extent of right hemisphere structures, including the right frontal operculum (Adolphs et al. 2002).

SUPERIOR MESIAL REGION

The superior mesial aspect of the frontal lobes comprises a set of structures that are critical for the initiation of movement and emotional expression. The supplementary motor area (the mesial aspect of area 6) and the anterior cingulate gyrus (area 24) are especially important (see Figure 2–16). Lesions in this region produce a syndrome known as *akinetic mutism* (A.R. Damasio and Van Hoesen 1983; Mega and Cohenour 1997), in which the patient makes no effort to communicate, either verbally or by gesture, and maintains an empty, noncommunicative facial expression. Movements are limited to tracking of moving targets with the eyes and performing body and arm movements connected with daily necessities such as eating, pulling up bedclothing, and going to the bathroom. Otherwise, the patient does not move or speak. The mutism can be distinguished from aphasia by the fact that, in the latter condition, patients will invariably express an intent to communicate. They will show frustration at their inability to speak and will seek compensatory strategies, such as gesturing or writing. By contrast, patients with akinetic mutism appear content to lie motionless and silent, and they do not respond to reasonable queries from the examiner or to other prompts. Functional neuroimaging studies in patients with this syndrome have found decreased signal in both the frontal and the anterior cingulate cortices (e.g., Tengvar et al. 2004). An example of the lesion in a patient with akinetic mutism is illustrated in Figure 2–19.

There does not appear to be a significant difference in the profile of akinetic mutism as a function of the side of the lesion; left- and right-sided lesions lead to more or less equivalent defects. However, the defects are more severe, and persist longer, with bilateral lesions. Patients with unilateral lesions may recover very quickly, sometimes within a few weeks.

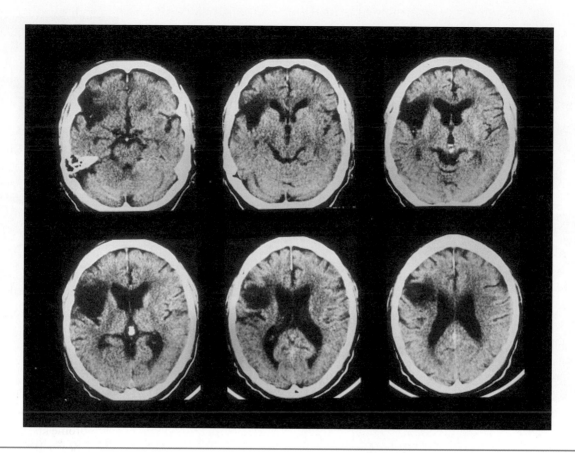

FIGURE 2–17. Computed tomographic scan of a 76-year-old right-handed man who developed Broca's aphasia after a left frontal infarction. The lesion, showing as a well-defined area of low density, is squarely in the heart of Broca's area—that is, the frontal opercular region formed by areas 44 and 45.

INFERIOR MESIAL REGION

Inferiorly, the mesial aspect of the frontal lobes is composed of the orbital region, which includes areas 11 and 12. The basal forebrain (not part of the frontal lobes proper) is situated immediately behind the posterior-most extension of the inferior mesial region (see Figure 2–16).

Basal Forebrain

The basal forebrain is composed of a set of bilateral para-midline gray nuclei that include the septal nuclei, the diagonal band of Broca, the nucleus accumbens, and the sub-stantia innominata. Lesions to this area, commonly caused by the rupture of aneurysms located in the anterior communicating artery or in the anterior cerebral artery, cause a distinctive neuropsychological syndrome in which memory defects figure most prominently (A.R. Damasio et al. 1985b, 1989a; O'Connor and Verfaellie 2002; Tranel et al. 2000b; Volpe and Hirst 1983). An example of this type of presentation is shown in Figure 2–20. Acutely, patients typically present with a confusional state and attentional problems, which resolve into an anterograde amnesia characterized by deficits in delayed free recall in the context of relatively better recognition, likely reflecting an underlying disruption of the neural mechanisms involved in strategic search processes. Evidence of temporally graded retrograde amnesia is also often seen. The amnesic profile of patients with basal forebrain lesions has several intriguing features. It is characterized by an impairment in the integration of different aspects of stimuli, wherein patients are able to learn and recall separate component features of entities and events but cannot associate those components into an integrated memory. For example, the patient may learn the name of a person, that person's face, and the person's personality traits. When attempting to recall the target individual, the patient will not bring this information together but will assign the individual the wrong name or the wrong personality traits. This modal mismatching defect affects the retrograde compartment as well.

Another frequent manifestation in patients with basal forebrain lesions is a proclivity for confabulation. The fabrications have a dreamlike quality and occur spontaneously. They are not prompted by the need to fill gaps of missing information in attempting to respond to an examiner's questions. In some instances, the internal experience of the

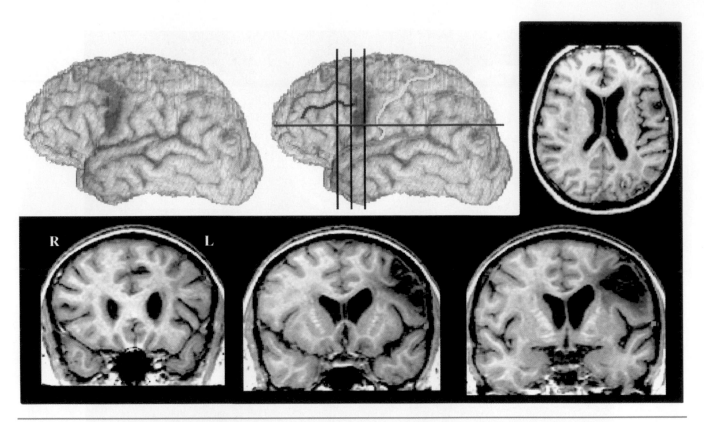

FIGURE 2–18.   Three-dimensional reconstruction of the brain of a patient with a lesion in the left premotor or prefrontal region. The patient had impaired retrieval of words for actions (verbs) but normal retrieval of words for concrete entities (nouns). This patient, and several others of this type whom we have studied, had a recovered nonfluent aphasia.

patient may even include fantasies that are not recognized as such. The patient will not be capable of distinguishing reality from nonreality in his or her own recall (A.R. Damasio et al. 1985b, 1989a; Tranel et al. 2000b). The memory defects of patients with basal forebrain lesions can persist well into the chronic phase of recovery; even after many years, patients continue to manifest learning and recall deficits and a tendency to confabulate. In the chronic phase, however, patients usually gain some insight into their difficulties. They learn to mistrust their own recall and to cross-check their own memories against an external source.

Ventromedial Region

The orbital and lower mesial frontal cortices (including Brodmann areas 11, 12, 25, and 32 and the mesial aspect of 10 and 9; see Figure 2–16) constitute the ventromedial frontal lobe, and several important neuropsychological correlates have been established for this region. Patients with ventromedial frontal lobe damage develop a severe disruption of social conduct, including defects in planning, judgment, and decision making (Bechara 2004; Bechara et al. 1994, 1996; A.R. Damasio 1994; Tranel 1994a; Tranel et al. 2000a), a condition that has been termed *acquired sociopathy* (Barrash et al. 2000b; A.R.

Damasio et al. 1990c, 1991). Preliminary evidence suggests that there may be functional asymmetries in the right and left ventromedial prefrontal sectors, with the right side being critical for mediating social conduct, decision making, and emotional processing and the left side playing a relatively minor role in these functions (Tranel et al. 2002). Provided that the lesion does not extend into the basal forebrain, such patients generally do not develop memory disturbances; in fact, such patients are remarkably free of conventional neuropsychological defects (A.R. Damasio and Anderson 2003; Stuss and Benson 1986; Tranel et al. 1994a). Patient EVR, initially described by Eslinger and Damasio (1985), is prototypical (Figure 2–21). However, more recent data suggest that in addition to well-documented emotional and behavioral dysregulation typically seen in these patients, the degree of cognitive dysfunction is greater than previously reported. Cato et al. (2004) suggested that this is the result of a lack of sensitivity of many traditional neuropsychological measures and presented data showing impaired performances on new neuropsychological measures that "tapped multiple executive functions simultaneously" (e.g., inhibition and set shifting) and "quantified and normed error types." The authors posited that these

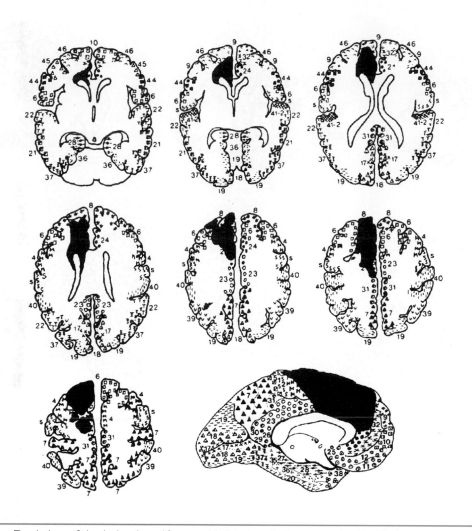

FIGURE 2–19. Depiction of the lesion in a 40-year-old right-handed man, marked in *black* on transverse templates and on the mesial brain. The lesion is in the left hemisphere and involves the mesial aspect of area 6 and the anterior part of the cingulate gyrus (area 24). Initially, the man had severe akinetic mutism, but by 3 months after onset, he had excellent recovery.

deficits reflect underlying problems in behavioral inflexibility (e.g., an inability to adjust response rate to increasing task demands) and a "liberal response style" characterized by set-loss errors and intrusions.

Throughout the history of neuropsychology, investigators have called attention to the seemingly bizarre development of abnormal social behavior following frontal brain injury, especially damage to the ventromedial sector (e.g., Ackerly and Benton 1948; Brickner 1934, 1936; Harlow 1868; Hebb and Penfield 1940). The patients have a few features in common (see A.R. Damasio and Anderson 2003), including the inability to organize future activity and hold gainful employment; diminished capacity to respond to punishment; a tendency to present an unrealistically favorable view of themselves; stereotyped but correct manners; a tendency to show inappropriate emotional reactions; and normal intelligence. It is crucial to keep in mind that in all cases, this personality

and behavioral profile developed after the onset of frontal lobe damage in individuals with previously normal personalities and socialization.

Other investigators have called attention to similar characteristics in patients with ventromedial frontal lobe damage. For example, Blumer and Benson (1975) noted a personality type that characterized patients with orbital damage (which the authors termed *pseudo-psychopathic*), in which salient features were puerility, a jocular attitude, sexually disinhibited humor, inappropriate and nearly total self-indulgence, and complete lack of concern for others. Stuss and Benson (1984, 1986) emphasized that such patients have a remarkable lack of empathy and a general lack of concern about others. The patients tend to show callous unconcern, boastfulness, and unrestrained and tactless behavior. Other descriptors include impulsiveness, facetiousness, and diminished anxiety and concern for the future. Mesulam (1986) emphasized the following personality features of

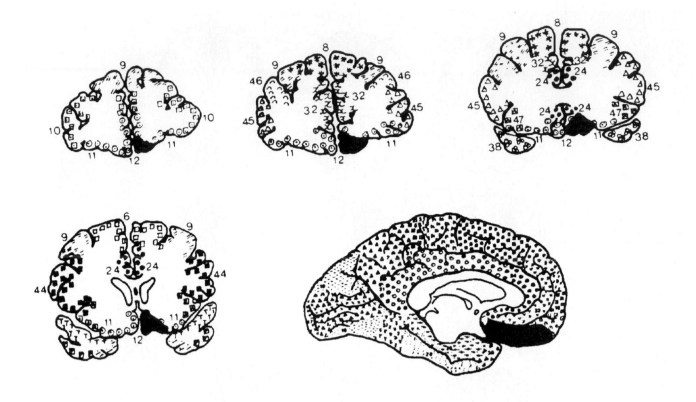

FIGURE 2–20.   Depiction of the lesion in a 32-year-old right-handed man who experienced rupture of an anterior communicating artery aneurysm. The lesion, shown in *black* on coronal sections (left hemisphere on the right) and on the mesial aspect of the hemisphere, involves the left gyrus rectus and the left basal forebrain. The man had a distinctive amnesic syndrome with confabulation and both anterograde and retrograde deficits.

patients with frontal lobe damage: puerile; profane; facetious; irresponsible; grandiose; irascible; erosion of foresight, judgment, and insight; loss of ability to delay gratification; loss of capacity for remorse; tendency to jump to premature conclusions; loss of capacity to grasp the context and gist of a complex situation; poor inhibition of immediate but inappropriate response tendencies; sustained shallowness; and impulsivity of thought and affect. More recently, Blair and Cipolotti (2000) described patient J.S., who, following bilateral damage to the orbitofrontal cortex, "became irritable and aggressive, failed to conform to social norms, was reckless regarding others' personal safety, showed a striking lack of remorse, and failed to plan ahead" (p. 1124).

A.R. Damasio (1994, 1995) has articulated a theory of emotion and feeling, which can be used to account for the somewhat enigmatic neuropsychological profiles of patients with a damaged ventromedial region. The theory posits that the response selection impairment in patients with ventromedial damage and acquired sociopathy is due to a defect in the activation of somatic markers that must accompany the internal and automatic processing of possible response options. The patients are deprived of a somatic marker that normally assists, both consciously

and covertly, with response selection, reducing their chances of responding in the most advantageous manner and increasing their chances of generating responses that will lead to negative consequences.

According to the theory, a somatic marker provides the individual with a conscious "gut feeling" on the merits of a given response. It would also force attention on the positive or negative nature of various response options based on their foreseeable consequences. Another effect, which would be covert, would be the modification of neural systems that propitiate appetitive or aversive behaviors, such as the dopamine and serotonin nonspecific systems that can alter processing in the cerebral cortex. This effect, activated by the somatic marker, would increase or decrease the chances of immediate response. For example, a negative somatic state would inhibit appetitive behaviors, whereas a positive somatic state would facilitate appetitive behaviors. This would occur even if the somatic state itself were not conscious.

In individuals without brain damage, the ventromedial frontal cortices receive signals from a large range of neural structures engaged by perception, including external information from vision, audition, and olfaction and

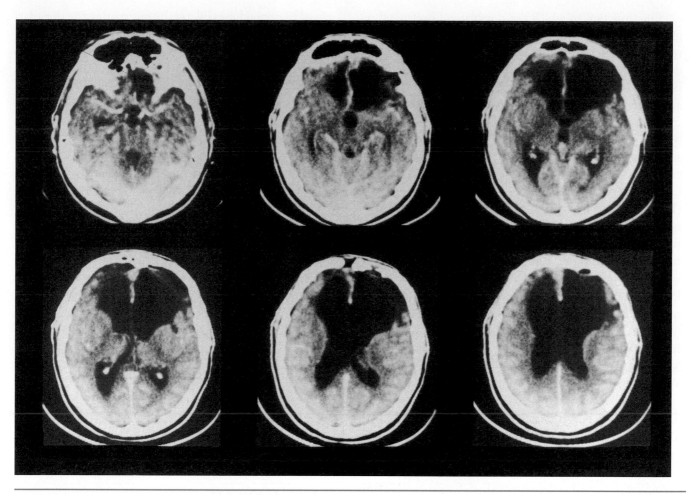

FIGURE 2–21. Computed tomographic scan of a 44-year-old right-handed man who underwent resection of a large orbitofrontal meningioma. The lesion, showing as an area of low density, encompasses bilateral destruction of the orbital and lower mesial frontal cortices. The basal forebrain is spared. The man developed severe changes in personality but did not manifest defects in conventional neuropsychological procedures.

internal somatic information from skeletal and visceral states. The signals arrive in the orbital region via projections from higher-order association cortices in temporal, parietal, and insular regions. In addition, the ventromedial cortices are a known source of projections from frontal regions toward central autonomic control structures; also, the ventromedial cortices receive and reciprocate projections from the hippocampus and amygdala (see A.R. Damasio et al. 1990c, 1991). Thus, the ventromedial cortices are in a position to form conjunctive records of concurrent signals hailing from external and internal stimuli, within neuron ensembles of the type that have been termed *convergence zones* (A.R. Damasio 1989a, 1989b). These cortices also can activate somatic effectors. A.R. Damasio (1994, 1995) has elaborated how this explanation can account for various facets of acquired sociopathy and other related conditions.

The ventromedial frontal region also may play a role in prospective memory, the capacity of "remembering in the future" (Schnyer et al. 2004). Take as an example the following scenario. You are supposed to remember to call your spouse around midday to arrange plans for picking up the children from school. You can appose a "somatic marker" to this stimulus configuration so that when noontime arrives, you are "reminded" by your brain via a signal from the ventromedial frontal region—which may come as the feeling that "something needs to be done"—to call your spouse.

DORSOLATERAL PREFRONTAL REGION

The dorsolateral aspect of the frontal lobes comprises a vast expanse of cortex that occupies Brodmann areas 8, 9, 10, and 46 (see Figure 2–16). The functions of the lateral prefrontal region (exclusive of the frontal operculum and other language-related structures discussed previously) in humans are not well understood. Some of the better-established correlates are reviewed below.

One function to which the dorsolateral prefrontal region has been linked is working memory. *Working memory* refers to a relatively short (on the order of minutes) window of mental processing during which information is held "online," and operations are performed on it. For example, the demands of the Digit Span backwards test from the Wechsler Adult Intelligence Scale—III, or of the serial 7s test, are examples of working memory. In essence, working memory is a temporary storage and processing system used for problem solving and other cognitive operations that take place over a limited time frame (Baddeley 1992). Working memory is used to bridge temporal gaps—that is, to hold representations in a mental workspace long enough so that we can make appropriate responses to stimulus configurations or contingencies in which some, or even all, of the basic ingredients are no longer extant in perceptual space. The prefrontal cortex has been implicated in the mediation of working memory (Alivisatos and Milner 1989; Fuster 1989; Goldman-Rakic 1987; Jonides et al. 1993; McCarthy et al. 1994; Milner et al. 1985; Petrides 2005; E.E. Smith et al. 1995; Wilson et al. 1993), and Goldman-Rakic (1987) has suggested that this is the exclusive memory function of the entire prefrontal cortex, each region being connected with a particular domain of operations. Evidence indicates left- and right-sided specialization of the prefrontal regions with regard to working memory, following the typical left–verbal/right–spatial arrangement (E.E. Smith et al. 1996).

Our work has yielded findings consistent with this notion. For example, we found that patients with damage to the dorsolateral prefrontal cortex had severe impairments in working memory tasks involving delayed responding but relatively preserved performance on decision-making tasks (Bechara et al. 1998). The reverse outcome—impaired decision making and normal working memory—was obtained in patients with ventromedial prefrontal damage, suggesting that different sectors of the frontal lobe are specialized for these two cognitive operations.

The dorsolateral prefrontal region also appears to be involved in higher-order integrative and executive control functions, and damage to this sector has been linked to intellectual deficits (see Stuss and Benson 1986; Stuss and Levine 2002). Several investigators have noted memory impairment that affects judgments of recency and frequency of events but not the content of the events. Patients fail to remember how often, or how recently, they have experienced a certain stimulus, but they do recognize the stimulus as familiar (Milner and Petrides 1984; Milner et al. 1985; M.L. Smith and Milner 1988). The reverse dissociation—impaired recognition of content but preserved recency and frequency discrimination—was reported in connection with a lesion involving the mesial temporal lobes bilaterally but sparing the dorsolateral prefrontal cortices (Sagar et al. 1990).

The dorsolateral frontal cortices have been linked to the verbal regulation of behavior (Luria 1969), and verbal fluency, as measured by the ability to generate word lists under certain stimulus constraints, is notably impaired in many patients with dorsolateral lesions, especially when those lesions are bilateral or on the left (Benton 1968; Stuss et al. 1998). Unilateral right dorsolateral lesions may impair fluency in the nonverbal domain. For instance, patients may lose the capacity to produce designs in a fluent manner (Jones-Gotman and Milner 1977). Finally, deficits on laboratory tests of executive function, which test the ability to form, maintain, and change cognitive sets, as well as the tendency to perseverate (the Wisconsin Card Sorting Test is a paradigmatic example), can be fairly pronounced in patients with dorsolateral lesions, although they are by no means specific (Anderson et al. 1991; Milner 1963; Stuss and Levine 2002; Tranel et al. 1994a).

SUBCORTICAL STRUCTURES

Two sets of subcortical structures are considered—the basal ganglia and the thalamus. A summary of some neuropsychological correlates of damage to these structures is presented in the table "Highlights for the Clinician."

BASAL GANGLIA

The basal ganglia are a set of deep gray nuclear structures, the caudate nucleus and the lenticular nucleus, with the latter being divided into the putamen and the globus pallidus. On the left side, lesions to these structures produce a speech and language disturbance that involves a mixture of manifestations that cannot be easily classified according to standard aphasia nomenclature; hence the pattern has come to be known as *atypical aphasia* (Alexander 1989; A.R. Damasio et al. 1982a; Naeser et al. 1982; for review, see Radanovic and Scaff 2003). In cases in which the lesion is a result of stroke caused by stenosis or occlusion of the left middle cerebral artery, it has been suggested that the variability of this syndrome may be due to the resultant cortical hypoperfusion (Hillis et al. 2004). Because damage in this region will almost invariably include the anterior limb of the internal capsule, right hemiparesis is a common accompanying manifestation. The aphasia is characterized by speech that is usually fluent but is paraphasic and dysarthric; (typically) poor auditory comprehension; and, in some cases, impaired repetition. An example of MR imagery from a patient with a basal ganglia lesion and atypical aphasia is shown in Figure 2–22.

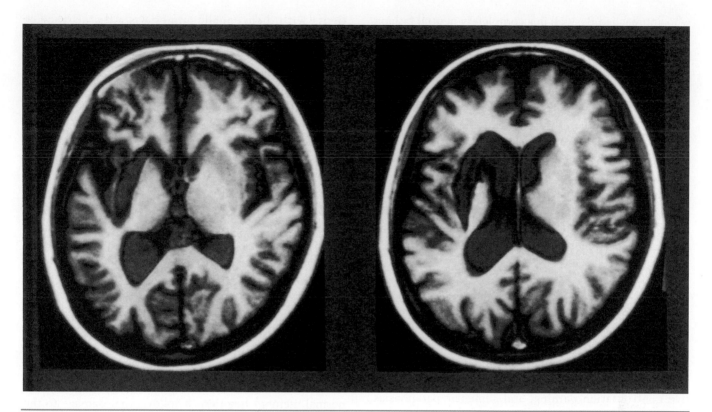

FIGURE 2–22.   T1-weighted magnetic resonance image of a 35-year-old right-handed woman who sustained a subcortical hemorrhage. The lesion, showing as an area of black on these transverse sectional images, involves the left basal ganglia, including the head and body of the caudate nucleus, and part of the putamen. The woman had a characteristic basal ganglia type of aphasia, with marked dysarthria and mixed linguistic impairments.

It has been noted that patients with basal ganglia lesions and atypical aphasia nearly always have lesions that involve the head of the caudate nucleus, together with the putamen and anterior limb of the internal capsule (H. Damasio 1989). Lesions confined to the putamen, or to laterally adjacent structures such as the anterior insula and subjacent white matter, do not produce an aphasic disturbance, although defects in articulation and prosody may be noted. Other authors, however, have pointed out that in the key reports of aphasia-producing lesions to the basal ganglia (Cappa et al. 1983; A.R. Damasio et al. 1982a; Naeser et al. 1982), the patients all had significant damage to white matter structures in addition to basal ganglia involvement (Alexander 1989). One additional note of importance is that patients with basal ganglia lesions and aphasia tend to show very good recovery (H. Damasio et al. 1984).

As alluded to earlier (see subsection "Mesial Temporal Region" earlier in this chapter), the basal ganglia also have been linked to various forms of nondeclarative memory, including learning of motor skills and other capacities that do not require any conscious mental inspection of the contents of memory (for review, see Packard and Knowlton 2002). The caudate nucleus, which together with the putamen forms the striatal component of the basal ganglia, may have nondeclarative memory functions that are related to the development of habits and other nonconscious response tendencies. The tendencies we develop to respond to certain situations in certain ways, behaviors such as following the same route home each day or repeatedly seeking out a particular person for moral support and encouragement, are examples of habits and response tendencies that we engage in on a fairly automatic basis with little or no conscious deliberation. These types of "memory" behavior have been linked to the striatum and, in particular, the caudate nucleus.

To illustrate this effect, consider a study we completed in patient Boswell (Tranel and Damasio 1993). We showed that Boswell, who had severe anterograde amnesia covering all aspects of declarative memory, could acquire new knowledge, covertly, if this knowledge was associated with positive or negative affective valence during the time of acquisition. During the course of several days, Boswell was exposed to three different stimulus persons: 1) a "Good Guy," who treated Boswell very kindly and granted requests for treats and rewards; 2) a "Bad Guy," who never gave Boswell treats and who was always responsible for having Boswell perform tedious neuropsychological experiments; and 3) a "Neutral Guy," who approached Boswell in a completely neutral fashion. At the end of a week of exposure, Boswell was tested for declarative knowledge of the three persons, of which he had none. However, in a forced-choice paradigm in which he was instructed to "Choose the person you would go to for a reward," Boswell systematically selected the Good Guy over unfamiliar foils and systematically selected against the Bad Guy. Because Boswell's lesions guaranteed that the entorhinal and perirhinal cortices, hippocampus, amygdala, and higher-order neocortices in the anterior temporal region are not required to support this form of covert learning and retrieval, we suggested that such learning might depend on neural circuits involving the basal ganglia, including the caudate nucleus.

THALAMUS

Disturbances of speech and language have been linked to damage in the dominant thalamus (e.g., Mohr et al. 1975; for review, see Radanovic and Scaff 2003). The language disorder tends to be primarily a deficit at the semantic level, with prominent word-finding impairment, defective confrontation naming, and semantic paraphasias. This pattern has some resemblances to the transcortical aphasias, and it has been linked in particular to damage in anterior thalamic nuclei (e.g., Graff-Radford and Damasio 1984; Graff-Radford et al. 1985).

Another well-studied neuropsychological correlate of thalamic lesions is memory impairment. In the setting of chronic alcoholism and the development of Korsakoff's syndrome, such lesions typically involve the dorsomedial nucleus of the thalamus along with other diencephalic structures such as the mammillary bodies. The amnesic profile associated with such lesions has been extensively investigated (Butters 1984; Butters and Stuss 1989; Victor et al. 1989). In general, such patients develop a severe anterograde amnesia that covers all forms of declarative knowledge. However, similar to patients such as HM and Boswell, nondeclarative learning, such as the acquisition of new perceptuomotor skills, is spared. A distinctive feature of Korsakoff's syndrome patients is their tendency to confabulate when asked direct questions about recent memory (Victor et al. 1989). Neuroimaging findings have been variable, ranging from general cortical atrophy to atrophy in diencephalic and frontal regions (Kopelman 2002).

Individuals with diencephalic amnesia generally show some defect in the retrograde compartment. The impairment typically shows a temporal gradient, so that recall and recognition improve steadily with increasing distance between the present and the time of initial learning. Remote memories are retrieved more successfully (e.g., Cohen and Squire 1981). Also relatively common in pa-

tients with diencephalic amnesia is a disturbance of problem solving, along with other characteristics reminiscent of frontal lobe defects (Butters and Stuss 1989).

Thalamic lesions occurring as a consequence of stroke can also produce significant amnesia (Graff-Radford et al. 1985). Observations have indicated that the memory impairment is most severe when the lesions are anterior and bilateral (Graff-Radford et al. 1990b). Such lesions, which may interfere with hippocampus-related neural systems such as the mammillothalamic tract and with amygdala-related systems such as the ventroamygdalofugal pathway, produce an amnesic profile characterized by severe anterograde amnesia that spares nondeclarative learning and a retrograde defect that is temporally graded. Posterior thalamic lesions, even when bilateral, were not associated with significant or lasting amnesia (Graff-Radford et al. 1990b).

The diencephalon gives rise to several important neurochemical systems that innervate widespread regions of cerebral cortex. Thus, structures such as the mammillary bodies and certain thalamic nuclei may provide to the cortex important neurotransmitters that are needed for normal memory function. It follows that damage to the diencephalon may not only disrupt important neuroanatomical connections between limbic regions (including the hippocampal complex) and the neocortex but also interfere with memory-related neurochemical influences on the cortex.

CONCLUSION

Understanding the principal neuropsychological correlates of variously placed cerebral lesions is of obvious importance for the accurate diagnosis and effective management of patients who experience brain injury. Another consideration, of no less importance, is the relevance of such understanding for the development of theoretical formulations regarding brain-behavior relations (e.g., A. R. Damasio 1989b). As our understanding advances, it becomes increasingly important to appreciate the significance of both sides of the brain-behavior equation.

We have focused here on the neuropsychological manifestations of focal brain damage and have not considered at any length various psychiatric features that are taken up elsewhere in this textbook. It should be mentioned that there are close interrelations between cognitive and psychiatric disabilities in patients with brain injuries. A patient who has had a stroke, for example, may be as handicapped by severe depression as by aphasia, perhaps even more so (e.g., Robinson et al. 1988). Psychiatric manifestations in patients with head injury are common and may constitute the major source of morbidity (see reviews in Rizzo and Tranel 1996). Understanding the types of cognitive defects that commonly arise in connection with damage to particular brain areas can facilitate the diagnosis and management of psychiatric manifestations and help avoid situations in which patients are mistakenly or carelessly labeled as "functional" or "organic."

Highlights for the Clinician

Neuropsychological manifestations of brain lesions			
Structures and major subdivisions	**Hemispheric side of lesion**		
	Left	Right	Bilateral
Temporal lobes			
Mesial	Anterograde amnesia for verbal material	Anterograde amnesia for nonverbal material	Severe anterograde amnesia for verbal and nonverbal material
Temporal pole	Impaired retrieval of proper nouns	Impaired retrieval of concepts for unique entities Impaired memory for episodic and declarative knowledge	Impaired retrieval of concepts and names for unique entities Impaired episodic memory
Inferotemporal	Impaired retrieval of common nouns	Impaired retrieval of concepts for some nonunique entities	Impaired retrieval of concepts and names for some nonunique entities
Occipito-temporal junction	"Deep" prosopagnosia Impaired retrieval of concepts for some nonunique entities	Transient or mild prosopagnosia Impaired retrieval of concepts for some nonunique entities	Severe, permanent prosopagnosia Visual object agnosia
Occipital lobes			
Dorsal	Partial or mild Balint's syndrome	Partial or mild Balint's syndrome	Balint's syndrome (visual disorientation, ocular apraxia, optic ataxia) Defective motion perception Astereopsis
Ventral	Right hemiachromatopsia "Pure" alexia Impaired mental imagery	Left hemiachromatopsia Apperceptive visual agnosia Defective facial imagery	Full-field achromatopsia Visual object agnosia Impaired mental imagery Prosopagnosia
Parietal lobes			
Temporoparietal junction	Wernicke's aphasia	Amusia Defective music recognition "Phonagnosia"	Auditory agnosia
Inferior parietal lobule	Conduction aphasia Tactile object agnosia Acalculia	Neglect Anosognosia Anosodiaphoria Tactile object agnosia	Body schema disturbances Anosognosia Anosodiaphoria

(continued)

Highlights for the Clinician (continued)

Neuropsychological manifestations of brain lesions			
Structures and major subdivisions	**Hemispheric side of lesion**		
	Left	Right	Bilateral
Frontal lobes			
Frontal operculum	Broca's aphasia Defective retrieval of words for actions (verbs)	"Expressive" aprosody	Broca's aphasia Defective retrieval of words for actions (verbs)
Superior mesial region	Akinetic mutism	Akinetic mutism	Severe akinetic mutism
Basal forebrain (inferior mesial region)	Anterograde and retrograde amnesia with confabulation (worse for verbal stimuli)	Anterograde and retrograde amnesia with confabulation (worse for nonverbal stimuli)	Anterograde and retrograde amnesia with confabulation for verbal and nonverbal stimuli
Orbital (inferior mesial region)	Defective social conduct "Acquired" sociopathy Prospective memory defects	Defective social conduct "Acquired" sociopathy Prospective memory defects	Defective social conduct "Acquired" sociopathy Prospective memory defects
Dorsolateral prefrontal region	Impaired working memory for verbal material Impaired verbal intellect Defective recency and frequency judgments for verbal material Defective verbal fluency Impaired "executive functions"	Impaired working memory for nonverbal spatial material Impaired nonverbal intellect Defective recency and frequency judgments for nonverbal material Defective design fluency Impaired "executive functions"	Impaired working memory for verbal and nonverbal spatial material Impaired verbal and nonverbal intellect Defective recency and frequency judgments for verbal and nonverbal material Defective verbal and design fluency Impaired "executive functions"
Subcortical structures			
Basal ganglia	Atypical aphasia Dysarthria Aprosody Impaired nondeclarative memory Defective motor skill learning	Dysarthria Aprosody Impaired nondeclarative memory Defective motor skill learning	Atypical aphasia Dysarthria Aprosody Impaired nondeclarative memory Defective motor skill learning
Thalamus	Thalamic aphasia Anterograde amnesia with confabulation Retrograde amnesia with temporal gradient Impairments in "executive functions" Attention or concentration defects	Anterograde amnesia with confabulation Retrograde amnesia with temporal gradient Impairments in "executive functions" Attention or concentration defects	Thalamic aphasia Anterograde amnesia with confabulation Retrograde amnesia with temporal gradient Impairments in "executive functions" Attention or concentration defects

RECOMMENDED READINGS

Damasio H: Human Brain Anatomy in Computerized Images, 2nd Edition. New York, Oxford University Press, 2005

Feinberg TE, Farah MJ (eds): Behavioral Neurology and Neuropsychology, 2nd Edition. New York, McGraw-Hill, 2003

Heilman KM, Valenstein E (eds): Clinical Neuropsychology, 4th Edition. New York, Oxford University Press, 2003

Kopelman MD: Disorders of memory. Brain 125:2152–2190, 2002

Mesulam MM (ed): Principles of Behavioral Neurology. Philadelphia, PA, FA Davis, 1985

Rizzo M, Eslinger PJ (eds): Principles and Practice of Behavioral Neurology and Neuropsychology. Philadelphia, PA, Elsevier, 2004

Squire LR, Stark CEL, Clark RE: The medial temporal lobe. Annu Rev Neurosci 27:279–306, 2004

Tranel D: The Iowa-Benton school of neuropsychological assessment, in Neuropsychological Assessment of Neuropsychiatric Disorders, 2nd Edition. Edited by Grant I, Adams KM. New York, Oxford University Press, 1996, pp 81–101

REFERENCES

Ackerly SS, Benton AL: Report of a case of bilateral frontal lobe defect. Research Publications—Association for Research in Nervous and Mental Disease 27:479–504, 1948

Adair JC, Schwartz RL, Barrett AM: Anosognosia, in Clinical Neuropsychology, 4th Edition. Edited by Heilman KM, Valenstein E. New York, Oxford University Press, 2003, pp 185–214

Adolphs R: Is the human amygdala specialized for processing social information? Ann N Y Acad Sci 985:326–340, 2003

Adolphs R, Tranel D: The amygdala and processing of facial emotional expressions, in The Amygdala, 2nd Edition. Edited by Aggleton J. New York, Wiley-Liss, 2000, pp 587–630

Adolphs R, Tranel D, Denburg N: Impaired emotional declarative memory following unilateral amygdala damage. Learn Mem 7:180–186, 2000

Adolphs R, Damasio H, Tranel D: Neural systems for recognition of emotional prosody: a 3-D lesions study. Emotion 2:23–51, 2002

Adolphs R, Tranel D, Damasio AR: Dissociable neural systems for recognizing emotions. Brain Cogn 52:61–69, 2003

Adolphs R, Gosselin F, Buchanan TW, et al: A mechanism for impaired fear recognition after amygdala damage. Nature 433:68–72, 2005a

Adolphs R, Tranel D, Buchanan TW: Amygdala damage impairs emotional memory for gist but not details of complex stimuli. Nat Neurosci 8:512–518, 2005b

Aguirre GK: Functional imaging in behavioral neurology and neuropsychology, in Behavioral Neurology and Neuropsychology, 2nd Edition. Edited by Feinberg TE, Farah MJ. New York, McGraw-Hill, 2003, pp 85–96

Alexander MP: Clinical-anatomical correlations of aphasia following predominantly subcortical lesions, in Handbook of Neuropsychology, Vol 2. Edited by Boller F, Grafman J. Amsterdam, Elsevier, 1989, pp 47–66

Alivisatos B, Milner B: Effects of frontal or temporal lobectomy on the use of advance information in a choice reaction time task. Neuropsychologia 27:495–503, 1989

Anderson SW, Tranel D: Awareness of disease states following cerebral infarction, dementia, and head trauma: standardized assessment. Clin Neuropsychol 3:327–339, 1989

Anderson SW, Damasio H, Jones RD, et al: Wisconsin Card Sorting Test performance as a measure of frontal lobe damage. J Clin Exp Neuropsychol 13:909–922, 1991

Arvanitakis Z, Graff-Radford ZR: The corpus callosum and callosal disconnection syndromes: a model for understanding brain connectivity, asymmetry, and function, in Principles and Practice of Behavioral Neurology and Neuropsychology. Edited by Rizzo M, Eslinger PJ. Philadelphia, PA, Elsevier, 2004, pp 423–433

Babinski J: Contribution a l'etude des troubles mentaux dans l'hemiplegie organique cerebrale (agnosognosie). Rev Neurol 27:845–847, 1914

Baddeley AD: Working memory. Science 255:566–569, 1992

Bar-On R, Tranel D, Denburg N, et al: Exploring the neurological substrate of emotional and social intelligence. Brain 126:1790–1800, 2003

Barrash J, Damasio H, Adolphs R, et al: The neuroanatomical correlates of route learning impairment. Neuropsychologia 38:820–836, 2000a

Barrash J, Tranel D, Anderson SW: Acquired personality changes associated with bilateral damage to the ventromedial prefrontal region. Dev Neuropsychol 18:355–381, 2000b

Bartels A, Zeki S: The architecture of the colour centre in the human visual brain: new results and a review. Eur J Neurosci 12:172–193, 2000

Barton JJS: Disorders of face perception and recognition. Neurol Clin N Am 21:521–548, 2003

Bauer RM: Autonomic recognition of names and faces in prosopagnosia: a neurophysiological application of the Guilty Knowledge Test. Neuropsychologia 22:457–469, 1984

Bauer RM, Demery JA: Agnosia, in Clinical Neuropsychology, 4th Edition. Edited by Heilman KM, Valenstein E. New York, Oxford University Press, 2003, pp 236–295

Beauvois MF, Saillant B: Optic aphasia for colours and colour agnosia: a distinction between visual and visuo-verbal impairments in the processing of colours. Cognitive Neuropsychology 2:1–48, 1985

Bechara A: The role of emotion in decision-making: evidence from neurological patients with orbitofrontal damage. Brain Cogn 55:30–40, 2004

Bechara A, Damasio AR, Damasio H, et al: Insensitivity to future consequences following damage to prefrontal cortex. Cognition 50:7–12, 1994

Bechara A, Tranel D, Damasio H, et al: Double dissociation of conditioning and declarative knowledge relative to the amygdala and hippocampus in humans. Science 269:1115–1118, 1995

Bechara A, Tranel D, Damasio H, et al: Failure to respond autonomically to anticipated future outcomes following damage to prefrontal cortex. Cereb Cortex 6:215–225, 1996

Bechara A, Damasio H, Tranel D, et al: Dissociation of working memory from decision making within the human prefrontal cortex. J Neurosci 18:428–437, 1998

Bechara A, Damasio H, Damasio AR: Role of the amygdale in decision-making. Ann N Y Acad Sci 985:356–369, 2003

Bellugi U, Poizner H, Klima E: Language, modality and the brain, in Brain Development and Cognition. Edited by Johnson MH. Cambridge, MA, Blackwell Publishers, 1989, pp 403–423

Benson DF, Geschwind N: Aphasia and related disorders: a clinical approach, in Principles of Behavioral Neurology. Edited by Mesulam MM. Philadelphia, PA, FA Davis, 1985, pp 193–238

Benson DF, Brown J, Tomlinson EB: Varieties of alexia. Neurology 21:951–957, 1971

Benton AL: Differential behavioral effects in frontal lobe disease. Neuropsychologia 6:53–60, 1968

Benton AL: Visuoperceptual, visuospatial, and visuoconstructive disorders, in Clinical Neuropsychology, 2nd Edition. Edited by Heilman KM, Valenstein E. New York, Oxford University Press, 1985, pp 151–186

Benton AL: Neuropsychology: past, present, and future, in Handbook of Neuropsychology, Vol 1. Edited by Boller F, Grafman J. Amsterdam, Elsevier, 1988, pp 1–27

Benton AL: Facial recognition 1990. Cortex 26:491–499, 1990

Benton AL: The Hecaen-Zangwill legacy: hemispheric dominance examined. Neuropsychol Rev 2:267–280, 1991

Benton AL: Neuropsychological assessment. Annu Rev Psychol 45:1–23, 1994

Benton AL, Tranel D: Visuoperceptual, visuospatial, and visuoconstructional disorders, in Clinical Neuropsychology, 3rd Edition. Edited by Heilman KM, Valenstein E. New York, Oxford University Press, 1993, pp 165–214

Bisiach E, Luzzatti C: Unilateral neglect of representation space. Cortex 14:129–133, 1978

Blair RJR, Cipolotti L: Impaired social response reversal: a case of "acquired sociopathy." Brain 123:1122–1141, 2000

Blumer D, Benson DF: Personality changes with frontal and temporal lobe lesions, in Psychiatric Aspects of Neurologic Disease. Edited by Benson DF, Blumer D. New York, Grune & Stratton, 1975, pp 151–169

Boller F, Spinnler H (eds): The frontal lobes, in Handbook of Neuropsychology, Vol 9. Edited by Boller F, Grafman J. Amsterdam, Elsevier, 1994, pp 3–255

Brickner RM: An interpretation of frontal lobe function based upon the study of a case of partial bilateral frontal lobectomy. Research Publications—Association for Research in Nervous and Mental Disease 13:259–351, 1934

Brickner RM: The Intellectual Functions of the Frontal Lobes: Study Based Upon Observation of a Man After Partial Bilateral Frontal Lobectomy. New York, Macmillan, 1936

Broca P: Localisation des fonctions cerebrales: siege du langage articule. Bulletin for the Society of Anthropology 4:200–204, 1863

Broca P: Sur la faculte du langage articule. Bulletin for the Society of Anthropology 6:337–393, 1865

Bruyer R, Laterre C, Seron X, et al: A case of prosopagnosia with some preserved covert remembrance of familiar faces. Brain Cogn 2:257–284, 1983

Burke DM, MacKay DG, Worthley JS, et al: On the tip of the tongue: what causes word finding failures in young and older adults? J Mem Lang 30:542–579, 1991

Burns M: Clinical management of agnosia. Top Stroke Rehabil 11:1–9, 2004

Butters N: Alcoholic Korsakoff's syndrome: an update. Semin Neurol 4:226–244, 1984

Butters N, Stuss DT: Diencephalic amnesia, in Handbook of Neuropsychology, Vol 3. Edited by Boller F, Grafman J. Amsterdam, Elsevier, 1989, pp 107–148

Butterworth B: What Counts: How Every Brain Is Hardwired for Math. New York, Free Press, 1999

Cabeza R, Nyberg L: Imaging cognition II: an empirical review of 275 PET and fMRI studies. J Cogn Neurosci 12:1–47, 2000

Cahill L, Babinsky R, Markowitsch HJ, et al: The amygdala and emotional memory. Nature 377:295–296, 1995

Cahill L, Haier RJ, Fallon J, et al: Amygdala activity at encoding correlated with long-term, free recall of emotional information. Proc Natl Acad Sci U S A 93:8016–8021, 1996

Caplan D: Aphasic syndromes, in Clinical Neuropsychology, 4th Edition. Edited by Heilman KM, Valenstein E. New York, Oxford University Press, 2003, pp 14–34

Cappa SF, Cavalotti G, Guidotti M, et al: Subcortical aphasia: two clinical-CT scan correlation studies. Cortex 19:227–241, 1983

Caramazza A: The organization of conceptual knowledge in the brain, in The New Cognitive Neurosciences, 2nd Edition. Edited by Gazzaniga MS. Cambridge, MA, MIT Press, 2000, pp 1037–1046

Caselli RJ: Rediscovering tactile agnosia. Mayo Clin Proc 66:129–241, 1991

Caselli RJ: Ventrolateral and dorsomedial somatosensory association cortex damage produces distinct somesthetic syndromes in humans. Neurology 43:762–771, 1993

Cato MA, Delis DC, Abildskov TJ, et al: Assessing the elusive cognitive deficits associated with ventromedial prefrontal damage: a case of modern-day Phineas Gage. J Int Neuropsychol Soc 10:453–465, 2004

Cermak LS, O'Connor M: The anterograde and retrograde retrieval ability of a patient with amnesia due to encephalitis. Neuropsychologia 21:213–234, 1983

Chao LL, Martin A: Cortical regions associated with perceiving, naming, and knowing about colors. J Cogn Neurosci 11:25–35, 1999

Clark VP, Parasuraman R, Keil K, et al: Selective attention to face identity and color studied with fMRI. Hum Brain Mapp 5:293–297, 1997

Cohen NJ, Eichenbaum H: Memory, Amnesia, and the Hippocampal System. Cambridge, MA, MIT Press, 1993

Cohen NJ, Squire LR: Retrograde amnesia and remote memory impairment. Neuropsychologia 19:337–356, 1981

Cohen NJ, Ryan J, Hunt C, et al: Hippocampal system and declarative (relational) memory: summarizing the data from functional neuroimaging studies. Hippocampus 9:83–98, 1999

Corbetta M, Miezin FM, Dobmeyer S, et al: Attentional modulation of neural processing of shape, color, and velocity in humans. Science 248:1556–1559, 1990

Corkin S: Tactually guided maze learning in man: effects of unilateral cortical excisions and bilateral hippocampal lesions. Neuropsychologia 3:339–351, 1965

Corkin S: Acquisition of motor skill after bilateral medial temporal-lobe excision. Neuropsychologia 6:255–264, 1968

Corkin S: Lasting consequences of bilateral medial temporal lobectomy: clinical course and experimental findings in HM. Semin Neurol 4:249–259, 1984

Corkin S: What's new with the amnesic patient HM? Nat Rev 3:153–160, 2002

Corkin S, Amaral DG, Johnson KA, et al: HM's MRI scan shows sparing of the posterior half of the hippocampus and parahippocampal gyrus. J Neurosci 17:3964–3979, 1997

Damasio AR: Disorders of complex visual processing: agnosias, achromatopsia, Balint's syndrome, and related difficulties of orientation and construction, in Principles of Behavioral Neurology. Edited by Mesulam M-M. Philadelphia, PA, FA Davis, 1985, pp 259–288

Damasio AR: The brain binds entities and events by multiregional activation from convergence zones. Neural Comput 1:123–132, 1989a

Damasio AR: Time-locked multiregional retroactivation: a systems-level proposal for the neural substrates of recall and recognition. Cognition 33:25–62, 1989b

Damasio AR: Descartes' Error: Emotion, Reason, and the Human Brain. New York, Grossett/Putnam, 1994

Damasio AR: Toward a neurobiology of emotion and feeling: operational concepts and hypotheses. The Neuroscientist 1:19–25, 1995

Damasio AR, Anderson SW: The frontal lobes, in Clinical Neuropsychology, 4th Edition. Edited by Heilman KM, Valenstein E. New York, Oxford University Press, 2003, pp 404–446

Damasio AR, Benton AL: Impairment of hand movements under visual guidance. Neurology 29:170–174, 1979

Damasio AR, Damasio H: The anatomic basis of pure alexia. Neurology 33:1573–1583, 1983

Damasio AR, Damasio H: Cortical systems underlying knowledge retrieval: evidence from human lesion studies, in Exploring Brain Functions: Models in Neuroscience. Edited by Poggio TA, Glaser DA. New York, Wiley, 1993, pp 233–248

Damasio AR, Damasio H: Cortical systems for retrieval of concrete knowledge: the convergence zone framework, in Large-Scale Neuronal Theories of the Brain. Edited by Koch C. Cambridge, MA, MIT Press, 1994, pp 61–74

Damasio AR, Tranel D: Nouns and verbs are retrieved with differently distributed neural systems. Proc Natl Acad Sci U S A 90:4957–4960, 1993

Damasio AR, Van Hoesen GW: Emotional disturbances associated with focal lesions of the limbic frontal lobe, in Neuropsychology of Human Emotion. Edited by Heilman KM, Satz P. New York, Guilford, 1983, pp 85–110

Damasio AR, Yamada T, Damasio H, et al: Central achromatopsia: behavioral, anatomical and physiologic aspects. Neurology 30:1064–1071, 1980

Damasio AR, Damasio H, Rizzo M, et al: Aphasia with lesions in the basal ganglia and internal capsule. Arch Neurol 39:15–20, 1982a

Damasio AR, Damasio H, Van Hoesen GW: Prosopagnosia: anatomic basis and behavioral mechanisms. Neurology 32:331–341, 1982b

Damasio AR, Eslinger P, Damasio H, et al: Multimodal amnesic syndrome following bilateral temporal and basal forebrain damage. Arch Neurol 42:252–259, 1985a

Damasio AR, Graff-Radford NR, Eslinger PG, et al: Amnesia following basal forebrain lesions. Arch Neurol 42:263–271, 1985b

Damasio AR, Tranel D, Damasio H: "Deep" prosopagnosia: a new form of acquired face recognition defect caused by left hemisphere damage. Neurology 38 (suppl 1):172, 1988

Damasio AR, Tranel D, Damasio H: Amnesia caused by herpes simplex encephalitis, infarctions in basal forebrain, Alzheimer's disease, and anoxia, in Handbook of Neuropsychology, Vol 3. Edited by Boller F, Grafman J. Amsterdam, Elsevier, 1989a, pp 149–166

Damasio AR, Tranel D, Damasio H: Disorders of visual recognition, in Handbook of Neuropsychology, Vol 2. Edited by Boller F, Grafman J. Amsterdam, Elsevier, 1989b, pp 317–332

Damasio AR, Damasio H, Tranel D, et al: Neural regionalization of knowledge access: preliminary evidence. Cold Spring Harb Symp Quant Biol 55:1039–1047, 1990a

Damasio AR, Tranel D, Damasio H: Face agnosia and the neural substrates of memory. Annu Rev Neurosci 13:89–109, 1990b

Damasio AR, Tranel D, Damasio H: Individuals with sociopathic behavior caused by frontal damage fail to respond autonomically to social stimuli. Behav Brain Res 41:81–94, 1990c

Damasio AR, Tranel D, Damasio H: Music and the Brain. Miami, FL, American Academy of Neurology, 1990d

Damasio AR, Tranel D, Damasio H: Somatic markers and the guidance of behavior: theory and preliminary testing, in Frontal Lobe Function and Dysfunction. Edited by Levin HS, Eisenberg HM, Benton AL. New York, Oxford University Press, 1991, pp 217–229

Damasio AR, Tranel D, Rizzo M: Disorders of complex visual processing, in Principles of Behavioral and Cognitive Neurology, 2nd Edition. Edited by Mesulam MM. New York, Oxford University Press, 2000, pp 332–372

Damasio H: Neuroimaging contributions to the understanding of aphasia, in Handbook of Neuropsychology, Vol 2. Edited by Boller F, Grafman J. Amsterdam, Elsevier, 1989, pp 3–46

Damasio H: Human Brain Anatomy in Computerized Images. New York, Oxford University Press, 1995

Damasio H: Neuroanatomical correlates of the aphasias, in Acquired Aphasia, 3rd Edition. Edited by Sarno MT. New York, Academic Press, 1998, pp 43–70

Damasio H: Human Brain Anatomy in Computerized Images, 2nd Edition. New York, Oxford University Press, 2005

Damasio H, Damasio AR: The anatomical basis of conduction aphasia. Brain 103:337–350, 1980

Damasio H, Damasio AR: The lesion method in behavioral neurology and neuropsychology, in Behavioral Neurology and Neuropsychology, 2nd Edition. Edited by Feinberg TE, Farah MJ. New York, McGraw-Hill, 2003, pp 71–84

Damasio H, Frank RJ: Three-dimensional in vivo mapping of brain lesions in humans. Arch Neurol 49:137–143, 1992

Damasio H, Eslinger P, Adams HP: Aphasia following basal ganglia lesions: new evidence. Semin Neurol 4:151–161, 1984

Damasio H, Grabowski TJ, Tranel D, et al: A neural basis for lexical retrieval. Nature 380:499–505, 1996

Damasio H, Tranel D, Grabowski T, et al: Neural systems behind word and concept retrieval. Cognition 92:179–229, 2004

Daniele A, Giustolisi L, Silveri MC, et al: Evidence for a possible neuroanatomical basis for lexical processing of nouns and verbs. Neuropsychologia 32:1325–1341, 1994

Davidoff JB, De Bleser R: Impaired picture recognition with preserved object naming and reading. Brain Cogn 24:1–23, 1994

Davidoff J, Landis T: Recognition of unfamiliar faces in prosopagnosia. Neuropsychologia 28:1143–1161, 1990

Denburg NL, Tranel D: Body schema and acalculia, in Clinical Neuropsychology, 4th Edition. Edited by Heilman KM, Valenstein E. New York, Oxford University Press, 2003, pp 161–184

Denburg NL, Jones RD, Adolphs R, et al: Recognition without awareness in a patient with simultanagnosia. J Int Neuropsychol Soc 6:115, 2000

Deouell LY, Ivry RB, Knight RT: Electrophysiologic methods and transcranial magnetic stimulation in behavioral neurology and neuropsychology, in Behavioral Neurology and Neuropsychology, 2nd Edition. Edited by Feinberg TE, Farah MJ. New York, McGraw-Hill, 2003, pp 105–134

De Renzi E: Prosopagnosia in two patients with CT scan evidence of damage confined to the right hemisphere. Neuropsychologia 24:385–389, 1986

De Renzi E, Lucchelli F: Dense retrograde amnesia, intact learning capability and abnormal forgetting rate: a consolidation deficit? Cortex 29:449–466, 1993

De Renzi E, Perani F, Carlesimo GA, et al: Prosopagnosia can be associated with damage confined to the right hemisphere: an MRI and PET study and a review of the literature. Neuropsychologia 32:893–902, 1994

Eichenbaum H, Cohen NJ: From Conditioning to Conscious Recollection: Memory Systems of the Brain. New York, Oxford University Press, 2001

Eslinger PJ, Damasio AR: Severe disturbance of higher cognition after bilateral frontal lobe ablation: patient EVR. Neurology 35:1731–1741, 1985

Eslinger PJ, Damasio AR: Preserved motor learning in Alzheimer's disease: implications for anatomy and behavior. J Neurosci 6:3006–3009, 1986

Etard O, Mellet E, Papathanassiou D, et al: Picture naming without Broca's and Wernicke's area. Neuroreport 11:617–622, 2000

Fabiani M, Gratton G, Coles MGH: Event-related brain potentials: methods, theory, and applications, in Handbook of Psychophysiology, 2nd Edition. Edited by Cacioppo JT, Tassinary LG, Berntson CG. Cambridge, UK, Cambridge University Press, 2000, pp 53–84

Farah MJ: The neuropsychology of mental imagery, in Handbook of Neuropsychology, Vol 2. Edited by Boller F, Grafman J. Amsterdam, Elsevier, 1989, pp 395–413

Farah MJ: Disorders of visual-spatial perception and cognition, in Clinical Neuropsychology, 4th Edition. Edited by Heilman KM, Valenstein E. New York, Oxford University Press, 2003, pp 146–160

Feinberg TE, Farah MJ: The development of modern behavioral neurology and neuropsychology, in Behavioral Neurology and Neuropsychology, 2nd Edition. Edited by Feinberg TE, Farah MJ. New York, McGraw-Hill, 2003, pp 3–23

Fiez JA, Petersen SE, Cheney MK, et al: Impaired non-motor learning and error detection associated with cerebellar damage. Brain 115:155–178, 1992

Forde EME, Humphreys GW: Category-specific recognition impairments: a review of important case studies and influential theories. Aphasiology 13:169–193, 1999

Frank RJ, Damasio H, Grabowski TJ: Brainvox: an interactive, multimodal, visualization and analysis system for neuroanatomical imaging. Neuroimage 5:13–30, 1997

Frisk V, Milner B: The relationship of working memory to the immediate recall of stories following unilateral temporal or frontal lobectomy. Neuropsychologia 28:121–135, 1990

Fuster JM: The Prefrontal Cortex: Anatomy, Physiology, and Neuropsychology of the Frontal Lobes. New York, Raven, 1989

Gabrieli JDE, Cohen NJ, Corkin S: The impaired learning of semantic knowledge following bilateral medial temporal-lobe resection. Brain Cogn 7:157–177, 1988

Gabrieli JDE, Corkin S, Mickel SF, et al: Intact acquisition and long-term retention of mirror-tracing skill in Alzheimer's disease and in global amnesia. Behav Neurosci 107:899–910, 1993

Gainotti G: What the locus of brain lesion tells us about the nature of the cognitive defect underlying category-specific disorders: a review. Cortex 36:539–559, 2000

Gainotti G, Silveri MC, Daniele A, et al: Neuroanatomical correlates of category-specific semantic disorders: a critical survey. Memory 3:247–264, 1995

Gainotti G, Barbier A, Marra C: Slowly progressive defect in recognition of familiar people in a patient with right anterior temporal atrophy. Brain 126:792–803, 2003

Gao J-H, Parsons LM, Bower JM, et al: Cerebellum implicated in sensory acquisition and discrimination rather than motor control. Science 272:545–547, 1996

Gazzaniga MS: Perceptual and attentional processes following callosal section in human. Neuropsychologia 25:119–133, 1987

Gazzaniga MS: Cerebral specialization and interhemispheric communication: does the corpus callosum enable the human condition? Brain 123:1293–1326, 2000

Geschwind N: Disconnexion syndromes in animals and man. Brain 88:237–294, 585–644, 1965

Giovanello KS, Schnyer DM, Verfaellie M: A critical role for the anterior hippocampus in relational memory: evidence from an fMRI study comparing associative and item recognition. Hippocampus 14:5–8, 2004

Goldman-Rakic PS: Circuitry of primate prefrontal cortex and regulation of behavior by representational memory, in Handbook of Physiology: The Nervous System. Edited by Plum F. Bethesda, MD, American Physiological Society, 1987, pp 373–417

Goodglass H, Wingfield A, Hyde MR, et al: Category specific dissociations in naming and recognition by aphasic patients. Cortex 22:87–102, 1986

Goodglass H, Christiansen JA, Gallagher RE: Syntactic constructions used by agrammatic speakers: comparison with conduction aphasics and normals. Neuropsychology 8:598–613, 1994

Gorno-Tempini M-L, Cipolotti L, Price CJ: Category differences in brain activation studies: where do they come from? Proc R Soc Lond B 267:1253–1258, 2000

Grabowski TJ, Damasio H, Frank RJ, et al: Neuroanatomical analysis of functional brain images: validation with retinotopic mapping. Hum Brain Mapp 2:134–148, 1995

Grabowski TJ, Damasio H, Tranel D: Physiologic correlates of retrieving names for unique entities. Neurology 54 (suppl 3):A397–A398, 2000a

Grabowski TJ, Damasio H, Tranel D: Retrieving names of unique entities engages the left temporal pole. Neuroimage 11:S262, 2000b

Grabowski TJ, Damasio H, Tranel D, et al: A role for left temporal pole in the retrieval of words for unique entities. Hum Brain Mapp 13:199–212, 2001

Grabowski TJ, Damasio H, Tranel D, et al: Residual naming after damage to the left temporal pole: a PET activation study. Neuroimage 19:846–860, 2003b

Graff-Radford NR, Damasio H: Disturbances of speech and language associated with thalamic dysfunction. Semin Neurol 4:162–168, 1984

Graff-Radford NR, Damasio H, Yamada T, et al: Nonhemorrhagic thalamic infarctions: clinical, neurophysiological and electrophysiological findings in four anatomical groups defined by CT. Brain 108:485–516, 1985

Graff-Radford NR, Damasio AR, Hyman BT, et al: Progressive aphasia in a patient with Pick's disease: a neuropsychological, radiologic, and anatomic study. Neurology 40:620–626, 1990a

Graff-Radford NR, Tranel D, Van Hoesen GW, et al: Diencephalic amnesia. Brain 113:1–25, 1990b

Grafman J, Litvan I, Massaquoi S, et al: Cognitive planning deficit in patients with cerebellar atrophy. Neurology 42:1493–1496, 1992

Greenblatt SH: Alexia without agraphia or hemianopia: anatomical analysis of an autopsied case. Brain 96:307–316, 1973

Greenblatt SH: Localization of lesions in alexia, in Localization in Neuropsychology. Edited by Kertesz A. New York, Academic Press, 1983, pp 323–356

Hallett M: Transcranial magnetic stimulation and the human brain. Nature 406:147–150, 2000

Hamann SB, Ely TD, Grafton ST, et al: Amygdala activity related to enhanced memory for pleasant and aversive stimuli. Nat Neurosci 2:289–293, 1999

Harlow JM: Recovery from the passage of an iron bar through the head. Publications of the Massachusetts Medical Society 2:327–347, 1868

Hart J, Berndt RS, Caramazza A: Category-specific naming deficit following cerebral infarction. Nature 316:439–440, 1985

Hebb DO, Penfield W: Human behavior after extensive bilateral removals from the frontal lobes. Archives of Neurology and Psychiatry 44:421–438, 1940

Heilman KM, Wilder BJ, Malzone WF: Anomic aphasia following anterior temporal lobectomy. Transactions of the American Neurological Association 97:291–293, 1972

Heilman KM, Watson RT, Valenstein E: Neglect and related disorders, in Clinical Neuropsychology, 4th Edition. Edited by Heilman KM, Valenstein E. New York, Oxford University Press, 2003, pp 296–346

Heindel WC, Salmon DP, Butters N: Cognitive approaches to the memory disorders of demented patients, in Comprehensive Handbook of Psychopathology, 2nd Edition. Edited by Sutker PB, Adams HE. New York, Plenum, 1993, pp 735–761

Herscovitch P: Functional neuroimaging, in Principles and Practice of Behavioral Neurology and Neuropsychology. Edited by Rizzo M, Eslinger PJ. Philadelphia, PA, Elsevier, 2004, pp 115–143

Heywood CA, Kentridge RW: Achromatopsia, color vision, and cortex. Neurol Clin N Am 21:483–500, 2003

Hickok G, Bellugi U, Klima E: The neurobiology of sign language and its implications for the neural basis of language. Nature 381:699–702, 1996

Hillis AE, Caramazza A: Representations of grammatical categories of words in the brain. J Cogn Neurosci 7:396–407, 1995

Hillis AE, Tuffiash E, Caramazza A: Modality-specific deterioration in naming verbs in nonfluent primary progressive aphasia. J Cogn Neurosci 14:1099–1108, 2002a

Hillis AE, Tuffiash E, Wityk RJ, et al: Regions of neural dysfunction associated with impaired naming of actions and objects in acute stroke. Cogn Neuropsychol 19:523–534, 2002b

Hillis AE, Barker PB, Wityk RJ, et al: Variability in subcortical aphasia is due to variable sites of cortical hypoperfusion. Brain Lang 89:524–530, 2004

Horel JA: The neuroanatomy of amnesia: a critique of the hippocampal memory hypothesis. Brain 101:403–445, 1978

Hubel DH, Livingstone MS: Segregation of form, color, and stereopsis in primate area 18. J Neurosci 7:3378–3415, 1987

Humphreys GW, Forde EME: Hierarchies, similarity, and interactivity in object recognition: "category-specific" neuropsychological deficits. Behav Brain Sci 24:453–509, 2001

Hunkin NM, Parkin AJ, Bradley VA, et al: Focal retrograde amnesia following closed head injury: a case study and theoretical account. Neuropsychologia 33:509–523, 1995

Hyman BT, Tranel D: Hemianesthesia and aphasia: an anatomical and behavioral study. Arch Neurol 46:816–819, 1989

Hyman BT, Damasio AR, Van Hoesen GW, et al: Alzheimer's disease: cell specific pathology isolates the hippocampal formation. Science 225:1168–1170, 1984

Hyman BT, Kromer LJ, Van Hoesen GW: A direct demonstration of the perforant pathway terminal zone in Alzheimer's disease using the monoclonal antibody Alz-50. Brain Res 450:392–397, 1988

Jones RD, Tranel D: Visual disorders, in Encyclopedia of the Human Brain, Vol 4. Edited by Ramachandran VS. Amsterdam, Elsevier, 2002, pp 775–789

Jones RD, Grabowski TG, Tranel D: The neural basis of retrograde memory: evidence from positron emission tomography for the role of non-mesial temporal lobe structures. Neurocase 4:471–479, 1998

Jones-Gotman M, Milner B: Design fluency: the invention of nonsense drawings after focal cortical lesions. Neuropsychologia 15:653–674, 1977

Jonides J, Smith EE, Koeppe RA, et al: Spatial working memory in humans as revealed by PET. Nature 363:623–625, 1993

Kanwisher N, Moscovitch M: The cognitive neuroscience of face processing: an introduction. Cognitive Neuropsychology 17:1–11, 2000

Kapur N: Focal retrograde amnesia in neurological disease: a critical review. Cortex 29:217–234, 1993

Kapur N, Ellison D, Parkin AJ, et al: Bilateral temporal lobe pathology with sparing of medial temporal lobe structures: lesion profile and pattern of memory disorder. Neuropsychologia 32:23–38, 1994

Kemmerer D, Tranel D: A double dissociation between the meanings of action verbs and locative prepositions. Neurocase 9:421–435, 2003

Khedr EM, Hamed E, Said A, et al: Handedness and language cerebral lateralization. Eur J Appl Physiol 87:469–473, 2002

Kopelman MD: The neuropsychology of remote memory, in Handbook of Neuropsychology, Vol 8. Edited by Boller F, Grafman J. Amsterdam, Elsevier, 1992, pp 215–238

Kopelman MD: Disorders of memory. Brain 125:2152–2190, 2002

Kopelman MD, Lasserson D, Kingsley D, et al: Structural MRI volumetric analysis in patients with organic amnesia, 2: correlations with anterograde memory and executive tests in 40 patients. J Neurol Neurosurg Psychiatry 71:23–28, 2001

Kosslyn SM: Aspects of a cognitive neuroscience of mental imagery. Science 240:1621–1626, 1988

Kosslyn SM, Koenig O: Wet Mind: The New Cognitive Neuroscience. New York, Free Press, 1995

Kourtzi Z, Kanwisher N: Activation in human MT/MST by static images with implied motion. J Cogn Neurosci 12:48–55, 2000

LaBar KS, Gatenby C, Gore JC, et al: Human amygdale activation during conditioned fear acquisition and extinction: a mixed-trial fMRI study. Neuron 20:937–945, 1998

Landis T, Cummings JL, Christen L, et al: Are unilateral right posterior cerebral lesions sufficient to cause prosopagnosia? Clinical and radiological findings in six additional patients. Cortex 22:243–252, 1986

Lavenex P, Amaral DG: Hippocampal neocortical interaction: a hierarchy of associativity. Hippocampus 10:420–430, 2000

Lee GP, Arena JG, Meador KJ, et al: Changes in autonomic responsiveness following bilateral amygdalotomy in humans. Neuropsychiatry Neuropsychol Behav Neurol 1:119–129, 1988a

Lee GP, Meador KJ, Smith JR, et al: Clinical case report: preserved crossmodal association following bilateral amygdalotomy in man. Int J Neurosci 40:47–55, 1988b

Lee GP, Bechara A, Adolphs R, et al: Clinical and physiological effects of stereotaxic bilateral amygdalotomy for intractable aggression. J Neuropsychiatry Clin Neurosci 10:413–420, 1998

Levin HS, Eisenberg HM, Benton AL (eds): Frontal Lobe Function and Dysfunction. New York, Oxford University Press, 1991

Levy J: Regulation and generation of perception in the asymmetric brain, in Brain Circuits and Functions of the Mind. Edited by Trevarthen C. Cambridge, UK, Cambridge University Press, 1990, pp 231–246

Lezak MD, Howieson DB, Loring DW: Neuropsychological Assessment, 4th Edition. New York, Oxford University Press, 2004

Lissauer H: Ein fall von Seelenblindheit nebst einem Beitrag zur theorie derselben. Archiv für Psychiatrie und Nervenkrankheiten 21:22–70, 1890

Livingstone MS, Hubel DH: Segregation of form, color, movement, and depth: anatomy, physiology, and perception. Science 240:740–749, 1988

Luria AR: Frontal lobe syndromes, in Handbook of Clinical Neurology, Vol 2. Edited by Vinken PG, Bruyn GW. Amsterdam, North Holland, 1969, pp 725–757

Luzzatti C, Davidoff J: Impaired retrieval of object-colour knowledge with preserved colour naming. Neuropsychologia 32:933–950, 1994

Markowitsch HJ, Calabrese P, Haupts M, et al: Searching for the anatomical basis of retrograde amnesia. J Clin Exp Neuropsychol 15:947–967, 1993

Markowitsch HJ, Calabrese P, Wuerker M, et al: The amygdala's contribution to memory: a study on two patients with Urbach-Wiethe disease. Neuroreport 5:1349–1352, 1994

Martin A, Haxby JV, Lalonde FM, et al: Discrete cortical regions associated with knowledge of color and knowledge of action. Science 270:102–105, 1995

Martin A, Ungerleider LG, Haxby JV: Category specificity and the brain: the sensory/motor model of semantic representations of objects, in The New Cognitive Neurosciences, 2nd Edition. Edited by Gazzaniga MS. Cambridge, MA, MIT Press, 2000, pp 1023–1036

McCarthy G: Functional neuroimaging of memory. The Neuroscientist 1:155–163, 1995

McCarthy G, Blamire AM, Puce A, et al: Functional magnetic resonance imaging of human prefrontal cortex activation during a spatial working memory task. Proc Natl Acad Sci U S A 91:8690–8694, 1994

McClelland JL, McNaughton BL, O'Reilly RC: Why are there complementary learning systems in the hippocampus and neocortex: insights from the successes and failures of connectionist models of learning and memory. Psychol Rev 102:419–457, 1995

McCormick DA, Thompson RF: Cerebellum: essential involvement in the classically conditioned eyelid response. Science 223:296–299, 1984

Meadows JC: The anatomical basis of prosopagnosia. J Neurol Neurosurg Psychiatry 37:489–501, 1974a

Meadows JC: Disturbed perception of colors associated with localized cerebral lesions. Brain 97:615–632, 1974b

Mega MS, Cohenour RC: Akinetic mutism: disconnection of frontal-subcortical circuits. Neuropsychiatry Neuropsychol Behav Neurol 10:254–259, 1997

Mesad S, Laff R, Devinsky O: Transient postoperative prosopagnosia. Epilepsy Behav 4:567–570, 2003

Mesulam MM: Frontal cortex and behavior. Ann Neurol 19:320–325, 1986

Miceli G, Silveri MC, Nocentini U, et al: Patterns of dissociation in comprehension and production of nouns and verbs. Aphasiology 2:351–358, 1988

Michel F, Perenin MT, Sieroff E: Prosopagnosie sans hemianopsie apres lesion unilaterale occipito-temporale droite. Revue Neurologique 142:545–549, 1986

Milner B: Effects of different brain lesions on card sorting: the role of the frontal lobes. Arch Neurol 9:90–100, 1963

Milner B: Visual recognition and recall after right temporal-lobe excision in man. Neuropsychologia 6:191–209, 1968

Milner B: Disorders of learning and memory after temporal lobe lesions in man. Clin Neurosurg 19:421–446, 1972

Milner B, Petrides M: Behavioural effects of frontal-lobe lesions in man. Trends Neurosci 7:403–407, 1984

Milner B, Petrides M, Smith ML: Frontal lobes and the temporal organization of memory. Hum Neurobiol 4:137–142, 1985

Miozzo A, Soardi S, Cappa SF: Pure anomia with spared action naming due to a left temporal lesion. Neuropsychologia 32:1101–1109, 1994

Mishkin M: Memory in monkeys severely impaired by combined but not separate removal of amygdala and hippocampus. Nature 273:297–298, 1978

Mohr JP, Watters WC, Duncan GW: Thalamic hemorrhage and aphasia. Brain Lang 2:3–17, 1975

Mohr JP, Pessin MS, Finkelstein S, et al: Broca aphasia: pathologic and clinical aspects. Neurology 28:311–324, 1978

Murray EA: Representational memory in nonhuman primates, in Neurobiology of Comparative Cognition. Edited by Kesner RP, Olton DS. Hillsdale, NJ, Erlbaum, 1990, pp 127–155

Murray EA, Mishkin M: Amygdalectomy impairs crossmodal association in monkeys. Science 228:604–606, 1985

Murray EA, Mishkin M: Visual recognition in monkeys following rhinal cortical ablations combined with either amygdalectomy or hippocampectomy. J Neurosci 6:1991–2003, 1986

Nadel L, Moscovitch M: The hippocampal complex and long-term memory revisited. Trends Cogn Sci 5:228–230, 2001

Nadel L, Samsonovich A, Ryan L, et al: Multiple trace theory of human memory: computational, neuroimaging, and neuropsychological results. Hippocampus 10:352–368, 2000

Naeser MA, Alexander MP, Helm-Estabrooks N, et al: Aphasia with predominantly subcortical lesion sites. Arch Neurol 39:2–14, 1982

Nahm FKD, Tranel D, Damasio H, et al: Cross-modal associations and the human amygdala. Neuropsychologia 31:727–744, 1993

Newcombe F: The processing of visual information in prosopagnosia and acquired dyslexia: functional versus physiological interpretation, in Research in Psychology and Medicine. Edited by Osborne DJ, Bruneberg MM, Eiser JR. London, Academic Press, 1979, pp 315–322

Newcombe F, Ratcliff G: Disorders of visuospatial analysis, in Handbook of Neuropsychology, Vol 2. Edited by Boller F, Grafman J. Amsterdam, Elsevier, 1989, pp 333–356

Nyberg L, McIntosh AR, Houle S, et al: Activation of medial temporal structures during episodic memory retrieval. Nature 380:715–717, 1996

O'Connor M, Verfaellie M: The amnesic syndrome: overview and subtypes, in The Handbook of Memory Disorders. Edited by Baddeley AD, Kopelman MD, Wilson BA. Chichester, UK, Wiley, 2002, pp 145–166

O'Connor M, Butters N, Miliotis P, et al: The dissociation of anterograde and retrograde amnesia in a patient with herpes encephalitis. J Clin Exp Neuropsychol 14:159–178, 1992

Oliveira-Souza R, Moll J, Eslinger PJ: Neuropsychological assessment, in Principles and Practice of Behavioral Neurology and Neuropsychology. Edited by Rizzo M, Eslinger PJ. Philadelphia, PA, Elsevier, 2004, pp 47–64

Packard MG, Knowlton BJ: Learning and memory functions of the basal ganglia. Annu Rev Neurosci 25:563–593, 2002

Paulson HL, Galetta SL, Grossman M, et al: Hemiachromatopsia of unilateral occipitotemporal infarcts. Am J Ophthalmol 118:518–523, 1994

Petrides M: Lateral prefrontal cortex: architectonic and functional organization. Phil Trans R Soc B 360:781–795, 2005

Phelps EA, LaBar K, Anderson AK, et al: Specifying the contributions of the human amygdala to emotional memory: a case study. Neurocase 4:527–540, 1998

Poizner H, Klima ES, Bellugi U: What the Hands Reveal About the Brain. Cambridge, MA, Harvard University Press, 1987

Polich J: Clinical application of the P300 event-related brain potential. Phys Med Rehabil Clin N Am 15:133–161, 2004

Poolos NP: Magnetoencephalography as a noninvasive probe of brain activity: the state of the art. The Neuroscientist 1:127–129, 1995

Posner MI, Petersen SE, Fox PT, et al: Localization of cognitive operations in the human brain. Science 240:1627–1631, 1988

Price CJ, Friston KJ: Functional neuroimaging studies of neuropsychological patients, in Behavioral Neurology and Neuropsychology, 2nd Edition. Edited by Feinberg TE, Farah MJ. New York, McGraw-Hill, 2003, pp 97–104

Radanovic M, Scaff M: Speech and language disturbances due to subcortical lesions. Brain Lang 84:337–352, 2003

Raichle ME: Exploring the mind with dynamic imaging. Seminars in Neurosciences 2:307–315, 1990

Raichle ME: Functional imaging in behavioral neurology and neuropsychology, in Behavioral Neurology and Neuropsychology. Edited by Feinberg TE, Farah MJ. New York, McGraw-Hill, 1997, pp 83–100

Rapcsak SZ, Kaszniak AW, Rubens AB: Anomia for facial expressions: evidence for a category specific visual-verbal disconnection syndrome. Neuropsychologia 27:1031–1041, 1989

Rapcsak SZ, Comer JF, Rubens AB: Anomia for facial expressions: neuropsychological mechanisms and anatomical correlates. Brain Lang 45:233–252, 1993

Reed CL, Caselli RJ: The nature of tactile agnosia: a case study. Neuropsychologia 32:527–539, 1994

Reed JM, Squire LR: Retrograde amnesia for facts and events: findings from four new cases. J Neurosci 18:3943–3954, 1998

Rempel-Clower NL, Zola-Morgan SM, Squire LR, et al: Three cases of enduring memory impairment after bilateral damage limited to the hippocampal formation. J Neurosci 16:5233–5255, 1996

Richardson MP, Strange BA, Dolan RJ: Encoding of emotional memories depends on amygdala and hippocampus and their interactions. Nat Neurosci 7:278–285, 2004

Riddoch MJ, Humphreys GW: Visual agnosia. Neurol Clin N Am 21:501–520, 2003

Rizzo M: Astereopsis, in Handbook of Neuropsychology, Vol 2. Edited by Boller F, Grafman J. Amsterdam, Elsevier, 1989, pp 415–427

Rizzo M: "Balint's syndrome" and associated visuospatial disorders, in Bailliere's International Practice and Research. Edited by Kennard C. London, WB Saunders, 1993, pp 415–437

Rizzo M, Hurtig R: Looking but not seeing: attention, perception, and eye movements in simultanagnosia. Neurology 37:1642–1648, 1987

Rizzo M, Nawrot M: Human visual cortex and its disorders. Curr Opin Ophthalmol 4:38–47, 1993

Rizzo M, Tranel D (eds): Head Injury and Postconcussive Syndrome. New York, Churchill Livingstone, 1996

Rizzo M, Vecera SP: Psychoanatomical substrates of Balint's syndrome. J Neurol Neurosurg Psychiatry 72:162–178, 2002

Rizzo M, Smith V, Pokorny J, et al: Color perception profiles in central achromatopsia. Neurology 43:995–1001, 1993

Roberts TPL, McGonigle DJ: fMRI and related techniques, in Principles and Practice of Behavioral Neurology and Neuropsychology. Edited by Rizzo M, Eslinger PJ. Philadelphia, PA, Elsevier, 2004, pp 145–171

Robertson IH, Marshall JC (eds): Unilateral Neglect: Clinical and Experimental Studies. Hillsdale, NJ, Erlbaum, 1993

Robin DA, Tranel D, Damasio H: Auditory perception of temporal and spectral events in patients with focal left and right cerebral lesions. Brain Lang 39:539–555, 1990

Robinson RG, Boston JD, Starkstein SE, et al: Comparison of mania and depression after brain injury: causal factors. Am J Psychiatry 145:172–178, 1988

Roland PE: Brain Activation. New York, Wiley-Liss, 1993

Rosler F, Heil M, Henninghausen E: Distinct cortical activation patterns during long-term memory retrieval of verbal, spatial, and color information. J Cogn Neurosci 7:51–65, 1995

Ross ED: The aprosodias: functional-anatomic organization of the affective components of language in the right hemisphere. Arch Neurol 38:561–569, 1981

Rubens AB: Transcortical motor aphasia, in Studies in Neurolinguistics, Vol 1. Edited by Whitaker H, Whitaker HA. New York, Academic Press, 1976, pp 293–303

Rugg MD: Functional neuroimaging of memory, in Handbook of Memory Disorders, 2nd Edition. Edited by Baddeley AD, Kopelman MD, Wilson BA. Chichester, UK, Wiley, 2002, pp 57–80

Ryan JD, Cohen NJ: Processing and short-term retention of relational information in amnesia. Neuropsychologia 42:497–511, 2004

Ryan JD, Althoff RR, Whitlow S, et al: Amnesia is a deficit in relational memory. Psychol Sci 11:454–461, 2000

Sagar HJ, Gabrieli JDE, Sullivan EV, et al: Recency and frequency discrimination in the amnesic patient HM. Brain 113:581–602, 1990

Saint-Cyr JA, Taylor AE, Lang AE: Procedural learning and neostriatal dysfunction in man. Brain 111:941–959, 1988

Sakai K, Watanabe E, Onodera Y, et al: Functional mapping of the human colour centre with echo-planar magnetic resonance imaging. Proc R Soc Lond B 261:89–98, 1995

Schiff HB, Alexander MP, Naeser MA, et al: Aphemia: clinic-anatomic correlations. Arch Neurol 40:720–727, 1983

Schmahmann JD: An emerging concept: the cerebellar contribution to higher function. Arch Neurol 48:1178–1187, 1991

Schnider A, Landis T, Regard M, et al: Dissociation of color from object in amnesia. Arch Neurol 49:982–985, 1992

Schnyer DM, Verfaellie M, Alexander MP, et al: A role for right medial prefrontal cortex in accurate feeling-of-knowing judgments: evidence from patients with lesions to frontal cortex. Neuropsychologia 42:957–966, 2004

Scoville WB, Milner B: Loss of recent memory after bilateral hippocampal lesions. J Neurol Neurosurg Psychiatry 20:11–21, 1957

Semenza C, Zettin M: Evidence from aphasia for the role of proper names as pure referring expressions. Nature 342:678–679, 1989

Sergent J, Villemure J-G: Prosopagnosia in a right hemispherectomized patient. Brain 112:975–995, 1989

Silverman DH, Alavi A: PET imaging in the assessment of normal and impaired cognitive function. Radiol Clin North Am 43:67–77, 2005

Smith EE, Jonides J, Koeppe RA, et al: Spatial versus object working memory: PET investigations. J Cogn Neurosci 7:337–356, 1995

Smith EE, Jonides J, Koeppe RA: Dissociating verbal and spatial working memory using PET. Cereb Cortex 6:11–20, 1996

Smith ML, Milner B: Estimation of frequency of occurrence of abstract designs after frontal or temporal lobectomy. Neuropsychologia 26:297–306, 1988

Smith ML, Milner B: Right hippocampal impairment in the recall of spatial location: encoding deficit or rapid forgetting? Neuropsychologia 27:71–81, 1989

Sperry RW: The great cerebral commissure. Sci Am 210:42–52, 1968

Squire LR: Memory and hippocampus: a synthesis from findings with rats, monkeys, and humans. Psychol Rev 99:195–231, 1992

Squire LR, Zola SM: Ischemic brain damage and memory impairment: a commentary. Hippocampus 6:546–552, 1996

Squire LR, Stark CEL, Clark RE: The medial temporal lobe. Annu Rev Neurosci 27:279–306, 2004

Stafiniak P, Saykin AJ, Sperling MR, et al: Acute naming deficits following dominant temporal lobectomy: prediction by age at 1st risk for seizures. Neurology 40:1509–1512, 1990

Stefanacci L, Buffalo EA, Schmolck H, et al: Profound amnesia after damage to the medial temporal lobe: a neuroanatomical and neuropsychological profile of patient EP. J Neurosci 20:7024–7036, 2000

Stephan KE: On the role of general system theory for functional neuroimaging. J Anat 205:443–470, 2004

Stuss DT, Benson DF: Neuropsychological studies of the frontal lobes. Psychol Bull 95:3–28, 1984

Stuss DT, Benson DF: The Frontal Lobes. New York, Raven, 1986

Stuss DT, Levine B: Adult clinical neuropsychology: lessons from studies of the frontal lobes. Annu Rev Psychol 53:401–433, 2002

Stuss DT, Alexander MP, Hamer L, et al: The effects of focal anterior and posterior brain lesions on verbal fluency. J Int Neuropsychol Soc 4:265–278, 1998

Sugiura M, Watanabe J, Satoh T, et al: Differential activation of temporoparietal structures during recognition of famous names and that of personally familiar names: an event-related fMRI study. Neuroimage 16:S281, 2001

Tengvar C, Johansson B, Sorensen J: Frontal lobe and cingulated cortical metabolic dysfunction in acquired akinetic mutism: a PET study of the interval form of carbon monoxide poisoning. Brain Inj 18:615–625, 2004

Teuber H-L: Alteration of perception and memory in man: reflections on methods, in Analysis of Behavioral Change. Edited by Weiskrantz L. New York, Harper & Row, 1968, pp 274–328

Thompson RFL: The neurobiology of learning and memory. Science 233:941–947, 1986

Tootell RBH, Reppas JB, Kwong KK, et al: Functional analysis of human MT and related visual cortical areas using functional magnetic resonance imaging. J Neurosci 15:3215–3230, 1995

Tranel D: Dissociated verbal and nonverbal retrieval and learning following left anterior temporal damage. Brain Cogn 15:187–200, 1991a

Tranel D: What has been rediscovered in "Rediscovering tactile agnosia"? Mayo Clin Proc 66:210–214, 1991b

Tranel D: "Acquired sociopathy": the development of sociopathic behavior following focal brain damage, in Progress in Experimental Personality and Psychopathology Research, Vol 17. Edited by Fowles DC, Sutker P, Goodman SH. New York, Springer, 1994a, pp 285–311

Tranel D: Assessment of higher-order visual function. Curr Opin Ophthalmol 5:29–37, 1994b

Tranel D: Higher brain function, in Neuroscience in Medicine. Edited by Conn PM. Philadelphia, PA, JB Lippincott, 1995a, pp 555–580

Tranel D: Where did my arm go? Contemporary Psychology 40:885–887, 1995b

Tranel D: The Iowa-Benton school of neuropsychological assessment, in Neuropsychological Assessment of Neuropsychiatric Disorders, 2nd Edition. Edited by Grant I, Adams KM. New York, Oxford University Press, 1996, pp 81–101

Tranel D: Non-conscious brain processing indexed by psychophysiological measures, in Progress in Brain Research: The Biological Basis for Mind Body Interactions, Vol 122. Edited by Mayer EA, Saper C. Amsterdam, Elsevier Science, 2000, pp 315–330

Tranel D: Central color processing and its disorders, in Handbook of Neuropsychology, 2nd Edition, Vol 4. Edited by Boller F, Grafman J. Amsterdam, Elsevier Science, 2001, pp 1–14

Tranel D, Anderson SW: Syndromes of aphasia, in Concise Encyclopedia of Language Pathology. Edited by Fabbro F. Amsterdam, Elsevier, 1999, pp 305–319

Tranel D, Damasio AR: Knowledge without awareness: an autonomic index of facial recognition by prosopagnosics. Science 228:1453–1454, 1985

Tranel D, Damasio AR: The covert learning of affective valence does not require structures in hippocampal system or amygdala. J Cogn Neurosci 5:79–88, 1993

Tranel D, Damasio AR: The agnosias and apraxias, in Neurology in Clinical Practice, 2nd Edition. Edited by Bradley WG, Daroff RB, Fenichel GM, et al. Stoneham, MA, Butterworth, 1996, pp 119–129

Tranel D, Hyman BT: Neuropsychological correlates of bilateral amygdala damage. Arch Neurol 47:349–355, 1990

Tranel D, Damasio AR, Damasio H: Intact recognition of facial expression, gender, and age in patients with impaired recognition of face identity. Neurology 38:690–696, 1988

Tranel D, Anderson SW, Benton AL: Development of the concept of "executive function" and its relationship to the frontal lobes, in Handbook of Neuropsychology, Vol 9. Edited by Boller F, Grafman J. Amsterdam, Elsevier, 1994a, pp 125–148

Tranel D, Damasio AR, Damasio H, et al: Sensorimotor skill learning in amnesia: additional evidence for the neural basis of nondeclarative memory. Learn Mem 1:165–179, 1994b

Tranel D, Damasio H, Damasio AR: Double dissociation between overt and covert face recognition. J Cogn Neurosci 7:425–432, 1995

Tranel D, Damasio H, Damasio AR: A neural basis for the retrieval of conceptual knowledge. Neuropsychologia 35:1319–1327, 1997a

Tranel D, Damasio H, Damasio AR: On the neurology of naming, in Anomia: Neuroanatomical and Cognitive Correlates. Edited by Goodglass H, Wingfield A. New York, Academic Press, 1997b, pp 65–90

Tranel D, Bechara A, Damasio AR: Decision making and the somatic marker hypothesis, in The New Cognitive Neurosciences, 2nd Edition. Edited by Gazzaniga MS. Cambridge, MA, MIT Press, 2000a, pp 1047–1061

Tranel D, Damasio AR, Damasio H: Amnesia caused by herpes simplex encephalitis, infarctions in basal forebrain, and anoxia/ischemia, in Handbook of Neuropsychology, 2nd Edition, Vol 1. Edited by Boller F, Grafman J. Amsterdam, Elsevier Science, 2000b, pp 37–62

Tranel D, Adolphs R, Damasio H, et al: A neural basis for the retrieval of words for actions. Cognitive Neuropsychology 18:655–670, 2001

Tranel D, Bechara A, Denburg NL: Asymmetric functional roles of right and left ventromedial prefrontal cortices in social conduct, decision-making, and emotional processing. Cortex 38:589–612, 2002

Tranel D, Martin C, Damasio H, et al: Effects of noun-verb homonymy on the neural correlates of naming concrete entities and actions. Brain Lang 92:288–299, 2005

Trevarthen C (ed): Brain Circuits and Functions of the Mind: Essays in Honor of R.W. Sperry. Cambridge, MA, Cambridge University Press, 1990

Tsukiura T, Fujii T, Okuda J, et al: Contribution of the rostral part of the left temporal lobe to retrieving people's names: a functional MRI study. Neuroimage 11:S373, 2000

Tulving E, Schacter DL, McLachlan DR, et al: Priming of semantic autobiographical knowledge: a case study of retrograde amnesia. Brain Cogn 8:3–20, 1988

Valenza N, Murray M, Ptak R, et al: The space of senses: impaired crossmodal interactions in a patient with Balint syndrome after bilateral parietal damage. Neuropsychologia 42:1737–1748, 2004

Vallar G, Bottini G, Paulesu E: Neglect syndromes: the role of the parietal cortex. Adv Neurol 93:293–319, 2003

Van Essen CD, Maunsell JHR: Hierarchical organization and functional streams in the visual cortex. Trends Neurosci 6:370–375, 1983

Van Hoesen GW: The parahippocampal gyrus. Trends Neurosci 5:345–350, 1982

Van Hoesen GW, Damasio AR: Neural correlates of cognitive impairment in Alzheimer's disease, in Handbook of Physiology: Higher Functions of the Nervous System. Edited by Mountcastle V, Plum F. Bethesda, MD, American Physiological Society, 1987, pp 871–898

Van Hoesen GW, Hyman BT, Damasio AR: Cell-specific pathology in neural systems of the temporal lobe in Alzheimer's disease, in Progress in Brain Research. Edited by Swaab D. Amsterdam, Elsevier, 1986, pp 361–375

Van Lancker D, Kreiman J: Unfamiliar voice discrimination and familiar voice recognition are independent and unordered abilities. Neuropsychologia 25:829–834, 1988

Van Lancker D, Cummings J, Kreiman J, et al: Phonagnosia: a dissociation between familiar and unfamiliar voices. Cortex 24:195–209, 1988

Van Lancker D, Kreiman J, Cummings J: Voice perception deficits: neuroanatomical correlates of phonagnosia. J Clin Exp Neuropsychol 11:665–674, 1989

Venneri A, Shanks MF: Belief and awareness: reflections on a case of persistent anosognosia. Neuropsychologia 42:230–238, 2004

Victor M, Adams RD, Collins GH: The Wernicke-Korsakoff Syndrome and Related Neurologic Disorders Due to Alcoholism and Malnutrition, 2nd Edition. Philadelphia, PA, FA Davis, 1989

Vignolo LA: Auditory agnosia. Philos Trans R Soc Lond B Biol Sci 298:49–57, 1982

Vogel JJ, Bowers CA, Vogel DS: Cerebral lateralization of spatial abilities: a meta-analysis. Brain Cogn 52:197–204, 2003

Volpe BT, Hirst W: Amnesia following the rupture and repair of an anterior communicating artery aneurysm. J Neurol Neurosurg Psychiatry 46:704–709, 1983

Wada Y, Yamamoto T: Selective impairment of facial recognition due to a hematoma restricted to the right fusiform and lateral occipital region. J Neurol Neurosurg Psychiatry 71:254–257, 2001

Warrington EK, McCarthy RA: Category-specific access dysphasia. Brain 106:859–878, 1983

Weintraub S, Mesulam M-M: Neglect: hemispheric specialization, behavioral components and anatomical correlates, in Handbook of Neuropsychology, Vol 2. Edited by Boller F, Grafman J. Amsterdam, Elsevier, 1989, pp 357–374

Wernicke C: Der aphasische Symptomencomplex. Breslau, Cohn und Weigert, 1874

Whatnough C, Chertkow H, Murtha S, et al: Dissociable brain regions process object meaning and object structure during picture naming. Neuropsychologia 40:174–186, 2002

Wilson FAW, O'Scalaidhe SP, Goldman-Rakic PS: Dissociation of object and spatial processing domains in primate prefrontal cortex. Science 260:1955–1958, 1993

Young AW, Aggleton JP, Hellawell DJ, et al: Face processing impairments after amygdalotomy. Brain 118:15–24, 1995

Zaidel E, Iacoboni M, Zaidel DW, et al: The callosal syndromes, in Clinical Neuropsychology, 4th Edition. Edited by Heilman KM, Valenstein E. New York, Oxford University Press, 2003, pp 347–403

Zeki SM: Colour coding in rhesus monkey prestriate cortex. Brain Res 53:422–427, 1973

Zeki SM: A century of cerebral achromatopsia. Brain 113:1727–1777, 1990

Zihl J, Von Cramon Z, Mai N: Selective disturbances of movement vision after bilateral brain damage. Brain 106:313–340, 1983

Zola-Morgan S, Squire LR: Memory impairment in monkeys following lesions of hippocampus. Behav Neurosci 100:165–170, 1986

Zola-Morgan S, Squire LR, Amaral DG: Human amnesia and the medial temporal region: enduring memory impairment following a bilateral lesions limited to field CA1 of the hippocampus. J Neurosci 6:2950–2967, 1986

Zola-Morgan S, Squire LR, Amaral DG, et al: Lesions of perirhinal and parahippocampal cortex that spare the amygdala and hippocampal formation produce severe memory impairment. J Neurosci 9:4355–4370, 1989

3

NERVOUS, ENDOCRINE, AND IMMUNE SYSTEM INTERACTIONS IN PSYCHIATRY

Oyetunde O. Alagbe, M.D.

Dwight L. Evans, M.D.

Andrew H. Miller, M.D.

During the past several decades, great strides have been made toward understanding the pathways by which the central nervous system (CNS) and the immune system interact. Data indicate that immune cells and tissues have the capacity to receive signals from the brain and endocrine system, and immune-derived molecules (cytokines) have potent effects on nervous system function. In addition to elucidating the details of these communication pathways at a biochemical and molecular biological level, a major challenge has been to place interactions among the nervous, endocrine, and immune systems into a clinical context. Investigators have examined the relevant impact of neuropsychiatric conditions and stress on immune-related disorders as well as the role of the immune system in neuropsychiatric disease. This chapter provides an overview of the results of these investigations along with information on the mechanisms involved.

OVERVIEW OF THE IMMUNE SYSTEM

Before considering the relationship among the nervous, endocrine, and immune systems, it is important to review the general purpose and internal organization of the immune response.

The immune system is a group of tissues, cells, and cell products such as antibodies and cytokines that protect the body from invading pathogens and malignantly transformed cells. The immune system also helps clear the body of damaged and dead cells and mobilizes subsequent repair pathways. Thus, the immune system protects the organism from invading external threats such as bacteria, viruses, fungi, and parasites as well as from internal threats such as neoplasms and tissue damage and destruction.

The immune system is made of solid tissues and circulating cells that are distributed throughout the body. Solid tissues are organized into specific structures classified as either central lymphoid tissues (bone marrow, thymus) or peripheral lymphoid tissues (lymph nodes, spleen mucosa, associated lymphoid tissue). Areas of high exposure to external pathogens—such as the digestive tract, pulmonary tract, and skin—contain specialized lymphoid tissues, such as Peyer's patches in the gut.

All immune cells originate from hematopoietic stem cells in bone marrow. Under the influence of signaling molecules such as cytokines and hormones, these cells develop along myeloid or lymphoid paths of differentiation.

The myeloid cell line includes monocytes and granulocytes such as neutrophils, basophils, and eosinophils. Monocytes and basophils differentiate further into macrophages and mast cells, respectively, and take up residence in tissues throughout the body. The lymphoid cell line includes B cells, T cells, and natural killer (NK) cells.

After production in the bone marrow, the cells that will become B lymphocytes mature in the bone marrow, whereas T lymphocytes travel to the thymus, where they will mature (Abbas and Lichtman 2003). The bone marrow and thymus are for this reason termed primary immune tissues. Because immune cells are constantly being produced with random recognition sites for an enormous variety of antigens, an important part of the maturational process for both types of lymphocytes is the elimination of cells that would react with self antigens. This essential and complex step occurs in the primary immune tissues. After maturation, cells circulate and take up residence in the secondary immune tissues (such as the spleen and lymph nodes), which provide sites for interaction with circulating pathogens.

Both the differentiation of the progenitor cell lines into either myeloid or lymphoid immune cells and the overall regulation of the immune system depend on many mediators, including immune signaling factors called cytokines. Cytokines are produced by a number of cells, including activated leukocytes, microglia, endothelial cells, fibroblasts, and adipocytes. The word *cytokine* (*cyto*, cell; *kinesis*, movement) derives from the original identification of these factors as important regulators of cell movement. However, cytokines have been found to have local and systemic effects on a wide variety of body functions not limited to the immune system.

As shown in Table 3–1, different cytokines have overlapping immunologic functions, and a cytokine may exert different effects on different target cells. A cytokine can act on the cell producing it, cells nearby, or distant cells (autocrine, paracrine, and endocrine activity, respectively). Cytokines are broadly classified according to their function and the sequence homology of the receptors to which they bind (Abbas and Lichtman 2003). In general, three functional categories have been defined: mediators and regulators of innate immunity, mediators and regulators of acquired immunity, and stimulators of hematopoiesis (including the colony-stimulating factors interleukin 3 [IL-3], IL-7, IL-9, and IL-11).

NATURAL IMMUNITY

For simplicity, the immune system may be divided into two functional arms: natural (or innate) immunity and specific (or acquired) immunity. Features of these functional arms are summarized in Table 3–2. Natural immunity is the body's frontline defense against pathogen inva-

sion and disruption of tissue integrity. Natural immunity does not require previous exposure to antigen. In contrast, acquired immunity is more specialized, depends on previous exposure to antigen, and typically is magnified on the body's reexposure to antigen. Despite the pedantic distinction between innate and acquired immune functions, these two parts of the immune system constantly finetune the immune response by mutual cellular interactions and soluble factors such as cytokines and hormones.

Innate immunity is mediated in large part by phagocytes (e.g., monocytes/macrophages, neutrophils) and NK cells. Phagocytes (especially macrophages) are concentrated in the lungs, the Kupffer cells of the liver, and the lining of the lymph nodes and spleen. Macrophage equivalents in the brain are referred to as microglia. Macrophages and other cells that mediate innate immunity detect microorganisms through nonspecific pattern recognition receptors. These receptors recognize a relatively small repertoire ($\sim 10^3$) of conserved elements of invading pathogens and also can recognize components of damaged cells. One set of pattern recognition receptors is the toll-like receptors that serve to potently activate the inflammatory response, including activation of the inflammatory signaling molecule nuclear factor-kappa B (NFkB) (as described in the following paragraph). Binding of the toll-like receptors also constitutes a "danger signal" to the immune system, and it is believed that the recognition of danger in combination with the recognition that an "invader" is "foreign" (e.g., not self) is fundamental to activating a full-blown immunologic assault (the so-called Danger Theory) (Matzinger 2001). On recognition of pathogens, macrophages and their equivalents (e.g., dendritic cells) engulf or lyse the invader and then express small pieces of the pathogen's proteins, called epitopes, on their cell surface (Abbas and Lichtman 2003). These epitopes (or antigens) then serve to interact with other immune cells (typically cells resulting from the acquired immune response—see next paragraph), which become activated when antigens are recognized. For this reason, macrophages and cells with similar capacities are referred to as antigen-presenting cells. Interaction between antigen-presenting cells and cells resulting from the acquired immune response is one example of the cooperation between the innate and acquired immunity.

Cytokines that mediate innate immunity include type I interferons (IFN) α and β, tumor necrosis factor α (TNF-α), and IL-1, IL-6, IL-10, IL-12, and IL-15. IL-1, IL-6, and TNF-α also are referred to as proinflammatory cytokines. These cytokines, along with chemokines (which attract other cell types), are produced early in the process of infection or inflammation, especially by macrophages, and are involved in the amplification of early innate immune re-

TABLE 3–1. Representative cytokines and their function

Cytokine	Made by	Activities
Interleukin 1	Activated macrophages, B cells, neutrophils, astrocytes, epithelial and endothelial cells	Activates B cells, helper T cells, endothelial cells Stimulates acute phase protein production Promotes inflammation and hematopoiesis Centrally induces fever, somnolence, anorexia
Interleukin 2	Antigen-activated Th1 cells	Promotes growth and differentiation of T and B lymphocytes Promotes NK cell proliferation
Interleukin 4	Th2 cells, mast cells, basophils, eosinophils	Promotes B cell growth and differentiation Promotes production of immunoglobulin E
Interleukin 5	Th2 cells, mast cells, eosinophils	Promotes B cell growth and differentiation Promotes eosinophil differentiation
Interleukin 6	Th2 cells, macrophages, fibroblasts, epithelium, adipocytes	Promotes B cell growth and differentiation Promotes antibody secretion Stimulates hepatocytes to produce acute phase proteins
Interleukin 8	T cells, macrophages, epithelium	Promotes activation and chemotaxis of neutrophils, basophils, T cells
Interleukin 10	Th2 cells, macrophages, epithelium, monocytes	Suppresses Th1-produced cytokines (interleukin 1, tumor necrosis factor α, interleukin 2)
Interleukin 12	B cells, macrophages	Stimulates production of interferon γ by helper T and NK cells Promotes induction of helper T cells
Tumor necrosis factor α	Macrophages, NK cells, T cells, B cells, mast cells	Promotes inflammation Activates monocytes and neutrophils Induces fever
Tumor necrosis factor α	Th1 cells, B cells	Promotes angiogenesis Promotes inflammation
Transforming growth factor β	Macrophages, T cells, B cells, mast cells	Promotes immunosuppression
Granulocyte-macrophage colony-stimulating factor	T cells, macrophages, NK cells, B cells	Promotes granulocyte and monocyte growth
Interferon α	Macrophages, fibroblasts, lymphoblastoid cells, virally infected cells, epithelial cells	Increases expression of major histocompatibility molecules Induces fever, reduces appetite Induces resistance to virus Stimulates NK cell activity
Interferon β	Fibroblasts, endothelial cells, virally infected cells	Stimulates NK cell activity Induces resistance to virus
Interferon γ	Activated Th1 cells, NK cells, B cells, macrophages	Activates macrophages Inhibits Th2 cells Blocks interleukin 4 effects on B cells Prevents class switching

Note. Th1 = T helper 1; Th2 = T helper 2; NK = natural killer.

TABLE 3–2.   Features of innate and acquired immunity

	Innate (natural) immunity	Acquired immunity
Circulating molecules	Complement Acute phase proteins	Antibodies
Cell types	Phagocytes (macrophages, neutrophils) Natural killer cells	T and B lymphocytes
Recognition	Pattern recognition receptors broadly (with limited specificity) recognize pathogens, dead cells, and cellular debris	B and T cell receptors have very narrow specificity (i.e., recognize specific molecular sequences derived from pathogens and pathogen-infected cells)
Soluble mediators	Type I interferons (α, β) Tumor necrosis factor, IL-1, IL-6	Interferon γ IL-2, IL-4, IL-10
Other	Surface barriers, cilia, lysozyme, secretions (tears, mucus, saliva), pH, normal flora	

Note.   IL=interleukin.

sponses. Two major intracellular signaling pathways that are triggered by proinflammatory cytokines include mitogen-activated protein kinase and NFkB. The mitogen-activated protein kinase signaling cascade includes three interactive subfamilies (c-Jun N-terminal kinase, extracellular signal-related kinases, and p38 mitogen-activated protein kinase), which regulate cell survival and proliferation as well as cytokine production (Johnson and Lapadat 2002). NFkB is one of the fundamental inflammatory signaling pathways; in addition to promoting cell survival and proliferation, it leads to increased expression of proinflammatory cytokines, chemokines, adhesion molecules, and reactive oxygen species (Kumar et al. 2004). Together, these factors attract other inflammatory cells to the site of invasion, stimulate a response by the liver called the acute phase response, and signal systemic neural and hormonal feedback mechanisms in the brain (see Figure 3–1). TNF and IL-1 induce fever by activating prostaglandin pathways that stimulate hypothalamic cells involved in the regulation of body temperature. These cytokines also have effects on other hypothalamic functions, including the regulation of sleep, appetite, and sexual drive (described later in this chapter in the subsection "Pathways of Immune System to Brain Signaling"). Notably, increased NFkB activity has been implicated in the pathogenesis of a number of illnesses, including cardiovascular disease, diabetes, and cancer (Kumar et al. 2004). Of relevance to regulation by the nervous and endocrine systems, NFkB is potently negatively regulated by glucocorticoids (Rhen and Cidlowski 2005).

The acute phase response is primarily mediated by IL-6, which stimulates the liver to produce proteins called acute phase reactants that help isolate and destroy invading pathogens, control damage to self tissues, and stimu-

late repair pathways (Baumann and Gauldie 1994). These proteins include C-reactive protein, macroglobulin, fibrinogen, and antiproteases. C-reactive protein coats bacteria for phagocytosis, whereas fibrinogen aids in clotting. Elevated fibrinogen contributes in part to the elevated sedimentation rate in inflammatory disorders by enhancing rouleaux formation (stacking/clustering of red blood cells). Antiproteases control tissue destruction by inactivating destructive proteases produced by immune cells. The activation of the acute phase response is a good example of the regulation and counterregulation that occurs both to stimulate and to control the immune response; immune cells produce proinflammatory cytokines and proteases, stimulating production of acute phase proteins by the liver, which in turn control immune-induced tissue destruction. Feedback of this kind occurs at many levels of immune function and is discussed in greater detail later in this chapter. Notably, acute phase reactants such as C-reactive proteins are relatively stable and persistent in the blood and therefore have been used as biomarkers of an activated innate immune response (inflammation) in a number of disease states. Indeed, C-reactive protein has become an important prognostic marker of poor outcome in patients with cardiovascular disease (Ridker 2004).

Finally, the system of complement proteins is another important component of innate, or nonspecific, immunity. These proteins are produced by the liver and interact in a sequential "cascade," which can amplify the immune response at the site of injury (Abbas and Lichtman 2003; Delves and Roitt 2000a, 2000b). Complement proteins have effects on cell lysis and opsonization and can attract other immune cells and stimulate their activity. They also can help neutralize antigen-antibody complexes. The NK

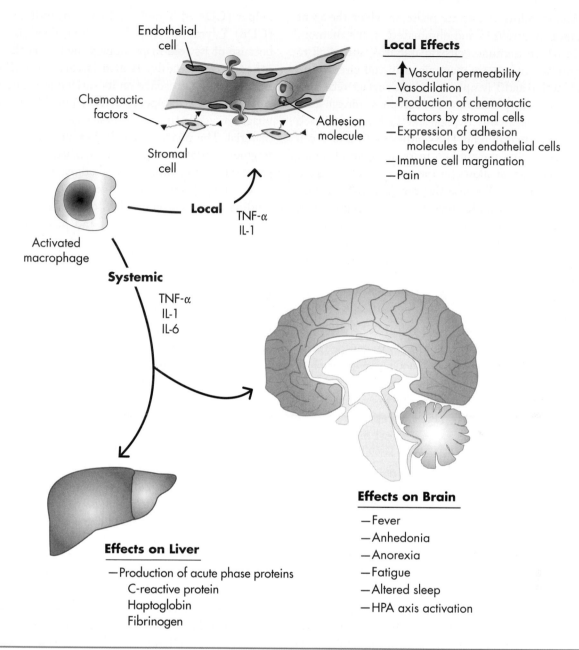

Local Effects

— ↑ Vascular permeability
— Vasodilation
— Production of chemotactic
    factors by stromal cells
— Expression of adhesion
    molecules by endothelial cells
— Immune cell margination
— Pain

Effects on Liver

— Production of acute phase proteins
    C-reactive protein
    Haptoglobin
    Fibrinogen

Effects on Brain

— Fever
— Anhedonia
— Anorexia
— Fatigue
— Altered sleep
— HPA axis activation

FIGURE 3–1. Innate immunity. Activated macrophages release cytokines at the site of tissue injury or infection. Locally, these cytokines act on endothelial and tissue stromal cells. Tissue stromal cells produce chemotactic factors, recruiting other immune cells to the site of injury. The endothelial cells produce adhesion molecules, enhancing immune cell margination and diapedesis. In the brain, proinflammatory cytokines—including interleukin 1 (IL-1), IL-6, and tumor necrosis factor α (TNF-α)—activate the hypothalamic-pituitary-adrenal (HPA) axis and induce sickness behavior and fever. The proinflammatory cytokines also induce the liver to produce acute-phase proteins.

cells, phagocytes, cytokines, and complement proteins all make up the branch of innate immunity that produces the body's first-line, nonspecific response to threat.

ACQUIRED IMMUNITY

Acquired immunity (also called specific or adaptive immunity) is provided by a complex set of cells and signaling molecules that enable the body to discriminate between very specific antigenic components of foreign antigens and "remember" them so that a more robust response is mobilized on reexposure. Several features of the acquired immune response are illustrated in Figure 3–2. Acquired immunity occurs in four conceptually distinct phases: an induction phase, in which an infectious agent or antigen is detected; an activation phase, in which immune cells proliferate and mobilize; an effector phase, in which the agent or antigen is neutralized and eliminated; and a memory phase, in which immune cells capable of responding to reexposure to antigen are maintained in the circulation. Although both B and T lymphocytes have surface receptors that are genetically programmed to recognize foreign antigens, the mechanisms of activation and the function of each cell type are quite different. The synthesis of a B or T cell receptor depends on the random rearrangement of multiple gene products that allows for the potential to recognize 10^8 distinct antigens. Because this rearrangement is random, this process allows for production of receptors that might react with self antigens. As mentioned previously, elimination of these autoimmune cells is an important step in lymphocyte maturation in the primary immune tissues.

B CELLS

Acquired immunity mediated by B cells has been termed *humoral immunity*, because this immunity can be transferred by transfusion of cell-free blood products such as plasma. The B cell first recognizes a foreign antigen when that antigen binds to the B cell surface receptor that specifically matches that antigen. The B cell receptor is a surface immunoglobulin, which has two identical binding sites, each of which can recognize the tertiary structure of a foreign antigen. In addition to binding the antigen, the B cell also requires a signal (generally a cytokine) from a helper T cell to become fully activated (Delves and Roitt 2000a, 2000b). The activated B cell then proliferates into clonally identical cells that differentiate further into plasma cells that produce soluble antibodies of the same binding specificity as the surface receptor (Figure 3–2A). Although antibodies produced by a specific B cell or its clone are identical in structure at the antigen-binding site, other portions of the antibody can vary depending on the antibody's class. Different classes of antibody (e.g., immunoglobulin M [IgM], IgA, IgG, IgD) have specific class-dependent functions. For example, IgM, a large immunoglobulin, has five identical antigen-binding sites and is capable of activating the complement system. In a similar way, other classes of antibodies have their own class-specific functions.

T CELLS

The activation of T cells is more complex, and the immunity conferred by T cell–dependent processes is termed *cell mediated*, because it depends on cellular functions rather than antibody production and can be transferred from one individual to the next only through the passage of cells. There are different functionally distinct populations of T lymphocytes; the best characterized are the

helper (CD4+) T cells and the cytolytic or cytotoxic (CD8) T lymphocytes. The helper T cell is so named because of its role in producing mediators that activate other immune cells. It also is termed a CD4+ cell because of the presence on its surface of a particular cell surface protein. Helper T cells require the assistance of phagocytic cells that must first ingest and digest foreign material. The phagocytic cell then presents the digested fragments on its surface in association with a particular set of self surface molecules called major histocompatibility complex (MHC) molecules. The CD4+ T cell, on binding to the antigen-MHC complex on a phagocytic cell, then becomes activated and produces cytokines, such as IL-2 and IL-4, which in turn promote growth and activation of other immune cells. CD4+ cells also may become memory cells that remain latent and help the body respond more rapidly and efficiently when reexposed to the same stimulus. The presence of circulating soluble CD4 and CD8 molecules represents immune activation. Other markers of immune activation are indirect and represent negative feedback mechanisms by which the body attempts to control the immune response. IL-10 and transforming growth factor β are two cytokines that are involved in negatively modulating immunity. IL-1 receptor antagonist is another circulating mediator that binds to the IL-1 receptor, thus limiting the effects of the cytokine IL-1. Finally, CD25 T cells also are involved in immune regulation and immune suppression.

Cell-mediated immunity provides mechanisms for fighting viral infection and malignancy. Cells of the body, when virally infected or malignantly transformed, may present antigen such as virus particles on their surface in association with a different class of MHC molecules. When the cytotoxic T lymphocyte detects this antigen–MHC molecule complex on a cell, the cytotoxic cell releases enzymes that kill the affected cell (Figure 3–2B). The cytotoxic T lymphocyte also is called a CD8+ cell because it has a cell surface protein called CD8, analogous to the CD4 protein on helper T lymphocytes. CD8 cells play a critical role in the clearance of viruses such as HIV. Cell-mediated immunity thus depends on a complex set of cellular and molecular interactions. The surface MHC molecules, which are genetically coded, play a key role in this complex interaction. The effectiveness of one's MHC in the process of binding and presenting antigen depends on the individual's genetic endowment. The particular set of MHC genes an individual carries will thus play a key role in determining resistance to disease and susceptibility to autoimmune disorder.

Data indicate that T helper cell subclasses, identified as T helper 1 (Th1) and T helper 2 (Th2) cells, show distinct patterns of immune activation within cell-mediated immu-

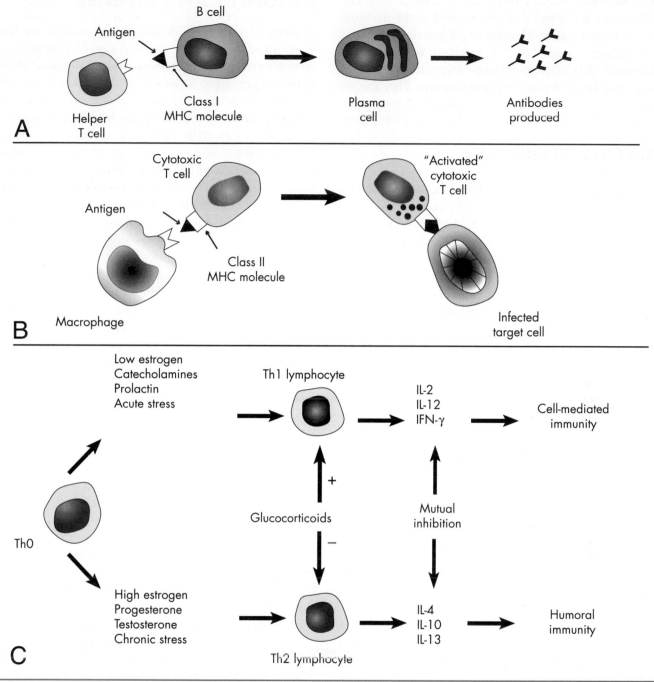

FIGURE 3–2.   Processes of acquired immunity. *Panel A.* B cell activation. The B cell presents antigen to a helper T cell, which then secretes cytokines that stimulate development of the B cell into an antibody-producing plasma cell. The helper T cell recognizes antigen in association with a major histocompatibility complex (MHC) molecule. *Panel B.* Cell killing by cytotoxic T cell. A cytotoxic T cell becomes activated by an encounter with an antigen-presenting cell (such as a macrophage) in the presence of stimulating cytokines. The activated cytotoxic T cell produces toxic granules. When the cytotoxic T cell binds to the target cell, the granules are released, killing the target cell. *Panel C.* T helper (Th) lymphocytes develop along Th1 and Th2 pathways. Naive helper T lymphocytes (Th0) develop along Th1 or Th2 pathways under the influence of stimulating factors such as hormones and catecholamines. Th1 and Th2 cells produce characteristic cytokine profiles with specific immune system effects. Th1 cells generally stimulate forms of cell-mediated immunity such as the delayed-type hypersensitivity response and natural killer cell activity, whereas Th2 cells stimulate humoral immunity. Glucocorticoids inhibit the Th1 response and stimulate the Th2 response. The Th1 and Th2 pathways mutually inhibit each other.

nity (see Figure 3–2C) (Abbas and Lichtman 2003). Th1 cells secrete IFN-γ and IL-2, are involved in cell-mediated immunity, and assist with cytotoxic T lymphocyte activation. Th2 cells secrete IL-4, IL-6, and IL-10 and are involved in antibody formation and allergic responses. These subclasses thus have different functional patterns. They also appear to have different responses to neuroendocrine control.

TESTS OF IMMUNITY

Several laboratory approaches have been used to study the relationship between immune function and stress or psychiatric illness. They can be divided into enumerative and functional tests. Enumerative studies count circulating immune cells of various types and subtypes (e.g., neutrophils, CD4+ lymphocytes). Cells can be identified by morphologic characteristics (as determined in a complete blood cell count and differential) or by expression of unique cell surface molecules (referred to as clusters of differentiation, or CD markers). Cell surface molecules as well as intracellular content of relevant proteins can be determined by using flow cytometry. Flow cytometry is a powerful technique tailored for examining cells such as human blood cells that grow in a nonadherent manner and are in single-cell suspension. Cells are labeled with fluorochrome-conjugated antibodies to relevant surface markers (CD markers) or intracellular proteins. Indeed, labeling of phosphorylated proteins can provide more specific information about activation of relevant immune or other postreceptor signaling pathways.

Functional studies examine different in vivo and in vitro measures of immune function. For example, white blood cells taken from patients diagnosed with illness have been tested in vitro for their ability to proliferate/divide or produce cytokines in response to various mitogens or bacterial products (e.g., lipopolysaccharide). Mitogens are plant lectins that have the capacity to crosslink receptors on various immune cell types (including T cells, B cells, and macrophages), thereby activating cellular function (Abbas and Lichtman 2003). Lipopolysaccharide binds to toll-like receptors (pattern recognition receptors) and activates multiple proinflammatory cytokines, including IL-1, IL-6, and TNF-α. NK cell activity is another type of in vitro functional immune assay in which isolated NK cells are incubated with radiolabeled tumor cells, and the amount of tumor cell killing is measured by the amount of radioactivity released. In vivo functional tests of immunity include measures of cytokines or acute phase proteins in the blood or cerebrospinal fluid (CSF), response to antigens such as in the delayed-type hypersensitivity reaction, or antibody production against vaccines or latent viruses.

IMMUNITY AND DISEASE

Diseases of immune dysfunction help to illustrate how finely tuned the system is and how essential the immune system's role is in maintaining health. Diseases of the immune system can be subclassified into immune deficiencies, allergic diseases, and autoimmune disorders. In diseases of immune deficiency, the body is unable either to identify or to fight pathogens or malignancies. An example is the syndrome of severe combined immunodeficiency, in which both B and T cell functions are grossly impaired. Usually congenital, this disorder of both humoral and cell-mediated immunity prevents the body from fighting off infections of all sorts. Without treatment, affected individuals typically succumb rapidly to bacterial, viral, or fungal infection (or a combination of these). Other immune deficiencies are more specific. For example, certain cancer chemotherapy regimens that preferentially cause neutropenia make patients especially vulnerable to infection by extracellular bacteria. AIDS, associated with infection with HIV, demonstrates how deficiency in one component of the immune system can cause widespread pathology. The virus binds to the CD4+ protein on the surface of the helper T lymphocyte, enters the cell, and interferes with the cell's functioning in a variety of ways. Because the helper T lymphocyte plays such a pivotal role in immunity, loss of helper T cell function predisposes affected individuals to a variety of immune-related disorders. Patients are susceptible to opportunistic infections with organisms such as *Cryptococcus*, *Mycobacterium* species, and *Toxoplasma*. Reactivation or severe infection with cytomegalovirus or herpes viruses can occur. Patients with HIV infection also are at risk for cancers such as Kaposi's sarcoma and CNS lymphoma. The syndrome of HIV/AIDS demonstrates how dysfunction of one immune cell type reverberates throughout a number of immune processes.

Disorders of immunity also include those of excessive immunity. These diseases fall into two types: allergic diseases, in which the immune system responds excessively to nonpathogenic environmental antigens, and autoimmune diseases, in which the system fails to prevent reaction to self antigens. These processes have multiple pathological consequences. They can waste body energy resources, injure self tissues, and keep the immune system from functioning at an efficient level against external pathogens. The main immunopathology in all allergic diseases is degranulation of mast cells, which are particularly abundant in the skin and the mucosa of the respiratory and gastrointestinal tracts. The pathophysiology of allergic reactions involves the activation of mast cells in response to antigens binding to IgE and an overactive Th2 cell response. Histamines are released by mast cells, leading to increased capillary permeability and smooth muscle contraction. The most severe form of allergy is the anaphylactic reaction, occurring when exposure to an antigen induces bronchospasm or a hypotensive reaction (Abbas and Lichtman 2003).

Autoimmune diseases occur when the system misidentifies self cells as foreign and the cascade of immune events results in damage of self tissue. These multifactorial illnesses arise from a combination of events, including individual genetic predisposition, exposure to an antigen, and hormonal patterns. Lymphocytes that should be eliminated for binding too robustly to self antigens may survive to maturity. Viral infections or other stimuli may cause surface changes of self cells, which cause immune cells to identify these cells as foreign and attack them. By these mechanisms, direct tissue damage can occur. Secondary effects also can occur, as in systemic lupus erythematosus (SLE), when circulating antigen-antibody complexes are deposited in and damage renal tissue and microvasculature. These examples of immune deficiency states and autoimmune disorders reflect the variety and severity of diseases that can occur when immune regulation is impaired.

Although immunologists have elucidated many of the intricacies of internal regulation of the immune response, a growing database has led to an increasing appreciation that factors and pathways external to the immune system, including those involving the nervous and endocrine systems, are intimately involved in immune regulation. The foundation for this expanded consideration of immune regulation derives from multiple studies demonstrating meaningful communication among the nervous, endocrine, and immune systems. Relevant areas of research include 1) the impact of stress and psychiatric disease on immune function and immune-related disorders, 2) the influence of the immune system and immune-related disorders on the brain and neuropsychiatric disorders, and 3) shared pathways of communication among nervous, endocrine, and immune systems, including nervous innervation of lymphoid tissue and shared expression of receptors for multiple transmitters.

STRESS AND IMMUNITY

One of the most well-studied areas of the relationship among the nervous, endocrine, and immune systems is the impact of stress on immune function.

STRESS AND IMMUNITY IN LABORATORY ANIMALS

Early investigators exposed laboratory animals to various stressors and measured susceptibility to disease induced by infection or inoculation with tumor cells. Rasmussen and colleagues (1957) performed some of the first of these experiments in the 1950s and 1960s. For example, mice exposed to stressors such as shock, restraint, and loud noise were found to exhibit increased susceptibility to a number of viral infections, especially if the stressor was applied after virus exposure. Ader and Friedman (1965) demonstrated that handling and mild electric shock administered during the first few weeks of life also modified the rates of tumor development and survival in rats injected with Walker 256 sarcoma cells as adults. These investigations confirmed an association between stress and disease susceptibility, leading researchers to examine what specific changes in immune system parameters might be involved.

One of the first studies documenting the impact of stress on the immune system was conducted by Keller and colleagues (1981), who exposed adult rats to 19 hours of tail shock. The animals exhibited profound reductions in the proliferation of peripheral blood T cells in response to in vitro stimulation by the nonspecific T cell mitogen phytohemagglutinin. Subsequent studies have shown that a wide variety of stressors—including handling, foot shock, restraint, rotation, crowding, noise, forced exercise, light-dark cycle inversion, and exposure to a predator—are capable of altering a similarly wide variety of immune parameters, including decreases in peripheral blood lymphocytes, lymphocyte proliferation, cytokine production, NK cell activity, phagocytic function, and antibody formation (Weiss and Sundar 1992). In most of this research, the stressors were acute and led to immune findings that suggest immune suppression. Nevertheless, the data in large part were derived from immune compartments of the blood and spleen, which represent a fraction of the immune processes occurring in the body at any particular time. Indeed, elegant work by Dhabhar and colleagues demonstrated that during acute stress, immune cells traffic out of the blood and into peripheral tissues (including most notably the skin), where immune responses are, if anything, more vigorous (Dhabhar and McEwen 2001; Dhabhar et al. 2000). It was suggested that this redistribution of lymphocytes and other immune cells during acute stress may serve to enhance the ability to fight off pathogens in the case of wounding.

Although early studies primarily focused on measures of acquired immune responses, more recent studies indicate that innate immune responses may be activated by both acute and chronic stress (Grippo et al. 2005). Stress-induced increases in circulating levels of acute phase proteins such as $\alpha 1$-antitrypsin, C-reactive protein, and haptoglobin have been reported, along with increases in the proinflammatory cytokines IL-6, IL-1, and TNF-α. Increased cytokine expression was apparent both in the periphery and in the brain (O'Connor et al. 2003). Interestingly, data suggest that stress-induced reductions in brain-derived neurotrophic factor, which is believed to be involved in synaptic plasticity and mood regulation, are in part mediated by stress-induced increases in IL-1 (Barrientos 2003). Acute stress also has been associated with the activation of NFkB in both mice and humans. Thus, decreases in cell-mediated immunity appear to be paradoxically accompanied by increases in innate immunity during stress (LeMay et al. 1990; Zhou et al. 1993). One possibility is that activation of innate immune responses during stress may contribute to stress-induced decreases in acquired immune responses. Of note in this regard, Moraska (2002) found that administration of IL-1 receptor antagonist before stressor exposure was able to reverse the effects of stress on antibody responses to keyhole limpet hemocyanin. Finally, chronic stress was associated with resistance to the inhibitory effects of glucocorticoids in macrophages, which may further contribute to unrestrained activation of innate inflammatory responses (Bailey et al. 2004).

Table 3–3 summarizes immune changes in laboratory animals in response to stress.

STRESS AND IMMUNITY IN HUMANS: LABORATORY STRESSORS

Laboratory stressors are generally mild, acute stressors, including cognitive tasks such as public speaking or mental arithmetic. Although some alterations in immune parameters are similar between studies of naturalistic and experimentally induced stressors, other immune changes after stress in the laboratory are distinct. Laboratory stressors have been associated with decreased lymphocyte proliferative responses to mitogen stimulation, similar to changes found with chronic life stress. However, in contrast to naturalistic stressors, laboratory stressors have been associated with increased NK cell number and in vitro NK cell activity. These NK cell findings were transient and were correlated with increased cardiovascular reactivity (Benschop et al. 1995, 1996; Herbert et al. 1994).

Work by Pike and colleagues (1997) evaluated immune responses to acute psychological stress (mental arithmetic) in individuals who were or were not undergoing chronic life stress. Although the subjects exhibited no baseline differences in NK cell number or activity, when subjects were exposed to an acute stressor, individuals experiencing chronic stress in daily life had neuroendocrine and immune responses different from those under low stress. Chronically stressed individuals exhibited increased peak epinephrine responses and blunted peak

TABLE 3–3.   Stress-induced changes in immune function: studies in laboratory animals

Immune responses to acute stress

Decreased number of circulating lymphocytes

Decreased lymphocyte proliferative responses to mitogens

Decreased phagocyte function

Decreased/increased natural killer cell activity

Increased number of natural killer cells in circulation

Increased antibody production

Increased cutaneous delayed-type hypersensitivity

Increased acute phase proteins (α1-antitrypsin, C-reactive protein, haptoglobin)

Increased proinflammatory cytokines (interleukin 1, interleukin 6, tumor necrosis factor α)

Activation of nuclear factor-kappa B (NFkB)

Immune responses to chronic stress

Decreased numbers of circulating lymphocytes and monocytes

Decreased lymphocyte proliferative response to mitogens

Decreased natural killer cell activity

Decreased number of natural killer cells

Increased susceptibility to viral infection

Increased rate of tumor development

Decreased antibody production

Decreased delayed-type hypersensitivity

Increased proinflammatory cytokines (interleukin 1, interleukin 6, tumor necrosis factor α)

levels of β-endorphin in response to the task. Both groups responded to the acute stressor with increased NK cell numbers, but the NK activity per cell was decreased in the subjects under chronic stress. Chronic stress thus appears to cause changes in the immune system that alter the individual's responses to acute stress. These findings may be especially relevant to the role of stress in the chronically mentally ill or medically ill.

Some work exists addressing issues of how psychological or dispositional attitudes and controllability of a stressor interact to affect the immune response to laboratory stressors (G.E. Miller et al. 1999a, 1999b). Peters and colleagues (1999) reported experiments in humans in which effort and controllability were separated experimentally. The amount of effort expended in performing a task was associated with transient increases in CD8 and CD16 cell numbers and NK cell activity, whereas uncontrollability was associated with increased serum cortisol and decreased production of IL-6 by stimulated lymphocytes. Similarly, the expectation of success (optimism) in law students was found to be associated with increased CD4 cell number and increased NK cell activity during students' first semester of law school (Segerstrom et al. 1998). These findings suggest an interaction among psychological characteristics, stress, and immune function.

Like laboratory animals, human subjects exposed to acute experimental stressors also exhibit activation of the innate immune response. For example, in one study in humans undergoing a public speaking and mental arithmetic task, significant increases in the inflammatory signaling molecule NFkB were found, indicating that effects of stress on the immune system are apparent at the most fundamental level of inflammatory signaling (Bierhaus et al. 2003). Given the previously noted relationship between NFkB and a number of diseases including cancer, cardiovascular disease, and diabetes (Kumar et al. 2004), these data suggest that activation of NFkB may serve as a fundamental link between stress and a variety of illnesses.

STRESS AND IMMUNITY IN HUMANS: NATURALISTIC STRESSORS

Researchers have examined a variety of immune parameters in apparently healthy humans undergoing naturalistic or laboratory stressors. Table 3–4 summarizes immune findings in humans during acute and chronic stress. Naturalistic stressors such as caregiving for patients with Alzheimer's disease and undergoing academic examinations have been studied extensively. Elderly caregivers of spouses with Alzheimer's disease, presumably experiencing chronic stress, were found to exhibit a variety of immune abnormalities, including decreased lymphocyte proliferation and IL-2 production, decreased ratio of T helper to T suppressor cells (Pariante et al. 1997), and decreased NK cell activity (Esterling et al. 1996). Medical students experiencing examination stress also showed a variety of altered immune responses, including changes in cytokine production that indicate a shift from Th1 to Th2 immune responses (Segerstrom and Miller 2004). A large meta-analysis by Herbert and Cohen (1993) examined studies of stress effects on human immune variables. Immunologic effects observed across studies of long-term naturalistic stressors include increased white blood cells, decreased peripheral blood lymphocytes, decreased cytotoxic/suppressor T cells, decreased lym-

TABLE 3–4. Stress-induced changes in immune function: human studies

Immune responses to acute stress

Increased white blood cell count

Increased natural killer cell number

Decreased number of T lymphocytes

Decreased proliferative responses to mitogens

Increased natural killer cell activity

Increased production of proinflammatory cytokines (IL-6)

Increased antibody titers to viruses

Increased secretion of immunoglobin A

Decreased antibody response to vaccine

Immune responses to chronic stress

Increased white blood cell count

Decreased number of lymphocytes

Decreased ratio of helper T cells to suppressor T cells

Decreased lymphocyte proliferative responses to mitogens

Decreased lymphocyte production of IL-2 by stimulated lymphocytes

Increased production of proinflammatory cytokines (IL-6)

Decreased natural killer cell activity

Increased antibody titers to viruses

Decreased antibody response to vaccine

Delayed wound healing

Note. IL=interleukin.

phocyte responses to phytohemagglutinin and concanavalin A, and increased antibody titers to herpes simplex virus type 1 and Epstein-Barr virus. Increased viral antibody titers presumably reflect virus reactivation secondary to altered cell-mediated (acquired) immune function. Probably the most reproducible stress-induced change was decreased NK cell cytotoxicity. The type of stressor seems to play a role also, with social (interpersonal) stressors having more profound effects than nonsocial ones.

Like animal study subjects, human subjects also exhibit increased activity of the innate immune response during exposure to naturalistic stressors. Indeed, in a study by Kiecolt-Glaser and colleagues (2003), elderly individuals undergoing caregiving stress exhibited a fourfold greater increase in IL-6 over time compared with the level observed in a noncaregiver control population.

Data suggest that the immunologic changes associated with stress may have implications for health and disease. A study of spousal caregivers of dementia patients found impaired wound healing compared with age-matched control subjects (Kiecolt-Glaser et al. 1995). Investigations of healthy subjects also demonstrated that stress increases the likelihood of both infection and symptom development after standardized inoculation with several rhinoviruses (S. Cohen et al. 1991). Finally, decreased antibody responses to hepatitis B and influenza vaccines, respectively, were found in medical students experiencing acute examination stress (Glaser et al. 1992) and in spousal caregivers of Alzheimer's disease patients (Kiecolt-Glaser et al. 1996). Overall, these data indicate that humans undergoing naturalistic stressors exhibit evidence of immune dysfunction, generally consistent with decreased acquired immune system responsiveness, increased susceptibility to infection, and impaired wound healing.

STRESS, DEPRESSION, AND IMMUNITY: IMPACT ON DISEASE

Physicians have long been interested in the effects of stress, depression, and other psychological factors on the onset and course of illnesses related to the immune system, including cancer, infectious diseases, and autoimmune disorders.

CANCER

Anecdotal reports have suggested an association between the development of cancer and preceding stressful life events. Findings included an increase in stressful life events before the development of colorectal cancer (Courtney et al. 1993) but no such association between stressful life events and the development of breast cancer (Roberts et al. 1996). In general, studies of this type have been retrospective and examine only patients with one type of cancer. Retrospective investigations are confounded by the fact that the diagnosis of cancer itself can alter the patient's recall of events preceding diagnosis.

Because of the small number of new cases and the long period over which many diseases develop, prospective epidemiological studies with large numbers of subjects and lengthy follow-up periods must be performed before an association between stress and the incidence of disease can be demonstrated. A survey of more than 11,000 parents of children diagnosed with cancer was conducted on Danish national health registries to examine the impact of the severe stressor—the diagnosis of cancer in one's child—on

the development of disease in their parents. This survey found no association between the diagnosis of cancer in one's child and an increased odds ratio for the development of cancer, allergies, or autoimmune disease during a period ranging from 7 to 49 years after the child's cancer diagnosis (Johansen and Olsen 1997). Few studies of this sort are available that provide such strong data about the association between stress and the development of disease.

Regarding the impact of depression on the development of cancer, the data have been somewhat mixed (Raison and Miller 2003a). In a meta-analysis of prospective studies by McGee and colleagues (1994), a small but statistically significant increased risk of cancer in patients with depression was revealed. In a more recent review of more than 50 studies on mortality and depression by Wulsin and colleagues (1999), the authors concluded that although depression seems to increase the risk of death by cardiovascular disease, especially in men, depression does not seem to increase the risk of death by cancer. Both reviews comment on the lack of high-quality studies controlling for potential mediating variables. Of note are studies finding an increased incidence of cancer in depressed smokers (Linkins and Comstock 1990), an increased incidence of lung cancer in depressed men (Knekt et al. 1996), and an increased incidence of cancer in men with high levels of hopelessness (Everson et al. 1996). Taken together, the data suggest that depression may not in itself put individuals at substantially higher risk but may increase the risk of cancer in individuals with other risk factors, especially smoking.

Although the impact of stress and/or depression on the development of cancer may be relatively small, data support the notion that psychological factors may have a greater effect once cancer is diagnosed. Mounting evidence suggests that susceptibility to immune-related diseases, including cancer, is related to genetic factors. Therefore, if stress, depression, and other psychological factors are associated with altered immune function, then the impact of these factors may be the greatest on patients with immune-related disorders and genetic predisposition to immune dysfunction. Ramirez and colleagues (1989) reported that severe life events and difficulties are associated with increased risk of breast cancer relapse. In addition, depression is relatively common in cancer patients (Evans et al. 1986), and depressive symptoms have been associated with decreased survival in patients with lung cancer (Buccheri 1998; Faller et al. 1999). Hopelessness also has been found to be associated with decreased survival in women with early-stage breast cancer (Watson et al. 1999, 2005). In a study by Walker and colleagues (1999), scores on depression and anxiety rating scales were independent predictors of therapeutic outcome in patients with newly diagnosed breast cancer. Because stress or psychiatric symptoms may predispose cancer patients to worse outcomes, clinicians have wondered whether psychosocial interventions that address these factors might alter the disease outcome. To test these notions, Spiegel and colleagues (1989) and Fawzy and colleagues (1993) treated cancer patients with group psychotherapy under controlled conditions and found improved outcomes in the intervention group compared with those receiving standard therapy. These outcomes included lengthened survival in patients with metastatic breast cancer and decreased recurrence in patients with malignant melanoma. Not all studies have reproduced these findings. Two studies that used cognitive-behavior therapy in patients with metastatic breast cancer found no improved survival in the intervention group (A.J. Cunningham et al. 1998; Edelman et al. 1999). A problem with the few studies in this area is that all patients have been included, not simply those who might be psychiatrically vulnerable to stress-related immune alterations. It remains to be determined whether more powerful treatment effects would be observed if studies targeted patients with psychosocial risk factors, including depressive symptoms, reduced social support, or impaired coping strategies.

Regarding potential mechanisms of the effects of distress, depression, and hopelessness on outcome in cancer patients, there is evidence to suggest that the hypothalamic-pituitary-adrenal (HPA) axis may be involved. HPA axis hormones (e.g., cortisol) have potent immunoregulatory effects and therefore may be a link between psychosocial status, immune function, and disease in cancer patients. Studies have shown that loss of normal circadian variation in cortisol secretion, similar to the pattern seen in patients with major depression, predicts earlier mortality among patients with metastatic breast cancer (Sephton et al. 2001). This impact of altered cortisol rhythms on cancer outcome has been modeled in laboratory animals. For example, Filipski and colleagues (2002) ablated the suprachiasmatic nucleus of mice (resulting in altered cortisol rhythms) and implanted osteosarcoma and pancreatic adenoma cells. Cancer cells grew significantly more rapidly in the mice with suprachiasmatic nucleus lesions (who also exhibited shortened survival) compared with sham-operated animals. Notably, it was found that cognitive-behavioral stress management therapy had significant effects on cortisol secretion in cancer patients (Cruess et al. 2000), and thereby this therapy may have an effect on disease outcome (Carver et al. 2003).

AIDS INFECTION

Infection with HIV is a worldwide epidemic. However, because of increasing availability of antiretroviral medications in developed countries, large numbers of patients are living longer with the illness. Of particular interest has been the neuropsychiatric aspects of HIV infection, including the relationship among psychosocial factors in infected individuals, their immune functioning, and clinical status. Although one study found no differences in immune variables in patients with HIV infection who are experiencing increased life stress (Rabkin et al. 1991), other research has found altered immune parameters in HIV-infected, stressed individuals (Evans et al. 1995; Leserman et al. 1997; Perry et al. 1992; Petitto et al. 2000). More recently, Leserman and colleagues (2000) reported an association of faster progression from HIV disease to AIDS with stressful life events and higher serum cortisol levels. Investigators also reported that life event stress, including bereavement, leads to more rapid early HIV disease progression as well as progression to AIDS (Evans et al. 1997; Leserman et al. 1997, 1999). Moreover, bereavement combined with negative expectations about one's future health status has been found to predict shorter survival in men with AIDS and increased likelihood of the development of HIV-related symptoms in men with HIV infection (Cole and Kemeny 2001; Reed et al. 1999). The effects of stress on HIV disease progression may be related to the influence of increased autonomic nervous system activity and catecholamines on relevant immune endpoints and viral replication. For example, Cole and colleagues (2001) found that increased autonomic nervous system activity in HIV-infected subjects was associated with an impaired response to highly active antiretroviral therapy, including poorer suppression of plasma viral load and poorer CD4+ T cell recovery over 3–11 months of treatment.

In addition to life stress, the relevance of depressive symptoms to HIV disease also has been explored. Some researchers found an association between depressive symptoms and HIV disease progression without increased mortality (Burack et al. 1993; Lyketsos et al. 1993; Page-Schafer et al. 1996), and others reported both disease progression and increased mortality (Mayne et al. 1996). Other work reported no association between depression and disease progression (Lyketsos et al. 1996; Perry et al. 1992; Rabkin et al. 1991). A meta-analysis by Zorrilla and colleagues (1996) reported an association between depressive symptoms and symptoms of HIV infection but not lymphocyte subsets. More recently, stress and depressive symptoms, particularly when they occurred jointly, were found to be associated with decreased cytotoxic (CD8+) T lymphocyte subsets as well as NK cells in men and women with HIV (Cruess et al. 2003; Evans et al. 2002; Leserman et al. 1997). Data from up to 7.5 years of a prospective study of HIV-infected men provide evidence that stress, social support, coping style, and depression can affect disease progression (Leserman et al. 1999, 2000). Interestingly, hopelessness as an individual variable was shown to affect disease progression, at least by CD4 count measures (Perry et al. 1992). Overall, it appears that life event stress (particularly bereavement) as well as depression can affect disease-relevant immunologic parameters in addition to disease progression in HIV patients. Nevertheless, it remains unclear whether treatment of depression and/or life stress can prolong survival. Of note in this regard, a cognitive-behavioral stress management intervention was shown to reduce depressive symptoms and cortisol secretion in association with evidence of increased CD4+CD45RA+CD29+ lymphocytes (Antoni et al. 2005).

OTHER VIRAL INFECTIONS

Several viral infections of humans, such as herpes simplex and herpes zoster viruses, cause initial infection and then enter into a state of latency, becoming reactivated at later times. The reactivation of these viruses is known to be associated with immune compromise, such as occurs in patients on chemotherapy or in those with AIDS. However, the data are mixed regarding how psychological factors—including stress, depression, and coping style—affect the body's interaction with these viruses. Elevated titers of antibodies against herpes viruses have been reported in stressed individuals, and although some clinicians suggest that this indicates decreased containment of latent viruses by the immune system, the clinical relevance remains unclear. A large meta-analytic review by Zorrilla and colleagues (1996) concluded that depressive symptoms were related to increased risk of recurrence of herpes simplex virus, whereas stress was not. In contrast, a prospective study of women with genital herpes found that persistent stress was associated with increased risk of recurrence, whereas short-term stress or depressed mood showed no such association (F. Cohen et al. 1999). Irwin and colleagues (1998) reported that patients with major depression demonstrated a decreased number of varicella zoster virus responder cells compared with controls. Interestingly, this pattern resembles the immunity pattern found in older patients (age >60 years). These findings of changes in viral activity provide further evidence for the clinical significance of the altered immune parameters found during stress and depression.

AUTOIMMUNE DISEASES

Autoimmune diseases are thought to result from a process of self antigens being misidentified as nonself, with subsequent proliferation of immune responses against self tis-

sues. The mechanisms by which this misidentification occurs are unknown, but a combination of genetic predisposition, environmental stimuli such as physical stressors and viral exposures, and psychological factors is believed to be involved. Work in the last decade identified particular patterns of immune activation associated with the various systemic autoimmune illnesses. For example, rheumatoid arthritis (RA) is characterized by increased cellular, or Th1, immunity, whereas excessive humoral, or Th2, immunity is associated with SLE (see Figure 3–2C for a summary of Th1 and Th2 immune processes). The interactions among an individual's human leukocyte antigen (HLA) makeup, environmental exposures to antigens, and hormonal pathways seem to be crucial to initiating and maintaining these illnesses. Important hormonal pathways involved in autoimmune disorders include the adrenal and gonadal steroids; in particular, the immunoregulatory activity of estrogen is thought to contribute to the high prevalence of autoimmune disease in women (see Figure 3–2C). Because both immune suppression and immune activation can occur in response to various stressors, the interactions among psychological factors and the clinical course of these diseases are complex. This section presents evidence for how stress and depression affect the onset and course of autoimmune diseases, including multiple sclerosis (MS), SLE, RA, and Graves' disease.

Multiple Sclerosis

MS is a relapsing and remitting neurological disease characterized by focal areas of CNS demyelination. Although the precise etiology of MS is unknown, autoimmunity against myelin and probably other CNS antigens appears to be involved. The course of MS typically waxes as new lesions (accompanied by inflammation) appear and wanes as the inflammation resolves. In general, though, the disease is progressive as new areas of demyelination continue to appear and neurologic impairment increases.

Clinicians have long debated how psychological factors affect the course of MS and have speculated that stress, negative life events, or psychological factors might be associated with clinical exacerbations of the illness. Results of studies have been mixed. Some studies reported an association between stressors and the onset or exacerbation of MS, whereas others found no such association. A particularly well-constructed study by Grant and colleagues (1989) found that patients with MS reported more life difficulties in the year preceding the onset of MS or within several months before exacerbations of the illness. In this study, only patients who were recently diagnosed or did not yet have a confirmed diagnosis of MS were included; thus, the subjects had only limited symptomatology at the time of study. In addition, structured interviews of adverse life events were complemented by a consensus rating of the severity of the stressor, thus avoiding inclusion of trivial events. Mohr and colleagues (2000) reported results of a prospective 2-year study examining the relationship between life stress, conflict, or psychological distress and new MS lesions on magnetic resonance images. They found that an increase in conflict and disruption of life routine (but not psychological distress) were associated with new lesions found on magnetic resonance images 4 and 8 weeks later; however, conflict, disruption of routine, and psychological distress were not related to clinical exacerbation of symptoms. These data suggest that certain psychological factors are associated with pathophysiological changes of MS, although not necessarily with clinical findings. An interesting prospective study evaluated 32 patients with MS exposed to the threat of missile attacks during the Persian Gulf War (Nisipeanu and Korczyn 1993). The researchers reported a decrease in the number of relapses in these patients during this period of extremely high stress. Therefore, it is possible that very high levels of stress are associated with marked increases in cortisol that inhibit disease activity. Further suggestion of a role for the HPA axis in MS patients was provided by Then Bergh and colleagues (1999), who found that MS patients exhibited glucocorticoid resistance, as manifested by altered results on dexamethasone/corticotropin-releasing hormone (CRH) challenge.

Relevant to the treatment implications of the impact of psychosocial factors on disease parameters in MS patients, it has been shown that treatment of depression in MS patients is associated with decreases in IFN-γ production by T cells, an effect that is modulated in part by social support (Mohr and Genain 2004; Mohr et al. 2001). Notably, IFN-γ production by T cells is believed to be a critical factor in MS pathogenesis, preceding and causing exacerbation.

Rheumatoid Arthritis

RA is an inflammatory disease manifested by chronic and disabling destruction of the joints. Like other autoimmune diseases, RA is more common in women, and hormonal mechanisms appear to be important to the development and progression of the disease. RA is accompanied by an excess of Th1 cell activation. A variety of psychosocial factors also appear to be related to the disease course, including acute and chronic stressors, individual personality variables, and social support (Herrmann et al. 2000). Some evidence suggests that major life events are associated with the onset of RA in predisposed individuals. One serologic marker for RA is the presence of rheumatoid factors (RFs). Stewart and colleagues (1994) evaluated

RA patients who were either RF positive or RF negative. They found that the RF-negative patients had higher scores on scales reporting negative life events before the onset of disease, whereas RF-positive patients did not exhibit such a strong association. In addition, objective measures of disease activity correlated with stress levels in the RF-negative group but not in the RF-positive group. This work suggests that stress may influence the onset and course of disease in different subgroups of patients. Furthermore, the role of stress may vary depending on one's predisposition to the disease, which may be determined by genetic or other constitutional factors. It may be that the RF-positive patients have a lower threshold for development of the disease and that therefore, stress is not required for the development of the disorder. For patients who are RF negative, however, larger amounts of stress may be necessary to drive disease activity.

Other research evaluating the effects of stress on the course of RA found no clear answer regarding the role of stress in the illness. Thomason and colleagues (1992) examined major and minor stressors, pain, disability, and erythrocyte sedimentation rate, a common serologic marker of inflammation. The researchers found no association between major stressors and RA status. However, after controlling for global disease status and major stressors, they found that minor stress did correlate with inflammation.

It is believed that RA may be related to dysregulation of negative feedback to the immune system by the glucocorticoid hormone cortisol. Chikanza and colleagues (1992) compared hormonal and immune responses to the physical stress of surgery in patients with RA, osteoarthritis, and osteomyelitis. Patients with osteomyelitis exhibited increases in IL-1β, IL-6, and cortisol after surgery. In contrast, although surgery was associated with elevations in IL-1β and IL-6 in RA patients, there was no corresponding increase of cortisol. Both groups of patients had similarly elevated erythrocyte sedimentation rates, suggesting that although both had inflammation, the adrenal production of cortisol was not appropriately elevated given the level of inflammation in the patients with RA. A similar finding was reported by Kanik and colleagues (2000), who found no relationship between inflammatory indices and cortisol levels in RA patients at baseline. In addition to cortisol, altered responses to catecholamines also were reported in RA patients (Kittner et al. 2002), possibly related to alterations in adrenergic receptor signaling (Lombardi et al. 1999).

Depression is commonly comorbid with RA and may relate to psychosocial factors such as pain and disability. Depression in patients with RA also was shown to be associated with increased mortality (Ang et al. 2005), and treatment with antidepressants led to improvements in RA-associated pain and disability (Bird and Broggini

2000). Depression in RA patients may be related to circulating immune factors released as part of the inflammatory process of the illness. In fact, studies reported increases in the proinflammatory cytokines IL-1, IL-6, and TNF-α in the joint spaces and serum of RA patients, which may mediate the depression that commonly occurs in RA (Steiner et al. 1999). The soluble IL-2 receptor (sIL-2R) is a marker for immune activation, and its presence was correlated with increased disease activity in RA. Harrington and colleagues (1993) examined the relationships among joint inflammation, mood, and levels of sIL-2R. Although the researchers found that joint swelling corresponded to increased sIL-2R levels, disturbed mood was surprisingly associated with decreased sIL-2R levels. More work is needed to explore the relationships among stress, depression, and disease activity in RA, paying attention to immune, HPA axis, and autonomic nervous system alterations that mediate these relationships.

Systemic Lupus Erythematosus

SLE is an autoimmune disorder with multiple systemic manifestations. The pathology of SLE has been identified as primarily antibody mediated, resulting in deposition of antigen-antibody immune complexes in tissues. Because SLE is approximately 10 times more common in women than in men, hormonal mechanisms are thought to play a critical role in the initiation and perpetuation of the illness. The proinflammatory effect of estrogen seems to influence the course of disease, as flares of the disease increase during pregnancy and drop off after menopause. Pregnancy is accompanied by a shift from Th1 to Th2 activity that seems to exacerbate SLE. Estrogen replacement therapy also increases the risk of development of SLE. The question of stress or other psychosocial factors in exacerbating the illness has been of interest to clinicians and researchers over the years. For example, DaCosta and colleagues (1999) found that a history of stressful life events in the 6 months before evaluation correlated with reduced functional ability 8 months after evaluation. Increasing severity of depression scores also was correlated with changes in functional ability 8 months after evaluation. Research on a large cohort of patients with SLE indicated that greater disease activity in SLE patients was associated with less social support and that increased physical disability was associated with depression in these patients (Ward et al. 1999). A possible mechanism for effects of psychosocial status on disease activity may involve stress-induced activation of autoreactive B cell clones via an increase in IL-4–producing cells (Jacobs et al. 2001). Taken together, the evidence suggests that stress and depression play a role in the clinical course of SLE.

Graves' Disease

Graves' disease is an antibody-mediated autoimmune disorder in which antibody to the thyroid-stimulating hormone (TSH) receptor stimulates the gland to produce thyroid hormone. Despite markedly increased levels of circulating thyroid hormones and accompanying decreases in thyrotropin-releasing hormone and TSH, the thyroid gland continues to produce hormone. The illness is accompanied by an increased likelihood of possessing the HLA type DR3. As with other autoimmune illnesses, clinicians have been interested in investigating the role of stress and psychological functioning in precipitating or exacerbating the illness. One factor that must be considered in these studies is that elevated thyroid hormone levels may alter retrospective recall of stressful events, perception of current stress, or behavior that might precipitate stressful events. Some studies have found an increase in stressful life events to be associated with the onset of the disease. Sonino and colleagues (1993) reported that an increase in multiple types of life events—positive and negative, controlled and uncontrolled—was associated with the onset of the illness. One strength of this study was that the patients were interviewed regarding stressful events after they were in remission from the disease. Another group found that stressful life events and smoking both were associated with the development of Graves' disease in women but not in men (Yoshiuchi et al. 1998). Because the disease is more prevalent in women and estrogen is thought to play a role because of its immunostimulatory effects (similar to what occurs in SLE), it is possible that development of the disease in men is associated with a stronger genetic predisposition than in women. Thus, although the disease is multifactorial, there is evidence for the role of stress and psychological factors in its onset, especially in women.

PANDAS

An immune-related disorder with neuropsychiatric manifestations occurring in children has been identified; it is called pediatric autoimmune neuropsychiatric disorder associated with streptococcal infections (PANDAS). The disorder, which has been characterized in case series and in well-controlled epidemiological studies, is associated with the immune response to infection with group A β-hemolytic streptococcus and involves the development of neuropsychiatric syndromes, including obsessive-compulsive disorder and tic disorder, after a primary infection with group A β-hemolytic streptococcus (Mell et al. 2005; Swedo et al. 1998). The symptom course is relapsing and remitting with exacerbations on reinfection with group A β-hemolytic streptococcus. The pathophysiology of this disorder is thought to be the result of antibodies against the group A β-hemolytic streptococcus, which cross-react with neuronal antigens, particularly in the basal ganglia. Both intravenous immunoglobulin and plasma exchange have been shown to produce clinical improvement, and data indicate that prophylaxis of streptococcal infections with relevant antibiotics can prevent symptom exacerbations in vulnerable patients (Snider et al. 2005). These intriguing data suggest that brain antigens may become direct targets of autoimmune processes, leading to neuropsychiatric disorders with protean manifestations.

PSYCHIATRIC ILLNESS AND IMMUNE FUNCTION

During the past several decades, a tremendous amount of information has been amassed from investigations of immune parameters in the major psychiatric illnesses. Results indicate that the immune system may play a role in many of the major psychiatric disorders, with important treatment implications.

DEPRESSION

The question of altered immunity in major depression has received the most attention with regard to the relationship among the nervous, endocrine, and immune systems in psychiatric disorders. Early work suggested that major depression is accompanied by impaired immunity, but subsequent studies present a more complicated picture. Immune changes accompanying depression include decreased lymphocyte count, increased neutrophil number, decreased mitogen responses of peripheral blood lymphocytes, and decreased NK cell activity (Table 3–5). At least two meta-analyses have confirmed these findings (Herbert and Cohen 1993; Segerstrom and Miller 2004).

Nevertheless, although the results in toto suggest immune alterations in depressed patients, important exceptions are apparent, indicating that the findings are not reproducible across studies. For example, Schleifer et al. (1989) and Andreoli et al. (1993) failed to detect differences in immune function in depressed patients who were compared with carefully matched control subjects. These two studies controlled for a number of relevant variables, including age, sex, severity of depression, level of physical activity, and alcohol and tobacco use. Although no mean differences between groups of depressed and nondepressed patients were found, particular subgroups of depressed patients in these and other studies have been shown to exhibit immune abnormalities. When immune

TABLE 3–5. Summary of immune changes in major depression

Peripheral blood

Decreased lymphocyte number

Increased neutrophil number

Decreased peripheral blood lymphocyte responses to mitogens

Decreased natural killer cell activity

Increased IL-6, soluble IL-6 receptor, soluble IL-2 receptor

Decreased IL-2

Increased acute phase proteins (C-reactive protein, α1-acid glycoprotein, haptoglobin, α1-antitrypsin, complement protein C4)

Cerebrospinal fluid

Decreased IL-6, soluble IL-6 receptor

Increased IL-1β

Note. IL = interleukin.

changes are found in depression, they typically accompany other characteristics of depressed patients. For example, although Schleifer and colleagues (1989) found no differences in mean values for immune measures between depressed and nondepressed groups, greater age and more severe depression were associated with decreases in CD4+ cell numbers and mitogen responsiveness of peripheral blood lymphocytes. A 1994 study reported that decreased NK cell activity in depressed patients was associated with sleep disturbance (Cover and Irwin 1994). Several studies have reported that male patients with depression are more likely than female patients with depression to have decreases in NK cells (Evans et al. 1992). Decreased circulating levels of NK cells also were associated with greater severity of depression (Evans et al. 1992). Thus, although depression as a factor in itself may not explain alterations in immune parameters, depression in the context of greater age, altered sleep, male sex, or more severe symptoms may be most likely to be associated with altered immune parameters.

More recent research has addressed the possibility that certain aspects of the immune response may become activated in depressed patients, particularly innate immunity as measured by acute phase proteins and proinflammatory cytokines (Raison et al. 2006). This possibility is consistent with the clinical observation of a high rate of depression in patients with autoimmune and other immune-related diseases, demonstrating that depression can coexist with immune activation. Moreover, a syndrome of "sickness behavior" resembling major depression occurs with the administration of cytokine therapies such as IFN-α and IL-2 (Capuron and Miller 2004; Dantzer 2004). Prominent features of this syndrome include depressed mood, anhedonia, sleep and appetite disturbances, malaise, and poor concentration. Because of the resemblance of the syndrome of sickness behavior to major depression, levels of serum cytokines and acute phase proteins in depressed patients have received special attention. A variety of results have been reported regarding abnormalities in serum levels of cytokines and acute phase proteins in patients with major depression (see Table 3–5). Overall patterns found in serum cytokine levels include increases in the proinflammatory cytokine IL-6, increases in soluble IL-6 receptor (sIL-6R) and sIL-2R, and a decrease in IL-2. Increases in acute phase proteins such as C-reactive protein, serum haptoglobin, the complement protein C4, α1-acid glycoprotein, and α1-antitrypsin also have been reported in several well-controlled studies. Not all studies have confirmed the findings of serum cytokine alterations, however. A large study examined serum cytokine levels in 361 psychiatric inpatients with a variety of diagnoses compared with healthy control subjects (Haack et al. 1999). After accounting for many individual variables such as sex, smoking status, and body mass index, the only differences found in major depression were slightly decreased serum levels of TNF-α and soluble TNF-α receptor p55.

Stubner and colleagues (1999) measured cytokine levels in the CSF of patients with depression and compared these levels with those measured in control subjects. They studied 20 elderly patients and 20 matched control subjects. It should be noted that all patients except one were taking psychotropic medication. This study found decreased levels of IL-6 and sIL-6R in the CSF of the depressed patients compared with the control subjects. When the CSF of hospitalized depressed patients was compared with that of 10 control subjects, higher levels of IL-1β, lower levels of IL-6, and no change in TNF-α levels were found in the depressed patients (Levine et al. 1999).

Several studies have examined measures of immune activation after recovery from depression. Significantly higher mitogen-induced production of IFN-γ and sIL-2R was found in hospitalized patients with depression compared with control subjects (Seidel et al. 1995). These parameters normalized over 6 weeks of successful treatment. Initially increased serum levels of C-reactive protein, haptoglobin, and α2-macroglobulin also normalized over this time period. Interestingly, patients with treatment-resistant depression may be especially likely to exhibit immune activation, as reflected by increased plasma concentrations

of IL-6 and sIL-6R (Maes 1999). These data suggest that cytokine antagonists may offer an intriguing alternative to standard antidepressant therapy in treatment-resistant patients. Indeed, animal studies have indicated that cytokine-induced depressive-like symptoms can be reversed or attenuated by pretreatment with cytokine synthesis inhibitors and cytokine antagonists or by genetic manipulation (e.g., knockout) of cytokine gene expression (Meyers 1999; Yirmiya et al. 2000). Moreover, depressive symptoms have been found to be reversed in RA patients treated with a drug that antagonizes TNF (Mathias et al. 2000).

Finally, the genetics of the immune system in relation to major depression have been explored. The data suggest that certain gene polymorphisms (e.g., genes encoding for IL-1 and TNF-α) may predict susceptibility to depressive illness and antidepressant responsiveness (Fertuzinhos et al. 2004; Jun et al. 2003; Rosa et al. 2004).

SCHIZOPHRENIA

The search for a cause of schizophrenia has led to the immune system for several reasons. First, the possibility of a viral (or bacterial) infection (superinfection) during neural development has been suggested by several epidemiological studies (Yolken and Torrey 1995). Findings include 1) an increased likelihood that schizophrenic patients were born in late winter or spring; 2) an association between viral epidemics during pregnancy and later development of schizophrenia in the offspring; and 3) an increased likelihood of older siblings being in the household during pregnancies (siblings are thought to be a potential source for viral infections). Moreover, the clinical presentation of schizophrenia, particularly the early prodromal symptoms, neurological "soft signs," and the global dysfunction caused by the disease suggest the possibility of early disruption in brain development.

Specific measures of immune function in schizophrenic patients have presented an overall pattern of immune activation in this illness. Table 3–6 summarizes immune alterations that have been reported in patients with schizophrenia. Increased numbers of immune cells such as B cells, CD4+ lymphocytes, and monocytes have been reported in multiple studies. In at least two studies, a subset of patients have exhibited increased numbers of CD5+ B cells, a B cell subset associated with autoimmune disease (McAllister et al. 1989; Printz et al. 1999).

Despite the changes in cell numbers, there have been conflicting reports regarding alterations in lymphocyte responses to mitogens and NK cell activity. Studies have reported increases (Yovel et al. 2000), decreases (Abdeljaber et al. 1994; Ganguli et al. 1995; Sasaki et al. 1994), and no change (Caldwell et al. 1991). Factors such as

TABLE 3–6. Summary of immune changes in schizophrenia

Peripheral blood

Increased number of B cells, CD4+ lymphocytes, monocytes

Increased number of CD5+ cells

Increased soluble IL-2 receptor

Increased IL-2 levels in serum

Decreased IL-2 production by mitogen-stimulated lymphocytes

Decreased sICAM-1

Increased levels of haptoglobin, fibrinogen, complement proteins C3C and C4, α1-acid glycoprotein, hemopexin

Cerebrospinal fluid

Increased IL-2

Increased soluble IL-6 receptor

Increased IL-10

Increased α2-haptoglobin

Increased soluble intercellular adhesion molecule

Increased albumin

Note. IL=interleukin; sICAM-1=soluble intercellular adhesion molecule 1.

---

smoking status may confound the results of these functional studies, particularly NK cell activity.

Several specific cytokines, including IL-6 and IL-2, have been implicated in schizophrenia. Increases in serum IL-6 levels have been reported in schizophrenic patients, particularly in those with longer duration of illness or more severe symptomatology. Increases in serum sIL-2R concentrations also have been found, possibly representing a state marker for schizophrenia, because the increases were seen only in the affected twin of nonconcordant twin pairs (Ganguli and Rabin 1989). The involvement of IL-2 in schizophrenia is further suggested by the observation that IL-2 administration can provoke psychotic symptoms and cognitive impairment in nonpsychiatric patients. An increased IL-2 level in the serum also was reported (Kim et al. 2000); however, in vitro production of IL-2 by stimulated lymphocytes was decreased, possibly representing lymphocyte "exhaustion" due to sustained in vivo IL-2 production versus a decreased capacity of lymphocytes to produce IL-2. In contrast to these abnormalities, a large study of immune factors in psychiatric inpatients and psychiatrically healthy control subjects found that the only abnormality in schizophrenic patients was a slightly decreased soluble TNF-α receptor p55 subunit (Haack et al. 1999).

Elevations in serum acute phase proteins, which are nonspecific accompaniments to inflammation, also have been reported in patients with schizophrenia. Elevations have been reported in haptoglobin, fibrinogen, the complement proteins C3C and C4, α1-acid glycoprotein, and hemopexin in schizophrenia (Maes et al. 1997). Other groups have found similar elevations in multiple acute phase proteins. A small postmortem study of brain tissue from schizophrenic patients found elevated levels of fibrinogen split products (Korschenhausen et al. 1996).

Studies of immune measures, including cytokines and their receptors and acute phase proteins, in the CSF of schizophrenic patients have produced inconsistent results, but taken together they suggest the presence of immune activation. An increase in CSF IL-2 has been reported in untreated schizophrenic patients (Licinio et al. 1993), although no change has been found in other studies. An increased sIL-6R concentration in the CSF suggests immune activation, because the IL-6 receptor when bound to IL-6 increases its activity. A relationship has been suggested between high levels of sIL-6R in the CSF and positive symptoms of psychosis. Increased IL-10 in the CSF has been correlated to an increase in negative symptoms of psychosis. Other studied cytokines that have yielded conflicting results include IL-1 and TNF. An increase in the acute phase protein α2-haptoglobin was found in the CSF of schizophrenic patients. Elevated CSF levels of soluble intercellular adhesion molecules and albumin in schizophrenic patients suggest an impairment of the integrity of the blood-brain barrier in at least a subset of patients with schizophrenia. Impairment of blood-brain barrier integrity can accompany a process of immune activation. More recent studies have focused on the balance between Th1 and Th2 cytokines in schizophrenic patients, with some data indicating a higher Th1/Th2 ratio, which is attenuated by effective neuroleptic treatment (Kim et al. 2004).

The evidence of activation of aspects of the immune system, particularly the elevations in proinflammatory cytokines and IL-2, suggests that inflammation in response to infection or as part of an autoimmune process may contribute to schizophrenia. However, neither infectious agents nor autoantibodies to CNS antigens have been consistently identified in patients with schizophrenia (Yolken and Torrey 1995). Another possible explanation for the development of schizophrenia is exposure to a viral infection early in development that disrupts neural development and is subsequently cleared from the body. In addition, an environmental stimulus may trigger a temporary autoimmune response similar to the cardiac injury that occurs in patients with rheumatic fever after infection with β-hemolytic streptococci (Delves and Roitt 2000a, 2000b). Clearly, more research in this area is required before any role of the immune system can be substantiated. Nevertheless, data indicating that addition of the anti-inflammatory agent celecoxib (a cyclooxygenase 2 inhibitor) to standard therapy with an antipsychotic agent can improve treatment outcome in schizophrenic patients are intriguing and provide some indication of the potential translational promise of this line of inquiry (Muller et al. 2002; Riedel et al. 2005).

BIPOLAR DISORDER

Bipolar disorder has not received as much attention as depression or schizophrenia in the search for immune alterations. Presentations of the illness vary dramatically, and studies similarly vary as to the clinical status of the patients studied. The relapsing and remitting, chronic nature of the disorder highlights the question of state versus trait abnormalities in this illness in particular and in psychiatric illnesses in general.

Tsai and colleagues (1999) used a case–control design to investigate several functional measures of immunity in patients with bipolar disorder during mania and after remission. Lymphocyte proliferative responses to the mitogen phytohemagglutinin were increased during the manic phase, as were plasma sIL-2R levels. These findings normalized after remission of the disease. One group reported increased levels of sIL-2R and sIL-6R in symptomatic patients with rapid-cycling bipolar disorder, which normalized after 30 days of treatment with lithium (Rapaport et al. 1999). Interestingly, levels of IL-2, sIL-2R, and sIL-6R also were increased in psychiatrically healthy volunteers who took lithium. Other findings in manic patients have included significantly elevated levels of total immunoglobulins and complement proteins, and lower levels of serum IgD (Wadee et al. 2002). In addition, manic patients were found to exhibit increased levels of organ-specific autoantibodies (Padmos et al. 2004). These findings suggest that immune abnormalities occur in bipolar disorder, perhaps during acute phases of the illness. More work is needed in this area to determine what, if any, immune alterations reliably occur in this disease, if these alterations represent state or trait changes, and whether observed immune changes represent viable therapeutic targets.

MECHANISMS OF BRAIN-IMMUNE INTERACTIONS

There are many pathways through which the immune system and brain interact and mediate the complex relationships observed in various clinical conditions. These pathways involve nervous system innervation of lymphoid tissue, the expression of relevant receptors on immune cells for transmitters derived from the nervous system, and access to and presence of cytokines and their receptors in the brain.

NEURAL INNERVATION OF IMMUNE TISSUES

A primary mechanism by which the nervous and immune systems interact is via autonomic nervous system innervation of lymphoid tissues. Nerve fibers of the sympathetic branch of the autonomic nervous system have been best described and are found in the bone marrow, thymus, spleen, and lymph nodes (Felten et al. 1984; Giron et al. 1980; Williams et al. 1981). Nerve fibers arising from the vagus, phrenic, and recurrent laryngeal nerves, with contributions from the stellate ganglia of the thoracic sympathetic chain, innervate the thymus gland. The celiac ganglion provides sympathetic nerves to the spleen, and the bone marrow is innervated by nerve fibers arising from the level of the spinal cord associated with the location of the bone. Autonomic nervous system innervation of the lymph nodes is not as dense or as uniquely distributed as that of the spleen or thymus. In general, sympathetic nerve fibers enter lymphoid tissues in association with the vascular supply. Although autonomic nerve fibers play an important role in regulating vascular tone, sympathetic (noradrenergic) nerve terminals, as identified by tyrosine hydroxylase staining, have been found deep in the parenchyma of immune tissues in close association with immune cells (Figure 3–3). Aside from catecholamines, other relevant neurotransmitters (neuropeptides) are expressed in nerve fibers innervating immune tissues, including neuropeptide Y, substance P, vasoactive intestinal peptide, calcitonin gene–related peptide, and CRH. Interruption of autonomic nervous system fibers by pharmacologic or surgical means has been shown to attenuate inhibitory influences of catecholamines on acquired immune responses and NK cell activity and to block the effects of stress on immune function in the spleen.

As an example of the bidirectional nature of nervous-immune system interactions, data suggest that locally released cytokines can influence neurotransmitter release from nerve fibers in immune tissues. Finally, stimulation of the vagus nerve (motor branch of the vagus) was shown to reduce the release of inflammatory cytokines in response to immune stimulation and protect animals from the lethality of septic shock (Borovikova et al. 2000). These effects are mediated via activation of acetylcholine α7 nicotinic receptors, which in turn was shown to reduce the induction of NFkB and subsequently the inflammatory response, including the production of TNF-α (Pavlov and Tracey 2005).

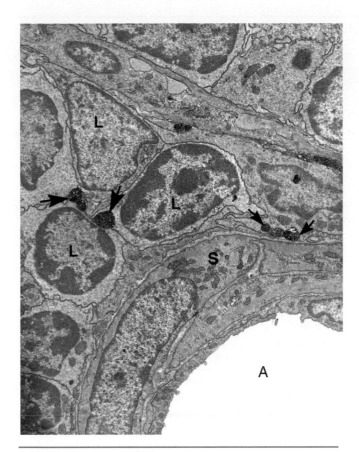

FIGURE 3–3. Sympathetic nervous system innervation of lymphoid tissue. Tyrosine hydroxylase-immunoreactive nerve processes (*small arrowheads*) in contact with the smooth muscle (S) of the central arteriole (A), and nerve processes (*large arrowheads*) in direct contact with lymphocytes (L) in the periarteriolar lymphatic sheath of the rat spleen. (Transmission electron micrograph, 6,732×.)

Source. Courtesy of Denise L. Bellinger, Department of Neurology and Anatomy, University of Rochester School of Medicine and Dentistry, Rochester, NY. Reprinted with permission from Miller AH, Pariante CM, Pearce BD: "Immune System and Central Nervous System Interactions," in *Comprehensive Textbook of Psychiatry/VII.* Edited by Kaplan HI, Sadock BJ. Philadelphia, PA, Lippincott Williams and Wilkins, 2000, p. 123.

These data suggest that the α7 nicotinic receptor may serve as a novel therapeutic target for anti-inflammatory agents.

IMMUNE CELL RECEPTORS FOR NEURALLY DERIVED MOLECULES

Cells of the immune system express receptors for a variety of molecules that are regulated or produced by the nervous system. The β-adrenergic receptor was one of the first receptors identified on lymphocytes, and over the years receptors for virtually all of the major neurotransmitters, hormones, and neuropeptides have been characterized on immune cells (Table 3–7).

Several important concepts are relevant to understanding the effects of neurally derived molecules on immune function. First, the expression of receptors is heterogeneous. For example, of the two types of receptors for adrenal steroids—mineralocorticoid receptors and glucocorticoid receptors—only glucocorticoid receptors are expressed in the thymus, whereas both glucocorticoid and mineralocorticoid receptors are expressed in the spleen. Related to heterogeneity in receptor expression in immune cells and tissues is heterogeneity in receptor density. For example, of the three subsets of T cells, the number of β-adrenergic receptors is highest for T suppressor cells, followed by T cytotoxic cells and then T helper cells.

Heterogeneity of both receptor expression and receptor density is important for understanding the sensitivities of the various immune cells and tissues to circulating hormones and is important for determining the net effect of those agents on immune function in vivo.

A second important concept is that the microenvironment of any given tissue is critical in determining hormonal or neurotransmitter influences on immune function. This concept even applies to circulating factors whose access to receptors of local immune cells depends on a host of tissue enzymes and binding proteins. Thus, the influence of any given molecule on the immune system is a function of 1) the type of cell that exhibits the relevant receptor, 2) the density of the receptors on that cell, and 3) whether that cell is located in an immune compartment that allows access of the relevant molecule to the receptor under the conditions being studied. Finally, crosstalk between receptor-associated signal transduction pathways is an important biochemical mechanism by which neurally derived or regulated molecules influence the immune response.

MAJOR PATHWAYS OF BRAIN TO IMMUNE SIGNALING

Given the above-noted capacity of the immune system to receive signals from the nervous and endocrine systems, investigators have begun to tease apart the relative contributions of the two major outflow pathways activated by stress: the HPA axis and the sympathetic nervous system (SNS) (Figure 3–4).

Hypothalamic-Pituitary-Adrenal Axis

Glucocorticoids, the final product of HPA axis activation, have well-documented effects on multiple aspects of the immune system (Dhabhar and McEwen 2001; McEwen et al. 1997; Schleimer et al. 1989; Wilckens and DeRijk 1997). Glucocorticoids influence the immune response by 1) modulating the trafficking of immune cells throughout the body (Dhabhar et al. 1995, 1996; Miller et al. 1994);

TABLE 3–7.   Receptors expressed on immune cells for neurotransmitters, hormones, and peptides

Neurotransmitters	Hormones	Peptides
Acetylcholine	Corticosteroids	ACTH
Dopamine	(glucocorticoids,	α-MSH
Histamine	mineralocorticoids)	AVP
Norepinephrine	Gonadal steroids	Calcitonin
Serotonin	(estrogen,	CGRP
	progesterone,	CRH
	testosterone)	GHRH
	Growth hormone	GnRH
	Opioids (endorphins,	IGF-I
	enkephalins)	Melatonin
	Prolactin	NPY
	Thyroid hormone	PTH
		Somatostatin
		Substance P
		TRH
		TSH
		VIP

Note.   ACTH = adrenocorticotropin; α-MSH = α-melanocyte-stimulating hormone; AVP = arginine vasopressin; CGRP = calcitonin gene–related peptide; CRH = corticotropin-releasing hormone; GHRH = growth hormone–releasing hormone; GnRH = gonado-tropin-releasing hormone; IGF-I = insulin-like growth factor 1; NPY = neuropeptide Y; PTH = parathyroid hormone; TRH = thyro-tropin-releasing hormone; TSH = thyroid-stimulating hormone; VIP = vasoactive intestinal peptide.

2) inhibiting cytokine production and function through interaction of glucocorticoid receptors with transcription factors (e.g., AP-1, NFkB), which in turn regulate cytokine gene expression and/or the expression of cytokine-inducible genes (Almawi et al. 1990; Auphan et al. 1995; Rhen and Cidlowski 2005; Vacca et al. 1992); 3) inhibiting the generation of products of the arachidonic acid pathway, which mediate inflammation (Goldstein et al. 1992; Schleimer et al. 1989); 4) inhibiting T cell–mediated and NK cell–mediated cytotoxicity (Nair and Schwartz 1984); 5) modulating cell death pathways in immature and mature cell types (J.J. Cohen 1989; Gonzalo et al. 1993; McEwen et al. 1997; Wyllie 1980); and 6) modulating the Th1/Th2 phenotype of the immune response by inhibiting Th1 (cell-mediated) responses and enhancing Th2 (antibody) responses (see Figure 3–2C).

Glucocorticoids mediate some of the acute effects of stress on the immune system, including the effects of stress on peripheral blood immune cell distribution and lymphocyte proliferative responses to mitogens in rodents, as well as the inhibitory effects of stress on lymph node cellularity during viral infections in mice (Cunnick et al. 1990; Dhabhar et al. 1995, 1996; Hermann et al. 1995). Finally, as discussed in the next paragraph, glucocorticoids appear to mediate some of the effects of CRH on immune responses.

Although glucocorticoids are best known for their ability to mediate the immunosuppressive effects of stress, it is important to mention that glucocorticoid hormones also play an important role in maintaining bodily homeostasis and protecting the body against an overshoot of potentially damaging immune activation (Munck and Guyre 1991). For example, neutralization of endogenous glucocorticoid function results in increases in pathological symptoms and mortality rate in animals exposed to endotoxin (e.g., lipopolysaccharide) and autoimmunity-inducing stimuli (e.g., streptococcal cell wall antigen or myelin basic protein) (Bertini et al. 1988; Sternberg et al. 1989). Similar increases in pathological symptoms (as well as death) have been found to occur after viral infections in the absence of glucocorticoids (Miller et al. 2000; Price et al. 1996; Ruzek et al. 1999). Regarding inflammatory responses in the brain, glucocorticoids have been shown to have an essential role in protecting the brain against innate immune responses (Nadeau and Rivest 2003). These data support the notion that glucocorticoids are immunomodulators and that the ultimate effects of stress-induced elevations in glucocorticoids are a function of the context within which they occur.

Sympathetic Nervous System

As might be anticipated by the pattern of nervous innervation of lymphoid tissues, abrogation of stress-induced

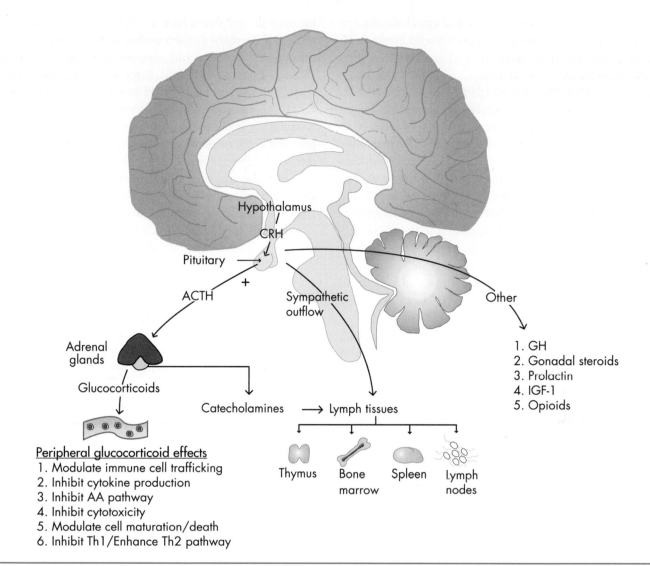

Hypothalamus

CRH

Pituitary

+

ACTH

Sympathetic
outflow

Other

Adrenal
glands

Glucocorticoids

Catecholamines → Lymph tissues

1. GH
2. Gonadal steroids
3. Prolactin
4. IGF-1
5. Opioids

Peripheral glucocorticoid effects
1. Modulate immune cell trafficking
2. Inhibit cytokine production
3. Inhibit AA pathway
4. Inhibit cytotoxicity
5. Modulate cell maturation/death
6. Inhibit Th1/Enhance Th2 pathway

Thymus   Bone   Spleen   Lymph
          marrow   nodes

FIGURE 3–4. Neuroendocrine mechanisms by which the brain influences the immune system. Activation of the hypothalamic-pituitary-adrenal (HPA) axis and the sympathetic nervous system (SNS) by corticotropin-releasing hormone (CRH) results in the release of glucocorticoids and catecholamines by the adrenal glands and norepinephrine by SNS fibers that innervate immune tissues. Glucocorticoids have multiple immune-mediating effects: mobilizing cells to peripheral immune compartments (e.g., the skin), shaping the relative balance between helper T cell (Th) subtypes, and containing inflammation. Glucocorticoids also provide negative feedback on the HPA axis at several levels, including CRH. Activation of SNS fibers in lymphoid tissues also influences cellular migration and function and helps shape Th cell development. Opioids, sexually dimorphic hormones, growth hormone (GH), and insulin-like growth factor 1 (IGF-1) released from the brain and pituitary also have multiple effects on immunity and in turn can interact with HPA axis and SNS influences. AA=arachidonic acid; ACTH=adrenocorticotropic hormone.

immune changes by antagonizing the SNS (see Figure 3–4) is most apparent in solid immune tissues such as the spleen. For example, Cunnick and colleagues (1990) showed that stress-induced suppression of splenic lymphocyte proliferation to polyclonal mitogens is not influenced by adrenalectomy but is markedly attenuated by β-adrenergic receptor antagonists. Based on this and other studies (Cunnick et al. 1992; A.H. Miller et al. 1990), it is apparent that different neuroendocrine mechanisms can be operative in different immune compartments. Specifically,

immune responses in the peripheral blood seem to be more influenced by glucocorticoids, whereas immune responses in the spleen seem to be more sensitive to catecholamines.

In humans, the SNS appears to play an important role in the immune changes induced by brief experimental stressors, as suggested by the rapid onset of these changes and the higher sensitivity of subjects with increased cardiovascular responses (Herbert et al. 1994). Moreover, the majority of the effects of acute laboratory stressors are blocked by pretreatment with α-adrenergic receptor antagonists

(Bachen et al. 1995). Administration of catecholamines to humans transiently produces immune changes similar both qualitatively and quantitatively to those observed with acute stress (Benschop et al. 1996; Crary et al. 1983; Landmann et al. 1984; Maisel et al. 1989). Catecholamines also were shown to decrease the number of adhesion molecules on lymphocytes (Mills and Dimsdale 1996; Rogers et al. 1999), suggesting that increased SNS activity may alter numbers of circulating lymphocytes by decreasing endothelial adhesion of these cells. Interestingly, acute stress has likewise been shown to decrease the adhesion molecule L-selectin on lymphocytes (Mills and Dimsdale 1996).

Evidence of increased sympathetic activity was described in subjects experiencing chronic life stress (Uchino et al. 1992); therefore, it is likely that the SNS plays a role in certain of the immune changes occurring in association with naturalistic stressors as well. Indeed, data suggest that activation of SNS pathways and release of catecholamines play an important role in the capacity of stress to stimulate inflammatory signaling pathways leading to induction of NFkB and the release of IL-6 (see earlier section "Stress and Immunity in Humans: Laboratory Stressors"). Of relevance in this regard, IL-6 elevations secondary to increases in altitude in humans and induction of NFkB by immobilization stress in mice can be blocked by pretreatment with the α-adrenergic antagonist prazosin (Bierhaus et al. 2003; Mazzeo et al. 2001). Interestingly, while α-adrenergic antagonists abrogate effects of stress-induced activation of proinflammatory cytokines in the periphery, SNS-induced cytokine expression in the brain during stress appears to be mediated by β-adrenergic receptors (Johnson et al. 2005).

Corticotropin-Releasing Hormone

CRH is one of the major factors that regulate interactions between the nervous and immune systems during stress and neuropsychiatric disorders, including both affective and anxiety disorders. CRH released from the paraventricular nucleus in the hypothalamus is a central regulatory neuropeptide in the coordination of the neuroendocrine response to stress and in turn activates both the pituitary-adrenal axis and the SNS. Figure 3–5 presents an overview of feedback pathways among the HPA axis, the SNS, and the immune system. The immunologic effects of CRH on a wide range of immune functions were extensively characterized (Irwin 1993; Irwin et al. 1988, 1990). Intracerebroventricular administration of CRH to laboratory animals was found to suppress NK cell activity in the spleen (Irwin et al. 1988) and to inhibit in vivo and in vitro antibody formation, including the generation of an IgG response to immunization with keyhole-limpet hemocyanin (Irwin 1993; Leu and Singh 1993). CRH-overproduc-

ing mice also exhibited immune deficits characterized by a profound decrease in the number of B cells and severely diminished primary and memory antibody responses (Stenzel-Poore et al. 1996). Long-term intracerebroventricular administration of CRH and short-term infusion of CRH into the locus coeruleus were shown to suppress lymphocyte proliferative responses to nonspecific mitogens and T cell responses to T cell receptor antibody (Caroleo et al. 1993; Labeur et al. 1995; Rassnick et al. 1994).

CRH also has been found to stimulate the release of proinflammatory cytokines in both laboratory animals and humans. For example, long-term intracerebroventricular administration of CRH to rats led to induction of IL-1β mRNA in splenocytes, and short-term intravenous infusion of CRH in humans led to an almost fourfold induction of IL-1β (Labeur et al. 1995; Schulte et al. 1994). Both treatments also led to significant increases in the immunoregulatory cytokine IL-2 (Labeur et al. 1995; Schulte et al. 1994). In addition, CRH was found to induce the release of IL-1 and IL-6 from human mononuclear cells in vitro (Leu and Singh 1992; Paez Pereda et al. 1995). Interestingly, data show that CRH may play a critical role in inflammatory disorders. For example, CRH contributes to the inflammatory response in experimental autoimmune encephalomyelitis. Indeed, CRH-deficient animals are resistant to the disease (Benou et al. 2005).

In the periphery, CRH may play a role in inflammatory responses (Karalis et al. 1991, 1997). Local production of CRH was demonstrated in inflammatory diseases such as ulcerative colitis (Kawahito et al. 1995) and arthritis, in which it was suggested that it acts as a local proinflammatory agent (Nishioka et al. 1996). Evidence also suggests that CRH may act as a protective factor against inflammation-induced pain (Lariviere and Melzack 2000; Schafer et al. 1994) and plasma extravasation (Yoshihara et al. 1995).

Taken together, these results indicate that CRH has immunosuppressive effects on in vivo cellular and humoral responses while having a stimulatory effect on cytokine production and local inflammation.

As for mechanisms by which CRH influences immune responses, the sympathetic ganglionic blocker chlorisondamine was shown to reverse CRH-induced inhibition of NK cell activity in the spleen (Irwin et al. 1988), indicating that the SNS plays a major role in this effect. The HPA axis also is involved, as was shown by Labeur and colleagues (1995), who demonstrated that the effects of long-term intracerebroventricular CRH administration on splenocyte proliferative responses are eliminated by adrenalectomy. In addition, the B cell decreases found in CRH-overproducing mice are very consistent with the marked reduction in rodent B cells found after long-term exposure to glucocorticoids (Miller et al. 1994).

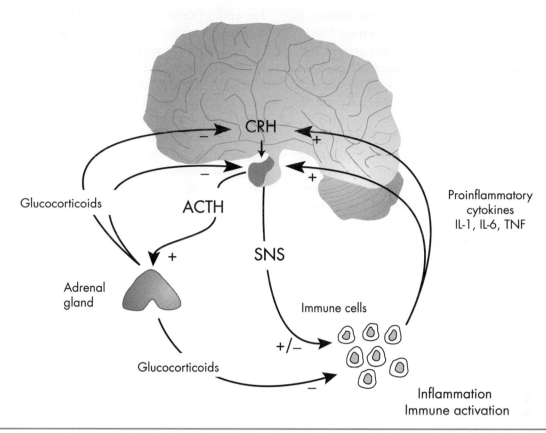

FIGURE 3–5. Bidirectional interactions between the immune system and brain. Immune cells produce cytokines, which stimulate the hypothalamic-pituitary-adrenal (HPA) axis at both the hypothalamus and pituitary. HPA activation results in glucocorticoid release by the adrenal glands via stimulation of pituitary adrenocorticotropic hormone (ACTH). Glucocorticoids, in turn, provide negative feedback to the HPA axis and generally inhibit inflammation. Sympathetic nervous system (SNS) outflow—particularly to lymph tissues such as spleen, bone marrow, and lymph nodes—has a variety of effects on immune cell trafficking and function.

Other Factors

Aside from glucocorticoids and catecholamines, numerous other mediators have been examined for their relevance to interactions among the nervous, endocrine, and immune systems. Of these, opioids, the gonadal steroids, growth hormone, and prolactin are briefly described in this section.

Opioids have well-known effects on the immune system, as determined both in vitro and in vivo (Eisenstein and Hilburger 1998; Hall et al. 1998; Mellon and Bayer 1998; Sharp et al. 1998). Some of the most compelling findings are the profound suppression of a wide range of immune parameters after in vivo administration of morphine (Eisenstein and Hilburger 1998). Morphine inhibits several peripheral immune functions, including NK cell activity, mitogen-induced lymphocyte proliferation, and phagocytic cell function; and these effects are mediated by activation of central opioid receptors (primarily the mu receptor) (Eisenstein and Hilburger 1998; Hall et al. 1998; Mellon and Bayer 1998; Sharp et al. 1998). Short-term effects of morphine are mediated in large

part by the SNS, whereas more chronic effects are mediated by activation of the HPA axis (Mellon and Bayer 1998). Direct effects of morphine on immune cell function also are involved (Sharp et al. 1998). In addition, endogenous opioids appear to play a role in modulating immune responses after stress (Sharp et al. 1998). For example, rats subjected to a foot-shock paradigm known to be associated with opioid analgesia exhibited decreased NK cell activity, which was prevented by administration of the opioid antagonist naltrexone (Shavit et al. 1984). Notably, Yin and colleagues (2000) reported that the effects of endogenous opioids in mediating the immunologic effects of stress were independent of the HPA axis and occurred through induction of increased cell loss (apoptosis) in the spleen. Interestingly, withdrawal of laboratory animals from morphine was found to sensitize them to the effects of lipopolysaccharide, leading to greater lethality and greater induction of inflammatory markers including TNF-α and nitric oxide (Feng et al. 2005).

The role of gonadal steroids in regulating immune responses is exemplified by the sexual dimorphism in immune function (Martin 2000; Whitacre et al. 1999). Adult women have more exuberant antibody responses to immune challenge, reject transplanted tissues more vigorously, are more susceptible to allergies, and live longer than adult men (Martin 2000). The majority of the approximately 40 autoimmune disorders are more common in women. In part, it is believed that the differences in immune responsiveness are secondary to a greater propensity in women to develop a Th1 response after infectious challenge or antigen exposure (except during pregnancy, when a Th2 propensity prevails) (Whitacre et al. 1999). The etiology of these sex differences in immune function is secondary to a combination of the direct effects of sexually dimorphic hormones—including estrogens, progesterone, androgens, prolactin, growth hormone, and insulin-like growth factor 1—on immune function and the influence of gonadal steroids on the development of nervous and immune system cells and tissues (Martin 2000). As noted, immune cells express receptors for these sexually dimorphic hormones, and evidence suggests that the enzymes that synthesize gonadal steroids are expressed in immune tissues (Martin 2000). Estrogens tend to promote Th1-type responses, whereas progesterone tends to promote Th2-type responses (Whitacre et al. 1999). Testosterone exhibits anti-inflammatory and immunosuppressive properties, as determined in animal models of autoimmunity (Whitacre et al. 1999). During pregnancy, when progesterone predominates, Th2-type immune responses prevail and autoimmune disorders related to excessive Th1-like activity (MS and RA) improve (Whitacre et al. 1999). Diseases related to Th2-like activity (e.g., SLE) are exacerbated during pregnancy (Martin 2000; Whitacre et al. 1999). In a related fashion, studies indicate that periods of high estrogen levels correlate with increased susceptibility to stress-induced lung tumor colonization in laboratory animals. This increased vulnerability to a tumor challenge is mediated by an increased sensitivity to adrenergic (catecholamine) suppression of NK cell activity (Ben-Eliyahu et al. 2000).

In addition to direct effects on the immune system, gonadal steroids also were shown to modulate the HPA axis response to stress (Torpy and Chrousos 1996). Thus, gonadal hormones also may influence immune responses indirectly through effects on HPA axis–immune pathways.

Finally, studies conducted on hypophysectomized rats show that the stress-induced suppression of peripheral blood lymphocyte proliferative responses to the mitogen phytohemagglutinin is more pronounced in stressed hypophysectomized animals than in stressed intact animals

(controls) (Keller et al. 1988). These findings suggest that pituitary hormones may be involved in counteracting stress-induced immunosuppressive mechanisms. The specific pituitary-dependent mitigating or compensating hormones are not known, but they likely include growth hormone or prolactin, both of which were shown to have immune-enhancing properties and to maintain basal immunocompetence (Ader et al. 2001; Venters et al. 2001; Yu-Lee 1997). Other endogenous hormones, including dehydroepiandrosterone (DHEA) and its metabolite androstenediol, also may be involved in counteracting stress-induced immune changes (Padgett and Sheridan 1999; Padgett et al. 1997; Regelson et al. 1994).

Biochemical Pathways

As far as the biochemical mechanisms of the effects of stress on the immune system are concerned, it is important to note that nitric oxide has been shown to be involved in the physiological and pathological responses to stress in various tissues, including tissues of the immune system. Nitric oxide is a ubiquitous molecule that is involved in very different phenomena (e.g., blood vessel tone, gastric mucosa protection, neurotoxicity, macrophage function) and acts mainly by forming covalent linkages to several targets such as enzymes. Nitric oxide production in the immune system was shown to be induced in acutely stressed rats (Persoons et al. 1995). Moreover, it has been found that stress-induced nitric oxide production by macrophages is involved in stress-induced decreases in the lymphocyte proliferative response, because both the depletion of macrophages and the addition of the nitric oxide synthesis inhibitor N(G)-methyl-L-arginine acetate (L-NMMA) attenuate stress-induced immune changes (Coussons-Read et al. 1994).

PATHWAYS OF IMMUNE SYSTEM TO BRAIN SIGNALING

Research lending support to the importance of interactions between the immune system and the CNS includes the discovery that cytokines can exert profound effects on the nervous and endocrine systems. Because cytokines do not freely cross the blood-brain barrier under usual circumstances (i.e., in the absence of CNS infection), considerable attention has been paid to how peripheral immune signals are transmitted to the brain (Watkins et al. 1995). Several mechanisms have been proposed (Table 3–8). For example, it has been suggested that local (peripheral) production of proinflammatory cytokines can stimulate visceral afferent nerve fibers, which in turn communicate with the brain through the vagus nerve. This mechanism modulates a number of CNS functions, including both neuroendocrine function and behavior. For example, vagal mediation of CRH release from the hypothalamus occurs via interconnected neuronal circuits involving ascending catecholaminergic fibers (A2 and C2 cell groups) of the nucleus of the solitary tract, which project to the parvocellular division of the paraventricular nucleus of the hypothalamus (E.T. Cunningham Jr et al. 1990; Ericsson et al. 1994; Watkins et al. 1995). Lending support to the idea that the vagus nerve mediates communication between peripheral cytokines and the CNS is the observation that the hyperthermia induced by intraperitoneally administered IL-1β can be blocked by transection of the subdiaphragmatic vagus nerve (Watkins et al. 1995). Moreover, data indicate that afferent signals traveling through the vagus nerve also may mediate the effects of local cytokines on social behavior (via the dorsal vagal complex), hyperalgesia, and conditioned taste aversion (Maier et al. 1998; Marvel et al. 2004).

Circulating cytokines also may enter the brain in regions where the blood-brain barrier is leaky, allowing passive diffusion into the brain parenchyma and entry into CSF flow pathways (Rivest et al. 2000; Schobitz et al. 1994). For example, a high dose of IL-1 causes the induction of the early immediate gene c-fos in two such leaky regions, the area postrema and the vascular organ of the lamina terminalis (Brady et al. 1994; Ericsson et al. 1994). Cytokines also can communicate with the brain through intermediates without themselves entering the CNS parenchyma, for example, by acting on cells of the brain endothelium or choroid plexus and inducing the release of secondary messengers, including prostaglandins and nitric oxide (Schobitz et al. 1994). Recently, work by Nadjar and colleagues (2005) demonstrated that induction of prostaglandins in the brain by peripherally administered IL-1 depends on the initial activation of NFkB in the microvasculature. This induction of central NFkB by peripheral cytokines may serve as an essential step in transducing peripheral inflammatory signals into the CNS.

Active transport mechanisms for proinflammatory cytokines provide another means by which small quantities of proinflammatory cytokines may reach neuroendocrine regulatory circuits (Banks 2005; Plotkin et al. 1996). Finally, immune activation and possibly stress can disrupt the blood-brain barrier and may upregulate the active transport of proinflammatory cytokines into the brain, thereby facilitating the communication of peripheral immune signals with CNS targets.

Once cytokines enter the brain, the signals can be transmitted and amplified within the context of the cytokine network in the brain (Benveniste 1998; Quan et al. 1999; Rothwell et al. 1996). Receptors for proinflammatory cytokines are located in the brain, including brain regions that play important roles in vegetative functions, emotional regulation, and memory (Benveniste 1998; Besedovsky and del Rey 1996; Schobitz et al. 1994). IL-1β and its mRNA have been found in nerve cell bodies and nerve fibers within the hypothalamus, the hippocampus, and other regions in human and rodent brains.

Furthermore, there is accumulating evidence that several cytokines derived from neural cells may act as intermediaries in communicating peripheral inflammatory signals to the brain. For example, peripheral injection of lipopolysaccharide and circulating cytokines such as IL-1 was shown to induce neural cells within the hypothalamus and other brain regions to produce proinflammatory cytokines such as IL-1, IL-6, and TNF (Gatti and Bartfai 1993; Laye et al. 1994; Quan et al. 1994; Spangelo et al. 1990; van Dam et al. 1992). Furthermore, studies suggest that such autoinduction of cytokines can be transmitted indirectly through vagal pathways, as discussed earlier in this section (Laye et al. 1995; Watkins et al. 1995). For example, direct stimulation of the vagus nerve was shown to induce IL-1β mRNA in the hypothalamus and hippocampus (Hosoi et al. 2000). Thus, during immune activation, peripherally released cytokines could either cross the blood-brain barrier (e.g., at leaky sites or through active transport mechanisms) or activate peripheral afferents and consequently recruit local neural cells to produce other cytokines such as IL-1, IL-6, or TNF, thereby amplifying cytokine signals in relevant brain areas. Among neural cells, activated glia (especially microglia) are rich sources of proinflammatory cytokines. Activated microglia and astrocytes can produce large quantities of IL-1, and virus-induced proinflammatory cytokines are potent stimulants of glial activation (Schobitz et al. 1994).

TABLE 3–8.   Mechanisms by which cytokines signal the brain

- Stimulation of peripheral afferent nerve fibers by local cytokines (in periphery)
- Passive diffusion at leaky regions in the blood-brain barrier
- Active transport across blood-brain barrier
- Stimulation of endothelium or choroid plexus to produce secondary messengers

Notably, data suggest that nonimmunologic stressors can induce cytokine expression in the brain, suggesting that the behavioral and neuroendocrine responses to stress may involve cytokine signaling pathways (Nguyen et al. 1998). Aside from cytokine receptors, receptors for a rich array of chemokines have also been described, allowing for trafficking of multiple immunologic cell types in and out of the brain (Cartier et al. 2005).

The impact of cytokines on CNS function was examined in numerous in vitro and in vivo studies. Cytokines were shown to influence neurotransmitter turnover and electrophysiological responses in the CNS (Brebner et al. 2000; Dunn 2001; Dunn and Wang 1995; Dunn et al. 1999). For example, after short-term administration, IL-1 has been shown to increase the release and metabolism of several monoamines, including norepinephrine and serotonin. In addition, both IL-2 and IFN-α have been shown to alter dopamine metabolism. Because most studies focused on short-term administration of cytokines, very little is known about the long-term effects of cytokine exposure (as might occur in chronic inflammatory disorders). It is of note that cytokines also appear to have significant effects on long-term potentiation (Jankowsky and Patterson 1999), raising the intriguing hypothesis that cytokines can have lasting influences on memory, behavior, and endocrine responses by affecting the synaptic plasticity of relevant neuronal circuits.

Acting at the level of the hypothalamus, the pituitary, and the adrenal glands, immune system products—including IL-1, IL-2, IL-6, leukemia inhibitory factor, and TNF—appear to play a role in the regulation of sleep, temperature, feeding behavior, and secretion of multiple hormones, most notably glucocorticoids (Besedovsky and del Rey 1996; Chesnokova and Melmed 2000). Based on a series of studies examining the mechanisms by which proinflammatory cytokines such as IL-1 and IL-6 lead to HPA axis activation, a major final common pathway involves cytokine induction of CRH in the paraventricular nucleus of the hypothalamus (Berkenbosch et al. 1987; Besedovsky and del Rey 1996; Bethin et al. 2000; Kovacs and Elenkov 1995; Matta et al. 1992; Naitoh et al. 1988; Rivier 1995; Schmidt et al. 1995; Spinedi et al. 1992; Suda et al. 1990). In addition to actions through CRH secretion, cytokines may regulate glucocorticoid release through multiple alternate pathways, including direct effects on the pituitary or adrenal glands (Besedovsky and del Rey 1996; Callahan and Piekut 1997; Kovacs and Elenkov 1995; Matta et al. 1992; Naitoh et al. 1988; Perlstein et al. 1993; Silverman et al. 2005; Spinedi et al. 1992). The simultaneous release of adrenocorticotropic hormone (ACTH)–like and β-endorphin-like products in response to a variety of stimuli, including CRH, indicates that immunocytes (probably macrophages), like pituitary cells, are capable of transcribing the proopiomelanocortin gene, which is responsible for coding the precursor protein from which ACTH and β-endorphin are derived. Other hormones found to be secreted by immunocytes include somatostatin, vasoactive intestinal polypeptide, thyrotropin, and prolactin.

Behavioral effects of cytokines include the induction in humans and laboratory animals of a syndrome referred to as *sickness behavior*, which has many features in common with major depression, including anhedonia, listlessness, altered sleep patterns, reduced appetite, and social withdrawal (see next section) (Bluthe et al. 1997; Connor and Leonard 1998; Kelley et al. 1997; Kent et al. 1992; Krueger et al. 1995; Plata-Salaman et al. 1996). There are several pathways by which cytokines (especially proinflammatory cytokines) could contribute to the development of major depression during cytokine therapies or medical illnesses associated with significant inflammatory processes (Figure 3–6). First, IL-1, IL-6, and TNF-α all were shown to be potent inducers of CRH (Besedovsky and del Rey 1996; Besedovsky et al. 1986; Ericsson et al. 1994; Rivier 1995; Schobitz et al. 1994). CRH hypersecretion is believed to play a central role in the pathophysiology of depression, both in terms of the effects of CRH on behaviors that are known to be altered in depression (including activity, sleep, and feeding) and in terms of the role of CRH in the hyperactivity of the HPA axis, which characterizes a significant proportion of depressed patients (Owens and Nemeroff 1993). Second, proinflammatory cytokines were shown to have significant effects on monamine turnover and availability in key brain regions believed to be involved in mood disorders, including the hippocampus and hypothalamus (Brebner et al. 2000; Dunn and Wang 1995; Dunn et al. 1999). Interestingly in this regard, data have indicated that activation of p38 mitogen-activated protein kinase increases the activity of the serotonin transporter, and as a result it may constitute a pathway whereby cytokines can decrease serotonin availability in the synapse (Zhu et al. 2005). Third, cytokines have the capacity to induce the euthyroid sick syndrome, which is characterized by normal TSH and T4 levels but a reduced T3 level in the early stage, and a normal TSH level but reduced T4 and T3 levels in the later stage (Papanicolaou 2000). Fourth, activation of the immune system by cytokines was associated with activation of the enzyme indolamine 2,3-dioxygenase, which metabolizes tryptophan and leads to reduced tryptophan availability (Brown et al. 1991; Song et al. 1998). Depletion of tryptophan was shown to precipitate depressive symptoms in vulnerable individuals (Moore et al. 2000). Finally, cytokines (especially IL-1) were shown to disrupt glucocorticoid receptor function

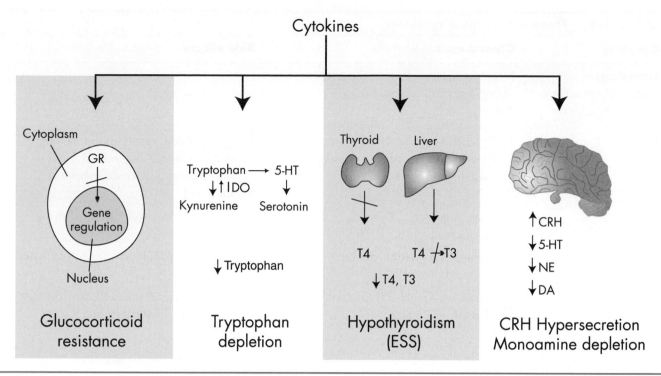

FIGURE 3–6. Potential mechanisms by which cytokines cause sickness behavior/depression. There are several potential mechanisms by which cytokines may induce behavioral symptoms in humans. At a cellular level, cytokines can induce glucocorticoid resistance by inhibiting glucocorticoid receptor (GR) translocation. Glucocorticoid resistance in turn releases corticotropin-releasing hormone (CRH) and proinflammatory cytokines from negative regulation by glucocorticoids. Cytokines can deplete tryptophan by increasing its conversion into kynurenine by the enzyme indolamine 2,3-dioxygenase (IDO). Tryptophan is the primary precursor of serotonin, and tryptophan depletion has been shown to precipitate depression in vulnerable individuals. Cytokines can inhibit production of T4 by the thyroid gland and the conversion of T4 to active T3 by the liver, leading to the euthyroid sick syndrome (ESS). In the brain, cytokines can stimulate secretion of CRH (which is elevated in the brains of patients with depression) and cause depletion of the monoamine neurotransmitters norepinephrine (NE), dopamine (DA), and 5-hydroxytryptophan (5-HT).

through activation of p38 mitogen-activated protein kinase and NFkB signaling pathways (Wang et al. 2004). Such cytokine-induced glucocorticoid receptor impairment in turn could disrupt negative feedback pathways on CRH, contributing to CRH hypersecretion, and further release of cytokines, contributing to runaway inflammation (Miller et al. 1999; Pariante and Miller 2001; Raison and Miller 2003b). Similar effects of cytokine signaling pathways were found on other hormone systems, including insulin-like growth factor 1 and vitamin D (Lu et al. 2004; Shen et al. 2004).

Immune System to Brain: Clinical Effects of Cytokines

Cytokines such as IFN-α, IFN-β, and IL-2 are used to treat viral illnesses, including chronic hepatitis B and C, and malignancies such as malignant melanoma and renal cell carcinoma (Table 3–9) (Lerner et al. 1999; Meyers and Valentine 1995). These cytokines are known for a variety of constitutional and psychiatric side effects that

frequently limit the dose and duration of treatment. Human recombinant forms of these immune mediators typically are administered in doses much higher than physiological ones. The pattern of their side effects may be divided into acute and chronic phases. The acute phase follows a single pattern of symptoms for different cytokines. Often described as a flu-like syndrome, these effects are characterized by fever, chills, myalgias, nausea, vomiting, and malaise. The group of symptoms in the later phase of toxicity for the interferons is referred to as *sickness behavior,* a syndrome of behavioral manifestations that resembles depression in humans (Dantzer 2004). Symptoms can include psychomotor slowing, depressed mood, decreased concentration, fatigue, and altered sleep. This syndrome has become of interest to psychiatry because it so closely resembles major depression and suggests some potential mechanisms involved in depression, especially in medically ill patients who have multiple sources of inflammation (and inflammatory cytokines) and high rates of depressive disorders. Other

TABLE 3–9.   Therapeutic uses of cytokines

Cytokine	Clinical uses	Side effects
Granulocyte-macrophage colony-stimulating factor	Neutropenia from cancer, chemotherapy, or bone marrow transplantation AIDS	
IFN-α	Malignancies—malignant melanoma, Kaposi's sarcoma, hairy cell leukemia Chronic hepatitis B and C	Fatigue, malaise, psychomotor slowing, cognitive changes (decreased concentration, decreased memory) Mania (rare)
IFN-β	Multiple sclerosis Malignancies	Fatigue, malaise, psychomotor slowing
IFN-γ	Chronic granulomatous disease Malignancies	Mild fatigue, malaise, dizziness, confusion
IL-2	Malignancies—renal cell carcinoma, malignant melanoma HIV	Fatigue, malaise, depression, neurotoxicity, somnolence, disorientation
Transforming growth factor β	Multiple sclerosis Myasthenia gravis	

Note.   IFN = interferon; IL = interleukin.

side effects of the therapeutic cytokines included mania, psychotic symptoms, and disorientation occasionally to the point of delirium (Meyers 1999).

Much information about the behavioral effects of cytokines and the mechanisms involved has been derived from the study of patients undergoing treatment with the cytokine IFN-α. IFN-α is a cytokine released early in viral infection. It has both antiviral and antiproliferative effects and therefore is used to treat both viral infections and cancer. Although a successful therapy, IFN-α is notorious for causing behavioral alterations, including depression in 20%–50% of patients, depending on the dose. Studies on IFN-α-treated patients reveal at least two distinct syndromes: 1) a mood/cognitive syndrome that appears late during IFN-α therapy, is responsive to antidepressants, and is associated with activation of neuroendocrine (CRH) pathways and altered serotonin metabolism (decreased tryptophan); and 2) a neurovegetative syndrome characterized by psychomotor slowing, fatigue, and anorexia that appears early during IFN-α treatment, is not responsive to antidepressants, and may be mediated by alterations in basal ganglia dopamine metabolism (Capuron and Miller 2004). Interestingly, it appears that IFN-α (and possibly other cytokines) has a direct effect on brain areas that involve information processing. Such effects are manifest in the dorsal region of the anterior cingulate cortex in humans, an area that also was found to be overactive in subjects with high trait anxiety, neuroticism, and

obsessive-compulsive disorder (Capuron et al. 2005). Findings from IFN-α research may provide important clues regarding the pathophysiology and treatment of cytokine-induced behavioral changes in medically ill patients, while also potentially modeling the involvement of the immune system in the development of neuropsychiatric symptoms in patients without medical disorders.

PSYCHOPHARMACOLOGY AND IMMUNE FUNCTION

Given the presence of relevant neurotransmitter receptors on immune cells, there logically has been interest in the relative impact on the immune system of psychopharmacological agents that alter neurotransmitter availability and function.

ANTIDEPRESSANTS

A number of investigators have examined in vitro and in vivo immune function after treatment with antidepressants. In vitro studies indicate that antidepressants generally reduce immune responsiveness (Maes et al. 1999). For example, tricyclic antidepressants were found to inhibit mitogen-induced lymphocyte proliferation and NK cell activity (Miller et al. 1986), although at least one report has suggested that selective serotonin reuptake inhibitors (SSRIs) may increase NK cell function (Frank et al. 1999). Both tricyclic antidepressants and SSRIs have been associated with decreased monocyte or lymphocyte production of several cytokines, including TNF-α, IL-1β, IL-2, and IFN-γ. Release of the inhibitory cytokine IL-10 has been shown to be increased in these cell types after in vitro administration of an antidepressant. Notably, one study found that tricyclic antidepressants have a similar inhibitory effect on proinflammatory (IL-1) production from activated glial cells, including microglia (Obuchowicz et al. 2006).

In vivo studies have given more mixed results, likely due to the fact that immune changes during antidepressant therapy are a conglomeration of the direct effects of drugs on immune cell activity and the indirect effects of drugs on physiology and mood. Results of in vivo studies ranged from no immunologic effect of antidepressant treatment (Brambilla and Maggioni 1998; Landmann et al. 1997; Schleifer et al. 1999) to normalization of altered immune parameters (Frank et al. 1999; Maes et al. 1997; Pariante and Miller 1995; Ravindran et al. 1998; Sluzewska et al. 1995) to decreases or increases in immune function during treatment. For example, Weizman and colleagues (1994) reported that IL-1β production increased during antidepressant treatment, whereas Seidel and colleagues (1995) reported that initially increased levels of acute phase proteins did not change during treatment, although initially increased levels of IL-2, IL-10, and IFN-γ returned to normal. Interestingly, data from both humans and laboratory animals indicate that pretreatment with antidepressants can block the development of sickness behavior during cytokine administration (Musselman et al. 2001). Whether these clinical effects are mediated by direct effects of antidepressants on the release of proinflammatory cytokines remains to be determined. Nevertheless, it was shown in laboratory animals that chronic treatment with the antidepressant tianeptine attenuates lipopolysaccharide-induced expression of TNF-α in the spleen and plasma, and alters the central balance between proinflammatory and anti-inflammatory (IL-1β, IL-10) cytokines (Castanon et al. 2004). In addition, in a study by Reynolds and colleagues (2004), the capacity of desipramine to reverse immobility in the forced swim test was associated with a decrease in TNF-α culminating in an increase in noradrenergic neurotransmission. These results suggest that proinflammatory cytokines may be involved in the therapeutic effects of antidepressant drugs.

ANTIPSYCHOTICS

The most well-known effect of antipsychotic drugs on the immune system is clozapine-induced agranulocytosis, which is believed to be related to alterations in granulocyte-macrophage colony-stimulating factor, an important signaling molecule in cell development in the bone marrow. Nevertheless, altered peripheral blood cytokine and cytokine receptor levels associated with antipsychotic treatment suggest that these agents have an effect on the cytokine network. Examples include an association between antipsychotics and decreased concentrations of TNF and sIL-6R. In contrast to the effects on TNF and sIL-6R, increased levels of sIL-2R have been reported with antipsychotic administration. In a study by van Kammen et al. (1999), schizophrenic patients exhibited no statistically significant changes in concentrations of CSF IL-6 at baseline and no effects of antipsychotic drugs on CSF IL-6 levels during treatment. In a study by Zhang and colleagues (2005), schizophrenic patients were treated with either typical or atypical antipsychotics; cortisol, IL-2, and IL-6 were then measured in the peripheral blood of these patients. It is of note that reductions in cortisol were associated with improvement in negative symptoms in patients treated with the atypical antipsychotic. However, both atypical and conventional drugs were associated with reductions in IL-2 and IL-6 as well as reductions in positive symptoms.

CONCLUSION

This chapter has provided a necessarily simplified overview of the fundamental concepts regarding interactions among the nervous, endocrine, and immune systems. The immune system has a documented capacity to receive signals from nervous system–derived transmitters, and more recent data indicate that immune signaling molecules (cytokines) have a profound impact on the CNS and endocrine system. Data from clinical studies indicate that these pathways of communication between the brain and immune system are relevant to the development, course, and outcome of both immunologically based diseases and neuropsychiatric disorders. Stress and depression have been shown to alter the development and course of cancer, infectious diseases, and autoimmune disorders, and activation of the immune system has been associated with depression and schizophrenia.

Nervous and immune system interactions represent an exciting new frontier in the understanding of the influence of the environment (internal and external) on the expression of genetic vulnerability to disease. New concepts of gene regulation coupled with elucidation of the specific neuroendocrine-immune pathways involved will undoubtedly lead to novel approaches to the prevention and treatment of immune and nervous system diseases. Appreciation of the complex interactions between bodily systems that mediate internal regulation is a critical component in understanding the development and outcome of all diseases.

Highlights for the Clinician

- ✦ A bidirectional communication network exists between the immune system and the nervous system.

- ✦ Chronic stress and depression have been associated with altered immune responses, including decreased NK cell activity and T cell proliferation, as well as activation of innate inflammatory immune responses.

- ✦ Chronic stress and depression have been associated with a worse outcome in infectious diseases, cancer, and autoimmune disorders—as well as impaired responses to vaccination and delayed wound healing, possibly due to direct effects on the immune response.

- ✦ Cytokines released during activation of the immune system (especially during innate inflammatory immune responses) can access the brain and alter monoamine metabolism, neuroendocrine function, synaptic plasticity, and behavior.

- ✦ Through their effects on the brain, cytokines may contribute to behavioral comorbidities in medically ill individuals and may play a role in the pathophysiology of neuropsychiatric disorders, including depression and schizophrenia.

RECOMMENDED READINGS

Ader R, Felten D, Cohen N (eds): Psychoneuroimmunology, 4th Edition. New York, Academic Press, 2006

Raison CL, Capuron C, Miller AH: Cytokines sing the blues: inflammation and the pathogenesis of depression. Trends Immunol 24–31, 2006

REFERENCES

Abbas AK, Lichtman AH: Cellular and Molecular Immunology, 5th Edition. Philadelphia, PA, WB Saunders, 2003

Abdeljaber MH, Nair MP, Schork MA, et al: Depressed natural killer cell activity in schizophrenic patients. Immunol Invest 23:259–268, 1994

Ader R, Friedman SB: Differential early experiences and susceptibility to transplanted tumors in the rat. J Comp Physiol 59:361–364, 1965

Ader R, Felten D, Cohen N (eds): Psychoneuroimmunology, 3rd Edition. New York, Academic Press, 2001

Almawi WY, Sewell KL, Hadro ET, et al: Mode of action of the glucocorticosteroids as immunosuppressive agents, in Molecular and Cellular Biology of Cytokines, Progress in Leukocyte Biology, Vol 10A. Edited by Oppenheim J, Powanda MC, Kluger MJ, et al. New York, Wiley-Liss, 1990, pp 321–326

Andreoli AV, Keller SE, Rabaeus M, et al: Depression and immunity: age, severity, and clinical course. Brain Behav Immun 7:279–292, 1993

Ang DC, Choi H, Kroenke K, et al: Comorbid depression is an independent risk factor for mortality in patients with rheumatoid arthritis. J Rheumatol 32:1013–1019, 2005

Antoni MH, Cruess DG, Klimas N, et al: Increases in a marker of immune system reconstitution are predated by decreases in 24-h urinary cortisol output and depressed mood during a 10-week stress management intervention in symptomatic HIV-infected men. J Psychosom Res 58:3–13, 2005

Auphan N, DiDonato JA, Rosette C, et al: Immunosuppression by glucocorticoids: inhibition of NF-kappa B activity through induction of I kappa B synthesis. Science 270:286–290, 1995

Bachen EA, Manuck SB, Cohen S, et al: Adrenergic blockade ameliorates cellular immune responses to mental stress in humans. Psychosom Med 57:366–372, 1995

Bailey MT, Avitsur R, Engler H, et al: Physical defeat reduces the sensitivity of murine splenocytes to the suppressive effects of corticosterone. Brain Behav Immun 18:416–424, 2004

Banks WA: Blood-brain barrier transport of cytokines: a mechanism for neuropathology. Curr Pharm Des 11:973–984, 2005

Barrientos RM: Brain-derived neurotrophic factor mRNA downregulation produced by social isolation is blocked by intrahippocampal interleukin-1 receptor antagonist. Neuroscience 121:847–853, 2003

Baumann H, Gauldie J: The acute phase response. Immunol Today 15:74–80, 1994

Ben-Eliyahu S, Shakhar G, Shakhar K, et al: Timing within the oestrous cycle modulates adrenergic suppression of NK activity and resistance to metastasis: possible clinical implications. Br J Cancer 83:1747–1754, 2000

Benou C, Wang Y, Imitola J, et al: Corticotropin-releasing hormone contributes to the peripheral inflammatory response in experimental autoimmune encephalomyelitis. J Immunol 174:5407–5413, 2005

Benschop RJ, Godaert GL, Geenen R, et al: Relationships between cardiovascular and immunological changes in an experimental stress model. Psychol Med 25:323–327, 1995

Benschop RJ, Rodriguez-Feuerhahn M, Schedlowski M: Catecholamine-induced leukocytosis: early observations, current research, and future directions. Brain Behav Immun 10:77–91, 1996

Benveniste EN: Cytokine actions in the central nervous system. Cytokine Growth Factor Rev 9:259–275, 1998

Berkenbosch F, van Oers J, del Rey A, et al: Corticotropin-releasing factor–producing neurons in the rat activated by interleukin-1. Science 238:524–526, 1987

Bertini R, Bianchi M, Ghezzi P: Adrenalectomy sensitizes mice to the lethal effects of interleukin 1 and tumor necrosis factor. J Exp Med 167:1708–1712, 1988

Besedovsky HO, del Rey A: Immune-neuro-endocrine interactions: facts and hypotheses. Endocr Rev 17:64–102, 1996

Besedovsky H, del Rey A, Sorkin E, et al: Immunoregulatory feedback between interleukin-1 and glucocorticoid hormones. Science 233:652–654, 1986

Bethin KE, Vogt SK, Muglia LJ: Interleukin-6 is an essential, corticotropin-releasing hormone–independent stimulator of the adrenal axis during immune system activation. Proc Natl Acad Sci U S A 97:9317–9322, 2000

Bierhaus A, Wolf J, Andrassy M, et al: A mechanism converting psychosocial stress into mononuclear cell activation. Proc Natl Acad Sci U S A 100:9090–9095, 2003

Bird H, Broggini M: Paroxetine versus amitriptyline for treatment of depression associated with rheumatoid arthritis: a randomized, double blind, parallel group study. J Rheumatol 27:2791–2797, 2000

Bluthe RM, Dantzer R, Kelley KW: Central mediation of the effects of interleukin-1 on social exploration and body weight in mice. Psychoneuroendocrinology 22:1–11, 1997

Borovikova LV, Ivanova S, Zhang M, et al: Vagus nerve stimulation attenuates the systemic inflammatory response to endotoxin. Nature 405:458–462, 2000

Brady LS, Lynn AB, Herkenham M, et al: Systemic interleukin-1 induces early and late patterns of c-fos mRNA expression in brain. J Neurosci 14:4951–4964, 1994

Brambilla F, Maggioni M: Blood levels of cytokines in elderly patients with major depressive disorder. Acta Psychiatr Scand 97:309–313, 1998

Brebner K, Hayley S, Zacharko R, et al: Synergistic effects of interleukin-1 beta, interleukin-6, and tumor necrosis factor-alpha: central monoamine, corticosterone, and behavioral variations. Neuropsychopharmacology 22:566–580, 2000

Brown RR, Ozaki Y, Datta SP, et al: Implications of interferon-induced tryptophan catabolism in cancer, auto-immune diseases and AIDS. Adv Exp Med Biol 294:425–435, 1991

Buccheri G: Depressive reactions to lung cancer are common and often followed by a poor outcome. Eur Respir J 11:173–178, 1998

Burack JH, Barrett DC, Stall RD, et al: Depressive symptoms and CD4 lymphocyte decline among HIV-infected men. JAMA 270:2568–2573, 1993

Caldwell CL, Irwin M, Lohr J: Reduced natural killer cell cytotoxicity in depression but not in schizophrenia. Biol Psychiatry 30:1131–1138, 1991

Callahan TA, Piekut DT: Differential fos expression induced by IL-1 beta and IL-6 in rat hypothalamus and pituitary gland. J Neuroimmunol 73:207–211, 1997

Capuron L, Miller AH: Cytokines and psychopathology: lessons from interferon alpha. Biol Psychiatry 56:819–824, 2004

Capuron L, Pagnoni G, Demetrashvili M, et al: Anterior cingulate activation and error processing during interferon-alpha treatment. Biol Psychiatry 58:190–196, 2005

Caroleo MC, Pulvirenti L, Arbitrio M, et al: Evidence that CRH microinfused into the locus coeruleus decreases cell-mediated immune response in rats. Funct Neurol 8:271–277, 1993

Cartier L, Hartley O, Dubois-Dauphin M, et al: Chemokine receptors in the central nervous system: role in brain inflammation and neurodegenerative diseases. Brain Res Brain Res Rev 48:16–42, 2005

Carver CS, Lehman JM, Antoni MH: Dispositional pessimism predicts illness-related disruption of social and recreational activities among breast cancer patients. J Pers Soc Psychol 84:813–821, 2003

Castanon N, Medina C, Mormede C, et al: Chronic administration of tianeptine balances lipopolysaccharide-induced expression of cytokines in the spleen and hypothalamus of rats. Psychoneuroendocrinology 29:778–790, 2004

Chesnokova V, Melmed S: Leukemia inhibitory factor mediates the hypothalamic pituitary adrenal axis response to inflammation. Endocrinology 141:4032–4040, 2000

Chikanza IC, Petrou P, Kingsley G, et al: Defective hypothalamic response to immune and inflammatory stimuli in patients with rheumatoid arthritis. Arthritis Rheum 35:1281–1288, 1992

Cohen F, Kemeny ME, Kearney KA, et al: Persistent stress as a predictor of genital herpes recurrence. Arch Intern Med 159:2430–2436, 1999

Cohen JJ: Lymphocyte death induced by glucocorticoids, in Anti-inflammatory Steroid Action, Basic and Clinical Aspects. Edited by Schleimer RP, Claman HN, Oronsky AL. San Diego, CA, Academic Press, 1989, pp 110–131

Cohen S, Tyrrell DA, Smith AP: Psychological stress and susceptibility to the common cold. N Engl J Med 325:606–612, 1991

Cole SW, Kemeny ME: Psychosocial influences on the progression of HIV infection, in Psychoneuroimmunology. Edited by Ader R, Felton DL, Cohen N. San Diego, CA, Academic Press, 2001, pp 583–612

Cole SW, Naliboff BD, Kemeny ME, et al: Impaired response to HAART in HIV-infected individuals with high autonomic nervous system activity. Proc Natl Acad Sci U S A 98:12695–12700, 2001

Connor TJ, Leonard BE: Depression, stress and immunological activation: the role of cytokines in depressive disorders. Life Sci 62:583–606, 1998

Courtney JG, Longnecker MP, Theorell T, et al: Stressful life events and the risk of colorectal cancer. Epidemiology 4:407–414, 1993

Coussons-Read ME, Maslonek KA, Fecho K, et al: Evidence for the involvement of macrophage-derived nitric oxide in the modulation of immune status by a conditioned aversive stimulus. J Neuroimmunol 50:51–58, 1994

Cover H, Irwin M: Immunity and depression: insomnia, retardation, and reduction of natural killer cell activity. J Behav Med 17:217–223, 1994

Crary B, Borysenko M, Sutherland DC, et al: Decrease in mitogen responsiveness of mononuclear cells from peripheral blood after epinephrine administration in humans. J Immunol 130:694–697, 1983

Cruess DG, Antoni MH, McGregor BA, et al: Cognitive-behavioral stress management reduces serum cortisol by enhancing benefit finding among women being treated for early stage breast cancer. Psychosom Med 62: 304–308, 2000

Cruess DG, Douglas SD, Petitto JM, et al: Association of depression, CD8+ T lymphocytes, and natural killer cell activity: implications for morbidity and mortality in human immunodeficiency virus disease. Curr Psychiatry Rep 5:445–450, 2003

Cunnick JE, Lysle DT, Kucinski BJ, et al: Evidence that shock-induced immune suppression is mediated by adrenal hormones and peripheral beta-adrenergic receptors. Pharmacol Biochem Behav 36:645–651, 1990

Cunnick JE, Lysle DT, Kucinski BJ, et al: Stress-induced alteration of immune function. Diversity of effects and mechanisms. Ann N Y Acad Sci 650:283–287, 1992

Cunningham AJ, Edmonds CV, Jenkins GP, et al: A randomized controlled trial of the effects of group psychological therapy on survival in women with metastatic breast cancer. Psychooncology 7:508–517, 1998

Cunningham ET Jr, Bohn MC, Sawchenko PE: Organization of adrenergic inputs to the paraventricular and supraoptic nuclei of the hypothalamus in the rat. J Comp Neurol 292:651–667, 1990

DaCosta D, Dobkin PL, Pinard L, et al: The role of stress in functional disability among women with systemic lupus erythematosus: a prospective study. Arthritis Care Research 12:112–119, 1999

Dantzer R: Cytokine-induced sickness behaviour: a neuroimmune response to activation of innate immunity. Eur J Pharmacol 500(1–3):399–411, 2004

Delves PJ, Roitt IM: The immune system. First of two parts. N Engl J Med 343:37–49, 2000a

Delves PJ, Roitt IM: The immune system. Second of two parts. N Engl J Med 343:108–117, 2000b

Dhabhar FS, McEwen BS: Bidirectional effects of stress and glucocorticoid hormones on immune function: possible explanations for paradoxical observations, in Psychoneuroimmunology, 2nd Edition. Edited by Ader R, Felten D, Cohen N. New York, Academic Press, 2001, pp 301–338

Dhabhar FS, Miller AH, McEwen BS, et al: Effects of stress on immune cell distribution: dynamics and hormonal mechanisms. J Immunol 154:5511–5527, 1995

Dhabhar FS, Miller AH, McEwen BS, et al: Stress-induced changes in blood leukocyte distribution: role of adrenal steroid hormones. J Immunol 157:1638–1644, 1996

Dhabhar FS, Satoskar AR, Bluethmann H, et al: Stress-induced enhancement of skin immune function: a role for gamma interferon. Proc Natl Acad Sci U S A 97:2846–2851, 2000

Dunn AJ: Effects of cytokines and infections on brain neurochemistry, in Psychoneuroimmunology. Edited by Ader R, Felten DL, Cohen N. San Diego, CA, Academic Press, 2001, pp 649–666

Dunn AJ, Wang J: Cytokine effects on CNS biogenic amines. Neuroimmunomodulation 2:319–328, 1995

Dunn AJ, Wang J, Ando T: Effects of cytokines on cerebral neurotransmission: comparison with the effects of stress. Adv Exp Med Biol 461:117–127, 1999

Edelman S, Lemon J, Bell DR, et al: Effects of group CBT on the survival time of patients with metastatic breast cancer. Psychooncology 8:474–481, 1999

Eisenstein TK, Hilburger ME: Opioid modulation of immune responses: effects on phagocyte and lymphoid cell populations. J Neuroimmunol 83:36–44, 1998

Ericsson A, Kovacs KJ, Sawchenko PE: A functional anatomical analysis of central pathways subserving the effects of interleukin-1 on stress-related neuroendocrine neurons. J Neurosci 14:897–913, 1994

Esterling BA, Kiecolt-Glaser JK, Glaser R: Psychosocial modulation of cytokine-induced natural killer cell activity in older adults. Psychosom Med 58:264–272, 1996

Evans DL, McCartney CF, Nemeroff CB, et al: Depression in women treated for gynecological cancer: clinical and neuroendocrine assessment. Am J Psychiatry 143:447–451, 1986

Evans DL, Folds JD, Petitto J, et al: Circulating natural killer cell phenotypes in males and females with major depression: relation to cytotoxic activity and severity of depression. Arch Gen Psychiatry 49:388–395, 1992

Evans DL, Leserman J, Perkins DO, et al: Stress-associated reductions of cytotoxic T lymphocytes and natural killer cells in asymptomatic HIV infection. Am J Psychiatry 152:543–550, 1995

Evans DL, Leserman J, Perkins DO, et al: Severe life stress as a predictor of early disease progression in HIV infection. Am J Psychiatry 154:630–634, 1997

Evans DL, Mason K, Bauer R, et al: Neuropsychiatric manifestations of HIV-1 infection and AIDS, in Psychopharmacology: The Fifth Generation of Progress. Edited by Charney D, Coyle J, Davis K, et al. New York, Raven, 2002, pp 1281–1300

Everson SA, Goldberg DE, Kaplan GA, et al: Hopelessness and risk of mortality and incidence of myocardial infarction and cancer. Psychosom Med 58:113–121, 1996

Faller H, Bulzebruck H, Drings P, et al: Coping, distress, and survival among patients with lung cancer. Arch Gen Psychiatry 56:756–762, 1999

Fawzy FI, Fawzy NW, Hyun CS, et al: Malignant melanoma: effects of an early structured psychiatric intervention, coping, and affective state on recurrence and survival 6 years later. Arch Gen Psychiatry 50:681–689, 1993

Felten DL, Livnats, Felten SY, et al: Sympathetic innervation of lymph nodes in mice. Brain Res Bull 13:693–699, 1984

Feng P, Meissler JJ Jr, Adler MW, et al: Morphine withdrawal sensitizes mice to lipopolysaccharide: elevated TNF-alpha and nitric oxide with decreased IL-12. J Neuroimmunol 164:57–65, 2005

Fertuzinhos SM, Oliveira JR, Nishimura AL, et al: Analysis of IL-1alpha, IL-1beta, and IL-1RA [correction of IL-RA] polymorphisms in dysthymia. J Mol Neurosci 22:251–256, 2004

Filipski E, King VM, Li X, et al: Host circadian clock as a control point in tumor progression. J Natl Cancer Inst 94:690–697, 2002

Frank MG, Hendricks SE, Johnson DR, et al: Antidepressants augment natural killer cell activity: in vivo and in vitro. Neuropsychobiology 39:18–24, 1999

Ganguli R, Rabin BS: Increased serum interleukin 2 receptor concentration in schizophrenic and brain-damaged subjects (letter). Arch Gen Psychiatry 46:292, 1989

Ganguli R, Brar JS, Chengappa KR, et al: Mitogen-stimulated interleukin-2 production in never-medicated, first-episode schizophrenic patients: the influence of age at onset and negative symptoms. Arch Gen Psychiatry 52:668–672, 1995

Gatti S, Bartfai T: Induction of tumor necrosis factor-alpha mRNA in the brain after peripheral endotoxin treatment: comparison with interleukin-1 family and interleukin-6. Brain Res 624:291–294, 1993

Giron LT Jr, Crutcher KA, Davis JN: Lymph nodes: a possible site for sympathetic neuronal regulation of immune responses. Ann Neurol 8:520–525, 1980

Glaser R, Kiecolt-Glaser JK, Bonneau RH, et al: Stress-induced modulation of the immune response to recombinant hepatitis B vaccine. Psychosom Med 54:22–29, 1992

Goldstein RA, Bowen DL, Fauci AS: Adrenal corticosteroids, in Inflammation: Basic Principles and Clinical Correlates. Edited by Gallin JI, Snyderman R. New York, Raven, 1992, pp 1061–1081

Gonzalo JA, Gonzalez-Garcia A, Martinez C, et al: Glucocorticoid-mediated control of the activation and clonal deletion of peripheral T cells in vivo. J Exp Med 177:1239–1246, 1993

Grant I, Brown GW, Harris T, et al: Severely threatening events and marked life difficulties preceding onset or exacerbation of multiple sclerosis. J Neurol Neurosurg Psychiatry 52:8–13, 1989

Grippo AJ, Francis J, Beltz TG, et al: Neuro endocrine and cytokine profile of chronic mild stress-induced anhedonia. Physiol Behav 84:697–706, 2005

Haack M, Hinze-Selch D, Fenzel T, et al: Plasma levels of cytokines and soluble cytokine receptors in psychiatric patients upon hospital admission: effects of confounding factors and diagnosis. J Psychiatr Res 33:407–418, 1999

Hall DM, Suo JL, Weber RJ: Opioid mediated effects on the immune system: sympathetic nervous system involvement. J Neuroimmunol 83:29–35, 1998

Harrington L, Affleck G, Urrows S, et al: Temporal covariation of soluble interleukin-2 receptor levels, daily stress, and disease activity in rheumatoid arthritis. Arthritis Rheum 36:199–203, 1993

Herbert TB, Cohen S: Depression and immunity: a meta-analytic review. Psychol Bull 113:472–486, 1993

Herbert TB, Cohen S, Marsland AL: Cardiovascular reactivity and the course of immune response to an acute psychological stressor. Psychosom Med 56:337–344, 1994

Hermann G, Beck FM, Sheridan JF: Stress-induced glucocorticoid response modulates mononuclear cell trafficking during an experimental influenza viral infection. J Neuroimmunol 56:179–186, 1995

Herrmann M, Scholmerich J, Straub RH: Stress and rheumatic diseases. Rheum Dis Clin North Am 26:737–763, 2000

Hosoi T, Okuma Y, Nomura Y: Electrical stimulation of afferent vagus nerve induces IL-1 beta expression in the brain and activates HPA axis. Am J Physiol Regul Integr Comp Physiol 279:R141–147, 2000

Irwin M: Brain corticotropin-releasing-hormone- and interleukin-1-beta-induced suppression of specific antibody production. Endocrinology 133:1352–1360, 1993

Irwin M, Hauger RL, Brown M, et al: CRF activates autonomic nervous system and reduces natural killer cell cytotoxicity. Am J Physiol Regul Integr Comp Physiol 255:R744–R747, 1988

Irwin M, Vale W, Rivier C: Central corticotropin-releasing factor mediates the suppressive effect of stress on natural killer cell cytotoxicity. Endocrinology 126:2837–2844, 1990

Irwin M, Costlow C, Williams H, et al: Cellular immunity to varicella-zoster virus in patients with major depression. J Infect Dis 178(suppl):S104–S108, 1998

Jacobs R, Pawlak CR, Mikeska E, et al: Systemic lupus erythematosus and rheumatoid arthritis patients differ from healthy controls in their cytokine pattern after stress exposure. Rheumatology (Oxford) 40:868–875, 2001

Jankowsky JL, Patterson PH: Cytokine and growth factor involvement in long-term potentiation [published correction appears in Mol Cell Neurosci 14:529, 1999]. Mol Cell Neurosci 14:273–286, 1999

Johansen C, Olsen JH: Psychological stress, cancer incidence and mortality from non-malignant diseases. Br J Cancer 75:144–148, 1997

Johnson GL, Lapadat R: Mitogen-activated protein kinase pathways mediated by ERK, JNK, and p38 protein kinases. Science 298:1911–1912, 2002

Johnson JD, Campisi J, Sharkey CM, et al: Catecholamines mediate stress-induced increases in peripheral and central inflammatory cytokines. Neuroscience 135:1295–1307, 2005

Jun TY, Pae CU, Hoon-Han, et al: Possible association between -G308A tumour necrosis factor-alpha gene polymorphism and major depressive disorder in the Korean population. Psychiatr Genet 13:179–181, 2003

Kanik KS, Chrousos GP, Schumacher HR, et al: Adrenocorticotropin, glucocorticoid, and androgen secretion in patients with new onset synovitis/rheumatoid arthritis: relations with indices of inflammation. J Clin Endocrinol Metab 85:1461–1466, 2000

Karalis K, Sano H, Redwine J, et al: Autocrine or paracrine inflammatory actions of corticotropin-releasing hormone in vivo. Science 254:421–423, 1991

Karalis K, Muglia LJ, Bae D, et al: CRH and the immune system. J Neuroimmunol 72:131–136, 1997

Kawahito Y, Sano H, Mukai S, et al: Corticotropin releasing hormone in colonic mucosa in patients with ulcerative colitis. Gut 37:544–551, 1995

Keller SE, Weiss JM, Schleifer SJ, et al: Suppression of immunity by stress: effect of a graded series of stressors on lymphocyte stimulation in the rat. Science 213:1397–1400, 1981

Keller SE, Schleifer SJ, Liotta AS, et al: Stress-induced alterations of immunity in hypophysectomized rats. Proc Natl Acad Sci U S A 85:9297–9301, 1988

Kelley KW, Hutchison K, French R, et al: Central interleukin-1 receptors as mediators of sickness. Ann N Y Acad Sci 823:234–246, 1997

Kent S, Bluthe RM, Kelley KW, et al: Sickness behavior as a new target for drug development. Trends Pharmacol Sci 13:24–28, 1992

Kiecolt-Glaser JK, Marucha PT, Malarkey WB, et al: Slowing of wound healing by psychological stress. Lancet 346:1194–1196, 1995

Kiecolt-Glaser JK, Glaser R, Gravenstein S, et al: Chronic stress alters the immune response to influenza virus vaccine in older adults. Proc Natl Acad Sci U S A 93:3043–3047, 1996

Kiecolt-Glaser JK, Preacher KJ, MacCallum RC, et al: Chronic stress and age related increases in proinflammatory cytokine IL-6. Proc Natl Acad Sci U S A 100:9090–9095, 2003

Kim YK, Kim L, Lee MS: Relationships between interleukins, neurotransmitters and psychopathology in drug-free male schizophrenics. Schizophr Res 44:165–175, 2000

Kim YK, Myint AM, Lee BH, et al: Th1, Th2 and Th3 cytokine alteration in schizophrenia. Prog Neuropsychopharmacol Biol Psychiatry 28:1129–1134, 2004

Kittner JM, Jacobs R, Pawlak CR, et al: Adrenaline-induced immunological changes are altered in patients with rheumatoid arthritis. Rheumatology (Oxford) 41:1031–1039, 2002

Knekt P, Raitasalo R, Heliovaara M, et al: Elevated lung cancer risk among persons with depressed mood. Am J Epidemiol 144:1096–1103, 1996

Korschenhausen DA, Hampel HJ, Ackenheil M, et al: Fibrin degradation products in postmortem brain tissue of schizophrenics: a possible marker for underlying inflammatory processes. Schizophr Res 19:103–109, 1996

Kovacs KJ, Elenkov IJ: Differential dependence of ACTH secretion induced by various cytokines on the integrity of the paraventricular nucleus. J Neuroendocrinol 7:15–23, 1995

Kumar A, Takada Y, Boriek AM, et al: Nuclear factor-kappaB: its role in health and disease. J Mol Med 82:434–448, 2004

Krueger JM, Takahashi S, Kapas L, et al: Cytokines in sleep regulation. Adv Neuroimmunol 5:171–188, 1995

Labeur MS, Arzt E, Wiegers GJ, et al: Long-term intracerebroventricular corticotropin-releasing hormone administration induces distinct changes in rat splenocyte activation and cytokine expression. Endocrinology 136:2678–2688, 1995

Landmann RM, Muller FB, Perini C, et al: Changes of immunoregulatory cells induced by psychological and physical stress: relationship to plasma catecholamines. Clin Exp Immunol 58:127–135, 1984

Landmann R, Schaub B, Link S, et al: Unaltered monocyte function in patients with major depression before and after three months of antidepressive therapy. Biol Psychiatry 41:675–681, 1997

Lariviere WR, Melzack R: The role of corticotropin-releasing factor in pain and analgesia. Pain 84:1–12, 2000

Laye S, Parnet P, Goujon E, et al: Peripheral administration of lipopolysaccharide induces the expression of cytokine transcripts in the brain and pituitary of mice. Brain Res Mol Brain Res 27:157–162, 1994

Laye S, Bluthe RM, Kent S, et al: Subdiaphragmatic vagotomy blocks induction of IL-1 beta mRNA in mice brain in response to peripheral LPS. Am J Physiol 268:R1327–1331, 1995

LeMay LG, Vander AJ, Kluger MJ: The effects of psychological stress on plasma interleukin-6 activity in rats. Physiol Behav 47:957–961, 1990

Lerner DM, Stoudemire A, Rosenstein DL: Neuropsychiatric toxicity associated with cytokine therapies. Psychosomatics 40:428–435, 1999

Leserman J, Petitto JM, Perkins DO, et al: Severe stress, depressive symptoms, and changes in lymphocyte subsets in human immunodeficiency virus–infected men: a 2-year follow-up study. Arch Gen Psychiatry 54:279–285, 1997

Leserman J, Jackson ED, Petitto JM, et al: Progression to AIDS: the effects of stress, depressive symptoms, and social support. Psychosom Med 61:397–406, 1999

Leserman J, Petitto JM, Golden RN, et al: Impact of stressful life events, depression, social support, coping, and cortisol on progression to AIDS. Am J Psychiatry 157:1221–1228, 2000

Leu SJ, Singh VK: Stimulation of interleukin-6 production by corticotropin-releasing factor. Cell Immunol 143:220–227, 1992

Leu SJ, Singh VK: Suppression of in vitro antibody production by corticotropin-releasing factor neurohormone. J Neuroimmunol 45:23–29, 1993

Levine J, Barak Y, Chengappa KN, et al: Cerebrospinal cytokine levels in patients with acute depression. Neuropsychobiology 40:171–176, 1999

Licinio J, Seibyl JP, Altemus M, et al: Elevated CSF levels of interleukin-2 in neuroleptic-free schizophrenic patients. Am J Psychiatry 150:1408–1410, 1993

Linkins RW, Comstock GW: Depressed mood and development of cancer. Am J Epidemiol 132:962–972, 1990

Lombardi MS, Kavelaars A, Schedlowski M, et al: Decreased expression and activity of G-protein-coupled receptor kinases in peripheral blood mononuclear cells of patients with rheumatoid arthritis. FASEB J 13:715–725, 1999

Lu X, Farmer P, Rubin J, et al: Integration of the NfkappaB p65 subunit into the vitamin D receptor transcriptional complex: identification of p65 domains that inhibit 1,25-dihydroxyvitamin D3-stimulated transcription. J Cell Biochem 92:833–848, 2004

Lyketsos CG, Hoover DR, Guccione M, et al: Depressive symptoms as predictors of medical outcomes in HIV infection. Multicenter AIDS Cohort Study. JAMA 270:2563–2567, 1993

Lyketsos CG, Hoover DR, Guccione M: Depression and survival among HIV-infected persons. JAMA 275:35–36, 1996

Maes M: Major depression and activation of the inflammatory response system. Adv Exp Med Biol 461:25–46, 1999

Maes M, Delange J, Ranjan R, et al: Acute phase proteins in schizophrenia, mania and major depression: modulation by psychotropic drugs. Psychiatry Res 66:1–11, 1997

Maes M, Song C, Lin AH, et al: Negative immunoregulatory effects of antidepressants: inhibition of interferon-gamma and stimulation of interleukin-10 secretion. Neuropsychopharmacology 20:370–379, 1999

Maier SF, Watkins LR: Cytokines for psychologists: implications of bidirectional immune-to-brain communication for understanding behavior, mood, and cognition. Psychol Rev 105:83–107, 1998

Maisel AS, Wright CM, Carter SM, et al: Tachyphylaxis with amrinone therapy: association with sequestration and down-regulation of lymphocyte beta-adrenergic receptors. Ann Intern Med 110:195–201, 1989

Martin J: Sexual dimorphism in immune function: the role of prenatal exposure to androgens and estrogens. Eur J Pharmacol 405:251–261, 2000

Marvel FA, Chen CC, Badr N, et al: Reversible inactivation of the dorsal vagal complex blocks lipopolysaccharide-induced social withdrawal and c-Fos expression in central autonomic nuclei. Brain Behav Immun 18:123–134, 2004

Mathias SD, Colwell HH, Miller DP, et al: Health-related quality of life and functional status of patients with rheumatoid arthritis randomly assigned to receive etanercept or placebo. Clin Ther 22:128–139, 2000

Matta SG, Weatherbee J, Sharp BM: A central mechanism is involved in the secretion of ACTH in response to IL-6 in rats: comparison to and interaction with IL-1b. Neuroendocrinology 56:516–525, 1992

Matzinger P: The danger model in its historical context. Scand J Immunol 54:4–9, 2001

Mayne TJ, Vittinghoff E, Chesney MA, et al: Depressive affect and survival among gay and bisexual men infected with HIV. Arch Intern Med 156:2233–2238, 1996

Mazzeo RS, Donovan D, Fleshner M, et al: Interleukin-6 response to exercise and high-altitude exposure: influence of alpha-adrenergic blockade. J Appl Physiol 91:2143–2149, 2001

McAllister CG, Rapaport MH, Pickar D, et al: Increased numbers of CD5+ B lymphocytes in schizophrenic patients. Arch Gen Psychiatry 46:890–894, 1989

McEwen BS, Biron CA, Brunson KW, et al: The role of adrenocorticoids as modulators of immune function in health and disease: neural, endocrine and immune interactions. Brain Res Brain Res Rev 23:79–133, 1997

McGee R, Williams S, Elwood M: Depression and the development of cancer: a meta-analysis. Soc Sci Med 38:187–192, 1994

Mell LK, Davis RL, Owens D: Association between streptococcal infection and obsessive-compulsive disorder, Tourette's syndrome, and tic disorder. Pediatrics 116:56–60, 2005

Mellon RD, Bayer BM: Evidence for central opioid receptors in the immunomodulatory effects of morphine: review of potential mechanism(s) of action. J Neuroimmunol 83:19–28, 1998

Meyers CA: Mood and cognitive disorders in cancer patients receiving cytokine therapy. Adv Exp Med Biol 461:75–81, 1999

Meyers CA, Valentine AD: Neurological and psychiatric adverse effects of immunological therapy. CNS Drugs 3:56–68, 1995

Miller AH, Asnis GM, van Praag HM, et al: Influence of desmethylimipramine on natural killer cell activity. Psychiatry Res 19:9–15, 1986

Miller AH, Spencer RL, Stein M, et al: Adrenal steroid receptor binding in spleen and thymus after stress or dexamethasone. Am J Physiol Endocrinol Metab 259:E405–412, 1990

Miller AH, Spencer RL, Hassett J, et al: Effects of selective type I and II adrenal steroid agonists on immune cell distribution. Endocrinology 135:1934–1944, 1994

Miller AH, Pariante CM, Pearce BD: Effects of cytokines on glucocorticoid receptor expression and function. Glucocorticoid resistance and relevance to depression. Adv Exp Med Biol 461:107–116, 1999

Miller AH, Pearce BD, Ruzek MC, et al: Interactions between the hypothalamic-pituitary-adrenal axis and immune system during viral infection: pathways for environmental effects on disease expression, in Handbook of Physiology, Vol IV. New York, Oxford University Press, 2000, pp 425–450

Miller GE, Cohen S, Rabin BS, et al: Personality and tonic cardiovascular, neuroendocrine, and immune parameters. Brain Behav Immun 13:109–123, 1999a

Miller GE, Dopp JM, Myers HF, et al: Psychosocial predictors of natural killer cell mobilization during marital conflict. Health Psychol 18:262–271, 1999b

Mills PJ, Dimsdale JE: The effects of acute psychologic stress on cellular adhesion molecules. J Psychosom Res 41:49–53, 1996

Mohr DC, Genain C: Social support as a buffer in the relationship between treatment for depression and T-cell production of interferon gamma in patients with multiple sclerosis. J Psychosom Res 57:155–158, 2004

Mohr DC, Goodkin DE, Bacchetti P, et al: Psychological stress and the subsequent appearance of new brain MRI lesions in MS. Neurology 55:55–61, 2000

Mohr DC, Goodkin DE, Islar J, et al: Treatment of depression is associated with suppression of nonspecific and antigen-specific T(H)1 responses in multiple sclerosis. Arch Neurol 58:1081–1086, 2001

Moore P, Landolt H, Seifritz E, et al: Clinical and physiological consequences of rapid tryptophan depletion. Neuropsychopharmacology 23:601–622, 2000

Moraska A: Elevated IL-1b contributes to antibody suppression produced by stress. J Appl Physiol 93:207–215, 2002

Muller N, Riedel M, Scheppach C, et al: Beneficial antipsychotic effects of celecoxib add-on therapy compared to risperidone alone in schizophrenia. Am J Psychiatry 159:1029–1034, 2002

Munck A, Guyre PM, Holbrook NJ: Physiological functions of glucocorticoids in stress and their relation to pharmacological actions. Endocr Rev 5:25–44

Musselman DL, Lawson DH, Gumnick JF, et al: Paroxetine for the prevention of depression induced by high-dose interferon alfa. N Engl J Med 29:961–966, 2001

Nadeau S, Rivest S: Glucocorticoids play a fundamental role in protecting the brain during innate immune response. J Neurosci 23:5536–5544, 2003

Nadjar A, Tridon V, May MJ, et al: NFkappaB activates in vivo the synthesis of inducible Cox-2 in the brain. J Cereb Blood Flow Metab 25:1047–1059, 2005

Nair MP, Schwartz SA: Immunomodulatory effects of corticosteroids on natural killer and antibody-dependent cellular cytotoxic activities of human lymphocytes. J Immunol 132:2876–2882, 1984

Naitoh Y, Fukata J, Tominaga T, et al: Interleukin-6 stimulates the secretion of adrenocorticotropic hormone in conscious, freely moving rats. Biochem Biophys Res Commun 155:1459–1463, 1988

Nguyen KT, Deak T, Owens SM, et al: Exposure to acute stress induces brain interleukin-1 beta protein in the rat. J Neurosci 18:2239–2246, 1998

Nishioka T, Kurokawa H, Takao T, et al: Differential changes of corticotropin releasing hormone (CRH) concentrations in plasma and synovial fluids of patients with rheumatoid arthritis (RA). Endocr J 43:241–247, 1996

Nisipeanu P, Korczyn AD: Psychological stress as risk factor for exacerbations in multiple sclerosis. Neurology 43:1311–1312, 1993

Obuchowicz E, Kowalski J, Labuzek K, et al: Amitriptyline and nortriptyline inhibit interleukin-1 release by rat mixed glial and microglial cell cultures. Int J Neuropsychopharmacol 9:27–35, 2006

O'Connor KA, Johnson JD, Hansen MK, et al: Peripheral and central proinflammatory cytokine response to a severe acute stressor. Brain Res 991:123–132, 2003

Owens MJ, Nemeroff CB: The role of corticotropin-releasing factor in the pathophysiology of affective and anxiety disorders: laboratory and clinical studies. Ciba Foundation Symposium 172:296–308, 1993; discussion 308–316, 1993

Padgett DA, Sheridan JF: Androstenediol (AED) prevents neuroendocrine-mediated suppression of the immune response to an influenza viral infection. J Neuroimmunol 98:121–129, 1999

Padgett DA, Loria RM, Sheridan JF: Endocrine regulation of the immune response to influenza virus infection with a metabolite of DHEA-androstenediol. J Neuroimmunol 78:203–211, 1997

Padmos RC, Bekris L, Knijff EM, et al: A high prevalence of organ-specific autoimmunity in patients with bipolar disorder. Biol Psychiatry 56:476–482, 2004

Paez Pereda M, Sauer J, Perez Castro C, et al: Corticotropin-releasing hormone differentially modulates the interleukin-1 system according to the level of monocyte activation by endotoxin. Endocrinology 136:5504–5510, 1995

Page-Schafer K, Delorenze GN, Satariano WA, et al: Comorbidity and survival in HIV-infected men in the San Francisco Men's Health Survey. Ann Epidemiol 6:420–430, 1996

Papanicolaou D: Euthyroid sick syndrome and the role of cytokines. Rev Endocr Metab Disord 1:43–48, 2000

Pariante CM, Miller AH: Natural killer cell activity in major depression: a prospective study of the in vivo effects of desmethylimipramine treatment. Eur Neuropsychopharmacol 5(suppl):83–88, 1995

Pariante CM, Miller AH: Glucocorticoid receptors in major depression: relevance to pathophysiology and treatment. Biol Psychiatry 49:391–404, 2001

Pariante CM, Carpiniello B, Orru MG, et al: Chronic caregiving stress alters peripheral blood immune parameters: the role of age and severity of stress. Psychother Psychosom 66:199–207, 1997

Pavlov VA, Tracey KJ: The cholinergic anti-inflammatory pathway. Brain Behav Immun 19:493–499, 2005

Perlstein RS, Whitnall MH, Abrams JS, et al: Synergistic roles of interleukin-6, interleukin-1, and tumor necrosis factor in the adrenocorticotropin response to bacterial lipopolysaccharide in vivo. Endocrinology 132:946–952, 1993

Perry S, Fishman B, Jacobsberg L, et al: Relationships over 1 year between lymphocyte subsets and psychosocial variables among adults with infection by human immunodeficiency virus. Arch Gen Psychiatry 49:396–401, 1992

Persoons JH, Schornagel K, Breve J, et al: Acute stress affects cytokines and nitric oxide production by alveolar macrophages differently. Am J Respir Crit Care Med 152:619–624, 1995

Peters ML, Godaert GL, Ballieux RE, et al: Immune responses to experimental stress: effects of mental effort and uncontrollability. Psychosom Med 61:513–524, 1999

Petitto JM, Leserman J, Perkins DO, et al: High versus low basal cortisol secretion in asymptomatic, medication-free HIV-infected men: differential effects of severe life stress on parameters of immune status. Behav Med 25:143–151, 2000

Pike JL, Smith TL, Hauger RL, et al: Chronic life stress alters sympathetic, neuroendocrine, and immune responsivity to an acute psychological stressor in humans. Psychosom Med 59:447–457, 1997

Plata-Salaman CR, Sonti G, Borkoski JP, et al: Anorexia induced by chronic central administration of cytokines at estimated pathophysiological concentrations. Physiol Behav 60:867–875, 1996

Plotkin SR, Banks WA, Kastin AJ: Comparison of saturable transport and extracellular pathways in the passage of interleukin-1 alpha across the blood-brain barrier. J Neuroimmunol 67:41–47, 1996

Price P, Olver SD, Silich M, et al: Adrenalitis and the adrenocortical response of resistant and susceptible mice to acute murine cytomegalovirus infection. Eur J Clin Invest 26:811–819, 1996

Printz DJ, Strauss DH, Goetz R, et al: Elevation of CD5+ B lymphocytes in schizophrenia. Biol Psychiatry 46:110–118, 1999

Quan N, Sundar SK, Weiss JM: Induction of interleukin-1 in various brain regions after peripheral and central injections of lipopolysaccharide. J Neuroimmunol 49:125–134, 1994

Quan N, Stern EL, Whiteside MB, et al: Induction of proinflammatory cytokine mRNAs in the brain after peripheral injection of subseptic doses of lipopolysaccharide in the rat. J Neuroimmunology 93:72–80, 1999

Rabkin JG, Williams JB, Remien RH, et al: Depression, distress, lymphocyte subsets, and human immunodeficiency virus symptoms on two occasions in HIV-positive homosexual men. Arch Gen Psychiatry 48:111–119, 1991

Raison CL, Miller AH: Cancer and depression: new developments regarding diagnosis and treatment. Biol Psychiatry 54:283–294, 2003a

Raison CL, Miller AH: When not enough is too much: the role of insufficient glucocorticoid signaling in the pathophysiology of stress-related disorders. Am J Psychiatry 160:1554–1565, 2003b

Raison CL, Capuron C, Miller AH: Cytokines sing the blues: inflammation and the pathogenesis of depression. Trends Immunol 27:24–31, 2006

Ramirez AJ, Craig TK, Watson JP, et al: Stress and relapse of breast cancer. BMJ 298:291–293, 1989

Rapaport MH, Guylai L, Whybrow P: Immune parameters in rapid cycling bipolar patients before and after lithium treatment. J Psychiatr Res 33:335–340, 1999

Rasmussen AF Jr, Marsh JT, Brill NQ: Increased susceptibility to herpes simplex in mice subjected to avoidance-learning stress or restraint. Proc Soc Exp Biol Med 96:183–189, 1957

Rassnick S, Sved AF, Rabin BS: Locus coeruleus stimulation by corticotropin-releasing hormone suppresses in vitro cellular immune responses. J Neurosci 14:6033–6040, 1994

Ravindran AV, Griffiths J, Merali Z, et al: Circulating lymphocyte subsets in major depression and dysthymia with typical or atypical features. Psychosom Med 60:283–289, 1998

Reed GM, Kemeny ME, Taylor SE, et al: Negative HIV-specific expectancies and AIDS-related bereavement as predictors of symptom onset in asymptomatic HIV-positive gay men. Health Psychol 18:354–363, 1999

Regelson W, Loria R, Kalimi M: Dehydroepiandrosterone (DHEA)—the "mother steroid," I: immunologic action. Ann N Y Acad Sci 719:553–563, 1994

Reynolds JL, Ignatowski TA, Sud R, et al: Brain-derived tumor necrosis factor-alpha and its involvement in noradrenergic neuron functioning involved in the mechanism of action of an antidepressant. J Pharmacol Exp Ther 10:1216–1225, 2004

Rhen T, Cidlowski JA: Antiinflammatory action of glucocorticoids—new mechanisms for old drugs. N Engl J Med 353:1711–1723, 2005

Ridker PM: High-sensitivity C-reactive protein, inflammation, and cardiovascular risk: from concept to clinical practice to clinical benefit. Am Heart J 148 (1 suppl):S19–26, 2004

Riedel M, Strassnig M, Schwarz MJ, et al: COX-2 inhibitors as adjunctive therapy in schizophrenia: rationale for use and evidence to date. CNS Drugs 19:805–819, 2005

Rivest S, Lacroix S, Vallieres L, et al: How the blood talks to the brain parenchyma and the paraventricular nucleus of the hypothalamus during systemic inflammatory and infectious stimuli. Proc Soc Exp Biol Med 223:22–38, 2000

Rivier C: Influence of immune signals on the hypothalamic-pituitary axis of the rodent. Front Neuroendocrinol 16:151–182, 1995

Roberts FD, Newcomb PA, Trentham-Dietz A, et al: Self-reported stress and risk of breast cancer. Cancer 77:1089–1093, 1996

Rogers CJ, Brissette-Storkus CS, Chambers WH, et al: Acute stress impairs NK cell adhesion and cytotoxicity through CD2, but not LFA-1. J Neuroimmunol 99:230–241, 1999

Rosa A, Peralta V, Papiol S, et al: Interleukin-1beta (IL-1beta) gene and increased risk for the depressive symptom-dimension in schizophrenia spectrum disorders. Am J Med Genet B Neuropsychiatr Genet 124:10–14, 2004

Rothwell NJ, Luheshi G, Toulmond S: Cytokines and their receptors in the central nervous system: physiology, pharmacology, and pathology. Pharmacol Ther 69:85–95, 1996

Ruzek MC, Pearce BD, Miller AH, et al: Endogenous glucocorticoids protect against cytokine-mediated lethality during viral infection. J Immunol 162:3527–3533, 1999

Sasaki T, Nanko S, Fukuda R, et al: Changes of immunological functions after acute exacerbation in schizophrenia. Biol Psychiatry 35:173–178, 1994

Schafer M, Carter L, Stein C: Interleukin 1 beta and corticotropin-releasing factor inhibit pain by releasing opioids from immune cells in inflamed tissue. Proc Natl Acad Sci U S A 91:4219–4223, 1994

Schleifer SJ, Keller SE, Bond RN, et al: Major depressive disorder and immunity. Role of age, sex, severity, and hospitalization. Arch Gen Psychiatry 46:81–87, 1989

Schleifer SJ, Keller SE, Bartlett JA: Depression and immunity: clinical factors and therapeutic course. Psychiatry Res 85:63–69, 1999

Schleimer RP, Claman HN, Oronsky AL: Anti-inflammatory Steroid Action: Basic and Clinical Aspects. San Diego, CA, Academic Press, 1989

Schmidt ED, Janszen AW, Wouterlood FG, et al: Interleukin-1–induced long-lasting changes in hypothalamic corticotropin-releasing hormone (CRH)-neurons and hyperresponsiveness of the hypothalamus-pituitary-adrenal axis. J Neurosci 15:7417–7426, 1995

Schobitz B, De Kloet ER, Holsboer F: Gene expression and function of interleukin 1, interleukin 6 and tumor necrosis factor in the brain. Prog Neurobiol 44:397–432, 1994

Schulte HM, Bamberger CM, Elsen H, et al: Systemic interleukin-1 alpha and interleukin-2 secretion in response to acute stress and to corticotropin-releasing hormone in humans. Eur J Clin Invest 24:773–777, 1994

Segerstrom SC, Miller GE: Psychological stress and the human immune system: a meta-analytic study of 30 years of inquiry. Psychol Bull 130:601–630, 2004

Segerstrom SC, Taylor SE, Kemeny ME, et al: Optimism is associated with mood, coping, and immune change in response to stress. J Pers Soc Psychol 74:1646–1655, 1998

Seidel A, Arolt V, Hunstiger M, et al: Cytokine production and serum proteins in depression. Scand J Immunol 41:534–538, 1995

Sephton SE, Sapolsky RM, Kraemer HC, et al: Diurnal cortisol rhythm as a predictor of breast cancer survival. J Nat Cancer Inst 92:994–1000, 2000

Sharp BM, Roy S, Bidlack JM: Evidence for opioid receptors on cells involved in host defense and the immune system. J Neuroimmunol 83:45–56, 1998

Shavit Y, Lewis JW, Terman GW, et al: Opioid peptides mediate the suppressive effect of stress on natural killer cell cytotoxicity. Science 223:188–190, 1984

Shen WH, Zhou JH, Broussard SR, et al: Tumor necrosis factor alpha inhibits insulin-like growth factor I-induced hematopoietic cell survival and proliferation. Endocrinology 145:3101–3105, 2004

Silverman MN, Pearce BD, Biron CA, et al: Immune modulation of the hypothalamic-pituitary-adrenal (HPA) axis during viral infection. Viral Immunol 18:41–78, 2005

Sluzewska A, Rybakowski JK, Laciak M, et al: Interleukin-6 serum levels in depressed patients before and after treatment with fluoxetine. Ann N Y Acad Sci 762:474–476, 1995

Snider LA, Lougee L, Slattery M, et al: Antibiotic prophylaxis with azithromycin or penicillin for childhood-onset neuropsychiatric disorders. Biol Psychiatry 57:788–792, 2005

Song C, Lin A, Bonaccorso S, et al: The inflammatory response system and the availability of plasma tryptophan in patients with primary sleep disorders and major depression. J Affect Disord 49:211–219, 1998

Sonino N, Girelli ME, Boscaro M, et al: Life events in the pathogenesis of Graves' disease: a controlled study. Acta Endocrinol (Copenh) 128:293–296, 1993

Spangelo BL, Judd AM, MacLeod RM, et al: Endotoxin-induced release of interleukin-6 from rat medial basal hypothalami. Endocrinology 127:1779–1785, 1990

Spiegel D, Bloom JR, Kraemer HC, et al: Effect of psychosocial treatment on survival of patients with metastatic breast cancer. Lancet 2:888–891, 1989

Spinedi E, Hadid R, Daneva T, et al: Cytokines stimulate the CRH but not the vasopressin neuronal system: evidence for a median eminence site of interleukin-6 action. Neuroendocrinology 56:46–53, 1992

Steiner G, Tohidast-Akrad M, Witzmann G, et al: Cytokine production by synovial T cells in rheumatoid arthritis. Rheumatology 38:202–213, 1999

Stenzel-Poore MP, Duncan JE, Rittenberg MB, et al: CRH overproduction in transgenic mice: behavioral and immune system modulation. Ann N Y Acad Sci 780:36–48, 1996

Sternberg EM, Hill JM, Chrousos GP, et al: Inflammatory mediator-induced hypothalamic-pituitary-adrenal axis activation is defective in streptococcal cell wall arthritis-susceptible Lewis rats. Proc Natl Acad Sci U S A 86:2374–2378, 1989

Stewart MW, Knight RG, Palmer DG, et al: Differential relationships between stress and disease activity for immunologically distinct subgroups of people with rheumatoid arthritis. J Abnorm Psychol 103:251–258, 1994

Stubner S, Schon T, Padberg F, et al: Interleukin-6 and the soluble IL-6 receptor are decreased in cerebrospinal fluid of geriatric patients with major depression: no alteration of soluble gp130. Neurosci Lett 259:145–148, 1999

Suda T, Tozawa F, Ushiyama T, et al: Interleukin-1 stimulates corticotropin-releasing factor gene expression in rat hypothalamus. Endocrinology 126:1223–1228, 1990

Swedo SE, Leonard HL, Garvey M, et al: Pediatric autoimmune neuropsychiatric disorders associated with streptococcal infections: clinical description of the first 50 cases. Am J Psychiatry 155:264–271, 1998

Then Bergh F, Kumpfel T, Trenkwalder C, et al: Dysregulation of the hypothalamo-pituitary-adrenal axis is related to the clinical course of MS. Neurology 53:772–777, 1999

Thomason BT, Brantley PJ, Jones GN, et al: The relation between stress and disease activity in rheumatoid arthritis. J Behav Med 15:215–220, 1992

Torpy DJ, Chrousos GP: The three-way interactions between the hypothalamic-pituitary-adrenal and gonadal axes and the immune system. Baillieres Clin Rheumatol 10:181–198, 1996

Tsai SY, Chen KP, Yang YY, et al: Activation of indices of cell-mediated immunity in bipolar mania. Biol Psychiatry 45:989–994, 1999

Uchino BN, Kiecolt-Glaser JK, Cacioppo JT: Age-related changes in cardiovascular response as a function of a chronic stressor and social support. J Pers Soc Psychol 63:839–846, 1992

Vacca A, Felli MP, Farina AR, et al: Glucocorticoid receptor-mediated suppression of the interleukin 2 gene expression through impairment of the cooperativity between nuclear factor of activated T cells and AP-1 enhancer elements. J Exp Med 175:637–646, 1992

van Dam AM, Brouns M, Louisse S, et al: Appearance of interleukin-1 in macrophages and in ramified microglia in the brain of endotoxin-treated rats: a pathway for the induction of non-specific symptoms of sickness? Brain Res 588:291–296, 1992

van Kammen DP, McAllister-Sistilli CG, Kelley ME, et al: Elevated interleukin-6 in schizophrenia. Psychiatry Res 87:129–136, 1999

Venters HD, Dantzer R, Freund GG, et al: Growth hormone and insulin-like growth factor as cytokines in the immune system, in Psychoneuroimmunology, 3rd Edition. Edited by Alder R, Felten D, Cohen N. New York, Academic Press, 2001, pp 339–362

Wadee AA, Kuschke RH, Wood LA, et al: Serological observations in patients suffering from acute manic episodes. Hum Psychopharmacol 17:175–179, 2002

Walker LG, Heys SD, Walker MB, et al: Psychological factors can predict the response to primary chemotherapy in patients with locally advanced breast cancer. Eur J Cancer 35:1783–1788, 1999

Wang X, Wu H, Miller AH: Interleukin-1 alpha-induced activation of p38 mitogen-activated kinase inhibits glucocorticoid receptor function. Mol Psychiatry 9:65–75, 2004

Ward MM, Lotstein DS, Bush TM, et al: Psychosocial correlates of morbidity in women with systemic lupus erythematosus. J Rheumatol 26:2153–2158, 1999

Watkins LR, Goehler LE, Relton JK, et al: Blockade of interleukin-1 induced hyperthermia by subdiaphragmatic vagotomy: evidence for vagal mediation of immune-brain communication. Neurosci Lett 183:27–31, 1995

Watson M, Haviland JS, Greer S, et al: Influence of psychological response on survival in breast cancer: a population-based cohort study. Lancet 354:1331–1336, 1999

Watson M, Homewood J, Haviland J, et al: Influence of psychological response on breast cancer survival: 10-year follow-up of a population-based cohort. Eur J Cancer 41:1710–1714, 2005

Weiss JM, Sundar S: Effects of stress on cellular immune responses in animals, in American Psychiatric Press Review of Psychiatry, Vol 11. Edited by Tasman A, Riba MB. Washington, DC, American Psychiatric Press, 1992, pp 145–168

Weizman R, Laor N, Podliszewski E, et al: Cytokine production in major depressed patients before and after clomipramine treatment. Biol Psychiatry 35:42–47, 1994

Whitacre CC, Reingold SC, O'Looney PA: A gender gap in autoimmunity. Science 283:1277–1278, 1999

Wilckens T, DeRijk R: Glucocorticoids and immune function: unknown dimensions and new frontiers. Immunol Today 18:418–424, 1997

Williams JM, Peterson RG, Shea PA: Sympathetic innervation of murine thymus and spleen: evidence for a functional link between the nervous and immune systems. Brain Res Bull 6:83–94, 1981

Wulsin LR, Vaillant GE, Wells VE: A systematic review of the mortality of depression. Psychosom Med 61:6–17, 1999

Wyllie AH: Glucocorticoid-induced thymocyte apoptosis is associated with endogenous endonuclease activation. Nature 284:555–556, 1980

Yin D, Tuthill D, Mufson RA, et al: Chronic restraint stress promotes lymphocyte apoptosis by modulating CD95 expression. J Exp Med 191:1423–1428, 2000

Yirmiya R, Pollak Y, Morag M, et al: Illness, cytokines, and depression. Ann N Y Acad Sci 917:478–487, 2000

Yolken RH, Torrey EF: Viruses, schizophrenia, and bipolar disorder. Clin Microbiol Rev 8:131–145, 1995

Yoshihara S, Ricciardolo FL, Geppetti P, et al: Corticotropin-releasing factor inhibits antigen-induced plasma extravasation in airways. Eur J Pharmacol 280:113–118, 1995

Yoshiuchi K, Kumano H, Nomura S, et al: Stressful life events and smoking were associated with Graves' disease in women, but not in men. Psychosom Med 60:182–185, 1998

Yovel G, Sirota P, Mazeh D, et al: Higher natural killer cell activity in schizophrenic patients: the impact of serum factors, medication, and smoking. Brain Behav Immun 14:153–169, 2000

Yu-Lee LY: Molecular actions of prolactin in the immune system. Exp Biol Med 215:35–52, 1997

Zhang XY, Zhou DF, Cao LY, et al: Cortisol and cytokines in chronic and treatment-resistant patients with schizophrenia: association with psychopathology and response to antipsychotics. Neuropsychopharmacology 30:1532–1538, 2005

Zhou D, Kusnecov AW, Shurin MR, et al: Exposure to physical and psychological stressors elevates plasma interleukin 6: relationship to the activation of hypothalamic-pituitary-adrenal axis. Endocrinology 133:2523–2530, 1993

Zhu CB, Carneiro AM, Dostmann WR, et al: p38 MAPK activation elevates serotonin transport activity via a trafficking-independent, protein phosphatase 2A-dependent process. J Biol Chem 280:15649–15658, 2005

Zorrilla EP, McKay JR, Luborsky L, et al: Relation of stressors and depressive symptoms to clinical progression of viral illness. Am J Psychiatry 153:626–635, 1996

Part II

Neuropsychiatric Assessment

4

BEDSIDE NEUROPSYCHIATRY

Eliciting the Clinical Phenomena of Neuropsychiatric Illness

Fred Ovsiew, M.D.

Unless we take pains to be accurate in our examinations as to the question propounded, our observations will be of little value. The investigator who simply asks leading questions...is not accumulating "facts," but is "organising confusion." He will make errors enough without adopting a clumsy plan of investigating which renders blundering certain.

—*John Hughlings-Jackson, 1880*

In this chapter, I review the tools offered by history-taking and examination for discovering the contribution of cerebral dysfunction to psychological abnormality and behavioral disturbance. The focus is on methods of filling in a matrix of clinical information; clinical correlates of the symptoms and signs discussed are mentioned but not comprehensively reviewed. The focus also is on the manifestations of cerebral disease rather than on systemic disorders and the signs to which they may give rise in the general physical examination. Fortunately, excellent coverage of the latter is available in general (McGee 2001; Orient and Sapira 2005) or as specifically applied to neuropsychiatry (Garden 2005; Ovsiew 2004; Sanders and Keshavan 2002).

A focus on the phenomenology of cerebral disease should not be mistaken for a commitment to a localizationist paradigm of cerebral function. Focal neurobehavioral syndromes are clinical facts and have been of substantial heuristic value in the cognitive neurosciences (D'Esposito 2003). The power of the cognitive neurosciences is being brought to bear on the deconstruction of psychiatric syndromes into disruptions of well-understood normal cognitive processes, the discipline of cognitive neuropsychiatry (Halligan and David 2001; Pantelis and Maruff 2002). This likely will lead to expansion of the mutual territory of psychiatry and the cognitive neurosciences, a welcome development. However, some clinicians appear to be waiting for the arrival of a psychiatric taxonomy in which behavioral signs carry the localizing power of focal neurological signs. In what is, so to speak, a best-case scenario for neuropsychiatric localizationism, understanding of psychopathology would provide "clues as to the cerebral location of functional pathology....The challenge for neuropsychiatry is to develop the neurobiology of the auditory system, of delusion formation and of disordered thinking to interpret the associations between psychotic symptoms encountered clinically" (Santhouse et al. 2000, p. 2062). For reasons discussed at length elsewhere, this is likely to represent a false hope (Ovsiew 2005).

TAKING THE HISTORY

Obtaining a history is an active process on the part of the interviewer, who must have in mind a matrix to be filled in with information. The excuse "the patient is a poor historian" has no place in neuropsychiatry. The examiner must realize that he or she, and not the patient, is the "historian," responsible for gathering information from all necessary sources and forming a coherent narrative. Discovering that the patient is unable to give an adequate account of his or her life and illness should prompt a search, first, for other informants and, second, for an explanation of the incapacity.

BIRTH

The neuropsychiatric history begins with events that took place even before the birth of the patient. Maternal illness in pregnancy and the process of labor and delivery should be reviewed for untoward events associated with fetal maldevelopment, including bleeding and substance abuse during pregnancy, the course of labor, low birth weight, and fetal distress at birth and in the immediate postnatal period. Obstetric complications are associated with schizophrenia and probably other psychiatric syndromes, potentially including mood disorder and anorexia nervosa (Verdoux and Sutter 2002).

DEVELOPMENT

At times, the historian can gather information from the first minutes of extrauterine life; for example, when Apgar scores are available in hospital records. More commonly, parental recollection of milestones must be relied on. The ages at which the child walked, spoke words, spoke sentences, went to school, and so on often can be elicited from parents. Parents may be able to compare the patient with a "control" sibling. The infant's temperament—shy, active, cuddly, fussy, and so on—may give

clues to persisting traits. School performance is an important marker of both the intellectual and the social competence of the child and often is the only information available about premorbid intellectual level. Of particular interest is an anomalous pattern of intellectual strengths and weaknesses. Relative weakness in reading (dyslexia) is well recognized. Low capacities in nonverbal skills along with arithmetic impairment suggest a nonverbal learning disability (Sundheim and Voeller 2004). Childhood illness, including febrile convulsions, head injury, and central nervous system infection, is sometimes the precursor of adult neuropsychiatric disorder (Cendes 2004; Koponen et al. 2004; Leask et al. 2002).

HANDEDNESS

Assessment of handedness provides an essential bedside clue to cerebral organization. Several questionnaires are available (Bryden 1977; Peters 1998). Fortunately, a few simple inquiries—asking the patient which hand he or she uses to write, throw, draw, and hold scissors or a toothbrush—serve well to establish handedness (Bryden 1977). With some nonverbal patients (e.g., the severely mentally retarded), watching the patient catch and throw a ball or a crumpled piece of paper is a simple examination for handedness. The "torque test" of drawing circles (Demarest and Demarest 1980), examination of the angle formed by the opposed thumb and little finger (Metzig et al. 1975), and observation of handwriting posture (Duckett et al. 1993; J. Levy and Reid 1976) have advocates as ways to establish cerebral dominance at the bedside.

ICTAL EVENTS

Many "spells" or "attacks" occur in neuropsychiatric patients, and taking the history of a paroxysmal event has certain requirements regardless of the nature of the event. The clinician should track through the phases of the paroxysm, starting with the prodrome, then the aura, then the remainder of the ictus (the aura being the onset or core of the ictus), and then the aftermath. For any attack disorder, how frequent and how stereotyped the events are should be determined. Rapidity of onset and cessation; disturbance of consciousness or of language; occurrence of autochthonous sensations, ideas, and emotions and of lateralized motor or cognitive dysfunction; purposefulness and coordination of actions; injury sustained during the attack; memory for the spell; and duration of the recovery period should be ascertained. Beginning an inquiry about seizures by asking if the patient has just one sort of spell or more than one reduces confusion as history-taking proceeds with a patient who has both partial and generalized seizures. Some patients with pseudoseizures will say that they have epileptic spells and then another sort that happens when they are upset.

Prodromal phases of epileptic attacks were formerly well known, when epileptic patients resided in colonies and were under observation as they "built up" to a seizure. Adverse mood changes commonly occur on the days preceding a seizure (Blanchet and Frommer 1986). Prodromes occur in migraine as well (Sacks 1971).

Some of the abnormal experiences well known in temporal lobe epilepsy—the "voluminous" mental state described by Hughlings-Jackson (Bancaud et al. 1994; Gloor et al. 1982)—occur in mood disorders and in other psychiatric states as a putative marker of limbic dysfunction (Ardila et al. 1993; Atre-Vaidya et al. 1994; C.L. Harris et al. 2002; Persinger and Makarec 1993; Roberts et al. 1990, 1992; Silberman et al. 1985; Teicher et al. 1993). These phenomena in nonepileptic populations are associated with markers of brain injury, such as a history of perinatal hypoxia, fever with delirium, or head trauma (Ardila et al. 1993; Verduyn et al. 1992); with childhood abuse (Teicher et al. 1993); and with beliefs in the paranormal (Skirda and Persinger 1993). Hermann et al. (1982) reported that patients with fear as a part of the seizure ictus are at elevated risk for psychopathology. The phenomena of the voluminous mental state can be elicited by questions about *déjà vu* and *jamais vu*, depersonalization and derealization, autoscopy, micropsia and macropsia, metamorphopsia, other visual illusions, paranormal experiences such as clairvoyance or precognition or a sensed presence, and other paroxysmal experiences. Persinger and Makarec (1987), Roberts et al. (1992), and Teicher et al. (1993) developed questionnaires to take an inventory of these experiences.

HEAD INJURY

Discerning the role of cerebral dysfunction in posttraumatic states is a common diagnostic challenge. The length of the anterograde amnesia, from the moment of trauma to the recovery of the capacity for consecutive memory, can be learned either from the patient or from hospital records. The patient can state what the last memories before the accident are; from last memory to injury is the period of retrograde amnesia. The lengths of these intervals and the duration of coma are correlated with the severity of brain damage. Usually, posttraumatic amnesia is the best indicator (Lishman 1998). The nature of the trauma, including its psychosocial setting and whether impulsive or reckless behavior led to the injury, should be learned.

ALCOHOL AND DRUG USE

A substance abuse history must be taken from all patients. Questions about vocational, family, and medical impairment attributable to abuse; shame and guilt over abuse and efforts to control it; morning or secret drinking; blackouts; and other familiar issues help the clinician identify pathological behavior in this sphere. Cocaine and alcohol abuse in particular are associated with a variety of neuropsychiatric consequences, including cognitive impairment, movement disorders, seizures, and stroke (Marshall 1999).

MILD COGNITIVE IMPAIRMENT

Some patients with mild cognitive disturbance not meeting the criteria for a diagnosis of dementia are unlike those now considered as in a prodromal stage of amnestic (Alzheimer's) or vascular dementia in that the impairment is chronic and stable; traumatic brain injury frequently gives rise to this state (M.P. Alexander 1995). Some features in these patients, such as emotional lability and irritability, are characteristic of, but not specific to, organic states. In my experience, certain cognitive symptoms reported by patients are so distinctive that they are nearly diagnostic of organic illness.

For example, before undergoing resection of an arteriovenous malformation, a successful businesswoman had been accustomed to reading the newspaper carefully over breakfast. After the procedure, she discovered that although she was able to read a newspaper and absorb its import adequately, she was not able to do so while eating breakfast. She could do only one thing at a time. This loss of the capacity for divided attention is highly characteristic of mild cerebral disease. Distractibility is heightened, and automatic tasks require attention and effort. An interesting example of this deficit is the "stops walking when talking" phenomenon (Lundin-Olsson et al. 1997; Parker et al. 2005; Sheridan et al. 2003). Impairment of gait (manifested clinically by cessation of walking but measurable in the laboratory) when attention is divided may presage falls or indicate encroaching cognitive dysfunction. Burgess et al. (2000) reviewed the features of focal lesions producing disturbances of "multitasking."

Sensitive descriptions by neurobiologically sophisticated self-observers of their own disorders leave little doubt that even limited brain lesions have effects not explicable on a localizationist model of brain function (Brodal 1973; Cole 1999). Lezak (1978) emphasized the patient's experience of perplexity and fatigue in mild and severe brain injury. These subtle features of mild cerebral dysfunction were clearly described and experimentally elucidated many years ago (Chapman and Wolff 1958; Chapman et al. 1958).

APPETITIVE FUNCTIONS

Appetitive functions include sleeping, eating, and sexual interest and performance. Disturbed sleep is common in patients with psychiatric disorders of any origin and in the general population as well. In a search for clues to organic factors in psychiatric illness, the clinician inquires about the pattern of disturbance: early waking in depressive illness, nighttime wakings related to pain or nocturnal myoclonus, excessive daytime sleepiness in narcolepsy and sleep apnea, sleep attacks in narcolepsy, and periodic excessive somnolence in Kleine-Levin syndrome and related disorders. Simple observation of a hospitalized patient by night nursing staff, or at home by family members, can identify snoring, apneas, or abnormal movements. Solms (1997) analyzed dreaming in a large series of brain-injured patients. He found that loss of dreaming occurs with parietal lesions in either hemisphere and with deep bifrontal injury. Dreams devoid of visual imagery occur with ventral occipitotemporal lesions.

Patterns of abnormal eating behavior in organic cerebral disease include the hyperphagia of medial hypothalamic disease, in which food exerts an irresistible attraction, or reduced eating with lateral hypothalamic lesions; the mouthing and eating of nonfood objects in bilateral amygdalar disease (part of the Klüver-Bucy syndrome); and the impulsive stuffing of food into the mouth irrespective of hunger in frontal disease (Mendez and Foti 1997; G. Smith et al. 1998). The full syndromal picture of anorexia nervosa results rarely from organic disease, usually involving right frontal and temporal regions (Uher and Treasure 2005). Regard and Landis (1997) described an accentuation of interest in fine cuisine—the "gourmand syndrome"—after anterior right hemisphere lesions.

Drinking behavior is markedly increased in "psychogenic" polydipsia, a disorder of unknown pathogenesis seen in schizophrenia (de Leon 2003). Peri-ictal drinking is associated with right hemisphere ictal onset, as is peri-ictal urination (Baumgartner et al. 2000; Trinka et al. 2003).

Sexual interest, sexual performance, and reproductive health are commonly disturbed in brain disease. A change in a person's habitual sexual interests, either quantitative or qualitative, occurring de novo in adult life, suggests organic disease (Cummings 1999). Hyposexuality is reportedly a feature of epilepsy, and either antiepileptic drugs or epilepsy itself may disturb sex hormones, in a fashion that may depend on the laterality of the seizure focus (Herzog et al. 2003; Morrell et al. 2005).

AGGRESSION

Patterns of aggressive behavior in brain disease relate to the locus of injury (Benjamin 1999a; Devinsky and Bear 1984).

Features of aggressive behavior such as its onset and cessation; the patient's mental state and especially clarity of consciousness during the violent period; the patient's capacity for planned, coordinated, and well-organized action as shown in the act; the patient's regret, or otherwise, afterward; and any associated symptoms may yield clues about the contribution of cerebral dysfunction to the behavior.

PERSONALITY CHANGE

Changes in sexual preference with onset in adult life have already been mentioned as pointers to organic mental disorder. Persisting alterations in or exaggerations of other personality traits, if not related to an abnormal mood state or psychosis, may be important indicators of the development of cerebral disease. Lability and shallowness of emotion, irritability, aggressiveness, loss of sense of humor, and coarsening of the sensibilities are often mentioned. However, the warning of Syz (1937) issued more than 70 years ago still applies:

> Whenever those nervous structures which control the personality-organization are damaged it may become particularly difficult to discriminate between alterations of function due to organic lesions and alterations due to reactive tendencies of the total organism in its adaptation to the environment. So that we may be confronted with combinations or fusions of the two types of processes which are difficult to untangle. (p. 374)

A set of personality traits said to be distinctive for temporal lobe epilepsy includes hypergraphia, mystical or religious interests, "humorless sobriety," tendency toward rage, interpersonal stickiness or "viscosity," and hyposexuality. Whether these traits are related to epilepsy, to the temporal lobe injury underlying epilepsy, or merely to psychopathology remains controversial (Bear et al. 1989; Blumer 1999; Devinsky and Najjar 1999; Trimble et al. 1997).

OCCUPATION

Exposures to heavy metals or volatile hydrocarbons and repeated blows to the head in boxers are examples of occupational causes of neuropsychiatric illness. Apart from gathering etiological information, the clinician needs to know about the patient's work to gauge premorbid capacities and to assess disability.

FAMILY HISTORY

Genetic contributions to many neuropsychiatric illnesses are well delineated (e.g., in Huntington's disease); in other illnesses, the contribution is probable but its nature less clear (e.g., in Tourette syndrome). Inquiry about the family history of neuropsychiatric illness is most rewarding when pursued relative by relative, even constructing a family tree. Although genetic epilepsy syndromes exist and the risk of idiopathic epilepsy is familial, risk for symptomatic epilepsy after postnatal insults seems, for the most part, to be independent of family history of epilepsy (Johnson and Sander 2001; Schaumann et al. 1994).

EXAMINING THE PATIENT

The British neurologist Henry Miller (1975) referred to psychiatry as "neurology without physical signs" (p. 462). Geoffrey Lloyd (1983) called psychosomatics "medicine without signs" (p. 539). We may consider neuropsychiatry to be "psychiatry with signs." Unfortunately, the sensitivity and specificity of many findings are unknown, even for signs that are routine or traditional in the clinical examination. Too often, the clinical examination proceeds by ritual. The clinician who asks the patient with right hemisphere stroke to interpret proverbs but not to copy figures, or asks him or her to remember three words but not three shapes, is bowing to tradition and ignoring the physiology of the brain disease. Moreover, the tasks may lack discernible relation to cognitive or anatomical systems: what underlies the ability to recall the names of the last four presidents? Probes of mental function should be chosen with reference to the structure of the mind, as best understood.

Sometimes, clinicians attempt to elicit not signs of brain disease but so-called positive signs of nonorganic states. Vibratory sensation that shows lateralized deficit on the sternum is an example. Most such signs are of limited utility, not because they are uncommon in hysteria but because suggestibility is common in organic mental states as well (Fishbain et al. 2003; Gould et al. 1986; Rolak 1988). These signs cannot be relied on for differential diagnosis. However, the Hoover and abductor signs may offer more specificity (Sonoo 2004; Stone et al. 2002).

ASYMMETRY AND
MINOR PHYSICAL ANOMALIES

Abnormal development of a hemisphere may be betrayed by slight differences in the size of the thumbs or thumbnails. A postcentral location of cortical lesions causing asymmetry is characteristic (Penfield and Robertson 1943). A small hemiface or hemicranium is usually ipsilateral to an epileptic focus (Tinuper et al. 1992).

Other physical anomalies are stable through childhood and give clues to abnormal neurodevelopment even in adulthood. The Waldrop scale is in common use, but minor anomalies not included in that scale may be relevant

(Ismail et al. 1998) (Table 4–1). They may occur in healthy individuals, and only an excessive number, not an individual anomaly, correlates with psychopathology. The deviant development can be traced to the first 4 months of fetal life, and either genetic or environmental factors can give rise to the disturbance of gestation (McNeil et al. 2000). Presumably, the relation of the anomalies to the brain disorder lies in a disturbance of contemporaneous cerebral development. Head circumference, however, differs from the other anomalies, both in its having significance as a sole finding and in the timing of its occurrence. Both microcephaly and macrocephaly are of clinical significance, the latter especially in the instance of autism spectrum disorders (Gillberg and de Souza 2002; Herbert et al. 2004).

Such anomalies are associated with schizophrenia (McNeil et al. 2000), even late-onset schizophrenia (Lohr et al. 1997). The evidence less conclusively associates them with other psychotic disorders (McGrath et al. 1995), schizophrenia spectrum disorders including schizotypal personality disorder (Schiffman et al. 2002; Weinstein et al. 1999), mood disorder (Lohr et al. 1997; Tenyi et al. 2004), tardive dyskinesia (Waddington et al. 1995), autism (Rodier et al. 1997), violent delinquency in boys (Arseneault et al. 2000), inhibited behavior in girls (C.A. Fogel et al. 1985), and violent behavior in criminals (Kandel et al. 1989). Thus, they are best regarded as a nonspecific indicator of abnormal neurodevelopment, maldevelopment that may interact with psychosocial factors in the genesis of psychopathology (Ismail et al. 2000; Pine et al. 1997; Tarrant and Jones 1999). Dysmorphic features in a mentally retarded patient should lead to investigations to identify the cause of the retardation (Ryan and Sunada 1997), in particular to consideration of a subtelomeric deletion, an increasingly recognized cause of nonsyndromal mental retardation (de Vries et al. 2001).

OLFACTION

Hyposmia or anosmia can be detected in Alzheimer's disease, Parkinson's disease, normal aging, schizophrenia, multiple sclerosis, subfrontal tumor, human immunodeficiency virus (HIV) infection, migraine, and traumatic brain injury (Martzke et al. 1997; Pinching 1977). The most common cause of hyposmia, however, is local disease of the nasal mucosa, and the examiner must exclude local disease before regarding the finding as having neuropsychiatric significance.

Pinching (1977) provided an assessment of what test odors are most sensitive and specific for olfactory defects. Stimuli that cause trigeminal irritation (such as ammonia) are not suitable. Floral and musk odors provide the greatest sensitivity. I use raspberry- and cherry-

TABLE 4–1.   Selected minor physical anomalies

Head and face

Head circumference[a]

≥ 2 Hair whorls

Fine, "electric" hair that will not comb down

Frontal bossing

Eyes

Wide-spaced eyes

Epicanthus

Short palpebral fissures

Iris discoloration or defect

Ears

Adherent lobes

Malformation

Asymmetry

Soft and pliable

Low-seated

Preauricular skin tag

Mouth

High arch of palate

Furrowed tongue

Geographic tongue

Abnormal philtrum

Cleft uvula

Extremities

Clinodactyly

Abnormal palm crease

Third toe longer than second toe

Partial syndactyly

Gap between first and second toes

Small nails

Single crease on fifth finger

Note.   *Italicized* items are included in Waldrop scale.
[a]The normal range of head circumference in adults is governed by a complex relation to height, weight, and sex. Roughly, for males the range is 54–60 cm (21.25–23.5 in) and for females, 52–58 cm (20.5–22.75 in) (Bushby et al. 1992).

scented lip balm to test for olfactory defects; these scents are simple and strong, and the containers can be easily carried in a coat pocket. More sophisticated equipment is available for clinical use and may be of diagnostic value (Katzenschlager and Lees 2004; Savic et al. 1997).

EYES

Dilated pupils associated with anticholinergic toxicity may be a clue to the cause of delirium, and small pupils associated with opiate intoxication may be a clue to substance abuse. Argyll Robertson pupils—bilaterally small, irregular, and reactive to accommodation but not to light—characteristically accompany neurosyphilis (Burke and Schaberg 1985; Luxon et al. 1979), but they also occur in sarcoidosis, Lyme disease, and other conditions (Dasco and Bortz 1989; Koudstaal et al. 1987). Pupillary abnormalities other than Argyll Robertson pupils, such as bilateral tonic pupils, also may occur in neurosyphilis (Fletcher and Sharpe 1986).

A Kayser-Fleischer ring is nearly always present when Wilson's disease affects the brain (Brewer 2005; Makharia et al. 2002). This brownish-green discoloration of the cornea begins at the limbus, at 12 o'clock and then at 6 o'clock, spreading from each location medially and laterally until a complete ring is formed. It can be difficult to discern in patients with dark irises, so slit-lamp examination should supplement bedside inspection.

Iris pigmentation is linked to the temperamental trait of behavioral inhibition: inhibited children are more apt to be blue-eyed than are their uninhibited peers (Coplan et al. 1998). Korein (1981) reported that pale (blue, green, gray, or hazel) irises are more common in patients with dystonia than in control subjects. An attempt to replicate the finding failed (Lang et al. 1982).

VISUAL FIELDS

When lesions disrupt the white matter of the temporal lobe, a homonymous superior quadrantanopsia or even a full homonymous hemianopsia can result from involvement of Meyer's loop, the portion of the optic radiation that dips into the temporal lobe (Cushing 1922; Hughes et al. 1999). (Meyer, incidentally, was the psychiatrist-neuropathologist Adolf Meyer, whose collaboration on ward rounds the neurosurgeon Cushing acknowledged.) The finding can be an important pointer to an otherwise neurologically silent temporal lobe lesion. In cases of delirium from posterior cerebral or right middle cerebral artery infarction, hemianopsia may be the only pointer to a structural cause rather than a toxic-metabolic encephalopathy (Caplan et al. 1986; Devinsky et al. 1988).

BLINKING

The normal response to regular one-per-second taps on the glabella (with the examiner behind the patient so that the striking finger is not within the patient's visual field and the patient is not responding to visual threat) is blinking to the first few taps, followed by habituation and no blinking. Failure to habituate to glabellar tap (Myerson's sign) is seen in parkinsonism. The normal spontaneous blink rate increases through childhood but is stable in adulthood at a rate of about 16±8 (Zametkin et al. 1979).

Stevens (1978a, 1978b) reminded us that Emil Kraepelin, among other early investigators, had commented on abnormalities of blinking in schizophrenia. She found high rates of spontaneous blinking, paroxysms of rapid rhythmic blinking during episodes of abnormal behavior, and abnormal responses to glabellar tap. On glabellar tap, Stevens's patients either failed to blink, produced a shower of blinks, or failed to habituate. Although Stevens's patients were drug-free, few were neuroleptic-naïve, so she could not distinguish between an abnormality intrinsic to schizophrenia and tardive dyskinesia. Others confirmed the findings (Helms and Godwin 1985; Karson 1979).

The matter is of particular interest because the rate of spontaneous blinking is quite insensitive to peripheral stimuli (ambient light, humidity, even deafferentation of the fifth nerve) but is under dopaminergic control (Ellsworth et al. 1991; Freed et al. 1980). Clinically, dopaminergic influence produces a low blink rate in parkinsonism and an increase in blink rate with effective levodopa treatment (Karson et al. 1984). Thus, blink rate provides a simple quantitative index of central dopamine activity.

EYE MOVEMENTS

Stevens (1978a) also called attention to early observations by Kraepelin and others of several abnormal eye movements seen in psychotic patients. She noted gaze abnormalities, abnormality in eye contact with the examiner (e.g., fixed staring or no eye contact), impaired convergence movements, and irregular smooth pursuit movements. Clinicians' descriptions of eye movements are often inferential (e.g., "looking at the voices"), but an attempt at phenomenological description is useful (e.g., "unexplained episodic lateral glances").

Stevens's finding of irregular smooth pursuit movements in schizophrenic patients can be compared with laboratory investigations of abnormal smooth pursuit movements in psychotic patients. This abnormality is thought to be a trait under genetic control and related to abnormal attentional function and vulnerability to psychosis (D.L. Levy et al. 1993). However, jerky smooth pursuit movements are a common and nonspecific finding on bedside examination and do not reliably distinguish schizophrenic patients from healthy control subjects (Chen et al. 1995).

Elucidating abnormalities of eye movement in neuropsychiatric patients requires separate examination of voluntary eye movements without fixation ("look to the left"), generation of saccades to a target ("look at my finger, now back at my face"), and smooth pursuit ("follow my finger"). Failure of voluntary downgaze is a hallmark of progressive supranuclear palsy but is not always present early in the course (Collins et al. 1995). Limitation of voluntary upgaze is common in the healthy elderly. Slowed saccades and abnormal initiation of saccades (e.g., inability to make a saccade without moving the head or blinking) are important early abnormalities in Huntington's disease (Blekher et al. 2004). Slowed saccades are also a feature of early progressive supranuclear palsy, distinguishing it from other parkinsonian syndromes (Leigh and Riley 2000). Abnormalities of eye movement (nystagmus, a sixth nerve palsy, or a gaze palsy) in a confused patient may indicate Wernicke's encephalopathy (Victor et al. 1989).

When the head is moved in the same direction as the visual target (e.g., the head is passively turned to the right as the examiner's hand moves from the midline to the patient's right), the eyes follow the visual target as instructed only when the patient is able to inhibit the vestibulo-ocular reflex; failure to inhibit this reflex leads to eye movements in the opposite direction (doll's eyes) in supranuclear disorders such as progressive supranuclear palsy and schizophrenia (S. Warren and Ross 1998). However, excessive synkinesia of head and eye movement (i.e., the head moves involuntarily when the patient is instructed to move only the eyes to a target) on voluntary initiation of gaze occurs in schizophrenia and dementia (Chen et al. 1995; Kolada and Pitman 1983).

Inability to inhibit reflexive saccades to a target is characteristic of frontal disease and is seen *inter alia* in schizophrenia (Kennard et al. 1994); in its extreme, when any moving object captures the patient's gaze, this phenomenon is visual grasping (Ghika et al. 1995b). Subtler manifestations can be elicited by instructing the patient to look at the examiner's finger when the fist moves, and vice versa, with one hand on each side of the patient—an antisaccade task (Currie et al. 1991). A human face is a particularly potent stimulus to visual grasping (Riestra and Heilman 2004), and this fact can be applied in the inattentive patient by using one's own face as a fixation point in testing pursuit movements (i.e., moving one's head from side to side in front of the patient rather than just a hand).

Apraxia of gaze, like other apraxias, refers to a failure of voluntary movement with the preserved capacity for spontaneous movement. Congenital ocular motor apraxia (Cogan's syndrome), in which saccadic shifts of gaze are abnormal and often require initiation by head thrusting, is often associated with other neurodevelopmental abnormalities—notably, truncal ataxia and apraxia of speech. Despite the customary term, congenital ocular motor apraxia is not truly an apraxia because the nonvolitional saccadic system is abnormal (C.M. Harris et al. 1996). This abnormality is commonly associated with hypoplasia of the cerebellar vermis (Jan et al. 1998; Sargent et al. 1997). In spasm of fixation, intentional saccades are severely impaired, but the quick phase of vestibular nystagmus is preserved, thus more exactly meeting the definition of apraxia. Saccades can be performed more normally if fixation is eliminated. Such cases are associated with bilateral frontoparietal lesions (Pierrot-Deseilligny et al. 1997). Apraxia of gaze is a feature in Balint's syndrome (see subsection "Disordered Reaching and Simultanagnosia" later in this chapter), but here too the term *apraxia* is questionable because even though visually guided saccades are severely impaired, saccades to command may be intact (Pierrot-Deseilligny et al. 1997). *Psychic paralysis of gaze*, Balint's original term, is a more accurate designation (Moreaud 2003). The dysfunction relates to a disorder of spatial attention; classically, although not necessarily, the patients show bilateral posterior parietal lesions (Rizzo and Vecera 2002).

In so-called apraxia of eyelid opening, patients have difficulty in initiating lid elevation. This disorder occurs in extrapyramidal disease—notably, progressive supranuclear palsy (Grandas and Esteban 1994)—and as an isolated finding (Defazio et al. 1998). Eye closure and reflex eye opening are normal. In apraxia of lid opening, as distinct from blepharospasm, the orbicularis oculi are not excessively contracted; in blepharospasm, the brows are lowered below the superior orbital margins (Charcot's sign) (Esteban et al. 2004). Sensory tricks may be effective in initiating eye opening (Defazio et al. 1998), probably an indicator of extrapyramidal dysfunction in the disorder (thus making the term *apraxia* incorrect). Some (Esteban et al. 2004) but not all (Algoed et al. 1992) authors distinguish the phenomenon from ptosis of cerebral origin, which occurs with frontal lesions, especially right hemisphere infarction. Supranuclear disorders of eyelid closure may occur with bilateral frontal lesions, either structural (Ghika et al. 1988) or functional, as in the case of progressive supranuclear palsy (Grandas and Esteban 1994). Spontaneous blinking is intact. Often, other bulbar musculature is involved (Ross Russell 1980).

FACIAL MOVEMENT

A double dissociation in the realm of facial movement shows that emotional movements and volitional movements are separately organized (Monrad-Krohn 1924; Wilson 1924). A paresis seen in movements in response to a command ("show me your teeth") is sometimes overcome in spontaneous smiling; this indicates disease in pyramidal pathways (Hopf et al. 1992). A severe impairment of voluntary control of the bulbar musculature with preservation of automatic movements is seen in bilateral opercular lesions, the anterior opercular or Foix-Chavany-Marie syndrome (Bakar et al. 1998). The inverse phenomenon—normal movement in response to a command but asymmetry of spontaneous emotional movements—is seen with disease in the supplementary motor area (Laplane et al. 1976), anterior thalamus (Bogousslavsky et al. 1988; Graff-Radford et al. 1984), amygdala (Guimaraes et al. 2005), striatum and internal capsule (Trosch et al. 1990), and brain stem (Cerrato et al. 2003). Damasio and Maurer (1978) reported the occurrence of this sign in autism and argued that it indicates disease in limbic regions. Emotional facial weakness is contralateral to the seizure focus in temporal lobe epilepsy (Jacob et al. 2003).

SPEECH

Dysarthria

Disorders of articulation are difficult to describe, although they often are easily recognized when heard. In pyramidal disorders, the speech output is slow, strained, and slurred. Often accompanying the speech disorder are other features of pseudobulbar palsy, including dysphagia, drooling, and disturbance of the expression of emotions. Usually, the causative lesions are bilateral. Bulbar, or flaccid, dysarthria is marked by breathiness and nasality, as well as impaired articulation. Signs of lower motor neuron involvement can be found in the bulbar musculature. The lesion is in the lower brain stem. Scanning speech is a characteristic sign of disease of the cerebellum and its connections; the rate of speech output is irregular, with equalized stress on the syllables. In parkinsonism and in depression, speech is hypophonic and monotonous, often tailing off with longer phrases.

Darley et al. (1975) described in detail a scheme for examining the motor aspects of speech. It begins with assessment of the elements of speech production (e.g., facial musculature, tongue, palate) at rest and during voluntary movement. The patient is asked to produce the vowel "ah" steadily for as long as possible; the performance is assessed for voice quality, duration, pitch, steadiness, and loudness. Production of strings of individual consonants (e.g., "puh-puh-puh-puh") and alternated consonants (e.g., "puh-tuh-kuh-puh-tuh-kuh") is assessed for rate and rhythm. Extended utterances also are examined to observe the effects of fatigue and context.

Stuttering and Cluttering

Common developmental stuttering, or stammering, is familiar to everyone's ear. The rhythm of speech is disturbed by the repetition, prolongation, or arrest of sounds. Acquired stuttering, subtly different from the developmental variety (Helm-Estabrooks 1999; Van Borsel and Taillieu 2001), is unusual but can be caused by stroke (Carluer et al. 2000; Ciabarra et al. 2000; Hamano et al. 2005; Kakishita et al. 2004), traumatic brain injury (Ardila et al. 1999), psychotropic drugs (Bär et al. 2004), and extrapyramidal disease (Benke et al. 2000; Leder 1996; Nicholas et al. 2005). Although ictal or postictal stuttering occurs rarely in epilepsy, the more common occurrence is in pseudoseizures (Chung et al. 2004; Michel et al. 2004; Vossler et al. 2004). In developmental but not acquired stuttering, involuntary movements of the face and head resembling those of cranial dystonia—such as excessive blinking, forced eye closure, clonic jaw movements, and head tilt—are characteristically seen (Kiziltan and Akalin 1996). Alternatively, such movements can be interpreted as being akin to tics; this view is supported by an increased prevalence of obsessive-compulsive behaviors in persons with developmental stuttering (Abwender et al. 1998). Rarely, developmental stuttering that had been overcome returns after a brain injury, or developmental stuttering disappears after a brain injury (Helm-Estabrooks 1999). Psychogenic stuttering—marked by dramatic response to psychological treatment, atypical or "bizarre" speech features, multiple concurrent pseudoneurological complaints, and variability or situation specificity in presentation—may occur with or without concomitant organic disease (Duffy and Baumgartner 1997).

Cluttering is a disorder of fluency in which discourse, rather than purely articulation, is disturbed by a range of deficits in speech pragmatics, motor control, and attention (Daly and Burnett 1999). Speech output is abnormal because of rapid rate, disturbed prosody, sound transpositions or slips of the tongue, poor narrative skills, and impaired management of the social interaction encompassing speech. Thoughts may be expressed in fragments; words or phrases may be repeated. In sharp contrast to developmental stuttering, patients with cluttering are characteristically unconcerned about their impairment. Stuttering may be mistakenly diagnosed or occur in association. Some features of the disorder are replicated by festinant speech in parkinsonism (Lebrun 1996), and rare instances of acquired cluttering have been reported (Thacker and De Nil 1996).

Foreign Accent Syndrome

In 1947, the Scandinavian neurologist Monrad-Krohn (1947) described a patient with a wartime missile injury of the left frontotemporal region. She was a noncombatant, in fact a woman who had never been out of her small Norwegian town. She showed aphasia, mild right-sided signs, and slight personality change. The most distressing factor in wartime Scandinavia was that her speech pattern had changed so that she sounded like a German when she spoke her native Norwegian. Several similar cases of "foreign accent syndrome" have been described (Carbary and Patterson 2000). All showed pathology in the language-dominant hemisphere involving motor or premotor cortex or subjacent white matter; one dextral patient had a foreign accent after a crossed aphemia with right hemisphere infarction (Berthier et al. 1991). What distinguishes these patients from those with cortical dysarthria or apraxia of speech seems to be that the phonetic and prosodic alterations lead to characteristics that occur in natural languages. Thus, listeners hear the speech as "foreign" rather than abnormal, although often the foreign accent is generic and listeners cannot agree on its apparent provenance (Christoph et al. 2004).

Aprosodia

Ross and Mesulam (1979), following the work of Heilman and his colleagues on "auditory affective agnosia" (Heilman et al. 1975; Tucker et al. 1977), reported cases in which right hemisphere lesions led to loss of the production or recognition of affective elements of speech. Analysis of the cases led to recognition of syndromes of loss of prosody in expression and of impaired decoding of prosodic information in speech. Ross (1981) later schematized these syndromes—the "aprosodias"—as mirror images of left hemisphere aphasic syndromes, although others failed to confirm this schema (Cancelliere and Kertesz 1990; Wertz et al. 1998).

Lesions of either the left or the right hemisphere may disturb prosody, the "melody of language," which conveys both propositional and affective information. Left hemisphere lesions may be marked by prosodic abnormality, along with aphasia and cortical dysarthria; right hemisphere lesions may produce alterations in the affective component of speech, sometimes with dysarthria as well (Wertz et al. 1998). Often, appropriate test materials also disclose disturbed recognition of the affective component of material presented visually to the right hemisphere patients. Unless the primary prosodic alteration is recognized, the abnormality may appear to lie in mood or social relatedness. The examiner should listen to spontaneous speech for prosodic elements; ask the patient to produce statements in various emotional tones, such as anger, sadness, surprise, and joy; produce such emotional phrasings himself or herself, using a neutral sentence (e.g., "I am going to the store") while turning his or her face away from the patient, and ask the patient to identify the emotion; and ask the patient to reproduce an emotional phrasing the examiner has generated (Ross 1993).

Echolalia

In echolalia, the patient repeats the speech of another person automatically, without communicative intent or effect (Ford 1989). Often, the speech repeated is the examiner's and the phenomenon is immediately apparent without being specifically elicited. However, at times other verbalizations in the environment are repeated; for example, patients may repeat words overheard from the corridor or the television. Sometimes the patient repeats only the last portion of what he or she hears, beginning with a natural break in the utterance. Sometimes grammatical corrections are made when the examiner deliberately utters an ungrammatical sentence. The patient may reverse pronouns (e.g., "I" for "you") in the interlocutor's utterance, altering the sentence in a grammatically appropriate way. These corrections and alterations evince intactness of the patient's syntactic capabilities. The patient may automatically complete a well-known phrase uttered by the examiner (the completion phenomenon): "Roses are red," says the examiner. "Roses are red, violets are blue," responds the patient. Speaking to the patient in a foreign language may elicit obviously automatic echolalic speech.

Echolalia is a normal phenomenon in the learning of language in infancy (Lecours et al. 1983). Echolalia in transcortical aphasia marks the intactness of primary language areas in the frontal and temporal lobes, with syntax thus unimpaired but disconnected from control by other language functions (Hadano et al. 1998; Mendez 2002). Other underlying disorders include autism, Tourette syndrome, dementia of the frontal type and other degenerative disorders, catatonia, and startle-reaction disorders (McPherson et al. 1994). In all these situations, it may represent an environmental-dependency reaction, in which verbal responding is tightly stimulus-bound, echolalia representing the converse of failure of normal initiation of speech much as perseveration represents the converse of impersistence (see subsections "Perseveration" and "Impersistence" later in this chapter).

Palilalia

Palilalia is the patient's automatic repetition of his or her own word or phrase. Commonly, the volume of the patient's voice trails off and the rate of speech is festinant; less frequently, in *palilalie atonique*, repetitions of the utterance without acceleration alternate with silence

(Benke and Butterworth 2001). Despite claims to the contrary, repetition need not be confined to elements at the end of the utterance (Van Borsel et al. 2001). Palilalia occurs with extrapyramidal diseases, including progressive supranuclear palsy (Kluin et al. 1993) and postencephalitic or idiopathic parkinsonism (Benke et al. 2000), but thalamic lesions (Dietl et al. 2003), general paresis (Geschwind 1964), Tourette syndrome (Serra-Mestres et al. 1998; Van Borsel et al. 2004), traumatic brain injury (Ardila et al. 1999), and epilepsy (Linetsky et al. 2000; Yankovsky and Treves 2002) have been implicated as well.

"Blurting"

I have seen a few patients whose speech was marked by impulsive utterances of stereotyped or simple responses with no aphasic or echolalic features. For example, an elderly woman had the clinical features of progressive supranuclear palsy with no elementary cognitive abnormality. When questioned, she often replied "yes, yes" or "no, no" even before the questioner finished speaking and regardless of her intended answer to the question. She could then correct herself and give the reply she wished to give. She was unable to explain the behavior. These personal cases evinced disease in the frontostriatal circuit. The phenomenon seems to be related to echolalia and palilalia as well as to the environment-driven, impulsive (but not stereotyped) utterances of patients with frontal lobe disease (Ghika et al. 1995b). The phenomenon occurs in dementia of the frontal type (Snowden and Neary 1993). Similar phenomena, with similar correlates, were called "echoing approval" by Ghika et al. (1996) and "yes-no reversals" by Frattali et al. (2003; Ovsiew 2003).

Mutism

The term *mutism* should be reserved for the situation "in which a person does not speak and does not make any attempt at spoken communication despite preservation of an adequate level of consciousness" (Departments of Psychiatry and Child Psychiatry, The Institute of Psychiatry, and The Maudsley Hospital London 1987, p. 33). The first order of business in assessing an alert patient who does not speak is to examine phonation, articulation, and nonspeech movements of the relevant musculature (e.g., swallowing and coughing) to determine whether the disorder is due to elementary sensorimotor abnormalities involving the apparatus of speech.

If an elementary disorder is not at fault, the examination proceeds to a search for specific disturbances of verbal communication. Does the patient make any spontaneous attempt at communication through means other than speech? Does the patient gesture? Can the patient write, or, if hemiplegic, can he or she write with the non-dominant hand? Can he or she arrange cut-out paper letters or letters from a child's set of spelling toys? Or, if familiar with sign language, can he or she sign?

Some patients with acute vascular lesions restricted to the lower primary motor cortex and the adjacent frontal operculum have transient mutism and then recover through severe dysarthria without agrammatism, a disorder known as *aphemia* (Fox et al. 2001). The same syndrome can arise from right hemisphere disease, testifying to its nature as an articulatory rather than a language disorder (Mendez 2004; Vitali et al. 2004). Transcortical motor aphasia features a prominent disturbance of spontaneous speech, occasionally beginning as mutism (M.P. Alexander 1989). Damasio and Van Hoesen (1983) described such a patient with a lesion in the dominant supplementary motor area; after recovery, the patient reported that she lacked the urge to speak. Mutism commonly develops in patients with frontotemporal dementia or primary progressive aphasia (Snowden et al. 1992). A restricted disturbance of verbal communication must be distinguished from a more global disorder of the initiation of activity. At its extreme, the latter is the state of akinetic mutism. M.P. Alexander (1999) pointed out that mutism has its "lesser forms": long latencies, terseness, and simplification of utterances.

ABNORMALITIES OF MOVEMENT

Weakness

The findings associated with lesions of the pyramidal tracts, spinal cord, peripheral nerves, and muscles are described in texts of neurology (Duus 1998). Several simple maneuvers allow recognition of the motor effects of cerebral lesions (N.E. Anderson et al. 2005; Teitelbaum et al. 2002). Pronator drift is assessed by asking the patient to keep the arms outstretched and supinated, with the fingers together and then with the fingers apart. Abduction of the fingers in the first portion of the test and pronation, elbow flexion, or lateral and downward drift in the second portion indicate pyramidal disease (Weaver 2000). Testing should last at least 30 seconds. Upward drift indicates a parietal lesion. (By asking the patient to hold the arms pronated, the examiner can conveniently seek asterixis and tremor at this point in the examination.) In the finger-rolling test, the patient is asked to rotate each index finger around the other for 5 seconds in each direction. The tendency for one finger to orbit the other indicates a subtle pyramidal lesion on the stationary side. Fine finger movements are assessed by asking the patient, with the hands supinated in the lap, to touch the thumb to each of the other four fingers in

turn, one hand at a time. Mirror movements (discussed in the subsection "Synkinesia and Mirror Movements" later in this chapter) are conveniently observed incidentally at this point in the examination.

Greater awareness of the findings in nonpyramidal syndromes may help the clinician identify neurobehavioral syndromes associated with cerebral disease outside the primary motor regions. Caplan et al. (1990) described the features of a "nonpyramidal hemimotor" syndrome with caudate nucleus lesions. Patients show clumsiness and decreased spontaneous use of the affected limbs; associated movements are decreased as well. What appears at first glance to be paresis proves to be a slow development of full strength; if coaxed and given time, the patient shows mild weakness at worst. Freund and Hummelsheim (1985) explored the motor consequences of lesions of the premotor cortex. They observed a decrease in spontaneous use of the arm and attributed it to a failure of postural fixation; when supported, the arm showed at worst mild slowing of finger movements. The defect in elevation and abduction of the arm was best demonstrated by asking the patient to swing the arms in a windmill movement, both arms rotating forward or backward; the same defect can be found in cycling movements of the legs, especially backward cycling (Freund 1992). Movement rapidly decomposed when such coordination was required. Pyramidal signs—increased tendon jerks, Babinski's sign, and spasticity—may be absent in patients with these findings. In acute parietal lesions, "motor helplessness" due to loss of sensory input is regularly seen (Ghika et al. 1998).

Disordered Gait

Assessment of gait is a central feature of the neuropsychiatric physical examination. Alterations in gait are common in subcortical vascular disease, for example, and may provide crucial diagnostic information. The examiner must scrutinize the patient's rising from a chair, standing posture, postural reflexes, initiation of gait, stride length and base, and turning (Nutt et al. 1993). Failures of gait ignition (initiation), locomotion, and postural control can be distinguished (Baezner and Hennerici 2005). In mild gait ignition failure, start hesitation and occasional freezing are seen. In mild locomotion failure, slow and short strides on a widened base are present, with mild unsteadiness. In postural control failure, falling is seen in conjunction with turning impairment, ultimately leading to an inability to stand unsupported. Stressed gait (e.g., walking heel to toe or on the outer aspects of the feet) may reveal asymmetric posturing of the upper extremity in patients without other signs.

Frontal gait disorder is characterized by short, shuffling steps on either a wide or a narrow base, with hesitation at starts and turns. Postural equilibrium is impaired, although not as much as in Parkinson's disease, and the trunk is held upright on stiff, straight legs. Festination is not a feature, and the upper extremities are unimpaired or far less affected. This is the gait disorder of subcortical vascular dementia (FitzGerald and Jankovic 1989; Thompson and Marsden 1987), and it must be distinguished from Parkinson's disease (Kurlan et al. 2000). A widened base strongly points away from idiopathic Parkinson's disease and toward subcortical vascular disease or a parkinsonian-plus syndrome. Thalamic, basal ganglia, and cortical lesions can produce balance disorders with falling and unfamiliar derangements of station and gait, easily mistaken for psychogenic disorders (Nutt 2005).

Falls also occur in patients with dementia or delirious patients whose executive dysfunction leads to carelessness with regard to walking rather than specific gait impairment. Contrariwise, cautious gait occurs in healthy people in treacherous footing (e.g., on ice) or in the frail and anxious elderly. Features of cautious gait include short stride length at a slow pace, a widened base, excessive knee flexion, and decreased arm swing. Such patients are often anxious and depressed and evince an excess of extrapyramidal and frontal release—but not pyramidal or cerebellar—physical signs, as well as a reduction in muscle strength (Giladi et al. 2005). Although anxiety may play an important role in the genesis of the gait pattern, the organic factors must not be ignored, even though the gait disorder is not a classically localizable one.

Akinesia

Akinesia has several aspects: delay in the initiation of movement, slowness in the execution of movement, and special difficulty with complex movements. The disturbance is established by requiring the patient to perform a repeated action, such as tapping thumb to forefinger, or two actions at once. A decrement in amplitude or freezing in the midst of the act is observed. When established, akinesia is unmistakable in the patient's visage and demeanor and in the way he or she sits motionlessly and has trouble arising from the chair. A distinction between parkinsonian akinesia and depressive psychomotor retardation is not easy to make, but the associated features of tremor, rigidity, and postural instability are generally absent in depressive illness (Rogers et al. 1987).

Agitation

The term *agitation* is often misused to refer to the behavior of aggression or the affect of anxiety. "The preferred definition of psychomotor agitation is of a disorder of motor activity associated with mental distress which is characterized by a restricted range of repetitive, nonprogressive ('to-and-fro'), non-goal directed activity" (Day 1999, p. 95). In distinction from akathisia, the excessive movement characteristically involves the upper extremities. Agitation in the verbal sphere is manifested in repetitive questioning or complaining, screaming, or attention seeking (Cohen-Mansfield and Libin 2005). In some patients with Alzheimer's disease, wandering is associated with depressive and anxiety symptoms and may represent agitation in this cognitively impaired population (Klein et al. 1999; Logsdon et al. 1998). Why certain causes of confusion regularly produce agitation—alcohol withdrawal, hypoxemia, postictal twilight state, and infarction in the territory of the left posterior cerebral artery—and others do not is uncertain.

Roaming, differentiated from wandering by being purposeful and exploratory, is characteristic of frontotemporal dementia (Mendez et al. 1993). In my experience, the excessive activity may be stereotyped, as, for example, the patient who roamed the hospital unit in rectilinear fashion, just so far from each wall with precise turns at each corner.

Akathisia

Motor restlessness accompanied by an urge to move is referred to as *akathisia* (Sachdev 1995). Although akathisia is most familiar as a side effect of psychotropic drugs, the phenomenon occurs often in idiopathic Parkinson's disease (Comella and Goetz 1994) and occasionally with extensive destruction of the orbitofrontal cortex, as in traumatic brain injury (Stewart 1991) or herpes simplex encephalitis (Brazzelli et al. 1994). In a few cases, it has been associated with restricted basal ganglion lesions, even occurring unilaterally with a contralateral lesion (Carrazana et al. 1989; Hermesh and Munitz 1990; Stuppaeck et al. 1995). Akathisia also may occur after withdrawal from dopamine-blocking drugs or as a tardive movement disorder (Sachdev 1995).

Eliciting the account of subjective restlessness from a psychotic patient may be difficult. Complaints specifically referable to the legs are more characteristic of akathisia than of anxiety (Sachdev and Kruk 1994). Although by derivation the term refers to an inability to sit, its objective manifestations are most prominent when the patient attempts to stand still. The patient "marches in place," shifting weight from foot to foot. Seated, the patient may shuffle or tap his or her feet or repeatedly cross his or her legs. When the disorder is severe, the recumbent patient may show myoclonic jerks or a coarse tremor of the legs. One patient of mine with severe withdrawal akathisia caused an ulcer of the heel of her foot by constantly rubbing it against the bedsheets.

Hypertonus

Three forms of increased muscle tone concern the neuropsychiatrist. In *spasticity*, tone is increased in flexors in the upper extremity and extensors in the lower but not in the antagonists. The hypertonus shows an increase in resistance followed by an immediate decrease (the clasp-knife phenomenon) and depends on the velocity of the passive movement. This is the typical hemiplegic pattern of hemisphere stroke, universally called pyramidal, which indicates a lesion actually not in the pyramidal tract but in the corticoreticulospinal tract (G.E. Alexander and DeLong 1992; Brodal 1981). In *rigidity*, tone is increased in both agonists and antagonists throughout the range of motion; the increase is not velocity dependent. This is the characteristic hypertonus of extrapyramidal disease.

In *paratonia*, or *Gegenhalten*, increased tone is erratic and depends on the intensity of the imposed movement. This pattern of hypertonus is usually related to extensive brain dysfunction, typically with frontosubcortical involvement. The erratic quality is related to the presence of both oppositional and facilatory aspects of the patient's motor performance. Beversdorf and Heilman (1998) described a test for facilatory paratonia: the patient's arm is repeatedly flexed to 90° and extended to 180° at the elbow, then the examiner's hand is withdrawn at the point of arm extension. In the abnormal response, the patient lifts or even continues to flex and extend the arm. Sudo et al. (2002) described the same phenomenon under the designation "elbow flexion response." A cogwheel feel to increased muscle tone is not intrinsic to the hypertonus; the cogwheeling in parkinsonism is imparted by postural (not rest) tremor superimposed on rigidity (Findley et al. 1981). In delirium and dementia, the paratonia of diffuse brain dysfunction can be mistaken for extrapyramidal rigidity when the examiner feels cogwheeling, which actually indicates the additional presence of the common tremor of metabolic encephalopathy or postural tremor of some other etiology (Kurlan et al. 2000). Striking variability in muscle tone ("poikilotonia") can occur in the acute phase of parietal stroke (Ghika et al. 1998).

Dystonia

Dystonia constitutes "sustained muscle contractions, frequently causing twisting and repetitive movements, or abnormal postures" (Fahn et al. 1987, p. 335). The contractions may be generalized or focal. Typically, the dystonic arm hyperpronates, with a flexed wrist and extended fingers; the dystonic lower extremity shows an inverted foot with plantar flexion. Several syndromes of focal dystonia are well recognized, such as torticollis, writer's cramp, and blepharospasm with jaw and mouth movements (Meige syndrome). A dystonic pattern of particular interest is oculogyric crisis, in which forced thinking or other psychological disturbance accompanies forced deviation of the eyes (Benjamin 1999b; Leigh et al. 1987).

Dystonic movements characteristically worsen with voluntary action and may be evoked only by very specific action patterns. Dystonic movements, especially in an early stage or mild form of the illness, can produce apparently bizarre symptoms, such as a patient who cannot walk because of twisting feet and legs but who is able to run or a patient who can do everything with his or her hands except write. Adding to the oddness is the frequent capacity of the patient to reduce the involuntary movement by using "sensory tricks" (*le geste antagoniste*); in torticollis, for example, the neck contractions that are forceful enough to break restraining devices may yield to the patient's simply touching the chin with his or her own finger. Eliciting a history of such tricks or observing the patient's use of them is diagnostic.

Tremor

Tremors are rhythmic, regular, oscillating movements. Three major forms of tremor are distinguished. In *rest tremor*, the movement is present distally when the limb is supported and relaxed; action reduces the intensity of the tremor. The frequency is usually low, about 4–8 cps. This is the well-known tremor of Parkinson's disease. Because the amplitude of the tremor diminishes with action, rest tremor is usually less disabling than it might appear. In *postural tremor*, the outstretched limb oscillates. At times, this can be better visualized by placing a piece of paper over the outstretched hand. Postural tremor is produced by anxiety, by certain drugs (e.g., caffeine, lithium, steroids, and adrenergic agonists), and by hereditary essential tremor. A coarse, irregular, postural tremor is frequently seen in metabolic encephalopathy (Young 2002). In *intention tremor* (also called *kinetic tremor*), the active limb oscillates more prominently as the limb approaches its target during goal-directed movements, but the tremor is present throughout the movement. *Rubral*, or *midbrain*, *tremor* is a low-frequency, large-amplitude, predominantly proximal, sometimes unilateral tremor with rest, postural, and intention components (Vidailhet et al. 1998). In a few reported cases, tardive tremor has had both rest and postural components (Tarsy and Indorf 2002).

Observing the patient with arms supported and fully at rest, then with arms outstretched, and then with arms abducted to 90° at the shoulders and bent at the elbows while the hands are held palms down with the fingers pointing at each other in front of the chest, will identify most upper-extremity tremors (Jankovic and Lang 2004). A given patient's organic tremor may vary in amplitude, for example, with anxiety when the patient is aware of being observed. However, anxiety and other factors do not alter tremor frequency. Thus, if the patient's tremor slows or accelerates when the examiner asks him or her to tap slowly or quickly with the opposite limb, hysteria should be suspected (Koller et al. 1989).

Chorea

Chorea refers to "irregular, rapid, flowing, nonstereotyped, and random involuntary movements" (Higgins 2001, p. 707) that dance over the patient's body. The more proximal, writhing component to these movements is termed *athetosis*. The patient may incorporate the movements into purposeful ones in an effort to hide the chorea when it is mild. As with dystonia, chorea may become more evident when elicited by gait or other activity. Choreic disturbance of respiratory movements probably often goes unrecognized, especially in tardive dyskinesia (Komatsu et al. 2005; Rich and Radwany 1994). Predominantly proximal movements, large in amplitude and violent in force, are called ballistic. Usually, ballism is unilateral (hemiballism), but it can be bilateral (Vila and Chamorro 1997). Despite the common expectation of a lesion in the subthalamic nucleus, lesions elsewhere in the basal ganglia are more frequently culpable (Postuma and Lang 2003).

The differential diagnosis of chorea is wide (Higgins 2001). Late-onset abnormal movements due to dopamine-blocking drugs—tardive dyskinesia—may be choreic, although the oral movements may be considered stereotypies (Stacy et al. 1993). If the patient has psychosis, the clinician must not assume that chorea is tardive dyskinesia but must consider a differential diagnosis of diseases that can produce both chorea and psychosis (e.g., Wilson's disease, systemic lupus erythematosus, Huntington's disease, and Fahr's syndrome). Furthermore, abnormal movements similar to those of tardive dyskinesia can be seen in untreated severe psychiatric illness (McCreadie et al. 2005; Turner 1992). Antiepileptic drugs, antidepressants, lithium, levodopa, and nonantipsychotic antidopaminergic drugs such as metoclopramide and prochlorperazine also can produce abnormal movements (Podskalny and Factor 1996; Sewell and Jeste 1992; Zaatreh et al. 2001).

Many elderly patients with oral dyskinesia are edentulous. In edentulous dyskinesia, abnormality of tongue movement is minimal; in contrast, vermicular (wormlike) movements of the tongue inside the mouth are prominent in tardive dyskinesia. In Huntington's disease, impersistence of tongue protrusion is prominent, whereas in tardive dyskinesia, voluntary protrusion of the tongue markedly reduces the abnormal oral movements. Abnormal movements of the upper face are much more prominent in Huntington's disease than in tardive dyskinesia (Jankovic and Lang 2004).

Myoclonus

Myoclonus comprises sudden, jerky, shocklike movements, which can originate at various levels in the nervous system (Caviness and Brown 2004). Certain forms of myoclonus are within normal experience; the hiccup and the jerk that awakens one just as one drifts off to sleep (the hypnic jerk) are myoclonic phenomena. Myoclonus does not show the continuous, dancelike flow of movement that characterizes chorea. When myoclonus is rhythmic, it differs from tremor in having an interval between individual movements, a "square wave" rather than a "sine wave." The distinction of myoclonus from tic is partly based on subjective features: the tiqueur reports a wish to move, a sense of relief after the movement, and the ability to delay the movement (albeit at the cost of increasing subjective tension) (Lang 1992). Also, tics can be more complex and stereotyped than myoclonic jerks. Various psychoactive medicines, notably lithium, can cause myoclonus (Caviness and Brown 2004). Myoclonus is a prominent feature of Creutzfeldt-Jakob disease (in which cortical myoclonus is often elicited by auditory stimuli), dementia with Lewy bodies, and corticobasal degeneration. Myoclonus can accompany dystonia (Obeso et al. 1983), including tardive dystonia (Abad and Ovsiew 1993), and tardive myoclonus without dystonia is also recognized (Little and Jankovic 1987). Myoclonus occurring in a confused patient is usually a feature of toxic-metabolic encephalopathy but should raise the question of nonconvulsive status epilepticus, an easily overlooked condition (Kaplan 2002). Gaze deviation, lateralized dystonic posturing, and automatisms should be red flags for the latter condition.

Asterixis

Repeated momentary loss of postural tone produces a flapping movement of the outstretched hands originally described in the setting of liver failure but subsequently recognized in many or all states of metabolic encephalopathy and in all muscle groups. Young and Shahani (1986) recommended eliciting it by asking the patient to dorsiflex the index fingers for 30 seconds while the hands and arms are outstretched, with the patient watching to ensure maximum voluntary contraction. Physiologically, asterixis is the inverse of multifocal myoclonus; the electromyogram shows brief silence on the background of sustained discharge (Young and Shahani 1986). The coarse tremor of delirium is a slower version of asterixis. Bilateral asterixis is a valuable sign because it points reliably to a toxic-metabolic confusional state. Asterixis, to my knowledge, has never been described in the idiopathic psychoses and is thus pathognomonic for an organic encephalopathy. Occasionally, asterixis is unilateral and reflects a lesion of the contralateral thalamic, parietal, or medial frontal structures (usually thalamic) (Tatu et al. 2000); rarely, bilateral asterixis is of structural origin (Rio et al. 1995).

Startle

The normal reaction to an unexpected auditory stimulus invariably includes an eye blink and then predominantly flexor muscle jerks that are most intense cranially, tapering caudally (Brown et al. 1991). A rare, usually familial, disorder in which this reflex is disturbed is called hyperexplexia. It features hyperreflexia, hypertonus, and abnormal gait in infancy; myoclonus; and exaggerated startle, frequently causing falls. Abnormal startle reactions are also seen in posttraumatic stress disorder, Tourette syndrome, some epilepsies, certain culture-bound syndromes such as latah and the "jumping Frenchmen of Maine," brain stem encephalitis, postanoxic encephalopathy, and hexosaminidase A deficiency (Brown 1999).

Tics and Compulsions

Some of the key features of tics were described earlier in this chapter in differentiating tics from myoclonus. Tics are sudden jerks, sometimes simple (a blink or a grunt) but sometimes as complex as a well-organized voluntary movement (e.g., repeatedly touching an object or speaking a word) (Lees 1985; Lennox 1999). In addition to the important subjective differences noted previously, tics differ from many other abnormal movements in that they may persist during sleep (Jankovic and Lang 2004). (Some myoclonic disorders and some dyskinetic movements also may persist during sleep [Sawle 1999].) Despite the quasivoluntary quality of some tics, electrophysiological evidence shows that tics differ from identical movements produced voluntarily by the same person in that they lack the readiness potential *(Bereitschaftspotential)* that normally precedes a voluntary movement (Obeso et al. 1981).

A distinction between complex tics and compulsions rests partly on the subjective experience of the patient (Holzer et al. 1994). Compulsions are taken to be voluntary, but tics may be experienced as deliberate responses to an urge (like scratching because of an itch) or be given a post hoc meaning by the patient, so the distinction between "voluntary" and "involuntary" movements and actions may be obscured. Organic obsessions and compulsions are similar phenomenologically to those in the idiopathic disorder (Berthier et al. 1996; Chacko et al. 2000). Some apparent compulsions represent utilization behavior rather than activity driven by anxiety (Destée et al. 1990).

Stereotypy and Mannerisms

Stereotypies are purposeless and repetitive movements that may be performed in lieu of other motor activity for long periods (Lees 1988). Ridley (1994) distinguished stereotypy from perseveration, noting that in the former, the amount of one type of behavior is excessive, and in the latter, the range of behavior is reduced so that behavior is repetitive but not excessive. Stereotypies include movements such as crossing and uncrossing the legs, clasping and unclasping the hands, picking at clothes or at the nails or skin, head banging, and rocking. In schizophrenia, a delusional idea associated with stereotyped movements can sometimes, but not always, be elicited (I.H. Jones 1965).

Stereotyped movements are seen in schizophrenia, autism, mental retardation, Rett syndrome, Tourette syndrome, neuroacanthocytosis, congenital blindness (but not in those whose blindness is acquired late; Fazzi et al. 1999), and numerous other psychopathological states (Frith and Done 1990; Ridley and Baker 1982; Stein et al. 1998). They are particularly characteristic of frontotemporal dementia (Mendez et al. 2005; Nyatsanza et al. 2003). Nonautistic children may show repetitive complex movements. These are phenomenologically distinct from tics in that they are more rhythmic, patterned, and prolonged; lack premonitory urges or internal tension; are easily abolished by distraction but are not disturbing to the child and thus are not intentionally controlled; and start earlier, often before age 2 years (Mahone et al. 2004). They may persist into adulthood and may be associated with obsessive and compulsive symptoms (Niehaus et al. 2000). At times, especially in the mentally retarded, a distinction of stereotypies from epileptic events may be difficult (Paul 1997). Many of the abnormal movements of tardive dyskinesia (e.g., chewing movements and pelvic rocking) are patterned and repetitive, not random as is chorea, and are best described as stereotypies (Kaneko et al. 1993; Stacy et al. 1993).

Amphetamine intoxication is a well-recognized cause of stereotypy, known in this setting as *punding*, a Swedish word introduced during a Scandinavian epidemic of amphetamine abuse (Rylander 1972). Similarly, cocaine and levodopa can cause stereotyped movements (Evans et al.

TABLE 4–2.   Selected catatonic signs

Sign	Definition
Grimacing	Maintenance of odd facial movement
Posturing	Maintenance of odd postures without rigidity
Excitement	Increased motor activity, excluding akathisia or goal-directed action
Mitgehen	Exaggerated cooperative movements in response to light pressure
Waxy flexibility	Slight resistance to passive movement like that of warm wax with maintenance of uncomfortable postures
Verbigeration	Stereotyped repetition of words or phrases

2004). Stereotypies occur occasionally ipsilateral or contralateral to a motor deficit during the acute phase of stroke (Ghika et al. 1995a; Ghika-Schmidt et al. 1997) and rarely with other focal lesions (Edwards et al. 2004; Maraganore et al. 1991; McGrath et al. 2002).

Manneristic movements are purposeful movements carried out in a bizarre way. They may result from the incorporation of stereotypies into goal-directed movements (Lees 1985, 1988).

Catatonia

The syndrome described by Kahlbaum in the nineteenth century and absorbed into the concept of dementia praecox by Kraepelin occurs in a wide variety of organic states as well as in the classic idiopathic psychoses (Barnes et al. 1986; Taylor and Fink 2003). Catatonia comprises a large number of behaviors ("incomprehensible motor phenomena"; Jaspers 1963, p. 181), some of which are listed and described in Table 4–2. Such signs are common in severe mental disorder (Rogers 1985; Ungvari et al. 2005; van der Heijden et al. 2005), and several scales for their assessment have been devised and validated (Braunig et al. 2000; Bush et al. 1996; McKenna et al. 1991; Northoff et al. 1999). Many of the signs are seen with frontosubcortical lesions (Northoff 2002), and cataleptic postures (waxy flexibility) can occur with contralateral parietal lesions (Ghika et al. 1998; Saver et al. 1993).

The catatonic syndrome can be defined broadly as abnormality of movement or muscle tone associated with psychosis (C.M. Fisher 1989); this was essentially Jaspers's definition ("psychotic disturbances of motor activity"; Jaspers 1963, p. 180). A more specific delineation required "at least one motor sign (catalepsy, posturing, or waxy flexibility) in combination with at least one sign of psychosocial withdrawal or excitement and/or bizarre repetitious movement (mutism, negativism, impulsiveness, grimacing, stereotypies, mannerisms, command automatism, echopraxia/echolalia or verbigeration)" (Barnes et al. 1986, p. 991). Taylor and Fink (2003) pro-

posed formal criteria for the syndrome: 1) immobility, mutism, or stupor of at least an hour's duration accompanied by catalepsy, automatic obedience, or posturing observed on two occasions, or 2) two or more observations of two or more of the following motor features: stereotypy, echophenomena, catalepsy, automatic obedience, posturing, negativism, *Gegenhalten*, or ambitendency.

Synkinesia and Mirror Movements

Excessive synkinesia—automatic movement accompanying intended voluntary movement—occurs in a variety of states (Zulch and Muller 1969). Obligatory, congenital bimanual synkinesia ("mirror movements") persisting into adulthood occurs with cerebral palsy due to a lesion predating 24 weeks of gestation, cervical spine disease (such as Klippel-Feil syndrome), agenesis of the corpus callosum, and Kallmann's syndrome (Krampfl et al. 2004; Krams et al. 1999; G.D. Schott and Wyke 1981). Often no definite malformation or injury can be identified (Rasmussen 1993). The pathophysiology involves abnormal ipsilateral motor pathways or diminished transcallosal inhibition (Arányi and Rösler 2002; Ueki et al. 2005). Asymmetric parkinsonism also gives rise to mirror movements (Espay et al. 2005). To observe the phenomenon, the examiner asks the patient to touch, repeatedly and in turn, the fingers of the right hand to the right thumb, and then the left fingers to the left thumb, as the hands rest supine in front of the patient; along with watching the active hand for fine motor coordination, the examiner watches the contralateral hand for mirror movements.

PRIMITIVE REFLEXES

The received wisdom is that the signs listed in Table 4–3 are brought about by cortical disease, especially frontal, which disinhibits primitive movement patterns (Walterfang and Velakoulis 2005). The various signs differ in their sensitivity and specificity for brain disease and in many instances may not be of pathological significance

TABLE 4–3. Primitive reflexes

Reflex	Elicitation	Abnormal response
Suck	Insert object (e.g., tongue blade) between patient's lips	Lips show sucking action
Snout	Press on patient's nasal philtrum	Lips purse
Rooting	Bring object (e.g., reflex hammer) toward patient's mouth and then to side	Mouth opens and turns toward moving object
Grasp	Stroke patient's palm from proximal to distal while not touching dorsum of hand	Fingers flex and hold examiner's finger
Avoidance	Same as grasp, or stroke ulnar aspect of patient's hand	Fingers extend or hand moves away
Palmomental	Scrape thenar eminence	Ipsilateral mentalis muscle contracts so chin twitches
Nuchocephalic	Briskly turn shoulders of standing patient whose eyes are closed	Head remains in initial position

(Landau 1989). For example, Jacobs and Grossman (1980) found that the palmomental sign could be elicited in more than 20% of healthy subjects in their third and fourth decades and in more than 50% in their ninth decade; the snout sign could be found in more than 30% of subjects older than 60. Similarly, Koller et al. (1982) found the snout sign in more than half, and Vreeling et al. (1995) in just fewer than half, of healthy elderly subjects.

The presence of multiple primitive reflexes that fail to habituate on repeated stimulation more reliably suggests pathology (Owen and Mulley 2002). In one study, the presence of more than two primitive reflexes (of the four sought) showed 93% specificity in distinguishing vascular dementia patients from age-matched control subjects (Di Legge et al. 2001). Similarly, in a study of patients infected with HIV, 92% of the subjects but no control subject had more than two primitive reflexes (of six sought) (Tremont-Lukats et al. 1999). Thus, the examiner should place little weight on a single primitive reflex, especially if it fatigues on repeated stimulation. The exception is the grasp reflex, which in the two studies just cited was present in no healthy subject and in only rare patients with vascular disease but not dementia—and thus reliably indicates disease when present.

The localizing value of these signs is also variable. Some authors have included the Babinski, Hoffmann, or Rossolimo signs in the category of primitive reflexes. To be sure, these pyramidal signs reflect disinhibition of early motor synergies, but because of their specificity for the pyramidal tract, it is reasonable to consider them separately from primitive reflexes. The grasp reflex is a genuine frontal sign: in a study of 491 patients, grasping was never associated with a postcentral lesion (De Renzi and Barbieri

1992). The locus of damage is characteristically medial, involving supplementary motor area and cingulate gyrus (De Renzi and Barbieri 1992; Hashimoto and Tanaka 1998). Often, it occurs bilaterally with a unilateral lesion (De Renzi and Barbieri 1992). A similar response is elicitable in the sole of the foot, but the plantar grasp is present only when the palmar grasp is present, so its diagnostic utility is limited. Awareness of the plantar grasp reflex, however, may keep the examiner from missing an extensor plantar response when this is masked by the plantar grasp.

The glabellar and palmomental signs are commonly but nonspecifically present in parkinsonian disorders (Brodsky et al. 2004). The palmomental reflex has no lateralizing value (Gotkine et al. 2005). A snout reflex must be distinguished from a pathologically brisk stretch reflex of the orbicularis oris, the latter forming part of a pyramidal syndrome that includes other brisk jerks in the face (J.M. Schott and Rossor 2003).

Primitive reflexes may be more common in frontotemporal dementia than in vascular dementia with frontal predominance (Sjögren et al. 1997) or Alzheimer's disease (Hogan and Ebly 1995). They are commonly present in schizophrenia (Walterfang and Velakoulis 2005) and in late-onset depressive illness (Baldwin et al. 2005). Some less familiar signs, such as the nuchocephalic (Jenkyn et al. 1975), avoidance (Denny-Brown 1958), and self-grasping (Ropper 1982) signs, may prove to be relatively specific or of localizing value.

SOFT SIGNS

Under the rubric of soft signs is grouped a varied set of findings taken to show impairment in sensorimotor integration and motor control. Unfortunately, the many studies of these signs have not used the same test batteries (Sanders and Keshavan 1998) (Table 4–4). A focus on soft signs in psychiatric patients should not blind the examiner to "hard signs" and extrapyramidal signs unrelated to medication in patients with idiopathic psychiatric illness (Griffiths et al. 1998; Kinney et al. 1993; McCreadie et al. 2005).

Schizophrenia is unquestionably associated with an excess of abnormal findings. They are independent of neuroleptic treatment and are present in first-episode cases (Browne et al. 2000; Shibre et al. 2002; Venkata-subramanian et al. 2003), indeed in high-risk subjects prior to the onset of psychosis (Lawrie et al. 2001). Data conflict as to correlation with genetic risk for the illness (Gourion et al. 2004; Lawrie et al. 2001). A relation to perinatal injury is possible as well (Cantor-Graae et al. 2000). A high level of neurological soft signs is associated with low IQ (Dazzan et al. 2004), negative symptoms (Chen et al. 2005), neuropsychological deficits (Arango et al. 1999; Wong et al. 1997), and poor response to treatment (R.C. Smith et al. 1999). In a group of first-episode psychotic patients, the presence of neurological soft signs was correlated with reductions in volume of striatum, thalamus, and (for sensory integration signs) cerebral cortex (Dazzan et al. 2004).

Although the bulk of studies have examined the occurrence of soft signs in schizophrenia, these signs are not specific to this disorder, being found in homeless persons (Douyon et al. 1998); violent psychopathic persons (Lindberg et al. 2004); and patients with mood disorder (Negash et al. 2004), obsessive-compulsive disorder (Bolton et al. 1998), borderline personality disorder (Gardner et al. 1987; Stein et al. 1993), and posttraumatic stress disorder (Gurvits et al. 2000). However, the pattern of abnormal findings may differ between disorders (Boks et al. 2004; Bolton et al. 1998). In summary, soft signs should be considered to provide a nonspecific index of vulnerability to idiopathic psychiatric disorder (Johnstone et al. 2005).

SIGNS OF CALLOSAL DISCONNECTION

Simple maneuvers suffice to elicit many of the crucial elements of the disconnection syndrome (Bogen 1993). On examination, the patient with callosal lesions shows an inability to name odors presented to the right nostril. In visual field testing, a hemianopsia appears to be present in each hemifield alternately, opposite to the hand the patient uses to point to stimuli. Thus, when the patient is using the right hand, he or she responds only to stimuli in the right hemifield, but when the patient is using the left hand, he or she responds only to stimuli in the left hemifield.

Apraxia of the left hand can be shown by the usual testing maneuvers. Because verbal information processed in the left hemisphere cannot be transferred to the right, and because the right hemisphere has limited capacity to understand spoken commands, the patient is not able to produce appropriate responses with the left hand to spoken commands. Similarly, writing with the left hand is impossible. Geschwind and Kaplan (1962) emphasized these features of the "deconnection syndrome" in work that initiated the modern era of clinical disconnection studies and in considerable measure initiated the development of behavioral neurology (Absher and Benson 1993). For reciprocal reasons, the right hand shows a constructional disorder.

The patient has an anomia for unseen objects felt with the left hand. If the examiner places one of the patient's hands (again unseen) into a given posture, the patient is unable to match the posture with the other hand. Similarly, the patient cannot touch with the left thumb the finger of the left hand that corresponds to the finger of the right hand touched by the examiner, and vice versa.

No doubt the most dramatic feature of callosal disconnection is behavioral conflict between the hands or the patient's sense that the left hand behaves in an "alien" fashion. Brion and Jedynak (1972) described "le signe de la main étrangère," translated in the English summary of the article as the "strange hand sign" but subsequently (and better) as the "alien hand sign." The original description clearly conveyed a sensory phenomenon, akin to neglect and in fact considered a "hemisomatagnosia specific for touch" (Brion and Jedynak 1972, p. 262). For example, one patient felt his left hand with his right behind his back while dressing. He recognized it as a hand but not as his own hand. The authors emphasized the unawareness specifically of ownership of the hand, that is, the sense of "strangeness" or alienation. In all four cases reported by Brion and Jedynak (1972), the patients had posterior callosal lesions. Many subsequent patients with intermanual conflict have had lesions in various positions in the callosum (Scepkowski and Cronin-Golomb 2003).

However, not all patients with the alien hand phenomenon have callosal disconnection. The phenomenon of directed though unwilled behavior by the hand—the "anarchic hand"—associated with frontal lobe pathology is described later in this chapter (see subsection "Anarchic Hand"). A posterior alien hand syndrome seen after noncallosal lesions producing a disturbance of the body schema in addition to abnormal movements has been described (Ay et al. 1998; Bundick and Spinella 2000). Other patients without callosal lesions may have the alien hand syndrome through a combination of deficits involving praxis and proprioception (MacGowan et al. 1997). The alien hand seen in corticobasal degeneration (C.M. Fisher 2000) may fit this pattern in some instances; in others, it may be more closely akin to the levitation of the

TABLE 4–4. Comparison of batteries of soft signs

Element	NES	Modified NES	CNI	Griffiths
Gait and balance				
Casual gait			√	
Tandem gait	√	√	√	√
Romberg	√	√	√	√
Complex movements				
Ring/fist	√	√		√
Fist/edge/palm	√	√	√	√
Oseretsky (alternating fists)	√	√	√	√
Finger/thumb opposition	√		√	√
Rhythm tapping	√		√	
Tap reproduction	√	√		
Dysdiadochokinesia	√	√	√	√
Extraocular movements				
Visual tracking			√	√
Convergence	√			√
Gaze persistence	√		√	
Other motor				
Drift			√	
Motor persistence			√	
Finger–nose	√		√	√
Mirror movements	√		√	√
Synkinesia of head	√		√	
Tremor	√		√	√
Choreoathetosis	√		√	√
Sensory				
Audiovisual integration	√	√		√
Stereognosis	√		√	√
Graphesthesia	√	√	√	√
Face-hand test	√	√	√	√
Right-left orientation	√	√	√	√
Primitive reflexes				
Glabellar	√		√	√
Snout	√		√	√
Palmomental		√	√	
Grasp	√		√	√
Suck	√			√

Note. NES = Neurological Evaluation Scale—see Buchanan and Heinrichs 1989. Modified NES—see Sanders et al. 1998. CNI = Cambridge Neurological Inventory—see Chen et al. 1995. Griffiths—see Griffiths et al. 1998.

upper extremity seen with contralateral parietal lesions (Barclay et al. 1999; Ghika et al. 1998; Gondim et al. 2005; Saver et al. 1993).

ORIENTATION

Disorientation is the shibboleth of the cognitive examination for the non-neuropsychiatrist. In common psychiatric parlance, *disorientation* means organic disease, but the shortcomings of this definition are twofold. First, many patients have organic cognitive disorders without disorientation, particularly focal cognitive disorders such as alexia or constructional disorder. Even in the syndromes of delirium and dementia, disorientation is far from invariable. Cutting (1980) found in his series of 74 cases of "acute organic reaction" that only 36% were disoriented to the year, 43% to the month, and 34% to the name of the hospital. By contrast, 85% had abnormalities of mood, and 46% had abnormal beliefs. Similarly, in a study of disorientation after stroke, the sensitivity of disorientation for dementia was only 59% and for defective attention by neuropsychological assessment only 34% (Desmond et al. 1994). Second, disorientation is a nonspecific indicator. A patient may be unable to give the date or place because of impairment in attention, memory, language, or content of thought. The neuropsychiatrist probes these mechanisms by using more specific tasks.

The pattern of disorientation can have diagnostic importance. Disorientation to place can carry an entirely different significance from disorientation to date (see below). Delirious disorientation was distinguished from delusional disorientation in Jacksonian terms by M. Levin (1951, 1956), who pointed out that the delirious patient mistakes the unfamiliar for the familiar—reducing the novel to the automatic—as when the patient reports that the hospital is "a factory," where he or she formerly worked. By contrast, the schizophrenic patient mistakes the familiar for the unfamiliar, as when the patient identifies his or her location as Mars. Schnider et al. (1996) argued that in amnestic patients, disorientation reflects confusion in temporal context due to orbitofrontal dysfunction. However, this mechanism does not apply to disorientation in dementia (Joray et al. 2004).

ATTENTION

Full alertness with normal attention lies at one end of a continuum, the other end of which is coma. Where the patient is on this continuum can be assessed by observing the reaction to a graded series of probes: entering the room, speaking the patient's name, touching the patient without speaking, shouting, and so on through painful stim-

ulation. The proper recording of the response is by specific notation of the probe and the reaction (e.g., "makes no response to examiner's entrance but orients to examiner's voice; speaks only when shaken by the shoulder").

Deficits occur in the capacity to maintain attention to external stimuli (vigilance), the capacity to attend consistently to internal stimuli (concentration), and the capacity to shift attention from one stimulus to another. Vigilance can be assessed by the patient's capacity to carry out a continuous-performance task; such tasks have been extensively used in the psychological laboratory. In a bedside adaptation, the "A test," the patient is presented with a string of letters, one per second, and is required to signal at each occurrence of the letter A (Strub and Black 1988). A single error of omission or of commission is considered an abnormal response. Concentration can be assessed by the patient's capacity to recite the numbers from 20 to 1 or to give the days of the week or the months of the year in reverse order. A pathognomonic error is the intrusion of the ordinary forward order: "20, 19, 18, 17, 18, 19, …." This amounts to a failure to inhibit the intrusion of the more familiar "set."

Digit span is a classic psychological test of attention, easily performed at the bedside. The examiner recites strings of numbers, slowly, clearly, and without phrasing into chunks. The patient is required to repeat them immediately. Subsequently, the patient can be asked to repeat strings of digits after reversing them in his or her head. The normal forward digit span is usually considered to be a minimum of five. The backward digit span may depend on visuospatial processing as well as attention (Black 1986). A related task of working memory is asking the patient to alphabetize the letters of the word *world* (Leopold and Borson 1997). Testing working memory by number-letter alternation is discussed later in this chapter (see section "Screening Batteries and Rating Scales").

Neglect

The patient who pays no attention to the left side of his or her body and the left side of space is one of the most dramatic phenomena in neuropsychiatry. The bedside clinician can readily identify the patient who leaves his or her left arm out of the sleeve of a gown, leaves the left side of breakfast uneaten, and so on. Neglect can further be recognized during a line-bisection task (the patient must place an X at the midpoint of a line drawn by the examiner) or a cancellation task (in which the patient crosses out letters or other items for which he or she must search in an array). A line made up of tiny letters (perhaps because it activates the left hemisphere) creates a more sensitive test than an ordinary line (Lee et al.

2004). However, careful attention to neglect in behavior—grooming, dressing, moving about, knowledge of left limbs—is even more sensitive than paper-and-pencil tasks (Azouvi et al. 2002).

Neglect may occur not only in external space but also in "representational space" (i.e., the patient may neglect the left half of an imagined object). Indeed, representational and perceptual neglect doubly dissociate (Ortigue et al. 2003). Bisiach and Luzzatti (1978) demonstrated representational neglect by asking patients to describe a well-known piazza as it appeared from one direction, thereby eliciting a description that neglected the left side of the piazza, and then asking the patients to describe the piazza as it appeared from the opposite direction, thereby eliciting a description that neglected the previously described side of the piazza and included the previously neglected side. A patient who showed left neglect in near space but not in far space provides evidence of the multiple representations of space; when "far" was reinterpreted as "near"—the patient used a stick instead of a light pen to bisect a distant line—neglect reappeared (Berti and Frassinetti 2000). In a related simple but telling demonstration of the flexibility or task-specificity of internal representations, Poizner et al. (1984) found that a deaf patient fluent in sign language who developed left visuospatial hemineglect from right hemisphere stroke did not neglect left hemispace in sign.

Mesulam (1981) constructed a network theory in which the parietal cortex, frontal cortex, and cingulate cortex interact to generate attention to the opposite side of space. Lesions in these cortices produce distinguishable contralateral sensory neglect, directional hypokinesia, and reduced motivational value, respectively. Thus, Daffner et al. (1990) described a patient whose capacity for spatial exploration in left hemispace was reduced after a right frontal infarction, as shown by failure on a letter-cancellation task, despite the absence of sensory abnormality. Following a subsequent right parietal lesion, visual and auditory extinction on the left emerged, and the exploratory defect was accentuated. Inventive experimental paradigms confirmed this distinction between the input and output ends of a sensorimotor processing continuum (Bisiach 1993; Tegnér and Levander 1991). Rarely, neglect occurs not on the left-right axis but on a vertical or radial (near-far) axis (Adair et al. 1995).

An inverse syndrome of "acute hemiconcern" was described as occurring after right parietal stroke producing pseudothalamic sensory loss without neglect. The patients transiently concentrated attention on the left side of the body and manipulated it actively (Bogousslavsky et al. 1995).

Hypermetamorphosis

Wernicke coined the term *hypermetamorphosis* to refer to an excessive and automatic attention to environmental stimuli. Klüver and Bucy (1937, 1939; Nahm 1997) documented this phenomenon in monkeys with bilateral temporal lobectomy. The human Klüver-Bucy syndrome depends critically on involvement of the amygdala bilaterally (Poeck 1985a). One patient, an elderly man, presented to the hospital with serial seizures. On awakening, he showed a postictal twilight state. In this period, he compulsively attended to elements of the environment and kept up a remarkable running commentary on them: "You're wearing a tie, there's a picture on the wall," and so on. Electroencephalography showed bilateral posterior temporal spike foci. Perhaps this is related to the Schneiderian symptom of auditory hallucinations that provide a running commentary on the schizophrenic patient's activity.

An inverse syndrome of rejection behavior, with intolerance of and withdrawal from sensory stimuli, can be seen with parietal disease (J.D. Warren et al. 2004). The avoidance reflex, already described, is putatively a fragment of this withdrawal syndrome.

MEMORY

Bedside testing of verbal memory can be done briefly and validly (Kopelman 1986). Recall of paragraph-length material after a 45-minute delay may be an ideal test, but recall of a name and an address or three words after several minutes is simple and satisfactory (Bowers et al. 1989; Katzman et al. 1983; Kopelman 1986). Addition of a cueing procedure at the learning stage as well as the retrieval stage in memory testing adds specificity to the diagnosis of memory impairment by controlling for attention and semantic processing (Buschke et al. 1999; Kuslansky et al. 2002; Yuspeh et al. 1998). Thus, at presentation of target words for recall, the examiner can provide a category cue, to be used several minutes later if free recall fails. Failure at this point strongly suggests impairment in hippocampal memory systems. The improvement of verbal recall with semantic cues suggests a disorder of retrieval mechanisms, such as is seen in frontal-subcortical disease. Memory failure is a sensitive indicator of attentional dysfunction, in which case the basis is not in memory systems proper.

Similar testing of figural memory at the bedside is also easily done. For example, the "three words–three shapes" test of Weintraub and Mesulam (Weintraub 2000; Weintraub and Mesulam 1985) quickly and simply compares verbal and figural memory side by side. I sometimes ask patients to recall three pointed directions (e.g., up at a 45° angle, to the right, and to the left).

The testing of verbal and nonverbal short-term memory does not cover all the memory subroutines that have been identified by neuropsychologists. Whether remote memory can be validly assessed at the bedside is uncertain. Can we briefly and validly, without specialized materials, make assessments of memory for source and temporal context, functions especially impaired in frontal lobe lesions? In frontal amnesia, recognition memory is relatively spared for a given level of memory by free recall. Can we reliably discern this disparity at the bedside? Can we assess procedural memory—for example, the learning of a motor task? Developing and validating bedside methods for these domains are goals for the future.

LANGUAGE AND PRAXIS

Aphasia

The term *aphasia* refers to acquired deficits in lexical and syntactic capacities. Goodglass and Kaplan (1983) presented a scheme for examination that has been widely adopted. Higher-level disorders of language, such as pragmatic deficits and thought disorder, are discussed elsewhere in this chapter.

Spontaneous speech.   Although the clinician hears the patient's spontaneous speech during the interview, it is nonetheless essential to listen for a period of time with an ear to language abnormalities. One listens for fluency—melody, effortfulness, rate, and phrase length—and for errors, both of syntax and of word choice (lexicon).

Repetition.   Language disorders with spared repetition (or even excessive echolalic repetition) and disproportionately impaired repetition both occur. Repetition is tested by offering the patient phrases of increasing length and grammatical complexity. For example, one may start with single words and continue with simple phrases, then invert the phrases into questions, and then use phrases made up of grammatical function words (e.g., "no ifs, ands, or buts").

Naming.   Naming can be tested by using items at hand: a watch and its parts; parts of the body; shirt, sleeve, and cuff; and so on. Naming is dependent on the frequency of occurrence of the target word in the vocabulary, so testing must employ less frequently used items to detect mild but clinically meaningful deficits. Occasionally, alternative methods are required, as with a blind patient (or a patient with optic aphasia or visual agnosia), for whom tactile naming can be used. One also can ask the patient to name items based on a description (e.g., "What do you call the four-legged animal that barks? What is the

vehicle that travels underwater?"). Some patients have extraordinary domain-specific dissociations in naming ability (category-specific anomia); for example, the ability to name vegetables may be intact while the ability to name animals is devastated (Gainotti 2000).

Comprehension.   Preferably the output demands are minimized in testing comprehension, so motor responses should not be required. Asking yes-or-no questions of progressive difficulty (e.g., "Am I wearing a hat, is there a tree in the room, does lunch come before dinner, is ice cream hotter than coffee?") is simple and is systematized in the Boston Diagnostic Aphasia Examination (BDAE) (Goodglass and Kaplan 1983). Patients with anterior aphasia often have mild disorders of comprehension of syntactically complex material. This can be observed by asking patients to interpret sentences in which the passive voice and similarly difficult constructions are used (e.g., "The lion was killed by the tiger. Which animal was dead?").

Reading.   Reading comprehension can be tested conveniently by offering the same stimuli as were used orally. Before diagnosing alexia, one must establish the patient's premorbid literacy. Alexia can be present with no other abnormality of language (alexia without agraphia or pure alexia) (Coslett 2000).

Writing.   Writing is most conveniently tested by asking the patient spontaneously to write a short paragraph about his or her illness or about being in the hospital. Agraphia is a constant accompaniment of aphasic syndromes, so the writing sample is a good screening test of language function (assuming premorbid literacy). It is a particularly sensitive test in identifying confusional states (Chédru and Geschwind 1972a, 1972b). One study found that delirious patients produce jagged, angular segments of letters that should be curved (Baranowski and Patten 2000). Similarly, agraphic errors can be seen in writing samples of patients with Alzheimer's disease earlier in the course than are aphasic errors in spontaneous speech (Faber-Langendoen et al. 1988; Horner et al. 1988). Isolated defects of writing ability (pure agraphia) also occur (Luzzi and Piccirilli 2003).

Ideomotor Apraxia

Incapacity to perform skilled movements in the absence of elementary sensory or motor dysfunction that explains the defect is known as *apraxia*. Limb-kinetic apraxia amounts to cortical clumsiness, especially of finger coordination (Zadikoff and Lang 2005). Ideational apraxia is discussed later in this chapter. Ideomotor apraxia is discussed here because of its close relation to language disorders.

Requesting that the patient perform skilled transitive (i.e., on an imagined object) movements most sensitively detects ideomotor apraxia (Leiguarda 2005). Thus, in the presence of auditory comprehension difficulties, the presence of apraxia is difficult to establish. Deficits in motor performance may differ across several dimensions: transitive versus intransitive, meaningful versus non-meaningful, outward-directed versus self-directed, single versus repetitive, or novel versus overlearned (Leiguarda and Marsden 2000). Furthermore, performance of axial, orofacial, and limb movements may be differentially affected. Thus, a screening examination should use several tasks that differ in these respects. Disorders of performing pantomimed transitive movements predominantly occur in patients with left hemisphere lesions.

For oral apraxia, suitable tests are "Show me how you would blow out a match" and "How do you lick a postage stamp?" For limb apraxia, the patient should demonstrate movements such as waving good-bye; thumbing a ride; and using a hammer, comb, or toothbrush. Responses in which the patient uses a body part in lieu of the pantomimed object are often considered defective. Thus, if the patient continues to use his or her fingers as the comb despite instruction to pretend that he or she is holding a comb, the body-part-as-object response is taken as parapraxic (Peigneux and van der Linden 1999). As with other tasks in the cognitive examination, errors in performing skilled movements are more telling than simple failures, and the patient who shows how to hammer with a flat palm is unequivocally apraxic. For some forms of apraxia, patients do not complain of apraxic deficits and are not disabled by them because the deficits do not appear in a natural context. However, this may not always be so, and exploration of the motor performance deficit across contexts is appropriate (Hanna-Pladdy et al. 2003). Recognition, naming, and other aspects of gesture performance also can be assessed (Crutch 2005).

Visuospatial Function

Visuospatial Analysis

The traditional probes for impairment with regard to spatial relations are drawing and copying tasks. Copying a Greek cross, intersecting pentagons, a figure from the Bender-Gestalt test, or the figures in Mesulam's and Weintraub's three-shapes test (Weintraub 2000) or drawing a clock face serves as a suitable screen; more subtle abnormality may be identified with use of the Rey Complex Figure. The complexity of the Rey figure offers the opportunity to assess not only the final performance but also the patient's strategy. Having the patient change the color of ink several times during the copying process

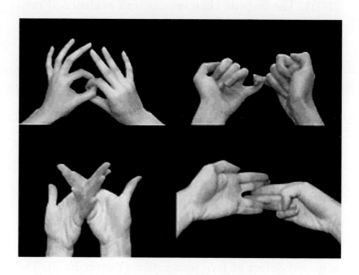

FIGURE 4–1. Interlocking finger positions.

Source. Reprinted from Moo LR, Slotnick SD, Tesoro MA, et al.: "Interlocking Finger Test: A Bedside Screen for Parietal Lobe Dysfunction." *Journal of Neurology, Neurosurgery and Psychiatry* 74:530–532, 2003. Used with permission.

shows the steps taken to produce the final drawing (Milberg et al. 1996). Both left-sided and right-sided lesions impair copying performance, although differently. The difference between a piecemeal approach (the patient slavishly copies element by element) and a gestalt approach (the patient grasps the major structures, such as the large rectangle) can be noted, with the former suggesting right-sided disease. Neglect of the left side of the figure likewise strongly suggests right hemisphere disease.

Another screening approach to the recognition of parietal lobe disease, on either side, is asking the patient to copy meaningless finger positions (see Figure 4–1) (Moo et al. 2003). This task presumably requires intact praxis as well as visuospatial function and has been shown to depend on bilateral supramarginal gyrus activation (S. Tanaka et al. 2001).

Other tasks probe visuospatial analysis without the same output demand. Elements of neuropsychological instruments can be used, for example, in asking the patient to discern overlapping figures or to identify objects photographed from noncanonical views. Even if vision is impaired, it is possible to test related functions by topographical skills: "If I go from Chicago to New York, is the Atlantic Ocean in front of me, behind me, or to my left or right?"

Visual Agnosia

The relative importance of elementary perceptual processes in the agnosias has been debated; certainly, in many cases (the apperceptive agnosias), subtle defects of form perception can be identified (Riddoch and Humphreys

2003). The bedside clinician can seek evidence of relatively intact elementary visual processing (e.g., copying the picture of an object may be possible). Although the patient's language is intact (e.g., he or she is able to name the object in the picture from a description or from tactile data), his or her capacity to recognize the object visually—either by naming it or by demonstrating its use—is strikingly abnormal. Such patients are often markedly impaired in activities of daily living. Visual agnosia results from a ventral lesion of the "what" stream of processing.

Disorders of Complex Visual Processing

Alert to the patient's and family's reports and equipped with photographs of a few famous people, the bedside examiner can identify clinical cases of prosopagnosia, an acquired defect of face recognition (Barton 2003). The lesion is ventral occipitotemporal, either on the right or bilaterally. Disordered recognition not of facial identity but of features such as gaze direction or expression may be associated with more dorsal lesions. Some prosopagnostic patients show not only an inability to recognize specific faces (while knowing that they are looking at a face) but also an inability to recognize individual exemplars of other classes of items; such patients may not be able to identify their own car or farm animal.

Developmental prosopagnosia differs subtly from the acquired form: concurrent visuospatial deficits are less likely; covert recognition is equally affected, whereas in acquired prosopagnosia, it may be spared (Kress and Daum 2003). Although reviews suggested that developmental prosopagnosia is rare, recent Web-based case ascertainment may indicate otherwise (Duchaine and Nakayama 2004). The defect often associates with social-emotional processing problems in disorders such as Asperger's syndrome (Barton et al. 2004) and should be sought as part of the neuropsychiatric approach to patients with personality deviation in this realm.

Defective color vision due to cerebral disease (central achromatopsia) is caused by ventral occipital damage contralateral to the defective field (Bouvier and Engel 2006). Superior field defects, prosopagnosia, and other visual disorders commonly co-occur. Presenting colored stimuli in each hemifield is essential to its detection; patients with hemiachromatopsia may not report a loss of color vision and may do well at naming colors in central vision (Rizzo 2000). Akinetopsia, the impairment of the perception of motion, is rare; it results from dorsal lesions in extrastriate visual cortex (Zeki 1991).

Isolated defects of topographical skill occur, although the usual patient with trouble finding his or her way around home or hospital unit has a broader right hemisphere syndrome (Aguirre and D'Esposito 1999; Barrash 1998). The focal cases generally show either an agnosia for landmarks or scenes, related to a ventral lesion, or an inability to orient in egocentric space despite preserved recognition, a dorsal deficit (Aguirre and D'Esposito 1999). Other patterns may occur as well. The former patients often have achromatopsia or prosopagnosia, and the latter patients have reaching deficits (see below). Several authors have described transient disorders of topographical skill, putatively similar pathogenetically to transient global amnesia (Gil-Néciga et al. 2002; Stracciari 2003). Developmental impairments of topographical skill also occur (Dutton 2003).

Disordered Reaching and Simultanagnosia

Rare patients are unable to guide the movements of the hand and arm by vision (Rizzo and Vecera 2002). This phenomenon, known as *optic ataxia*, is seen along with apraxia of voluntary gaze (ocular apraxia) and an impairment of the simultaneous perception of multiple objects (simultanagnosia) in the triad composing Balint's syndrome. If the patient's reaching under visual guidance (within a field of normal vision) is disturbed, arm movement without visual guidance must be examined (e.g., by observing the patient, with the patient's eyes closed, dressing, pointing to parts of his or her body, or reaching with the right hand to grasp the outstretched left thumb and vice versa).

Simultanagnosia is detected by asking the patient to describe a visually complex array; the Cookie Theft picture from the BDAE is suitable. Simultanagnosia is a rare and incompletely characterized defect, and its association with optic ataxia and psychic paralysis of gaze is inconstant. These disorders result from dorsal lesions of the "where" processing stream. Focal cortical degenerations or Alzheimer's disease may produce dysfunction of posterodorsal or posteroventral cortices, with disturbed spatial processing or object recognition (Caselli 2000).

FORM OF THOUGHT

Thought Disorder

Features of thought disorder in the idiopathic psychoses—poverty of speech, pressure of speech, derailment, tangentiality, incoherence, and so on—have been carefully defined (Andreasen 1979). Cutting and Murphy (1988) differentiated among intrinsic thinking disturbances, including loose associations, concreteness, overinclusiveness, and illogicality; disorders of the expression of thought, including disturbed pragmatics of language; and deficits in real-world knowledge, which can produce odd conversational interchange. They argued that the distinctive pattern of schizophrenic thought is suggestive of right hemisphere dysfunction. However, the group of schizophrenic patients with thought disorder may be heterogeneous (Kuperberg et al. 2000), and lesions elsewhere may produce abnormal expression of thought (Chatterjee et al. 1997). Both executive and semantic dysfunction may participate in the pathogenesis of formal thought disorder (Barrera et al. 2005).

Many authors have noted the similarity between the "negative" features of thought disorder and the characteristics of the frontal lobe syndrome. Cutting (1987) contrasted the "positive" features of thought disorder in schizophrenia with the thinking process of delirious patients. The latter was prominently illogical or slowed and impoverished in output; more distinctively, delirious patients gave occasional irrelevant replies amid competent responses. The form of thought in mentally retarded patients and in patients with dementia has not been well characterized.

Confabulation

The confabulating patient fabricates material in response to the examiner's queries and may tell tales spontaneously as well. Although this disorder is linked with amnesia, elaborate or spontaneous confabulation betokens additional disease outside memory systems, particularly the disturbance of the temporal context of memories that is characteristic of orbitofrontal lesions (Schnider 2003). Schizophrenic patients produce confabulations in narrative speech, probably because of difficulty suppressing abnormal ideas and insensitivity to context and the listener's expectations (Kramer et al. 1998; Nathaniel-James et al. 1996). Akin to confabulation is a phenomenon Geschwind (1964) called "wild paraphasia." He offered the example of a patient who calls an intravenous pole a Christmas tree decoration. In this case, the failure lies not within language systems but in impaired visual perception as well as in the cerebral apparatus for self-monitoring; disruption of attention in a confusional state is the usual setting (Wallesch and Hundsalz 1994). Delusional memories in psychotic patients appear to be neuropsychologically distinct from confabulation (Kopelman 1999; Kopelman et al. 1995).

Vorbeireden (Vorbeigehen)

Vorbeireden (Vorbeigehen), the symptom of approximate answers, is the defining feature of the Ganser state (Dwyer and Reid 2004). The patient's responses show that he or she understands the questions, but the lack of knowledge implied by the mistaken replies is implausible (e.g., the patient reports that a horse has three legs). This phenomenon is rare. The remainder of the syndrome includes confusion, hallucinations, and conversion symptoms. Whether it rests on organic foundations has been controversial from the outset. Ganser (1974) described three patients (of four he had seen); two had experienced head injury, and one was recovering from typhus. Subsequently, some regarded the behavior as dissociative (Feinstein and Hattersley 1988; Heron et al. 1991), and others emphasized the neuropsychological underpinnings (Cutting 1990).

Narrative Process in the Interview Setting

Patients who do not have elementary disorders of language function may nonetheless have macrolinguistic deficits. When words and sentences—lexicon and syntax—are normal, paragraphs and discourse may not be. Patients with right hemisphere disease, despite the adequacy of their lexical-semantic and syntactical performance, have deficits in the capacity to tell a story or recognize the point of a joke (Brownell and Martino 1998; Paradis 1998). These patients rarely give "I don't know" responses; rather, they contrive some answer even if implausible; they fail to draw appropriate inferences, especially from emotional data, so that incongruity is not recognized; and their sense of humor is impaired (Wapner et al. 1981). People who have temporal lobe epilepsy or who have had traumatic brain injury show deficits in planning, producing, and monitoring discourse; their narratives may be verbose and inefficient or contain insufficient or irrelevant information, requiring the listener to expend extra effort to understand them (Biddle et al. 1996; Field et al. 2000).

These findings emphasize the value of open-ended inquiries (e.g., "What brings you to the hospital?"), with attention to the patient's discourse taken as a whole as a sign of cerebral function. Disorders at the level of discourse are well recognized phenomenologically in psychiatry. Patients who experienced attachment disorganization in childhood show disturbances of the form of thought when discussing emotionally powerful material; this may relate to the characteristic vagueness and inconsistency of the medical accounts provided by hysterical patients (Ovsiew 2006). One patient with compulsive personality disorder and a remarkably circumstantial communicative style, who had an advanced degree in linguistics, acknowledged to me that people had a hard time talking with her because she "violated the Gricean maxims," referring to the work of the logician Grice on meaning and communication. (The maxims are: give as much information as required and no more; be truthful; be relevant; and be perspicuous.) The neural substrates of verbosity, circumstantiality, irrelevancy, and vagueness have not been carefully considered.

CONTENT OF THOUGHT

Delusions

Misidentification syndromes, such as Capgras' and Frégoli's syndromes, and states seemingly related to misidentification, such as the phantom boarder syndrome, are common in dementia (Hwang et al. 2003; Nagaratnam et al. 2003). These states raise the questions of focal brain dysfunction, especially impairment of facial recognition, and many patients with misidentification delusions have right or bilateral frontolimbic lesions, sometimes with prominent memory and executive cognitive dysfunction (Barton 2003; Edelstyn et al. 2001; Hudson and Grace 2000). However, not all patients with misidentification syndromes—or nonsyndromal misidentification phenomena, which are quite common in psychosis (Mojtabai 1998)—have a recognizable organic contribution to the disorder (Signer 1994). The presence of persecutory delusions before the advent of misidentification speaks against evident organic factors (Fleminger and Burns 1993).

Several terms designate patients who, with delusional intensity, mistake their location, including *reduplicative paramnesia* (Pick 1903), *disorientation for place* (C.M. Fisher 1982), and *délire spatial* (spatial delusion) (Vighetto et al. 1985). One of my patients, for example, insisted that he was in his own house, thanked me for bringing all the doctors to visit him at home, and, when skeptically confronted with features of the environment, explained that he kept poles for intravenous lines and the like at home in case he needed them. These patients generally have evident organic disease with defects of visuospatial analysis and executive function (Fleminger and Burns 1993; Sellal et al. 1996).

Malloy and Richardson (1994) argued that delusions confined to a single topic suggest frontal lobe disorder, but again, as Kopelman et al. (1995) emphasized, by no means can organic disease always be identified. Complex psychotic phenomena, such as first-rank symptoms, are associated with preservation of cognitive capacity (Almeida et al. 1995); patients with frank dementia show unsystematized abnormal beliefs that often arise ad hoc from situations of cognitive failure.

Cutting (1987) pointed out that themes of "imminent misadventure to others" and "bizarre happenings in the immediate vicinity" characterize delirium rather than acute schizophrenic psychosis.

Hallucinations

Visual hallucinations suggest organic states, especially if auditory hallucinations are absent, but visual hallucinations occur commonly in idiopathic schizophrenia (Bracha et al. 1989; Goodwin et al. 1971). Elementary visual hallucinations may arise from ocular disease or occipital disease; migraine auras or migraine accompaniments without headache are a common cause. Complex, or formed, visual hallucinations arise from a variety of pathological bases (Manford and Andermann 1998), including narcolepsy, epilepsy, and deafferentation of the visual system due to stroke.

Visual hallucinations without other psychopathology (the Charles Bonnet syndrome), usually in the presence of ocular disease with visual loss, are also common, especially in the elderly (Menon et al. 2003). The hallucinations are usually vivid images of animals or human beings or of faces (Santhouse et al. 2000), and the patient is aware of their unreality. The visual experience exceeds veridical perception in clarity. Characteristically, patients with these symptoms do not report them spontaneously (Menon 2005). Visual hallucinations in a hemifield blind from cerebral disease occur with small occipital strokes or occasionally other posterior lesions (Cole 1999). Because the pathogenesis of hallucinations in ocular disease may differ from that in occipital disease, the eponym probably is best reserved for hallucinations associated with peripheral visual impairment (Cole 2001; ffytche and Howard 1999).

Vivid, elaborate, and well-formed visual hallucinations may occur with disease in the upper brain stem or thalamus (peduncular hallucinosis) (Manford and Andermann 1998). Such hallucinations often worsen in the evening (crepuscular) or when the patient is sleepy, and again the patient is generally aware of their unreality. A dreamlike state may accompany the hallucinosis. Similar hallucinations occur as hypnagogic phenomena in narcolepsy and in response to dopaminergic drugs in Parkinson's disease, and the brain stem mechanism may be related (C.M. Fisher 1991). Visual hallucinations early in a degenerative dementia suggest a diagnosis of dementia with Lewy bodies (Ballard et al. 1999). A lilliputian character is present in visual hallucinations of various etiologies without apparent specificity (Cohen et al. 1994).

Auditory hallucinations have resulted from pontine lesions, with characteristics in some ways similar to peduncular visual hallucinations, as well as from lesions in the temporal lobes (Braun et al. 2003). Musical hallucinations are associated with hearing impairment, especially in depressed elderly women (Evers and Ellger 2004). Musical hallucinations also occur in idiopathic psychiatric disorder (Baba and Hamada 1999). Unilateral auditory hallucinations are characteristically ipsilateral to a deaf (or the more deaf) ear (Almeida et al. 1993).

Olfactory hallucinations, often taken to imply epilepsy or temporal lobe disease, are common in idiopathic psychiatric disorders (Kopala et al. 1994). Rarely, the olfactory reference syndrome—a patient's belief that he or she emits an aversive odor, with accompanying social withdrawal—can arise from organic causes, perhaps especially right hemisphere lesions (Devinsky et al. 1998; Lochner and Stein 2003; Toone 1978).

Palinopsia refers to persisting or recurrent visual images after the stimulus is gone. Responsible lesions are typically parieto-occipital, perhaps related to a role for abnormal parietal spatial representations in pathogenesis (Santhouse et al. 2000). The physiology of this phenomenon may be epilepsy or disinhibition of the short-term visual memory system (Maillot et al. 1993). The analogous phenomenon in auditory experience is palinacousis, which is due to temporal lobe lesions on either side (Jacobs et al. 1973). David (1994) proposed that thought-echo is due to a disturbance in short-term auditory verbal memory (the phonological loop).

EMOTION

Assessment of emotion and its modulation is performed by the clinician as a natural part of observing the patient during the examination; in addition, the examiner asks questions about the patient's emotional experience. Nothing substitutes for extended and sensitive conversation.

Pathological laughter and crying are defined not only by the lack of congruent inner experience but also by their elicitation through nonemotional stimuli (e.g., waving a hand before the patient's face) and by the all-or-none character of the response (Poeck 1985b). These signs may result from lesions of the descending tracts modulating brain stem centers or may be better understood as reflecting failure of the cerebellar contribution to regulation of affect (Parvizi et al. 2001). *Pathological affect*, defined as requiring incongruent subjective experience, may be on a continuum with the affective dyscontrol, lability, and shallowness that occur in frontal disease or dementia. This latter state, also called *emotionalism*, comprises increased tearfulness (or, more rarely, laughter) and sudden, unexpected, and uncontrollable tears (Calvert et al. 1998). So defined, emotionalism is common, associated with cognitive impairment, and related to left frontal and temporal lesions, but affect is not dissociated from the patient's emotional experience or situation. Rating scales for pathological emotion and a self-report measure are available (Allman et al. 1992; Moore et al. 1997; Newsom-Davis et al. 1999; R.A. Smith et al. 2004). Pathological affect can disguise a major depressive syndrome, so the examiner should seek not only the signs of pseudobulbar palsy but also the symptoms and signs of melancholia (Calvert et al. 1998; Ross and Stewart 1987).

The catastrophic reaction is a sudden access of dysphoria and anger in a patient facing a task beyond his or her capacities; the patient conveys frustration, often cries, and is unable to go on with other tasks for a period of time (Goldstein 1952; Reinhold 1953). This behavioral response is associated with left hemisphere lesions, especially left opercular lesions (Carota et al. 2001).

A sudden display of laughter—*le fou rire prodromique* (mad prodromal laughter)—is a rare antecedent to a catastrophic vascular event, usually in the brain stem or thalamus (Coelho and Ferro 2003). Laughing (gelastic) and crying (dacrystic) seizures are unusual (Luciano et al. 1993), although ictal emotion, especially fear, is common (Williams 1956). Gelastic epilepsy is associated with hypothalamic hamartomas and left-sided lesions (Arroyo et al. 1993), and dacrystic epilepsy is associated with right-sided lesions (Luciano et al. 1993). Although crying is more common than laughter in pathological affect, laughing seizures are more common than crying seizures (Sackeim et al. 1982). Weeping during an ictus, in fact, suggests pseudoseizure (Walczak and Bogolioubov 1996).

Apathy is the absence or quantitative reduction of affect or motivation. It differs from depression; even the slowed, unexpressive depressed patient reports unpleasant emotional experience if the mental state is carefully explored. The term *apathy* has been in recent use for the phenomenon called *abulia*, which is discussed further later in this chapter (see subsection "Abulia"). Manes and Leiguarda (2005) argued that the addition of a cognitive component—a lack of interest or concern—to the motivational defect of apathy implicates dorsolateral along with medial frontal systems and would reserve the term *abulia* for these cases. *Euphoria*, a persistent and unreasonable sense of well-being without the increased mental and motor rates of a manic state, is often alluded to in connection with multiple sclerosis. Actually, euphoria is unusual, and its occurrence almost always signals extensive disease and cognitive impairment (Ron and Logsdail 1989).

INITIATION AND ORGANIZATION OF ACTION

The capacity for initiation and organization of action corresponds to a major aspect of the concept of executive cognitive function. Disorders of activation, planning, sequencing, self-monitoring, and flexible attention are important causes of functional disability (B.S. Fogel 1994). Moreover, such disturbances may be more evident during clinical examination than during formal neuropsychometric assessment because the structure of the formal assessment enhances the defective capacity of the patient to ignore distracting stimuli and direct and organize action toward adaptive goals. This problem in the "ecological validity" of neuropsychological assessment applies particularly to deficits due to orbitofrontal injury.

Elucidating deficits in the patient's planning and organizing of adaptive behavior may require inventive testing methods, such as those described by Shallice and Burgess (Burgess 2000; Shallice and Burgess 1991). An interesting verbal bedside probe is asking the patient to estimate quantities with which the patient is familiar but which may never have been explicitly quantitated (e.g., the length of a person's spine or the cost of a refrigerator) (Shallice and Evans 1978; M.L. Smith and Milner 1984). Unable to draw on rote knowledge, the patient with executive dysfunction may generate implausible responses that he or she is unable to monitor and correct.

Abulia

C.M. Fisher (1984) resurrected the old term *abulia* (Berrios and Gili 1995)—etymologically, a lack of will—to describe loss of spontaneity due to cerebral disease, of which the extreme case is akinetic mutism. In a less severe form of abulia, the phenomena include slowness, delayed response, laconic speech, and reduced initiative and effort, the patient perhaps performing only one of a series of requested actions. C.M. Fisher (1968) described a transient but repeated lack of response as "intermittent interruption of behavior." Apathy often accompanies abulia, and in recent years, the term *apathy* has come to subsume the disorder of will and action to which *abulia* had referred as well as the disorder of affect or motivation to which *apathy* primarily refers. Other terms used for this phenomenon are *pure psychic akinesia* (Laplane et al. 1984), *loss of psychic self-activation* (Laplane 1990), and *athymhormia* (Habib 2004). Laplane and colleagues (Laplane 1994; Laplane et al. 1989) emphasized its occurrence after basal ganglia lesions, with a subjective sense of mental emptiness, in which context obsessive-compulsive phenomena may co-occur.

At times, even severe abulia can be overcome by stimuli that elicit automatic responses. For example, in the "telephone test," the clinician whose hospital patient is making no response to queries goes to a nearby room and telephones the patient, who astonishingly may be capable of having a conversation on the telephone (L.R. Caplan, personal communication, 1981). One of my patients who replied to no more than one question out of a dozen, not even to simple inquiries as to the place or her name, readily recited a whole stanza of *The Rubáiyát of Omar Khayyám*, her favorite poem. More prosaically, such a patient may generate automatic sequences, such as the alphabet, when spontaneous speech is impossible.

Generating lists of words by categories (e.g., "Name all the animals you can think of," or all modes of transportation, or items one might buy in a supermarket) requires

sustained attention to a task, ability to organize an effective search of memory, intact language, and, of course, a certain amount of real-world knowledge. Equivocal data support the supposition that this task (semantic fluency) is more severely affected in Alzheimer's disease than is generating a list of words beginning with a given letter (phonemic fluency) as a putative manifestation of the breakdown of semantic networks reflective of temporo-parietal disease (Duff Canning et al. 2004). However, the presence of depressive symptoms also affects performance in these domains, and whether the disproportion between performance on the two tasks can be used in neuropsychological differential diagnosis is uncertain (Duff Canning et al. 2004; Ravdin et al. 2003).

The data univocally indicate that semantic fluency is the more sensitive bedside task. At the bedside, quantitative scoring—available data suggest 15 animals in 1 minute as a cutoff for normal performance (Duff Canning et al. 2004)—can be supplemented by assessing the strategy the patient applies. Normally, a patient may name all the animals that come to mind from one class (e.g., barnyard animals) and then switch to another class (e.g., jungle animals). The patient with a disorder of spontaneity and flexible attention has trouble picking a productive strategy and switching it when necessary.

Perseveration

Perseveration refers to the patient's continuing into present activity the elements of previous actions. Luria (1965) devised several bedside tasks to probe the programming of action and to detect perseveration. For example, the patient is asked to form alternately a ring and a fist with his or her hand. Luria noted that in the most characteristic form of abnormality, the patient perseverates on one position or the other, even while correctly saying aloud, "ring-fist-ring-fist." Luria and Homskaya (1963) regarded this disconnection of action from verbal mediation as the essence of frontal dysfunction. A similar but harder task is alternating from fist to edge of hand to palm, or the patient can be asked to alternate repeatedly from outstretched left fist and right palm to outstretched right fist and left palm (the Oseretsky test).

If similar tasks in the graphomotor sphere are given to the patient, a permanent record of the patient's performance results. Simply obtaining a writing sample often elicits perseveration. In Figure 4–2, a patient's response to the request to write a note to a family member is shown. She looked at the upper line, wondered aloud why she kept repeating things, and produced the lower line. Other tasks include asking for repeated sequences of two crosses and a circle or three triangles and two squares.

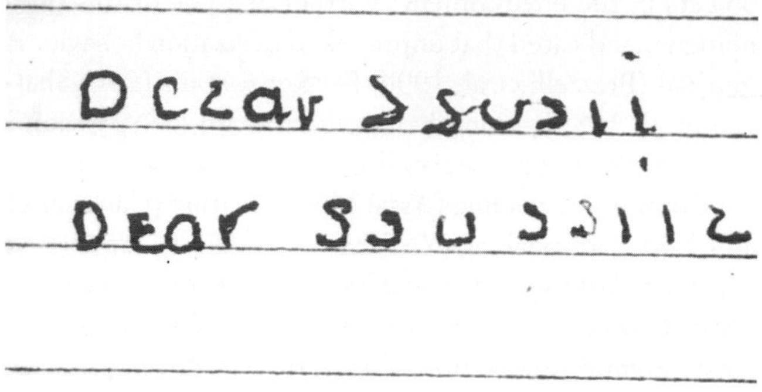

FIGURE 4–2. Perseveration. The patient was asked to write a note to a family member. She wrote the first line, wondered aloud why she hadn't gotten it right, then tried again on the second line.

Sandson and Albert (1987) described several forms of perseveration. In *recurrent* perseveration, a prior response occurs in the context of a new set or demand for action (e.g., the patient names a pen correctly but then calls the point a pen, a watch a pen, and so on). In *stuck-in-set* perseveration, the patient maintains a category or set inappropriately, indicating a disorder of conceptual shifting or flexibility. The task posed by Sandson and Albert involved asking the patient to shift from responding with a circle or square to specified stimuli to responding with a square or circle to those stimuli (i.e., to reverse the response). Others have used tasks of reciprocal action programs. For example, the patient is asked to point with one finger when the examiner points with two, and vice versa. *Continuous* perseveration, in the Sandson and Albert terminology, entails continuation or prolongation of a response without cessation. Asking the patient to produce alternately the cursive letters *m* and *n* may provoke this continuation.

Perseveration can be seen in diseases of various brain regions, but when related to diseases outside frontal regions, it is characteristically limited to a specific modality of processing or response (Goldberg 1987). For example, a patient with disease in the temporoparietal language area may make perseverative errors in naming. Ghika-Schmidt and Bogousslavsky (2000) described palipsychism, a phenomenon seen in anterior thalamic infarction in which perseveration led to overlapping of categories of thought ordinarily easily kept separate. As an example, they cited a woman who ascribed her illness to "a triangle," which she had just been shown. Sandson and Albert (1987) claimed that continuous perseveration is related to nondominant hemisphere disease, but this finding has not been con-

firmed (Annoni et al. 1998). Indeed, the localizing value of mild perseverative errors is questionable (Ruchinskas and Giuliano 2003). Motor perseveration may take the form of stereotyped abnormal movements reminiscent of focal motor status epilepticus (Fung et al. 1997).

A simple bedside sign of perseveration, the applause sign, is evoked by asking the patient to clap three times as quickly as possible, but only three times, after the examiner demonstrates the action (Dubois et al. 2005). Patients with progressive supranuclear palsy, who evince a combination of frontal and subcortical deficits, have strikingly poor performance on this "three-clap test."

Disinhibition

Loss of the capacity for planful action leaves the patient with organic cerebral disease prey to impulses; impulsive behavior is the reverse of the coin of which perseveration is the obverse. The clinician learns about such deficits primarily from the history. The questions often used to examine the patient's judgment (e.g., "What would you do if you found a stamped, addressed envelope in the street?") are not useful, in my opinion. The issue under examination is not the patient's knowledge of social norms; rather, it is his or her ability to use this knowledge to direct behavior. Eslinger and Damasio (1985) argued that a disconnection between such knowledge and its use characterizes orbitofrontal disease—so-called acquired sociopathy.

Usually, but not always, the structure of the interview and examination prevents display of impulsive behavior. For example, one middle-aged patient, being interviewed in his wife's presence, took advantage of my attention to his wife as she spoke to remove chewing gum from his mouth and carefully place it underneath the radiator cover. Few formal tests identify this functional defect. Failure to inhibit reflexive gaze was discussed earlier. Go/no-go tasks are commonly used to explore the effects of frontal lesions in animals (Drewe 1975). A simple bedside adaptation is a tapping task in which the patient is instructed to tap for one stimulus and to refrain for another: "When I tap once, I want you to tap twice; when I tap twice, you do nothing at all." After a practice trial, a single error of commission represents a failure (Leimkuhler and Mesulam 1985). Heilman and Watson (1991) described other ways of specifying deficits in various forms of "defective response inhibition."

Ideational Apraxia

The phenomenon of ideational apraxia is the incapacity to carry out a sequential or ordered set of actions toward a unitary goal in the presence of the necessary objects (Leiguarda and Marsden 2000). For example, the patient may be able to carry out the individual acts involved in preparing a letter to be sent—folding the letter, placing it in the envelope, sealing the envelope—but not be able to do them in the proper order to produce a useful result. Focal lesions involving the left temporoparietal and frontal cortex may impair the use of simple familiar tools as well as the pantomiming of their use. However, disturbance of naturalistic actions involving more complex implements may occur with lesions of either hemisphere and is characteristically associated with confusional states or dementia. It represents a global disorder of the organization of behavior: "It takes the whole brain to make a cup of coffee" (Hartmann et al. 2005).

Impersistence

M. Fisher (1956) described the incapacity of certain patients to sustain activities they were quite capable of beginning. The patient with impersistence peeks when asked to keep the eyes closed or the gaze averted. Maintaining eyelid closure, tongue protrusion, mouth opening, and lateral gaze to the left may be the tasks most sensitive to this incapacity (Jenkyn et al. 1977; Kertesz et al. 1985). In most but not all studies, impersistence has been an indicator of right hemisphere disease (De Renzi et al. 1986; Jenkyn et al. 1977; Joynt et al. 1962; Kertesz et al. 1985). Inability to carry out two simultaneous simple actions ("simultanapraxia") is strongly associated with right frontal injury and with impersistence (Sakai et al. 2000).

Environment-Driven Responses

An important concept in thinking about dysexecutive syndromes is environmental dependency (Bindschaedler and Assal 1992; Lhermitte 1986). When the organism cannot generate plans for behavior toward self-initiated goals, behavior directed by the environment results. Blurting, echolalia, disinhibition, and hypermetamorphosis were discussed earlier, as was the tendency of the patient with frontal disease to stuff food into the mouth. Visual grasping, manual groping, and the "rush toward rewarding objects" are related environment-driven responses (Ghika et al. 1995b).

Imitation behavior or echopraxia can be incidentally observed during the interview and examination; for instance, the examiner incidentally rubs his or her nose, or puts hands on hips, or the like, and the patient—without instruction—imitates the behavior (De Renzi et al. 1996). The two phenomena—imitation behavior and echopraxia—seem to differ along a continuum of deliberation. In the milder form (imitation behavior), patients may withhold imitation of certain gestures, although the imitation behavior may resume after a distraction; in the most severe cases, echopraxic imitation occurs even while the patient is verbalizing the instruction not to imitate (Pillon

and Dubois 2005). Lhermitte et al. (1986) described utilization behavior as an automatic tendency to make use of objects in the environment. Further analysis of this phenomenon indicated that unprovoked utilization behavior is unusual (Brazzelli et al. 1994; De Renzi et al. 1996; Shallice et al. 1989). Nonetheless, Lhermitte (1993) found this behavior to be associated with major depression.

Compulsive reading (Assal 1985), writing (Cambier et al. 1988), and speaking (Y. Tanaka et al. 2000) are related behaviors, but hyperlexia and hypergraphia of this type are distinct from similar phenomena described in limbic epilepsy, mental retardation, and pervasive developmental disorder (Grigorenko et al. 2003; Jancar and Kettle 1984; Okamura et al. 1993; van Vugt et al. 1996). Collecting behavior, or hoarding, is another behavior mediated by the failure of frontal inhibition; patients with frontotemporal dementia or frontal injury may accumulate, with greater or lesser specificity and planning, desired items despite their uselessness and adverse consequences (S.W. Anderson et al. 2005; Pillon and Dubois 2005).

Anarchic Hand

The sense of "alienation" of the hand seen in posterior callosal injury was described earlier. Sometimes, the dramatic manifestation of unwilled acts undertaken by the limb is anatomically and physiologically different. The acts of the "wayward" (Goldberg 1987) or "anarchic" (Della Sala and Marchetti 2005) hand are elicited by the environment; they are well organized and recognized as abnormal by the patient, who does not disclaim ownership of the hand. This phenomenon is due to medial frontal injury with or without callosal involvement and may represent a complex form of grasping or groping; in another sense, it is unilateral utilization behavior (Della Sala et al. 1994; Gasquoine 1993). It represents disinhibition of the lateral motor system responsive to external stimuli from the control of the medial motor system responsible for self-generated action.

AWARENESS OF DEFICIT

The patient who lacks awareness of a deficit obvious to everyone else is a common phenomenon in neuropsychiatry, one with important implications for treatment. The demented patient with Alzheimer's disease often lacks awareness of the reason his or her spouse wants to visit the doctor (Migliorelli et al. 1995). In Anton's syndrome, the patient is unaware of blindness, typically cortical blindness (Förstl et al. 1993). Patients with tardive dyskinesia are often unaware of the abnormal movements, probably because of a schizophrenic defect state (Collis and Macpherson 1992).

The classical—and common—circumstance is right hemisphere damage giving rise to denial of a left hemiparesis. This disturbance of awareness depends on the combination of parietal and frontal lesions (Berti et al. 2005; Pia et al. 2004). A range of states can be seen, from minimization of the gravity of the deficit (anosodiaphoria) through simple unawareness (anosognosia) to bizarre denial of ownership of the affected body part or delusional beliefs about it (somatoparaphrenia) (Halligan et al. 1995). Unawareness of incapacity to perform bimanual tasks is particularly common (Nimmo-Smith et al. 2005). Surprisingly (from the perspective of currently dominant paradigms), not only the denial but also the presumably elementary sensory impairment may depend on operations in the patient's inner representational world, including defensive operations (Bottini et al. 2002; Solms and Turnbull 2002). Such defensive processes appear to contribute to lack of insight in psychosis, along with cognitive impairment (Subotnik et al. 2005). Individual differences in the normal tendency to mislocate stimuli on the basis of attention may provide the substrate for pathological neglect (Marcel et al. 2004).

A purely motivational explanation of anosognosia is inadequate, however, as is shown by the rarity of denial of illness when the lesion is peripheral and by the lack of denial of other deficits in the patient with anosognosia for hemiplegia. As Vuilleumier (2004, p. 13) put it, "Some particular brain states seem required to permit anosognosia." However, the disordered brain state may not always consist in denial; disturbances of discovery of anomalous functioning (because of neglect or deafferentation) or of the formation of beliefs in circumstances of uncertainty may lie at the root of anosognosia.

PSYCHOLOGICAL MANAGEMENT IN THE NEUROPSYCHIATRIC EXAMINATION

In neuropsychiatry—as in all of medicine—the diagnostic evaluation is also part of the psychological treatment. The interest and concern shown by the examiner, the rapport formed with the patient and the family, and the laying on of hands all form the basis of subsequent treatment and must be attended to from the beginning of the consultation.

A common difficulty for beginners is how to introduce the formal cognitive inquiry. All too often, one hears the examiner apologize for the "silly but routine" questions he or she is about to ask. (One never hears a cardiologist apologize for the silly but routine instrument be-

ing applied to the patient's precordium.) This is rarely the best way to gain the patient's full cooperation and best effort. Most of the time, patients report symptoms that can lead naturally (i.e., naturally from the patient's point of view) to a cognitive examination. For example, a patient with depressive symptoms may report trouble concentrating. If the examiner then says, "Let me ask you some questions to check your concentration," the patient is more likely to collaborate and less likely to be offended. Nearly any tasks can then be introduced.

At what point in the interview should this be done? If the initial few minutes of history-taking give reason to suspect substantial cognitive difficulty, one may wish to do at least some of the testing promptly. Not all of the cognitive examination needs to be done at once. Fatigue is an important factor in the cognitive performance of many patients, and long examinations may not elicit their best performance. Caplan (1978) pointed out that variability in performance is characteristic of patients with cerebral lesions and that perseveration may lead to drastic declines as tasks proceed. For this reason, short periods of probing may yield new perspectives on a patient's capacities. Shorter periods of questioning also may help prevent the catastrophic reaction that ensues when a patient's capacities are exceeded. This reaction of agitation and disorganization (Goldstein 1952; Reinhold 1953) is suggestive of organic disease but certainly counterproductive for emotional rapport. Moreover, for a period after such a reaction, the patient is incapable of tasks that are otherwise within his or her capacities, so the data subsequently collected are limited in their significance.

Who should be present for the diagnostic inquiry? Usually, it is necessary to interview ancillary informants to gather a neuropsychiatric history. Frequently, one discovers that a family member has misjudged the nature or severity of the patient's impairment. Testing the patient in front of the family to show impairments allows consensual validation and mutual discussion. This testing requires tact and occasionally requires that the examination be discontinued.

SCREENING BATTERIES AND RATING SCALES

Several investigators have developed brief screening tests of cognitive functioning (Lorentz et al. 2002; Malloy et al. 1997; Ruchinskas and Curyto 2003). These have the advantages of being repeatable, quantitative, and reliable. They are most useful for the recognition of dementia; focal cognitive syndromes may easily escape detection. The widely used Mini-Mental State Examination (MMSE; Fol-

TABLE 4–5.   Behavioral Dyscontrol Scale

1. Patient taps twice with the dominant hand and once with the nondominant hand, repetitively.

2. Patient taps twice with the nondominant hand and once with the dominant hand, repetitively.

3. Patient squeezes examiner's hand when examiner says "red," does nothing when examiner says "green."

4. If examiner taps twice, patient taps once; if examiner taps once, patient taps twice.

5. Patient alternates between touching the thumb and each finger of dominant hand, in succession, to table top, repetitively.

6. Patient makes a fist with knuckles turned down, places the edge of the extended hand on the table, places the palm on the table, repetitively.

7. Facing the examiner, patient duplicates positions of the examiner's hands, using the same hand as the examiner (i.e., without mirroring). Positions include left fist beside left ear, right index finger pointing to right eye, "T" with left hand vertical and right hand horizontal, left hand on left ear, and fingers of right hand under chin with fingers bent at 90°.

8. Patient alternates counting with recitation of the alphabet through the letter *L*.

9. Examiner rates patient's insight.

Note.   All items except rating of insight scored 0 points (failure), 1 point (impaired), or 2 points (normal). Insight is given 0 points (complete inability to judge own performance) to 3 points (intact insight).
Source.   Adapted from Grigsby et al. 1992 and Grigsby et al. 1998.

stein et al. 1975) has important limitations, notably, that executive cognitive dysfunction is not tested. An expansion of the MMSE, called the Modified Mini-Mental State (3MS) Examination (Teng and Chui 1987), which includes elements of executive function, may be more sensitive and specific (Grace et al. 1995). Supplementing the memory item of the MMSE by a cued-recall procedure provides the benefit of distinguishing between retrieval and storage deficits (Yuspeh et al. 1998); a simple cued-recall memory test serves well to screen for Alzheimer's disease (Kuslansky et al. 2002). Katzman et al. (1983) offered a simple screening examination for dementia; it consists of questions probing orientation, attention, and memory. Like the MMSE, it serves best as a screen for cortical dementing disorders.

Other instruments may be more appropriate as screens for subcortical disorders. Power et al. (1995) devised a screening test for HIV-related dementia. Along with a memory task and a test of inhibition of reflexive saccades, it contains timed construction and writing tasks. Even the memory and the timed tasks, without the inhibition task, can identify HIV-related cognitive impairment (Berghuis et al. 1999), although some findings question whether sensitivity is adequate (C.A. Smith et al. 2003). Because vascular dementia and vascular mild cognitive impairment feature mental slowing, reduced working memory, and executive dysfunction, screening for these common disorders has different requirements from screening for Alzheimer's disease or amnestic mild

cognitive impairment (Galluzzi et al. 2005; Sachdev et al. 2004); some data suggest that the HIV Dementia Scale may fit into this niche (van Harten et al. 2004). A particularly simple screen, also validated in a population of patients with AIDS, is an oral modification of the Trail Making B Test, called the Mental Alternation Test (B.N. Jones et al. 1993). The patient is asked to alternate between numbers and letters: "1-A, 2-B, 3-C,…." The number of correct alternations in 30 seconds is the score; incorrect items are not counted. A cutoff of 14/15 gave a sensitivity of 95% and a specificity of 93% in a population of HIV-positive patients being evaluated for encephalopathy. Grigsby and colleagues reported on the utility of this measure for assessing information processing and working memory in various other populations (Grigsby and Kaye 1995; Grigsby et al. 1994).

The choice of an appropriate screening instrument thus depends on the population being screened and the goals of screening. However, the assessment of executive cognitive dysfunction is of paramount importance in neuropsychiatry, and in all neuropsychiatric patients a screen for cognitive deficit is incomplete without attention to this domain. The sole use of the MMSE or a comparable instrument is insufficient for assessment of the skills required for independent functioning (Dymek et al. 2000; Schillerstrom et al. 2003). The Executive Interview (EXIT; Royall et al. 1992) is a screening test for executive cognitive dysfunction. A simpler measure is the Behavioral Dyscontrol Scale (Table 4–5). Both scales show better cor-

Similarities: "In what way are they alike?"

✦ banana and orange (in the event of total failure, e.g., "they are not alike," or partial failure, e.g., "both have peel," help the patient by saying, "both a banana and an orange are" but credit 0 for the item; do not help the patient for the two following items)

✦ table and chair

✦ tulip, rose, and daisy

Score only category response (fruits, furniture, flower) correct:

    3 correct = 3

    2 correct = 2

    1 correct = 1

    0 correct = 0   [___]

Lexical fluency: "Say as many words as you can beginning with the letter *S*, any words except surnames or proper nouns." If the patient gives no response during the first 5 seconds, say, "for instance, snake." If the patient pauses 10 seconds, stimulate him by saying, "any word beginning with the letter *S*." The time allowed is 60 seconds.

Score (word repetitions or variations, surnames, or proper nouns are not counted)

    More than nine words = 3

    Six to nine = 2

    Three to five = 1

    Fewer than three = 0   [___]

Motor series: "Look carefully at what I'm doing." The examiner, seated in front of the patient, performs alone three times with his left hand the series of Luria "fist-edge-palm." "Now, with your right hand do the same series, first with me, then alone." The examiner performs the series three times with the patient, then says to him or her: "Now, do it on your own."

    Six correct consecutive series alone = 3

    At least three correct consecutive series alone = 2

    Fails alone, but performs three correct consecutive series with the examiner = 1

    Cannot perform three correct consecutive series even with the examiner = 0   [___]

Conflicting instructions: "Tap twice when I tap once." To be sure that the patient has understood the instruction, a series of three trials is run: 1-1-1. "Tap once when I tap twice." To be sure that the patient has understood the instruction, a series of three trials is run: 2-2-2. The examiner performs the following series 1-1-2-1-2-2-2-1-1-2.

    No error = 3

    One or two errors = 2

    More than two errors = 1

    Patient taps like the examiner at least four consecutive times = 0   [___]

Go/no-go: "Tap once when I tap once." To be sure that the patient has understood the instruction, a series of three trials is run: 1-1-1. "Do not tap when I tap twice." To be sure that the patient has understood the instruction, a series of three trials is run: 2-2-2. The examiner performs the following series: 1-1-2-1-2-2-2-1-1-2.

    No error = 3

    One or two errors = 2

    More than two errors = 1

    Patient taps like the examiner at least four consecutive times = 0   [___]

Prehension behavior: The examiner is seated in front of the patient. Place the patient's hands palm up on his or her knees. Without saying anything or looking at the patient, the examiner brings his or her hands close to the patient's hands and touches the palms of both the patient's hands, to see if he or she will spontaneously take them. If the patient takes the hands, the examiner will try again after asking him or her: "Now do not take my hands."

    Patient does not take the examiner's hands = 3

    Patient hesitates and asks what he or she has to do = 2

    Patient takes the hands without hesitation = 1   [___]

    Patient takes the examiner's hand even after being told not to do so = 0

                                           Total = ____

FIGURE 4–3. Frontal Assessment Battery.

Source. Reprinted with permission from Dubois B, Slachevsky A, Litvan I, et al.: "The FAB: A Frontal Assessment Battery at Bedside." *Neurology* 55:1621–1626, 2000.

relation with functional status, such as the ability to live independently, than the MMSE (Grigsby et al. 1998; Royall et al. 2005). Dubois et al. (2000) devised the Frontal Assessment Battery (Figure 4–3) for identifying executive dysfunction at the bedside in several domains in patients with extrapyramidal disorders. Individual items of the scale address motor sequencing, verbal fluency, response inhibition, and other executive functions. The scale, which requires less than 5 minutes to administer, promises to be useful (Slachevsky et al. 2004). Freehand drawing of a clock is sensitive to executive cognitive dysfunction (Royall et al. 1998, 1999, 2004). For clock drawing to be used as a screening instrument for executive dysfunction, scoring must reflect organizational elements of the drawing performance, subtracting out problems related to visuospatial function (Royall et al. 1998, 1999).

Scales for quantifying noncognitive aspects of organic dysfunction also exist. Inventories of comportmental disturbance related to executive dysfunction include the Middelheim Frontality Score (De Deyn et al. 2005), the Frontal Systems Behavior Scale, and others (Malloy and Grace 2005). These make use of caregiver reports or clinical observations to assess "frontal" behaviors and personality change. Some, such as the Frontal Behavioral Inventory, showed good performance at separating Alzheimer's disease from frontotemporal dementia (Kertesz et al. 2003). The Neuropsychiatric Inventory and the Neurobehavioral Rating Scale cast a broader net. The Neuropsychiatric Inventory comprises assessments of psychosis, mood and affective disorders, aggression, disinhibition, and aberrant motor activity (Cummings et al. 1994). A screen and metric approach is used; 10 screening questions invoke supplementary questions to rate frequency and severity. A modification allows its use as a questionnaire for relatives or caregivers (Kaufer et al. 2000). The Neurobehavioral Rating Scale is a modification of the well-known Brief Psychiatric Rating Scale, with the addition of items thought relevant for a population with head injuries but also appropriate for patients with dementia and other disorders (H.S. Levin et al. 1987; McCauley et al. 2001; Sultzer et al. 1995).

CONCLUSION

The "complete examination" is a figment. No practical examination can include all possible elements. The expert clinician is constantly generating hypotheses and constructing an examination to confirm or refute them (Caplan 1990). The diagnostician as historian constantly strives to write the patient's biography: How did this person arrive at this predicament at this time? This biographical endeavor is far more complex than attaching a DSM-IV-TR (American Psychiatric Association 2000) label to a patient. Diagnosis in neuropsychiatry does not mean the search only for cause, or only for localization, or only for functional capacity. It means, along with those aims, constructing a pathophysiological and psychopathological formulation from cause to effect, from etiological factor to symptomatic complaint or performance. This formulation of pathogenetic mechanisms provides a rational framework for intervention.

Cognitive examination is the traditional psychiatric method for making a nonidiopathic mental diagnosis, and reliance on hard signs on physical examination is the traditional neurological method. The material reviewed in this chapter shows the broad array of tools that can implicate brain impairment in the pathogenesis of mental disorder. The clinician should maximize use of the means available in this difficult task, ideally without interference from disciplinary boundaries.

Highlights for the Clinician

- ✦ Organic contributors to psychopathology can be recognized at the bedside through skillful history-taking and examination.

- ✦ Only knowledge of the psychiatric features of epilepsy, traumatic brain injury, and other common pathologies allows the clinician to know what questions to ask and what findings to look for. These features may differ from the characteristic phenomena of idiopathic psychiatric illness.

- ✦ Listening to the patient tell the story of the illness is part of the examination (because narrative skills may be subtly altered by brain disease) and is also part of the psychological management of a brain-injured patient.

- ✦ Similarly, physical examination plays both an irreplaceable practical role in eliciting clinical information and a helpful psychological role in establishing the medical context of the clinical encounter.

RECOMMENDED READINGS

Cutting J: Principles of Psychopathology: Two Worlds, Two Minds, Two Hemispheres. New York, Oxford University Press, 1997

Ovsiew F: Neuropsychiatric approach to the patient, in Comprehensive Textbook of Psychiatry, Vol 1. Edited by Sadock BJ, Sadock VA. Philadelphia, PA, Lippincott Williams & Wilkins, 2005, pp 323–349

Sanders RD, Keshavan MS: Physical and neurologic examinations in neuropsychiatry. Semin Clin Neuropsychiatry 7:18–29, 2002

REFERENCES

Abad V, Ovsiew F: Treatment of persistent myoclonic tardive dystonia with verapamil. Br J Psychiatry 162:554–556, 1993

Absher JR, Benson DF: Disconnection syndromes: an overview of Geschwind's contributions. Neurology 43:862–867, 1993

Abwender DA, Trinidad KS, Jones KR, et al: Features resembling Tourette syndrome in developmental stutterers. Brain Lang 62:455–464, 1998

Adair JC, Williamson DJ, Jacobs DH, et al: Neglect of radial and vertical space: importance of the retinotopic reference frame. J Neurol Neurosurg Psychiatry 58:724–728, 1995

Aguirre GK, D'Esposito M: Topographical disorientation: a synthesis and taxonomy. Brain 122:1613–1628, 1999

Alexander GE, DeLong MR: Central mechanisms of initiation and control of movement, in Diseases of the Nervous System/Clinical Neurobiology, 2nd Edition, Vol 1. Edited by Asbury AK, McKhann GM, McDonald WI. Philadelphia, PA, WB Saunders, 1992, pp 285–308

Alexander MP: Frontal lobes and language. Brain Lang 37:656–691, 1989

Alexander MP: Mild traumatic brain injury: pathophysiology, natural history, and clinical management. Neurology 45:1253–1260, 1995

Alexander MP: Disturbances in language initiation: mutism and its lesser forms, in Movement Disorders in Neurology and Psychiatry, 2nd Edition. Edited by Joseph AB, Young RR. Oxford, UK, Blackwell Science, 1999, pp 366–371

Algoed L, Janssens J, Vanhooren G: Apraxia of eyelid opening secondary to right frontal infarction. Acta Neurol Belg 92:228–233, 1992

Allman P, Marshall M, Hope T, et al: Emotionalism following stroke: development and reliability of a semi-structured interview. Int J Methods Psychiatr Res 2:125–131, 1992

Almeida OP, Förstl H, Howard R, et al: Unilateral auditory hallucinations. Br J Psychiatry 162:262–264, 1993

Almeida OP, Howard RJ, Levy R, et al: Psychotic states arising in late life (late paraphrenia): the role of risk factors. Br J Psychiatry 166:215–228, 1995

American Psychiatric Association: Diagnostic and Statistical Manual of Mental Disorders, 4th Edition, Text Revision. Washington, DC, American Psychiatric Association, 2000

Anderson NE, Mason DF, Fink JN, et al: Detection of focal cerebral hemisphere lesions using the neurological examination. J Neurol Neurosurg Psychiatry 76:545–549, 2005

Anderson SW, Damasio H, Damasio AR: A neural basis for collecting behaviour in humans. Brain 128:201–212, 2005

Andreasen NC: Thought, language, and communication disorders. Arch Gen Psychiatry 36:1315–1321, 1979

Annoni GM, Pegna AJ, Michel CM, et al: Motor perseverations: a function of the side and the site of a cerebral lesion. Eur Neurol 40:84–90, 1998

Arango C, Bartko JJ, Gold JM, et al: Prediction of neuropsychological performance by neurological signs in schizophrenia. Am J Psychiatry 156:1349–1357, 1999

Arányi Z, Rösler K: Effort-induced mirror movements. Exp Brain Res 145:76–82, 2002

Ardila A, Niño CR, Pulido E, et al: Episodic psychic symptoms in the general population. Epilepsia 34:133–140, 1993

Ardila A, Rosselli M, Surloff C, et al: Transient paligraphia associated with severe palilalia and stuttering: a single case report. Neurocase 5:435–440, 1999

Arroyo S, Lesser RP, Gordon B, et al: Mirth, laughter and gelastic seizures. Brain 116:757–780, 1993

Arseneault L, Tremblay RE, Boulerice B, et al: Minor physical anomalies and family adversity as risk factors for violent delinquency in adolescence. Am J Psychiatry 157:917–923, 2000

Assal G: Un aspect du comportement d'utilisation: la dépendance vis-à-vis du langage écrit. Rev Neurol (Paris) 141:493–495, 1985

Atre-Vaidya N, Taylor MA, Jampala VC, et al: Psychosensory features in mood disorder: a preliminary report. Compr Psychiatry 35:286–289, 1994

Ay H, Buonanno FS, Price BH, et al: Sensory alien hand syndrome: case report and review of the literature. J Neurol Neurosurg Psychiatry 65:366–369, 1998

Azouvi P, Samuel C, Louis-Dreyfus A, et al: Sensitivity of clinical and behavioural tests of spatial neglect after right hemisphere stroke. J Neurol Neurosurg Psychiatry 73:160–166, 2002

Baba A, Hamada H: Musical hallucinations in schizophrenia. Psychopathology 32:242–251, 1999

Baezner H, Hennerici M: From trepidant abasia to motor network failure—gait disorders as a consequence of subcortical vascular encephalopathy (SVE): review of historical and contemporary concepts. J Neurol Sci 229–230:81–88, 2005

Bakar M, Kirshner HS, Niaz F: The opercular-subopercular syndrome: four cases with review of the literature. Behav Neurol 11:97–103, 1998

Baldwin R, Jeffries S, Jackson A, et al: Neurological findings in late-onset depressive disorder: comparison of individuals with and without depression. Br J Psychiatry 186:308–313, 2005

Ballard C, Holmes C, McKeith I, et al: Psychiatric morbidity in dementia with Lewy bodies: a prospective clinical and neuropathological comparative study with Alzheimer's disease. Am J Psychiatry 156:1039–1045, 1999

Bancaud J, Brunet-Bourgin F, Chauvel P, et al: Anatomic origin of *déjà vu* and vivid "memories" in human temporal lobe epilepsy. Brain 117:71–90, 1994

Bär KJ, Häger F, Sauer H: Olanzapine- and clozapine-induced stuttering: a case series. Pharmacopsychiatry 37:131–134, 2004

Baranowski SL, Patten SB: The predictive value of dysgraphia and constructional apraxia for delirium in psychiatric inpatients. Can J Psychiatry 45:75–78, 2000

Barclay CL, Bergeron C, Lang AE: Arm levitation in progressive supranuclear palsy. Neurology 52:879–882, 1999

Barnes MP, Saunders M, Walls TJ, et al: The syndrome of Karl Ludwig Kahlbaum. J Neurol Neurosurg Psychiatry 49:991–996, 1986

Barrash J: A historical review of topographical disorientation and its neuroanatomical correlates. J Clin Exp Neuropsychol 20:807–827, 1998

Barrera A, McKenna PJ, Berrios GE: Formal thought disorder in schizophrenia: an executive or a semantic deficit? Psychol Med 35:121–132, 2005

Barton JJ: Disorders of face perception and recognition. Neurol Clin 21:521–548, 2003

Barton JJS, Cherkasova MV, Hefter R, et al: Are patients with social developmental disorders prosopagnosic? Perceptual heterogeneity in the Asperger and socio-emotional processing disorders. Brain 127:1706–1716, 2004

Baumgartner C, Gröppel G, Leutmezer F, et al: Ictal urinary urge indicates seizure onset in the nondominant temporal lobe. Neurology 55:432–434, 2000

Bear D, Hermann B, Fogel B: Interictal behavior syndrome in temporal lobe epilepsy: the views of three experts. J Neuropsychiatry Clin Neurosci 1:308–318, 1989

Benjamin S: A neuropsychiatric approach to aggressive behavior, in Neuropsychiatry and Mental Health Services. Edited by Ovsiew F. Washington, DC, American Psychiatric Press, 1999a, pp 149–196

Benjamin S: Oculogyric crisis, in Movement Disorders in Neurology and Neuropsychiatry, 2nd Edition. Edited by Joseph AB, Young RR. Boston, MA, Blackwell Scientific, 1999b, pp 92–103

Benke T, Butterworth B: Palilalia and repetitive speech: two case studies. Brain Lang 78:62–81, 2001

Benke T, Hohenstein C, Poewe W, et al: Repetitive speech phenomena in Parkinson's disease. J Neurol Neurosurg Psychiatry 69:319–325, 2000

Berghuis JP, Uldall KK, Lalonde B: Validity of two scales in identifying HIV-associated dementia. J Acquir Immune Defic Syndr 21:134–140, 1999

Berrios GE, Gili M: Abulia and impulsiveness revisited: a conceptual history. Acta Psychiatr Scand 92:161–167, 1995

Berthier ML, Ruiz A, Massone MI, et al: Foreign accent syndrome: behavioural and anatomic findings in recovered and non-recovered patients. Aphasiology 5:129–147, 1991

Berthier ML, Kulisevsky J, Gironell A, et al: Obsessive-compulsive disorder associated with brain lesions: clinical phenomenology, cognitive function, and anatomic correlates. Neurology 47:353–361, 1996

Berti A, Frassinetti F: When far becomes near: remapping of space by tool use. J Cogn Neurosci 12:415–420, 2000

Berti A, Bottini G, Gandola M, et al: Shared cortical anatomy for motor awareness and motor control. Science 309:488–491, 2005

Beversdorf DQ, Heilman KM: Facilatory paratonia and frontal lobe functioning. Neurology 51:968–971, 1998

Biddle KR, McCabe A, Bliss LS: Narrative skills following traumatic brain injury in children and adults. J Commun Disord 29:447–469, 1996

Bindschaedler C, Assal G: La dépendance à l'égard de l'environnement lors de lésions cérébrales: conduites d'imitation, de préhension et d'utilisation. Schweiz Archiv fur Neurologie und Psychiatrie 143:175–187, 1992

Bisiach E: Mental representation in unilateral neglect and related disorders: the twentieth Barlett Memorial Lecture. Q J Exp Psychol 46A:435–461, 1993

Bisiach E, Luzzatti C: Unilateral neglect of representational space. Cortex 14:129–133, 1978

Black FW: Digit repetition in brain-damaged adults: clinical and theoretical implications. J Clin Psychol 42:770–782, 1986

Blanchet P, Frommer GP: Mood change preceding epileptic seizures. J Nerv Ment Dis 174:471–476, 1986

Blekher TM, Yee RD, Kirkwood SC, et al: Oculomotor control in asymptomatic and recently diagnosed individuals with the genetic marker for Huntington's disease. Vision Res 44:2729–2736, 2004

Blumer D: Evidence supporting the temporal lobe epilepsy personality syndrome. Neurology 53:S9–12, 1999

Bogen JE: The callosal syndromes, in Clinical Neuropsychology, 3rd Edition. Edited by Heilman KM, Valenstein E. New York, Oxford University Press, 1993, pp 337–407

Bogousslavsky J, Regli F, Uske A: Thalamic infarcts: clinical syndromes, etiology, and prognosis. Neurology 38:837–848, 1988

Bogousslavsky J, Kumral E, Regli F, et al: Acute hemiconcern: a right anterior parietotemporal syndrome. J Neurol Neurosurg Psychiatry 58:428–432, 1995

Boks MPM, Liddle PF, Burgerhof JGM, et al: Neurological soft signs discriminating mood disorders from first episode schizophrenia. Acta Psychiatr Scand 110:29–35, 2004

Bolton D, Gibb W, Lees A, et al: Neurological soft signs in obsessive compulsive disorder: standardised assessment and comparison with schizophrenia. Behav Neurol 11:197–204, 1998

Bottini G, Bisiach E, Sterzi R, et al: Feeling touches in someone else's hand. Neuroreport 13:249–252, 2002

Bouvier SE, Engel SA: Behavioral deficits and cortical damage loci in cerebral achromatopsia. Cereb Cortex 16:183–191, 2006

Bowers D, White T, Bauer RM: Recall of three words after 5 minutes: its relationship to performance on neuropsychological memory tests (abstract). Neurology 39 (suppl 1):176, 1989

Bracha HS, Wolkowitz OM, Lohr JB, et al: High prevalence of visual hallucinations in research subjects with chronic schizophrenia. Am J Psychiatry 146:526–528, 1989

Braun CM, Dumont M, Duval J, et al: Brain modules of hallucination: an analysis of multiple patients with brain lesions. J Psychiatry Neurosci 28:432–449, 2003

Braunig P, Kruger S, Shugar G, et al: The Catatonia Rating Scale—development, reliability and use. Compr Psychiatry 41:147–158, 2000

Brazzelli M, Colombo N, Della Sala S, et al: Spared and impaired cognitive abilities after bilateral frontal damage. Cortex 30:27–51, 1994

Brewer GJ: Neurologically presenting Wilson's disease: epidemiology, pathophysiology and treatment. CNS Drugs 19:185–192, 2005

Brion S, Jedynak C-P: Troubles du transfert interhémisphérique: à propos de trois observations de tumeurs du corps calleux. Le signe de la main étrangère. Rev Neurol (Paris) 126:257–266, 1972

Brodal A: Self-observations and neuro-anatomical considerations after a stroke. Brain 96:675–694, 1973

Brodal A: Neurological Anatomy in Relation to Clinical Medicine, 3rd Edition. New York, Oxford University Press, 1981

Brodsky H, Dat Vuong K, Thomas M, et al: Glabellar and palmomental reflexes in parkinsonian disorders. Neurology 63:1096–1098, 2004

Brown P: Myoclonus, in Movement Disorders in Clinical Practice. Edited by Sawle G. Oxford, UK, Isis Medical Media, 1999, pp 147–157

Brown P, Rothwell JC, Thompson PD, et al: New observations on the normal auditory startle reflex in man. Brain 114:1891–1902, 1991

Browne S, Clarke M, Gervin M, et al: Determinants of neurological dysfunction in first episode schizophrenia. Psychol Med 30:1433–1441, 2000

Brownell H, Martino G: Deficits in inference and social cognition: the effects of right hemisphere brain damage on discourse, in Right Hemisphere Language Comprehension: Perspectives From Cognitive Neuroscience. Edited by Beeman M, Chiarello C. Mahwah, NJ, Lawrence Erlbaum, 1998, pp 309–328

Bryden MP: Measuring handedness with questionnaires. Neuropsychologia 15:617–624, 1977

Buchanan RW, Heinrichs DW: The Neurological Evaluation Scale (NES): a structured instrument for the assessment of neurological signs in schizophrenia. Psychiatry Res 27:335–350, 1989

Bundick T, Spinella M: Subjective experience, involuntary movement, and posterior alien hand syndrome. J Neurol Neurosurg Psychiatry 68:83–85, 2000

Burgess PW: Strategy application disorder: the role of the frontal lobes in human multitasking. Psychol Res 63:279–288, 2000

Burgess PW, Veitch E, de Lacy Costello A, et al: The cognitive and neuroanatomical correlates of multitasking. Neuropsychologia 38:848–863, 2000

Burke JM, Schaberg DR: Neurosyphilis in the antibiotic era. Neurology 35:1368–1371, 1985

Buschke H, Kuslansky G, Katz M, et al: Screening for dementia with the Memory Impairment Screen. Neurology 52:231–238, 1999

Bush G, Fink M, Petrides G, et al: Catatonia, I: rating scale and standardized examination. Acta Psychiatr Scand 93:129–136, 1996

Bushby KMD, Cole T, Matthews JNS, et al: Centiles for adult head circumference. Arch Dis Child 67:1286–1287, 1992

Calvert T, Knapp P, House A: Psychological associations with emotionalism after stroke. J Neurol Neurosurg Psychiatry 65:928–929, 1998

Cambier J, Masson C, Benammou S, et al: La graphomanie: activité graphique compulsive manifestation d'un gliome fronto-calleux. Rev Neurol (Paris) 144:158–164, 1988

Cancelliere AEB, Kertesz A: Lesion localization in acquired deficits of emotional expression and comprehension. Brain Cogn 13:133–147, 1990

Cantor-Graae E, Ismail B, McNeil TF: Are neurological abnormalities in schizophrenic patients and their siblings the result of perinatal trauma? Acta Psychiatr Scand 101:142–147, 2000

Caplan LR: Variability of perceptual function: the sensory cortex as a "categorizer" and "deducer." Brain Lang 6:1–13, 1978

Caplan LR: The Effective Clinical Neurologist. Cambridge, MA, Blackwell Scientific, 1990

Caplan LR, Kelly M, Kase CS, et al: Infarcts of the inferior division of the right middle cerebral artery: mirror image of Wernicke's aphasia. Neurology 36:1015–1020, 1986

Caplan LR, Schmahmann JD, Kase CS, et al: Caudate infarcts. Arch Neurol 47:133–143, 1990

Carbary TJ, Patterson JP: Foreign accent syndrome following a catastrophic second injury: MRI correlates, linguistic and voice pattern analysis. Brain Cogn 43:78–85, 2000

Carluer L, Marié R-M, Lambert J, et al: Acquired and persistent stuttering as the main symptom of striatal infarction. Mov Disord 15:343–346, 2000

Carota A, Rossetti AO, Karapanayiotides T, et al: Catastrophic reaction in acute stroke: a reflex behavior in aphasic patients. Neurology 57:1902–1905, 2001

Carrazana E, Rossitch E, Martinez J: Unilateral "akathisia" in a patient with AIDS and a toxoplasmosis subthalamic abscess. Neurology 39:449–450, 1989

Caselli RJ: Visual syndromes as the presenting feature of degenerative brain disease. Semin Neurol 20:139–144, 2000

Caviness JN, Brown P: Myoclonus: current concepts and recent advances. Lancet Neurol 3:598–607, 2004

Cendes F: Febrile seizures and mesial temporal sclerosis. Curr Opin Neurol 17:161–164, 2004

Cerrato P, Imperiale D, Bergui M, et al: Emotional facial paresis in a patient with a lateral medullary infarction. Neurology 60:723–724, 2003

Chacko RC, Corbin MA, Harper RG: Acquired obsessive-compulsive disorder associated with basal ganglia lesions. J Neuropsychiatry Clin Neurosci 12:269–272, 2000

Chapman LF, Wolff HG: Disease of the neopallium and impairment of the highest integrative functions. Med Clin North Am 42:677–689, 1958

Chapman LF, Thetford WN, Berlin L, et al: Highest integrative functions in man during stress, in Brain and Human Behavior, Vol XXXVI. Edited by Solomon HC, Cobb S, Penfield W. Baltimore, MD, Williams & Wilkins, 1958, pp 491–534

Chatterjee A, Yapundich R, Mennemeier M, et al: Thalamic thought disorder: on being "a bit addled." Cortex 33:419–440, 1997

Chédru F, Geschwind N: Disorders of higher cortical functions in acute confusional states. Cortex 8:395–411, 1972a

Chédru F, Geschwind N: Writing disturbances in acute confusional states. Neuropsychologia 10:343–353, 1972b

Chen EYH, Shapleske J, Luque R, et al: The Cambridge Neurological Inventory: a clinical instrument for assessment of soft neurological signs in psychiatric patients. Psychiatry Res 56:183–204, 1995

Chen EY-H, Hui CL-M, Chan RC-K, et al: A 3-year prospective study of neurological soft signs in first-episode schizophrenia. Schizophr Res 75:45–54, 2005

Christoph DH, de Freitas GR, dos Santos DP, et al: Different perceived foreign accents in one patient after prerolandic hematoma. Eur Neurol 52:198–201, 2004

Chung SJ, Im JH, Lee JH, et al: Stuttering and gait disturbance after supplementary motor area seizure. Mov Disord 19:1106–1109, 2004

Ciabarra AM, Elkind MS, Roberts JK, et al: Subcortical infarction resulting in acquired stuttering. J Neurol Neurosurg Psychiatry 69:546–549, 2000

Coelho M, Ferro JM: Fou rire prodromique: case report and systematic review of literature. Cerebrovasc Dis 16:101–104, 2003

Cohen MAA, Alfonso CA, Haque MM: Lilliputian hallucinations and medical illness. Gen Hosp Psychiatry 16:141–143, 1994

Cohen-Mansfield J, Libin A: Verbal and physical non-aggressive agitated behaviors in elderly persons with dementia: robustness of syndromes. J Psychiatr Res 39:325–332, 2005

Cole M: When the left brain is not right the right brain may be left: report of personal experience of occipital hemianopia. J Neurol Neurosurg Psychiatry 67:169–173, 1999

Cole M: Charles Bonnet syndrome: an example of cortical dissociation syndrome affecting vision? (letter). J Neurol Neurosurg Psychiatry 71:134, 2001

Collins SJ, Ahlskog JE, Parisi JE, et al: Progressive supranuclear palsy: neuropathologically based diagnostic clinical criteria. J Neurol Neurosurg Psychiatry 58:167–173, 1995

Collis RJ, Macpherson R: Tardive dyskinesia: patients' lack of awareness of movement disorder. Br J Psychiatry 160:110–112, 1992

Comella CL, Goetz CG: Akathisia in Parkinson's disease. Mov Disord 9:545–549, 1994

Coplan RJ, Coleman B, Rubin KH: Shyness and little boy blue: iris pigmentation, gender, and social wariness in preschoolers. Dev Psychobiol 32:37–44, 1998

Coslett HB: Acquired dyslexia. Semin Neurol 20:419–426, 2000

Crutch S: Apraxia. ACNR Advances in Clinical Neuroscience and Rehabilitation 5:16–17, 2005

Cummings JL: Neuropsychiatry of sexual deviations, in Neuropsychiatry and Mental Health Services. Edited by Ovsiew F. Washington, DC, American Psychiatric Press, 1999, pp 363–384

Cummings JL, Mega M, Gray K, et al: The Neuropsychiatric Inventory: comprehensive assessment of psychopathology in dementia. Neurology 44:2308–2314, 1994

Currie J, Ramsden B, McArthur C, et al: Validation of a clinical antisaccadic eye movement test in the assessment of dementia. Arch Neurol 48:644–648, 1991

Cushing H: Distortions of the visual fields in cases of brain tumour: the field defects produced by temporal lobe lesions. Brain 44:341–396, 1922

Cutting J: Physical illness and psychosis. Br J Psychiatry 136:109–119, 1980

Cutting J: The phenomenology of acute organic psychosis: comparison with acute schizophrenia. Br J Psychiatry 151:324–332, 1987

Cutting J: The Right Cerebral Hemisphere and Psychiatric Disorders. Oxford, UK, Oxford University Press, 1990

Cutting J, Murphy D: Schizophrenic thought disorder: a psychological and organic interpretation. Br J Psychiatry 152:310–319, 1988

Daffner KR, Ahern GL, Weintraub S, et al: Dissociated neglect behavior following sequential strokes in the right hemisphere. Neurology 28:97–101, 1990

Daly DA, Burnett ML: Cluttering: traditional views and new perspectives, in Stuttering and Related Disorders of Fluency, 2nd Edition. Edited by Curlee RF. New York, Thieme Medical Publishing, 1999, pp 222–254

Damasio AR, Maurer RG: A neurological model for childhood autism. Arch Neurol 35:777–786, 1978

Damasio AR, Van Hoesen GW: Emotional disturbances associated with focal lesions of the limbic frontal lobe, in Neuropsychology of Human Emotion. Edited by Heilman KM, Satz P. New York, Guilford, 1983, pp 85–110

Darley FL, Aronson AE, Brown JR: Motor Speech Disorders. Philadelphia, PA, WB Saunders, 1975

Dasco CC, Bortz DL: Significance of the Argyll Robertson pupil in clinical medicine. Am J Med 86:199–202, 1989

David AS: Thought echo reflects the activity of the phonological loop. Br J Clin Psychol 33:81–83, 1994

Day RK: Psychomotor agitation: poorly defined and badly measured. J Affect Disord 55:89–98, 1999

Dazzan P, Morgan KD, Orr KG, et al: The structural brain correlates of neurological soft signs in AeSOP first-episode psychoses study. Brain 127:143–153, 2004

De Deyn PP, Engelborghs S, Saerens J, et al: The Middelheim Frontality Score: a behavioural assessment scale that discriminates frontotemporal dementia from Alzheimer's disease. Int J Geriatr Psychiatry 20:70–79, 2005

Defazio G, Livrea P, Lamberti P, et al: Isolated so-called apraxia of eyelid opening: report of 10 cases and a review of the literature. Eur Neurol 39:204–210, 1998

de Leon J: Polydipsia: a study in a long-term psychiatric unit. Eur Arch Psychiatry Clin Neurosci 253:37–39, 2003

Della Sala S, Marchetti C: Anarchic hand, in Higher-Order Motor Disorders. Edited by Freund HJ, Jeannerod M, Hallett M, et al. Oxford, UK, Oxford University Press, 2005, pp 291–301

Della Sala S, Marchetti C, Spinnler H: The anarchic hand: a fronto-mesial sign, in Handbook of Neuropsychology, Vol 9. Edited by Boller F, Grafman J. Amsterdam, The Netherlands, Elsevier, 1994, pp 233–255

Demarest J, Demarest L: Does the "torque test" measure cerebral dominance in adults? Percept Mot Skills 50:155–158, 1980

Denny-Brown D: The nature of apraxia. J Nerv Ment Dis 126:9–32, 1958

Departments of Psychiatry and Child Psychiatry, The Institute of Psychiatry, and The Maudsley Hospital London: Psychiatric Examination: Notes on Eliciting and Recording Clinical Information in Psychiatric Patients, 2nd Edition. Oxford, UK, Oxford University Press, 1987

De Renzi E, Barbieri C: The incidence of the grasp reflex following hemispheric lesion and its relation to frontal damage. Brain 115:243–313, 1992

De Renzi E, Gentilini M, Bazolli M: Eyelid movement disorders and motor impersistence in acute hemisphere disease. Neurology 36:414–418, 1986

De Renzi E, Cavalleri F, Facchini S: Imitation and utilisation behaviour. J Neurol Neurosurg Psychiatry 61:396–400, 1996

Desmond DW, Tatemichi TK, Figueroa M, et al: Disorientation following stroke: frequency, course, and clinical correlates. J Neurol 241:585–591, 1994

D'Esposito M: Neurological Foundations of Cognitive Neuroscience. Cambridge, MA, MIT Press, 2003

Destée A, Gray F, Parent M, et al: Comportement compulsif d'allure obsessionnelle et paralysie supranucléaire progressive. Rev Neurol (Paris) 146:12–18, 1990

Devinsky O, Bear D: Varieties of aggressive behavior in temporal lobe epilepsy. Am J Psychiatry 141:651–656, 1984

Devinsky O, Najjar S: Evidence against the existence of a temporal lobe epilepsy personality syndrome. Neurology 53:S13–25, 1999

Devinsky O, Bear D, Volpe BT: Confusional states following posterior cerebral artery infarction. Arch Neurol 45:160–163, 1988

Devinsky O, Khan S, Alper K: Olfactory reference syndrome in a patient with partial epilepsy. Neuropsychiatry Neuropsychol Behav Neurol 11:103–105, 1998

de Vries BBA, White SM, Knight SJL, et al: Clinical studies on submicroscopic subtelomeric rearrangements: a checklist. J Med Genet 38:145–150, 2001

Dietl T, Auer DP, Modell S, et al: Involuntary vocalisations and a complex hyperkinetic movement disorder following left side thalamic haemorrhage. Behav Neurol 14:99–102, 2003

Di Legge S, Di Piero V, Altieri M, et al: Usefulness of primitive reflexes in demented and non-demented cerebrovascular patients in daily clinical practice. Eur Neurol 45:104–110, 2001

Douyon R, Guzman P, Romain G, et al: Subtle neurological deficits and psychopathological findings in substance-abusing homeless and non-homeless veterans. J Neuropsychiatry Clin Neurosci 10:210–215, 1998

Drewe EA: Go-no go learning after frontal lobe lesions in humans. Cortex 11:8–16, 1975

Dubois B, Slachevsky A, Litvan I, et al: The FAB: a frontal assessment battery at bedside. Neurology 55:1621–1626, 2000

Dubois B, Slachevsky A, Pillon B, et al: "Applause sign" helps to discriminate PSP from FTD and PD. Neurology 64:2132–2133, 2005

Duchaine BC, Nakayama K: Developmental prosopagnosia and the Benton Facial Recognition Test. Neurology 62:1219–1220, 2004

Duckett S, Gibson W, Salama M: Levy-Reid hypothesis. Brain Lang 45:121–124, 1993

Duff Canning SJ, Leach L, Stuss D, et al: Diagnostic utility of abbreviated fluency measures in Alzheimer disease and vascular dementia. Neurology 62:556–562, 2004

Duffy JR, Baumgartner J: Psychogenic stuttering in adults with and without neurologic disease. J Med Speech Lang Pathol 5:75–96, 1997

Dutton GN: Cognitive vision, its disorders and differential diagnosis in adults and children: knowing where and what things are. Eye 17:289–304, 2003

Duus P: Topical Diagnosis in Neurology, 3rd Edition. New York, Thieme, 1998

Dwyer J, Reid S: Ganser's syndrome. Lancet 364:471–473, 2004

Dymek MP, Atchison P, Harrell L, et al: Competency to consent to medical treatment in cognitively impaired patients with Parkinson's disease. Neurology 56:17–24, 2000

Edelstyn NM, Oyebode F, Barrett K: The delusions of Capgras and intermetamorphosis in a patient with right-hemisphere white-matter pathology. Psychopathology 34:299–304, 2001

Edwards MJ, Dale RC, Church AJ, et al: Adult-onset tic disorder, motor stereotypies, and behavioural disturbance associated with antibasal ganglia antibodies. Mov Disord 19:1190–1196, 2004

Ellsworth JD, Lawrence MS, Roth RH, et al: D_1 and D_2 dopamine receptors independently regulate spontaneous blink rate in the vervet monkey. J Pharmacol Exp Ther 259:595–600, 1991

Eslinger PJ, Damasio AR: Severe disturbance of higher cognition after bilateral frontal lobe ablation: patient EVR. Neurology 35:1731–1741, 1985

Espay AJ, Li JY, Johnston L, et al: Mirror movements in parkinsonism: evaluation of a new clinical sign. J Neurol Neurosurg Psychiatry 76:1355–1358, 2005

Esteban A, Traba A, Prieto J: Eyelid movements in health and disease: the supranuclear impairment of the palpebral motility. Neurophysiol Clin 34:3–15, 2004

Evans AH, Katzenschlager R, Paviour D, et al: Punding in Parkinson's disease: its relation to the dopamine dysregulation syndrome. Mov Disord 19:397–405, 2004

Evers S, Ellger T: The clinical spectrum of musical hallucinations. J Neurol Sci 227:55–65, 2004

Faber-Langendoen K, Morris JC, Knesevich JW, et al: Aphasia in senile dementia of the Alzheimer type. Neurology 23:365–370, 1988

Fahn S, Marsden CD, Calne DB: Classification and investigation of dystonia, in Movement Disorders 2. Edited by Marsden CD, Fahn S. London, Butterworths, 1987, pp 332–358

Fazzi E, Lanners J, Danova S, et al: Stereotyped behaviours in blind children. Brain Dev 21:522–528, 1999

Feinstein A, Hattersley A: Ganser symptoms, dissociation, and dysprosody. J Nerv Ment Dis 176:692–693, 1988

ffytche DH, Howard RJ: The perceptual consequences of visual loss: "positive" pathologies of vision. Brain 122:1247–1260, 1999

Field SJ, Saling MM, Berkovic SF: Interictal discourse production in temporal lobe epilepsy. Brain Lang 74:213–222, 2000

Findley LJ, Gresty MA, Halmagyi GM: Tremor, the cogwheel phenomenon and clonus in Parkinson's disease. J Neurol Neurosurg Psychiatry 44:534–546, 1981

Fishbain DA, Cole B, Cutler RB, et al: A structured evidence-based review on the meaning of nonorganic physical signs: Waddell signs. Pain Med 4:141–181, 2003

Fisher CM: Intermittent interruption of behavior. Trans Am Neurol Assoc 93:209–210, 1968

Fisher CM: Disorientation for place. Arch Neurol 39:33–36, 1982

Fisher CM: Abulia minor vs. agitated behavior. Clin Neurosurg 31:9–31, 1984

Fisher CM: "Catatonia" due to disulfiram toxicity. Arch Neurol 46:798–804, 1989

Fisher CM: Visual hallucinations on eye closure associated with atropine toxicity: a neurological analysis and comparison with other visual hallucinations. Can J Neurol Sci 18:18–27, 1991

Fisher CM: Alien hand phenomena: a review with the addition of six personal cases. Can J Neurol Sci 27:192–203, 2000

Fisher M: Left hemiplegia and motor impersistence. J Nerv Ment Dis 123:201–218, 1956

FitzGerald PM, Jankovic J: Lower body parkinsonism: evidence for vascular etiology. Mov Disord 4:249–260, 1989

Fleminger S, Burns A: The delusional misidentification syndromes in patients with and without evidence of organic cerebral disorder: a structured review of case reports. Biol Psychiatry 33:22–32, 1993

Fletcher WA, Sharpe JA: Tonic pupils in neurosyphilis. Neurology 36:188–192, 1986

Fogel BS: The significance of frontal system disorders for medical practice and health policy. J Neuropsychiatry Clin Neurosci 6:343–347, 1994

Fogel CA, Mednick SA, Michelsen N: Hyperactive behavior and minor physical anomalies. Acta Psychiatr Scand 72:551–556, 1985

Folstein MF, Folstein SE, McHugh PR: "Mini-Mental State": a practical method for grading the cognitive state of patients for the clinician. J Psychiatr Res 12:189–198, 1975

Ford RA: The psychopathology of echophenomena. Psychol Med 19:627–635, 1989

Förstl H, Owen AM, David AS: Gabriel Anton and "Anton's symptom": on focal diseases of the brain which are not perceived by the patient (1898). Neuropsychiatry Neuropsychol Behav Neurol 6:1–8, 1993

Fox RJ, Kasner SE, Chatterjee A, et al: Aphemia: an isolated disorder of articulation. Clin Neurol Neurosurg 103:123–126, 2001

Frattali C, Duffy JR, Litvan I, et al: Yes/no reversals as neurobehavioral sequela: a disorder of language, praxis, or inhibitory control? Eur J Neurol 10:103–106, 2003

Freed WJ, Kleinman JE, Karson CN, et al: Eye-blink rates and platelet monoamine oxidase activity in chronic schizophrenic patients. Biol Psychiatry 15:329–332, 1980

Freund H-J: Apraxia, in Diseases of the Nervous System/Clinical Neurobiology, 2nd Edition, Vol 1. Edited by Asbury AK, McKhann GM, McDonald WI. Philadelphia, PA, WB Saunders, 1992, pp 751–767

Freund H-J, Hummelsheim H: Lesions of premotor cortex in man. Brain 108:697–733, 1985

Frith CD, Done DJ: Stereotyped behaviour in madness and in health, in Neurobiology of Stereotyped Behaviour. Edited by Cooper SJ, Dourish CT. Oxford, UK, Clarendon Press, 1990, pp 232–259

Fung VSC, Morris JGL, Leicester J, et al: Clonic perseveration following thalamofrontal disconnection: a distinctive movement disorder. Mov Disord 12:378–385, 1997

Gainotti G: What the locus of brain lesion tells us about the nature of the cognitive defect underlying category-specific disorders: a review. Cortex 36:539–559, 2000

Galluzzi S, Sheu C-F, Zanetti O, et al: Distinctive clinical features of mild cognitive impairment with subcortical cerebrovascular disease. Dement Geriatr Cogn Disord 19:196–203, 2005

Ganser SJM: A peculiar hysterical state (1898), in Themes and Variations in European Psychiatry. Edited by Hirsch SR, Shepherd M. Bristol, UK, John Wright & Sons, 1974, pp 67–73

Garden G: Physical examination in psychiatric practice. Advances in Psychiatric Treatment 11:142–149, 2005

Gardner D, Lucas PB, Cowdry RW: Soft sign neurological abnormalities in borderline personality disorder and normal control subjects. J Nerv Ment Dis 175:177–180, 1987

Gasquoine PG: Alien hand sign. J Clin Exp Neuropsychol 15:653–667, 1993

Geschwind N: Non-aphasic disorders of speech. Int J Neurol 4:207–214, 1964

Geschwind N, Kaplan E: A human cerebral deconnection syndrome: a preliminary report. Neurology 12:675–685, 1962

Ghika J, Regli F, Assal G, et al: Impossibilité à la fermeture volontaire des paupières: discussion sur les troubles supranucléaires de la fermeture palpébrale à partir de 2 cas, avec revue de la littérature. Schweiz Arch Neurol Psychiatr 139:5–21, 1988

Ghika J, Bogousslavsky J, van Melle G, et al: Hyperkinetic motor behaviors contralateral to hemiplegia in acute stroke. Eur Neurol 35:27–32, 1995a

Ghika J, Tennis M, Growdon J, et al: Environment-driven responses in progressive supranuclear palsy. J Neurol Sci 130:104–111, 1995b

Ghika J, Bogousslavsky J, Ghika-Schmidt F, et al: "Echoing approval": a new speech disorder. J Neurol 243:633–637, 1996

Ghika J, Ghika-Schmid F, Bogousslasvky J: Parietal motor syndrome: a clinical description in 32 patients in the acute phase of pure parietal strokes studied prospectively. Clin Neurol Neurosurg 100:271–282, 1998

Ghika-Schmidt F, Bogousslavsky J: The acute behavioral syndrome of anterior thalamic infarction: a prospective study of 12 cases. Ann Neurol 48:220–227, 2000

Ghika-Schmidt F, Ghika J, Regli F, et al: Hyperkinetic movement disorders during and after acute stroke: the Lausanne Stroke Registry. J Neurol Sci 146:109–116, 1997

Giladi N, Herman T, Reider G II, et al: Clinical characteristics of elderly patients with a cautious gait of unknown origin. J Neurol 252:300–306, 2005

Gillberg C, de Souza L: Head circumference in autism, Asperger syndrome, and ADHD: a comparative study. Dev Med Child Neurol 44:296–300, 2002

Gil-Néciga E, Alberca R, Boza F, et al: Transient topographical disorientation. Eur Neurol 48:191–199, 2002

Gloor P, Olivier A, Quesny LF, et al: The role of the limbic system in experiential phenomena of temporal lobe epilepsy. Ann Neurol 12:129–140, 1982

Goldberg G: From intent to action: evolution and function of the premotor systems of the frontal lobe, in The Frontal Lobes Revisited. Edited by Perecman E. Hillsdale, NJ, Erlbaum, 1987, pp 273–306

Goldstein K: The effect of brain damage on the personality. Psychiatry 15:245–260, 1952

Gondim FA, Oliveira GR, Cruz-Flores S: Position-dependent levitation of the dominant arm after left parietal stroke: an unreported feature of posterior alien limb syndrome? Mov Disord 20:632–633, 2005

Goodglass H, Kaplan E: The Assessment of Aphasia and Related Disorders, 2nd Edition. Philadelphia, PA, Lea & Febiger, 1983

Goodwin DW, Alderson P, Rosenthal R: Clinical significance of hallucinations in psychiatric disorders: a study of 116 hallucinatory patients. Arch Gen Psychiatry 24:76–80, 1971

Gotkine M, Haggiag S, Abramsky O, et al: Lack of hemispheric localizing value of the palmomental reflex. Neurology 64:1656, 2005

Gould R, Miller BL, Goldberg MA, et al: The validity of hysterical signs and symptoms. J Nerv Ment Dis 174:593–597, 1986

Gourion D, Goldberger C, Olie JP, et al: Neurological and morphological anomalies and the genetic liability to schizophrenia: a composite phenotype. Schizophr Res 67:23–31, 2004

Grace J, Nadler JD, White DA, et al: Folstein vs Modified Mini-Mental State Examination in geriatric stroke. Arch Neurol 52:477–484, 1995

Graff-Radford NR, Eslinger PJ, Damasio AR, et al: Nonhemorrhagic infarction of the thalamus: behavioral, anatomic, and physiologic correlates. Neurology 34:14–23, 1984

Grandas F, Esteban A: Eyelid motor abnormalities in progressive supranuclear palsy. J Neural Transm 42(suppl):33–41, 1994

Griffiths TD, Sigmundsson T, Takei N, et al: Neurological abnormalities in familial and sporadic schizophrenia. Brain 121:191–203, 1998

Grigorenko EL, Klin A, Volkmar F: Annotation: Hyperlexia: disability or superability? J Child Psychol Psychiatry 44:1079–1091, 2003

Grigsby J, Kaye K: Alphanumeric sequencing and cognitive impairment among elderly persons. Percept Mot Skills 80:732–734, 1995

Grigsby J, Kaye K, Robbins LJ: Reliabilities, norms and factor structure of the Behavioral Dyscontrol Scale. Percept Mot Skills 74:883–892, 1992

Grigsby J, Kaye K, Busenbark D: Alphanumeric sequencing: a report on a brief measure of information processing used among persons with multiple sclerosis. Percept Mot Skills 78:883–887, 1994

Grigsby J, Kaye K, Baxter J, et al: Executive cognitive abilities and functional status among community-dwelling older persons in the San Luis Valley Health and Aging Study. J Am Geriatr Soc 46:590–596, 1998

Guimaraes J, Simoes-Ribeiro F, Mendes-Ribeiro JA, et al: Eating seizures and emotional facial paresis: evidence suggesting the amygdala is a common anatomophysiological substratum. Epilepsy Behav 6:266–269, 2005

Gurvits TV, Gilbertson MW, Lasko NB, et al: Neurologic soft signs in chronic posttraumatic stress disorder. Arch Gen Psychiatry 57:181–186, 2000

Habib M: Athymhormia and disorders of motivation in basal ganglia disease. J Neuropsychiatry Clin Neurosci 16:509–524, 2004

Hadano K, Nakamura H, Hamanaka T: Effortful echolalia. Cortex 34:67–82, 1998

Halligan PW, David AS: Cognitive neuropsychiatry: towards a scientific psychopathology. Nat Rev Neurosci 2:209–215, 2001

Halligan PW, Marshall JC, Wade DT: Unilateral somatoparaphrenia after right hemisphere stroke: a case description. Cortex 31:173–182, 1995

Hamano T, Hiraki S, Kawamura Y, et al: Acquired stuttering secondary to callosal infarction. Neurology 64:1092–1093, 2005

Hanna-Pladdy B, Heilman KM, Foundas AL: Ecological implications of ideomotor apraxia: evidence from physical activities of daily living. Neurology 60:487–490, 2003

Harris CL, Dinn WM, Marcinkiewicz JA: Partial seizure-like symptoms in borderline personality disorder. Epilepsy Behav 3:433–438, 2002

Harris CM, Shawkat F, Russell-Eggitt I, et al: Intermittent horizontal saccade failure ("ocular motor apraxia") in children. Br J Ophthalmol 80:151–158, 1996

Hartmann K, Goldenberg G, Daumuller M, et al: It takes the whole brain to make a cup of coffee: the neuropsychology of naturalistic actions involving technical devices. Neuropsychologia 43:625–637, 2005

Hashimoto R, Tanaka Y: Contribution of the supplementary motor area and anterior cingulate gyrus to pathological grasping phenomena. Eur Neurol 40:151–158, 1998

Heilman KM, Watson RT: Intentional motor disorders, in Frontal Lobe Function and Dysfunction. Edited by Levin HS, Eisenberg HM, Benton AL. New York, Oxford University Press, 1991, pp 199–213

Heilman KM, Scholes R, Watson RT: Auditory affective agnosia: disturbed comprehension of affective speech. J Neurol Neurosurg Psychiatry 38:69–72, 1975

Helm-Estabrooks N: Stuttering associated with acquired neurological disorders, in Stuttering and Related Disorders of Fluency, 2nd Edition. Edited by Curlee RF. New York, Thieme Medical Publishers, 1999, pp 255–268

Helms PM, Godwin CD: Abnormalities of blink rate in psychoses: a preliminary report. Biol Psychiatry 20:103–106, 1985

Herbert MR, Ziegler DA, Makris N, et al: Localization of white matter volume increase in autism and developmental language disorder. Ann Neurol 55:530–540, 2004

Hermann BP, Dikmen S, Schwartz MS, et al: Interictal psychopathology in patients with ictal fear: a quantitative investigation. Neurology 32:7–11, 1982

Hermesh H, Munitz H: Unilateral neuroleptic-induced akathisia. Clin Neuropharmacol 13:253–258, 1990

Heron EA, Kritchevsky M, Delis DC: Neuropsychological presentation of Ganser symptoms. J Clin Exp Neuropsychol 13:652–666, 1991

Herzog AG, Coleman AE, Jacobs AR, et al: Relationship of sexual dysfunction to epilepsy laterality and reproductive hormone levels in women. Epilepsy Behav 4:407–413, 2003

Higgins DS Jr: Chorea and its disorders. Neurol Clin 19:707–722, 2001

Hogan DB, Ebly EM: Primitive reflexes and dementia: results from the Canadian Study of Health and Aging. Age Ageing 24:375–381, 1995

Holzer JC, Goodman WK, McDougle CJ, et al: Obsessive-compulsive disorder with and without a chronic tic disorder: a comparison of symptoms in 70 patients. Br J Psychiatry 164:469–473, 1994

Hopf HC, Müller-Forell W, Hopf NJ: Localization of emotional and volitional facial paresis. Neurology 42:1918–1923, 1992

Horner J, Heyman A, Dawson D, et al: The relationship of agraphia to the severity of dementia in Alzheimer's disease. Arch Neurol 45:760–763, 1988

Hudson AJ, Grace GM: Misidentification syndromes related to face specific area in the fusiform gyrus. J Neurol Neurosurg Psychiatry 69:645–648, 2000

Hughes TS, Abou-Khalil B, Lavin PJM, et al: Visual field defects after temporal lobe resection: a prospective quantitative analysis. Neurology 53:167–172, 1999

Hughlings-Jackson J: On right- or left-sided spasm at the onset of epileptic paroxysms, and on crude sensation warnings and elaborate mental states. Brain 3:192–214, 1880–1881

Hwang JP, Yang CH, Tsai SJ: Phantom boarder symptom in dementia. Int J Geriatr Psychiatry 18:417–420, 2003

Ismail B, Cantor-Graae E, McNeil TF: Minor physical anomalies in schizophrenic patients and their siblings. Am J Psychiatry 155:1695–1702, 1998

Ismail B, Cantor-Graae E, McNeil TF: Minor physical anomalies in schizophrenia: cognitive, neurological and other clinical correlates. J Psychiatr Res 34:45–56, 2000

Jacob A, Cherian PJ, Radhakrishnan K, et al: Emotional facial paresis in temporal lobe epilepsy: its prevalence and lateralizing value. Seizure 12:60–64, 2003

Jacobs L, Grossman MD: Three primitive reflexes in normal adults. Neurology 30:184–188, 1980

Jacobs L, Feldman M, Diamond SP, et al: Palinacousis: persistent or recurring auditory sensations. Cortex 9:275–287, 1973

Jan JE, Kearney S, Groenveld M, et al: Speech, cognition, and imaging studies in congenital ocular motor apraxia. Dev Med Child Neurol 40:95–99, 1998

Jancar J, Kettle LB: Hypergraphia and mental handicap. J Ment Defic Res 28:151–158, 1984

Jankovic J, Lang AE: Movement disorders: diagnosis and assessment, in Neurology in Clinical Practice, 4th Edition, Vol 1. Edited by Bradley WG, Daroff RB, Fenichel G, et al. Philadelphia, PA, Butterworth-Heinemann, 2004, pp 293–322

Jaspers K: General Psychopathology. Chicago, IL, University of Chicago Press, 1963

Jenkyn L, Walsh D, Walsh B, et al: The nuchocephalic reflex. J Neurol Neurosurg Psychiatry 38:561–566, 1975

Jenkyn LR, Walsh DB, Culver CM, et al: Clinical signs in diffuse cerebral dysfunction. J Neurol Neurosurg Psychiatry 40:956–966, 1977

Johnson MR, Sander JW: The clinical impact of epilepsy genetics. J Neurol Neurosurg Psychiatry 70:428–430, 2001

Johnstone EC, Ebmeier KP, Miller P, et al: Predicting schizophrenia: findings from the Edinburgh High-Risk Study. Br J Psychiatry 186:18–25, 2005

Jones BN, Teng EL, Folstein MF, et al: A new bedside test of cognition for patients with HIV infection. Ann Intern Med 119:1001–1004, 1993

Jones IH: Observations on schizophrenic stereotypies. Compr Psychiatry 6:323–335, 1965

Joray S, Herrmann F, Mulligan R, et al: Mechanism of disorientation in Alzheimer's disease. Eur Neurol 52:193–197, 2004

Joynt RJ, Benton AL, Fogel ML: Behavioral and pathological correlates of motor impersistence. Neurology 12:876–881, 1962

Kakishita K, Sekiguchi E, Maeshima S, et al: Stuttering without callosal apraxia resulting from infarction in the anterior corpus callosum. J Neurol 251:1140–1141, 2004

Kandel E, Brennan PA, Mednick SA, et al: Minor physical anomalies and recidivistic adult criminal behavior. Acta Psychiatr Scand 79:103–107, 1989

Kaneko K, Yuasa T, Miyatake T, et al: Stereotyped hand clasping: an unusual tardive movement disorder. Mov Disord 8:230–231, 1993

Kaplan PW: Behavioral manifestations of nonconvulsive status epilepticus. Epilepsy Behav 3:122–139, 2002

Karson CN: Oculomotor signs in a psychiatric population: a preliminary report. Am J Psychiatry 136:1057–1060, 1979

Karson CN, Burns RS, LeWitt PA, et al: Blink rates and disorders of movement. Neurology 34:677–678, 1984

Katzenschlager R, Lees AJ: Olfaction and Parkinson's syndromes: its role in differential diagnosis. Curr Opin Neurol 17:417–423, 2004

Katzman R, Brown T, Fuld P, et al: Validation of a short orientation-memory-concentration test of cognitive impairment. Am J Psychiatry 140:734–739, 1983

Kaufer DI, Cummings JL, Ketchel P, et al: Validation of the NPI-Q, a brief clinical form of the Neuropsychiatric Inventory. J Neuropsychiatry Clin Neurosci 12:233–239, 2000

Kennard C, Crawford TJ, Henderson I: A pathophysiological approach to saccadic eye movements in neurological and psychiatric disease. J Neurol Neurosurg Psychiatry 57:881–885, 1994

Kertesz A, Nicholson I, Cancelliere A, et al: Motor impersistence: a right-hemisphere syndrome. Neurology 35:662–666, 1985

Kertesz A, Davidson W, McCabe P, et al: Behavioral quantitation is more sensitive than cognitive testing in frontotemporal dementia. Alzheimer Dis Assoc Disord 17:223–229, 2003

Kinney DK, Yurgelun-Todd DA, Woods BT: Neurological hard signs in schizophrenia and major mood disorders. J Nerv Ment Dis 181:202–204, 1993

Kiziltan G, Akalin MA: Stuttering may be a type of action dystonia. Mov Disord 11:278–282, 1996

Klein DA, Steinberg M, Galik E, et al: Wandering behaviour in community-residing persons with dementia. Int J Geriatr Psychiatry 14:272–279, 1999

Kluin KJ, Foster NL, Berent S, et al: Perceptual analysis of speech disorders in progressive supranuclear palsy. Neurology 43:563–566, 1993

Klüver H, Bucy PC: Psychic blindness and other symptoms following bilateral temporal lobectomy in rhesus monkeys. Am J Physiol 119:352–353, 1937

Klüver H, Bucy PC: Preliminary analysis of functions of the temporal lobes in monkeys. AMA Arch Neurol Psychiatry 42:979–1000, 1939

Kolada SJ, Pitman RK: Eye-head synkinesia in schizophrenic adults during a repetitive visual search task. Biol Psychiatry 18:675–684, 1983

Koller WC, Glatt S, Wilson RS, et al: Primitive reflexes and cognitive function in the elderly. Ann Neurol 12:302–304, 1982

Koller W, Lang A, Vetere-Overfield B, et al: Psychogenic tremors. Neurology 39:1094–1099, 1989

Komatsu S, Kirino E, Inoue Y, et al: Risperidone withdrawal-related respiratory dyskinesia: a case diagnosed by spirography and fibroscopy. Clin Neuropharmacol 28:90–93, 2005

Kopala LC, Good KP, Honer WG: Olfactory hallucinations and olfactory identification ability in patients with schizophrenia and other psychiatric disorders. Schizophr Res 12:205–211, 1994

Kopelman MD: Clinical tests of memory. Br J Psychiatry 148:517–525, 1986

Kopelman MD: Varieties of false memory. Cogn Neuropsychol 16:197–214, 1999

Kopelman MD, Guinan EM, Lewis PDR: Delusional memory, confabulation, and frontal lobe dysfunction: a case study in De Clérambault's syndrome. Neurocase 1:71–77, 1995

Koponen H, Rantakallio P, Veijola J, et al: Childhood central nervous system infections and risk for schizophrenia. Eur Arch Psychiatry Clin Neurosci 254:9–13, 2004

Korein J: Iris pigmentation (melanin) in idiopathic dystonic syndromes including torticollis. Ann Neurol 10:53–55, 1981

Koudstaal PJ, Vermeulen M, Wokke JH: Argyll Robertson pupils in lymphocytic meningoradiculitis (Bannwarth's syndrome). J Neurol Neurosurg Psychiatry 50:363–365, 1987

Kramer S, Bryan KL, Frith CD: "Confabulation" in narrative discourse by schizophrenic patients. Int J Lang Commun Disord 33(suppl):202–207, 1998

Krampfl K, Mohammadi B, Komissarow L, et al: Mirror movements and ipsilateral motor evoked potentials in ALS. Amyotroph Lateral Scler Other Motor Neuron Disord 5:154–163, 2004

Krams M, Quinton R, Ashburner J, et al: Kallmann's syndrome: mirror movements associated with bilateral corticospinal tract hypertrophy. Neurology 52:816–822, 1999

Kress T, Daum I: Developmental prosopagnosia: a review. Behav Neurol 14:109–121, 2003

Kuperberg GR, McGuire PK, David AS: Sensitivity to linguistic anomalies in spoken sentences: a case study approach to understanding thought disorder in schizophrenia. Psychol Med 30:345–357, 2000

Kurlan R, Richard IH, Papka M, et al: Movement disorders in Alzheimer's disease: more rigidity of definitions is needed. Mov Disord 15:24–29, 2000

Kuslansky G, Buschke H, Katz M, et al: Screening for Alzheimer's disease: the Memory Impairment Screen versus the conventional three-word memory test. J Am Geriatr Soc 50:1086–1091, 2002

Landau WM: Reflex dementia: disinhibited primitive thinking. Neurology 39:133–137, 1989

Lang AE: Clinical phenomenology of tic disorders: selected aspects. Adv Neurol 58:25–32, 1992

Lang AE, Ellis C, Kingon H, et al: Iris pigmentation in idiopathic dystonia. Ann Neurol 12:585–586, 1982

Laplane D: La perte d'auto-activation psychique. Rev Neurol (Paris) 146:397–404, 1990

Laplane D: Obsessions et compulsions par lésions des noyaux gris centraux. Rev Neurol (Paris) 150:594–598, 1994

Laplane D, Orgogozo JM, Meininger V, et al: Paralysie faciale avec dissociation automatico-volontaire inverse par lesion frontale: son origine corticale. Ses relations avec l'A. M. S. Rev Neurol (Paris) 132:725–734, 1976

Laplane D, Baulac M, Widlöcher D, et al: Pure psychic akinesia with bilateral lesions of basal ganglia. J Neurol Neurosurg Psychiatry 47:377–385, 1984

Laplane D, Levasseur M, Pillon B, et al: Obsessive-compulsive and other behavioural changes with bilateral basal ganglia lesions: a neuropsychological, magnetic resonance imaging and positron tomographic study. Brain 112:699–725, 1989

Lawrie SM, Byrne M, Miller P, et al: Neurodevelopmental indices and the development of psychotic symptoms in subjects at high risk of schizophrenia. Br J Psychiatry 178:524–530, 2001

Leask SJ, Done DJ, Crow TJ: Adult psychosis, common childhood infections and neurological soft signs in a national birth cohort. Br J Psychiatry 181:387–392, 2002

Lebrun Y: Cluttering after brain damage. J Fluency Disord 21:289–295, 1996

Lecours AR, Lhermitte F, Bryans B: Aphasiology. London, Ballière Tindall, 1983

Leder SB: Adult onset of stuttering as a presenting sign in a parkinsonian-like syndrome: a case report. J Commun Disord 29:471–478, 1996

Lee BH, Kang SJ, Park JM, et al: The Character-Line Bisection Task: a new test for hemispatial neglect. Neuropsychologia 42:1715–1724, 2004

Lees AJ: Tics and Related Disorders. Edinburgh, UK, Churchill Livingstone, 1985

Lees AJ: Facial mannerisms and tics. Adv Neurol 49:255–261, 1988

Leigh RJ, Riley DE: Eye movements in parkinsonism: it's saccadic speed that counts. Neurology 54:1018–1019, 2000

Leigh RJ, Foley JM, Remler BF, et al: Oculogyric crisis: a syndrome of thought disorder and ocular deviation. Ann Neurol 22:13–17, 1987

Leiguarda R: Apraxias as traditionally defined, in Higher-Order Motor Disorders. Edited by Freund HJ, Jeannerod M, Hallett M, et al. Oxford, UK, Oxford University Press, 2005, pp 303–338

Leiguarda RC, Marsden CD: Limb apraxias: higher-order disorders of sensorimotor integration. Brain 123:860–879, 2000

Leimkuhler ME, Mesulam M-M: Reversible go-no go deficits in a case of frontal lobe tumor. Ann Neurol 18:617–619, 1985

Lennox G: Tics and related disorders, in Movement Disorders in Clinical Practice. Edited by Sawle G. Oxford, UK, Isis Medical Media, 1999, pp 135–146

Leopold NA, Borson AJ: An alphabetical "WORLD": a new version of an old test. Neurology 49:1521–1524, 1997

Levin HS, High WM, Goethe KE, et al: The Neurobehavioural Rating Scale: assessment of the behavioural sequelae of head injury by the clinician. J Neurol Neurosurg Psychiatry 50:183–193, 1987

Levin M: Delirium: a gap in psychiatric teaching. Am J Psychiatry 107:689–694, 1951

Levin M: Thinking disturbances in delirium. AMA Arch Neurol Psychiatry 75:62–66, 1956

Levy DL, Holzman PS, Matthysse S, et al: Eye tracking dysfunction and schizophrenia: a critical perspective. Schizophr Bull 19:461–536, 1993

Levy J, Reid M: Variations in writing posture and cerebral organization. Science 194:614–615, 1976

Lezak MD: Subtle sequelae of brain damage: perplexity, distractibility, and fatigue. Am J Phys Med 57:9–15, 1978

Lhermitte F: Human autonomy and the frontal lobes, part II: patient behavior in complex and social situations: the "environmental dependency syndrome." Ann Neurol 19:335–343, 1986

Lhermitte F: Les comportements d'imitation et d'utilisation dans les états dépressifs majeurs. Bull Acad Natl Med 177:883–892, 1993

Lhermitte F, Pillon B, Serdaru M: Human autonomy and the frontal lobes, I: imitation and utilization behavior: a neuropsychological study of 75 patients. Ann Neurol 19:326–334, 1986

Lindberg N, Tani P, Stenberg J-H, et al: Neurological soft signs in homicidal men with antisocial personality disorder. Eur Psychiatry 19:433–437, 2004

Linetsky E, Planer D, Ben-Hur T: Echolalia-palilalia as the sole manifestation of nonconvulsive status epilepticus. Neurology 55:733–734, 2000

Lishman WA: Organic Psychiatry: The Psychological Consequences of Cerebral Disorder, 3rd Edition. Oxford, UK, Blackwell Science, 1998

Little JT, Jankovic J: Tardive myoclonus: a case report. Mov Disord 2:307–311, 1987

Lloyd G: Medicine without signs. BMJ 287:539–542, 1983

Lochner C, Stein D: Olfactory reference syndrome: diagnostic criteria and differential diagnosis. J Postgrad Med 49:328–331, 2003

Logsdon RG, Teri L, McCurry SM, et al: Wandering: a significant problem among community-residing individuals with Alzheimer's disease. J Gerontol 53B:294–299, 1998

Lohr JB, Alder M, Flynn K, et al: Minor physical anomalies in older patients with late-onset schizophrenia, early onset schizophrenia, depression, and Alzheimer's disease. Am J Geriatr Psychiatry 5:318–323, 1997

Lorentz WJ, Scanlan JM, Borson S: Brief screening tests for dementia. Can J Psychiatry 47:723–733, 2002

Luciano D, Devinsky O, Perrine K: Crying seizures. Neurology 43:2113–2117, 1993

Lundin-Olsson L, Nyberg L, Gustafson Y: "Stops walking when talking" as a predictor of falls in elderly people (letter). Lancet 349:617, 1997

Luria AR: Two kinds of motor perseveration in massive injury of the frontal lobes. Brain 88:1–10, 1965

Luria AR, Homskaya ED: Le trouble du role régulateur du langage au cours des lésions du lobe frontal. Neuropsychologia 1:9–26, 1963

Luxon L, Lees AJ, Greenwood RJ: Neurosyphilis today. Lancet i:90–93, 1979

Luzzi S, Piccirilli M: Slowly progressive pure dysgraphia with late apraxia of speech: a further variant of the focal cerebral degeneration. Brain Lang 87:355–360, 2003

MacGowan DJL, Delanty N, Petito F, et al: Isolated myoclonic alien hand as the sole presentation of pathologically established Creutzfeldt-Jakob disease: a report of two patients. J Neurol Neurosurg Psychiatry 63:404–407, 1997

Mahone EM, Bridges D, Prahme C, et al: Repetitive arm and hand movements (complex motor stereotypies) in children. J Pediatr 145:391–395, 2004

Maillot F, Belin C, Perrier D, et al: Persévération visuelle et palinopsie: une pathologie de la mémoire visuelle? Rev Neurol (Paris) 149:794–796, 1993

Makharia GK, Nandi B, Garg PK, et al: Wilson's disease with neuropsychiatric manifestations and liver disease but no Kayser-Fleischer ring. J Clin Gastroenterol 35:101–102, 2002

Malloy P, Grace J: A review of rating scales for measuring behavior change due to frontal systems damage. Cogn Behav Neurol 18:18–27, 2005

Malloy PF, Richardson ED: The frontal lobes and content-specific delusions. J Neuropsychiatry Clin Neurosci 6:455–466, 1994

Malloy PF, Cummings JL, Coffey CE, et al: Cognitive screening instruments in neuropsychiatry: a report of the Committee on Research of the American Neuropsychiatric Association. J Neuropsychiatry Clin Neurosci 9:189–197, 1997

Manes F, Leiguarda R: Frontostriatal circuits and disorders of goal-directed actions, in Higher-Order Motor Disorders. Edited by Freund HJ, Jeannerod M, Hallett M, et al. Oxford, UK, Oxford University Press, 2005, pp 413–439

Manford M, Andermann F: Complex visual hallucinations: clinical and neurobiological insights. Brain 121:1819–1840, 1998

Maraganore DM, Lees AJ, Marsden CD: Complex stereotypies after right putaminal infarction: a case report. Mov Disord 6:358–361, 1991

Marcel A, Postma P, Gillmeister H, et al: Migration and fusion of tactile sensation—premorbid susceptibility to allochiria, neglect and extinction? Neuropsychologia 42:1749–1767, 2004

Marshall EJ: Neuropsychiatry of substance abuse, in Neuropsychiatry and Mental Health Services. Edited by Ovsiew F. Washington, DC, American Psychiatric Press, 1999, pp 105–148

Martzke JS, Kopala LC, Good KP: Olfactory dysfunction in neuropsychiatric disorders: review and methodological considerations. Biol Psychiatry 42:721–732, 1997

McCauley SR, Levin HS, Vanier M, et al: The Neurobehavioural Rating Scale—Revised: sensitivity and validity in closed head injury assessment. J Neurol Neurosurg Psychiatry 71:643–651, 2001

McCreadie RG, Srinivasan TN, Padmavati R, et al: Extrapyramidal symptoms in unmedicated schizophrenia. J Psychiatr Res 39:261–266, 2005

McGee SR: Evidence-Based Physical Diagnosis. Philadelphia, PA, WB Saunders, 2001

McGrath JJ, van Os J, Hoyos C, et al: Minor physical anomalies in psychoses: associations with clinical and putative aetiological variables. Schizophr Res 18:9–20, 1995

McGrath CM, Kennedy RE, Hoye W, et al: Stereotypic movement disorder after acquired brain injury. Brain Inj 16:447–451, 2002

McKenna PJ, Lund CE, Mortimer AM, et al: Motor, volitional and behavioural disorders in schizophrenia, 2: the "conflict of paradigms" hypothesis. Br J Psychiatry 158:328–336, 1991

McNeil TF, Cantor-Graae E, Ismail B: Obstetric complications and congenital malformation in schizophrenia. Brain Res Rev 31:166–178, 2000

McPherson SE, Kuratani JD, Cummings JL, et al: Creutzfeldt-Jakob disease with mixed transcortical aphasia: insights into echolalia. Behav Neurol 7:197–203, 1994

Mendez MF: Prominent echolalia from isolation of the speech area. J Neuropsychiatry Clin Neurosci 14:356–357, 2002

Mendez MF: Aphemia-like syndrome from a right supplementary motor area lesion. Clin Neurol Neurosurg 106:337–339, 2004

Mendez MF, Foti DJ: Lethal hyperoral behaviour from the Kluver-Bucy syndrome. J Neurol Neurosurg Psychiatry 62:293–294, 1997

Mendez MF, Selwood A, Mastri AR, et al: Pick's disease versus Alzheimer's disease: a comparison of clinical characteristics. Neurology 43:289–292, 1993

Mendez MF, Shapira JS, Miller BL: Stereotypical movements and frontotemporal dementia. Mov Disord 20:742–745, 2005

Menon GJ: Complex visual hallucinations in the visually impaired: a structured history-taking approach. Arch Ophthalmol 123:349–355, 2005

Menon GJ, Rahman I, Menon SJ, et al: Complex visual hallucinations in the visually impaired: the Charles Bonnet Syndrome. Surv Ophthalmol 48:58–72, 2003

Mesulam M-M: A cortical network for directed attention and unilateral neglect. Ann Neurol 10:309–325, 1981

Metzig E, Rosenberg S, Ast M: Lateral asymmetry in patients with nervous and mental disease: a preliminary study. Neuropsychobiology 1:197–202, 1975

Michel V, Burbaud P, Taillard J, et al: Stuttering or reflex seizure? A case report. Epileptic Disord 6:181–185, 2004

Migliorelli R, Tesón A, Sabe L, et al: Anosognosia in Alzheimer's disease: a study of associated factors. J Neuropsychiatry Clin Neurosci 7:338–344, 1995

Milberg WP, Hebben N, Kaplan E: The Boston Process Approach to neuropsychological assessment, in Neuropsychological Assessment of Neuropsychiatric Disorders, 2nd Edition. Edited by Grant I, Adams KM. New York, Oxford University Press, 1996, pp 65–86

Miller H: Psychiatry—medicine or magic? In Contemporary Psychiatry: Selected Reviews From the British Journal of Hospital Medicine, Vol 5. Edited by Silverstone T, Barraclough B. London, Ashford, Kent, Headley, 1975, pp 462–466

Mojtabai R: Identifying misidentifications: a phenomenological study. Psychopathology 31:90–95, 1998

Monrad-Krohn GH: On the dissociation of voluntary and emotional innervation in facial paresis of central origin. Brain 47:22–35, 1924

Monrad-Krohn GH: Dysprosody or altered "melody of language." Brain 70:405–415, 1947

Moo LR, Slotnick SD, Tesoro MA, et al: Interlocking finger test: a bedside screen for parietal lobe dysfunction. J Neurol Neurosurg Psychiatry 74:530–532, 2003

Moore SR, Gresham LS, Bromberg MB, et al: A self report measure of affective lability. J Neurol Neurosurg Psychiatry 63:89–93, 1997

Moreaud O: Balint syndrome. Arch Neurol 60:1329–1331, 2003

Morrell MJ, Flynn KL, Done S, et al: Sexual dysfunction, sex steroid hormone abnormalities, and depression in women with epilepsy treated with antiepileptic drugs. Epilepsy Behav 6:360–365, 2005

Nagaratnam N, Irving J, Kalouche H: Misidentification in patients with dementia. Arch Gerontol Geriatr 37:195–202, 2003

Nahm FK: Heinrich Klüver and the temporal lobe syndrome. J Hist Neurosci 6:193–208, 1997

Nathaniel-James DA, Foong J, Frith CD: The mechanism of confabulation in schizophrenia. Neurocase 2:475–483, 1996

Negash A, Kebede D, Alem A, et al: Neurological soft signs in bipolar I disorder patients. J Affect Disord 80:221–230, 2004

Newsom-Davis IC, Abrahams S, Goldstein LH, et al: The emotional lability questionnaire: a new measure of emotional lability in amyotrophic lateral sclerosis. J Neurol Sci 169:22–25, 1999

Nicholas AP, Earnst KS, Marson DC: Atypical Hallervorden-Spatz disease with preserved cognition and obtrusive obsessions and compulsions. Mov Disord 20:880–886, 2005

Niehaus DJ, Emsley RA, Brink P, et al: Stereotypies: prevalence and association with compulsive and impulsive symptoms in college students. Psychopathology 33:31–35, 2000

Nimmo-Smith I, Marcel AJ, Tegner R: A diagnostic test of unawareness of bilateral motor task abilities in anosognosia for hemiplegia. J Neurol Neurosurg Psychiatry 76:1167–1169, 2005

Northoff G: What catatonia can tell us about "top-down modulation": a neuropsychiatric hypothesis. Behav Brain Sci 25:555–577; discussion 578–604, 2002

Northoff G, Koch A, Wenke J, et al: Catatonia as a psychomotor syndrome: a rating scale and extrapyramidal motor symptoms. Mov Disord 14:404–416, 1999

Nutt JG: Higher-order disorders of gait, in Higher-Order Motor Disorders. Edited by Freund HJ, Jeannerod M, Hallett M, et al. Oxford, UK, Oxford University Press, 2005, pp 237–248

Nutt JG, Marsden CD, Thompson PD: Human walking and higher-level gait disorders, particularly in the elderly. Neurology 43:268–279, 1993

Nyatsanza S, Shetty T, Gregory C, et al: A study of stereotypic behaviours in Alzheimer's disease and frontal and temporal variant frontotemporal dementia. J Neurol Neurosurg Psychiatry 74:1398–1402, 2003

Obeso JA, Rothwell JC, Marsden CD: Simple tics in Gilles de la Tourette's syndrome are not prefaced by a normal premovement EEG potential. J Neurol Neurosurg Psychiatry 44:735–738, 1981

Obeso JA, Rothwell JC, Lang AE, et al: Myoclonic dystonia. Neurology 33:825–830, 1983

Okamura T, Fukai M, Yamadori A, et al: A clinical study of hypergraphia in epilepsy. J Neurol Neurosurg Psychiatry 56:556–559, 1993

Orient JM, Sapira JD: Sapira's Art and Science of Bedside Diagnosis, 3rd Edition. Philadelphia, PA, Lippincott Williams & Wilkins, 2005

Ortigue S, Viaud-Delmon I, Michel CM, et al: Pure imagery hemi-neglect of far space. Neurology 60:2000–2002, 2003

Ovsiew F: Yes/no reversals (letter). Eur J Neurol 10:464; author reply 464, 2003

Ovsiew F: Neuropsychiatric physical diagnosis in context, in Neuropsychiatric Assessment. Edited by Yudofsky SC, Kim HF. Washington, DC, American Psychiatric Publishing, 2004, pp 1–38

Ovsiew F: Neuropsychiatric approach to the patient, in Comprehensive Textbook of Psychiatry, Vol 1. Edited by Sadock BJ, Sadock VA. Philadelphia, PA, Lippincott Williams & Wilkins, 2005, pp 323–349

Ovsiew F: An overview of the psychiatric approach to conversion disorder, in Psychogenic Movement Disorders: Neurology and Neuropsychiatry. Edited by Hallett M, Fahn S, Jankovic J, et al. Philadelphia, PA, Lippincott Williams & Wilkins, 2006, pp 115–121

Owen G, Mulley GP: The palmomental reflex: a useful clinical sign? J Neurol Neurosurg Psychiatry 73:113–115, 2002

Pantelis C, Maruff P: The cognitive neuropsychiatric approach to investigating the neurobiology of schizophrenia and other disorders. J Psychosom Res 53:655–664, 2002

Paradis M: The other side of language: pragmatic competence. Journal of Neurolinguistics 11:1–10, 1998

Parker TM, Osternig LR, Lee HJ, et al: The effect of divided attention on gait stability following concussion. Clin Biomech (Bristol, Avon) 20:389–395, 2005

Parvizi J, Anderson SW, Martin CO, et al: Pathological laughter and crying: a link to the cerebellum. Brain 124:1708–1719, 2001

Paul A: Epilepsy or stereotypy? Diagnostic issues in learning disabilities. Seizure 6:111–120, 1997

Peigneux P, van der Linden M: Influence of ageing and educational level on the prevalence of body-part-as-objects in normal subjects. J Clin Exp Neuropsychol 21:547–552, 1999

Penfield W, Robertson JSM: Growth asymmetry due to lesions of the postcentral cerebral cortex. AMA Arch Neurol Psychiatry 50:405–430, 1943

Persinger MA, Makarec K: Temporal lobe epileptic signs and correlative behaviors displayed by normal populations. J Gen Psychol 114:179–195, 1987

Persinger MA, Makarec K: Complex partial epileptic signs as a continuum from normals to epileptics: normative data and clinical populations. J Clin Psychol 49:33–45, 1993

Peters M: Description and validation of a flexible and broadly usable handedness questionnaire. Laterality 3:77–96, 1998

Pia L, Neppi-Modona M, Ricci R, et al: The anatomy of anosognosia for hemiplegia: a meta-analysis. Cortex 40:367–377, 2004

Pick A: Clinical studies, III: on reduplicative paramnesia. Brain 26:260–267, 1903

Pierrot-Deseilligny C, Gaymard B, Muri R, et al: Cerebral ocular motor signs. J Neurol 244:65–70, 1997

Pillon B, Dubois B: From the grasping reflex to the environmental dependency syndrome, in Higher-Order Motor Disorders. Edited by Freund HJ, Jeannerod M, Hallett M, et al. Oxford, UK, Oxford University Press, 2005, pp 373–382

Pinching AJ: Clinical testing of olfaction reassessed. Brain 100:377–388, 1977

Pine DS, Shaffer D, Schonfeld IS, et al: Minor physical anomalies: modifiers of environmental risks for psychiatric impairment? J Am Acad Child Adolesc Psychiatry 36:395–403, 1997

Podskalny GD, Factor SA: Chorea caused by lithium intoxication: a case report and literature review. Mov Disord 11:733–737, 1996

Poeck K: The Kluver-Bucy syndrome in man, in Handbook of Clinical Neurology, Vol 45: Clinical Neuropsychology. Edited by Frederiks JAM. Amsterdam, The Netherlands, Elsevier, 1985a, pp 257–263

Poeck K: Pathological laughter and crying, in Handbook of Clinical Neurology, Vol 45: Clinical Neuropsychology. Edited by Frederiks JAM. Amsterdam, The Netherlands, Elsevier, 1985b, pp 219–225

Poizner H, Kaplan E, Bellugi U, et al: Visual-spatial processing in deaf brain-damaged signers. Brain Cogn 3:281–306, 1984

Postuma RB, Lang AE: Hemiballism: revisiting a classic disorder. Lancet Neurol 2:661–668, 2003

Power C, Selnes OA, Grim JA, et al: HIV Dementia Scale: a rapid screening test. J Acquir Immune Defic Syndr Hum Retrovirol 8:273–278, 1995

Rasmussen P: Persistent mirror movements: a clinical study of 17 children, adolescents and young adults. Dev Med Child Neurol 35:699–707, 1993

Ravdin LD, Katzen HL, Agrawal P, et al: Letter and semantic fluency in older adults: effects of mild depressive symptoms and age-stratified normative data. Clin Neuropsychol 17:195–202, 2003

Regard M, Landis T: "Gourmand syndrome": eating passion associated with right anterior lesions. Neurology 48:1185–1190, 1997

Reinhold M: Human behaviour reactions to organic cerebral disease. J Ment Sci 99:130–136, 1953

Rich MW, Radwany SM: Respiratory dyskinesia: an underrecognized phenomenon. Chest 105:1826–1832, 1994

Riddoch MJ, Humphreys GW: Visual agnosia. Neurol Clin 21:501–520, 2003

Ridley RM: The psychology of perseverative and stereotyped behaviour. Prog Neurobiol 44:221–231, 1994

Ridley RM, Baker HF: Stereotypy in monkeys and humans. Psychol Med 12:61–72, 1982

Riestra AR, Heilman KM: Visual facial grasp. Neurocase 10:363–365, 2004

Rio J, Montalbán J, Pujadas F, et al: Asterixis associated with anatomic cerebral lesions: a study of 45 cases. Acta Neurol Scand 91:377–381, 1995

Rizzo M: Clinical assessment of complex visual dysfunction. Semin Neurol 20:75–87, 2000

Rizzo M, Vecera SP: Psychoanatomical substrates of Balint's syndrome. J Neurol Neurosurg Psychiatry 72:162–178, 2002

Roberts RJ, Varney NR, Hulbert JR, et al: The neuropathology of everyday life: the frequency of partial seizure symptoms among normals. Neuropsychology 4:65–85, 1990

Roberts RJ, Gorman LL, Lee GP, et al: The phenomenology of multiple partial seizure-like symptoms without stereotyped spells: an epilepsy spectrum disorder? Epilepsy Res 13:167–177, 1992

Rodier PM, Bryson SE, Welch JP: Minor malformations and physical measurements in autism: data from Nova Scotia. Teratology 55:319–325, 1997

Rogers D: The motor disorders of severe psychiatric illness: a conflict of paradigms. Br J Psychiatry 147:221–232, 1985

Rogers D, Lees AJ, Smith E, et al: Bradyphrenia in Parkinson's disease and psychomotor retardation in depressive illness. Brain 110:761–776, 1987

Rolak LA: Psychogenic sensory loss. J Nerv Ment Dis 176:686–687, 1988

Ron MA, Logsdail SJ: Psychiatric morbidity in multiple sclerosis: a clinical and MRI study. Psychol Med 19:887–895, 1989

Ropper AH: Self-grasping: a focal neurological sign. Ann Neurol 12:575–577, 1982

Ross ED: The aprosodias: functional-anatomic organization of the affective components of language in the right hemisphere. Arch Neurol 38:561–569, 1981

Ross ED: Nonverbal aspects of language. Neurol Clin 11:9–23, 1993

Ross ED, Mesulam M-M: Dominant language functions of the right hemisphere? Arch Neurol 36:144–148, 1979

Ross ED, Stewart RS: Pathological display of affect in patients with depression and right frontal brain damage: an alternative mechanism. J Nerv Ment Dis 175:165–172, 1987

Ross Russell RW: Supranuclear palsy of eyelid closure. Brain 103:71–82, 1980

Royall DR, Mahurin RK, Gray KF: Bedside assessment of executive cognitive impairment: the Executive Interview. J Am Geriatr Soc 40:1221–1226, 1992

Royall DR, Cordes JA, Polk MJ: CLOX: an executive clock drawing test. J Neurol Neurosurg Psychiatry 64:588–594, 1998

Royall DR, Mulroy AR, Chiodo LK, et al: Clock drawing is sensitive to executive control: a comparison of six methods. J Gerontol 54B:P328–P333, 1999

Royall DR, Espino DV, Polk MJ, et al: Prevalence and patterns of executive impairment in community dwelling Mexican Americans: results from the Hispanic EPESE Study. Int J Geriatr Psychiatry 19:926–934, 2004

Royall DR, Palmer R, Chiodo LK, et al: Executive control mediates memory's association with change in instrumental activities of daily living: the Freedom House Study. J Am Geriatr Soc 53:11–17, 2005

Ruchinskas RA, Curyto KJ: Cognitive screening in geriatric rehabilitation. Rehabil Psychol 48:14–22, 2003

Ruchinskas RA, Giuliano AJ: Motor perseveration in geriatric medical patients. Arch Clin Neuropsychol 18:455–461, 2003

Ryan R, Sunada K: Medical evaluation of persons with mental retardation referred for psychiatric assessment. Gen Hosp Psychiatry 19:274–280, 1997

Rylander G: Psychoses and the punding and choreiform syndromes in addiction to central stimulant drugs. Psychiatr Neurol Neurochir 75:203–212, 1972

Sachdev P: Akathisia and Restless Legs. Cambridge, UK, Cambridge University Press, 1995

Sachdev P, Kruk J: Clinical characteristics and predisposing factors in acute drug-induced akathisia. Arch Gen Psychiatry 51:963–974, 1994

Sachdev PS, Brodaty H, Valenzuela MJ, et al: The neuropsychological profile of vascular cognitive impairment in stroke and TIA patients. Neurology 62:912–919, 2004

Sackeim HA, Greenberg MS, Weiman AL, et al: Hemispheric asymmetry in the expression of positive and negative emotions. Arch Neurol 39:210–218, 1982

Sacks O: Migraine: Evolution of a Common Disorder. London, Faber & Faber, 1971

Sakai Y, Nakamura T, Sakurai A, et al: Right frontal areas 6 and 8 are associated with simultanapraxia, a subset of motor impersistence. Neurology 54:522–524, 2000

Sanders RD, Keshavan MS: The neurologic examination in adult psychiatry: from soft signs to hard science. J Neuropsychiatry Clin Neurosci 10:395–404, 1998

Sanders RD, Keshavan MS: Physical and neurologic examinations in neuropsychiatry. Semin Clin Neuropsychiatry 7:18–29, 2002

Sanders RD, Forman SD, Pierri JN, et al: Inter-rater reliability of the neurological examination in schizophrenia. Schizophr Res 29:287–292, 1998

Sandson J, Albert ML: Perseveration in behavioral neurology. Neurology 37:1736–1741, 1987

Santhouse AM, Howard RJ, ffytche DH: Visual hallucinatory syndromes and the anatomy of the visual brain. Brain 123 (pt 10):2055–2064, 2000

Sargent MA, Poskitt KJ, Jan JE: Congenital ocular motor apraxia: imaging findings. AJNR Am J Neuroradiol 18:1915–1922, 1997

Saver J, Greenstein P, Ronthal M, et al: Asymmetric catalepsy after right hemisphere stroke. Mov Disord 8:69–73, 1993

Savic I, Bookheimer SY, Fried I, et al: Olfactory bedside test: a simple approach to identify temporo-orbitofrontal dysfunction. Arch Neurol 54:162–168, 1997

Sawle G: Movement disorders during sleep, in Movement Disorders in Clinical Practice. Edited by Sawle G. Oxford, UK, Isis Medical Media, 1999, pp 159–163

Scepkowski LA, Cronin-Golomb A: The alien hand: cases, categorizations, and anatomical correlates. Behav Cogn Neurosci Rev 2:261–277, 2003

Schaumann BA, Annegers JF, Johnson B, et al: Family history of seizures in posttraumatic and alcohol-associated seizures disorders. Epilepsia 35:48–52, 1994

Schiffman J, Ekstrom M, LaBrie J, et al: Minor physical anomalies and schizophrenia spectrum disorders: a prospective investigation. Am J Psychiatry 159:238–243, 2002

Schillerstrom JE, Deuter MS, Wyatt R, et al: Prevalence of executive impairment in patients seen by a psychiatry consultation service. Psychosomatics 44:290–297, 2003

Schnider A: Spontaneous confabulation and the adaptation of thought to ongoing reality. Nat Rev Neurosci 4:662–671, 2003

Schnider A, von Däniken C, Gutbrod K: Disorientation in amnesia: a confusion of memory traces. Brain 119:1627–1632, 1996

Schott GD, Wyke MA: Congenital mirror movements. J Neurol Neurosurg Psychiatry 44:586–599, 1981

Schott JM, Rossor MN: The grasp and other primitive reflexes. J Neurol Neurosurg Psychiatry 74:558–560, 2003

Sellal F, Fontaine SF, Van Der Linden M, et al: To be or not to be at home? A neuropsychological approach to delusion for place. J Clin Exp Neuropsychol 18:234–248, 1996

Serra-Mestres J, Robertson MM, Shetty T: Palicoprolalia: an unusual variant of palilalia in Gilles de la Tourette's syndrome. J Neuropsychiatry Clin Neurosci 10:117–118, 1998

Sewell DD, Jeste DV: Metoclopramide-associated tardive dyskinesia: an analysis of 67 cases. Arch Fam Med 1:271–278, 1992

Shallice T, Burgess PW: Deficits in strategy application following frontal lobe damage in man. Brain 114:727–741, 1991

Shallice T, Evans ME: The involvement of the frontal lobes in cognitive estimation. Cortex 4:294–303, 1978

Shallice T, Burgess PW, Schon F, et al: The origins of utilization behavior. Brain 112:1587–1598, 1989

Sheridan PL, Solomont J, Kowall N, et al: Influence of executive function on locomotor function: divided attention increases gait variability in Alzheimer's disease. J Am Geriatr Soc 51:1633–1637, 2003

Shibre T, Kebede D, Alem A, et al: Neurological soft signs (NSS) in 200 treatment-naive cases with schizophrenia: a community-based study in a rural setting. Nord J Psychiatry 56:425–431, 2002

Signer SF: Localization and lateralization in the delusion of substitution: Capgras symptom and its variants. Psychopathology 27:168–176, 1994

Silberman EK, Post RM, Nurnberger J, et al: Transient sensory, cognitive and affective phenomena in affective illness: a comparison with complex partial epilepsy. Br J Psychiatry 146:81–89, 1985

Sjögren M, Wallin A, Edman A: Symptomatological characteristics distinguish between frontotemporal dementia and vascular dementia with a dominant frontal lobe syndrome. Int J Geriatr Psychiatry 12:656–661, 1997

Skirda RJ, Persinger MA: Positive associations among dichotic listening errors, complex partial epileptic-like signs, and paranormal beliefs. J Nerv Ment Dis 181:663–667, 1993

Slachevsky A, Villalpando JM, Sarazin M, et al: Frontal Assessment Battery and differential diagnosis of frontotemporal dementia and Alzheimer disease. Arch Neurol 61:1104–1107, 2004

Smith CA, van Gorp WG, Ryan ER, et al: Screening subtle HIV-related cognitive dysfunction: the clinical utility of the HIV dementia scale. J Acquir Immune Defic Syndr 33:116–118, 2003

Smith G, Vigen V, Evans J, et al: Patterns and associates of hyperphagia in patients with dementia. Neuropsychiatry Neuropsychol Behav Neurol 11:97–102, 1998

Smith ML, Milner B: Differential effects of frontal-lobe lesions on cognitive estimation and spatial memory. Neuropsychologia 22:697–705, 1984

Smith RA, Berg JE, Pope LE, et al: Validation of the CNS Emotional Lability Scale for pseudobulbar affect (pathological laughing and crying) in multiple sclerosis patients. Mult Scler 10:679–685, 2004

Smith RC, Kadewari RP, Rosenberger JR, et al: Nonresponding schizophrenia: differentiation by neurological soft signs and neuropsychological tests. Schizophr Bull 25:813–825, 1999

Snowden JS, Neary D: Progressive language dysfunction and lobar atrophy. Dementia 4:226–231, 1993

Snowden JS, Neary D, Mann DM, et al: Progressive language disorder due to lobar atrophy. Ann Neurol 31:174–183, 1992

Solms M: The Neuropsychology of Dreams: A Clinico-Anatomical Study. Mahwah, NJ, Lawrence Erlbaum, 1997

Solms M, Turnbull O: The Brain and the Inner World: An Introduction to the Neuroscience of Subjective Experience. New York, Other Press, 2002

Sonoo M: Abductor sign: a reliable new sign to detect unilateral non-organic paresis of the lower limb. J Neurol Neurosurg Psychiatry 75:121–125, 2004

Stacy M, Cardoso F, Jankovic J: Tardive stereotypy and other movement disorders in tardive dyskinesias. Neurology 43:937–941, 1993

Stein DJ, Hollander E, Cohen L, et al: Neuropsychiatric impairment in impulsive personality disorders. Psychiatry Res 48:257–266, 1993

Stein DJ, Niehaus DJII, Seedat S, et al: Phenomenology of stereotypic movement disorder. Psychiatr Ann 28:397–312, 1998

Stevens JR: Disturbances of ocular movements and blinking in schizophrenia. J Neurol Neurosurg Psychiatry 41:1024–1030, 1978a

Stevens JR: Eye blink and schizophrenia: psychosis or tardive dyskinesia. Am J Psychiatry 135:223–226, 1978b

Stewart JT: Akathisia following traumatic brain injury: treatment with bromocriptine. J Neurol Neurosurg Psychiatry 52:1200–1201, 1991

Stone J, Zeman A, Sharpe M: Functional weakness and sensory disturbance. J Neurol Neurosurg Psychiatry 73:241–245, 2002

Stracciari A: Transient global amnesia and transient topographical amnesia. J Neurol 250:633–634, 2003

Strub RL, Black FW: The bedside mental status examination, in Handbook of Neuropsychology, Vol I. Edited by Boller F, Grafman J. Amsterdam, The Netherlands, Elsevier, 1988, pp 29–46

Stuppaeck CH, Miller CH, Ehrmann H, et al: Akathisia induced by necrosis of the basal ganglia after carbon monoxide intoxication. Mov Disord 10:229–231, 1995

Subotnik KL, Nuechterlein KH, Irzhevsky V, et al: Is unawareness of psychotic disorder a neurocognitive or psychological defensiveness problem? Schizophr Res 75:147–157, 2005

Sudo K, Matsuyama T, Goto Y, et al: Elbow flexion response as another primitive reflex. Psychiatry Clin Neurosci 56:131–137, 2002

Sultzer DL, Berisford MA, Gunay I: The Neurobehavioral Rating Scale: reliability in patients with dementia. J Psychiatr Res 29:185–191, 1995

Sundheim ST, Voeller KK: Psychiatric implications of language disorders and learning disabilities: risks and management. J Child Neurol 19:814–826, 2004

Syz H: Recovery from loss of mnemic retention after head trauma. J Gen Psychol 17:355–387, 1937

Tanaka S, Inui T, Iwaki S, et al: Neural substrates involved in imitating finger configurations: an fMRI study. Neuroreport 12:1171–1174, 2001

Tanaka Y, Albert ML, Hara H, et al: Forced hyperphasia and environmental dependency syndrome. J Neurol Neurosurg Psychiatry 68:224–226, 2000

Tarrant CJ, Jones PB: Precursors to schizophrenia: do biological markers have specificity? Can J Psychiatry 44:335–349, 1999

Tarsy D, Indorf G: Tardive tremor due to metoclopramide. Mov Disord 17:620–621, 2002

Tatu L, Moulin T, Monnier G, et al: Unilateral pure thalamic asterixis: clinical, electromyographic, and topographic patterns. Neurology 54:2339–2342, 2000

Taylor MA, Fink M: Catatonia in psychiatric classification: a home of its own. Am J Psychiatry 160:1233–1241, 2003

Tegnér R, Levander M: Through a looking glass: a new technique to demonstrate directional hypokinesia in unilateral neglect. Brain 114:1943–1951, 1991

Teicher MH, Glod CA, Surrey J, et al: Early childhood abuse and limbic system ratings in adult psychiatric outpatients. J Neuropsychiatry Clin Neurosci 5:301–306, 1993

Teitelbaum JS, Eliasziw M, Garner M: Tests of motor function in patients suspected of having mild unilateral cerebral lesions. Can J Neurol Sci 29:337–344, 2002

Teng EL, Chui HC: The Modified Mini-Mental State (3MS) Examination. J Clin Psychiatry 48:314–318, 1987

Tenyi T, Trixler M, Csabi G, et al: Minor physical anomalies in non-familial unipolar recurrent major depression. J Affect Disord 79:259–262, 2004

Thacker RC, De Nil LF: Neurogenic cluttering. J Fluency Disord 21:227–238, 1996

Thompson PD, Marsden CD: Gait disorder of subcortical arteriosclerotic encephalopathy: Binswanger's disease. Mov Disord 2:1–8, 1987

Tinuper P, Plazzi G, Provini F, et al: Facial asymmetry in partial epilepsies. Epilepsia 33:1097–1100, 1992

Toone BK: Psychomotor seizures, arterio-venous malformation and the olfactory reference syndrome: a case report. Acta Psychiatr Scand 58:61–66, 1978

Tremont-Lukats IW, Teixeira GM, Hernández DE: Primitive reflexes in a case-control study of patients with advanced human immunodeficiency virus type 1. J Neurol 246:540–543, 1999

Trimble M, Mendez M, Cummings J: Neuropsychiatric symptoms from the temporolimbic lobes. J Neuropsychiatry Clin Neurosci 9:429–438, 1997

Trinka E, Walser G, Unterberger I, et al: Peri-ictal water drinking lateralizes seizure onset to the nondominant temporal lobe. Neurology 60:873–876, 2003

Trosch RM, Sze G, Brass LM, et al: Emotional facial paresis with striatocapsular infarction. J Neurol Sci 98:195–201, 1990

Tucker DM, Watson RT, Heilman KM: Discrimination and evocation of affectively intoned speech in patients with right parietal disease. Neurology 27:947–950, 1977

Turner TH: A diagnostic analysis of the Casebooks of Ticehurst House Asylum, 1845–1890. Psychol Med Monogr Suppl 21:1–70, 1992

Ueki Y, Mima T, Oga T, et al: Dominance of ipsilateral corticospinal pathway in congenital mirror movements. J Neurol Neurosurg Psychiatry 76:276–279, 2005

Uher R, Treasure J: Brain lesions and eating disorders. J Neurol Neurosurg Psychiatry 76:852–857, 2005

Ungvari GS, Leung SK, Ng FS, et al: Schizophrenia with prominent catatonic features ("catatonic schizophrenia"), I: demographic and clinical correlates in the chronic phase. Prog Neuropsychopharmacol Biol Psychiatry 29:27–38, 2005

Van Borsel J, Taillieu C: Neurogenic stuttering versus developmental stuttering: an observer judgement study. J Commun Disord 34:385–395, 2001

Van Borsel J, Schelpe L, Santens P, et al: Linguistic features in palilalia: two case studies. Clin Linguist Phon 15:663–677, 2001

Van Borsel J, Goethals L, Vanryckeghem M: Disfluency in Tourette syndrome: observational study in three cases. Folia Phoniatr Logop 56:358–366, 2004

van der Heijden FMMA, Tuinier S, Arts NJM, et al: Catatonia: disappeared or under-diagnosed? Psychopathology 38:3–8, 2005

van Harten B, Courant MNJ, Scheltens P, et al: Validation of the HIV Dementia Scale in an elderly cohort of patients with subcortical cognitive impairment caused by subcortical ischaemic vascular disease or a normal pressure hydrocephalus. Dement Geriatr Cogn Disord 18:109–114, 2004

van Vugt P, Paquier P, Kees L, et al: Increased writing activity in neurological conditions: a review and clinical study. J Neurol Neurosurg Psychiatry 61:510–514, 1996

Venkatasubramanian G, Latha V, Gangadhar BN, et al: Neurological soft signs in never-treated schizophrenia. Acta Psychiatr Scand 108:144–146, 2003

Verdoux H, Sutter AL: Perinatal risk factors for schizophrenia: diagnostic specificity and relationships with maternal psychopathology. Am J Med Genet 114:898–905, 2002

Verduyn WH, Hilt J, Roberts MA, et al: Multiple partial seizure-like symptoms following "minor" closed head injury. Brain Inj 6:245–260, 1992

Victor M, Adams RD, Collins GH: The Wernicke-Korsakoff Syndrome and Related Neurological Diseases Due to Alcoholism and Malnutrition, 2nd Edition. Philadelphia, PA, FA Davis, 1989

Vidailhet M, Jedynak CP, Pollak P, et al: Pathology of symptomatic tremors. Mov Disord 13 (suppl 3):49–54, 1998

Vighetto A, Henry E, Garde P, et al: Le délire spatial: une manifestation des lésions de l'hémisphère mineur. Rev Neurol (Paris) 141:476–481, 1985

Vila N, Chamorro A: Ballistic movements due to ischemic infarcts after intravenous heroin overdose: report of two cases. Clin Neurol Neurosurg 99:259–262, 1997

Vitali P, Nobili F, Raiteri U, et al: Right hemispheric dysfunction in a case of pure progressive aphemia: fusion of multimodal neuroimaging. Psychiatry Res 130:97–107, 2004

Vossler DG, Haltiner AM, Schepp SK, et al: Ictal stuttering: a sign suggestive of psychogenic nonepileptic seizures. Neurology 63:516–519, 2004

Vreeling FW, Houx PJ, Jolles J, et al: Primitive reflexes in Alzheimer's disease and vascular dementia. J Geriatr Psychiatry Neurol 8:111–117, 1995

Vuilleumier P: Anosognosia: the neurology of beliefs and uncertainties. Cortex 40:9–17, 2004

Waddington JL, O'Callaghan E, Buckley P, et al: Tardive dyskinesia in schizophrenia: relationship to minor physical anomalies, frontal lobe dysfunction and cerebral structure on magnetic resonance imaging. Br J Psychiatry 167:41–45, 1995

Walczak TS, Bogolioubov A: Weeping during psychogenic nonepileptic seizures. Epilepsia 37:208–210, 1996

Wallesch C-W, Hundsalz A: Language function in delirium: a comparison of single word processing in acute confusional states and probable Alzheimer's disease. Brain Lang 46:592–606, 1994

Walterfang M, Velakoulis D: Cortical release signs in psychiatry. Aust N Z J Psychiatry 39:317–327, 2005

Wapner W, Hamby S, Gardner H: The role of the right hemisphere in the apprehension of complex linguistic materials. Brain Lang 14:15–33, 1981

Warren JD, Hu MT, Galloway M, et al: Observations on the human rejection behaviour syndrome: Denny-Brown revisited. Mov Disord 19:860–862, 2004

Warren S, Ross RG: Deficient cancellation of the vestibular ocular reflex in schizophrenia. Schizophr Res 34:187–193, 1998

Weaver DF: A clinical examination technique for mild upper motor neuron paresis of the arm. Neurology 54:531–532, 2000

Weinstein DD, Diforio D, Schiffman J, et al: Minor physical anomalies, dermatoglyphic asymmetries, and cortisol levels in adolescents with schizotypal personality disorder. Am J Psychiatry 156:617–623, 1999

Weintraub S: Neuropsychological assessment of mental state, in Principles of Cognitive and Behavioral Neurology, 2nd Edition. Edited by Mesulam M-M. Oxford, UK, Oxford University Press, 2000, pp 121–173

Weintraub S, Mesulam M-M: Mental state assessment of young and elderly adults in behavioral neurology, in Principles of Behavioral Neurology. Edited by Mesulam M-M. Philadelphia, PA, FA Davis, 1985, pp 71–123

Wertz RT, Henschel CR, Auther LL, et al: Affective prosodic disturbance subsequent to right hemisphere stroke: a clinical application. J Neurolinguistics 11:89–102, 1998

Williams D: The structure of emotions reflected in epileptic experiences. Brain 79:29–67, 1956

Wilson SAK: Some problems in neurology: no. II—pathological laughing and crying. J Neurol Psychopathol 4:299–333, 1924

Wong AHC, Voruganti LNP, Heslegrave RJ, et al: Neurocognitive deficits and neurological signs in schizophrenia. Schizophr Res 23:139–146, 1997

Yankovsky AE, Treves TA: Postictal mixed transcortical aphasia. Seizure 11:278–279, 2002

Young RR: What is a tremor? Neurology 58:165–166, 2002

Young RR, Shahani BT: Asterixis: one type of negative myoclonus. Adv Neurol 43:137–156, 1986

Yuspeh RL, Vanderploeg RD, Kershaw DA: Validity of a semantically cued recall procedure for the Mini-Mental State Examination. Neuropsychiatry Neuropsychol Behav Neurol 11:207–211, 1998

Zaatreh M, Tennison M, D'Cruz O, et al: Anticonvulsants-induced chorea: a role for pharmacodynamic drug interaction? Seizure 10:596–599, 2001

Zadikoff C, Lang AE: Apraxia in movement disorders. Brain 128:1480–1497, 2005

Zametkin AJ, Stevens JR, Pittman R: Ontogeny of spontaneous blinking and of habituation of the blink reflex. Ann Neurol 5:453–457, 1979

Zeki S: Cerebral akinetopsia (visual motion blindness): a review. Brain 114 (pt 2):811–824, 1991

Zulch KJ, Muller N: Associated movements in man, in Handbook of Clinical Neurology, Vol 1. Edited by Vinken PJ, Bruyn GW. Amsterdam, The Netherlands, North-Holland, 1969, pp 404–426

5

ELECTRODIAGNOSTIC TECHNIQUES IN NEUROPSYCHIATRY

Nash N. Boutros, M.D.
Robert W. Thatcher, Ph.D.
Silvana Galderisi, M.D.

Electrophysiological techniques are powerful tools for measuring brain dysfunction that cannot be detected by anatomical brain imaging. Electrophysiological techniques have the advantages of being largely noninvasive, widely available, and relatively inexpensive. They complement positron emission tomography (PET) and functional and anatomical magnetic resonance imaging (MRI) techniques by providing noninvasive measures of physiology with exquisite temporal resolution. At the current state of knowledge, the main clinical use of electrophysiological tests is to rule out epilepsy and gross brain pathology.

The recent evolution of neuropsychiatry as a subspecialty of psychiatry represents a paradigmatic shift in the responsibilities of psychiatrists in diagnosing and managing behavioral disorders with concomitant and demonstrable brain pathology. Disorders such as dementia, head injury, and attention deficit–related disorders, as well as psychiatric manifestations accompanying many neurolog-

ical disorders like epilepsy, cerebrovascular accidents, and movement and degenerative disorders, are the province of neuropsychiatry. Psychiatrists who deal with such disorders must become familiar with organic neuroevaluative tools like electroencephalography (EEG), evoked potentials, and polysomnography, as well as functional and structural neuroimaging techniques and neuropsychological evaluations. For many decades, once organicity was suspected, the case became the province of neurology. In fact, this general attitude resulted in the recategorization of a number of disorders from the field of psychiatry to the field of neurology, and these changes led to a significant decrease in the interest and training of psychiatrists in diagnosing and managing such disorders. The best-known example is "epilepsy." Consequently, the role of epileptic brain activity in generating or contributing to psychiatric syndromes has received little attention in the last few decades. As a general rule, psychiatrists are not

Supported by the following grant: R01 MH58784.

exposed to EEG in their training. This trend has led directly to psychiatrists not being skilled in using this technology in the workup or management of their patients.

Moreover, advances in computer analysis have led to an expanded role of electrophysiological tests in probing the diagnosis and management of patients whose pathology lies on a more functional than structural level (e.g., schizophrenia and affective, anxiety, personality, and addictive disorders). Indeed, as electrophysiology continues to be a powerful research tool in the exploration of the biological substrate for neuropsychiatric disorders, it is progressively apparent that electrophysiological techniques will likely play a major role in the everyday diagnostic and therapeutic work of all professionals dealing with behavioral aberration syndromes. This chapter provides a broad overview of the clinical electrophysiological diagnostic tests, as well as research findings with significant promise for becoming clinically useful. It should be emphasized that a number of electrophysiological techniques are used solely for research purposes, such as eye-movement tracking, pupillary responses, electromyographic startle response, and startle prepulse inhibition. These methods are not covered in this chapter, but they have generated a plethora of important findings and could possibly find their way to clinical application in the not-too-distant future.

As the role of diagnostic testing expands, it is increasingly crucial that clinicians develop the ability to evaluate the clinical value of a diagnostic test. The field of evaluating the usefulness of diagnostic tests is indeed evolving in all branches of medicine and not just in psychiatry (Bruns 2003). In brief, in determining whether a particular test is useful, the clinician must balance the information that the test yields with the degree of invasiveness and discomfort associated with it and the cost of the test. The test's sensitivity (i.e., its ability to detect an abnormality when one exists), specificity (the possibility of a negative test when an abnormality does not exist), and reliability (the presence of the abnormality in repeated testing) are all factors that contribute to the value of the information that the test provides. No test should be disseminated for wide use before these three factors are known. Once these factors are known and a standardized method for performing the test is developed, then the value of the information yielded should be balanced against the cost and degree of invasiveness of the test. For example, a test that yields some information (e.g., gives a hint about prognosis without influencing management) may still be worth performing if it is completely noninvasive and of low cost. Here the judgment of a knowledgeable clinician becomes crucial. As another example, a test that yields life-saving information (e.g., cardiac catheterization) is usually recommended even though the degree of invasiveness is considerable and

the cost is substantial. Clearly, if an alternative test with either less invasiveness or lower cost can be developed to provide the same or comparable information, then such an alternative should be seriously considered.

ELECTROENCEPHALOGRAPHY

HISTORY

Electrical brain signals were first discovered in 1875 in England by Richard Caton, who demonstrated that oscillating electrical potentials could be detected by electrodes placed on the cerebral cortex of animal brains (Brazier 1986). Caton demonstrated that the cerebral cortex has a baseline or tonic level of electrical activity. He also showed that phasic electrical activity could be evoked in response to sensory stimulation (Caton 1875). In Russia, Kaufman (1912) discovered abnormal electroencephalographic discharges in experimentally induced epilepsy in animals. Years later, the use of the electroencephalogram in humans was pioneered in Germany by Hans Berger, a neuropsychiatrist. In his original report, Berger (1929) described the posterior alpha rhythm and its disappearance with eye opening. Soon thereafter, spike and wave discharges were described in epileptic patients, heralding the rapid growth of the field of epileptology (Gibbs et al. 1935) and the wide use of EEG in clinical practice (Table 5–1).

THEORETICAL OVERVIEW

The electrical signal detected by the electroencephalograph is the final summation of a multitude of potentials generated by the cerebral cortex. The structural organization of the cerebral cortex can be conceptualized as a mosaic of vertical columns with apical dendrites oriented toward the surface and axons projecting to deeper structures (Fenton 1989). Thus, the signal detected by the scalp electrode is predominated by the excitatory and inhibitory postsynaptic potentials on dendrites and neuronal cell bodies, and not the deeper axon action potentials (Goff et al. 1978; Goldensohn 1979). The superficial cortical layers are influenced by projections from the thalamus, which in turn receives input from the reticular activating system. Thus, the cortical electroencephalographic signal is regulated by brain stem structures controlling arousal and sleep. For example, during waking, the brisk tonic activity of the reticular activating system leads to the desynchronization of the cortical electroencephalographic signal. At sleep onset, the thalamocortical rhythms are unmasked and synchronized, leading to a slower, higher-amplitude signal (Andersen and Andersson 1968; Fenton 1989).

TABLE 5–1. History of electroencephalography in neuropsychiatry

1791	Galvani experiments with frog nerve preparations and speculates that nervous tissue has intrinsic electrical activity.
1848	Du Bois-Reymond discovers the action potential of nerve tissue.
1875	Caton demonstrates the presence of electrical brain signals in animals. He shows that the brain is electrically active at rest and that sensory stimulation evokes cortical potential changes.
1912	Kaufman reports abnormal electroencephalographic discharges in experimentally induced epilepsy in animals.
1929	Berger presents the first human electroencephalographic study.
1935	Gibbs and colleagues describe the spike and wave discharge in human epilepsy.
1938	Grass and Gibbs provide the early work on quantification of the EEG.
1947	The American EEG Society (AES) is founded.
1965	The American Medical EEG Association (AMEEGA) is founded (Khoshbin 2000).
1992	The American Psychiatric Electrophysiology Association (APEA) is founded (Boutros 2000). Turan Itil is elected as first president.
1998	AMEEGA and APEA merge to form the EEG and Clinical Neuroscience Society (ECNS). Dr. Norman Moore is elected as first president.

Although brain potentials may range in frequency from 0.1 to 1,000 Hz (Niedermeyer and Lopes da Silva 2005), the scalp electroencephalographic signal has an upper frequency range of approximately 70 Hz. The naked eye can only resolve activity up to about 40 Hz. This range is subdivided into frequency bands defined as gamma (> 30 Hz), beta (12–30 Hz), alpha (8–12 Hz), theta (4–7 Hz), and delta (0.1–4.0 Hz). When the brain is at rest, large areas of cortex may fire in relative synchrony. Therefore, lower frequencies, such as the alpha rhythm, are better detected than higher frequencies, which are highly asynchronous and are attenuated by transmission through the skull and scalp (Cooper et al. 1965).

CLINICAL ELECTROENCEPHALOGRAPHY

Routine EEG is performed when the subject is awake and at rest. Activation procedures such as hyperventilation and photic stimulation may be used to elicit abnormal activity. Sleep deprivation can increase the sensitivity for detecting epileptiform activity. The electrode placement generally follows the standard 10–20 montage (Jasper 1958). Figure 5–1 shows the standard placement. Note that odd numbers are on the subject's left side and smaller numbers are toward the front of the head.

Special electrodes—such as nasopharyngeal, anterior temporal, or sphenoidal electrodes—may be used to increase sensitivity or further enhance localization of abnormal discharges. Nasopharyngeal electrodes have proven to be difficult to apply and maintain in psychiatric patients. These electrodes are usually placed through the nostrils and tend to be uncomfortable and prevent patients from falling asleep during the procedure (this is a serious limitation, as discussed below in this section) (Struve and Feigenbaum 1981). Conversely, the anterior temporal electrodes are completely noninvasive. Nonepileptiform abnormalities in patients over age 40 were enhanced by these electrodes (Nowack et al. 1988).

Sphenoidal electrodes were introduced in the early 1950s. Using a hollow needle, a fine electrode insulated except at the tip is inserted between the zygoma and the sigmoid notch in the mandible until the electrode contacts the base of the skull lateral to the foramen ovale. Sphenoidal electrodes can be placed through a fine needle rather closely to important structures such as the amygdala and hippocampus. The electrodes can be tolerated for a number of days (as is done in epileptic patients being monitored). Some studies of sphenoidal electrodes show an increase in abnormality in as many as 40.5% of seizure patients who had no other specific changes in waking or sleep electroencephalograms (Kristensen and Sindrup 1978). Almost all clinical neurophysiology laboratories are familiar with these special electrode placements.

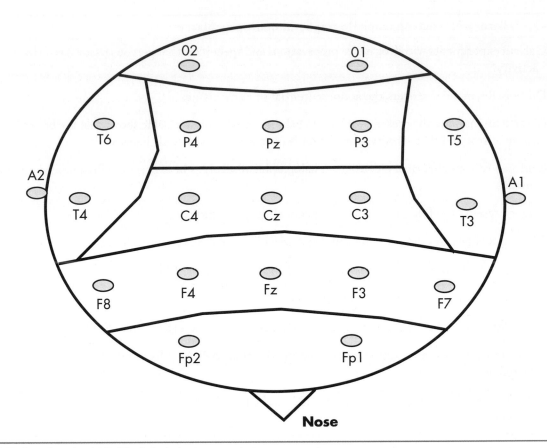

FIGURE 5–1. Standard 10–20 clinical electroencephalogram montage.

The most prevalent method of electroencephalogram analysis in the clinical setting is the visual analysis by the electroencephalographer. We emphasize here that while the visual inspection of the electroencephalogram remains an essential first step, much can be learned from further quantification of the activity. Hence, it is important that the electroencephalogram be recorded to allow such additional processing.

The record is first examined for the background activity, which should be 8–13 Hz in a relaxed, awake adult whose eyes are closed. Symmetry of the activity between the hemispheres is also evaluated. Once the background and symmetry are evaluated, the electroencephalographer looks for abnormal activities. The two main categories of abnormalities are abnormal slow-wave activity and abnormal paroxysmal (or epileptiform) activity. The "abnormal" qualification is important, because under certain conditions both slowing and paroxysmal activity normally can be seen. This observation highlights the absolute necessity that electroencephalograms be interpreted by well-trained clinicians only. Slow activity that is seen only on one side or in a specific region is almost always abnormal and should lead the clinician to consider further workup. Diffuse slowing of the background rhythm

is the hallmark of a diffuse encephalopathic process (Struve and Boutros 2005). In cases of delirium, diffuse (and possibly paroxysmal) slow activity can be superimposed on a more or less normal background activity. Evaluation of slow activity is best done while the patient is awake and relaxed. Epileptiform (i.e., paroxysmal) activity can also be localized (in which case it is almost always abnormal) or bilateral. Only vertex sharp waves seen during Stage II sleep are a definite normal activity. With a few exceptions (so-called controversial waveforms; see the section "Controversial Waveforms" later in this chapter), paroxysmal activity should be considered abnormal and indicative of an epileptic process. However, it should be emphasized that the presence of an epileptic discharge does not itself satisfy the diagnosis of epilepsy. For an adequate evaluation of epileptiform activity, sleep tracing is essential (Struve and Pike 1974).

Although the human visual association cortex remains far superior to any computer method of detecting epileptiform or paroxysmal activity, when there are large amounts of data (e.g., 24 hours of recording), a spike-detection computer program becomes indispensable for eliminating most of the record and leaving only a few epochs for the human eye's final determination. Activation

TABLE 5–2. Electroencephalographic findings in a sample of neuropsychiatric disorders

Disorder	Electroencephalographic findings
Epilepsy	Focal and generalized spikes, sharp waves, polyspikes, and spike-wave complexes
Delirium	Generalized slowing and irregular high-voltage delta activity
Encephalitis	Background slowing, diffuse epileptiform activity, and periodic lateralized epileptiform discharges
Barbiturate or benzodiazepine intoxication	Background slowing and diffuse superimposed beta activity
Tumor or infarction	Focal slowing at border of infarction or tumor; necrotic tissue is electrically silent
Aging	Generalized slowing of alpha rhythm, diffuse theta and delta activity, decline of low-voltage beta activity, and focal delta activity in temporal areas
Dementia	Accelerated development of electroencephalographic changes of normal aging, paroxysmal bifrontal delta activity, and asymmetry between hemispheres
Creutzfeldt-Jakob disease and subacute sclerosing panencephalitis	Periodic complexes
Uremic or hepatic encephalopathy	Triphasic waves

Source. Adapted from Fenton 1989.

methods are routinely used to increase the yield of an electroencephalogram and include photic stimulation, hyperventilation, and sleep deprivation.

The electroencephalogram is a nonspecific indicator of cerebral function. Any pathophysiological insult to the central nervous system (CNS) can result in electrophysiological alterations. For example, a large variety of pharmacological, metabolic, and neurodegenerative processes can result in diffuse slowing of electroencephalographic rhythms. Thus, with few exceptions (see Table 5–2), EEG provides nonspecific evidence of brain abnormality. Disorders that affect deep brain structures or that result in a chronic indolent loss of neurons typically show diffuse electroencephalographic changes (Fenton 1989; Niedermeyer and Lopes da Silva 2005). Electroencephalographic abnormalities are most pronounced with acute injuries of the outer cortex. EEG can detect focal or localized abnormalities, allowing clinical–electrophysiological correlations (Niedermeyer and Lopes da Silva 2005).

After the visual examination, the background activity is quantified with respect to frequency and amplitude. Quantitative electroencephalographic analysis perhaps holds the most promise in electrophysiological research in neuropsychiatry. Because there are no specific waveforms seen in neuropsychiatric disorders, electrophysiological differentiation of patients from control subjects may be obtainable only by demonstrating a quantitative

difference between the two groups (Pfefferbaum et al. 1995; Shagass 1977). More details regarding the quantification of the electroencephalogram are provided later in this chapter, in "Quantitative Electroencephalography."

Among the more standard psychiatric disorders, panic disorder, episodic aggression, attention-deficit/hyperactivity disorder (ADHD), dementia, and epilepsy have demonstrated a high prevalence of electroencephalographic abnormalities. These topics, as well as screening electroencephalograms, are discussed in the following sections.

Panic Disorder

Panic symptoms significantly resemble symptoms induced by temporolimbic epileptic activity, particularly from activity originating in the insular cortex in the temporal lobes (Reiman et al. 1989). Fear, derealization, tachycardia, diaphoresis, and abdominal discomfort are characteristic symptoms of simple partial seizures with psychiatric and autonomic symptomatology. Evidence from population surveys suggests that panic disorder is significantly more prevalent in epileptic patients than in the general public (Pariente et al. 1991).

In another report, Young et al. (1995) described five patients with brief simple partial seizures that mimicked panic attacks. The investigators concluded that the most common psychiatric disorder that must be differentiated from temporal lobe epilepsy is panic disorder. In their sample, seizures were briefer and more stereotyped than panic attacks. Additionally, aphasia and dysmnesia accompanied seizure activity in some patients. This differentiation could be diagnostically challenging as patients with documented complex partial seizures of temporal lobe origin may have concomitant nonictal episodic emotional symptoms, including phobia, true panic attacks, and anxiety (Signer 1988).

A number of reports provide evidence that electroencephalographic abnormalities are not infrequent in panic disorder patients. However, the findings differ from study to study and range from paroxysmal epileptiform discharges to asymmetric increases in slow-wave activity (Bystritsky et al. 1999). Weilburg et al. (1995) reported on 15 subjects with atypical panic attacks who met DSM-III-R criteria (American Psychiatric Association 1987) for panic disorder and who underwent routine EEG, followed by prolonged ambulatory electroencephalographic monitoring using sphenoidal electrodes. The investigators found focal paroxysmal electroencephalographic changes consistent with partial seizure activity and occurring during a panic attack in 33% ($n = 5$) of the subjects. It is important to note that multiple attacks were recorded before panic-related electroencephalographic changes were demonstrated. Moreover, 2 of the 5 subjects with demonstrated electroencephalographic abnormalities during panic attacks had perfectly normal baseline EEGs. Jabourian et al (1992) compared the EEGs of unmedicated patients with panic attacks and depressive disorders. They reported 63% of the EEGs of panic patients to be abnormal ($n = 50$), while only 18% of the EEGs of depressive patients were abnormal ($n = 50$).

Episodic Aggression

The prevalence of abnormal electroencephalograms in association with episodic aggression varies widely among studies, ranging from as low as 6.6% in patients with rage attacks and episodic violent behavior (Riley and Niedermeyer 1978) to as high as 53% in patients diagnosed with antisocial personality disorder (Harper et al. 1972). Williams (1969) compared the electroencephalograms of 206 habitual aggressors and 127 persons who committed isolated acts of violence. He reported a fivefold increase in electroencephalographic abnormalities in habitual aggressors (57%) versus nonhabitual aggressors (12%). Williams also found more frontal region abnormalities in the habitual aggressors but more diffuse and epileptic activity in the nonhabitual aggressors. Howard (1984) showed that patients who had committed violent offenses against strangers, as opposed to people known to them, tended to have bilateral paroxysmal electroencephalographic features, with 70% of subjects with bilateral paroxysmal discharges having attacked strangers.

The appearance of an abnormal electroencephalogram may predict a favorable therapeutic response to anticonvulsant medications. Monroe (1975) showed that anticonvulsants can block electroencephalographic epileptiform discharges and can lead to dramatic clinical improvement in individuals exhibiting repeated and frequent aggressive behavior. An earlier study by Boelhouwer et al. (1968) found that adolescents or young adults exhibiting the 14 and 6 positive spikes responded favorably to the combination of anticonvulsants and antipsychotic medications. Tunks and Dermer (1977) reported a detailed case where, other than deafness, there were no obvious neurological abnormalities in a female with episodic aggression who responded extremely well to carbamazepine therapy. Neppe (1983) provided evidence that the addition of carbamazepine can be clinically useful in the treatment of schizophrenia patients who exhibit temporal lobe abnormalities on the electroencephalogram and who do not have a history of a seizure disorder. Earlier, Hakola and Laulumaa (1982) noted a reduction of aggressive episodes when carbamazepine was added to the neuroleptic regime of 8 highly aggressive women with schizophrenia who also had electroencephalographic abnormalities. However, other studies suggest that anticonvulsant therapy may have a beneficial effect on aggressive tendencies, irrespective of the presence or absence of electroencephalographic abnormalities (Luchins 1984). Until definitive studies are performed, patients should be given a trial of an anticonvulsant when an electroencephalogram proves to be abnormal—particularly if the abnormality is focal and paroxysmal.

It should be emphasized that it is well documented that a single negative electroencephalogram does *not* rule out epilepsy, even in patients with well-documented seizures. Moreover, the necessity for obtaining sleep during the recording cannot be overemphasized (Boutros and Struve 2002). Finally, it is possible that electroencephalographic abnormalities can be detected only during actual panic or aggressive episodes, requiring more prolonged ambulatory electroencephalographic monitoring.

Attention-Deficit/Hyperactivity Disorder

An important point needs to be emphasized before discussing the role of the routine electroencephalogram in the diagnosis and management of attention deficit disorder (ADD) and ADHD: it is essential that each individual (child or adult) being considered for the diagnosis of ADD or ADHD receive a full neurological history and examination, with additional neurological workup (electroencephalogram or imaging) if the exam gives any indication of abnormality (Millichap 1997; Niedermeyer and Naidu 1998). Phillips et al. (1993) reported on routine electroencephalographic screening of 86 children hospitalized over an 18-month period for behavioral problems (conduct disorder or conduct disorder plus ADHD, $n = 75$, breakdown not provided; ADHD alone, $n = 11$). Eight (9%) records exhibited definite abnormalities, showing background slowing or paroxysmal discharges. Hughes et al. (2000) examined the electroencephalograms of 176 children with ADHD. The investigators reported an overall rate of "definite, noncontroversial, epileptiform activity" in 30.1% of subjects, mainly focal (usually occipital or temporal). Less often the epileptic activity was generalized, with bilaterally synchronous spike and wave complexes seen in 11 children. In the entire group, only 27.8% of electroencephalograms were completely normal, and an additional 18.8% had positive spikes (see below under "Controversial Waveforms") as the only abnormality. The investigators concluded that ADHD is a condition that often has organic changes in the form of electroencephalographic abnormalities; at times, these abnormalities are of epileptiform character. Such activity could contribute to either a deficit in attention or a plethora of movements (Hughes et al. 2000). Millichap (2000) described the electroencephalographic findings from 100 consecutive children with ADHD, reporting an incidence of 7% with "definite abnormalities" suggestive of epilepsy and an additional 19% with moderately abnormal dysrhythmias not diagnostic of epilepsy. On the basis of these findings, Millichap suggested six specific indications for obtaining an electroencephalogram in children presenting with ADHD—specifically, 1) personal or family history of seizures; 2) inattentive episodes characterized by excessive daydreaming and/or periodic confused states; 3) comorbid, episodic, unprovoked temper or rage attacks; 4) frequently recurrent headaches; 5) a history of head trauma, encephalitis, or meningitis preceding the onset of ADHD; and 6) abnormalities on neurological examination.

Age, Dementia, and Delirium

The background alpha rhythm changes very little with normal aging (Visser 1985) and is extremely useful in longitudinal studies. A drop of 1 Hz over a short period of time may indicate a significant encephalopathic process even though the alpha rhythm remains in the normal range (Pro and Wells 1977). Low-voltage beta activity increases in adults up to age 60 and declines thereafter. Mild diffuse slowing is found in approximately 20% of healthy elders over age 75. Focal delta activity, particu-

larly in the anterior temporal areas, is seen in 30%–40% of the normal population over age 60 (Fenton 1989).

The electroencephalogram is useful in the study and diagnosis of cognitive disorders. For example, electroencephalographic slowing has been found to be correlated with the severity of dementia (Fenton 1986) and the number of senile plaques (Deisenhammer and Jellinger 1974) in Alzheimer's disease. Robinson et al. (1994) reported that 92% of subjects with Alzheimer's disease, confirmed prospectively by histopathology, had abnormal electroencephalograms, in contrast to 35% of age-matched control subjects. Similarly, the severity of delirium has been found to be correlated with electroencephalographic abnormalities (Matsushima et al. 1997). The electroencephalogram is a valuable tool in hospital psychiatry, because it can help distinguish a mild delirium from major depression and remains the only tool capable of accurately diagnosing cases of nonconvulsive ambulatory status epilepticus (Riggio 2005) and nonmotoric presentations of frontal lobe seizures (Jobst and Williamson 2005).

Epilepsy and Epileptiform Activity

The most important use of EEG continues to be in the diagnosis of seizure disorders. No other brain abnormality has an electrophysiological pattern as distinctive as epilepsy (Duffy 1988). Epilepsy is found in approximately 0.3%–0.6% of adults in the general population (Anderson et al. 1999). The presence of spikes (defined as a potential with a duration less than 70 msec), sharp waves (duration of 70–200 msec), and polyspikes, frequently followed by a slow wave, are often seen interictally in epileptic patients (Aminoff 1986; Goodin and Aminoff 1984). The study of the behavioral consequences of epilepsy has a rich history and is discussed in detail in Chapter 16, "Neuropsychiatric Aspects of Seizure Disorders."

Epileptiform activity is found in 1%–10% of the nonepileptic general population (Zivin and Marsan 1968). The prevalence of electroencephalographic abnormalities in healthy populations is a controversial issue (see the section "Controversial Waveforms" for more discussion of this important issue). Epileptiform electroencephalographic variants are seen in approximately 30% of patients with schizophrenia and psychotic mood disorders (Inui et al. 1998). Electroencephalographic spikes are occasionally seen in nonepileptic patients who are taking antidepressant or antipsychotic medications (Fenton 1989). For example, 13% of patients with schizophrenia in one sample developed electroencephalographic spikes after initiating clozapine therapy (Freudenreich et al. 1997). More frequently, nonepileptic patients may have paroxysmal electroencephalographic activity during sedative-hypnotic withdrawal states.

Controversial Waveforms

Deserving a specific mention is what is termed *controversial sharp waves* or *spikes* (for a more expanded discussion, please refer to Hughes and Wilson 1983). Four EEG patterns are consistently observed to be more prevalent in psychiatric populations than in either healthy or nonpsychiatric patient–control populations (Struve and Pike 1974). Despite the increased prevalence in psychiatric patients, defining the patterns' exact neurobiological basis and clinical correlates has proved to be an elusive goal. It should be noted that none of the following patterns predictably correlate with an epileptic disorder. The four patterns in EEG are 1) the 14 and 6 positive spikes; 2) the rhythmic midtemporal discharges; 3) the 6/second spike and waves; and 4) the small, sharp spikes. Currently available literature strongly suggests that much well-designed research is necessary to resolve the issues surrounding these phenomena. Meanwhile, until the correlates of these patterns (physiological or pathological) are identified, the assertion that these patterns are completely irrelevant to neuropsychiatric conditions is not fully supportable.

Usefulness of clinical EEG in psychiatric research is hampered by the reported prevalence of abnormalities in normal adults, ranging from 4% to 57.5%. We have recently examined the criteria used for selecting healthy individuals in available literature. Seven criteria for choosing healthy control subjects were used as the bases for this review. The majority of studies met none, one, or two criteria. We conclude that the boundaries for a normal, unquantified electroencephalogram are poorly defined. Reports of the prevalence of electroencephalographic abnormalities in healthy individuals should be interpreted with caution until more recent and better-designed studies are performed (Boutros et al. 2005b).

Screening Electroencephalograms

The routine use of screening electroencephalograms in psychiatric patients remains controversial. Data from the 1989 National Hospital Discharge Survey (Pokras 1990) showed that 2.8% of the 1.51 million patients discharged from general hospitals with a primary diagnosis of mental disorder undergo an electroencephalogram (Olfson 1992). In contrast, 18%–33% of patients with mental disorders treated at university hospitals undergo an electroencephalogram (Lam et al. 1988; van Sweden and de Bruecker 1986). Van Sweden and de Bruecker (1986) reported that 42.5% of patients with mental disorders referred for EEG have significant abnormalities. Unsuspected abnormal electroencephalograms have been found in approximately 20% of psychiatric patients (Struve 1983). However, an abnormal electroencephalo-

gram may not redirect treatment choices or lead to an improvement in clinical outcome. A retrospective study of 698 psychiatric inpatients found that a screening electroencephalogram altered the clinical diagnosis in only 1.7% of cases (Warner et al. 1990).

QUANTITATIVE ELECTROENCEPHALOGRAPHY

The electroencephalographer makes a visual inspection of the background electroencephalographic rhythm. However, it is impossible for the unaided human eye to appreciate or analyze the time-dependent changes in frequency content, particularly when there are multiple leads. Techniques of quantitative electroencephalography (QEEG) include power spectral analysis and period amplitude analysis. Often, electroencephalographic parameters are assigned a visual analog, such as color, which allows for formation of topographical maps. All quantitative electroencephalographic techniques effectively make the enormous amount of data contained in a typical electrophysiological recording more accessible.

Spectral analysis is a computer-based method of analyzing the electroencephalographic frequency spectrum over time. It allows for the determination of the relative predominance (usually termed *relative power* and reported in percentages of the total absolute EEG power), or absolute power of any single frequency band. Spectral analysis takes advantage of the analytic power of the computer and its ability to translate an enormous quantity of background electroencephalographic frequency data into concise parameters by a method called the *fast Fourier transform* (Press et al. 1986). The correlation between the spectra of contralateral or adjacent leads provides a measure of electroencephalographic coherence. A subtle neuropathological process may be detected only from observing a change in coherence or relative electroencephalographic power of specific frequency bands. For example, Leuchter et al. (1987) found that analysis of electroencephalographic spectra and coherence could distinguish patients with Alzheimer's disease from those with multi-infarct dementia, as well as from healthy control subjects. John et al. (1988) have shown that electroencephalographic coherence measures are important discriminators of schizophrenia and that coherence is often diagnostically valuable in discriminating schizophrenia from bipolar depressed patients (Hughes and John 1999). Studies of ADHD and ADD have consistently shown that electroencephalographic coherence and phase delays are important discriminating variables (Chabot et al. 1996, 2001; Clarke et al. 1998, 2001).

Since the 1980s, QEEG has evolved into a neuroimaging technique that accurately quantifies the three-dimensional current sources of the electroencephalogram (Thatcher et al. 1994). Methods such as spatiotemporal source localization (Scherg and Von Cramon 1985) and distributed source localization (Michel et al. 2004; Pascual Marqui et al. 1994) can be used to identify three-dimensional current sources of the surface electroencephalogram and coregister the sources with other imaging modalities such as the MRI, PET, and functional MRI (Thatcher et al. 1994, 2005). QEEG source localization, such as Low Resolution Electromagnetic Tomography (LORETA), is useful in identifying focal disorders and relating such focal abnormalities to neuropsychiatric disorders including schizophrenia, depression, and dementia; mild traumatic brain injury; and measures of intelligence. The advantage of QEEG source localization is the millisecond time resolution in comparison to other neuroimaging modalities such as MRI and PET and SPECT.

Other forms of electroencephalographically derived data can be condensed into a topographical map. For example, derivative statistics such as the coefficient of variation can be topographically mapped, giving the neurophysiologist an immediate visual impression of the variability of spectral content (Duffy 1986). Electrophysiological data from multiple subjects can be summarized into a consolidated group map. Group maps of various patient groups and control subjects can be visually and statistically compared (Rosse et al. 1987). Finally, maps demonstrating the functional activation of electrical activity secondary to performing specific neuropsychological tasks can be compared to the resting state (Gruzelier and Liddiard 1989).

QEEG has been used in clinical research to determine whether patients with psychiatric disorders can be distinguished electrophysiologically from healthy control subjects. For example, several studies have shown that patients with schizophrenia have more delta activity, particularly over the frontal cortex, compared with control subjects (Guenther et al. 1986; Morihisa et al. 1983). Subsequent studies that have controlled for eye movement artifact have replicated the finding of increased diffuse delta activity in patients with schizophrenia but have failed to find a tendency for frontal localization (Karson et al. 1987). A possible role of neuroleptic treatment in the increase of slower rhythms (i.e., delta and theta) was ruled out by studies showing that slower rhythms are even more pronounced in untreated patients (Galderisi et al. 1992), and it is also present in children at genetic risk for schizophrenia (Itil 1977). Preliminary findings in studies of dementia have shown significant differences in alpha power between presenile and senile-onset patients, whereas little difference is seen between healthy young and old subjects (Gueguen et al. 1989). Alpha and beta power during photic stimulation are significantly decreased in patients with presenile dementia, compared with age-matched control subjects (Wada et al. 1997). Quantitative electroencephalographic studies have shown regional asymmetries in alpha power in depressed and anxious subjects (Bruder et al. 1997). Frontal asymmetry is associated with traitlike fearful temperament and increased activity of brain corticotropin-releasing factor (Kalin et al. 2000). Multiple studies have reported increased delta activity in intoxication, delirium, and dementia. Hence, quantitative electroencephalographic measures are indicative of both state and trait characteristics of brain function.

QEEG has been successfully used to detect age-related changes in electroencephalographic activity in normal and clinical populations (Bresnahan et al. 1999; John et al. 1977; Matousek and Petersen 1973; Thatcher et al. 2003, 2005); brain ischemia during surgery (Edmonds et al. 1992); subtle cerebral anomalies in carbon monoxide poisoning (Denays et al. 1994); and cerebral manifestations of systemic lupus erythematosus (Ritchlin et al. 1992). However, a pervasive problem in the clinical applicability of QEEG to neuropsychiatry is that issues of sensitivity, specificity, reliability, and validity have yet to be clearly established for the various clinical situations in which QEEG may be indicated. This problem was illustrated when Adams et al. (1995) conducted a controlled reliability study measuring quantitative electroencephalographic versus standard electroencephalographic measures of cerebral ischemia in surgical procedures. QEEG showed anomalies suggestive of ischemia during control procedures that were presumed to have little risk for ischemia. Another concern regarding the use of QEEG is that the transformation of extremely complex data into a simple image can distort the underlying data and present features that appear to be grounded in fact (Brodie 1996).

A review of the diagnostic value of QEEG to the field of neuropsychiatry concluded that "the method of QEEG has progressed well beyond the technology demonstration stage, and is evolving into a tool that may aid in the prediction of the clinical course of a disorder as well as a patient's response to certain medications" (Cunningham and Price 2004, p. 204). Table 5–3 shows the published diagnostic accuracy of QEEG for the evaluation of different neuropsychiatric disorders. The citations to the literature for each of these areas of diagnostic accuracy are in Hughes and John (1999).

Use of QEEG in schizophrenia, mood disorders, anxiety disorders, and mild head injury or postconcussion syndrome is discussed below. Not discussed in this chapter are electroencephalographic abnormalities often seen

TABLE 5–3.   The accuracy of QEEG in classifying neuropsychiatric disorders

Diagnostic class	Neuropsychiatric disorder	Accuracy (%)
Learning disorders, attention-deficit problems	ADD/ADHD vs. control	82
	ATT vs. control	95
	LD vs. control	74
	SLD vs. control	66
	ADD/ADHD vs. LD	92
	ADD vs. ADHD	69
Dementing disorders	Dementia (AD, MID, FTD) vs. control	80
	AD vs. MID	75
	AD vs. FID	84
	Vascular vs. nonvascular dementia	88
	Dementia vs. depression	77
Mood disorders	Depressed vs. control	80
	Depression vs. dementia	81
	Unipolar vs. bipolar depression	85
	Depression vs. schizophrenia	80

Note.   AD = Alzheimer's disease; ADD = attention-deficit disorder; ADHD = attention-deficit/hyperactivity disorder; ATT = attention disorder not meeting criteria for ADD or ADHD; FTD = frontotemporal dementia; LD = learning disability; MID = multi-infarct dementia; QEEG = quantitative electroencephalography; SLD = speech and language developmental disability.

Source.   Hughes and John 1999.

in other categories of psychiatric disorders, such as anorexia nervosa and other eating disorders (Hughes and John 1999). Translating such findings to clinical applications is a complicated process that requires focused research effort (Boutros et al. 2005a).

SCHIZOPHRENIA

Most studies show that patients with schizophrenia have more abnormalities than are found in healthy control subjects. Despite the large number of reported electroencephalographic abnormalities in schizophrenia populations, middle-aged subjects with schizophrenia do not appear to have more clinical seizures than age-matched control subjects (Gelisse et al. 1999). Several studies have documented electroencephalographic asymmetries in subjects with schizophrenia, particularly in the left hemisphere (Abrams and Taylor 1979; Nasrallah 1986). The lack of a family history of schizophrenia is associated with an increased likelihood of abnormal electroencephalographic activity in patients with schizophrenia (Kendler and Hays 1982). Although an abnormal electroencephalogram may be a predictor of resistance to neuroleptic medications (Itil 1982), the principal clinical utility of

the electroencephalogram in schizophrenia is as a screening tool for gross neuropathology or seizure disorder.

The electroencephalographic evaluation of schizophrenia is complicated by the heterogeneity of the illness and the diversity of medication histories and dosages at the time of examination. Common electroencephalographic abnormalities in patients with schizophrenia include decreased alpha and increased delta and beta activity (Dierks et al. 1989; Gattaz et al. 1992). Several patterns seem to characterize different subtypes of schizophrenia (Hughes and John 1999). Cluster analyses of electroencephalographic variables suggests at least five subtypes, each with different electroencephalographic profiles characterized as follows: 1) decrease of absolute delta and beta power posteriorly and a generalized increase in relative theta power; 2) decrease of absolute delta and theta power posteriorly and generalized increase of relative beta; 3) increase of absolute and relative theta power anteriorly and a generalized decrease of relative beta power; 4) generalized decrease of absolute delta, and to a lesser degree beta, power accompanied by a decrease of delta, theta, and beta and an increase of alpha relative power anteriorly; and 5) a generalized increase of theta and decrease of beta of both absolute and relative power measures (John et al. 1994). Some of the patients with schizophrenia whose electroencephalographic profiles were identified by cluster analysis displayed differential responses to treatment with haloperidol (Lifshitz and Gradijan 1974) or risperidone (Czobor and Volavka 1993). Increased interhemispheric coherence in frontal regions in all frequency bands was observed in all five subtypes of schizophrenia. In contrast, depressed patients typically exhibit decreased coherence (John et al. 1988). This finding again emphasizes that electroencephalographic coherence, especially in the gamma frequency band, is an important differential diagnostic measure when considering bipolar depression versus schizophrenia (Hughes and John 1999; Spencer et al. 2004; Symond et al. 2005). Recent studies by Lehmann et al. (2005) used quantitative electroencephalographic measures to evaluate brief spatiotemporal organizations of neural populations called *microstates* in subjects with schizophrenia. The researchers found that microstate concatenation was disturbed in patients with schizophrenia, whose electroencephalograms showed early termination of microstates as well as abnormal current density (LORETA).

MOOD DISORDERS

The incidence of abnormal EEG findings in mood disorders ranges from 20% to 40% (Taylor and Abrams 1981). Clinical depression is often associated with right hemisphere foci and more activation of the right frontal area, including an increased incidence of sharp waves (Flor-Henry 1976; Schaffer et al. 1982). Increased alpha and/or theta power is often present in unipolar depressed patients (John et al. 1988; Pollock and Schneider 1990). Decreased coherence and increased interhemispheric asymmetry in anterior regions are also commonly reported in depressed patients (Hughes and John 1999). In bipolar depression, in contrast to unipolar depression, alpha activity is often decreased and beta activity is increased (Clementz et al. 1994; Hughes and John 1999). The prevalence of sharp waves and spike activity in bipolar patients and the use of anticonvulsant medication for the treatment of bipolar disorders have led Hughes and John (1999) to suggest an overlap between convulsive disorders and bipolar illness, and they encourage clinicians to evaluate the electroencephalogram of depressed and bipolar patients for possible sharp waves and epileptiform activity.

ANXIETY DISORDERS

There is a high incidence of electroencephalographic abnormalities in patients with anxiety disorders, particularly in patients with panic attacks (see "Panic Disorder" earlier in this chapter). In line with other brain imaging investigations, most quantitative electroencephalographic and event-related potential studies have confirmed the involvement of frontal or temporal regions (Abraham and Duffy 1991; Wiedemann et al. 1999).

Quantitative electroencephalographic findings in patients with obsessive-compulsive disorder (OCD) have often involved the anterior region of the scalp; frequency characteristics, however, have been inconsistent—for both slow and fast activities, either a decrease or an increase over the anterior regions has been described (Khanna 1988; Molina et al. 1995). Hughes and John (1999) postulate two subtypes of OCD patients, one with increased alpha relative power and the second with increased theta activity. The former responded positively (82%) to serotonergic antidepressants, while the latter failed to improve (Prichep et al. 1993). Abnormalities of the alpha band over the anterior regions have been interpreted as an index of increased activation of the frontal regions, in line with findings of other studies (Bucci et al. 2004; Simpson et al. 2000).

MILD HEAD INJURY OR POSTCONCUSSION SYNDROME

Rapid acceleration/deceleration brain injuries are often accompanied by diffuse axonal injury from shear and rotational forces and contusions to the gray matter (Ommaya 1995). Even mild levels of force—in which there is either no loss of consciousness or less than 20 minutes of unconsciousness—can result in reduced attention span, reduced short-term memory capacity, depression, mood disorders, word-finding problems, and slowness of thought. Electroencephalographic changes that often accompany mild head injury are 1) reduced beta and/or alpha activity and increased theta activity (Korn et al. 2005; Rowe et al. 2004; Tebano et al. 1988; Thatcher et al. 1989, 1998a) and 2) changes in coherence and phase delays (Thatcher et al. 1989, 1998b, 2001b). Frontal and temporal lobe electroencephalographic abnormalities are commonly reported in patients with mild head injury. Electroencephalographic discriminant analyses of a group of patients with mild head injury compared with age-matched controls were > 95% accurate (Thatcher et al. 1989), and a follow-up study of 103 patients with mild versus severe head injury predicted Glasgow Coma Scale scores at the time of hospital admission ($r = 0.849$) with discriminant accuracy of > 95% (Thatcher et al. 2001b). Validation of the electroencephalographic changes observed in patients with mild head injury includes correlations with MRI T2 relaxation time (Thatcher et al. 1998a, 1998b, 2001a), neuropsychological tests (Thatcher et al. 2001a), and PET scan measures (Korn et al. 2005). Similar electroencephalographic findings have been reported in boxers and athletes who have had a mild concussion (Thompson et al. 2005). Useful reviews of quantitative electroencephalographic measures of mild traumatic brain injury, including therapeutic methods, have been provided by Duff (2004) and Thatcher (2006).

PHARMACO-ELECTROENCEPHALOGRAPHY

An important application of QEEG is its use in detecting drug-induced changes electroencephalographically, a technique called pharmaco-encephalography (pharmaco-EEG). Drug-induced modifications of the electroencephalogram were first described by Hans Berger in the early 1930s. He noticed, by visual inspection, that drugs influencing behavior also produced electroencephalographic changes. In 1933, he described electroencephalographic changes following the administration of barbiturates, morphine, and scopolamine (Berger 1933). Later, on the basis of one electroencephalographic channel recording and analysis, Max Fink (1963) identified nine different electroencephalographic change profiles associated with psychoactive drugs showing different behavioral effects. The advent of quantitative electroencephalographic analysis stimulated a large body of research on the use of electrophysiological methodology to detect and analyze drug effects on brain functioning and led to the development of pharmaco-EEG.

DRUG DEVELOPMENT

The sensitivity of pharmaco-EEG in detecting drug effects on the brain led several drug companies to include pharmaco-electroencephalographic investigations in preclinical studies. During the 1970s and the 1980s, double-blind, placebo-controlled studies (e.g., rising doses, reference compound, multiple rising doses) enabled the discovery of the antidepressant activity of mianserin (identified as an anti-allergic compound in animal studies) and doxepin (an anxiolytic according to preclinical prediction) and the discovery of the sedative activity of fenfluramine (characterized as a psychostimulant by other preclinical data) (Fink 1974). The discovery of the unpredicted antidepressant activity of mianserin stimulated the development of new animal tests, which in turn allowed the identification of the antidepressant properties of fluvoxamine and fluoxetine.

Pharmaco-electroencephalographic studies were also used in early stages of drug development to identify therapeutic doses of new psychotropic drugs (e.g., fluvoxamine and sertraline). The large amount of collected data led to the creation of databases in which psychoactive drugs were classified according to their quantitative electroencephalographic profiles (i.e., changes induced by the drug in the different frequency bands, based on single-lead analysis). Methodology and results of such investigations have been described in several publications (Herrmann 1982; Kikutchi et al. 2005; Saletu 1987). Attempts at revising the pharmaco-electroencephalographic classifications based on single-lead analysis by using multilead recording and electroencephalographic mapping techniques did not yield significant advances in the field. Preliminary studies based on source analysis methods have been carried out (Saletu et al. 2002a).

In addition, use of pharmaco-electroencephalographic methods in preclinical studies enable early detection of possible CNS effects of new compounds developed for peripheral target organs. The use of pharmaco-EEG avoids late discovery of CNS toxicity. An anti-inflammatory drug, for example, was first found to produce behavioral abnormalities and epileptic seizures and then was submitted to electroencephalographic investigation, which revealed spike-waves potentials and general slowing (Itil and Itil 1986). For these studies, appropriate experimental designs include single- and repeated-dose administration schedules evaluating the new drug versus placebo and versus other drugs with the same indication.

CLINICAL APPLICATIONS

Pharmaco-electroencephalographic studies using QEEG to identify early predictors of clinical response to psychotropic drugs are of great potential interest to clinical psychiatry. In fact, too often the right drug for the right patient is identified by trial and error and, as a consequence, a delay in the patient's appropriate treatment occurs, with an obvious increase of costs and further deterioration of clinical condition.

Two different approaches can be distinguished within pharmaco-electroencephalographic research attempting to predict clinical response to treatment: 1) studies investigating subjects' pretreatment electroencephalographic characteristics and 2) pharmaco-electroencephalographic studies examining sensu stricto drug-induced electroencephalographic changes occurring early in the course of treatment, even after a single dose of the drug.

In schizophrenia, some authors have described the presence of a "hypernormal" electroencephalogram, characterized by the prevalence of a highly stable and synchronized alpha rhythm. Such a pattern has been found in patients with an unfavorable response to treatment with standard neuroleptics (Czobor and Volavka 1991; Galderisi et al. 1994; Itil et al. 1981). However, it was never demonstrated that pretreatment characteristics of QEEG provide a good discrimination between patients with schizophrenia who do and do not have a favorable response to treatment.

Auditory evoked potentials have also been used to predict clinical response to antidepressant treatment. Hegerl and Juckel (1993) proposed that the loudness dependence of auditory evoked potentials (LDAEP) is a valid indicator of central serotonergic system activity. Patients with a strong LDAEP before treatment show a favorable response to selective serotonin reuptake inhibitors and lithium (Gallinat et al. 2000; Hegerl et al. 1992; Paige et al. 1994).

For neuroleptics, several pharmaco-electroencephalographic studies have been carried out with the aim of identifying early predictors of treatment response. Increased theta and alpha activity in QEEG, more often in the slow alpha range (7.5–9.5 Hz), has been reported in patients with schizophrenia following high-potency neuroleptic administration (Galderisi et al. 1992; Saletu et al. 1986). Several independent groups have reported a relationship between increased alpha activity in QEEG and a favorable clinical response (Jin et al. 1995; Moore et al. 1997; Schellenberg et al. 1994). It has been found that slow alpha changes enable the identification of responders and nonresponders with an overall accuracy ranging from 89.3% to 91.3%, depending on the analyzed sample (Galderisi 2002; Galderisi et al. 1994). Attempts to identify early predictors of response to second-generation antipsychotics have not yielded consistent findings so far (Knott et al. 2001; Mucci et al. 2006). Further studies should consider the opportunity to integrate traditional pharmaco-electroencephalographic indices, such as changes in either absolute or relative power, with topographic and connectivity indices (Lacroix et al. 1995).

Few studies have used the test-dose procedure to predict clinical response to antidepressants and to anxiolytics. Galderisi et al. (1996) used a test-dose procedure to study quantitative electroencephalographic changes associated with clinical response to moclobemide in unipolar depressed patients. A drug-induced increase of beta was found to correlate with the decrease of depression psychopathological ratings observed after 42 days of treatment. Knott et al. (1996) found that depressed patients who responded to imipramine differed from nonresponders in quantitative electroencephalographic theta power before treatment, after a single dose of the drug, and after 2 weeks of active drug treatment. Leuchter and colleagues (Cook and Leuchter 2001; Leuchter et al. 1999) introduced a new QEEG measure, *cordance*, which is correlated with regional cortical perfusion, and suggested the clinical utility of this index in predicting clinical response in major depression.

A quantitative electroencephalographic profile after a single dose of an acetylcholinesterase inhibitor was found to be a good predictor of cognitive modifications in patients with Alzheimer's disease. Quantitative electroencephalographic changes induced by a single dose of tacrine predicted the clinical response to short-term (4 weeks) and medium-term (7–12 weeks) treatment with the same drug (Alhainen et al. 1991; Knott et al. 2000). Responders to tacrine treatment showed a drug-induced increase of alpha and of the alpha-theta ratio, while nonresponders failed to show the same changes.

Saletu et al. (2002b) hypothesized that psychotropic drugs successfully treat patients when the drugs reverse electroencephalographic abnormalities observed in those patients at baseline (a key-lock principle). The hypothesis is attractive and supported by several empirical observations. However, the premise is at odds with the clinical observation that, in some instances (e.g., in treatment with clozapine), the increase of electroencephalographic abnormalities is positively related to favorable clinical response (Koukkou et al. 1979; Stevens et al. 1996) and no normalization of brain functional activity occurs during neuroleptic treatment (Cohen et al. 1997).

In conclusion, quantitative electroencephalographic and evoked-potential indices might represent valuable tools to complement clinical assessment (see also "Evoked Potentials" later in this chapter) and to guide the clinician's choice of appropriate drug treatment. However, much of the available evidence comes from studies including either drug-naïve or drug-free subjects. A largely diffuse application in the clinical routine requires replication of findings in drug-treated populations and a larger number of studies testing drugs that were recently introduced in the clinical practice.

OTHER APPLICATIONS

Further potential clinical applications of electrophysiological techniques include long-term monitoring of CNS drug effects using indices of functional connectivity (e.g., coherence) and defining the threshold at which therapeutic electroencephalographic modifications become toxic electroencephalographic abnormalities. However, none of these applications has received sufficient empirical validation so far.

EVOKED POTENTIALS

The earliest studies of electroencephalograms demonstrated that sensory stimuli provoked a measurable electrophysiological response (Caton 1875). *Event-related potentials* (ERPs) are measured by signal averaging techniques, in which the potentials elicited from repeated stimulation are superimposed by computer analysis. These techniques enhance the stimulus-specific response (i.e., the evoked potential) and cause the background activity to average to zero (Knight 1985).

The development of these techniques quickly led to the characterization of the somatosensory, visual, and brain stem auditory evoked potentials. These potentials, which have well-defined positive and negative peaks and occur within the first 20 msec after the stimulus, represent the electrical activity of the primary neural pathway from the sensory receptor to the cortex. The primary sensory evoked potentials are useful for determining if the sensory pathways are intact. Structural damage, as may result from multiple sclerosis (Levine et al. 1994), or functional impairment, as may result from delirium (Trzepacz et al. 1989), will result in abnormal primary sensory evoked potentials. A logical application of the primary sensory evoked responses (visual, auditory, or somatosensory) is in the assessment of patients with suspected conversion symptoms manifesting in a specific sensory modality. For instance, if an individual is experiencing a total hemianesthesia, his or her somatosensory evoked responses from the affected side should not be normal. Given that extensive research, particularly with longitudinal follow-up of such conditions, is sparse, such findings should be taken as suggestive, and the clinician will have to decide how to utilize the information.

The early mid-latency components (20–50 msec) have not been thoroughly examined. The later middle (50–250 msec or later) and late (250 msec or later) potentials are of particular interest in neuropsychiatry because they represent higher cognitive processes and hence are sensitive to psychological factors such as attention and vigilance. Cognitions take place in milliseconds and are often manifested electrophysiologically in high-frequency cortical activity (Knight 1985).

The late mid-latency auditory evoked responses (MLAERs) have been extensively studied. There are three main components in this range: a positive component occurring between 40 and 80 msec (P50), a negative component occurring between 75 and 150 msec (N100) and a positive component occurring between 150 and 250 msec (P200) (Buchsbaum 1977). The P50 has recently attracted much attention because a deficit in the attenuation of its amplitude with stimulus repetition has been strongly linked with schizophrenia (Bramon et al. 2004).

ERPs index the electrical activity of the neural pathways involved in attention and cognition (Pfefferbaum et al. 1995) and therefore have advantages in the study of information processing. The term *ERP* refers to both the late mid-latency and late components of the evoked response. Several ERPs are named with reference to the experimental condition that elicits the response, such as the contingent negative variation and selective attention effect; others are named for electrophysiological characteristics, such as the P300 (positive wave, 300 msec).

P300

The P300 potential has received a great deal of attention in psychiatric electrophysiology. This potential is elicited when a subject is asked to identify rare target stimuli interspersed with frequent nontarget stimuli. P300 can also be measured in a three-stimulus oddball task, in which subjects are instructed to respond to an infrequent target auditory or visual stimulus that is presented interspersed with frequent nontarget stimuli and infrequent nontarget distractors (Donchin and Coles 1988).

The evidence to date suggests that P300 has several subcomponents generated by multiple neural sources (Johnson 1993; Polich and Kok 1995); the P300 subcomponents P3a and P3b will be discussed here. The P3a is seen when a novel unexpected stimulus is presented. The P3a is thought to be an orienting response that is mediated by frontal structures (Courchesne et al. 1975; Snyder and Hillyard 1976; Squires et al. 1975). The P3a is decreased in subjects with lesions in the prefrontal cortex (Knight 1984), subjects with human immunodeficiency virus (HIV) disease with cognitive impairment (Fein et al. 1995b), and subjects with chronic drug (Biggins et al. 1997) or alcohol (Fein et al. 1995a) abuse. The P3b is seen with attended target stimuli and is mediated by central and parietal structures (Knight et al. 1989). Most studies have reported changes in P300 latency and amplitude associated with different patient groups. P300 latency and amplitude conceptually represent the speed and magnitude of information processing handled by the brain in response to a stimulus.

Several studies have found that patients with schizophrenia have abnormal P300 potentials. The most consistent finding is a reduction in amplitude (Javitt et al. 1995; Levit et al. 1973; Roth et al. 1980). P300 abnormalities are evident in both medicated and drug-free patients and are associated with several clinical features of schizophrenia, including negative symptoms, thought disorder, illness duration, and age at onset (Hirayasu et al. 1998; Mathalon et al. 2000; Pfefferbaum et al. 1989). Asymmetrical auditory P300 reduction has been frequently reported, with smaller amplitudes over the left temporal regions (McCarley et al. 1991, 1993; Salisbury et al. 1998). P300 amplitude reduction or left-lateralized deficit has also been reported in first-degree relatives of patients with schizophrenia, in high-risk subjects, and in psychosis-prone groups (Nuchpongsai et al. 1999). Not all studies, however, have found significant auditory P300 amplitude reductions either bilaterally or asymmetrically (Mathalon et al. 2000; Weisbrod et al. 2000).

P300 abnormalities are not unique to schizophrenia. Interestingly, Kutcher et al. (1987) found that P300 abnormalities were prevalent in patients with borderline personality disorder and could distinguish these patients from those with other personality disorders; however, the P300 abnormalities were indistinguishable from those of patients with schizophrenia. O'Donnell et al. (1995) reported that prolongation of P300 latency, which is normally associated with aging, is exaggerated in subjects with schizophrenia. The researchers suggested that this finding is electrophysiological evidence that schizophrenia is a neurodegenerative disorder. More recently, Mathalon and colleagues (2000) reported that P300 latency is delayed as a function of duration of illness in schizophrenia. The P300 latency is a possible measure of cognitive processing speed (Polich 1996). Javitt et al. (1995) found a reduced amplitude of the mismatch negativity component of the auditory ERP preceding the P300 in schizophrenia subjects. Because the mismatch negativity is the earliest cortical response to stimulus novelty (Kazmerski et al. 1997) and requires frontal lobe involvement, abnormal information processing in schizophrenia may be related to impaired functioning of the frontal cortex.

These findings about P300 abnormalities have been linked to cognitive deficits in schizophrenia. For example, evoked-potential studies of information processing using the P300 response have shown that patients with schizophrenia have difficulties in screening out distracting stimuli (Grillon et al. 1990). This finding is strong support for the hypothesis that persons with schizophrenia have impaired sensorimotor gating or filtering of internal and external stimuli (Braff and Geyer 1990; McGhie and Chapman 1961). P300 abnormalities in patients with schizophrenia have been found to be correlated with left sylvian fissure enlargement on computed tomography scans, as well as with positive symptoms (McCarley et al. 1989). Additional studies are needed to validate the correlational data so far obtained in addition to clarifying inconsistencies in the reported findings. In the most comprehensive meta-analysis of P300 in schizophrenia published to date, Jeon and Polich (2003) address most of these issues and provide a theoretical framework for further studies. These investigators further conclude that stimulus parameters, task conditions, and measurement methods need to be better established empirically before clinical applications can become a reliable index of disease state.

As mentioned above, P300 abnormalities are not exclusive to schizophrenia. Polich (2004) suggested that the P300 can provide information about cognition that is quantitatively comparable to other clinically used biomedical assays. Causes of P300 variability regarding task and biological determinants have been well characterized so that refinement of P300 assessment methods for clinical applications is possible.

The relationship between posttraumatic stress disorder (PTSD) and P300 has been studied in several reports. Studies have found P300 amplitude to be both increased and decreased in subjects with PTSD relative to control subjects without PTSD. The studies that found decreases in P300 amplitude attributed the results to concentration and memory impairments (McFarlane et al. 1993) or attention deficits (Charles et al. 1995; Metzger et al. 1997). Those investigators finding increases in P300 amplitude suggest that their results are due to altered selective attention (Attias et al. 1996), heightened neurophysiological response (Kounios et al. 1997), or heightened orienting response (Kimble et al. 2000). Except for Kimball et al. (2000), all of the studies that found a reduced P300 in subjects with PTSD utilized the auditory modality (Charles et al. 1995; McFarlane et al. 1993; Metzger et al. 1997), whereas those studies finding an increased P300 in PTSD were conducted in the visual modality (Attias et al. 1996; Kounios et al. 1997). These findings raise the question of whether information processing abnormalities, as indexed by the P300 component, are modality specific.

Middle (e.g., P50) and late (e.g., P300) evoked potentials may provide important insights to the physiology of attention, categorization, and filtering of sensory stimuli. However, unlike the earlier peaks, these potentials are more prone to experimental artifact. Motivation, level of consciousness, medications, sensory acuity, and movement artifact all can confound the data (Rosse et al. 1989).

POLYSOMNOGRAPHY

Among neuropsychiatrists, interest in the study of sleep began with a fascination about dreams. Griesinger (1868) speculated that dreams were occurring when sleeping subjects had eye movements. Freud (1895/1954) suggested that dreaming was associated with profound relaxation to prevent the physical expression of dreams. Eight years after the first published human electroencephalographic study, the first all-night electroencephalographic study showed that sleep was composed of discrete stages (Loomis et al. 1937). Then, Aserinsky and Kleitman

TABLE 5–4.   Physiological variables frequently recorded during polysomnography

Physiological variable	Recording medium (utility)
Sleep stage	Electroencephalogram (multiple leads may be used to diagnose sleep-associated seizures)
Eye movements	Electro-oculogram (helpful in defining Stage I and REM sleep and in detecting eye movement artifact in the electroencephalographic signal)
Muscle contractions	Electromyogram Submentalis (detects muscle atonia seen in REM sleep) Anterior tibialis (detects periodic leg movements [nocturnal myoclonus]) Intercostal and diaphragm (detects respiratory effort)
Respiratory effort	Thoracic or abdominal strain gauge Esophageal pressure balloon
Nasal and oral airflow	Throat microphone (detects snoring) Nasal or oral thermistors (helps in diagnosing sleep apnea)
Oxygen saturation	Oximetry
Carbon dioxide content	Transcutaneous carbon dioxide monitor
Cardiac rate and arrhythmias	Electrocardiogram
Sleeping position	Video camera (documents presence of abnormal movements)
Nocturnal penile tumescence	Penile strain gauges
Gastroesophageal reflux	Esophageal pH probe

Note.   REM = rapid eye movement.

(1953) discovered and electrographically characterized rapid eye movement (REM) sleep. Since that discovery, there has been a tremendous growth in sleep research as well as the emergence of the field of sleep medicine. Perhaps the most important result of this development has been the recognition that symptoms of insomnia and excessive sleepiness have broad differential diagnoses and warrant a thorough assessment.

Polysomnography remains the principal diagnostic tool in the field of sleep medicine. The term *polysomnography* is progressively becoming ambiguous because the physiological variables that can be measured during all-night recordings are numerous (Table 5–4). A thorough polysomnographic study provides data on sleep continuity, sleep architecture, REM sleep physiology, sleep-related respiratory impairment, oxygen desaturation, cardiac arrhythmias, and periodic movements. Additional measures may include nocturnal penile tumescence and temperature and infrared video monitoring. For a detailed discussion of sleep disorders, please see Chapter 17, "Neuropsychiatric Aspects of Sleep and Sleep Disorders."

Quantitative analysis of sleep EEG has been utilized to characterize sleep microarchitecture in depressed subjects (Armitage et al. 1992; Reynolds and Kupfer 1987). These studies have utilized spectral analysis and period amplitude analysis to describe differences in delta-wave activity in depressed subjects compared with healthy and psychiatric control subjects (Armitage 1995). These two techniques complement each other by yielding different quantitative information about the electroencephalographic signal. Spectral analysis is achieved through fast Fourier transform, a frequency-domain technique that combines information about wave amplitude and incidence into power spectra for all frequency components. *Period amplitude analysis* is a time-domain technique that measures amplitude and counts EEG frequencies within predetermined bandwidths (Armitage 1995; Reynolds and Brunner 1995). Both techniques have a high degree of overlap (Pigeau et al. 1981). Quantitative electroencephalographic studies in the sleep electroencephalogram have shown that diminished interhemispheric and intrahemispheric coherence is associated with major depression, suggesting an underlying disturbance of ultradian regulation of electroencephalographic rhythms (Fulton et al. 2000).

The majority of psychiatric disorders are accompanied by subjective and objective sleep disturbances. For the most part, however, the findings are relatively nonspecific and the cost of studies remains too high for routine clinical diagnostic and/or prognostic use. Where sleep studies are likely to become clinically useful in the foreseeable future is in the workup of mood disorders. A number of review articles outlined the sleep architectural abnormalities frequently associated with mood disorders. The sensitivity and specificity of electroencephalographic sleep-measure abnormalities as markers of depression vary according to the criteria value used, the statistical analysis utilized, and the reference groups included (Buysse and Kupfer 1990). Polysomnography, on the other hand, can be quite useful in differentiating nocturnal nonepileptic attacks from epileptic seizures (Roberts 1998).

ACTIVITY MONITORING

Motion activity monitoring (actigraphy) is increasingly being used in studies of sleep-wake patterns. Wrist-worn activity monitors provide continuous activity data using a battery-operated wristwatch-size microprocessor that senses motion and detects movement in all three axes. A signal is generated that is processed and stored in the unit's memory. Frequency, sensitivity, and threshold parameters are adjustable, and data can be stored in an ASCII file according to specified time intervals that range from 1 second to 1 hour. There is also an event marker for participants to indicate "lights out" and "lights on" time, as well as other salient events. The unit weighs 2 ounces and is worn comfortably around the wrist. Data can be presented in the form of percentage of time spent awake and asleep for a variety of time frames.

There is an excellent correlation (0.89–0.98) between polysomnographic and actigraphic estimates of sleep time in healthy persons (Kripke et al. 1978; Mullaney et al. 1980). Furthermore, actigraphy allows for an extended period of data collection in the home environment. In addition, actigraphy is excellent for detecting longitudinal changes or treatment effects (Brooks et al. 1993; Chambers 1994). A principal disadvantage of actigraphy is that it is not a true measure of sleep and does not give information about sleep architecture. Furthermore, the actigraphic accuracy in estimating sleep time diminishes the more disturbed the sleep is (Hauri and Wisbey 1994; B. Levine et al. 1986), and actigraphy may have some disadvantages in disorders associated with increased nocturnal locomotor activity. Sadeh et al. (1995) have emphasized the need to conduct validation studies of actigraphic sleep assessment in specific populations' natural environments.

MAGNETOENCEPHALOGRAPHY

Magnetoencephalography (MEG) is the recording of the magnetic fields generated by intraneuronal electric current. The *right-hand rule* of electromagnetism is that magnetic fields occur at right angles to the direction of current flow (Zimmerman 1983). Thus the magnetoencephalographic signal, which is a billionfold weaker than the earth's magnetic field (Reeve et al. 1989), can be conceptualized as the magnetic counterpart to the electroencephalographic or evoked-potential signal. MEG naturally complements EEG and has potential advantages in localization and a broader range in frequency resolution (Cuffin and Cohen 1979; Rose et al. 1987). Magnetic fields are not appreciably affected by the scalp and skull. For example, high frequencies are poorly resolved by scalp electrodes in EEG (Pfurtscheller and Cooper 1975) but may be better detected with MEG. MEG is also more accurate in detecting deep-brain sources and can detect tangential current sources, such as from neurons in the sulci, whose axial orientation is parallel to the scalp (Reite et al. 1989). The recent availability of large-array superconducting biomagnetometer systems has made MEG a feasible diagnostic test to perform (Gallen et al. 1995). Perhaps its greatest promise is to accurately detect the neuronal sources of known electroencephalographic and evoked-potential signals (Reeve et al. 1989; Reite et al. 1989) and to more precisely localize epileptic foci in the brain (Baumgartner et al. 2000). Magnetic source imaging, which combines MEG with anatomical MRI, has been used to produce neuromagnetic maps of somatosensory and auditory evoked potentials in healthy subjects (Gallen et al. 1993). Magnetic source imaging is also used to evaluate seizure foci in patients who are neurosurgical candidates (Aung et al. 1995). The principal disadvantage of MEG is that the magnetometer must contend with a low signal-to-noise ratio, necessitating the use of expensive shielding to eliminate ambient magnetic noise.

CONCLUSION

Neuropsychiatric electrophysiology continues to be a powerful clinical and research tool. It remains one of the few noninvasive probes of brain function. The future advances in this field will likely come from combining quantitative electrophysiological data with anatomical imaging obtained from well-defined clinical populations and well-selected control groups. The clinical applicability of quantitative electroencephalographic and electrophysiological techniques continues to hold much promise.

Highlights for the Clinician

Testing modality	Indications	Caveats
Standard EEG	✦ With episodic behavior (e.g., aggression or panic attacks), epileptic discharges may be seen and may indicate that a trial of anticonvulsant is warranted.	✦ Sleep must be attained before the study is considered negative.
QEEG	✦ To detect subtle abnormalities. Could be useful in evaluating cases of postconcussive syndrome. ✦ QEEG is likely to become very useful in psychiatry, and clinicians should stay abreast of developments in this area.	✦ Requires specialized training for analysis and interpretation
Evoked potentials	✦ To test the integrity of the sensory pathways.	
Cognitive evoked potentials	✦ Could be used to assess attentional and cognitive capacity.	✦ Requires specialized laboratories
All-night EEG	✦ Could be used to assess nocturnal episodes (to differentiate panic from epileptic attacks).	
Pharmaco-EEG	✦ To predict clinical response using a test dose of a psychotropic medication.	✦ An evolving field; clinicians should stay abreast of developments.

Note.   EEG = electroencephalography; QEEG = quantitative electroencephalography.

RECOMMENDED READINGS

Coburn KL, Lauterbach EC, Boutros NN, et al: The value of quantitative electroencephalography in clinical psychiatry: a report by the committee on research of the American Neuropsychiatric Association. J Neuropsychiatry Clin Neurosci 18:460–500, 2006

Duffy FH: Long latency evoked potential database for clinical applications: justification and examples. Clin EEG Neurosci 36:88–98, 2005

Niedermeyer E, Lopes da Silva F: Electroencephalography: Basic Principles, Clinical Applications and Related Fields. Baltimore, MD, Lippincott Williams & Wilkins, 2005

REFERENCES

Abraham HD, Duffy FH: Computed EEG abnormalities in panic disorder with and without premorbid drug abuse. Biol Psychiatry 29:687–690, 1991

Abrams R, Taylor MA: Laboratory studies in the validation of psychiatric diagnoses, in Hemisphere Asymmetries of Function in Psychopathology. Edited by Gruzelier JH, Flor-Henry P. New York, Elsevier North-Holland, 1979, pp 363–372

Adams DC, Heyer EJ, Emerson RG, et al: The reliability of quantitative electroencephalography as an indicator of cerebral ischemia. Anesth Analg 81:80–83, 1995

Alhainen K, Partanen J, Reinikainen K, et al: Discrimination of tetrahydroaminoacridine responders by a single dose pharmaco-EEG in patients with Alzheimer's disease. Neurosci Lett, 127:113–116, 1991

American Psychiatric Association: Diagnostic and Statistical Manual of Mental Disorders, 3rd Edition, Revised. Washington, DC, American Psychiatric Association, 1987

Aminoff MJ: Electroencephalography: general principles and clinical applications, in Electrodiagnosis in Clinical Neurology. Edited by Aminoff MJ. New York, Churchill Livingstone, 1986, pp 21–75

Andersen P, Andersson SA: Physiologic Basis of the Alpha Rhythm. New York, Appleton-Century-Crofts, 1968

Anderson VE, Hauser WA, Rich SS: Genetic heterogeneity and epidemiology of the epilepsies. Adv Neurol 79:59–73, 1999

Armitage R: Microarchitectural findings in sleep EEG in depression: diagnostic implications. Biol Psychiatry 37:72–84, 1995

Armitage R, Roffwarg HP, Rush AJ, et al: Digital period analysis of sleep EEG in depression. Biol Psychiatry 31:52–68, 1992

Aserinsky E, Kleitman N: Regularly occurring periods of eye motility and concomitant phenomena during sleep. Science 118:273–274, 1953

Attias J, Bleich A, Furman V, et al: Event-related potentials in post-traumatic stress disorder of combat origin. Biol Psychiatry 40:373–381, 1996

Aung M, Sobel DF, Gallen CC, et al: Potential contribution of bilateral magnetic source imaging to the evaluation of epilepsy surgery candidates. Neurosurgery 37:1113–1120, 1995

Baumgartner C, Pataraia E, Lindinger G, et al: Magnetoencephalography in focal epilepsy. Epilepsia 41 (suppl 3):S39–S47, 2000

Berger H: Uber das Elektrenkephalogramm des Menschen. Archiv fur Psychiatrie und Nervenkrankheiten 87:527–570, 1929

Berger H: Uber das Elektroencephalogramm des Menschen. VIII. Mitteilung. Archiv fur Psychiatrie und Nervenkrankheiten 101:452–469, 1933

Biggins CA, MacKay S, Clark W: Event-related potential evidence for frontal cortex effects of chronic cocaine dependence. Biol Psych 42:472–485, 1997

Boelhouwer C, Henry C, Glueck BC Jr: Positive spiking: a double-blind control study on its significance in behavior disorders, both diagnostically and therapeutically. Am J Psychiatry 125:473–480, 1968

Boutros NN: The American Psychiatric Electrophysiology Association (APEA): history and mission. Clin Electroencephalogr 31:67–70, 2000

Boutros NN, Struve F: Electrophysiological assessment of neuropsychiatric disorders. Semin Clin Neuropsychiatry 7:30–41, 2002

Boutros N, Fraenkel L, Feingold A: A four-step approach for developing diagnostic tests in psychiatry: EEG in ADHD as a test case. J Neuropsychiatry Clin Neurosci 17:455–464, 2005a

Boutros N, Mirolo HA, Struve F: Normative data for the unquantified EEG: examination of adequacy for neuropsychiatric research. J Neuropsychiatry Clin Neurosci 17:84–90, 2005b

Braff DL, Geyer MA: Sensorimotor gating and schizophrenia. Arch Gen Psychiatry 47:181–188, 1990

Bramon E, Rabe-Hesketh S, Sham P, et al: Meta-analysis of the P300 and P50 waveforms in schizophrenia. Schizophr Res 70:315–329, 2004

Brazier MAB: The emergence of electrophysiology as an aid to neurology, in Electrodiagnosis in Clinical Neurology. Edited by Aminoff MJ. New York, Churchill Livingstone, 1986, pp 1–19

Bresnahan SM, Anderson JW, Barry RJ: Age-related changes in quantitative EEG in attention-deficit/hyperactivity disorder. Biol Psychiatry 46:1690–1697, 1999

Brodie JD: Imaging for the clinical psychiatrist: facts, fantasies, and other musings. Am J Psychiatry 153:145–149, 1996

Brooks JO III, Friedman L, Bliwise DL, et al: Use of the wrist actigraph to study insomnia in older adults. Sleep 16:151–155, 1993

Bruder GE, Fong R, Tenke CE, et al: Regional brain asymmetries in major depression with or without an anxiety disorder: a quantitative electroencephalographic study. Biol Psychiatry 41:939–948, 1997

Bruns DE: The STARD initiative and the reporting of studies of diagnostic accuracy. Clin Chemistry 49:19–20, 2003

Bucci P, Mucci A, Volpe U, et al: Executive hypercontrol in obsessive-compulsive disorder: electrophysiological and neuropsychological indices. Clin Neurophysiol 115:1340–1348, 2004

Buchsbaum MS: The middle evoked response components and schizophrenia. Schizophr Bull 3:93–104, 1977

Buysse DJ, Kupfer DJ: Diagnostic and research applications of electroencephalographic sleep studies in depression: conceptual and methodological issues. J Nerv Ment Dis 178:405–414, 1990

Bystritsky A, Leuchter AF, Vapnik T: EEG abnormalities in nonmedicated panic disorder. J Nerv Ment Dis 187:113–114, 1999

Caton R: The electric currents of the brain. BMJ 2:278, 1875

Chabot RJ, Merkin H, Wood LM, et al: Sensitivity and specificity of QEEG in children with attention deficit or specific developmental learning disorders. Clin Electroencephalogr 27:26–34, 1996

Chabot RJ, di Michele F, Prichep L, et al: The clinical role of computerized EEG in the evaluation and treatment of learning and attention disorders in children and adolescents. J Neuropsychiatry Clin Neurosci 13:171–186, 2001

Chambers MJ: Actigraphy and insomnia: a closer look, 1. Sleep 17:405–408, 1994

Charles G, Hansenne M, Ansseau M, et al: P300 in posttraumatic stress disorder. Neuropsychobiology 32:72–74, 1995

Clarke AR, Barry RJ, McCarthy R, et al: EEG analysis in attention-deficit/hyperactivity disorder: a comparative study of two subtypes. Psychiatr Res 81:19–29, 1998

Clarke AR, Barry RJ, McCarthy R, et al: EEG-defined subtypes of children with attention-deficit/hyperactivity disorder. Clin Neurophysiol 112:2098–2105, 2001

Clementz BA, Sponheim SR, Iacono WG, et al: Resting EEG in first-episode schizophrenia patients, bipolar psychosis patients, and their first-degree relatives. Psychophysiology 31:486–494, 1994

Cohen RM, Nordahl TE, Semple WE, et al: The brain metabolic patterns of clozapine- and fluphenazine-treated patients with schizophrenia during a continuous performance task. Arch Gen Psychiatry 54:481–486, 1997

Cook IA, Leuchter AF: Prefrontal changes and treatment response prediction in depression. Semin Clin Neuropsychiatry 6:113–120, 2001

Cooper R, Winter AL, Crow HJ, et al: Comparison of subcortical, cortical and scalp activity using chronically indwelling electrodes in man. Electroencephalogr Clin Neurophysiol 18:217–228, 1965

Courchesne E, Hillyard SA, Galambos R: Stimulus novelty, task relevance and the visual evoked potential in man. Electroencephalogr Clin Neurophysiol 39:131–143, 1975

Cuffin BN, Cohen D: Comparison of the magnetoencephalogram and electroencephalogram. Electroencephalogr Clin Neurophysiol 47:132–146, 1979

Cunningham MG, Price BH: Architecture of neuropsychiatric disease: highlights of the 15th Annual Meeting of the American Neuropsychiatric Association, February 21–24, 2004, Bal Harbour, FL. Rev Neurol Dis 1:202–206, 2004

Czobor P, Volavka J: Pretreatment EEG predicts short-term response to haloperidol treatment. Biol Psychiatry 30:927–942, 1991

Deisenhammer E, Jellinger K: EEG in senile dementia. Electroencephalogr Clin Neurophysiol 36:91, 1974

Denays R, Makhoul E, Dachy B, et al: Electroencephalographic mapping and 99mTc HMPAO single photon emission computed tomography in carbon monoxide poisoning. Ann Emerg Med 24:947–952, 1994

Dierks T, Maurer K, Ihl R, et al: Evaluation and interpretation of topographic EEG data in schizophrenic patients, in Topographic Brain Mapping of EEG and Evoked Potentials. Edited by Maurer K. Berlin-Heidelberg, Springer-Verlag, 1989, pp 507–517

Donchin E, Coles MG: Is the P300 component a manifestation of context updating? Behav Brain Sci 11:357–427, 1988

Duff J: The usefulness of quantitative EEG (QEEG) and neurotherapy in the assessment and treatment of post-concussion syndrome. Clin EEG Neurosci 35:198–209, 2004

Duffy FH: Topographic Mapping of Brain Electrical Activity. Boston, MA, Butterworth, 1986

Duffy FH: Issues facing the clinical use of brain electrical activity mapping, in Functional Brain Imaging. Edited by Pfurtscheller G, Lopes da Silva FH. Toronto, ON, Hans Huber, 1988, pp 149–160

Edmonds HL Jr, Griffiths LK, van der Laken J, et al: Quantitative electroencephalographic monitoring during myocardial revascularization predicts postoperative disorientation and improves outcome (comments). J Thorac Cardiovasc Surg 103:555–563, 1992

Fein G, Biggins CA, MacKay S: Alcohol abuse and HIV infection have additive effects on frontal cortex function as measured by auditory evoked potential P3A latency. Biol Psychiatry 37:183–195, 1995a

Fein G, Biggins CA, MacKay S: Delayed latency of the event-related brain potential P3A component in HIV disease: progressive effects with increasing cognitive impairment. Arch Neurol 52:1109–1118, 1995b

Fenton GW: The electrophysiology of Alzheimer's disease. Br Med Bull 42:29–33, 1986

Fenton GW: The EEG in neuropsychiatry, in The Bridge Between Neurology and Psychiatry. Edited by Reynolds EH, Trimble MR. Edinburgh, UK, Churchill Livingstone, 1989, pp 302–333

Fink M: Quantitative electroencephalography in human psychopharmacology, II: drug patterns, in EEG and Behavior. Edited by Glaser GH. New York, Basic Books, 1963, pp 177–197

Fink M: EEG profiles and bioavailability measures of psychoactive drugs, in Psychotropic Drugs and the Human EEG (Modern Problems in Pharmacopsychiatry, Vol 8). Edited by Itil TM. New York, Karger, 1974, pp 43–75

Flor-Henry P: Lateralized temporal-limbic dysfunction and psychopathology. Ann N Y Acad Sci 280:777–797, 1976

Freud S: Project for a scientific psychology (1895), in The Origins of Psychoanalysis: Letters to Wilhelm Fliess, Drafts and Notes, 1887–1902. Edited by Bonaparte M, Freud A, Kres E. New York, Basic Books, 1954, p 400

Freudenreich O, Weiner RD, McEvoy JP: Clozapine-induced electroencephalogram changes as a function of clozapine serum levels. Biol Psychiatry 42:132–137, 1997

Fulton MK, Armitage R, Rush AJ: Sleep electroencephalographic coherence abnormalities in individuals at high risk for depression: a pilot study. Biol Psychiatry 47:618–625, 2000

Galderisi S: Clinical applications of pharmaco-EEG in psychiatry: the prediction of response to treatment with antipsychotics. Methods Find Exp Clin Pharmacol 24 (suppl C):85–89, 2002

Galderisi S, Mucci A, Mignone ML, et al: CEEG mapping in drug-free schizophrenics: differences from healthy subjects and changes induced by haloperidol treatment. Schizophr Res 6:15–24, 1992

Galderisi S, Maj M, Mucci A, et al: QEEG alpha1 changes after a single dose of high potency neuroleptics as a predictor of short term response to treatment in schizophrenic patients. Biol Psychiatry 35:367–374, 1994

Galderisi S, Mucci A, Bucci P, et al: Influence of moclobemide on cognitive functions of nine depressed patients: pilot trial with neurophysiological and neuropsychological indices. Neuropsychobiology 33:48–54, 1996

Gallen CC, Sobel DF, Lewine JD, et al: Neuromagnetic mapping of brain function. Radiology 187:863–867, 1993

Gallen CC, Hirschkoff EC, Buchanan DS: Magnetoencephalography and magnetic source imaging: capabilities and limitations. Neuroimaging Clin N Am 5:227–249, 1995

Gallinat J, Bottlender R, Juckel G, et al: The loudness dependency of the auditory evoked N1/P2 component as a predictor of the acute SSRI response in depression. Psychopharmacology 148:404–411, 2000

Gattaz W, Mayer S, Ziegler P, et al: Hypofrontality on topographic EEG in schizophrenia: correlations with neuropsychological and psychopathological parameters. Eur Arch Psychiatry Clin Neurosci 241:328–332, 1992

Gelisse P, Samuelian JC, Genton P: Is schizophrenia a risk factor for epilepsy or acute symptomatic seizures? Epilepsia 40:1566–1571, 1999

Gibbs FA, Davis H, Lennox WG: The electroencephalogram in epilepsy and in conditions of impaired consciousness. Arch Neurol Psychiatry 34:1133–1135, 1935

Goff WR, Allison T, Vaughan HG: The functional neuroanatomy of event-related potentials, in Event-Related Potentials in Man. Edited by Callaway E, Tueting P, Koslow SH. New York, Academic Press, 1978, pp 1–79

Goldensohn ES: Neurophysiologic substrates of EEG activity, in Current Practice of Electroencephalography. Edited by Klass DW, Daly DD. New York, Raven Press, 1979, pp 421–439

Goodin DS, Aminoff MJ: Does the interictal EEG have a role in the diagnosis of epilepsy? Lancet 1:837, 1984

Grass AM, Gibbs FA: A Fourier transform of the electroencephalogram. J Neurophysiol 1:521–526, 1938

Griesinger W: Berliner medicinisch-psychologische Gesellschaft. Archiv für Psychiatrie und Nervenkrankeiten 1:200–204, 1868

Grillon C, Courchesne E, Ameli R, et al: Increased distractibility in schizophrenic patients. Arch Gen Psychiatry 47:171–179, 1990

Gruzelier J, Liddiard D: The neuropsychology of schizophrenia in the context of topographical mapping of electrocortical activity, in Topographic Brain Mapping of EEG and Evoked Potentials. Edited by Maurer K. Berlin, Springer-Verlag, 1989, pp 421–437

Gueguen B, Etevenon P, Plancon D, et al: EEG mapping in pathological aging and dementia: utility for diagnosis and therapeutic evaluation, in Topographic Brain Mapping of EEG and Evoked Potentials. Edited by Maurer K. Berlin, Springer-Verlag, 1989, pp 219–225

Guenther W, Breitling D, Banquet JP, et al: EEG mapping of left hemisphere dysfunction during motor performance in schizophrenia. Biol Psychiatry 21:249–262, 1986

Hakola HP, Laulumaa VA: Carbamazepine in the treatment of violent schizophrenics. Lancet 1:1358, 1982

Harper MA, Morris M, Bleyerveld J: The significance of an abnormal EEG in psychopathic personalities. Aust N Z J Psychiatry 6:215–224, 1972

Hauri PJ, Wisbey J: Actigraphy and insomnia: a closer look. Part 2. Sleep 17:408–410, 1994

Hegerl U, Juckel G: Intensity dependence of auditory evoked potentials as an indicator of central serotonergic neurotransmission: a new hypothesis. Biol Psychiatry 33:173–187, 1993

Hegerl U, Wulff H, Muller-Oerlinghausen B: Intensity dependence of auditory evoked potentials and clinical response to prophylactic lithium medication: a replication study. Psychiatry Res 44:181–190, 1992

Herrmann W: Development and critical evaluation of an objective procedure for the electroencephalographic classification of psychotropic drugs, in Electroencephalography in Drug Research. Edited by Herrmann WM. Stuttgart, Fischer, 1982, pp 249–351

Hirayasu Y, Asato N, Ohta H, et al: Abnormalities of auditory event-related potentials in schizophrenia prior to treatment. Biol Psychiatry 43:244–253, 1998

Howard RC: The clinical EEG and personality in mentally abnormal offenders. Psychol Med 14:569–580, 1984

Hughes JR, John E: Conventional and quantitative electroencephalography in psychiatry. J Neuropsychiatry Clin Neurosci 11:190–208, 1999

Hughes JR, Wilson WP (eds): EEG and Evoked Potentials in Psychiatry and Behavioral Neurology. Boston, MA, Butterworths, 1983

Hughes JR, DeLeo AJ, Melyn MA: The electroencephalogram in attention deficit-hyperactivity disorder: emphasis on epileptiform discharges. Epilepsy Behav 1:271–277, 2000

Inui K, Motomura E, Okushima R, et al: Electroencephalographic findings in patients with DSM-IV mood disorder, schizophrenia, and other psychotic disorders. Biol Psychiatry 43:69–75, 1998

Itil TM: Qualitative and quantitative EEG findings in schizophrenia. Schizophr Bull 3:61–79, 1977

Itil TM: The use of electroencephalography in the practice of psychiatry. Psychosomatics 23:799–813, 1982

Itil TM, Itil KZ: The significance of pharmacodynamic measurement in the assessment of bioavailability and bioequivalence of psychotropic drugs using CEEG and dynamic brain mapping. J Clin Psychiatry 47(suppl):20–27, 1986

Itil TM, Shapiro DM, Schneider SJ, et al: Computerized EEG as a predictor of drug response in treatment resistant schizophrenics. J Nerv Ment Dis 169:629–637, 1981

Jabourian AP, Erlich M, Desvignes C, et al: Panic-attacks and 24-hour ambulatory EEG monitoring. Ann Med Psychol 150:240–245, 1992

Jasper HH: The ten-twenty electrode system of the International Federation. Electroencephalogr Clin Neurophysiol 10:371–375, 1958

Javitt DC, Doneshka P, Grochowski S, et al: Impaired mismatch negativity generation reflects widespread dysfunction of working memory in schizophrenia. Arch Gen Psychiatry 52:550–558, 1995

Jeon YW, Polich J: Meta-analysis of P300 and schizophrenia: patients, paradigms, and practical implications. Psychophysiology 40:684–701, 2003

Jin Y, Potkin SG, Sandman C: Clozapine increases EEG photic driving in clinical responders. Schizophr Bull 21:263–268, 1995

Jobst BC, Williamson PD: Frontal lobe seizures. Psychiatr Clin North Am 28:635–651, 2005

John ER, Karmel BZ, Corning WC, et al: Neurometrics: numerical taxonomy identifies different profiles of brain functions within groups of behaviorally similar people. Science 196:1393–1410, 1977

John ER, Prichep LS, Fridman J: Neurometrics: computer assisted differential diagnosis of brain dysfunctions. Science 293:162–169, 1988

John ER, Prichep LS, Alper KR, et al: Quantitative electrophysiological characteristics and subtyping of schizophrenia. Biol Psychiatry 36:801–826, 1994

Johnson R: On the neural generators of the P300 component of the event-related potential. Psychophysiology 30:90–97, 1993

Kalin NH, Shelton SE, Davidson RJ: Cerebrospinal fluid corticotropin-releasing hormone levels are elevated in monkeys with patterns of brain activity associated with fearful temperament. Biol Psychiatry 47:579–585, 2000

Karson CN, Coppola R, Morihisa JM, et al: Computed electroencephalographic activity mapping in schizophrenia. Arch Gen Psychiatry 44:514–517, 1987

Kaufman PY: Electrical phenomenon in cerebral cortex. Obzory Psikhiatrii Nevrologii i Eksperimental'noi Psikhologii 7–8:403, 1912

Kazmerski VA, Friedman D, Ritter W: Mismatch negativity during attend and ignore conditions in Alzheimer's disease. Biol Psychiatry 42:382–402, 1997

Kendler KS, Hays P: Familial and sporadic schizophrenia: a symptomatic, prognostic, and EEG comparison. Am J Psychiatry 139:1557–1562, 1982

Khanna S: Obsessive-compulsive disorder: is there a frontal lobe dysfunction? Biol Psychiatry 24:602–613, 1988

Khoshbin S: The history of the Electroencephalography and Clinical Neuroscience Society (ECNS). Part I: A brief history of the American Medical Electroencephalographic Association (AMEEGA). Clin Electroencephalogr 31:63–66, 2000

Kikuchi M, Wada Y, Higashima M, et al: Individual analysis of EEG band power and clinical drug response in schizophrenia. Neuropsychobiology 51:183–190, 2005

Kimble M, Kaloupek D, Kaufman M, et al: Stimulus novelty differentially affects attentional allocation in PTSD. Biol Psychiatry 47:880–890, 2000

Knight RT: Decreased response to novel stimuli after prefrontal lesions in man. Electroencephalogr Clin Neurophysiol 59:9–20, 1984

Knight RT: Electrophysiology in behavioral neurology, in Principles of Behavioral Neurology. Edited by Mesulam M-M. Philadelphia, PA, FA Davis, 1985, pp 327–346

Knight R, Scabini D, Woods D, et al: Contributions of temporal-parietal junction to the human auditory P3. Brain Res 502:109–116, 1989

Knott VJ, Telner JI, Lapierre YD, et al: Quantitative EEG in the prediction of antidepressant response to imipramine. J Affect Disord 39:175–184, 1996

Knott V, Mohr E, Mahoney C, et al: Pharmaco-EEG test dose response predicts cholinesterase inhibitor treatment outcome in Alzheimer's disease. Methods Find Exp Clin Pharmacol 22:115–122, 2000

Knott V, Labelle A, Jones B, et al: Quantitative EEG in schizophrenia and in response to acute and chronic clozapine treatment. Schizophr Res 50:41–53, 2001

Korn A, Golan H, Melamed I, et al: Focal cortical dysfunction and blood-brain barrier disruption in patients with Postconcussion syndrome. J Clin Neurophysiol 22:1–9, 2005

Koukkou M, Angst J, Zimmer D: Paroxysmal EEG activity and psychopathology during the treatment with clozapine. Pharmakopsychiatr Neuropsychopharmakol 12:173–183, 1979

Kounios J, Litz B, Kaloupek D, et al: Electrophysiology of combat-related PTSD. Ann N Y Acad Sci 821:504–507, 1997

Kripke DF, Mullaney DJ, Messin S, et al: Wrist actigraphic measures of sleep and rhythms. Electroencephalogr Clin Neurophysiol 44:674–676, 1978

Kristensen O, Sindrup EH: Psychomotor epilepsy and psychosis II: electroencephalographic findings (sphenoidal electrode recordings). Acta Neurol Scand 57:370–379, 1978

Kutcher SP, Blackwood DHR, St Clair D, et al: Auditory P300 in borderline personality disorder and schizophrenia. Arch Gen Psychiatry 44:645–650, 1987

Lacroix D, Chaput Y, Rodriguez JP, et al: Quantified EEG changes associated with a positive clinical response to clozapine in schizophrenia. Prog Neuropsychopharmacol Biol Psychiatry 19:861–876, 1995

Lam RW, Hurwitz TA, Wada JA: The clinical use of EEG in a general psychiatric setting. Hospital and Community Psychiatry 39:533–536, 1988

Lehmann D, Faber PL, Galderisi S, et al: EEG microstate duration and syntax in acute, medication-naive, first-episode schizophrenia: a multi-center study. Psychiatry Res 138:141–156, 2005

Leuchter AF, Spar JE, Walter DO, et al: Electroencephalographic spectra and coherence in the diagnosis of Alzheimer's type and multi-infarct dementia. Arch Gen Psychiatry 44:993–998, 1987

Leuchter AF, Uijtdehaage SH, Cook IA, et al: Relationship between brain electrical activity and cortical perfusion in normal subjects. Psychiatry Res 90:125–140, 1999

Levine B, Moyles T, Roehrs T, et al: Actigraphic monitoring and polygraphic recording in determination of sleep and wake, in Sleep Research, Vol 15. Edited by Chase MH, McGinty DJ, Crane G. Los Angeles, CA, UCLA Brain Information Service/Brain Research Institute, 1986, p 247

Levine RA, Gardner JC, Fullerton BC, et al: Multiple sclerosis lesions of the auditory pons are not silent. Brain 117:1127–1141, 1994

Levit AL, Sutton S, Zubin J: Evoked potential correlates of information processing in psychiatric patients. Psychol Med 3:487–494, 1973

Lifshitz K, Gradijan J: Spectral evaluation of the electroencephalogram: power and variability in chronic schizophrenics and control subjects. Psychophysiology 11:479–490, 1974

Loomis AL, Harvey EN, Hobart GA: Cerebral states during sleep, as studied by human brain potentials. J Exp Psychol 21:127–144, 1937

Luchins DJ: Carbamazepine in violent non-epileptic schizophrenics. Psychopharmacol Bull 20:569–571, 1984

Mathalon DH, Ford JM, Rosenbloom M, et al: P300 reduction and prolongation with illness duration in schizophrenia. Biol Psychiatry 47:413–427, 2000

Matousek M, Petersen I: Norms for the EEG, in Automation of Clinical Electroencephalography. Edited by Kellaway P, Petersen I. New York, Raven Press, 1973, pp 75–102

Matsushima E, Nakajima K, Moriya H, et al: A psychophysiological study of the development of delirium in coronary care units. Biol Psychiatry 41:1211–1217, 1997

McCarley RW, Faux SF, Shenton M, et al: CT abnormalities in schizophrenia: a preliminary study of their correlations with P300/P200 electrophysiological features and positive/negative symptoms. Arch Gen Psychiatry 46:698–708, 1989

McCarley RW, Faux SF, Shenton ME, et al: Event-related potentials in schizophrenia: their biological and clinical correlates and a new model of schizophrenic pathophysiology. Schizophr Res 4:209–231, 1991

McCarley RW, Shenton ME, O'Donnell BF, et al: Uniting Kraepelin and Bleuler: the psychology of schizophrenia and the biology of temporal lobe abnormalities. Harv Rev Psychiatry 1:36–56, 1993

McFarlane AC, Weber DL, Clark CR: Abnormal stimulus processing in posttraumatic stress disorder. Biol Psychiatry 34:311–320, 1993

McGhie A, Chapman J: Disorders of attention and perception in early schizophrenia. Br J Med Psychol 34:103–116, 1961

Metzger LJ, Orr SP, Lasko NB, et al: Auditory event-related potentials to tone stimuli in combat-related posttraumatic stress disorder. Biol Psychiatry 42:1006–1015, 1997

Michel CM, Murray MM, Lantz G, et al: EEG source imaging. Clin Neurophysiol 115:2195–2222, 2004

Millichap JG: Temporal lobe arachnoid cyst-attention deficit disorder syndrome: role of the electroencephalogram in diagnosis. Neurology 48:1435–1439, 1997

Millichap JG: Attention deficit-hyperactivity disorder and the electroencephalogram. Epilepsy Behav 1:453–454, 2000

Molina V, Montz R, Perez-Castejon MJ, et al: Cerebral perfusion, electrical activity and effects of serotonergic treatment in obsessive-compulsive disorder: a preliminary study. Neuropsychobiology 32:139–148, 1995

Monroe RR: Anticonvulsants in the treatment of aggression. J Nerv Mental Dis 160:119–126, 1975

Moore NC, Tucker KA, Brin FB, et al: Positive symptoms of schizophrenia: response to haloperidol and remoxipride is associated with increased alpha EEG activity. Hum Psychopharmacol 12:75–80, 1997

Morihisa JM, Duffy FH, Wyatt RJ: Brain electrical activity mapping in schizophrenic patients. Arch Gen Psychiatry 40:719–728, 1983

Mucci A, Volpe U, Merlotti E, et al: Pharmaco-EEG in Psychiatry. Clin EEG Neurosci 37:81–98, 2006

Mullaney DJ, Kripke DF, Messin S: Wrist-actigraphic estimation of sleep time. Sleep 3:83–92, 1980

Nasrallah HA: Is schizophrenia a left hemisphere disease? in Can Schizophrenia Be Localized in the Brain? Edited by Andreasen NC. Washington, DC, American Psychiatric Press, 1986, pp 55–74

Neppe VM: Carbamazepine as adjunctive treatment in nonepileptic chronic inpatients with EEG temporal lobe abnormalities. J Clin Psychiatry 44:326–331, 1983

Niedermeyer E, Lopes da Silva F: Electroencephalography: Basic Principles, Clinical Applications, and Related Fields. Baltimore, MD, Lippincott Williams and Wilkins, 2005

Niedermeyer E, Naidu SB: Rett syndrome, EEG and the motor cortex as a model for better understanding of attention deficit hyperactivity disorder (ADHD). Eur Child Adolesc Psychiatry 7:69–72, 1998

Nowack WJ, Janati A, Metzer WS, et al: The anterior temporal electrode in the EEG of the adult. Clin Electroencephalogr 19:199–204, 1988

Nuchpongsai P, Arakaki H, Langman P, et al: N2 and P3b components of the event-related potential in students at risk for psychosis. Psychiatry Res 88:131–141, 1999

O'Donnell BF, Faux SF, McCarley RW, et al: Increased rate of P300 latency prolongation with age in schizophrenia: electrophysiological evidence for a neurodegenerative process. Arch Gen Psychiatry 52:544–549, 1995

Olfson M: Utilization of neuropsychiatric diagnostic tests for general hospital patients with mental disorders. Am J Psychiatry 149:1711–1717, 1992

Ommaya AK: Head injury mechanisms and the concept of preventive management: a review and critical synthesis. J Neurotrauma 12:527–546, 1995

Paige SR, Fitzpatrick DF, Kline JP, et al: Event-related potential amplitude/intensity slopes predict response to antidepressants. Neuropsychobiology 30:197–201, 1994

Pascual-Marqui R, Michel CM, Lehmann D: Low resolution brain electromagnetic tomography: a new method for localizing electrical activity in the brain. Int J Psychophysiol 18:49–65, 1994

Pariente D, Lepine JP, Lellouch J: Life time history of panic attacks and epilepsy: an association from a general population survey. J Clin Psychiatry 52:88–89, 1991

Pfefferbaum A, Ford JM, White PM, et al: P3 in schizophrenia is affected by stimulus modality, response requirements, medication status, and negative symptoms. Arch Gen Psychiatry 46:1035–1044, 1989

Pfefferbaum A, Roth WT, Ford JM: Event-related potentials in the study of psychiatric disorders. Arch Gen Psychiatry 52:559–563, 1995

Pfurtscheller G, Cooper R: Frequency dependence of the transmission of the EEG from cortex to scalp. Electroencephalogr Clin Neurophysiol 38:93–96, 1975

Phillips BB, Drake ME Jr, Hietter SA, et al: Electroencephalography in childhood conduct and behavior disorders. Clin Electroencephalogr 24:25–30, 1993

Pigeau RA, Hoffmann RF, Moffitt AR: A multivariate comparison between two EEG analysis techniques: period analysis and fast Fourier transform. Electroencephalogr Clin Neurophysiol 52:656–658, 1981

Pokras R: National Hospital Discharge Survey Data Tape Documentation, 1989. Hyattsville, MD, National Center for Health Statistics, 1990

Polich J: Meta-analysis of P300 normative aging studies. Psychophysiology 33:334–353, 1996

Polich J: Clinical application of the P300 event-related brain potential. Phys Med Rehabil Clin N Am 15:133–161, 2004

Polich J, Kok A: Cognitive and biological determinants of P300: an integrative review. Biol Psychology 41:103–146, 1995

Pollock VE, Schneider LS: Quantitative, waking EEG research on depression. Biol Psychiatry 27:757–780, 1990

Press WH, Flannery BP, Teukolsky SA, et al: Numerical Recipes: The Art of Scientific Computing. New York, Cambridge University Press, 1986

Prichep LS, Mas F, Hollander E: Quantitative electroencephalographic subtyping of obsessive-compulsive disorder. Psychiatry Res 50:25–32, 1993

Pro JD, Wells CE: The use of the electroencephalogram in the diagnosis of delirium. Dis Nerv Syst 38:804–808, 1977

Reeve A, Rose DF, Weinberger DR: Magnetoencephalography: applications in psychiatry. Arch Gen Psychiatry 46:573–576, 1989

Reiman EM, Raichle ME, Robins E, et al: Neuroanatomical correlates of lactate-induced anxiety attacks. Arch Gen Psychiatry 46:493–500, 1989

Reite M, Teale P, Goldstein L, et al: Late auditory magnetic sources may differ in the left hemisphere of schizophrenic patients. Arch Gen Psychiatry 46:565–572, 1989

Reynolds CF III, Brunner D: Sleep microarchitecture in depression: commentary. Biol Psychiatry 37:71, 1995

Reynolds CF III, Kupfer DJ: Sleep research in affective illness: state of the art circa 1987. Sleep 10:199–215, 1987

Riggio S: Nonconvulsive status epilepticus: clinical features and diagnostic challenges. Psychiatr Clin North Am 28:653–664, 2005

Riley T, Niedermeyer E: Rage attacks and episodic violent behavior: electroencephalographic findings and general considerations. Clin Electroencephalogr 9:131–139, 1978

Ritchlin CT, Chabot RJ, Alper K, et al: Quantitative electroencephalography: a new approach to the diagnosis of cerebral dysfunction in systemic lupus erythematosus. Arthritis Rheum 35:1330–1342, 1992

Roberts R: Differential diagnosis of sleep disorders, nonepileptic attacks and epileptic seizures. Curr Opin Neurol 11:135–139, 1998

Robinson DJ, Merskey H, Blume WT, et al: Electroencephalography as an aid in the exclusion of Alzheimer's disease. Arch Neurol 51:280–284, 1994

Rose DF, Smith PD, Sato S: Magnetoencephalography and epilepsy research. Science 238:329–335, 1987

Rosse RB, Owen CM, Morihisa JM: Brain imaging and laboratory testing in neuropsychiatry, in The American Psychiatric Press Textbook of Neuropsychiatry. Edited by Hales RE, Yudofsky SC. Washington DC, American Psychiatric Press, 1987, pp 17–39

Rosse RB, Warden DL, Morihisa JM: Applied electrophysiology, in Comprehensive Textbook of Psychiatry, 5th Edition. Edited by Kaplan HI, Sadock BJ. Baltimore, MD, Williams and Wilkins, 1989, pp 74–85

Roth WT, Horvath TB, Pfefferbaum A, et al: Event related potentials in schizophrenics. Electroencephalogr Clin Neurophysiol 48:127–139, 1980

Rowe DL, Robinson PA, Rennie CJ, et al: Neurophysiologically based mean-field modelling of tonic cortical activity in post-traumatic stress disorder (PTSD), schizophrenia, first episode schizophrenia and attention deficit hyperactivity disorder (ADHD). J Integr Neurosci 3:453–487, 2004

Sadeh A, Hauri PJ, Kripke DF, et al: The role of actigraphy in the evaluation of sleep disorders. Sleep 18:288–302, 1995

Saletu B: The use of pharmaco-EEG in drug profiling, in Human Psychopharmacology Measures and Methods. Edited by Hindmarch I, Stonier PD. New York, Wiley, pp 173–200, 1987

Saletu B, Küfferle B, Grünberger J, et al: Quantitative EEG, SPEM, and psychometric studies in schizophrenics before and during differential neuroleptic therapy. Pharmacopsychiatry 19:434–437, 1986

Saletu B, Anderer P, Saletu-Zyhlarz GM, et al: Classification and evaluation of the pharmacodynamics of psychotropic drugs by single-lead pharmaco-EEG, EEG mapping and tomography (LORETA). Methods Find Exp Clin Pharmacol 24 (suppl C):97–120, 2002a

Saletu B, Anderer P, Saletu-Zyhlarz GM, et al: EEG topography and tomography in diagnosis and treatment of mental disorders: evidence for a key-lock principle. Methods Find Exp Clin Pharmacol 24 (suppl D):97–106, 2002b

Salisbury DF, Shenton ME, Sherwood AR, et al: First-episode schizophrenic psychosis differs from first-episode affective psychosis and controls in P300 amplitude over left temporal lobe. Arch Gen Psychiatry 55:173–180, 1998

Schaffer CE, Davidson RH, Saron C: Frontal and parietal electroencephalogram asymmetry in depressed and nondepressed subjects. Biol Psychiatry 18:753–762, 1982

Schellenberg R, Milch W, Schwarz A, et al: Quantitative EEG and BPRS data following Haldol-Decanoate administration in schizophrenics. Int Clin Psychopharmacol 9:17–24, 1994

Scherg M, Von Cramon D: Two bilateral sources of the late AEP as identified by a spatio-temporal dipole model. Electroencephalogr Clin Neurophysiol 62:32–44, 1985

Shagass C: Twisted thoughts, twisted brain waves? in Psychopathology and Brain Dysfunction. Edited by Shagass C, Gershon S, Friedhoff AJ. New York, Raven, 1977, pp 353–378

Signer SF: Seizure disorder or panic disorder? Am J Psychiatry 145:275–276, 1988

Simpson HB, Tenke CE, Towey JB, et al: Symptom provocation alters behavioral ratings and brain electrical activity in obsessive-compulsive disorder: a preliminary study. Psychiatry Res 95:149–155, 2000

Snyder E, Hillyard SA: Long-latency evoked potentials to irrelevant, deviant stimuli. Behav Biol 16:319–331, 1976

Spencer KM, Nestor PG, Perlmutter R, et al: Neural synchrony indexes disordered perception and cognition in schizophrenia. Proc Natl Acad Sci U S A 101:17288–17293, 2004

Squires NK, Squires KC, Hillyard SA: Two varieties of long-latency positive waves evoked by unpredictable auditory stimuli in man. Electroencephalogr Clin Neurophysiol 38:387–401, 1975

Stevens JR, Denney D, Szot P: Kindling with clozapine: behavioral and molecular consequences. Epilepsy Res 26:295–304, 1996

Struve FA: Selective referral versus routine screening in clinical EEG assessment of psychiatric inpatients. Psychiatr Med 1:317–343, 1983

Struve FA, Boutros NN: Somatic implications of generalized and/or focal slowing in psychiatric patients. Clin EEG Neurosci 36:171–175, 2005

Struve FA, Feigenbaum S: Experience with nasopharyngeal electrode recording with psychiatric patients: a clinical note. Clin Electroencephalogr 12:84–88, 1981

Struve FA, Pike LE: Routine admission electroencephalograms of adolescent and adult psychiatric patients awake and asleep. Clin Electroencephalogr 5:56–71, 1974

Symond MP, Harris AW, Gordon E, et al: "Gamma synchrony" in first-episode schizophrenia: a disorder of temporal connectivity? Am J Psychiatry 162:459–465, 2005

Taylor MA, Abrams R: Prediction of treatment response in mania. Arch Gen Psychiatry 38:800–803, 1981

Tebano MT, Cameroni M, Gallozzi GA, et al: EEG spectral analysis after minor head injury in man. Electroencephalogr Clin Neurophysiol 70:185–189, 1988

Thatcher RW: Electroencephalography and mild traumatic brain injury, in Foundations of Sport-Related Brain Injuries. Edited by Slobounov S, Sebastianelli W. New York, Springer-Verlag, 2006, pp 241–265

Thatcher RW, Walker RA, Gerson I, et al: EEG discriminant analyses of mild head trauma. Electroencephalogr Clin Neurophysiol 73:94–106, 1989

Thatcher RW, Hallet M, Zeffiro T, et al (eds): Functional Neuroimaging: Technical Foundations, New York, Academic Press, 1994, pp 209–299

Thatcher RW, Biver C, McAlaster R, et al: Biophysical linkage between MRI and EEG amplitude in closed head injury. Neuroimage 7:352–367, 1998a

Thatcher RW, Biver C, McAlaster R, et al: Biophysical linkage between MRI and EEG coherence in closed head injury. Neuroimage 8:307–326, 1998b

Thatcher RW, Biver C, Gomez JF, et al: Estimation of the EEG power spectrum using MRI T2 relaxation time in traumatic brain injury. Clin Neurophysiol 112:1729–1745, 2001a

Thatcher RW, North DM, Curtin RT, et al: An EEG severity index of traumatic brain injury. J Neuropsychiatry Clin Neurosci 13:77–87, 2001b

Thatcher RW, Walker RA, Biver C, et al: Quantitative EEG normative databases: validation and clinical correlation. Journal of Neurotherapy 7:87–122, 2003

Thatcher RW, North D, Biver C: Evaluation and validity of a LORETA normative EEG database. Clin EEG Neurosci 36:116–122, 2005

Thompson J, Sebastianelli W, Slobounov S: EEG and postural correlates of mild traumatic brain injury in athletes. Neurosci Lett 377:158–163, 2005

Trzepacz PT, Sclabassi RJ, Van Thiel DH: Delirium: a subcortical phenomenon? J Neuropsychiatry Clin Neurosci 1:283–290, 1989

Tunks ER, Dermer SW: Carbamazepine in the dyscontrol syndrome associated with limbic system dysfunction. J Nerv Ment Dis 164:56–63, 1977

van Sweden B, de Bruecker G: Patterns of EEG dysfunction in general hospital psychiatry. Neuropsychobiology 16:131–134, 1986

Visser SL: EEG and evoked potentials in the diagnosis of dementia, in Senile Dementia of the Alzheimer Type. Edited by Traber J, Gispen WH. Berlin, Springer, 1985, pp 102–116

Wada Y, Nanbu Y, Jiang ZY, et al: Electroencephalographic abnormalities in patients with presenile dementia of the Alzheimer type: quantitative analysis at rest and during photic stimulation. Biol Psychiatry 41:217–225, 1997

Warner MD, Boutros NN, Peabody CA: Usefulness of screening EEGs in a psychiatric inpatient population. J Clin Psychiatry 51:363–364, 1990

Weilburg JB, Schachter S, Worth J, et al: EEG abnormalities in patients with atypical panic attacks. J Clin Psychiatry 56:358–362, 1995

Weisbrod M, Kiefer M, Marzinzik F, et al: Executive control is disturbed in schizophrenia: evidence from event-related potentials in a Go/NoGo task. Biol Psychiatry 47:51–60, 2000

Wiedemann G, Pauli P, Dengler W, et al: Frontal brain asymmetry as a biological substrate of emotions in patients with panic disorders. Arch Gen Psychiatry 56:78–84, 1999

Williams D: Neural factors related to habitual aggression: consideration of differences between those habitual aggressives and others who have committed crimes of violence. Brain 92:503–520, 1969

Young GB, Chandarana PC, Blume WT, et al: Mesial temporal lobe seizures presenting as anxiety disorders. J Neuropsychiatry Clin Neuroscience 7:352–357, 1995

Zimmerman JE: Magnetic quantities, units, materials, and measurements, in Biomagnetism: An Interdisciplinary Approach. Edited by Williamson SJ, Romani GL, Kaufman L, et al. New York, Plenum, 1983, pp 17–42

Zivin L, Marsan CA: Incidence and prognostic significance of "epileptiform" activity in the EEG of non-epileptic subjects. Brain 91:751–778, 1968

6

THE NEUROPSYCHOLOGICAL EVALUATION

Diane B. Howieson, Ph.D.
Muriel D. Lezak, Ph.D.

Neuropsychologists assess brain function by making inferences from an individual's cognitive, sensorimotor, emotional, and social behavior. During the early history of neuropsychology, these assessments were often the most direct measure of brain integrity in persons who did not have localizing neurological signs and symptoms and who had problems confined to higher mental functions (Hebb 1942; Teuber 1948). Neuropsychological measures are useful diagnostic indicators of brain dysfunction for many conditions and will remain the major diagnostic modality for some (Bigler 1999; Farah and Feinberg 2000; Lezak et al. 2004; Mesulam 2000; Petersen et al. 2001). However, methods for determining brain structure and function have become increasingly accurate in recent decades (e.g., Kamitani and Tong 2005). Advances in quantitative and functional neuroimaging have enriched our understanding of pathological disturbances of the brain (Aine 1995; Damasio and Damasio 2003; J.M. Levin et al. 1996; Menon and Kim 1999; Stern and Silbersweig 2001; Tilak Ratnanather et al. 2004). It is even possible to produce precisely placed, reversible "lesions" to study how the remainder of the brain functions without a designated cortical area (Deouell et al. 2003; Grafman and Wassermann 1999; V. Walsh and Rushworth 1999). These developments have allowed a shift in the focus of neuropsychological assessment from the diagnosis of possible brain damage to a better understand-

ing of specific brain-behavior relations and the psychosocial consequences of brain damage.

INDICATIONS FOR A NEUROPSYCHOLOGICAL EVALUATION

Patients referred to a neuropsychologist for assessment typically fall into one of three groups. The first, and probably largest, group consists of patients with known brain disorders. The more common neurological disorders are cerebrovascular disorders, developmental disorders, traumatic brain injury, Alzheimer's disease and related dementing disorders, progressive diseases primarily involving subcortical structures (e.g., Parkinson's disease, multiple sclerosis, Huntington's chorea), tumors, seizures, and infections. Psychiatric disorders also may be associated with brain dysfunction; chief among them are schizophrenia, obsessive-compulsive disorder, and depression.

A neuropsychological evaluation can be useful in defining the nature and severity of the associated behavior and emotional problems. The assessment provides information about patients' cognition, personality characteristics, social behavior, emotional status, and adaptation to their conditions. Patients' potential for independent living and productive activity can be inferred from these data. Information about their behavioral strengths and weaknesses provides a foundation for treatment planning, vocational training, competency determination, and counseling for both patients and their families (Bennett and Raymond 2003; Diller 2000; Kalechstein et al. 2003; Sloan and Ponsford 1995).

> A 52-year-old real estate agent had a left hemisphere stroke producing mild aphasia and right-sided hemiparesis. A neuropsychological examination conducted several months later showed that she had good language comprehension and reading skills, mild word-finding problems, mild visuospatial deficits, and moderate impairment in verbal memory. Like many patients who have had strokes (Astrom et al. 1993; Cullum and Bigler 1991; Niemi et al. 1988; Robinson 1998), she was also depressed. Information from the examination was used to make decisions about the likelihood of returning successfully to her previous job, to plan rehabilitation and strategies to help her compensate for persistent cognitive deficits, to make recommendations regarding treatment of her depression, and to begin family counseling.

The second group of patients is composed of persons with a known risk factor for brain disorder in whom a change in behavior might be the result of such a disorder. In these cases, a neuropsychological evaluation might be used both to provide evidence of brain dysfunction and to describe the nature and severity of problems. A person who has sustained a blow to the head from an automobile accident that produces a brief loss of consciousness, even with no apparent further neurological complications, might experience disruption in cognitive efficiency. On returning to work after 1 week, this individual might be unable to keep up with job demands. After several weeks of on-the-job difficulties, the physician may refer the patient to a neuropsychologist for evaluation of possible brain injury from the accident. The examiner would look for evidence of problems with divided attention, sustained concentration and mental tracking, and memory, all of which are common findings in the weeks or months following mild head injury (Bennett and Raymond 1997; Varney and Roberts 1999; Wrightson and Gronwall 1999). The neuropsychologist can advise the patient that these problems frequently occur after head injury and that considerable improvement might be expected during the next month or two. Recommendations about how to structure work activities to minimize both these difficulties and the equally common problem of fatigue provide both aid and comfort to the concerned patient. The neuropsychologist might repeat the examination several months after the injury to determine whether these predictions held true and to assess the individual's adjustment and possible need for further counseling or other treatment.

Many depressed older persons may complain of poor memory, raising concern about the onset of a possible dementing disorder.

> A 55-year-old rancher noticed problems remembering to carry out activities and difficulty retaining information. He had an aunt with Alzheimer's disease and was worried that he might have this disease. His emotional stressors included concern about his son's substance abuse. His cognitive testing showed memory performance typical of his age and argued for a diagnosis of anxiety and depression rather than dementia.

In patients such as this, it is not unusual to observe attention and memory problems based on depression alone. For most of them, the history and nature and degree of cognitive problems would differentiate the diagnoses.

Many medical conditions can affect brain function (Lezak et al. 2004; Tarter et al. 2001). Brain function can be disrupted by systemic illnesses: endocrinopathies; metabolic and electrolyte disturbances associated with diseases of the kidney, liver, and pancreas; nutritional deficiencies; and conditions that compromise blood supply to the brain. These latter include vascular disorders, cardiac and pulmonary diseases, anemia, and complications of anesthesia or surgery. Age and health habits also must be taken into consideration when evaluating a person's behavioral alterations because they affect the probability of cerebral disorder (Payami et al. 1997; Perfect and Maylor 2000). In addition, many medicines can disrupt cognition through their subtle and sometimes not so subtle effects on alertness, attention, and memory (Pagliaro and Pagliaro 1998; Stein and Strickland 1998).

In this third group, brain disease or dysfunction may be suspected when a person's behavior changes without an identifiable cause: that is, the patient has no known risk factors for brain disorder, so this possible diagnosis is based on exclusion of other diagnoses. Frequently, psychiatrists are asked to evaluate adults with no psychiatric history who have had an uncharacteristic change in behavior or personality and for whom no obvious sources of current emotional distress can be identified. An explanation is sought because behavior patterns and personality are relatively stable characteristics of adults, and these changes require an explanation. The list of diagnoses that could account for a late-onset psychiatric disturbance is long because it may include a wide variety of brain disorders such as metabolic disturbance, vitamin deficiency, endocrine disorder, and heavy metal poisoning to neoplasm, infection, and multiple small strokes. The psychiatric literature contains numerous examples of individuals (notably, George Gershwin) who were treated for psychiatric illness before it was discovered that they had brain disease, such as a tumor (Duwe and Turetsky 2002; Lisanby et al. 1998; Teasell and Shapiro 2002).

The most common application of the neuropsychological evaluation of older adults without obvious risk factors for brain disease—other than age—is for early detection of progressive dementia, such as Alzheimer's disease (Howieson et al. 1997; Knopman and Selnes 2003; Kramer et al. 2003; Rentz and Weintraub 2000). Most persons have symptoms associated with dementia for at least 1 year before they see a health care provider because the problems initially are minor and easily attributed to factors such as aging, a concurrent illness, or recent emotional stress. The progression of these symptoms is insidious, especially because many patients have "good" as well as "bad" days during the early stages of a dementing disorder. Neuropsychological assessment is useful in evaluating whether problems noted by the family or the individual are age-related, are attributable to other factors such as depression, or are suggestive of early dementia. During the past decade, human immunodeficiency virus (HIV) infection and the complications of drug abuse have been added as conditions that can produce an insidious dementia in younger persons (Dore et al. 2003; I. Grant et al. 1995; Kelly et al. 1996; Rogers and Robbins 2003).

Another clinical condition that produces no clinical clues for brain damage except for a change in behavior is the so-called silent stroke. Without obvious sensory, motor, or speech problems, a stroke may go undetected yet produce persistent behavioral alterations. Silent stokes can produce subtle cognitive impairment (Armstrong et al. 1996; Pohjasvaara et al. 1999; W.P. Schmidt et al. 2004); a series of small strokes may generate an insidious dementia over time (O'Connell et al. 1998; Vermeer et al. 2003). Silent strokes and white matter hyperintensities observed on magnetic resonance imaging (MRI) scans (Nebes et al. 2001) and cerebrovascular risk factors (Mast et al. 2005) of elderly persons also may be associated with depression. Exposure to environmental toxins also can result in common patterns of neuropsychological impairment (Morrow et al. 2001; Reif et al. 2003).

In cases with no known explanation for mental deterioration, it becomes important to search for possible risk factors or other reasons for brain disease through history taking, the physical examination, laboratory tests, and interviews with the patient's family or close associates. Should this search produce no basis for the mental deterioration, a diagnostic neuropsychological study can be useful. The neuropsychological examination of persons with or without known risk factors for brain damage is diagnostically useful if it identifies cognitive or behavioral deficits, particularly if these deficits occur in a meaningful pattern. A pattern is considered meaningful when it is specific to one, or only a few, diagnoses such as a pattern of cognitive disruption suggestive of a lateralized or focal brain lesion.

> A man with HIV infection had a 2-week history of "feeling odd." He became easily lost, even in familiar settings, and complained of an inability to perform a task as simple as making his sheets "fit the bed." He said that he could not read because he was unable to follow a line consistently across the page. He had stopped working as a barber after giving a poor haircut. He had no established symptoms of his infection. Although he was known to have an appropriate reactive depression related to his infection, his complaints were atypical for depression. A neuropsychological evaluation showed that he had severe and circumscribed visuospatial and constructional deficits, a pattern of cognitive deficits usually associated with right parietal dysfunction. A subsequent MRI scan showed white matter disease involving a large area of the right parietal lobe and several small areas elsewhere in the right hemisphere. A biopsy confirmed the diagnosis of multifocal progressive leukoencephalopathy.

Neuropsychological signs and symptoms that are possible indicators of a pathological brain disorder are presented in Table 6–1. Confidence in diagnoses based on neuropsychological evidence will be greater when risk factors for brain dysfunction exist or the patient shows signs and symptoms of brain dysfunction than when neuropsychological diagnoses rely solely on exclusion of other diagnoses.

One of the greatest challenges for a neuropsychologist is to determine whether patients with psychiatric illness show evidence of an underlying brain disorder. Many psychiatric patients without neurological disease have cognitive disruptions and behavioral or emotional aberrations. Cognitive impairment is highly prevalent in schizophrenia (Heinrichs and Zakzanis 1998; Hill et al. 2001), particularly for attention, processing speed, memory, problem solving, cognitive flexibility, and organizational and planning abilities (Goldman et al. 1996). Because considerable heterogeneity exists for symptoms of schizophrenia (Binks and Gold 1998; Goldstein et al. 1998; Seaton et al. 2001), some patients appear cognitively normal (Allen et al. 2003; Palmer et al. 1997). Obsessive-compulsive disorders are often accompanied by mild cognitive impairment. Areas of difficulty may include nonverbal memory, use of strategies, visuospatial skills, and selected executive functions (Deckersbach et al. 2000; Greisberg and McKay 2003; Mataix-Cols et al. 1999; Savage et al. 2000; K.D. Wilson 1998). Both schizophrenia and obsessive-compulsive behavior have been linked to dysfunction of frontal subcortical circuits (Abbruzzese et al. 1995; Chamberlain et al. 2005), and temporal lobe structures also have been implicated (Adler et al. 2000; Post 2000).

TABLE 6–1.   Neuropsychological signs and symptoms that may indicate a pathological brain process

Functional class	Symptoms and signs
Speech and language	Dysarthria Dysfluency Marked change in amount of speech output Paraphasias Word-finding problems
Academic skills	Alterations in reading, writing, calculating, and number abilities Frequent letter or number reversals
Thinking	Perseveration of speech Simplified or confused mental tracking, reasoning, and concept formation
Motor	Weakness or clumsiness, particularly if lateralized Impaired fine motor coordination (e.g., changes in handwriting) Apraxias Perseveration of action components
Memory[a]	Impaired recent memory for verbal or visuospatial material or both Disorientation
Perception	Diplopia or visual field alterations Inattention (usually left-sided) Somatosensory alterations (particularly if lateralized) Inability to recognize familiar stimuli (agnosia)
Visuospatial abilities	Diminished ability to perform manual skills (e.g., mechanical repairs and sewing) Spatial disorientation Left-right disorientation Impaired spatial judgment (e.g., angulation of distances)
Emotions[b]	Diminished emotional control with temper outburst and antisocial behavior Diminished empathy or interest in interpersonal relationships Affective changes Irritability without evident precipitating factors Personality change
Comportment[b]	Altered appetites and appetitive activities Altered grooming habits (excessive fastidiousness or carelessness) Hyperactivity or hypoactivity Social inappropriateness

[a]Many emotionally disturbed persons complain of memory deficits, which most typically reflect the person's self-preoccupation, distractibility, or anxiety rather than a dysfunctional brain. Thus, memory complaints in themselves do not necessarily warrant neuropsychological evaluation.

[b]Some of these changes are most likely to be neuropsychologically relevant in the absence of depression, although they can also be mistaken for depression.

Depressed patients often underperform on measures of speed of processing, mental flexibility, and executive function compared with control subjects (Veiel 1997; Weiland-Fiedler et al. 2004). Memory impairment occurs less consistently (Basso and Bornstein 1999b; Boone et al. 1995; Palmer et al. 1996), and memory performance may be intact even when memory complaints are present (Dalgleish and Cox 2000; Kalska et al. 1999).

Cognitive deficits, including memory, are more common in depressed patients with psychotic features than in those with no psychotic features (Basso and Bornstein 1999a; McKenna et al. 2000). Compared with control subjects, euthymic bipolar patients may have difficulty with attention, memory, abstraction (Denicoff et al. 1999; Quraishi and Frangou 2002), and executive functions (Ferrier et al. 1999; Malhi et al. 2004). The degree of cognitive impairment appears to be related to the number of prior depressive episodes (Denicoff et al. 1999; Van Gorp et al. 1998). Although several psychological explanations have been proposed to explain cognitive deficits in mood disorders, such as self-focused rumination associated with dysphoria (Hertel 1998), underlying structural and functional abnormalities have been reported in the neural pathways that modulate mood (Ali et al. 2000; Caetano et al. 2004; Liotti and Mayberg 2001; Neumeister et al. 2005; Strakowski et al. 1999).

Conversely, neurological diseases can present with prominent psychiatric features (Cummings 1999; Lezak et al. 2004). Confabulations associated with undiagnosed brain lesions, such as Korsakoff's syndrome, may be misinterpreted as a psychotic illness (Benson et al. 1996). An assortment of delusional misidentification syndromes have been associated with neurological diseases (Feinberg and Roane 2003). Hallucinations may be an early feature of Lewy body dementia and may occur with Parkinson's disease, Alzheimer's disease, other neurodegenerative diseases, stroke, epilepsy, migraine, and toxic-metabolic encephalopathies (Tekin and Cummings 2003).

Although neuropsychological assessment provides a measure of the type and degree of cognitive disorder, it often cannot specify the cause of the disturbance. Cognitive deficits appearing in an adult patient who previously functioned well and has no history of psychiatric illness or recent stress should raise suspicions of a neurological disorder.

ROLE OF THE REFERRING PSYCHIATRIST

The referring psychiatrist has the tasks of identifying patients who might benefit from a neuropsychological evaluation, preparing the patient, and formulating referral questions that best define the needed information. A valid evaluation depends on obtaining the patient's best performance. It is nearly impossible to obtain satisfactory evaluations of patients who are uncooperative, fatigued, actively psychotic, seriously depressed, highly anxious, or physically uncomfortable (Lezak et al. 2004). For example, seriously depressed patients may appear to have dementia, and the evaluation may underestimate the individual's full potential (Chaves and Izquierdo 1992; King and Caine 1996; Yousef et al. 1998). Whenever possible, severely depressed or actively psychotic patients should be referred after they have shown clinical improvement, when the findings may be more representative of their true ability uncontaminated by reversible emotional or behavioral disturbances.

To obtain the patient's cooperation and alleviate unnecessary anxiety, it is important to prepare the patient for the evaluation (Lezak et al. 2004). The patient should understand the purpose and nature of the evaluation. The explanation usually includes a statement that the evaluation is requested to assess how the brain is functioning by looking at activities that the brain processes, such as mental abilities. In most cases, patients should know that the examiner will look for mental and emotional strengths as well as problem areas to obtain information that will assist in counseling and planning.

The more explicit the referral question, the more likely it is that the evaluation will be conducted to provide the needed information. The referral question should include

- Identifying information about the patient
- Reasons that the evaluation is requested
- Description of the problem to be assessed
- Pertinent history

The neuropsychologist will design a different examination when the referral question asks whether the patient is a candidate for psychotherapy than when an evaluation is requested for a personal injury lawsuit. Some appropriate referrals seek behavioral descriptions, such as "Does this individual who has multiple sclerosis show evidence of cognitive deficits, and, if so, what are they? Could they interfere with treatment compliance?" Other referral questions may be framed around problems with patient management, counseling, and educational or vocational planning. In some instances, the neuropsychologist may identify a problem—or competencies—that adds to or negates the referral question, in which case the experienced neuropsychologist will reformulate the examination goals to conform to the needs of the patient in the light of the original referral question (e.g., see Lezak et al. 2004, pp. 112–113).

ASSESSMENT PROCESS

Interview and observation provide the data of neuropsychological evaluations. The interview is the basic component of the evaluation (Lezak et al. 2004; Luria 1980; Sbordone 2000). Its main purposes are to elicit the patient's and family's complaints, understand the circumstances in which these problems occur, and evaluate the patient's attitude toward these problems. Understanding the range of the patient's complaints, as well as which ones the patient views as most troublesome, contributes to the framework on which the assessment and recommendations are based. A thorough history of complaints and pertinent background is essential.

The presenting problems and the patient's attitude toward them also may provide important diagnostic information. Patients with certain neuropsychological conditions lack awareness of their problems or belittle their significance (Markova and Berrios 2000; Prigatano and Schacter 1991). Many patients with right hemisphere stroke, Alzheimer's disease, and frontal lobe damage are unaware of or unable to appreciate the problems resulting from their brain injury. In the extreme form of right hemisphere stroke, some patients with hemiplegia are unable to comprehend that the left side of their body is part of them, let alone that they cannot use it. In a more muted form, many patients with dementia attribute their memory problems to aging and minimize their significance (see Strub and Black 2000). Conversely, patients, families, or caregivers sometimes attribute problems to brain damage when a careful history suggests otherwise.

The interview provides an opportunity to observe the patient's appearance, attention, speech, thought content, and motor abilities and to evaluate affect, appropriateness of behavior, orientation, insight, and judgment. The interview can provide information about the patient's premorbid intellectual ability and personality, occupational and school background, social situation, and ability to use leisure time.

The tests used by neuropsychologists are simply standardized observational tools that, in many instances, have the added advantage of providing normative data to aid in interpreting the observations. Various assessment approaches are available, but they all have in common the goals of determining whether the patient shows evidence of brain dysfunction, identifying the nature of problems detected, and determining which functions have been preserved and, thus, what are the patient's cognitive strengths. The two main methods are individually tailored examinations and fixed battery assessments. The former is often referred to as the *hypothesis-testing* approach because hypotheses about the source(s) and nature of the brain dysfunction derived from information acquired before and during the assessment determine test selection (Kaplan 1988; Lezak et al. 2004; Milberg et al. 1996). In this approach, information about the patients' medical and psychological backgrounds and their activities generates the hypotheses to be tested regarding neuropsychological deficits. For example, the assessment request may involve an individual known to have had a heart attack who sustained brief and unremarked hypoxia. The family reports that the individual appears depressed because he sits all day without showing an interest in other people or activities. Several hypotheses could be generated from this information to explain the behavior. The patient may indeed be depressed. Alternatively, the individual may have inertia secondary to cerebral damage. The examiner may decide to include tests that are relatively unstructured and require active initiation and de novo organization. Other hypotheses that might be considered and tested include

the presence of confusion that prevents the patient from responding to the situations that the family describes, or of serious memory difficulties that interfere with the patient's intention to initiate or maintain ongoing activities.

The more information that can be gained before beginning the assessment, the more efficiently specific hypotheses can be generated. Moreover, hypothesis testing continues throughout the assessment. When a problem is observed on a particular test, new hypotheses are generated or old ones are modified with regard to the nature of the observed problem. Typically the examination focuses on the problem areas while briefly screening other areas that appear to be relatively intact, except when detailed information about residual competencies is required, as when developing a remediation program or helping a patient to regain self-confidence.

A second approach to neuropsychological testing is to use a fixed battery of tests (Broshek and Barth 2000; Reitan and Wolfson 1996). This approach involves examining the same range of cognitive and behavioral functioning in every individual. It is analogous to a physician conducting a standard physical examination on all patients. These fixed battery examinations frequently last 6–8 hours. The advantage of a fixed battery is that the patient receives a fairly broad-based examination. The consistency of the administration procedures and normative data and the relatively wide range of data make fixed batteries useful for research purposes. Although these advantages might lure the examiner into using this approach clinically, this fixed approach does not focus on specific areas of difficulty for most patients nor can it cover all areas relevant to either a reliable diagnosis or practical counseling. In some cases, it might be unclear why performance is impaired without additional testing outside of the battery. Time may be wasted in testing areas of cognition or sensorimotor functioning that are not problems, and subtle problems can be overlooked. Moreover, aspects of neuropsychological functioning not included in a fixed battery will not be examined. In this era of tightening health care budgets, good neuropsychological service must be provided at reasonable cost. Tailoring the examination to the patient's requirements rather than using a fixed battery allows the examiner to learn what is needed about the patient with a minimum of time and cost.

Cognitive performance is only one aspect of an assessment. A full evaluation of the individual assesses emotional and social characteristics as well. Many patients with brain injuries experience changes in personality, mood, or ability to control emotional states (Gainotti 2003; Heilman et al. 2003; Ochoa et al. 2003) and problems with social relationships (Dikmen et al. 1996; Lezak 1988a). Depression is a common and sometimes serious complication of brain disease. An unusually high incidence of depression occurs with certain neurodegenerative disorders, such as Parkinson's disease and Huntington's disease (Brandstadter and Oertel 2003; Levy et al. 1998; Rickards 2005). Other neurological diseases in which depression is common are tumors (particularly those of the orbitofrontal and temporoparietal cortex), multiple sclerosis, Wilson's disease, HIV encephalopathy, Alzheimer's disease, vascular dementia, and Lewy body dementia (Cummings 1994). At least 30% of stroke patients experience depression at some time (Paradiso et al. 1997; Pohjasvaara et al. 1998; Singh et al. 2000). Factors that appear to determine the presence of depression include the location of the brain injury and its recency, the degree of disability, and the patient's level of social activity (Gustafson et al. 1995; Robinson 1998). In some cases, these changes may be secondary to cognitive impairment (Andersen et al. 1995). Patients who have had a right hemisphere stroke may show impaired processing of emotional material and complex social situations, which leads to interpersonal problems (Lezak 1994). Although the history and observers' reports will inform the examiner of changes in these characteristics, current emotional status and personality also can be evaluated by standard psychological questionnaires and inventories (Gass 1992; Lezak et al. 2004).

As computers have become valuable aids in many fields, there has been increasing interest in using computerized testing procedures (Bleiberg et al. 2000; De Luca et al. 2003; Fowler et al. 1997; Kane and Kay 1992; Tornatore et al. 2005). This technology offers the possibility of obtaining test data under highly standardized conditions with minimal time expenditure by the examiner. These features make it valuable in circumstances when many individuals need to be screened for potential problems. Computers also have timing and scoring features and can plot the data graphically. In addition, computer programs are available in some cases for interpreting test responses. The Minnesota Multiphasic Personality Inventory–2 (MMPI-2) is available with computer scoring and, if purchased separately, interpretation (Butcher 1989). Computerized interpretations of the MMPI-2 and other tests presumably provide the most common interpretations of test patterns but are not applicable to every case, especially for individuals with brain disorders (Cripe 1999; Lezak et al. 2004). Therefore, they should be used only as a source of hypotheses about individuals to be confirmed or negated by data from other sources (Butcher et al. 2000).

Although many adults with brain injuries can tolerate responding to the computer format, and some may even enjoy it, these methods lose important information about the way the individual approaches cognitive tasks or why errors are made, unless the examiner monitors the process (Lezak

et al. 2004). Some brain-damaged patients are impulsive, and others overly cautious. Either factor could greatly alter a test score without providing information about the particular function that is the object of investigation.

THE NATURE OF NEUROPSYCHOLOGICAL TESTS

An important component of neuropsychological evaluations is psychological testing, in which an individual's cognitive and often emotional status and executive functioning are assessed with standardized formats. Neuropsychological assessment differs from psychological assessment in its basic assumptions. The latter compares the individual's responses with normative data from a sample of healthy individuals taking the same test (Lezak et al. 2004; Urbina 2004). The neuropsychological assessment of adults relies on comparisons between the patient's current level of functioning and the known or estimated level of premorbid functioning according to demographically similar individuals and current performance on tests of functions less likely to be affected by brain disorders. Thus, much of clinical neuropsychological assessment involves *intraindividual* comparisons of the abilities and skills under consideration.

Two types of standardized neuropsychological tests are available. Some tests involve cognitive or sensorimotor tasks that can be accomplished by all intact adults within the culture. They are designed so that all individuals are expected to be able to perform the task, and thus failure to do so may be interpreted as impairment. Examples of this approach include many aphasia tests of basic language skills. Anyone from an English-speaking Western cultural background would be expected to name, describe, and demonstrate the use of common objects as tested by the Porch Index of Communicative Ability (Porch 1981). The Dementia Rating Scale–2 (Mattis et al. 2001) is based on the assumption that adults will be able to perform most of the cognitive tasks used in this test. The manual specifies the small number of errors considered normal. Most individuals achieve a nearly perfect score on the Mini-Mental State Examination (MMSE; Folstein et al. 1975).

However, most tests of cognitive abilities are designed with the expectation that only very few persons will obtain a perfect score and that most scores will cluster in a middle range. For these tests, scores are conceptualized as continuous variables. The scores of many persons taking the test can be plotted as a distribution curve. Most scores on tests of complex learned behaviors fall into a characteristic bell-shaped curve called a normal distribution curve (Figure 6–1). The statistical descriptors of the curve are the *mean*, or average score; the degree of spread of scores about the

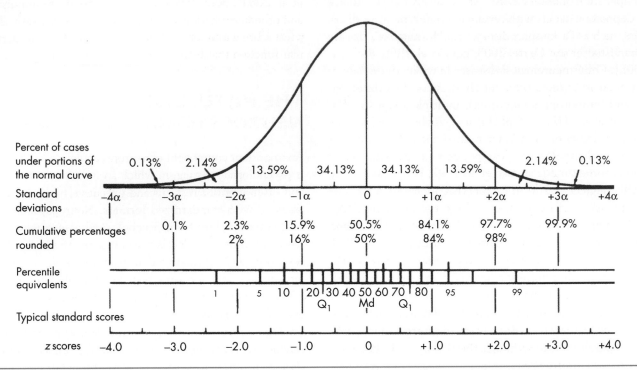

FIGURE 6–1. A normal distribution curve, showing the percentage of cases between −4 standard deviations (−σ) and +4 standard deviations (+σ). The average range is defined as −0.6 to +0.6 standard deviation or the 25th to the 75th percentiles.

Source. Adapted from the Test Service Bulletin of The Psychological Corporation, 1955.

mean, expressed as the *standard deviation;* and the *range,* or the distance from the highest to the lowest scores.

The level of competence in different cognitive functions as well as other behaviors varies from individual to individual and also within the same individual at different times. This variability also has the characteristics of a normal curve, as in Figure 6–1. Because of the normal variability of performance on cognitive tests, any single score can be considered only as representative of a normal performance range and must not be taken as a precise value. For example, the statistical properties of a score at the 75th percentile (the equivalent of a scaled score of 12 on a test in the Wechsler Intelligence Scale [WIS] battery) must be understood as likely representing a range of scores from the 50th to the 90th percentile. For this reason, many neuropsychologists are reluctant to report scores, but rather describe their findings in terms of ability levels. See Table 6–2 for interpretations of ability levels expressed as deviations from the mean of the normative sample.

An individual's score is compared with the normative data, often by calculating a standard or z score, which describes the individual's performance in terms of statistically regular distances (i.e., standard deviations). In this framework, scores within ±0.66 standard deviation are considered average because 50% of a normative sample scores within this range. The z scores are used to describe the

probability that a deviant response occurs by chance or because of an impairment. A performance in the below average direction that is greater than two standard deviations from the mean is usually described as falling in the impaired range because 98% of the normative sample taking the test achieve better scores. Figure 6–2 shows the performance of 34 men with schizophrenia on a set of neuropsychological tests. The z scores are calculated on the basis of the performance of a control group (the 0 line). The patient group had poorer performance than the control group on all measures.

TABLE 6–2. Ability test classifications expressed as deviations from the mean calculated from the normative sample

z Score range	Percentile	Classification
> +2.0	98–100	Very superior
+1.3 to +2.0	91–97	Superior
+0.67 to +1.3	75–90	High average
−0.66 to +0.66	26–74	Average
−0.67 to −1.3	10–25	Low average
−1.3 to −2.0	3–9	Borderline
< −2.0	0–2	Defective

Some test makers recommend "cut" or "cutoff" scores to evaluate certain test performances. The cutoff scores are those exceeded by most neuropsychologically intact persons; scores below the cutoff point are typically achieved by persons with impairment in the relevant abilities (e.g., Benton et al. 1994). Cutoff scores are usually derived on the basis of the distribution of scores of a healthy control sample. The threshold for "normal" is typically set at 1.5 standard deviations below the mean to include the top 95% of the normal sample. One difficulty with many fixed cutoff scores is that they are not based on normative samples that are appropriate for the individual being studied. For example, calculation of the cutoff score may not take into account level of education or age (Bornstein 1986; Prigatano and Parsons 1976). A score that is satisfactory for a person of *average* ability may be unsatisfactory for a person of *superior* ability. Or the cutoff score may derive from a biased sample, such as unselected psychiatric patients, in whom brain impairment occurs more frequently than in the population generally. The use of cutoff scores imposes an artificial dichotomy in describing a performance or an ability that is actually a continuous distribution (Dwyer 1996). Cutoff scores work best on tests of abilities normally expected in all adults, such as basic language or motor skills.

Psychological tests should be constructed to satisfy both reliability and validity criteria (Urbina 2004). The *reliability* of a test refers to the consistency of test scores when the test is given to the same individual at different times or with different sets of equivalent items. Because perfect reliability cannot be achieved for any test, each individual score represents a range of variability, which narrows to the degree that the reliability of the test approaches the ideal (Anastasi and Urbina 1997). Tests have *validity* when they measure what they purport to measure. If a test is designed to measure an attentional disorder, then patient groups known to have attention deficits should perform more poorly on the test than should persons from the population at large. Tests also should be constructed with large normative samples of individuals with similar demographic characteristics, particularly for age and education (Heaton et al. 2003; Steinberg and Bieliauskas 2005). For example, the Wechsler Adult Intelligence Scale–III has normative data for 2,450 adults stratified for age, sex, race, geographic region, occupation, and education according to U.S. census information (Psychological Corporation 1997), although test norms account only for age. Most tests have much smaller normative samples in the range of 30–200 individuals.

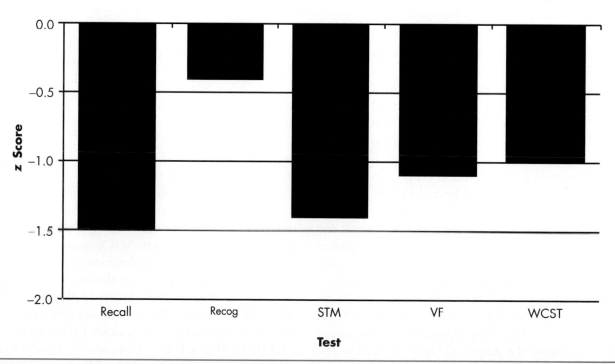

FIGURE 6–2.   Mean performance of patients with schizophrenia compared with control subjects on cognitive tests: delayed recall of words and stories (Recall); recognition of words when targets were mixed with distractors (Recog); short-term memory (STM) measured by the Brown-Peterson technique; verbal fluency (VF); and Wisconsin Card Sorting Test (WCST) categories achieved.

Source.   Adapted from Sullivan et al. 1994.

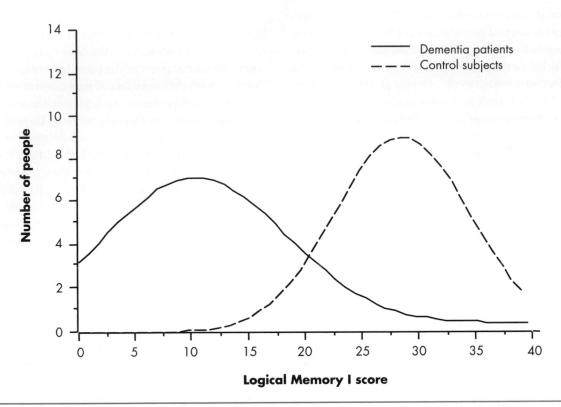

FIGURE 6–3.   Distribution of test scores by a group with mild dementia and age-matched control subjects on the Wechsler Memory Scale–Revised Logical Memory I, a story-recall test. Scores ranging from 15 to 39 occurred in both groups, whereas scores below 15 occurred in only the dementia group. The smaller the areas of overlapping curves, the higher the test specificity.

Some psychological tests detect subtle deficits better than do others. A simple signal detection test of attention, such as crossing out all the letters *A* on a page, is a less sensitive test of attention than is a divided attention task, such as crossing out all letters *A* and C. Tests involving complex tasks, such as problem solving requiring abstract thinking and cognitive flexibility, are more sensitive for reflecting brain dysfunction than many other cognitive tests because a wide variety of brain disorders can easily disrupt performance on them. However, other factors such as depression, anxiety, medicine side effects, and low energy level due to systemic illness also may disrupt cognition on these sensitive tests. Therefore, they are sensitive to cognitive disruption but not specific to one type of cognitive disturbance. The specificity of a test in detecting a disorder depends on the overlap between the distributions of the scores for persons who are intact and persons who have the disorder (Figure 6–3). The less overlap there is, the better the test can differentiate normal and abnormal performances. A test that is highly specific, such as the Token Test (Boller and Vignolo 1966; De Renzi and Vignolo 1962), which assesses language comprehension, produces few abnormal test scores in nonaphasic persons; that is, few false-positive findings. How-

ever, for such a test, false-negative results (i.e., that an impaired patient has normal findings) will be considerable because many persons with brain disorders have good language comprehension. Many neuropsychological tests offer a tradeoff between sensitivity and specificity.

Test selection involves a careful consideration of which tests are most likely to provide useful information for a given patient. Performance on any test may yield false-positive or false-negative information. Interpretation of neuropsychological tests by experienced clinicians involves consideration of a variety of data evaluated in light of meaningful patterns and inconsistencies.

Indications of brain dysfunction come from qualitative features of the patient's performance as well as from test scores (Lezak et al. 2004; Malloy et al. 2003; Pankratz and Taplin 1982). There are many ways of failing a test, and a poor score does not tell the means to the end (K.W. Walsh 1987). Occasionally, a patient gives a "far out" response to a question. The examiner asks the patient to repeat the question and, often in this circumstance, finds that the patient has misunderstood the question or instruction rather than lacked the ability to produce a correct response. Some features of behavioral disturbance are best recognized by the manner in which the patient approaches the testing situation or behaves with the examiner. Brain-injured patients are prone to problems with short attention span, distractibility, impulsivity, poor self-monitoring, disorganization, irritability, perplexity, and suspiciousness.

INTERPRETATION: PRINCIPLES AND CAUTIONS

The interpretation of test performance is based on an assumption that the patient is expected to perform in a particular way on tasks; deviations from expectation require evaluation (Lezak 1986; Lezak et al. 2004). Most healthy people perform within a statistically definable range on cognitive tests, and this range of performance levels is considered to be characteristic of healthy people. Deviations below this expected range raise the question of an impairment. A person may have scores in the high average range on many tests except for low average performance in one functional area.

> A 91-year-old former artist was referred by her family, who asked whether her gradual functional decline was related to aging or to a progressive dementia. Her performance, expressed in z scores, was compared with the scores of neuropsychologically normal persons of her age and educational background. Her scores were within expectations on some tests, including reasoning, constructions, and fund of information, but were deficient on tests of memory and confrontational naming. The deviations were significantly below expectations for her age group. The impaired performance and history were interpreted as supporting a diagnosis of mild dementia. She eventually progressed to show a full dementia syndrome with broad cognitive impairment.

The assumption of deficit is valid in most instances in which one or a set of scores fall significantly below expectations, although a few persons show an unusual variability on cognitive tasks (Lezak et al. 2004). Multiple measures involving similar or related abilities increase the reliability of findings. Thus, if a deviant score occurs on one task, other tests requiring similar skills are used to determine whether the deviant finding persists across tasks. If so, the finding is considered reliable. If similar tasks do not elicit a deviant performance, either the finding was spurious or the additional tasks varied in important features that did not involve the patient's problem area. The need to have multiple measures of many cognitive functions is the reason that some neuropsychological examinations may be lengthy.

Interpretation of test performances also must take into account demographic variables. When estimating the premorbid ability levels necessary for making intraindividual comparisons, the patients' educational and occupational background, sex, and race must be considered along with their level of test performance (Lezak et al. 2004; Vanderploeg et al. 1996). In cases in which educational level may not represent premorbid ability, reading level is often used as a best indicator (Manly et al. 2004). The more severely impaired the patients, the more unlikely it is that they will be performing at premorbid levels on any of the tests. This increases the examiner's reliance on demographic and historical data to estimate premorbid functioning. Some tests are fairly resistant to disruption by brain damage and may offer the best estimates of premorbid ability. Good examples are fund of information and reading vocabulary tests, such as the National Adult Reading Test (Nelson 1982) and a revision for American English, the North American Adult Reading Test, or NAART (Spreen and Strauss 1998).

For meaningful interpretations of neuropsychological test performance, examiners not only rely on many tests but also search for a performance pattern (test scores plus qualitative features) that makes neuropsychological sense. Because there are few pathognomonic findings in neuropsychology (or in most other branches of medical science for that matter) (Hertzman et al. 2001; Sox et al. 1988), a performance pattern often can suggest several diagnoses. For example, a cluster of documented deficits including slowed thinking and mild impairment of concentration and memory is a nonspecific finding associated with several conditions: very mild dementia, a mild postconcussion syndrome, mild toxic encephalopathy, depression, and fatigue, to name a few. Other patterns may be highly specific for certain conditions. The finding of left-sided neglect and visuospatial distortions is highly suggestive of brain dysfunction and specifically occurs with right hemisphere damage. For many neuropsychological conditions, typical deficit patterns are known, allowing the examiner to evaluate the patient's performances in light of these known patterns for a possible match.

The quality of a neuropsychological evaluation depends on many factors. In general, one should beware of conclusions from evaluations in which test scores alone (i.e., without information from history, interview, and observations of examination behavior) are used to make diagnostic decisions, and of dogmatic statements offered without strongly supportive evidence. It is also important to remember that neuropsychological tests do not measure "brain damage." Rather, the finding of impaired mental functioning implies an underlying brain disorder. However, other possible interpretations may exist.

MAJOR TEST CATEGORIES

In this section, we present a brief review of tests used for assessment of major areas of cognition and personality. Many useful neuropsychological tests are not described in this summary. Please refer to *Neuropsychological Assessment*, 4th Edition (Lezak et al. 2004), for a relatively complete review and to *A Compendium of Neuropsychological Tests*, 2nd Edition (Spreen and Strauss 1998), for more detailed normative data on many frequently used tests.

MENTAL ABILITY

The most commonly used set of tests of general intellectual function of adults in the Western world is contained in the various versions and translations of the WIS (Wechsler 1944, 1955, 1981, 1997a). These batteries of brief tests provide scores on a variety of cognitive tasks covering a range of skills. Each version was originally developed as an "intelligence" test to predict academic and vocational performance of neurologically intact adults by giving an IQ (intelligence quotient) score, which is based on the mean performance on the tests in this battery. The entire test battery may provide the bulk of the tests included in a neuropsychological examination. The individual tests were designed to assess relatively distinct areas of cognition, such as arithmetic, abstract thinking, and visuospatial organization, and thus are differentially sensitive to dysfunction of various areas of the brain. Therefore, these tests are often used to screen for specific areas of cognitive deficits. Many experienced neuropsychologists use and interpret these tests discretely, administering only those deemed relevant for each patient and treating the findings as they treat data obtained from individually developed tests.

When given to neuropsychologically impaired persons, the summary IQ scores can be very misleading because individual test scores lowered by specific cognitive deficits, when averaged in with scores relatively unaffected by the brain dysfunction, can result in IQ scores associated with ability levels that represent neither the severity of deficits nor the patient's residual competencies (Lezak 1988b). For example, a patient with a visuospatial deficit consisting of an inability to appreciate the structure of visual patterns would have difficulty performing the Block Design test, which requires copying pictured designs with blocks. When such a patient performs well above average on other tests, a summation of all the scores would both hide the important data and be lower than the other test scores in the battery would warrant. Therefore, neuropsychologists focus on the pattern of the Wechsler scores rather than the summed or average performance on all the tests in the battery.

In some cases, neuropsychologists have used discrepancies between summed scores on what Wechsler called the Verbal scale of the WIS (i.e., Verbal IQ) and summed scores on the so-called Performance scale (Performance IQ) to indicate a specific area of cognitive deficit. The procedure has developed because left hemisphere lesions tend to produce a relatively depressed Verbal IQ score, whereas both right hemisphere lesions and diffuse damage, as in dementia or any problem resulting in response slowing, produce a depressed Performance IQ score. Even this lesser amount of summation can mask important data (Bornstein 1983; Crawford 1992; Grossman 1983; Iverson et al. 2004). In the earlier example, impaired performance on one test would not be likely to produce sufficient relative lowering of the Performance IQ score to detect the cognitive deficit. Moreover, the Arithmetic and Digit Span tests of the Verbal scale are very sensitive to attentional deficits, and only three of the Performance scale measures involve motor response: one (Picture Completion) calls for a purely verbal response and loads significantly on the verbal factor in factor analytic studies.

A similar battery for assessing children is the Wechsler Intelligence Scale–III (WISC-III; Wechsler 1991). It contains tests analogous to those in the Wechsler Adult Intelligence Scale–III but appropriate for children ages 6–16 years.

LANGUAGE

Lesions to the hemisphere dominant for speech and language, which is the left hemisphere in 95%–97% of right-handed persons and 60%–70% of left-handed ones (Corballis 1991; Strauss and Goldsmith 1987), can produce any of a variety of disorders of symbol formulation and use—the aphasias (Spreen and Risser 2003). Although many aphasiologists argue against attempting to classify all patients into one of the standard aphasia syndromes because of so many individual differences, persons with aphasia tend to be grouped according to whether the main disorder is in language comprehension (receptive aphasia), expression (expressive aphasia), repetition (conduction aphasia), or naming (anomic aphasia). Many comprehensive language assessment tests are available, such as the Multilingual Aphasia Examination (Benton and Hamsher 1989). Comprehensive aphasia test batteries are best administered by speech pathologists or other clinicians with special training in this field. These batteries usually include measures of spontaneous speech, speech comprehension, repetition, naming, reading, and writing.

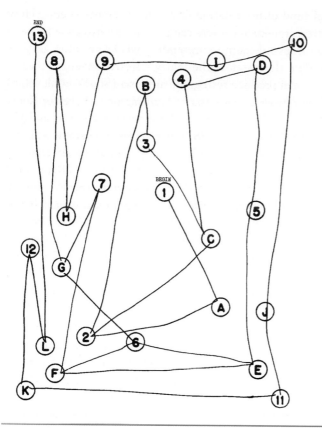

FIGURE 6–4.   Trail Making Test (Armitage 1946) Part B performance by a 61-year-old man with normal pressure hydrocephalus. Two types of errors are shown: erroneous sequencing (1→A→2→C) and failure to alternate between numbers and letters (D→5→E→F).

Test selection may be based on whether the information is to be used for diagnostic, prognostic, or rehabilitation purposes. For example, the Boston Diagnostic Aphasia Examination, 3rd Edition (BDAE-3; Goodglass et al. 2000), might be selected as an aid for treatment planning because of its wide scope and sensitivity to different aphasic characteristics. The Porch Index of Communicative Ability (Porch 1981) best measures treatment progress because of its sensitivity to small changes in performance. A language screening examination is the Bedside Evaluation Screening Test, 2nd Edition (BEST-2; West et al. 1998). This approximately 20-minute examination provides measures of comprehension, talking, and reading.

ATTENTION AND MENTAL TRACKING

A frequent consequence of brain disorders is slowed mental processing and impaired ability for focused behavior (Duncan and Mirsky 2004; Leclercq and Zimmermann 2002). Damage to the brain stem or diffuse damage involving the cerebral hemispheres, especially the white matter interconnections, can produce a variety of atten-

tional deficits. Attentional deficits are very common in neuropsychiatric disorders. Most neuropsychological assessments will include measures of these abilities. The Wechsler scales contain several relevant tests. Digit Span measures attention span or short-term memory for numbers in two ways: forward and backward digit repetition. Backward digit repetition is a more demanding task because it requires concentration and mental tracking plus the short-term memory component. It is not uncommon for moderately to severely brain-damaged patients to perform poorly on only the backward repetition portion of this test. Because Digits Forward and Digits Backward measure different functions, assessment data for each should be reported separately. Digit Symbol also requires concentration plus motor and mental speed for successful performance. The patient must accurately and rapidly code numbers into symbols. The Arithmetic test in the Wechsler battery is very sensitive to attentional disorders because it requires short-term auditory memory and rapid mental juggling of arithmetic problem elements. Poor performance on this test must be evaluated for the nature of the failures. Another commonly used measure of concentration and mental tracking is the Trail Making Test (Armitage 1946). In the first part of this test (Part A), the patient is asked to draw rapidly and accurately a line connecting in sequence a random display of numbered circles on a page. The level of difficulty is increased in the second part (Part B) by having the patient again sequence a random display of circles, this time alternating numbers and letters (Figure 6–4). This test requires concentration, visual scanning, and flexibility in shifting cognitive sets (Cicerone and Azulay 2002). It shares with many attention tests vulnerability to other kinds of deficits such as motor slowing, which could be based on peripheral factors such as nerve or muscle damage, and diminished visual acuity. It is also sensitive to educational deprivation and cannot be used with persons not well versed in the alphabet common to Western languages (e.g., English, French, Dutch, Italian).

In cases of subtle brain injury, assessment sensitivity can be increased by selecting a more difficult measure of concentration and mental tracking in which material must be held in mind while information is manipulated for the performance of complex cognitive activities such as comprehension, learning, and reasoning. When patients perform poorly on the WIS Arithmetic test, the examiner must determine whether the failure results from attentional deficits or lack of arithmetic skills. The ability to hold information in mind while performing a mental task is called *working memory* (Baddeley 1994). As such, working memory requires attention and short-term memory. The Self Ordered Pointing Task (Petrides and Milner 1982; Spreen and Strauss 1998) instructs patients to point to one item in a set ranging from 6 to 18 varied items. On each trial, in which the positions of the items are randomly changed, patients are told to point to a different item than they had previously pointed to, and then another, until they have pointed to all the items. The successful performance of this working memory task depends on keeping in mind which items have already been eliminated. Another example of a difficult attentional task is the Paced Auditory Serial Addition Task (PASAT; Gronwall 1977; Gronwall and Sampson 1974). The patient is required to add consecutive pairs of numbers rapidly under an interference condition. As numbers are presented at a fixed rate, the patient must always add the last two numbers presented and ignore the number that represents the last summation. For example, if the numbers "3–5–2–7" are presented, the patient must respond "8" after the number 5, and then "7" after the number 2, and then "9." It is a difficult test of divided attention because of the strong tendency to add the last number presented to the last summation. The level of difficulty can be heightened by speeding up the rate of presentation of numbers. The PASAT is among those tests that are most sensitive to attentional disorders (Cicerone and Azulay 2002). However, because most persons taking this test, even those who achieve good scores, believe that they have done poorly, its negative effect on a patient's mood and test-taking attitude must be taken into account before selecting it (Feldner et al. 2006).

MEMORY

Memory is another cognitive function that is frequently impaired by brain disorders. Many diffuse brain injuries produce general impairments in abilities for new learning and retention. Many focal brain injuries also produce memory impairment; left hemisphere lesions are most likely to produce primarily verbal memory deficits, whereas visuospatial memory impairments tend to be associated with right hemisphere lesions (Abrahams et al. 1997; Ojemann and Dodrill 1985; Wagner et al. 1998), although not all visuospatial tests show a right hemisphere advantage (Raspall et al. 2005). Memory impairment often is a prominent feature of herpes encephalitis, Huntington's chorea, Korsakoff's syndrome, hypoxia, closed head injury, and a variety of neurological degenerative diseases such as Alzheimer's disease (Baddeley et al. 2002; Bauer et al. 2003; Mayes 2000).

In most cases of brain injury, memory for information learned before the injury is relatively preserved compared with new learning. For this reason, many patients with memory impairment will perform relatively well on tests of fund of information or recall of remote events. However, amnesic disorders can produce a retrograde amnesia, with loss of memory extending weeks, months, or years before the onset of the injury. Electroconvulsive therapy also can produce retrograde amnesia (Squire et al. 1975). The retrograde amnesia of Huntington's chorea or Korsakoff's syndrome can go back for decades (Butters and Miliotis 1985; Cermak 1982). In rare cases, a patient will have retrograde amnesia without significant anterograde amnesia; that is, new learning ability remains intact (Kapur et al. 1996; Reed and Squire 1998). Isolated retrograde amnesia may include amnesia for autobiographical events (Della Sala et al. 1993; Evans et al. 1996; Kapur 1997; Levine et al. 1998). However, cases of isolated amnesia for personal identity often have a psychogenic cause (Hodges 1991).

The Wechsler Memory Scale (WMS) batteries (Wechsler 1987, 1997b) are the most commonly used set of tests of new learning and retention in the United States. These batteries are composed of a variety of tests measuring free recall or recognition of both verbal and visual material. In addition, these tests include measures of recall of personal information and attention, concentration, and mental tracking. Several of the tests provide measures of both immediate and delayed (approximately 30 minutes) recall.

Other memory tests frequently used include word-list learning tasks, such as the Rey Auditory Verbal Learning Test (Lezak et al. 2004; Rey 1964; M. Schmidt 1996) or the California Verbal Learning Test (Delis et al. 1986, 2000), and visuospatial tasks, such the Complex Figure Test (Mitrushina et al. 2005; Osterrieth 1944; Rey 1941; Spreen and Strauss 1998). When patients are unable to give verbal responses or to use their preferred hand for drawing, recognition memory tests requiring a simple "yes" or "no" response are useful. Representative of these learning tests are the Continuous Visual Memory Test (Trahan and Larrabee 1988) and the Recognition Memory Test (Warrington 1984).

PERCEPTION

Perception in any of the sensory modalities can be affected by brain disease. Perceptional inattention (sometimes called neglect) is one of the major perceptual syndromes because it occurs frequently with focal brain damage (Bisiach and Vallar 1988; Heilman et al. 2000b; Rafal 2000; Lezak 1994). This phenomenon involves diminished or absent awareness of stimuli in one side of personal space by a patient with an intact sensory system. Unilateral inattention is often most prominent immediately after acute-onset brain injury such as stroke. Most commonly seen is left-sided inattention associated with right hemisphere lesions.

Several techniques can be used to detect unilateral inattention. Visual inattention can be assessed by using a Line Bisection Test (Schenkenberg et al. 1980), in which the patient is asked to bisect a series of uneven lines on a page, or by using a cancellation task requiring the patient to cross out a designated symbol distributed among other similar symbols over a page (Haeske-Dewick et al. 1996; Mesulam 2000). A commonly used test for tactile inattention is the Face-Hand Test (G. Berg et al. 1987; Smith 1983). With eyes closed, the patient is instructed to indicate when points on the face (cheeks) or hands or both are touched by the examiner. Each side is touched singly and then in combination with the other side, such as left cheek and right hand. The patient should have no difficulty reporting a single point of stimulation. Failure to report stimulation to one side when both sides are stimulated is referred to as *tactile inattention* or *double simultaneous extinction*.

The most commonly used forms of perceptual tests assess perceptual discrimination among similar stimuli. These visual tests may include discrimination of geometric forms, angulation, color, faces, or familiar objects (Lezak et al. 2004; McCarthy and Warrington 1990; Newcombe and Ratcliff 1989). Some perceptual tasks assess the ability to integrate isolated percepts. The Hooper Visual Organization Test (Hooper 1958) presents line drawings of familiar objects in fragmented, disarranged pieces and asks for the name of each object. Some standard cognitive tests also can be administered in tactile version (Beauvais et al. 2004; Van Lancker et al. 1989; Varney 1986). Frequently used tactile tests include form recognition and letter or number recognition (Reitan and Wolfson 1993).

Another important area of perceptual assessment is recognition of familiar visual stimuli. Although the syndromes are rare and often occur independently of one another, a brain injury can produce an inability to recognize visually familiar objects (visual object agnosia) or faces (prosopagnosia) (Barton et al. 2004; Bauer and Demery 2003; McCarthy and Warrington 1990). Assessment involves testing the recognition—often in the form of naming—of real objects or representations of objects, sometimes in a masked or distorted form. For facial recognition, "same or different" questions have been used. The WIS batteries include a perceptual task in which the subject must identify missing features of drawings of familiar objects.

Some patients with brain injury have difficulty discriminating sounds even with good hearing and no aphasia. Therefore, tests have been devised to measure discrimination of speech sounds (Benton et al. 1994; Wepman and Reynolds 1987) and nonsymbolic sound patterns (Seashore et al. 1960). Discrimination of speech tends to be associated with left temporal lobe lesions, whereas nonsymbolic sounds such as sirens, bells, and doors closing seem to be associated with right temporal lobe lesions (Milner 1971; Polster and Rose 1998). In interpreting patients' performances on certain tests involving auditory discrimination, the examiner must be sensitive to the possible effects of attentional deficits because low scores on these tests can result from a constricted auditory span or compromised ability to concentrate. This potential for misinterpretation of examination findings is always present and is one of the reasons that valid neuropsychological assessment requires knowledgeable and experienced examiners.

PRAXIS

Many patients with left hemisphere damage have at least one form of apraxia, and apraxia is common in progressed stages of Alzheimer's disease, Parkinson's disease, Pick's disease, and progressive supranuclear palsy (Dobigny-Roman et al. 1998; Fukui et al. 1996; Leiguarda et al. 1997). Apraxic patients' inability to perform a desired sequence of motor activities is not the result of motor weakness. Rather, the deficit is in planning and carrying out the required activities (De Renzi et al. 1983; Heilman et al. 2000a; Jason 1990) and is associated with disruption of neural representations for extrapersonal (e.g., spatial location) and intrapersonal (e.g., hand position) features of movement (Haaland et al. 1999). Tests for apraxia assess the patient's ability to reproduce learned movements of the face or limbs. These learned movements can include the use of objects (usually pantomime use of objects) and gestures (Goodglass et al. 2000; Rothi et al. 1997; Strub and Black 2000) or sequences of movements demonstrated by the examiner (Christensen 1979; Haaland and Flaherty 1984).

CONSTRUCTIONAL ABILITY

Although constructional problems were once considered a form of apraxia, more recent analysis has shown that the underlying deficits involve impaired appreciation of one or more aspects of spatial relationships. These can include distortions in perspective, angulation, size, and distance judgment. Thus, unlike apraxia, the problem is not an inability to organize a motor response for drawing lines or assembling constructions but rather misperceptions and misjudgments involving spatial relationships. Neuropsychological assessments may include any of a number of measures of visuospatial processing. Patients may be asked to copy geometric designs, such as the Complex Figure (Mitrushina et al. 2005; Osterrieth 1944; Rey 1941; Spreen and Strauss 1998) presented in Figure 6–5 or one of the alternative forms (Lezak et al. 2004; Loring et al. 1988). The WIS battery includes constructional tasks involving copying pictured designs with blocks and assembling puzzle pieces (Wechsler 1944, 1955, 1981, 1997a). Lesions of the posterior cerebral cortex are associated with the greatest difficulty with constructions, and right hemisphere lesions produce greater deficits than do left hemisphere lesions (Benton and Tranel 1993).

CONCEPTUAL FUNCTIONS

Tests of concept formation measure aspects of thinking including reasoning, abstraction, and problem solving. Conceptual dysfunction tends to occur with serious brain injury regardless of site. Most neuropsychological tests require that simple conceptual functioning be intact. For example, reasoning skills are required for the successful performance of most WIS tests: Comprehension assesses commonsense verbal reasoning and interpretation of proverbs; Similarities measures ability to make verbal abstractions by asking for similarities between objects or concepts; Arithmetic involves arithmetic problem solving; Picture Completion requires perceptual reasoning; Picture Arrangement examines sequential reasoning for thematic pictures; Block Design and Object Assembly test visuospatial analysis and synthesis, respectively; and Matrix Reasoning depends on pattern, spatial, and numerical relationships as well as verbal components.

Other commonly used tests of concept formation include the Category Test (Halstead 1947), the Wisconsin Card Sorting Test (WCST; E.A. Berg 1948; D.A. Grant and Berg 1948; Spreen and Strauss 1998), and the California Sorting Test (Hartman et al. 2004). These tests measure concept formation, hypothesis testing, problem solving, flexibility of thinking, and short-term memory. The Category Test presents patterns of stimuli and requires the patient to figure out a principle or concept that is true for each item within the set based on feedback about the correctness of each response. The patient is told that the correct principle may be the same for all sets or different for each set. For example, the correct principle in one set is position (first, second, etc.) of the stimulus on the page, whereas for another, it is the number of items on the page.

The WCST is similar to the Category Test in requiring the patient to figure out a principle that is true for items within a set. This test differs in several ways. One of the main ways is that without warning the patient, the examiner changes the correct principle as the test proceeds. Therefore, the patient must figure out independently that a shift in principles has occurred and act accordingly. The California Sorting Test asks patients to sort cards with multiple features into sets with common features and to repeat the sorting with as many new sorting criteria as possible.

Tests of conceptualization and reasoning illustrate some of the interpretation problems inherent in most neuropsychological tests because they require complex mental activity. Thus, patients with recent memory disorders and those who are highly distractible may be able to solve the conceptual problems presented by these tests but fail because of inability to keep the correct solution in mind.

EXECUTIVE FUNCTIONS

Executive functions include abilities to formulate a goal, to plan, to carry out goal-directed plans effectively, and to monitor and self-correct spontaneously and reliably (Lezak 1982). Perseveration (as shown in Figure 6–5, Panel C) occurs when the response is repeated inappropriately and may involve motor acts (as shown), speech, or thoughts. Open-ended tests that permit the patient to decide how to perform the task and when it is complete are difficult tasks for many patients with frontal lobe or diffuse brain injuries (Lezak 1982; Luria 1980). Yet the abilities these tasks test are essential for fulfilling most adult responsibilities and maintaining socially appropriate conduct. An example of a class of tests that assess executive functions are tests of planning, such as mazes. The patient must plan an exit from the maze, which involves foresight to minimize trial-and-error behavior. The Tower of London (Shallice 1982) and Tower of Hanoi tests also assess planning and foresight, as disks are moved from stack to stack to reach a stated goal. Patients with frontal lobe lesions have particular difficulty with planning tests (Carlin et al. 2000; Goel and Grafman 1995). Other tasks that rely heavily on planning for successful completion are multistep tasks calling for decision-making or priority-setting abilities. Few neuropsychological tests are specifically designed to assess these aspects of behavior, yet many complex tasks depend on this analysis. An exception is a set of real-world tasks developed for this purpose called the Behavioral Assessment of the Dysexecutive Syndrome (BADS) (B.A. Wilson et al. 1996), which has been shown to bring out problems with flexibility, planning, and priority setting in patients with brain injury (Norris and Tate 2000), and schizophrenia (Krabbendam et al. 1999).

One example of a priority-setting task is the Twenty Questions test, which is known as a popular game. In the test version (Laine and Butters 1982), the patient is shown an array of 48 drawings of familiar objects and told to identify the one the examiner is thinking of by asking only "yes-or-no" questions. The goal is to identify the specified objects with as few questions as possible. The quality of the questions asked varies according to the number of objects they include or exclude as a possible target. Many patients with frontal lobe injuries begin questioning with low-priority questions or even by asking whether the target is a specific object (Baldo et al. 2004;

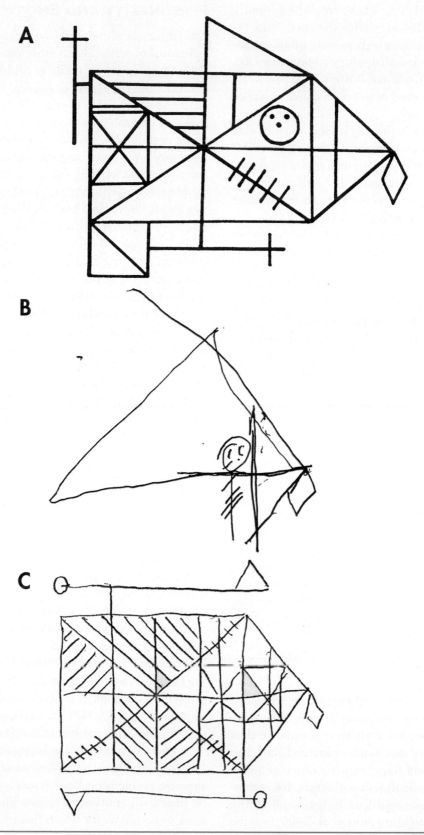

FIGURE 6–5. Rey Complex Figure (*Panel A*) and copy (*Panel B*) drawn by a 77-year-old man who had a right hemisphere stroke 2 days before, which produced left-sided neglect and delayed recall. *Panel C* was drawn by a 72-year-old man with strong perseverative tendencies.

Upton and Thompson 1999). These frontal lobe injury patients also can have difficulty with the conceptual requirement of the test because high-priority questions are more abstract. Detoxified alcoholic patients also have difficulty on this task (Laine and Butters 1982).

Adaptive behavior often requires changing behavior according to new demands. The WCST also measures adaptive decision making in that the patient must be able to recognize the changed sorting principle and adjust his or her responses accordingly. Many patients with dorsolateral frontal lobe lesions recognize that a change has occurred but either are slow or never alter their responses according to the new demands (Stuss et al. 2000).

Inertia presents one of the most difficult assessment problems for neuropsychologists. Few open-ended tests measure initiation or ability to carry out purposeful behavior. By their very nature, most tests are structured and require little initiation by the patient (Lezak 1982). Examples of less structured tests include the Tinker Toy Test, in which the patient decides what to build and how to design it (Bayless et al. 1989; Lezak 1982). Because there are few rules, the patient's level of productivity on this task typically reflects his or her level of productivity in the real world (Lezak et al. 2004). Tests of verbal fluency are used to measure initiation of concepts and persistence on a task. Patients are asked to name as many items as they can in a category, such as animals, or produce as many words as they can beginning with a specified letter of the alphabet (Mitrushina et al. 2005; Spreen and Strauss 1998). These tasks are performed best if the examinee initiates effective and varied strategies. The Executive Function Route-Finding task of Boyd and Sautter (1993) is a practical technique for examining initiative and resourcefulness by asking the patient to find a specified place in the hospital or building complex (e.g., a cafeteria in the building) located two floors from the clinic or a smoking zone outside.

MOTOR FUNCTIONS

Neuropsychological tests can supplement the neurological examination of motor functions by providing standardized measures of motor activities. Normative data have been developed for commonly measured functions such as grip strength and finger tapping; more complex tests of fine motor coordination include tests that require patients to place pegs rapidly in holes, such as the Grooved Pegboard Test (Mitrushina et al. 2005) and the Purdue Pegboard Test (Spreen and Strauss 1998). These tests examine absolute performance and compare the preferred hand against the nonpreferred hand to measure the possibility of lateralized motor deficit.

PERSONALITY AND EMOTIONAL STATUS

Numerous questionnaires have been devised to measure symptoms of physical and emotional distress of patients with neurological or medical problems (Fischer et al. 2004; Lezak 1989). As examples, the Neurobehavioral Rating Scale (H. S. Levin et al. 1987) is an examiner-rated measure of problems commonly associated with traumatic brain injury, and the Mayo-Portland Adaptability Inventory provides for ratings from clinicians, the patient, and the patient's family members (Malec et al. 2000).

Many tests devised to measure psychological distress or psychiatric illness have been used with persons with brain disorders. The Symptom Checklist–90—Revised (SCL-90-R; Derogatis 1983) is a self-report of symptoms associated with psychiatric disorders when they occur at high frequency levels. The MMPI (Dahlstrom et al. 1975; Hathaway and McKinley 1951; G. S. Welsh and Dahlstrom 1956) and the revised version, the MMPI-2 (Butcher 1989; Butcher and Pope 1990; Butcher et al. 1989), have been used extensively with patients with brain disorders (Chelune et al. 1986; Dahlstrom et al. 1975; Mueller and Girace 1988). In general, these patients tend to have elevated MMPI and MMPI-2 profiles, which may reflect the relatively frequent incidence of emotional disturbance (Filskov and Leli 1981), patients' accurate reporting of symptoms and deficits (Lezak et al. 2004), or their compromised ability to read or understand the test questions. Elevations in scales Hs ("Hypochondriasis"), Hy ("Hysteria"), and Sc ("Schizophrenia") are common because many "neurological" symptoms appear on these scales (Cripe 1999; Gass 1992; Gass and Apple 1997; Lachapelle and Alfano 2005). The interpretation of data from persons with brain disorders must take into account the contributions of neurological symptoms, the patient's emotional reactions to the condition, and the patient's premorbid personality.

Many attempts have been made to use the MMPI to differentiate diagnoses of psychiatric and neurological illness. Results generally have been unsatisfactory, probably due to the extreme variety of brain disorders and their associated problems (Glassmire et al. 2003; Lezak et al. 2004). It is not surprising that the MMPI also has been an inefficient instrument for localizing cerebral lesions (Lezak et al. 2004).

Neuropsychologists are frequently asked to evaluate "psychological overlay" or functional complaints. The diagnostic problem occurs because some individuals may be financially motivated to establish injuries related to work or accidents for which financial compensation may be sought. In addition, some individuals receive emotional or social rewards for invalidism, leading to malingering and functional disabilities. It is difficult to establish with complete certainty that a person's complaints are functional. To add to the complexity of the diagnosis, patients with established brain injury sometimes embellish their symptoms, wittingly or unwittingly, so that the range of problems may represent a combination of true deficits and exaggeration. The clinician usually must search for a combination of factors that would support or discredit a functional diagnosis (Lezak et al. 2004). General factors include evidence of inconsistency in history, reporting of symptoms, or test performance; the individual's emotional predisposition; the probability of secondary gain; and the patient's emotional reactions to his or her complaints, such as the classic *la belle indifférence*.

Psychological tests may be helpful in establishing evidence of exaggeration of symptoms. Responses to the MMPI and MMPI-2 validity scales (L, F, and K) can provide information about the patient's cooperativeness while taking this test and the likelihood that symptoms are exaggerated—or minimized. Because people faking brain damage tend to exaggerate poor performance on testing, another useful diagnostic approach has been the Symptom Validity Test (Pankratz 1979). The fundamental procedure examines the patient's complaints of inability by forcing a response to a simple, two-alternative problem involving the complaint. The examiner uses many trials to calculate the likelihood that the performance deviates from chance or from expected performance. The Hiscock and Hiscock Digit Memory Test (Hiscock et al. 1994) tests the validity of memory complaints by requiring the patient to recall a short series of numbers during a forced-choice, two-item recognition task. The Test of Memory Malingering also evaluates complaint validity by asking the patient to choose which pictures had been shown to him or her previously with a similar forced-choice technique (Spreen and Strauss 1998; Tombaugh 1996).

SPECIAL ASSESSMENT TOOLS

BATTERIES

Many neuropsychologists use a formalized battery of tests, in which case they may develop considerable skill and familiarity with this preselected set of tests. The WIS battery of tests, described earlier, is commonly used for this purpose.

Of the commercial batteries designed for neuropsychological evaluations, by far the most popular in the United States is the Halstead-Reitan Battery. This battery was designed to assess frontal lobe disorders by Ward C. Halstead (1947) and was subsequently taken on by Ralph Reitan (1969), who added some tests and recommended this battery as a diagnostic test for all kinds of brain damage. The tests include the Category Test, described earlier; the Tactual Performance Test, a tactile spatial performance

and memory test; the Rhythm Test, purported to be a nonverbal auditory perception test; the Speech Sounds Perception Test, purported to be a phoneme discrimination test; the Finger Tapping Test, a motor speed test; the Trail Making Test, described earlier; the Aphasia Screening Test, which was originally developed by the aphasiologist Wepman but later discarded by him for being both ineffectual and misleading; a sensory examination; and a measure of grip strength (see Lezak et al. 2004). Examiners using this battery currently administer it with one of the forms of the WIS, the WMS, and the MMPI-2. A newer "all-purpose" battery is the Kaplan-Baycrest Neurocognitive Assessment (Leach et al. 2000). As this is a new test battery, limited clinical data have been reported.

Examinations designed to address specific diagnostic questions are available. Several dementia examinations have been devised. The Dementia Rating Scale (Mattis et al. 2001) contains items assessing attention, initiation/perseveration, construction, conceptualization, and memory and is useful in distinguishing dementia from cognitive decline associated with aging. A brief examination for dementia by the Consortium to Establish a Registry for Alzheimer's Disease (CERAD) uses the MMSE and tests of category fluency, confrontational naming, verbal learning, and design copy (K.A. Welsh et al. 1992). Batteries for assessing executive deficits include the BADS (B.A. Wilson et al. 1998), the Behavioral Dyscontrol Scale (Grigsby et al. 1992), and the Executive Interview (Royall et al. 1992).

SCREENING TESTS

Many clinicians would like to have a brief, reliable screening examination with good sensitivity for brain damage of unknown cause or when it is only suspected. However, there is a tradeoff between the amount of information obtained in an assessment and its actual usefulness in the detection of brain dysfunction. Brief examinations are often too restricted in range or too simple to be sensitive to subtle or circumscribed areas of dysfunction. The commonly used MMSE contains only 11 simple tasks. It is useful for examining patients with global confusion, poor memory, or dementia. However, many brain-injured patients, such as those with stroke, mild to moderate head injury, and even early dementia, perform adequately on this examination (Benedict and Brandt 1992).

The Neurobehavioral Cognitive Status Examination, also called COGNISTAT (Kiernan et al. 1987; Mysiw et al. 1989; Schwamm et al. 1987), takes about 30 minutes to administer and contains reasonably difficult items of attention, language comprehension, repetition and naming, constructional ability, memory, calculations, reasoning, and judgment, thereby increasing its sensitivity. It is a screening examination, however, and not a substitute for a thorough neuropsychological examination. It may be used to acquire information to decide whether further evaluation is warranted. As with any screening examination, intact performance does not exclude the possibility of brain dysfunction. The Repeatable Battery for the Assessment of Neuropsychological Status (Randolph et al. 1998) also takes about 30 minutes to administer and is useful in screening patients with neurological and psychiatric disease (Hobart et al. 1999; Larson et al. 2005).

COMPETENCY

A cognitive competency determination is usually based on a specialized interview in which a patient's ability to handle financial matters and make decisions about his or her well-being is assessed by asking questions about the individual's personal situation. The patient's understanding of his or her personal needs is more relevant to a competency determination than is a score on a formal test. Patients' consent to medical treatment under different legal standards is assessed by asking patients to make decisions after they evaluate the associated risks and benefits of hypothetical medical problems and treatment alternatives (Marson et al. 1995a, 1995b, 2001). Examinations of legal competencies also are used for issues such as parenting capacity and competence to stand trial (Grisso 2002).

TREATMENT AND PLANNING

Examination findings are used to assess an individual's strengths and weaknesses and to formulate treatment interventions (Christensen and Uzzell 2000; Lezak 1987; Raskin and Mateer 1999; B.A. Wilson et al. 2002). Clinical interventions vary according to the individual's specific needs. Many patients with brain disorders have

primary or secondary emotional problems for which psychotherapy or counseling is advisable. However, brain-injured patients frequently have problems that require special consideration. Foremost among these problems are cognitive rigidity, impaired learning ability, and diminished self-awareness, any one of which may limit the patient's adaptability and capacity to benefit from rehabilitation. Therefore, neuropsychological evaluations provide important information about treatment possibilities and strategies. The evaluation is also used to consider patients' capability for independence in society and their educational or vocational potential.

QUALIFICATIONS FOR PERFORMING NEUROPSYCHOLOGICAL EVALUATIONS

The field of neuropsychology is enriched by the diversity of areas of expertise of those interested in the study of brain-behavior relations. Professionals in this field come from backgrounds in psychology, psychiatry, neurology, neurosurgery, and language pathology, to name the most common contributing disciplines. In psychology alone, practitioners come from backgrounds in clinical, cognitive, developmental, and physiological psychology.

Professionals qualified to provide clinical evaluations have both expertise in brain-behavior relations and skills in diagnostic assessment and counseling (Barth et al. 2003; Hannay et al. 1998). A growing number of neuropsychologists have qualified for proficiency in this subspecialty area, earning the American Board of Professional Psychology's award of Diploma in Clinical Neuropsychology (Bieliauskas and Matthews 1987).

Highlights for the Clinician

Indications for a neuropsychological evaluation

✦ Assess nature and severity of known brain disorders
✦ Assess potential brain disorder in people with known risk factors
✦ Diagnose behavioral or cognitive changes of unknown etiology

Role of the referring clinician

✦ Identify patients who might benefit from a neuropsychological evaluation
✦ Prepare the patient through education about the reasons for and nature of the examination
✦ Provide an explicit and thorough referral question

Assessment process

✦ Interview
✦ Use standardized cognitive, behavioral, and emotional tests
✦ Interpret results on the basis of comparisons with appropriate normative data

Highlights for the Clinician *(continued)*

Major test categories

+ Language
+ Attention and mental tracking
+ Memory
+ Perception
+ Praxis
+ Constructional ability
+ Conceptual functions
+ Executive functions
+ Motor functions
+ Personality and emotional status

Uses of data

+ Identify patient's strengths and weaknesses
+ Provide a diagnosis
+ Formulate a treatment or an intervention
+ Determine competency

RECOMMENDED READINGS

Heilman K, Valenstein E (eds): Clinical Neuropsychology, 4th Edition. New York, Oxford University Press, 2003

Lezak M, Howieson D, Loring D: Neuropsychological Assessment, 4th Edition. New York, Oxford University Press, 2004

REFERENCES

Abbruzzese M, Bellodi L, Ferri S, et al: Frontal lobe dysfunction in schizophrenia and obsessive-compulsive disorder: a neuropsychological study. Brain Cogn 27:202–212, 1995

Abrahams S, Pickering A, Polkey CE, et al: Spatial memory deficits in patients with unilateral damage to the right hippocampal formation. Neuropsychologia 35:11–24, 1997

Adler CM, McDonough-Ryan P, Sax KW, et al: fMRI of neuronal activation with symptom provocation in unmedicated patients with obsessive compulsive disorder. J Psychiatr Res 34:317–324, 2000

Aine CJ: A conceptual overview and critiques of functional neuroimaging techniques in humans, I: MRI/FMRI and PET. Crit Rev Neurobiol 9:229–309, 1995

Ali SO, Denicoff KD, Altshuler LL, et al: A preliminary study of the relation of neuropsychological performance to neuroanatomic structures in bipolar disorder. Neuropsychiatry Neuropsychol Behav Neurol 13:20–28, 2000

Allen DN, Goldstein G, Warnick E: A consideration of neuropsychologically normal schizophrenia. J Int Neuropsychol Soc 9:56–63, 2003

Anastasi A, Urbina S: Psychological Testing. Upper Saddle River, NJ, Prentice-Hall, 1997

Andersen G, Vestergaard K, Ingemann-Nielsen M, et al: Risk factors for post-stroke depression. Acta Psychiatr Scand 92:193–198, 1995

Armitage SG: An analysis of certain psychological tests used for the evaluation of brain injury. Psychol Monogr (No 277) 60:1–48, 1946

Armstrong FD, Thompson RJ Jr, Wang W, et al: Cognitive functioning and brain magnetic resonance imaging in children with sickle cell disease. Neuropsychology Committee of the Cooperative Study of Sickle Cell Disease. Pediatrics 97:864–870, 1996

Astrom M, Adolfsson R, Asplund K: Major depression in stroke patients: a 3-year longitudinal study. Stroke 24:976–982, 1993

Baddeley A: Working memory: the interface between memory and cognition, in Memory Systems 1994. Edited by Schacter DL, Tulving E. Cambridge, MA, MIT Press, 1994, pp 351–367

Baddeley A, Kopelman M, Wilson B (eds): The Handbook of Memory Disorders, 2nd Edition. West Sussex, England, Wiley, 2002

Baldo JV, Delis DC, Wilkins DP, et al: Is it bigger than a breadbox? Performance of patients with prefrontal lesions on a new executive function test. Arch Clin Neuropsychol 19:407–419, 2004

Barth J, Ryan T, Hawk G, et al: Introduction to the NAN 2001 definition of a clinical neuropsychologist. Arch Clin Neuropsychol 18:551–555, 2003

Barton JJ, Cherkasova MV, Press DZ, et al: Perceptual functions in prosopagnosia. Perception 33:939–956, 2004

Basso MR, Bornstein RA: Neuropsychological deficits in psychotic versus nonpsychotic unipolar depression. Neuropsychology 13:69–75, 1999a

Basso MR, Bornstein RA: Relative memory deficits in recurrent versus first-episode major depression on a word-list learning task. Neuropsychology 13:557–563, 1999b

Bauer R, Demery J: Agnosia, in Clinical Neuropsychology. Edited by Heilman K, Valenstein E. New York, Oxford University Press, 2003, pp 236–295

Bauer R, Grande L, Valenstein E: Amnesic disorders, in Clinical Neuropsychology. Edited by Heilman K, Valenstein E. New York, Oxford University Press, 2003, pp 495–573

Bayless JD, Varney NR, Roberts RJ: Tinker Toy Test performance and vocational outcome in patients with closed head injuries. J Clin Exp Neuropsychol 11:913–917, 1989

Beauvais J, Woods S, Delaney R, et al: Development of a tactile Wisconsin Card Sorting Test. Rehabil Psychol 49:282–287, 2004

Benedict RH, Brandt J: Limitation of the Mini-Mental State Examination for the detection of amnesia. J Geriatr Psychiatry Neurol 5:233–237, 1992

Bennett TL, Raymond MJ: Mild brain injury: an overview. Appl Neuropsychol 4:1–5, 1997

Bennett T, Raymond M: Utilizing neuropsychological assessment in disability determination and rehabilitation planning, in Handbook of Forensic Neuropsychology. Edited by Horton AJ, Hartlage L. New York, Springer, 2003, pp 237–257

Benson DF, Djenderedjian A, Miller BL, et al: Neural basis of confabulation. Neurology 46:1239–1243, 1996

Benton AL, Hamsher K de S: Multilingual Aphasia Examination. Iowa City, IO, AJA Associates, 1989

Benton AL, Tranel D: Visuoperceptual, visuospatial, and visuoconstructive disorders, in Clinical Neuropsychology. Edited by Heilman KM, Valenstein E. New York, Oxford University Press, 1993, pp 461–497

Benton AL, Silvan AB, Hamsher K de S, et al: Contributions to Neuropsychological Assessment. New York, Oxford University Press, 1994

Berg EA: A simple objective test for measuring flexibility in thinking. J Gen Psychol 39:15–22, 1948

Berg G, Edwards DR, Danzinger WL, et al: Longitudinal change in three brief assessments of SDAT. J Am Geriatr Soc 35:205–212, 1987

Bieliauskas LA, Matthews CG: American Board of Clinical Neuropsychology: policies and procedures. Clin Neuropsychol 1:21–28, 1987

Bigler ED: Neuroimaging in mild TBI, in The Evaluation and Treatment of Mild Traumatic Brain Injury. Edited by Varney NR, Roberts RJ. Hillsdale, NJ, Erlbaum, 1999, pp 63–80

Binks SW, Gold JJ: Differential cognitive deficits in the neuropsychology of schizophrenia. Clin Neuropsychol 12:8–20, 1998

Bisiach E, Vallar G: Hemineglect in humans, in Handbook of Neuropsychology, Vol 1. Edited by Boller F, Grafman J. Amsterdam, The Netherlands, Elsevier, 1988, pp 195–222

Bleiberg J, Kane RL, Reeves DL, et al: Factor analysis of computerized and traditional tests used in mild brain injury research. Clin Neuropsychol 14:287–294, 2000

Boller F, Vignolo LA: Latent sensory aphasia in hemisphere-damaged patients: an experimental study with the Token Test. Brain 89:815–831, 1966

Boone KB, Lesser IM, Miller BL, et al: Cognitive functioning in older depressed outpatients: relationship of presence and severity of depression to neuropsychological test scores. Neuropsychology 9:390–398, 1995

Bornstein RA: Verbal IQ–Performance IQ discrepancies on the Wechsler Adult Intelligence Scale–Revised in patients with unilateral or bilateral cerebral dysfunction. J Consult Clin Psychol 51:779–780, 1983

Bornstein RA: Classification rates obtained with "standard" cutoff scores on selected neuropsychological measures. J Clin Exp Neuropsychol 8:413–420, 1986

Boyd TM, Sautter SW: Route-finding: a measure of everyday executive functioning in the head-injured adult. Appl Cogn Psychol 7:171–181, 1993

Brandstadter D, Oertel WH: Depression in Parkinson's disease. Adv Neurol 91:371–381, 2003

Broshek DK, Barth JT: The Halstead-Reitan Neuropsychological Test Battery, in Neuropsychological Assessment in Clinical Practice. Edited by Groth-Marnet G. New York, Wiley, 2000, pp 223–262

Butcher JN: User's Guide for the MMPI-2 Minnesota Report: Adult Clinical System. Minneapolis, MN, National Computer Systems, 1989

Butcher JN, Pope KS: MMPI-2: a practical guide to clinical, psychometric, and ethical issues. Independent Practitioner 10:20–25, 1990

Butcher JN, Dahlstrom WG, Graham JR, et al: Minnesota Multiphasic Personality Inventory (MMPI-2): Manual for Administration and Scoring. Minneapolis, University of Minnesota Press, 1989

Butcher JN, Perry JN, Atlis MM: Validity and utility of computer-based test interpretation. Psychol Assess 12:6–18, 2000

Butters J, Miliotis P: Amnesic disorders, in Clinical Neuropsychology, 2nd Edition. Edited by Heilman KM, Valenstein E. New York, Oxford University Press, 1985, pp 403–451

Caetano SC, Hatch JP, Brambilla P, et al: Anatomical MRI study of hippocampus and amygdala in patients with current and remitted major depression. Psychiatry Res 132:141–147, 2004

Carlin D, Bonerba J, Phipps M, et al: Planning impairments in frontal lobe dementia and frontal lobe lesion patients. Neuropsychologia 38:655–665, 2000

Cermak LS (ed): Human Memory and Amnesia. Hillsdale, NJ, Erlbaum, 1982

Chamberlain SR, Blackwell AD, Fineberg NA, et al: The neuropsychology of obsessive compulsive disorder: the importance of failures in cognitive and behavioural inhibition as candidate endophenotypic markers. Neurosci Biobehav Rev 29:399–419, 2005

Chaves ML, Izquierdo I: Differential diagnosis between dementia and depression: a study of efficiency increment. Acta Neurol Scand 85:378–382, 1992

Chelune GJ, Ferguson W, Moehle K: The role of standard cognitive and personality tests in neuropsychological assessment, in Clinical Application of Neuropsychological Test Batteries. Edited by Incagnoli T, Goldstein G, Golden CJ. New York, Plenum, 1986, pp 75–119

Christensen A-L: Luria's Neuropsychological Investigation Test, 2nd Edition. Copenhagen, Denmark, Munksgaard, 1979

Christensen A-L, Uzzell B (eds): International Handbook of Neuropsychological Rehabilitation. Dordrecht, The Netherlands, Kluwer Academic Publishers, 2000

Cicerone K, Azulay J: Diagnostic utility of attention measures in postconcussion syndrome. Clin Neuropsychol 16:280–289, 2002

Corballis MC: The Lopsided Ape. New York, Oxford University Press, 1991

Crawford JR: Current and premorbid intelligence measures in neuropsychological assessment, in A Handbook of Neuropsychological Assessment. Edited by Crawford JR, Parker DM, McKinlay WW. Hove, UK, Erlbaum, 1992, pp 21–49

Cripe LI: Use of the MMPI with mild closed head injury, in The Evaluation and Treatment of Mild Traumatic Brain Injury. Edited by Varney NR, Roberts RJ. Hillsdale, NJ, Erlbaum, 1999, pp 291–314

Cullum CM, Bigler ED: Short- and long-term psychological status following stroke: short form MMPI results. J Nerv Ment Dis 179:274–278, 1991

Cummings JL: Depression in neurologic diseases. Psychiatr Ann 24:525–531, 1994

Cummings JL: Principles of neuropsychiatry: towards a neuropsychiatric epistemology. Neurocase 5:181–188, 1999

Dahlstrom WG, Welsh GS, Dahlstrom LE: An MMPI Handbook, Vol 1: Clinical Interpretation, Revised. Minneapolis, University of Minnesota Press, 1975

Dalgleish R, Cox SG: Mood and memory, in Memory Disorders in Psychiatric Practice. Edited by Berrios GE, Hodges JR. New York, Cambridge University Press, 2000, pp 34–46

Damasio H, Damasio A: The lesion method in behavioral neurology and neuropsychology, in Behavioral Neurology and Neuropsychology. Edited by Feinberg T, Farah M. New York, McGraw-Hill, 2003, pp 71–84

Deckersbach T, Otto MW, Savage CR, et al: The relationship between semantic organization and memory in obsessive-compulsive disorder. Psychother Psychosom 69:101–107, 2000

Delis DC, Kramer JH, Kaplan E, et al: California Verbal Learning Test. San Antonio, TX, Psychological Corporation, 1986

Delis DC, Kaplan E, Kramer JH, et al: California Verbal Learning Test, 2nd Edition (CVLT-II) Manual. San Antonio, TX, Harcourt Brace, 2000

Della Sala S, Laiacona M, Spinnler H, et al: Autobiographical recollection and frontal damage. Neuropsychologia 31:823–839, 1993

De Luca CR, Wood SJ, Anderson V, et al: Normative data from the CANTAB, I: development of executive function over the lifespan. J Clin Exp Neuropsychol 25:242–254, 2003

Denicoff KD, Ali SO, Mirsky AF, et al: Relationship between prior course of illness and neuropsychological functioning in patients with bipolar disorder. J Affect Disord 56:67–73, 1999

Deouell L, Ivry R, Knight R: Electrophysiologic methods and transcranial magnetic stimulation in behavioral neurology and neuropsychology, in Behavioral Neurology and Neuropsychology. Edited by Feinberg T, Farah M. New York, McGraw-Hill, 2003, pp 105–134

De Renzi E, Vignolo LA: The Token Test: a sensitive test to detect disturbances in aphasics. Brain 85:665–678, 1962

De Renzi E, Faglioni P, Lodesani M, et al: Performance of left brain–damaged patients on imitation of single movements and motor sequences. Cortex 19:333–343, 1983

Derogatis LR: Symptom Checklist 90–Revised (SCL-90-R). Towson, MD, Clinical Psychometric Research, 1983

Dikmen S, Machamer J, Savoie T, et al: Life quality outcome in head injury, in Neuropsychological Assessment of Neuropsychiatric Disorders, 2nd Edition. Edited by Grant I, Adams KM. New York, Oxford University Press, 1996, pp 552–576

Diller L: Poststroke rehabilitation practice guidelines, in International Handbook of Neuropsychological Rehabilitation. Edited by Christensen A-L, Uzzell BP. New York, Kluwer Academic/Plenum, 2000, pp 167–182

Dobigny-Roman N, Dieudonne-Moinet B, Verny M, et al: Ideomotor apraxia test: a new test of imitation of gestures for elderly people. Eur J Neurol 5:571–578, 1998

Dore GJ, McDonald A, Li Y, et al: Marked improvement in survival following AIDS dementia complex in the era of highly active antiretroviral therapy. AIDS 17:1539–1545, 2003

Duncan C, Mirsky A: The Attention Battery for Adults: a systematic approach to assessment, in Comprehensive Handbook of Psychological Assessment, Vol 1: Intellectual and Neuropsychological Assessment. Edited by Goldstein G, Beers S, Hersen M. Hoboken, NJ, Wiley, 2004, pp 263–276

Duwe BV, Turetsky BI: Misdiagnosis of schizophrenia in a patient with psychotic symptoms. Neuropsychiatry Neuropsychol Behav Neurol 15:252–260, 2002

Dwyer CA: Cut scores and testing: statistics, judgment, truth, and error. Psychol Assess 8:360–362, 1996

Evans JJ, Breen EK, Antoun N, et al: Focal retrograde amnesia for autobiographical events following cerebral vasculitis: a connectionist account. Neurocase 2:1–11, 1996

Farah MJ, Feinberg TE (eds): Patient-Based Approaches to Cognitive Neuroscience. Cambridge, MA, MIT Press, 2000

Feinberg T, Roane D: Misidentification syndromes, in Behavioral Neurology and Neuropsychology. Edited by Feinberg T, Farah M. New York, McGraw-Hill, 2003, pp 373–381

Feldner MT, Leen-Feldner EW, Zvolensky MJ, et al: Examining the association between rumination, negative affectivity, and negative affect induced by a paced auditory serial addition task. J Behav Ther Exp Psychiatry 37:171–187, 2006

Ferrier IN, Stanton BR, Kelly TP, et al: Neuropsychological function in euthymic patients with bipolar disorder. Br J Psychiatry 175:246–251, 1999

Filskov SB, Leli DA: Assessment of the individual in neuropsychological practice, in Handbook of Clinical Neuropsychology. Edited by Filskov SB, Boll TJ. New York, Wiley-Interscience, 1981, pp 545–576

Fischer J, Hannay J, Loring D, et al: Observational methods, rating scales, and inventories, in Neuropsychological Assessment. Edited by Lezak M, Howieson D, Loring D. New York, Oxford University Press, 2004, pp 698–737

Folstein MF, Folstein SE, McHugh PR: Mini-Mental State: a practical method for grading the cognitive state of patients for the clinician. J Psychiatr Res 12:189–198, 1975

Fowler KS, Saling MM, Conway EL, et al: Computerized neuropsychological tests in the early detection of dementia: prospective findings. J Int Neuropsychol Soc 3:139–146, 1997

Fukui T, Sugita K, Kawamura M, et al: Primary progressive apraxia in Pick's disease: a clinicopathologic study. Neurology 47:467–473, 1996

Gainotti G: Emotional disorders in relation to unilateral brain damage, in Behavioral Neurology and Neuropsychology. Edited by Feinberg T, Farah M. New York, McGraw-Hill, 2003, pp 725–734

Gass CS: MMPI-2 interpretation of patients with cerebrovascular disease: a correction factor. Arch Clin Neuropsychol 7:17–27, 1992

Gass CS, Apple C: Cognitive complaints in closed-head injury: relationship to memory test performance and emotional disturbance. J Clin Exp Neuropsychol 19:290–299, 1997

Glassmire DM, Kinney DI, Greene RL, et al: Sensitivity and specificity of MMPI-2 neurologic correction factors: receiver operating characteristic analysis. Assessment 10:299–309, 2003

Goel V, Grafman J: Are the frontal lobes implicated in "planning" functions? Interpreting data from the Tower of Hanoi. Neuropsychologia 33:623–642, 1995

Goldman RS, Axelrod BN, Taylor SF: Neuropsychological aspects of schizophrenia, in Neuropsychological Assessment of Neuropsychiatric Disorders. Edited by Grant I, Adams KM. New York, Oxford University Press, 1996, pp 504–528

Goldstein G, Allen DN, Seaton BE: A comparison of clustering solutions for cognitive heterogeneity in schizophrenia. J Int Neuropsychol Soc 4:353–362, 1998

Goodglass H, Kaplan E, Barresi B: Boston Diagnostic Aphasia Examination, 3rd Edition. Philadelphia, PA, Lippincott Williams & Wilkins, 2000

Grafman J, Wassermann E: Transcranial magnetic stimulation can measure and modulate learning and memory. Neuropsychologia 37:159–167, 1999

Grant DA, Berg EA: A behavioral analysis of degree of reinforcement and ease of shifting to new responses on a Weigl-type card-sorting problem. J Exp Psychol 38:404–411, 1948

Grant I, Heaton RK, Atkinson JH: Neurocognitive disorders in HIV-1 infection. HNRC Group. HIV Neurobehavioral Research Center. Curr Top Microbiol Immunol 202:11–32, 1995

Greisberg S, McKay D: Neuropsychology of obsessive-compulsive disorder: a review and treatment implications. Clin Psychol Rev 23:95–117, 2003

Grigsby J, Kaye K, Robbins LJ: Reliabilities, norms and factor structure of the Behavioral Dyscontrol Scale. Percept Mot Skills 74:883–892, 1992

Grisso T: Evaluating Competencies: Forensic Assessments and Instruments, 2nd Edition. New York, Plenum, 2002

Gronwall DMA: Paced auditory serial-addition task: a measure of recovery from concussion. Percept Mot Skills 44:367–373, 1977

Gronwall DMA, Sampson H: The Psychological Effects of Concussion. Auckland, New Zealand, University Press, 1974

Grossman FM: Percentage of WAIS-R standardization sample obtaining verbal-performance discrepancies. J Consult Clin Psychol 51:641–642, 1983

Gustafson Y, Nilsson I, Mattsson M, et al: Epidemiology and treatment of post-stroke depression. Drugs Aging 7:298–309, 1995

Haaland KY, Flaherty D: The different types of limb apraxia made by patients with left vs. right hemisphere damage. Brain Cogn 3:370–384, 1984

Haaland KY, Harrington DL, Kneight RT: Spatial deficits in ideomotor limb apraxia: a kinematic analysis of aiming movements. Brain 122:1169–1182, 1999

Haeske-Dewick HC, Canavan AG, Homberg V: Directional hyperattention in tactile neglect within grasping space. J Clin Exp Neuropsychol 18:724–732, 1996

Halstead WC: Brain and Intelligence. Chicago, IL, University of Chicago Press, 1947

Hannay H, Bieliauskas L, Crosson B, et al: Policy statement. Proceedings of the Houston Conference on Specialty Education and Training in Clinical Neuropsychology. Arch Clin Neuropsychol 13:160–166, 1998

Hartman M, Nielsen C, Stratton B: The contributions of attention and working memory to age differences in concept identification. J Clin Exp Neuropsychol 26:227–245, 2004

Hathaway SR, McKinley JC: The Minnesota Multiphasic Personality Inventory Manual, Revised. New York, Psychological Corporation, 1951

Heaton RK, Taylor M, Manly J: Demographic effects and use of demographically corrected norms with the WAIS-III and WMS-III, in Clinical Interpretation of the WAIS-III and WMS-III. Edited by Tulsky D, Saklofske D. San Diego, CA, Academic Press, 2003, pp 181–210

Hebb DO: The effect of early and late brain injury upon test scores, and the nature of adult intelligence. Proceedings of the American Philosophical Society 85:275–292, 1942

Heilman KM, Watson RT, Rothi LJG: Disorders of skilled movement, in Patient-Based Approaches to Cognitive Neuroscience. Edited by Farah MJ, Feinberg TE. Cambridge, MA, MIT Press, 2000a, pp 335–343

Heilman KM, Watson RT, Valenstein E: Neglect, I: clinical and anatomic issues, in Patient-Based Approaches to Cognitive Neuroscience. Edited by Farah MJ, Feinberg TE. Cambridge, MA, MIT Press, 2000b, pp 115–123

Heilman K, Blonder L, Bowers D, et al: Emotional disorders associated with neurological diseases, in Clinical Neuropsychology. Edited by Heilman K, Valenstein E. New York, Oxford University Press, 2003, pp 447–478

Heinrichs RW, Zakzanis KK: Neurocognitive deficit in schizophrenia: a quantitative review of the evidence. Neuropsychology 12:426–445, 1998

Hertel PT: Relation between rumination and impaired memory in dysphoric moods. J Abnorm Psychol 107:166–172, 1998

Hertzman PA, Clauw DJ, Duffy J, et al: Rigorous new approach to constructing a gold standard for validating new diagnostic criteria, as exemplified by the eosinophilia-myalgia syndrome. Arch Intern Med 161:2301–2306, 2001

Hill SK, Ragland JD, Gur RC, et al: Neuropsychological differences among empirically derived clinical subtypes of schizophrenia. Neuropsychology 15:492–501, 2001

Hiscock CK, Branham JD, Hiscock M: Detection of feigned cognitive impairment: the two-alternative forced-choice method compared with selected conventional tests. J Psychopathol Behav Assess 16:95–110, 1994

Hobart MP, Goldberg R, Bartko JJ, et al: Repeatable battery for the assessment of neuropsychological status as a screening test in schizophrenia, II: convergent/discriminant validity and diagnostic group comparisons. Am J Psychiatry 156:1951–1957, 1999

Hodges JR: Transient Amnesia: Clinical and Neuropsychological Aspects. London, WB Saunders, 1991

Hooper HE: The Hooper Visual Organization Test Manual. Los Angeles, CA, Western Psychological Services, 1958

Howieson DB, Dame A, Camicioli R, et al: Cognitive markers preceding Alzheimer's dementia in the healthy oldest old. J Am Geriatr Soc 45:584–589, 1997

Iverson GL, Mendrek A, Adams RL: The persistent belief that VIQ-PIQ splits suggest lateralized brain damage. Appl Neuropsychol 11:85–90, 2004

Jason GW: Disorders of motor function following cortical lesions: review and theoretical considerations, in Cerebral Control of Speech and Limb Movements. Edited by Hammond GR. Amsterdam, The Netherlands, Elsevier, 1990, pp 141–168

Kalechstein AD, Newton TF, van Gorp WG: Neurocognitive functioning is associated with employment status: a quantitative review. J Clin Exp Neuropsychol 25:1186–1191, 2003

Kalska H, Punamaki RL, Makinen-Belli T, et al: Memory and metamemory functioning among depressed patients. Appl Neuropsychol 6:96–107, 1999

Kamitani Y, Tong F: Decoding the visual and subjective contents of the human brain. Nat Neurosci 8:679–685, 2005

Kane RL, Kay GG: Computerized assessment in neuropsychology: a review of tests and test batteries. Neuropsychol Rev 3:1–117, 1992

Kaplan E: A process approach to neuropsychological assessment, in Clinical Neuropsychological and Brain Function: Research, Measurement, and Practice. Edited by Boll T, Bryant BK. Washington, DC, American Psychological Association, 1988, pp 125–167

Kapur N: How can we best explain retrograde amnesia in human memory disorder? Memory 5:115–129, 1997

Kapur N, Scholey K, Moore E, et al: Long-term retention deficits in two cases of disproportionate retrograde amnesia. J Cogn Neurosci 8:416–434, 1996

Kelly MD, Grant I, Heaton RK: Neuropsychological findings in HIV infection and AIDS, in Neuropsychological Assessment of Psychiatric Disorders. Edited by Grant I, Adams KM. New York, Oxford University Press, 1996, pp 403–422

Kiernan RJ, Mueller J, Langston JW, et al: The Neurobehavioral Cognitive Status Examination: a brief but differentiated approach to cognitive assessment. Ann Intern Med 107:481–485, 1987

King DA, Caine ED: Cognitive impairment and major depression: beyond the pseudodementia syndrome, in Neuropsychological Assessment of Neuropsychiatric Disorders, 2nd Edition. Edited by Grant I, Adams KM. New York, Oxford University Press, 1996, pp 200–217

Knopman D, Selnes O: Neuropsychology of dementia, in Clinical Neuropsychology. Edited by Heilman K, Valenstein E. New York, Oxford University Press, 2003, pp 574–616

Krabbendam L, de Vugt ME, Derix MM, et al: The behavioural assessment of the dysexecutive syndrome as a tool to assess executive functions in schizophrenia. Clin Neuropsychol 13:370–375, 1999

Kramer JH, Jurik J, Sha SJ, et al: Distinctive neuropsychological patterns in frontotemporal dementia, semantic dementia, and Alzheimer disease. Cogn Behav Neurol 16:211–218, 2003

Lachapelle DL, Alfano DP: Revised Neurobehavioral Scales of the MMPI: sensitivity and specificity in traumatic brain injury. Appl Neuropsychol 12:143–150, 2005

Laine M, Butters N: A preliminary study of problem solving strategies of detoxified long-term alcoholics. Drug Alcohol Depend 10:235–242, 1982

Larson E, Kirschner K, Bode R, et al: Construct and predictive validity of the repeatable battery for the assessment of neuropsychological status in the evaluation of stroke patients. J Clin Exp Neuropsychol 27:16–32, 2005

Leach L, Kaplan E, Rewilak D, et al: Kaplan-Baycrest Neurocognitive Assessment Manual. San Antonio, TX, Psychological Corporation, 2000

Leclercq M, Zimmermann P (eds): Applied Neuropsychology of Attention: Theory, Diagnosis, and Rehabilitation. New York, Psychology Press, 2002

Leiguarda RC, Pramstaller PP, Merello M, et al: Apraxia in Parkinson's disease, progressive supranuclear palsy, multiple system atrophy and neuroleptic-induced parkinsonism. Brain 120:75–90, 1997

Levin HS, High WM, Goethe KE, et al: The Neurobehavioral Rating Scale assessment of behavioural sequelae of head injury by the clinician. J Neurol Neurosurg Psychiatry 50:183–193, 1987

Levin JM, Ross MH, Harris G, et al: Applications of dynamic susceptibility contrast magnetic resonance imaging in neuropsychiatry. Neuroimage 4:S147–162, 1996

Levine B, Black SE, Cabeza R, et al: Episodic memory and the self in a case of isolated retrograde amnesia. Brain 121:1951–1973, 1998

Levy ML, Cummings JL, Fairbanks LA, et al: Apathy is not depression. J Neuropsychiatry Clin Neurosci 10:314–319, 1998

Lezak MD: The problem of assessing executive functions. Int J Psychol 17:281–297, 1982

Lezak MD: An individual approach to neuropsychological assessment, in Clinical Neuropsychology. Edited by Logue PE, Schear JM. Springfield, IL, Charles C Thomas, 1986, pp 29–49

Lezak MD: Assessment for rehabilitation planning, in Neuropsychological Rehabilitation. Edited by Meier M, Benton AL, Diller L. Edinburgh, UK, Churchill Livingstone, 1987, pp 41–58

Lezak MD: Brain damage is a family affair. J Clin Exp Neuropsychol 10:111–123, 1988a

Lezak MD: IQ: R.I.P. J Clin Exp Neuropsychol 10:351–361, 1988b

Lezak MD: Assessment of psychosocial dysfunctions resulting from head trauma, in Assessment of the Behavioral Consequences of Head Trauma, Vol 7: Frontiers of Clinical Neuroscience. Edited by Lezak MD. New York, Alan R Liss, 1989, pp 113–144

Lezak MD: Domains of behavior from a neuropsychological perspective: the whole story, in Integrative Views of Motivation, Cognition, and Emotion. Nebraska Symposium on Motivation. Edited by Spaulding WD. Lincoln, University of Nebraska Press, 1994, pp 23–55

Lezak M, Howieson D, Loring D: Neuropsychological Assessment, 4th Edition. New York, Oxford University Press, 2004

Liotti M, Mayberg HS: The role of functional neuroimaging in the neuropsychology of depression. J Clin Exp Neuropsychol 23:121–136, 2001

Lisanby SH, Kohler C, Swanson CL, et al: Psychosis secondary to brain tumor. Semin Clin Neuropsychiatry 3:12–22, 1998

Loring DW, Lee GP, Meador KJ: Revising the Rey-Osterrieth: rating right hemisphere recall. Arch Clin Neuropsychol 3:239–247, 1988

Luria AR: Higher Cortical Functions in Man, 2nd Edition. New York, Basic Books, 1980

Malec JF, Moessner AM, Kragness M, et al: Refining a measure of brain injury sequelae to predict postacute rehabilitation outcome: rating scale analysis of the Mayo-Portland Adaptability Inventory. J Head Trauma Rehabil 15:670–682, 2000

Malhi GS, Ivanovski B, Szekeres V, et al: Bipolar disorder: it's all in your mind? The neuropsychological profile of a biological disorder. Can J Psychiatry 49:813–819, 2004

Malloy P, Belanger H, Hall S, et al: Assessing visuoconstructional performance in AD, MCI and normal elderly using the Beery Visual-Motor Integration Test. Clin Neuropsychol 17:544–550, 2003

Manly JJ, Byrd DA, Touradji P, et al: Acculturation, reading level, and neuropsychological test performance among African American elders. Appl Neuropsychol 11:37–46, 2004

Markova IS, Berrios GE: Insight into memory deficits, in Memory Disorders in Psychiatric Practice. Edited by Berrios GE, Hodges JR. New York, Cambridge University Press, 2000, pp 34–46

Marson DC, Cody HA, Ingram KK, et al: Neuropsychologic predictors of competency in Alzheimer's disease using a rational reasons legal standard. Arch Neurol 52:955–959, 1995a

Marson DC, Ingram KK, Cody HA, et al: Assessing the competency of patients with Alzheimer's disease under different legal standards: a prototype instrument. Arch Neurol 52:949–954, 1995b

Marson D, Dymek M, Geyer J: Informed consent, competency, and the neurologist. Neurologist 7:317–326, 2001

Mast BT, Azar AR, Murrell SA: The vascular depression hypothesis: the influence of age on the relationship between cerebrovascular risk factors and depressive symptoms in community dwelling elders. Aging Ment Health 9:146–152, 2005

Mataix-Cols D, Junque C, Sanchez-Turet M, et al: Neuropsychological functioning in a subclinical obsessive-compulsive sample. Biol Psychiatry 45:898–904, 1999

Mattis S, Jurica P, Leitten C: Dementia Rating Scale–2. Lutz, FL, Psychological Assessment Resources, 2001

Mayes AR: Selective memory disorders, in The Oxford Handbook of Memory. Edited by Tulving E, Craik FIM. Oxford, UK, Oxford University Press, 2000, pp 427–440

McCarthy RA, Warrington EK: Cognitive Neuropsychology: A Clinical Introduction. San Diego, CA, Academic Press, 1990

McKenna PJ, McKay AP, Laws K: Memory in functional psychosis, in Memory Disorders in Psychiatric Practice. Edited by Berrios GE, Hodges JR. New York, Cambridge University Press, 2000, pp 234–267

Menon RS, Kim SG: Spatial and temporal limits in cognitive neuroimaging with fMRI. Trends Cogn Sci 3:207–216, 1999

Mesulam M-M: Principles of Behavioral and Cognitive Neurology, 2nd Edition. New York, Oxford University Press, 2000

Milberg WP, Hebben N, Kaplan E: The Boston approach to neuropsychological assessment, in Neuropsychological Assessment of Neuropsychiatric Disorders. Edited by Grant I, Adams KM. New York, Oxford University Press, 1996, pp 58–80

Milner B: Interhemispheric differences in the localization of psychological processes in man. Br Med Bull 27:272–277, 1971

Mitrushina M, Boone K, Razani J, et al: Handbook of Normative Data for Neuropsychological Assessment, 2nd Edition. New York, Oxford University Press, 2005

Morrow L, Muldoon S, Sandstrom D: Neuropsychological sequelae associated with occupational and environmental exposure to chemicals, in Medical Neuropsychology. Edited by Tarter R, Butters M, Beers S. New York, Kluwer Academic/Plenum Press, 2001, pp 199–246

Mueller SR, Girace M: Use and misuse of the MMPI, a reconsideration. Psychol Rep 63:483–491, 1988

Mysiw WJ, Beegan JG, Gatens PF: Prospective cognitive assessment of stroke patients before inpatient rehabilitation: the relationship of the Neurobehavioral Cognitive Status Examination to functional improvement. Am J Phys Med Rehabil 68:168–171, 1989

Nebes RD, Vora IJ, Meltzer CC, et al: Relationship of deep white matter hyperintensities and apolipoprotein E genotype to depressive symptoms in older adults without clinical depression. Am J Psychiatry 158:878–884, 2001

Nelson HE: The National Adult Reading Test (NART): Test Manual. Windsor, UK, UK:NFER-Nelson, 1982

Neumeister A, Wood S, Bonne O, et al: Reduced hippocampal volume in unmedicated, remitted patients with major depression versus control subjects. Biol Psychiatry 57:935–937, 2005

Newcombe F, Ratcliff G: Disorders of visuospatial analysis, in Handbook of Neuropsychology, Vol 2. Edited by Boller F, Grafman J. Amsterdam, The Netherlands, Elsevier, 1989, pp 333–356

Niemi M-L, Laaksonen R, Kotila M, et al: Quality of life 4 years after stroke. Stroke 19:1101–1107, 1988

Norris G, Tate RL: The Behavioural Assessment of the Dysexecutive Syndrome (BADS): ecological, concurrent and construct validity. Neuropsychol Rehabil 10:33–45, 2000

O'Connell JE, Gray CS, French JM, et al: Atrial fibrillation and cognitive function: case-control study. J Neurol Neurosurg Psychiatry 65:386–389, 1998

Ochoa E, Erhan H, Feinberg T: Emotional disorders in relation to nonfocal brain damage, in Behavioral Neurology and Neuropsychology. Edited by Feinberg T, Farah M. New York, McGraw-Hill, 2003, pp 735–742

Ojemann GA, Dodrill CB: Verbal memory deficits after left temporal lobectomy for epilepsy. J Neurosurg 62:101–107, 1985

Osterrieth PA: Le test de copie d'une figure complex. Archives de Psychologie 30:206–356, 1944

Pagliaro LA, Pagliaro AM: Psychologists' Neuropsychotropic Drug Reference. Philadelphia, PA, Brunner/Mazel, 1998

Palmer BW, Boone KB, Lesser IM, et al: Neuropsychological deficits among older depressed patients with predominantly psychological or vegetative symptoms. J Affect Disord 41:17–24, 1996

Palmer BW, Heaton RK, Paulsen JS, et al: Is it possible to be schizophrenic yet neuropsychologically normal? Neuropsychology 11:437–446, 1997

Pankratz L: Symptom validity testing and symptom retraining: procedures for the assessment and treatment of functional sensory deficits. J Consult Clin Psychol 47:409–410, 1979

Pankratz LD, Taplin JD: Issues in psychological assessment, in Critical Issues, Developments, and Trends in Professional Psychology. Edited by McNamara JR, Barclay AG. New York, Praeger, 1982, pp 115–151

Paradiso S, Ohkubo T, Robinson RG: Vegetative and psychological symptoms associated with depressed mood over the first two years after stroke. Int J Psychiatry Med 27:137–157, 1997

Payami H, Grimslid H, Oken B, et al: A prospective study of cognitive health in the elderly (Oregon Brain Aging Study): effects of family history and apolipoprotein E genotype. Am J Hum Genet 60:948–956, 1997

Perfect TJ, Maylor EA (eds): Models of Cognitive Aging. Oxford, UK, Oxford University Press, 2000

Petersen RC, Stevens JC, Ganguli M, et al: Practice parameter: early detection of dementia: mild cognitive impairment (an evidence-based review). Report of the Quality Standards Subcommittee of the American Academy of Neurology. Neurology 56:1133–1142, 2001

Petrides M, Milner B: Deficits on subject-ordered tasks after frontal- and temporal-lobe lesions in man. Neuropsychologia 20:249–262, 1982

Pohjasvaara T, Leppavuori A, Siira I, et al: Frequency and clinical determinants of poststroke depression. Stroke 29:2311–2317, 1998

Pohjasvaara T, Mantyla R, Aronen HJ, et al: Clinical and radiological determinants of prestroke cognitive decline in a stroke cohort. J Neurol Neurosurg Psychiatry 67:742–748, 1999

Polster MR, Rose SB: Disorders of auditory processing: evidence for modularity in audition. Cortex 34:47–65, 1998

Porch BE: Porch Index of Communicative Ability: Manual. Austin, TX, Pro-Ed, 1981

Post RM: Neural substrates of psychiatric syndromes, in Principles of Behavioral and Cognitive Neurology. Edited by Mesulam M-M. New York, Oxford University Press, 2000, pp 406–438

Prigatano GP, Parsons OA: Relationship of age and education to Halstead test performance in different patient populations. J Consult Clin Psychol 44:527–533, 1976

Prigatano GP, Schacter DL (eds): Awareness of Deficit After Brain Injury. New York, Oxford University Press, 1991

Psychological Corporation: WAIS-III and WMS-III Technical Manual. San Antonio, TX, Psychological Corporation, 1997

Quraishi S, Frangou S: Neuropsychology of bipolar disorder: a review. J Affect Disord 72:209–226, 2002

Rafal RD: Neglect II: cognitive neuropsychological issues, in Patient-Based Approaches to Cognitive Neuroscience. Edited by Farah MJ, Feinberg TE. Cambridge, MA, MIT Press, 2000, pp 115–123

Randolph C, Tierney MC, Mohr E, et al: The Repeatable Battery for the Assessment of Neuropsychological Status (RBANS): preliminary clinical validity. J Clin Exp Neuropsychol 20:310–319, 1998

Raskin SA, Mateer CA: Neuropsychological Management of Mild Traumatic Brain Injury. New York, Oxford University Press, 1999

Raspall T, Donate M, Boget T, et al: Neuropsychological tests with lateralizing value in patients with temporal lobe epilepsy: reconsidering material-specific theory. Seizure 14:569–576, 2005

Reed JM, Squire LR: Retrograde amnesia for facts and events: findings from four new cases. J Neurosci 18:3943–3954, 1998

Reif JS, Burch JB, Nuckols JR, et al: Neurobehavioral effects of exposure to trichloroethylene through a municipal water supply. Environ Res 93:248–258, 2003

Reitan RM: Manual for the Administration of Neuropsychological Test Batteries for Adults and Children. Indianapolis, IN, Author, 1969

Reitan RM, Wolfson D: The Halstead-Reitan Neuropsychological Test Battery: Theory and Clinical Interpretation, 2nd Edition. Tucson, AZ, Neuropsychology Press, 1993

Reitan R, Wolfson D: Theoretical, methodological, and validational basis of the Halstead-Reitan Neuropsychological Battery, in Neuropsychological Assessment of Neuropsychiatric Disorders. Edited by Grant I, Adams K. New York, Oxford University Press, 1996, pp 3–42

Rentz DM, Weintraub S: Neuropsychological detection of early probable Alzheimer's disease, in Early Diagnosis of Alzheimer's Disease. Edited by Scinto LFM, Daffner KR. Totowa, NJ, Humana Press, 2000, pp 169–189

Rey A: L'examen psychologique dans les cas d'encephalopathie traumatique. Archives de Psychologie 28:286–340, 1941

Rey A: L'examen Clinique en Psychologie. Paris, France, Presses Universitaries de France, 1964

Rickards H: Depression in neurological disorders: Parkinson's disease, multiple sclerosis, and stroke. J Neurol Neurosurg Psychiatry 76 (suppl 1):i48–52, 2005

Robinson RG: The Clinical Neuropsychiatry of Stroke. New York, Cambridge University Press, 1998

Rogers R, Robbins T: The neuropsychology of chronic drug abuse, in Disorders of Brain and Mind. Edited by Ron M, Robbins T. New York, Cambridge University Press, 2003, pp 447–467

Rothi LJG, Raymer AM, Heilman KM: Limb praxis assessment, in Apraxia: The Neuropsychology of Action. Edited by Rothi LJG, Heilman KM. Hove, UK, Psychology Press, 1997, pp 61–73

Royall DR, Mahurin RK, Gray KF: Bedside assessment of executive cognitive impairment: the Executive Interview. J Am Geriatr Soc 40:1221–1226, 1992

Savage CR, Deckersbach T, Wilhelm S, et al: Strategic processing and episodic memory impairment in obsessive compulsive disorder. Neuropsychology 14:141–151, 2000

Sbordone RJ: The assessment interview in clinical neuropsychology, in Neuropsychological Assessment in Clinical Practice. Edited by Groth-Marnat G. New York, Wiley, 2000, pp 94–126

Schenkenberg T, Bradford DC, Ajax ET: Line bisection and unilateral visual neglect in patients with neurologic impairment. Neurology 30:509–517, 1980

Schmidt M: Rey Auditory Verbal Learning Test (RAVLT): A Handbook. Los Angeles, CA, Western Psychological Services, 1996

Schmidt WP, Roesler A, Kretzschmar K, et al: Functional and cognitive consequences of silent stroke discovered using brain magnetic resonance imaging in an elderly population. J Am Geriatr Soc 52:1045–1050, 2004

Schwamm LH, Van Dyke C, Kiernan RJ, et al: The Neurobehavioral Cognitive Status Examination: comparison with the Cognitive Capacity Screening Examination and the Mini-Mental State Examination in a neurosurgical population. Ann Intern Med 107:486–491, 1987

Seashore CE, Lewis D, Saetveit DL: Seashore Measures of Musical Talents, Revised. New York, Psychological Corporation, 1960

Seaton BE, Goldstein G, Allen DN: Sources of heterogeneity in schizophrenia: the role of neuropsychological functioning. Neuropsychol Rev 11:45–67, 2001

Shallice T: Specific impairments of planning. Philos Trans R Soc Lond B Biol Sci 298:199–209, 1982

Singh A, Black SE, Herrmann N, et al: Functional and neuroanatomic correlations in poststroke depression: the Sunnybrook Stroke Study. Stroke 31:637–644, 2000

Sloan S, Ponsford J: Assessment of cognitive difficulties following TBI, in Traumatic Brain Injury: Rehabilitation for Everyday Adaptive Living. Edited by Ponsford J. Hillsdale, NJ, Erlbaum, 1995, pp 65–101

Smith A: Clinical psychological practice and principles of neuropsychological assessment, in Handbook of Clinical Psychology: Theory, Research and Practice. Edited by Walker CE. Homewood, IL, Dorsey Press, 1983, pp 445–500

Sox HC, Blatt MA, Higgins MC, et al: Medical Decision Making. Boston, MA, Butterworth, 1988

Spreen O, Risser AH: Assessment of Aphasia. New York, Oxford University Press, 2003

Spreen O, Strauss E: A Compendium of Neuropsychological Tests, 2nd Edition. New York, Oxford University Press, 1998

Squire LR, Slater PC, Chase PM: Retrograde amnesia: temporal gradient in very long-term memory following electroconvulsive therapy. Science 187:77–79, 1975

Stein RA, Strickland TL: A review of the neuropsychological effects of commonly used prescription medicines. Arch Clin Neuropsychol 13:259–284, 1998

Steinberg B, Bieliauskas L: Introduction to the special edition: IQ-based MOANS norms for multiple neuropsychological instruments. Clin Neuropsychol 19:277–279, 2005

Stern E, Silbersweig DA: Advances in functional neuroimaging methodology for the study of brain systems underlying human neuropsychological function and dysfunction. J Clin Exp Neuropsychol 23:3–18, 2001

Strakowski SM, Del Bello MP, Sax KW, et al: Brain magnetic resonance imaging of structural abnormalities in bipolar disorder. Arch Gen Psychiatry 56:254–260, 1999

Strauss E, Goldsmith SM: Lateral preferences and performance on non-verbal laterality tests in a normal population. Cortex 23:495–503, 1987

Strub RL, Black FW: The Mental Status Examination in Neurology. Philadelphia, PA, FA Davis, 2000

Stuss DT, Levine B, Alexander MP, et al: Wisconsin Card Sorting Test performance in patients with focal frontal and posterior brain damage: effects of lesion location and test structure on separable cognitive processes. Neuropsychologia 38:388–402, 2000

Sullivan EV, Shear PK, Zipursky RB, et al: A deficit profile of executive, memory, and motor functions in schizophrenia. Biol Psychiatry 36:641–653, 1994

Tarter R, Butters M, Beers S (eds): Medical Neuropsychology, 2nd Edition. New York, Kluwer Academic/Plenum, 2001

Teasell RW, Shapiro AP: Misdiagnosis of conversion disorders. Am J Phys Med Rehabil 81:236–240, 2002

Tekin S, Cummings JL: Hallucinations and related conditions, in Clinical Neuropsychology. Edited by Heilman K, Valenstein E. New York, Oxford University Press, 2003, pp 479–494

Teuber H-L: Neuropsychology, in Recent Advances in Diagnostic Psychological Testing. Edited by Harrower MR. Springfield, IL, Charles C Thomas, 1948, pp 30–52

Tilak Ratnanather J, Wang L, Nebel MB, et al: Validation of semiautomated methods for quantifying cingulate cortical metrics in schizophrenia. Psychiatry Res 132:53–68, 2004

Tombaugh TN: Test of Memory Malingering (TOMM). New York, Multi Health Systems, 1996

Tornatore JB, Hill E, Laboff JA, et al: Self-administered screening for mild cognitive impairment: initial validation of a computerized test battery. J Neuropsychiatry Clin Neurosci 17:98–105, 2005

Trahan DE, Larrabee GJ: Continuous Visual Memory Test. Odessa, FL, Psychological Assessment Resources, 1988

Upton D, Thompson PJ: Twenty questions task and frontal lobe dysfunction. Arch Clin Neuropsychol 14:203–216, 1999

Urbina S: Essentials of Psychological Testing. New York, Wiley, 2004

Vanderploeg RD, Schinka JA, Axelrod BN, et al: Estimation of WAIS-R premorbid intelligence: current ability and demographic data used in a best-performance fashion. Psychol Assess 8:404–411, 1996

Van Gorp WG, Altshuler L, Theberge DC, et al: Cognitive impairment in euthymic bipolar patients with and without prior alcohol dependence: a preliminary study. Arch Gen Psychiatry 55:41–46, 1998

Van Lancker DR, Dreiman J, Cummings J: Voice perception deficits: neuroanatomical correlates of phonagnosia. J Clin Exp Neuropsychol 11:665–674, 1989

Varney NR: Somesthesis, in Experimental Techniques in Human Neuropsychology. Edited by Hannay HJ. New York, Oxford University Press, 1986, pp 212–237

Varney NR, Roberts RJ (eds): The Evaluation and Treatment of Mild Traumatic Brain Injury. Hillsdale, NJ, Erlbaum, 1999

Veiel HO: A preliminary profile of neuropsychological deficits associated with major depression. J Clin Exp Neuropsychol 19:587–603, 1997

Vermeer SE, Prins ND, den Heijer T, et al: Silent brain infarcts and the risk of dementia and cognitive decline. N Engl J Med 348:1215–1222, 2003

Wagner AD, Poldrack RA, Eldridge LL, et al: Material-specific lateralization of prefrontal activation during episodic encoding and retrieval. Neuroreport 9:3711–3717, 1998

Walsh KW: Neuropsychology, 2nd Edition. Edinburgh, UK, Churchill Livingstone, 1987

Walsh V, Rushworth M: A primer of magnetic stimulation as a tool for neuropsychology. Neuropsychologia 37:125–135, 1999

Warrington EK: Recognition Memory Test. Windsor, UK, NFER-Nelson, 1984

Wechsler D: The Measurement of Adult Intelligence, 3rd Edition. Baltimore, MD, Williams & Wilkins, 1944

Wechsler D: WAIS Manual. New York, Psychological Corporation, 1955

Wechsler D: WAIS-R Manual. New York, Psychological Corporation, 1981

Wechsler D: Wechsler Memory Scale—Revised Manual. San Antonio, TX, Psychological Corporation, 1987

Wechsler D: WISC-III Manual: Wechsler Intelligence Scale for Children–III. New York, Psychological Corporation, 1991

Wechsler D: WAIS-III: Administration and Scoring Manual. San Antonio, TX, Psychological Corporation, 1997a

Wechsler D: WMS-III: Administration and Scoring Manual. San Antonio, TX, Psychological Corporation, 1997b

Weiland-Fiedler P, Erickson K, Waldeck T, et al: Evidence for continuing neuropsychological impairments in depression. J Affect Disord 82:253–258, 2004

Welsh GS, Dahlstrom WG (eds): Basic Readings on the MMPI in Psychology and Medicine. Minneapolis, University of Minnesota Press, 1956

Welsh KA, Butters N, Hughes JP, et al: Detection and staging of dementia in Alzheimer's disease: use of the neuropsychological measures developed for the Consortium to Establish a Registry for Alzheimer's Disease. Arch Neurol 49:448–452, 1992

Wepman JM, Reynolds WM: Wepman's Auditory Discrimination Test, 2nd Edition. Los Angeles, CA, Western Psychological Services, 1987

West JF, Sands E, Ross-Swain D: Bedside Evaluation Screening Test, Austin, TX, Pro-Ed, 1998

Wilson BA, Alderman N, Burgess PW, et al: Behavioural Assessment of the Dysexecutive Syndrome. Bury St Edmunds, England, Thames Valley Test Co, 1996

Wilson BA, Evans JJ, Emslie H, et al: The development of an ecologically valid test for assessing patients with a dysexecutive syndrome. Neuropsychol Rehabil 8:213–228, 1998

Wilson BA, Evans JJ, Keohane C: Cognitive rehabilitation: a goal-planning approach. J Head Trauma Rehabil 17:542–555, 2002

Wilson KD: Issues surrounding the cognitive neuroscience of obsessive-compulsive disorder. Psychon Bull Rev 5:161–172, 1998

Wrightson P, Gronwall D: Mild Head Injury. Oxford, UK, Oxford University Press, 1999

Yousef G, Ryan WJ, Lambert T, et al: A preliminary report: a new scale to identify the pseudodementia syndrome. Int J Geriatr Psychiatry 13:389–399, 1998

CLINICAL AND FUNCTIONAL IMAGING IN NEUROPSYCHIATRY

Robin A. Hurley, M.D.
Ronald E. Fisher, M.D., Ph.D.
Katherine H. Taber, Ph.D.

Modern medicine has embraced technology in almost every field. Although it is slightly more challenging to adapt the marvels of engineering and physics to emotion and behavior, psychiatry has seen the influence. Neuropsychiatry, as a subspecialty, developed to assess and treat cognitive or emotional disturbances caused by brain dysfunction. This concept could not have evolved without the influence of brain imaging, engineering, and physics. In the short time span of one century, imaging technology advanced from a primitive skull X ray to real-time pictures of brain changes as we perform a task or feel an emotion such as sadness or happiness. Cutting-edge imaging contributions are found not only in the diagnostic arena but also in estimating the course of illness and the expected treatment response and in the development of new neurotransmitter-specific medications.

Currently, brain imaging is divided into two categories: structural and functional (Table 7–1). Structural imaging is defined as information regarding the physical appearance of the brain that is independent of thought, neuronal or motor activity, or mood. Computed tomography (CT) and magnetic resonance imaging (MRI) are the standard tools. Functional imaging of the brain measures changes related to neuronal activity. The most common functional imaging techniques use indirect measures, such as blood flow, metabolism, and oxygen extraction. Functional imaging techniques currently used in clinical practice include single-photon emission computed tomography (SPECT), positron emission tomography (PET), and magnetic resonance spectroscopy (MRS). Other functional imaging techniques under development for clinical use or for research include functional magnetic resonance imaging (fMRI), xenon-enhanced computed tomography (Xe/CT), and magnetoencephalography (MEG).

In the first section of this chapter, we review structural imaging concepts and basic technologies; we then discuss the functional techniques most used in psychiatric patients and conclude with a brief discussion of functional neuroanatomy and an imaging atlas. We do not summarize the imaging findings of all neuropsychiatric diseases or all of the potential research applications. We do, however, review the basics of how and why to image and how to understand the findings; thus, this chapter provides the reader with a knowledge base for using neuroimaging in clinical practice.

TABLE 7–1.   Brain imaging modalities

Type of imaging	Parameter measured
Anatomical and pathological	
Computed tomography (CT)	Tissue density
Magnetic resonance imaging (MRI)	Many properties of tissue (T1 and T2 relaxation times, spin density, magnetic susceptibility, water diffusion, blood flow)
Functional	
(resting brain activity, brain activation, neurotransmitter receptors)	
Positron emission tomography (PET)	Radioactive tracers in blood or tissue
Single-photon emission computed tomography (SPECT)	Radioactive tracers in tissue
Xenon-enhanced computed tomography (Xe/CT)	Xenon concentration in blood
Functional magnetic resonance imaging (fMRI)	Deoxyhemoglobin levels in blood
Magnetoencephalography (MEG)	Magnetic fields induced by neuronal discharges
Magnetic resonance spectroscopy (MRS)	Metabolite concentrations in tissue

GENERAL PRINCIPLES OF STRUCTURAL IMAGING

Early studies in the 1980s promoted the limited use of CT scanning in psychiatric patients only after focal neurological findings had been developed (Larson et al. 1981). Studies in the late 1980s and 1990s encouraged a broader use of diagnostic CT in psychiatric patients (Beresford et al. 1986; Kaplan et al. 1994; Rauch and Renshaw 1995; Weinberger 1984). With the advent of utilization review and cost containment in the late 1990s, once again more narrow criteria were proposed that recommended use of CT only when reversible pathology was suspected (Branton 1999; Erhart et al. 2005). Diagnostic imaging has advanced considerably in the last decade, with multiple new brain imaging techniques coming into common clinical use. In addition, our understanding of functional anatomy, as it relates to psychiatric conditions, has increased enormously. A study of nondemented psychiatric patients found that treatment was changed in 15% of patients as a result of imaging examinations (Erhart et al. 2005). Clinical indications for neuroimaging include sustained confusion or delirium, subtle cognitive deficits, unusual age at symptom onset or evolution, atypical clinical findings, or abrupt personality changes with accompanying neurological signs or symptoms (Erhart et al. 2005; Hurley et al. 2002). In addition, neuroimaging is recommended following poison or toxin exposures (including significant alcohol abuse) and brain injuries of any kind (traumatic or "organic") (Table 7–2). The information obtained from brain imaging studies may assist with differential diagnosis, alter a treatment plan, and inform prognosis.

TABLE 7–2.   Indications for imaging

Diagnosis or medical condition

Traumatic brain injury

Significant alcohol abuse

Seizure disorders with psychiatric symptoms

Movement disorders

Autoimmune disorders

Eating disorders

Poison or toxin exposure

Delirium

Clinical signs and symptoms

Dementia or cognitive decline

New-onset mental illness after age 50

Initial psychotic break

Presentation at an atypical age for diagnosis

Focal neurological signs

Catatonia

Sudden personality changes

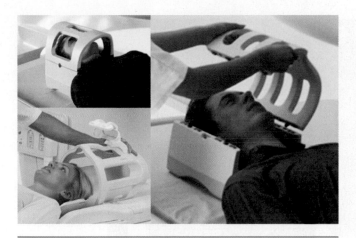

FIGURE 7–1.   The head coil used in magnetic resonance imaging fits rather snugly, which can be difficult for some patients. Openings have been included in modern head coils to improve patient tolerance.

Source.   Pictures courtesy of Phillips Medical Systems.

PRACTICAL CONSIDERATIONS

ORDERING THE EXAMINATION

The neuroradiologist needs very clear clinical information on the imaging request form (not just "rule out pathology" or "new-onset mental status changes"). If a lesion is suspected in a particular location, the neuroradiologist should be informed of this or given enough clinical data for selection of the best imaging method and parameters to view suspicious areas. The clinician should ask the neuroradiologist about any special imaging techniques that may enhance visualization of the limbic circuits (see subsection "Common Pulse Sequences" later in this chapter). The neuroradiologist and technical staff also need information on the patient's current condition (e.g., delirious, psychotic, easily agitated, paranoid). This may eliminate difficulties with patient management during the scan.

CONTRAST-ENHANCED STUDIES

When ordering a CT or an MRI, the physician can request that an additional set of images be gathered after intravenous administration of a contrast agent. This process, although different physical principles are used for CT or MRI (see later sections for full discussion), is required for identification of lesions that are the same signal intensity as surrounding brain tissue. Contrast agents travel in the vascular system and normally do not cross into the brain parenchyma because they cannot pass through the blood-brain barrier. The blood-brain barrier is formed by tight junctions in the capillaries that serve as a structural barrier and func-

tion like a plasma membrane. The ability of a substance to pass through these junctions depends on several factors, including the substance's affinity for plasma proteins, its lipophilic nature, and its size. (An excellent review of the physiology of the blood-brain barrier and the basics of contrast enhancement can be found in Sage et al. 1998.)

In some disease processes, the blood-brain barrier is broken or damaged. As a result, contrast agents can diffuse into brain tissue. Pathological processes in which the blood-brain barrier is disrupted include autoimmune diseases, infections, and tumors. Contrast enhancement also can be useful in the case of vascular abnormalities (such as arteriovenous malformations and aneurysms), although the contrast agent remains intravascular. When ordering the imaging procedure, the psychiatrist should be mindful to request a study with contrast enhancement if one of the above disease states is suspected.

PATIENT PREPARATION

The psychiatrist should always explain the procedure to the patient shortly beforehand, being mindful to mention the loud noises of the scanner (MRI), the tightly enclosing imaging coil (MRI) (Figure 7–1), and the requirement for absolute immobility during the test (MRI and CT). If the psychiatrist suspects that the patient may become agitated or be unable to remain still for the length of the examination, then sedation may be necessary. A clinician may select a regimen that he or she is familiar and comfortable with. We have found that for patients with agitation and psychosis, a sedating antipsychotic with lorazepam 1–2 mg intramuscularly 30 minutes before scanning usually works well in a physically healthy nongeriatric adult.

UNDERSTANDING THE SCAN

The psychiatrist should review the scan and radiology report with the neuroradiologist. It is important to remember that the radiographic view places the patient's right on the reader's left and the patient's left on the reader's right. The first points to observe on a scan are the demographics: the hospital name; the date; the scanner number; and the patient's name, age, sex, and identification number. It is also important to note whether the scan was done with or without contrast enhancement. If an MRI has been obtained, the weighting parameters are important. The locations of these factors on CT and MRI scans are illustrated later in the chapter. Next, the psychiatrist should ask the neuroradiologist to point out the normal anatomical markers and any pathology observed on the films. Prior understanding of the limbic system anatomy is essential and is reviewed later in this chapter.

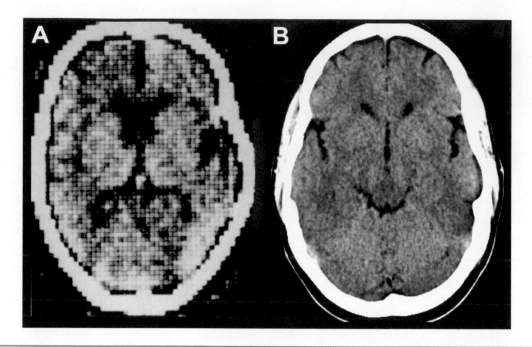

FIGURE 7–2. A first-generation computed tomography (CT) scanner, circa 1975, created (A) crude axial brain images that still were superior to other imaging techniques available at the time. (B) Modern CT scanners produce images of much higher resolution.

WHAT CAN BE LEARNED FROM STRUCTURAL IMAGING?

Soon after the advent of CT and MRI, scientists began to image patients with psychotic and mood disorders hoping to demonstrate concrete proof that these illnesses were indeed brain disorders and not conditions of "weak personalities" or "poor parenting." Initial studies in the classic conditions of bipolar disorder, major depression, and schizophrenia met with disappointing results—with, at most, nonspecific findings that occur in many disease states (e.g., ventricular enlargement or generalized atrophy). As neuropsychiatry matures, so has the knowledge that can be attained from structural images. Researchers studying conditions such as cerebral vascular accidents, ruptured aneurysms, traumatic brain injury, and multiple sclerosis were among the first to document that psychiatric symptoms do occur as a result of brain injury; that emotion, memory, and thought processing happen by way of tracts or circuits (Mega and Cummings 1994); and that indeed many patients do have subtle lesions that account for their symptoms. Not only has this information led to a further understanding of brain function, but it has provided prognostic information for patients and has led to treatment plan changes (Diwadkar and Keshavan 2002; Erhart et al. 2005; Gupta et al. 2004; Symms et al. 2004).

COMPUTED TOMOGRAPHIC IMAGING

The first computed tomographic image, obtained in 1972, required 9 days to collect the data and more than 2 hours to process it on a mainframe computer (Figure 7–2A) (Orrison and Sanders 1995). The multiple detector scanners of today can capture multiple slices in less than one half second, with the entire brain scanned in about 5 seconds (Figure 7–2B).

TECHNICAL CONSIDERATIONS

Standard Two-Dimensional CT

Like a conventional radiograph, CT uses an X-ray tube as a source of photons. When a conventional radiograph is acquired, the photons directly expose X-ray film. When a CT image is acquired, the photons are collected by detectors. The latest-generation CT scanners split the X-ray beam and add multiple detectors, allowing collection of multiple slices simultaneously ("multislice scanners"). These data are relayed to a computer that places the data in a two-dimensional grid to form the image (Rauch and Renshaw 1995). Many hospitals now display and store the resultant images digitally via a Picture Archiving and Communication System, although some still print to X-ray film (De Backer et al. 2004a, 2004b). CT scans deliver a radiation dose of about 5 rads to the lens

TABLE 7–3. Relative gray-scale appearance on a noncontrast computed tomography scan

Tissue	Appearance
Bone	White
Calcified tissue	White
Clotted blood	White[a]
Gray matter	Light gray
White matter	Medium gray
Cerebrospinal fluid	Nearly black
Water	Nearly black
Air	Black

[a]Becomes isointense to brain as clot ages approximately 1–2 weeks.

of the eye. Although a minimum of 200 rads is thought to be necessary to induce cataracts, many patients receive multiple scans, and pediatric patients are more sensitive than are adults (Hopper et al. 2001). To avoid even this small dose of radiation to the lens of the eye, some institutions use a line drawn between the orbit and the external auditory meatus (referred to as the *orbitomeatal line*) as the inferior boundary of the brain CT scans, thereby avoiding most of the exposure to the lens. The dose to the brain is about 7 rads in adults and about 10 rads in infants; although this amount was long believed to be quite safe, some controversy has arisen regarding data suggesting a possible long-term decrease in cognitive function following this level of radiation to the brain of infants (Hall et al. 2004). Although no appreciable radiation is deposited outside the head, a lead apron is often placed over the abdomen of a pregnant woman during a head CT scan.

The patient lies on a table that is advanced between acquisition of each CT slice. To acquire each CT slice, a beam of photons rotates around the head. As the photons pass through the head, some are absorbed by the tissues of the head. Detectors located opposite the beam source measure the attenuation of the photons (Figure 7–3A). Thus, the CT images of the brain record tissue density as measured by the variable attenuation of X-ray photons. High-density tissues such as bone appear white, indicating an almost complete absorption of the X rays (high attenuation). Air has the lowest rate of attenuation (or absorption of radiation) and appears black. The appearance of other tissues is given in Table 7–3.

Modern CT scanners generate brain images with slice thickness typically in the 2.5–5.0 mm range. The slice thickness of a CT image is an important variable in clinical scanning. Thinner slices allow visualization of smaller le-

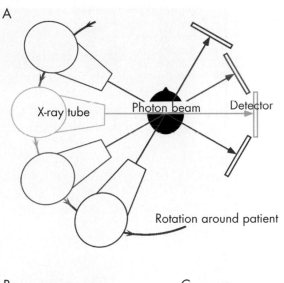

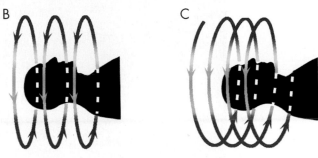

FIGURE 7–3. (A) Schematic of a conventional computed tomography X-ray tube and detector. Note the simultaneous circular movement of both devices about the head. (B) The scanning path in conventional computed tomography is made up of separate closed loops. (C) The scanning path in spiral (helical) computed tomography follows a continuous overlapping spiral path.

sions. However, the thinnest sections have less contrast (i.e., the signal intensity difference between gray and white matter is less) because the signal-to-noise ratio is lower. It also takes longer to complete the examination because more slices must be acquired. Thus, there is more chance of patient motion degrading the images. Thicker sections (or slices) have greater contrast, but smaller lesions may be missed. Also, the incidence of artifacts is greater as a result of increased volume averaging (averaging of two adjacent, but very different, parts of the brain within a single CT slice). This is particularly true in the base of the skull, and this may obscure brainstem and mesial temporal structures. See Figure 7–4 for an explanation of scan parameters.

Three-Dimensional CT (Single-Slice and Multislice Helical CT)

As CT imaging became an integral part of medical diagnostics, faster and more advanced technologies were

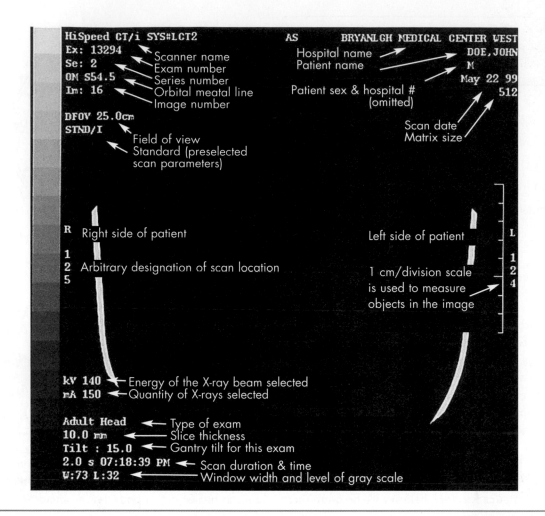

FIGURE 7–4. Computed tomography header information and arbitrary gray scale. Explanations for abbreviations used on the image are also included.

invented. The 1990s brought the clinical introduction of helical (spiral) CT, in which the detector rotates continuously around the patient during scanning (Figure 7–3C). This is much faster than the older "scan—stop—move the table and reset the detector—scan again" sequence used for standard two-dimensional CT (Figure 7–3B). Even more recently, multiple-detector helical CT scanners have come into clinical use; they produce multiple slices as multiple detectors rotate together around the patient. Sixty-four-slice (64-detector) scanners are now clinically available. These allow for extremely rapid imaging, the most important advantage of which is capturing contrast flowing through arteries, thereby creating superb CT angiograms, which are likely to replace most traditional invasive diagnostic angiography in the near future (Willmann and Wildermuth 2005). On all CT scanners, two-dimensional images are obtained, from which reconstructions in coronal or sagittal planes can be made in a few minutes, if desired. Three-dimensional reconstructions can also be done (Figure 7–5).

Initially, single-slice helical CT was principally useful in body scanning. It had limited use in the brain because of skull thickness (i.e., it produced grainy images that did not discriminate between gray and white matter very well) (Bahner et al. 1998; Coleman and Zimmerman 1994). Applications for the head included evaluations of pediatric patients (thinner cranium), adult carotid stenosis, aneurysms, arteriovenous malformations, and vessel occlusions in acute stroke and as a tool for intravenous angiography (Coleman and Zimmerman 1994; Kuszyk et al. 1998; Schwartz 1995). The newest helical CT scanners provide images of similar quality to the standard single-slice CT and are now the standard of care for brain CT imaging (Kuntz et al. 1998).

CONTRAST AGENTS

The administration of intravenous iodinated contrast medium immediately before obtaining a CT scan greatly improves the detection of many brain lesions that are

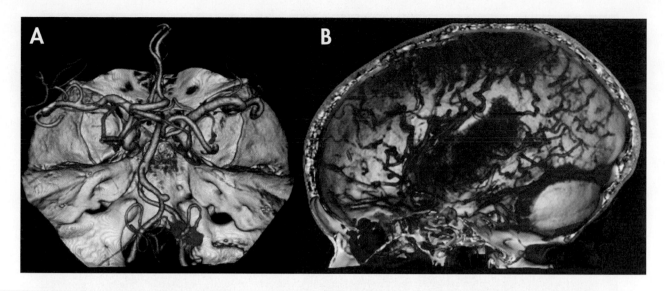

FIGURE 7–5. Three-dimensional reconstruction from helical (spiral) computed tomography allows viewing of data sets from any desired angle. (A) Vertebral artery aneurysm. (B) Aneurysm with hemorrhage. Reconstructions of vasculature are particularly valuable for both diagnosis and surgical planning.

Source. Images courtesy of Toshiba America Medical Systems, Inc.

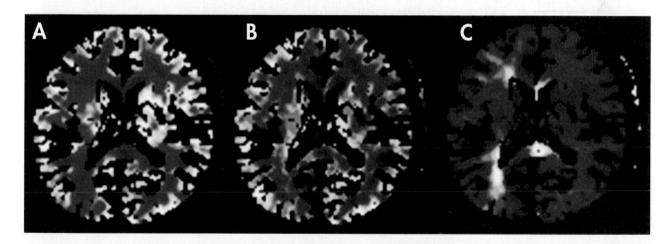

FIGURE 7–6. Contrast agents, when administered as a fast bolus, can be used to measure several aspects of cerebral perfusion, including (A) cerebral blood flow, (B) cerebral blood volume, and (C) mean transit time.

Source. Images courtesy of Toshiba America Medical Systems, Inc.

isodense on noncontrast CT. Contrast agents are useful when a breakdown of the blood-brain barrier occurs. Under normal circumstances, the blood-brain barrier does not allow passage of contrast medium into the extravascular spaces of the brain. When a break in this barrier occurs, the contrast agent enters the damaged area and collects in or around the lesion. The *increased* density of the contrast agent will appear as a white area on the scan. Without a companion noncontrast CT scan, preexisting dense areas (calcified or hemorrhagic) might be mistaken for contrast-enhanced lesions. In difficult cases, a double dose of con-

trast agent may be used to improve detection of lesions with minimal blood-brain barrier impairment. Contrast agents, when administered as a fast bolus, can also be used to measure several aspects of cerebral perfusion, including cerebral blood flow, cerebral blood volume, and mean transit time (Figure 7–6) (Halpin 2004).

Currently, there are two types of iodinated CT contrast agents: ionic or high osmolality and nonionic or low osmolality. Both types are associated with allergic reactions, and contraindications for both exist. Allergic reactions to contrast agents are defined by two types in two

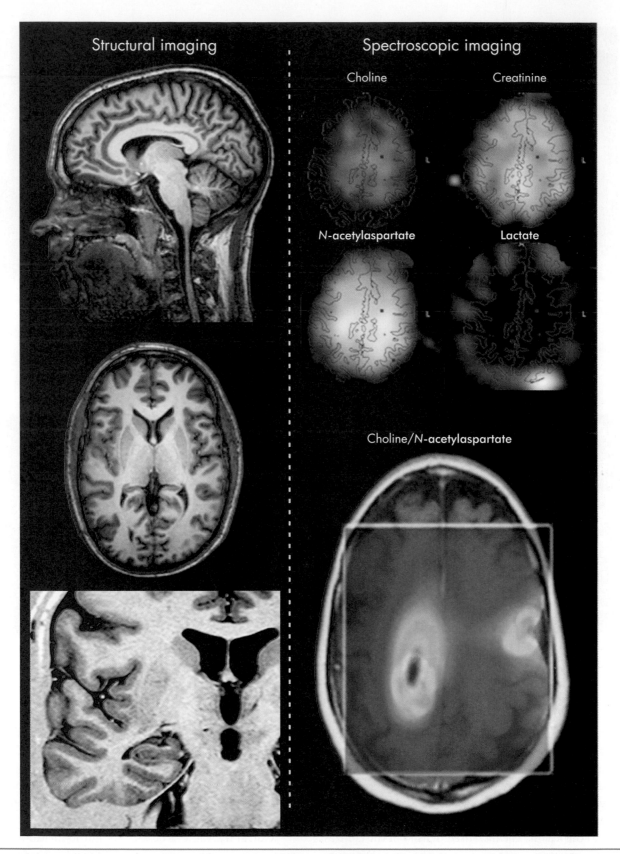

FIGURE 7–7.   Higher-field (>1.5 T) magnetic resonance scanners are becoming increasingly available. The higher magnetic field strength provides more signal, making higher-resolution structural imaging (*left*) and chemical shift imaging (*right*) practical.

Source.   Pictures courtesy of Phillips Medical Systems.

time frames: anaphylactoid or nonanaphylactoid (chemotoxic) and immediate or delayed (Detre and Alsop 2005; Federle et al. 1998; Jacobs et al. 1998; Oi et al. 1997; Yasuda and Munechika 1998). Anaphylactoid reactions include hives, rhinitis, bronchospasm, laryngeal edema, hypotension, and death. Chemotoxic reactions include nausea, vomiting, warmth or pain at the injection site, hypotension, tachycardia, and arrhythmias (Cohan et al. 1998; Federle et al. 1998; Mortele et al. 2005). Immediate reactions occur within 1 hour of injection; delayed reactions, within 7 days but usually within 24 hours. The overall mortality rate from any contrast dye is reported to be 1 per 100,000. Data suggest that ionic contrast reactions occur at a rate of 4%–12% (most commonly mild) and nonionic reactions occur at a rate of 1%–3% (Cochran 2005; Cochran et al. 2002). One study reviewed approximately 20,000 contrast-enhanced CT examinations and found the rate of mild and moderate ionic dye reactions to be 2.2% and 0.08%, respectively, with 0.59% mild and 0.05% moderate with the nonionic (Valls et al. 2003).

The ionic agents are significantly less expensive, but they are less often used because of the greater risk of allergic reactions. The American College of Radiology standards recommend the use of nonionic dye in patients with histories of significant contrast media reactions; any previous serious allergic reaction to any material; asthma; sickle cell disease; diabetes; renal insufficiency (creatinine ≥1.5 mg/dL); cardiac diseases; inability to communicate; geriatric age; or other debilitating health problems (including myasthenia gravis, multiple myeloma, and pheochromocytoma) (Cohan et al. 1998; Halpern et al. 1999; Konen et al. 2002). Patients who are receiving dialysis or who have histories of milder reactions to shellfish require the use of nonionic dyes when contrast CT is unavoidable. The older ionic agents are not used in these patients.

Extravasation (leakage of the contrast dye at the injection site) is generally a mild problem associated with some stinging or burning. However, in infrequent cases, patients have developed tissue ulceration or necrosis. If a patient has had a previous episode of extravasation, then nonionic dye should be used because it is associated with fewer reactions.

Other areas of caution include patients with histories of anaphylaxis. These patients should be considered for other types of imaging rather than contrast-enhanced CT. If contrast-enhanced CT is necessary, then premedication with steroids and antihistamines and the use of nonionic dye are recommended. Metformin, an oral antihyperglycemic agent, must be withheld before iodinated dye is given. It can be restarted after 48 hours with laboratory evidence of normal renal function. Metformin can

cause lactic acidosis, especially in patients with a history of renal or hepatic dysfunction, alcohol abuse, or cardiac disease (Cohan et al. 1998).

MAGNETIC RESONANCE IMAGING

In 1946, the phenomenon of nuclear magnetic resonance was discovered. The discovery led to the development of a powerful new technique for studying matter by using radio waves together with a static magnetic field. This development, combined with other important insights and emerging technologies in the 1970s, led to the first magnetic resonance image of a living patient. By the 1980s, commercial MRI scanners were becoming more common. Although the physics that make MRI possible are complex, a grasp of the basic principles will help the clinician understand the results of the imaging examination and explain this procedure to anxious patients.

PHYSICAL PRINCIPLES

Reconstructing an Image

Clinical MRI is based on manipulating the small magnetic field around the nucleus of the hydrogen atom (proton), a major component of water in soft tissue. To make a magnetic resonance image of a patient's soft tissues, the patient must be placed inside a large magnet. The strength of the magnet is measured in teslas (T). A high-field clinical system has a field strength of 1.5 or 3.0 T (Figure 7–7). (More powerful systems are often used in research settings.) A mid-field system is generally 0.5 T, and low-field units range from 0.1 to 0.5 T (Figure 7–8) (Scarabino et al. 2003).

The magnetic field of the MRI scanner slightly magnetizes the hydrogen atoms in the body, changing their alignment. The stronger the magnetic field, the more magnetized the hydrogen atoms in tissue become and the more signal they will produce. The stronger signal available with 1.5-T and 3.0-T systems allows images of higher resolution to be collected. Some patients feel uncomfortable or frankly claustrophobic while lying inside these huge enclosing magnets (Figure 7–9A). Open-design magnets are now available that help the patient feel less confined (Figure 7–9B) (Scarabino et al. 2003). These are increasingly popular, constituting an estimated 40% of sales in the last 5 years, although the image quality is lower than in closed systems (Moseley et al. 2005).

To create a magnetic resonance image, the patient is placed in the center of the magnetic resonance scanner's powerful magnetic field. This strong magnetic field (usually 1.5 or 3.0 T) is always on and is perfectly uniform across the

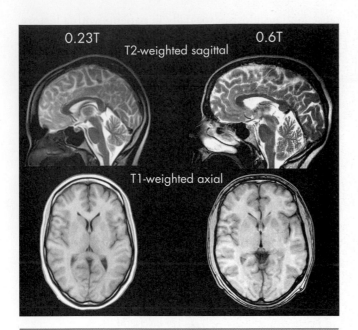

FIGURE 7–8.   Magnetic resonance scanners come in a variety of magnetic field strengths (measured in tesla, T). Most clinical systems are 1.5 T and higher, but lower field strengths are also clinically useful.

Source.   Pictures courtesy of Phillips Medical Systems.

patient. The nuclei of the hydrogen atoms in the patient's body possess tiny magnetic fields, which instantly align with the strong magnetic field of the scanner. A series of precisely calculated radio frequency (RF) pulses is then applied. The hydrogen nuclei absorb this RF energy, which causes them to temporarily lose their alignment with the strong magnetic field. They gradually relax back into magnetic alignment, releasing the absorbed energy in a characteristic temporal pattern, depending on the nature of the tissue containing the hydrogen atoms. This electromagnetic energy is detected by the same coils used to generate the RF pulses and is converted into an electrical signal that is sent to a computer. For some body regions, such as the brain or knee, a coil is placed directly around the body region to improve delivery and reception of the electromagnetic pulses and signals. The scanner's computer converts these signals into a spatial map, the magnetic resonance image. The final output is a matrix consisting of a three-dimensional image composed of many small blocks, or voxels. The voxel size on a 1.5-T scan of the brain is variable but approximately 1 mm on each side.

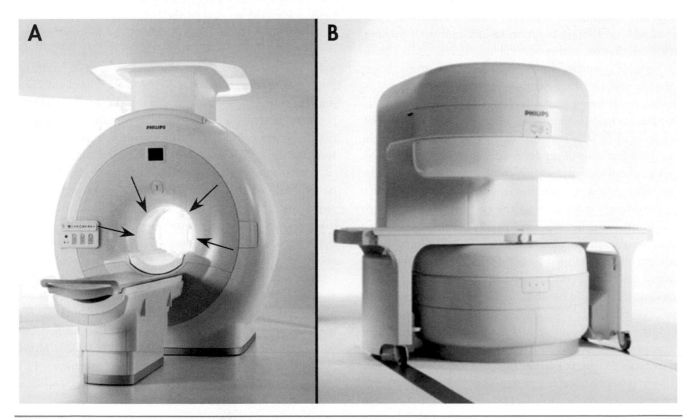

FIGURE 7–9.   *(A)* The traditional magnetic resonance scanner is an enclosing tunnel *(arrows)*. *(B)* Open designs are gaining in popularity.

Source.   Pictures courtesy of Phillips Medical Systems.

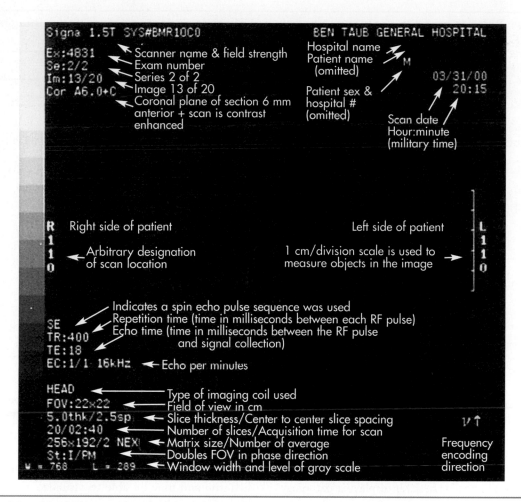

FIGURE 7–10. Magnetic resonance imaging header information and arbitrary gray scale. Explanations for abbreviations used on the image are also included. RF=radio frequency.

Creation of a magnetic resonance image requires the application of small magnetic field gradients across the patient in addition to the constant, more powerful field. This allows the scanner to tell which part of the body is emitting what signal. The magnetic field gradients needed to acquire the image are created by huge coils of wire embedded in the magnet. These are driven with large-current audio amplifiers similar to those used for musical concerts. The current in these coils must be switched on and off very rapidly. This causes the coils to vibrate and creates loud noises during the scan that may occasionally distress the unprepared patient, although patients are always given earplugs, which greatly dampen the noise.

Common Pulse Sequences

The combination of RF and magnetic field pulses used by the computer to create the image is called the *pulse sequence*. Pulse sequences have been developed that result in images sensitive to different aspects of the hydrogen atom's behavior in a high magnetic field. Thus, each image type contains unique information about the tissue. A pulse sequence is repeated many times to form an image.

The pulse sequence used most commonly in clinical MRI is the *spin echo* (SE) sequence. Most centers now use a faster variant of this sequence, the *fast spin echo* (FSE). These pulse sequences emphasize different tissue properties by varying two factors. One is the time between applying each repetition of the sequence, referred to as the *repetition time* or *time to recovery* (TR). The other is the time at which the receiver coil collects signal after the RF pulses have been given. This is called the *echo time* or *time until the echo* (TE). Images collected using a short TR and short TE are most heavily influenced by the T1 relaxation times of the tissues and so are called *T1 weighted*. Locations of scan parameters on study images are indicated in Figure 7–10. Traditionally, this type of image is considered best for displaying anatomy because there are sharply marginated boundaries between the gray matter of the brain (medium gray), the white matter of the brain (very light gray), and cerebrospinal fluid (CSF) (black). Images collected using a

TABLE 7–4.   Relative gray-scale values present in tissues visible on magnetic resonance imaging scans (non-contrast-enhanced)

	Spin echo pulse sequences		
Tissue	**T1-weighted**	**T2-weighted**	**FLAIR**
Bone	Black	Black	Black
Calcified tissue	Variable, usually gray	Variable, usually gray	Variable, usually gray
Gray matter	Medium gray	Medium gray	Medium gray
White matter	Light gray	Dark gray	Dark gray
Cerebrospinal fluid	Black	White	Black
Water	Black	White	Black
Air	Black	Black	Black
Pathology (excluding blood)	Gray	White	White
Blood			
Acute	Dark gray	Black	Black
Subacute	White	White	White

Note.   FLAIR = fluid-attenuated inversion recovery.

long TR and a long TE are most heavily influenced by the T2 relaxation times of the tissues and so are called *T2 weighted*. Boundaries between the gray matter of the brain (medium gray), the white matter of the brain (dark gray), and CSF (white) are more blurred than on T1-weighted images. This type of image is best for displaying pathology, which most commonly appears bright, often similar in intensity to CSF. A very useful variant on the T2-weighted scan, called a *fluid-attenuated inversion recovery* (FLAIR) image, allows the intense signal from CSF to be nullified (CSF appears dark). This makes pathology near CSF-filled spaces much easier to see (Arakia et al. 1999; Bergin et al. 1995; Brant-Zawadzki et al. 1996; Rydberg et al. 1994). FLAIR improves identification of subtle lesions, making it useful for neuropsychiatric imaging. A summary of the expected imaging appearance of various tissues on commonly used types of magnetic resonance images is given in Table 7–4. The appearance of the brain is illustrated in Figure 7–11.

The next most commonly used pulse sequence in clinical imaging is the *gradient echo* (GE or GRE) sequence. In this type of image acquisition, a gradient-reversing RF pulse is used to generate the echo. This technique is very sensitive to anything in the tissue causing magnetic field inhomogeneity, such as hemorrhage or calcium. These images are sometimes called *susceptibility weighted* because differences in magnetic susceptibility between tissues cause localized magnetic field inhomogeneity and signal loss. As a result, gradient echo images have artifacts at the interfaces between tissues with very

different magnetic susceptibility, such as bone and brain. The artifacts at the skull base are sometimes severe. A more recently developed method of MRI that is finding increasing clinical use is diffusion-weighted imaging. Diffusion-weighted MRI is sensitive to the speed of water diffusion and may be able to visualize areas of ischemic stroke in the critical first few hours after onset (Huisman 2003; Kuhl et al. 2005; Mascalchi et al. 2005; Nakamura et al. 2005; Symms et al. 2004). It is also showing potential in the imaging of other conditions, such as hypoglycemic encephalopathy, infection, neurodegenerative conditions, traumatic brain injury, and metabolic diseases (Jung et al. 2005; Mascalchi et al. 2005; Symms et al. 2004).

New Pulse Sequences

Two pulse sequences that are sensitive to other aspects of tissue state are being tested for clinical work. Magnetization transfer imaging is sensitive to interactions between free protons (unbound water in tissue) and bound protons (water bound to macromolecules such as those in myelin membranes) (Hanyu et al. 1999; Tanabe et al. 1999). It may be able to differentiate white matter lesions from different causes and thus provide insight into pathological processes (Filippi and Rocca 2004; Hanyu et al. 1999; Hurley et al. 2003; Symms et al. 2004; Tanabe et al. 1999). Diffusion tensor imaging is a more complex version of diffusion-weighted imaging (Dong et al. 2004; Kubicki et al. 2002; Sundgren et al. 2004; Taber et al. 2002b; Taylor et al. 2004). A set of images is collected that allows calculation of

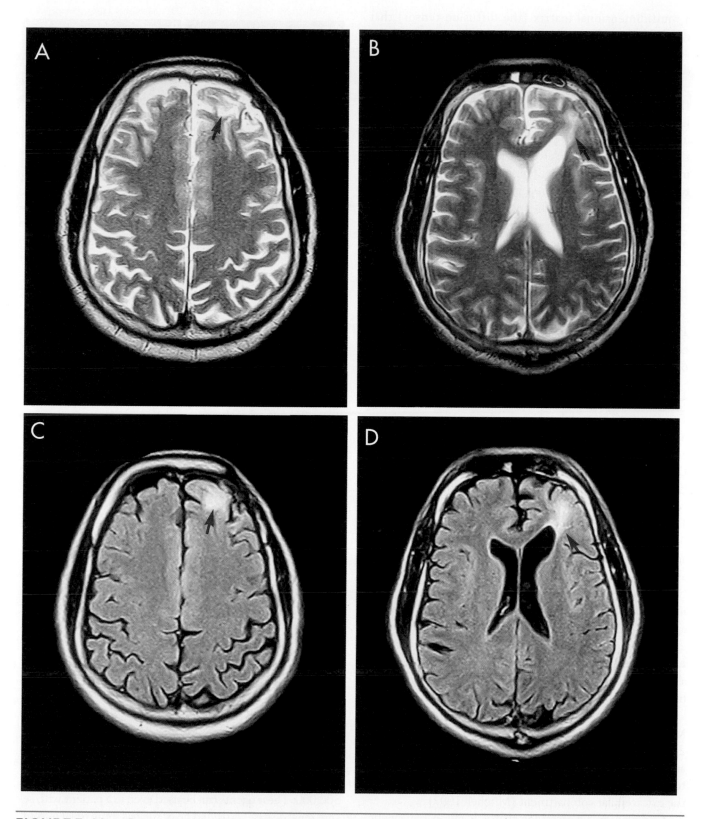

FIGURE 7–11. Comparison of axial T2-weighted (T2W) and fluid-attenuated inversion recovery (FLAIR) magnetic resonance imaging (MRI) in a 36-year-old man who presented for admission with nausea, vomiting, and hyponatremia. Two days later, the patient was agitated, sexually inappropriate, and wandering incoherently. Neuropsychiatric workup identified status epilepticus. Subsequent MRI detected a previous left frontal traumatic brain injury (*arrows*). Although the injury is visible on T2W images (*A, B*), the extent of the injury is much more easily appreciated on the FLAIR images (*C, D*).

a multidimensional matrix (the diffusion tensor) that describes the diffusional speed in each direction for every voxel in the image. The speed of diffusion is similar in all directions in gray matter (isotropic diffusion) but is faster parallel to axons in white matter (anisotropic diffusion) (Figure 7–12). This technique is sensitive to many processes that alter diffusion, including ischemia and gliosis. It can be used to identify areas of pathology or damage, such as those that occur in multiple sclerosis or following traumatic brain injury. It also has potential for studying very subtle structural changes, such as altered brain connectivity in neuropsychiatric disorders. Another promising new magnetic resonance technique provides a method for imaging of cerebral blood flow by "tagging" water molecules in the carotid arteries with RF pulses (arterial spin labeling), which changes the signal intensity of the blood as it flows up into the brain (Detre and Alsop 2005). This technique has great potential because it does not require administration of a contrast agent or exposure to any form of radiation. In the future, a combination of some of these newer methods of MRI may provide important information for differential diagnosis.

CONTRAST AGENTS

The first experimental contrast-enhanced magnetic resonance image was made in 1982 using a gadolinium complex, gadolinium-diethylenetriamine penta-acetic acid (Gd-DTPA), now called gadopentetate dimeglumine. Six years later, gadopentetate dimeglumine was approved as an intravenous contrast agent for human clinical MRI scans (Wolf 1991). Metal ions such as gadolinium are quite toxic to the body if they are in a free state. To make an MRI contrast agent, the metal ion is attached to a very strong ligand (such as DTPA) that prevents any interaction with surrounding tissue. This allows the gadolinium complex to be excreted intact by the kidneys. Several gadolinium-based contrast agents are currently in common use for brain imaging, including gadopentetate dimeglumine (Magnevist, Berlex Laboratories), gadodiamide (Omniscan, Nycomed Amersham), gadoteridol (ProHance, Bracco Diagnostics), gadobenate dimeglumine (MultiHance, Bracco Diagnostics), and gadoversetamide (OptiMARK, Tyco Healthcare/ Mallinckrodt Inc) (Baker et al. 2004; Kirchin and Runge 2003; Runge 2001; Shellock and Kanal 1999). These agents are administered intravenously, whereupon they distribute to the vascular compartment and then diffuse throughout the extracellular compartment (Mitchell 1997).

Gadolinium is a metal ion that is highly paramagnetic, with a natural magnetic field 657 times greater than that of the hydrogen atom. Unlike the iodinated contrast agents used in CT, the currently used clinical MRI contrast agents are not imaged directly. Rather, the presence of the contrast agent changes the T1 and T2 properties of hydrogen atoms

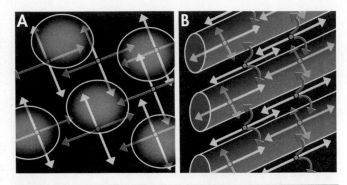

FIGURE 7–12.   Gray matter contains cell bodies and processes and is quite heterogeneous. Water diffusion is the same in all directions (isotropic), as indicated by (A) the similar length of the green and pink arrows. White matter contains tightly packed axons. Water diffusion is faster (B, green arrows) along the length of (parallel to) axons than it is (B, pink arrows) across axons.

(protons) in nearby tissue (Runge et al. 1997). Like CT contrast agents, MRI contrast agents do not enter the brain under normal conditions because they cannot pass through the blood-brain barrier. When the blood-brain barrier is damaged, these agents accumulate in tissue around the breakdown. The effect of this accumulation is most easily seen on a T1-weighted scan. It results in an increase in signal (seen as a white or bright area; see Figure 7–13) (Runge et al. 1997). Like CT, cerebral blood flow can be assessed if images are acquired very quickly after administration of a contrast agent (this technique is variously called dynamic susceptibility contrast, first-pass perfusion MRI, or bolus perfusion MRI) (Latchaw 2004; Sunshine 2004).

On a worldwide basis, 30%–40% of MRI studies include contrast enhancement (Shellock and Kanal 1999). The total incidence of adverse side effects appears to be less than 3%–5%, with any single type of side effect occurring in fewer than 1% of patients (Kirchin and Runge 2003; Runge 2001; Runge et al. 1997; Shellock and Kanal 1999). Immediate reactions at the injection site include warmth or a burning sensation, pain, and local edema. Delayed reactions (including erythema, swelling, and pain) appear 1–4 days after the injection. Immediate systemic reactions include nausea (sometimes vomiting) and headache. Anaphylactoid reactions have been reported, particularly in patients with a history of allergic respiratory disease. The incidence of these reactions appears to be somewhere between 1 and 5 in 500,000. These agents can be used even in a patient with severe renal disease, provided he or she has some renal output. This allows contrast-enhanced MRI scans to be obtained in dialysis patients. The presence of some of these contrast agents (Omniscan, OptiMARK) has been reported to interfere with colorimetric assays for serum calcium, resulting in an incorrect diagnosis of hypocalcemia in 15% of patients in

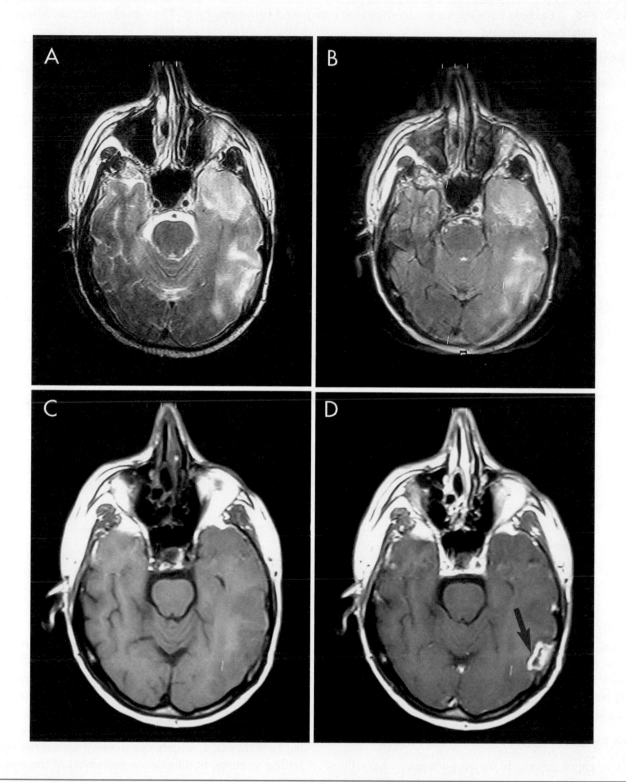

FIGURE 7–13.   Some types of pathology are much more easily visualized following administration of a contrast agent. A 69-year-old man presented with acute confusion and status post a generalized tonic-clonic seizure. Sequential magnetic resonance imaging showed left temporal mass, most probably an astrocytoma (infiltrating type). The tumor is more easily seen on (A) T2-weighted and (B) fluid-attenuated inversion recovery (FLAIR) images than on (C) T1-weighted images. (D) After administration of contrast, an area of blood-brain barrier breakdown within the tumor becomes visible (*arrow*).

TABLE 7–5. Factors considered when choosing computed tomography (CT) or magnetic resonance imaging (MRI) examination

Clinical considerations	CT	MRI
Availability	Universal	Limited
Sensitivity	Good	Superior
Resolution	1.0 mm	1.0 mm
Average examination time	4–5 minutes	30–35 minutes
Plane of section	Axial only	Any plane of section
Conditions for which it is the preferred procedure	Screening examination Acute hemorrhage Calcified lesions Bone injury	All subcortical lesions Poison or toxin exposure Demyelinating disorders Eating disorders Examination requiring anatomical detail, especially temporal lobe or cerebellum Any condition best viewed in nonaxial plane
Contraindications	History of anaphylaxis or severe allergic reaction (contrast-enhanced CT) Creatinine≥1.5 mg/dL (contrast-enhanced CT) Metformin administration on day of scan (contrast-enhanced CT)	Any magnetic metal in the body, including surgical clips and sutures Implanted electrical, mechanical, or magnetic devices Claustrophobia History of welding (requires skull films before MRI) Pregnancy (legal contraindication)
Medicare reimbursement per scan without contrast medium	~$240	~$540
Medicare reimbursement with and without contrast medium[a]	~$380	~$1,150

[a]A scan without contrast media is always acquired before the contrast-enhanced scan.

one study (Kirchin and Runge 2003). (For a more extensive review of the biosafety aspects of MRI contrast agents, see Shellock and Kanal 1999.) Many new MRI contrast agents are under development (Bulte 2004). As new contrast agents become available for MRI of the brain, the range of applications in neuropsychiatry may well expand.

SAFETY AND CONTRAINDICATIONS

To date, there appear to be no permanent hazardous effects from short-term exposure to magnetic fields and RF pulses generated in clinical MRI scanners (Price 1999; Shellock and Crues 2004). Volunteers scanned in systems with higher field strength (4 T) have reported effects including headaches, dizziness, and nausea (Shellock 1991). With very intense gradients, it is possible to stimulate peripheral nerves directly, but this is not a con-

cern at clinical field strengths (Bourland et al. 1999; Hoffmann et al. 2000; Shellock and Crues 2004).

There are, however, important contraindications to the use of MRI (see Table 7–5 for summary). The magnetic field can damage electrical, mechanical, or magnetic devices implanted in or attached to the patient. Pacemakers can be damaged by programming changes, possibly inducing arrhythmias. Currents can develop within the wires, leading to burns, fibrillation, or movement of the wires or the pacemaker unit itself. Cochlear implants, dental implants, magnetic stoma plugs, bone-growth stimulators, and implanted medication-infusion pumps can all be demagnetized or injure the patient by movement during exposure to the scanner's magnetic field. In addition, metallic implants, shrapnel, bullets, or metal shavings within the eye (e.g., from welding) can conduct a current and/or move, injuring the eye. All of these devices distort the magnetic resonance image locally and may decrease diagnostic accuracy. Metallic objects near the magnet can be drawn into the magnet at high speed, injuring the patient or staff (Price 1999; Shellock 1991, 2002; Shellock and Crues 2004).

Although there is no evidence of damage to the developing fetus, most authorities recommend caution. Judgment should be exercised when considering MRI of a pregnant woman. When possible, express written consent might be obtained from the patient, especially in the first trimester (Shellock 1991; Shellock and Crues 2004; Shellock and Kanal 1991; Wilde et al. 2005). Difficulties also have been encountered when a patient requires physiological monitoring during the procedure. Several manufacturers have developed MRI-compatible respirators and monitors for blood pressure and heart rate. If these are not available, then the standard monitoring devices must be placed at least 8 feet from the magnet. Otherwise, the readout may be altered or the devices may interfere with obtaining the MRI scan.

MRI VERSUS CT

The choice of imaging modality should be based on the anatomy and/or pathology that one desires to view (see Table 7–5). CT is used as an inexpensive screening examination. Also, a few conditions are best viewed with CT, including calcification, acute hemorrhage, and any bone injury, because these pathologies are not yet reliably imaged with MRI (Figure 7–14). However, in the vast majority of cases, MRI is the preferred modality (Figure 7–15). The anatomical detail is much better, more types of pathology are visible, and the brain can be imaged in any plane of section. For example, subcortical lesions are consistently better visualized with MRI because of the greater gray-white contrast and the ability to image in planes other than axial. Thus, most temporal lobe structures, especially the hippocampal formation and amygdala, are most easily evaluated with the coronal and sagittal planes of section rather than axial. Demyelination resulting from poison exposure or autoimmune disease (such as multiple sclerosis) is also better visualized on MRI, especially when many small lesions are present (Figure 7–16). MRI does not produce the artifacts from bone that are seen in CT, so all lesions near bone (e.g., brain stem, posterior fossa, pituitary, hypothalamus) are better visualized on MRI.

GENERAL PRINCIPLES OF FUNCTIONAL IMAGING

Functional brain imaging techniques provide several ways of assessing brain physiology. Regional cerebral

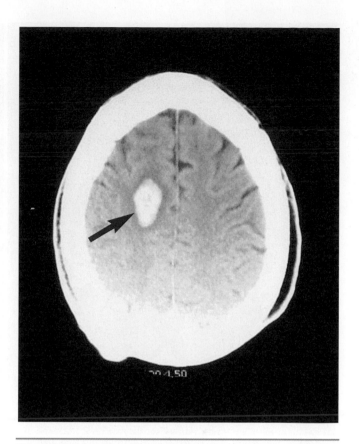

FIGURE 7–14.   Computed tomography is the preferred imaging method for acute head injury. This axial image is from a 56-year-old man taking warfarin who presented with left-sided weakness a few hours after being involved in a motorcycle accident. He experienced a brief loss of consciousness following the accident. Note the well-visualized area of hyperdense hemorrhage (*arrow*).

blood flow (rCBF) and regional cerebral metabolic rate (rCMR) are the most broadly used measures (SPECT and PET). These both provide an indirect measure of brain activity. Neuronal activity consumes oxygen and metabolites and induces vasodilation of the nearby muscular arterioles, leading to a prompt increase in blood flow. A close coupling occurs between neuronal activity, rCBF, and rCMR, although the increase in blood flow, for unknown reasons, is more than is necessary to supply the increased demand for oxygen and glucose.

If acquired under resting conditions, both rCMR and rCBF provide a way to assess the baseline functional state of brain areas. Many of these techniques can also be used during performance of a mental or physical task designed to activate specific neuronal pathways or structures. This allows brain activity under specific cognitive or affective conditions to be measured. Pharmacological challenges are also used. Neuronal activity can be directly assessed during activation tasks via measures of electrical activity

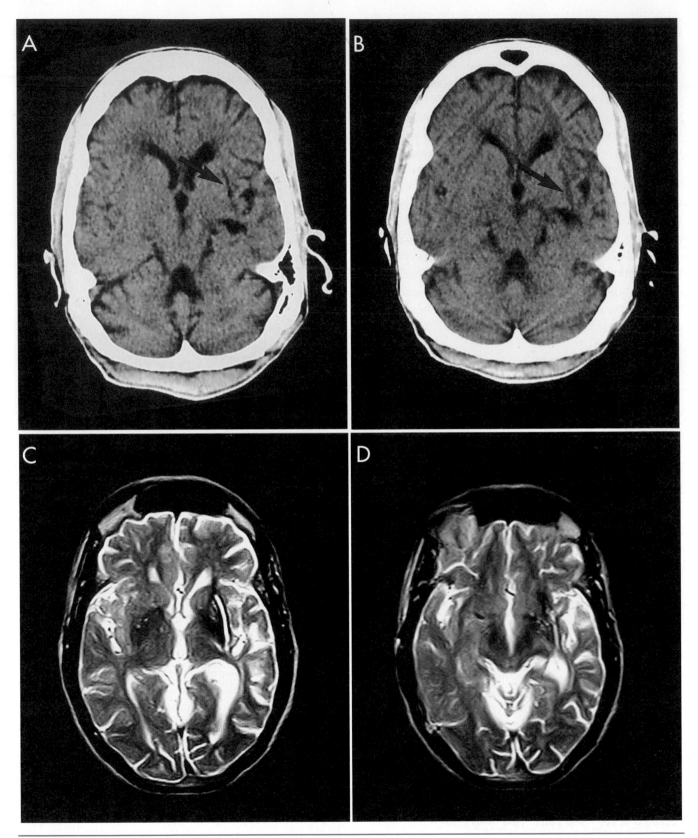

FIGURE 7–15.   Many types of pathology are more easily seen on magnetic resonance imaging (MRI) than on computed tomographic (CT) imaging. These axial images are from a 69-year-old man who presented status post a generalized tonic-clonic seizure. Abnormal areas indicative of subcortical ischemia are evident on (A, B) the conventional CT images (*arrows*). Areas of ischemic injury and old hemorrhage as well as normal anatomy are much better visualized on (C, D) T2-weighted MRI.

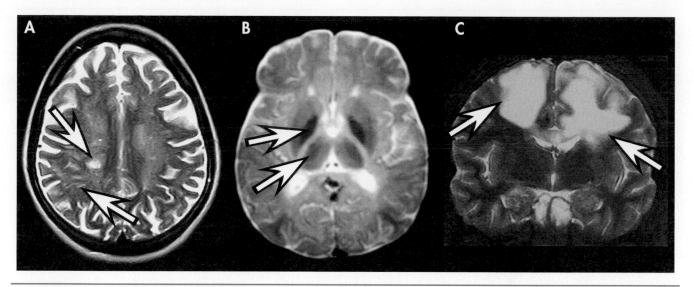

FIGURE 7–16. Magnetic resonance imaging (MRI) has many clinical applications. (A) Multiple sclerosis is characterized by ovoid hyperintense demyelinating lesions parallel to the subependymal veins (*arrows*) on T2-weighted MRI. (B) Chronic toluene abuse causes hypointensity in the basal ganglia and thalamus on both T1- and T2-weighted (*arrows*) images. (C) Acute disseminated encephalomyelitis causes extensive white matter damage, resulting in areas of hyperintensity (*arrows*) on T2-weighted images.

(electroencephalography [EEG]) or magnetic activity (MEG). In addition, functional imaging techniques are available to measure various neurotransmitter receptor systems and regional brain metabolites. These techniques have been immensely helpful in laboratory study of multiple aspects of cognitive and emotional functioning, including learning, memory, emotional regulation, control of attention, and modulation of behavior. Differences between specific patient groups and healthy individuals have provided important insights into functional impairments that occur in some psychiatric diseases. There are many research studies of common psychiatric conditions such as major depressive disorder, schizophrenia, obsessive-compulsive disorder, and attention-deficit/hyperactivity disorder. Results have been quite variable; thus, clinical applications of functional imaging have been limited by the translation of this understanding to the individual patient.

Unlike structural imaging, functional imaging is dynamic and state-dependent. Many factors can influence scan results of a particular individual on a particular day. Thus, its penetrance into the clinical arena has been slower to evolve. Functional imaging is particularly useful for identification of "hidden" lesions, areas that are dysfunctional but do not look abnormal on structural imaging. Evaluation of the resting state also has shown potential for prediction of treatment response in some conditions. In general, patients whose clinical symptoms do not fit the classic historical picture for the working diagnosis should be considered for some form of functional imaging.

NUCLEAR BRAIN IMAGING: POSITRON EMISSION TOMOGRAPHY AND SINGLE-PHOTON EMISSION COMPUTED TOMOGRAPHY

Both PET and SPECT involve intravenous injection of a radioactive compound that distributes in the brain and emits (indirectly, in the case of PET) photons that are detected and used to form an image. The tracer is a molecule whose chemical properties determine its distribution in the body (e.g., fluorodeoxyglucose distributes in cells in proportion to their glucose metabolic rate) and which contains one radioactive atom, called a *radionuclide*. Depending on what compound was injected, the distribution of radioactivity indicates regional blood flow, metabolism, number of available neurotransmitter receptors, and so forth. Regional cerebral metabolism and cerebral perfusion are tightly linked under most physiological and pathophysiological conditions (Raichle 2003). Both types of imaging studies provide very similar functional information. It is important to note that, in principle, almost any cellular function can be imaged by synthesizing a radioactive compound that crosses the blood-brain barrier and binds to a component of the relevant cellular machinery. For example, this has already been accomplished for adenylyl cyclase, protein kinase C, more than a dozen neurotransmitter receptors and transporters, and many other components of cellular biochemistry and physiology (see Table

TABLE 7–6.   Radiotracers for functional brain imaging

Parameter measured	SPECT radiotracers	PET radiotracers
Glucose uptake (regional cerebral metabolic rate; rCMR)	None	$[^{18}F]$-fluorodeoxyglucose (FDG)
Blood flow (regional cerebral blood flow; rCBF)	$[^{99m}Tc]$-HMPAO $[^{99m}Tc]$-ECD $[^{123}I]$-IMP[a]	$[^{15}O]$-water
Serotonin transporter binding	$[^{123}I]$-β-CIT $[^{123}I]$-ADAM	$[^{11}C]$-McN-5652 $[^{11}C]$-DASB $[^{11}C]$-ADAM
Serotonin type 1A (5-HT$_{1A}$) receptor binding	Under development	$[^{11}C]$-WAY-100635
Serotonin 5-HT$_{2A}$ receptor binding	$[^{123}I]$-5-I-R91150	$[^{11}C]$-N-methylspiperone $[^{18}F]$-setoperone
Dopamine D$_2$ receptor binding	$[^{123}I]$-IBZM	$[^{11}C]$-raclopride $[^{11}C]$-N-methylspiperone
Dopamine D$_1$ receptor binding	None	$[^{11}C]$-SCH23390 $[^{11}C]$-NNC112
DOPA decarboxylase activity	None	$[^{18}F]$-6-fluoro-L-dopa (F-DOPA) $[^{11}C]$–DOPA
Dopamine transporter (DAT) binding	$[^{123}I]$-β-CIT $[^{123}I]$-FP-CIT $[^{123}I]$-Altropane $[^{99m}Tc]$-Altropane	$[^{18}F]$-CFT
Acetylcholine nicotinic receptor binding	$[^{123}I]$-5-IA-85380	2$[^{18}F]$F-A-85380
Acetylcholine muscarinic receptor binding	$[^{123}I]$-IQNB $[^{123}I]$-IDEX	$[^{11}C]$-methyl benztropine $[^{18}F]$FP-TZTP

Note.   ADAM = 2-[2-(dimethylaminomethylphenylthio)]-5-iodophenylamine; CFT = 2β-carbomethoxy-3β-(4-[^{18}F]-fluorophenyl)tropane; β-CIT = 2β-carbomethoxy-3β-(4-iodophenyl)-tropane; DASB = 3-amino-4-(2-dimethylaminomethylphenylsulfanyl)benzonitrile; ECD = ethyl cysteinate dimer; F-A-85380 = fluoro-3-2(S)-azetidinylmethoxy pyridine; FP-CIT = N-(3-fluoropropyl)-2ss-carbomethoxy-3ss-(4-iodophenyl)nortropane; FP-TZTP = fluoropropyl-thio-thiadiazo-tetrahydro-methylpyridine; HMPAO = d,l-hexamethylpropylene amine oxime; 5-IA-85380 = 5-iodo-3-2(S)-azetidinylmethoxy pyridine; IBZM = 3-iodo-6-methoxybenzamine; IDEX = iododexitimide; IMP = iodoamphetamine; IQNB = iodoquinuclidinyl benzilate; PET = positron emission tomography; SPECT = single-photon emission computed tomography.
[a]No longer available in the United States.

7–6). Although these tracers are most useful in research, clinical applications for some are under development.

PRACTICAL CONSIDERATIONS

Ordering the Examination

The nuclear medicine physician needs very clear clinical information on the imaging request form (not just "rule out pathology" or "new-onset mental status changes"). If a lesion is suspected in a particular location, this should be noted. The imaging physician and technical staff also need information on the patient's current condition (e.g., delirious, psychotic, easily agitated, paranoid). This may

eliminate difficulties with patient management during tracer administration or scanning.

Patient Preparation

The psychiatrist should always explain the procedure to the patient shortly beforehand, being mindful to mention the requirement for absolute immobility during the approximately 30 minutes of scanning. Nuclear cameras are not nearly as confining as magnetic resonance scanners are and very rarely cause claustrophobic reactions (Figure 7–17). Nonetheless, the scanning table is quite hard and can be uncomfortable for patients with back pain; pain

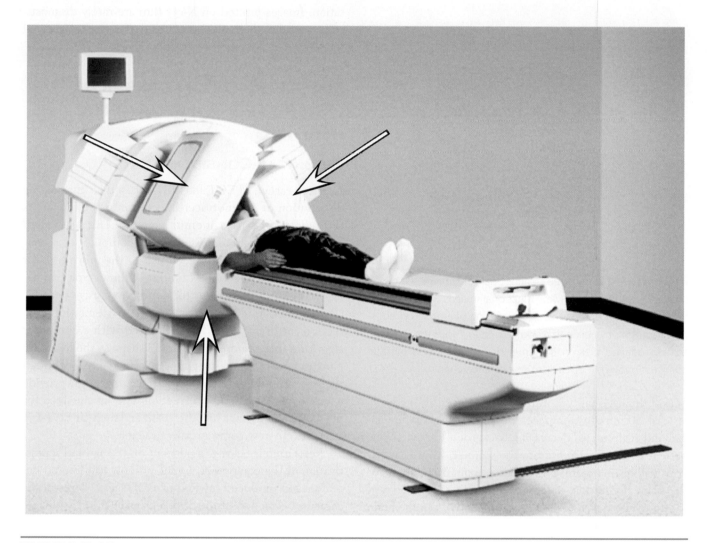

FIGURE 7–17.   Two of the three cameras of this multidetector single-photon emission computed tomography (SPECT) system are indicated by *arrows*. The cameras rotate around the patient's head during the imaging examination. Data are collected from multiple positions as the cameras rotate around the patient's head.

Source.   Pictures courtesy of Phillips Medical Systems.

medication may be worthwhile in some patients. If the psychiatrist suspects that the patient may become agitated or be unable to remain still for the length of the examination, then sedation may be necessary. Because of unknown effects on cerebral activity and blood flow, antianxiety medications and other sedative medications are best given after the tracer distribution in the brain has become fixed. This occurs approximately 5–10 minutes after injection for SPECT and 20–30 minutes after injection for PET. Such medications can be critical to achieving a successful scan in selected patients. A clinician may select a regimen that he or she is familiar and comfortable with. We have found that for patients with agitation and psychosis, a sedating antipsychotic with lorazepam 1–2 mg intramuscularly 30 minutes before scanning usually works well in a physically healthy nongeriatric adult. During

imaging, the head is generally held still with support from a head-holder attachment on the imaging table, sometimes with additional support from light taping.

In preparation for scanning, an intravenous line is inserted, and the patient is placed in a quiet and darkened room. Ten to 20 minutes later, a technologist enters the room quietly and injects the radioactive tracer. This procedure allows for decreased visual and auditory stimulation during tracer uptake. The patient typically remains in the room for 30–60 minutes, although the darkness and quiet are essential only during the tracer uptake period. For clinical SPECT, uptake occurs within 1–2 minutes of injection; for clinical PET, uptake requires 20–30 minutes. During the uptake period, the tracer distributes and is trapped in the tissue of interest. Theoretically, the patient could be imaged immediately following the uptake

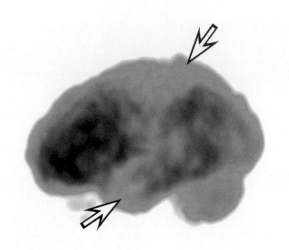

FIGURE 7–18.   Three-dimensional (3D) reconstructions provide another way to view functional images. The areas of highest flow are dark in this 3D rendering of a positron emission tomography cerebral blood flow scan. Note the large areas of reduced flow in the anterior temporal and parietal cortices (*arrows*), the result of severe anoxic injury.

period. Image quality is improved, however, if one waits at least 30 minutes for tracer washout from adjacent facial and scalp areas, decreasing background activity. The patient is then transported to the scanner, where the patient will lie on the imaging table for about 30 minutes for the scan. If clinically necessary, scanning can be delayed for up to about 4 hours, although the activity in the brain is gradually decreasing from radioactive decay, resulting in gradually worsening image quality.

Understanding the Scan

Cerebral blood flow and cerebral metabolism are high in gray matter where synapses and cell bodies are located. They are lower in white matter, composed of axons. Thus, tracer uptake is high in cellular areas, such as the thalami, basal ganglia, and cortex, and lower in white matter. Consequently, SPECT and PET are not good for evaluating white matter diseases.

The psychiatrist should review the images and radiology report with the nuclear medicine physician. It is important to remember that the radiographic view places the patient's right on the reader's left and the patient's left on the reader's right. After confirmation of patient identification, the psychiatrist should ask the nuclear medicine physician to point out normal anatomical markers and any pathology observed on the images. Note that PET and SPECT scans are always interpreted as digital images. Reasonable copies can be printed on photographic paper. However, paper reproductions are often quite suboptimal for image interpretation. Images printed on X-ray film are rarely diagnostically useful and should be avoided. Three-dimensional renderings are sometimes available (Figure 7–18).

SINGLE-PHOTON EMISSION COMPUTED TOMOGRAPHIC IMAGING

TECHNICAL CONSIDERATIONS

As noted earlier, SPECT, like PET, is based on imaging the distribution of a radiotracer injected into the blood. As the radiotracer decays, it emits a photon. This is detected by a gamma camera and used by the computer to reconstruct a tomographic image, similar to the procedure for standard CT (see section "Computed Tomographic Imaging" earlier in this chapter for a more extensive description of technique) (Warwick 2004). Attenuation correction for brain SPECT is estimated with a computer algorithm that assumes an ellipsoid shape of the head and constant water-density tissue attenuation. Although these assumptions are not entirely accurate, they provide a reasonable attenuation correction without the need for delivering X rays within the scanner (such SPECT-CT scanners are now commercially available).

Resolution is heavily dependent on the age and sophistication of the equipment. Older systems had limited detectors and produced lower-quality images. "Triple-head" cameras developed in the 1990s provide the best images because they acquire more counts and can be positioned very close to the patient's head. Unfortunately, the commercial market for SPECT cameras is dominated by cardiac and oncological applications, and triple-head cameras are no longer sold. Most modern SPECT cameras have a theoretical resolution of about 6–7 mm. In practice, the shoulders physically prevent the camera heads from being positioned close enough to the patient's head, reducing clinical resolution to about 1–1.3 cm (Van Heertum et al. 2004).

The two SPECT tracers approved for clinical use in the United States are [^{99m}Tc]-HMPAO (Ceretec; *d,l*-hexamethylpropylene amine oxime) and [^{99m}Tc]-ECD (Neurolite; ethyl cysteinate dimer). Both provide very comparable measures of cerebral blood flow (perfusion), with regional uptake roughly proportional to flow. Uptake occurs during the first 1–2 minutes after injection. After that, the tracer is "fixed" in the brain. These are lipophilic compounds that diffuse across the blood-brain barrier and into neurons and glia, where they are converted into hydrophilic compounds that cannot diffuse out of the cell. Abnormalities in intracellular esterase or glutathione metabolism, in neurons or glia, might lead to SPECT abnormalities indepen-

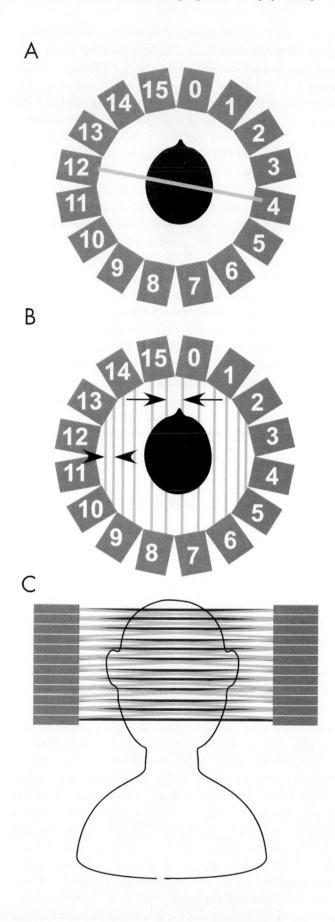

A

B

C

FIGURE 7–19. (A) A ring of detectors (*numbered blocks*) is used to acquire a positron emission tomography (PET) image. A 16-detector ring is illustrated. The detectors are arranged in pairs on opposite sides of the ring to allow simultaneous detection of the photon pair (annihilation coincidence detection). (B) The curved nature of the detector ring results in closer spacing of the lines of coincidence detection toward the periphery (*arrowheads*) compared with the center (*arrows*). Arc correction is applied before reconstruction to make spacing uniform in the image. (C) The number of image slices and the image resolution can be increased by combining detections from within a detector ring (*dark gray lines*, direct coincidences) with detections between adjacent detector rings (*light gray lines*, cross coincidences).

dent of blood flow changes. In fact, evidence suggests that most tracer uptake, at least for HMPAO, may be in glial cells rather than in neurons (Slosman et al. 2001). It must be remembered that the uptake of tracer does not have to be within neurons to be useful. Uptake is used as an indirect indicator of neuronal electrochemical activity. Even if the uptake is mainly in glia, it has been shown to clearly reflect local cerebral blood flow, which is tightly linked to neuronal activity (Magistretti and Pellerin 1996).

Although several differences between these two tracers have been described (Inoue et al. 2003), the two remain very comparable in terms of their clinical utility. A previously used perfusion tracer, $[^{123}I]$-IMP (iodoamphetamine), is no longer commercially available in the United States and is infrequently used elsewhere. SPECT tracers are commonly available for imaging the dopamine transporter (DAT) in Europe and Asia, but this technique has not been approved by the U.S. Food and Drug Administration (Warwick 2004).

SAFETY AND CONTRAINDICATIONS

The only contraindication to a nuclear medicine scan is pregnancy, and even this is only a relative indication. If the brain scan can be postponed until after delivery, a small radiation dose to the fetus can be avoided. Although very rarely necessary, the study could be performed in uncommon situations in which the scan result is critical. It is important to recognize that the tracers used in all diagnostic nuclear medicine examinations are 1,000 to 1 million times too low a concentration to have any pharmacological effects or allergenic side effects (other than placebo effects). They disappear by radioactive decay, so renal and hepatic function are irrelevant. The radiation dose to the patient as a result of a nuclear brain scan is comparable to that of a CT scan and is generally considered to be without long-term consequences, although some controversy over this issue has arisen (see discussion in subsection "Standard Two-Dimensional CT" earlier in this chapter).

POSITRON EMISSION TOMOGRAPHIC IMAGING

TECHNICAL CONSIDERATIONS

PET is based on imaging the distribution of a short-lived radioactive tracer (radiotracer) that has been introduced into the bloodstream (Cherry 2001; Fahey 2002; Paans et al. 2002; Turner and Jones 2003; Van Heertum et al. 2004). Several positron-emitting radionuclides are available for incorporation into tracers, but virtually all current clinical PET tracers use fluorine 18 (^{18}F). The most important PET tracer is [^{18}F]-fluorodeoxyglucose (FDG), which provides a map of glucose metabolism.

Positrons are released as the radiotracer decays. These travel a very short distance in tissue (about a millimeter on average for fluorine 18) before encountering an electron, and the two mutually annihilate. The mass of the two particles is converted into pure energy in the form of two high-energy photons. These travel away from each other in a straight line at the speed of light (line of response). Most of these photon pairs pass through the body and strike detectors on opposite sides of the scanner nearly simultaneously (Figure 7–19). The PET scanner recognizes when two photons have struck the ring simultaneously (annihilation coincidence detection) and estimates the site of origin of the photons as lying somewhere on a path between the two involved detectors. The object to be imaged (the head) is surrounded by several parallel rings containing thousands of these detector pairs. By combining the results of millions of such coincidence detection events, the scanner's computer can generate a high-resolution image of the distribution of radiotracer in the body, with areas of relatively high concentration appearing as "hot spots" in the image.

PET scanners contain retractable septa made of lead or tungsten between detector rings. These septa reduce detection of photons that have changed direction while in the body (such scattered photons exit the body at a location that causes the scanner to miscalculate their sites of origin). The septa allow imaging in one plane at a time, a two-dimensional acquisition. This mode is preferred on some scanner systems for whole-body imaging. The septa can be removed to yield a higher count rate. This is called three-dimensional acquisition and is much faster than two-dimensional acquisition because of the higher count rate. The increase in scattered photons striking the detector and the increase in random counts that also occur when the septa are removed can be reasonably well cor-rected with various software algorithms. Most centers prefer a three-dimensional acquisition for brain PET scanning. It allows a high-quality brain PET scan to be acquired in as little as 6–8 minutes. A comparable two-dimensional brain scan would take approximately 15–20 minutes. The theoretical limit for spatial resolution is about 2.5 mm (Turner and Jones 2003), whereas the resolution of clinical PET is on the order of 4–5 mm.

The only approved PET tracer for clinical use in the United States is [^{18}F]-FDG. It is taken up into cells similarly to glucose and undergoes metabolism to FDG-6-phosphate. It does not undergo further metabolism and is trapped within these cells, providing a measure of cerebral metabolic activity (rCMR glucose). Glucose uptake in PET images is likely to reside predominantly in glial cells, which convert glucose into lactate and provide the lactate to neurons as a key energy source for neurons (Magistretti and Pellerin 1996). It must be remembered that the uptake of tracer does not have to be within neurons: uptake is used as an indirect indicator of neuronal electrochemical activity. Even if the uptake is mainly in glia, it has been shown to clearly reflect local cerebral glucose metabolism, which is tightly linked to neuronal activity.

SAFETY AND CONTRAINDICATIONS

The safety considerations and contraindications are the same as for SPECT (see prior section).

CLINICAL APPLICATIONS

SPECT VERSUS PET

Nuclear brain imaging is coming into increasing use for the clinical evaluation and case formulation of psychiatric patients. These techniques can contribute to differential diagnosis, assist treatment planning, and provide information for prognostic decisions. PET has the advantages of higher spatial resolution and true attenuation correction (nearly eliminating attenuation artifacts). SPECT has the advantages of being more widely available, less expensive (approximately $1,200 for SPECT vs. approximately $1,800 for PET), and reimbursable for most conditions. Reimbursement for brain PET in the United States is currently limited to distinguishing frontotemporal dementia from Alzheimer's disease, doing presurgical evaluation of intractable epilepsy (seizure focus localization), and distinguishing radiation necrosis from recurrent brain tumors. SPECT imaging is considered a standard clinical investigative tool for neuropsychiatric evaluation. However, PET scanners are rapidly becoming more common-place, and reimbursement for other indications is likely to

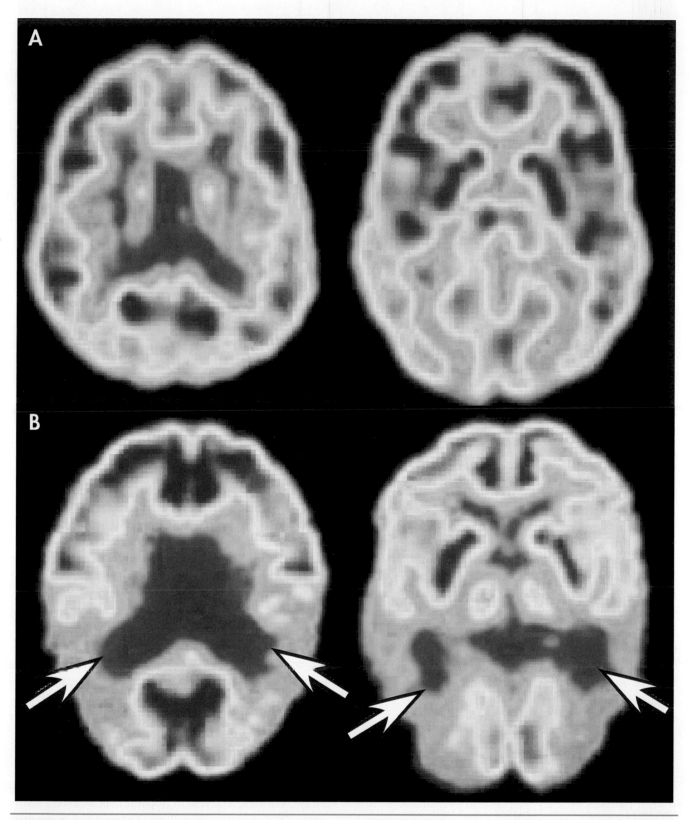

FIGURE 7–20. Positron emission tomographic imaging of cerebral metabolism is quite useful in diagnosis of Alzheimer's disease. (*A*) In individuals without Alzheimer's disease, uptake of [^{18}F]-fluorodeoxyglucose (FDG) is high (*orange-red*) throughout the cerebral cortex. (*B*) Uptake is reduced (*blue*) regionally, usually symmetrically (*arrows*), in patients with Alzheimer's disease.

Source. Pictures courtesy of Siemens Medical.

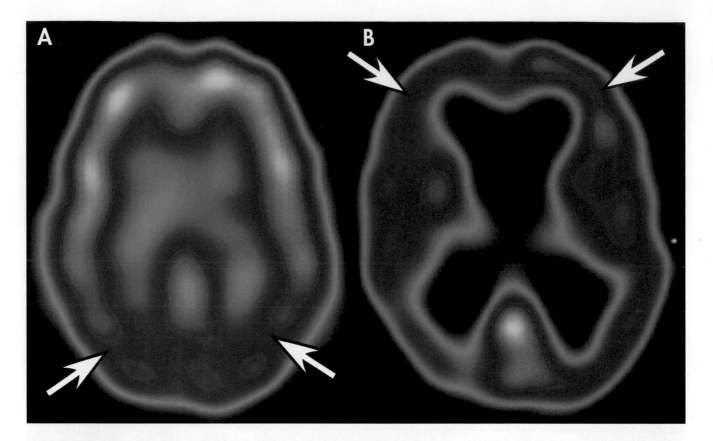

FIGURE 7–21.   Regional cerebral blood flow (rCBF) in Alzheimer's disease. (A) As imaged here with single-photon emission computed tomography, rCBF is decreased in posterior temporoparietal cortex in early Alzheimer's disease (*arrows*). (B) As the disease progresses, frontal lobe involvement is common (*arrows*).

occur in the near future. The old requirement for an on-site cyclotron has been obviated by the establishment of numerous commercial cyclotrons throughout the United States, many of which can deliver an ^{18}F tracer (110-minute half-life) great distances by airplane. Virtually any hospital in the United States with a PET scanner can have [^{18}F]-FDG delivered to it relatively inexpensively. Tracers that use carbon 11 (20-minute half-life), oxygen 15 (2-minute half-life), or nitrogen 13 (10-minute half-life) require an on-site cyclotron facility. Common nuclear medicine findings in selected clinical conditions are discussed in the following subsections.

PRIMARY DEMENTIAS

Dementia is the most common clinical reason for nuclear brain imaging. Scanning is particularly helpful in the evaluation of patients with atypical clinical presentations. It is expected to play a more significant role as better treatment options become available for different etiologies. For Alzheimer's disease, bilateral, symmetrical posterior temporoparietal decreased perfusion or metabolism is the classic pattern (Figure 7–20B and Figure 7–21A). However, this is seen in

approximately one-third of the patients with Alzheimer's disease. Frequently, the abnormalities are asymmetrical and may initially involve only temporal or parietal cortex. As the disease progresses, the frontal (and occasionally occipital) lobes become involved, with decreased perfusion (Figure 7–21B). Uptake in the subcortical structures, primary visual cortex, and primary sensorimotor cortex is usually preserved even in late-stage disease. The defects are always diffuse, over a large area of cortex, and easily recognizable as neurodegenerative in origin, although not necessarily specific to Alzheimer's disease.

Clinical SPECT and PET findings in dementia with Lewy bodies (DLB) overlap those of Alzheimer's disease, although the abnormalities are more likely to be asymmetrical and to involve the occipital cortex (Figure 7–22). DAT imaging has shown more promise in distinguishing the two entities. The loss of dopamine neurons is significant in DLB, resulting in striking abnormalities in the striatum in these patients compared with those who have Alzheimer's disease (Figure 7–23) (Walker et al. 2002).

SPECT or PET scanning shows reduced perfusion of the frontal and/or anterior temporal cortex (usually bilat-

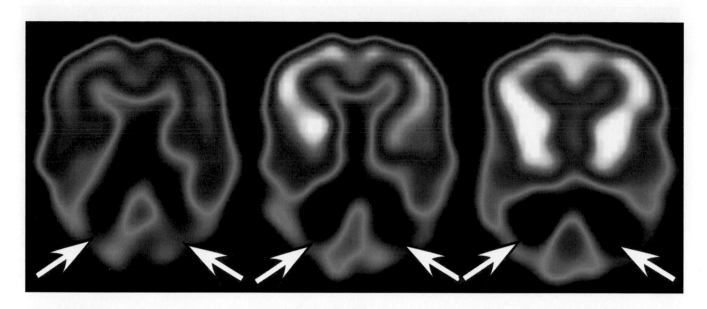

FIGURE 7–22. A common finding in dementia with Lewy bodies is decreased perfusion in occipital cortex *(arrows)*, here imaged with single-photon emission computed tomography.

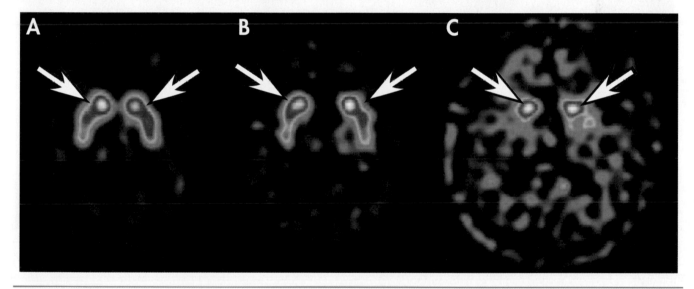

FIGURE 7–23. The dopamine transporter (DAT) is a presynaptic receptor that ferries dopamine back into the presynaptic terminal. Imaging DAT provides a way to assess the integrity of the dopaminergic nigrostriatal pathway. In this example, single-photon emission computed tomographic imaging with the radiotracer [^{123}I]-2β-carbomethoxy-3β-(4-iodophenyl)-N-(3-fluoro-propyl) nortropane (FP-CIT) has been used. Note that activity is high *(yellow-orange)* throughout the striatum in (A) nonimpaired individuals and in (B) patients with Alzheimer's disease. (C) It is greatly reduced in dementia with Lewy bodies.

Source. Reprinted from Walker Z, Costa DC, Walker RW, et al.: "Differentiation of Dementia With Lewy Bodies From Alzheimer's Disease Using a Dopaminergic Presynaptic Ligand." *Journal of Neurology, Neurosurgery, and Psychiatry* 73:134–140, 2002. Used with permission.

erally) in frontotemporal dementia (e.g., Pick's disease), which is usually readily distinguished from Alzheimer's disease and DLB (Figure 7–24). Parkinson's patients often develop dementia that may be etiologically distinct from DLB, but the SPECT and PET appearance has not been well characterized and likely overlaps significantly with both Alzheimer's disease and DLB. Clinical SPECT and PET imaging in Creutzfeldt-Jakob disease identifies large areas of severely reduced perfusion (Figure 7–25). These are usually symmetrical. This appearance overlaps

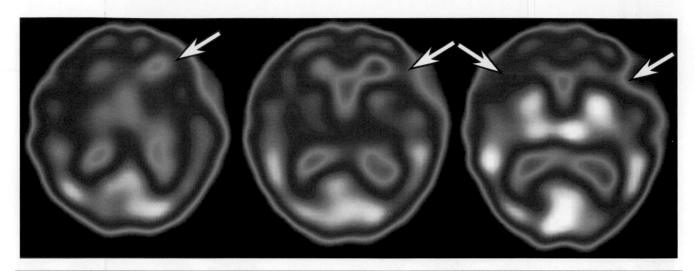

FIGURE 7–24. A common finding in frontotemporal dementia (e.g., Pick's disease) is decreased perfusion in frontal and temporal cortex (*arrows*), here imaged with single-photon emission computed tomography.

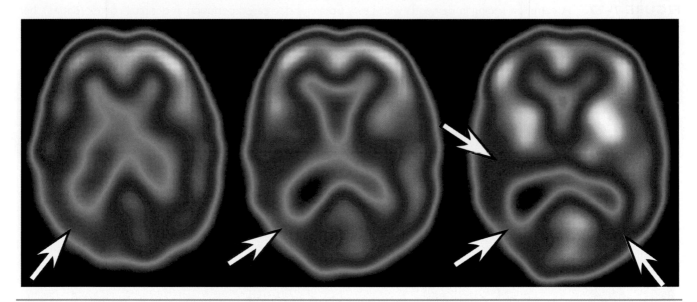

FIGURE 7–25. A common finding in Creutzfeldt-Jakob disease is large asymmetrical areas of decreased perfusion in cortex (*arrows*), here imaged with single-photon emission computed tomography.

with Alzheimer's disease and DLB, so clinical correlation is needed. Sequential SPECT and PET scans (performed about 2 months apart) often show dramatic progression (Taber et al. 2002a). In Huntington's disease, SPECT and PET imaging shows characteristic reduced perfusion to the basal ganglia, especially the head of the caudate, often early in the course of the illness (Figure 7–26). Nuclear imaging is quite sensitive and reasonably specific but is rarely used for diagnosis (diagnosis is made very accurately by sequence analysis of the Huntington's disease gene). It may be useful in predicting progression of disease (Hurley et al. 1999a). As dementia progresses, many patients develop large regions of reduced cortical perfu-

sion or metabolism on SPECT and PET in a pattern similar to that for other neurodegenerative diseases.

EPILEPSY

SPECT and PET are used along with MRI and EEG in patients with medically refractory seizures to determine the optimum site for stereotaxic placement of depth electrodes. The implanted electrodes, in turn, usually provide the definitive localization of the seizure focus and the boundaries of the tissue to be surgically resected. Nuclear medicine examinations are obtained either in the presence of seizure activity (ictal examination, blood flow increased

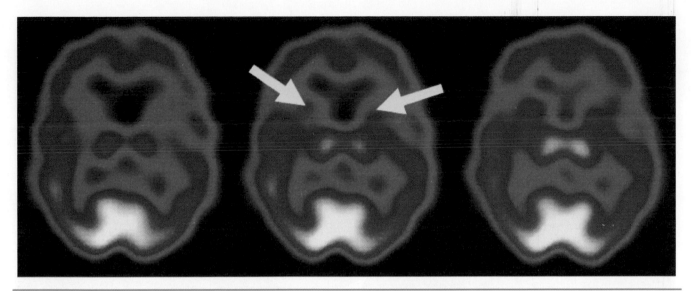

FIGURE 7–26. A characteristic finding early in Huntington's disease is decreased perfusion in the basal ganglia, particularly caudate (*arrows*), here imaged with single-photon emission computed tomography.

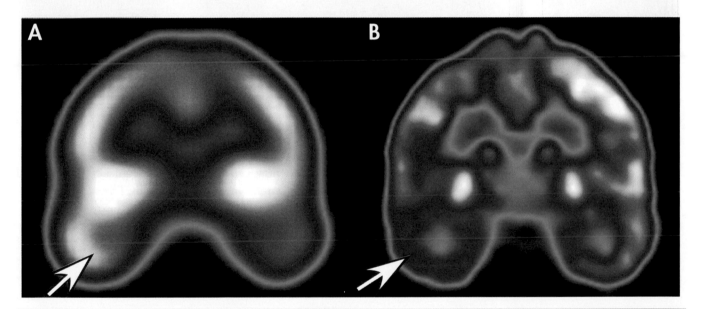

FIGURE 7–27. Nuclear medicine imaging is useful for visualizing the area of an epileptic focus. (A) Scans obtained during a seizure (ictal scan) will show increased perfusion or metabolism, as illustrated here with a coronal single-photon emission computed tomographic image of cerebral blood flow (*arrow*). (B) Scans obtained in the absence of seizure will show decreased perfusion or metabolism, as illustrated here with a coronal positron emission tomographic image of cerebral metabolism (*arrow*).

in the focus) or in the absence of seizure activity (interictal examination, blood flow decreased in the focus) (Figure 7–27). Ictal examinations can only be performed with SPECT because it has rapid tracer uptake (seizures tend to last only a few minutes). This provides an accurate picture of cerebral blood flow as it was during the seizure. Ictal imaging is the better method but requires that the tracer be injected at the beginning of a seizure, less than 1 minute after onset. This necessitates that the patient be admitted to a surveillance room with EEG and videotape monitoring. The tracer is kept in a syringe attached to the patient's intravenous line. When EEG confirms onset of a seizure, tracer is immediately injected. Most centers now perform both ictal and interictal studies on every patient, looking for regions that are hot on the ictal scan but normal or cold on the interictal scan. Sensitivity and accuracy of emission tomographic imaging have been reported to be approximately 80% (Henry and Van Heertum 2003).

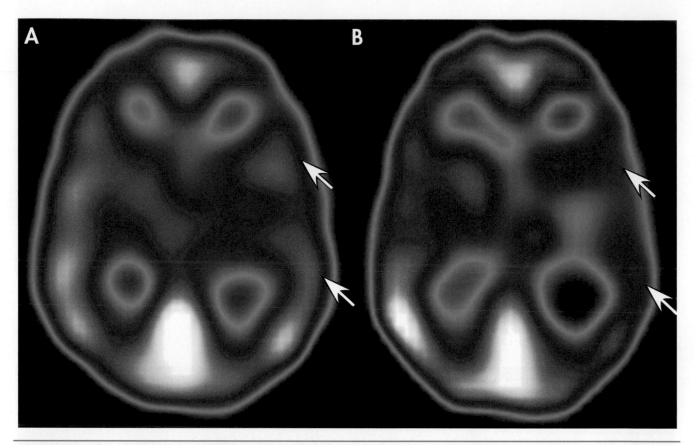

FIGURE 7–28.   Areas that are compromised but still functional in acute stroke can be identified by comparing (A) resting single-photon emission computed tomography cerebral blood flow images with (B) those obtained following administration of acetazolamide. Blood flow will not increase in areas in which arterioles were already fully dilated at baseline (*arrows*).

However, most studies include large numbers of patients with seizure foci easily determined from structural lesions on MRI or by EEG. In practice, nuclear imaging is needed primarily in patients with normal MRI results and non-localizing or equivocal EEG findings. Accuracy of SPECT and PET in this subset of patients is likely much lower, although fewer data are available.

VASCULAR DISEASE

Although multi-infarct dementia is commonly diagnosed by structural imaging, the pattern of SPECT and PET abnormalities is often quite distinctive, with multiple moderate-sized perfusion defects that have well-defined boundaries. Small vessel disease (e.g., Binswanger's disease) is not associated with a specific SPECT or PET pattern, although basal ganglia and frontal cortex lesions often have been reported (Hurley et al. 2000b). Areas of cerebral infarction are easily identified on clinical SPECT, but it is rarely clinically useful in this regard. In acute stroke, the essential information that is needed from neuroimaging is whether the stroke is hemorrhagic prior to initiating throm-

bolytic therapy. CT scanning is much quicker to obtain and is quite accurate in this regard. SPECT is superior to CT and MRI in predicting outcome of acute stroke and defining the size of viable but at-risk tissue but not sufficiently so to warrant routine clinical use (Barthel et al. 2001; Guadagno et al. 2003). Areas of compromised vascular reserve (partially occluded vessels), which often appear normal on a resting SPECT scan, can be visualized on a SPECT scan performed following intravenous injection of acetazolamide. Acetazolamide raises blood carbon dioxide levels, causing normal arterioles to dilate. Arterioles distal to an arterial stenosis or obstruction are already fully dilated as a physiological compensatory mechanism and cannot dilate further in response to acetazolamide (Figure 7–28). Brain regions supplied by such arterioles thus appear relatively hypoperfused, compared with normal tissue, on a postacetazolamide SPECT perfusion scan indicating decreased vascular reserve. Such findings are thought to predict impending ischemic events that may warrant therapeutic intervention (e.g., carotid endarterectomy), although well-controlled studies with long-term clinical follow-up are not available (Marti-Fabregas et al. 2001).

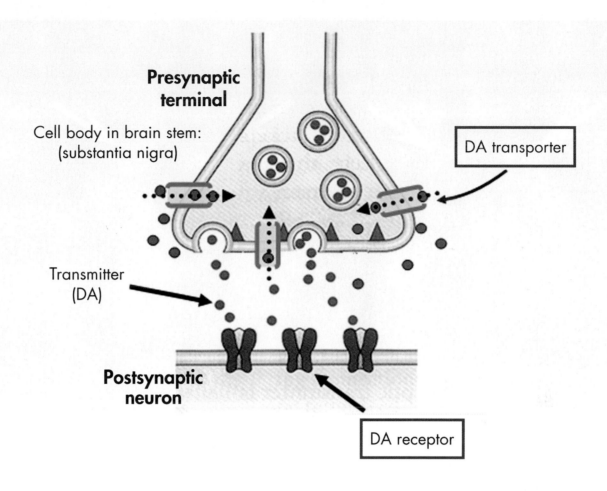

Presynaptic terminal

Cell body in brain stem: (substantia nigra)

DA transporter

Transmitter (DA)

Postsynaptic neuron

DA receptor

FIGURE 7–29. This schematic diagram of a dopamine (DA) synapse in the striatum illustrates the function of presynaptic DA transporters (DATs). DAT carries DA back into the presynaptic terminal. Here it is immediately degraded (by monoamine oxidase) into 3,4-dihydroxyphenylacetic acid (DOPAC) prior to recycling.

TRAUMATIC BRAIN INJURY

Many studies have reported that SPECT is more sensitive than CT or MRI for traumatic brain injury. SPECT often shows abnormal findings (areas of reduced perfusion) in symptomatic patients even when structural imaging shows negative results (Anderson et al. 2005). It must always be borne in mind, however, that many nonimpaired subjects have some limited areas of mildly reduced perfusion. Patient motion during imaging also can produce abnormalities. False-positive studies are an important concern because almost any abnormality, even relatively small or mild ones, would have to be called positive in the scenario of traumatic brain injury. Perhaps the most useful result at this time is that a few studies have indicated that a negative (normal) brain SPECT result after mild traumatic brain injury predicts an excellent long-term neurological outcome (Anderson et al. 2005; Bonne et al. 2003).

SPECT AND PET: IMAGING NEUROTRANSMITTER SYSTEMS

Radioligands that bind to neurotransmitter receptors have been developed to image multiple neurotransmitter systems. The same principles of radioligand development for SPECT and PET imaging can be applied to almost any type of synapse in the brain (Figure 7–29). Examples of available radioligands include dopamine and serotonin receptors and transporters, acetylcholine (muscarinic and nicotinic) receptors, histamine receptors, $GABA_A$ receptors, adenosine receptors, and opiate receptors (see Table 7–6). SPECT and PET imaging of neurotransmitter systems has shown promise for clinical applications. In particular, radioligands for the dopamine system have been very widely studied and are already in clinical use in Europe and Asia.

DATs are located on presynaptic terminals (see Figure 7–29). They serve to transport dopamine from the synaptic

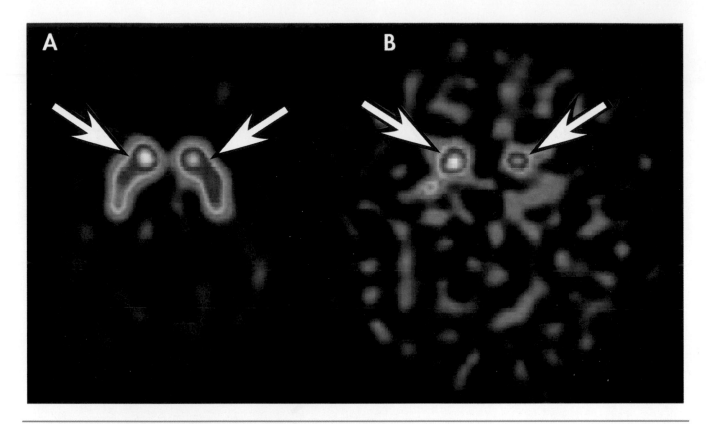

FIGURE 7–30. The primary clinical use of dopamine transporter (DAT) imaging is in the diagnostic evaluation of early Parkinson's disease. In this example, single-photon emission computed tomographic imaging with the radiotracer [^{123}I]-2β-carbomethoxy-3β-(4-iodophenyl)-*N*-(3-fluoropropyl) nortropane (FP-CIT) has been performed. (*A*) Note that activity is high (*yellow-orange*) throughout the striatum in nonimpaired individuals (*arrows*). (*B*) Activity is greatly reduced in the patient with Parkinson's disease (*arrows*).

Source.   Reprinted from Walker Z, Costa DC, Walker RW, et al.: "Differentiation of Dementia With Lewy Bodies From Alzheimer's Disease Using a Dopaminergic Presynaptic Ligand." *Journal of Neurology, Neurosurgery, and Psychiatry* 73:134–140, 2002. Used with permission.

space back into the terminal. This halts the action of the transmitter (thereby preparing the synapse for the next electrochemical message) and recycles it. Many ligands have been developed that bind to DATs. All are analogues of cocaine. Cocaine's mechanism of action is to bind to and inhibit the closely related transporters for dopamine, norepinephrine, and serotonin. Molecules structurally similar to cocaine have been developed for imaging that are more specific for the DAT. Activity on SPECT DAT scans is mainly in the striatum, consistent with the known high density of dopamine synapses in this region (see Figure 7–23). SPECT yields a good semiquantitative estimate of DAT density. The primary clinical use of SPECT DAT imaging is in the diagnostic evaluation of early Parkinson's disease, for which it has been shown in repeated studies to be quite sensitive and specific (Figure 7–30) (Benamer et al. 2003; Leenders 2003). DAT SPECT is already in routine clinical use in Europe and Asia for this purpose. A normal DAT SPECT result in a patient with early parkinsonian symptoms suggests that classic Parkinson's disease is not present. Possible alter-

native diagnoses include vascular Parkinson's disease, essential tremor, drug-induced parkinsonism, and somatization disorder. DAT SPECT sometimes has positive results in asymptomatic siblings who go on to develop Parkinson's disease. Imaging of the postsynaptic D$_2$ receptor, another approach to assessing the dopaminergic system, is normal in Parkinson's disease and reduced in multiple system atrophy (Kim et al. 2002; Knudsen et al. 2004). This is an emerging application in Europe. PET imaging of [^{18}F]-6-fluoro-L-dopa (F-DOPA) also may be useful (Figure 7–31).

CONCLUSION: SPECT AND PET IN NEUROPSYCHIATRY

In summary, perfusion SPECT and glucose metabolism PET find their primary use in the diagnostic workup of patients with dementia. Both types of imaging produce reasonably high diagnostic accuracy in distinguishing Alzheimer's disease from frontotemporal dementia (currently

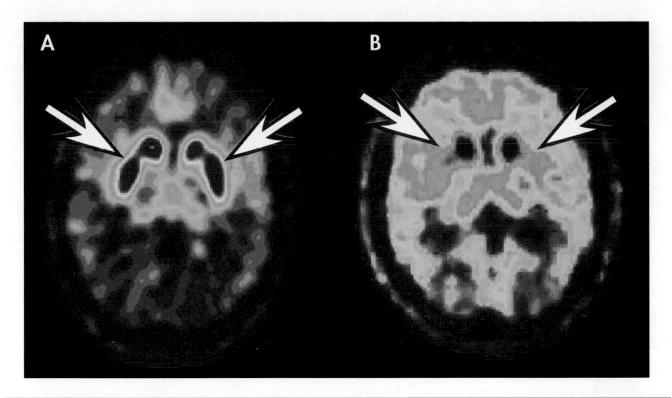

FIGURE 7–31. Positron emission tomography can be used to image nigrostriatal dopaminergic function. In Following cerebral uptake, [^{18}F]-6-fluoro-L-dopa (F-DOPA) is converted to [^{18}F]-fluorodopamine by dopamine decarboxylase. Compared with (A) individuals without Parkinson's disease, (B) patients with Parkinson's disease have reduced uptake in the basal ganglia (*arrows*).

Source. Pictures courtesy of Siemens Medical.

the only reimbursable indication for a brain PET in dementia) and in distinguishing neurodegenerative disease from other causes of dementia and from pseudodementia. PET is generally superior to SPECT because of higher resolution and better attenuation correction. It is more expensive and less widely available than SPECT, but both of these issues are rapidly improving. Both modalities have a clearly defined role in the preoperative evaluation of patients with medically refractory epilepsy, with ictal perfusion SPECT showing the best results. Both tests are sensitive and reasonably specific for vascular disease, but a specific clinical role has yet to be defined. Acetazolamide stress perfusion SPECT shows promise for determining clinical significance of borderline vascular obstructions and for selecting patients who need intervention. Clinical benefit for these potential indications, however, has yet to be proven. Both modalities are very sensitive in detecting neuronal injury in patients with mild traumatic brain injuries. However, false-positive scans are a concern, and the clinical significance of positive scans in patients with brain trauma has yet to be fully determined. The routine clinical application of nuclear imaging to patients with mood disorders, attention-deficit/hyperactivity disorder, schizophrenia, obsessive-compulsive disorder, and other psychiatric disorders

has been disappointing, despite numerous abnormalities reported in research studies. Perhaps more promising in these disorders is the use of neurotransmitter SPECT and PET. Such studies, particularly DAT SPECT, have already shown excellent accuracy and clinical utility in patients with movement disorders, especially Parkinson's disease and related disorders. Imaging of receptors and transporters may eventually play an important role in the diagnosis and management of many neuropsychiatric illnesses.

XENON-ENHANCED COMPUTED TOMOGRAPHY (XE/CT)

Xe/CT uses stable xenon gas, which is radiodense, as a contrast agent. Xenon gas is lipid soluble, so once it dissolves into blood, it enters the brain. After obtaining baseline standard CT images, the patient inhales a mixture of xenon (26%–33%) and oxygen (Figure 7–32). A second set of images is then collected in which the distribution of the xenon shows regional blood flow, allowing areas of abnormality to be identified (Latchaw 2004). At this range of concentration, transient side effects of xenon inhalation include euphoria, dysphoria, sedation, nausea, and apnea (reversible with instructions to breathe). These side effects can be problematic in psychiatric patients. Advantages of Xe/CT over other methods of imaging blood flow include lack of radiotracer exposure, good image resolution, and direct anatomical correlation. It is inexpensive, can be repeated frequently (e.g., after a drug challenge), and adds no more than a few minutes to the total examination time. In February 2001, the use of xenon as an X-ray contrast agent was temporarily halted by the U.S. Food and Drug Administration, pending completion of required studies for labeling purposes. These studies are currently under way. Xe/CT proved clinically useful for cerebrovascular accidents, bleeds, aneurysms, and evaluation of blood flow after traumatic brain injury (Figure 7–33) (Kilpatrick et al. 2001; Kushi et al. 1999; Latchaw 2004; Taber et al. 1999; von Oettingen et al. 2002).

FUNCTIONAL MAGNETIC RESONANCE IMAGING

fMRI is based on the modulation of image intensity by the oxygenation state of blood. Deoxygenated hemoglobin (deoxyhemoglobin) is highly paramagnetic. It distorts the local magnetic field in its immediate vicinity. This causes a loss of magnetic resonance signal, particularly on gradient echo and other susceptibility-weighted pulse sequences. Thus, it is a natural magnetic resonance contrast agent. Image intensity is dependent on the local balance between oxygenated and deoxygenated hemoglobin. This is the origin of the acronym BOLD (blood oxygen level dependent) for the fMRI technique (Taber et al. 2003; Turner and Jones 2003).

An area of brain suddenly becomes more active when it is participating in a cognitive task. The increase in local blood flow is larger than is required to meet the activity-related increase in oxygen consumption. As a result, the venous blood becomes slightly *more* oxygenated. This decrease in local deoxyhemoglobin concentration causes a slight (1%–5%) increase in signal intensity in the activated area of brain on the magnetic resonance image. The change is too small to see by eye. It is measured by comparing signal intensity under a baseline (resting or control) condition with the signal intensity under an activated condition. Unlike PET, SPECT, or Xe/CT, all fMRI measures depend on comparison of two conditions (e.g., baseline and activated).

Activations will be seen in many areas when a subject performs a task in a scanner. Defining and creating a baseline state for comparison can be a considerable challenge. Ideally, the subject is scanned under two conditions that differ only in the cognitive function under study. For example, to identify the brain regions involved in verbal

short-term memory, the subject might be scanned while viewing words projected onto a screen and then clicking with a mouse on those recently seen (test scan). For comparison, the same subject might be scanned while viewing words and clicking on all words beginning with a particular letter (control scan). When the areas of activity on the control scan are subtracted from the areas of activity on the test scan, the remaining areas of activation should primarily reflect verbal short-term memory. However, if a brain area of interest is abnormally active under the baseline (control) condition, further activation may not be measurable, resulting in an apparent absence of activation when the image sets are analyzed.

A problem with the most commonly used fMRI methods is presence of susceptibility-related artifacts in areas of magnetic field inhomogeneity, such as the interfaces between brain, bone, and air. Thus, regions of importance to neuropsychiatry adjacent to bone, such as the orbitofrontal cortex and the inferior temporal region, may be difficult to assess. It is also important to differentiate areas of increased signal within activated tissue itself from increased signal in the veins that drain the activated area. Motion artifacts can also be a problem. Any movement (minor head movement, respiration, speech related) can create spurious areas of activation and mask areas of true activation. Head restraints and post processing are both important in this regard (Bizzi et al. 1993; Desmond and Annabel Chen 2002; Matthews and Jezzard 2004; Taber et al. 2003; Turner and Jones 2003).

fMRI has several advantages over other methods of imaging brain activity. Most important, it is totally noninvasive and requires no ionizing radiation or radiopharmaceuticals. Minimal risk makes it appropriate for use in both children and adults and for use in longitudinal studies requiring multiple scanning sessions for each subject. High-resolution structural images are acquired in the same session, providing much better localization of areas of interest than is possible with PET or SPECT. In addition, most clinical MRI scanners can be modified without great expense to enable fMRI. However, fMRI is neither simple nor easy to implement and analyze, which may limit its clinical usefulness. At present, it should be considered a research technique.

The most common application of fMRI is in the field of cognitive neuroscience with psychiatrically healthy volunteers. However, interest in using fMRI to assess patients with neurological and/or neuropsychiatric disorders is increasing. Evaluation of brain function, recovery, and reorganization (adaptive plasticity, compensatory recruitment) after stroke is a promising potential area for its use (Cao et al. 1998; Marshall et al. 2000; Matthews and Jezzard 2004; Pineiro et al. 2002). It also may be of value prior to surgical brain resection in patients with epilepsy

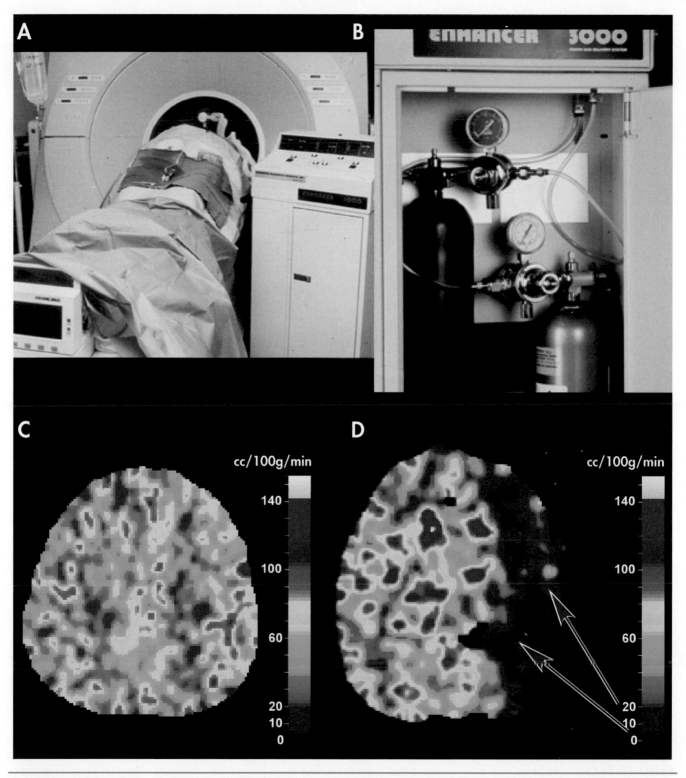

FIGURE 7–32. (A) A standard computed tomography (CT) scanner is used for xenon-enhanced computed tomographic (Xe/CT) imaging of cerebral blood flow. (B) Accessory equipment is used to blend xenon gas (28%) with oxygen (40%) for the patient to breathe. The gas enters the blood and acts as a contrast agent. Xe/CT provides quantitative images of cerebral blood flow. (C) In a healthy individual, cerebral blood flow is high (*yellow-red*) throughout cerebral cortex. Following stroke (D), Xe/CT allows differentiation of areas of irreversible ischemia (flow<8 cc/100 g/min=core, *purple arrow*) from areas in which ischemia is still reversible (flow between 8 and 20 cc/100 g/min=penumbra, *blue arrow*).

Source. Pictures courtesy of Diversified Diagnostic Products, Inc.

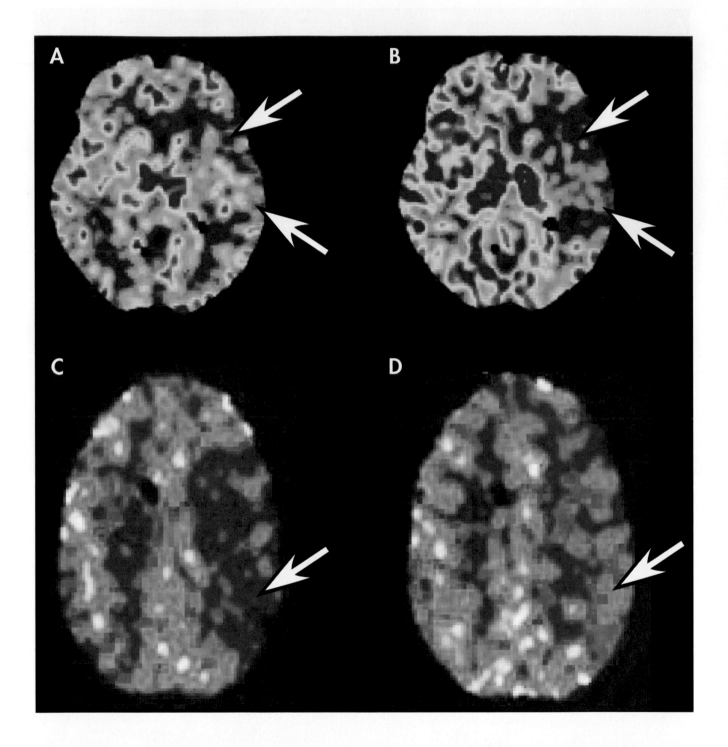

FIGURE 7–33. (A) Areas at risk for ischemic injury are not always obvious on baseline xenon-enhanced computed tomographic (Xe/CT) images (arrows). (B) Administration of an agent that briefly increases global cerebral blood flow, such as acetazolamide, provides a way to identify areas with impaired capacity (arrows). Xe/CT also provides a way to monitor the effectiveness of therapy intended to improve cerebral blood flow in areas of ischemia. (C) In this case, an initial administration of dopamine increased the patient's blood pressure (to 170/110 mm Hg) but did not reverse the perfusion deficit (arrow). (D) Raising the blood pressure further (to 220/125 mm Hg) restored blood flow to the area (arrow).

Source. Pictures courtesy of Diversified Diagnostic Products, Inc.

or brain tumors for definition of the exact boundaries of the primary motor areas and for lateralization of language function. The language area is now identified with the Wada test. The Wada test is both invasive and expensive, so this will be an important clinical application for fMRI if validation studies support its use (Desmond and Annabel Chen 2002; Matthews and Jezzard 2004). Preliminary studies found amygdala hyperactivity in depression, which normalized with antidepressant treatment (Sheline et al. 2001). Abnormalities in prefrontal and parietal cortex activity while performing cognitive tasks have been reported in patients with schizophrenia (Holmes et al. 2005; Menon et al. 2001). Studies also have been done in substance abuse populations (Garavan et al. 2000). Identification of early (perhaps even preclinical) disease may be possible, as indicated by differences in activation to a memory task in patients who later developed Alzheimer's disease and abnormalities of activation during a semantic categorization task in asymptomatic apolipoprotein ε4 carriers (who are genetically at risk to develop Alzheimer's disease) (Bookheimer et al. 2000; Lind et al. 2006). Evaluation of the effects of genetic polymorphisms on information processing and emotional function as measured by fMRI (imaging genomics) is of increasing interest (Hariri et al. 2002). However, development of standardized protocols and comparison groups will be critical for clinical use (Desmond and Annabel Chen 2002).

It is important to note that all of the previously mentioned studies averaged data from multiple patients and compared these data with averaged data from control subjects to find general differences in brain activity. These are all research experiments designed to probe the pathophysiology of a disease. They do not yet provide a useful diagnostic or prognostic test for an individual clinical patient. Data from individual subjects, however, are increasingly appearing in fMRI reports. With carefully designed and analyzed studies, it is quite possible that fMRI will eventually be applied clinically in specialized centers. As mentioned previously, implementation and analysis of fMRI require considerable expertise. This technique is unlikely to become a routine hospital procedure in the near future.

MAGNETIC RESONANCE SPECTROSCOPY

MRS is a technique used to measure brain metabolites. This measurement is commonly displayed as a spectrum rather than an image. MRS uses the same scanners and magnets as clinical MRI but requires specialized hardware and software. The most commonly used method is proton (^{1}H) MRS, which provides a measure of several substances. Primary markers of importance include N-acetylaspartate (NAA; located primarily in neurons, a marker for neuron and axon viability), choline (principally phosphatidyl choline, a membrane constituent), and creatine (used as an internal standard because its level is usually stable). An additional peak may be present from lactate (metabolite associated with inflammation or neuronal mitochondrial dysfunction and related to activated anaerobic glycolytic metabolism). If a short echo-time acquisition is used, it is possible to observe myo-inositol (a putative glial marker). The absolute amount of signal in each spectral peak is highly dependent on the acquisition parameters, so for comparison purposes, the signals of interest (NAA, choline) are commonly expressed relative to creatine. It is also possible to measure absolute metabolite concentrations, but the acquisition is more complex. The choline/creatine peak reflects membrane metabolism and has been found to be elevated during both degradation (demyelination) and rapid synthesis. The NAA/creatine peak reflects neuronal and axonal density.

MRS is a useful research technique for neuropsychiatry and is beginning to enter the clinical realm. It has been used to study carbon monoxide poisoning and the resultant white matter degeneration (Sakamoto et al. 1998; Sohn et al. 2000). Some interesting clinical applications have been published. In combination with diffusion-weighted MRI, proton MRS can be used to better identify abscesses in postinfectious acute cerebellar ataxias (Ramandeep et al. 2005). It also may identify areas of irreversible encephalopathy (Murata et al. 2001).

MAGNETOENCEPHALOGRAPHIC IMAGING

MEG involves noninvasive measurement of the magnetic signal generated by the brain's neuroelectric activity. It offers an attractive alternative to EEG because these magnetic fields are only minimally altered by the different electrical conductivities of the brain, CSF, skull, and scalp. A cognitive task is used to stimulate neuronal activity, creating localized neuromagnetic fields that are recorded by sensors. These data are used to calculate the temporal and spatial patterns of the neuronal activation. An additional advantage is that the activities of right and left cortical areas are easily distinguished. Furthermore, MEG data can be integrated with MRI data to generate magnetic source localization images showing exactly the brain regions involved. Currently, this is primarily a research technique (Hurley et al. 2000a; Parra et al. 2004; Wheless et al. 2004).

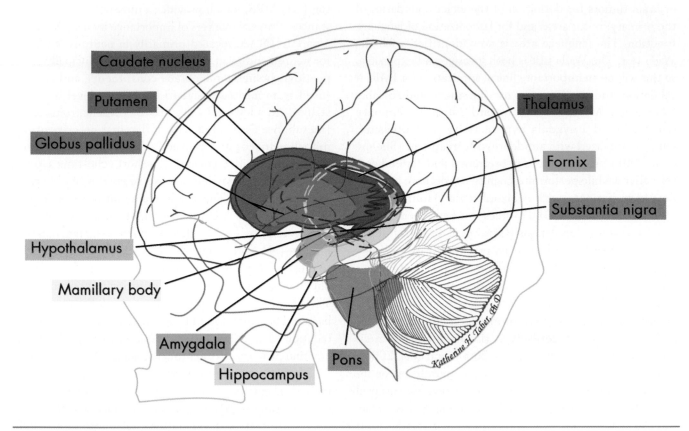

FIGURE 7–34.   This cartoon of a lateral view of the brain and skull shows the approximate positions and configurations of the major subcortical structures. The colors assigned in this figure are used in the axial atlas (Figures 7–35 through 7–41) and sagittal atlas (Figures 7–42 and 7–43) to facilitate structure identification.

NORMAL IMAGING ANATOMY

It is essential for the practicing psychiatrist to have a basic understanding of the cortical and subcortical anatomy involved in thought, memory, and emotion if he or she is to use information gathered from imaging. This includes sufficient knowledge to identify these structures on neuroimaging in the various planes of section. In addition, the psychiatrist must have the ability to identify clinical scenarios that warrant imaging investigation for lesions (e.g., traumatic brain injury, stroke, poison and toxin exposure).

In this section, we present an introductory overview of the functional neuroanatomy of executive function, memory, and emotion, as well as clinical examples and references for further reading. An illustration of the key subcortical structures is given in Figure 7–34. These structures are color-coded within the axial imaging atlas to promote understanding (Figures 7–35 through 7–41). It is important to realize that in many cases, lesions within these structures are best viewed in the coronal and sagittal planes of section—thus, MRI is often preferable to CT (see Figures 7–42 and 7–43 for the sagittal atlas). In addi-

tion, both T2-weighted sagittal and FLAIR sequences may provide details of lesions not seen on other sequences. However, the attending physician may need to specifically request these pulse sequences before imaging. This atlas and the accompanying brief descriptive material can not only familiarize the clinician with normal imaging anatomy pertinent to a psychiatrist but also serve as a base for more in-depth study. The cranial nerves, motor pathways, and peripheral sensory tracts are not discussed.

Thought, memory, and emotion are believed to occur by way of complicated circuits or networks of interconnected areas of brain. Lesions at any point in a circuit can potentially give rise to identical symptoms (Burruss et al. 2000; Dalgleish 2004; Taber et al. 2004; Tekin and Cummings 2002). The reader should be mindful that although the larger brain structures are mentioned in the following discussion, any lesion along the small tracts between regions can also produce similar deficits. A comprehensive review of these circuits is beyond the scope of this chapter. With the advent of graphic programs and computer technology, many three-dimensional models are available that make these circuits easier to understand. The major

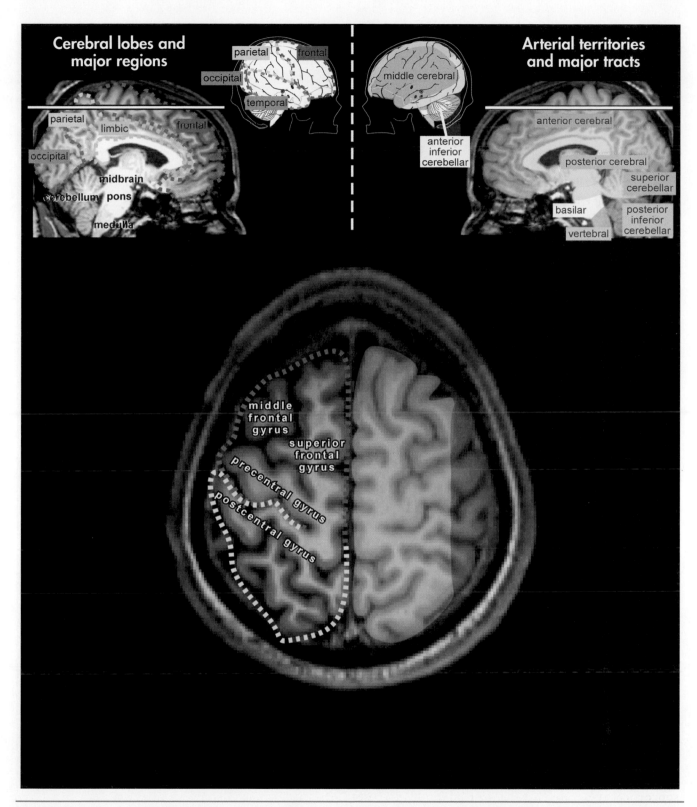

FIGURE 7–35.   T1-weighted axial magnetic resonance image (MRI) with major tracts (*right side*) and brain regions (*left side*) labeled. Major subcortical structures are color-coded to match Figure 7–34. Vascular territories (*right side*) and lobes (*left side*) are color-coded to match the key.

Source.   MRI courtesy of Phillips Medical Systems. Atlas section used with permission of Veterans Health Administration Mid-Atlantic Mental Illness Research, Education, and Clinical Center.

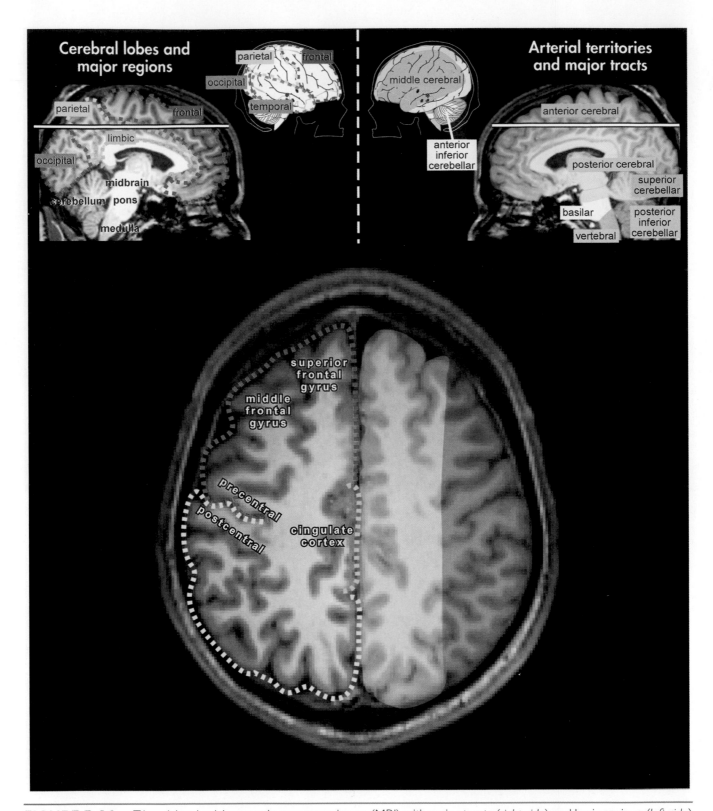

FIGURE 7–36.   T1-weighted axial magnetic resonance image (MRI) with major tracts (*right side*) and brain regions (*left side*) labeled. Major subcortical structures are color-coded to match Figure 7–34. Vascular territories (*right side*) and lobes (*left side*) are color-coded to match the key.

Source.   MRI courtesy of Phillips Medical Systems. Atlas section used with permission of Veterans Health Administration Mid-Atlantic Mental Illness Research, Education, and Clinical Center.

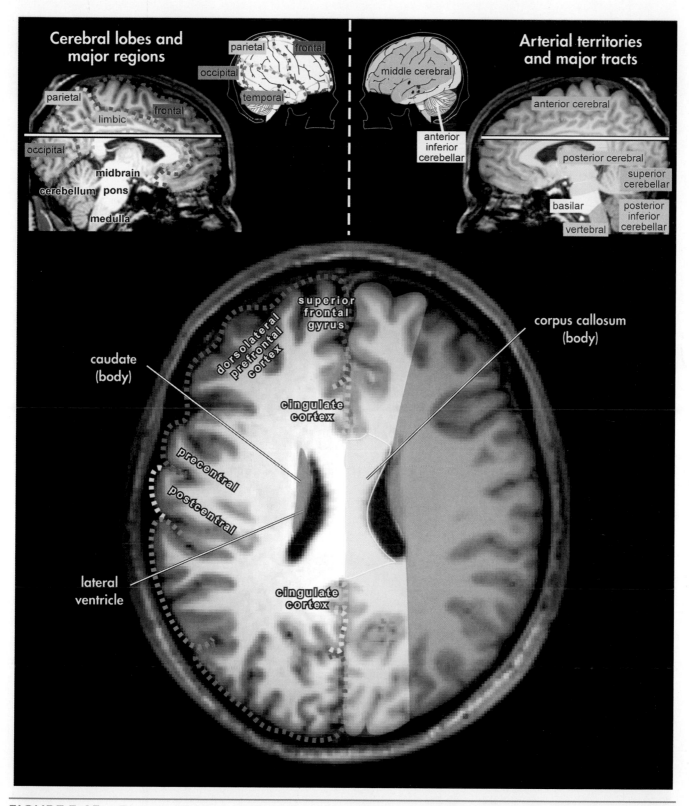

FIGURE 7–37. T1-weighted axial magnetic resonance image (MRI) with major tracts (*right side*) and brain regions (*left side*) labeled. Major subcortical structures are color-coded to match Figure 7–34. Vascular territories (*right side*) and lobes (*left side*) are color-coded to match the key.

Source. MRI courtesy of Phillips Medical Systems. Atlas section used with permission of Veterans Health Administration Mid-Atlantic Mental Illness Research, Education, and Clinical Center.

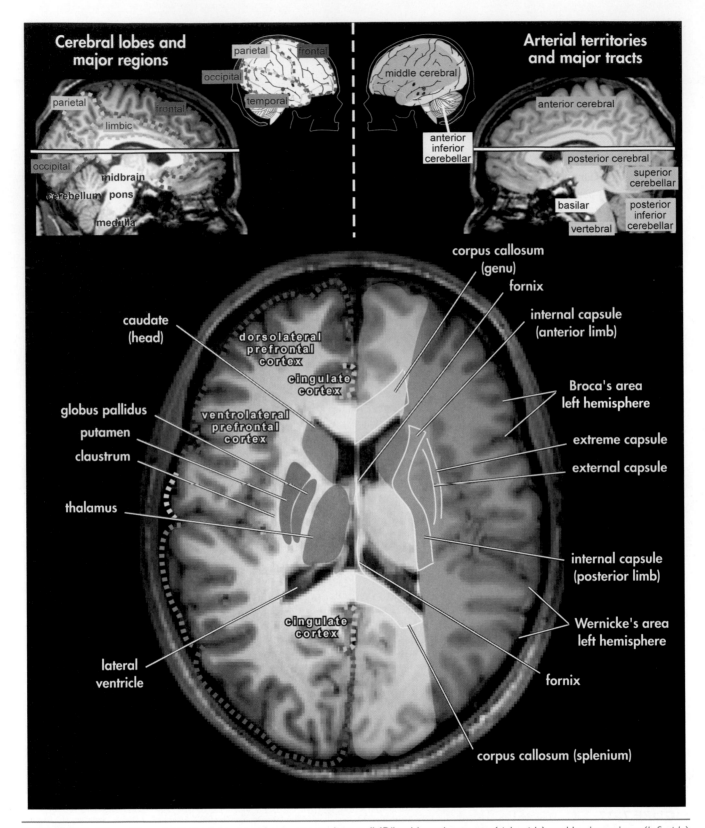

FIGURE 7–38. T1-weighted axial magnetic resonance image (MRI) with major tracts (*right side*) and brain regions (*left side*) labeled. Major subcortical structures are color-coded to match Figure 7–34. Vascular territories (*right side*) and lobes (*left side*) are color-coded to match the key.

Source. MRI courtesy of Phillips Medical Systems. Atlas section used with permission of Veterans Health Administration Mid-Atlantic Mental Illness Research, Education, and Clinical Center.

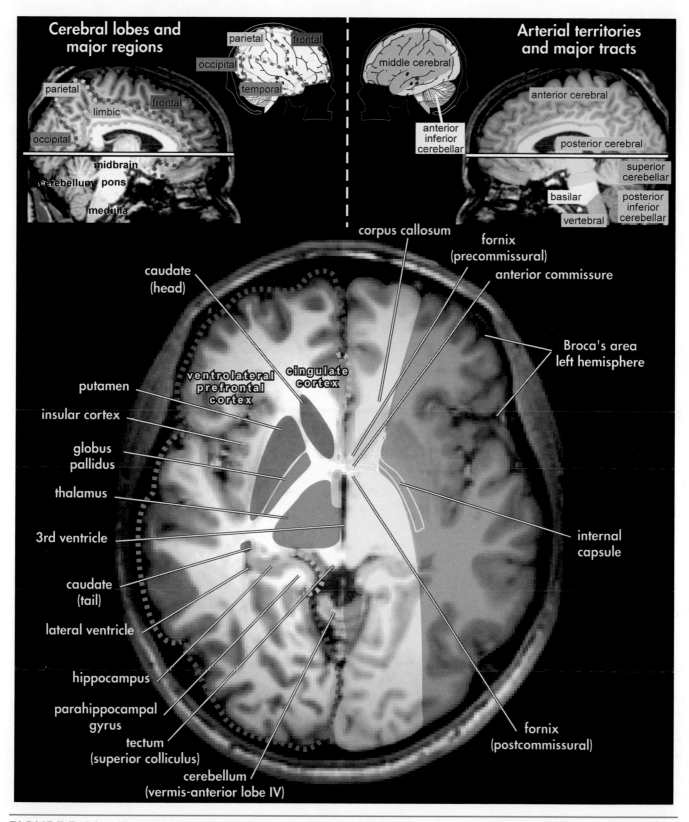

FIGURE 7–39. T1-weighted axial magnetic resonance image (MRI) with major tracts (*right side*) and brain regions (*left side*) labeled. Major subcortical structures are color-coded to match Figure 7–34. Vascular territories (*right side*) and lobes (*left side*) are color-coded to match the key.

Source. MRI courtesy of Phillips Medical Systems. Atlas section used with permission of Veterans Health Administration Mid-Atlantic Mental Illness Research, Education, and Clinical Center.

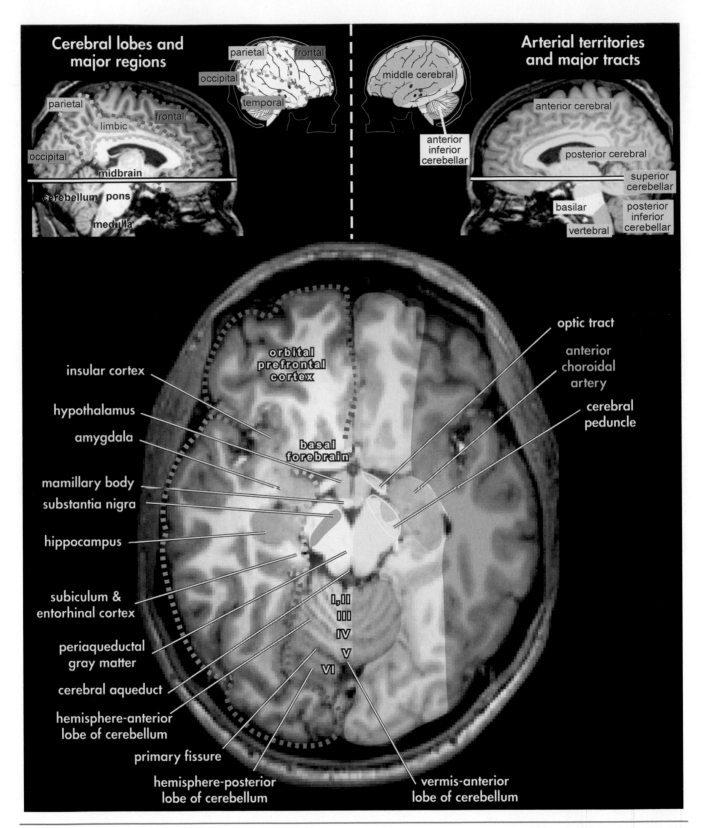

FIGURE 7–40.   T1-weighted axial magnetic resonance image (MRI) with major tracts (*right side*) and brain regions (*left side*) labeled. Major subcortical structures are color-coded to match Figure 7–34. Vascular territories (*right side*) and lobes (*left side*) are color-coded to match the key.

Source.   MRI courtesy of Phillips Medical Systems. Atlas section used with permission of Veterans Health Administration Mid-Atlantic Mental Illness Research, Education, and Clinical Center.

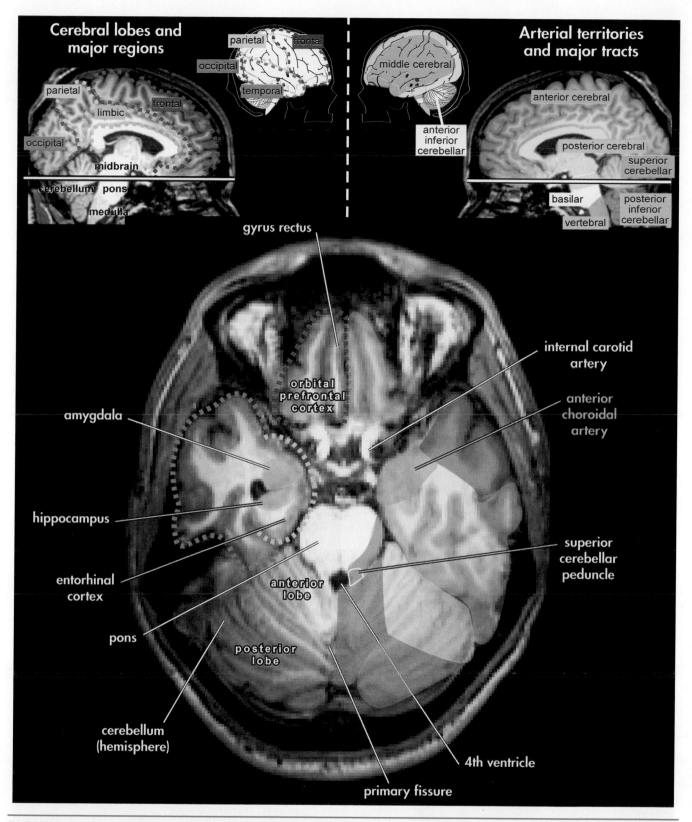

FIGURE 7–41. T1-weighted axial magnetic resonance image (MRI) with major tracts *(right side)* and brain regions *(left side)* labeled. Major subcortical structures are color-coded to match Figure 7–34. Vascular territories *(right side)* and lobes *(left side)* are color-coded to match the key.

Source. MRI courtesy of Phillips Medical Systems. Atlas section used with permission of Veterans Health Administration Mid-Atlantic Mental Illness Research, Education, and Clinical Center.

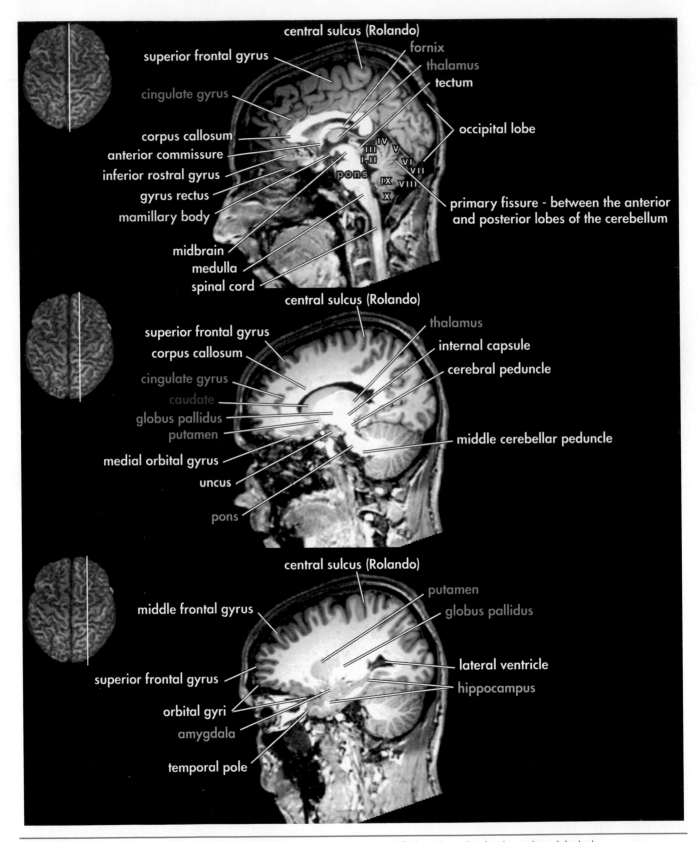

FIGURE 7–42.   T1-weighted sagittal magnetic resonance images (MRIs) with major brain regions labeled.

Source.   MRI courtesy of Phillips Medical Systems. Atlas section used with permission of Veterans Health Administration Mid-Atlantic Mental Illness Research, Education, and Clinical Center.

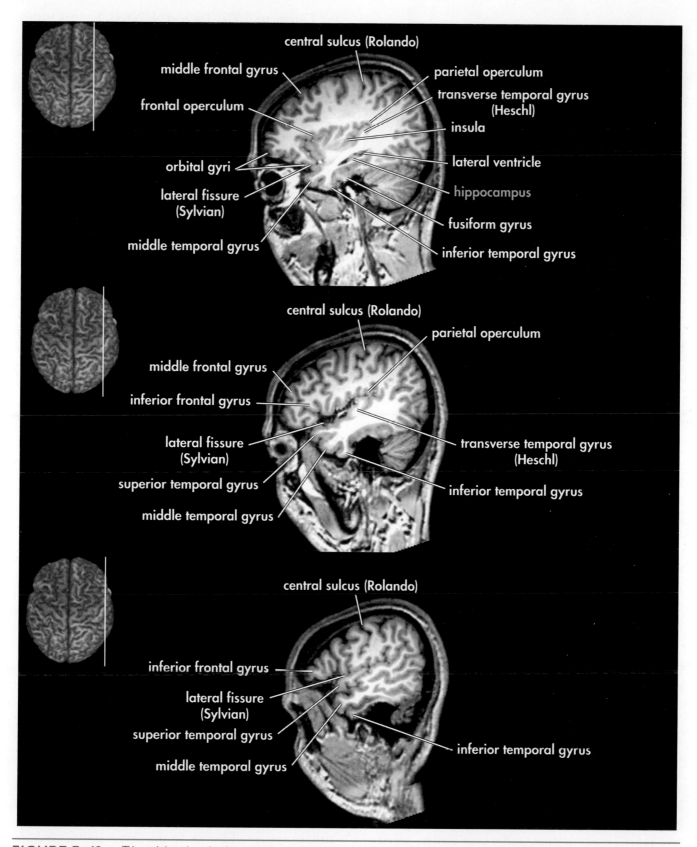

FIGURE 7–43. T1-weighted sagittal magnetic resonance images (MRIs) with major brain regions labeled.

Source. MRI courtesy of Phillips Medical Systems. Atlas section used with permission of Veterans Health Administration Mid-Atlantic Mental Illness Research, Education, and Clinical Center.

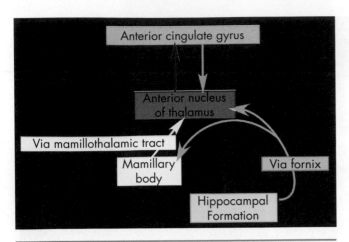

FIGURE 7–44. Schematic diagram of the emotion and memory circuit of Papez.

neuropsychiatric symptoms associated with damage to various subcortical structures are summarized in the following subsections. These summaries were derived from a more comprehensive review, which can be consulted for more detail (Naumescu et al. 1999).

CEREBRAL CORTEX

The largest division of the human brain is the cerebral cortex. Anatomists divide the cerebral cortex into either four or five lobes. All recognize the frontal, temporal, parietal, and occipital lobes. Some consider the limbic lobe a fifth lobe; others consider it to be contained within the temporal and frontal lobes and diencephalon (see Figures 7–34 through 7–41). The cerebral cortex and its associated functions are discussed by Harel and Tranel in Chapter 2 of this volume.

BASAL GANGLIA

The basal ganglia are a group of small, interconnected subcortical nuclei made up of the caudate nucleus, putamen, globus pallidus, claustrum, subthalamus, and substantia nigra (see Figures 7–34, 7–37, 7–38, 7–39, 7–40, and 7–42). The caudate nucleus and putamen are often called the *corpus striatum*, and the globus pallidus and putamen are called the *lentiform nucleus*. Together, the structures of the basal ganglia are familiar to psychiatrists from disorders such as Huntington's chorea and Parkinson's disease or as the targets of many poison and toxin exposures. These nuclei serve a key role as a site for bringing emotion, executive function, motivation, and motor activity together. Many input and output circuits traverse these areas, including the three frontal lobe circuits of dorsolateral, orbitofrontal, and anterior cingulate gyrus (Burruss et al. 2000; Tekin

and Cummings 2002; Tisch et al. 2004). Lesions within these structures result in syndromes of hypokinetic or hyperkinetic movements as well as cognitive and emotional dysfunction. The basal ganglia contain significant acetylcholine, dopamine, GABA, and neuropeptide projections. The dopaminergic projections have been pharmacological targets for schizophrenia and Parkinson's disease.

Caudate Nucleus

The caudate nuclei are C-shaped structures, each having a head, body, and tail. They arch to follow the walls of the lateral ventricles and terminate into the amygdaloid nuclei bilaterally (see Figures 7–34, 7–37, 7–38, 7–39, and 7–42). The caudate nucleus and putamen together are thought of as the input nuclei receiving projections from the cerebral cortex, thalamus, and substantia nigra pars compacta. The major outputs for the caudate nucleus and putamen are the globus pallidus and substantia nigra pars reticulata. Neuropsychiatric symptoms of damage to the caudate nucleus are numerous and can be divided into behavioral, emotional, memory, language, and other symptoms. More commonly reported deficits include disinhibition, disorganization, executive dysfunction, apathy, depression, memory loss, atypical aphasia, psychosis, personality changes, and predisposition for delirium.

Putamen

The putamen is the most lateral of the basal ganglia structures. It is separated from the caudate nucleus by the anterior limb of the internal capsule (see Figures 7–34, 7–38, 7–39, and 7–42). The putamen and the caudate nucleus are considered input nuclei. See the preceding "Caudate Nucleus" subsection for afferent and efferent projections. Neuropsychiatric symptoms of lesions to the putamen include primarily language and behavioral deficits (e.g., atypical aphasia, obsessive-compulsive traits, executive dysfunction). However, hemineglect, depression, and memory loss have been reported.

Globus Pallidus

The globus pallidus lies medial to the putamen and has two divisions (internal and external) (see Figures 7–34, 7–38, 7–39, and 7–42). The globus pallidus is functionally considered an output nucleus. Primary output is to the subthalamus and thalamus via GABAergic pathways. (For a further discussion of the afferent and efferent connections of the globus pallidus, see Crossman 1995.) Neuropsychiatric symptoms of lesions to the globus pallidus include primarily emotional and other types (e.g., anxiety, depression, apathy, psychosis, and central pain). Other less often reported symptoms include amnesia and cognitive deficits.

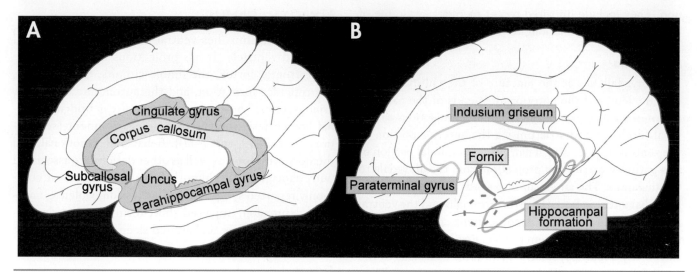

FIGURE 7–45.   Schematic diagrams of the medial surface of the right cerebral hemisphere showing the (A) outer and (B) inner limbic lobes.

Substantia Nigra

The substantia nigra nuclei of the midbrain are dark because they contain melanin. They are divided into the pars compacta and the pars reticulata. The first sends dopaminergic projections to the caudate nucleus and putamen. The latter receives input from the striatum and sends efferents to the thalamus, subthalamus, and reticular formation (see Figures 7–34 and 7–40). Reported neuropsychiatric symptoms of lesions to the substantia nigra include primarily behavioral and emotional deficits (e.g., apraxia, ataxia, aggression, and depression), with less frequent reports of memory and cognitive deficits.

LIMBIC SYSTEM

The term *limbic system* is most often used to describe the areas of brain involved in the production of emotion, memory, or aggression (Dalgleish 2004; Morgane and Mokler 2006). Originally suggested by Broca ("*le grand lobe limbique*"), the name is purely descriptive of the anatomical location of these structures (*limbus* means "border," and these structures border the neocortex). Papez suggested that these areas were important for memory and emotion, rather than just smell as had been previously believed. MacLean applied the name "limbic system" to the circuit of Papez, reasoning that these structures are placed to integrate signals from the external and internal worlds (Figure 7–44). Commonly, these structures are divided into an outer and an inner lobe (Figure 7–45). The outer lobe is composed of the cingulate, subcallosal, parahippocampal, and uncal cortices. The inner lobe consists of the paraterminal gyrus, the indusium griseum (supracallosal gyrus), and the hippocampal complex. Other areas

closely associated with these and often considered part of the limbic system include the mamillary bodies and parts of the thalamus. Some authors also include other areas, such as the orbitofrontal cortex and hypothalamus. (See Mega et al. 1997 for an excellent review of the anatomical and phylogenetic development of the limbic system.)

Hippocampal Formation and Parahippocampal Cortex

The hippocampal formation and parahippocampal cortex (or gyrus) are collectively considered to be the "memory structures." They function in essence to form and direct the storage of memories. The parahippocampus extends from the cingulate cortex to the amygdala (see Figure 7–45). The main body of the hippocampal formation extends from the crus of the fornix to the amygdala located in the medial temporal lobe. The fornix is the major fiber tract of the hippocampal formation (see Figures 7–34, 7–38, 7–39, 7–42, and 7–43). Neuropsychiatric symptoms of lesions to the hippocampal formation are primarily memory deficits. These include anterograde and retrograde amnesia, inability to form new memories, and temporally graded amnesia.

The fornix is made up of afferent and efferent hippocampal fibers. It forms from the fibers (fimbria) that course on the ventricular surface of the hippocampus. The fimbria become the crus of the fornix. The crus join to form the body of the fornix. The body then passes between the lateral ventricles in the septum pellucidum. The body divides around the anterior commissure to form the anterior (precommissural) and posterior (postcommissural) columns of the fornix (see Figure 7–39). Neuropsychiatric symptoms of lesions to the fornix are memory deficits and overlap those following damage to the hippocampal formation. They include impaired recent memory, syndrome of transitory amnesia, and long-term anterograde amnesia.

Amygdala

The amygdala lies at the juncture of the tail of the caudate nucleus and the anterior-most ends of the parahippocampus and hippocampus. It sends projections to the basal forebrain and striatum via the anterior portion of the ventral amygdalofugal pathway. The caudal portion of this pathway carries the projection from the amygdala to the thalamus. The amygdala also sends projections to the hypothalamus via both the stria terminalis and the ventral amygdalofugal pathway. A component continues on to the midbrain and brain stem (see Figures 7–34, 7–40, 7–41, and 7–42). Neuropsychiatric symptoms of lesions to the amygdala are primarily behavioral and emotional. They include passivity or aggression, hypersexuality, hyperorality, hyperphagia, decreased fear, anxiety or startle, and decreased link between emotion and memory.

Mamillary Body

The mamillary bodies are two small round nuclei that lie in the posterior portion of the diencephalon. They receive afferents from the hippocampus and send efferents to the brain stem and thalamus (see Figures 7–34, 7–40, and 7–42). The mamillothalamic tract is the projection from the mamillary bodies to the anterior nucleus of the thalamus. Neuropsychiatric symptoms of lesions to the mamillary body or its tract are primarily memory deficits and psychosis. Confabulation and anterograde memory loss are most common.

Thalamus

The thalamus is medial to the caudate nucleus and putamen and lateral to the third ventricle. The superior and medial portions contain the anterior nucleus, medial dorsal nucleus, and lateral dorsal nucleus (see Figures 7–34, 7–38, 7–39, and 7–42) (Taber et al. 2004). These nuclei have intimate interconnections with the limbic system. Damage to the medial portion of the left thalamus is associated with deficits in language, verbal intellect, and verbal memory. Damage to the right is associated with deficits in visuospatial and nonverbal intellect and visual memory. Medial thalamus may be important for temporal aspects of memory. Bilateral damage is associated with severe memory impairment ("thalamic amnesia") as well as dementia. The memory deficits may result from destruction of the tracts (mamillothalamic tract, amygdalofugal tract) connecting these thalamic nuclei with limbic structures. Damage to the anterior and medial thalamus can also result in disturbances of autonomic functions, mood, and the sleep-wake cycle.

HYPOTHALAMUS

The hypothalamus lies ventral to the thalamus around the third ventricle. It has projections to and from the orbitofrontal cortex, the limbic circuits, the thalamus, the reticular formation, and the autonomic and endocrine systems. Thus, it is a key structure in bridging internal homeostasis and the outside environment (see Figures 7–34, 7–39, and 7–40). Behavioral, emotional, and memory symptoms as well as other deficits are associated with damage to the hypothalamus. Examples of commonly reported symptoms are aggression, violence, anorexia, depression, impaired short-term memory, dementia, gelastic seizures, and altered sleep-wake cycle.

PONS

The pons lies in the posterior fossa between the midbrain and the medulla oblongata. It contains nuclei and tracts that are necessary for arousal (reticular formation) and affective stability (see Figures 7–34, 7–41, and 7–42). The raphe nuclei (found at the midline along the entire brain stem) send serotonergic projections to structures throughout the brain, including the thalamus, hippocampus, basal ganglia, and frontal cortex. The locus coeruleus is also found in the pons. It sends noradrenergic projections to the limbic system, hypothalamus, thalamus, cerebellum, and cerebral cortex. Neuropsychiatric symptoms of pontine lesions include behavioral, emotional, language, memory, and other deficits. Commonly reported deficits include disinhibition, disturbed sleep-wake cycles, anxiety, depression, emotional lability, cognitive deficits, central pain, personality changes, and psychosis.

CEREBELLUM

The cerebellum lies ventral to the temporal and occipital lobes and the pons, surrounding the fourth ventricle (see Figures 7–39, 7–40, and 7–42). In addition to its extensive connections with the motor system, the cerebellum projects (via the thalamus) to cingulate, dorsomedial prefrontal, and dorsolateral prefrontal cortices (Middleton and Strick 2000, 2001; Schmahmann and Pandya 1997a, 1997b; Taber et al. 2005). Recent work indicates that cerebellar lesions, particularly to the posterior cerebellum and vermis, can result in a range of cognitive and emotional deficits, including executive dysfunction, visual-spatial deficits, personality changes, and linguistic abnormalities (Konarski et al. 2005; Rapoport et al. 2000; Schmahmann 2004; Taber et al. 2005; Turner and Schiavetto 2004).

Highlights for the Clinician

Testing modality	Indications	Caveats
Structural neuroimaging		
Computed tomography (CT)	✦ Screening examination ✦ Acute hemorrhage ✦ Calcified lesions ✦ Bone injury	*Contraindications for use of contrast enhancement:* ✦ History of anaphylaxis or severe allergic reaction ✦ Creatinine level ≥15 mg/dL ✦ Metformin administration on day of scan
Magnetic resonance imaging (MRI)	✦ Sustained confusion/delirium ✦ Subtle cognitive deficits ✦ Unusual age at symptom onset or evolution ✦ Atypical clinical findings ✦ Abrupt personality changes with accompanying neurological signs/symptoms ✦ Following poison or toxin exposures (including significant alcohol abuse) ✦ Following brain injuries of any kind (traumatic or "organic")	*Contraindications for use of MRI:* ✦ Any magnetic metal in the body, including surgical clips and sutures ✦ Implanted electrical, mechanical, or magnetic devices ✦ Claustrophobia ✦ History of welding (requires skull films before MRI) ✦ Pregnancy (legal contraindication)
Functional neuroimaging		
Positron emission tomography (PET)	✦ Particularly useful for identification of "hidden" lesions (areas that are dysfunctional but do not look abnormal on structural imaging) ✦ Particularly useful also for patients whose clinical symptoms do not fit the classic historical picture for the working diagnosis ✦ Evaluation of resting state has shown potential for prediction of treatment response in some conditions ✦ PET has the advantages of higher spatial resolution than SPECT and true attenuaton correction (nearly eliminating attenuation artifacts)	✦ Reimbursement limited to dementia, presurgical evaluation of epilepsy, and distinguishing radiation necrosis from recurrent brain tumors
Single-photon emission computed tomography (SPECT)	✦ Same indications as for PET ✦ SPECT has the advantages of being more widely available than PET, less expensive, and reimbursable for most conditions	✦ Lower spatial resolution, more artifacts

RECOMMENDED READINGS

Anderson KE, Taber KH, Hurley RA: Functional imaging, in Textbook of Traumatic Brain Injury. Edited by Silver JM, McAllister TW, Yudofsky SC. Washington, DC, American Psychiatric Publishing, 2005, pp 107–133

Dalgleish T: The emotional brain. Nat Rev Neurosci 5:583–589, 2004

Erhart SM, Young AS, Marder SR, et al: Clinical utility of magnetic resonance imaging radiographs for suspected organic syndromes in adult psychiatry. J Clin Psychiatry 66:968–973, 2005

Gupta A, Elheis M, Pansari K: Imaging in psychiatric illness. Int J Clin Pract 58:850–858, 2004

Schmahmann JD: Disorders of the cerebellum: ataxia, dysmetria of thought, and the cerebellar cognitive affective syndrome. J Neuropsychiatry Clin Neurosci 16:367–378, 2004

Tekin S, Cummings JL: Frontal-subcortical neuronal circuits and clinical neuropsychiatry—an update. J Psychosom Res 53:647–654, 2002

REFERENCES

Anderson KE, Taber KH, Hurley RA: Functional imaging, in Textbook of Traumatic Brain Injury. Edited by Silver JM, McAllister TW, Yudofsky SC. Washington, DC, American Psychiatric Publishing, 2005, pp 107–133

Arakia Y, Ashikaga R, Fujii K, et al: MR fluid-attenuated inversion recovery imaging as routine brain T2-weighted imaging. Eur J Radiol 32:136–143, 1999

Bahner MLRW, Zuna I, Engenhart-Cabillic R, et al: Spiral CT vs incremental CT: is spiral CT superior in imaging of the brain? Eur Radiol 8:416–420, 1998

Baker JF, Kratz LC, Stevens GR, et al: Pharmacokinetics and safety of the MRI contrast agent gadoversetamide injection (Optimark) in healthy pediatric subjects. Invest Radiol 39:334–339, 2004

Barthel H, Hesse S, Dannenberg C, et al: Prospective value of perfusion and X-ray attenuation imaging with single-photon emission and transmission computed tomography in acute cerebral ischemia. Stroke 32:1558–1597, 2001

Benamer HT, Oerel WH, Patterson J, et al: Prospective study of presynaptic dopaminergic imaging in patients with mild parkinsonism and tremor disorders, 1: baseline and 3-month observations. Mov Disord 18:977–984, 2003

Beresford TP, Blow FC, Hall RCW, et al: CT scanning in psychiatric inpatients: clinical yield. Psychosomatics 27:105–112, 1986

Bergin PS, Fish DR, Shorvon SD, et al: Magnetic resonance imaging in partial epilepsy: additional abnormalities shown with the fluid attenuate inversion recovery (FLAIR) pulse sequence. J Neurol Neurosurg Psychiatry 58:439–443, 1995

Bizzi A, Righini A, Turner R, et al: MR of diffusion slowing in global cerebral ischemia. AJNR Am J Neuroradiol 14:1347–1354, 1993

Bonne O, Gilboa A, Louzoun Y, et al: Cerebral blood flow in chronic symptomatic mild traumatic brain injury. Psychiatry Res 124:141–152, 2003

Bookheimer SY, Strojwas MH, Cohen MS, et al: Patterns of brain activation in people at risk for Alzheimer's disease. N Engl J Med 343:450–456, 2000

Bourland JD, Nyenhuis JA, Schaefer DJ: Physiologic effects of intense MR imaging gradient fields. Neuroimaging Clin N Am 9:363–377, 1999

Branton T: Use of computerized tomography by old age psychiatrists: an examination of criteria for investigation of cognitive impairment. Int J Geriatr Psychiatry 14:567–571, 1999

Brant-Zawadzki M, Atkinson D, Detrick M, et al: Fluid-attenuated inversion recovery (FLAIR) for assessment of cerebral infarction. Stroke 27:1187–1191, 1996

Bulte JW: MR contrast agents for molecular and cellular imaging (editorial). Curr Pharm Biotechnol 5:483–483(1), 2004

Burruss JW, Hurley RA, Taber KH, et al: Functional neuroanatomy of the frontal lobe circuits. Radiology 214:227–230, 2000

Cao Y, D'Olhaberriague L, Vikingstad EM, et al: Pilot study of functional MRI to assess cerebral activation of motor function after poststroke hemiparesis. Stroke 29:112–122, 1998

Cherry S: Fundamentals of positron emission tomography and applications in preclinical drug development. J Clin Pharmacol 41:482–491, 2001

Cochran ST: Anaphylactoid reactions to radiocontrast media. Curr Allergy Asthma Rep 5:28–31, 2005

Cochran ST, Bomyea K, Sayre JW: Trends in adverse events after IV administration of contrast media. AJR Am J Roentgenol 178:1385–1388, 2002

Cohan RH, Matsumoto JS, Quaglianao PV: ACR Manual on Contrast Media, 4th Edition. Reston, VA, American College of Radiology, 1998

Coleman LT, Zimmerman RA: Pediatric craniospinal spiral CT: current applications and future potential. Semin Ultrasound CT MR 15:148–155, 1994

Crossman AR: Neuroanatomy: An Illustration Colour Text. Edinburgh, Scotland, Churchill Livingstone, 1995, p 69

Dalgleish T: The emotional brain. Nat Rev Neurosci 5:583–589, 2004

De Backer AI, Mortele KJ, De Keulenaer BL: Considerations for planning and implementation. JBR-BTR 87:241–246, 2004a

De Backer AI, Mortele KJ, De Keulenaer BL: Picture archiving and communication system—part one: filmless radiology and distance radiology. JBR-BTR 87:234–241, 2004b

Desmond JE, Annabel Chen SH: Ethical issues in the clinical application of fMRI: factors affecting the validity and interpretation of activations. Brain Cogn 50:482–497, 2002

Detre JA, Alsop DC: Arterial spin labeled perfusion magnetic resonance imaging, in Imaging of the Nervous System. Edited by Latchaw RE, Kucharczyk J, Moseley ME. Philadelphia, PA, Elsevier Mosby, 2005, pp 323–331

Diwadkar VA, Keshavan MS: Newer techniques in magnetic resonance imaging and their potential for neuropsychiatric research. J Psychosom Res 53:677–685, 2002

Dong Q, Welsh RC, Chenevert TL, et al: Clinical applications of diffusion tensor imaging. J Magn Reson Imaging 19:6–18, 2004

Erhart SM, Young AS, Marder SR, et al: Clinical utility of magnetic resonance imaging radiographs for suspected organic syndromes in adult psychiatry. J Clin Psychiatry 66:968–973, 2005

Fahey FH: Data acquisition in PET imaging. J Nucl Med Technol 30:39–40, 2002

Federle MP, Willis LL, Swanson DP: Ionic versus nonionic contrast media: a prospective study of the effect of rapid bolus injection on nausea and anaphylactoid reaction. J Neurol Sci 22:341–345, 1998

Filippi M, Rocca MA: Magnetization transfer magnetic resonance imaging in the assessment of neurological diseases. J Neuroimaging 14:303–313, 2004

Garavan H, Pankiewicz J, Bloom A, et al: Cue-induced cocaine craving: neuroanatomical specificity for drug users and drug stimuli. Am J Psychiatry 157:1789–1798, 2000

Guadagno JV, Calautti C, Baron JC: Progress in imaging stroke: emerging clinical applications. Br Med Bull 65:145–157, 2003

Gupta A, Elheis M, Pansari K: Imaging in psychiatric illness. Int J Clin Pract 58:850–858, 2004

Hall P, Adami HO, Trichopoulos D, et al: Effect of low doses of ionising radiation in infancy on cognitive function in adulthood: Swedish population based cohort study. BMJ 328:19, 2004

Halpern JD, Hopper KD, Arredondo MG, et al: Patient allergies: role in selective use of nonionic contrast material. Radiology 199:359–362, 1999

Halpin SF: Brain imaging using multislice CT: a personal perspective. Br J Radiol 77:S20–S26, 2004

Hanyu H, Asano T, Sakurai H, et al: Magnetization transfer ratio in cerebral white matter lesions of Binswanger's disease. J Neurol Sci 1:87–89, 1999

Hariri AR, Mattay VS, Tessitore A, et al: Serotonin transporter genetic variation and the response of the human amygdala. Science 297:400–403, 2002

Henry TR, Van Heertum RL: Positron emission tomography and single photon emission computed tomography in epilepsy care. Semin Nucl Med 33:88–104, 2003

Hoffmann A, Faber SC, Werhahn KJ, et al: Electromyography in MRI—first recordings of peripheral nerve activation caused by fast magnetic field gradients. Magn Reson Med 43:534–539, 2000

Holmes AJ, MacDonald A 3rd, Carter CS, et al: Prefrontal functioning during context processing in schizophrenia and major depression: an event-related fMRI study. Schizophr Res 76:199–206, 2005

Hopper KD, Neuman JD, King SH, et al: Radioprotection to the eye during CT scanning. AJNR Am J Neuroradiol 22:1194–1198, 2001

Huisman TAGM: Diffusion-weighted imaging basic concepts and application in cerebral stroke and head trauma. Eur Radiol 13:2283–2297, 2003

Hurley RA, Jackson EF, Fisher RE, et al: New techniques for understanding Huntington's disease. J Neuropsychiatry Clin Neurosci 11:173–175, 1999a

Hurley RA, Taber KH, Zhang J, et al: Neuropsychiatric presentation of multiple sclerosis. J Neuropsychiatry Clinical Neurosci 11:5–7, 1999b

Hurley RA, Lewine JD, Jones GM, et al: Applications of magnetoencephalography to the study of autism. J Neuropsychiatry Clin Neurosci 12:1–5, 2000a

Hurley RA, Tomimoto H, Akiguchi I, et al: Binswanger's disease: an ongoing controversy. J Neuropsychiatry Clin Neurosci 12:301–304, 2000b

Hurley RA, Hayman LA, Taber KH: Clinical imaging in neuropsychiatry, in The American Psychiatric Publishing Textbook of Neuropsychiatry and Clinical Neurosciences, 4th Edition. Edited by Yudofsky SC, Hales RE. Washington, DC, American Psychiatric Publishing, 2002, pp 245–283

Hurley RA, Ernst T, Khalili K, et al: Identification of HIV associated progressive multifocal leukoencephalopathy: magnetic resonance imaging and spectroscopy. J Neuropsychiatry Clin Neurosci 15:1–6, 2003

Inoue E, Nakagawa M, Goto R, et al: Regional differences between 99mTC-ECD and 99mTc-HMPAO SPET in perfusion changes with age and gender in healthy adults. Eur J Nucl Med Mol Imaging 30:489–497, 2003

Jacobs JE, Birnbaum BA, Langlotz CP: Contrast media reactions and extravasation: relationship to intravenous injection rates. Radiology 209:411–416, 1998

Jung SL, Kim BS, Lee KS, et al: Magnetic resonance imaging and diffusion-weighted imaging changes after hypoglycemic coma. J Neuroimaging 15:193–196, 2005

Kaplan H, Sadock B, Grebb J: The brain and behavior, in Kaplan and Sadock's Synopsis of Psychiatry: Behavioral Sciences Clinical Psychiatry, 7th Edition. Edited by Kaplan H, Sadock BJ, Graff JA. Baltimore, MD, Williams & Wilkins, 1994, pp 112–125

Kilpatrick MM, Yonas H, Goldstein S, et al: CT-based assessment of acute stroke: CT, CT angiography, and xenon-enhanced CT cerebral blood flow. Stroke 32:2543–2549, 2001

Kim YJ, Ishise M, Ballinger JR, et al: Combination of dopamine transporter and D2 receptor SPECT in the diagnostic evaluation of PD, MSA, and PSP. Mov Disord 17:303–312, 2002

Kirchin MA, Runge VM: Contrast agents for magnetic resonance imaging safety update. Top Magn Reson Imaging 14:426–435, 2003

Knudsen GM, Karlsborg M, Thomsen G, et al: Imaging of dopamine transporters and D_2 receptors in patients with Parkinson's disease and multiple system atrophy. Eur J Nucl Med Mol Imaging 31:1631–1638, 2004

Konarski JZ, McIntyre RS, Grupp LA, et al: Is the cerebellum relevant in the circuitry of neuropsychiatric disorders? J Psychiatry Neurosci 30:178–186, 2005

Konen E, Konen O, Katz M, et al: Are referring clinicians aware of patients at risk from intravenous injection of iodinated contrast media? Clin Radiol 57:132–135, 2002

Kubicki M, Westin CF, Maier SE, et al: Uncinate fasciculus findings in schizophrenia: a magnetic resonance diffusion tensor imaging study. Am J Psychiatry 159:813–820, 2002

Kuhl CK, Textor J, Gieseke J, et al: Acute and subacute ischemic stroke at high-field-strength (3.0.T) diffusion-weighted MR imaging: intraindividual comparative study. Radiology 234:509–516, 2005

Kuntz R, Skalej M, Stefanou A: Image quality of spiral CT versus conventional CT in routine brain imaging. Eur J Radiol 26:235–240, 1998

Kushi H, Moriya T, Saito T, et al: Importance of metabolic monitoring systems as an early prognostic indicator in severe head injured patients. Acta Neurochir Suppl 75:67–68, 1999

Kuszyk BS, Beauchamp NJ, Fishman EK: Neurovascular applications of CT angiography. Semin Ultrasound CT MR 19:394–404, 1998

Larson EB, Mack LA, Watts B, et al: Computed tomography in patients with psychiatric illnesses: advantage of a "rule-in" approach. Ann Intern Med 95:360–364, 1981

Latchaw RE: Cerebral perfusion imaging in acute stroke. J Vasc Interv Radiol 15(1 pt 2):S29–S46, 2004

Leenders KL: Significance of non-presynaptic SPECT tracer methods in Parkinson's disease. Mov Disord 18:S39–S42, 2003

Lind J, Persson J, Ingvar M, et al: Reduced functional brain activity response in cognitively intact apolipoprotein E epsilon4 carriers. Brain 129:1240–1248, 2006

Magistretti PL, Pellerin L: The contribution of astrocytes to the 18F-2-deoxyglucose signal in PET activation studies. Mol Psychiatry 1:445–452, 1996

Marshall RS, Perera GM, Lazar RM, et al: Evolution of cortical activation during recovery from corticospinal tract infarction. Stroke 31:656–661, 2000

Marti-Fabregas JA, Catafau AM, Mari C, et al: Cerebral perfusion and haemodynamics measured by SPET in symptom-free patients with transient ischaemic attack: clinical implications. Eur J Nucl Med 28:1828–1835, 2001

Mascalchi M, Filippi M, Floris R, et al: Diffusion-weighted MR of the brain: methodology and clinical application. Radiol Med (Torino) 109:155–197, 2005

Matthews PM, Jezzard P: Functional magnetic resonance imaging. J Neurol Neurosurg Psychiatry 75:6–12, 2004

Mega MS, Cummings JL: Frontal-subcortical circuits and neuropsychiatric disorders. J Neuropsychiatry Clin Neurosci 6:358–370, 1994

Mega MS, Cummings JL, Salloway S, et al: The limbic system: an anatomic, phylogenetic, and clinical perspective [see comments]. J Neuropsychiatry Clin Neurosci 9:315–330, 1997

Menon V, Anagnoson RT, Mathalon DH, et al: Functional neuroanatomy of auditory working memory in schizophrenia: relation to positive and negative symptoms. Neuroimage 13:433–446, 2001

Middleton FA, Strick PL: Basal ganglia and cerebellar loops: motor and cognitive circuits. Brain Res Rev 31:236–250, 2000

Middleton FA, Strick PL: Cerebellar projections to the prefrontal cortex of the primate. J Neurosci 21:700–712, 2001

Mitchell DG: MR imaging contrast agents—what's in a name? J Magn Reson Imaging 7:1–4, 1997

Morgane PJ, Mokler DJ: The limbic brain: continuing resolution. Neurosci Biobehav Rev 30:119–125, 2006

Mortele KJ, Olivia MR, Ondategui S, et al: Universal use of nonionic iodinated contrast medium for CT: evaluation of safety in a large urban teaching hospital. AJR Am J Roentgenol 184:31–34, 2005

Moseley ME, Sawyer-Glover A, Kucharczyk J: Magnetic resonance imaging principles and techniques, in Imaging of the Nervous System. Edited by Latchaw RE, Kucharczyk J, Moseley ME. Philadelphia, PA, Elsevier Mosby, 2005, pp 3–30

Murata T, Fujito T, Kimura H, et al: Serial MRI and H-MRS of Wernicke's encephalopathy: report of a case with remarkable cerebellar lesions on MRI. Psychiatry Res 108:49–55, 2001

Nakamura H, Yamada K, Kizu O, et al: Effect of thin-section diffusion-weighted MR imaging on stroke diagnosis. AJNR Am J Neuroradiol 26:560–565, 2005

Naumescu I, Hurley RA, Hayman LA, et al: Neuropsychiatric symptoms associated with subcortical brain injuries. Int J Neuroradiol 5:51–59, 1999

Oi H, Yamazaki H, Matsushita M: Delayed vs. immediate adverse reactions to ionic and non-ionic low-osmolality contrast media. Radiat Med 15:23–27, 1997

Orrison WW Jr, Sanders JA: Clinical brain imaging: computerized axial tomography and magnetic resonance imaging, in Functional Brain Imaging. Edited by Orrison WW Jr, Lewine JD, Sanders JA, et al. St. Louis, MO, Mosby-Year Book, 1995, pp 97–144

Paans AMJ, van Waarde A, Elsinga PH, et al: Positron emission tomography: the conceptual idea using a multidisciplinary approach. Methods 27:195–207, 2002

Parra J, Kalitzin SN, Lopes De Silva FH: Magnetoencephalography: an investigational tool or a routine clinical technique? Epilepsy Behav 510:277–285, 2004

Pineiro R, Pendlebury S, Johansen-Berg H, et al: Altered hemodynamics responses in patients after subcortical stroke measured by functional MRI. Stroke 33:103–109, 2002

Price RR: The AAPM/RSNA physics tutorial for residents: MR imaging safety consideration. Radiological Society of North America. Radiographics 19:1641–1651, 1999

Raichle ME: Functional brain imaging and human brain function. J Neurosci 23:3959–3962, 2003

Ramandeep S, Jaggi MS, Husain M, et al: Diagnosis of bacterial cerebellitis: diffusion imaging and proton magnetic resonance spectroscopy. Pediatr Neurol 31:72–74, 2005

Rapoport M, van Reekum R, Mayberg H: The role of the cerebellum in cognition and behavior: a selective review. J Neuropsychiatry Clin Neurosci 12:193–198, 2000

Rauch S, Renshaw PF: Clinical neuroimaging in psychiatry. Harv Rev Psychiatry 2:297–312, 1995

Runge VM: Safety of magnetic resonance contrast media. Top Magn Reson Imaging 12:309–314, 2001

Runge VM, Lawrence RM, Wells JW: Principles of contrast enhancement in the evaluation of brain diseases: an overview. J Magn Reson Imaging 7:5–13, 1997

Rydberg JN, Hammond CA, Grimm RC, et al: Initial clinical experience in MR imaging of the brain with a fast fluid-attenuated inversion-recovery pulse sequence. Radiology 193:173–180, 1994

Sage MR, Wilson AJ, Scroop R: Contrast media and the brain: the basis of CT and MR imaging enhancement. Neuroimaging Clin N Am 8:695–707, 1998

Sakamoto K, Murata T, Omori M, et al: Clinical studies on three cases of the interval form of carbon monoxide poisoning: serial proton magnetic resonance spectroscopy as prognostic predictor. Psychiatry Res 83:179–198, 1998

Scarabino T, Nemore F, Giannatempo GM, et al: 3.0 T Magnetic resonance in neuroradiology. Eur J Radiol 48:154–164, 2003

Schmahmann JD: Disorders of the cerebellum: ataxia, dysmetria of thought, and the cerebellar cognitive affective syndrome. J Neuropsychiatry Clin Neurosci 16:367–378, 2004

Schmahmann JD, Pandya DN: Anatomic organization of the basilar pontine projections from prefrontal cortices in rhesus monkey. J Neurosci 17:438–458, 1997a

Schmahmann JD, Pandya DN: The cerebrocerebellar system. Int Rev Neurobiol 41:31–60, 1997b

Schwartz RB: Helical (spiral) CT in neuroradioliogic diagnosis. Radiol Clin North Am 33:981–995, 1995

Sheline YI, Barch DM, Donnelly JM, et al: Increased amygdala response to masked emotional faces in depressed subjects resolves with antidepressant treatment: an fMRI study. Biol Psychiatry 50:651–658, 2001

Shellock FG: Bioeffects and safety considerations, in Magnetic Resonance Imaging of the Brain and Spine. Edited by Atlas SW. New York, Raven, 1991, pp 87–107

Shellock FG: Magnetic resonance safety update 2002: implants and devices. J Magn Reson Imaging 16:485–496, 2002

Shellock FG, Crues JV: MR procedures: biologic effects, safety, and patient care. Radiology 232:635–652, 2004

Shellock FG, Kanal E: Policies, guidelines, and recommendations for MR imaging safety and patient management. SMRI Safety Committee. J Magn Reson Imaging 1:97–101, 1991

Shellock FG, Kanal E: Safety of magnetic resonance imaging contrast agents. J Magn Reson Imaging 10:477–484, 1999

Slosman DO, Ludwig C, Zerarka S, et al: Brain energy metabolism in Alzheimer's disease: 99mTe-HMPAO SPECT imaging during verbal fluency and role of astrocytes in the cellular mechanism of 99mTc-HMPAO retention. Brain Res Brain Res Rev 36:230–240, 2001

Sohn YH, Jeong Y, Kim HS, et al: The brain lesion responsible for parkinsonism after carbon monoxide poisoning. Arch Neurol 57:1214–1218, 2000

Sundgren PC, Dong Q, Gomez-Hasssan DM, et al: Diffusion tensor imaging of the brain: review of clinical applications. Neuroradiology 46:339–350, 2004

Sunshine JL: CT, MR imaging, and MR angiography in the evaluation of patients with acute stroke. J Vasc Interv Radiol 15:S47–S55, 2004

Symms M, Jäger HR, Schmierer K, et al: A review of structural magnetic resonance neuroimaging. J Neurol Neurosurg Psychiatry 75:1235–1244, 2004

Taber KH, Zimmerman JG, Yonas H, et al: Applications of xenon CT in clinical practice: detection of hidden lesions. J Neuropsychiatry Clin Neurosci 11:423–425, 1999

Taber KH, Cortelli P, Staffen W, et al: Expanding the role of imaging in prion disease. J Neuropsychiatry Clin Neurosci 14:371–376, 2002a

Taber KH, Pierpaoli C, Rose SE, et al: The future for diffusion tensor imaging in neuropsychiatry. J Neuropsychiatry Clin Neurosci 14:1–5, 2002b

Taber KH, Rauch SL, Lanius RA, et al: Functional magnetic resonance imaging: application to post traumatic stress disorder. J Neuropsychiatry Clin Neurosci 15:125–129, 2003

Taber KH, Wen C, Khan A, et al: The limbic thalamus. J Neuropsychiatry Clin Neurosci 16:127–132, 2004

Taber KH, Strick PL, Hurley RA: Rabies and the cerebellum: new methods for tracing circuits in the brain. J Neuropsychiatry Clin Neurosci 17:133–139, 2005

Tanabe JL, Ezekeil F, Jagust WJ, et al: Magnetization transfer ratio of white matter hyperintensities in subcortical ischemic vascular dementia. AJNR Am J Neuroradiol 20:839–844, 1999

Taylor WD, Hsu E, Krishnan KRR, et al: Diffusion tensor imaging: background, potential, and utility in psychiatric research. Biol Psychiatry 55:201–207, 2004

Tekin S, Cummings JL: Frontal-subcortical neuronal circuits and clinical neuropsychiatry—an update. J Psychosom Res 53:647–654, 2002

Tisch S, Silberstein P, Limousin-Dowsey P, et al: The basal ganglia: anatomy, physiology, and pharmacology. Psychiatr Clin North Am 27:757–799, 2004

Turner R, Jones T: Techniques for imaging neuroscience. Br Med Bull 65:3–20, 2003

Turner R, Schiavetto A: The cerebellum in schizophrenia: a case of intermittent ataxia and psychosis—clinical, cognitive, and neuroanatomical correlates. J Neuropsychiatry Clin Neurosci 16:400–408, 2004

Valls C, Andria E, Sanchez A, et al: Selective use of low-osmolality contrast media in computed tomography. Eur Radiol 13:2000–2005, 2003

Van Heertum RL, Greenstein EA, Tikofsky RS: 2-Deoxy-fluoro-glucose-positron emission tomography imaging of the brain: current clinical applications with emphasis on the dementias. Semin Nucl Med 34:300–312, 2004

von Oettingen G, Bergholt B, Gyldensted C, et al: Blood flow and ischemia within traumatic cerebral contusions. Neurosurgery 50:781–788, 2002

Walker Z, Costa DC, Walker RW, et al: Differentiation of dementia with Lewy bodies from Alzheimer's disease using a dopaminergic presynaptic ligand. J Neurol Neurosurg Psychiatry 73:134–140, 2002

Warwick JM: Imaging of brain function using SPECT. Metab Brain Dis 19:113–123, 2004

Weinberger DR: Brain disease and psychiatric illness: when should a psychiatrist order a CAT scan? Am J Psychiatry 141:1521–1527, 1984

Wheless JW, Castillo E, Maggio V, et al: Magnetoencephalography (MEG) and magnetic source imaging (MSI). Neurologist 10:138–153, 2004

Wilde JP, Rivers AW, Price DL: A review of the current use of magnetic resonance imaging in pregnancy and safety implication for the fetus. Prog Biophys Mol Biol 87:335–353, 2005

Willmann JK, Wildermuth S: Multidetector-row CT angiography of upper- and lower-extremity peripheral arteries. Eur Radiol 15:D3–D98, 2005

Wolf GL: Paramagnetic contrast agents for MR imaging of the brain, in MR and CT Imaging of the Head, Neck, and Spine. Edited by Latchaw RE. St. Louis, MO, Mosby-Year Book, 1991, pp 95–108

Yasuda M, Munechika H: Delayed adverse reaction to nonionic monomeric contrast enhanced media. Invest Radiol 33:1–5, 1998

8

EPIDEMIOLOGICAL AND GENETIC ASPECTS OF NEUROPSYCHIATRIC DISORDERS

Dolores Malaspina, M.D., M.S.P.H.

Cheryl Corcoran, M.D., M.S.P.H.

Scott Schobel, M.D.

Steven P. Hamilton, M.D., Ph.D.

The last decade has witnessed a revolution in our understanding of the etiology of many neuropsychiatric disorders. Advances in statistical genetics, genetic epidemiology, and molecular biology have provided new insights and avenues for conducting genetic and epidemiological studies and for analyzing gene-environment interactions. The recent sequencing of the human genome now sets the stage for even greater progress in the coming years. In this chapter, we first focus on the methods of genetic epidemiology and then review some of the recent findings of these disciplines in the study of neuropsychiatric disorders.

EPIDEMIOLOGICAL STUDIES

Epidemiology is based on the fundamental assumption that factors causal to human disease can be identified through the systematic examination of different populations, or of subgroups within a population, in different places or at different times (Hennekens and Buring 1987). Epidemiological research may be viewed as a directed series of questions:

- What is the frequency of a disorder?
- Are there subgroups in which the disorder is more frequent?
- What specific risk factors are associated with the disorder?
- Are these risk factors consistently and specifically related to the disorder?
- Does exposure to these factors precede the development of disease?

A variety of epidemiological strategies have been developed to address these questions.

The authors would like to thank Jessica MacDonald, Kristin Van Heertum, and Caitlin Warinsky for their assistance in the preparation of this chapter.

MEASURES OF DISEASE FREQUENCY

Measures of disease frequency serve as the basis for formulating and testing etiological hypotheses because they permit a comparison of frequencies between different populations or among individuals within a population with particular exposures or characteristics. The two measures of disease frequency used most often are *prevalence* and *incidence*. The former refers to the number of existing cases of a disease at a given point in time as a proportion of the total population. The latter refers to the number of new cases of a disease during a given period as a proportion of the total population at risk. The two measures are interrelated: the prevalence of a disease depends on both its incidence and its duration. One can compare two populations with and without a factor suspected of contributing to the development of disease through the calculation of the ratio of disease frequency in the two populations; this is known as the *relative risk*.

Disease incidence can be defined in several ways. *Risk* refers to the probability that an individual will develop a disease over a specified time and thus can vary from zero (no risk) to one (an individual will develop the disease). A common difficulty in long-term studies is that subjects become lost to follow-up, thus distorting the risk estimate upward if the subject remains disease-free or downward if the subject develops the disease. The alternative measure of incidence, called the *rate*, is used to address this problem. The rate is the instantaneous measure of individuals newly developing the disease in relation to the subject number that remain at risk (i.e., new cases per person-years of follow-up).

DESCRIPTIVE STUDIES

Descriptive studies contribute to formulating etiological hypotheses by showing a statistical association between exposure to specific risk factors and occurrence of the disease in single individuals or groups of individuals. Descriptive studies are conducted when little is known about the occurrence or antecedents of a disease. Hypotheses regarding risk factors then may emerge from studying several characteristics of affected individuals (e.g., sex, age, birth cohort), their place of residence, or the timing of their exposure. Descriptive studies, however, cannot be used to test etiological hypotheses: they lack adequate comparison groups, making it difficult to determine the specificity of exposure to the disease, and they are cross-sectional, making it difficult to determine the temporal relation between an exposure and the development of disease.

ANALYTIC STUDIES

An analytic study commences when enough is known about a disease that specific a priori hypotheses can be examined. Such etiological hypotheses may be tested through various analytic strategies. In a prospective cohort study, information is obtained about exposure status to selected variables at the time the study begins. New cases of illness are then identified from among those who did and those who did not have the exposure to the selected variables. This contrasts with retrospective cohort studies, in which prior exposure status is established on the basis of available information, usually obtained from available documentation and/or subject interviews. Disease incidence is determined from the time chosen by the investigator until the defined end point of the study. Case–control studies begin with the designation of disease status, and then past exposure to a risk factor is compared in those individuals who have a disease (case subjects) and in the appropriate control subjects. Procedures for matching control subjects to case subjects involve attempting to control for confounding variables and other biases.

BIRTH COHORT STUDIES

Another important type of epidemiological study is the birth cohort study, in which all individuals born in a certain location at a certain time are followed up. Correlations between hypothetical causes and disease expression can then be explored.

GENETIC STUDIES

Genetic research is concerned with identifying inherited factors that contribute to the development of disease. It, too, may be conceptualized as a directed series of questions:

- Is the disorder familial?
- Is it inherited?
- What is being inherited in the disorder; that is, what constitutes predisposition to the disorder, and what are the earliest manifestations of such predisposition?
- What additional ("epigenetic") variables increase or decrease the chances of genetically predisposed individuals developing the disorder?
- How is the disorder inherited?
- Where and what are the abnormal genes conferring genetic risk?
- What are the molecular and, ultimately, the pathological consequences of these abnormal genes?

TABLE 8–1. Relative risk for neuropsychiatric disorders

Disease	Population prevalence per 100,000	Morbid risk in first-degree relatives (%)	Relative risk (%)
Narcolepsy	10–100	30–50	5,000
Huntington's disease	19	50	2,630
Wilson's disease	10	25	2,500
Parkinson's disease	133	8.3	62.4
Autism	50–100	2–4	45–90
Bipolar disorder	500–1,500	8	16
Schizophrenia	900	12.8	14.2
Panic disorder	2,700	31	10
Obsessive-compulsive disorder	1,000–2,000	10	4.5
Alzheimer's disease	7,700	14.4	1.9
Prion diseases	<0.1	?	?

A variety of genetic strategies have been developed to address these questions (see "Highlights for the Clinician" at end of chapter).

FAMILY, TWIN, AND ADOPTION STUDIES

Family studies are a type of relative-risk study in which patterns of disease distributions within families are examined and the variability of the disease within families is compared with the variability between families. These studies may show an elevated risk for an illness in first-degree relatives of an affected individual in comparison with that in the general population (Table 8–1), but they cannot distinguish whether this elevated risk is due primarily to shared genetic or environmental factors.

Twin studies can further be used to resolve the genetic contribution to a disorder. Although they are exposed to the same familial environment, monozygotic (MZ) and dizygotic (DZ) twin pairs differ in their genetic endowment (sharing 100% and 50% of their genes, respectively). Thus, when genetic factors are important in etiology, the MZ and DZ co-twins of probands differ in their risk for the disorder. As a result, the comparison of relative concordance rates for MZ and DZ twins is an index of the disorder's heritability, or the proportion of variability that can be attributed to genetic, as opposed to environmental and other random, variables. It is still conceivable that environmental as well as genetic differences may influence the relative risk of diseases in MZ and DZ twins.

Adoption studies offer still another strategy for disentangling genetic and environmental influences, and they are particularly useful for the study of psychiatric disorders, in which cultural influences might otherwise allow for vertical transmission of behaviors. There are several types of adoption studies. In the adoptee study method, offspring separated at birth from their affected mothers are compared with the adopted-away offspring of control mothers. This can be considered a special form of cohort study. Cross-fostering studies examine adoptees whose biological parents are without illness and contrast the rates of illness in those reared by affected and unaffected adoptive parents. In the adoptee's family method, the biological relatives of affected adoptees are matched with the biological relatives of control adoptees, and their rates of illness are compared. Such studies are examples of the case–control paradigm.

HIGH-RISK STUDIES

The high-risk approach represents another form of cohort study. Individuals who are at genetic risk for a disorder (e.g., those with affected parents) are followed up prospectively, from early in life through the period of maximum risk for the disorder. This strategy permits the identification of features that are of primary pathogenic significance to the disorder, in contrast to those that are secondary to the illness or to its treatment. Moreover, by contrasting characteristics of at-risk individuals who go on to develop the disorder with characteristics of those who do not, this strategy allows for the identification of additional genetic and environmental influences that contribute to disease expression.

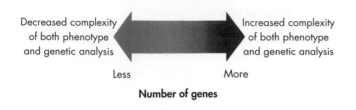

FIGURE 8–1.   Complex genetic risk. The number of genes involved in a phenotype is theorized to be directly related to both the complexity of the phenotype and the difficulty of genetic analysis.

Source.   Reprinted from Gottessman II, Gould TD: "The Endophenotype Concept in Psychiatry: Etymology and Strategic Intentions." *American Journal of Psychiatry* 160:636–645, 2003. Used with permission.

IDENTIFYING MODE OF INHERITANCE

Even when family, twin, and adoption studies suggest a role for genetic factors, they say nothing of which, or even how many, genes are involved. Single-gene mutations are inherited in a mendelian dominant, recessive, or sex-linked manner. They can produce thousands of *monogenic* disorders, many of which affect mental functioning, but any particular monogenic disorder is rare, and common diseases are likely to be *polygenic*—representing the combined small effects of many genes (Figure 8–1). Even with genetic liability, environmental influences may be necessary for an illness to be expressed.

Segregation analysis tests explicit models about the inheritance of disease genes on existing family data by comparing the distribution of illness observed in family members with that predicted by a given genetic hypothesis. The detection of mendelian ratios in a sibship can provide support for single-locus inheritance of the genes that confer susceptibility to a disease. Segregation analysis also can be conducted in other pedigree structures, including complex genealogies, to test models of inheritance from single-gene to polygenic inheritance. Segregation analysis (of nuclear family data) allows estimation of model parameters (such as gene frequency and penetrance) by treating each family as a separate observation (Kidd 1981). Its power is limited because it assumes that the same genetic disorder is present in all families. Pedigree analysis, on the other hand, examines more (multigenerational) relationships and is less likely to result in a type I error (a falsely attributed relation to disease) but is more likely to result in a type II error (an overlooked relation to disease) because an individual pedigree may manifest an idiosyncratic form of the disorder. Examina-

tion of *multiplex* sibships, in which two or more sibs are affected, represents a compromise approach.

COMPLEX DISORDERS

Genetic causation can range from a point mutation in single genes to polygenic causes that entail epistasis (interaction) among the several genes involved and/or environmental factors. Many, if not all, of the neuropsychiatric disorders have a complex pattern of inheritance. Qualities of complex disorders include the following:

- An unknown mode of inheritance
- Incomplete penetrance, wherein additional genetic or environmental factors may be necessary for the final expression of the disorder
- Epistasis, whereby the disorder may result from the interaction of several major genes
- Variable expressivity, in which a single form of the disorder may have several phenotypic expressions, making it difficult to define who is affected
- Diagnostic instability, such that a subject's affection status may change over time
- Etiological heterogeneity, under which an ordinarily genetic syndrome may have sporadic (environmentally produced) forms—known as *phenocopies*—as well as a variety of genetic forms resulting from disruption in several different genes—a condition known as *nonallelic heterogeneity*

The enormous growth in elucidating the genetics of some neuropsychiatric disorders in the last decade is chiefly the result of recent advances in statistical methods and molecular approaches designed to overcome these complexities.

LINKAGE ANALYSIS

Linkage analysis, also called positional cloning, is a strategy for isolating a gene of unknown structure or function based on its chromosomal location. It is based on establishing, within pedigrees, the coinheritance of the disorder with identifiable genetic markers of known chromosomal location. Mendel's second law (the law of independent assortment) implies that the disease gene, and hence the disorder, will not be consistently coinherited with a marker allele derived from a different chromosome. Moreover, even if the disease and marker alleles originally lie on the same parental chromosome (are *syntenic*), they may become separated during gametogenesis through the process of recombination or crossing over, wherein genetic material on homologous chromosomes is

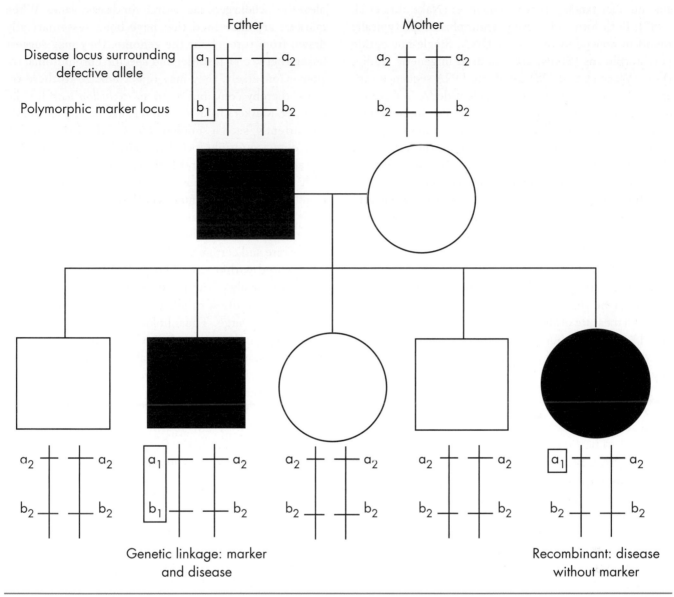

FIGURE 8–2. Genetic linkage and recombination. Depicted is a hypothetical family (*circles=females; squares=males*) segregating an autosomal dominant disease. The disease locus a (containing either the defective allele a_1 or its normal counterpart a_2) lies close to a polymorphic marker locus b (containing marker alleles b_1 and b_2). The father is affected by the disease (*top filled square*) and is heterozygous at both the disease and the marker loci. The mother is unaffected (*top unfilled circle*) and is homozygous at both loci. Because the disease and marker loci are genetically linked (i.e., they lie near one another), crossing over rarely occurs between them. Most children who inherit the disease allele, a_1, will also receive the b_1 allele from their mothers. Occasionally, a recombination event will occur in the father, and he will transfer a chromosome bearing the b_2 marker allele along with the disease allele (as has occurred in the daughter represented by the circle labeled "recombinant").

Source. Adapted from Rieder RO, Kaufmann CA: "Genetics," in *The American Psychiatric Press Textbook of Psychiatry, 2nd Edition.* Edited by Talbott JA, Hales RE, Yudofsky SC. Washington, DC, American Psychiatric Press, 1994, pp. 35–79. Used with permission.

exchanged (Figure 8–2). These rearranged chromosomes are ultimately passed on to the offspring.

Disease genes are mapped to the human chromosomes with linkage maps of the human genome. These maps were constructed according to DNA polymorphisms, which are the numerous loci in the genome that

vary in sequence among individuals, which can be identified by simple laboratory techniques. Types of polymorphisms that are used for genetic studies originally included restriction fragment length polymorphisms (RFLPs), which result from a mutation in a restriction enzyme site (Botstein et al. 1980), and later included variable-number tandem repeat sequences (Nakamura et al. 1987). Both forms of these polymorphisms are typically found in noncoded regions of DNA. Single-nucleotide polymorphisms (SNPs) are also used in genetic studies (D.G. Wang et al. 1998). SNPs are DNA sequence variations that occur when a single nucleotide (A, T, C, or G) in the genome sequence is altered. SNPs can be in non-coding regions or in genes that affect disease susceptibility or drug response and are becoming the marker of choice for genetic studies, given that they are the most common form of variation in the human genome.

When the polymorphism and disease gene are close to each other on the chromosome, there is a low chance of their being separated by recombination at meiosis (i.e., they are linked). The probability that a disease and marker allele will recombine depends on their distance from each other. In fact, the frequency with which the two alleles recombine (the recombination rate, or θ [theta]) can be used as a measure of the distance between their respective loci: 1% recombination is synonymous with a genetic distance of 1 centimorgan (cM) and roughly corresponds to a physical distance of 10^6 base pairs (bp) of DNA.

If disease and marker alleles lie near one another, crossing over will occur only rarely, and parental gametes will be overrepresented. The disease and marker loci are then said to be *linked*. Statistical support for linkage is obtained by examining the cosegregation of disease and marker phenotypes within a pedigree, determining the likelihood (Z) of achieving the observed distribution of phenotypes given estimates for the recombination fraction, θ, ranging from 0.00 to 0.50 (the latter representing no linkage), and calculating the odds ratio [defined as the ratio $Z(\theta)/Z(\theta = 0.50)$], that is, the relative likelihood of there being linkage versus no linkage. This odds ratio depends on the particular genetic parameters chosen in determining the likelihood. These parameters include the mode of inheritance, the frequency of the disease allele, and the probability of the disease given the presence of 0, 1, or 2 disease alleles. To the extent that evidence for linkage depends on such parameters, likelihood-based calculations are referred to as *parametric* linkage analyses. By convention, the odds ratio is expressed as its base 10 logarithm and is known as a *lod score*. In this way, the linkage data from several pedigrees can be pooled and their respective contributions added to obtain a combined probability of linkage. Also by convention, when the lod score at the best estimate of θ (defined as that estimate yielding the highest lod score) is greater than +3, linkage is confirmed; when it is less than −2, linkage is rejected for the data set supported for that set of pedigrees.

The thousands of DNA markers that encompass the genetic map of the entire genome can be used to com-plete the "whole genome" search for disease genes. When markers are examined that have been systematically drawn from throughout the genome, they may suggest linkage between a disorder and specific chromosomal regions. Conversely, they may reject linkage to these regions, thereby contributing to an *exclusion map* for the disorder. Markers from several regions may be examined concurrently; such a simultaneous search of the genome may detect multiple loci that contribute to a disorder. Notably, because several loci are tested as candidates with whole genome scans, *P* values must be made lower than 0.05 to reject the null hypothesis.

It is worth emphasizing that linkage refers to the two loci and not to their associated alleles. Even if crossing over is rare and certain allele pairs are disproportionately represented within any given pedigree, recombination does occasionally occur and eventually results in a more random distribution of allele combinations within the population at large. Thus, linkage of two loci does not necessarily imply an association of specific disease and marker phenotypes in the general population. An exception occurs when disease and marker loci lie so near to each other that it takes many generations for the allele combinations to equilibrate. For example, if the two loci are separated by 1 cM, it will take 69 generations, or about 2,000 years, until the frequency of an allele combination goes halfway to its equilibrium value (Ott 1985).

NONPARAMETRIC APPROACHES

Genetic linkage studies have been successful in identifying genes that have a large effect on illness risk. But such studies are problematic when several genes of small effect cause a disorder, as is true in most psychiatric conditions. It is also difficult to find enough large families with members who are willing to take part in the study. In addition, when the mode of inheritance is unknown, then many different models and assumptions must be applied to the data, leading to significant statistical problems.

Nonparametric analyses represent alternative methods for evaluating genetic linkage. These studies can be conducted without making assumptions about the mode of inheritance. One commonly used nonparametric approach is the *affected sib-pair* strategy (McCarthy et al. 1998). This method compares siblings who are definitely affected or unaffected, so the boundary of the condition does not need to be defined. It examines the frequency with which two siblings, both affected with the disorder of interest, share 0, 1, or 2 alleles coinherited from a common ancestor at the locus of interest; such alleles are said to be *identical by descent*. Under the null hypothesis of no linkage, these frequencies are 1/4, 1/2, and 1/4, respectively. Statistically significant deviations from this distribution of frequencies suggest linkage.

Association studies can examine if a particular DNA polymorphism is associated with a disorder by comparing unrelated affected and unaffected individuals. Association studies can even identify genes of very small effect or those that participate in gene-environment interactions and may provide stronger statistical power than traditional linkage approaches (Risch and Merikangas 1996). A candidate gene study is a type of association study. Hypothesis-dependent candidate genes (those nominated by neurobiological clues to disease pathogenesis) and hypothesis-independent candidate genes (those put forward without regard to pathogenic hypotheses) may be explored. A method that is widely used to test candidate genes is allelic association, also called *linkage disequilibrium*. It can be used when most of the individuals with the disease are descended from a common ancestor in whom the disease mutation originated. Different allele frequencies will be found between individuals with the disease and the general population for markers that are very close to the disease gene. Methods have now been developed for testing association between hundreds of thousands of markers across the genome and phenotypes of interest. Figure 8–3 shows the theoretical risk of disease conferred by the assumption of allelic heterogeneity of additive effect of rare alleles versus that of multiple common interacting alleles. Figure 8–4 shows the genetic risk of schizophrenia as inferred in family studies of the disorder. Note the similarity of the curve produced by the family study data to that of the multiple common interacting alleles model shown in Figure 8–3.

ANTICIPATION, IMPRINTING, AND MITOCHONDRIAL INHERITANCE

A clinical phenomenon called *anticipation,* wherein the age at onset of disease decreases and the severity of disease increases in successive generations, has been recognized for many decades. With the discovery of expanding trinucleotide repeats in the early 1990s (Richards and Sutherland 1992), a convincing molecular mechanism was provided for this phenomenon. The phenomenon is now well described for several neuropsychiatric disorders, including myotonic dystrophy, fragile X syndrome, and Huntington's disease (HD), and there has been some evidence for anticipation in schizophrenia and bipolar disorder. Differences in the offspring's liability for illness due to the sex of the transmitting parent may be the result of genomic imprinting (Langlois 1994) or of mitochondrial inheritance. Genomic imprinting is the selective methylation of inherited chromosomes. Methylation

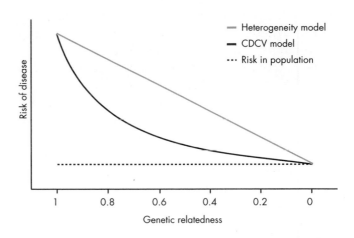

FIGURE 8–3. The common disease/common variant model. The risk of disease as a function of genetic relatedness to affected individuals is shown. Two hypothetical common diseases are considered (*blue and black lines*), each having the same monozygotic risk and the same underlying risk in the population (*red dashed line*). For the disease represented by the blue line, the risk of disease falls linearly with decreased genetic relatedness, consistent with disease heterogeneity, owing to the reduction in the number of shared rare alleles—the disease heterogeneity model. For the disease indicated by the black line, the fall in risk as a function of genetic relatedness is more rapid, as can occur when multiple common interacting alleles contribute to disease—an example of the common disease/common variant (CDCV) model.

Source. Reprinted from Wang WY, Barratt BJ, Clayton DG, et al.: "Genome-Wide Association Studies: Theoretical and Practical Concerns." *Nature Reviews Genetics* 6:109–118, 2005. Copyright 2005, Macmillan Magazines, Ltd. Used with permission.

affects the likelihood that genes will be transcribed and that correlating proteins will be made.

MOLECULAR APPROACHES

Once linkage analysis has implicated a particular chromosomal region in the etiology of a disorder, a variety of molecular genetic approaches may be used for identifying the disease gene and its pathological consequences. Thus, markers in linkage disequilibrium with, and thus in close proximity to, the disease gene may be identified. Genetic markers flanking the disease gene also may be recognized, thereby defining the minimal genetic region containing the disease gene. Overlapping cytogenetic anomalies producing the disease may then narrow this minimal genetic region. Alternatively, a more refined location for the putative disease locus may be provided by multilocus marker *haplotypes* surrounding the locus in genetically isolated populations (through a strategy known as *shared segment mapping*). The sequencing of the gene requires

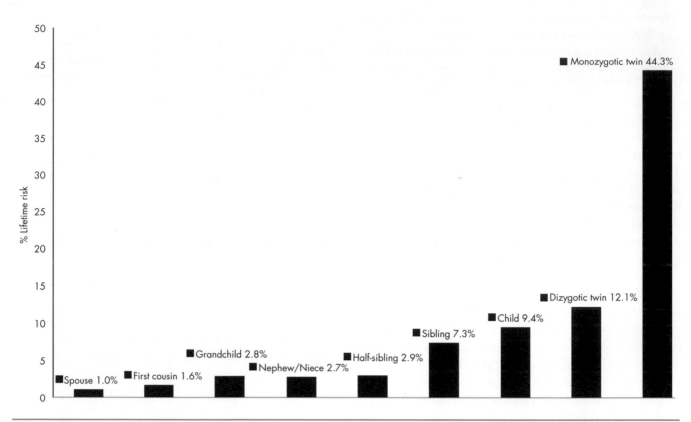

FIGURE 8–4. Family rates of schizophrenia.

Source. Data from McGue and Gottesman 1991.

advanced gene sequencing and analytic technology. Specific molecular abnormalities (insertions, deletions, and base substitutions) within the disease gene then may be discovered, and research then focuses on determining how the genetic malfunction causes disease. Genetically modified animals, particularly mice, which breed rapidly, have been used to study human genetics. Introducing the normal or disease gene into appropriate in vitro and in vivo model systems may determine the pathological consequences of the disease mutation (Figure 8–5).

Although there are no clear animal models for human psychiatric diseases, certain traits that vary continuously (and are likely polygenic) can be studied with quantitative trait loci analysis (Flint et al. 2005).

HUMAN GENOME

The sequencing of the human genome provides an enormous technical advance for the understanding of human disease (Collins et al. 2003). A draft sequence map of about 90% of the DNA in the human genome was completed in 2000 (International Human Genome Sequencing Consortium 2001; Venter et al. 2001), and the "finished" sequence (2.85 billion nucleotides, representing 99% of the euchromatic genome) was reported several years later (International Human Genome Sequencing Consortium 2004). The initial analysis supports the existence of approximately 20,000–25,000 genes in the human genome. This estimate is similar to that of other mammals and only somewhat larger than that of metazoan model system genomes, such as the fruitfly *Drosophila melanogaster* (M.D. Adams et al. 2000) and nematode *Caenorhabditis elegans* (C. elegans Sequencing Consortium 1998). Allied mammalian sequencing projects in the mouse (Mouse Genome Sequencing Consortium 2002), rat (Rat Genome Sequencing Project Consortium 2004), dog (Lindblad-Toh et al. 2005), and chimpanzee (Chimpanzee Sequencing and Analysis Consortium 2005) have been carried out, with more under way. Sequences from diverse mammals such as the rabbit, elephant, armadillo, tenrec, and hedgehog will assist in understanding the evolution of the mammalian lineage. The frog, chicken, and several species of fish have also been sequenced and will provide information about vertebrate evolution. The large amount of data from vertebrate species will provide much useful information in terms of comparative genomics. For example, highly conserved sequences not coding for proteins that are shared across the vertebrate phylogeny may suggest important regulatory functions (Boffelli et al. 2004; Dermitzakis et al. 2003).

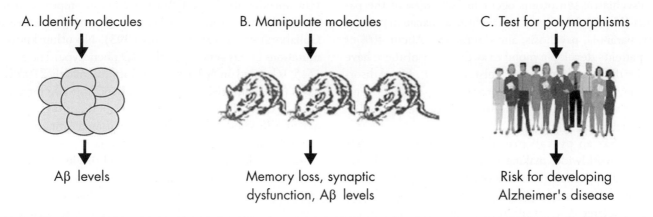

A. Identify molecules

Aβ levels

B. Manipulate molecules

Memory loss, synaptic
dysfunction, Aβ levels

C. Test for polymorphisms

Risk for developing
Alzheimer's disease

FIGURE 8–5. Alzheimer's disease genetic research strategy. The candidate molecule (A), or the molecular pathway to which it belongs, can be manipulated in animal models using transgenic technologies (B). In the case of Alzheimer's disease, this manipulation should phenocopy the behavioral, electrophysiological, and biochemical phenotype of Alzheimer's disease. Genomic screens can be performed in humans, testing whether polymorphisms in the molecular pathway increase the risk of Alzheimer's disease (C).

Source. Reprinted from Lewandowski NM, Small SA: "Brain Microarray: Finding Needles in Molecular Haystacks." *The Journal of Neuroscience* 25:10341–10346, 2005. Used with permission.

A particularly interesting component of the effort to sequence the human genome was the discovery of vast numbers of genetic variants in the form of SNPs. These single base changes (e.g., an "A" is substituted by a "G") in genomic sequence occur every few hundred base pairs throughout the genome. Some occur in all human populations, reflecting their ancient age, whereas others occur in individual populations, evidence of a more recent origin. It is estimated that 10 million of these variants occur within the genome. Some occur in functional regions of genes, often altering gene function, but the vast majority occur in intronic regions or in areas between genes and are less likely to have a biological effect. Given their density, SNPs are useful markers for linkage and association studies (Martin et al. 2000). The discovery that SNPs that are close to one another are often inherited in blocks of low genetic diversity led to the idea that analyzing a select set of these SNPs would allow researchers to analyze a large segment of the genome without having to examine all DNA variation while attempting to map diseases in humans (Gabriel et al. 2002; Johnson et al. 2001). The International HapMap Project was initiated to understand the patterns of DNA variation across major human populations (The International HapMap Consortium 2003). This project genotyped some 5.8 million SNPs in 270 persons from Utah; Nigeria; Tokyo, Japan; and Beijing, China, and found patterns of genetic diversity common to all populations, as well as those unique to each group (The International HapMap Consortium 2005). This freely available data can be used by investigators to identify genetic determinants of common diseases and has led to reports of association to genes for age-related macular degeneration and Parkinson's disease (PD)

(R.J. Klein et al. 2005; Maraganore et al. 2005). The prospect of using these tools for discovery of genes for many of the disorders described in this chapter is reasonable.

BASAL GANGLIA DISEASE

HUNTINGTON'S DISEASE

In 1872, George Huntington described a familial illness he found in his Long Island, New York, practice: it was characterized by dancelike movements and "insanity." The illness appeared in midlife, afflicted men and women equally, did not skip generations, and led to early death. In 1908, the famed physician William Osler described HD as having an autosomal dominant mode of inheritance with complete penetrance: he noted that affected individuals usually had an affected parent, and conversely, approximately one-half of the offspring of affected parents were themselves affected. As early as 1932, Vessie noted that HD was prevalent throughout the world. Over the ensuing century, HD has been more completely described and its mutant gene and gene product identified, isolated, and well studied.

HD is characterized by progressive dementia, chorea, and psychiatric symptoms. The mean age at onset is about 40 years, but its symptoms can occur as early as age 2 and as late as age 80–90. HD usually causes death within 15–20 years of onset (Margolis and Ross 2003). In about 10% of the individuals with HD, the onset of symptoms occurs before age 20 (Gusella et al. 1993). Juvenile-onset HD or the "Westphal variant" is characterized by akinesia and rigidity instead of chorea, as well as a more rapid and severe course of illness.

Psychiatric symptoms occur in 70%–80% of the patients (Harper 1996) and can include a change in personality, paranoia, psychosis, and depression. About 40% of the patients develop a mood disorder; 25% of these have bipolar disorder (Peyser and Folstein 1990). Mood disorder may antedate other symptoms by 2–20 years (Folstein et al. 1983). In HD, the suicide rate is estimated to be as high as 12% (Harper 1996).

HD has an overall prevalence of 5–10 cases per 100,000 worldwide, making it the most common neurodegenerative disorder (Landles and Bates 2004). However, prevalence has been found to be higher in some places because of a large concentration of affected families; for example, the prevalence is more than 100 per 100,000 in a specific region of Venezuela (Wexler et al. 2004).

The age at onset of HD is variable and depends on the sex and the age at onset of the transmitting parent. Anticipation, which means that each successive generation tends to develop HD at an earlier age than did the previous one, occurs and is most striking with paternal inheritance. Many individuals with early-onset disease inherit the *HD* gene from their father and show anticipation; that is, a significantly earlier age at onset compared with their father (Ridley et al. 1988), whereas many individuals with late-onset disease inherit the gene from their mother.

With the advent of genetic testing, it became possible to stratify at-risk relatives into gene-positive and gene-negative subgroups. A well-designed longitudinal study with multiple comparisons showed no cognitive differences between these two groups, suggesting that factors other than genetic susceptibility to HD account for differences in cognition between nominally at-risk persons and healthy control subjects (Giordani et al. 1995). However, genetic testing enables study of putative preclinical HD: asymptomatic gene carriers have declines in putamen volume (G.J. Harris et al. 1999) and mean annual striatal loss of dopamine receptors (T.C. Andrews et al. 1999) intermediate between HD patients and gene-negative at-risk individuals.

Genetics

HD is transmitted in an autosomal dominant fashion. Heterozygous inactivation of the *HD* gene as a result of chromosomal translocation is not associated with an abnormal phenotype (Ambrose et al. 1994).

In 1983, the gene responsible for HD was mapped to the short arm of chromosome 4 by the use of a linked polymorphic marker (Gusella et al. 1983). This evidence made it possible to detect HD allele carriers presymptomatically and also confirmed that HD is truly a dominant genetic condition (R.H. Myers et al. 1989; Wexler et al. 1987). Ten years later, in 1993, the genetic abnormality responsible for

HD was identified as a CAG trinucleotide-repeat expansion in the first exon of a novel gene (Huntington Disease Collaborative Research Group 1993). No other known mutations in this gene cause the HD phenotype. The gene, *IT15*, is located on 4p16.3; it spans approximately 210 kilobases (kb), comprises 67 exons, and encodes two messenger RNA (mRNA) species with a predicted protein product of 348 kilodaltons (kDa), known as huntingtin (see the following subsection "Huntingtin").

The explanation for the "parental origin effect" became clear when the *HD* gene was identified and cloned and its nature of mutation understood. Age at onset was found to be inversely related to the length of trinucleotide repeats in the gene (Figure 8–6) (Margolis and Ross 2003). The sex of the transmitting parent is a major factor influencing the trinucleotide expansion (Telenius et al. 1993). CAG repeats tend to expand modestly from one generation to the next but can double in length when passed from father to child. These dramatic expansions occur during spermatogenesis; examination of sperm DNA shows variation in trinucleotide repeat length among individual sperm (Leeflang et al. 1995; MacDonald et al. 1993). CAG expansions likely propagate through the formation of stable hairpin structures and mismatched duplexes during gametogenesis (Mariappan et al. 1998).

The CAG repeat is highly polymorphic in the general population and ranges from 6 to 35 copies (Margolis and Ross 2003); 99% of people have fewer than 30 repeats. Individuals with HD, however, have more than 39 repeats and a median of 44 repeats (Kremer et al. 1994). Almost all individuals (>99%) with a clinical diagnosis of HD have CAG trinucleotide expansion of the *HD* gene. Adult-onset HD (ages 35–55) is associated with 40–50 CAG repeats; juvenile-onset HD is associated with repeat lengths of more than 64 CAG units. Spontaneous HD occurs when trinucleotide repeats expand beyond a threshold length of about 37 copies. Individuals with 36–39 repeats may or may not develop HD (Margolis and Ross 2003).

Multiple studies have shown that the CAG repeat size and the age at onset of HD are inversely correlated but that for a given repeat size, there is a wide range of onset ages. Thus, the use of repeat size to predict the age at onset is not particularly useful (Gusella et al. 1993). This suggests the influence of as-yet-unknown genetic, environmental, and stochastic modifying factors, as does the fact that individuals with 36–39 CAG repeats may develop the disease late in life or not at all. CAG repeat lengths also are associated with the age at onset of psychiatric symptoms and the presence of intranuclear inclusions but not with disease duration, which is invariably 15–20 years. The CAG expansion within the *HD* gene is thus a highly sensitive and specific marker for the inherit-

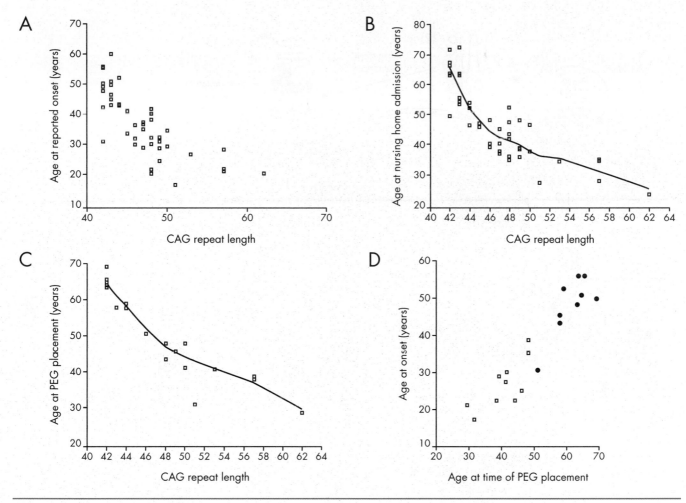

FIGURE 8–6. CAG repeats in Huntington's disease. (*A*) Relationship between CAG repeat length and age at onset of Huntington's disease (HD). CAG repeat length is inversely correlated with age at onset of HD; $r=-0.77$. (*B*) Relationship between CAG repeat length and age at nursing home admission. CAG repeat length is inversely correlated with age at nursing home admission; $r=-0.81$. (*C*) Relationship between CAG repeat length and age at percutaneous endoscopic gastrostomy (PEG) placement. CAG repeat length is inversely correlated with age at PEG placement; $r=-0.91$. (*D*) Relationship between age at onset of HD and age at PEG, stratified by the median CAG repeat length. *Boxes* represent individuals with CAG repeat length >46. *Filled circles* represent individuals with CAG repeat length ≤46. In a regression model, both age at onset ($P=0.001$) and CAG repeat length ($P=0.001$) were associated with age at PEG placement.

Source Reprinted from Marder K, Sandler S, Lechich A, et al.: "Relationship Between CAG Repeat Length and Late Stage Outcomes in Huntington's Disease." *Neurology* 59:1622–1624. Used with permission.

ance of the HD mutation (Kremer et al. 1994). Rapid and accurate diagnosis can be made with polymerase chain reaction–based tests, even in utero (Alford et al. 1996).

Huntingtin. The *HD* gene codes for huntingtin, a protein that bears no significant similarity to any known protein. Its known functions include transcriptional regulation, intracellular transport, and protection against neuronal apoptosis, and it is also involved in the endosome-lysosome pathway (Landles and Bates 2004). It is highly conserved across species and is expressed broadly across the organism during all stages of development. It

is found in the cell body, nucleus, dendrites and nerve terminals of neurons as well as mitochondria, Golgi apparatus, and endoplasmic reticulum (Landles and Bates 2004). Homozygous inactivation of huntingtin in mouse models was found to be lethal: embryos did not develop organs and died before embryonic day 8.5. Neuropathological analysis of these embryos showed apoptotic cell death in the embryonic ectoderm (Duyao et al. 1995), thus confirming huntingtin's involvement in prevention of neuronal apoptosis (Figure 8–7).

In another investigation (Mangiarini et al. 1996), a mouse model with a transgene of the huntingtin gene

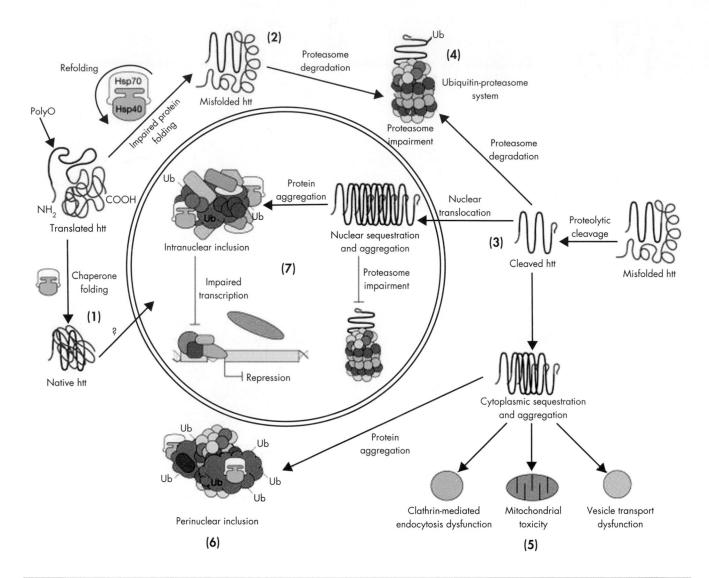

FIGURE 8–7.   Model for cellular pathogenesis in Huntington's disease. The molecular chaperones Hsp70 and Hsp40 promote the folding of newly synthesized huntingtin (htt) into a native structure. Wild-type htt is predominantly cytoplasmic and probably functions in vesicle transport, cytoskeletal anchoring, clathrin-mediated endocytosis, neuronal transport, or postsynaptic signaling. htt may be transported into the nucleus and have a role in transcriptional regulation (1). Chaperones can facilitate the recognition of abnormal proteins, promoting either their refolding or ubiquitination (Ub) and subsequent degradation by the 26S proteasome. The HD mutation induces conformational changes and is likely to cause the abnormal folding of htt, which, if not corrected by chaperones, leads to the accumulation of misfolded htt in the cytoplasm (2). Alternatively, mutant htt might also be proteolytically cleaved, giving rise to amino-terminal fragments that form sheet structures (3). Ultimately, toxicity might be elicited by mutant full-length htt or by cleaved N-terminal fragments, which may form soluble monomers, oligomers, or large insoluble aggregates. In the cytoplasm, mutant forms of htt may impair the ubiquitin-proteasome system (UPS), leading to the accumulation of more proteins that are misfolded (4). These toxic proteins might also impair normal vesicle transport and clathrin-mediated endocytosis. Also, the presence of mutant htt could activate proapoptotic proteins directly or indirectly by mitochondrial damage, leading to greater cellular toxicity and other deleterious effects (5). In an effort to protect itself, the cell accumulates toxic fragments into ubiquitinated cytoplasmic perinuclear aggregates (6). In addition, mutant htt can be translocated into the nucleus to form nuclear inclusions, which may disrupt transcription and the UPS (7).

Source.   Reprinted from Landles C, Bates GP: "Huntingtin and the Molecular Pathogenesis of Huntington's Disease." *EMBO Report* 5:958–963, 2004. Copyright 2004, Macmillan Publishers, Ltd. Used with permission.

with 115–150 CAG repeats yielded a phenotype that included progressive involuntary stereotypies, tremors, seizures, reduction in brain and body weight, and early death. These mice did not show neurodegeneration but had early signs of neural apoptosis and selective reductions in receptors (dopamine, acetylcholine, and glutamate receptors) in the brain. In a third attempt, transgenic mice were created with full huntingtin complementary DNA (cDNA) with 89 CAG repeats. The phenotype of these mice more closely resembled human HD, with initial hyperactivity yielding to hypoactivity, subsequent akinesia, and death; neuropathological analysis showed selective neurodegeneration in the striatum and cortex, gliosis, and neuronal loss of about 20% (Reddy et al. 1999).

The critical pathogenic event in HD may be accelerated apoptosis. Apoptotic DNA fragments have been found in postmortem striatal tissue of HD patients (Butterworth et al. 1998). Mutant huntingtin is cleaved by caspase-3, an apoptotic enzyme, and this cleavage is enhanced by polyglutamate length (Martindale et al. 1998; Wellington et al. 1998). Mutant huntingtin is expressed abundantly by presynaptic cholinergic interneurons and cortical pyramidal cells that activate the striatal neurons that die (Fusco et al. 1999). This lends credence to the idea that excessive synaptic release of glutamate leads to excitotoxic striatal cell death (Sapp et al. 1999).

Potential Treatment

Thus far, only palliative treatment of symptoms exists for HD. A novel approach to therapy is to introduce trophic factors that may delay or retard excitotoxic damage of striatal neurons. In a nongenetic animal model for HD, in which rodents received intrastriatal injection of excitatory amino acids, selective destruction of medium spiny neurons and motor and cognitive changes resulted, similar to what occurs in HD. When these animals received fibroblast grafts that secrete trophic factors, degeneration of striatal neurons was retarded, and motor and cognitive defects were prevented (Kordower et al. 1999). Small grafts induce widespread expression of catalase, a free radical scavenger, throughout the striatum. Neuroprotection is likely conferred by nerve growth factors' antioxidative properties or their effect on adenosine triphosphate (ATP) production. Simple infusion of trophic factors themselves was not effective.

Another potential therapy is the use of antioxidants (such as coenzyme Q10 and ubiquinone) that protect against glutamate toxicity and rescue mitochondrial metabolism and administration of creatine to buffer against energy depletion (Grunewald and Beal 1999). Others have proposed antiapoptosis agents, immunosuppressants, and fetal cell transplant as possible therapeutic approaches for this fatal disease that as yet has no clear treatment.

PARKINSON'S DISEASE

PD is a progressive neurological disorder that is caused by the loss of dopaminergic neurons in the substantia nigra and nigrostriatal pathway of the midbrain. It was first described as "Shaking Palsy" in 1817 by James Parkinson because of the presence of a resting tremor and rigidity. The cardinal symptoms are poverty or slowness of movement (akinesia or bradykinesia), rigidity of the trunk and limb muscles, tremor or trembling that typically begins in the hands ("pill rolling"), and postural instability with impaired balance and coordination. Other common symptoms are a waxy facial expression, stooped posture, shuffling gait, and micrographia. The motor deficits arise from impairments in initiation, planning, and sequencing of voluntary movements. Some patients additionally experience difficulty in swallowing and chewing, speech impairments, and sleep disturbances. An associated dysfunction of the autonomic nervous system can cause urinary incontinence, constipation, sexual dysfunction, hypotension, and skin problems.

Many PD patients develop psychiatric syndromes, particularly depression, emotionality, and panic attacks, even in advance of the neurological signs. Treatment-emergent symptoms can include visual hallucinations, paranoid delusions, mania, and delirium. A sizable minority of patients develop cognitive slowing ("bradyphrenia"), and up to 40% of end-stage patients have dementia (Cedarbaum and McDowell 1987).

The onset is often subtle and gradual. Thereafter, the symptoms and their progression are quite variable, but PD frequently progresses to curtail walking, talking, and performing even simple tasks of daily living. There is no laboratory test for PD, which is diagnosed on the basis of the history and physical findings. The neuropathology includes a loss of pigmented (dopaminergic) neurons in the zona compacta of the substantia nigra and the presence of Lewy bodies in the remaining neurons. Noninvasive neuroimaging techniques can be used to examine the nigrostriatal pathophysiology (see Fischman 2005). Lewy bodies in other areas (cortex, amygdala, locus coeruleus, hypothalamus, dorsal medial nucleus of the vagus, and nucleus basalis of Meynert) may explain the nonmotor symptoms.

Epidemiological Studies

PD is a common condition, affecting about 1% of adults older than 60 years. Differences in case ascertainment and diagnostic criteria limit the ability to compare the incidence and prevalence of PD, but substantial variability is found between and within countries. The prevalence estimate is 133 in 100,000; the average age at onset is 63 years but may be increasing. The incidence of the disorder has been reported as 11 in 100,000 person-years (see Checkoway and Nelson 1999). PD may affect men at a slightly higher rate than women. Early-onset PD begins between age 21 and 40 and accounts for 5%–10% of patients. The prevalence of PD increases with age, but it is not just an acceleration of normal aging; age is associated with a decline in striatal dopamine but not with changes in the caudate and putamen (van Dyck et al. 2002).

Secondary PD that is drug induced by dopamine antagonists (neuroleptics, antiemetics) or, less often, by calcium channel blockers is symmetric and resolves with drug discontinuation. PD can also be secondary to cerebrovascular disease that causes multiple lacunar strokes.

Family Studies

Most PD patients have no family history, although a 2- to 14-fold increase in PD is seen in close relatives of affected individuals (Gasser et al. 1998). The greatest risk is found for the relatives of young probands; thus, 8.3% of the sibs of probands ages 35–44 were affected compared with 1.4% of the sibs of probands ages 65–74 years. Interestingly, PD is also increased in the relatives of probands with Alzheimer's disease, suggesting an etiological overlap between these disorders (Hofman et al. 1989). A strong familial nature for a syndrome is consistent with either shared genes or shared environments. Twin studies can be used to better disentangle these etiologies. Twin studies show that MZ and DZ twins of PD patients older than 60 have a similar concordance, consistent with the importance of environmental exposures, while for those with PD whose age at onset was 50 or younger, increased concordance in MZ twins was found (see Tanner et al. 1999). This suggests that, as in other diseases, there may be an early-onset form that has a greater genetic component. Some cases of PD can be attributed to specific gene mutations and toxic exposures, but the etiology of most cases is unknown. PD is a complex genetic disorder that probably results from the actions of multiple factors, including vulnerability genes, environmental exposures, aging, and gene-environment interactions.

Environmental Exposures

Research examining a role for environmental toxins in the etiology of PD was stimulated by the finding that exposure to MPTP (1-methyl-4-phenyl-1,2,3,6-tetrahydropyridine), a toxic by-product made in the clandestine synthesis of a recreational drug, caused persistent PD in very young substance abusers (Langston et al. 1983) and in higher primates (Marsden and Jenner 1987). MPTP freely crosses the blood-brain barrier, where it is converted to a metabolite that is selectively taken up into dopaminergic neurons. The metabolite inhibits mitochondrial metabolism, leading to a decline in ATP and an accumulation of free radicals and oxidative damage. Investigation of the pathophysiology of MPTP yielded hypotheses about the etiology and pathophysiology of sporadic PD.

The risk for PD is also associated with other neurotoxins, including trace metals, cyanide, lacquer thinner, organic solvents, carbon monoxide, mercury, and carbon disulfide. In North America and Europe, early-onset PD appears to be associated with rural residence, perhaps reflecting exposure to pesticides, well water, or other toxins (Olanow and Tatton 1999). Preclinical parkinsonian symptoms are more common in regions of Israel where carbamates and organophosphates are detected (Herishanu et al. 1998). As reviewed by Kamel and Hoppin (2004), the accumulated data are compelling that pesticide exposure is associated with a significantly increased risk of PD, with risk estimates ranging from 1.6- to 7-fold (D.G. Le Couteur et al. 1999). The greatest evidence for association with a specific pesticide may be for paraquat (Liou et al. 1997), which produces selective degeneration of neurons (McCormack et al. 2002). Most studies focus on organopesticides, but other types of pesticides, including organochlorines, carbamates, fungicides, and fumigants, are known to be neurotoxic and may have similar effects. These toxins need not be selective for dopaminergic neurons because dopaminergic neurons may be comparatively more vulnerable than others in the brain. In sporadic PD, it may be that oxidant damage interferes with proteasomal cleavage of key gene products (synuclein), therefore leading to Lewy body formation (Jenner and Olanow 1998).

Infection may also increase the risk for PD, although these cases may be clinically and pathologically distinct from other PD (Gamboa et al. 1974). The great influenza pandemic of 1918 was linked to postencephalitic PD. Population studies also suggest that the risk for PD is increased by intrauterine influenza virus exposure, perhaps by the depletion of neurons in the developing substantia nigra (Mattock et al. 1988).

Cigarette smoking and tobacco use have an apparently protective effect against PD according to numerous designs that showed lower relative risks for smokers than for nonsmokers (reviewed in Checkoway and Nelson 1999). However, Allam et al. (2004) recently reviewed these studies and concluded that the apparently protective effect of cigarette smoking against PD actually resulted from reverse causation. Those individuals who developed PD were less likely to have strong smoking habits at younger ages, perhaps because of prodromal condition. This line of research remains undetermined. Certainly, cigarette smoking would not be advanced as a protective strategy, in any case. Caffeine also may be protective against PD (G.W. Ross et al. 2000).

There are no consistent findings regarding PD and diet, despite expectations that vitamins A, C, and E would be protective given their antioxidant properties and that a high-fat diet would increase risk because of the potential for free radical generation (Checkoway and Nelson 1999). One study found an odds ratio of 9.0 for very high intake of animal fat (Logroscino et al. 1998).

Susceptibility Genes

Although strong familial patterns may also arise from shared exposures to toxins, several genes have been identified for patients with juvenile familial PD. These account for a small minority of cases but have illuminated pathology in the ubiquitin-proteasome system as the mechanism of neurodegeneration that may underlie PD in both familial and sporadic disease (reviewed by Samii et al. 2004). *PARK1* was the first gene linked to autosomal dominant PD. It codes for α-synuclein protein,

which is the major component of Lewy bodies. The gene may be involved in synaptic vesicle transport or uptake. In addition, elevation of this protein by a triplication of the normal gene (*PARK4*) was shown to precipitate early-onset PD in other families. The excessive or mutant α-synuclein protein may misfold or aggregate, causing it to be resistant to degradation by the ubiquitin-proteasome system (Figure 8–8). The most common gene defects may be in the *PARK2* gene, initially identified in recessive familial cases (Lucking et al. 2000). It codes for parkin, an enzyme (ubiquitin ligase) that is required for normal protein degradation. There are several parkin mutations, which may explain a half or more of the early-onset and juvenile-onset cases (see West et al. 2002), with other cases arising in parkin mutation heterozygotes. This defect leads to cell loss that typically is unaccompanied by Lewy bodies. Other mutations are described in the ubiquitin C-terminal hydrolase, which participates in the ubiquitin metabolism (Leroy et al. 1998): the DJ1 protein, which might be implicated in the response to oxidative stress (Bonifati et al. 2003); and *PINK1* (PTEN [phosphatase and tensin homologue deleted on chromosome 10]-induced kinase 1), which is a mitochondrial gene (Valente et al. 2004).

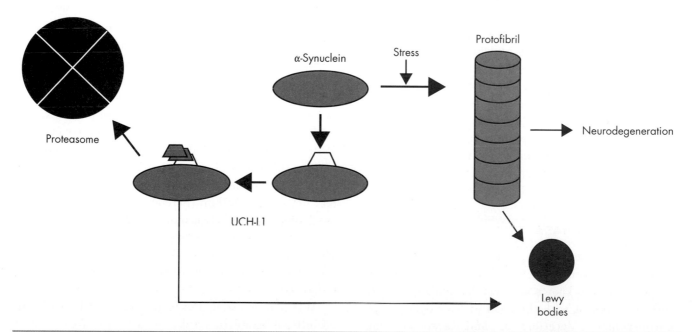

FIGURE 8–8. Processing of α-synuclein, the major component of Lewy bodies, in Parkinson's disease. The processing of α-synuclein by the ubiquitin-proteasome system can be potentially neurotoxic. In Parkinson's disease (PD), α-synuclein can oligomerize into protofibrils that in turn are potentially neurotoxic. The α-synuclein molecule can also be monoubiquitinated or polyubiquinated; in either form, it can be processed by the proteasome and is involved in various mechanisms of pathogenesis of PD. UCH-L1 = ubiquitin carboxy-terminal hydrolase L1.

Source. Adapted from Hasimoto M, Kawahara K, Bar-On P, et al.: "The Role of α-Synuclein Assembly and Metabolism in the Pathogenesis of Lewy Body Disease." *Journal of Molecular Neuroscience* 24(3):343–352, 2004. Used with permission.

Molecular Mechanisms

Overall, the genetic findings provide strong evidence that the pathophysiology of PD involves a dysregulation of protein degradation by the ubiquitin-proteasome system. The ubiquitin-proteasome pathway affects many cellular processes and is a fundamental component of cell cycle regulation, although how it leads to cell death of dopaminergic neurons is still under investigation. Ubiquitin molecules are normally attached to damaged proteins as a signal for degradation.

Most cases do not involve gene defects in this pathway, suggesting that the damage is extrinsically determined. Such damage may arise from mitochondrial toxicity, oxidative stress, excitotoxicity, apoptosis, and inflammation (Gasser 2001). In some individuals, the genetic susceptibility may be related to diminished detoxification of external agents by endogenous enzymes (Kuhn and Muller 1997; Langston 1998). Reports have linked PD to several metabolic enzymes. Cytochrome P450 (CYP) D6, a hepatic enzyme, and variants in CYPD6 weakly increase the risk for PD but may interact with glutathione S-transferase to elevate the risk for PD by 11- to 14-fold above that of the general population (Foley and Riederer 1999). An association between slow acetylation (N-acetyltransferase) and PD has been reported (Bandmann et al. 1997); slow acetylators may metabolize toxins more slowly, therefore potentiating their effect on vulnerable neurons. Also, in individuals with pesticide exposure, an association was found between PD and polymorphisms in a glutathione transferase locus (Menegon et al. 1998); the glutathione pathway plays a role in scavenging free radicals. Together, these observations suggest that many PD cases arise through a two-hit gene-environment interaction pathway. In this model, risk entails both the genetic vulnerability and the toxic exposure, and neither factor is a sufficient cause of the disease.

WILSON'S DISEASE

In 1912, Wilson described a familial nervous disease associated with cirrhosis of the liver. Patients with this disorder (which is also known as hepatolenticular degeneration) may present with the triad of liver dysfunction, neuropsychiatric deterioration, and Kayser-Fleischer rings of the cornea. Renal impairment in patients with Wilson's disease (WD) also may be present. The prevalence of WD is 1 in 30,000 (Schilsky 2002). Onset may be as early as age 4 or as late as the fifth decade.

WD occurs as a result of excessive copper accumulation and failure of copper excretion. Normally, copper is extracted from the portal circulation by hepatocytes and then either used for cellular metabolism, incorporated into ceruloplasmin, or excreted into bile. These last two pathways are impaired in WD. WD is diagnosed by measuring ceruloplasmin oxidase activity and hepatic copper content. A standard for disease diagnosis is the presence of more than 250 μg of copper per gram of liver (dry weight).

In WD, toxic amounts of copper accumulate first in the liver, where it leads to impaired protein synthesis, lipid peroxidation of membranes, DNA oxidative damage, and a reduced amount of cellular antioxidants. Mitochondria are especially vulnerable to this free radical damage and show early structural damage. Hepatocellular necrosis and apoptosis occur. Excess copper then spills out from damaged hepatocytes into the serum to infiltrate the brain, kidneys, and corneas. The basal ganglia are especially susceptible to the toxic effects of copper, possibly because the copper-containing enzyme dopamine β-hydroxylase is synthesized there (Ferenci 2004).

Neurological features in WD include spasticity, rigidity, dysarthria, dysphagia, apraxia, and a flapping tremor of the wrist and shoulder. Psychiatric manifestations are frequent and include personality changes, depressive episodes, cognitive dysfunction, and psychosis (Akil et al. 1991; Dening 1991). About one-third of the patients have psychiatric symptoms at the time of initial diagnosis (Ferenci 2004), and 10% of the patients present initially with only psychiatric symptoms (Akil et al. 1991). Although neuropsychiatric symptoms are nearly always accompanied by ocular Kayser-Fleischer rings (Schilsky 2002), they are not correlated with serum copper levels (Rathbun 1996) and hence may reflect active neurotoxicity rather than total copper load (Estrov et al. 2000). Interestingly, psychiatric symptoms are often exacerbated with chelation therapy of excess copper (Dening 1991; McDonald and Lake 1995). Magnetic resonance imaging shows loss of gray and white matter throughout the brain, including the caudate nucleus, brain stem, cerebrum, and cerebellum (Ferenci 2004).

Earlier onset of WD is more likely to be characterized by hepatic rather than neuropsychiatric signs (Cox et al. 1972). Nonetheless, many patients with signs of intellectual deterioration and movement disorder may present before age 10.

WD is progressive and fatal if untreated; death can occur from hemolytic crisis or liver failure. Treatment of WD involves removal of excess copper, either by using a chelating agent such as penicillamine (Walshe 1956) or trientine or by blocking intestinal copper absorption with zinc salts (Hoogenraad et al. 1979). Liver transplant is also an effective treatment and cure for end-stage WD. Possible therapies in the future include liver cell transplantation and gene therapy with adenoviral vectors carrying the normal WD gene.

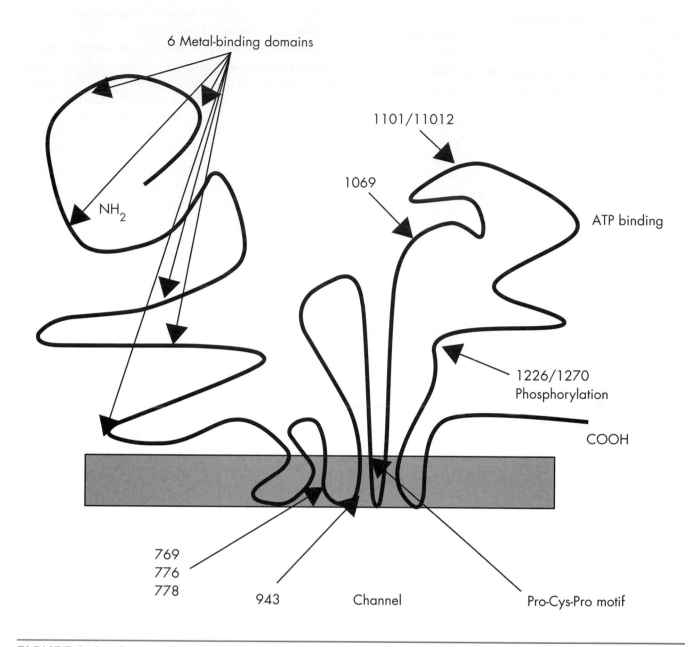

FIGURE 8–9. P-type adenosine triphosphatase (ATPase) in Wilson's disease. P-type adenosine triphosphatase (ATPase) is responsible for the binding and transport of copper. Note the six copper-binding domains, the adenosine triphosphate (ATP)-binding domain, the phosphorylation domain, and the channel domain. ATP=adenosine triphosphate; Pro-Cys-Pro=proline-cysteine-proline.

Source. Reprinted from El-Youssef M: "Wilson Disease." *Mayo Clinic Proceedings* 78(9):1126–1136, 2003. Used with permission.

Genetics

WD is an autosomal recessive disorder. The *WD* locus (*WND*) was assigned to the long arm of chromosome 13 by close linkage with the red cell esterase D locus in a large Israeli-Arab kindred (Frydman et al. 1985). Bonne-Tamir et al. (1986) confirmed this linkage in two unrelated Druze kindreds and placed the *WND* locus distal to esterase D on chromosome 13. Haplotype analysis of 13q14.3 further defined the region surrounding the *WND* locus (G.R. Thomas et al. 1994). The identification of the

WD gene, named *ATP7B*, was enabled by genetic study of Menkes' syndrome, which entails mutation in a related but different copper transporter (and which leads to copper deficiency rather than excess) (Daniel et al. 2004). Hence Petrukhin et al. (1994) reported the complete exon/intron structure of the *WD* gene, and individuals with WD were confirmed to have mutations at this locus. *ATP7B* has been cloned and found to encode a putative copper-transporting P-type ATPase (Figure 8–9) (Bull et al. 1993; Tanzi et al. 1993; Yamaguchi et al. 1993).

Identification and Diagnosis

More than 200 disease-specific mutations have been identified in WD (Schilsky 2002), including point mutations, deletions, insertions, and missense and splice site mutations. Most mutations occur either in transmembranous regions or at a site involved in ATP binding. The most frequent mutation (30% of patients of European descent) is a point mutation at position 1069, in which glutamine replaces histamine (H1069Q), which may be associated with later presentation and primarily neurological manifestation (Schiefermeier et al. 2000). The large number of mutations reduces the feasibility of a general screening test at this time. However, newer sequence analysis methodologies that screen the entire coding system of *ATP7B* may make such general screening plausible in the future. This will depend on differentiating disease-specific mutations from normal polymorphisms of the gene. At this time, haplotype analysis can be used for screening family members of patients with WD. At-risk siblings can have genetic and biochemical testing as toddlers; minimally toxic zinc therapy can begin as early as age 3 years to reduce copper absorption.

ILLNESSES OF CHILDHOOD

AUTISM

Autism is an uncommon neuropsychiatric disorder that is manifested by profound impairments in verbal and nonverbal communication and reciprocal social interrelationships and by interests and behaviors that are often repetitive and restrictive (American Psychiatric Association 2000). Onset of autism typically occurs before age 3 years, and the disorder persists throughout the life of the patient. Estimates of the population prevalence of autism are on the order of 5–10 per 10,000 (Bryson et al. 1988; Fombonne 1999). A consistently observed male-to-female ratio of 3–4:1 has been noted, with females often having more severe impairment, particularly in IQ (Volkmar et al. 1993).

Family Studies

Beginning in the 1980s, family studies in which siblings of autistic probands were directly assessed showed rates of autism in the siblings of 2%–6% (Ritvo et al. 1989; Tsai et al. 1981). Another 20 subsequent studies continued to support these findings (Bailey et al. 1998). Szatmari (1999) pooled many such studies and estimated the risk to siblings as 2.2% (95% confidence interval [CI] = 1.1%–3.3%). Second- and third-degree relatives of autistic probands also have been assessed (DeLong and Dwyer 1988; Jorde et al. 1991; Pickles et al. 1995; Szatmari et al. 1995). These studies suggested an overall rate of autism of 0.2% in second-degree relatives and 0.1% in third-degree relatives. This dramatic decline in relative risk compared with that of first-degree relatives suggests a polygenic complex disorder. Family study data have been examined to determine whether a broader phenotype of pervasive developmental disorders (PDDs), of which autism is one, or other traits that occur in the relatives of autistic probands should be considered as phenotypes. On the whole, this research indicated that relatives of autistic probands can have a spectrum of behavioral traits, from isolated communication impairments and social difficulties to more severe disorders in the PDD spectrum (reviewed in Bailey et al. 1998). Although suggestive, this area of investigation has not been completely resolved, and it is clear that no evidence exists for "a behavioral or cognitive profile that is either universal or specific" (Bailey et al. 1998).

Twin Studies

To determine whether the familial component of autism is genetic, several twin studies have been performed (Bailey et al. 1995; Folstein et al. 1977; Ritvo et al. 1985; Steffenburg et al. 1989). These investigations, with a total of 108 twin pairs, reported a concordance rate of 36%–91% for MZ twins and 0%–24% for DZ twins. Only one group saw any concordance between DZ pairs (Ritvo et al. 1985). The observed nonconcordance in the DZ twins was probably secondary to the small sample number and low recurrence rate seen in siblings in family studies. These concordance rates yield heritability estimates in the range of 90%. This suggests that a substantial portion of the liability to autism is genetic in origin. These data also highlight the nonmendelian nature of its inheritance, implying multiple genes and epistatic gene interactions. Twin studies also support the inheritance of a broader phenotype. In an early study involving 21 twin pairs, concordance for cognitive and social abnormalities was 82% for MZ pairs and 10% for DZ pairs (Folstein et al. 1977). In a follow-up study that included the original group plus 28 new twin pairs, concordance for cognitive and social disorders was 92% for MZ pairs and again 10% for DZ pairs (Bailey et al. 1995). Imaging of MZ twins concordant or discordant for autism suggests a complex picture, with discordant twins showing cerebral white matter volumes similar to each other yet different from nonautistic control subjects (Kates et al. 2004). Epidemiological data suggest that the process of twinning itself is not related to the high concordance rate (Hallmayer et al. 2002).

Adoption Studies

There are no known adoption studies for autistic disorder, although one study suggests that PDD-like traits are more common in biological relatives of PDD probands than in nonbiological (including adoptive) relatives (Szatmari et al. 2000).

High-Risk Studies

For several decades, clinicians have been describing the co-incidence of autism and various medical disorders. Depending on the stringency of the diagnostic criteria for autism and the comprehensiveness of the medical workup, this association is between 10% and 37% (Barton and Volkmar 1998; Gillberg and Coleman 1996; Rutter et al. 1994). Despite this variability in estimates and the ongoing debate on how they are derived, it is clear that the likelihood of a coexisting medical condition is related to a decreasing IQ (Ritvo et al. 1990; Steffenburg 1991). For example, one retrospective study that assessed 211 autistic subjects found that 24% of the subjects with an IQ greater than 50 had a broadly defined medical condition, whereas a full 40% of the individuals with an IQ less than 50 met the broad criteria for a medical condition (Barton and Volkmar 1998). Steffenburg (1991) used this association to propose potentially etiological subgroups of autism on the basis of the associated medical condition. These groupings included 1) pure hereditary autism, 2) other hereditary conditions (e.g., neurofibromatosis, tuberous sclerosis, fragile X syndrome), 3) other specific brain damage conditions (e.g., Möbius' syndrome, Rett's disorder), 4) nonspecific brain damage (e.g., epilepsy; hearing deficiencies; altered cerebrospinal fluid [CSF], electroencephalogram [EEG], computed tomography [CT] scan), and 5) unknown brain damage or genetic factors.

One well-documented disease association occurs with tuberous sclerosis. This condition is an autosomal dominant disorder involving the growth of hamartomas, which are abnormal benign lesions, in several organs, including the brain. The central nervous system (CNS) involvement is characterized by cortical and subependymal lesions, as well as seizures and mental retardation. Twenty-five percent of the patients with tuberous sclerosis also have autism, and up to 40% have a disorder in the PDD spectrum (Smalley et al. 1998). Tuberous sclerosis has been reported to occur in 1%–2% of the patients with autism (Smalley et al. 1992), and the rate is even higher in autistic individuals with a seizure disorder (Gillberg 1991). This co-occurrence between autism and tuberous sclerosis is much higher than would be predicted by prevalence rates of both of these rare disorders. Two genes have been identified—*TSC1* (Kandt et al. 1992) and *TSC2* (van Slegtenhorst et al. 1997)—whose gene products are known as hamartin and tuberin, respectively. The gene

products of both genes are thought to be tumor suppressors (A.J. Green et al. 1994; van Slegtenhorst et al. 1997).

Smalley et al. (1998) developed several hypotheses that may explain why genes thought to govern regulation of growth and differentiation could be associated with autism. First, and most favored, loss of tuberous sclerosis complex (TSC) protein function may lead to abnormal neural development in regions possibly related to autism. Second, TSC genes may actually be in close proximity, or linkage disequilibrium, to true autism genes. Finally, neuroanatomical and neuropsychological sequelae of tuberous sclerosis gene dysfunction, like seizures or tubers, may indirectly damage areas of the brain associated with autism. Further investigation of TSC gene products in neuronal function (Astrinidis et al. 2002; R.F. Lamb et al. 2000) may provide intriguing insights into one of a potential number of etiologies of autism.

Mode of Inheritance

Several patterns of inheritance have been offered for autism, most deriving from particular clinical findings. The observation that the prevalence among girls is lower than among boys, yet female probands often have more autistic relatives, suggested a multifactorial hypothesis composed of genetic and nongenetic factors (Tsai et al. 1981). Likewise, the high male-to-female ratio and association with fragile X syndrome have suggested X-linked mechanisms, although enthusiasm for this theory has been tempered by the lack of linkage findings on the X chromosome (see following subsection "Linkage Analysis"). Genomic imprinting also has been suggested as a mode of inheritance that attempts to solve the problem of unequal sex prevalence (Skuse 2000).

More formal attempts at understanding the mode of inheritance have had varied results. Ritvo et al. (1985) performed a classical segregation analysis on 46 multiple nuclear families (i.e., two or three autistic probands per family) and reported a segregation ratio close to that expected for an autosomal recessive mode of inheritance. They rejected both dominant and polygenic inheritance in these families. These data must be interpreted in light of the multiply affected ascertainment bias of the study. The same group produced different conclusions when they carried out a segregation analysis on all cases in a "well-defined" population (Jorde et al. 1991). Jorde et al. used a mixed model in 185 families and determined that the only inconsistent model was a single major locus model. Other analyses ruled out simple X-linked or imprinted X-linked segregation (Pickles et al. 2000). Pickles et al. (1995) used an analytic strategy that focused on the decrease in relative risk with degree of relatedness and estimated that three loci were most likely involved (range = 2–10). Together, these studies suggest that the interaction of multiple genes is more likely to cause autism than is a single major locus. The issues of selection resulting from low reproduction rates, phenotypic uncertainty, and genetic heterogeneity all complicate the elucidation of the mode of inheritance of autism. Attempts to determine clinical markers of heterogeneity have proven frustrating. One group found no obvious indicators of heterogeneity with estimations of clinical variability between and within MZ twin pairs (A. Le Couteur et al. 1996). A similar approach was used in 37 multiplex families, and again there was no concordance for IQ or specific autistic symptoms, although some repetitive and ritualistic behaviors seemed to show some intrafamily concordance (Spiker et al. 1994).

Linkage Analysis

The last decade has seen the first attempts to identify susceptibility loci for autism. Multiple international multicenter genome scans have been published. Genetic linkage has been reported on the X chromosome and all but 5 of the 22 autosomes (Folstein and Rosen-Sheidley 2001; Wassink et al. 2005). Our brief review focuses on 7q and 2q, two genomic regions that have been most consistently observed between the various linkage studies. The first region is on the long arm of chromosome 7.

The International Molecular Genetic Study of Autism Consortium (IMGSAC) examined 87 European affected sibling pairs and observed a high score of 2.53 on 7q, with the score increasing to 3.55 in a subgroup of 56 of 66 families from the United Kingdom (International Molecular Genetic Study of Autism Consortium 1998). Subsequent analyses that used more markers and sibling pairs continued to support linkage to this region (International Molecular Genetic Study of Autism Consortium 2001a, 2001b). These analyses also suggest parent of origin and sex-limited effects on several chromosomes, including chromosome 7 (J.A. Lamb et al. 2005). The Collaborative Linkage Study of Autism, which included 75 multiplex families and 416 markers (Collaborative Linkage Study of Autism 2001), found maximum multipoint heterogeneity lod scores of 2.2 for a 7q marker, under a recessive model with 29% of the families being linked to this region. Another group focused on a segment of 7q in 76 families and found some evidence for linkage in this region (Ashley-Koch et al. 1999), a finding that remained when more families were genotyped (Shao et al. 2002b). An independent study of 110 families initially found no support for 7q until the authors genotyped additional markers in the area after adding 50 more families, result-

ing in a multipoint lod score of 2.13 (J. Liu et al. 2001). Increasing the number of families to 345 led to somewhat diminished support for 7q (Yonan et al. 2003). The same family set was used to link the 7q region to quantitative phenotypes involving repetitive behaviors and language in 152 families (Alarcon et al. 2002), although adding 235 additional families diminished this finding (Alarcon et al. 2005). These families also yielded evidence for a sex-limited effect in these linkage analyses, although not on chromosome 7 (Stone et al. 2004). Other genome scans provide minimal support for the 7q region (Auranen et al. 2000; Philippe et al. 1999), but some do not (Risch et al. 1999).

Chromosome arm 2q has also emerged as a potential location for an autism gene or genes. IMGSAC has found varying levels of support for linkage on 2q, from a multipoint maximum lod score of 0.65 in 99 families at 103 cM (International Molecular Genetic Study of Autism Consortium 1998), increasing to 1.6 at 111 cM and to 3.74 at a more telomeric marker (206 cM), and using a broader phenotypic definition in a total of 152 families (International Molecular Genetic Study of Autism Consortium 2001a). Another group reported a multipoint heterogeneity lod score of 1.98 at 183 cM in 95 families (Buxbaum et al. 2001). A genome screen in 99 families showed a maximum lod score of 2.12 at 198 cM (Shao et al. 2002b), which increased to 2.86 in a subset of 45 families also segregating delays in phrase speech (Shao et al. 2002a).

From these studies, the region of 7q is clearly the most interesting. Other studies have focused linkage analyses on a region of common chromosomal abnormalities in autism and are discussed later in this chapter. The initial lack of consistent linkage findings on the X chromosome in some of the earliest genome scans mentioned earlier was of interest given the noted sex imbalance in prevalence. One older study in which 38 multiplex families were genotyped with 35 X chromosome markers showed no significant findings, with a single marker showing a maximum lod score of 1.24 (Hallmayer et al. 1996). More recently, the work of J. Liu et al. (2001) reported a finding on the X chromosome as their second highest (maximum lod score of 2.56), which decreased to 1.78 when an additional 235 families were added (Yonan et al. 2003). A subsequent study of 99 families again was linked to the X chromosome with a multipoint score of 2.54, although very distant from the previously discussed studies (Shao et al. 2002b), whereas a Finnish study observed a maximum score of 2.75 in 38 families at another point on the X chromosome (Auranen et al. 2002). Finally, 22 families were genotyped with X chromosome markers and showed modest support for linkage on the distal portion of the X chromosome.

In summary, these studies suggest evidence for autism susceptibility loci on 7q and 2q, even though several different samples with differing geographic origin and diagnostic classification were used. Positional cloning of candidate genes and higher-density marker scans will determine whether these remarkable findings hold true.

Chromosomal Abnormalities

Chromosomal abnormalities have long been associated with autism. In a thorough review, Gillberg (1998) catalogs much of what has been described. On the basis of diagnostic criteria from DSM-III, DSM-III-R, DSM-IV (American Psychiatric Association 1980, 1987, 1994), and ICD-10 (World Health Organization 1992), some 49 individuals with autism have been reported to have abnormalities of 16 of 22 autosomes and both sex chromosomes. With less stringent criteria, only chromosomes 14 and 20 have not been associated with autism (Gillberg 1998). One survey found that 5% of autistic individuals had a major chromosomal abnormality (Ritvo et al. 1990). Anomalies occur most often in patients with mental retardation, with chromosome 15 abnormalities being particularly common and showing deletions and partial trisomy or tetrasomy in the 15q11–13 region. There appears to be some specificity to this region, as one study showed that 20 of 29 individuals selected for inverted duplications of chromosome 15 had "a high probability" of being autistic (Rineer et al. 1998). This is especially interesting in that deletions in this region are also implicated in Angelman syndrome, a behavioral syndrome that is characterized by prominent mental retardation, ataxic gait, and episodic smiling and laughing. In one survey of a population of 49,000 children, all 4 children diagnosed with Angelman syndrome also met the criteria for autism (Steffenburg et al. 1996). Interest in this region has spawned focused linkage studies, which have produced promising results (Bass et al. 1999; Cook et al. 1998), as well as successful efforts in physical mapping of the region (Maddox et al. 1999). Although it is still unclear what role chromosomal anomalies may play in autism, the strength of their association appears strong and thus will catalyze further investigation (Castermans et al. 2004).

Candidate Genes

A recent review stated that at least 89 genes have been reported as candidate genes for autism (Wassink et al. 2005). Many genes are chosen on the basis of hypothesized pathways thought to be involved with autism or from observations in laboratory animal models of neurodevelopment (Bartlett et al. 2005). An example of this line of research stems from investigations that showed elevated blood serotonin levels in autistic individuals, when compared with control subjects (Abramson et al. 1989; J.C. Anderson et al. 1987). Serotonin levels were higher in autistic persons with autistic siblings, compared with autistic probands with no affected siblings, suggesting a relation between serotonin and a genetic diathesis for autism (Piven et al. 1991). The utility of serotonergic drugs in autism has rekindled interest in the serotonin system, particularly the serotonin transporter. A family-based study of 86 parent-proband trios showed significant linkage disequilibrium with a functional promoter polymorphism in the serotonin transporter gene (SLC6A4), the protein responsible for recycling synaptic serotonin and the target of many psychoactive medications (Cook et al. 1997). A dozen studies with similar design have been carried out, with ambiguous results rendering the role of this particular gene in autism still obscure.

A second strategy is an extension of the linkage studies described earlier, in which genes within regions of chromosomes linked to autism are further genotyped as polymorphic markers to assess association to that gene or are directly sequenced for disease or susceptibility variants. Some of these studies have not had positive results (Bacchelli et al. 2003; Bonora et al. 2002, 2005), although one gene, a mitochondrial aspartate/glutamate transporter located in the 2q interval, shows association with autism (Ramoz et al. 2004).

A third approach capitalizes on the rich catalog of cytogenetic abnormalities in autism, as described in the previous section. Examples include the neuroligin 3 and neuroligin 4 genes, which are found on the X chromosome and are involved with synaptogenesis. These genes lie in a region of the chromosome reported to be deleted in some autism patients (N.S. Thomas et al. 1999). Mutations in these genes have been described in carefully chosen autism families (Jamain et al. 2003; Laumonnier et al. 2004; Yan et al. 2005), although these mutations may be present in only a small subset of autism families (Gauthier et al. 2005; Vincent et al. 2004; Ylisaukko-oja et al. 2005). Another example involves the region of chromosome 15q11–13 that harbors several genes that may be interesting autism candidate genes (J.A. Lamb et al. 2000). A cluster of genes comprising the α_5, β_3, and γ_3 subunits of the γ-aminobutyric acid (GABA) receptor lies in the region. GABA is the chief inhibitory neurotransmitter in the CNS, and the GABA system is thought to be involved in seizure disorders. Mice deficient for the β_3 subunit show abnormal EEG findings, experience seizures, and engage in behavior reported to be similar to that in patients with Angelman syndrome (learning deficits, hyperactivity, poor motor coordination, and disturbed rest–activity patterns) (DeLorey et al. 1998).

Cook et al. (1998) used a microsatellite marker located in the third intron of the human β₃ gene (*GABRB3*), as well as eight other markers in the region, to genotype 140 autistic families. The *GABRB3* marker was in significant linkage disequilibrium with autism, an observation confirmed by another group as well (Buxbaum et al. 2002). Linkage in this region was enhanced when phenotypic subtypes were used (Shao et al. 2003) but not with other subtypes (Ma et al. 2005a). Other groups have not replicated association to the region (Ma et al. 2005b; Maestrini et al. 1999).

In summary, despite extensive efforts to screen genes conjectured to be related to autism, very few have been unequivocally identified. Given the high genetic character of autism or "autisms," it is safe to conclude that genes that influence the phenotype will be identified. Efforts are being made to increase further the likelihood of identifying these genetic determinants. Such advances include developments in statistical genetics and refinements of the autism phenotype (Wassink et al. 2005). Laboratory innovations, such as use of whole genome association designs, use of microarray-based expression and DNA copy number analysis, screening of noncoding DNA based on comparative genomic data, and assessment of epigenetic modification, also may contribute to a better understanding of autism.

DEMENTIA

ALZHEIMER'S DISEASE

Alzheimer's disease is the most common cause of dementia, accounting for 50%–70% of all cases. It is a neurodegenerative disease that usually begins after age 65 years, although early-onset cases also occur. Alzheimer's disease is characterized by a progressive deterioration of mental abilities, particularly memory, language, abstract thought, and judgment. Psychiatric and behavioral disturbances are among its earliest symptoms, with overt neurological signs dominating the clinical picture as the illness progresses, including rigid limbs, frontal release findings, and seizures. The course leads inevitably to the loss of independent living and death over an average course of 8–10 years. The clinical picture, history, and laboratory studies permit a probable diagnosis of Alzheimer's disease, but the definitive diagnosis depends on postmortem studies.

The genetic discoveries in Alzheimer's disease have uncommonly complemented and extended what was known about the neuropathology of the disease. The pathognomonic neuropathology shows selective neuronal loss, with neurofibrillary tangles in the neurons and amyloid substance deposited in senile plaques and cerebral blood vessels. The neurofibrillary tangles consist of microtubule-associated tau proteins. These normally stabilize the microtubules of the neuronal cytoskeleton and are regulated by phosphorylation and dephosphorylation processes. In Alzheimer's disease, the microtubule-associated tau proteins become abnormally hyperphosphorylated and accumulate as paired helical filament tangles in degenerating neurons. The plaques are mainly built up by the deposition of β-amyloid protein, which is a proteolytic fragment of the larger precursor, β-amyloid precursor protein (β-APP).

Inflammation appears to be an important feature in many cases, perhaps initiated by immune reactions to β-amyloid plaques or tangles or reactions to the local vasculature or from systemic conditions. Alzheimer's disease and vascular dementia are not mutually exclusive, and pathological features of both disorders commonly coexist.

Epidemiological Studies

The prevalence estimates of Alzheimer's disease depend on the population sampled (community or nursing home residents), age, and diagnostic criteria (definition of "significant impairment"). Age at onset before 65 distinguishes presenile (types 1, 3, 4) from senile (type 2) dementia, although the cutoff ages are indistinct. Presenile cases are more likely to be familial, to be rapidly progressive, and to show prominent temporal and parietal lobe features, including dysphasia or dyspraxia. Later-onset cases (type 2) have a more insidious course and generalized cognitive impairments.

About 3% of those ages 65–74 years and half of the population older than 85 have Alzheimer's disease. Alzheimer's disease rates approximately double every 5 years after age 40 years (Hendrie 1998); the prevalence is expected to swell as the average life span increases. Although age is the most important illness predictor, Alzheimer's disease pathology is not an expected feature of aging.

Geographic variations in the prevalence of Alzheimer's disease suggest the importance of environmental and lifestyle factors or variability in diagnosis and research methodology. Studies of migrant populations confirm the former. For example, the prevalence of Alzheimer's disease in Japan is 1.5%, whereas ethnic Japanese persons in Honolulu, Hawaii, have a prevalence of Alzheimer's disease of 5.4%, a rate comparable to that of white people in Hawaii (White et al. 1996).

Most Alzheimer's disease cases are sporadic, particularly the senile forms, and several demographic measures, lifestyle choices, environmental exposures, and medical conditions are associated with Alzheimer's disease risk. Even in the nonfamilial cases, it is expected that genetic susceptibility plays an important role. In particular, risk is associated with alleles of *APOE* (apolipoprotein E), which is a major component of very-low-density lipoproteins (VLDL). The Alzheimer's disease risk for the ε4 homozygotes (*APOE*E4*) is especially elevated, although not all patients with Alzheimer's disease have *APOE*E4*, and many people with the ε4 allele remain free of disease. The *APOE*E4* allele is associated with an increased number of amyloid plaques, and it may interact with other susceptibility genes and environmental factors.

Females have a greater risk for Alzheimer's disease, even after accounting for their longer life span, with males showing a higher rate of vascular dementias. It was hypothesized that the risk for women could be due to menopause, and many long-term studies suggested that women who take estrogen-based hormone replacement therapy (HRT) had a lower risk of developing Alzheimer's disease. For example, the relative risk (RR) of Alzheimer's disease for HRT users versus nonusers was 0.46 (95% CI = 0.21–1.00) in the Baltimore Longitudinal Study (Kawas et al. 1997) and 0.24 (95% CI = 0.07–0.77) in the Italian Longitudinal Study on Aging (Baldereschi et al. 1998). These associations remained significant after adjustment for age, education, age at menarche, age at menopause, smoking, alcohol use, body weight, and number of children. However, because HRT use was not random among these subjects, it is possible that women who are less likely to develop Alzheimer's disease for other reasons are just more likely to use HRT. Zandi et al. (2002) found no benefit of current HRT use except for those whose use exceeded 10 years. Recently, the Women's Health Initiative Memory Study surprised investigators by showing a doubling of the risk of all-cause dementia in women randomly assigned to receive Prempro, a specific form of combination hormone therapy, after age 64 years (Shumaker et al. 2003). This study was abruptly halted because the risks of HRT were found to "outweigh the benefits." Consequently, estrogen and progesterone combination therapy is not currently recommended for prevention of cognitive decline or dementia, and studies examining estrogen alone are being reexamined. There is new speculation that gonadotropins, rather than estrogen and progesterone, may play the key role in determining the risk for and progression of Alzheimer's disease. As recently reviewed (see Webber et al. 2005), women with Alzheimer's disease have higher levels of luteinizing hormone (LH) than do control subjects. Both LH and its receptor are expressed in brain regions that are susceptible to Alzheimer's disease pathology. Furthermore, because LH is mitogenic, it could dysregulate cell cycles as described in Alzheimer's disease neurons (see Casadesus et al. 2005).

A higher educational level is a protective factor (Launer et al. 1999), perhaps because of increased synaptic and/or dendritic complexity attendant to learning demands. A well-controlled prospective study of at-risk individuals confirmed that low educational attainment was associated with a doubling of Alzheimer's disease incidence (Stern et al. 1994). The effect of education may be a result of higher socioeconomic status or linked to other factors that influence risk for Alzheimer's disease, such as lower stress or better diet. Determining whether education may directly mitigate the risk of developing Alzheimer's disease has implications for the prevention and treatment of Alzheimer's disease, such as using cognitive training to lower the risk for vulnerable individuals (Hendrie 1998).

Traumatic brain injury (TBI) has been related to Alzheimer's disease risk. A prospective study showed that TBI increased the incidence of Alzheimer's disease by fourfold over the next 5 years (RR = 4.1; 95% CI = 1.3–12.7), particularly in cases with *APOE*E4* (Mayeux et al. 1995; Tang et al. 1996). The association between TBI and Alzheimer's disease risk may be affected by the severity of the TBI (loss of consciousness or not) and by family history (Guo et al. 2000). One study suggested that TBI does not increase absolute risk but shortens the time to onset in those patients who will otherwise develop the disease (Nemetz et al. 1999). As reviewed by Jellinger (2004), some research findings support the plausibility of this association; *APOE* alleles are associated with prognosis following TBI, and neuropathological studies show that TBI can cause apolipoprotein β deposition and tau pathology.

Strong evidence supports a role for chronic inflammation in initiating and worsening Alzheimer's disease. Amyloid is a proinflammatory substance, and neuropathological examination shows that plaques are surrounded by signs of inflammation. Use of nonsteroidal anti-inflammatory drugs (NSAIDs), such as ibuprofen, has shown protective effects (see Gasparini et al. 2005). Support for the inflammation hypothesis, reviewed by Finch (2005), includes C-reactive protein elevations, participation of activated brain microglia in amyloid plaque formation, and roles of the *APOE*E4* allele, which may exacerbate brain vascular abnormalities.

Cigarette smoking has been purported to have protective effects, but a pooled analysis of four prospective studies showed that it actually increased Alzheimer's disease risk, especially in men (Launer et al. 1999), and chronic nicotine exposure appears to enhance Alzheimer's disease pathology (Oddo et al. 2005). Oxidative stress may play a role in cellular damage, and antioxidants, such as vitamin E, are purported to slow the progression of Alzheimer's disease. In addition, low levels of vitamin B_{12} or folate may increase Alzheimer's disease risk, perhaps by increasing the amino acid homocysteine, which is also a cardiovascular disease risk factor that may cause inflammation. Aluminum exposure received a great deal of early attention as a risk factor, but this has not held up in controlled studies.

Hypertension also significantly elevates Alzheimer's disease risk, an effect that may be mediated by vascular injury and inflammation. In their review, Luchsinger and Mayeux (2004) highlighted the possible mechanisms linking cerebrovascular diseases with Alzheimer's disease. Diabetes and hyperinsulinemia are also likely to be important risk factors. Dysregulation of insulin or insulin-like growth factor pathway, from either genetic mutations or metabolic derangements, could also mediate the disease risk (de la Monte and Wands 2005; Launer 2005).

Family and Twin Studies

Approximately a quarter of patients with Alzheimer's disease have another first-degree relative with Alzheimer's disease, and the familial nature of Alzheimer's disease has been established in case–control, family, and twin studies (reviewed in Richard and Amouyel 2001). The recurrence risks in family studies are small and variable: 0%–14.4% for parents and 3.8%–13.9% for siblings. The familial recurrences are more prominent in early-onset disease, although such cases may be just more easily ascertained, and both early- and late-onset cases frequently occur within a single family. Family studies are hindered by the late age at onset of Alzheimer's disease because vulnerable individuals often die from other conditions before the incidence age of Alzheimer's disease or may even develop dementia from another etiology.

Because family members have similar types of environmental exposures, twin studies are needed to determine whether familial factors are the result of shared genes. These studies consistently show higher concordance rates for MZ than for DZ twin pairs, ranging from 21% to 67% for MZ twin pairs and 8% to 50% for DZ twin pairs. For example, Raiha et al. (1996) showed pairwise concordance rates of 18.6% and 4.7% for MZ and DZ twins, respectively, with corresponding probandswise concordance rates of 31.3% and 9.3%. These results show that heritability is a factor for at least some forms of Alzheimer's disease. Because of the late onset and strong environmental component to Alzheimer's disease risk, discordance among DZ twins may arise from different environmental influences or variation in incidence ages as well as from genetic differences. Variation in age at onset in MZ twins has been linked to events such as hysterectomy and infection (Nee and Lippa 1999).

Molecular Genetic Studies

Evidence has continued to accumulate that early- and later-onset forms differ in their underlying pathophysiol-ogy. The familial early-onset autosomal dominant forms, which explain less than 2% of Alzheimer's disease, are linked to mutations in three genes, as reviewed by Rubinsztein (1997): the *APP* gene on chromosome 21 (Goate et al. 1991), the presenilin 1 (*PSEN1*) gene on chromosome 14 (Sherrington et al. 1995), and the presenilin 2 (*PSEN2*) gene on chromosome 1 (Levy-Lehad et al. 1995; Rogaev et al. 1995).

The *APP* mutation on chromosome 21 causes "type 1" Alzheimer's disease. It explains about 15% of early-onset cases and is also the type of Alzheimer's disease that universally develops in individuals with Down syndrome, in whom the excess APP activity is due to a trisomy of the entire chromosome 21 rather than just the *APP* mutation. Another 18%–50% of the early-onset cases are from *PSEN1* mutations (type 3); this type has its onset during midlife, typically in the 40s, and progresses rapidly. Type 4 is caused by mutations in the *PSEN2* gene, which accounts for fewer than 1% of these cases. It presents at ages 40–75 and follows a slowly deteriorating course that averages 11 years. Although these three loci are uncommon causes of Alzheimer's disease, their identification has shed light on the biochemistry of amyloid formation and deposition in the human brain. Each of these mutations causes dysregulation of APP processing, leading to an increased production of β-amyloid peptide. This accumulation leads to misprocessing of the tau protein, which accumulates in amyloid plaques, explaining the typical neuropathology of Alzheimer's disease.

Most cases are late onset and sporadic (type 2), although clusters of late-onset cases in families exist. Except for the small percentage of patients with Alzheimer's disease who have mendelian inheritance patterns, the genetic component in most cases likely entails complex interactions between other genes and environmental exposures. APOE (chromosome 19) appears to play a role in all forms of Alzheimer's disease, both early-onset and late-onset familial and sporadic cases. *APOE* alleles act to modify the influence of other genotypes and exposures on the risk for Alzheimer's disease. Risk is increased by the ε4 allele and may be decreased by the ε2 allele. The most common allele (ε3) does not appear to influence risk. These effects are age-dependent and nonmendelian and vary between population samples, in keeping with the variability of genes and exposures.

Other purported susceptibility regions that could modulate the APOE effects include the APOE receptors. Of particular interest are the LDL receptor-related protein and the VLDL receptor gene (Okuizumi et al. 1995) of the LDL receptor superfamily. Additional evidence shows associations between Alzheimer's disease and other genes, such as the α_1-antichymotrypsin gene (Kamboh et al. 1995), major histocompatibility genes, CYP450 genes (*CYP2D6*), and the gene encoding the nonamyloid component of senile plaques (*NACP*) (reviewed in Cruts et al. 1998).

The genetic and epidemiological research findings in Alzheimer's disease make an intriguing story that is gaining coherence as it progresses. These findings will almost certainly lead to advancements in the prevention, early detection, and treatment of Alzheimer's disease.

PRION DISEASES

Prions are proteinaceous infectious agents that cause a group of rare and fatal neurodegenerative disorders that were initially recognized as "transmissible spongiform encephalopathies." By the 1960s, it was recognized that the infectious agent was a protein because its infectivity was resistant to normal sterilization procedures and was susceptible to protein degradation (Alper 1967). Stanley B. Prusiner (1982) subsequently discovered the prion protein, for which he received a Nobel Prize in 1997.

Prions are normal cellular membrane proteins that become infectious simply by changing shape, without a change in their nucleic acid sequence. When misfolded, they undergo a conformational change from an α-helix to a β-pleated sheet. These misfolded prions (PrPRES) induce normal prion proteins (PrP) to change shape. The abnormal prion proteins can be transmitted from an exogenous source (consumed human flesh or beef, human endocrine injections, or dura mater transplants) or may derive from germline or somatic mutations in the *PRNP* gene. Although much has now been learned about prions, the mechanisms whereby a self-reproducing protein structure can cause infection remain intriguing and unknown.

The various prion diseases differ somewhat in their clinical profiles, but their presentation commonly includes impaired cognition, behavior changes, insomnia, and ataxia that progresses to include extrapyramidal and pyramidal symptoms, myoclonus, and akinetic mutism. Prion diseases have no effective treatments, but laboratory studies are conducted to verify that the symptoms have no treatable explanation. The definitive diagnosis is made by a brain biopsy. The neuropathology shows spongiform degeneration, with microglial activation, and a protease-resistant form of the host-derived prion protein.

Epidemiological Studies

Sporadic Creutzfeldt-Jakob disease. The sporadic form of Creutzfeldt-Jakob disease (CJD) is the most common prion disease, accounting for approximately 60%–70% of all cases (see review of CJD variants by Gambetti et al. 2003). Its prevalence is 1 in 1 million.

Sex ratios are nearly equal, although there may be an excess risk in men older than 60. Seventy-five percent of patients die within 6 months, although many die within a few weeks of the diagnosis (Knight 1998). CJD usually begins with a rapidly progressive dementia, although abnormal behavior or gait imbalance is the presenting symptom in about one-third of patients. The autopsy findings show gliosis, neuron loss, and spongiform change. Prion-containing amyloid deposits are identified by immunochemical staining.

Familial CJD. The familial form of CJD shows autosomal dominant inheritance, but laboratory studies confirm that even these prion diseases are potentially transmissible. In affected families, about half of those with the mutant gene develop CJD. The clinical presentation of familial CJD varies, depending on the site of mutation within the *PRNP* gene. It can closely resemble the classic sporadic form of CJD or present a variant phenotype.

Gerstmann-Sträussler-Sheinker syndrome. Gerstmann-Sträussler-Sheinker syndrome (GSS) is a rare familial autosomal dominant neurodegenerative disorder with an earlier age at onset than nonfamilial CJD. Its prevalence is estimated to be about 5 in 100 million (Belay 1999). Patients initially present with ataxia and later develop dementia; they also have dysarthria, oculodysmetria, and hyporeflexia. Death ensues within 1–10 years. Neuropathological examination identifies neuronal vacuolation, astrocytic gliosis, and deposition of amyloid plaques. Although it is a familial condition, GSS can also be transmitted to subhuman primates and rodents via intracerebral inoculation as an infectious disease; infectivity is associated with the 27- to 30-kDa protein known as the *scrapie prion protein* (PrP^{Sc}). Antibodies to PrP^{Sc} react with the amyloid plaques seen in GSS.

Fatal familial insomnia. Fatal familial insomnia is extremely rare and has been identified in fewer than 20 families. As with other familial prion diseases, it has an autosomal dominant inheritance pattern. The mean age at onset in fatal familial insomnia is 49, and the disease lasts about a year. The course includes progressive insomnia, dementia, and motor findings of ataxia, dysphagia, dysarthria, tremor, and myoclonus. Autonomic abnormalities are common; psychiatric symptoms are also frequent and include panic attacks, phobias, and hallucinations. Late-appearing symptoms include primitive reflexes, breathing disorders, weight loss, mutism, and coma. Both slow-wave and rapid eye movement phases of sleep are lost, patients have enacted dream states, and the insomnia is near-total. Fatal familial insomnia involves nearly exclusive bilateral degeneration of the thalamus without spongiform changes or amyloid seen at postmortem examination. Despite its atypical presentation, the finding of abnormal prion protein on neuropathological examination confirmed that fatal familial insomnia is a prion disease (Medori et al. 1992).

Acquired Prion Diseases

Iatrogenic CJD depends on human-to-human transmission, typically via medical procedures. Its period of incubation depends on route of transmission: 12 years for peripheral hormone administration and 6 years for direct transplant of brain tissue. Unlike other forms of CJD, the iatrogenic disease presents with ataxia and gait abnormalities, and only mild dementia is found in the late illness course (Belay 1999).

Other acquired prion diseases include kuru, now extinct, which was transmitted by cannibalism in New Guinea, and the recently defined new variant, or nvCJD. This variant is a new disease first identified in Great Britain that is thought to have derived from the infectious agent of bovine spongiform encephalopathy (BSE), more popularly known as "mad cow disease" (see Zeidler and Ironside 2000). The average age at onset in nvCJD is much younger, at 27 years, than that of sporadic CJD. The duration of illness (14 months) is longer than in classic sporadic CJD. Common presenting symptoms are psychiatric, such as agitation, aggression, anxiety, depression, lability, and social withdrawal. Hallucinations, delusions, insomnia, and sensory distortions are not uncommon. Most patients do not show clear neurological signs until months after initial presentation. Many have had upgaze paresis, a symptom uncommon in sporadic CJD. Progressive dementia, ataxia, and myoclonus do occur, although later in the illness, and then in the context of delusions. Neuropathologically, nvCJD differs from the classic sporadic form: it has "daisy" or "florid" amyloid plaques surrounded by "petals" of spongiosis, which is also typical of sheep scrapie. It is of note that nvCJD can be detected in tonsils, appendix, spleen, and lymph nodes, as well as in the brain. Transmission across other mammalian species had previously been reported, with house cats (Pearson et al. 1991), ungulates (Kirkwood et al. 1990), and primates contracting spongiform encephalopathies after presumably eating contaminated food.

Molecular Studies

The inherited prion diseases are associated with autosomal mutations in the *PRNP* gene (Oesch et al. 1985), which encodes the prion protein. The human gene is located on chromosome 20 (see Glatzel et al. 2005). It has three exons, but its entire open reading frame is contained in only one exon. More than two dozen different amino acid–changing mutations have been identified in the coding region for these disorders. It is unclear what accounts for different types of prion activity, which have been described as strains that modify the course of illness. Some investigators hypothesize that an informational molecular component in addition to prion protein, perhaps a nucleic acid, accounts for different strains (Almond 1998).

Prion protein is expressed at its highest levels in the CNS and less so in the lymphoreticular system, heart, and skeleton. The normal protein is a copper-binding molecule, 33–35 kDa, which is localized to cell membranes in the CNS. Mice genetically engineered to have no prion protein have only subtle findings, other than being resistant to the development of prion diseases, which has complicated studies aimed at elucidating its normal biology (Weissmann and Flechsig 2003). The misfolded disease-associated prion protein PrP^{Sc} has a growing list of putative physiological roles, which include signal transduction, long-term memory, neuronal cell adhesion and neurite extension, and participation in cascades that resist cell death. Evidence suggests an ancient evolutionary past for prion-based inheritance because it is observed across phylogeny. Yet other research considers the possible role of prion proteins in modifying genomewide gene expression through epigenetic mechanisms (Shorter and Lindquist 2005). Prion diseases have illuminated a fascinating aspect of biology that is now being aggressively investigated.

PSYCHIATRIC DISORDERS

BIPOLAR DISORDER

Bipolar I disorder is an episodic disturbance in mood characterized by mania (elevated or irritable mood, increased psychomotor activity, distractibility, diminished need for sleep, and often psychosis) alternating with depression (dysphoric mood, diminished psychomotor activity, decreased concentration, sleep and appetite disturbances, and often suicidality). Bipolar II disorder consists of hypomanic rather than manic episodes; hypomania is a discrete change in mood observable by others that is less severe than mania and does not require hospitalization.

Epidemiological Studies

General population estimates of the prevalence of bipolar I disorder range from 1% to 1.6% in the United States and from 0.3% to 1.5% worldwide (Weissman et al. 1996). The risk for bipolar and other mood disorders has increased in successive cohorts over the course of the last century; this increase may be due to the effect of some exogenous pathogenic factor over a limited period or to genetic anticipation (see subsection "Anticipation" later in this chapter).

Family Studies

A meta-analysis of eight family studies showed a sevenfold increase in lifetime risk for bipolar disorder in family members of bipolar probands compared with family members of control subjects (Craddock and Jones 1999). The risk for bipolar disorder appears to be especially elevated for the relatives of probands with early-onset disorder, and the risk also increases with the number of psychiatrically ill relatives (Gershon et al. 1982). Recurrence risks do not vary with the gender of either the relative or the bipolar proband (Heun and Maier 1993). Other psychiatric conditions that aggregate in the relatives of probands with bipolar disorder are bipolar II disorder, recurrent unipolar disorder, schizoaffective disorder (bipolar type), and suicide.

The age at onset of the first manic or depressive episode has been shown to be earlier, and the frequency of episodes greater, in the younger generation of two generations of affected relative pairs (McInnis et al. 1993; Nylander et al. 1994). Genetic anticipation has been associated with the pathogenic expansion of trinucleotide repeat sequences in several neuropsychiatric disorders. Observed anticipation in bipolar disorder may be the result of such genetic factors, environmental changes, or ascertainment issues.

Furthermore, it has been observed that some pedigrees have primarily paternal transmission, whereas others have mostly maternal transmission of the illness to offspring. Sex differences in transmission may implicate vulnerability genes on sex chromosomes, mitochondrial inheritance in some families, or the role of genomic imprinting, in which genes are differentially methylated depending on which parent they are inherited from.

Twin Studies

Ten twin studies of mood disorders that have been conducted since 1928, in which affected twins had either bipolar or unipolar disorder, have suggested higher concordance rates in MZ pairs (58%–74%) than in same-sex DZ pairs (17%–29%) (see Tsuang and Faraone 1990). A relative scarcity of unipolar-bipolar pairs argues against these disorders being genotypically identical, although a relation between the two disorders seems to exist. Six twin studies have focused on bipolar disorder alone; each showed greater concordance among MZ than among DZ twins. Pooling of data from these studies yielded an MZ concordance rate of about 50% (Craddock and Jones 1999). Interestingly, as in schizophrenia, among discor-

dant MZ twin pairs, offspring of the affected and nonaffected twin have identical risk of developing bipolar disorder; this supports the role of environmental factors in the expression of the bipolar phenotype for those who are genetically vulnerable.

Adoption Studies

A significantly greater risk of affective disorder (unipolar, bipolar, and schizoaffective) was found in the biological parents (18%) than in the adoptive parents (7%) of adopted bipolar probands (Mendlewicz and Rainer 1977). The risk for illness in biological parents of adopted and nonadopted bipolar probands was similar. Another study of biological and adopted relatives of probands with mood disorders and control probands also showed that the biological relatives of affected probands had increased risk for the same broad spectrum of affective disorder; the biological relatives of affected probands were 8 times more likely to have unipolar depression and 15 times more likely to have completed suicide (Wender et al. 1986). Wender's study also found that several environmental factors in an adoptive family appear to play a role in the development of mood disorders, including parental alcohol problems, other parental psychiatric problems, and parental death (Cadoret et al. 1985).

High-Risk Studies

Structured diagnostic interviews of 60 offspring who had at least one parent with bipolar disorder yielded a 51% prevalence of psychiatric disorder, predominantly attention-deficit, unipolar, and bipolar disorders (Chang et al. 2000). The risk of bipolar disorder in offspring was associated with early age at onset of bipolar disorder in the parent. Bilineal risk was associated in affected children with greater severity of depression and irritability. In a single extended pedigree identified by a bipolar proband, the risk of early-onset affective disorder was correlated with degree of relatedness to affected adults (Todd et al. 1994). In a series of National Institute of Mental Health (NIMH) bipolar pedigrees, children of parents with affective disorder were five times more likely to have an affective disorder than were children of healthy parents (Todd et al. 1996). Children of bipolar parents may have greater degrees of aggressiveness, obsessionality, and affective expression than do age-matched control subjects (reviewed in Goodwin and Jamison 1990). High-risk children have been found to have cognitive deficits, especially on performance subtests of the Wechsler Intelligence Scale for Children, that are suggestive of right hemisphere dysfunction and also are reminiscent of deficits seen in adult bipolar patients (Kestenbaum 1979).

Linkage Analysis

The last decade has seen numerous genome scans in bipolar disorder performed on several continents in many populations. Initial reports supported loci on chromosome 4 (Blackwood et al. 1996), chromosome 12 (Detera-Wadleigh et al. 1999; Ewald et al. 1998a; Morissette et al. 1999), chromosome 13 (Detera-Wadleigh et al. 1999), chromosome 18 in outbred and isolated populations (Berrettini et al. 1994; Freimer et al. 1996; Stine et al. 1995), chromosome 21 (Smyth et al. 1997; Straub et al. 1994), and chromosome X (Pekkarinen et al. 1995; Stine et al. 1997). Some of these findings have been subsequently replicated, but many have not. Examples of nonreplication do not necessarily disprove linkage because replicating linkage results for oligogenic disorders is difficult (Suarez et al. 1994), and different susceptibility loci may be important in different populations.

Given the number of linkage scans, bipolar disorder, like schizophrenia, is amenable to meta-analysis. Badner and Gershon (2002) used a multiple scan probability approach in 353 families with 1,230 affected patients from 11 studies and reported the most significant linkage to chromosome arms 13q and 22q. Another group used a different approach—an overlapping set of scans and varying levels of bipolar disorder phenotype (347 or 512 pedigrees, 948 or 1,733 cases, in 9 or 14 studies, respectively, for very narrow or narrow phenotypes). The most significant findings across these studies occurred on chromosomes 9, 10, and 14 (Segurado et al. 2003), none of which reached the level of significance required for whole genome studies.

These meta-analyses do not imply that genes for bipolar disorder exist in the many reported linkage regions; they may simply suggest that many of these loci may not be linked to the disorder across all of the populations studied. The genetic heterogeneity between populations and the locus (i.e., gene) heterogeneity within populations represent a challenge for using a linkage-based approach for gene finding in bipolar disorder. Nevertheless, the body of genome scan data has provided plentiful leads for further investigation.

Molecular Approaches

Candidate genes.   A leading theory of pathophysiology in bipolar disorder is the catecholamine hypothesis, in which mania is caused by an excess, and depression is caused by a deficit, of catecholamines; roles for norepinephrine and dopamine are supported by the pharmacological effects on mood of antidepressants, L-dopa, amphetamines, and antipsychotics. Therefore, numerous candidate gene studies in bipolar disorder have focused on genes involved in catecholamine synthesis, degradation, and transduction. For an illustrative example, initial case–control studies showed an allelic association between monoamine oxidase A (on the X chromosome) and bipolar disorder (Kawada et al. 1995; Lim et al. 1994b), but a third study that used a more conservative, within-family control (haplotype relative risk) design did not confirm this association (Nothen et al. 1995). Subsequent studies also showed no association (Furlong et al. 1999; Kirov et al. 1999a; Preisig et al. 2000; Turecki et al. 1999). Similarly, catechol-O-methyltransferase (*COMT*) is an important candidate gene because its protein methylates and inactivates dopamine and norepinephrine. *COMT* maps to 22q11, a region associated with velocardiofacial syndrome and increased incidence of schizophrenia and bipolar disorder. Early suggestive but not conclusive evidence indicates that *COMT* may be linked to bipolar disorder in select populations, such as Irish women (Mynett-Johnson et al. 1998), Han Chinese (Li et al. 1997), and patients with velocardiofacial syndrome (Lachman et al. 1996). It also may be a modifying gene for susceptibility to ultrarapid cycling in bipolar disorder in adults (Kirov et al. 1998; Lachman et al. 1996; Papolos et al. 1998). Subsequent studies have supported the association between *COMT* and bipolar disorder (Rotondo et al. 2002; Shifman et al. 2004); however, several studies found no linkage between bipolar disorder and *COMT* in either general white or other subpopulations.

The serotonin transporter has been extensively studied, with meta-analyses of case–control and family-based studies showing a slight, although significant, elevation in risk for bipolar disorder depending on genotype at the serotonin transporter–linked promoter region (*5-HTTLPR*) polymorphism or intron 2 tandem repeat polymorphism (Cho et al. 2005; Lasky-Su et al. 2005). A similar review of 25 studies analyzing serotonin receptors in bipolar disorder found no consistent evidence of association (Anguelova et al. 2003).

Other theories of pathogenesis in bipolar disorder inform the choice of candidate genes. Disruption of circadian rhythms has been implicated in bipolar disorder (S.H. Jones et al. 2005; Mansour et al. 2005b), leading to assessment of how genetic variation in circadian genes such as *TIMELESS*, *CLOCK*, *CRY1*, *GSKB3*, and *PER3* may influence bipolar disorder and lithium responsiveness (Bailer et al. 2005; Benedetti et al. 2004; Mansour et al. 2005a; Nievergelt et al. 2005).

With the increasingly apparent role of neurotrophic factors in mood disorders (Hashimoto et al. 2004), many groups have focused on genes such as that for brain-derived neurotrophic factor (BDNF), with promising evidence for association (Lohoff et al. 2005; Sklar et al.

2002), although not in all populations (Kunugi et al. 2004; Nakata et al. 2003). The finding of association between a gene on chromosome 13, D-amino acid oxidase activator (*DAOA*), and schizophrenia (Chumakov et al. 2002) led to efforts to investigate this gene in bipolar disorder. This was partly motivated by this region also showing linkage to bipolar disorder in several studies. Several studies have supported an association between *DAOA* and bipolar disorder (Fallin et al. 2005; Hattori et al. 2003; Schumacher et al. 2004). This raises the possibility that there may be shared genetic influences between bipolar disorder and schizophrenia and has led to analysis of bipolar samples with other genes associated with schizophrenia (Fallin et al. 2005; Green et al. 2005; Raybould et al. 2005), such as *NRG1* (neuregulin-1) and *DTNBP1* (dystrobrevin binding protein-1).

Alternative endophenotypes for bipolar disorder genetic studies have been proposed as a result of clinical and biological observations. These include seasonality and puerperal psychosis (Craddock and Jones 1999), as well as serotonin transporter binding (Leboyer et al. 1999), cognitive function after manipulation of central serotonin function (Sobczak et al. 2002, 2003), and brain hyperintensities found with imaging (Ahearn et al. 1998). Finally, a set of some 252 genes has been proposed to represent the likeliest candidate genes for mood disorders based on functional pathways representing neurotransmitter systems, neuroendocrine systems, neurotrophic pathways, circadian biology, and miscellaneous CNS functions (Hattori et al. 2005).

Anticipation. In the light of intergenerational differences in disease expression that are consistent with anticipation, several groups have sought evidence for trinucleotide repeat expansion in bipolar disorder. O'Donovan et al. (1995) used a repeat expansion detection assay and reported significantly larger CAG repeats among 49 unrelated bipolar subjects than among 74 control subjects. The finding of expanded repeats has been replicated by some investigators but not others (O'Donovan et al. 2003) and may not represent a strong influence on bipolar disorder (Tsutsumi et al. 2004). Note that the number of repeats is not associated with age at onset or disease severity (Craddock et al. 1997). However, the number of repeats has been found to be associated with change in phenotype from unipolar depression to bipolar disorder across generations (Mendlewicz et al. 1997).

PANIC DISORDER

Panic disorder is a common anxiety disorder that has come under increasing scrutiny by neuropsychiatric geneticists. Panic disorder is characterized by panic attacks, the spontaneous occurrence of intense anxiety accompanied by somatic symptoms, including dyspnea, palpitations, sweating, and chest pain. Panic disorder is diagnosed in the setting of recurrent panic attacks with 1 month of anticipatory anxiety, worry about the implications of the attacks, or significant attack-related behavior changes (American Psychiatric Association 2000). Understanding of the genetics of panic disorder was initially hampered by earlier approaches of studying anxiety disorders as a class. Only with the pharmacological dissection of anxiety syndromes (D.F. Klein 1964) and the development of operational criteria for panic disorder (DSM-III) could reliable diagnoses be made and thus grant genetic studies more phenotypic certainty.

Epidemiological Studies

An international epidemiological study of 40,000 persons reported a lifetime prevalence of panic disorder of 1.4%–2.9% (Weissman et al. 1997). This study found an exception to this in Taiwan, where the rate was 0.4% and where the rates of other psychiatric disorders were equally reduced. The replication of this study reported a 12-month prevalence of 2.7% (Kessler et al. 2003). The prevalence of panic disorder in females is about twice that in males (Eaton et al. 1994). The age at highest risk is 25–44 years (Robins et al. 1984), with a mean age at onset of 24; the hazard rates are highest at 25–34 for females and 30–44 for males (Burke et al. 1990).

Family Studies

Investigations from the first half of the twentieth century focusing on the diagnostic precursors to modern panic disorder suggested a familial component to panic (Cohen and White 1951; Oppenheimer and Rothschild 1918). Subsequent studies have relied on two advances in family genetic studies—criteria-based diagnoses and direct interview of relatives. The first study to use DSM-III diagnoses showed that 31% of the first-degree relatives of panic probands were affected, compared with 4% of the relatives of control subjects (Crowe et al. 1980) (relative risk = 7.8). An extension of this study with twice the number of probands and relatives confirmed this finding, with a relative risk on the order of 9.9–10.7, depending on the diagnostic criteria used (Crowe et al. 1983). Among 41 families with panic disorder, 25 (61.0%) had at least one affected relative, compared with 4 of 41 (9.8%) control families. The risk was double for female relatives compared with male relatives. Several subsequent studies confirmed these findings (Fyer et al. 1995; Hopper et al. 1987; Maier et al. 1993; Mendlewicz et al. 1993; Noyes et al. 1986; Weissman 1993). One group found that specific smothering symptoms increased the risk of panic disorder (Horwath et al. 1997) and that early age at onset increased the risk of panic in the first-degree relatives of panic probands to 17 (Goldstein et al. 1997). On the whole, family studies of first-degree relatives of panic disorder probands suggested a relative risk of 2.6–20 (mean = 7.8) (Knowles and Weissman 1995). Similar work in second-degree relatives of panic probands showed a sevenfold relative risk (Pauls et al. 1979b), similar to studies in first-degree relatives. Also consistent with the first-degree relative studies, female second-degree relatives were at higher risk for panic disorder. Overall, these studies indicate that panic disorder clearly aggregates in a familial pattern, but whether that pattern is due to genetic factors is undetermined.

Twin Studies

Before 1970, six twin studies were published in which the clinical entity "neurosis" was investigated. The largest found that the ICD diagnosis of "anxiety state" led to concordance rates of 41% for MZ twin and 4% for DZ twin pairs (Slater and Shields 1969). It was not until the 1980s that twin studies that used rigorous diagnostic criteria were published. Torgerson (1983) used DSM-III diagnostic criteria and interviewed 299 Norwegian twin pairs; in 11 twin pairs, 1 co-twin had panic disorder, and in 18 twin pairs, 1 person had panic disorder with agoraphobia. No co-twin shared the same diagnosis in this group, although in 2 MZ twin pairs, 1 twin had panic disorder, and the other twin had panic disorder with agoraphobia. When criteria were loosened to include any anxiety disorder with panic attacks, concordances of 31% and 0% were found for MZ and DZ pairs, respectively. A larger study that used DSM-III-R diagnoses identified 49 twin pairs in which 1 twin had an anxiety disorder and 32 comparison pairs without an anxiety disorder. When the co-twins were assessed, 5 of 20 (25.0%) of the MZ co-twins and 3 of 29 (10.3%) of the DZ twins were found to have panic disorder (Skre et al. 1993). The concordance rates for the comparison group were 8% and 10% in MZ and DZ twin pairs, respectively.

A much larger analysis of 1,030 female twin pairs derived from the Virginia Twin Registry was carried out by Kendler's group (Kendler et al. 1993). DSM-III-R diagnoses were made with varying levels of certainty, and 5.8% of the 2,163 interviewed twins met lifetime criteria for panic disorder. The concordance rates were 24% and 11% for MZ and DZ twins, respectively. The best-fitting model for the narrowest diagnostic scheme implied that the variance in susceptibility to panic disorder was due to

individual-specific environment and additive genes, and the heritability was estimated at 46%. Analysis of 6,724 male-male twin pairs from the Vietnam Era Twin Registry supports this estimate (Scherrer et al. 2000). These estimates lie at the middle of the 30%–62% heritabilities extrapolated from the older Norwegian twin studies. One potential explanation for this discrepancy is the ascertainment methods used in the different sets of studies. Kendler and colleagues (1993) used a population-based approach, whereas the work of Torgersen (1983) and Skre and colleagues (1993) relied on treatment samples, which conceivably can be considered more severe and potentially more genetically liable. An argument against this notion was offered in a study in which familial rates of panic disorder did not differ when probands were ascertained from a specialty anxiety clinic, specialty depression clinic, or population survey (Wickramaratne et al. 1994). Indeed, a study that used population-recruited twin pairs found high concordance rates for MZ twins (73%) but not for DZ pairs (0%) (Perna et al. 1997). Other explanations include differences in clinician blindness and the sex difference between studies (i.e., all female vs. female and male twin pairs). Another observation that comes from the twin literature involves the low DZ concordance rate. DZ twins should have a morbid risk similar to that of other first-degree relatives. Across the twin studies of panic disorder, risk to a DZ co-twin of a panic proband is 0%–11, which is much lower than the 8%–41% reported in family studies for first-degree relatives. The nature of this inconsistency is unclear, but it certainly warrants caution in attempting to estimate heritability of panic disorder. Despite this caveat, twin studies support a modest genetic component of panic disorder.

Adoption Studies

There are no known adoption studies for panic disorder.

High-Risk Studies

Panic disorder is often comorbid with other psychiatric conditions, raising an interest in whether these comorbidities may provide insight into the genetics of panic disorder. Depression occurs in at least one-third of the persons with panic disorder (Markowitz et al. 1989). Investigation of the families of depressed patients showed evidence for (Weissman et al. 1984) and against (Coryell et al. 1988) the hypothesis that panic disorder would increase the risk of depression in relatives. A family study that collected patients from treatment clinics and population-based surveys showed that panic disorder itself did not increase risk for depression in relatives per se, and vice versa, whereas comorbid panic and depression increased the risk of both panic alone and depression alone, as well as comorbid panic and depression, in relatives (Weissman 1993). These authors concluded that depression and panic are separate disorders, agreeing with many of the existing family studies (Crowe et al. 1983; Mendlewicz et al. 1993) and twin studies (Skre et al. 1993) of panic disorder. This conclusion was reinforced by the finding that children who are at high risk for developing panic include children whose parents have panic disorder, but not if they have depression alone (Biederman et al. 2001).

Comorbidity between alcohol disorder and panic is a well-known clinical phenomenon. Relatives of panic probands have been reported to be at higher risk for alcohol or substance abuse (E.L. Harris et al. 1983). Other family investigations indicate that panic does not increase risk for an alcohol disorder any more than do several other psychiatric disorders (Coryell et al. 1988; Mendlewicz et al. 1993).

Another interesting observation about comorbid conditions derives from linkage studies in bipolar disorder. In one study, 57 bipolar families collected for linkage analysis were found to have 41 persons with panic disorder among 528 relatives. Of these 41 persons, 36 also had bipolar disorder (MacKinnon et al. 1997). Nearly 18% of the original bipolar probands and relatives who received diagnoses of bipolar disorder had panic disorder as well, suggesting a potential familial subtype of panic disorder and/or bipolar disorder. This group analyzed 203 additional families and found similar results (MacKinnon et al. 2002). The same group stratified 28 of the original families by whether the identified bipolar proband had panic disorder (5 families), panic attacks (6 families), or no panic attacks or disorder (17 families) and performed a linkage study with 31 markers on chromosome 18, where previous evidence of linkage for bipolar disorder had been detected (Stine et al. 1995). Multipoint nonparametric linkage analysis determined that the 5 bipolar/panic *disorder* families showed z scores of greater than 4.0 ($P<0.0001$) over five consecutive markers on chromosome 18, whereas the bipolar/panic *attack* families showed intermediate scores, and the bipolar/no panic group showed low or negative scores (MacKinnon et al. 1998). Further work suggests that in this pedigree, mania is characterized by rapid mood switching (MacKinnon et al. 2003). These data provide intriguing, but limited, evidence for a subgroup of both disorders that may share a common genetic mechanism.

Another avenue of research has identified a potential biological marker for panic disorder in high-risk individuals. Numerous groups have used inhaled carbon dioxide (CO_2) or infused lactate, among other compounds, to induce panic attacks in persons with panic disorder (Balon et al. 1988; Gorman et al. 1990). Children with anxiety disorders have markedly different responses to CO_2 when compared with control subjects (Pine et al. 2000). Subsequent work by Balon et al. (1989) has shown that when family histories of healthy subjects were taken, subjects with a high prevalence of anxiety disorders in their first-degree relatives had panic attacks after lactate infusion, whereas those who did not panic showed a lower risk in their relatives. One group showed that the psychiatrically healthy first-degree relatives of panic probands had CO_2-induced panic attacks at significantly higher rates than did control subjects with no family history of panic disorder, although at rates lower than the identified probands (Perna et al. 1995). The same group studied prevalence rates of panic disorder in 895 first-degree relatives of 203 panic probands. A positive reaction to CO_2 inhalation in the proband conferred a morbid risk of 14.4% among first-degree relatives, whereas the rate in the families of probands with negative responses was 3.9% (Perna et al. 1996). In another study (Coryell 1997), a total of 39 persons with and without family histories of panic disorder had CO_2 inhalation; those with a positive family history were more likely to experience panic attacks. Bellodi et al. (1998) evaluated 20 MZ and 25 DZ twin pairs obtained from an Italian twin registry to test for concordance of the panic response to CO_2 inhalation and found concordance rates of 55.6% and 12.5% for MZ and DZ pairs, respectively. A segregation analysis of 165 families found that the 134 families in which a panic proband was hypersensitive to CO_2 fit a dominant single major locus model of inheritance (Cavallini et al. 1999b). Subsequent studies showed that genetic determinants of CO_2 response are not necessarily enriched in panic disorder (Philibert et al. 2003) and that history of panic disorder in a parent does not predict CO_2 response (Pine et al. 2005). Overall, these data suggest that genetic mechanisms may determine CO_2 and lactate hypersensitivity. It is not clear whether these determinants also influence the development of panic disorder. Challenges with these agents may still provide a tool to identify more familial forms of panic disorder.

Mode of Inheritance

The first attempt to define mode of inheritance for panic disorder came from an early family study of 139 patients, mostly servicemen, with neurocirculatory asthenia (Cohen and White 1951). Family histories were obtained from the probands, and the observed rates of neurocirculatory asthenia were compared with expected rates under several genetic models. The data fit a so-called double-dominant inheritance pattern, in which two dominant genes of equal frequency occurred. Simple dominant, recessive, and sex-linked models of inheritance were ruled out. This syndrome, characterized by nervousness, dyspnea (in 99% of the individuals), palpitations, fatigability, and a host of other somatic symptoms (Cohen and White 1949), is clearly a precursor diagnosis to the modern conception of panic disorder. But the imprecision of the diagnosis and the method of data collection limit useful conclusions from the data.

In the first study to address the mode of inheritance of panic disorder based on DSM criteria, Pauls and colleagues (1979a) compared rates of unilineal and bilineal inheritance in their family data and suggested a single-gene dominant model, a finding supported by additional data showing a dropoff in risk in second-degree relatives (Pauls et al. 1979b). These same investigators carried out a segregation analysis on their data set, which also suggested a dominant model, albeit with an unrealistic phenocopy rate of zero (Pauls et al. 1980), whereas further model-fitting work on their expanding family collection determined that neither dominant nor polygenic models could be ruled out (Crowe et al. 1983). One segregation analysis estimated that dominant and recessive models were equally likely, and more important, the phenocopy rate of 1% suggested that a quarter to half of all cases would be nongenetic, depicting a complex, heterogeneous picture (Vieland et al. 1993). This finding was replicated in an independent sample (Vieland et al. 1996) and predicted the twin concordance rate observed by Kendler et al. (1993). Interestingly, a segregation analysis of panic disorder families selected for CO_2 sensitivity suggested that a single locus may explain the genetic propensity to panic disorder in those particular families (Cavallini et al. 1999b. Overall, segregation analyses agree on the genetic contribution to panic disorder but have not resolved the specific model of inheritance, giving weight to autosomal dominant, autosomal recessive, and polygenic etiologies.

Linkage Analysis

In the setting of positive evidence from family studies for a familial component to panic disorder, and confirmation from twin studies and segregation analyses that the familial factor is genetic, several genetic linkage studies of panic disorder have been performed. The first of these tested 26 families comprising 198 interviewed relatives with 29 polymorphic red cell antigens and blood proteins, covering 10 chromosomes (Crowe et al. 1987). Crowe and colleagues used a dominant model derived from their earlier segregation analysis and found that one marker, α-haptoglobin (16q22), had a maximum lod score of 2.27. Nonparametric sib-pair analysis supported this finding ($P = 0.02$). The

same group followed up this suggestive, although nonsignificant, linkage finding (Crowe et al. 1990). Ten new families were tested for linkage at the α-haptoglobin locus, this time with a DNA-based RFLP to detect two polymorphisms with the locus, and linkage was excluded. When the 10 families were combined with the previous 26 families and analyzed, the maximum lod score was 0.67, largely excluding the α-haptoglobin locus in panic disorder.

One group procured a large collection of multiply affected pedigrees, with 2–12 affected members per family (Fyer and Weissman 1999). This group performed a two-stage genome scan on 23 families (Knowles et al. 1998). One marker on chromosome arm 7p15 mapped to a region also showing positive scores in the work of Crowe and colleagues, as described later in this subsection. While collecting these pedigrees, the investigators observed that certain medical conditions, particularly renal and bladder problems, thyroid conditions, and mitral valve prolapse, seemed to be enriched in these families. Considering these families a potential subgroup, they carried out a linkage analysis comparing 19 families with this "syndrome" with 15 families without the "syndrome" (Weissman et al. 2000). A maximum lod score was 3.3 for a chromosome 13 marker in a model of heterogeneity; this score rose to 4.22 when observing the families with bladder involvement and setting any proband with bladder problems as affected. This group confirmed their chromosome 13 findings when expanding the number of families from 19 to 60 (Hamilton et al. 2003). This bladder-related phenotype was thought to be reminiscent of the urological condition interstitial cystitis. These same investigators assessed the prevalence of panic disorder in relatives of persons with interstitial cystitis ascertained through urology clinics and found the rate significantly elevated over that found in probands with other urological disorders (Weissman et al. 2004). Although preliminary, these studies suggest the utility of developing potential syndromic subtypes for sharpening genetic analysis.

In a second genome scan, 253 persons from 23 multiplex panic disorder pedigrees were analyzed (Crowe et al. 2001). A lod score of 2.23 was observed in close proximity to the 7p15 finding described in the previous paragraph. Subsequent analysis with an innovative Bayesian linkage approach confirmed linkage to 7p15 in the same sample (Logue et al. 2003). A third genome screen was carried out in 20 pedigrees containing 153 persons, and both panic disorder and agoraphobia were used as phenotypes. For panic disorder, the authors observed a maximal lod score of 2.04 located on chromosome arm 1q (Gelernter et al. 2001) in a region showing modest linkage in the scan of Crowe et al. The analysis for agoraphobia reported positive scores in regions not overlapping with the panic findings. When subsequent studies used these panic disorder pedigrees to test for linkage to simple phobia or social phobia, again areas of modest linkage were observed that did not overlap with the panic disorder findings (Gelernter et al. 2003, 2004).

A fourth scan of 25 families was carried out in Iceland and used a broad phenotype that included panic disorder, as well as generalized anxiety disorder, phobias, and somatoform pain (Thorgeirsson et al. 2003). A maximum multipoint lod score of 4.18 was observed on 9q31, a region that had not been observed in the previous screens. The lack of overlap between these linkage studies may be explained as positive scores due to chance. More likely, they may represent prominent genetic heterogeneity. This possibility suggests that efforts focusing on genetic subgroups defined by co-occurring mental disorders or medical conditions may lead to more homogeneous phenotypes. An example of this is shown by an analysis of a single large pedigree in which 75 of 99 members were genotyped in 11 regions on 9 chromosomes chosen by synteny to mouse regions identified as quantitative trait loci for anxiety behaviors. A parametric lod score of 2.38 was found on chromosome arm 10q for a novel phenotype that included panic disorder and childhood-onset anxiety disorders.

In summary, linkage studies have not provided strong evidence of genomic regions that are highly likely to be related to panic disorder, possibly reflective of the lower sensitivity of parametric linkage studies in diseases of uncertain mode of inheritance and in which multiple genes of small effect may be operative.

Molecular Approaches

Several lines of evidence provide theoretical candidate genes for panic disorder. The pharmacological efficacy of drugs that affect various neurotransmitter receptors, transporters, and catabolic enzymes, as well as challenge studies with specific panicogens and pathways investigated in animal models of fear and anxiety, all point toward several genes of neuropsychiatric interest. Unfortunately, most investigations attempting to associate panic disorder with variants on these genes have provided little support for the candidates (Finn and Smoller 2001). Early linkage studies focusing on the polymorphic genes for tyrosine hydroxylase, α- and β-adrenergic receptors, GABA receptors, and pro-opiomelanocortin did not support the association of these genes with panic disorder. Similarly, negative results were found for the dopamine types 2 and 4 (D_2 and D_4) receptors and the dopamine transporter. Numerous case–control studies and several family-based association and linkage studies of the serotonin system found no role for serotonin-

related genes in panic disorder. One exception involves the serotonin type 2A receptor, for which more than one group found association, albeit other groups did not (Inada et al. 2003; Maron et al. 2005; Rothe et al. 2004). Genes found to be positive in at least two studies include those encoding the adenosine 2A receptor and COMT. Two studies of the adenosine 2A receptor found association or linkage in white populations (Deckert et al. 1998; Hamilton et al. 2004), but two studies in Asian populations did not observe an association (Lam et al. 2005; Yamada et al. 2001). COMT is interesting because at least four studies support the role of this gene in panic disorder (Domschke et al. 2004; Hamilton et al. 2002; Woo et al. 2002, 2004) in white and Asian populations.

This rather uneven history of candidate gene studies in panic disorder points to several problems plaguing psychiatric genetics in general: 1) low power from limited sample sizes for detecting genes of small effect; 2) low prior probability and multiple testing; 3) population admixture, affecting case–control studies; and 4) phenotypic heterogeneity. As in studies of other disorders, an ideal solution would include a very large, family-based sample with a subtype population (e.g., those with CO_2 hypersensitivity or an endophenotypic medical syndrome) such as that described earlier.

OBSESSIVE-COMPULSIVE DISORDER

Obsessive-compulsive disorder (OCD) is a common anxiety disorder in which the patient has persistent intrusive thoughts, or obsessions, typically involving concerns about contamination, symmetry, or checking. Patients with OCD also perform ritualistic tasks, or compulsions, that interfere with normal daily function. OCD has been well characterized in children and adolescents and has been found to lead to substantial impairment and social isolation.

Epidemiological Studies

Prior to the large epidemiological studies of the 1980s, OCD was thought to be relatively uncommon, with a prevalence of about 0.05% (Rasmussen and Eisen 1992). It is likely that the traditional study of inpatients and, to a lesser extent, outpatients led to the dramatic underestimation of prevalence of a disorder for which treatment was often not sought or was provided by nonpsychiatric physicians (S. Shapiro et al. 1984).

As part of the Epidemiologic Catchment Area (ECA) study, more than 9,500 persons across three sites in the United States were interviewed for 15 DSM-III disorders, for which lifetime and 6-month prevalence data were obtained. OCD was found to have a lifetime prevalence of 1.9%–3.0% among the three sites (Robins et al.

1984), whereas 6-month prevalence was estimated to be 1.3%–2.0% (J.K. Myers et al. 1984). A subsequent study extended the ECA findings to more than 18,500 persons across all five ECA sites and confirmed a lifetime prevalence of 1.9%–3.3% (Karno et al. 1988). Some caution is warranted regarding these results. Analysis of the temporal stability of the diagnosis of OCD with the ECA data reported that only 19.2% of those meeting diagnostic criteria for OCD continued to do so when reinterviewed 1 year later (E. Nelson and Rice 1997). Those persons whose diagnosis remained stable reported an earlier age at onset and had stable comorbid conditions (particularly other anxiety disorders). The authors interpreted these results as a combination of false positive and false negative findings and questioned the validity of the instrument used, the Diagnostic Interview Schedule.

In a population-based study of 356 adolescents selected from an original screening set of 5,600, the DSM-III diagnosis of OCD had current and lifetime prevalences of 1.0% and 1.9%, respectively (Flament et al. 1988). Community survey data from seven countries obtained by the Cross National Collaborative Group indicated an annual prevalence rate of 1.1%–1.8% and a lifetime rate of 1.9%–2.5% (Weissman et al. 1994). One country, Taiwan, was clearly an outlier, with corresponding rates of 0.4% and 0.7%, respectively. This finding was consonant with the observed low rates of all psychiatric disorders in Taiwan. Finally, a replication sample for the National Comorbidity Survey found a lifetime prevalence of 1.6% (Kessler et al. 2005).

There appears to be a slight excess of females with OCD compared with males. In a review of 11 studies performed before 1970 of treatment populations totaling 1,336 persons, 51% of the patients were women (Black 1974). Other epidemiological evidence suggests a larger female-to-male ratio, with five of the seven countries in the Cross National Collaborative Group having ratios of 1.2–1.6, with two outlying countries with proportions of 0.8 and 3.8 (Weissman et al. 1994). The difference between the epidemiological and treatment populations, possibly reflecting gender difference in treatment-seeking behaviors, may explain the discrepancy between the estimates. One striking finding has been the reversal of the sex ratio in children. In one clinic-based sample, 76.5% (13 of 17) of the patients were boys (Hollingsworth et al. 1980), and a cohort of 70 patients followed up at the NIMH showed a male-to-female ratio of 2:1 (Swedo et al. 1989b). The ratio during adolescence seems to revert to that seen with adults (Flament et al. 1988). The mean age at onset is 20.9 years, with a significant difference between sexes (male 19.5, female 22.0, $P<0.003$) (Rasmussen and Eisen 1992).

Family Studies

Until the 1930s, very little was known about the heredity of OCD. Beginning with 50 obsessional patients from the Maudsley Hospital in London, A. Lewis (1936) collected detailed information about 100 parents and 206 siblings. Thirty-seven of the parents had "obsessional traits" (e.g., methodicalness, strong religious feelings, strictness), as did 20 of the siblings. Another British study, comparing first-degree relatives of probands with several psychoneurotic states with control subjects, found a prevalence of obsessional states of 7.1%–7.5% in the 96 relatives of the 20 probands with obsessional states (F.W. Brown 1942). The prevalence in the 189 relatives of the 31 control subjects was 0%.

More than a dozen family studies have been published since the 1960s and have been comprehensively reviewed (Pauls and Alsobrook 1999; Sobin and Karayiorgou 2000). Methodological considerations distinguish many of these studies. The use of the family history method, in which a proband provides historical information about relatives, predominated among the older studies. The family study method, in which direct interviews of all first-degree relatives are used, came to the fore in more recent studies. Some studies combine both approaches. Because persons with OCD may be less forthcoming about embarrassing or shameful symptoms in a direct interview, the family history method may identify affected relatives. Conversely, direct interview may detect affected relatives with symptoms unknown to the family history informant. One review of 11 OCD family studies published since 1965 illustrates this methodological problem (Sobin and Karayiorgou 2000). Nine adult studies with 686 probands and 2,427 first-degree relatives showed OCD or obsessive-compulsive symptoms at rates ranging from 0% to 20%. Two child and adolescent studies with a total of 66 probands and 186 first-degree relatives showed OCD rates of 9.5%–25%. Sobin and Karayiorgou noted that the studies that used more direct interviews reported high morbid risk rates, although several of those also were family studies of children and adolescents, enriching for the early-onset form of the disorder. This is important in the context of studies indicating that the age at onset modifies risk for OCD in relatives (Pauls et al. 1995). Indeed, when family studies are designed to utilize children as probands, the rates of OCD in first-degree relatives are particularly elevated (Hanna et al. 2005) when compared with studies in which probands are older than 18 (Nestadt et al. 2000b). Despite the wide range of estimates of morbid risk to first-degree relatives from studies facing a variety of methodological challenges, family studies suggest a familial aggregation of OCD.

Twin Studies

The number of twin studies focusing on OCD is not large. In 1936, A. Lewis described three sets of MZ twins with concordant obsessional traits but drew few conclusions from his data, opining "two or three pairs tell very little: it is a pity that twins are so rare" (pp. 325–326). A later review of the largely anecdotal intervening literature calculated a concordance of 56.9% (29 of 51) among MZ pairs, with an adjusted rate of 65.0% (13 of 20) after removing 30 pairs with questionable zygosity (Rasmussen and Tsuang 1984). Unfortunately, data for direct comparison to DZ twin rates were not presented, preventing any conclusions about the contribution of genetic factors.

Three subsequent studies have been published, all including DZ twins and totaling 233 MZ and 328 DZ pairs (G. Andrews et al. 1990; Carey and Gottesman 1981; Torgersen 1983). In 30 twin pairs with pre-DSM-III diagnoses (15 MZ and 15 DZ), one group found MZ and DZ concordances of 87% and 47%, respectively, for obsessional symptoms but found no difference for OCD (Carey and Gottesman 1981). A twin registry–based study (446 pairs, 186 MZ and 260 DZ) and a clinically derived sample (85 pairs, 32 MZ and 53 DZ) both looked at concordance of a variety of anxiety disorders among twins (G. Andrews et al. 1990; Torgersen 1983). Both found no concordant DSM-III OCD, but both did note higher concordances when OCD was grouped together with other anxiety and affective disorders. For example, Torgersen observed in his clinical sample that when OCD was grouped with agoraphobia, panic disorder, and social phobia, but not with generalized anxiety disorder, respective MZ and DZ concordances of 45.0% (9 of 20) and 15.2% (5 of 33) were seen. This effect was lost when generalized anxiety disorder was added to the diagnostic grouping. In the population-based study, 19 of 186 (10.2%) MZ twins were concordant for a "neurotic" cluster of disorders, including depression, dysthymia, generalized anxiety disorder, panic disorder, and OCD, compared with 25 of 260 (9.6%) DZ pairs (G. Andrews et al. 1990). This difference was not significant. The authors still concluded that their twin study suggested a genetic component to these disorders because their population prevalences predicted a nongenetic concordance rate on the order of 7%. A sample of more than 10,000 twin pairs, all children, was analyzed for obsessive-compulsive symptoms; a prominent additive genetic influence on symptomatology was found (Hudziak et al. 2004). A smaller study of 527 adult female twin pairs suggested a smaller genetic influence on obsessive-compulsive symptoms based on the Padua Inventory (Jonnal et al. 2000).

One group used a different diagnostic approach to assess obsessional traits and symptoms with the Leyton Obsessional Inventory (Clifford et al. 1984). They studied 419 twin pairs derived from a British normal twin registry and found heritabilities of 44% and 47% for obsessional traits and symptoms, respectively. It is difficult to draw firm conclusions from the OCD twin literature. As a group, these studies are characterized by heterogeneous diagnostic schemes, interviewer knowledge of co-twin diagnosis and zygosity, and analytic strategies often based on combining diagnostic entities into larger groups. Given these disparities, it has not been possible to carry out a meta-analysis of these twin studies (Hettema et al. 2001). Despite all of these differences, this literature does argue that OCD has a genetic component.

Adoption Studies

There are no known adoption studies for OCD.

High-Risk Studies

The striking differences in male-to-female ratios in OCD patients with prepubertal childhood-onset (3:1) and postpubertal adolescent-onset (1:1) disorder derive from the wide differences in age at onset between males and females. Males with early-onset OCD have been reported to have persistent and severe symptoms (Flament et al. 1990) as well as a higher incidence of birth complications compared with females (Lensi et al. 1996), suggesting that males may be more vulnerable to CNS damage resulting in OCD than are females.

The study of OCD in children and adolescents has provided other useful insights into high-risk populations and the heterogeneous nature of the disorder (Leonard 1999). It has long been observed that OCD co-occurs with tics and Tourette's disorder (Pauls et al. 1986), particularly in males and those with early-onset OCD (Leonard et al. 1992). Early-onset OCD also predicts Tourette's disorder and tics in relatives, suggesting a distinct risk group for OCD (Pauls et al. 1995). Even after excluding Tourette's disorder from OCD probands in a family study, tics were more prevalent in OCD families (Grados et al. 2001). It has been proposed that the use of phenotypes such as these may strengthen gene-finding efforts (Miguel et al. 2004). Obsessive-compulsive symptoms can be used as a tool for narrowing other phenotypes, as was shown by using these symptoms to define a subset of autism pedigrees and assess genetic linkage and association (Buxbaum et al. 2004; McCauley et al. 2004).

Studies of children with Sydenham's chorea, a neurological manifestation of rheumatic fever, led to the discovery that many children with this poststreptococcal autoimmune syndrome showed higher rates of obsessive-compulsive symptoms (Swedo et al. 1989a). In cohorts of children with OCD, some children were described as having acute and dramatic development of symptoms, associated with choreiform movements and other neurological abnormalities, prepubertal onset, and frequent streptococcal infections (Snider and Swedo 2004). Continued investigation into this phenomenon has resulted in the definition of PANDAS (pediatric autoimmune neuropsychiatric disorder associated with streptococcal infections) (Swedo et al. 1998). Swedo's group used a monoclonal antibody (D8/17) against a B-cell antigen previously found to identify probands with rheumatic fever (Khanna et al. 1989) to assay children with PANDAS, children with Sydenham's chorea, and 24 control children (Swedo et al. 1997). They found that the PANDAS and Sydenham's chorea groups were D8/17-positive significantly more often than were control subjects (85% and 89%, respectively, vs. 17%). These data suggest that being D8/17-positive may increase susceptibility to these two disorders. A subsequent study appears to generalize this finding to early-onset OCD and Tourette's disorder, showing that these groups also expressed the D8/17 antigen more frequently than did control samples (T.K. Murphy et al. 1997). The original description of this marker suggested the intriguing possibility that the increased susceptibility to PANDAS, OCD, and Tourette's disorder may be genetically mediated. Khanna et al. found that 100% of the rheumatic fever probands were D8/17 positive, expressing the antigen on 33% of their B cells. Unaffected siblings and parents expressed the marker on 15% and 13% of their cells, respectively, a rate approximately twice that of control subjects (Khanna et al. 1989). The authors assessed the pattern of marker expression in their pedigrees and concluded that this was consistent with autosomal recessive inheritance. Assessment of the first-degree relatives of children with PANDAS showed rates of OCD higher than those seen in the general population (Lougee et al. 2000).

Mode of Inheritance

Only in the past decade have efforts focused on the mode of transmission in OCD. Cavallini et al. (1999a) performed a segregation analysis of 107 Italian families with DSM-III-R OCD and focused on the phenotypes of OCD or OCD plus Tourette's disorder and tics. For the OCD-only analysis, the model of no genetic transmission was rejected but general mendelian inheritance was not. Within the mendelian model, the dominant model was the best fitting according to Akaike's Information Content. Interestingly, the analysis of the OCD plus Tourette's disorder and tics group rejected both the no

genetic transmission and the general mendelian models. More than half (54 of 107) of the families in this study had a single member with OCD, a finding noted consistently in family studies. The importance of this observation was addressed in another segregation analysis of 96 DSM-III-R OCD probands and their 453 first-degree relatives (Alsobrook et al. 1999). Fifty-one families had a family history of OCD, meaning an affected member besides the index proband, whereas 45 of 96 (46.9%) did not. In all of the families, segregation analysis rejected only the model of no genetic transmission. When analyzing only those with a positive family history of OCD, all models were rejected except for a mixed model. This group then stratified their families with a four-factor structure for obsessive symptoms (Leckman et al. 1997). Segregation analysis was performed on the subsets of families in which the proband scored in one of the four factors, and all analyses rejected the no genetic transmission model. In the analysis that used factor 3, corresponding to symmetry, ordering, counting, and ritual obsessions and compulsions, polygenic transmission also was rejected, suggesting a general mendelian model. A segregation analysis of 153 families suggested a single gene for OCD but also showed that the sex of the chosen OCD proband influenced the aggregation pattern in the pedigrees (Nestadt et al. 2000a). Although a single major locus model appears possible, the prominent clinical heterogeneity seen in OCD, as well as the limited set of genetic models tested in these segregation analyses, argues for a more complicated mode of transmission. The factor analysis approach of Alsobrook et al. (1999), the use of potential biological markers such as D8/17, and the development of more sophisticated modeling may provide further insights into the genetic mode of inheritance for OCD.

Linkage Analysis

The first genome scan in OCD analyzed seven families containing a childhood-onset proband (Hanna et al. 2002). Thirty-two of the 65 interviewed and genotyped individuals had OCD. The investigators observed a maximum multipoint linkage score of 2.25 on chromosome arm 9p for the first 56 subjects. The score decreased to 1.97 when an additional 14 markers were genotyped in the whole sample. A study that used a sib-pair analysis, a potentially less powerful method that omits models of transmission, was subsequently performed. In this study, 41 affected sibling pairs defined by a narrow phenotype showed linkage to chromosome arm 9p with a heterogeneity lod score of 2.26 (Willour et al. 2004). Nonparametric analysis yielded a score of 2.52 in this region as well. The linkage interval corresponds directly to the region found by Hanna et al., suggesting that this region may harbor an OCD locus. Sib-pair analysis may prove useful but will require the collection of families far larger than most extant studies, providing a rationale for collaborative OCD genetic studies.

Molecular Approaches

Several candidate gene association studies, mostly case–control, have been carried out with OCD populations. Most of these studies investigated genes involved with serotonin and dopamine function, a result of hypotheses derived from pharmacological studies and clinical observations (W.K. Goodman et al. 1990a, 1990b).

Genes involved in serotonin function have received the most attention. The serotonin transporter gene (*SLC6A4*), the molecular target for serotonin reuptake inhibitors, has been studied extensively. Probes of transporter availability in blood have suggested that serotonin transporter function is compromised in OCD (Delorme et al. 2005; Marazziti et al. 1999) and in the brain (Hesse et al. 2005). Sequence analysis of cDNAs isolated from 22 OCD patients and 4 control subjects showed no changes in amino acid sequence at this locus (Altemus et al. 1996). The coding sequence of *SLC6A4* was scanned with denaturing gradient gel electrophoresis in 45 OCD patients, and again no variants were seen (Di Bella et al. 1996). Several studies, both family-based and case–control, have used a repeat sequence (*5-HTTLPR*) in the promoter region of *SLC6A4* that altered transcription activity depending on the number of repeats (Lesch et al. 1996). These studies in aggregate do not support a prominent role for this gene in OCD.

Serotonin receptors also have been studied. Several groups have reported on polymorphisms in the serotonin type 2A (5-HT$_{2A}$) receptor (*HTR2A*) and OCD (Enoch et al. 1998; Meira-Lima et al. 2004; Nicolini et al. 1996; Tot et al. 2003), although with inconsistent results. Association studies of modest sizes reported negative results for the 5-HT$_{2C}$ receptor (*HTR2C*) (Cavallini et al. 1998; Frisch et al. 2000) and positive results for the 5-HT$_{1D\beta}$ receptor (*HTR1D*) (Camarena et al. 2004; Mundo et al. 2002).

The first candidate gene studies in OCD involved genes for dopamine receptors, given the association between OCD and Tourette's disorder, a disorder commonly treated with dopamine receptor antagonists. Several case–control studies found no association between OCD and the *DRD2*, *DRD3*, and *DRD4* genes (D$_2$, D$_3$, and D$_4$ dopamine receptor genes). Likewise, negative associations have been found for the dopamine transporter, despite alterations in brain dopamine transporter binding (Hesse et al. 2005).

The final candidate gene, *COMT*, is an enzyme involved in the catabolism of several neurotransmitters, including dopamine. This gene was studied in light of data suggesting that persons with a microdeletion of 22q11 frequently had obsessive and compulsive symptoms (Papolos et al. 1996). *COMT* lies within this region and is commonly deleted in persons with this chromosomal aberration (Karayiorgou et al. 1995). Karayiorgou et al. (1997) studied a common SNP in the coding region of *COMT* that led to a change in amino acid sequence and three- to fourfold difference in enzyme activity. Seventy-three OCD probands were compared with 148 control subjects, and the low-activity allele of *COMT* was associated with OCD in males but not in females. In particular, the strong association with the homozygous low-activity genotype suggested a recessive effect. This finding was replicated in a follow-up family-based study that used 110 probands (Karayiorgou et al. 1999). Further, this study reported similar significant male-specific associations between OCD and a polymorphism in the monoamine oxidase A gene, a gene on the X chromosome whose protein product also is involved with the enzymatic degradation of neurotransmitters and is the target of one class of medications. Subsequent studies (Alsobrook et al. 2002; Erdal et al. 2003; Niehaus et al. 2001) and a meta-analysis of extant literature (Azzam and Mathews 2003) suggested that this gene likely has a small effect on OCD.

As with other complex disorders discussed in this chapter, association studies like many of those described above present some problems. Often, candidate genes are chosen on the basis of hypotheses derived from the indirect evidence of psychopharmacological treatment studies. The role of pharmacologically relevant candidate genes may prove to be an epiphenomenon and not shed light on the etiologies of these disorders. Problems of disease heterogeneity, without the judicious use of clinical or biological subtypes, may only ensure false-negative results, whereas issues of population admixture in case–control studies will continue to foster false-positive results. Nevertheless, linkage and candidate gene studies still hold promise.

SCHIZOPHRENIA

Schizophrenia comprises a group of serious psychiatric disorders that are characterized by "positive" (psychotic) symptoms, "negative" (deficit) symptoms, and cognitive impairment. Most patients are initially affected in young adulthood; 50% go on to experience some disability throughout their lives, and an additional 25% never recover and require lifelong care. The lifetime risk for schizophrenia is 0.9% (McGue and Gottesman 1991), and this risk is approximately equal for men and women, although women have a later mean onset by about 5 years and have a second and smaller postmenopausal peak of incidence (Häfner et al. 1993).

Pathophysiology

Excessive subcortical transmission of dopamine has consistently been linked to the positive symptoms of schizophrenia (Abi-Dargham et al. 2000), whereas a deficit in dopamine activity in the prefrontal cortex is associated with negative symptoms. Hypofunction of both excitatory N-methyl-D-aspartate (NMDA) glutamate (Heresco-Levy and Javitt 1998) and inhibitory GABA receptors is also believed to be involved in schizophrenia. Alterations of GABA neurotransmission in the dorsolateral prefrontal cortex may underlie the working memory deficits commonly seen in schizophrenic patients (D.A. Lewis et al. 2004).

In addition to neurotransmitter abnormalities, disruptions of synapses may underlie the clinical picture of schizophrenia. This theory is supported by postmortem studies in schizophrenia that reported increased packing of neuron cell bodies, with a decrease in the neuropil that composes the connections between neurons—specifically, dendritic branches and their spines, where synapses are concentrated (Glantz and Lewis 2000; Harrison 1999; Rosoklija et al. 2000). Postmortem studies also showed abnormal expression of a host of synaptic proteins and their corresponding mRNA (Harrison 1999). The idea of excessive synaptic pruning as the underlying mechanism for schizophrenia symptoms gains support from computer simulations of neuronal networks (McGlashan and Hoffman 2000). Reduction in neuropil also may explain the reduced brain volumes evident in schizophrenia (Harrison 1999).

The timing of pathophysiological processes in schizophrenia is not entirely clear. A common model of schizophrenia is that it results from abnormal prenatal neural development that remains latent until the affected region matures and is required to function optimally (Weinberger 1987). This model is consistent with the fact that schizophrenic patients have an excess of minor physical anomalies, which originate in utero, compared with control subjects (M.F. Green et al. 1994; Lohr and Flynn 1993). A neurodevelopmental model is also supported by the finding of subtle cognitive and motor abnormalities in the premorbid period during childhood (Done et al. 1994; P. Jones et al. 1994). Fish and colleagues (Fish 1977; Fish et al. 1992) coined the phrase *pandevelopmental retardation*, which refers to these premorbid subtle abnormalities found in multiple domains, including motor, sensory, cognitive, and cerebellar function, in children who go on to develop schizophrenia. Other studies confirm the presence of early and subtle abnormalities in at-risk children,

such as compromised psychomotor performance and cognitive and motor dysfunction by age 10 years (Marcus et al. 1981). An innovative blinded review of home videotapes showed that raters could accurately identify which children would later develop schizophrenia by examining their motor skills (Walker et al. 1994). Other precursors of schizophrenia (albeit nonspecific) include delays in developmental milestones (e.g., walking and talking), more isolated play at ages 4 and 6 years, speech problems and clumsiness at ages 7 and 11 years, and poor school performance and social anxiety during the teen years (reviewed in P. Jones and Cannon 1998; Tarrant and Jones 1999). Global attentional dysfunction may be a biobehavioral marker for genetic liability to schizophrenia because attentional deficits exist in nearly half of all schizophrenic patients and in the offspring of parents with schizophrenia (Erlenmeyer-Kimling and Cornblatt 1978, 1992). Abnormal social behavior (e.g., trouble making friends, disciplinary problems, and unusual behavior in childhood and adolescence) may be another nonspecific indicator of risk for schizophrenia (Parnas et al. 1982a, 1982b).

However, evidence also indicates that patients are not "doomed from the womb" and that some postnatal exposures, including TBI and the use of drugs, such as cannabis, may increase the risk for schizophrenia (Malaspina et al. 2001) (Arseneault et al. 2004). Dynamic changes in brain volumes over time in schizophrenic patients also provide support for the theory that progressive deteriorative processes occur in this putatively neurodevelopmental disorder. Cross-sectional imaging studies show increased ventricle size and reduced frontal and temporal lobe volumes in schizophrenic patients (Wright et al. 2000), abnormalities that are often evident by illness onset (Pantelis et al. 2003) and also present to some extent in those with increased genetic risk for illness (Lawrie et al. 1999). However, volumetric changes may be an active process that continues beyond the onset of illness (Pantelis et al. 2003): for example, the superior temporal gyrus decreases in volume after onset of first psychosis (Kasai et al. 2003). These progressive reductions in brain volumes may be amenable to pharmacological intervention (Lieberman et al. 2005).

Genetics and Mode of Inheritance

Evidence from family, twin, and adoption studies suggests that the liability to schizophrenia is at least in part inherited. First-degree relatives of schizophrenic probands have an increased risk of schizophrenia, with estimated risk rates of 6% for parents, 10% for siblings, and 13% and 46% for children with, respectively, one or two affected parents (McGue and Gottesman 1991). Identical twins have a concordance rate of 53%, whereas fraternal twins have a concordance rate of 15% (Kendler and Gardner 1997); the disparity in these rates suggests that 60%–90% of the liability to schizophrenia can be attributed to genes (Cannon et al. 1998; P. Jones and Cannon 1998). Of interest, offspring of affected and unaffected (discordant) MZ twins have equal risk for schizophrenia (about 16%–18%), consistent with either incomplete penetrance or gene-environment interaction.

Adoption studies also support inheritance of schizophrenia liability (Heston 1966; Kety et al. 1994; Rosenthal et al. 1968) but cannot determine whether such effects are genetic or environmental (in utero) if mothers are the parent of comparison. When fathers are the parent in common (paternal half-siblings), however, the same increased risk in biological (vs. adopted) relatives holds (Kety 1988). Adoption studies also provide evidence for a gene-environment interaction, because adopted-away children of biological mothers with schizophrenia are even more likely to develop schizophrenia if they are raised in an adverse environment (Tienari et al. 1991; Wahlberg et al. 1997).

Increased familial risk exists not only for schizophrenia but also for its spectrum disorders, such as schizotypal personality disorder (Battaglia and Torgersen 1996; Siever et al. 1993), and for features characteristic of schizophrenia (i.e., endophenotypes), including smooth-pursuit eye movement (Levy et al. 1994), neurological soft signs (Kinney et al. 1986), and gating impairments (Myles-Worsley et al. 1999).

Although schizophrenia is a genetic disorder, the nature of the genetic diathesis remains unclear. It is not simply a mendelian disorder (O'Donovan and Owen 1999). Most likely, schizophrenia results from epistasis, the interaction of multiple genes of small effect. A three-locus epistasis model can optimally account for the rapidly decreasing recurrence risk data for individuals with lowering degrees of relatedness to probands with schizophrenia (Risch 1990). As described, schizophrenia is likely etiologically heterogeneous, with various genetic, environmental, and interactive etiologies resulting in a common phenotype. Alleles that confer risk may be highly prevalent in the population, and illness may result from some constellation of disease genes when none or few may be sufficient by themselves.

Because the phenotype of schizophrenia is heterogeneous, some studies have focused on examining putative "endophenotypes" or "intermediate phenotypes" of schizophrenia genes. These lie on the pathway between genotype and disease and are usually measured differently (physiology, anatomy, neuropsychology). Endophenotypes are associated with illness, heritable, traitlike, and found also in family members without the disease. These may be

easier to define than the diagnosis itself and may have a higher penetrance in humans. Also, endophenotypes can be studied in animal models to delineate pathophysiology. Promising candidate endophenotypes include aberrant smooth-pursuit eye movement (Crawford et al. 1998; O'Driscoll et al. 1998; R.G. Ross et al. 1998), N-acetyl-aspartate concentrations in the hippocampus (Callicott et al. 1998), abnormal hippocampal morphology (Csernansky et al. 1998), the P50 gating deficit (see "Chromosome 15: α_7 nicotinic receptor" subsection later in this chapter), and abnormalities in working memory.

There is some evidence for anticipation in schizophrenia, which is the successive decrease in age at onset in newer generations of multiply affected pedigrees (Petronis and Kennedy 1995), as well as some evidence of increased trinucleotide repeat expansions, which account for anticipation in other illnesses such as Huntington's disease (Morris et al. 1995; O'Donovan et al. 1995). However, the location of these repeats and their relevance to schizophrenia etiology remain unknown (O'Donovan and Owen 1999).

The intriguing notion that schizophrenia can result from de novo genetic events in the paternal germ line was first suggested by Malaspina et al. (2001) to explain the strong relation of paternal age to the risk for schizophrenia. Since then, multiple studies in diverse populations have replicated the paternal age effect (A.S. Brown et al. 2002; Byrne 2003; Dalman 2002; El-Saadi 2004; Sipos et al. 2004; Zammit 2003). In the Malaspina cohort, paternal age, overall, explained more than 25% of the risk for schizophrenia. Comparably, in Sweden, Rasmussen et al. estimated that 15% of the cases were attributable to paternal age greater than 30 years. The paternal age effect appears to be restricted to patients without a family history of psychosis (Byrne et al. 2003; Malaspina et al. 2002; Sipos et al. 2004). Sipos and colleagues found that paternal age was unrelated to the risk for familial cases, whereas the offspring of the oldest fathers showed a 5.5-fold increased risk for sporadic (nonfamilial) schizophrenia. The epidemiological evidence is convincing. There is a "dosage effect" of increasing paternal age on the relative risk for schizophrenia, and each cohort study has shown a tripling of risk for the offspring of the oldest fathers (>45–55 years). The studies have used prospective exposure data and validated psychiatric diagnoses, and they have together controlled for potential confounding factors, such as family history, maternal age, parental education and social ability, social class, birth order, birth weight, and birth complications. Furthermore, the studies showed specificity of late paternal age on the risk for schizophrenia compared with other psychiatric disorders, which is not the case for any other schizophrenia risk factor, including most of the susceptibility alleles (see the subsections later in this section). Furthermore, accumulating evidence suggests that sporadic (paternal age–related) schizophrenia may be a separate variant of the disease from familial cases (Malaspina et al. 1998, 2000a, 2000b, 2005).

Early linkage studies in schizophrenia were disappointing because of type I error, failures to replicate, small sample sizes, and the likelihood that each susceptibility gene has only a small effect. Two meta-analyses of linkage studies have supported 8p and 22q most strongly, among others, as regions associated with schizophrenia (Badner and Gershon 2002; C.M. Lewis et al. 2003). Candidate gene analysis focusing particularly on dopamine pathways also has provided a low yield for identifying schizophrenia genes. Of the many dopamine-related genes, evidence is strongest for the D_3 receptor, located on chromosome 3, which may confer some risk for schizophrenia (Kirov et al. 2005).

However, in the past few years, several putative susceptibility genes have been identified for schizophrenia, and they are listed here by chromosome number. Most of these genes code for proteins involved in excitatory glutamatergic pathways, and many influence synaptic function. With most of the genes identified thus far, specific mutant alleles or changes in the coding frame have not been identified as associated with increased schizophrenia risk. Overall, dysbindin and neuregulin have the greatest support as susceptibility genes, and good evidence supports disrupted-in-schizophrenia-1 (*DISC1*), *DAO/DAOA*, and regulator of G-protein signaling-4 (*RGS4*). Some of these regions and genes have been associated with bipolar disorder as well, including *DISC1*, neuregulin, and *DAOA* (Table 8–2) (Craddock et al. 2005).

Chromosome 1: *DISC1*.   The major susceptibility gene for schizophrenia identified on chromosome 1 is *DISC1*. Its region—1q42—was initially identified as a potential locus for schizophrenia risk on the basis of an extended pedigree that had a balanced chromosomal translocation that involved this region (St. Clair et al. 1990). *DISC1* has shown linkage with schizophrenia in extended pedigrees (Ekelund et al. 2004) and has been associated with a broad phenotype that includes not only schizophrenia but also schizoaffective and bipolar disorders. The specific gene was identified as *DISC1* and was found in animal models to be associated with the putative endophenotype of electrophysiological abnormalities—specifically, reduced P300 (Blackwood et al. 2001). DISC1 protein is associated with the development and function of the hippocampus, particularly the growth of neuritis (Miyoshi et al. 2003), which is of interest as a leading model for schizophrenia pathophysiology as reduced neuropil and abnormal connectivity. *DISC1* also appears to be involved in cell migration, scaffolding and formation of the cytoskeleton, intracellular transport, mitochondrial function, and distribution of receptors in the membrane (Harrison and Weinberger 2005). The distribution of *DISC1* within the cell is altered in the orbitofrontal cortex in patients with psychosis (Sawamura et al. 2005). One allele has specifically been associated with hippocampal structure, neurochemistry, and function in both nonschizophrenic individuals and schizophrenic patients (Callicott et al. 2005).

TABLE 8–2.   Schizophrenia susceptibility genes

Gene	Name	Gene locus
NRG1	Neuregulin-1	8p12–21
DTNBP1	Dysbindin	6p22
DAOA	D-Amino acid oxidase activator	12q24
G72	Interacts with *DAOA*	13q32–34
RGS4	Regulator of G-protein signaling-4	1q21–22
PRODH2	Proline dehydrogenase	22q11
COMT	Catechol-O-methyltransferase	22q11
GRM3	Metabotropic glutamate receptor-3	7q21–22
DISC1	Disrupted-in-schizophrenia-1	1q42
PPP3CC	Calcineurin	8p21
Akt1	Protein kinase B	14q22–32
CHRNA7	α_7 Nicotinic receptor	15q13–14

RGS4. *RGS4*, located at 1q22, was targeted as a potential susceptibility gene because it had decreased gene expression in schizophrenia, as identified by postmortem microarray studies (Mirnics et al. 2001). Linkage was also established to this region in extended schizophrenia pedigrees, with a highly significant lod score of 6.50 (Brzustowicz et al. 2000). The expression of *RGS4* is regulated by dopaminergic activity, and itself modulates 5-HT$_{1A}$ activity. *RGS4* also interacts with an *NRG1* receptor, ErbB3, whose expression is downregulated in schizophrenia.

Chromosome 6: dysbindin or *DTNBP1*. The region of 6p22.3 was first identified as a region of interest in schizophrenia through extensive association mapping of illness with SNPs and haplotypes in extended German schizophrenia pedigrees (Straub et al. 2002). Association was also supported by studies of sibling pairs and parent-offspring trios (Kirov et al. 2004; Schwab et al. 2003) and other pedigrees (N.M. Williams et al. 2004), and significant associations have been found in more than 10 independent samples (Kirov et al. 2005). Specific risk alleles and haplotypes have not been identified, and susceptibility may be conferred by changes in message expression or processing. Reduced levels of dysbindin message have been found in the prefrontal cortex (Weickert et al. 2004), and dysbindin protein was reduced in glutamatergic terminals of the hippocampal formation (Talbot et al. 2004) in postmortem studies of schizophrenia. Mutant alleles are associated with differences in working and episodic memory in both patients and at-risk individuals (Harrison and Weinberger 2005). Dysbindin is part of the dystrophin glycoprotein complex, which is located in postsynaptic densities, especially in the mossy fiber synaptic terminals in the hippocampus (and cerebellum). Dysbindin may regulate presynaptic proteins, such as SNAP25 and synapsin 1 (Numakawa et al. 2004) (which have differential neural expression in schizophrenia), and hence influence the presynaptic exocytotic release of glutamate.

Chromosome 8: *NRG1*. The association of the region of 8p21–22 with schizophrenia was first identified in a study in Iceland (Stefansson et al. 2002) and then replicated in diverse samples, including from Scotland, United Kingdom, Ireland, China, South Africa, and Portugal (Petryshen et al. 2005). Several potential schizophrenia genes are found in this region, including frizzled-3 and calcineurin A (Tosato et al. 2005), but the most promising candidate gene in the region is neuregulin. Neuregulin has been implicated in animal studies in a range of functions, including cell signaling, axon guidance, synaptogenesis, glial differentiation, myelination, and neurotransmission (Corfas et al. 2004; Michailov et

al. 2004). Of interest, hypomorphic mice have increased ventricular volume, changes in α$_7$ nicotinic receptors, and failures of prepulse inhibition, all features that are characteristic of schizophrenia. Neuregulin also modifies expression of NMDA receptors, both through its own ErbB receptors and via actin. As with other putative susceptibility genes for schizophrenia, neuregulin also appears to be associated with bipolar disorder (with psychotic features) (E.K. Green et al. 2005).

Chromosomes 12 (*DAO*) and 13 (*DAOA*). In French Canadian and Russian populations, novel susceptibility genes for schizophrenia were located on chromosome 13; one of these, identified as *G72*, was found to be primate-specific and to be expressed particularly in the caudate and amydala (Kirov et al. 2005). *G72* was localized to 13q33 (Addington et al. 2004), and polymorphisms of this gene have been associated with structural and functional abnormalities in both the prefrontal cortex and the hippocampus in patients with schizophrenia (Harrison and Weinberger 2005). *G72* was subsequently renamed *DAOA* because it was found to be an activator of *DAO* (D-amino acid oxidase), a susceptibility gene on chromosome 12. *DAO* oxidizes D-serine, a potent endogenous agonist of the NMDA glutamatergic receptor. Notably, *DAOA* has been associated in bipolar patients with persecutory delusions in particular (Schulze et al. 2005).

Chromosome 15: α$_7$ nicotinic receptor. Common in schizophrenia is a failure in sensory gating—namely, the failure to inhibit the P50 auditory evoked response to repeated stimuli, which appears to be inherited in an autosomal dominant fashion in schizophrenia pedigrees (Siegel et al. 1984). The endophenotype of this auditory evoked potential deficit has been linked to the α$_7$ subunit of the nicotinic acetylcholine receptor gene on 15q14 (Freedman et al. 1999).

Chromosome 22: *COMT*. The region of 22q11 has been of interest for several years because microdeletions in this region lead to a phenotype known as velocardiofacial syndrome, which frequently includes schizophrenia-like psychosis (about 24%) (Ivanov et al. 2003; K.C. Murphy et al. 1999). Linkage to this region has been found for schizophrenia (Badner and Gershon 2002; C.M. Lewis et al. 2003). Several genes within this region are part of the usual deletion zone and are plausible candidates for increasing schizophrenia susceptibility, including *COMT*, proline dehydrogenase (*PRODH*), and zinc DHHC domain-containing protein 8 (*ZDHHC8*) (Kirov et al. 2005). Proline dehydrogenase mutations in mice are associated with abnormalities in sensorimotor gating analogous to schizophrenia (Gogos et al. 1999), as well as decreased levels of glutamate and GABA. Also, mutations are associated with hyperprolinemia, which has been found in schizophrenia. However, despite a finding of association of *PRODH* with schizophrenia in a Chinese sample (Li et al. 2004) and a microdeletion in this region in a schizophrenia pedigree (Jacquet et al. 2002), there have been several negative studies, and the association is not clear (Kirov et al. 2005). *ZDHHC8* codes for a transmembranous palmitoyl transferase and has been little studied (Kirov et al. 2005). In contrast, *COMT* has been extensively studied as a putative schizophrenia allele.

COMT is a methylating enzyme that effectively inactivates dopamine and other catecholamines. It is largely responsible for dopamine clearance in the prefrontal cortex, which has a dearth of dopamine transporter in comparison to more subcortical brain regions. Alleles of interest vary at codon 148 of the brain-predominant membrane-bound form of COMT: the allele with valine at this position has higher activity and is associated with worse cognition (Egan et al. 2001; Malhotra et al. 2002).

The two alleles of interest are Val-*COMT* (valine) and Met-*COMT* (methionine), resulting from a substitution in a single base pair in the gene (codon 148). Val-*COMT* has higher enzyme activity and hence depletes more prefrontal dopamine; it is not surprising then that Val-*COMT* is associated with worse cognition (Egan et al. 2001; Malhotra et al. 2002). However, no clear association of the valine allele alone with schizophrenia was found in a meta-analysis (Fan et al. 2005; Glatt et al. 2003). The association of specific haplotypes suggests that other codons in *COMT* or nearby genes may be responsible for the association (Kirov et al. 2005). However, among putative schizophrenia alleles, *COMT* alone has been implicated in a gene-environment interaction (Val-*COMT* × cannabis) in schizophrenia etiology (Caspi et al. 2005).

Environment

Several prenatal and early life environment factors contribute to schizophrenia in conjunction with genetic predisposition and family history. A 5%–8% excess of schizophrenia is seen among individuals born in the winter and early spring (Bembenek 2005), consistent with associations of maternal infections during pregnancy with schizophrenia risk (up to sevenfold), including rubella (A.S. Brown et al. 2001), influenza (Brown et al. 2004), and toxoplasmosis (Brown et al. 2005; Strous and Shoenfeld 2005). Postnatal infections (especially neonatal coxsackie B meningitis) are also associated with later schizophrenia (Rantakallio et al. 1997).

Other intrauterine and obstetrical risk factors besides infection associated with later schizophrenia include preeclampsia, low birth weight, hypoxic events (Canon et al. 2002), maternal cigarette smoking (O'Dwyer 1997; Sacker et al. 1995), Rh incompatibility (Hollister et al. 1996), maternal stress (Huttunen and Niskanen 1978; Van Os and Selten 1998), and exposure to famine or malnutrition early in gestation (e.g., the Dutch Hunger Winter of 1944–1945) (Dalman et al. 1999; Susser et al. 1996).

Other variables associated with schizophrenia risk include urban residence and upbringing (Pederson and Mortensen 2001), immigration (Cantor-Graae et al. 2005), TBI (Malaspina et al. 1999), and use of drugs, particularly cannabis (Arseneault et al. 2004). Most exposures have small effects, with typical odds ratios or risk ratios of approximately 2. Questions of causation remain because premorbid or prodromal symptoms could increase risk of exposure (e.g., to head injury or drug use).

Immigration is associated with somewhat higher risk, compared with other exposures, because migration from poor countries to wealthy countries is associated with a 3- to 10-fold increase in schizophrenia risk, compared with both the host country and the country of origin (reviewed in P. Jones and Cannon 1998). This effect is greater for second-generation than for first-generation migrants, arguing against selective migration of at-risk individuals. It is not clear whether this finding reflects the effect of urbanization, stress, racism, or exposure to some new infectious or other environmental agent.

Gene-Environment Interaction

Increasingly, it is clear that gene-environment interactions must be considered for illness risk, with changes in gene expression as the likely mechanism (Quirion and Insel 2005). Data that support models of interaction between genetic vulnerability and the environment result from adoption studies. For adopted-away children of mothers with schizophrenia, adversity and poor family functioning in the adoptive home increase the risk for schizophrenia; however, no such effect is seen for adopted-away children of healthy mothers (Tienari 1991). In an Israeli study, children of mothers with schizophrenia had a higher risk of developing the illness themselves if raised in a kibbutz instead of a family home; again, this effect was not seen for children without genetic risk (Mirsky et al. 1985). Among the most exciting findings of gene-environment interaction for schizophrenia is the interaction of a specific allele of a susceptibility gene (i.e., Val-*COMT*) with an exposure (specifically, cannabis abuse) in increasing schizophrenia risk (Caspi et al. 2005).

NARCOLEPSY

The interesting scientific story of narcolepsy began more than a century ago, when the association of muscle weakness triggered by excitement (cataplexy) and excessive daytime sleepiness with sleep attacks was first described, as reviewed by Mignot (2001). These symptoms remain the hallmark criteria for classic narcolepsy. Other common features include hypnagogic hallucinations (dreamlike sequences experienced while awake, often involving visual or auditory hallucinations) and sleep paralysis (inability to move when falling asleep or awakening), with blackouts and automatic behaviors occurring less frequently. Periodic leg movements, sleep apnea, and rapid eye movement (REM) sleep behavior disorders become increasingly common in older narcoleptic patients, but cataplexy is the only symptom with a very high specificity for narcolepsy.

The definitive clinical diagnosis is based on polysomnographic evidence of abnormal REM sleep on the Multiple Sleep Latency Test (Carskadon and Dement 1975) consisting of short sleep latencies (<8 minutes) and at least two naps with sleep-onset REM sleep. Nocturnal polysomnography may be normal or show short nocturnal REM sleep latency, unexplained arousals, or periodic leg movements. The symptoms of narcolepsy are the physiological sequelae of impaired wakefulness and REM sleep dysregulation; cataplexy and sleep paralysis are REM sleep atonia that intrude into wakefulness, and hypnagogic and hypnopompic hallucinations arise from dream imagery that emerges during wakefulness. The narcolepsy-cataplexy complex is associated with hypofunction of the centrally mediated hypocretin (orexin) pathway, which promotes wakefulness and stabilizes sleep-wake cycles.

Epidemiological Studies

The prevalence of narcolepsy with cataplexy is approximately 1 in 2,000 individuals in the United States and Europe but may be as high as 1 in 625 in Japan (Mignot 2001). The excessive sleepiness of narcolepsy typically begins in the second or third decade. A delay in the onset of cataplexy and auxiliary symptoms is typical. Misdiagnosis is common, and most cases are never diagnosed or treated. The diagnosis often is not made until after age 40 years.

Narcolepsy is a heterogeneous disorder with multigenic, human leukocyte antigen (HLA)–associated, and environmentally influenced forms (Mignot 2004). The symptoms of narcolepsy emerge after a cerebrovascular accident or TBI in about half of the cases and are also observed in association with other neurological disorders, such as multiple sclerosis, encephalitis, myotonic dystrophy, and epilepsy.

Family Studies

Although familial transmission of narcolepsy is uncommon (Aldrich 1990), first-degree relatives of affected individuals are 20–40 times more likely to have narcolepsy than is the general population, consistent with genetic transmissibility (Mignot 1998). Twin studies confirm the familial nature of the condition but also highlight the importance of nongenetic factors. The clinical expression of narcolepsy can vary markedly, even within the same family.

Early evidence of a genetic susceptibility for narcolepsy was derived from the correlation between the frequency of narcolepsy and geographic variation of class II HLA antigens on chromosome 6. This association is among the highest known for HLA-linked syndromes. There is also a strong month-of-birth effect for narcolepsy, consistent with an environmentally influenced risk (Dauvilliers et al. 2003), but this appears to be a severe form that is independent of the HLA loci (Picchioni et al. 2004).

Linkage Analysis

Mignot's group (Lin et al. 1999) used positional cloning in a well-established canine colony to identify carnac-1 as an autosomal recessive gene for narcolepsy. The susceptibility allele was a mutation in the G-protein-coupled orexin-2 receptor. A role for this gene in narcolepsy was further confirmed when Yanagisawa and colleagues reported narcoleptic-like attacks in mice with an orexin knockout mutation (Chemelli et al. 1999). This linkage finding led directly to the identification of a candidate gene for human narcolepsy, orexin (hypocretin), and the possibility of new insights into the neurophysiology of sleep and wakefulness. Although mutations and polymorphisms in hypocretin-related genes are rare causes of the complex in humans, it rapidly became evident that abnormalities in hypothalamic hypocretin (orexin) neurotransmission are key features of narcolepsy with cataplexy.

Recent studies confirmed that narcolepsy-cataplexy is tightly associated with *HLA-DQB1*0602* in all studied ethnic groups (see Mignot et al. 2001). Illness risk in heterozygotes is moderated by numerous other class II alleles, several of which are protective (*DQB1*0601*, *DQB1*0501*, and *DQA1*01*), and epigenetic effects of additional loci are likely to be involved as well. For example, a recent genomewide linkage analysis in a large multiplex French family showed strong linkage to chromosome 21 (maximum two-point lod score = 3.36 at *D21S1245*) explained by a single haplotype that was between markers *D21S267* and *ABCG1* in a 5.15-Mb region of 21q (Dauvilliers et al. 2004).

Molecular Approaches

Human narcolepsy appears to be caused largely by a loss of hypocretin cells in the lateral hypothalamus rather than hypocretin ligand or receptor mutations, as observed in canines (Mignot 2004). Hypocretin neurons arise in the lateral and posterior hypothalamus and project to the limbic system, thalamus, brain stem, and spinal cord (Reid et al. 1998). The narcolepsy-cataplexy symptoms arise from the diminished neuroexcitatory signals from the hypothalamus. Hypocretin has additional effects on metabolism, appetite, and feeding behaviors (Sakurai et al. 1998).

According to the HLA data, Mignot et al. (2001) proposed that immunologically mediated damage to hypocretin-containing cells is a common cause of narcolepsy-cataplexy. An immune basis for narcolepsy seems likely even in non-HLA-linked cases. Dauvilliers et al. (2003) suggested that the month-of-birth study effect may derive from modification of immune system functioning by fetal development or early exposures. Furthermore, clinical improvement in an early-onset case by immunoglobulin treatment supports an antibody-mediated pathophysiology (Lecendreux et al. 2003).

Reduced or absent hypocretin levels are found in the cerebrospinal fluid in most human cases of narcolepsy. Even myotonic dystrophy (Martinez-Rodriguez et al. 2003) and Prader-Willi syndrome (Mignot et al. 2002) patients with excessive daytime sleepiness show hypocretin abnormalities. These findings have added greatly to research in the physiology and treatment of sleep disorders.

Highlights for the Clinician

Paradigms of psychiatric and genetic research				
Paradigm	Questions	Samples studied	Method of inquiry	Scientific goals
Basic genetic epidemiology	✦ Is the disorder familial? Is it inherited?	Family, twin, and adoption studies	Statistical	To quantify the degree of familial aggregation and/or heritability
Advanced genetic epidemiology	✦ What is being inherited? Are there epigenetic factors?	Family, twin, and adoption studies	Statistical	To explore the nature and mode of action of genetic risk factors
Gene finding	✦ How is the disorder inherited? Where are the abnormal genes?	High-density families, trios, case–control samples	Statistical	To determine the genomic location and identity of susceptibility genes
Molecular genetics	✦ What is (are) their molecular and pathological effect(s)?	Humans, animals	Biological	To identify critical DNA variants and trace the biological pathways from DNA to disorder

Adapted from Kendler KS: "Psychiatric Genetics: A Methodologic Critique." *American Journal of Psychiatry* 162:3–11, 2005.

RECOMMENDED READINGS

McGuffin P, Owen M, Gottesman I: Psychiatric Genetics and Genomics. Oxford, UK, Oxford University Press, 2002

Zorumski C, Rubin E: Psychopathology in the Genome and Neuroscience Era. Washington, DC, American Psychiatric Publishing, 2005

REFERENCES

Abi-Dargham A, Rodenhiser J, Printz D, et al: Increased baseline occupancy of D_2 receptors by dopamine in schizophrenia. Proc Natl Acad Sci U S A 97:8104–8109, 2000

Abramson RK, Wright HH, Carpenter R, et al: Elevated blood serotonin in autistic probands and their first-degree relatives. J Autism Dev Disord 19:397–407, 1989

Adams MD, Celniker SE, Holt RA, et al: The genome sequence of Drosophila melanogaster. Science 287:2185–2195, 2000

Addington AM, Gornick M, Sporn AL, et al: Polymorphisms in the 13q33.2 gene G70/G30 are associated with childhood-onset schizophrenia and psychosis not otherwise specified. Biol Psychiatry 10:976–980, 2004

Ahearn EP, Steffens DC, Cassidy F, et al: Familial leukoencephalopathy in bipolar disorder. Am J Psychiatry 155:1605–1607, 1998

Akil M, Schwartz JA, Dutchak D, et al: The psychiatric presentations of Wilson's disease [see comments]. J Neuropsychiatry Clin Neurosci 3:377–382, 1991

Alarcon M, Cantor RM, Liu J, et al: Evidence for a language quantitative trait locus on chromosome 7q in multiplex autism families. Am J Hum Genet 70:60–71, 2002

Alarcon M, Yonan AL, Gilliam TC, et al: Quantitative genome scan and Ordered-Subsets Analysis of autism endophenotypes support language QTLs. Mol Psychiatry 10:747–757, 2005

Aldrich MS: Narcolepsy. N Engl J Med 323:389–394, 1990

Alford RL, Ashizawa T, Jankovic J, et al: Molecular detection of new mutations, resolution of ambiguous results and complex genetic counseling issues in Huntington disease. Am J Med Genet 66:281–286, 1996

Allam MF, Campbell MJ, Del Castillo AS, et al: Parkinson's disease protects against smoking? Behav Neurol 15:65–71, 2004

Almond JW: Bovine spongiform encephalopathy and new variant Creutzfeldt-Jakob disease. Br Med Bull 54:749–759, 1998

Alper T, Cramp WA, Haig DA, et al: Does the agent of scrapie replicate without nucleic acid? Nature 214:764–766, 1967

Alsobrook [II] JP, Leckman JF, Goodman WK, et al: Segregation analysis of obsessive-compulsive disorder using symptom-based factor scores. Am J Med Genet 88:669–675, 1999

Alsobrook JP, Zohar AH, Leboyer M, et al: Association between the COMT locus and obsessive-compulsive disorder in females but not males. Am J Med Genet 114:116–120, 2002

Altemus M, Murphy DL, Greenberg B, et al: Intact coding region of the serotonin transporter gene in obsessive-compulsive disorder. Am J Med Genet 67:409–411, 1996

Ambrose CM, Duyao MP, Barnes G, et al: Structure and expression of the Huntington's disease gene: evidence against simple inactivation due to an expanded CAG repeat. Somat Cell Mol Genet 20:27–38, 1994

American Psychiatric Association: Diagnostic and Statistical Manual of Mental Disorders, 3rd Edition. Washington, DC, American Psychiatric Association, 1980

American Psychiatric Association: Diagnostic and Statistical Manual of Mental Disorders, 3rd Edition, Revised. Washington, DC, American Psychiatric Association, 1987

American Psychiatric Association: Diagnostic and Statistical Manual of Mental Disorders, 4th Edition. Washington, DC, American Psychiatric Association, 1994

American Psychiatric Association: Diagnostic and Statistical Manual of Mental Disorders, 4th Edition, Text Revision. Washington, DC, American Psychiatric Association, 2000

Anderson GM, Freedman DX, Cohen DJ, et al: Whole blood serotonin in autistic and normal subjects. J Child Psychol Psychiatry 28:885–900, 1987

Andrews G, Stewart G, Allen R, et al: The genetics of six neurotic disorders: a twin study. J Affect Disord 19:23–29, 1990

Andrews TC, Weeks RA, Turjanski N, et al: Huntington's disease progression: PET and clinical observations. Brain 122 (pt 12):2353–2363, 1999

Anguelova M, Benkelfat C, Turecki G: A systematic review of association studies investigating genes coding for serotonin receptors and the serotonin transporter, I: affective disorders. Mol Psychiatry 8:574–591, 2003

Arseneault L, Cannon M, Witton J, et al: Causal association between cannabis and psychosis: examination of the evidence. Br J Psychiatry 184:110–117, 2004

Ashley-Koch A, Wolpert CM, Menold MM, et al: Genetic studies of autistic disorder and chromosome 7. Genomics 61:227–236, 1999

Astrinidis A, Cash TP, Hunter DS, et al: Tuberin, the tuberous sclerosis complex 2 tumor suppressor gene product, regulates Rho activation, cell adhesion and migration. Oncogene 21:8470–8476, 2002

Auranen M, Nieminen T, Majuri S, et al: Analysis of autism susceptibility gene loci on chromosomes 1p, 4p, 6q, 7q, 13q, 15q, 16p, 17q, 19q and 22q in Finnish multiplex families. Mol Psychiatry 5:320–322, 2000

Auranen M, Vanhala R, Varilo T, et al: A genomewide screen for autism-spectrum disorders: evidence for a major susceptibility locus on chromosome 3q25–27. Am J Hum Genet 71:777–790, 2002

Azzam A, Mathews CA: Meta-analysis of the association between the catecholamine-O-methyl-transferase gene and obsessive-compulsive disorder. Am J Med Genet B Neuropsychiatr Genet 123:64–69, 2003

Bacchelli E, Blasi F, Biondolillo M, et al: Screening of nine candidate genes for autism on chromosome 2q reveals rare nonsynonymous variants in the cAMP-GEFII gene. Mol Psychiatry 8:916–924, 2003

Bacon BR, Schilsky ML: New knowledge of genetic pathogenesis of hemochromatosis and Wilson's disease. Adv Intern Med 44:91–116, 1999

Badner JA, Gershon ES: Meta-analysis of whole-genome linkage scans of bipolar disorder and schizophrenia. Mol Psychiatry 7:405–411, 2002

Bailer U, Wiesegger G, Leisch F, et al: No association of clock gene T3111C polymorphism and affective disorders. Eur Neuropsychopharmacol 15:51–55, 2005

Bailey A, Le Couteur A, Gottesman I, et al: Autism as a strongly genetic disorder: evidence from a British twin study. Psychol Med 25:63–77, 1995

Bailey A, Palferman S, Heavey L, et al: Autism: the phenotype in relatives. J Autism Dev Disord 28:369–392, 1998

Baldereschi M, Di Carlo A, Lepore V, et al: Estrogen-replacement therapy and Alzheimer's disease in the Italian Longitudinal Study on Aging. Neurology 50:996–1002, 1998

Balon R, Pohl R, Yeragani VK, et al: Lactate- and isoproterenol-induced panic attacks in panic disorder patients and controls. Psychiatry Res 23:153–160, 1988

Balon R, Jordan M, Pohl R, et al: Family history of anxiety disorders in control subjects with lactate-induced panic attacks. Am J Psychiatry 146:1304–1306, 1989

Bandmann O, Vaughan J, Holmans P, et al: Association of slow acetylator genotype for N-acetyltransferase 2 with familial Parkinson's disease [see comments]. Lancet 350:1136–1139, 1997

Bartlett CW, Gharani N, Millonig JH, et al: Three autism candidate genes: a synthesis of human genetic analysis with other disciplines. Int J Dev Neurosci 23:221–234, 2005

Barton M, Volkmar F: How commonly are known medical conditions associated with autism? J Autism Dev Disord 28:273–278, 1998

Bass MP, Menold MM, Wolpert CM, et al: Genetic studies in autistic disorder and chromosome 15. Neurogenetics 2219–2226, 1999

Battaglia M, Torgersen S: Schizotypal disorder: at the crossroads of genetics and nosology. Acta Psychiatr Scand 94:303–310, 1996

Belay ED: Transmissible spongiform encephalopathies in humans. Annu Rev Microbiol 53:283–314, 1999

Bellodi L, Perna G, Caldirola D, et al: CO_2-induced panic attacks: a twin study. Am J Psychiatry 155:1184–1188, 1998

Bembenek A: Seasonality of birth in schizophrenia patients. Psychiatr Pol 39:259–270, 2005

Benedetti F, Bernasconi A, Lorenzi C, et al: A single nucleotide polymorphism in glycogen synthase kinase 3-beta promoter gene influences onset of illness in patients affected by bipolar disorder. Neurosci Lett 355:37–40, 2004

Berrettini WH, Ferraro TN, Goldin LR, et al: Chromosome 18 DNA markers and manic-depressive illness: evidence for a susceptibility gene. Proc Natl Acad Sci U S A 91:5918–5921, 1994

Bickeboller H, Kistler M, Scholz M: Investigation of the candidate genes ACTHR and golf for bipolar illness by the transmission/disequilibrium test. Genet Epidemiol 14:575–580, 1997

Black A: The natural history of obsessional neurosis, in Obsessional States. Edited by Beech HR. London, Methuen, 1974, pp 19–54

Blackwood DH, He L, Morris SW, et al: A locus for bipolar affective disorder on chromosome 4p. Nat Genet 12:427–430, 1996

Blackwood DH, Fordyce A, Walker MT, et al: Schizophrenia and affective disorders: cosegregation with a translocation at chromosome 1q42 that directly disrupts brain-expressed genes: clinical and P300 findings in a family. Am J Hum Genet 69:428–433, 2001

Boffelli D, Nobrega MA, Rubin EM: Comparative genomics at the vertebrate extremes. Nat Rev Genet 5:456–465, 2004

Bonifati V, Rizzu P, van Baren MJ, et al: Mutations in the DJ-1 gene associated with autosomal recessive early onset parkinsonism. Science 299:256–259, 2003

Bonne-Tamir B, Farrer LA, Frydman M, et al: Evidence for linkage between Wilson disease and esterase D in three kindreds: detection of linkage for an autosomal recessive disorder by the family study method. Genet Epidemiol 3:201–209, 1986

Bonora E, Bacchelli E, Levy ER, et al: Mutation screening and imprinting analysis of four candidate genes for autism in the 7q32 region. Mol Psychiatry 7:289–301, 2002

Bonora E, Lamb JA, Barnby G, et al: Mutation screening and association analysis of six candidate genes for autism on chromosome 7q. Eur J Hum Genet 13:198–207, 2005

Botstein D, White RL, Skolnick M, et al: Construction of a genetic linkage map using restriction fragment length polymorphisms. Am J Hum Genet 32:314–331, 1980

Brown AS, Cohen P, Harkavy-Friedman J, et al: A.E. Bennett Research Award: prenatal rubella, premorbid abnormalities, and adult schizophrenia. Biol Psychiatry 49:473–486, 2001

Brown AS, Schaefer CA, Wyatt RJ, et al: Paternal age and risk of schizophrenia in adult offspring. Am J Psychiatry 159:1528–1533, 2002

Brown AS, Begg MD, Gravenstein S, et al: Serologic evidence of prenatal influenza in the etiology of schizophrenia. Arch Gen Psychiatry 61:774–780, 2004

Brown AS, Schaefer CA, Quesenberry CP Jr, et al: Maternal exposure to toxoplasmosis and risk of schizophrenia in adult offspring. Am J Psychiatry 162:767–773, 2005

Brown FW: Heredity in the psychoneuroses. Proc R Soc Med 35785–35790, 1942

Bryson SE, Clark BS, Smith IM: First report of a Canadian epidemiological study of autistic syndromes. J Child Psychol Psychiatry 29:433–445, 1988

Brzustowicz LM, Hodgkinson KA, Chow EW, et al: Location of a major susceptibility locus for familial schizophrenia on chromosome 1q21-q22. Science 288:678–682, 2000

Bull PC, Thomas GR, Rommens M, et al: The Wilson disease gene is a putative copper transporting ATPase similar to the Menkes disease gene. Nat Genet 5:327–337, 1993

Burke KC, Burke JD Jr, Regier DA, et al: Age at onset of selected mental disorders in five community populations. Arch Gen Psychiatry 47:511–518, 1990

Butterworth NJ, Williams L, Bullock JY, et al: Trinucleotide (CAG) repeat length is positively correlated with the degree of DNA fragmentation in Huntington's disease striatum. Neuroscience 87:49–53, 1998

Buxbaum JD, Silverman JM, Smith CJ, et al: Evidence for a susceptibility gene for autism on chromosome 2 and for genetic heterogeneity. Am J Hum Genet 68:1514–1520, 2001

Buxbaum JD, Silverman JM, Smith CJ, et al: Association between a GABRB3 polymorphism and autism. Mol Psychiatry 7:311–316, 2002

Buxbaum JD, Silverman J, Keddache M, et al: Linkage analysis for autism in a subset of families with obsessive-compulsive behaviors: evidence for an autism susceptibility gene on chromosome 1 and further support for susceptibility genes on chromosome 6 and 19. Mol Psychiatry 9:144–150, 2004

Byrne M, Agerbo E, Ewald H, et al: Parental age and risk of schizophrenia: a case-control study. Arch Gen Psychiatry 60:673–678, 2003

Cadoret RJ, O'Gorman TW, Heywood E, et al: Genetic and environmental factors in major depression. J Affect Disord 9:155–164, 1985

Callicott JH, Egan MF, Bertolino A, et al: Hippocampal N-acetyl aspartate in unaffected siblings of patients with schizophrenia: a possible intermediate neurobiological phenotype. Biol Psychiatry 44:941–950, 1998

Callicott JH, Straub RE, Pezawas L, et al: Variation in DISC1 affects hippocampal structure and function and increases risk for schizophrenia. Proc Natl Acad Sci U S A 102:8627–8632, 2005

Camarena B, Aguilar A, Loyzaga C, et al: A family based association study of the 5-HT-1Dbeta receptor gene in obsessive-compulsive disorder. Int J Neuropsychopharmacol 7:49–53, 2004

Cannon TD, Kaprio J, Lonnqvist J, et al: The genetic epidemiology of schizophrenia in a Finnish twin cohort: a population-based modeling study. Arch Gen Psychiatry 55:67–74, 1998

Canon M, Jones PB, Murray RM: Obstetric complications and schizophrenia. Am J Psychiatry 159:1080–1092, 2002

Cantor-Graae E, Zolkowska K, McNeil TF: Increased risk of psychotic disorder among immigrants in Malmo: a 3-year first-contact study. Psychol Med 35:1155–1163, 2005

Carey G, Gottesman II: Twin and family studies of anxiety, phobic, and obsessive disorders, in Anxiety: New Research and Changing Concepts. Edited by Klein DF, Rabkin JD. New York, Raven, 1981, pp 117–136

Carskadon MA, Dement WC: Sleep studies on a 90-minute day. Electroencephalogr Clin Neurophysiol 39:145–155, 1975

Casadesus G, Atwood CS, Zhu X, et al: Evidence for the role of gonadotropin hormones in the development of Alzheimer disease. Cell Mol Life Sci 62:293–298, 2005

Caspi A, Moffitt TE, Cannon M, et al: Moderation of the effect of adolescent-onset cannabis use on adult psychosis by a functional polymorphism in the catechol-O-methyltransferase gene: longitudinal evidence of a gene x environment interaction. Biol Psychiatry 57:1117–1127, 2005

Castermans D, Wilquet V, Steyaert J, et al: Chromosomal anomalies in individuals with autism: a strategy towards the identification of genes involved in autism. Autism 8:141–161, 2004

Cavallini MC, Di Bella D, Pasquale L, et al: 5HT2C CYS23/SER23 polymorphism is not associated with obsessive-compulsive disorder. Psychiatry Res 77:97–104, 1998

Cavallini MC, Pasquale L, Bellodi L, et al: Complex segregation analysis for obsessive compulsive disorder and related disorders. Am J Med Genet 88:38–43, 1999a

Cavallini MC, Perna G, Caldirola D, et al: A segregation study of panic disorder in families of panic patients responsive to the 35% CO$_2$ challenge. Biol Psychiatry 46:815–820, 1999b

Cedarbaum JM, McDowell FH: Sixteen-year follow-up of 100 patients begun on levodopa in 1968: emerging problems. Adv Neurol 45:469–472, 1987

C. elegans Sequencing Consortium: Genome sequence of the nematode C. elegans: a platform for investigating biology [published erratum appears in Science 283:35, 1999; 283:2103, 1999; 285:1493, 1999]. Science 282:2012–2018, 1998

Chang KD, Steiner H, Ketter TA: Psychiatric phenomenology of child and adolescent bipolar offspring. J Am Acad Child Adolesc Psychiatry 39:453–460, 2000

Checkoway H, Nelson LM: Epidemiologic approaches to the study of Parkinson's disease etiology. Epidemiology 10:327–336, 1999

Chemelli RM, Willie JT, Sinton CM, et al: Narcolepsy in orexin knockout mice: molecular genetics of sleep regulation. Cell 98:437–451, 1999

Chimpanzee Sequencing and Analysis Consortium: Initial sequence of the chimpanzee genome and comparison with the human genome. Nature 437:69–87, 2005

Cho HJ, Meira-Lima I, Cordeiro Q, et al: Population-based and family based studies on the serotonin transporter gene polymorphisms and bipolar disorder: a systematic review and meta-analysis. Mol Psychiatry 10:771–781, 2005

Chumakov I, Blumenfeld M, Guerassimenko O, et al: Genetic and physiological data implicating the new human gene G72 and the gene for D-amino acid oxidase in schizophrenia. Proc Natl Acad Sci U S A 99:13675–13680, 2002

Clifford CA, Murray RM, Fulker DW: Genetic and environmental influences on obsessional traits and symptoms. Psychol Med 14:791–800, 1984

Cohen ME, White PD: Life situations, emotions and neurocirculatory asthenia (anxiety neurosis, neurasthenia, effort syndrome). Res Publ Assoc Res Nerv Ment Dis 29:832–869, 1949

Cohen ME, White PD: Life situations, emotions, and neurocirculatory asthenia (anxiety neurosis, neurasthenia, effort syndrome). Psychosom Med 13:335–357, 1951

Cohen ME, Badal DW, Kilpatrick A, et al: The high familial prevalence of neurocirculatory asthenia (anxiety neurosis, effort syndrome). Am J Hum Genet 3:126–158, 1951

Collaborative Linkage Study of Autism: An autosomal genomic screen for autism. Am J Med Genet 105:609–615, 2001

Collins FS, Morgan M, Patrinos A: The Human Genome Project: lessons from large-scale biology. Science 300:286–290, 2003

Cook EH Jr, Courchesne R, Lord C, et al: Evidence of linkage between the serotonin transporter and autistic disorder. Mol Psychiatry 2:247–250, 1997

Cook EH Jr, Courchesne RY, Cox NJ, et al: Linkage-disequilibrium mapping of autistic disorder, with 15q11-13 markers. Am J Hum Genet 62:1077–1083, 1998

Corfas G, Roy K, Buxbaum JD: Neuregulin 1-erbB signaling and the molecular/cellular basis of schizophrenia. Nat Neurosci 7:575–580, 2004

Coryell W: Hypersensitivity to carbon dioxide as a disease-specific trait marker. Biol Psychiatry 41:259–263, 1997

Coryell W, Endicott J, Andreasen NC, et al: Depression and panic attacks: the significance of overlap as reflected in follow-up and family study data. Am J Psychiatry 145:293–300, 1988

Cox DW, Fraser FC, Sass-Kortsak A: A genetic study of Wilson's disease: evidence for heterogeneity. Am J Hum Genet 24:646–666, 1972

Craddock N, Jones I: Genetics of bipolar disorder. J Med Genet 36:585–594, 1999

Craddock N, McKeon P, Moorhead S, et al: Expanded CAG/CTG repeats in bipolar disorder: no correlation with phenotypic measures of illness severity. Biol Psychiatry 42:876–881, 1997

Craddock N, O'Donovan MC, Owen MJ: The genetics of schizophrenia and bipolar disorder: dissecting psychosis. J Med Genet 42:193–204, 2005

Crawford TJ, Sharma T, Puri BK, et al: Saccadic eye movements in families multiply affected with schizophrenia: the Maudsley Family Study. Am J Psychiatry 155:1703–1710, 1998

Crowe RC, Pauls DL, Slymen DJ, et al: A family study of anxiety neurosis. Morbidity risk in families of patients with and without mitral valve prolapse. Arch Gen Psychiatry 37:77–79, 1980

Crowe RR, Noyes R, Pauls DL, et al: A family study of panic disorder. Arch Gen Psychiatry 40:1065–1069, 1983

Crowe RR, Noyes R, Jr., Wilson AF, et al: A linkage study of panic disorder. Arch Gen Psychiatry 44:933–937, 1987

Crowe RR, Noyes R, Jr., Samuelson S, et al: Close linkage between panic disorder and alpha-haptoglobin excluded in 10 families. Arch Gen Psychiatry 47:377–380, 1990

Crowe RR, Goedken R, Samuelson S, et al: Genomewide survey of panic disorder. Am J Med Genet 105:105–109, 2001

Cruts M, van Duijn CM, Backhovens H, et al: Estimation of the genetic contribution of presenilin-1 and -2 mutations in a population-based study of presenile Alzheimer disease. Hum Mol Genet 7:43–51, 1998

Csernansky JG, Joshi S, Wang L, et al: Hippocampal morphometry in schizophrenia by high dimensional brain mapping. Proc Natl Acad Sci U S A 95:11406–11411, 1998

Dalman C, Allebeck P, Cullberg J, et al: Obstetric complications and the risk of schizophrenia: a longitudinal study of a national birth cohort. Arch Gen Psychiatry 56:234–240, 1999

Dalman C, Allebeck P: Paternal age and schizophrenia: further support for an association. Am J Psychiatry 159:1591–1592, 2002

Daniel KG, Harbach RH, Guida WC, et al: Copper storage diseases: Menkes, Wilsons, and cancer. Front Biosci 9:2652–2662, 2004

Dauvilliers Y, Carlander B, Molinari N: Month of birth as a risk factor for narcolepsy. Sleep 26:663–665, 2003

Dauvilliers Y, Blouin JL, Neidhart E, et al: A narcolepsy susceptibility locus maps to a 5 Mb region of chromosome 21q. Ann Neurol 56:382–388, 2004

de la Monte SM, Wands JR: Review of insulin and insulin-like growth factor expression, signaling, and malfunction in the central nervous system: relevance to Alzheimer's disease. J Alzheimers Dis 7:45–61, 2005

Deckert J, Nothen MM, Franke P, et al: Systematic mutation screening and association study of the A1 and A2a adenosine receptor genes in panic disorder suggest a contribution of the A2a gene to the development of disease. Mol Psychiatry 3:81–85, 1998

DeLong GR, Dwyer JT: Correlation of family history with specific autistic subgroups: Asperger's syndrome and bipolar affective disease. J Autism Dev Disord 18:593–600, 1988

DeLorey TM, Handforth A, Anagnostaras SG, et al: Mice lacking the beta$_3$ subunit of the GABA$_A$ receptor have the epilepsy phenotype and many of the behavioral characteristics of Angelman syndrome. J Neurosci 18:8505–8514, 1998

Delorme R, Betancur C, Callebert J, et al: Platelet serotonergic markers as endophenotypes for obsessive-compulsive disorder. Neuropsychopharmacology 30:1539–1547, 2005

Dening TR: The neuropsychiatry of Wilson's disease: a review. Int J Psychiatry Med 21:135–148, 1991

Dermitzakis ET, Reymond A, Scamuffa N, et al: Evolutionary discrimination of mammalian conserved non-genic sequences (CNGs). Science 302:1033–1035, 2003

Detera-Wadleigh SD, Badner JA, Berrettini WH, et al: A high-density genome scan detects evidence for a bipolar-disorder susceptibility locus on 13q32 and other potential loci on 1q32 and 18p11.2. Proc Natl Acad Sci U S A 96:5604–5609, 1999

Di Bella D, Catalano M, Balling U, et al: Systematic screening for mutations in the coding region of the human serotonin transporter (5-HTT) gene using PCR and DGGE. Am J Med Genet 67:541–545, 1996

Domschke K, Freitag CM, Kuhlenbaumer G, et al: Association of the functional V158M catechol-O-methyl-transferase polymorphism with panic disorder in women. Int J Neuropsychopharmacol 7:183–188, 2004

Done DJ, Crow TJ, Johnstone EC, et al: Childhood antecedents of schizophrenia and affective illness: social adjustment at ages 7 and 11. BMJ 309:699–703, 1994

Duyao MP, Auerbach AB, Ryan A, et al: Inactivation of the mouse Huntington's disease gene homolog Hdh. Science 269:407–410, 1995

Eaton WW, Kessler RC, Wittchen HU, et al: Panic and panic disorder in the United States. Am J Psychiatry 151:413–420, 1994

Egan MF, Goldberg TE, Kolachana BS, et al: Effect of COMT Val 108/158 Met genotype on frontal lobe function and risk for schizophrenia. Proc Natl Acad Sci U S A 98:6917–6922, 2001

Ekelund J, Hennah W, Hiekkalinna T, et al: Replication of 1q42 linkage in Finnish schizophrenia pedigrees. Mol Psychiatry 9:1037–1041, 2004

El-Saadi O, Pedersen CB, McNeil TF, et al: Paternal and maternal age as risk factors for psychosis: findings from Denmark, Sweden and Australia. Schizophr Res 67:227–236, 2004

Enoch MA, Kaye WH, Rotondo A, et al: 5-HT2A promoter polymorphism -1438G/A, anorexia nervosa, and obsessive-compulsive disorder. Lancet 351:1785–1786, 1998

Erdal ME, Tot S, Yazici K, et al: Lack of association of catechol-O-methyltransferase gene polymorphism in obsessive-compulsive disorder. Depress Anxiety 18:41–45, 2003

Erlenmeyer-Kimling L, Cornblatt B: Attentional measure in the study of children at high risk for schizophrenia. J Psychiatr Res 114:93–98, 1978

Erlenmeyer-Kimling L, Cornblatt BA: A summary of attentional findings in the New York High-Risk Project. J Psychiatr Res 26:405–426, 1992

Estrov Y, Scaglia F, Bodamer OA: Psychiatric symptoms of inherited metabolic disease. J Inherit Metab Dis 23:2–6, 2000

Ewald H, Degn B, Mors O, et al: Significant linkage between bipolar affective disorder and chromosome 12q24. Psychiatr Genet 8:131–140, 1998a

Fallin MD, Lasseter VK, Avramopoulos D, et al: Bipolar I disorder and schizophrenia: a 440-single-nucleotide polymorphism screen of 64 candidate genes among Ashkenazi Jewish case-parent trios. Am J Hum Genet 77:918–936, 2005

Fan JB, Zhang CS, Gu NF, et al: Catechol-O-methyltransferase gene Val/Met functional polymorphism and risk of schizophrenia: a large-scale association study plus meta-analysis. Biol Psychiatry 57:139–144, 2005

Ferenci P: Review article: diagnosis and current therapy of Wilson's disease. Aliment Pharmacol Ther 19:157–165, 2004

Finch CE: Developmental origins of aging in brain and blood vessels: an overview. Neurobiol Aging 26:281–291, 2005

Finn CT, Smoller JW: The genetics of panic disorder. Curr Psychiatry Rep 3:131–137, 2001

Fischman AJ: Role of [18F]-dopa-PET imaging in assessing movement disorders. Radiol Clin North Am 43:93–106, 2005

Fish B: Neurobiologic antecedents of schizophrenia in children: evidence for an inherited, congenital neurointegrative defect. Arch Gen Psychiatry 34:1297–1313, 1977

Fish B, Marcus J, Hans SL, et al: Infants at risk for schizophrenia: sequelae of a genetic neurointegrative defect: a review and replication analysis of pandysmaturation in the Jerusalem Infant Development Study. Arch Gen Psychiatry 49:221–235, 1992

Flament MF, Whitaker A, Rapoport JL, et al: Obsessive compulsive disorder in adolescence: an epidemiological study. J Am Acad Child Adolesc Psychiatry 27:764–771, 1988

Flament MF, Koby E, Rapoport JL, et al: Childhood obsessive-compulsive disorder: a prospective follow-up study. J Child Psychol Psychiatry 31:363–380, 1990

Flint J, Valdar W, Shifman S, et al: Strategies for mapping and cloning quantitative trait genes in rodents. Nat Rev Genet 6:271–286, 2005

Foley P, Riederer P: Pathogenesis and preclinical course of Parkinson's disease. J Neural Transm Suppl 56:31–74, 1999

Folstein S, Rutter M: Infantile autism: a genetic study of 21 twin pairs. J Child Psychol Psychiatry 18:297–321, 1977

Folstein SE, Rosen-Sheidley B: Genetics of autism: complex aetiology for a heterogeneous disorder. Nat Rev Genet 2:943–955, 2001

Folstein SE, Abbott MH, Chase GA, et al: The association of affective disorder with Huntington's disease in a case series and in families. Psychol Med 13:537–542, 1983

Fombonne E: The epidemiology of autism: a review. Psychol Med 29:769–786, 1999

Freedman R, Adler LE, Leonard S: Alternative phenotypes for the complex genetics of schizophrenia. Biol Psychiatry 45:551–558, 1999

Freimer NB, Reus VI, Escamilla MA, et al: Genetic mapping using haplotype, association and linkage methods suggests a locus for severe bipolar (BPI) at 18q22-q23. Nat Genet 12:436–441, 1996

Frisch A, Michaelovsky E, Rockah R, et al: Association between obsessive-compulsive disorder and polymorphisms of genes encoding components of the serotonergic and dopaminergic pathways. Eur Neuropsychopharmacol 10:205–209, 2000

Frydman M, Bonne-Tamir B, Farrer LA, et al: Assignment of the gene for Wilson disease to chromosome 13: linkage to esterase D locus. Proc Natl Acad Sci U S A 82:1819–1821, 1985

Furlong RA, Ho L, Rubinsztein JS, et al: Analysis of the monoamine oxidase A (MAOA) gene in bipolar affective disorder by association studies, meta-analyses, and sequencing of the promoter. Am J Med Genet 88:398–406, 1999

Fusco FR, Chen Q, Lamoreaux WJ, et al: Cellular localization of huntingtin in striatal and cortical neurons in rats: lack of correlation with neuronal vulnerability in Huntington's disease. J Neurosci 19:1189–1202, 1999

Fyer AJ, Weissman MM: Genetic linkage study of panic: clinical methodology and description of pedigrees. Am J Med Genet 88:173–181, 1999

Fyer AJ, Mannuzza S, Chapman TF, et al: Specificity in familial aggregation of phobic disorders. Arch Gen Psychiatry 52:564–573, 1995

Gabriel SB, Schaffner SF, Nguyen H, et al: The structure of haplotype blocks in the human genome. Science 296:2225–2229, 2002

Gambetti P, Kong Q, Zou W, et al: Sporadic and familial CJD: classification and characterisation. Br Med Bull 66:213–239, 2003

Gamboa ET, Wolf A, Yahr MD, et al: Influenza virus antigen in postencephalitic parkinsonism brain: detection by immunofluorescence. Arch Neurol 31:228–232, 1974

Gasparini L, Ongini E, Wilcock D, et al: Activity of flurbiprofen and chemically related anti-inflammatory drugs in models of Alzheimer's disease. Brain Res Brain Res Rev 48:400–408, 2005

Gasser T: Genetics of Parkinson's disease. J Neurol 248:833–840, 2001

Gasser T, Muller-Myhsok B, Wszolek ZK, et al: A susceptibility locus for Parkinson's disease maps to chromosome 2p13. Nat Genet 18:262–265, 1998

Gauthier J, Bonnel A, St-Onge J, et al: *NLGN3/NLGN4* gene mutations are not responsible for autism in the Quebec population. Am J Med Genet B Neuropsychiatr Genet 132:74–75, 2005

Gelernter J, Bonvicini K, Page G, et al: Linkage genome scan for loci predisposing to panic disorder or agoraphobia. Am J Med Genet 105:548–557, 2001

Gelernter J, Page GP, Bonvicini K, et al: A chromosome 14 risk locus for simple phobia: results from a genomewide linkage scan. Mol Psychiatry 8:71–82, 2003

Gelernter J, Page GP, Stein MB, et al: Genome-wide linkage scan for loci predisposing to social phobia: evidence for a chromosome 16 risk locus. Am J Psychiatry 161:59–66, 2004

Gershon ES, Hamovit J, Guroff JJ, et al: A family study of schizoaffective, bipolar I, bipolar II, unipolar, and normal control probands. Arch Gen Psychiatry 39:1157–1167, 1982

Gillberg C: The treatment of epilepsy in autism. J Autism Dev Disord 21:61–77, 1991

Gillberg C: Chromosomal disorders and autism. J Autism Dev Disord 28:415–425, 1998

Gillberg C, Coleman M: Autism and medical disorders: a review of the literature. Dev Med Child Neurol 38:191–202, 1996

Giordani B, Berent S, Boivin MJ, et al: Longitudinal neuropsychological and genetic linkage analysis of persons at risk for Huntington's disease. Arch Neurol 52:59–64, 1995

Glantz LA, Lewis DA: Decreased dendritic spine density on prefrontal cortical pyramidal neurons in schizophrenia. Arch Gen Psychiatry 57:65–73, 2000

Glatt SJ, Faraone SV, Tsuang MT: Association between a functional catechol-O-methyltransferase gene polymorphism and schizophrenia: meta-analysis of case-control and family based studies. Am J Psychiatry 160:469–476, 2003

Glatzel M, Stoeck K, Seeger H, et al: Human prion diseases: molecular and clinical aspects. Arch Neurol 62:545–552, 2005

Goate A, Chartier-Harlin MC, Mullan M, et al: Segregation of a missense mutation in the amyloid precursor protein gene with familial Alzheimer's disease. Nature 349:704–706, 1991

Gogos JA, Santha M, Takacs Z, et al: The gene encoding proline dehydrogenase modulates sensorimotor gating in mice. Nat Genet 21:434–439, 1999

Goldstein RB, Wickramaratne PJ, Horwath E, et al: Familial aggregation and phenomenology of "early"-onset (at or before age 20 years) panic disorder. Arch Gen Psychiatry 54:271–278, 1997

Goodman WK, McDougle CJ, Price LH, et al: Beyond the serotonin hypothesis: a role for dopamine in some forms of obsessive compulsive disorder? J Clin Psychiatry 51(suppl): 36–43; discussion 55–58, 1990

Goodwin FK, Jamison KR: Manic-Depressive Illness. New York, Oxford University Press, 1990

Gorman JM, Papp LA, Martinez J, et al: High-dose carbon dioxide challenge test in anxiety disorder patients. Biol Psychiatry 28:743–757, 1990

Grados MA, Riddle MA, Samuels JF, et al: The familial phenotype of obsessive-compulsive disorder in relation to tic disorders: the Hopkins OCD family study. Biol Psychiatry 50:559–565, 2001

Green AJ, Johnson PH, Yates JR: The tuberous sclerosis gene on chromosome 9q34 acts as a growth suppressor. Hum Mol Genet 3:1833–1834, 1994

Green EK, Raybould R, Macgregor S, et al: Operation of the schizophrenia susceptibility gene, neuregulin 1, across traditional diagnostic boundaries to increase risk for bipolar disorder. Arch Gen Psychiatry 62:642–648, 2005

Green MF, Bracha HS, Satz P, et al: Preliminary evidence for an association between minor physical anomalies and second trimester neurodevelopment in schizophrenia. Psychiatry Res 53:119–127, 1994

Grunewald T, Beal MF: Bioenergetics in Huntington's disease. Ann N Y Acad Sci 893:203–213, 1999

Guo Z, Cupples LA, Kurz A, et al: Head injury and the risk of AD in the MIRAGE study. Neurology 54:1316–1323, 2000

Gusella JF, Wexler NS, Conneally PM, et al: A polymorphic DNA marker genetically linked to Huntington's disease. Nature 306:234–238, 1983

Gusella JF, MacDonald ME, Ambrose CM, et al: Molecular genetics of Huntington's disease. Arch Neurol 50:1157–1163, 1993

Häfner H, Maurer K, Löffler W, et al: The influence of age and sex on the onset and early course of schizophrenia. Br J Psychiatry 162:80–86, 1993

Hallmayer J, Hebert JM, Spiker D, et al: Autism and the X chromosome: multipoint sib-pair analysis. Arch Gen Psychiatry 53:985–989, 1996

Hallmayer J, Glasson EJ, Bower C, et al: On the twin risk in autism. Am J Hum Genet 71:941–946, 2002

Hamilton SP, Slager SL, Heiman GA, et al: Evidence for a susceptibility locus for panic disorder near the catechol-O-methyltransferase gene on chromosome 22. Biol Psychiatry 51:591–601, 2002

Hamilton SP, Fyer AJ, Durner M, et al: Further genetic evidence for a panic disorder syndrome mapping to chromosome 13q. Proc Natl Acad Sci U S A 100:2550–2555, 2003

Hamilton SP, Slager SL, De Leon AB, et al: Evidence for genetic linkage between a polymorphism in the adenosine 2A receptor and panic disorder. Neuropsychopharmacology 29:558–565, 2004

Hanna GL, Veenstra-VanderWeele J, Cox NJ, et al: Genome-wide linkage analysis of families with obsessive-compulsive disorder ascertained through pediatric probands. Am J Med Genet 114:541–552, 2002

Hanna GL, Himle JA, Curtis GC, et al: A family study of obsessive-compulsive disorder with pediatric probands. Am J Med Genet B Neuropsychiatr Genet 134:13–19, 2005

Harper PS: New genes for old diseases: the molecular basis of myotonic dystrophy and Huntington's disease: the Lumleian Lecture 1995. J R Coll Physicians Lond 30:221–231, 1996

Harris EL, Noyes R Jr, Crowe RR, et al: Family study of agoraphobia. Report of a pilot study. Arch Gen Psychiatry 40:1061–1064, 1983

Harris GJ, Codori AM, Lewis RF, et al: Reduced basal ganglia blood flow and volume in pre-symptomatic, gene-tested persons at-risk for Huntington's disease. Brain 122 (pt 9):1667–1678, 1999

Harrison PJ: The neuropathology of schizophrenia: a critical review of the data and their interpretation. Brain 122 (pt 4):593–624, 1999

Harrison PJ, Weinberger DR: Schizophrenia genes, gene expression, and neuropathology: on the matter of their convergence. Mol Psychiatry 10:40–68, 2005

Hashimoto K, Shimizu E, Iyo M: Critical role of brain-derived neurotrophic factor in mood disorders. Brain Res Brain Res Rev 45:104–114, 2004

Hattori E, Liu C, Badner JA, et al: Polymorphisms at the G72/G30 gene locus, on 13q33, are associated with bipolar disorder in two independent pedigree series. Am J Hum Genet 72:1131–1140, 2003

Hattori E, Liu C, Zhu H, et al: Genetic tests of biologic systems in affective disorders. Mol Psychiatry 10:719–740, 2005

Hendrie HC: Epidemiology of dementia and Alzheimer's disease. Am J Geriatr Psychiatry 6:S3–S18, 1998

Hennekens CH, Buring JE: Epidemiology in Medicine. Boston, MA, Little, Brown, 1987

Heresco-Levy U, Javitt DC: The role of N-methyl-D-aspartate (NMDA) receptor-mediated neurotransmission in the pathophysiology and therapeutics of psychiatric syndromes. Eur Neuropsychopharmacol 8:141–152, 1998

Herishanu YO, Kordysh E, Goldsmith JR: A case-referent study of extrapyramidal signs (preparkinsonism) in rural communities of Israel. Can J Neurol Sci 25:127–133, 1998

Hesse S, Muller U, Lincke T, et al: Serotonin and dopamine transporter imaging in patients with obsessive-compulsive disorder. Psychiatry Res 140:63–72, 2005

Heston LL: Psychiatric disorders in foster home reared children of schizophrenic mothers. Br J Psychiatry 112:819–825, 1966

Hettema JM, Neale MC, Kendler KS: A review and meta-analysis of the genetic epidemiology of anxiety disorders. Am J Psychiatry 158:1568–1578, 2001

Heun R, Maier W: The distinction of bipolar II disorder from bipolar I and recurrent unipolar depression: results of a controlled family study. Acta Psychiatr Scand 87:279–284, 1993

Hofman A, Collette HJ, Bartelds AI: Incidence and risk factors of Parkinson's disease in the Netherlands. Neuroepidemiology 8:296–299, 1989

Hollingsworth CE, Tanguay PE, Grossman L, et al: Long-term outcome of obsessive-compulsive disorder in childhood. J Am Acad Child Psychiatry 19:134–144, 1980

Hollister JM, Laing P, Mednick SA: Rhesus incompatibility as a risk factor for schizophrenia in male adults. Arch Gen Psychiatry 53:19–24, 1996

Hoogenraad HU, Koevoet R, de Ruyter Korver EGWM: Oral zinc sulphate as long term treatment in Wilson's disease. Eur Neurol 18:205–211, 1979

Hopper JL, Judd FK, Derrick PL, et al: A family study of panic disorder. Genet Epidemiol 4:33–41, 1987

Horwath E, Adams P, Wickramaratne P, et al: Panic disorder with smothering symptoms: evidence for increased risk in first-degree relatives. Depress Anxiety 6:147–153, 1997

Hudziak JJ, vanBeijsterveldt CEM, Althoff RR, et al: Genetic and environmental contributions to the Child Behavior Checklist Obsessive-Compulsive Scale: a cross-cultural twin study. Arch Gen Psychiatry 61:608–616, 2004

Huntington Disease Collaborative Research Group: A novel gene containing a trinucleotide repeat that is expanded and unstable on Huntington disease chromosomes. Cell 72:971–983, 1993

Huttunen MO, Niskanen P: Prenatal loss of father and psychiatric disorders. Arch Gen Psychiatry 35:429–431, 1978

Inada Y, Yoneda H, Koh J, et al: Positive association between panic disorder and polymorphism of the serotonin 2A receptor gene. Psychiatry Res 118:25–31, 2003

The International HapMap Consortium: The International HapMap Project. Nature 426:789–796, 2003

The International HapMap Consortium: A haplotype map of the human genome. Nature 437:1299–1320, 2005

International Human Genome Sequencing Consortium: Initial sequencing and analysis of the human genome. Nature 409:860–921, 2001

International Human Genome Sequencing Consortium: Finishing the euchromatic sequence of the human genome. Nature 431:931–945, 2004

International Molecular Genetic Study of Autism Consortium: A full genome screen for autism with evidence for linkage to a region on chromosome 7q. Hum Mol Genet 7:571–578, 1998

International Molecular Genetic Study of Autism Consortium: A genomewide screen for autism: strong evidence for linkage to chromosomes 2q, 7q, and 16p. Am J Hum Genet 69:570–581, 2001a

International Molecular Genetic Study of Autism Consortium: Further characterization of the autism susceptibility locus AUTS1 on chromosome 7q. Hum Mol Genet 10:973–982, 2001b

Ivanov D, Kirov G, Norton N, et al: Chromosome 22q11 deletions, velo-cardio-facial syndrome and early-onset psychosis: molecular genetic study. Br J Psychiatry 183:409–413, 2003

Jacquet H, Raux G, Thibaut F, et al: PRODH mutations and hyperprolinemia in a subset of schizophrenic patients. Hum Mol Genet 11:2243–2249, 2002

Jamain S, Quach H, Betancur C, et al: Mutations of the X-linked genes encoding neuroligins NLGN3 and NLGN4 are associated with autism. Nat Genet 34:27–29, 2003

Jellinger KA: Head injury and dementia. Curr Opin Neurol 17:719–723, 2004

Jenner P, Olanow CW: Understanding cell death in Parkinson's disease. Ann Neurol 44:S72–S84, 1998

Johnson GC, Esposito L, Barratt BJ, et al: Haplotype tagging for the identification of common disease genes. Nat Genet 29:233–237, 2001

Jones P, Cannon M: The new epidemiology of schizophrenia. Psychiatr Clin North Am 21:1–25, 1998

Jones P, Rodgers B, Murray R, et al: Child development risk factors for adult schizophrenia in the British 1946 birth cohort. Lancet 344:1398–1402, 1994

Jones SH, Hare DJ, Evershed K: Actigraphic assessment of circadian activity and sleep patterns in bipolar disorder. Bipolar Disord 7:176–186, 2005

Jonnal AH, Gardner CO, Prescott CA, et al: Obsessive and compulsive symptoms in a general population sample of female twins. Am J Med Genet 96:791–796, 2000

Jorde LB, Hasstedt SJ, Ritvo ER, et al: Complex segregation analysis of autism. Am J Hum Genet 49:932–938, 1991

Kamboh MI, Sanghera DK, Ferrell RE, et al: APOE*4-associated Alzheimer's disease risk is modified by alpha 1-antichymotrypsin polymorphism [published erratum appears in Nat Genet 11:104, 1995]. Nat Genet 10:486–488, 1995

Kamel F, Hoppin JA: Association of pesticide exposure with neurologic dysfunction and disease. Environ Health Perspect 112:950–958, 2004

Kandt RS, Haines JL, Smith M, et al: Linkage of an important gene locus for tuberous sclerosis to a chromosome 16 marker for polycystic kidney disease. Nat Genet 2:37–41, 1992

Karayiorgou M, Morris MA, Morrow B, et al: Schizophrenia susceptibility associated with interstitial deletions of chromosome 22q11. Proc Natl Acad Sci U S A 92:7612–7616, 1995

Karayiorgou M, Altemus M, Galke BL, et al: Genotype determining low catechol-O-methyltransferase activity as a risk factor for obsessive-compulsive disorder. Proc Natl Acad Sci U S A 94:4572–4575, 1997

Karayiorgou M, Sobin C, Blundell ML, et al: Family-based association studies support a sexually dimorphic effect of COMT and MAOA on genetic susceptibility to obsessive-compulsive disorder. Biol Psychiatry 45:1178–1189, 1999

Karno M, Golding JM, Sorenson SB, et al: The epidemiology of obsessive-compulsive disorder in five US communities. Arch Gen Psychiatry 45:1094–1099, 1988

Kasai K, Shenton ME, Salisbury DF, et al: Progressive decrease of left Heschl gyrus and planum temporale gray matter volume in first-episode schizophrenia: a longitudinal magnetic resonance imaging study. Arch Gen Psychiatry 60:766–775, 2003

Kates WR, Burnette C, Eliez S, et al: Neuroanatomic variation in monozygotic twin pairs discordant for the narrow phenotype for autism. Am J Psychiatry 161:539–546, 2004

Kawada Y, Hattori M, Dai XY, et al: Possible association between monoamine oxidase A gene and bipolar affective disorder. Am J Med Genet 56:335–336, 1995

Kawas C, Resnick S, Morrison A, et al: A prospective study of estrogen replacement therapy and the risk of developing Alzheimer's disease: the Baltimore Longitudinal Study of Aging [published erratum appears in Neurology 51:654, 1998]. Neurology 48:1517–1521, 1997

Kendler KS, Gardner CO: The risk for psychiatric disorders in relatives of schizophrenic and control probands: a comparison of three independent studies. Psychol Med 27:411–419, 1997

Kendler KS, Neale MC, Kessler RC, et al: Panic disorder in women: a population-based twin study. Psychol Med 23:397–406, 1993

Kessler RC, Berglund P, Demler O, et al: The epidemiology of major depressive disorder: results from the National Comorbidity Survey Replication (NCS-R). JAMA 289:3095–3105, 2003

Kessler RC, Berglund P, Demler O, et al: Lifetime prevalence and age-of-onset distributions of DSM-IV disorders in the National Comorbidity Survey Replication. Arch Gen Psychiatry 62:593–602, 2005

Kestenbaum CJ: Children at risk for manic-depressive illness: possible predictors. Am J Psychiatry 136:1206–1208, 1979

Kety SS: Schizophrenic illness in the families of schizophrenic adoptees: findings from the Danish national sample. Schizophr Bull 14:217–222, 1988

Kety SS, Wender PH, Jacobsen B, et al: Mental illness in the biological and adoptive relatives of schizophrenic adoptees: replication of the Copenhagen Study in the rest of Denmark. Arch Gen Psychiatry 51:442–455, 1994

Khanna AK, Buskirk DR, Williams RC Jr, et al: Presence of a non-HLA B cell antigen in rheumatic fever patients and their families as defined by a monoclonal antibody. J Clin Invest 83:1710–1716, 1989

Kidd KK: Genetic models for psychiatric disorders, in Genetic Research Strategies for Psychobiology and Psychiatry. Edited by Gershon ES, Matthysse S, Breakefield XO, et al. Pacific Grove, CA, Boxwood Press, 1981, pp 369–382

Kinney DK, Woods BT, Yurgelun-Todd D: Neurologic abnormalities in schizophrenic patients and their families; II: neurologic and psychiatric findings in relatives. Arch Gen Psychiatry 43:665–668, 1986

Kirkwood JK, Wells GA, Wilesmith JW, et al: Spongiform encephalopathy in an Arabian oryx (Oryx leucoryx) and a greater kudu (Tragelaphus strepsiceros) [see comments]. Vet Rec 127:418–420, 1990

Kirov G, Murphy KC, Arranz MJ, et al: Low activity allele of catechol-O-methyltransferase gene associated with rapid cycling bipolar disorder. Mol Psychiatry 3:342–345, 1998

Kirov G, Jones I, McCandless F, et al: Family based association studies of bipolar disorder with candidate genes involved in dopamine neurotransmission: DBH, DAT1, COMT, DRD2, DRD3 and DRD5. Mol Psychiatry 4:558–565, 1999a

Kirov G, Norton N, Jones I, et al: A functional polymorphism in the promoter of monoamine oxidase A gene and bipolar affective disorder. Int J Neuropsychopharmacol 2:293–298, 1999b

Kirov G, Ivanov D, Williams NM, et al: Strong evidence for association between the dystrobrevin binding protein 1 gene (DTNBP1) and schizophrenia in 488 parent-offspring trios from Bulgaria. Biol Psychiatry 55:971–975, 2004

Kirov G, Donovan MC, Owen MJ: Finding schizophrenia genes. J Clin Invest 115:1440–1448, 2005

Klein DF: Delineation of two drug-responsive anxiety syndromes. Psychopharmacologia 5:397–408, 1964

Klein RJ, Zeiss C, Chew EY, et al: Complement factor H polymorphism in age-related macular degeneration. Science 308:385–389, 2005

Knight R: Creutzfeldt-Jakob disease: clinical features, epidemiology and tests. Electrophoresis 19:1306–1310, 1998

Knowles JA, Weissman MM: Panic disorder and agoraphobia, in Review of Psychiatry, Volume 14. Edited by Oldham JM, Riba MB. Washington, DC, American Psychiatric Press, 1995, pp 383–404

Knowles JA, Fyer AJ, Vieland VJ, et al: Results of a genome-wide genetic screen for panic disorder. Am J Med Genet 81:139–147, 1998

Kordower JH, Isacson O, Emerich DF: Cellular delivery of trophic factors for the treatment of Huntington's disease: is neuroprotection possible? Exp Neurol 159:4–20, 1999

Kremer HPH, Goldberg YP, Andrew SE, et al: Worldwide study of the Huntington's disease mutation: the sensitivity and specificity of the repeated CAG sequences. N Engl J Med 330:1401–1406, 1994

Kuhn W, Muller T: [Therapy of Parkinson disease, 2: new therapy concepts for treating motor symptoms]. Fortschr Neurol Psychiatr 65:375–385, 1997

Kunugi H, Iijima Y, Tatsumi M, et al: No association between the Val66Met polymorphism of the brain-derived neurotrophic factor gene and bipolar disorder in a Japanese population: a multicenter study. Biol Psychiatry 56:376–378, 2004

Lachman HM, Morrow B, Shprintzen R, et al: Association of codon 108/158 catechol-O-methyltransferase gene polymorphism with the psychiatric manifestations of velo-cardio-facial syndrome. Am J Med Genet 67:468–472, 1996

Lam P, Hong CJ, Tsai SJ: Association study of A2a adenosine receptor genetic polymorphism in panic disorder. Neurosci Lett 378:98–101, 2005

Lamb JA, Moore J, Bailey A, et al: Autism: recent molecular genetic advances. Hum Mol Genet 9:861–868, 2000

Lamb JA, Barnby G, Bonora E, et al: Analysis of IMGSAC autism susceptibility loci: evidence for sex limited and parent of origin specific effects. J Med Genet 42:132–137, 2005

Lamb RF, Roy C, Diefenbach TJ, et al: The TSC1 tumour suppressor hamartin regulates cell adhesion through ERM proteins and the GTPase Rho. Nat Cell Biol 2:281–287, 2000

Landles C, Bates GP: Huntington and the molecular pathogenesis of Huntington's disease (Fourth in Molecular Medicine Review Series). EMBO Rep 5:958–963, 2004

Langlois S: Genomic imprinting: a new mechanism for disease. Pediatr Pathol 14:161–165, 1994

Langston JW: Epidemiology versus genetics in Parkinson's disease: progress in resolving an age-old debate. Ann Neurol 44 (3 suppl 1):S45–S52, 1998

Langston JW, Ballard P, Tetrud JW, et al: Chronic parkinsonism in humans due to a product of meperidine-analog synthesis. Science 219:979–980, 1983

Lasky-Su JA, Faraone SV, Glatt SJ, et al: Meta-analysis of the association between two polymorphisms in the serotonin transporter gene and affective disorders. Am J Med Genet B Neuropsychiatr Genet 133:110–115, 2005

Laumonnier F, Bonnet-Brilhault F, Gomot M, et al: X-linked mental retardation and autism are associated with a mutation in the NLGN4 gene, a member of the neuroligin family. Am J Hum Genet 74:552–557, 2004

Launer LJ: Diabetes and brain aging: epidemiologic evidence. Curr Diab Rep 5:59–63, 2005

Launer LJ, Andersen K, Dewey ME, et al: Rates and risk factors for dementia and Alzheimer's disease: results from EURO-DEM pooled analyses. EURODEM Incidence Research Group and Work Groups. European Studies of Dementia. Neurology 52:78–84, 1999

Lawrie SM, Whalley H, Kestelman JN, et al: Magnetic resonance imaging of brain in people at high risk of developing schizophrenia. Lancet 353(9146):30–33, 1999

Leboyer M, Quintin P, Manivet P, et al: Decreased serotonin transporter binding in unaffected relatives of manic depressive patients. Biol Psychiatry 46:1703–1706, 1999

Lecendreux M, Maret S, Bassetti C, et al: Clinical efficacy of high-dose intravenous immunoglobulins near the onset of narcolepsy in a 10-year-old boy. J Sleep Res 12:347–348, 2003

Leckman JF, Grice DE, Boardman J, et al: Symptoms of obsessive–compulsive disorder. Am J Psychiatry 154:911–917, 1997

Le Couteur A, Bailey A, Goode S, et al: A broader phenotype of autism: the clinical spectrum in twins. J Child Psychol Psychiatry 37:785–801, 1996

Le Couteur DG, McLean AJ, Taylor MC, et al: Pesticides and Parkinson's disease. Biomed Pharmacother 53:122–130, 1999

Leeflang EP, Zhang L, Tavare S, et al: Single sperm analysis of the trinucleotide repeats in the Huntington's disease gene: quantification of the mutation frequency spectrum. Hum Mol Genet 4:1519–1526, 1995

Lensi P, Cassano GB, Correddu G, et al: Obsessive-compulsive disorder. Familial-developmental history, symptomatology, comorbidity and course with special reference to gender-related differences. Br J Psychiatry 169:101–107, 1996

Leonard H: Childhood onset obsessive compulsive disorder: is there a unique subtype? Med Health R I 82:122, 1999

Leonard HL, Lenane MC, Swedo SE, et al: Tics and Tourette's disorder: a 2- to 7-year follow-up of 54 obsessive-compulsive children. Am J Psychiatry 149:1244–1251, 1992

Leroy E, Boyer R, Auburger G, et al: The ubiquitin pathway in Parkinson's disease (letter). Nature 395:451–452, 1998

Lesch KP, Bengel D, Heils A, et al: Association of anxiety-related traits with a polymorphism in the serotonin transporter gene regulatory region. Science 274:1527–1531, 1996

Levy DL, Holzman PS, Matthysse S, et al: Eye tracking and schizophrenia. Schizophr Bull 20:47–62, 1994

Levy-Lehad E, Lahad A, Wijsman EM, et al: Apolipoprotein E genotypes and age of onset in early onset familial Alzheimer's disease. Ann Neurol 38:678–680, 1995

Lewis A: Problems of obsessional illness. Proc R Soc Med 29325–29336, 1936

Lewis CM, Levinson DF, Wise LH, et al: Genome scan meta-analysis of schizophrenia and bipolar disorder, part II: schizophrenia. Am J Hum Genet 73:34–48, 2003

Lewis DA, Volk DW, Hashimoto T: Selective alterations in prefrontal cortical GABA neurotransmission in schizophrenia: a novel target for the treatment of working memory dysfunction. Psychopharmacology 174:143–150, 2004

Li T, Vallada H, Curtis D, et al: Catechol-O-methyltransferase Val158Met polymorphism: frequency analysis in Han Chinese subjects and allelic association of the low activity allele with bipolar affective disorder. Pharmacogenetics 7:349–353, 1997

Li T, Ma X, Sham PC, et al: Evidence for association between novel polymorphisms in the PRODH gene and schizophrenia in a Chinese population. Am J Med Genet B Neuropsychiatr Genet 129:13–15, 2004

Lieberman JA, Tollefson GD, Charles C, et al: Antipsychotic drug effects on brain morphology in first-episode psychosis. HGDH Study Group. Arch Gen Psychiatry 62:361–370, 2005

Lim LC, Powell JF, Murray R, et al: Monoamine oxidase A gene and bipolar affective disorder. Am J Hum Genet 54:1122–1124, 1994b

Lin L, Faraco J, Li R, et al: The sleep disorder canine narcolepsy is caused by a mutation in the hypocretin (orexin) receptor 2 gene. Cell 98:365–376, 1999

Lindblad-Toh K, Wade CM, Mikkelsen TS, et al: Genome sequence, comparative analysis and haplotype structure of the domestic dog. Nature 438:803–819, 2005

Liou HH, Tsai MC, Chen CJ, et al: Environmental risk factors and Parkinson's disease: a case-control study in Taiwan. Neurology 48:1583–1588, 1997

Liu J, Nyholt DR, Magnussen P, et al: A genomewide screen for autism susceptibility loci. Am J Hum Genet 69:327–340, 2001

Logroscino G, Marder K, Graziano J, et al: Dietary iron, animal fats, and risk of Parkinson's disease. Mov Disord 13 (suppl 1):13–16, 1998

Logue MW, Vieland VJ, Goedken RJ, et al: Bayesian analysis of a previously published genome screen for panic disorder reveals new and compelling evidence for linkage to chromosome 7. Am J Med Genet B Neuropsychiatr Genet 121:95–99, 2003

Lohoff FW, Sander T, Ferraro TN, et al: Confirmation of association between the Val66Met polymorphism in the brain-derived neurotrophic factor (BDNF) gene and bipolar I disorder. Am J Med Genet B Neuropsychiatr Genet 139:51–53, 2005

Lohr JB, Flynn K: Minor physical anomalies in schizophrenia and mood disorders. Schizophr Bull 19:551–556, 1993

Lougee L, Perlmutter SJ, Nicolson R, et al: Psychiatric disorders in first-degree relatives of children with pediatric autoimmune neuropsychiatric disorders associated with streptococcal infections (PANDAS). J Am Acad Child Adolesc Psychiatry 39:1120–1126, 2000

Luchsinger JA, Mayeux R: Cardiovascular risk factors and Alzheimer's disease. Curr Atheroscler Rep 6:261–266, 2004

Lucking CB, Durr A, Bonifati V, et al: Association between early onset Parkinson's disease and mutations in the parkin gene. N Engl J Med 342:1560–1567, 2000

Ma DQ, Jaworski J, Menold MM, et al: Ordered-subset analysis of savant skills in autism for 15q11-q13. Am J Med Genet B Neuropsychiatr Genet 135:38–41, 2005a

Ma DQ, Whitehead PL, Menold MM, et al: Identification of significant association and gene-gene interaction of GABA receptor subunit genes in autism. Am J Hum Genet 77:377–388, 2005b

MacDonald ME, Barnes G, Srinidhi J, et al: Gametic but not somatic instability of CAG repeat length in Huntington's disease. J Med Genet 30:982–986, 1993

MacKinnon DF, McMahon FJ, Simpson SG, et al: Panic disorder with familial bipolar disorder. Biol Psychiatry 42:90–95, 1997

MacKinnon DF, Xu J, McMahon FJ, et al: Bipolar disorder and panic disorder in families: an analysis of chromosome 18 data. Am J Psychiatry 155:829–831, 1998

MacKinnon DF, Zandi PP, Cooper J, et al: Comorbid bipolar disorder and panic disorder in families with a high prevalence of bipolar disorder. Am J Psychiatry 159:30–35, 2002

MacKinnon DF, Zandi PP, Gershon ES, et al: Association of rapid mood switching with panic disorder and familial panic risk in familial bipolar disorder. Am J Psychiatry 160:1696–1698, 2003

Maddox LO, Menold MM, Bass MP, et al: Autistic disorder and chromosome 15q11-q13: construction and analysis of a BAC/PAC contig. Genomics 62:325–331, 1999

Maestrini E, Lai C, Marlow A, et al: Serotonin transporter (5-HTT) and gamma-aminobutyric acid receptor subunit beta3 (GABRB3) gene polymorphisms are not associated with autism in the IMGSA families: the International Molecular Genetic Study of Autism Consortium. Am J Med Genet 88:492–496, 1999

Maier W, Lichtermann D, Minges J, et al: A controlled family study in panic disorder. J Psychiatr Res 27 (suppl 1):79–87, 1993

Malaspina D, Friedman JH, Kaufmann C, et al: Psychobiological heterogeneity of familial and sporadic schizophrenia. Biol Psychiatry 43:489–496, 1998

Malaspina D, Sohler NL, Susser E: Interaction of genes and prenatal exposures in schizophrenia, in Prenatal Exposures in Schizophrenia. Edited by Susser E, Brown AS, Gorman JM. Washington, DC, American Psychiatric Press, 1999, pp 35–61

Malaspina D, Bruder G, Furman V, et al: Schizophrenia subgroups differing in dichotic listening laterality also differ in neurometabolism and symptomatology. J Neuropsychiatry Clin Neurosci 12:485–492, 2000a

Malaspina D, Goetz RR, Yale S, et al: Relation of familial schizophrenia to negative symptoms but not to the deficit syndrome. Am J Psychiatry 157:994–1003, 2000b

Malaspina D, Goetz RR, Friedman JH, et al: Traumatic brain injury and schizophrenia in members of schizophrenia and bipolar disorder pedigrees. Am J Psychiatry 158:440–446, 2001

Malaspina D, Brown A, Goetz D, et al: Schizophrenia risk and paternal age: a potential role for de novo mutations in schizophrenia vulnerability genes. CNS Spectr 7:26–29, 2002

Malaspina D, Reichenberg A, Weiser M, et al: Paternal age and intelligence: implications for age-related genomic changes in male germ cells. Psychiatr Genet15:117–125, 2005

Malhotra AK, Kestler LJ, Mazzanti C, et al: A functional polymorphism in the COMT gene and performance on a test of prefrontal cognition. Am J Psychiatry 159:652–654, 2002

Mangiarini L, Sathasivam K, Seller M, et al: Exon 1 of the HD gene with an expanded CAG repeat is sufficient to cause a progressive neurological phenotype in transgenic mice. Cell 87:493–506, 1996

Mansour HA, Monk TH, Nimgaonkar VL: Circadian genes and bipolar disorder. Ann Med 37:196–205, 2005a

Mansour HA, Wood J, Chowdari KV, et al: Circadian phase variation in bipolar I disorder. Chronobiol Int 22:571–584, 2005b

Maraganore DM, de Andrade M, Lesnick TG, et al: High-resolution whole-genome association study of Parkinson disease. Am J Hum Genet 77:685–693, 2005

Marazziti D, Osso L, Presta S, et al: Platelet [3H]paroxetine binding in patients with OCD-related disorders. Psychiatry Res 89:223–228, 1999

Marcus J, Auerbach J, Wilkinson L, et al: Infants at risk for schizophrenia: the Jerusalem Infant Development Study. Arch Gen Psychiatry 38:703–713, 1981

Margolis RL, Ross CA: Diagnosis of Huntington disease. Clin Chem 49:1726–1732, 2003

Mariappan SV, Silks LA III, Chen X, et al: Solution structures of the Huntington's disease DNA triplets, (CAG)n. J Biomol Struct Dyn 15:723–744, 1998

Markowitz JS, Weissman MM, Ouellette R, et al: Quality of life in panic disorder. Arch Gen Psychiatry 46:984–992, 1989

Maron E, Nikopensius T, Koks S, et al: Association study of 90 candidate gene polymorphisms in panic disorder. Psychiatr Genet 15:17–24, 2005

Marsden CD, Jenner PG: The significance of 1-methyl-4-phenyl-1,2,3,6-tetrahydropyridine. Ciba Found Symp 126:239–256, 1987

Martin ER, Lai EH, Gilbert JR, et al: SNPing away at complex diseases: analysis of single-nucleotide polymorphisms around APOE in Alzheimer disease. Am J Hum Genet 67:383–394, 2000

Martindale D, Hackam A, Wieczorek A, et al: Length of huntingtin and its polyglutamine tract influences localization and frequency of intracellular aggregates. Nat Genet 18:150–154, 1998

Martinez-Rodriguez JE, Lin L, Iranzo A, et al: Decreased hypocretin-1 (Orexin-A) levels in the cerebrospinal fluid of patients with myotonic dystrophy and excessive daytime sleepiness. Sleep 26:287–290, 2003

Mattock C, Marmot M, Stern G: Could Parkinson's disease follow intra-uterine influenza? A speculative hypothesis. J Neurol Neurosurg Psychiatry 51:753–756, 1988

Mayeux R, Ottman R, Maestre G, et al: Synergistic effects of traumatic head injury and apolipoprotein-epsilon 4 in patients with Alzheimer's disease [see comments]. Neurology 45:555–557, 1995

McCarthy MI, Kruglyak L, Lander ES: Sib-pair collection strategies for complex diseases. Genet Epidemiol 15:317–340, 1998

McCauley JL, Olson LM, Dowd M, et al: Linkage and association analysis at the serotonin transporter (SLC6A4) locus in a rigid-compulsive subset of autism. Am J Med Genet Neuropsychiatr Genet 127:104–112, 2004

McCormack AL, Thiruchelvam M, Manning-Bog AB, et al: Environmental risk factors and Parkinson's disease: selective degeneration of nigral dopaminergic neurons caused by the herbicide paraquat. Neurobiol Dis 10:119–127, 2002

McDonald LV, Lake CR: Psychosis in an adolescent patient with Wilson's disease: effects of chelation therapy. Psychosom Med 57:202–204, 1995

McGlashan TH, Hoffman RE: Schizophrenia as a disorder of developmentally reduced synaptic connectivity. Arch Gen Psychiatry 57:637–648, 2000

McGue M, Gottesman II: The genetic epidemiology of schizophrenia and the design of linkage studies. Eur Arch Psychiatry Clin Neurosci 240:174–181, 1991

McInnis MG, McMahon FJ, Chase GA, et al: Anticipation in bipolar affective disorder. Am J Hum Genet 53:385–390, 1993

Medori R, Tritschler HJ, LeBlanc A, et al: Fatal familial insomnia, a prion disease with a mutation at codon 178 of the prion protein gene [see comments]. N Engl J Med 326:444–449, 1992

Meira-Lima I, Shavitt RG, Miguita K, et al: Association analysis of the catechol-O-methyltransferase (COMT), serotonin transporter (5-HTT) and serotonin 2A receptor (5HT2A) gene polymorphisms with obsessive-compulsive disorder. Genes Brain Behav 3:75–79, 2004

Mendlewicz J, Rainer JD: Adoption study supporting genetic transmission in manic-depressive illness. Nature 268:327–329, 1977

Mendlewicz J, Sevy S, Mendelbaum K: Minireview: Molecular genetics in affective illness. Life Sci 52:231–242, 1993

Mendlewicz J, Lindbald K, Souery D, et al: Expanded trinucleotide CAG repeats in families with bipolar affective disorder. Biol Psychiatry 42:1115–1122, 1997

Menegon A, Board PG, Blackburn AC, et al: Parkinson's disease, pesticides, and glutathione transferase polymorphisms [see comments]. Lancet 352:1344–1346, 1998

Michailov GV, Sereda MW, Brinkmann BG, et al: Axonal neuregulin-1 regulates myelin sheath thickness. Science 304:700–703, 2004

Mignot E: Genetic and familial aspects of narcolepsy. Neurology 50 (2 suppl 1):S16–S22, 1998

Mignot E: A hundred years of narcolepsy research. Arch Ital Biol 139:207–220, 2001

Mignot E: A year in review—basic science, narcolepsy, and sleep in neurologic diseases. Sleep 27:1209–1212, 2004

Mignot E, Lin L, Rogers W, et al: Complex HLA-DR and -DQ interactions confer risk of narcolepsy-cataplexy in three ethnic groups. Am J Hum Genet 68:686–699, 2001

Mignot E, Lammers GJ, Ripley B, et al: The role of cerebrospinal fluid hypocretin measurement in the diagnosis of narcolepsy and other hypersomnias. Arch Neurol 59:1553–1562, 2002

Miguel EC, Leckman JF, Rauch S, et al: Obsessive-compulsive disorder phenotypes: implications for genetic studies. Mol Psychiatry 10:258–275, 2004

Mirnics K, Middleton FA, Lewis DA, et al: Analysis of complex brain disorders with gene expression microarrays: schizophrenia as a disease of the synapse. Trends Neurosci 24:479–486, 2001

Mirsky AF, Silberman EK, Latz A, et al: Adult outcomes of high-risk children: differential effects of town and kibbutz rearing. Schizophr Bull 11:150–154, 1985

Miyoshi K, Honda A, Baba K, et al: Disrupted-In-Schizophrenia 1, a candidate gene for schizophrenia, participates in neurite outgrowth. Mol Psychiatry 8:685–694, 2003

Morissette J, Villeneuve A, Bordeleau L, et al: Genome-wide search for linkage of bipolar affective disorders in a very large pedigree derived from a homogeneous population in Quebec points to a locus of major effect on chromosome 12q23-q24. Am J Med Genet 88:567–587, 1999

Morris AG, Gaitonde E, McKenna PJ, et al: CAG repeat expansions and schizophrenia: association with disease in females and with early age-at-onset. Hum Mol Genet 4:1957–1961, 1995

Mouse Genome Sequencing Consortium: Initial sequencing and comparative analysis of the mouse genome. Nature 420:520–562, 2002

Mundo E, Richter MA, Zai G, et al: 5HT1Dbeta Receptor gene implicated in the pathogenesis of obsessive-compulsive disorder: further evidence from a family based association study. Mol Psychiatry 7:805–809, 2002

Murphy KC, Jones LA, Owen MJ: High rates of schizophrenia in adults with velo-cardio-facial syndrome. Arch Gen Psychiatry 56:940–945, 1999

Murphy TK, Goodman WK, Fudge MW, et al: B lymphocyte antigen D8/17: a peripheral marker for childhood-onset obsessive-compulsive disorder and Tourette's syndrome? Am J Psychiatry 154:402–407, 1997

Myers JK, Weissman MM, Tischler GL, et al: Six-month prevalence of psychiatric disorders in three communities 1980 to 1982. Arch Gen Psychiatry 41:959–967, 1984

Myers RH, Leavitt J, Farrer LA, et al: Homozygotes for Huntington's disease. Am J Hum Genet 45:614–618, 1989

Myles-Worsley M, Coon H, Tiobech J, et al: Genetic epidemiological study of schizophrenia in Palau, Micronesia: prevalence and familiality. Am J Med Genet 88:4–10, 1999

Mynett-Johnson LA, Murphy VE, Claffey E, et al: Preliminary evidence of an association between bipolar disorder in females and the catechol-O-methyltransferase gene. Psychiatr Genet 8:221–225, 1998

Nakamura Y, Leppert M, O'Connell P, et al: Variable number of tandem repeat (VNTR) markers for human gene mapping. Science 235:1616–1622, 1987

Nakata K, Ujike H, Sakai A, et al: Association study of the brain-derived neurotrophic factor (*BDNF*) gene with bipolar disorder. Neurosci Lett 337:17–20, 2003

Nee LE, Lippa CF: Alzheimer's disease in 22 twin pairs—13-year follow-up: hormonal, infectious and traumatic factors. Dement Geriatr Cogn Disord 10:148–151, 1999

Nelson E, Rice J: Stability of diagnosis of obsessive-compulsive disorder in the Epidemiologic Catchment Area study. Am J Psychiatry 154:826–831, 1997

Nemetz PN, Leibson C, Naessens JM, et al: Traumatic brain injury and time to onset of Alzheimer's disease: a population-based study. Am J Epidemiol 149:32–40, 1999

Nestadt G, Lan T, Samuels J, et al: Complex segregation analysis provides compelling evidence for a major gene underlying obsessive-compulsive disorder and for heterogeneity by sex. Am J Hum Genet 67:1611–1616, 2000a

Nestadt G, Samuels J, Riddle M, et al: A family study of obsessive-compulsive disorder. Arch Gen Psychiatry 57:358–363, 2000b

Nicolini H, Cruz C, Camarena B, et al: *DRD2*, *DRD3* and *5HT2A* receptor gene polymorphisms in obsessive-compulsive disorder. Mol Psychiatry 1:461–465, 1996

Niehaus DJH, Kinnear CJ, Corfield VA, et al: Association between a catechol-O-methyltransferase polymorphism and obsessive-compulsive disorder in the Afrikaner population. J Affect Disord 65:61–65, 2001

Nievergelt CM, Kripke DF, Remick RA, et al: Examination of the clock gene Cryptochrome 1 in bipolar disorder: mutational analysis and absence of evidence for linkage or association. Psychiatr Genet 15:45–52, 2005

Nothen MM, Eggerman K, Albus M, et al: Association analysis of the monoamine oxidase A gene in bipolar affective disorder by using family based internal controls. Am J Hum Genet 57:975–977, 1995

Noyes R Jr, Crowe RR, Harris EL, et al: Relationship between panic disorder and agoraphobia. A family study. Arch Gen Psychiatry 43:227–232, 1986

Numakawa T, Yagasaki Y, Ishimoto T, et al: Evidence of novel neuronal functions of dysbindin, a susceptibility gene for schizophrenia. Hum Mol Genet 13:2699–2708, 2004

Nylander PO, Engstrom C, Chotai J, et al: Anticipation in Swedish families with bipolar affective disorder. J Med Genet 31:686–689, 1994

Oddo S, Caccamo A, Green KN, et al: Chronic nicotine administration exacerbates tau pathology in a transgenic model of Alzheimer's disease. Proc Natl Acad Sci U S A 102:3046–3051, 2005

O'Donovan MC, Owen MJ: Candidate-gene association studies of schizophrenia. Am J Hum Genet 65:587–592, 1999

O'Donovan MC, Guy C, Craddock N, et al: Expanded CAG repeats in schizophrenia and bipolar disorder. Nat Genet 10:380–381, 1995

O'Donovan M, Jones I, Craddock N: Anticipation and repeat expansion in bipolar disorder. Am J Med Genet C Semin Med Genet 123:10–17, 2003

O'Driscoll GA, Lenzenweger MF, Holzman PS: Antisaccades and smooth pursuit eye tracking and schizotypy. Arch Gen Psychiatry 55:837–843, 1998

O'Dwyer JM: Schizophrenia in people with intellectual disability: the role of pregnancy and birth complications. J Intellect Disabil Res 41 (pt 3):238–251, 1997

Oesch B, Westaway D, Walchli M, et al: A cellular gene encodes scrapie PrP 27–30 protein. Cell 40:735–746, 1985

Okuizumi K, Onodera O, Namba Y, et al: Genetic association of the very low density lipoprotein (VLDL) receptor gene with sporadic Alzheimer's disease. Nat Genet 11:207–209, 1995

Olanow CW, Tatton WG: Etiology and pathogenesis of Parkinson's disease. Annu Rev Neurosci 22:123–144, 1999

Oppenheimer BS, Rothschild MA: The psychoneurotic factor in the irritable heart of soldiers. JAMA 70:1919–1922, 1918

Ott J: Analysis of Human Genetic Linkage. Baltimore, MD, Johns Hopkins University Press, 1985

Pantelis C, Velakoulis D, McGorry PD, et al: Neuroanatomical abnormalities before and after onset of psychosis: a cross-sectional and longitudinal MRI comparison. Lancet 361:281–288, 2003

Papolos DF, Faedda GL, Veit S, et al: Bipolar spectrum disorders in patients diagnosed with velo-cardio-facial syndrome: does a hemizygous deletion of chromosome 22q11 result in bipolar affective disorder? Am J Psychiatry 153:1541–1547, 1996

Papolos DF, Veit S, Faedda GL, et al: Ultra-ultra rapid cycling bipolar disorder is associated with the low activity catecholamine-O-methyltransferase allele. Mol Psychiatry 3:346–349, 1998

Parnas J, Schulsinger F, Schulsinger H, et al: Behavioral precursors of schizophrenia spectrum: a prospective study. Arch Gen Psychiatry 39:658–664, 1982a

Parnas J, Schulsinger F, Teasdale TW, et al: Perinatal complications and clinical outcome within the schizophrenia spectrum. Br J Psychiatry 140:416–420, 1982b

Pauls DL, Alsobrook JP 2nd: The inheritance of obsessive-compulsive disorder. Child Adolesc Psychiatr Clin N Am 8:481–496, 1999

Pauls DL, Crowe RR, Noyes R Jr: Distribution of ancestral secondary cases in anxiety neurosis (panic disorder). J Affect Disord 1:387–390, 1979a

Pauls DL, Noyes R Jr, Crowe RR: The familial prevalence in second-degree relatives of patients with anxiety neurosis (panic disorder). J Affect Disord 1:279–285, 1979b

Pauls DL, Bucher KD, Crowe RR, et al: A genetic study of panic disorder pedigrees. Am J Hum Genet 32:639–644, 1980

Pauls DL, Towbin KE, Leckman JF, et al: Gilles de la Tourette's syndrome and obsessive-compulsive disorder: evidence supporting a genetic relationship. Arch Gen Psychiatry 43:1180–1182, 1986

Pauls DL, Alsobrook JP 2nd, Goodman W, et al: A family study of obsessive-compulsive disorder. Am J Psychiatry 152:76–84, 1995

Pearson GR, Gruffydd-Jones TJ, Wyatt JM, et al: Feline spongiform encephalopathy (letter). Vet Rec 128:532, 1991

Pedersen CB, Mortensen PB: Family history, place and season of birth as risk factors for schizophrenia in Denmark: a replication and reanalysis. Br J Psychiatry 179:46–52, 2001

Pekkarinen P, Terwilliger J, Bredbacka PE, et al: Evidence of a predisposing locus to bipolar disorder on Xq24-q27.1 in an extended Finnish pedigree. Genome Res 5:105–115, 1995

Perna G, Cocchi S, Bertani A, et al: Sensitivity to 35% CO_2 in healthy first-degree relatives of patients with panic disorder. Am J Psychiatry 152:623–625, 1995

Perna G, Bertani A, Caldirola D, et al: Family history of panic disorder and hypersensitivity to CO_2 in patients with panic disorder. Am J Psychiatry 153:1060–1064, 1996

Perna G, Caldirola D, Arancio C, et al: Panic attacks: a twin study. Psychiatry Res 66:69–71, 1997

Petronis A, Kennedy JL: Unstable genes—unstable mind? Am J Psychiatry 152:164–172, 1995

Petrukhin K, Lutsenko S, Chernov I, et al: Characterization of the Wilson disease gene encoding a P-type copper transporting ATPase: genomic organization, alternative splicing, and structure/function predictions. Hum Mol Genet 3:1647–1656, 1994

Petryshen TL, Middleton FA, Kirby A, et al: Support for involvement of neuregulin 1 in schizophrenia pathophysiology. Mol Psychiatry 10:366–374, 328, 2005

Peyser CE, Folstein SE: Huntington's disease as a model for mood disorders: clues from neuropathology and neurochemistry. Mol Chem Neuropathol 12:99–119, 1990

Philibert RA, Nelson JJ, Sandhu HK, et al: Association of an exonic LDHA polymorphism with altered respiratory response in probands at high risk for panic disorder. Am J Med Genet B Neuropsychiatr Genet 117:11–17, 2003

Philippe A, Martinez M, Guilloud-Bataille M, et al: Genome-wide scan for autism susceptibility genes. Paris Autism Research International Sibpair Study. Hum Mol Genet 8:805–812, 1999

Picchioni D, Mignot EJ, Harsh JR: The month-of-birth pattern in narcolepsy is moderated by cataplexy severity and may be independent of HLA-DQB1*0602. Sleep 27:1471–1475, 2004

Pickles A, Bolton P, Macdonald H, et al: Latent-class analysis of recurrence risks for complex phenotypes with selection and measurement error: a twin and family history study of autism. Am J Hum Genet 57:717–726, 1995

Pickles A, Starr E, Kazak S, et al: Variable expression of the autism broader phenotype: findings from extended pedigrees. J Child Psychol Psychiatry 41:491–502, 2000

Pine DS, Klein RG, Coplan JD, et al: Differential carbon dioxide sensitivity in childhood anxiety disorders and nonill comparison group. Arch Gen Psychiatry 57:960–967, 2000

Pine DS, Klein RG, Roberson-Nay R, et al: Response to 5% carbon dioxide in children and adolescents: relationship to panic disorder in parents and anxiety disorders in subjects. Arch Gen Psychiatry 62:73–80, 2005

Piven J, Tsai GC, Nehme E, et al: Platelet serotonin, a possible marker for familial autism. J Autism Dev Disord 21:51–59, 1991

Preisig M, Bellivier F, Fenton BT, et al: Association between bipolar disorder and monoamine oxidase A gene polymorphisms: results of a multicenter study. Am J Psychiatry 157:948–955, 2000

Prusiner SB: Novel proteinaceous infectious particles cause scrapie. Science 216:136–144, 1982

Quirion R, Insel TR: Psychiatry as a clinical neuroscience discipline. JAMA 294:2221–2224, 2005

Raiha I, Kaprio J, Koskenvuo M, et al: Dementia in twins. Lancet 347:1706, 1996

Ramoz N, Reichert JG, Smith CJ, et al: Linkage and association of the mitochondrial aspartate/glutamate carrier SLC25A12 gene with autism. Am J Psychiatry 161:662–669, 2004

Rantakallio P, Jones P, Moring J, et al: Association between central nervous system infections during childhood and adult onset schizophrenia and other psychoses: a 28-year follow-up. Int J Epidemiol 26:837–843, 1997

Rasmussen SA, Eisen JL: The epidemiology and clinical features of obsessive compulsive disorder. Psychiatr Clin North Am 15:743–758, 1992

Rasmussen SA, Tsuang MT: The epidemiology of obsessive compulsive disorder. J Clin Psychiatry 45:450–457, 1984

Rat Genome Sequencing Project Consortium: Genome sequence of the Brown Norway rat yields insights into mammalian evolution. Nature 428:493–521, 2004

Rathbun JK: Neuropsychological aspects of Wilson's disease. Int J Neurosci 85:221–229, 1996

Raybould R, Green EK, Macgregor S, et al: Bipolar disorder and polymorphisms in the dysbindin gene (DTNBP1). Biol Psychiatry 57:696–701, 2005

Reddy PH, Charles V, Williams M, et al: Transgenic mice expressing mutated full-length HD cDNA: a paradigm for locomotor changes and selective neuronal loss in Huntington's disease. Philos Trans R Soc Lond B Biol Sci 354:1035–1045, 1999

Reid MS, Nishino S, Tafti M, et al: Neuropharmacological characterization of basal forebrain cholinergic stimulated cataplexy in narcoleptic canines. Exp Neurol 151:89–104, 1998

Richard F, Amouyel P: Genetic susceptibility factors for Alzheimer's disease. Eur J Pharmacol 412:1–12, 2001

Richards RI, Sutherland GR: Dynamic mutations: a new class of mutations causing human disease. Cell 70:709–712, 1992

Ridley RM, Frith CD, Crow TJ, et al: Anticipation in Huntington's disease is inherited through the male line but may originate in the female. J Med Genet 25:589–595, 1988

Rineer S, Finucane B, Simon EW: Autistic symptoms among children and young adults with isodicentric chromosome 15. Am J Med Genet 81:428–433, 1998

Risch N: Linkage strategies for genetically complex traits, I: multilocus models. Am J Hum Genet 46:222–228, 1990

Risch N, Merikangas K: The future of genetic studies of complex human diseases. Science 273:1516–1517, 1996

Risch N, Spiker D, Lotspeich L, et al: A genomic screen of autism: evidence for a multilocus etiology. Am J Hum Genet 65:493–507, 1999

Ritvo ER, Spence MA, Freeman BJ, et al: Evidence for autosomal recessive inheritance in 46 families with multiple incidences of autism. Am J Psychiatry 142:187–192, 1985

Ritvo ER, Freeman BJ, Pingree C, et al: The UCLA–University of Utah epidemiologic survey of autism: prevalence. Am J Psychiatry 146:194–199, 1989

Ritvo ER, Mason-Brothers A, Freeman BJ, et al: The UCLA-University of Utah epidemiologic survey of autism: the etiologic role of rare diseases. Am J Psychiatry 147:1614–1621, 1990

Robins LN, Helzer JE, Weissman MM, et al: Lifetime prevalence of specific psychiatric disorders in three sites. Arch Gen Psychiatry 41:949–958, 1984

Rogaev EI, Sherrington R, Rogaeva EA, et al: Familial Alzheimer's disease in kindreds with missense mutations in a gene on chromosome 1 related to the Alzheimer's disease type 3 gene. Nature 376:775–778, 1995

Rosenthal D, Wender PH, Kety SS, et al: Schizophrenics' offspring reared in adoptive homes. J Psychiatr Res 6:377–391, 1968

Rosoklija G, Toomayan G, Ellis SP, et al: Structural abnormalities of subicular dendrites in subjects with schizophrenia and mood disorders: preliminary findings. Arch Gen Psychiatry 57:349–356, 2000

Ross GW, Abbott RD, Petrovitch H, et al: Association of coffee and caffeine intake with the risk of Parkinson disease. JAMA 283:2674–2679, 2000

Ross RG, Olincy A, Harris JG, et al: Anticipatory saccades during smooth pursuit eye movements and familial transmission of schizophrenia. Biol Psychiatry 44:690–697, 1998

Rothe C, Koszycki D, Bradwejn J, et al: Association study of serotonin-2A receptor gene polymorphism and panic disorder in patients from Canada and Germany. Neurosci Lett 363:276–279, 2004

Rotondo A, Mazzanti C, Dell'Osso L, et al: Catechol-O-methyltransferase, serotonin transporter, and tryptophan hydroxylase gene polymorphisms in bipolar disorder patients with and without comorbid panic disorder. Am J Psychiatry 159:23–29, 2002

Rubinsztein DC: The genetics of Alzheimer's disease. Prog Neurobiol 52:447–454, 1997

Rutter M, Bailey A, Bolton P, et al: Autism and known medical conditions: myth and substance. J Child Psychol Psychiatry 35:311–322, 1994

Sacker A, Done DJ, Crow TJ, et al: Antecedents of schizophrenia and affective illness: obstetric complications. Br J Psychiatry 166:734–741, 1995

Sakurai T, Amemiya A, Ishii M, et al: Orexins and orexin receptors: a family of hypothalamic neuropeptides and G protein-coupled receptors that regulate feeding behavior. Cell 92:573–585, 1998

Samii A, Nutt JG, Ransom BR: Parkinson's disease. Lancet 363:1783–1793, 2004

Sapp E, Penney J, Young A, et al: Axonal transport of N-terminal huntingtin suggests early pathology of corticostriatal projections in Huntington disease. J Neuropathol Exp Neurol 58:165–173, 1999

Sawamura N, Sawamura-Yamamoto T, Ozeki Y, et al: A form of DISC1 enriched in nucleus: altered subcellular distribution in orbitofrontal cortex in psychosis and substance/alcohol abuse. Proc Natl Acad Sci U S A 102:1187–1192, 2005

Scherrer JF, True WR, Xian H, et al: Evidence for genetic influences common and specific to symptoms of generalized anxiety and panic. J Affect Disord 57:25–35, 2000

Schilsky ML: Diagnosis and treatment of Wilson's disease. Pediatr Transplant 6:15–19, 2002

Schiefermeier M, Kollegger H, Madl C, et al: The impact of apolipoprotein E genotypes on age at onset of symptoms and phenotypic expression in Wilson's disease. Brain 123 (pt 3):585–590, 2000

Schulze TG, Ohlraun S, Czerski PM, et al: Genotype-phenotype studies in bipolar disorder showing association between the DAOA/G30 locus and persecutory delusions: a first step toward a molecular genetic classification of psychiatric phenotypes. Am J Psychiatry 162:2101–2108, 2005

Schumacher J, Jamra RA, Freudenberg J, et al: Examination of G72 and D-amino-acid oxidase as genetic risk factors for schizophrenia and bipolar affective disorder. Mol Psychiatry 9:203–207, 2004

Schwab SG, Knapp M, Mondabon S, et al: Support for association of schizophrenia with genetic variation in the 6p22.3 gene, dysbindin, in sib-pair families with linkage and in an additional sample of triad families. Am J Hum Genet 72:185–190, 2003

Segurado R, Tera-Wadleigh SD, Levinson DF, et al: Genome scan meta-analysis of schizophrenia and bipolar disorder, part III: bipolar disorder. Am J Hum Genet 73:49–62, 2003

Shao Y, Raiford KL, Wolpert CM, et al: Phenotypic homogeneity provides increased support for linkage on chromosome 2 in autistic disorder. Am J Hum Genet 70:1058–1061, 2002a

Shao Y, Wolpert CM, Raiford KL, et al: Genomic screen and follow-up analysis for autistic disorder. Am J Med Genet 114:99–105, 2002b

Shao Y, Cuccaro ML, Hauser ER, et al: Fine mapping of autistic disorder to chromosome 15q11-q13 by use of phenotypic subtypes. Am J Hum Genet 72:539–548, 2003

Shapiro S, Skinner EA, Kessler LG, et al: Utilization of health and mental health services: three Epidemiologic Catchment Area sites. Arch Gen Psychiatry 41:971–978, 1984

Sherrington R, Rogaev EI, Liang Y, et al: Cloning of a gene bearing missense mutations in early onset familial Alzheimer's disease. Nature 375:754–760, 1995

Shifman S, Bronstein M, Sternfeld M, et al: COMT: a common susceptibility gene in bipolar disorder and schizophrenia. Am J Med Genet 128B:61–64, 2004

Shorter J, Lindquist S: Prions as adaptive conduits of memory and inheritance. Nat Rev Genet 6:435–450, 2005

Shumaker SA, Legault C, Rapp SR, et al: WHIMS Investigators. Estrogen plus progestin and the incidence of dementia and mild cognitive impairment in postmenopausal women: the Women's Health Initiative Memory Study: a randomized controlled trial. JAMA 289:2651–2662, 2003

Siegel C, Waldo M, Mizner G, et al: Deficits in sensory gating in schizophrenic patients and their relatives: evidence obtained with auditory evoked responses. Arch Gen Psychiatry 41:607–612, 1984

Siever LJ, Kalus OF, Keefe RS: The boundaries of schizophrenia. Psychiatr Clin North Am 16:217–244, 1993

Sipos A, Rasmussen F, Harrison G, et al: Paternal age and schizophrenia: a population based cohort study. BMJ 329:1070, 2004

Sklar P, Gabriel SB, McInnis MG, et al: Family based association study of 76 candidate genes in bipolar disorder: BDNF is a potential risk locus: brain-derived neutrophic factor. Mol Psychiatry 7:579–593, 2002

Skre I, Onstad S, Torgersen S, et al: A twin study of DSM-III-R anxiety disorders. Acta Psychiatr Scand 88:85–92, 1993

Skuse DH: Imprinting, the X-chromosome, and the male brain: explaining sex differences in the liability to autism. Pediatr Res 47:9–16, 2000

Slater E, Shields J: Genetical aspects of anxiety, in Studies of Anxiety. Edited by Lader MH. Ashford, Kent, UK, Headly Brothers, pp 62–71, 1969

Smalley SL: Autism and tuberous sclerosis. J Autism Dev Disord 28:407–414, 1998

Smalley SL, Tanguay PE, Smith M, et al: Autism and tuberous sclerosis. J Autism Dev Disord 22:339–355, 1992

Smyth C, Kalsi G, Curtis D, et al: Two-locus admixture linkage analysis of bipolar and unipolar affective disorder supports the presence of susceptibility loci on chromosomes 11p15 and 21q22. Genomics 39:271–278, 1997

Snider LA, Swedo SE: PANDAS: current status and directions for research. Mol Psychiatry 9:900–907, 2004

Sobczak S, Riedel WJ, Booij I, et al: Cognition following acute tryptophan depletion: difference between first-degree relatives of bipolar disorder patients and matched healthy control volunteers. Psychol Med 32:503–515, 2002

Sobczak S, Honig A, Schmitt JA, et al: Pronounced cognitive deficits following an intravenous L-tryptophan challenge in first-degree relatives of bipolar patients compared to healthy controls. Neuropsychopharmacology 28:711–719, 2003

Sobin C, Blundell ML, Karayiorgou M: Phenotypic differences in early- and late-onset obsessive-compulsive disorder. Compr Psychiatry 41:373–379, 2000

Spiker D, Lotspeich L, Kraemer HC, et al: Genetics of autism: characteristics of affected and unaffected children from 37 multiplex families. Am J Med Genet 54:27–35, 1994

St. Clair D, Blackwood D, Muir W, et al: Association within a family of a balanced autosomal translocation with major mental illness. Lancet 336:13–16, 1990

Stefansson H, Sigurdsson E, Steinthorsdottir V, et al: Neuregulin 1 and susceptibility to schizophrenia. Am J Hum Genet 71:877–892, 2002

Steffenburg S: Neuropsychiatric assessment of children with autism: a population-based study. Dev Med Child Neurol 33:495–511, 1991

Steffenburg S, Gillberg C, Hellgren L, et al: A twin study of autism in Denmark, Finland, Iceland, Norway and Sweden. J Child Psychol Psychiatry 30:405–416, 1989

Steffenburg S, Gillberg CL, Steffenburg U, et al: Autism in Angelman syndrome: a population-based study. Pediatr Neurol 14:131–136, 1996

Stern Y, Gurland B, Tatemichi TK, et al: Influence of education and occupation on the incidence of Alzheimer's disease [see comments]. JAMA 271:1004–1010, 1994

Stine OC, Xu J, Koskela R, et al: Evidence for linkage of bipolar disorder to chromosome 18 with a parent-of-origin effect. Am J Hum Genet 57:1384–1394, 1995

Stine OC, McMahon FJ, Chen L, et al: Initial genome screen for bipolar disorder in the NIMH genetics initiative pedigrees: chromosomes 2, 11, 13, 14, and X. Am J Med Genet 74:263–269, 1997

Stone JL, Merriman B, Cantor RM, et al: Evidence for sex-specific risk alleles in autism spectrum disorder. Am J Hum Genet 75:1117–1123, 2004

Straub RE, Lehner T, Luo Y, et al: A possible vulnerability locus for bipolar affective disorder on chromosome 21q22.3. Nat Genet 8:291–296, 1994

Straub RE, Jiang Y, MacLean CJ, et al: Genetic variation in the 6p22.3 gene DTNBP1, the human ortholog of the mouse dysbindin gene, is associated with schizophrenia. Am J Hum Genet 71:337–348, 2002

Strous RD, Shoenfeld Y: Revisiting old ghosts: prenatal viral exposure and schizophrenia. Isr Med Assoc J 7:43–45, 2005

Suarez BK, Hampe CL, Van Eerdewegh P: Problems of replicating linkage claims in psychiatry, in Genetic Approaches to Mental Disorders. Edited by Gershon ES, Cloninger CR. Washington, DC, American Psychiatric Press, 1994, pp 23–46

Susser E, Neugebauer R, Hoek HW, et al: Schizophrenia after prenatal famine: further evidence [see comments]. Arch Gen Psychiatry 53:25–31, 1996

Swedo SE, Rapoport JL, Cheslow DL, et al: High prevalence of obsessive-compulsive symptoms in patients with Sydenham's chorea. Am J Psychiatry 146:246–249, 1989a

Swedo SE, Rapoport JL, Leonard H, et al: Obsessive-compulsive disorder in children and adolescents: clinical phenomenology of 70 consecutive cases. Arch Gen Psychiatry 46:335–341, 1989b

Swedo SE, Leonard HL, Mittleman BB, et al: Identification of children with pediatric autoimmune neuropsychiatric disorders associated with streptococcal infections by a marker associated with rheumatic fever. Am J Psychiatry 154:110–112, 1997

Swedo SE, Leonard HL, Garvey M, et al: Pediatric autoimmune neuropsychiatric disorders associated with streptococcal infections: clinical description of the first 50 cases. [published erratum appears in Am J Psychiatry 155:578, 1998]. Am J Psychiatry 155:264–271, 1998

Szatmari P: Heterogeneity and the genetics of autism. J Psychiatry Neurosci 24:159–165, 1999

Szatmari P, Archer L, Fisman S, et al: Asperger's syndrome and autism: differences in behavior, cognition, and adaptive functioning. J Am Acad Child Adolesc Psychiatry 34:1662–1671, 1995

Szatmari P, MacLean JE, Jones MB, et al: The familial aggregation of the lesser variant in biological and nonbiological relatives of PDD probands: a family history study. J Child Psychol Psychiatry 41:579–586, 2000

Talbot K, Eidem WL, Tinsley CL, et al: Dysbindin-1 is reduced in intrinsic, glutamatergic terminals of the hippocampal formation in schizophrenia. J Clin Invest 113:1353–1363, 2004

Tang MX, Maestre G, Tsai WY, et al: Effect of age, ethnicity, and head injury on the association between APOE genotypes and Alzheimer's disease. Ann N Y Acad Sci 802:6–15, 1996

Tanner CM, Ottman R, Goldman SM, et al: Parkinson disease in twins: an etiologic study. JAMA 281:341–346, 1999

Tanzi RE, Petrukhin K, Chernov I, et al: The Wilson disease gene is a copper transporting ATPase with homology to the Menkes disease gene. Nat Genet 5:344–350, 1993

Tarrant CJ, Jones PB: Precursors to schizophrenia: do biological markers have specificity? [see comments]. Can J Psychiatry 44:335–349, 1999

Telenius H, Kremer HPH, Theilmann J, et al: Molecular analysis of juvenile Huntington's disease: the major influence on (CAG)n repeat length is the sex of the affected parent. Hum Mol Genet 2:1535–1540, 1993

Thomas GR, Bull PC, Roberts EA, et al: Haplotype studies in Wilson disease. Am J Hum Genet 54:71–78, 1994

Thomas NS, Sharp AJ, Browne CE, et al: Xp deletions associated with autism in three females. Hum Genet 104:43–48, 1999

Thorgeirsson TE, Oskarsson H, Desnica N, et al: Anxiety with panic disorder linked to chromosome 9q in Iceland. Am J Hum Genet 72:1221–1230, 2003

Tienari P: Interaction between genetic vulnerability and family environment: the Finnish adoptive family study of schizophrenia. Acta Psychiatr Scand 84:460–465, 1991

Todd RD, Reich W, Reich T: Prevalence of affective disorder in the child and adolescent offspring of a single kindred: a pilot study. J Am Acad Child Adolesc Psychiatry 33:198–207, 1994

Todd RD, Reich W, Petti TA, et al: Psychiatric diagnoses in the child and adolescent members of extended families identified through adult bipolar affective disorder probands. J Am Acad Child Adolesc Psychiatry 35:664–671, 1996

Torgersen S: Genetic factors in anxiety disorders. Arch Gen Psychiatry 40:1085–1089, 1983

Tosato S, Dazzan P, Collier D: Association between the neuregulin 1 gene and schizophrenia: a systematic review. Schizophr Bull 31:613–617, 2005

Tot S, Erdal ME, Yazici K, et al: T102C and -1438 G/A polymorphisms of the 5-HT2A receptor gene in Turkish patients with obsessive-compulsive disorder. Eur Psychiatry 18:249–254, 2003

Tsai L, Stewart MA, August G: Implication of sex differences in the familial transmission of infantile autism. J Autism Dev Disord 11:165–173, 1981

Tsuang MT, Faraone SV: The Genetics of Mood Disorders. Baltimore, MD, Johns Hopkins University Press, 1990

Tsutsumi T, Holmes SE, McInnis MG, et al: Novel CAG/CTG repeat expansion mutations do not contribute to the genetic risk for most cases of bipolar disorder or schizophrenia. Am J Med Genet B Neuropsychiatr Genet 124:15–19, 2004

Turecki G, Grof P, Cavazzoni P, et al: MAOA: association and linkage studies with lithium responsive bipolar disorder. Psychiatr Genet 9:13–16, 1999

Valente EM, Abou-Sleiman PM, Caputo V, et al: Hereditary early onset Parkinson's disease caused by mutations in PINK1. Science 304:1158–1160, 2004

van Dyck CH, Seibyl JP, Malison RT, et al: Age-related decline in dopamine transporters: analysis of striatal subregions, nonlinear effects, and hemispheric asymmetries. Am J Geriatr Psychiatry 10:36–43, 2002

Van Os J, Selten JP: Prenatal exposure to maternal stress and subsequent schizophrenia: the May 1940 invasion of The Netherlands [see comments]. Br J Psychiatry 172:324–326, 1998

van Slegtenhorst M, de Hoogt R, Hermans C, et al: Identification of the tuberous sclerosis gene TSC1 on chromosome 9q34. Science 277:805–808, 1997

Velakoulis D, Wood SJ, Wong MT, et al: Hippocampal and amygdala volumes according to psychosis stage and diagnosis: a magnetic resonance imaging study of chronic schizophrenia, first-episode psychosis, and ultra-high-risk individuals. Arch Gen Psychiatry 63:139–149, 2006

Venter JC, Adams MD, Myers EW, et al: The sequence of the human genome. Science 291:1304–1351, 2001

Vieland VJ, Hodge SE, Lish JD, et al: Segregation analysis of panic disorder. Psychiatr Genet 3:63–71, 1993

Vieland VJ, Goodman DW, Chapman T, et al: New segregation analysis of panic disorder. Am J Med Genet 67:147–153, 1996

Vincent JB, Kolozsvari D, Roberts WS, et al: Mutation screening of X-chromosomal neuroligin genes: no mutations in 196 autism probands. Am J Med Genet B Neuropsychiatr Genet 129:82–84, 2004

Volkmar FR, Szatmari P, Sparrow SS: Sex differences in pervasive developmental disorders. J Autism Dev Disord 23:579–591, 1993

Wahlberg KE, Wynne LC, Oja H, et al: Gene-environment interaction in vulnerability to schizophrenia: findings from the Finnish Adoptive Family Study of Schizophrenia. Am J Psychiatry 154:355–362, 1997

Walker EF, Savoie T, Davis D: Neuromotor precursors of schizophrenia. Schizophr Bull 20:441–451, 1994

Walshe JM: Penicillamine: a new oral therapy for Wilson's disease. Am J Med 21:487–495, 1956

Wang DG, Fan JB, Siao CJ, et al: Large-scale identification, mapping, and genotyping of single-nucleotide polymorphisms in the human genome. Science 280:1077–1082, 1998

Wassink TH, Brzustowicz LM, Bartlett CW, et al: The search for autism disease genes. Ment Retard Dev Disabil Res Rev 10:272–283, 2005

Webber KM, Casadesus G, Marlatt MW, et al: Estrogen bows to a new master: the role of gonadotropins in Alzheimer pathogenesis. Ann N Y Acad Sci 1052:201–209, 2005

Weickert CS, Straub RE, McClintock BW, et al: Human dysbindin (DTNBP1) gene expression in normal brain and in schizophrenic prefrontal cortex and midbrain. Arch Gen Psychiatry 61:544–555, 2004

Weinberger DR: Implications of normal brain development for the pathogenesis of schizophrenia. Arch Gen Psychiatry 44:660–669, 1987

Weissman MM: Family genetic studies of panic disorder. J Psychiatr Res 27 (suppl 1):69–78, 1993

Weissman MM, Leckman JF, Merikangas KR, et al: Depression and anxiety disorders in parents and children: results from the Yale family study. Arch Gen Psychiatry 41:845–852, 1984

Weissman MM, Bland RC, Canino GJ, et al: The cross national epidemiology of obsessive compulsive disorder. The Cross National Collaborative Group. J Clin Psychiatry 55(suppl): 5–10, 1994

Weissman MM, Bland RC, Canino GJ, et al: Cross-national epidemiology of major depression and bipolar disorder. JAMA 276:293–299, 1996

Weissman MM, Bland RC, Canino GJ, et al: The cross-national epidemiology of panic disorder. Arch Gen Psychiatry 54:305–309, 1997

Weissman MM, Fyer AJ, Haghighi F, et al: Potential panic disorder syndrome: clinical and genetic linkage evidence. Am J Med Genet 96:24–35, 2000

Weissman MM, Gross R, Fyer A, et al: Interstitial cystitis and panic disorder: a potential genetic syndrome. Arch Gen Psychiatry 61:273–279, 2004

Weissmann C, Flechsig E: PrP knock-out and PrP transgenic mice in prion research. Br Med Bull 66:43–60, 2003

Wellington CL, Ellerby LM, Hackam AS, et al: Caspase cleavage of gene products associated with triplet expansion disorders generates truncated fragments containing the polyglutamine tract. J Biol Chem 273:9158–9167, 1998

Wender PH, Kety SS, Rosenthal D, et al: Psychiatric disorders in the biological and adoptive families of adopted individuals with affective disorders. Arch Gen Psychiatry 43:923–929, 1986

West A, Periquet M, Lincoln S, et al: Complex relationship between Parkin mutations and Parkinson disease. Am J Med Genet 114:584–591, 2002

Wexler NS, Young AB, Tanzi R, et al: Homozygotes for Huntington's disease. Nature 3326:194–197, 1987

Wexler NS, Lorimer J, Porter J, et al: Venezuelan kindreds reveal that genetic and environmental factors modulate Huntington's disease age of onset. Project US-VCR. Proc Natl Acad Sci U S A 101:3498–3503, 2004

White L, Petrovitch H, Ross GW, et al: Prevalence of dementia in older Japanese-American men in Hawaii: the Honolulu-Asia Aging Study [see comments]. JAMA 276:955–960, 1996

Wickramaratne PJ, Weissman MM, Horwath E, et al: The familial aggregation of panic disorder by source of proband ascertainment. Psychiatr Genet 4:125–133, 1994

Williams NM, Preece A, Morris DW, et al: Identification in 2 independent samples of a novel schizophrenia risk haplotype of the dystrobrevin binding protein (DTNBP1). Arch Gen Psychiatry 61:336–344, 2004

Willour VL, Yao SY, Samuels J, et al: Replication study supports evidence for linkage to 9p24 in obsessive-compulsive disorder. Am J Hum Genet 75:508–513, 2004

Woo JM, Yoon KS, Yu BH: Catechol-O-methyltransferase genetic polymorphism in panic disorder. Am J Psychiatry 159:1785–1787, 2002

Woo JM, Yoon KS, Choi YH, et al: The association between panic disorder and the L/L genotype of catechol-O-methyltransferase. J Psychiatr Res 38:365–370, 2004

World Health Organization: The ICD-10 Classification of Mental and Behavioural Disorders. Geneva, Switzerland, World Health Organization, 1992

Wright IC, Rabe-Hesketh S, Woodruff PW, et al: Meta-analysis of regional brain volumes in schizophrenia. Am J Psychiatry 157:16–25, 2000

Yamada K, Hattori E, Shimizu M, et al: Association studies of the cholecystokinin B receptor and A2a adenosine receptor genes in panic disorder. J Neural Transm 108:837–848, 2001

Yamaguchi Y, Heiny ME, Gitlin JD: Isolation and characterization of a human liver cDNA as a candidate gene Wilson disease. Biochem Biophys Res Commun 197:271–277, 1993

Yan J, Oliveira G, Coutinho A, et al: Analysis of the neuroligin 3 and 4 genes in autism and other neuropsychiatric patients. Mol Psychiatry 10:329–332, 2005

Ylisaukko-oja T, Rehnstrom K, Auranen M, et al: Analysis of four neuroligin genes as candidates for autism. Eur J Hum Genet 13:1285–1292, 2005

Yonan AL, Alarcon M, Cheng R, et al: A genomewide screen of 345 families for autism-susceptibility loci. Am J Hum Genet 73:886–897, 2003

Zammit S, Allebeck P, Dalman C, et al: Paternal age and risk for schizophrenia. Br J Psychiatry 183:405–408, 2003

Zandi PP, Carlson MC, Plassman BL, et al, Cache County Memory Study Investigators. Hormone replacement therapy and incidence of Alzheimer disease in older women: the Cache County Study. JAMA 288:2123–2129, 2002

Zeidler M, Ironside JW: The new variant of Creutzfeldt-Jakob disease. Rev Sci Tech 19:98–120, 2000

Part III

Neuropsychiatric Symptomatologies

9

NEUROPSYCHIATRIC ASPECTS OF PAIN MANAGEMENT

Brenda Golianu, M.D.

Rashmi Bhandari, Ph.D.

Richard J. Shaw, M.D.

William G. Brose, M.D.

Raymond Gaeta, M.D.

David Spiegel, M.D.

Pain is a common, frustrating, and—though often undertreated—treatable problem. Because pain is affected by all the neural processes that modulate perception, it is a fascinating neuropsychiatric phenomenon.

PREVALENCE OF PAIN

Approximately one-third of all Americans, it is estimated, have some form of chronic pain. Back pain, arthritis, headaches, and musculoskeletal disorders, as well as pain due to neurological, cardiac, or oncological disease combined, affect an estimated 97 million people and lead to long-term disability in more than 50 million people (Brookoff 2000). Cancer pain affects approximately one-third of cancer patients with primary disease and two-thirds of those with metastatic disease. Chronic pain is a common symptom among patients seeking medical care and is often associated with frequent and costly treatments. The costs of chronic pain are not limited to medical care, however. Disability payments and lost productivity associated

with chronic pain create even more of a financial impact. Pain is the third leading cause of workplace absenteeism in the United States, according to a Louis Harris Poll ("Louis Harris Poll of Pain in the Workplace" 1996). In a follow-up survey conducted in 2006, there was a dramatic increase in chronic pain among the U.S. full-time workforce but a growing tendency for those affected to attend work: 89% of full-time employees living with chronic pain said they typically go to work rather than stay at home when they experience chronic pain ("Pain in the Workplace" 2006). The same poll showed that 75% of the population use over-the-counter medications for pain and 35% of the population use prescribed medications for pain. A chronic pain study performed in Sweden in 2005 concluded that 20% of people ages 18–39 years have chronic pain. In middle-aged people, ages 40–59, that percentage increases to 27%, and 31% of older adults ages 60–81 experience daily pain (Rustoen et al. 2005). A chronic pain study performed in Michigan in 1997 concluded that 20% of all adults have chronic pain. In addition, 70% of these Michigan pain patients reported that they continued to have pain despite treatment. Pain is also a leading reason patients seek alternative and complementary treatments (Astin 1998; Spiegel et al. 1998), a practice now engaged in by some 42% of Americans (Eisenberg et al. 1998). When we attempt to include the cost of lost productivity, the additive economic impact of pain is staggering, in excess of $100 billion annually (Gallagher 1999). The monetary cost of pain is not the only issue. From a social perspective, pain is a tremendous burden. This level of continued human suffering is unacceptable. The lost opportunities and hopes that every pain sufferer experiences have a tremendous impact on everyone.

CORTICAL MODULATION OF PAIN

The International Association for the Study of Pain (IASP) defines pain as "an unpleasant sensory and emotional experience associated with actual or potential tissue damage or described in terms of such damage" ("Pain Terms" 1979) The operational word *experience* in this definition places pain outside the realm of simple sensation. Unlike sight, smell, taste, hearing, and touch, pain has a more complicated perceptual foundation. The capacity for any of the five senses to provide the sensory component to pain further differentiates pain from a simple sensation. Functional brain imaging research has confirmed the in vivo presence of profound neurochemical changes in chronic pain states (Borsook and Becerra 2006; Craig et al. 1996; Kwan et al. 2000; Tolle et al. 1999). Whether these changes are uniquely associated with affective, sensory, cognitive, motor, inhibitory, learned, or autonomic responses to a painful stimulus is unclear. New and exciting research holds the promise of elucidating the specific connections between the sensory and experiential components of pain.

Pain is the ultimate psychosomatic phenomenon. It is composed of both a somatic signal that something is wrong with the body and a message or interpretation of the signal involving attentional, cognitive, affective, and social factors. The limbic system and the cortex provide means of modulating pain signals, either amplifying them through excessive attention or affective dysregulation or minimizing them through denial, inattention, relaxation, or attention control techniques. Like any other perceptual phenomenon, pain is modulated by attentional processes. Novelty tends to enhance pain perception, as with an acute injury, whereas chronic pain is often reported to be greater during evenings and weekends, when people are not distracted by routine activities. Although pain during sleep is reported less frequently than pain while awake, pain often

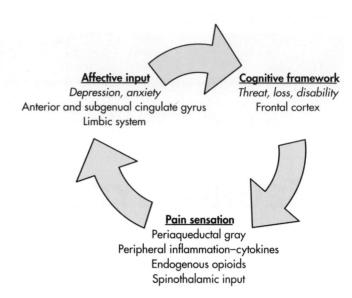

FIGURE 9–1. The circuitous, mutually reinforcing nature of the pain experience.

interferes with sleep, and severe pain can substantially reduce sleep efficiency. In addition, the medications that are employed to treat pain often reduce alertness and arousal and may cause daytime sleepiness or somnolence, compounding nighttime sleep difficulties. This and other undesired effects of analgesic medications—including the potential for abuse of opioid analgesics—further increase the suffering of those experiencing chronic pain.

Melzack and Wall (1965; Melzack 1982) explained pain phenomena as the existence of a gate-like mechanism that modulates whether physical pain sensation reaches the brain to be perceived as pain. Pain sensations are transmitted to this gate in the dorsal horn of the spinal column. If the gate is "open," the impulse continues to the brain, where it is then recognized as pain. If the gate is "closed," no signal is transmitted to the brain and consequently no pain sensation is perceived. According to this theory, both physical/sensory processes and cognitive/emotional (central) processes are able to open or shut this gate (Dahlquist 1999).

This model has now been replaced by the *neuromatrix* model, which states that the pain experience itself is created as a matrix of perception, modulated by multiple components within the central nervous system (CNS) (Melzack 1999). This matrix includes three key components: ascending modulation within the spinal cord, central processing, and descending inhibition (Figure 9–1). The cortical or central processing involves several key areas: the anterior cingulate gyrus and the insular, prefrontal, inferior parietal, primary and secondary somatosensory (SI and SII), primary motor, and premotor cortices (Ladabaum et al. 2000). Disruption of any of these pathways may lead to the perception of pain. In addition, the remodeling that may take place over time may make treatment of pain more difficult. The anterior cingulate and the insular cortex are thought to be a part of the "medial" pain system, involved in generating the affective/ emotional component of pain, while the somatosensory cortex, SI and SII, and parietal cortex have been postulated to be a part of the "lateral" pain system, thought to be involved in the discriminative sensory components of pain (Payron et al. 2000). Casey and colleagues (2003) used functional magnetic resonance imaging (fMRI) to explore allodynia induced by capsaicin and heat in normal male subjects and found significant evidence for frontal modulation of the pain experience. In addition, significant remodeling of the pain perception matrix may take place over time in patients who experience chronic pain, making treatment more difficult. In a study with patients with chronic back pain, Flor and colleagues (1997) showed that the brain's cortical representation of the "back" area shifted medially, possibly indicating an expansion of the "back" representation to the neighboring "foot" and "leg" areas of the cortex. There is also evidence that functional alterations in the neural matrix may occur in patients with fibromyalgia. Patients with fibromyalgia show augmentation of both cortical and subcortical pain processing on fMRI scans when compared with matched control subjects (Gracely et al. 2002).

It is well known that many athletes and soldiers incur serious injuries in the height of sport or combat and are unaware of the injury until someone points out bleeding or swelling. Even overwhelming and serious injury may sometimes be accompanied by a surprising absence of pain perception until hours after the injury. This traumatic dissociation has been observed in victims of natural disaster, combat, and motor vehicle accidents (Spiegel et al. 1988). On the other hand, some individuals with comparatively minor physical disturbance report being totally immobilized and demoralized by pain. Certain genetic phenotypes have been found recurrently in patients with certain chronic pain conditions (A. Mailis, personal communication, October 2000). fMRI and single-photon emission computed tomography (SPECT) are promising and powerful research tools that are revealing many of the mysteries of perception of acute and chronic pain (Borsook and Becerra 2006). However, the production of clinically meaningful effects on the integrated neurochemistry does not require our understanding of these interconnections. A single parent with a sarcoma complained of severe, unremitting pain that was interlaced with tearful concern about her failure to discuss her terminal prognosis with her adolescent son. When an appropriate meeting was arranged in which she could discuss

her prognosis with him and plan for his future, the pain resolved (Kuhn and Bradnan 1979). From this example one can clearly see that attending to both the physical injury and the emotional one makes strong physiological sense in the treatment of pain.

COGNITIVE FACTORS INFLUENCING PAIN

ATTENTION TO PAIN

Health perception is modulated by the cortex, which enhances or diminishes awareness of incoming signals. Neuropsychological and brain imaging research has demonstrated at least three attentional centers that modulate perception: a posterior parieto-occipital orienting system, a focusing system localized to the anterior cingulate gyrus, and an arousal-vigilance system in the right frontal lobe (Posner and Petersen 1990). These systems, among their other functions, provide for selective attention to incoming stimuli, allowing competing stimuli to be relegated to the periphery of awareness (Price 2000). Brain imaging research indicates that reduced pain perception produced through hypnotic analgesia is associated with activation of the anterior cingulate gyrus (Crawford et al. 1993; Rainville et al. 1997). Other studies indicate that alteration of perception with hypnosis also produces consonant changes in the primary sensory association cortex (Kosslyn et al. 2000). Thus, both naturally occurring and therapeutic factors that modulate attention may modulate pain perception via activation of brain centers of selective attention and modulating activity of the sensory cortex.

MEANING OF PAIN

It has been known for half a century that the meaning structure in which pain is embedded influences the intensity of pain experienced. Beecher (1956) had noted with initial surprise that soldiers on the Anzio beachhead in World War II who had been quite badly wounded seemed to require very little in the way of analgesic medication. In a classic study, he examined a matched set of surgical patients at Massachusetts General Hospital with equally or less serious surgically induced wounds. These patients demanded far higher levels of analgesic medication than did the combat soldiers, despite less serious injury. Beecher concluded that this difference was based on a difference in the meaning of the pain. To combat soldiers, the pain was almost welcome as an indication that they were likely to get out of combat alive, whereas to the surgical patients, pain represented an interference with life and a threat to survival. This means that patients who interpret pain signals as an ominous sign of the worsening of their disease are likely to experience a greater intensity of pain (D. Spiegel and Bloom 1983b).

Other factors that can amplify pain perception include the severity of the condition causing pain symptoms. For example, the proximity of death is associated with increased pain and distress among women with metastatic breast cancer (L. Butler et al. 2003). Pain is also strongly influenced by a past history of trauma experience, such as childhood sexual abuse (Arnow et al. 1999; Leserman et al. 1996, 1998). Such experiences sensitize individuals to subsequent trauma, both through activation of memories that can amplify pain perception (L.D. Butler et al. 1996) and through long-term effects on the hypothalamic-pituitary-adrenal axis response to stress (Heim et al. 1998). In infants and children, a prior history of a painful experience (such as circumcision) may sensitize the infant or child to subsequent noxious stimuli such as routine immunization in the doctor's office (Taddio et al. 1997). The nature of a traumatic incident can also influence the pain experience. This can include awareness of infliction of intentional harm or neglect—for example, by an employer who failed to provide adequate safety measures. Many who suffer pain after injury are extremely distressed by any residual pain at all, insisting that they be returned to their preinjury state of good health. Such an "all-or-none" attitude leads to the amplification of whatever pain remains. Secondary losses related to pain, such as loss of income, employment, social status, and social contact, are emotionally painful and may intensify the physical symptom of pain as a language of distress. Some feel that pain complaints are more socially acceptable than expressions of sadness, depression, or anxiety about an injury. Also, secondary gain, in the form of disability or veterans' benefits or an increase in attention from loved ones, friends, and caregivers, may make it emotionally rewarding to report continued pain.

MOOD DISORDERS

Descending influence of cortical function on pain is related to mood and anxiety disorders as well. Serotonergic and noradrenergic function influences pain processing (Yaksh 1988). The serotonergic and noradrenergic neurotransmitter systems are involved in depressive and anxiety disorders and are modulated by antidepressants. Bond and Pearson (1969) reported a correlation between neuroticism on the Maudsley Personality Inventory (Eysenck and Eysenck 1964) and pain among patients who had cervical carcinoma. This result was confirmed by Woodforde and Fielding (1970), who reported that cancer patients who sought treatment in a pain clinic were rated as being

more depressed and having more psychosomatic, gastrointestinal, and hypochondriacal symptoms than cancer patients who did not seek pain treatment. Several other studies (Ahles et al. 1983; Derogatis et al. 1983; Lansky et al. 1985; Massie and Holland 1987; D. Spiegel and Bloom 1983b) have reported that patients with pain score higher on measures of depression, anxiety, and other signs of mood disturbance than do those with little or no pain. In particular, depression and anxiety are frequent concomitants of pain, as found in earlier studies (Blumer and Heilbronn 1982; Bond 1973; Bond and Pearson 1969; Woodforde and Fielding 1970). This earlier work implied that patients with psychopathology complained more about pain than did psychiatrically healthy patients. Later work suggested that there is an interaction and that perhaps chronic pain amplifies or even produces depression (Peteet et al. 1986; Spiegel and Sands 1988). Indeed, the presence of significant pain among cancer patients is more strongly associated with major depressive symptoms than is a prior life history of depression (Spiegel 1994).

Depression is the most frequently reported psychiatric diagnosis among chronic pain patients. Reports of depression among chronic pain populations range from 10% to 87% (Dworkin et al. 1990; Pilowski et al. 1977; Reich et al. 1983). The relative severity of the depression observed in chronic pain patients is illustrated by the finding by Katon et al. (1985) that 32% of a sample of 37 pain patients met criteria for major depression and 43% had a past episode of major depression. In a large sample of health maintenance organization (HMO) patients (Dworkin et al. 1990), patients with two or more pain conditions were found to be at elevated risk for major depression, whereas patients with only one pain condition did not show such an elevated rate of mood disorder. Fishbain and colleagues (1997) found 60% of patients with chronic pain conditions had two or more Axis I disorders and 56% had depression. Clearly there is strong evidence of an association between depression and chronic pain. Fishbain posed three hypotheses in the form of questions about the timing of onset of depression: Was the depression present prior to the development of the pain condition (the *antecedent* hypothesis)? Was it a consequence of a chronic pain condition (the *consequence* hypothesis)? Or was the depression a reactivation of a previous depressive episode (the *scar* hypothesis)? Fishbain could not answer these questions. However, he did find that there was a statistical relationship between pain onset and the onset of depression, as well as between pain severity and the development of depression. Another pertinent issue in the discussion of mood disorders centers on the response to treatment. Wasan and colleagues (2004) found that in patients with low back pain, 48% of patients with a low level of psychiatric symptoms had a good response to opioid analgesia, while in the group with a high level of psychiatric symptoms, only 20% experienced relief. Katz and colleagues (2004) found that depressed patients showed significantly less improvement in physical functioning, vitality, and social functioning than did patients who did not suffer from depression.

Although pain patients referred for psychiatric treatment are clearly selected for a higher prevalence of depression and anxiety (Lansky et al. 1985), there is general agreement in the literature that pain and mood disorders co-occur and that therefore the treatment of pain from a neuropsychiatric point of view must include appropriate treatment of depression and anxiety. Anxiety is a frequent concomitant of acute pain. It may be an appropriate response to serious trauma, injury, or illness. Pain may serve a signal function or may be part of an anxious preoccupation, as in the case of the woman with the sarcoma cited earlier. Similarly, anxiety and pain may reinforce each other, producing a snowball effect of escalating and mutually reinforcing central and peripheral symptoms. There is growing evidence that pathways related to pain are anatomically close to those that mediate depression. Emotional aspects of pain are mediated by the anterior cingulate gyrus in conjunction with amygdala and limbic structures, while sensory aspects are controlled by parietal and insular cortices. The anterior cingulate is also a key portion of the anterior attention system, along with the frontal cortex (Posner and Petersen 1990). The unpleasantness of painful stimuli is associated with activity of the anterior cingulate, and hypnotic analgesia with suggestion of reduced unpleasantness works in proportion to reduced blood flow in the anterior cingulate cortex (Rainville et al. 1997, 2002). Similarly, depression is associated with limbic input, hyperactivity of the subgenual portion of the cingulate gyrus, and hypofrontality, which, especially on the right, regulates attention (Mayberg 1997; Mayberg et al. 1999). Thus, a circuit involving limbic and cingulate activity and reduced frontal activity reinforces both pain and depression and their interactions. In summary, it appears that not only are patients with chronic pain more susceptible to either develop depression or have a reactivation of a previous episode, but the presence of depression also may decrease their response to treatment of their pain.

NEUROBIOLOGICAL MECHANISMS OF PAIN

PERIPHERAL SENSORY RECEPTORS

Each individual can appreciate that when a potentially damaging stimulus is applied to a sensitive area of the body such as the skin, a chain of signals is initiated that results in identification of the stimulus as painful. Early

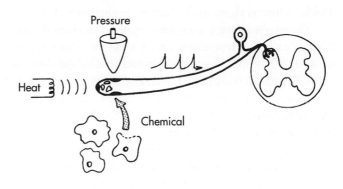

FIGURE 9–2. Sensitivity range of the polymodal C fiber nociceptor. Available evidence suggests that the terminals are sensitive to direct heat or mechanical distortion; thus, transduction can occur at the terminal. The terminals are also sensitive to chemicals released from damaged cells. In this manner, any tissue cell can serve as an intermediate in the transduction process. In a sense, all tissue cells are "receptors" for injury.

Source. Reprinted from Fields HL: *Pain.* New York, McGraw-Hill, 1987, p. 27. Copyright 1987 McGraw-Hill. Used with permission.

descriptions of peripheral nerves indicated that they were modality specific and that each class of nerve fiber was responsible for only one sensory modality (Müller 1844). This concept was not supported by anatomical studies of skin surface, which demonstrated that not every class of nerve ending is present in all skin areas. More recent neurophysiological work has established the existence of specific primary afferent nerves for signaling noxious stimulation. These nerves are termed *nociceptors.*

Nociceptors are activated by some form of energy (mechanical, thermal, or chemical) (Figure 9–2). They transduce that energy into an electrical impulse, which is conducted through the nerve axon toward the brain. The reflex response and the subjective reporting of pain associated with a noxious stimulus are the results of processing by the spinal cord, brain stem, midbrain, and higher cortex of signals from the numerous primary afferent nociceptors that were activated by the stimulus. Nociceptors are characterized by 1) having a high threshold for all naturally occurring stimuli compared with other receptors in the same tissue and 2) progressively augmenting response to repeated or increasingly noxious stimuli (sensitization).

Cutaneous Pain Sensation

Mechanosensory nociceptors respond when the pressure necessary for producing tissue damage has been achieved. Most of these receptors initiate impulses carried by thinly myelinated fibers (A fibers). The responses increase in proportion to the magnitude of the pressure applied.

These receptors in the trunk have fairly large receptive fields, whereas those in the face have smaller fields.

Thermoreceptive nociceptors respond to normal heating or cooling with sensitivity near 1°C when the temperature is 30°–40°C; they also respond to noxious thermal stimuli with an increasing frequency of discharge. High-frequency discharge can be seen in C fiber afferents after the application of intense heat (47°–51°C) to the small receptive fields near these receptors.

Mechanothermal nociceptors are activated by high-intensity heat or pressure sensation. They have small receptive fields and are probably responsible for the "first pain" transmitted by small myelinated Aδ fibers.

Polymodal C fiber nociceptors respond to many different noxious stimuli. These are the most common of all nociceptors. They are activated by pressure, temperature, and chemical stimuli supplied to their small receptive fields. These small unmyelinated fibers transmit at slower conduction velocities and are probably responsible for the phenomenon of "second pain."

Skeletal Muscle Pain

Nociceptors found in skeletal muscle respond to chemical agents that are released locally during muscle contraction. Metabolic by-products alone do not trigger these receptors. There appears to be a need for other algogenic agents, perhaps prostaglandins released during intense muscle contraction, to be present as well.

Cardiac Muscle Pain

Cardiac muscle afferents are activated by high-intensity mechanical stimulation, heat, and chemical agents. Humoral agents released locally may be responsible for the pain experienced in angina. Prostaglandins are released after myocardial hypoxia. Prostaglandins, histamine, bradykinin, and serotonin have each been shown to stimulate these receptors.

Joint Pain

Joint nociceptors activated by deformation or expansion within the joint relay pain messages via Aδ fiber afferents. These receptors also appear to be sensitized by certain chemical substances injected into the joint (e.g., urate crystals, endotoxin, and prostaglandins).

Visceral Pain

Viscera nociceptors have not been well identified. Pain is seen in response to mechanical (distention) as well as thermal and chemical stimuli. These receptors also appear to be sensitized by the presence of certain chemicals (e.g., prostaglandins).

MECHANISMS OF NOCICEPTION

Particular nociceptors respond only to particular types of stimuli. Although the exact pathways involved in the transduction of noxious-information nociceptors have not yet been elucidated, it appears that the peripheral terminal of the Aδ mechanical nociceptor is likely to function as a receptor (Fields 1987). Whether this is true for other nociceptors remains the subject of speculation. The presence of vesicles in primary nociceptive afferent terminals has been determined by electron microscopy. These vesicles probably provide the substrate for various peripherally active agents.

Substance P is an undecapeptide found in small-diameter primary afferent neurons. This peptide has been shown to be transmitted to the periphery by these nerves, and stimulation of these primary afferents leads to the release of substance P from the distal terminus of the nerve. However, local application of exogenous substance P to these nerve terminals does not induce a painful response. It does appear to activate local vasculature to cause extravasation of fluid into the tissues. Other chemicals present in the blood and tissues have been demonstrated to be algesic. Serotonin, histamine, acetylcholine, bradykinin, slow-reacting substance of anaphylaxis (SRS-A), calcitonin gene–related peptide (CGRP), and potassium all excite primary noxious afferents. At this time the definition of pain neuropeptide has not been specified. Prostaglandins alone do not excite pain fibers; however, they do appear to sensitize primary afferents to painful substances.

Direct tissue trauma results in potassium release, synthesis of bradykinin in plasma, and synthesis of prostaglandins in the region of damaged tissue (Figure 9–3A). Antidromic impulses in primary nociceptor afferents result in an increase in production of substance P from nerve endings. This increase is associated with an increase in vascular permeability and, in turn, results in the marked release of bradykinin. There is also an increase in histamine production from mast cells and an increase in serotonin production from platelets; both of these substances are capable of powerful activation of nociceptors (Figure 9–3B). Histamine release combines with substance P release to increase vascular permeability. Local increases in histamine and serotonin, via activation of nociceptors, result in a further increase in substance P; thus, a self-perpetuating cycle can be seen to develop at each region of the nociceptive afferent nerve fiber in the damaged tissue. In surrounding extracellular fluid, increases in histamine and serotonin result in activation of nearby nociceptors, which is one reason for secondary hyperalgesia (Figure 9–3C). Superimposed on all these events are the effects of the increased release of catecholamines from sympathetic nerve endings, which results in sensiti-

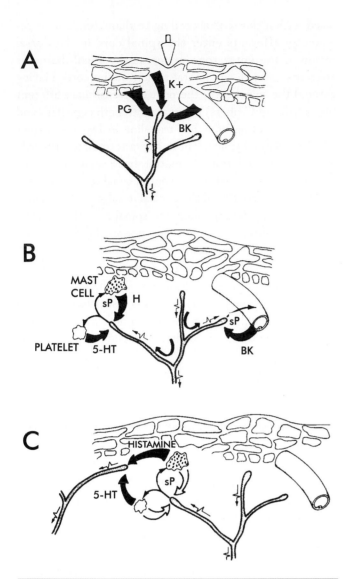

zation of nociceptors. Evidence from animal models of arthritis and various human data point to the sympathetic postganglionic neuron as being integral to the changes seen in vascular permeability in response to the activation of primary afferent nociceptors (Ladabaum et al. 2000).

PRIMARY AFFERENT TRANSMISSION

After a noxious stimulus has been detected by a nociceptor, the resultant impulse travels away from the point of origin via the primary afferent nerve. The primary afferent nerves that carry pain impulses are almost exclusively unmyelinated C fibers and finely myelinated Aδ fibers. Most C fiber afferents originate from polymodal nociceptors, which are activated by mechanical, chemical, and thermal noxious stimuli. The conduction velocity of these C fibers is approximately 1 m/sec, which probably explains the "slow pain" felt 1–2 seconds after the application of a noxious stimulus (Figure 9–4). The finely myelinated Aδ fibers also transmit pain impulses, but the conduction velocity of these neurons is much faster (12–30 m/sec). Aδ fibers are particularly sensitive to stimulation with sharp instruments. In addition, 20%–50% of Aδ fibers respond to heat as well as to mechanical stimulation. These fiber types carry the impulses that initially report a noxious stimulus. These primary afferent nociceptors make up the majority of fibers in any peripheral nerve.

FIGURE 9–3. Events leading to activation, sensitization, and spread of sensitization of primary afferent nociceptor terminals. *Panel A.* Direct activation by intense pressure and consequent cell damage. Cell damage leads to release of potassium (K$^+$) and to synthesis of prostaglandins (PG) and bradykinin (BK). Prostaglandins increase the sensitivity of the terminal to bradykinin and other pain-producing substances. *Panel B.* Secondary activation. Impulses generated in the stimulated terminal propagate not only to the spinal cord, but into other terminal branches, where they induce the release of peptides, including substance P (sP), which causes vasodilation and neurogenic edema with further accumulation of bradykinin. In addition, substance P causes the release of histamine (H) from mast cells and serotonin (5-HT) from platelets. *Panel C.* Histamine and serotonin levels rise in the extracellular space, secondarily sensitizing nearby nociceptors. This leads to a gradual spread of hyperalgesia and/or tenderness.

Source. Reprinted from Fields HL: *Pain.* New York, McGraw-Hill, 1987, p. 36. Copyright 1987 McGraw-Hill. Used with permission.

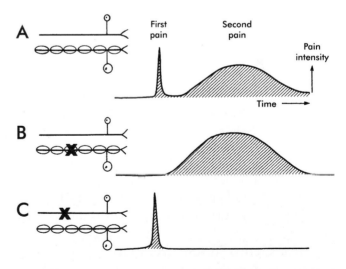

FIGURE 9–4. First and second pain fibers. *Panel A.* First pain and second pain are carried by two different primary afferent axons. *Panel B.* First pain is abolished by selective blockade of myelinated axons. *Panel C.* Second pain is abolished by blocking C fibers.

Source. Reprinted from Fields HL: *Pain.* New York, McGraw-Hill, 1987, p. 26. Copyright 1987 McGraw-Hill. Used with permission.

Lesion of these peripheral nerves does not necessarily correlate with the presence or absence of pain. The loss of large-fiber input in these cases may still create activation of cortical neurons, allowing perception of noxious stimuli that might otherwise be blocked by large-fiber afferent transmission were it intact. Pain that occurs in Fabry's disease—in which congenital absence of small-fiber afferents would predict abolition of painful sensation—also requires a more expansive definition of pain rather than a simple primary pain pathway. This type of pain is probably explained by altered modulation at high-processing centers. Thus it appears that single balance of large-fiber and small-fiber activity is far too simplistic a view of pain modulation.

Peripheral nerve injuries can also lead to pain. The proposed pathways by which such an injury could evoke a pain response include the following:

- Increased activity in sympathetic fibers that are near the damaged area
- Neuroma formation due to sprouting from damaged axons
- Collateral nerves sprouting from intact neighboring fibers
- Changes in dorsal root ganglion cells or in central terminals of damaged axons that have lost part of their dorsal input
- Stimulation of nociceptive nervi nervorum of peripheral nerves

Molecular genetics and cellular physiology research have led to a tremendous growth in knowledge about the structure and function of primary nociceptors (Wood et al. 2000). The presence of multiple receptors and various ion channels has suggested that a therapeutic target for analgesics could be elucidated within the primary afferent. Adenosine triphosphate–gated channels, proton-gated channels, heat-operated capsaicin-gated channels, and sensory-specific sodium channels join a plethora of receptors—including serotonins 5-HT$_{1A}$, 5-HT$_{1D}$, 5-HT$_2$, and 5-HT$_3$—that influence primary neuron activity.

SPINAL CORD TERMINALS OF PRIMARY AFFERENTS

Dorsal and Ventral Roots

The cell bodies of all somatic primary afferent fibers are in the dorsal root ganglia adjacent to the spinal cord. The only primary afferent cell body outside this position is the trigeminal ganglia, which is the rostral continuation of the dorsal root ganglia. Fibers from the dorsal root are organized within the root according to diameter. The large-diameter afferents enter the spinal cord in the dorsal region of the entry zone, whereas the small-diameter afferents enter in the lateral region of the cord. Having entered the spinal cord, the nociceptive primary afferent fibers (Aδ and C fibers) bifurcate into both cephalad- and caudad-projecting branches traveling in Lissauer's tract (the dorsolateral tract). These fibers terminate primarily in the ipsilateral dorsal gray matter, but a small number of the fibers cross dorsal to the central canal to terminate in the dorsal gray matter of the contralateral side. The majority of sensory afferents enter the spinal cord through the dorsal root entry zone. However, nonmyelinated C fiber afferents have also been discovered in the ventral root. The clinical relevance of the fibers that cross or those that enter the ventral root is not known. This heterogeneity in the pathway of the primary afferents associated with pain transmission helps explain the incomplete pain relief that is seen after ablation of a unilateral dorsal root entry zone.

Dorsal Horn

Once the impulses have entered the spinal cord via the dorsal or ventral roots, they terminate in the ipsilateral dorsal horn of the spinal cord. The dorsal horn is organized into distinct laminae, with specific primary afferent terminals found in individual laminae (Figure 9–5). Aδ fibers terminate primarily in lamina I, in ventral portions in lamina II, and through most of lamina III. Unmyelinated C fibers terminate in lamina II.

Lamina I

Lamina I is a thin, superficial layer of neurons that make up the marginal zone. The neurons with cell bodies in lamina I are termed *marginal cells*. These marginal cells receive projections from A and C fiber afferents responsive to noxious mechanical stimuli. In addition, they respond to some polymodal C fiber afferents as well as A temperature impulses. The neurons that respond to Aδ and C fiber noxious stimuli also show response to group III and group IV muscle afferents. This dual response accounts for a convergence of pain impulses from both skin and muscle. These neurons then project to one of several areas: to the thalamus by way of the contralateral spinothalamic tracts, to the ipsilateral dorsal white matter, or to the ipsilateral dorsal gray matter for an area of several segments.

Lamina II

Lamina II is also known as the substantia gelatinosa, owing to the clear appearance of this section of spinal matter in comparison with the surrounding marginal layer and nucleus proprius. This region has undergone

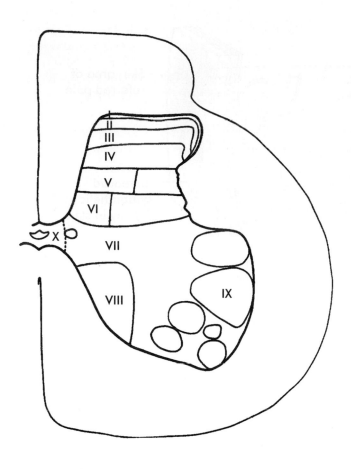

FIGURE 9–5. Schematic drawing of the lamination of the ventral cell column of the seventh lumbar spinal cord segment in the full-grown cat.

Source. Reprinted from Rexed B: "Cytoarchitectonic Organization of the Spinal Cord in the Cat." *Journal of Comparative Neurology* 96:415–495, 1952. Used with permission.

extensive evaluation. The neurons of lamina II act as a modulating center for afferent impulses of small and large fibers that terminate in this region. Afferent input is from noxious stimulation, as well as from light touch and pressure sensations. The area is densely packed with cells that make extensive synaptic connections with other cells in the area. The axons of most of these cells are short, and only a few of them project to the thalamus through the contralateral-anterolateral columns. The clinical phenomenon of selective spinal cord opioid analgesia is mediated through opioid receptors found in lamina II (Yaksh 1988). Stimulation of these receptors leads to inhibition of marginal cell firing in response to primary afferent signals. Similar inhibition has been postulated with other neurochemicals acting on this lamina, but much more work needs to be done to delineate the complex interactions involved in processing noxious stimuli here.

Laminae III and IV

The nucleus proprius is made up of the neurons located in laminae III and IV. One of the predominant populations of cells in the nucleus proprius responds to Aβ, Aδ, and C fiber input; these are termed *wide dynamic range neurons* (WDRs). Although the receptive fields of the individual afferents may be quite small, the corresponding WDR has a larger receptive field. Afferent input from closely related somatotopic fields is typically seen on a single WDR, accounting for the somatotopic convergence seen in stimulation of different areas. In addition to somatotopic convergence, there is also evidence that visceral afferents traveling with sympathetic neurons also converge on WDRs. WDRs project throughout the anterolateral funiculus to the thalamus.

The convergence of somatic nociceptive afferents and visceral nociceptive afferents on the same neuron in the dorsal horn probably explains the phenomenon of referred pain. The presence of visceral-somatic, muscular-somatic, and visceral-visceral convergence seen in the various laminae of the dorsal horn and the development of fairly large receptive fields in some of these second-order neurons also help to explain some of the peculiar characteristics of nonsomatic pain. Hyperexcitability in these dorsal horn neurons is proposed as one potential mechanism to account for central sensitivity seen in chronic pain states. The presence of *N*-methyl-D-aspartate (NMDA) receptor activity on these cell bodies shows increased participation in experimental models of nerve injury pain. These are shown schematically in Figure 9–6.

Lamina X (Central Canal)

The central canal has also been identified as receiving input from the Aδ fibers associated with noxious stimulation. These fibers terminate on cells with small receptive fields, like those seen in the marginal zone. The afferents are sensitive to temperature and pinch stimuli. The cells of the central canal are subsequently known to ascend ipsilaterally and contralaterally in the ventrolateral tract to the reticular formation.

Ascending Sensory Pathways

The second-order neurons that arise in the respective laminae of the dorsal horn of the spinal cord subsequently use several specific routes to carry their messages to higher brain centers (Figure 9–7). The specific routes are characterized as tracts and systems that include the neospinothalamic, paleospinothalamic, and spinoreticular systems and dorsal columns. The names given to these nociceptive pathways are derived from the point of origin and termination of their respective fibers. The spinothalamic and

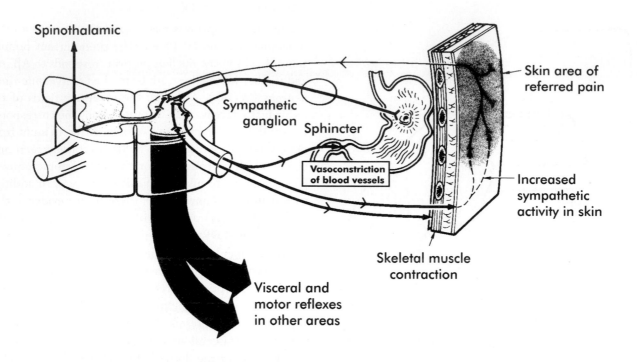

FIGURE 9–6. Visceral pain: convergence of visceral and somatic nociceptive afferents. Visceral sympathetic afferents converge on the same dorsal horn neuron as do somatic nociceptive afferents. Visceral noxious stimuli are then conveyed, together with somatic noxious stimuli, via the spinothalamic pathways to the brain. *Note.* 1) Referred pain is felt in the cutaneous area corresponding to the dorsal horn neurons on which visceral afferents converge; this is accompanied by allodynia and hyperalgesia in this skin area. 2) Reflex somatic motor activity results in muscle spasm, which may stimulate parietal peritoneum and initiate somatic noxious input to the dorsal horn. 3) Reflex sympathetic efferent activity may result in spasm of sphincters of viscera over a wide area, causing pain remote from the original stimulus. 4) Reflex sympathetic efferent activity may result in visceral ischemia and further noxious stimulation; also, visceral nociceptors may be sensitized by norepinephrine release and microcirculatory changes. 5) Increased sympathetic activity may influence cutaneous nociceptors, which may be at least partly responsible for referred pain. 6) Peripheral visceral afferents branch considerably, causing much overlap in the territory of individual dorsal roots; only a small number of visceral afferent fibers converge on dorsal horn neurons compared with somatic nociceptive fibers. Also, visceral afferents converge on the dorsal horn over a large number of segments. This dull, vague visceral pain is very poorly localized and is often called deep visceral pain.

Source. Reprinted from Cousins MJ, Bridenbaugh PO (eds.): *Neural Blockade in Clinical Anesthesia and Management of Pain,* 2nd Edition. Philadelphia, PA, JB Lippincott, 1988, p. 743. Used with permission.

spinoreticular systems represent the most important tracts associated with pain transmission in humans. The fibers from these tracts make up the anterolateral funiculus.

Axons from laminae I, IV, V, VII, and VIII make up the spinothalamic tract. These axons ascend predominantly in the contralateral ventral quadrant of the spinal cord. Crossed fibers predominate, but neuroanatomical studies have indicated that perhaps 25% of all fibers ascend in the ipsilateral ventral quadrant (Yaksh 1988). These spinothalamic fibers subsequently ascend to the thalamus.

Numerous other systems are also involved in the rostral projection of nociceptive information. Important among these other systems are the dorsal funicular systems and intersegmental systems, which are probably involved in descending inhibitory transmission as well.

Brain Stem Processing

The brain stem is involved in transmission of all ascending and descending information. Nociceptive afferent fibers relay to projection neurons in the dorsal horn, which ascend in the anterolateral funiculus to end in the thalamus. During the rostral conduction of these impulses, collateral neurons activate the nucleus reticularis gigantocellularis, which in turn sends projections to the thalamus, as well as to the periaqueductal gray matter (see Figure 9–7).

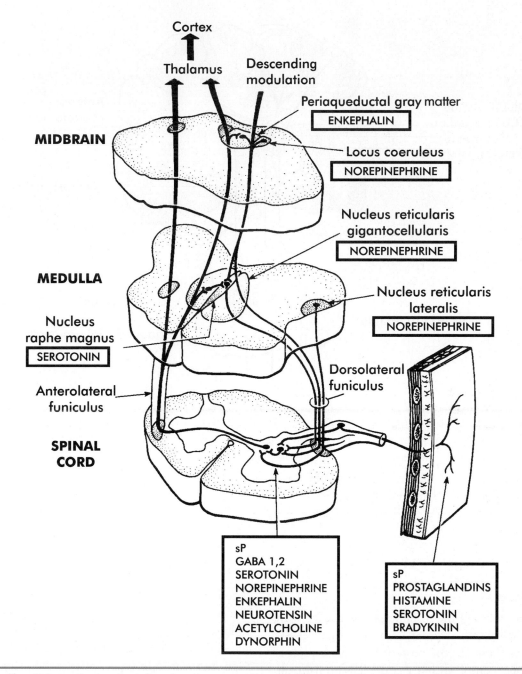

FIGURE 9–7. Schematic drawing of nociceptive processing, outlining ascending (*left side of diagram*) and descending (*right side of diagram*) pathways. Stimulation of nociceptors in the skin surface leads to impulse generation in the primary afferent. Concomitant with this impulse generation, increased levels of various endogenous algesic agents (substance P [sP], prostaglandins, histamine, serotonin, and bradykinin) are detected near the area of stimulation in the periphery. The noxious impulse is conducted to the dorsal horn of the spinal cord, where it is subjected to local factors and descending modulation. The endogenous neurochemical mediators of this interaction at the dorsal horn that have been characterized are listed in the figure. Primary nociceptive afferents relay to projection neurons in the dorsal horn that ascend in the anterolateral funiculus to end in the thalamus. En route, collaterals of the projection neurons activate the nucleus reticularis gigantocellularis, whose neurons project to the thalamus and also activate the periaqueductal gray matter of the midbrain. Enkephalinergic neurons from the periaqueductal gray matter and noradrenergic neurons from the nucleus reticularis gigantocellularis activate descending serotonergic neurons of the nucleus raphe magnus. These fibers join with noradrenergic fibers from the locus coeruleus reticularis lateralis to project descending modulatory impulses to the dorsal horn via the dorsolateral funiculus. GABA=γ-aminobutyric acid.

Source. Reprinted from Brose WG, Cousins MJ: "Gynecologic Pain," in *Gynecologic Oncology.* Edited by Coppelson M. Edinburgh, Churchill Livingstone, 1992, p. 1439. Used with permission.

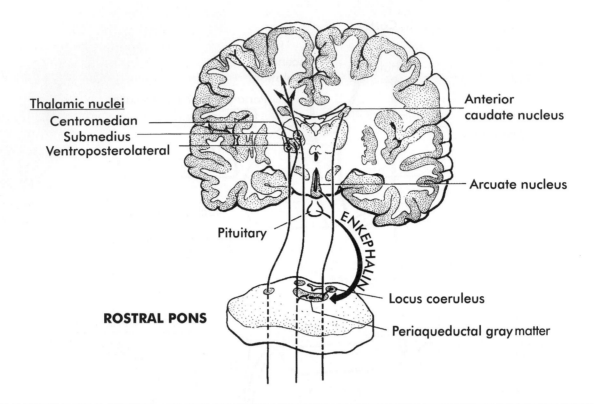

FIGURE 9–8. Rostral projections of nociceptive processing. Ascending stimuli (*left side of diagram*) traveling in the anterolateral funiculus—as well as impulses relayed from the medulla, pons, and midbrain—are projected to the thalamic nuclear complex. The centromedian, submedius, and ventroposterolateral nuclei receive nociceptive information. The ventroposterolateral nucleus projects discretely to the cortex. The centromedian nucleus projects more diffusely, particularly to the limbic region. The descending fibers (*right side of diagram*) inhibit the transmission of nociceptive information between primary afferents and the projection neurons in the dorsal horn. The periaqueductal gray matter is controlled by projections from the anterior caudate nucleus, the midline limbic nuclei, and the arcuate nucleus of the hypothalamus. In addition to direct neural connection, endorphins synthesized in the pituitary are released into the cerebrospinal fluid and the blood, where they can exert an inhibitory effect at multiple centers, including the periaqueductal gray matter.

Thalamic Relays

Several nuclear groups of the thalamus are associated with the relay of nociceptive afferent impulses (Figure 9–8). Included among these are the posterior nuclear complex, the ventrobasilar complex, and the medial intralaminar nuclear complex. In the thalamus, spinothalamic neurons terminate largely on the ventroposterolateral and centromedian nuclei. The ventrobasilar complex also receives input from the dorsal columns. The ventroposterolateral nucleus projects to areas 1, 2, and 3 of the parietal lobe, but these areas have not been found to be involved with aversive or emotional aspects of nociception. Consequently, it is currently believed that the ventroposterolateral nucleus is involved with localization of the impulse rather than with its qualitative aspects (Besson and Chaouch 1987; Willis 1985). The centromedian nucleus is believed to be involved in the qualitative aspects of nociception in that stimulation of this region triggers the unpleasantness asso-

ciated with tissue damage (Besson and Chaouch 1987). The projections of the centromedian nucleus are poorly understood, but presumably they activate the aversive centers in the limbic system. The nucleus submedius has also been implicated in nociceptive processing, because it receives all of its input from terminals of marginal projection neurons in the spinal cord. However, the physiological functions and connections of this nucleus are unknown.

Cerebral Cortex

The somatosensory cortex receives processed input from spinothalamic, spinoreticular, and dorsal column systems, as outlined earlier. Initially, the majority of attention was focused on SII as the principal cortical region involved with the reception and perception of noxious information. The anterior portion of SII receives input from the ventrobasilar thalamus, whereas the posterior portion of SII receives input from the posterior thalamus.

Berkley and Palmer (1974) demonstrated that bilateral ablation of the posterior region of SII produces an increase in nociceptive threshold. The application of non-invasive neural imaging techniques has created a new interest in this area of nociceptive processing. The current neuromatrix for pain expands beyond SI and SII to include the midbrain region and the periaqueductal gray matter, the lenticular complex, the insula, and the orbitofrontal, prefrontal, and motor areas (Kwan et al. 2000).

Descending Modulation

Up to this point, the discussion of pain pathways has been limited to the rostral projection of primary noxious stimuli. The failure of a particular painful stimulus to provoke given behavior in different individuals points out the uncoupling of a simple stimulus-response concept of pain processing. The uncoupling of pain stimulus and response is perhaps best identified by observing the absence of pain in some individuals who are injured in battle or in a sporting event. One of the primary focuses of research during the past two decades has been to delineate the physiological explanations for these observed differences in pain response. Through this investigation it has become apparent that the discussion of the afferent limb of the pain pathway mandates consideration of the modulating influences on that pain transmission.

Modulation of pain stimuli can occur at many different levels in the pathway. In their proposal of the gate theory, Melzack and Wall (1965) predicted modulation of small-fiber activity by the presence of large-fiber activity in the same region of the dorsal horn. Cutaneous activation of large-fiber afferents through transcutaneous nerve stimulation supports this peripheral modulation at the dorsal horn. In addition, the stimulation of dorsal columns that mimics the activation of descending inhibition has also been shown to inhibit the discharge of dorsal horn interneuron nociceptors. Earlier work by Hagbarth and Kerr (1954) demonstrated the existence of descending long-tract systems to modulate spinal evoked activity. Virtually every pathway carrying nociceptive information, including the spinothalamic and spinoreticular tracts, is under modulatory control from supraspinal systems. Experimental evidence of this supraspinal influence includes inhibition of nociceptive reflexes by electrical stimulation or microinjections of opioid at brain stem sites, both of which are naloxone reversible. Various nuclei of the medulla oblongata and the pons project caudally to the spinal gray matter and the spinal nucleus of the trigeminal nerve. Serotonergic neurons in the nucleus raphe magnus, the catecholaminergic neurons of the lateral reticular formation, and the locus coeruleus are all believed to play a role in descending modulation (Besson and Chaouch 1987; Fields and Basbaum 1984). Axons from these centers project to all levels of the spinal cord through the dorsolateral funiculus (Figure 9–6).

Stimulation of the medullary centers prevents the activation of second-order neurons in the dorsal horn or trigeminal gray matter by primary afferent fibers through this descending inhibition (Basbaum 1985; Besson and Chaouch 1987). The exact mechanism of this inhibition has not been characterized, but several models have been proposed (Basbaum 1985; Dubner 1985). In addition to the different modulating pathways that have been partially characterized (Figure 9–9), there are undoubtedly additional descending inhibitory influences that have yet to be evaluated. The depression of spinothalamic neurons by cortical and pyramidal stimulation is an example of such an uncharacterized pathway. Continued research in this area will help to unravel the complex reaction between pain stimulus and response and perhaps suggest additional therapeutic modalities that may be applied to the treatment of pain.

NEUROPHARMACOLOGY

PHARMACOLOGY OF PAIN

Basic research on the processing of nociceptive information by the CNS has led to an improved understanding of pain and pain treatment. Figure 9–7 summarizes the site of action of several of the chemical substances that have been identified with nociceptive processing. Using this simplified picture of the pain pathway, we can focus on pharmacological interventions at different points in the pathway and determine a clinical effect on the relief of pain.

PERIPHERAL DESENSITIZATION

A rough schematic drawing of the local circuitry involved in the detection of a noxious stimulus from the periphery is shown in Figure 9–10. After trauma to a peripheral site, an inflammatory reaction, including the activation of complement and coagulation-fibrinolytic pathways, begins. Local release of histamine, serotonin, prostaglandins, and substance P occurs. Subsequent changes in the local environment, such as decreased tissue pH, changes in the microcirculation, and an increase in efferent sympathetic activity, all appear to increase the response of peripheral nociceptors.

Attempts have been made through numerous drug therapies to interrupt these peripheral processes. Blockade of pain by aspirin-like drugs is one such peripheral action. Aspirin, indomethacin, ibuprofen, diclofenac, and ketorolac are all cyclooxygenase inhibitors. Cyclooxygenase is the en-

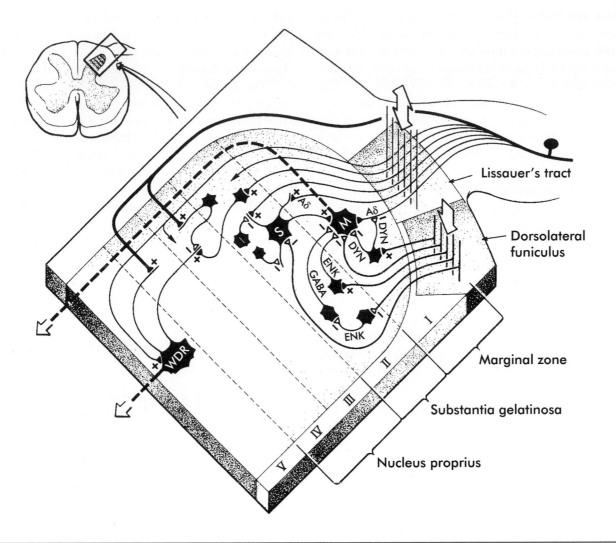

FIGURE 9–9.   Dorsal horn processing. Large- and small-diameter primary neurons have their cell bodies in the dorsal root ganglia. These fibers segregate as they approach the spinal cord. Large-diameter afferents *(thick solid lines)* travel in the medial portion, whereas small-diameter afferents *(thin solid lines:* C and Aδ) segregate to the lateral portions of the entry zone. The spinal terminals of the small fibers enter the cord, where they may ascend or descend for several segments in the dorsolateral tract (Lissauer's tract) and subsequently terminate throughout the dorsal horn of the spinal cord. Aδ fiber afferents terminate primarily in lamina I (marginal zone), whereas C fiber afferents terminate in lamina II (substantia gelatinosa). In lamina I, nociceptive fibers synapse on dendrites of the large marginal (M) neurons. Smaller neurons in lamina I may exert presynapse inhibition of the marginal neuron. Other nociceptive fibers (Aδ) synapse with stalked (S) neurons in lamina II. These S neurons stimulate M neurons in lamina I. The relay between primary afferent fibers and S neurons is also subject to modulation by inhibitory islet (I) neurons in lamina II. Central transmission is accomplished by M neurons directly, wide dynamic range neurons (WDRs) directly, or S neurons indirectly. M neurons are subject to inhibition by neurons in lamina II. Descending serotonergic neurons from the nucleus raphe magnus, which travel in the dorsolateral funiculus, are also shown. These neurons terminate throughout the spinal cord on interneurons (γ-aminobutyric acid [GABA] and enkephalins [ENK]) to provide inhibition of nociceptive transmission. DYN = dynorphin.

zyme responsible for the synthesis of prostaglandins, prostacyclins, and thromboxanes. All these endogenous substances have been proposed as mediators of the local pain response (Juan 1978). Clinical trials with topical capsaicin are also focused on peripheral action. This drug has been shown to deplete substance P from cutaneous nerve endings (Gamse et al. 1980). The initial effect is a burning pain, followed by insensitivity to subsequent painful stimuli.

The involvement of the sympathetic nervous system is also suspect. It is known that sympathetic fibers are present in large numbers near cutaneous nociceptors. Blockade of these sympathetic fibers can eliminate the pain of complex

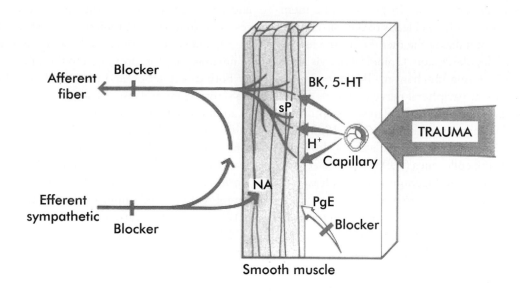

FIGURE 9–10. Local tissue factors and peripheral pain receptors. The physical stimuli of "trauma," the chemical environment (e.g., H+), algesic substances (e.g., serotonin [5-HT] and bradykinin [BK]), and microcirculatory changes may all modify peripheral receptor activity. Efferent sympathetic activity may increase the sensitivity of receptors by means of noradrenaline (NA) (norepinephrine) release. Substance P (sP) may be the peripheral pain transmitter. Points of potential blockade of nociception are shown as "Blocker"; other potential sites involve bradykinin, serotonin, noradrenaline, and substance P. PgE=prostaglandin E.

Source. Reprinted from Cousins MJ, Phillips GD (eds): *Acute Pain Management.* London, Churchill Livingstone, 1986, p. 742. Used with permission.

regional pain syndromes (CRPS) in some patients. The burning dysesthetic pain and hyperalgesia that are seen with this syndrome, which may be eliminated by sympathetic blockade, can be made to reappear with local application of norepinephrine, the sympathetic neurotransmitter.

NEURAL BLOCKADE

Early in the twentieth century, Cushing (1902) presented his theory that nerve blockade could prevent the pain and shock of amputation. Later, Crile (1910) proposed that disruption of the pain pathway might improve outcome from trauma. Indeed, a multitude of investigations have proved the beneficial effect of neural blockade with respect to neuroendocrine function after trauma and/or surgery (Kehlet and Dahl 1993).

Neural blockade can occur at any point along the pain pathway. The most common sites of neural blockade are peripheral nerves, somatic plexuses, and dorsal roots. These blockages can be performed with relatively short-acting agents such as local anesthetics for acute pain, whereas long-acting (permanent) blockade with alcohol or phenol are sometimes utilized for chronic pain. Surgical lesions at any of these points have also been suggested to provide long-lasting interruption of specific pain pathways. The disadvantage of permanent techniques is that they are neither specific to pain fibers nor reliable for protracted pain problems. The lack of anatomical separa-

tion of fibers carrying pain, motor, and other sensory information exposes the patient in whom neural blockade is employed to varying amounts of sympathetic, somatic, and perhaps motor dysfunction. In some chronic pain conditions, such as CRPS, even a "permanent" intervention such as a neurolytic blockade or surgical lesion may result in recurrence of pain due to CNS reorganization and redundancy of transmission. Therefore the use of these techniques is increasingly reserved for treatment of chronic pain toward the end of life, for example in end-stage cancer pain management.

OPIOID ANALGESIA

In recent years, researchers have identified multiple endogenous opioid chemicals that have analgesic effects (Yaksh 1988). Included among these are the enkephalins, dynorphins, and β-endorphin. The endogenous ligands for each receptor and exogenous agonists and antagonists are known (Dickenson 1991).

Mechanism of Action

Opioid receptors are synthesized in the cell body of the sensory neuron and are transported in both a central and peripheral direction. In the spinal cord, opioid receptors are found primarily in the substantia gelatinosa area of the spinal cord. Stimulation of these receptors leads to hyperpolarization of the nerve terminal and reduced excitatory neurotransmitter release. In postsynaptic membranes, activation of the channel leads to outward flow of potassium, thereby stabilizing the membrane and making it less sensitive to depolarization. Opioids work via a second messenger G protein mechanism. In the periphery, opioid receptors are at peripheral nerve terminals as well as on the surface of immune cells. These receptors are sensitized by inflammatory mediators (Stein 1993). The sensitivity of opioid receptors to modulation is also found in the CNS. Gray and colleagues (1998) found that some antidepressants induce endogenous opioid release and modulate the opioid response curve.

At least four different types of opioid receptors have also been located in the brain and spinal cord. Table 9–1 summarizes the pharmacodynamic effects obtained when each of these opioid receptors is stimulated. Pert and Snyder (1973) demonstrated opioid receptors in the brain and the brain stem. Later, Yaksh and Rudy (1976) reported long-lasting analgesia after the introduction of intrathecal opioids. The discovery that spinally administered opioids produced dose-dependent, stereospecific, naloxone-reversible analgesia has led to the development of an important clinical tool to combat pain.

Brain Receptors

It has been known for centuries that opium possesses analgesic properties. Despite the wide recognition of these properties, the location of the active sites for opium was not known. Microinjection techniques used in the 1960s identified the periaqueductal gray matter of the midbrain and the midline medullary nuclei to be the most sensitive sites. Through descending serotonergic and/or noradrenergic links with the spinal cord, morphine microinjections into these centers have been shown to inhibit spinal reflexes. This analgesic effect has also been shown to be similar to the effect achieved by systemically administered morphine. Further research has documented dose dependency, stereospecificity, naloxone reversibility, and well-defined structure activity relationships of these centers to other opioid agonists.

Spinal Cord Receptors

As interesting as the delineation of the descending inhibition of nociception initiated by centrally administered opioids is the growing appreciation of opioid systems in spinal function. Opioids administered systemically produce inhibition of nociceptive reflexes in animals with transected spinal cords. Also, administration of opioids to the dorsal horn of the spinal cord inhibits the discharge of nociceptive neurons. Multiple discrete populations of opioid receptors have been identified. Stimulation of μ

and κ systems present in the spinal cord depresses the response to noxious stimulation (Yaksh 1981).

Opioid systems appear to be active in the modulation of noxious impulses presented to the substantia gelatinosa by both direct action and indirect descending inhibition via serotonergic and noradrenergic systems (Yaksh 1988). In addition, nonopioid systems appear to be functioning at this level to produce analgesic effects. Baclofen and clonidine also rely on both ascending and descending effects for antinociception (Sawynok and Labella 1981). Newer work has focused on the NMDA receptor ion channel complex. Improved understanding of the complex interaction of the excitatory amino acids glutamate and NMDA with glycine activity and the nitric oxide intercellular pathways may yield novel agents that can be used in the future management of difficult painful syndromes.

In summary, it appears that the substantia gelatinosa receives collaterals of nociceptive information and that this information is subject to extensive modulation at the spinal level. Chemical mediators shown to be associated with analgesia at this level include opioids, serotonin, norepinephrine, γ-aminobutyric acid (GABA), neurotensin, and acetylcholine. Some of the proposed endogenous and exogenous ligands for these neurotransmitter systems are shown in Table 9–2.

NONSTEROIDAL ANTI-INFLAMMATORY DRUGS

The effect of nonsteroidal anti-inflammatory drugs (NSAIDs) in inhibiting synthesis of prostaglandins is currently thought to be the explanation of their pain-relieving properties. The prostaglandins, leukotrienes, and thromboxanes are oxygenated derivatives of arachidonic acid, an essential polyunsaturated fat. The term *eicosanoids* is often used to describe all the products of arachidonic acid metabolism. This inhibition occurs by the inactivation of cyclooxygenase, which catalyzes the formation of cyclic endoperoxides from arachidonic acid. Anti-inflammatory steroids act at an earlier step in the arachidonic acid metabolism pathway (Raja et al. 1988). Prostaglandins are formed in damaged tissue and appear to be involved in sensitizing the peripheral nociceptors to painful stimuli.

The indications for NSAIDs range from the treatment of aches and sprains to dysmenorrhea to long-term therapy for rheumatoid arthritis and osteoarthritis, as well as degenerative joint diseases (e.g., ankylosing spondylitis and gout). Their anti-inflammatory activities have also been shown to relieve pain in cancer patients with bone metastases. In contrast to the opioid drugs, there has not been a clear demonstration of a relationship between blood levels of NSAIDs and pain relief. The majority of NSAIDs can be

TABLE 9–1. Pharmacodynamic effects obtained when an opioid agonist interacts with the various types of opioid receptors

Effect	Receptor subtype			
	μ	κ	σ	δ
Pain relief	Yes	Yes, especially at spinal cord level	Yes	Yes
Sedation	Yes	Yes	—	—
Respiratory effects	Depression	Depression, but not as much as for μ (may reach plateau)	Stimulation	Depression
Affect	Euphoria	—	Dysphoria	—
Physical dependence	Marked	Less severe than with μ	—	Yes
Prototype agonist (other drugs with predominantly agonist activity)	Morphine (meperidine, methadone, fentanyl, heroin, codeine, propoxyphene, buprenorphine)	Ketocyclazocine (nalbuphine, dynorphin, butorphanol, nalorphine, pentazocine)	SKF 10,047	Enkephalins

Note. SKF = Smith, Kline, and French.
Source. Adapted from Gourlay GK, Cousins MJ, Cherry DA: "Drug Therapy," in *Handbook of Chronic Pain Management.* Edited by Burrows GD, Elton D, Stanley GV. Amsterdam, Elsevier, 1987, pp. 20–24. Used with permission.

classified into one of two groups based on their elimination half-lives (Table 9–3). The NSAIDs in the first group have half-lives between 2 and 4 hours. Acetaminophen is also included in this group, despite its lack of anti-inflammatory properties. The drugs in the second group have longer half-lives, ranging from 6 to 60 hours. Patients with renal insufficiency are thought to be at risk for toxicity due to these agents because they are excreted through the kidneys.

The use of NSAIDs alone has been supported through years of clinical practice. Dosing of the individual agents is covered in Table 9–3. These dosages have been derived from long-term therapy of rheumatological disease and represent near-maximal anti-inflammatory activity. Although these dosages are considered safe for long-term therapy, careful monitoring of side effects is appropriate. Side effects of NSAIDs include gastric irritation, salt and fluid retention, platelet inhibition, and tinnitus. The gastric damage is caused by decreased prostaglandin levels, which cause reduced production of gastric mucus, increased acid secretion, and decreased gastric mucosal blood supply. Acetaminophen does not share the potential for these prostaglandin-mediated side effects, but it carries the potential for liver damage with excessive doses.

Cyclooxygenase-2 (COX-2) inhibitors, which selectively target the COX-2 enzyme while sparing COX-1, were designed in an attempt to overcome the limitations of NSAIDs, especially gastric irritation and bleeding. Although very popular for several years, currently they have been recalled because of increased observed cardiovascular events.

ANALGESIC ADJUVANTS

The term *analgesic adjuvants* refers to the group of medications that have primary indications for nonpain diagnoses but have demonstrated efficacy for pain treatment. Although they are often used in combination with opioids and anti-inflammatory agents, these medications may have their own direct analgesic effects, and they may also be used as single agents for specific types of pain. The analgesic adjuvants are classified according to the category of medication to which they belong (Table 9–4).

Antidepressants

The involvement of neurotransmitters in the transmission of pain is discussed above in the section "Neurobiological Mechanisms of Pain." Tricyclic antidepressants (TCAs) and serotonin-norepinephrine reuptake inhibitors have been used as adjuncts in the pharmacological treatment of pain (Carter 2002). Although there has been interest in the use of the selective serotonin reuptake inhibitors

TABLE 9–2.   Spinal neurotransmitters, receptors, and ligands

Neurotransmitter system	Proposed receptor	Endogenous ligand	Exogenous ligand
Opioid	μ	β-Endorphin; Met/ Leuenkephalin	Morphine
	δ	Met/Leuenkephalin	
	κ	Dynorphin	
Adrenergic	α$_1$	Norepinephrine	Methoxamine
	α$_2$	Norepinephrine	Clonidine
	β	Epinephrine	Isoproterenol
Serotonergic	5-HT	Serotonin	Serotonin
GABAergic	A	GABA	Baclofen
	B	GABA	Muscimol
Neurotensin	—	Neurotensin	Neurotensin
Cholinergic	Muscarinic	Acetylcholine	Oxotremorine

Note.   GABA = γ-aminobutyric acid; 5-HT = 5-hydroxytryptamine (serotonin); — = unidentified.
Source.   Adapted from Yaksh TL: "Neurologic Mechanisms of Pain," in *Neural Blockade in Clinical Anesthesia and Management of Pain*, 2nd Edition. Edited by Cousins MJ, Bridenbaugh PO. Philadelphia, PA, JB Lippincott, 1988, pp. 791–844. Used with permission.

TABLE 9–3.   Terminal half-life, recommended dosage, influence of food on absorption, and incidence of gastric erosion from nonsteroidal anti-inflammatory drugs (NSAIDs)

Drug	Terminal half-life (hours)	Oral dosage (mg/hour)	Effect of food on absorption[a]	Incidence of gastric erosion (gastritis)
Aspirin	0.2–0.3	600–900/4	1	High
Salicylate	2–3	600/4	1	Intermediate
Diflunisal	8–12	500/12	1	Low
Diclofenac	1.5–2	25–50/8	1	Low
Ibuprofen	2–3	200–400/8	1	Low
Naproxen	12–15	250–375/12	3	Low
Fenoprofen	2–3	400–600/6	2	Low
Indomethacin	6–8	50–75/8	1	Intermediate
Sulindac	6–8	100–200/12	2	Low
Piroxicam	30–60	20–30/24	1	Low
Flufenamic acid	8–10	500/6	1	—
Mefenamic acid	3–4	250/6	1	Intermediate
Ketoprofen	1–4	50/6	1	Low
Ketorolac[b]	5	10–30/6	?	?

[a]1 = decrease in rate of absorption; no change in oral bioavailability; 2 = decrease in rate of absorption and oral bioavailability; 3 = no change in rate of absorption and oral bioavailability.
[b]Not currently available for clinical use; dosages based on review of scientific literature.
Source.   Adapted from Gourlay GK, Cousins MJ, Cherry DA: "Drug Therapy," in *Handbook of Chronic Pain Management*. Edited by Burrows GD, Elton D, Stanley GV. Amsterdam, Elsevier, 1987, pp. 20–24. Used with permission.

TABLE 9–4. Coanalgesic medications

Drugs, by classification	Indications	Comments
Antidepressant Amitriptyline Imipramine Venlafaxine Duloxetine Citalopram	Chronic pain, neuropathic pain associated with neuropathy and headache	Improves sleep, may improve appetite
Corticosteroid Dexamethasone Prednisolone Fludrocortisone	Neuropathic pain secondary to direct neural compression, pain secondary to increased intracranial pressure	May stimulate appetite; limit trial to 2 weeks and reassess efficacy
Anticonvulsant Carbamazepine Phenytoin Valproate Clonazepam Gabapentin Topiramate Lamotrigine	Neuropathic pain with paroxysmal character	Start slowly, increase gradually while observing for side effects
Clonidine	Neuropathic pain, spinal cord injury	Transdermal and intrathecal routes of administration Potential for sedation and hypotension
Phenothiazine Levomepromazine	Insomnia unresponsive to antidepressant or short-acting benzodiazepines	Increase dose slowly to achieve desired effect
Butyrophenone Haloperidol	Acute confusion, nausea, vomiting	Prolonged use may be complicated by tardive dyskinesia
Antihistamine Hydroxyzine	Nausea, pruritus, anxiety	Anticholinergic side effects
CNS stimulant Dextroamphetamine Cocaine Caffeine	Opioid-induced sedation, potentiation of NSAID, potentiation of opioid analgesia not proven in cancer	Should be used only as short-term therapeutic trial

Note. CNS = central nervous system; NSAID = nonsteroidal anti-inflammatory drug.
Source. Adapted from Ballantyne JC, Fishman SM, Salahadin A: *The Massachusetts General Hospital Handbook of Pain Management*, 3rd Edition. Philadelphia, PA, Lippincott Williams & Wilkins, 2006, pp. 127–140. Used with permission.

(SSRIs), they have generally not been found to be as effective in pain treatment. Although there is some indication of moderate selective efficacy (e.g., in diabetic neuropathy but not other neuropathic pain [Kishore-Kumar et al. 1990]), there is evidence of analgesic effects of SSRIs (Boyer 1992; Finley 1994), with clear clinical effects for problems such as fibromyalgia (Arnold et al. 2002). Citalopram has also been found to be effective in the treatment of recurrent abdominal pain in children (Campo 2004). Mirtazapine, a piperazinoapepine, is a

novel type of antidepressant with serotonergic and noradrenergic properties that has been found effective in case reports in reducing headache and other types of pain (Flores 2004). Many of the antidepressant drugs act by blocking the reuptake of norepinephrine and serotonin at synapses in the CNS. This effect may also occur in the medulla and increase the concentrations of these neurotransmitters at the synapses involved in the descending inhibition of dorsal horn cells. In addition, imipramine has been found to act by reducing expression of pain- and stress-invoked genetic changes in the hippocampus as well as spinal cord neurons at neurokinin-1 (NK-1) and brain-derived neurotrophic factor (BDNF) receptors (Duric and McCarson 2006a, 2006b). These mechanisms may represent some of the pathways behind the frequently observed clinical phenomenon of comorbid depression in the presence of chronic pain. It is unclear whether the effectiveness of TCAs is due to a reduction of comorbid depression or to specific neural effects on pain transmission and amplification pathways; however, they remain a valuable addition to analgesic treatment.

TCAs have been found to be superior to placebo in the treatment of pain (Carter 2002). Evidence suggests that TCAs have a direct analgesic effect that is separate from their efficacy in treating depression or insomnia. Different mechanisms have been suggested that include increased availability of serotonin, endogenous opioid peptide release, and a direct action on opioid receptors (Gray 1998). TCAs may also potentiate the action of opioids, allowing a reduction in chronic opioid requirements. The effect of TCAs for pain reduction and improved sleep is more rapid (3–7 days) and occurs at lower doses (0.1–0.2 mg/kg/day) than is expected in the treatment of depression.

Amitriptyline is one of the most widely studied TCAs and has been found to be effective in a wide range of pediatric pain syndromes, including migraine, peripheral neuropathies, phantom limb pain, fibromyalgia, and pain related to the invasion of nerves by tumors. Studies have emphasized the helpfulness of even low doses as well as benefit from sedation due to amitriptyline. Nevertheless, there is no theoretical or empirical basis to suggest that amitriptyline has any unique efficacy in pain management compared to other TCAs. Where sedation is problematic or the patient is particularly susceptible to anticholinergic side effects, imipramine and nortriptyline can be considered as alternatives.

TCAs are subject to anticholinergic side effects including dry mouth, constipation, blurred vision, urinary retention, confusion, and delirium. Autonomic side effects include orthostatic hypotension, profuse sweating, palpitations, tachycardia, and high blood pressure. Electrocardiographic (ECG) changes include flattened T-waves; prolonged Q-T, QRS, and PR intervals; and depressed S-T segments. Monitoring of the ECG is recommended at baseline and after the patient has been stabilized at a therapeutic dose. There has been increasing interest in the SSRIs, including venlafaxine and duloxetine, which some authors have suggested are as least as effective as the TCAs, with fewer side effects (Goldstein 2004). Venlafaxine has been used effectively in the treatment of adults with headache, neuropathic pain, fibromyalgia, diabetic peripheral neuropathy, and reflex sympathetic

dystrophy (Dwight 1998; Kiayias 2000; Taylor 1996). This group of medications may be of particular benefit to patients with comorbid mood and anxiety disorders.

Corticosteroids

Corticosteroids have been used successfully for the management of neuropathic pain from direct neural compression and from pain due to increased intracranial pressure. Systemic steroids are thought to reduce perineural edema and lymphatic edema that may be contributing to pain by compressing individual nerves. This treatment appears to be especially helpful in cases of spinal cord compression. Treatment of such neural compression involves relatively high doses of dexamethasone (near 30 mg/day). Steroids are best employed on a trial basis. A single morning dosage or twice-daily dosage of 2–4 mg/day of dexamethasone can be used over a 10- to 14-day period. An additional benefit of corticosteroids is that they often stimulate appetite; this effect may aid in the nutritional support of patients with malignancy. The use of steroids is not without problems, however. Attention needs to be focused on the possible development of oral and vaginal candidiasis; in addition, this treatment may worsen peripheral edema.

Anticonvulsants

Anticonvulsants are also often advocated as analgesic adjuvants. They suppress neuronal firing and have been successfully employed for the treatment of neuropathic pain states, including trigeminal neuralgia and peripheral neuropathies. Other indications include central pain states such as thalamic pain syndrome, postsympathectomy pain, diabetic neuropathy, migraine headaches, phantom limb pain, and peripheral neuropathies. Carbamazepine, clonazepam, and phenytoin have been widely used in the treatment of migraine and neuropathic pain, and divalproex sodium has been used for migraine prophylaxis. Newer agents such as topiramate and lamotrigine have been used for diabetic neuropathy and trigeminal neuralgia. Anticonvulsant drugs probably exert their effects by blocking voltage-dependent sodium channels and thereby interfering with the transduction and perhaps spontaneous depolarization seen in damaged neurons. Carbamazepine and phenytoin have been helpful in managing cancer pain with dysesthetic components. These drugs need to be started slowly and increased gradually, with particular attention to the development of possible side effects. With the exception of gabapentin, the anticonvulsants in general have multiple potential side effects, including behavioral changes, that may limit their use. Common side effects can include dizziness, ataxia, drowsiness, blurred vision, and gastrointestinal irritation. In addition, carbamazepine

TABLE 9–5. Anticonvulsants in common use

Drug	Mechanism of action	Adverse effects	Clinical applications
Gabapentin	Possible increase in total brain concentration of GABA	Somnolence, dizziness, ataxia, fatigue, concentration difficulties, GI disturbance, nystagmus, pedal edema	First-line drug for pain management Complex regional pain syndrome Postherpetic neuralgia Diabetic neuropathy Phantom limb pain
Carbamazepine	Inhibits NE uptake Prevents repeated discharges in neurons Blocks sodium channels	Sedation, nausea, diplopia, vertigo, hematological abnormalities, jaundice, oliguria, hypertension, acute left ventricular heart failure	Diabetic neuropathy Trigeminal neuralgia
Oxcarbazepine	Prevents repeated discharges in neurons Binds to sodium channels Increases potassium conductance	Dizziness, somnolence, diplopia, fatigue, ataxia, nausea, abnormal vision, hyponatremia	Trigeminal neuralgia Neuropathic pain syndromes
Topiramate	Blocks sodium channels Inhibits calcium channels Potentiates GABAergic inhibition	Kidney stones, somnolence, dizziness, ataxia, paresthesias, nervousness, abnormal vision, weight loss, cognitive slowing	Migraine headaches Neuropathic pain Diabetic neuropathy
Lamotrigine	Blocks sodium channels Inhibits glutamate release Modulates calcium and potassium currents	Dizziness, nausea, headache, ataxia, diplopia, blurred vision, somnolence, Stevens-Johnson syndrome	Complex regional pain syndrome Trigeminal neuralgia Spinal core injury Central poststroke pain
Levetiracetam	Reduces high-voltage calcium currents Opposes inhibition of GABA Affects potassium conductance	Somnolence, asthenia, dizziness, depression, nervousness	Migraine prophylaxis Postherpetic neuralgia Neuropathic pain
Pregabalin	Is GABA analog Increases neuronal GABA concentration	Dizziness, somnolence, headache	Diabetic neuropathy Postherpetic neuralgia
Zonisamide	Blocks sodium and calcium channels, facilitates 5-HT and DA transmission Increases GABA release	Somnolence, ataxia, anorexia, difficulty with concentration, agitation, headache, Stevens-Johnson syndrome	Neuropathic pain Migraine headaches

Note. GABA = γ-aminobutyric acid; GI = gastrointestinal; 5-HT = 5-hydroxytryptamine (serotonin); NE = norepinephrine.
Source. Adapted from Ballantyne JC, Fishman SM, Salahadin A: *The Massachusetts General Hospital Handbook of Pain Management*, 3rd Edition. Philadelphia, PA, Lippincott Williams & Wilkins, 2006, pp. 127–140. Used with permission.

has associated bone marrow toxicity, and sodium valproate is known to produce hepatic toxicity. Anticonvulsants also commonly have a requirement for serum level monitoring due to their narrow therapeutic window. Anticonvulsant drugs in common use are listed in Table 9–5.

Membrane Stabilizers

The use of lidocaine and 2-chloroprocaine in the treatment of certain peripheral neuropathies that have been refractory to other analgesic medications has led to the investigation of another group of drugs, which may be loosely clas sified as membrane stabilizers. In addition to intermittent intravenous infusion of these two local anesthetics, oral administration of the lidocaine congeners mexiletine and tocainide has been reported as useful in certain patients (Dejard et al. 1988; Lindstrom and Lindblom 1987). It is thought that these patients' pain typically has neuropathic components. In comparison to patients with episodic lancinating neuropathic pain, who benefit from antiepileptics, patients who benefit from membrane stabilizers may have a more constant pain. Lidocaine is used as an adjunct medication for mucositis pain related to chemotherapy agents, refractory cancer pain, and neuropathies, and to predict the potential efficacy of mexiletine. In a lidocaine test for tolerance, lidocaine is infused over 30 minutes, by continuous infusion, with close ECG and blood pressure monitoring. The infusion is stopped if the patient develops drowsiness or dysarthria or intolerable side effects such as tinnitus, dysphoria, dysrhythmias, or seizures. A reduction in pain during the lidocaine test suggests that mexiletine, the oral analog of lidocaine, may be useful in longer-term treatment of the patient's pain symptoms (Krane 2003). Mexiletine's most common side effects include nausea, vomiting, sedation, confusion, diplopia, and ataxia. Verapamil has been used to treat migraines and cluster headaches.

Antipsychotics

Antipsychotics have long been believed to potentiate the analgesic effect of opioids. Most studies employing these drugs are uncontrolled, however, and the enthusiasm for their continued use is in contrast to available literature. The phenothiazines are the most commonly employed antipsychotics for analgesia. Dundee and colleagues (Dundee et al. 1963; Moore and Dundee 1961a, 1961b) published data regarding the analgesic potency of 14 different phenothiazines. The results of these studies suggested that the action of a few potentially analgesic phenothiazines was initially antianalgesic and after 2–3 hours only mildly analgesic (Atkison et al. 1985). Antipsychotic agents have been used in the treatment of many chronic pain syndromes, including cancer, arthritis, migraine, neuropathy, and phantom limb pain. The mechanism of action is unknown, but these medications may have a local anesthetic action in spinal nerves. Chlorpromazine and haloperidol have been used to treat nausea associated with the use of opioids for pain.

Review of the use of phenothiazines in both experimental and clinical pain reveals that only levomepromazine (methotrimeprazine) has established analgesic properties. Haloperidol is a butyrophenone antipsychotic that has found a useful position in the management of acute confusional states associated with terminal cancer. Haloperidol also has useful antiemetic properties, which can be helpful in the management of cancer pain. The appropriate use of antipsychotics in the management of chronic cancer pain has not been established. Care must be taken in the long-term administration of these drugs because of the potential for tardive dyskinesia.

Benzodiazepines are often discussed as coanalgesics. These drugs do not have any demonstrated analgesic effect. Diazepam has been studied extensively with respect to analgesic activity, and it does not alter sensitivity to pain or potentiate the analgesic activity of opioids. These drugs do decrease affective responses to acute pain, however, and they may produce extended relief in chronic pain due to musculoskeletal disorders, perhaps as a result of their muscle-relaxant properties. Judicious use of benzodiazepines in cancer pain is appropriate for short-term relief of anxiety, but superior analgesic effects and nighttime sedation can be achieved by employing a TCA. Short-term use of benzodiazepines can be effective in postoperative pain and sickle cell crises.

Muscle Relaxants

The more general class of agents known as muscle relaxants is a diverse group with varied profiles but with the specific intent of providing muscle relaxation and hence relief from painful muscular conditions. The utility of these agents in the treatment of painful muscular conditions, however, is questionable; they may in general provide a nonspecific benefit from poorly characterized central effects.

The most specific of these agents is baclofen—an agent known to interact with the $GABA_B$ receptor, in distinction to the benzodiazepines, which interact with both the $GABA_A$ and the $GABA_B$ receptor sites. Although baclofen does have demonstrated efficacy in patients with spasticity from spinal cord injury or cerebral injury, the evidence that baclofen improves outcomes in chronic muscular syndromes such as fibromyalgia and myofascial pain is less convincing. Anecdotal reports suggest that baclofen may be a useful agent when used adjunctively with other agents in the management of chronic pain. Sedation is the primary limiting side effect. However, most patients acclimate rapidly.

Other agents in this class are more nonspecific in their actions, including cyclobenzaprine (Flexeril) and carisoprodol (Soma). These agents have CNS effects that allow skeletal muscle relaxation. Cyclobenzaprine has a higher side-effect profile that includes sedation, whereas carisoprodol is better tolerated.

Hydroxyzine is an antihistaminic agent. It has proven analgesic properties at high doses. It does not consistently improve analgesia obtained with opioids, but it does potentiate the effect of opioids on the affective components of pain. It appears that hydroxyzine administered intramuscularly has analgesic properties similar to those of low doses of morphine (Beaver and Feise 1976). In addition, the sedative and antipruritic properties of this drug are useful in the setting of chronic cancer pain. Hydroxyzine similarly may have an application in the augmentation of opioids in sickle cell crises.

Alpha-2 Agonists

Clonidine is an α-2-adrenergic agonist that decreases sympathetic outflow from the central nervous system, resulting in decreased heart rate and blood pressure. Clonidine may work both peripherally and centrally by increasing conduction of potassium. It appears to be particularly indicated for sympathetically maintained pain. Clonidine has been used in the treatment of diabetic neuropathy and postherpetic neuralgia. Intrathecal clonidine has also been used to reduce muscle spasms in patients with spinal cord injuries. Clonidine is generally considered a second-line drug after the use of antidepressants and anticonvulsants, but it does have some unique advantages, such as its transdermal formulation. Dosing of the patch starts with one Catapres TTS-1 patch increased to a maximum of two TTS-3 patches applied every 7 days. Side effects include dry mouth, drowsiness, fatigue, headaches, lethargy, dizziness, hypotension, sedation, and a rebound hypertension and nervousness following abrupt cessation.

Psychostimulants

The final group of analgesic adjuvants to be considered is the stimulants. This group includes amphetamines, cocaine, and caffeine. Psychostimulant medications are believed to have antinociceptive properties that may be mediated via norepinephrine, serotonin, or dopamine or by endogenous opioid mechanisms. Indications for psychostimulants include reduction of drowsiness caused by narcotic medications, as well as potential to reduce the dose of narcotics without diminution of analgesic effect. Methylphenidate and dextroamphetamine have been found to be safe and effective adjuncts to opioid analgesia and have also been used in the treatment of spasmodic torticollis, spastic colon, and headaches. Chronic cancer pain has been treated for nearly a century with combinations of opioid and stimulant in Brompton's cocktail. This mixture contains morphine, cocaine, and a phenothiazine. Despite years of clinical experience with such a mixture, no controlled studies have demonstrated superior analgesia with this combination compared with opioid alone. Potentiation of analgesia by sympathomimetics has been well described. Caffeine is known to increase the analgesic effects of aspirin and acetaminophen, and one study suggested that dextroamphetamine doubled the analgesic potency of morphine (Forrest et al. 1977). The long-term use of these stimulants in pain has not been systematically evaluated. The use of these drugs should probably be limited to a therapeutic trial period of several days to determine efficacy for individual patients.

OPIOIDS

Opioids are extremely effective agents in the treatment of nociceptive components of acute pain. Many misconceptions surround the use of opioid drugs, which results in a marked tendency toward inadequate doses and inappropriately long dosing intervals. Once a decision has been made to use opioid medications, it is both logical and essential to use an effective dosage regimen.

Although vast sums of money have been invested during the last decade in the development of new opioids, an increased understanding of the pharmacokinetics and pharmacodynamics involved in opioid administration has done more to improve the treatment of pain than has any new drug. The introduction of concepts such as the minimum effective analgesic concentration (MEC) has helped health care providers conceptualize the association between blood opioid concentrations and analgesic effect. Equally important to effective pain treatment has been the realization that there may be as much as a fivefold to sixfold interpatient variability in the value of MEC for any one agent. Many factors, both physical and psychological, influence MEC. It is impossible to predict the value of MEC for any patient-opioid combination. It is therefore necessary that the dose for each individual be adjusted to the desired effect. Although MEC and other pharmacokinetic variables cannot be used ahead of time to predict the exact analgesic doses of opioids necessary for obtaining analgesia, these concepts provide a good starting point. They also allow the prediction of the effect of certain disease states on opioid requirements.

In addition to planning effective analgesic therapy by individualizing opioids to a particular patient, the use of opioids often involves the management of side effects. The major side effects limiting the effectiveness of opioid therapy are nausea, vomiting, sedation, and respiratory depression. The incidence and severity of the side effects seen with the various μ agonists are probably similar at equianalgesic doses. Rather than restricting the dose of opioids to the point at which a patient is free from side effects but is experiencing pain, one should consider administering other medications to treat the side effects.

Methods of Administration

The continued reports of inadequate pain relief, despite the vast numbers of newly developed opioids, point to the problems associated with opioid delivery rather than to any defect in the individual drugs per se. There are many different delivery systems and dosing regimens that can provide good pain relief when used properly. The association between stable blood levels of opioids and continuous analgesia must be remembered when planning any systemic opioid therapy. The effective dose of opioid medication is the minimum dose that provides acceptable pain relief with a low incidence of side effects.

Oral administration.   The rapid clearance of the majority of opioids, combined with their extensive hepatic metabolism, has important implications for oral dosing. Drugs are absorbed from the gastrointestinal tract directly into the portal circulation, where they travel to the liver. Therefore, with oral dosing, a significant percentage of the dose is metabolized to inactive products before the opioids reach the systemic circulation (Mather and Gourlay 1984). This phenomenon is referred to as the *hepatic first-pass effect*. This effect and the poor bioavailability seen with certain opioids lead to perceptions that the oral administration of opioids is ineffective.

Oral bioavailability ranges from zero for heroin to 80% for methadone. The oral bioavailability of morphine ranges from 10% to 40%, leading to very wide fluctuations in oral dosing requirements between different patients. Similar variability is seen in meperidine (pethidine) and other opioids (Table 9–6). The high bioavailability of methadone and the long terminal half-life suggest that stable blood levels of the drug could be obtained from oral dosing.

Sublingual administration.   Ongoing interest in the improved pain management of patients with terminal malignancy has led to the investigation of sublingual administration. The sublingual route is particularly useful in patients who cannot tolerate oral medication because it causes nausea, vomiting, or dysphagia. This method of administration has theoretical advantages in that the oral cavity is well perfused, providing rapid onset of action; subsequent absorption results in systemic rather than portal drug delivery. The sublingual absorption of lipid-soluble drugs (methadone, fentanyl, and buprenorphine) from alkaline solution was shown to provide analgesic concentrations very quickly (Weinberg et al. 1988). The utility of this technique in comparison with other methods of administration still needs to be assessed.

Rectal administration.   Rectal administration of opioids has been advocated for patients who cannot swallow or those who have a high incidence of nausea or vomiting with oral administration. Studies of rectal administration of meperidine have indicated a bioavailability similar to that seen with oral dosing: 50% (Ripamonti and Bruera 1991). Prolonged pain relief of 6–8 hours is observed after large doses (400 mg) of rectal meperidine, but a significant latency of 2–3 hours after administration can be seen. Rectal oxycodone has also been shown to have clinical utility, providing pain relief for up to 8 hours.

Intramuscular administration.   The most commonly used approach to managing postoperative pain is intramuscular administration of morphine or meperidine. The typical prescription would read, "Morphine 10 mg (or meperidine 100 mg) intramuscularly every 3–4 hours as needed for pain." This approach has been shown to provide inadequate analgesia for many reasons: the patient may not request medication despite experiencing severe pain, the nurse may not administer the medication, the dose may not be adequate for the patient's needs. Even controlling all these potential problems, the variable blood levels seen after intramuscular dosing usually results in periods of pain alternating with periods of toxicity (Austin et al. 1980).

Subcutaneous administration.   Subcutaneous administration of opioids has been used for decades to provide analgesia. More recent attention has been focused on this technique with the availability of small infusion pumps for delivering continuous opioids to ambulatory patients. Recent applications include subcutaneous infusion for cancer pain and subcutaneous patient-controlled analgesia (PCA). Bruera et al. (1988b) presented data confirming the efficacy of subcutaneous infusion in treating patients with severe pain due to malignancy, both at home and in the hospital. The pharmacokinetic information available for subcutaneous administration of opioids is extremely limited. Continuous infusion of subcutaneous morphine has been demonstrated to provide analgesia and blood levels equivalent to those of intravenous infusion in postoperative patients (Waldeman et al. 1984). Other drugs have been delivered by this route, but no definitive information is available on blood levels achieved. Subcutaneous infusion appears to act clinically like a continuous infusion, but more carefully controlled trials need to be carried out to determine whether this similarity exists for all opioids.

Intravenous administration.   The use of intravenous opioids, by intermittent injection as well as continuous infusion, has been known for years to provide more rapid and effective analgesia. The clinical utility of this technique in the management of cancer pain was reviewed by the Sloan-Kettering Group (Portenoy et al. 1986). The pharmacokinetic support for this clinical observation has been developed over the last several years. Intravenous

TABLE 9–6. Doses, pharmacokinetic parameters, minimum effective concentration, and duration of pain relief for various opioid drugs

Opioid	Dose (mg) im/iv	Dose (mg) po	Terminal half-life (hours)	Bio-availability (%)	MEC (ng/ml)	Pain relief (hours)	Comments
Codeine	130	250	2–3	50	—	3–4	Weak opiate, frequently combined with aspirin. Useful for pain with visceral and integumentary components.
Propoxyphene	240	500	8–24	40	—	4–6	Weak opioid. Unacceptable incidence of side effects.
Oxycodone	10	30	—	30–50	—	4–6	Suppository (30 mg) can provide pain relief for 8–10 hours.
Diamorphine	5	15	0.05	—	—	2–3	Very soluble, rapidly converted to 6-mono-acetyl morphine and morphine in vivo. No oral bioavailability.
Morphine	10	40	2–4	10–40	10–40	3–4	Standard opiate to which new opioids are compared. New sustained-release formulation available in some countries is of considerable benefit in chronic cancer pain.
Methadone	10	10–15	10–80	70–95	20–80	10–60	Duration of pain relief ranges from 10 to 60 hours both postoperatively and for cancer pain. Variable half-life. Requires initial care to establish dose for each patient to avoid accumulation. Otherwise of great value.
Hydromorphone	2	4–6	2–3	50–60	4	3–4	More potent but shorter acting than morphine.
Levorphanol	2	4	12–16	40–60	—	4–6	Good oral availability, but long half-life compared to analgesia may lead to accumulation.

TABLE 9–6.   Doses, pharmacokinetic parameters, minimum effective concentration, and duration of pain relief for various opioid drugs *(continued)*

Opioid	Dose (mg)		Terminal half-life (hours)	Bio-availability (%)	MEC (ng/ml)	Pain relief (hours)	Comments
	im/iv	po					
Phenazocine	3	10–20	—	20–30	—	4–6	Similar to morphine, only more potent.
Oxymorphone	1	6	—	10–40	—	3–4	Similar to morphine, only more potent.
Meperidine	100	300	3–5	30–60	200–800	2–4	Not as effective in relieving anxiety as morphine. Suppositories (200–400 mg) have slow onset (2–3 hours) but can last for 6–8 hours. Normeperidine toxicity.
Dextromoramide	75	10	—	75	—	2–3	Methadone-like chemical structure. Short acting. Useful in covering exacerbation pain. Supplied in iv form.
Buprenorphine	0.3	0.2–1.2	2–3	30	—	6–8	Available in many countries as a sublingual tablet, which appears useful in treatment of cancer pain. Ceiling in analgesic effect at dosage near 5 mg/day. Should not be used with a pure opioid agonist.
Butorphanol	22	—	2.5–3.5	—	—	3–6	Oral form unavailable in many countries. Value in treatment of chronic pain not established.
Nalbuphine	10	40	4–6	20	—	3–6	Oral form unavailable in many countries. Value in treatment of chronic pain not established.

Note.   Data presented are estimates obtained from the literature. MEC=minimum effective analgesic concentration; —=not available.

Source.   Adapted from Gourlay GK, Cousins MJ, Cherry DA: "Drug Therapy," in *Handbook of Chronic Pain Management.* Edited by Burrows GD, Elton D, Stanley GV. Amsterdam, Elsevier, 1987, pp. 20–24. Used with permission.

administration of opioids can maintain analgesia as long as the blood opioid concentration is kept above the MEC in a given patient. Knowledge of the systemic clearance of a drug allows close approximation of the MEC value for a specific opioid to be delivered via continuous infusion. Using infusion alone, however, requires approximately four times the terminal half-life to achieve stable concentrations. The clinical use of continuous infusion opioids is best simplified by providing a loading dose followed by a continuous infusion. The amount of the loading dose and the initial infusion can be predicted if the MEC, volume of distribution (V_d), and clearance (Cl) are known. The practical steps in calculating such an analgesic infusion are

1. Loading dose = V_d MEC
2. Maintenance infusion = Cl MEC

Providing the loading dose as an infusion over 10–15 minutes (followed by the maintenance rate) will allow good analgesia to be rapidly established with a minimum of toxicity. Subsequently, the maintenance infusion rate should be adjusted to patient comfort.

Patient-controlled analgesia. The wide interpatient variability of the pharmacokinetic parameters discussed thus far is a primary reason that individual titration of opioid dosing is required in order to achieve adequate analgesia. Although the physician can do this by evaluating patients at a given time after the therapy has been initiated, the option of PCA is well suited to accommodating the differences between the theory and practice of pain relief. Using PCA, the physician decides the drug to be employed and the dose to be given. The patient can decide when a dose should be administered and the timing between doses.

Although there are several variants of PCA, the most commonly employed is a bolus demand form. With this type of PCA, the physician prescribes the drug on the basis of his or her personal preferences. The usual practice is to prescribe a bolus dose range that can be adjusted if toxicity or inadequate analgesia develops from a single demand. In addition, the minimum time between doses is also prescribed by the physician; this practice avoids potential toxicity from repeated demands being provided before the peak effect of each bolus has been seen.

The majority of pharmacokinetic information that has been applied to PCA has been inferred from the single-dose or continuous infusion of opioids. The applicability of this information to the multiple-dose system of PCA has yet to be investigated. Despite this theoretical uncertainty, the clinical practice of PCA is successful. Several investigators have reported higher patient satisfaction and lower pain scores with therapy, compared with other forms of parenteral opioid analgesia in acute pain management. The

efficacy of short-term subcutaneous PCA was also demonstrated in cancer pain management (Bruera et al. 1988a).

Spinal administration. The use of spinal opioids for acute pain management dates back only to the 1990s. Compared with all the delivery systems discussed above, which use indirect delivery of the opioid to the receptor site via the systemic circulation, spinal delivery is a system in which the opioids are delivered directly to the receptors in the spinal cord via local mechanisms. The presence of opioid receptors in the dorsal horn of the spinal cord was suggested by Calvillo and colleagues (1974). The localization of high concentrations of opioid receptors in the substantia gelatinosa followed (Atweh and Kuhar 1977). Behavioral analgesia from intrathecal administration of morphine in rats was reported by Yaksh and Rudy (1976). Large numbers of clinical reports of long-lasting analgesia obtained with spinal opioids followed, but these were accompanied by frequent reports of side effects, which included nausea, vomiting, sedation, pruritus, urinary retention, and respiratory depression. Fortunately, the identification of these side effects tempered the rampant application of this technique. Meanwhile, fundamental knowledge about the use of spinal opioids was obtained through extensive animal studies (Yaksh 1981; Yaksh and Noueihed 1985). The term *spinal opioid* as applied in this section is used to describe intrathecal, epidural, and intracerebroventricular administration of opioids.

The pharmacokinetics of epidurally administered morphine applied in the lumbar epidural space has been studied. After epidural injection of morphine, only low concentrations of lipid-soluble, un-ionized drug are present in the epidural space. Movement of the drug into the cerebrospinal fluid (CSF) by diffusion across the dura mater and transfer across the arachnoid granulation, as well as vascular uptake by spinal arteries and the epidural venous system, regulate the distribution of epidural morphine (Figure 9–11). Because only small concentrations of the morphine present in the CSF are un-ionized, the transfer across the spinal cord to the dorsal horn receptors is slow. Morphine is also available to move upward with the flow of CSF toward the brain. This explanation of epidural morphine distribution correlates well with the delayed onset of analgesia and the late respiratory depression seen.

Much of the existing concern about the use of spinal opioids has focused on concern for respiratory depression. This can be early (associated with the peak blood levels after epidural administration) or late (perhaps due to the rostral migration of morphine into sensitive respiratory centers). Outcome studies (Rawal et al. 1987) generated from large groups of patients in Sweden who

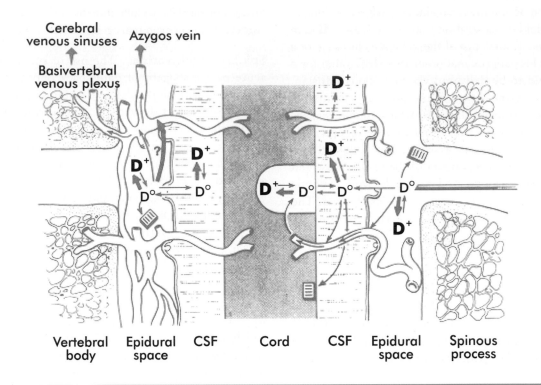

FIGURE 9–11. Pharmacokinetic model of an epidural injection of a hydrophilic opioid such as morphine. An epidural needle is shown delivering drug to the epidural space. The role of absorption by way of the radicular arteries remains speculative. The *shaded squares* represent nonspecific binding sites. D^0=un-ionized, lipophilic drug; D^+=ionized hydrophilic drug; CSF=cerebrospinal fluid.

Source. Reprinted from Cousins MJ, Bridenbaugh PO (eds.): *Neural Blockade in Clinical Anesthesia and Management of Pain,* 2nd Edition. Philadelphia, PA, JB Lippincott, 1988, p. 987. Used with permission.

received spinal opioids indicate that the incidence of severe delayed respiratory depression after epidural morphine administration is approximately 1/1,000 patients. Although certain demographic characteristics of at-risk populations have been identified, the inability to predict the occurrence of delayed respiratory depression in healthy patients points out the need for increased surveillance of all patients who are receiving opioid analgesia.

The spinal administration of opioids is appropriate for pain in virtually any region of the body. Spinally administered morphine has been shown to migrate over the entire distance of the spinal cord, even when injected in the lumbar epidural space (Gourlay et al. 1985, 1987). Pain relief from such spinal opioid systems has been demonstrated for pain in cervical dermatomes and even in the trigeminal system.

Multiple endogenous chemicals, which are thought to modulate nociceptive processing, have been identified in the region of the dorsal horn of the spinal cord. The clinical success of opioids in providing selective spinal analgesia has prompted the evaluation of analgesic agents other than morphine. Clonidine and baclofen have also been approved by the U.S. Food and Drug Administration for intraspinal administration. Clonidine is an adrenergic agonist

that can also be administered orally but appears to have selective benefits for certain patients when administered intrathecally, especially when coadministered with opioids. Baclofen is usually reserved for treatment of spinal injury muscle paroxysm. As further research and development of intraspinal medications is encouraged, the release of newer agents—including the selective N-type calcium channel blocker ziconotide—is likely. Intrathecal administration of multiple agents may be helpful where there is minimal or no response to one agent alone (Krames 2000).

In caring for such patients from a psychiatric perspective, it is important that they have a realistic understanding of the procedure planned and the degree of pain relief expected, and that they have strong psychological support for coping with the difficulties of the surgical procedure and any complications that may occur, as well as the possibility that pain relief may be incomplete following such an intervention.

Caveats in the Conversion of Opioids

In the conversion from one opioid form to another, several principles are germane. First, opioid conversion tables are designed based on the principle of single-dose administration. Consideration therefore must be given to the duration of the drug, and the quantity changed appropriately. For example, if a patient is receiving fentanyl PCA at 100 μg/h, that patient may use 2,400 μg within a 24-hour period. For conversion to methadone, what would an appropriate dose be? The half-life of fentanyl is 1 hour, whereas that of methadone is 12 hours. Therefore, the total initial dose of methadone for such a patient in a 24-hour period might be 10 mg bid. This would be accompanied by some short-acting medication, perhaps morphine soluble tablets on an as-needed basis, and the dosage would be adjusted over the subsequent days. Secondly, the exact conversion ratio may differ with the individual and with the previous history of opioid exposure. These are therefore general guidelines only. Pereira and colleagues (2001) performed a systematic search of published literature from 1966 to 1999 to critically appraise the emerging evidence on equianalgesic dose ratios derived from studies of chronic opioid administration. There were six major findings: 1) a paucity of data exists in long-term dosing studies, and they are heterogeneous in nature; 2) the ratios exhibit extremely wide ranges; 3) methadone is more potent than previously appreciated; 4) ratios related to methadone are highly correlated with the dose of the previous opioid; and 5) the ratio may change according to the direction of the opioid switch. In summary, satisfactory analgesia with oral dosing can be obtained if attention is focused on the pharmacokinetics of the particular opioid to be administered, the oral bioavailability of the drug, and a close titration of the drug to achieve adequate analgesia in each patient.

NONPHARMACOLOGICAL TREATMENTS

COGNITIVE-BEHAVIORAL TREATMENT

Cognitive-behavioral therapy (CBT) has been shown to enhance the prevention of long-term disability for chronic pain sufferers (Linton et al. 2005). In a meta-analysis, when CBT was compared to a heterogeneous collection of alternative treatments, it was found to be superior in reducing pain experience, increasing positive cognitive coping and appraisal, and reducing behavioral expression of pain (A.C. Butler et al. 2006).

CBT has a number of objectives. The first is to help patients change their view of their problem from overwhelming to manageable. Patients who are prone to catastrophize benefit from examining the way in which they view their situation. What has been perceived as a hopeless condition can be reframed as a difficult yet manageable one over which the patient can exercise some control.

The second objective is to convince patients that their treatment is relevant to their problem and that they must be actively involved both in that treatment and in their rehabilitation. They need to understand how relaxation training, cognitive restructuring, adaptive coping skills, and pacing behaviors can help decrease their pain. Patients must reorient their view away from that of passive victim to that of proactive, competent problem solver. When individuals are successful in managing painful episodes, their views change. They eventually begin to believe themselves capable of overcoming any acute flare-up of pain.

The third objective is to teach patients to monitor maladaptive thoughts and substitute positive thoughts. Persons with chronic pain are plagued, either consciously or unconsciously, by negative thoughts related to their condition. These negative thoughts have a way of perpetuating pain behaviors and feelings of hopelessness. Learning how and when to attack these negative thoughts and to substitute positive thoughts and adaptive management techniques is an important component of cognitive restructuring. Patients must be encouraged to attribute success to their own efforts; they need to feel that they are responsible for the gains they make. Finally, problems and lapses need to be discussed so that the patient will have an advance "game plan" to manage short-term setbacks.

STRESS MANAGEMENT/ RELAXATION TRAINING/ GUIDED IMAGERY

The psychological component of stress can include worrying, racing thoughts, anticipation, fear, obsessive planning, depression, and anxiety, as well as excessive cognitive rehearsal of expectations, evaluation of self and others involved in the life event, assessment of potential outcomes from the event, and assessment of the importance of the event (in either a positive or a negative sense) in our lives. The physical components of stress can include physiological arousal, sleep disturbance, fatigue, gastrointestinal disturbances, headaches, concentration problems, increased expression of irritability and anger, agitation, increased likelihood for illness, and reduced productivity. The impact and the expression of these stress symptoms vary with the individual and the stressful event. The psychological and physical components of stress interact and react with one another to produce additional stress. Direct evidence for the claim that psychological therapies may have a role to play in pediatric chronic pain management is provided in a number of review articles. Holden and colleagues (1999) reviewed 31 studies of treatments for children with chronic headache and found good evidence for the efficacy of relaxation and self-hypnosis in reducing pain.

Few effective treatments are available for children with recurrent abdominal pain. Relaxation and guided imagery have been shown to affect the autonomic nervous system, which tends to be altered in patients with functional gastrointestinal disorders. A pilot study (Ball et al. 2003) showed that 10 children who had previously had abdominal pain refractory to conventional treatment experienced a 67% decrease in pain during the therapy.

BIOFEEDBACK TRAINING

Biobehavioral biofeedback is a way to teach muscle relaxation. This technique helps people identify and regulate physiological factors that contribute to pain. Relaxation training lowers the response level, reduces symptoms, and minimizes the physical impact of stress. Electromyogram (EMG) training uses an EMG machine to monitor muscle tension. After specific muscles are identified as overly tense, electrodes are taped over them during EMG training to record function. This information immediately shows on a computer screen how the muscle responds to training. The techniques are practiced at home between sessions.

In their review of pediatric migraine, Hermann and Blanchard (1995) employed data-pooling techniques and found biofeedback and muscle relaxation to be more efficacious than placebo treatments and prophylactic drug treatments in controlling headache. A meta-analytic review of adult studies concluded that thermal biofeedback, in combination with relaxation training, was as efficacious as a commonly used daily prophylactic medication like propranolol (Holroyd and Penzien 1990). Morley and colleagues (1999) reviewed 25 articles on both adult and child literature and reported effect sizes for biofeedback to be around 0.70, suggesting that this is a promising intervention for chronic pain.

SLEEP EDUCATION

Insomnia and depression are common problems for people with chronic pain, and previous research found that each is correlated with measures of pain and disability. More recent studies concluded that patients with chronic pain and concurrent major depression and insomnia report the highest levels of pain-related impairment, but insomnia in the absence of major depression is also significantly associated with increased pain and distress (Wilson et al. 2002).

The pain management team helps people with insomnia make lifestyle adjustments to improve sleep. Sleep is critically important to health because it allows the body time to heal, replenishes the immune system, and invigorates the body and mind. Pain and insomnia negatively affect each other. As a person gets less sleep (or poor-

quality sleep), pain worsens; as pain worsens, sleep disturbances become more likely.

During the treatment phase, helpful recommendations are explored with the client. Some suggestions to improve sleep might include developing a consistent sleep schedule all seven days of the week; using imagery/relaxation strategies prior to bedtime; limiting intake of caffeine, salt, and nicotine; and not reading or watching TV in bed. Behavioral treatments of sleep difficulties that have been shown to have efficacy in treating children include fading and response cost. These easily incorporated changes often produce improvement in pain levels.

PARENTING TRAINING

With pediatric pain patients, parent training is one of the most important treatment approaches for pain management. Parent training is a particularly important strategy when working with pediatric chronic pain patients. Within a behavioral framework, a parental solicitous response style could be considered a reinforcing consequence of a pain behavior, thus serving to maintain or increase the likelihood of the behavior occurring. Support for this model could provide a foundation for contingency-based interventions within the family system for children with recurrent pain (B.A. Wall et al. 1997). More solicitous or encouraging responses from parents toward their children's pain or illness behaviors have been found to increase sick-role behaviors in children with recurrent and chronic pain (Gidron et al. 1995; Whitehead 1994). Greater parental reinforcement of children's pain was also associated with greater functional disability, independent of stress and pain severity (Gidron et al. 1995).

The bidirectional correlation between parenting and child factors should be considered. Walker and Greene (1989) noted that some children were more likely to be susceptible to developing chronic, potentially disabling responses to their recurrent pain than others because of underlying psychological characteristics, and children may respond differentially to parental reinforcement of their pain due to such characteristics. Walker later found that both positive consequences (e.g., positive attention, fewer chores) and negative consequences of pain (e.g., parent frustration) were associated with maintenance of somatization symptoms in children with recurrent abdominal pain, although this was moderated by the child's self-worth; that is, the relation of consequences of pain, both positive and negative, to more somatization was stronger for children with lower perceived self-worth (Walker et al. 2002).

DECREASING SECONDARY REINFORCEMENTS

Secondary gain is a major problem with chronic pain. The term refers to the secondary reinforcements that accompany a primary loss involving physical function, ability to work, ability to engage in sexual activity, or other concomitants of injury and illness. A pain syndrome can set off a downward social spiral in which a patient loses the ordinary reinforcement that comes from contact with colleagues at work and the self-esteem that comes from being productive. Increasing depression can result in a loss of energy and an inability to interact rewardingly with others, leading to social withdrawal. Social contact becomes increasingly organized around pain complaints. Patients who seem to lose the ability to elicit enjoyable and rewarding social interactions increasingly coerce attention from health care providers, family members, and friends over their disabilities, a process that contributes part of the secondary gain. Additional secondary gain may come in the form of being able to avoid unwanted responsibilities, such as the pressures of work, or unwelcome aspects of social interaction, such as sexual activity.

Another major form of secondary gain is financial reinforcement. Disability systems frequently intensify this form of secondary gain by creating an adversarial system in which any evidence of the patient's ability to return to normal function endangers financial support—a system that in essence requires complete disability. Thus, disability systems designed to provide a reasonable level of financial support for persons who have physical and psychiatric illness have become rather rigid and end up providing financial reinforcement for continued disability. In such an adversarial system, efforts at rehabilitation are used as evidence that there was never any serious disability in the first place. Furthermore, attaining disability status is often a protracted and unpleasant process. During a consolidation phase after an acute injury when patients might be able to return to some level of functioning despite continuing symptoms, they are instead engaged in a battle to prove the extent of their disability. Any improvement results in the reduction or elimination of disability payments.

Many patients are victims of this system. Others manipulate it, exaggerating their disability to obtain financial benefits, further reinforcing the system's adversarial nature. On the other hand, many more patients are accused of such exaggeration than actually commit it—in part because it is extremely difficult to communicate pain complaints in a rational and believable manner to others. Pain, after all, is not directly observable. It can only be interpreted through the reports, both verbal and nonverbal, of the patient. In their own desire to control their pain, patients tend to either overmodulate or undermodulate it. At times they seem perfectly composed and comfortable when in fact they are suffering; at other times they seem histrionic and disruptive and appear to be exaggerating the extent of their discomfort.

Secondary-gain factors, both social and financial, substantially complicate treatment, and it is best to do everything possible to minimize them. Useful social strategies include the behavior therapy principle of requesting health care personnel and family members to provide attention and positive reinforcement for non-pain-related behaviors (Fordyce et al. 1973) while diminishing reinforcement for pain-related interactions. For example, a nurse would be encouraged to walk up to a patient and say, "How nice to see you walking around," and to engage him or her in other conversation when the patient does in fact walk, but to minimize social contact when responding to a demand for more pain medication.

Many chronic pain patients seek multiple surgeries and other procedures in a vain hope of returning themselves to a preinjury, pain-free state. It is often important to help them change their goals from this all-or-none type of thinking to a more realistic goal of substantial pain reduction and improved function. This often involves helping them to accept the damage done to their lives by the injury or illness and to think more in terms of rehabilitation than restitution.

Interactions with the legal system can be handled by advising patients to discuss with their attorney the ways to obtain the largest lump-sum settlement possible as quickly as possible to prevent losing years in an emotionally and physically depleting struggle to prove how damaged they really are. Direct contact with attorneys (after a patient's permission has been obtained) is also a good way to reinforce the urgency of settling the complaint before the situation deteriorates further.

ELECTRICAL STIMULATION

Electrical stimulation seems to have found a place in pain management by exciting intrinsic mechanisms used for the modulation of nociceptive information. The prediction that large-fiber activity could block certain noxious information at the level of the dorsal horn resulted in the introduction of transcutaneous electrical nerve stimulation (TENS). Clinical utility of TENS has yet to be established for individual pain syndromes. Dorsal column stimulation (DCS) excites descending inhibitory pathways with electricity to provide analgesia. The success of DCS has been mixed, but it may have a place in certain deafferentation pain syndromes. The success of central morphine microinjection techniques to provide analgesia may have prompted Reynolds (1969) to demonstrate similar results in animals by electrical stimulation of the periaqueductal gray matter. Hosobuchi subsequently demonstrated naloxone-reversible analgesia in humans after implantation of brain stem electrodes (Bonica and Ventafridda 1979). Each of these applications of electrical stimulation was predicted on the basis of improved understanding of the pain pathway.

TENS, DCS, and spinal cord stimulation (SCS) are further discussed below.

Transcutaneous Electrical Nerve Stimulation

The origin of TENS in Western medical society dates back to Roman times, when the use of electric fish was ascribed analgesic properties. Publication of the gate theory of pain by Melzack and Wall (1965) renewed interest in electrical stimulation to produce analgesia. The excitation of large-fiber peripheral afferents by electrical stimulation at the periphery has been successful in treating nociceptive pain. TENS is a low-intensity stimulation, stimulating skin and muscle afferents in a specific segmental distribution. Numerous studies have documented the efficacy of TENS in certain pathological pain states. In addition, when used as an adjunct for postoperative analgesia, TENS has been shown to decrease the amount of opioid analgesia required.

Dorsal Column Stimulation

Many patients with deafferentation pain are candidates for dorsal column stimulation. This technique uses percutaneously positioned electrical leads that deliver a high-frequency current over the dorsal spinal cord in an effort to stimulate descending analgesic pathways. Effective electrical stimulation suggests that implantation of a self-contained battery-powered device may be efficacious in selected patients. There have been no prospective trials of this therapy in the management of neuropathic terminal cancer pain, but the responses achieved with other deafferentation pain syndromes point to possible efficacy in this difficult problem.

Spinal Cord Stimulation

Spinal cord stimulation is used for refractory neuropathic pain syndromes. It involves the insertion of a small electrode in the epidural space at the level of the perceived pain. The electrode is then stimulated with an electrical current. Usually a temporary trial is first performed, and if that is successful, a permanent lead is placed, accompanied by a battery-powered generator placed subcutaneously. Complications of the procedure include dural puncture and spinal headache, bleeding, infection, and displacement of leads leading to suboptimal pain control. SCS can provide significant pain relief for patients with complex regional pain syndromes (Kemler et al. 2000).

ACUPUNCTURE

The use of acupuncture in the treatment of painful conditions has seen increasing popularity in the last decade. Many studies are emerging that support the use of acupuncture for a variety of painful conditions such as headache and neck and back pain, while some negative studies are found as well (Coeytaux et al. 2005). Acupuncture involves the placement of needles at various locations in the body to stimulate a rebalancing of the body's own energy, called *chi*, for the purpose of eliciting a therapeutic response. Sometimes that results in decreased pain, although other applications have been found as well, such as decreased anxiety (Wang et al. 2001) and decreased depression. Some of the mechanisms of acupuncture analgesia have been elucidated. At low-frequency stimulation, acupuncture stimulates the production of endorphins, while high-frequency stimulation stimulates dynorphins (Han 2003). Much recent research in acupuncture has focused on the use of fMRI to explore changes in brain blood flow in response to needling of specific points on the body (Lewith et al. 2005). This is a promising area of research for increased understanding of some of the elusive mechanisms of action of acupuncture. In the treatment of painful conditions, acupuncture has been shown to be beneficial in cancer pain, osteoarthritis, neck and back pain, headache, dysmenorrhea, and tennis elbow, to name a few.

NEURAL BLOCKADE

Patients who exhaust the analgesics or who develop toxicity problems from other medications may benefit from techniques of neurolytic blockade. The most common approach is to proceed from the least invasive to the more invasive techniques, as required for pain management. In one major study undertaken in a comprehensive cancer care center, only 20% of patients required treatment with neurolytic blocks or other neurodestructive techniques (Ventafridda et al. 1987). The continued advancement of spinal opioid techniques, as well as the success of continuous subcutaneous opioid infusions, will probably continue to decrease the need for neurodestructive techniques. In cancer pain, local anesthetics may be used for diagnostic, prognostic, and therapeutic blocks.

Diagnostic blocks are used to localize the pain pathway and to pharmacologically differentiate the fiber type involved in mediating the pain. It is difficult to be certain that only a specific fiber type will be blocked by using differing concentrations of local anesthetics. Therefore, many pain clinicians prefer to use blockade at sites where the fibers are anatomically separated (e.g., lumbar sympathetic block and individual somatic nerve blocks). The interpretation of diagnostic neural blockade is both difficult and crucial to the appropriate use of these techniques. This interpretation is discussed in detail by Boas and Cousins (1988).

Prognostic blockades should always be carried out at least twice before neurolytic or surgical ablation. This permits confirmation that the pain is relieved and also gives the patient an opportunity to decide whether any side effects are acceptable.

Therapeutic blocks with local anesthetic cannot be expected to relieve pain permanently. However, pain may be due to muscle spasms, postoperative neuralgia, denervation phenomena, or neuroma formation. In some of these cases, a series of long-acting local anesthetic blocks will produce long-lasting or permanent pain relief.

NEURODESTRUCTIVE PROCEDURES

Continued progress in pain management with multidisciplinary therapies has decreased the use of neurodestructive procedures. Despite the continued success of less invasive and nondestructive techniques, however, neurolytic blockade still provides valuable adjunctive treatment of nociceptive and neuropathic pain in terminal cancer (Cousins 1988). Often, a properly performed neurodestructive procedure can markedly decrease medication use and control the unwanted side effects associated with high doses of analgesics. Virtually all neurodestructive techniques should be confined to the treatment of nociceptive pain. Not only are the CNS and peripheral changes associated with neuropathic pain never relieved by neurodestructive techniques, they are often aggravated by such procedures. Neurolytic blocks are mainly indicated for localized unilateral pain, except for pituitary ablation, which is suitable for diffuse areas of pain.

HYPNOSIS

Central psychological approaches to pain control can also be effective and are underutilized (Holroyd 1996). It has been known since the nineteenth century that hypnosis is effective in controlling even severe surgical pain (Esdaile 1846/1957). Hypnosis and similar techniques work through two primary mechanisms: peripheral muscle relaxation and a central combination of perceptual alteration and cognitive distraction. Pain is not infrequently accompanied by reactive muscle tension. Patients frequently splint the part of their body that hurts. Yet because muscle tension can by itself cause pain in normal tissue, and because traction on a painful part of the body can produce more pain, techniques that induce greater physical relaxation can reduce pain in the periphery. Therefore, having patients enter a state of hypnosis so they can concentrate on an image connoting physical relaxation, such as floating or lightness, often produces physical relaxation and reduces pain.

The second major component of hypnotic analgesia is perceptual alteration. Patients can be taught to imagine that the affected body part is warm or cool, tingling, light, or numb. This is especially useful for extremely hypnotizable individuals who can, for example, relive an experience of dental anesthesia and reproduce the drug-induced sensations of numbness in their cheek, which they can then transfer to the painful part of their body. They can also simply switch off perception of the pain with surprising effectiveness (Hargadon et al. 1995; Miller and Bowers 1993). Temperature metaphors are often especially useful, which is not surprising, given that pain and temperature sensations are part of the same sensory system. Thus, imagining that an affected body part is cooler or warmer (through an image of dipping it in ice water or heating it in the sun) can often help transform pain signals. Some patients prefer to imagine that the pain is a substance with dimensions that can be moved or that it can flow out of the body as if it were a viscous liquid. Others like to imagine that they can step outside their body—for example, to visit another room in the house. Less hypnotizable individuals often do better with distraction techniques that help them focus on competing sensations in another part of the body.

Hypnotic techniques can easily be taught to patients for self-administration (H. Spiegel and Spiegel 2004). Pain patients can be taught to enter a state of self-hypnosis in a matter of seconds with some simple induction strategies such as looking up while slowly closing their eyes; taking a deep breath and then letting the breath out; relaxing the eyes; imagining the body floating; and letting one hand float up in the air like a balloon. The patients are then instructed in the pain control exercise and are taught to bring themselves out by reversing the induction procedure, again looking up, letting the eyes open, and letting the raised hand float back down. Patients can use this exercise every 1–2 hours initially and anytime they experience an attack of pain. Patients can then evaluate their effectiveness in conducting the pain control exercise by rating on a scale from 0 to 10 the intensity of their pain before and after the self-hypnosis session. As with any pain treatment technique, hypnosis is more effective when employed early in the pain cycle, before the pain has become so overwhelming that it impairs concentration. Patients should be encouraged to use this technique early and often because it is simple and effective (D. Spiegel and Bloom 1983a) and has no side effects (H. Spiegel and Spiegel 2004). Indeed, it has been shown, in several randomized trials in interventional radiology, to produce better analgesia than that resulting from PCA with midazolam and fentanyl, with less anxiety, fewer side effects, and fewer procedural interruptions (Lang and Hamilton 1994; Lang et al. 1996). A large randomized trial demonstrated that patients taught self-hypnosis used half as much patient-controlled analgesic medication and had less pain and anxiety and fewer episodes of autonomic instability. In addition, the technique resulted in shortening procedure time by 18 minutes (Lang et al. 2000). Thus, hypnosis not only is an effective analgesic but can result in a shorter intervention with fewer procedural complications and be cost-effective as well (Lang and Rosen 2002).

Although not all patients are sufficiently hypnotizable to benefit from these techniques, two out of three adults are at least somewhat hypnotizable (H. Spiegel and Spiegel 2004), and it has been estimated that hypnotic capacity is correlated at a level of 0.5 with effectiveness in medical pain reduction. Highly hypnotizable individuals can use hypnosis as analgesia for surgery (Levitan and Harbaugh 1992), but clinically effective hypnotic analgesia is not confined to those with high hypnotizability (Holroyd 1996).

Hypnosis is especially effective in comforting children who are in pain (Kuttner et al. 1988), especially since they tend to be more hypnotizable than adults (H. Spiegel and Spiegel 2004). Several well-designed randomized, controlled studies have shown greater efficacy for hypnosis than for placebo attention control (Ellis and Spanos 1994; Hilgard and LeBaron 1982; Kellerman et al. 1983; Zeltzer and LeBaron 1982). This is probably due to the fact that children as a group are more hypnotizable than adults (Morgan and Hilgard 1973). Their imaginative capacities are so intense that separate relaxation exercises are not necessary. Children naturally relax when they mobilize their imagination during the sensory alteration component of hypnotic analgesia (Niven 1996). The use of hypnosis during a painful medical procedure, a voiding cystourethrogram, has been shown in a randomized trial to reduce pain, distress, and the length of the procedure by 14 minutes (L.D. Butler et al. 2005).

Other research indicates cortical effects of hypnotic alteration of perceptions, including reduced event-related potential (ERP) amplitude in response to somatosensory (Spiegel et al. 1989) and visual (Jasiukaitis et al. 1996) stimuli, and increased frontal and parietal blood flow (Crawford et al. 1993). Subjects who underwent hypnotic instruction that a painful stimulus will be less painful showed deactivation of anterior cingulate gyrus and reduced activity of somatosensory cortex demonstrated by positron emission tomography (PET) (Faymonville et al. 2000; Rainville et al. 1997). There is also PET evidence of alteration in activation of primary sensory cortex in the

visual system (color vision) in response to hypnotic modulation of perception (Kosslyn et al. 2000). Thus, hypnotic alteration of nociception seems to involve cortical modulation of attentional, affective, and somatosensory processes that directly affect pain perception.

CONCLUSION

The reality of pain is an inescapable consequence of our human condition. However, the experience of severe unrelenting pain related to various medical conditions can certainly be mitigated, and its treatment is a responsibility of all physicians. As we continue to enrich the knowledge base from which we understand the causes, transmission, and processing of pain signals, we can develop a more comprehensive and effective strategy that combines various approaches.

From the physiological viewpoint, we can work to remove the cause of pain at the periphery, perhaps with surgery. Inflammation can be reduced with anti-inflammatory agents. Muscle tension in accessory muscles can be reduced using physical therapy and nonmedical interventions. Pain transmission can be blocked through the use of local anesthetics, competitive electrical stimulation, or acupuncture. Opioids may be used orally, intravenously, or via spinal administration to decrease the intensity of transmission through activity in the spinal cord, as well as decrease the perception of pain in the central nervous system.

From the psychological viewpoint, it is important to address the significant personal, psychological, and social consequences of the pain. Comorbid depression and anxiety must be treated with appropriate antidepressant or other psychoactive medication and appropriate psychotherapy. Cognitive interventions such as hypnosis can help patients to reduce their focus on the pain and ameliorate their physiological response to it.

The old dichotomy between peripheral and central pain is being replaced by a more complex and interactive analysis—one that evaluates the central and the peripheral components of pain and designs interventions, taking advantage of therapeutic opportunities at all levels of pain perception processing. This point of view is important because it underscores that successful psychosocial interventions for reducing pain may occur via understandable neurological mechanisms, and that the success of these interventions does not prove that the pain is largely functional. In the same way, successful pharmacological intervention does not prove that the pain is completely peripheral in origin. Most pain syndromes are a combination of physical and neuropsychiatric distress and dysfunction and require a combination of biological and psychosocial intervention for optimally effective treatment. Although these interventions may not succeed in entirely eliminating the painful symptoms, they can offer patients great relief and significantly decrease the degree of suffering they experience.

Highlights for the Clinician

✦ The physiological and neurological bases of chronic pain are outlined.

✦ The mechanisms of the interrelationship between chronic pain and depression are described.

✦ A multidisciplinary method of treating severe chronic pain, using various modalities, is endorsed:

Pharmaceutical measures
- Tricyclic antidepressants
- Selective serotonin reuptake inhibitors
- Nonsteroidal agents
- Opioids
- Sodium channel blockers
- Anticonvulsants

Nonpharmaceutical interventions
- Psychotherapy
- Hypnosis
- Biofeedback
- Acupuncture
- Physical therapy
- Massage
- Diagnostic and therapeutic nerve blocks
- Implantation of intrathecal pumps and spinal cord stimulators

✦ Wherever possible, several of these therapies should be integrated as necessary to assist the patient in maximizing level of functioning while minimizing the painful experience.

✦ Care needs to be taken to ensure that all necessary diagnostic and therapeutic options have been pursued for the specific problem and an exact diagnostic is established.

✦ Pain and mood disorders co-occur, and therefore the treatment of pain from a neuropsychiatric point of view must include appropriate treatment of depression and anxiety.

RECOMMENDED READINGS

Bodnar RJ, Klein GE: Endogenous opiates and behavior: 2005. Peptides (2006), doi:10.1016/j.peptides.2006.07.011, 2006

Borsook D, Becerra LR: Breaking down the barriers: fMRI applications in pain, analgesia and analgesics. Mol Pain 2:30, 2006. Available at: http://www.molecular-pain.com.

Butler AC, Chapman JE, Forman EM, et al: The empirical status of cognitive-behavioral therapy: a review of meta-analyses. Clin Psychol Rev 26:17–31, 2006

Casey KL, Lorenz J, Minoshima S: Insights into the pathophysiology of neuropathic pain through functional brain imaging. Exp Neurol 184 (suppl 1):S80–S88, 2003

Fishbain DA, Cutler R, Rosomoff HL, et al: Do antidepressants have an analgesic effect in psychogenic pain and somatoform pain disorder? A meta-analysis. Psychosom Med 60:503–509, 1998

Melzack R: From the gate to the neuromatrix. Pain (suppl 6):S121–S126, 1999

Posner MI, Petersen SE: The attention system of the human brain. Annu Rev Neurosci 13:125–142, 1990

Price DD: Psychological and neural mechanisms of the affective dimension of pain. Science 288:1769–1772, 2000

Price DD, Zhou QQ, Moshiree B, et al: Peripheral and central contributions to hyperalgesia in irritable bowel syndrome. J Pain 7:529–535, 2006

Spiegel H, Spiegel D: Trance and Treatment: Clinical Uses of Hypnosis. Washington, DC, American Psychiatric Press, 2004

Wilson KG, Eriksson MY, D'Eon JL, et al: Major depression and insomnia in chronic pain. Clin J Pain 18 (suppl 2):77–83, 2002

REFERENCES

Ahles TA, Blanchard EB, Ruckdeschel JC: Multidimensional nature of cancer-related pain. Pain 17:277–288, 1983

Arnold LM, Hess EV, Hudson JI, et al: A randomized, placebo-controlled, double-blind, flexible-dose study of fluoxetine in the treatment of women with fibromyalgia. Am J Med 112:191–197, 2002

Arnow BA, Hart S, Scott C, et al: Childhood sexual abuse, psychological distress, and medical use among women. Psychosom Med 61:762–770, 1999

Astin JA: Why patients use alternative medicine: results of a national study. JAMA 279:1548–1552, 1998

Atkison JH, Kremer EF, Garfin SR: Current concepts review: psychopharmacologic agents in the treatment of pain. J Bone Joint Surg Am 67:337–339, 1985

Atweh SF, Kuhar MJ: Autoradiographic localization of opiate receptors in rat brain, I: spinal cord and lower medulla. Brain Res 124:53–67, 1977

Austin KL, Stapleton JV, Mather LE: Multiple intramuscular injections: a major source of variability in analgesic response to pethidine. Pain 8:4–19, 1980

Ball TM, Shapiro DE, Monheim CJ, et al: A pilot study of the use of guided imagery for the treatment of recurrent abdominal pain in children. Clin Pediatr 42 (suppl 6):527–532, 2003

Basbaum AI: Functional analysis of the cytochemistry of the spinal dorsal horn, in Advances in Pain Research and Therapy, Vol 9. Edited by Fields HL, Dubner R, Cervero F. New York, Raven, 1985, pp 149–171

Beaver WT, Feise G: Comparison of the analgesic effects of morphine, hydroxyzine, and their combination in patients with postoperative pain, in Advances in Pain Research and Therapy, Vol 1. Edited by Bonica JJ, Albe-Fessard DG. New York, Raven, 1976, pp 553–565

Beecher HK: Relationship of significance of wound to pain experienced. JAMA 161:1609–1616, 1956

Berkley KJ, Palmer R: Somatosensory cortical involvement in response to noxious stimulation in the cat. Exp Brain Res 20:363–374, 1974

Besson JM, Chaouch A: Peripheral and spinal mechanisms of nociception. Physiol Rev 67:67–186, 1987

Blumer D, Heilbronn M: Chronic pains as a variant of depressive disease: the pain prone disorder. J Nerv Ment Dis 170:381–406, 1982

Boas RA, Cousins MJ: Diagnostic neural blockade, in Neural Blockade in Clinical Anesthesia, 2nd Edition. Edited by Cousins MJ, Bridenbaugh PO. Philadelphia, PA, JB Lippincott, 1988

Bond MR: Personality studies in patients with pain secondary to organic disease. J Psychosom Res 17:257–263, 1973

Bond MR, Pearson IB: Psychological aspects of pain in women with advanced cancer of the cervix. J Psychosom Res 13:13–19, 1969

Bonica JJ, Ventafridda V: Advances in Pain Research and Therapy: International Symposium on Pain of Advanced Cancer. New York, Raven, 1979

Borsook D, Becerra LR: Breaking down the barriers: fMRI applications in pain, analgesia and analgesics. Mol Pain 2:30, 2006. Available at: http://www.molecularpain.com.

Boyer WF: Potential indications for the selective serotonin reuptake inhibitors. Int Clin Psychopharmacol 6 (suppl 5):5–12, 1992

Brookoff D. Chronic pain: a new disease? Hosp Pract (Off Ed) 35 (suppl 7):45–52, 2000

Bruera E, Brenneis C, Michaud M, et al: Patient controlled subcutaneous hydromorphone versus continuous subcutaneous infusion for the treatment of cancer pain. J Natl Cancer Inst 80:1152–1154, 1988a

Bruera E, Brenneis C, Michaud M, et al: Use of subcutaneous route for the administration of narcotics in patients with cancer pain. Cancer 62:407–411, 1988b

Butler AC, Chapman JE, Forman EM, et al: The empirical status of cognitive-behavioral therapy: a review of meta-analyses. Clin Psychol Rev 26:17–31, 2006

Butler L, Koopman C, Cordova M, et al: Psychological distress and pain significantly increase before death in metastatic breast cancer patients. Psychosom Med 65:416–426, 2003

Butler LD, Duran EFD, Jasiukatis P, et al: Hypnotizability and traumatic experience: a diathesis-stress model of dissociative symptomatology. Am J Psychiatry 153:42–63,1996

Butler LD, Symons BK, Henderson SL, et al: Hypnosis reduces distress and duration of an invasive medical procedure for children. Pediatrics 115:77–85, 2005

Calvillo O, Henry JL, Newman RS: Effects of morphine and naloxone on dorsal horn neurons in the cat. Can J Physiol Pharmacol 52:1207–1211, 1974

Campo JV, Perel J, Lucas A, et al: Citalopram treatment of pediatric recurrent abdominal pain and comorbid internalizing disorders: an exploratory study. J Am Acad Child Adolesc Psychiatry 43:1234–1242, 2004

Carter GT, Sullivan MD: Antidepressants in pain management. Curr Opin Investig Drugs 3:454–458, 2002

Casey KL, Lorenz J, Minoshima S: Insights into the pathophysiology of neuropathic pain through functional brain imaging. Exp Neurol 184 (suppl 1):S80–S88, 2003

Coeytaux RR, Kaufman JS, Kaptchuk TJ, et al: A randomized, controlled trial of acupuncture for chronic daily headache. Headache 45:1113–1123, 2005

Cousins MJ: Chronic pain and neurolytic blockade, in Neural Blockade in Clinical Anesthesia and Management of Pain, 2nd Edition. Edited by Cousins MJ, Bridenbaugh PO. Philadelphia, PA, JB Lippincott, 1988, pp 1053–1084

Crawford HJ, Gur RC, Skolnick B, et al: Effects of hypnosis on regional cerebral blood flow during ischemic pain with and without suggested hypnotic analgesia. Int J Psychophysiol 3:181–195, 1993

Crile GW: Phylogenetic association in relation to certain medical problems. Boston Medical and Surgical Journal 163:893, 1910

Cushing H: On the avoidance of shock in major amputations by cocainization of large nerve-trunks preliminary to their division. Ann Surg 36:321–345, 1902

Dahlquist LM: Pediatric Pain Management. New York, Plenum, 1999

Dejard A, Peterson P, Kestrup J: Mexiletine for the treatment of chronic painful diabetic neuropathy. Lancet 1:9–11, 1988

Derogatis LR, Morrow GR, Fetting J, et al: The prevalence of psychiatric disorders among cancer patients. JAMA 249: 751–757, 1983

Dickenson AH: Mechanisms of the analgesic actions of opiates and opioids. Br Med Bull 47:690–702, 1991

Dubner R: Specialization of nociceptive pathways: sensory discrimination, sensory modulation, and neural connectivity, in Advances in Pain Research and Therapy, Vol 9. Edited by Fields HL, Dubner R, Cervero F. New York, Raven, 1985, pp 111–117

Dundee JW, Love WJ, Moore J: Alterations in response to somatic pain associated with anesthesia, XV: further studies with phenothiazine derivatives and similar drugs. Br J Anaesth 35:597–610, 1963

Duric V, McCarson KE: Effects of analgesic or antidepressant drugs on pain- or stress-evoked hippocampal and spinal neurokinin-1 receptor and brain-derived neurotrophic factor gene expression in the rat. J Pharmacol Exp Ther 319:1235–1243, 2006a

Duric V, McCarson KE: Persistent pain produces stress-like alterations in hippocampal neurogenesis and gene expression. J Pain 7:544–555, 2006b

Dwight MM, Arnold LM, O'Brien H et al: An open clinical trial of venlafaxine treatment of fibromyalgia. Psychosomatics 39:14–17, 1998

Dworkin SF, Von Koroff M, LeResche L: Multiple pains and psychiatric disturbance: an epidemiologic investigation. Arch Gen Psychiatry 47:239–244, 1990

Eisenberg DM, Davis RB, Ettner SL, et al: Trends in alternative medicine use in the United States, 1990–1997: results of a follow-up national survey. JAMA 280:1569–1575, 1998

Ellis JA, Spanos NP: Cognitive-behavioral interventions for children's distress bone marrow aspirations and lumbar punctures: a critical review. J Pain Symptom Manage 9:96–108, 1994

Esdaile J: Hypnosis in Medicine and Surgery (1846). New York, Julian Press, 1957

Eysenck HJ, Eysenck BG: Manual of the Eysenck Personality Inventory. London, University of London Press, 1964

Faymonville ME, Laureys S, Degueldre C, et al: Neural mechanisms of antinociceptive effects of hypnosis. Anesthesiology 92:1257–1267, 2000

Fields HL: Pain. New York, McGraw-Hill, 1987

Fields HL, Basbaum AI: Endogenous pain control mechanisms, in Textbook of Pain. Edited by Wall PD, Melzack R. Edinburgh, UK, Churchill-Livingstone, 1984, pp 142–153

Finley PR: Selective serotonin reuptake inhibitors: pharmacologic profiles and potential therapeutic distinctions. Ann Pharmacother 28:1359–1369, 1994

Fishbain DA, Cutler R, Rosomoff HL, et al: Chronic pain-associated depression: antecedent or consequence of chronic pain? A review. Clin J Pain 13:116–137, 1997

Flor H, Braun C, Elbert T, et al: Extensive reorganization of primary somatosensory cortex in chronic back pain patients. Neurosci Lett 224:5–8, 1997

Flores C: Management of cancer pain. JAMA 291:1068 [author reply, 1068–1069], 2004

Fordyce WE, Fowler RS, Lehmann JR, et al: Operant conditioning in the treatment of chronic pain. Arch Phys Med Rehabil 54:399–408, 1973

Forrest WH, Brown BW, Brown CR, et al: Dextroamphetamine with morphine for the treatment of postoperative pain. N Engl J Med 296:712–715, 1977

Gallagher RM: Primary care and pain medicine. Med Clin North Am 83:555–583, 1999

Gamse R, Holzer P, Lembeck F: Decrease of substance P in primary afferent neurons and impairment of neurogenic plasma extravasation by capsaicin. Br J Pharmacol 68:207–213, 1980

Gidron Y, McGrath PJ, Goodday R: The physical and psychosocial predictors of adolescents' recovery from oral surgery. J Behav Med 18:385–399, 1995

Goldstein DJ, Lu Y, Detke MJ, et al: Duloxetine in the treatment of depression: a double-blind placebo-controlled comparison with paroxetine. J Clin Psychopharmacol 24:389–399, 2004

Gourlay GK, Cherry DA, Cousins MJ: Cephalad migration of morphine in CSF following lumbar epidural administration in patients with cancer pain. Pain 23:317–326, 1985

Gourlay GK, Cherry DA, Plummer JL, et al: The influence of drug polarity on the absorption of opioid drugs into the CSF and subsequent cephalad migration following lumbar epidural administration: application to morphine and pethidine. Pain 31:297–305, 1987

Gracely RH, Petzke F, Wolf JM, et al: Functional magnetic resonance imaging evidence of augmented pain processing in fibromyalgia. Arthritis Rheum 46:1333–1343, 2002

Gray AM, Spencer PS, Sewel RD: The involvement of the opioidergic system in the antinociceptive mechanism of action of antidepressant compounds. Br J Pharmacol 124:669–674, 1998

Hagbarth KE, Kerr DIB: Central influences on spinal afferent conduction. J Neurophysiol 17:295–300, 1954

Han Ji-Sheng: Acupuncture: neuropeptide release produced by electrical stimulation of different frequencies. Trends Neurosci 26 (suppl 1):17–22, 2003

Hargadon R, Bowers KS, Woody EZ: Does counterpain imagery mediate hypnotic analgesia? J Abnorm Psychol 104:508–516, 1995

Heim C, Ehlert U, Hanker J, et al: Abuse-related posttraumatic stress disorder and alterations of the hypothalamic-pituitary-adrenal axis in women with chronic pelvic pain. Psychosom Med 60:309–318, 1998

Hermann MK, Blanchard EB: Behavioral and prophylactic pharmacological intervention studies of pediatric migraine: an exploratory meta-analysis. Pain 60:239–256, 1995

Hilgard JR, LeBaron S: Relief of anxiety and pain in children and adolescents with cancer: quantitative measures and clinical observations. Int J Clin Exp Hypn 4:417–442, 1982

Holden EW, Deichmann MM, Levy J: Empirically supported treatments in pediatric psychology: recurrent pediatric headache. J Pediatr Psychol 24:91–109, 1999

Holroyd J: Hypnosis treatment of clinical pain: understanding why hypnosis is useful. Int J Clin Exp Hypn 441:33–51, 1996

Holroyd KA, Penzien DB: Pharmacological versus non-pharmacological prophylaxis of recurrent migraine headache: a meta-analytic review of clinical trials. Pain 42:1–13, 1990

Hosobuchi Y, Adams JE, Linchitz R: Pain relief by electrical stimulation of the central gray matter in humans and its reversal by naloxone. Science 197:183–186, 1977

Jasiukaitis P, Nouriani B, Spiegel D: Left hemisphere superiority for event-related potential effects of hypnotic obstruction. Neuropsychologia 34:661–668, 1996

Juan H: Prostaglandins as modulators of pain. Gen Pharmacol 9:403–409, 1978

Katon W, Egan K, Miller D: Chronic pain: lifetime psychiatric diagnosis and family history. Am J Psychiatry 142:1156–1160, 1985

Katz N, Kosinski M, Schein J, et al: Depression and pain: the relationship between chronic low back pain, depression, and opioid therapy (abstract). J Pain 5 (suppl 1):S70, 2004

Kehlet H, Dahl JB: The value of "multimodal" or "balanced analgesia" in postoperative pain treatment. Anesth Analg 77:1048–1056, 1993

Kellerman J, Zeltzer L, Ellenberg L, et al: Adolescents with cancer: hypnosis for the reduction of the acute pain and anxiety associated with medical procedures. J Adolesc Health Care 4:35–90, 1983

Kemler MA, Barendse GA, Van Kleef M, et al: Spinal cord stimulation in patients with chronic reflex sympathetic dystrophy. N Engl J Med 343:618–624, 2000

Kiayias JA, Vlachou ED, Lakka-Papadodima E: Venlafaxine HCl in the treatment of painful peripheral diabetic neuropathy. Diabetes Care 23:699, 2000

Kishore-Kumar R, Max MB, Schafer SC, et al: Desipramine relieves postherpetic neuralgia. Clin Pharmacol Ther 47:305–312, 1990

Kosslyn SM, Thompson WL, Costantini-Ferrando MF, et al: Hypnotic visual illusion alters color processing in the brain. Am J Psychiatry 157 (suppl 8):1279–1284, 2000

Krames ES: Intraspinal analgesia for nonmalignant pain, in Interventional Pain Management. Edited by Waldman SP, Philadelphia, PA, WB Saunders, 2000, pp 609–619

Krane EJ, Leong MS, Golianu B et al: Treatment of pediatric pain with nonconventional analgesics, in Pain in Infants, Children and Adolescents, 2nd edition. Edited by Schechter NL, Berde CB, Yaster M. Philadelphia, PA, Lippincott Williams & Wilkins, 2003, pp 225–240

Kuhn CC, Bradnan WA: Pain as a substitute for fear of death. Psychosomatics 20:494–495, 1979

Kuttner L, Bowman M, Teasdale M: Psychological treatment of distress, pain, and anxiety for young children with cancer. J Dev Behav Pediatr 9:374–381, 1988

Kwan CL, Crawley AP, Mikulis DJ, et al: An fMRI study of the anterior cingulate cortex and surrounding medial wall activations evoked by noxious cutaneous heat and cold stimuli. Pain 85:359–374, 2000

Ladabaum U, Minoshima S, Owyang CP: Pathobiology of visceral pain: molecular mechanisms and therapeutic implications, V: central nervous system processing of somatic and visceral sensory signals. Am J Physiol Gastrointest Liver Physiol 279:G1–G6, 2000

Lang EV, Hamilton D: Anodyne imagery: an alternative to iv sedation in interventional radiology. AJR Am J Roentgenol 162:1221–1226, 1994

Lang EV, Rosen MP: Cost analysis of adjunct hypnosis with sedation during outpatient interventional radiologic procedures. Radiology 222:375–382, 2002

Lang EV, Joyce JS, Spiegel D, et al: Self-hypnotic relaxation during interventional radiological procedures: effects on pain perception and intravenous drug use. Int J Clin Exp Hypn 44:106–119, 1996

Lang EV, Benotsch EG, Fick LJ, et al: Adjunctive non-pharmacological analgesia for invasive medical procedures: a randomised trial. Lancet 355:1486–1490, 2000

Lansky SB, List MA, Herrmann CA, et al: Absence of major depressive disorder in female cancer patients. J Clin Oncol 3:1553–1560, 1985

Leserman J, Drossman DA, Li Z, et al: Sexual and physical abuse history in gastroenterology practice: how types of abuse impact health status. Psychosom Med 58:4–15,1996

Leserman J, Li Z, Hu YJ, et al: How multiple types of stressors impact on health. Psychosom Med 60:175–181, 1998

Levitan AA, Harbaugh TE: Hypnotizability and hypnoanalgesia: hypnotizability of patients using hypnoanalgesia during surgery. Am J Clin Hypn 34:223–226, 1992

Lewith GT, White PJ, Pariente J: Investigating acupuncture using brain imaging techniques: the current state of play. Evid Based Complement Alternat Med 2 (suppl 3):315–319, 2005

Lindstrom P, Lindblom U: The analgesic effect of tocainide in trigeminal neuralgia. Pain 28:45–50, 1987

Linton SJ, Jansson M, Svärd L, et al: The effects of cognitive-behavioral and physical therapy preventive interventions on pain-related sick leave: a randomized controlled trial. Clin J Pain 21 (suppl 2):109–119, 2005

Louis Harris Poll of Pain in the Workplace. Sponsored by Ortho-McNeil Inc, 1996

Massie MJ, Holland JC: The cancer patient with pain: psychiatric complications and their management. Cancer Pain 71:243–258, 1987

Mather LE, Gourlay GK: The biotransformation of opioids, in Opioid Agonist/Antagonist Drugs in Clinical Practice. Edited by Nimmo WS, Smith G. Amsterdam, Excerpta Medica, 1984, pp 120–133

Mayberg HS: Limbic-cortical dysregulation: a proposed model of depression. J Neuropsychiatry Clin Neurosci 9:471–481, 1997

Mayberg HS, Liotti M, Brannan SK, et al: Reciprocal limbic-cortical function and negative mood: converging PET findings in depression and normal sadness. Am J Psychiatry 156:675–682,1999

Melzack R: Recent concepts of pain. J Med 13:147–160, 1982

Melzack R: From the gate to the neuromatrix. Pain (suppl 6):S121–S126, 1999

Melzack R, Wall PD: Pain mechanisms: a new theory. Science 150:971–979, 1965

Miller ME, Bowers KS: Hypnotic analgesia: dissociated experience or dissociated control? J Abnorm Psychol 102:29–39, 1993

Moore J, Dundee JW: Alterations in response to somatic pain associated with anesthesia, V: the effect of promethazine. Br J Anaesth 33:3–8, 1961a

Moore J, Dundee JW: Alterations in response to somatic pain associated with anesthesia, VII: the effects of nine phenothiazine derivatives. Br J Anaesth 33:422–431, 1961b

Morgan AH, Hilgard ER: Age differences in susceptibility to hypnosis. Int J Clin Exp Hypn 21:78–85, 1973

Morley S, Eccleston C, Williams A: Systematic review and meta-analysis of randomized controlled trials of cognitive behavior therapy and behavior therapy for chronic pain in adults, excluding headaches. Pain 80:1–13, 1999

Müller J: Von den Ergentumlichkeiten der ein zelnen Nerve [On the identification of a nerve cell], in Handbuch der Physiologie der Menschen. Edited by Kobling L. Coblenz, Germany, Holscher, 1844

Niven N: Theoretical concepts and practical applications of hypnosis in the treatment of children and adolescents with dental fear and anxiety. Br Dent J 180:11–16, 1996

Pain Terms: A List With Definitions and Notes on Usage. International Association for the Study of Pain. Pain 6:249–252, 1979

Pain in the Workplace: A 10-Year Update of Ortho-McNeil's Survey of the Impact of Pain on the Workplace. Sponsored by Pricara unit of Ortho-McNeil, Inc., in collaboration with the National Pain Foundation, 2006

Payron R, Garcia-Larrea, Gregoire MC, et al: Parietal and cingulated processes in central pain: a combined positron emission tomography (PET) and functional magnetic resonance imaging (fMRI) study of an unusual case. Pain 84:77–87, 2000

Pereira J, Lawlor P, Vigano A, et al: Equianalgesic dose ratios for opioids: a critical review and proposals for long-term dosing. J Pain Symptom Manage 22 (suppl 2):672–687, 2001

Pert CB, Snyder SH: Opiate receptors: demonstration in nervous tissue. Science 179:1011–1014, 1973

Peteet J, Tay V, Cohen G, et al: Pain characteristics and treatment in an outpatient cancer population. Cancer 57:1259–1265, 1986

Pilowski I, Chapman CR, Bonica JJ: Pain, depression and illness behavior in a pain clinic population. Pain 4:183–192, 1977

Portenoy RK, Moulin DE, Rodgers A, et al: IV infusion of opioids for cancer pain: clinical review and guidelines for use. Cancer Treat Rev 70:575–580, 1986

Posner MI, Petersen SE: The attention system of the human brain. Annu Rev Neurosci 13:125–142, 1990

Price DD: Psychological and neural mechanisms of the affective dimension of pain. Science 288:1769–1772, 2000

Rainville P, Duncan GH, Price DD, et al: Pain affect encoded in human anterior cingulate but not somatosensory cortex. Science 277:968–971, 1997

Rainville P, Hofbauer RK, Bushnell MC, et al: Hypnosis modulates activity in brain structures involved in the regulation of consciousness. J Cogn Neurosci 14:887–901, 2002

Raja SN, Meyer RA, Campbell JN: Peripheral mechanisms of somatic pain. Anesthesiology 68:571–590, 1988

Rawal N, Arner S, Gustaffson LL, et al: Present state of extradural and intrathecal opioid analgesia in Sweden: a nationwide follow-up survey. Br J Anaesth 59:791–799, 1987

Reich J, Tupin JP, Abramowitz SI: Psychiatric diagnosis of chronic pain patients. Am J Psychiatry 140:1495–1498, 1983

Reynolds DV: Surgery in the rat during electrical analgesia induced by focal brain stimulation. Science 164:444–445, 1969

Ripamonti C, Bruera E: Rectal, buccal and sublingual narcotics for the management of cancer pain. J Palliat Care 7:30–35, 1991

Rustoen T, Wahl AK, Hanestad BR, et al: Age and the experience of chronic pain. Clin J Pain 21 (suppl 6):513–523, 2005

Sawynok J, Labella L: GABA and baclofen potentiate the K^+-evoked release of methionine-enkephalin from rat striatal slices. Eur J Pharmacol 70:103–110, 1981

Spiegel D: Hypnosis, in The American Psychiatric Press Textbook of Psychiatry, 2nd Edition. Edited by Hales RE, Yudofsky SC, Talbott JA. Washington, DC, American Psychiatric Press, 1994, pp 1115–1142

Spiegel D: Oncological and pain syndromes, in Psychiatry Update: The American Psychiatric Association Annual Review, Vol 5. Edited by Frances AJ, Hales RE. Washington, DC, American Psychiatric Press, 1986, pp 561–579

Spiegel D, Bloom JR: Group therapy and hypnosis reduce metastatic breast carcinoma pain. Psychosom Med 45:333–339, 1983a

Spiegel D, Bloom JR: Pain in metastatic breast cancer. Cancer 52:341–345, 1983b

Spiegel D, Sands S: Pain management in the cancer patient. Journal of Psychosocial Oncology 6:205–216, 1988

Spiegel D, Hunt T, Dondershine H: Dissociation and hypnotizability in posttraumatic stress disorder. Am J Psychiatry 145:301–355, 1988

Spiegel D, Bierre P, Rootenberg J: Hypnotic alteration of somatosensory perception. Am J Psychiatry 146:749–754, 1989

Spiegel D, Stroud P, Fyfe A: Complementary medicine. West J Med 168:241–247, 1998

Spiegel H, Spiegel D: Trance and Treatment: Clinical Uses of Hypnosis. Washington, DC, American Psychiatric Press, 2004

Stein C: Neuro-immune interactions in pain. Crit Care Med 21 (9 suppl):S357–S358, 1993

Taddio A, Katz J, Ilersich AL, et al: Effect of neonatal circumcision on pain response during subsequent routing vaccination. Lancet 349:599–603, 1997

Taylor K, Rowbotham MC. Venlafaxine hydrochloride and chronic pain. West J Med 165:147–148, 1996

Tolle TR, Kaufmann T, Seissmeier T, et al: Region-specific encoding of sensory and affective components of pain in the human brain: a positron emission tomography correlation analysis. Ann Neurol 45:40–47, 1999

Ventafridda V, Tamburini M, Carceni A, et al: A validation study of the WHO method for cancer relief. Cancer 59:850–856, 1987

Waldeman C, Eason J, Rambohui E, et al: Serum morphine levels: a comparison between continuous subcutaneous and intravenous infusions in post-operative patients. Cancer Treat Rev 71:953–956, 1984

Walker L, Greene J: Children with recurrent abdominal pain and their parents: more somatic complaints, anxiety, and depression than other patient families? J Pediatr Psychol 14:231–293, 1989

Walker LS, Claar RC, Garber J: Social consequences of children's pain: when do they encourage symptom maintenance? J Pediatr Psychol 27:689–698, 2002

Wall BA, Holden EW, Gladstein J: Parent responses to pediatric headache. Headache 37:65–70, 1997

Wang SM, Peloquin C, Kain ZN: The use of auricular acupuncture to reduce preoperative anxiety. Anesth Analg 93:1178–1180, 2001

Wasan A, Davar G, Jamison R, et al: Psychiatric comorbidity diminishes opioid analgesia in patients with discogenic low back pain (abstract no 845). J Pain 5 (suppl 1):S70, 2004

Weinberg DS, Inturrisi CE, Reidenberg B, et al: Sublingual absorption of selected opioid analgesics. Clin Pharmacol Ther 44:335–342, 1988

Whitehead WE, Crowell MD, Heller BR, et al: Modelling and reinforcement of the sick role during childhood predicts adult illness behavior. Psychosom Med 56:541–550, 1994

Willis WD: Thalamocortical mechanisms of pain, in Advances in Pain Research and Therapy, Vol 9. Edited by Fields HL, Dubner R, Cervero F. New York, Raven, 1985, pp 175–200

Wilson KG, Eriksson MY, D'Eon JL, et al: Major depression and insomnia in chronic pain. Clin J Pain 18 (suppl 2):77–83, 2002

Wood JN, Akopian AN, Cesare P, et al: The primary nociceptor: special functions, special receptors, in Proceedings of the 9th World Congress on Pain, Vienna, 1999. Edited by Devor M, Rowbotham MC, Wiesenfeld-Hallin Z. Seattle, WA, IASP Press, 2000, pp 47–62

Woodforde JM, Fielding JR: Pain and cancer. J Psychosom Res 14:365–370, 1970

Yaksh TL: Spinal opiates analgesia: characteristics and principles of action. Pain 11:293–346, 1981

Yaksh TL: Neurologic mechanisms of pain, in Neural Blockade in Clinical Anesthesia and Management of Pain, 2nd Edition. Edited by Cousins MJ, Bridenbaugh PO. Philadelphia, PA, JB Lippincott, 1988, pp 791–844

Yaksh TL, Noueihed R: The physiology and pharmacology of spinal opiates. Annu Rev Pharmacol Toxicol 25:433–462, 1985

Yaksh TL, Rudy TA: Narcotic analgesia produced by a direct action on the spinal cord. Science 192:1357–1358, 1976

Zeltzer L, LeBaron S: Hypnosis and nonhypnotic techniques for reduction of pain and anxiety during painful procedures in children and adolescents with cancer. J Pediatr 101:1032–1035, 1982

10

NEUROPSYCHIATRIC ASPECTS OF DISORDERS OF ATTENTION

Ronald A. Cohen, Ph.D.

Stephen Salloway, M.D.

Lawrence H. Sweet, Ph.D.

Disorders of attention and consciousness often lead to requests for neuropsychiatric consultation. Attention-deficit/hyperactivity disorder (ADHD), in particular, has become prominent in public awareness. At the same time, advances in understanding attentional systems and treating attentional disorders are moving rapidly forward. Neuropsychiatrists need to understand the neural systems and neurochemistry involved in the mediation of attention and need to be familiar with assessment techniques and treatment strategies for attentional disorders.

In the first section of this chapter, we review the conceptual models of attentional systems in the brain and define terms that are commonly associated with attention and consciousness; in the second section, we review the assessment of attention; and in the third section, we discuss the clinical features and management of attentional disturbance seen in clinical practice with adults.

IMPORTANCE OF ATTENTION IN THE PRACTICE OF NEUROPSYCHIATRY

William James described attention in this way (James 1890):

> Everyone knows what attention is. It is the taking possession by the mind, in clear vivid form, of one out of what seems several simultaneous possible objects or trains of thought. Focalization, concentration of consciousness are of its essence. It implies withdrawal from some things in order to deal effectively with others.

Because the human mind cannot process at any one time all of the stimuli it receives from internal and external sources, processes must be present that can select, filter, and organize information into manageable and meaningful units. The term *attention* refers to that part of the cognitive apparatus that allows an individual to focus on selected features of sensory stimuli and ideas while keeping potentially distracting stimuli at bay.

The work of attention is essential to everyday existence and is part of our common vocabulary. At a cocktail party, people attempt to converse while simultaneously eating, drinking, listening to music, and being aware of other conversations and people nearby. Teachers instruct their students to "pay attention" in school, soldiers are ordered "to attention," and athletes may attribute a poor performance to a lack of concentration.

The terms *attention* and *consciousness* are closely related. Consciousness has been described as an alert state in which individuals are "aware of self and environment" (Adams and Victor 1981), whereas impaired consciousness implies diminished awareness and reactivity. The determination of an individual's level of consciousness is essential to the evaluation of attention. The neurobiology of consciousness is currently an area of active research. The interested reader should consult reviews in this area by Crick and Koch (1990), Hill (1989), and Picton and Stuss (1994).

ELEMENTS OF ATTENTION

Many terms have been used to describe aspects of attention. For the purpose of this review, attention depends on the interaction of four component processes: 1) *attentional capacity*, 2) *selective attention*, 3) *response selection and executive control*, and 4) *sustained attention*. These functional units are defined and discussed in the following paragraphs (R.A. Cohen 1993; Mirsky 1989; Posner and Boies 1971). A model depicting the flow of information through these four major components of attention is shown in Figure 10–1.

ATTENTIONAL CAPACITY AND FOCUS

Humans have a limited capacity for attention. We are able to perform only a small number of tasks concurrently. The intensity of attentional focus that can be allocated at one point in time is limited. Attentional capacity governs both the amount of information that can be handled and the intensity of cognitive processing that can be performed on that information.

Capacity limitations constrain other attentional processes, influencing the efficiency of both sensory and response selection in addition to control. In the light of this fact, some cognitive scientists have developed entire theories of attention based on the construct of a limited-capacity attentional system (Kahneman 1973).

Attentional capacity is not constant over time but fluctuates as a function of both extrinsic factors, such as the perceived value of stimuli and prevailing response demands, and intrinsic processes, such as energetic and structural factors (R.A. Cohen 1993; Kahneman 1973). *Energetic* factors include arousal, affective state, and drive and motivation. *Structural* factors include processing speed (e.g., reaction times), memory capacity, spatial dynamics, and temporal dynamics of the system. Structural capacity also varies in accordance with the individual's ability to perform specific cognitive operations. For instance, a chess expert is likely to find it easier than a novice to attend to a chess game. Structural factors represent more stable resource limitations that vary among individuals, whereas energetic factors fluctuate dramatically as a normal part of human functioning.

Focused attention is strongly dependent on attentional capacity. Attentional focus requires the ongoing allocation of available processing resources to a particular task or object. The intensity of focus is a function of requirements of the task but is constrained by capacity limitations.

It is relatively easy to identify examples of focused attention in everyday life. For instance, when one attempts to solve a mathematical problem, one may initially experience difficulty if one's abilities are not fully allocated to the task. Only when concentrated effort is directed toward the problem does a solution emerge. Focused attention is strongly associated with the subjective experience of concentration.

Processing speed is a function of the amount of information that an individual can register, integrate, and respond to per unit of time. The relationship between information processing speed and capacity is so dramatic that some investigators have argued that processing speed is a direct correlate of "intelligence." Correlations between reaction time and intelligence quotient (IQ) are between 0.6 and 0.9, depending on the sample characteristics and the type of IQ test utilized (Brand 1981; Vernon 1987). Information processing rate is therefore an important constraint on the capacity of attention as well as other aspects of cognition.

Reaction time reflects the time required to make an attentional selection or a response on tasks requiring attentional focus (Posner 1986). Tasks with greater processing demands tend to be associated with increased reaction times. From the standpoint of classic information processing theory, a system's information processing capacity is directly related to the rate of processing within the system: faster rates of processing are characteristic of larger-capacity systems (Broadbent 1958; Shannon and Weaver 1949).

Processing rate might be especially critical for tasks requiring manipulation of information within working memory (W. Schneider and Shiffrin 1977). Because the contents of working memory rapidly decay, information must be encoded into "chunks" and stored in long-term mem-

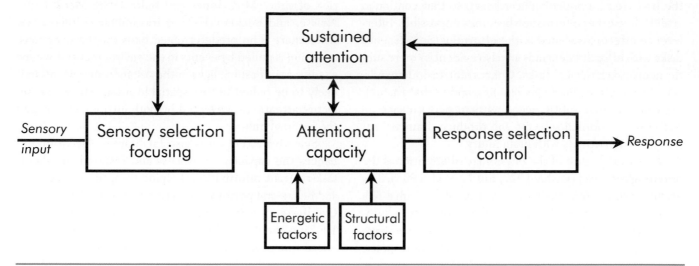

FIGURE 10–1. Primary factors underlying attention. This model depicts the flow of information through the four major components of attention: 1) sensory selection, 2) response selection control, 3) capacity, and 4) sustained attention. Attentional capacity is influenced by energetic and structural components. Sustained attention is the product of the information flow through the system and the resulting feedback, which affects each factor.

Source. Reprinted from Cohen RA: *Neuropsychology of Attention.* New York, Plenum, 1993, Figure 22.1, p. 470. Used with permission from Springer Science and Business Media.

ory before further information can be accepted into working memory. If the rate of stimulus presentation exceeds this processing capacity, the new information will not be processed adequately. Because the perceiver usually does not control the rate of information presentation, this is a relatively common occurrence. Most people have had the experience of finding a classroom lecture going too quickly for note-taking or assimilation. After asking for directions from a local person, we receive a rapid-paced description of distances, turns, and landmarks that becomes irretrievably jumbled by the time we take to the road again. In both cases, the rate of information presentation has exceeded the working memory's capacity and rate of processing, resulting in degradation of the information.

The capacity for focused attention is directly related to the difficulty of the task and the number of operations that must be performed simultaneously. Even under ordinary conditions, attention is subject to division among a multitude of processes and potential stimuli. A teenager who does homework while watching television is engaging in divided attention, as is someone who drives while listening to the radio.

Engaging in divided attention is difficult because of interference created by the competing stimuli. Attending to one object often makes focusing on another object impossible. Cognitive studies indicate that people have a limited capacity for divided attention that is dependent on the same factors that influence attentional capacity. As the number of simultaneous information sources to be processed increases,

attentional performance declines markedly, especially when task demands are made more difficult (Hasher and Zacks 1979; Kahneman and Treisman 1984; Navon 1985).

The quality of attentional performance on multiple simultaneous tasks is strongly dependent on how automatically the tasks can be performed. For instance, typists who are able to talk with people or carry out other activities while typing are demonstrating automatic attentional capacity for typing.

Cognitive scientists have demonstrated that automatic and controlled attentional processes can be dissociated by manipulating the parameters of particular tasks (W. Schneider and Shiffrin 1977). Memory load, spatial frame size, and number of targets to be detected are among the variables that influence an individual's ability to perform tasks automatically.

Some types of attention require much more effort than others. Tasks that require high levels of attentional effort have been characterized as *controlled-effortful attention.* Such tasks are also more apt to demand conscious awareness (Hasher and Zacks 1979; Kahneman and Treisman 1984). Effortful demands strongly influence the divided attentional capacity. This is obvious in cases of extreme physical exertion. It is not difficult to listen to a radio while engaging in moderate physical exercise, such as walking. However, it becomes increasingly difficult to maintain attentional focus when extreme physical exertion is required. At such times, people become increasingly aware of the signals being given out by the body (e.g., a pounding heartbeat), so that continued attention to other information becomes impossible. Interference effects associated with performing simultaneous tasks with effortful demands are also evident in more subtle neuropsychological tasks. Concurrent task demands, such as simultaneous finger tapping and verbal fluency, typically produce subtle decrements in performance on both tasks in normal subjects and produce dramatic impairments in patients with brain injury.

A central feature of the physiology of attention is the orienting response (Pavlov 1927; Siddle et al. 1983). The orienting response is the initial reaction of an animal to a novel stimulus and is characterized by activation in autonomic and motoric responses and brain electrical activity. Orienting responses are subject to decreases in response strength through a process of habituation. Habituation, an important element of attention, shifts attention and behavioral readiness away from stimuli that do not possess high levels of intrinsic salience to new stimuli. Sensitization is a process that opposes habituation and reflects an increased orienting response. Sensitization may occur due to an increase in generalized arousal or as a result of the introduction of other stimuli that increase the general readiness to respond to the habituated stimulus. There are now considerable data regarding the neural mechanisms underlying these responses (Kandel and Schwartz 1982), and it is likely that some of the mechanisms mediating these responses reflect brain events associated with attentional allocation.

SELECTIVE ATTENTION

Perhaps the most fundamental quality of all attentional processes is selectivity. Attention enables the selective deployment of cognitive resources toward salient information from either the external environment or the internal milieu. Attention also requires a shift from less salient information. Processes that enable or facilitate the selection of salient information for further cognitive processing are collectively referred to as *selective attention* (Treisman 1969; Triesman and Geffen 1967).

Selective attention influences the selection of particular target stimuli from the environment. Although selective attention is usually considered a phenomenon closely aligned with sensory processing and perception, it also facilitates the selection and control of response alternatives (R.A. Cohen and Waters 1985; J.A. Deutsch and Deutsch 1963; Jennings et al. 1980; Verfaellie et al. 1988). As a result of selective attention, some stimuli are given priority over others.

Selective attention always occurs relative to a temporal spatial frame of reference. Information that is processed is selected from a broad spatial array over a specified period of time (M.R. Jones and Boltz 1989; Meck 1984; Neisser and Becklen 1975; Parasuraman 1984). Even when there is no predetermined basis for the selections, attention is pulled by events in the environment. If we see a police car's flashing light in the distance, our attention is likely to be pulled to that spatial location. Therefore, selective attention is governed by both intrinsic factors and the external milieu.

Selective attention is also facilitative. Attention enhances the capacity to process and respond to salient, task-relevant information, helping to optimize cognitive and behavioral performance (Desimone and Gross 1979; Goldberg and Bushnell 1981; Goldberg and Wurtz 1972). Although attentional facilitation serves many beneficial functions, there are costs associated with attending. By attending to a particular stimulus, the likelihood of detecting other potentially relevant stimuli or choosing an alternative response strategy is reduced. Of course, this outcome is also adaptive. Individuals are constantly flooded with an infinite number of signals from both outside and within. By reducing the amount of information that will receive additional processing, attention constrains incoming information to the individual's available capacity at a given point in time, thereby keeping the level of information to be processed at a manageable level. Metaphorically, attention has often been compared to the aperture and lens system of a camera. By changing the depth of field and focal point, attention enables humans to direct themselves to appropriate aspects of external environmental events and internal operations. Attention thereby serves as a gating mechanism for the flow of information processing and the control of behavior.

RESPONSE SELECTION AND EXECUTIVE CONTROL

Although attention is often thought of as a process that prepares the individual for optimal sensory intake, perceptual analysis, and integration, it is also involved in response selection and control. Even when a task primarily requires selective attention, there are usually coexisting response demands (Heilman et al. 1985, 1988; Parasuraman 1975). To attend to information on the television, for example, we must first respond by turning on the television and then sitting down in a chair to look and listen. Although sensory selection may be elicited by the characteristics of the stimuli reaching our senses, more often than not the act of attending is linked to a planned, goal-directed course of action. We direct our behavior to obtain information that will allow us to select the most salient stimuli and optimal responses from available alternatives.

A wide variety of processes are associated with response selection and control, ranging from simple behavioral orienting (e.g., turning one's head in the direction of an auditory stimulus) to more complex cognitive processes involving intention, planning, and decision making. Response selection and control also form the basis for volitional action, as when a person who prepares to select and execute a response acts with deliberate focus in choosing the best response alternative.

Before responding, individuals generate a large number of response alternatives. The quality of these response alternatives is evaluated through trial and error or cognitively, without making an actual motor response. These responses form a response bias, which influences the probability of selecting specific responses. The process of establishing a response bias forms the attentional component of response intention (R.A. Cohen 1993; Heilman et al. 1988). Intention is influenced by the intrinsic salience of stimuli as well as the value placed on information or response alternatives within a specific context. In turn, intention influences the direction of attention, providing an impetus for both sensory and response selection.

The act of looking is an example of an intentional behavior. Looking not only involves the act of orienting one's head and eyes but also is associated with a readiness and preparation for future action (Neisser and Becklen 1975). For instance, a hunter who goes into the woods uses a wide range of tracking behaviors that may increase the likelihood of finding the target. The hunter's intentions guide his overt and covert responses and ultimately prime his level of vigilance to his target.

The attentional processes involved in response selection and control are related to a broader class of cognitive processes, commonly referred to as *executive functions* (Fuster 1989; Luria 1966). Several processes associated with response generation underlie executive control: intention, selection, initiation, inhibition, facilitation, and switching. Not only do these processes account for the control of simple motor responses, they also provide the foundation for more complex cognitive processes, such as planning, problem solving, and decision making, as well as conceptual processes such as categorization, organization, and abstraction. Executive control is strongly dependent on the actions of prefrontal-subcortical systems.

Attention is facilitated by neural mechanisms that suppress the probability of response to nontarget stimuli (inhibition) as well as by processes that increase the probability of response to targets (enhancement). Executive control is dependent on the ability to efficiently shift from one response alternative to another in accordance with changing environmental demands (switching).

SUSTAINED ATTENTION

Attention is also strongly influenced by the temporal dynamics of the prevailing task demands and is characterized by performance variability over time (M.R. Jones and Boltz 1989; Meck 1984; Parasuraman 1984). The centrality of temporal factors to attention distinguishes attentional processes from other cognitive operations. Attention is more variable than sensory processes, primary perception, and memory, which are characterized by relative consistency over time. We assume that if a perceptual system is working properly, it will always detect and recognize stimuli that meet certain psychophysical conditions. In contrast, attention is inherently inconsistent because the likelihood that a particular stimulus will be detected or will receive additional focused processing is constantly changing and depends on prevailing task conditions and the person's momentary disposition. The tendency for performance to vary as a function of the temporal characteristics of tasks is often a result of demands for sustained attention. Problems with sustained attention are commonly associated with tasks requiring attentional persistence for long durations, because sustained performance is accompanied by considerable processing demands. Although sustained attention varies as a function of the relationship between target stimuli and distractors as well as the cognitive operations that are required, time is by itself a central determinant of attention. Sustained attention depends on the cyclical reprocessing of information that provides positive and negative feedback from the results of prior action.

All people have limits in their capacity for sustained attention. Sitting in a 1-hour lecture is not a problem for most bright college students, but even the brightest students would encounter tremendous difficulties sustaining their focus for a lecture that lasted 12 consecutive hours.

Vigilance is sustained attention directed toward specific targets. It requires a state of readiness to detect and respond to small changes occurring at random intervals in the environment (Colquhoun and Baddeley 1967; Corcoran et al. 1977; Jerison 1967). Detecting rare targets with lengthy intervals between responses can be difficult. This type of sustained attention, which is usually referred to as *vigilance*, is actually quite common in everyday life. For example, a watchman may spend the entire night attending to the possibility of an intruder without this event ever occurring. Attention to low-frequency events has different processing requirements than responding to high-frequency events and, for many people, is more difficult. Vigilance and sustained attention are under the influence of sustained motivational level, boredom, and fatigue, which are sensitive to the dynamics of temporal tasks.

MODELS OF ATTENTION

Attention is not a unitary process; it spans multiple psychological domains and includes many neural systems. The boundaries of attention intersect with other constructs in common usage: memory, consciousness, vigilance, motivation, and alertness. Using examples of patients with distinctive lesions and information from basic neuroscience and neuroanatomy, a number of researchers have developed conceptual models of the cognitive constructs and neural systems involved in attention. There is considerable agreement among these conceptual systems (for greater detail, see R.A. Cohen 1993). There appears to be a consensus that attention is mediated through the interaction of neural networks (Mesulam 1981). The key structures involved in these neural networks are the reticular activating system (RAS), the thalamus and striatum, the nondominant posterior parietal cortex, the prefrontal cortex, and the anterior cingulate gyrus and limbic system.

Mesulam (1985) subdivided attention into two major categories: a matrix or state function and a vector or channel function. Matrix functions regulate overall information processing capacity, detection efficiency, focusing power, and vigilance, which he associated primarily with the RAS. The vector function regulates the direction or target of attention. This is analogous to selective attention and is associated with neocortical systems. In practice, these two systems are integrated (Figure 10–2).

Heilman et al. (1993) developed a model of a cortico-limbic-reticular formation network. This model accounts for hemiattention associated with neglect syndrome and provides a general neuroanatomical framework for attention. In this model, selective attention is considered to be dependent on arousal, sensory transmission, intact sensory association area projections, projections to the nucleus reticularis of the thalamus, sensory convergence to a heteromodal cortex, a supramodal cortex such as the inferior parietal lobule, and limbic connections (Figure 10–3). Neglect is considered to be an arousal-attentional disorder created by dysfunction of this network. Unilateral lesions affecting any part of the network may result in neglect.

A two-process model of attention has also been proposed by Posner and Cohen (1984) and Posner et al. (1987), who consider the parietal cortex and cingulate region to be the brain's two primary attentional systems. These researchers maintain that these two systems influence different attentional processes. The parietal cortex is involved in the covert disengagement of attention that is necessary for sensory selection, whereas the cingulate cortex is responsible for the intensity of attentional

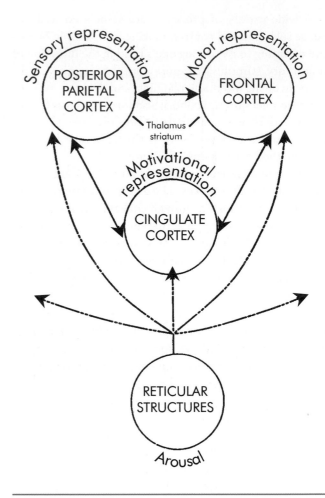

FIGURE 10–2.   A network involved in the distribution of attention to extrapersonal targets.

Source.   From Mesulam M-M: *Principles of Behavioral Neurology.* Philadelphia, PA, F.A. Davis, 1985, p. 157. Reprinted by permission of Oxford University Press.

focus. In the next section, we briefly describe the role of each of these systems in attention.

The RAS plays a major role in modulating arousal and provides global regulation of attentional tone for the forebrain (Moruzzi and Magoun 1949). Lesions of the midbrain reticular core may cause permanent stupor or coma. The midbrain reticular core projects to the intralaminar nuclei of the thalamus, which in turn project to the caudate nucleus, prefrontal cortex, and many other cortical regions but not to the primary sensory areas (E.G. Jones and Leavitt 1974; E.G. Jones et al. 1979; Steriade and Glenn 1982). The RAS-thalamic input to the cortex provides nonspecific priming for attention. The reticular nucleus of the thalamus has reciprocal connections with the midbrain RAS, the prefrontal cortex, and the sensory nuclei of the thalamus. The reticular nucleus appears to inhibit thalamic relay to the cortex, and Scheibel (1981) has proposed that the reticular nucleus acts as an attentional

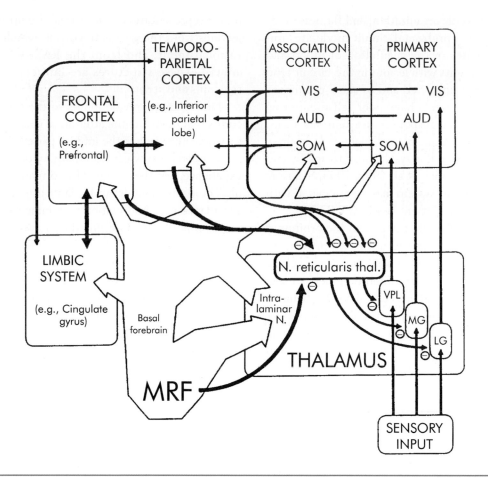

FIGURE 10–3. Schematic representation of pathways important in sensory attention and tonic arousal. MRF=mesencephalic reticular formation; VIS=visual; AUD=auditory; SOM=somasthetic. Thalamic sensory relay nuclei: VPL=ventralis posterolateralis; MG=medial geniculate; LG=lateral geniculate.

Source. From Heilman KM, Watson RT, Valenstein E: "Neglect and Related Disorders," in *Clinical Neuropsychology,* 3rd Edition. Edited by Heilman KM, Valenstein E. New York, Oxford University Press, 1993, pp. 279–336. Reprinted by permission of Oxford University Press.

gate or filter for sensory stimuli. Increased arousal or behavioral activation inhibits the reticular nucleus, facilitating transmission of sensory information to the cortex.

The intensity of arousal and direction of attention are strongly influenced by the hypothalamus through its regulation of the daily circadian rhythm and its role in the modulation of appetitive function (Folkard 1979; Hockey and Colquhoun 1972). Each individual has an internal circadian clock, which regulates the sleep-wake rhythm that is primarily under the control of the suprachiasmatic nucleus of the hypothalamus. Some individuals describe themselves as "morning persons" or "night persons" on the basis of consistently higher levels of alertness, energy, and attentional capacity at certain times of the day. This phenomenon is probably related to interactions between the RAS and the suprachiasmatic nucleus/extended circadian network. The circadian rhythm is a dynamic process that changes throughout the life cycle. Understanding the relationship between the circadian rhythm and attention is important for optimizing educational and occupational activities. This relationship is also important in clinical practice when a clinician advises patients with attentional disturbance regarding remedial academic and work programs and patients with Alzheimer's disease who experience disruption of the circadian rhythm and are vulnerable to attentional disturbance and confusion in the late afternoon and evening.

The frontal lobe is an essential component of the attentional matrix. The prefrontal cortex is linked with subcortical structures in three behaviorally relevant circuits (Alexander et al. 1986; Cummings 1993; Mega and Cummings 1994; Salloway and Cummings 1994). The dorsolateral prefrontal cortex circuit is involved in maintaining response flexibility and generating response alternatives, the working memory, and the temporal sequencing of information. Lesions affecting this system are associated with perseveration, distractibility, impersistence, slowing of cognitive speed, impairments in abstraction and memory retrieval, cognitive disorganization, and flatness of affect. The orbitomedial prefrontal circuit modulates impulses and participates in the regulation of mood and working memory. Patients with lesions in this circuit tend to be impulsive and disinhibited and to show prominent mood lability. These patients have poor self-monitoring and have trouble inhibiting responses on attentional tasks. The anterior cingulate circuit plays a major role in drive and motivation. Lesions in this system lead to apathy and poor motivation (R.A. Cohen et al. 1990, 1994; Salloway 1994). Dysfunction in this system may be associated with the easy boredom seen in patients with ADHD.

The dorsolateral prefrontal cortex and the orbitomedial prefrontal region are involved in the executive control of attention and cognition. These functions include intention and response initiation, inhibition, persistence, and switching, processes that are central to the planning and generation of behavior and to the direction of responding relative to goals. Executive control depends on the ability to inhibit responding to irrelevant stimuli and to facilitate goal-appropriate responses. A mechanism whereby "switching" between response alternatives can occur is necessary for executive control.

The clinical disorder of hemispatial inattention associated with hemineglect syndrome provides evidence that the nondominant parietal cortex plays a central role in visual selective attention. Subsequent neurophysiological investigations expand on these observations, yielding information about underlying mechanisms confirming that neurons in the inferior parietal lobule have specialized attentional functions. Single-unit neuron activity from inferior parietal cells of awake primates shows increased firing rates when attention is directed toward motivationally salient stimuli (Bushnell et al. 1981; Hyvarinen et al. 1980; Mountcastle et al. 1975). Neurons in area PG (angular gyrus) of the right inferior parietal lobule have the ability to facilitate future responding to expected stimuli at a particular spatial location. Neuronal activation of inferior parietal neurons occurs in the absence of motoric responding, including eye movements, but is associated with the task demands for future responding. Furthermore, firing rates of inferior parietal neurons can be modified by changing attentional and motivational parameters. These neurons in monkeys appear to activate before actual sensory analysis (Bushnell et al. 1981; Desimone and Gross 1979; Goldberg and Bushnell 1981; Goldberg and Wurtz 1972; Hyvarinen et al. 1980).

Many investigators have demonstrated that the right parietal lobe is dominant for directed attention to extrapersonal space. The posterior parietal cortex maintains a sensory representation of extrapersonal space, whereas the frontal eye fields and associated cortex maintain a motor representation. These areas are influenced by projections from the cingulate cortex, which provide motivational input, and from the RAS, which modulates arousal. These structures are interconnected with the thalamus and striatum.

Limbic areas provide inputs to the sensory association cortex that modulate the attentional response of sensory association areas such as the inferior parietal lobules. The mesial temporal cortex controls memory processes, emotional experience, and the binding of informational value to stimuli. These inputs inhibit or facilitate attentional response in accordance with information pertaining to stimulus significance, motivational state, and the goal orientation of the animal (Hyvarinen et al. 1980; Nauta 1986; Pribram 1969).

The anterior cingulate gyrus, a component of the limbic circuit, plays a pivotal role in attention by contributing important energetic components of drive and motivation. Bilateral lesions of the anterior cingulate region can produce a profound apathetic state of akinetic mutism. Such lesions may be seen after infarction of the bilateral anterior cerebral artery caused by rupture of an aneurysm of the anterior communicating artery. Individuals in this state are alert but demonstrate little interest in interacting with stimuli in the environment.

Evidence for the role of the cingulate gyrus in attention comes from cognitive studies in normal adults using functional imaging and from the evaluation of patients after cingulotomy (R.A. Cohen et al. 1990, 1994). The cingulate gyrus activates as a function of the intensity of attentional focus and effort. In two studies (Pardo et al. 1991; Petersen et al. 1989) of regional cerebral blood flow with positron emission tomography (PET) in subjects completing the Stroop task and a semantic activation task, the anterior cingulate region was found to activate during tasks that involve scrutinizing stimuli and selecting the correct response (Figure 10–4).

Obsessive-compulsive disorder may be a disorder of excessive vigilance involving dysregulation in frontostriatothalamic circuits (Baxter 1992; Baxter et al. 1992; Modell et al. 1989). Functional imaging studies have found increased activity in the orbital frontal gyrus, the cingulate gyrus, and the head of the caudate nucleus, particularly in the left hemisphere (Benkelfat et al. 1990; Swedo et al. 1992). Metabolism normalizes in these areas when symptoms are reduced after successful drug and behavioral treatments. This disorder highlights the role that the basal ganglia and thalamus play in modulating components of attention such as arousal, vigilance, executive control, and response selection (Mindus et al. 1994; Rapoport 1991; Salloway et al. 1995).

Although the neurochemistry underlying attention systems is not well understood, there is evidence that catecholaminergic, cholinergic, and, indirectly, serotonergic

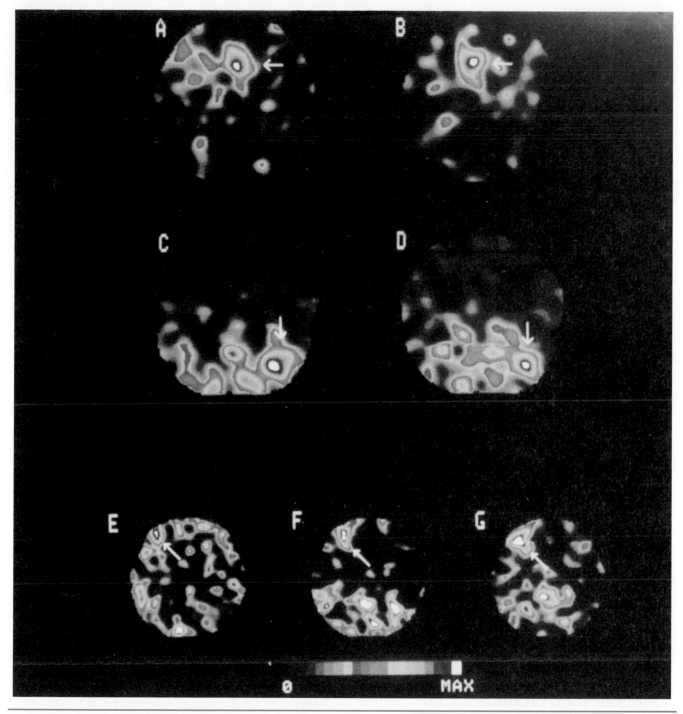

FIGURE 10–4. Positron emission tomographic imaging of visual (*A, C, F*) versus auditory (*B, D, G*) presentation of a semantic association task. These slices (except *E*) represent blood flow changes when blood flow response during repetition of presented words is subtracted from blood flow response during the subject's verbal statement of a use for the presented word (e.g., "cake"— "eat"). Slices *A* and *B* show activation near the midline in anterior cingulate cortex. Slices *C* and *D* show activation in right lateral cerebellum. Slices *E, F,* and *G* show activation in left anterior, inferior frontal cortex. Slices *F* and *G* are from the vocalize use association task; slice *E* is from a different semantic association task, in which subjects were asked to silently monitor a list of words for members of a semantic category. These findings demonstrate the role of anterior brain systems on tasks requiring focused semantic processing and increased attentional demands.

Source. Reprinted by permission from Macmillan Publishers Ltd, from Pardo JV, Fox PT, Raichle ME: "Localization of a Human System for Sustained Attention by Positron Emission Tomography." *Nature* 349:61–64, 1991. Copyright 1991.

systems are important in attentional processes (McCormick 1989; Sato et al. 1987; Shute and Lewis 1967). The RAS comprises a network of monoaminergic (norepinephrine, dopamine, and serotonin) and cholinergic neurotransmitters. Stimulation or blockade of these neurotransmitters can have a prominent effect on arousal and neuronal responsiveness to sensory input. The clinical efficacy of stimulant medication in treating ADHD provides indirect evidence for the role of catecholamines in attention. These medications promote catecholaminergic activity by increasing the presynaptic release and blocking the reuptake of dopamine and norepinephrine (Clemens and Fuller 1979; Shekim et al. 1994; Shenker 1992).

Ebstein and colleagues (1996) found that individuals with high levels of novelty-seeking behavior had abnormalities in the gene for the dopamine type 4 (D_4) receptor, suggesting that dopamine systems play a role in novelty seeking and reinforcement. In contrast, patients with Parkinson's disease have low levels of exploratory behavior (J.S. Schneider et al. 1994). In addition, dopamine has an effect on cognitive speed and reaction time. Patients with untreated Parkinson's disease have slower cognitive speed than patients taking levodopa, even after controlling for motor dysfunction (Lange et al. 1992; Owens et al. 1992). This effect is probably mediated through mesencephalic-prefrontal dopaminergic pathways.

A study of monkeys treated with 1-methyl-4-phenyl-1,2,3,6-tetrahydropyridine (MPTP), a drug toxic to dopaminergic neurons, demonstrated that dopamine agonists and stimulants increase task persistence (J.S. Schneider et al. 1994). Dopamine and norepinephrine also participate in prefrontal memory systems (Arnstein and Goldman-Rakic 1985). Serotonergic systems probably modulate the impulsive and hyperactive symptoms associated with attentional disturbance by directly affecting mood and by interacting with catecholaminergic systems in the nucleus accumbens and prefrontal cortex (Costall et al. 1979; Halperin et al. 1994).

ASSESSING DISORDERS OF ATTENTION

Although it is an essential part of human experience, attention is difficult to directly observe or measure. Attention fluctuates with changes in task conditions and in the processing capacity of the subject. Attentional performance is often situationally dependent. Patients may demonstrate good attentional ability in a structured office setting but be quite impaired in a school, work, or home environment with high stimulation and less structure. Consequently, attention is less amenable than many other cognitive functions to assessment by traditional standardized paper-and-pencil testing.

The ability to pay attention is fundamental to effective cognitive performance. When attentional processes are impaired, assessment of the mental status examination may be unreliable. Clinicians often reach conclusions regarding the presence of attentional disturbance by default. When reduced cognitive performance is observed in the absence of consistent deficits of memory, language, visual integration, or other cognitive functions, attentional problems are implicated. Yet methodological advances such as the advent of computer-based assessment paradigms, as well as increased knowledge regarding underlying attentional processes, have led to better methods for the assessment of attention.

In clinical practice, the evaluation of attention is often made quickly, at the bedside or in the office. Three sources of information are typically used in the assessment of attention: 1) clinical interview and self-report inventories, 2) direct behavioral observation, and 3) standardized tests of cognitive functions. In this section, we summarize these approaches to the clinical evaluation of attention. The reader is encouraged to review Lezak (1995) for a more detailed account of the actual test procedures and norms and R.A. Cohen (1993) for methodological issues in the assessment of attention.

The clinical interview and medical history can provide important information regarding possible attentional disturbance. DSM-IV-TR (American Psychiatric Association 2000) provides a foundation for the clinical interview and describes the criteria for a diagnosis of ADHD.

ADHD researchers have developed a number of specific inventories for rating attention and behavioral disturbances. Conners (1969) developed a teacher's rating system for measuring behavioral problems, including ADHD in children. (See Barkley et al. 1990 for a complete review of such inventories.)

Inventories developed for rating the cognitive and behavioral impairments of patients with brain damage may also prove useful. The Neurobehavioral Rating Scale (Levin et al. 1987) was developed for rating symptoms of closed head injury (CHI) and contains items pertaining to attention impairment. Although structured interviews and inventories provide useful clinical information about possible attentional disturbance, data from these sources must be considered with caution. These methods often require ratings from a family member or someone who may lack objectivity. ADHD is such a popular disorder that patients may be very quick to describe problems concentrating when their behavior is within normal limits. An adequate assessment of attention, therefore, requires data from multiple sources.

Clinical inferences regarding possible attentional disturbance are often based on behavioral observation. A patient who is well directed with eye contact and orientation toward a task is usually considered to be attending. Restlessness and an inability to stay seated during tasks are strong indicators of hyperactivity. Initial clinical judgments regarding attentional disturbance are often made on the basis of such observations. If greater measurement validity is desired, however, a number of methods for structured behavioral observation and quantification are available. These include event recording (frequency of undesirable behavior) and interval recording (duration of behaviors). Several excellent texts are available for a more detailed review of behavioral assessment methods (see Bellack and Hersen 1988).

Unlike most other cognitive processes, attention primarily serves a facilitative function (R.A. Cohen et al. 1998). Attention enhances or inhibits perception, memory, motor output, and executive functions, including problem solving. The following must be considered when assessing attention (R.A. Cohen et al. 1998):

- Pure tests of attention do not exist.
- Attention usually must be assessed within the context of performance on tasks that load on one or more of these other domains.
- Attentional performance is often a function of a derived measure obtained by comparing performance across tasks that load differentially with respect to key attentional parameters (e.g., target-distractor ratio).
- Absolute performance is often less informative than measures of performance inconsistencies in the assessment of attention. For example, how performance varies as a function of time, spatial characteristics, or memory load provides more information about attentional dynamics than simply considering total errors on a visual detection task.
- Attentional assessment requires a multifactorial approach. Given that attention is not the by-product of a unitary process, it cannot be adequately assessed on the basis of findings from one specific test. For example, conclusions about attention solely based on Digit Span performance are misguided.

NEUROPSYCHOLOGICAL TESTS OF ATTENTION

Neuropsychiatrists often request neuropsychological assessment to help in the evaluation of attentional disturbance. It is important for clinicians to be familiar with the tests commonly used to assess attention and the specific features of attention that they are designed to measure.

Attention comprises multiple processes, and the clinical evaluation of attention requires that data from multiple tasks be considered. Each task should be sensitive to a specific manifestation of attention. Although at times possible attentional disturbance can be inferred from the findings of a single test, a thorough assessment of attention requires the use of more than one test. A comprehensive assessment of attention necessitates the use of a neuropsychological battery containing several standardized paradigms that are capable of measuring specific impairments of attention. Table 10–1 lists the domains that should be evaluated in a comprehensive assessment of attention.

Many tests are designed to assess other cognitive functions but are also sensitive to attentional disturbance. The Mental Control and Digit Span subtests of the Wechsler Memory Scale (Wechsler 1945), as well as other memory measures, also provide indirect measures of attention. Comparison of the recall on Trial 1 relative to subsequent learning trials on word list learning tasks, such as Paired Associated Learning, indicates how well the patient is attending initially. Possible attentional problems may also be identified on the basis of the subject's response characteristics during testing. Excessive interitem variability may reflect fluctuations in attentional focus and problems with sustained attention. Intertest variability, particularly when inconsistencies are noted between subtests measuring the same cognitive function, may also suggest impaired attention. However, caution should be used when interpreting performance variability, because some variability may reflect the standard error of measurement and subtle differences in the nature of certain tasks.

When considering tests sensitive to specific processes of attention, it is important to recognize that the attentional components measured by these tests are not completely distinct. Tests that are particularly sensitive to impairments of sustained attention may also require executive control and attentional focus. Impairments affecting one element of attention may be associated with impairments of other attentional functions.

Attentional Capacity and Focus

A variety of structural and energetic factors influence attentional capacity. Tasks that tax energetic or structural capacity limitations typically require effortful, focused attention. Many tests are available for the assessment of attentional capacity and focus. Although these tasks are similar in requiring attentional focus, the actual cognitive operation necessary to perform the task may vary. Subjects may therefore exhibit performance inconsistencies across tasks according to their ability to perform certain cognitive operations.

TABLE 10–1.   Neuropsychological measures of attentional domains

Sensory selective attention

Double simultaneous stimulation

Letter or symbol cancellation

Line bisection

Spatial cueing paradigms

Dichotic listening

Wechsler Adult Intelligence Scale—Revised (WAIS-R): picture completion

Orienting response

Event-related potential (ERP) tasks

Response selection and control (executive control)

Motor impersistence task

Go/no-go task

Reciprocal motor programs

Trail Making Test

Wisconsin Card Sorting Test

Porteus Mazes Test

Controlled word generation

Design fluency

Spontaneous verbal generation

Attentional capacity—focus

Digit Span Forward, Digit Span Backwards

Corsi Blocks Test

Serial addition/subtraction

Consonant Trigrams Test

Symbol-digit tasks

Stroop Test

Reaction time paradigms

Paced Auditory Serial Addition Task (PASAT)

Dichotic Listening Test

Sustained performance and vigilance

Continuous Performance Test (CPT)

Motor Continuation Task

Cancellation tasks

Among the standard measures used to assess attentional focus are tests that require mental arithmetic and control. Digit Span Backwards, Backwards Spelling, the Arithmetic subtest of the Wechsler Adult Intelligence Scale—Revised

(WAIS-R) (Wechsler 1981), serial addition and subtraction tests, and asking the patient to recite the months of the year backwards are examples of such tasks. All of these tasks are also very sensitive to brain dysfunction.

The Digit Span test of the WAIS-R (Wechsler 1981) asks subjects to repeat digits. The length of the digit sequence is increased across trials until there has been a failure across two consecutive trials of a particular length. The average number of digits that normal adults can repeat is five to seven. In the Digit Span Backwards test, subjects are asked to repeat digits in reverse. This test requires attentional focus and controlled effort. The discrepancy between Digit Span Forward and Digit Span Backwards normally does not exceed two digits.

The Digit Span Forward test is often described as a test of attention. Yet performance on this test is strongly associated with short-term memory, working memory, and the language requirement of repetition. Performance is dependent on the ability to hold a string of items in mind for a short period of time until a response is requested. Encoding of the information into a more permanent memory storage is not necessary for completion of these tasks. Typically, individuals are unable to recall information from such tasks soon after initial recall. Therefore, tests of brief attention span bridge the functions of attention and short-term memory.

A weak score on the Digit Span test alone is not diagnostic of attentional disturbance. When analyzed in relation to other findings, however, this measure may provide useful clinical information. If performance on the digits backwards test exceeds that on the digits forward test, the possibility of inattention or motivational factors should be considered. Considerable interitem variability, such as missing some short sequences but then correctly repeating longer sequences, is significant because it suggests a lapse of attention.

The Corsi Blocks Test (Milner 1971) is a visual-spatial variation of the Digit Span test. The subject observes while the examiner points to a sequence of spatially distributed blocks. The subject is then asked to point to block sequences of various lengths in forward and reverse order. The normal nonverbal attention span should be equivalent to that seen in the Digit Span test. However, poor performance on spatial span tests may also reflect spatial attentional deficits (De Renzi et al. 1977).

The Consonant Trigrams Test (L.R. Peterson and Peterson 1959) is another test of attentional focus. Subjects are asked to repeat a string of three consonants. On some trials, the consonants are repeated immediately after they are presented, whereas on others, delays of 3, 9, and 18 seconds are used, during which subjects perform an interference task requiring mental arithmetic.

KEY

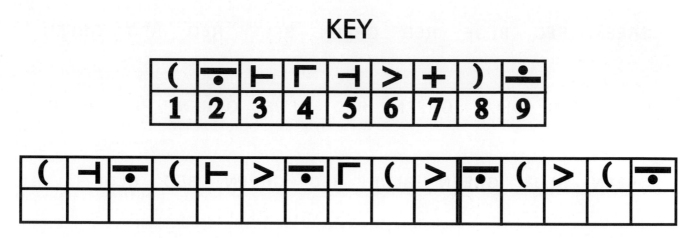

FIGURE 10–5. Symbol Digit Modalities Test.

Source. SDMT sample material copyright 1973 by Western Psychological Services. Reprinted for reference by permission WPS, 12031 Wilshire Boulevard, Los Angeles, CA 90025, U.S.A., www.wpspublish.com. Not to be reprinted in whole or in part for any additional purpose without the expressed written permission of the publisher. All rights reserved.

Slowed processing speed is a common manifestation of the attentional disturbance associated with brain damage, usually reflected by increased reaction times across a variety of information processing tasks (Gronwall and Sampson 1974; Gronwall and Wrightson 1974). Deficits in reaction times are strongly associated with the neuropsychological impairments of multiple sclerosis (MS), Parkinson's disease, and CHI, as discussed in the next section. Slowed processing speed and attentional disturbance often coexist in patients with relatively intact cognitive functions across other domains.

Measurement of reaction time is most easily achieved by computerized calculation of the time required to respond, via key press, to an auditory or visual stimulus. The complexity of reaction time can be increased by measuring the time required for an individual to make differential responses to different targets (e.g., right-hand key press to light, left-hand key press to sound). This test is referred to as choice reaction time.

The Paced Auditory Serial Addition Task (PASAT) (Gronwall and Sampson 1974; Gronwall and Wrightson 1974) is an example of a highly controlled test of attention that requires both focused and sustained attention. The PASAT is a variation of a serial arithmetic task. The subject is asked to add the first number presented to the second, the second number to the third, and so forth. Subjects must inhibit their tendency to add the new number to the prior sum. Performance is a function of the number of errors in calculation. The level of difficulty can be altered by varying the interstimulus interval.

The PASAT is sensitive to subtle attentional impairments. However, considerable effort is required for adequate performance, and the PASAT is difficult for patients with severe brain dysfunction. Poor motivation and reduced arousal also greatly affect performance on the PASAT.

The Symbol Digit Modalities Test (SDMT) (Smith 1973) and the Digit Symbol subtests of the WAIS-R are also excellent measures of focused attentional capacity. These tasks require rapid processing of symbolic information and the coding of symbol-number pairs. Collectively, they can be considered as symbol-coding tests. Subjects are presented with a template containing nine number and symbol pairs. Below the template is a random array of the symbols without numbers. The task is to write the appropriate number above the symbol, using the template as a guide. Performance is determined by the number of correct numbers transcribed in 90 seconds. Focused attention is required because the number-symbol pairs to be coded are not familiar to the subject (Figure 10–5).

A number of tasks place demands on attentional capacity and focus because of the requirement to divide attention or to inhibit interfering stimuli or responses. An example is the Stroop Test, in which the subject is required to name the color of a word while ignoring the actual word (Nehemkis and Lewinsohn 1972; Stroop 1935). Interference is created because the color and the meaning of the word are mismatched. The score is based on the number of colors named in 45 seconds and the number of errors produced by reading the word instead of naming the color (Figure 10–6). This test places strong demands on inhibitory systems, which must suppress both the other stimulus feature and a strong response tendency.

Concurrent production tasks (e.g., finger tapping while performing verbal fluency) provide a vehicle for assessing capacity limitations associated with divided attention. Such tasks are extremely effortful and require con-

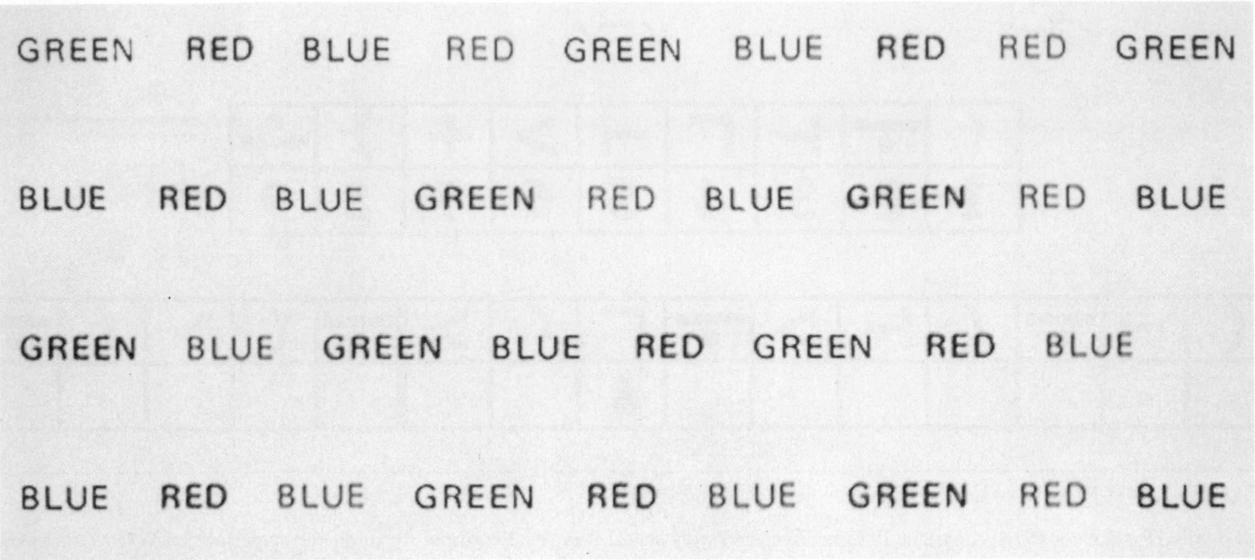

GREEN	RED	BLUE	RED	GREEN	BLUE	RED	RED	GREEN
BLUE	RED	BLUE	GREEN	RED	BLUE	GREEN	RED	BLUE
GREEN	BLUE	GREEN	BLUE	RED	GREEN	RED	BLUE	
BLUE	RED	BLUE	GREEN	RED	BLUE	GREEN	RED	BLUE

FIGURE 10–6. Stroop task-interference trial. The patient is required to scan down each column, naming the actual color of the word while ignoring the word itself. Each stimulus contains a mismatch between word and color, which creates distraction and demands for attentional focus. The number of colors named in 45 seconds is determined, as is the number of breaks in response set (i.e., reading the word).

Source. Adapted from Stroop 1935.

trolled, focused attention. The task of finger tapping with fluency is useful for assessing demands associated with two forms of response production. Dichotic listening paradigms provide another test for assessing focused attention in the context of sensory selective attention.

Sensory Selective Attention

Tests used in the assessment of neglect syndrome provide a foundation for the assessment of sensory selective attention. For instance, letter and symbol cancellation tasks are useful for detecting abnormalities in both the spatial distribution of visual attention and general signal detection capacity. On the symbol cancellation task, the subject scans an array of letters or symbols and marks a line through or circles all of the *A*'s, or any other designated target symbol (Kaplan et al. 1989) (Figure 10–7). The total time for detection and cancellation of all targets, along with the number of misses and false-positive errors, is determined. Information can also be obtained about the subject's ability to carry out a consistent detection strategy.

Line bisection may also provide evidence for a hemispatial attentional disturbance (Albert 1973). The paradigm of double simultaneous stimulation provides a method for detecting extinction and neglect of stimuli in the impaired hemispace. The analysis of the spontaneous drawings of objects and copying of figures may point to lateral differences in attention to detail or spatial quality.

All of these techniques are standard methods for assessing visual selective attention.

A number of experimental paradigms also exist that may facilitate the assessment of selective attention. For instance, dichotic listening paradigms that involve the presentation of different information to the two ears provide a way of assessing auditory attentional selection under different conditions of discrimination and response bias (Kimura 1967; Springer 1986). However, this paradigm also involves divided attention and reflects capacity limitations. Dichotic listening has been employed in shadowing paradigms, which require the subject to repeat material being presented in one ear (the shadowed ear) while processing a competing message in the other ear. Subjects typically have great difficulty extracting information from the nonshadowed ear during dichotic listening but can detect physical changes in the stimuli to that ear (Cherry 1953). Subjects also show little memory of material presented to the nonshadowed ear, although they attend better to the nonshadowed channel when different modalities are used (Treisman and Davies 1986) and after they have learned to attend to the nonshadowed channel (Underwood 1976).

A comprehensive assessment of selective attention requires the incorporation of signal detection and reaction time methods, either explicitly or implicitly (Green and Swets 1966). Signal detection methods enable the determination of attentional accuracy under different task conditions. A discriminability index (D´) can be derived on the basis of errors due to missing a target and false-positive errors due to responding to nontargets. A response bias (beta) can also be determined that indicates the systematic errors and response tendencies of the subject. Other indices can also be determined, which enable a parametric analysis of attentional performance.

Response Selection and Executive Control

Tests of executive functioning can be characterized by four factors: 1) the capacity to inhibit interference and maintain a pattern of responding; 2) the ability to alternate between response sets; 3) the ability to plan, organize, and derive solutions on tasks requiring hypothesis testing; and 4) the capacity for response generation. A large number of measures of response selection and executive functions are available. Double alternating movements, graphemic sequences (e.g., Rampart figures), motor impersistence, and the go/no-go paradigm (Christensen 1989; Stuss and Benson 1986) are useful for the assessment of simple motoric response control. Tests such as the Trail Making Test (Armitage 1946), the Stroop tasks (Stroop 1935), the Wisconsin Card Sorting Test (Heaton 1985), and the Porteus Mazes Test (Porteus 1965) provide a means of assessing higher-order executive functions, such as goal-directed behavior, response planning, and active switching of response set (Armitage 1946; Christensen 1989; Porteus 1965; Stuss and Benson 1986).

Intentionality is often inferred rather than measured directly, but there are ways of assessing impairments of intentionality. A failure to spontaneously initiate behaviors despite a capacity to respond on command suggests an intentional problem. Failure to persist with motor responding in the neglected hemispace is thought to reflect an intentional disturbance as well. However, more tests of intention need to be developed.

A subject's capacity for initiation, generation, and persistence can be measured in a number of ways. On the Controlled Word Association Test, subjects produce as many words as possible that start with a particular letter (*F*, *A*, or *S*) or that belong to a semantic category (animals) in 60 seconds (Benton et al. 1983; Spreen and Strauss 1991). The total number of words generated is then scored. The response norms vary with age and level of education. Normal young adults can generate 36 *F*, *A*, or *S* words in 3 minutes and the names of more than 20 animals in 1 minute. Normal geriatric subjects should be able to generate the names of more than 13 animals. Information about the subject's tendency to perseverate and self-monitoring capacity can be gained from this task.

Design fluency is a nonverbal alternative to the Controlled Word Association Test (Jones-Gotman and Milner

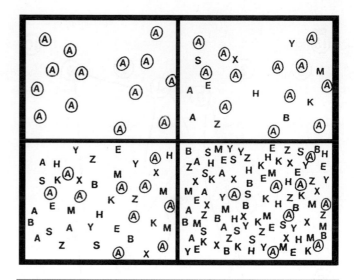

FIGURE 10–7. Letter cancellation. A subject with right subcortical infarction was asked to circle all the A's. Performance declined with increase in stimulus load. Note the relative inattention to the left side of each box.

Source. Reprinted from Kaplan RF, Verfaellie M, Meadows ME, et al.: "Changing Attentional Demands in Left Hemispatial Neglect." *Archives of Neurology* 48:1263–1266, 1991. Copyright 1991 American Medical Association. All rights reserved. Used with permission.

1977). This task requires subjects to draw as many different designs as possible using a set of dots, and the number of figures produced in a set time period is determined. Verbal and design fluency not only indicate the total quantity of response output for a circumscribed time period but also can point to problems with initiation and persistence.

Simple and choice reaction time may be helpful in characterizing latencies for response initiation. Tests of motor functioning such as the Grooved Pegboard Test (Klove 1963) measure the generation of fine motor responses. This test measures the time required for the sequential rotation and placement of 25 pegs in holes on a grooved board. Scores are calculated separately for both the right and left hand. Although motor speed and dexterity may be intact in patients with severe impairments of spontaneous response generation, impairment on pure motor tasks may correlate in some subjects with executive dysfunction, which affects other aspects of response generation. Motor system deficits need to be considered when assessing whether response generation deficits relate to attentional-executive impairments. Occasionally, problems in the motor domain may be a confounding variable in the interpretation of neuropsychological results. However, deficits in the ability to persist on motor tasks may also reflect secondary problems with executive functioning.

This capacity can be measured by interference tasks such as the Stroop Test. Intrusion errors across other cog-

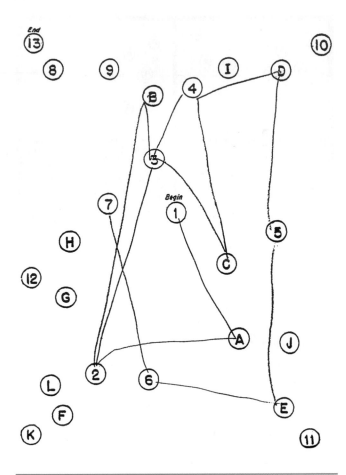

FIGURE 10–8.   Trail Making Test. This test requires the patient to connect the numbers and letters in alternating sequence. In this example, the patient, a 52-year-old man with a right thalamic stroke, failed to maintain the sequence (at numbers 2 and 3), indicating breaks in response set. Impersistence, with neglect of the left side of the page, is also evident.

ters or numbers or when there is a break in the sequence and a particular item is omitted. Each task is timed.

Sorting tasks, such as the Wisconsin Card Sorting Test, measure concept formation and hypothesis testing (Stuss and Benson 1986). Subjects are presented with cards containing features for color, shape, and number. The task is to determine the correct category for a response based on feedback provided by the examiner. Subjects sort cards to the appropriate category but must switch to a new category when the response criteria change. Failure on the Wisconsin Card Sorting Test is often associated with impairments of conceptual flexibility and switching and perseveration secondary to frontal lobe damage affecting the dorsolateral region.

Sustained Attention and Vigilance

Tests that measure performance over time provide a means of assessing sustained attention and vigilance. Currently, the task most widely used for this type of assessment is the Continuous Performance Test (CPT) (Rosvold et al. 1956), which measures signal detection performance over blocks of trials. There are many versions of the CPT, all consisting of the same basic paradigm. Visual or auditory stimuli (usually letters) are presented sequentially. Intermixed among distractor stimuli are particular target stimuli, such as the letter *A*. The task is to respond to the target and not to the distractors. The attentional demands of the task can be modified on many CPT versions by changing the ratio of targets to distractors, the total number of stimuli, the total time of the test, the perceptual complexity of the stimuli and background, the interstimulus interval, and the use of anticipatory stimuli. A variety of signal detection measures—such as misses, false-positives, inconsistency, and vigilance decrement—can be determined to help quantify impairments of sustained attention.

Symbol coding tasks, such as the Digit Symbol subtest, may be used to assess sustained attention by comparing performance during the early and late stages of the task. Similar task modifications can also be sensitive to tests requiring sustained attentional performance in completion of a task involving other cognitive operations. On the Sustained Motor Tapping Test (R.A. Cohen 1993), the subject is required to tap a finger on key for an extended period. Decrement in responding is measured as a function of the number of taps per 10-second interval. The Motor Continuation Task (Wing and Kristofferson 1973) requires the subject to maintain a set tapping rate for a given interval. Performance is determined on the basis of the variance in interbeat interval.

nitive tests may also point to problems with response inhibition. The go/no-go paradigm is a simple test in which the subject is asked to place a hand on the table and raise the index finger in response to a single tap while holding still in response to two taps. The taps should be made on the undersurface of the table to avoid the use of visual cues. Patients with prefrontal lesions have difficulty inhibiting the raising of the finger.

Several tasks require the alternation of response pattern. The Trail Making Test (Armitage 1946) is one of the most commonly used tests of response switching ability and mental control. Subjects are initially required to connect a sequence of numbers by drawing a line between numbers that are placed randomly on a sheet of paper (Trails A). On Trails B, subjects are required to alternate between numbers and letters in ascending order (Figure 10–8). Errors occur when the patient fails to alternate and connects two let-

Many sustained attentional tasks, such as the CPT and Symbol Cancellation, can be modified to increase the demand for focused attention and effort. On the CPT, this can be done by increasing the complexity of target selection (e.g., respond to *x* only when preceded by an *A*). By adjusting parameters such as memory load, interstimulus times, and the presence of more than one stimulus in a target field on a trial, other attentional factors in addition to sustained attention can be examined. This is particularly useful in experimental studies, although it is somewhat problematic for clinical use, because modifying the task demands changes the norms for these tests.

Steps in Decision Making When Assessing Attention

Regardless of the battery that is chosen, the assessment of attention depends on a logical, stepwise decision process (R.A. Cohen et al. 1998):

1. Is the patient fully alert? Is lethargy or fatigue evident?
2. Is activity level within normal limits, or is the patient slow or agitated?
3. Does the patient seem to exert adequate effort?
4. Are sensory, perceptual, and motor functions intact? If not, it is essential to factor in the contribution of these impairments.
5. Is attentional capacity reduced? Do impairments consistently appear on tasks requiring high levels of focus, working memory, or effort?
6. Is reduced capacity general or limited to specific operations or modalities? If it is operation specific, attentional effects may be secondary to the greater effort required for tasks that are more difficult cognitively for the patient.
7. If a general capacity problem is present, limiting factors should be examined in detail. This involves assessing factors such as processing speed and memory influence.
8. Is attentional performance temporally inconsistent? Is there a performance decrement? If so, a more thorough assessment of sustained attention is in order.
9. Is the attention problem limited to sensory selection or to response selection and control?
10. If sensory selective attention impairment is suggested, is spatial distribution of attention abnormal? Is attention also impaired in nonspatial visual or auditory tasks?
11. Are response selection problems related to specific problems with intention, initiation, inhibition, persistence, switching, or other executive functions?

Current Assessment Trends

Technological advances have provided the opportunity to overcome some of the primary disadvantages of reliance on a "paper-and-pencil" methodology. Although traditional neuropsychological methods typically provide useful data about error characteristics, they are not well suited for response time measurement, nor do such measures provide adequate information about interitem variability or change in performance across the task duration (R.A. Cohen et al. 1998). Therefore, employing computerized attention tasks allows for better control of stimulus and response parameters and provides more specific response characteristics. Optimally, signal detection and reaction time measures are analyzed simultaneously as a function of different attentional task demands to provide a more complete profile of attentional performance (R.A. Cohen et al. 1998).

PSYCHOPHYSIOLOGICAL METHODS

Psychophysiological testing provides a potentially rich source of information about the neurobiological substrates of attention. Demonstration of physiological reactivity associated with attention helps localize the brain regions involved in attentional processes and measures the intensity of attention. Although these methods are not widely used in standard clinical assessment, physiological methods are useful for studying normal attentional responses and characterizing disturbances of attention in patients with neuropsychiatric illness.

The two physiological methods most commonly used involve the measurement of either autonomic or central nervous system indices. Autonomic studies use skin conductance response and cardiovascular measures, such as changes in heart rate. Other peripheral responses, such as muscle activity (electromyography), have also been used (Coles and Duncan-Johnson 1975; Kahneman and Beatty 1966; Oscar-Berman and Gade 1979). Heart rate deceleration during sensory processing and selective attention versus heart rate acceleration during effortful attentional processing has been well demonstrated. Other autonomic measures such as pupil dilation, skin conductance, and electromyographic changes also reflect task-specific attentional activation. Studies of the central nervous system use electroencephalographic (EEG) measurement in conjunction with sensory or cognitive tasks leading to a sensory evoked potential response (Hansch et al. 1982; Hansen et al. 1983; Hillyard and Hansen 1986; Hillyard et al. 1973; Squires et al. 1980). The small EEG activation associated with a series of stimulus presentations is averaged to produce an event-related potential (ERP) that can be localized to specific brain regions. Both autonomic and ERP indices provide excellent measures of attentional allocation.

The ERP consists of a series of specific positive (P) and negative (N) voltage deflections. On attentional tasks, the first deflection occurs at approximately 100 milliseconds (N1) and is associated with passive attention to rare events (automatic selective attention). The most widely studied deflection usually occurs at approximately 300 milliseconds (P3 or P300) in normal subjects and reflects task-dependent factors such as stimulus probability, expectancy, and task relevance. The P300 has been linked to conscious deployment of limited-capacity attentional resources.

The N2 and P300 components have been studied extensively in relation to normal aging, psychopathology, and neurologic brain disorders. Slowing of the P300 component is seen in patients with dementia and other brain diseases, whereas psychiatric disorders most often result in decreased amplitude of particular ERP components (R.A. Cohen et al. 1995; O'Donnell et al. 1990). The measurement of changes in ERP in conjunction with different tasks provides a direct means of determining the effect of changing attentional task demands on brain activity.

NEUROIMAGING TECHNIQUES

Functional Magnetic Resonance Imaging

Technological advances in functional neuroimaging continue to provide exciting advances in the cognitive and affective neurosciences. Developments in functional magnetic resonance imaging (fMRI) in particular have enabled investigators to directly examine human brain function associated with neuroscientific constructs such as attention. In general, the paradigms used in these studies are similar to those employed for previous psychophysiological and functional neuroimaging (e.g., ERP, PET) studies, but yield better spatial resolution. In fMRI, brain responses to specific sensory, emotional, or cognitive challenges are contrasted with activity associated with an appropriate baseline control task to identify brain systems related to such operations and to quantify such responses for hypothesis testing across groups or experimental conditions. Although fMRI paradigms usually encompass more than one of these attentional categories, a brief review of some fMRI literature is provided below that highlights each.

Sensory selective attention, particularly visuospatial selective attention, is the attention type that has been studied most rigorously using fMRI. These attention tasks typically elicit frontal, parietal, and occipital lobe activity. Frontal regions center around the middle frontal and medial frontal gyri, frontal eye fields, and anterior cingulate, whereas parietal regions typically include the inferior and superior parietal lobule and the intraparietal sulci (Beauchamp et al. 2001; Brefczynski and DeYoe 1999; Corbetta et al. 1998; Culham et al. 1998, 2001; Gitelman et al. 1999; Kim et al. 1999; LaBar et al. 1999; Nobre et al. 2004; Rosen et al. 1999; Yantis et al. 2002). Others have reported similar frontal and parietal activity with temporal lobe activity during an auditory sensory selective at-

tention paradigm (Pugh et al. 1996). There is strong evidence that visual cortex activity during visual selective attention paradigms maps onto the same regions elicited during actual visual stimulation (Brefczynski and DeYoe 1999; Corbetta et al. 1998; Culham et al. 1998, 2001; Gitelman et al. 1999; Kim et al. 1999; Rosen et al. 1999), and the magnitude of the response in sensory regions may be manipulated by varying attentional focus (Johnson and Zatorre 2005). There have been attempts to dissociate sensory selective attention from related executive processes. For example, parietal areas have been implicated in shifting attention in space, and frontal regions may also be associated with maintaining task and with executing intentional shifts, such as eye saccades (Beauchamp et al. 2001; Nobre et al. 2004; Rosen et al. 1999; Yantis 2005). Findings from these studies suggest that modality-specific attentional activity occurs in the relevant bottom-up sensory processing regions, whereas frontal and parietal regions may be related to top-down attentional processing. Several research groups have examined this distinction by presenting endogenous (top-down) and exogenous (bottom-up) cues to shift attentional focus. Findings are mixed (e.g., Peelen et al. 2004) but suggest that endogenous attentional shifts elicit greater frontal-parietal activity consistent with top-down attentional control (Mayer et al. 2004; Nobre et al. 2004; Rosen et al. 1999).

Studies of *response selection and executive control* have revealed similar patterns of task-related activity. Visuomotor intention has been related to activity in regions known to be associated with the actual movement, in addition to the frontoparietal activation patterns noted in sensory selective attention paradigms (Luks and Simpson 2004). It has also been demonstrated that attended and nonattended movements result in different patterns of activity within primary motor cortices (Binkofski et al. 2002), and the frontal-motor intention network may be disrupted among Parkinson's patients (Rowe et al. 2002). These studies suggest that brain activity associated with attentional bias toward anticipated action may be detected by using fMRI, and that attention to action can be quantified (and may differ) before and during the actual response.

Attentional capacity and focus is frequently studied by variations in attentional load, including divided attention and interference paradigms. Findings from these fMRI studies also report increased activity in the same regions of the frontal and parietal lobes, in addition to areas related to the type of sensory selective attention that has been engaged (Chang et al. 2001; D'Esposito et al. 1995; Drummond et al. 2001; Herath et al. 2001; Jancke et al. 2003; Johnson and Zatorre 2005; Loose et al. 2003; E.E. Smith and Jonides 1997; Sweet et al. 2004, 2006). Activity in these regions has also shown positive relationships

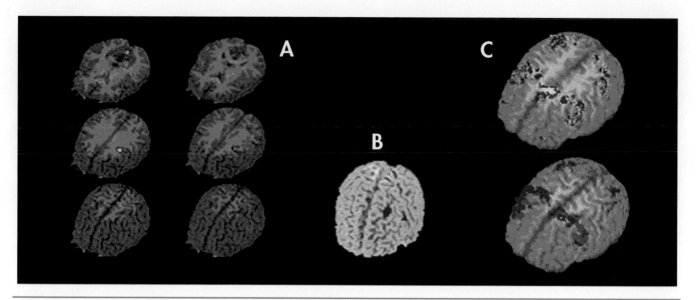

FIGURE 10–9. Brain activity associated with attentional demands. *Panel A.* Brain activity related to the WAIS-III Symbol Search (*red*) and a visuospatial control task (*blue;* Sweet et al. 2005). *Panel B.* Brain activity related to performance level during Symbol Search (Sweet et al. 2005). *Panel C. Top,* brain activity related to the n-Back task among multiple sclerosis patients (*red*), matched control subjects (*blue*), and both (*yellow*). *Bottom,* brain activity related to increased working memory demands (Sweet et al. 2004, 2006).

with increasing working memory load among human immunodeficiency virus (HIV) and MS patients, who are known to exhibit such attentional impairment (Chang et al. 2001; Sweet et al. 2004, 2005, 2006) (Figure 10–9).

Sustained attention and vigilance has often been studied in the context of a deficit among patient populations, such as patients with ADHD (Sunshine et al. 1997) and bipolar disorder (Strakowski et al. 2004). Although group differences have been reported in patient studies, task-associated activation patterns are generally consistent across patients and controls. In one study, healthy volunteers were presented with two continuous performance tasks. Frontal and parietal activity was apparent during both tasks, but dorsolateral frontal activity was significantly greater during the more difficult sustained-attention task (Strakowski et al. 2004).

Taken together, findings for a wide range of tasks support the role of a frontoparietal attentional network that may be reliably engaged, and the magnitude of response depends on the level of attentional demands. The parietal lobes are most implicated in attentional shifts in space, whereas the frontal cortices are thought to be involved in executive control processes, such as maintaining attention, intention, and inhibition. A growing fMRI literature distinguishes top-down and bottom-up attentional processes that remain to be fully articulated; however, it appears that motor and sensory modality-specific attentional processes may be localized to expected regions based on actual sensory and motor functions, while the parietal and frontal regions are responsible for the top-

down functions, such as shifting and controlling, that define each of these attentional domains.

Diffusion Tensor Imaging

Advances in other novel MRI-based methods, including diffusion tensor imaging (DTI), provide additional tools for studying structural subcortical changes underlying attention impairments. DTI measures the random thermal motion of water in brain tissue (Tuch et al. 2003). Water diffusion along directional pathways (e.g., white matter) occurs preferentially along the axis of the pathway (anisotropic diffusion) compared with equally distributed movement (isotropic diffusion) in nondirectional regions (e.g., gray matter). Alterations in myelin (e.g., MS) or changes to the microstructure of axonal projections reduce fractional anisotropy (Beaulieu 2002), and therefore DTI metrics are useful biomarkers of white matter integrity (Makris 1997; Tuch et al. 2001, 2002, 2003; Wiegell et al. 2000, 2003). More than 200 published studies have demonstrated the utility of DTI to examine brain dysfunction in clinical populations (as described in reviews by Lim and Helpern [2002] and Sundgren et al. [2004]), and results are consistent with the pathologies associated with the particular disorder being studied (Ahrens et al. 1998; Beaulieu 2002).

Studies of HIV patients illustrate the potential utility of DTI for studying attention impairments. DTI abnormalities in white matter pathways of the corpus callosum and subcortical white matter have been shown to be related to severity of systemic HIV disease. Diffusion in the

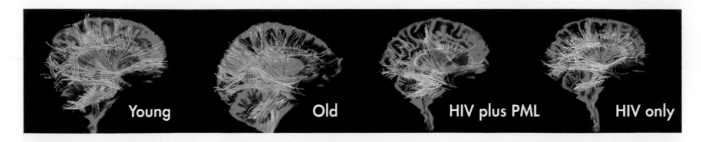

FIGURE 10–10.   Diffusion tensor imaging (DTI) tractography among four individuals who differ by age and HIV status. *From left:* In the first image, dense white matter fiber tracts are apparent in a young healthy adult. In the second image, a decrease in white matter tracts projecting to frontal brain regions is evident in an older healthy adult (age 66). The third image depicts the combined effects of HIV and progressive multifocal leukoencephalopathy (PML), with a dramatic reduction in frontal pathways and also evidence of white matter lesions. The fourth image shows reductions in frontal white matter pathways, without extensive white matter lesions, in a young patient with HIV without PML.

frontal white matter of HIV patients has also been shown to correlate significantly with performance on cognitive tests and glial markers in frontal white matter. Our group has characterized differences in DTI metrics in young (<45 years) and older (>50 years) healthy and HIV-infected adults. Linear declines in total stream tube numbers, length, and measures of coherence of white matter tracts relative to age and HIV status were found (Figure 10–10). Greater decrements in the coherence and integrity of white matter tracts suggest reductions in number, length, and integrity of subcortical pathways between the basal ganglia and frontal cortex among HIV infected patients with advanced age. Furthermore, DTI abnormalities among the older HIV infected patients corresponded with performance on tests of attention and processing efficiency, including Trail Making, 2-Back wording memory response times, and Stroop performance.

These DTI changes may precede more dramatic macroscopic structural brain changes evident on standard MRI. Furthermore, preliminary findings suggest that changes in these DTI metrics may correspond with changes in attention performance over time among HIV and other patient groups with subcortical disorders. In the future, coupling DTI methods with fMRI methods described previously may provide useful clinical approaches for simultaneously assessing the structural and functional brain underpinnings of attention disorders.

CLINICAL DISORDERS OF ATTENTION

In this section, we provide clinical examples of attentional disturbance seen in neurological and psychiatric disorders (see R.A. Cohen 1993).

Impairments of attention may present as relatively specific and well localized or as diffuse and nonlocalizing deficits. Both types of attentional disturbance provide insights into the cognitive processes of attention and the brain mechanisms that underlie these processes. Although localized lesions provide the best vehicle for analysis of the role of specific brain structures in attentional control, nonspecific attentional impairments associated with nonlocalized brain disorders illustrate the influence of metabolic and neurochemical abnormalities on information processing rate, arousal, and a host of other energetic and structural factors that may affect attentional capacity.

LEVELS OF CONSCIOUSNESS

A subject's level of consciousness must be determined before attention can be adequately assessed. Levels of consciousness range from normal consciousness to coma. A patient with normal consciousness is awake, alert, fully responsive, and aware of self and environment. Individuals in deep coma appear to be asleep, unarousable, and unresponsive to external and internal stimuli. With less severe forms of coma, brain stem reflexes are present, and posturing of the limbs may be seen. In a persistent vegetative state, patients may open their eyes spontaneously and in response to pain. They may have roving eye movements and may blink in response to threat. They may fix their gaze on an individual or an object in the environment, giving the false impression of conscious cognition. There is arousal or wakefulness without awareness or meaningful responsiveness. The locked-in syndrome is characterized by intact consciousness and awareness but inability to generate verbal and motor responses. It is usually caused by basilar artery infarction in the pons, causing quadriparesis and mutism while sparing most cortical function. Akinetic mutism, which is usually caused by bilateral infarction in the territory of the anterior cerebral artery, is characterized by a profound amotivational state in which the individual is alert but remains motionless and mute and reacts only minimally to environmental stimuli. Stupor is a level of consciousness in which the patient shows minimal cognitive or behavioral activity yet is arousable. With repeated stimulation, a stuporous patient will open his or her eyes and may even vocalize, but responses to verbal commands are minimal. Abnormal reflexes, tremor, restlessness, or other movement problems are common, and the patient is often described as "obtunded." With stupor, as with all deeper levels of coma, minimal awareness is evident.

Between normal consciousness and stupor, there are many levels of impaired consciousness, usually referred to as *confusional states*, *lethargy*, or *delirium*. The term *confusion* lacks precision but usually refers to a state of decreased clarity and speed of thinking. Confused patients may be able to engage in conversation but exhibit slowness and incoherence, disorientation, and extreme distractibility. Psychosis, agitation, irritability, and a fluctuating level of arousal is common. At higher levels of consciousness, patients may be responsive and able to communicate and may show no evidence of disorientation or confusion yet exhibit inattention or alteration in their quality of awareness.

METABOLIC ENCEPHALOPATHY

Alterations in level and quality of consciousness and attention are hallmark features of metabolic encephalopathy. Metabolic disorders are typically associated with diffuse neuronal dysregulation rather than structural brain lesions and often arise from systemic problems outside the brain. Metabolic disorders affect consciousness and attention by altering levels of oxygen, CO_2, glucose, electrolyte balance, proteins, or other biochemicals in the brain. The specific attentional disturbance depends on the type and severity of metabolic disturbance. Metabolic problems that produce activation are likely to produce restlessness in addition to distractibility and prominent shifting of attention. Psychomotor retardation and lethargy may occur with impaired sustained attention, decreased generative ability, and errors of omission of selective attention. Attentional performance is often quite variable because of the waxing and waning of consciousness.

ATTENTIONAL DISTURBANCE IN NEUROLOGICAL DISORDERS

Stroke

Stroke has long been considered one of the best neurological disorders for the study of brain-behavior relation-

ships because of its rapid onset and well-localized neuroanatomical involvement. Neglect syndrome is the most well-known and dramatic disorder of attention resulting from stroke. Most patients with neglect exhibit impairments of sensory selective attention, although some may have primary problems with response selection and control. Regardless of which attentional process is most affected, all patients with neglect syndrome have a fundamental disorder involving the spatial distribution and allocation of attention.

The defining feature of neglect syndrome is the failure to attend to, respond to, or be aware of stimuli on one side of space. Many variants of neglect syndrome may be observed clinically. Patients may fail to draw the left side of an object when copying figures or when producing spontaneous drawings. Drawings may also contain a shift of the object to the extreme right side of the page. Visual scanning is typically impaired because the patient looks only to the right hemispace, missing information on the left. On testing, patients with neglect often miss targets on cancellation tasks or fail at line bisection, even though they are capable of adequately perceiving these stimuli.

The underlying attentional disturbance of neglect can be demonstrated in a number of ways. Patients with primary sensory disturbances such as hemianopia usually direct their gaze to compensate for their field cut. In contrast, patients with neglect may have normal visual fields yet fail to look at certain spatial positions (i.e., spatial inattention). There is often a failure to direct visual search to one hemispace. In extreme cases, patients may appear to actively direct their gaze or even their entire body position away from the hemispace contralateral to the side of the lesion. They may be able to perceive the entire field but do not consistently attend to all stimuli that are perceived. Hemispatial neglect can be dissociated from primary sensory and perceptual disturbances, such as hemianopia or visual agnosia, on this basis.

Although visual-spatial neglect is most common, patients may exhibit inattention to stimuli presented across different modalities. Somatosensory neglect with inattention to tactile or proprioceptive stimulation to one side of the body is relatively common. Inaccurate reporting of spatial orientation, body position, or direction of movement may be given. Some patients exhibit neglect of one side of their own body, acting as though their left arm or leg does not belong to them. Others may report that their limb ipsilateral to the lesion site has been touched when stimulation was to the contralateral limb (allesthesia). Auditory neglect has also been reported in certain patients. Patients with allokinesia turn to the ipsilesional hemispace when addressed from the side contralateral to the lesion. These phenomena demonstrate that neglect syndrome is not only a disorder of spatial in-attention but often is also a disorder of altered awareness of spatial experience.

It is not uncommon for patients with neglect syndrome to exhibit disturbed emotional experience relative to their neglected side of space. A patient who was monitored in our clinic responded appropriately when approached from his intact side but became hostile and verbally combative when social interactions were attempted from the impaired side. Most patients, however, exhibit indifference toward the neglected hemispace, as well as apathy and denial or lack of awareness of their symptoms (anosognosia). Patients may confabulate and produce elaborate descriptions that are complete fabrications about their neglected side. This may even take the form of a depersonalization of the affected body part. Alterations in affective response and awareness in patients with neglect reflect important relationships among emotional experience, awareness, and attention.

Neglect was once attributed to impairments of sensory or perceptual processes, as well as body schema disturbance (Battersby et al. 1956; Brain 1941; Denny-Brown and Chambers 1958). Sensory hypotheses have been refuted by cases of neglect resulting from lesions outside of primary sensory pathways. Perceptual and body schema hypotheses appear somewhat more viable, because patients with neglect often exhibit coexisting perceptual or spatial impairments. Neglect cannot be explained fully on the basis of a perceptual defect alone but may result from lesions in brain regions directly involved in perception and in the absence of other sensory or perceptual impairments. The fact that neglect across different sensory modalities may coexist in a single patient tends to argue against a perceptual hypothesis, because perception is usually modality specific.

Experimental investigations have confirmed the role of attention in hemineglect syndrome. Manipulation of attentional parameters demonstrates that symptoms of hemineglect change as task demands are modified. For example, symbol detection performance in patients with right hemisphere lesions depends on both the relationship of the targets to distractors and the hemispace to be searched (Rapczak et al. 1989). Patients have greatest difficulty when they must both explore the left hemispace and perform difficult visual discriminations. Increasing the number of distractors relative to targets increases the severity of hemineglect on cancellation tasks (Kaplan et al. 1991) (see Figure 10–7).

The following are summary points for hemineglect, extinction, and hemi-inattention syndromes (R.A. Cohen et al. 1998):

1. Hemi-inattention and neglect are manifestations of unilateral brain lesions. Striking spatial asymmetry in attentional performance is a central feature of these syndromes.
2. Neglect usually occurs relative to the left side of space, which illustrates the importance of the nondominant hemisphere in spatial attention.
3. Although most patients with neglect have a number of common symptoms, the specific attentional disturbance depends on the exact location of the lesion:
   a. Lesions affecting the reticular system that produce neglect also involve significant arousal and activation impairments.
   b. Unilateral basal ganglia damage often results in both hemiattention and intention impairments, reflecting the importance of this system to sensorimotor integration.
   c. Cingulate lesions are more likely to affect intention than sensory selective attention.

Although hemineglect syndrome is one of the most dramatic forms of attentional disturbance, focal lesions secondary to stroke commonly produce disorders that do not involve hemineglect (R.A. Cohen et al. 1998):

1. Focal frontal lesions may produce impairments of focused attention in addition to the common finding of attentional impairments of response selection and control.
2. Thalamic lesions may result in problems with informational gating and selection regardless of whether unilateral neglect is present.
3. Subcortical lesions often produce impairments of arousal, activation, and information processing speed, which in turn may limit attentional capacity.
4. Subcortical small vessel disease secondary to cerebral hypoperfusion may result in dementia; this type of dementia seems to affect attention and information processing efficiency most dramatically.

Although impairments of attention are common sequelae of neurological diseases, attention has generally received less emphasis than other cognitive functions in neuropsychological investigations of brain disorders. This probably reflects the fact that attention cannot be localized to an individual brain system in the same way as can disorders of language or vision. Attention may be more difficult to measure in the normal clinical context than aphasia, apraxia, or other major neurobehavioral syndromes. However, attentional dysfunction is a defining characteristic of some neurological diseases and is an important feature in others, as outlined below.

Multiple Sclerosis

MS, one of the most common neurological diseases affecting young adults, is characterized by multifocal areas of demyelination. Studies of MS have focused primarily on the sensorimotor symptoms, although cognitive dysfunction is common. Approximately 10% of patients with MS exhibit a progressive decline in cognitive abilities that is indicative of subcortical dementia (Rao 1986). These patients have great difficulty on a wide range of neuropsychological tasks, including major problems with learning and memory.

Ten percent of patients with MS develop subcortical dementia, and more than 40% demonstrate cognitive impairment (Heaton et al. 1985). Learning, memory, and executive control are most commonly affected, and impairments of these functions are usually associated with reduced perceptual-motor speed, psychomotor slowing, and attentional difficulties. Many of the problems with learning and memory found in MS patients may be attributable to attentional factors (Kessler et al. 1992).

Patients with MS experience difficulty maintaining consistent effort on tasks. Under conditions of increased information load, they typically show performance decrements. They also experience slowing of processing and psychomotor speed. Although MS patients often have primary motor deficits that may partially account for their psychomotor slowing, it is unlikely that gross motor slowing alone explains the decrease in information processing speed. R.A. Cohen and Fisher (1988) found that the motor impairments of MS patients could be dissociated from the attentional difficulties of these patients.

Of the cognitive impairments that often accompany MS, the most common disorders involve attention (R.A. Cohen 1993; R.A. Cohen et al. 1998):

1. Fatigue is the most common of all symptoms in MS. Fatigue is associated not only with motor effort but also with attending to and performing cognitive tasks.
2. Subcortical lesions secondary to demyelination may disrupt attentional control.
3. Subcortical white matter lesions also reduce neural transmission speed. Slowed processing time reduces attentional capacity and creates processing bottlenecks.

CASE EXAMPLE

A 40-year-old man with a 5-year history of chronic progressive MS experiences waxing and symptoms of chronic fatigue. When fatigue is worse, his thinking slows down and he becomes confused. In this state, it is difficult for him to process information and to interpret events, particularly of an emotional nature. Attentional capacity is easily overwhelmed, which leads to frustration, irritability, and angry outbursts.

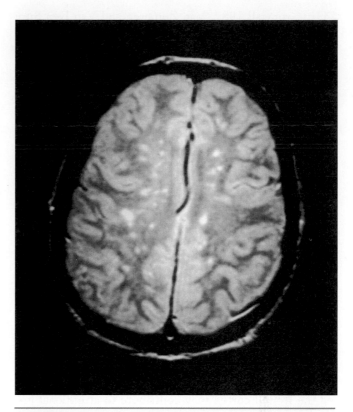

FIGURE 10–11. T2-weighted axial magnetic resonance imaging scan above the level of the lateral ventricles demonstrates multiple areas of high signal in the frontal subcortical white matter in a 40-year-old with multiple sclerosis and attentional disturbance.

Magnetic resonance imaging reveals extensive areas of high signal intensity on T_2-weighted scans in the midline frontal lobe white matter (Figure 10–11). The MS plaques interrupt pathways involved in speed of processing, focusing, and sustaining attention. Systems involved in regulation of mood and impulses are also affected.

Closed Head Injury

Primary brain damage associated with CHI is usually the result of contusions and diffuse axonal injury. Contusions, which are caused by the impact of the brain on the surface of the skull, occur most often on the basal surfaces of the frontal lobes and the poles of the temporal lobes, regardless of the site of the external impact on the head. Diffuse axonal damage occurs due to shearing of axons as they are stretched by the movement of surrounding brain tissue. Axons of the brain stem and cerebral hemispheres are both affected by rotational forces associated with CHI.

The cognitive processes most likely to be affected after CHI are attention and executive functions (Levin and Kraus 1994). Persistent distractibility, poor concentration, apathy, and fatigability are prominent sequelae of

CHI (Gronwall 1987; Van Zomeren and Van Den Burg 1985). Patients with CHI may perform poorly on tests of mental control, concentration, and performance speed. Timed tests are particularly sensitive to head trauma. Vigilance performance is often impaired. The classic tests of attention from the Wechsler Intelligence and Memory scales, Digit Symbol, Digit Span, and Mental Control, are often depressed (Gronwall 1987). Deficits of arousal, selective attention, divided attention, processing speed, and executive functions may contribute to poor performance on these measures. Problems with divided attention may reflect reduced information processing capacity and speed in addition to decreased ability to inhibit interference (Stuss 1987; Stuss et al. 1989; Van Zomeren and Van Den Burg 1985; Van Zomeren et al. 1984).

The attention and executive impairments of CHI usually reflect subcortical and frontal lobe dysfunction. Damage to subcortical midbrain systems impairs arousal. Damage to white matter pathways from shearing forces disrupts the spread of activation from the midbrain systems to higher cortical areas and contributes to slowing of information processing. Contusion and hematoma involving the frontal cortex may contribute to attentional impairment in patients with CHI. Frontal lobe damage is associated with executive dysfunction, including response intention selection and control, as discussed previously.

Epilepsy

Transient changes in the level and quality of consciousness are a common feature of seizure disorders. The acute impairment of awareness and attention is often seen in the ictal or postictal state. Cognitive impairments observed in the interictal state are highly variable and are influenced by a variety of factors, including location of the seizure focus, seizure frequency, and side effects of anticonvulsant medications. Memory impairment is common and may be related to mesial temporal and limbic system dysfunction (C.P. Deutsch 1953; Loiseau et al. 1980; Rausch et al. 1978).

Determination of attentional disturbance in epileptic patients is confounded by problems of seizure frequency and control, etiology of the seizures, and side effects of medication. There is considerable heterogeneity in the brain disorders that can cause seizures, and attentional performance is not consistent in patients with epilepsy. In a study that sought to minimize methodological confounding factors, Piccirilli et al. (1994) found that children with rolandic epilepsy who had right-sided or bilateral spikes had impairments on a letter cancellation task, whereas children with left-sided foci did as well as control subjects. Mirsky et al. (1960) found that patients

with generalized epilepsy had greater problems than those with focal seizures on a test of sustained attention. Several studies have found that patients with epilepsy are more impaired than control subjects on tests of divided attention (Glowinsky 1973). This impairment appears to be related to slowed speed of cognitive processing, which affects attentional capacity (Bruhn and Parsons 1977).

CASE EXAMPLE

An 8-year-old boy was doing poorly in English and mathematics classes. His teacher felt that he was a "daydreamer" because he often stared off into space and had trouble paying attention. She thought that he might have ADHD. His parents became frustrated because he had trouble explaining what went on in school and he was often confused about his homework assignments. Neurological evaluation was unremarkable. Electroencephalography revealed intermittent 3 Hz spike and wave discharges lasting 3–10 seconds, consistent with absence epilepsy.

This is a case of occult absence epilepsy presenting with learning problems caused by brief intermittent disturbances in awareness and attention. Making the diagnosis was crucial in this patient because his seizures were well controlled with sodium valproate, resulting in a marked improvement in school performance.

Alzheimer's Disease

Alzheimer's disease involves a progressive deterioration of most cognitive abilities, with impairments of learning and memory as cardinal features. By the time a patient with Alzheimer's disease is brought to medical attention, a marked anterograde amnesia is apparent. Attentional disturbance is not usually described as a primary feature of Alzheimer's disease, and some authors have emphasized that attention is largely spared in patients with this disorder. However, this conclusion may be somewhat misleading.

Patients with early-stage Alzheimer's disease typically do not exhibit overt behaviors indicative of inattention, such as restlessness, failure to look at the examiner, or diminished attention span on tasks such as Digit Span Forward. Patients with early Alzheimer's disease are usually alert, energetic, and motivated. Yet relatively early in the disease course, problems are evident in the areas of focused attention, capacity, and executive control.

Patients with Alzheimer's disease have difficulty performing concurrent tasks and consequently perform poorly on tasks such as the Stroop Test (R.A. Cohen 1993; Storandt et al. 1984). They also encounter great difficulty on tasks requiring concentration and focus, such as Digit Span Backwards and Symbol Coding Tasks. Simple executive control abilities may be adequate (e.g., double alternating movements), but failure occurs on more complex tasks requiring switching, such as Trail Making. Abnormal responses involving sudden lapses in accuracy are quite common, even on tasks involving sensory selective attention. Patients also show deficits of sustained attention early in the disease course, which may be secondary both to response impersistence caused by frontal lobe damage and to amnesia. Such a patient will begin a task or sentence, suffer a distraction or pause to find a word, and then forget the task requirements or the thread of discourse.

As the disease progresses, performance becomes impaired on most tasks requiring effortful attentional processing (Storandt et al. 1984). Pervasive disturbance eventually develops, affecting all attentional processes. Perhaps the only aspect of attention that is not greatly affected until the latest stages of Alzheimer's disease is arousal and automatic orienting to stimuli. Eventually, all areas of higher cognitive function deteriorate, and the patient is rendered mute and unresponsive, with no capacity to attend and with minimal self-awareness.

ATTENTIONAL DISTURBANCE ASSOCIATED WITH PSYCHIATRIC ILLNESS

Affective Disorders

Difficulties with concentration and sustained attention are commonly reported by patients with affective disorders and constitute key determinants for making the diagnosis of both major depression and bipolar affective disorder (American Psychiatric Association 2000). The opposing energetic and motivational states associated with major depression and mania have considerable bearing on the attentional disturbances that accompany these disorders. Depressed patients tend to exhibit behavioral withdrawal and anhedonia, with reduced verbal output, psychomotor speed, and motivation, as well as loss of interest. They have diminished goal-directed behavior and quickly fatigue on tasks that normally require little effort. In contrast, manic patients are usually very energized, with flight of ideas, pressured speech, and increases in goal-directed behaviors. Although the depressed patient has difficulty initiating and sustaining behaviors, the manic patient may have problems with response inhibition across a wide range of behavioral and social contexts.

Early neuropsychological studies of affective disorders found that cognitive impairments are associated with affective disorders. Learning problems are easily demonstrated in depressed patients, but the basis for these impairments has not been entirely clear (R.A. Cohen and Lohr 1995; R.M. Cohen et al. 1982). There is a strong relationship between expenditure of effort and

memory performance in patients with affective disorders (R.M. Cohen et al. 1982). Difficulty exerting sufficient effort may account for problems in performance across a range of tasks, from difficulties with learning and memory to actual decrements in motor strength.

Impairments on tests of verbal and nonverbal memory also tend to coexist with problems in the area of mental control and attention (Breslow et al. 1977; Stromgren 1977). Depressed patients typically exhibit considerable variability in memory performance. For instance, Breslow et al. (1977) found that depressed patients did not differ from control subjects in performance on paired associate learning tasks, even though performance on the mental control subtest of the Wechsler Memory Scale was significantly weaker for the affective disorder patients. Such findings argue against a primary amnestic disorder in these patients and for an inefficient learning process.

The most consistently demonstrated attentional impairment in patients with affective disorders is in the area of sustained attention and vigilance. Sustained attention performance is proportional to the level of depression and improves when depression resolves (Byrne 1977; Malone and Hemsley 1977). Therefore, the deficits in sustained attention in patients with affective disorders are state dependent (Firth et al. 1983).

Diminished attentional capacity is particularly evident on tasks that require psychomotor speed, attentional focus, and effortful demands for mental control. Deficits are common on Digit Span Backwards, serial arithmetic tasks such as the PASAT, Digit Symbol Substitution, and other tasks that require focused attention and concentration (R.A. Cohen and Lohr 1995; R.M. Cohen et al. 1982). Impaired attentional capacity in depressed patients is most likely a by-product of alterations in behavioral energetics, including arousal, appetitive, and motivational states.

Slowing on the finger-tapping test has been shown to correlate with impaired performance on the Stroop interference test and on other measures of mental control (Raskin et al. 1969). Sustained effort, attention, and cognitive flexibility were found to be impaired in these patients. A relationship between psychomotor, executive, and attentional functioning has also been reported by other investigators (Breslow et al. 1977; R.M. Cohen et al. 1982).

Although effortful expenditure is clearly a problem for depressed patients, a paradoxical relationship between effort and performance has occasionally been described. Depressed patients occasionally fail to show an advantage on Digit Span Forward over Digit Span Backwards, which has been interpreted as evidence that depressed patients fail to exert sufficient effort on less demanding tasks. The assumption is that easier tasks are not sufficiently motivating to activate the depressed patient's attention. Although undoubtedly some depressed patients may benefit from attentional activation by increasing the motivating quality of tasks, most studies do not support the hypothesis that depressed patients perform better on effortful tasks. To the contrary, the performance of depressed patients usually decreases as effortful task demands increase (R.A. Cohen and Lohr 1995; R.M. Cohen et al. 1982). Although diminished psychomotor speed may result in slowed scanning and response times, depressed patients do not typically exhibit major impairments on most sensory selective-attention paradigms. Such patients may occasionally miss targets, particularly over sustained periods of time, but neglect or inattention to specific spatial locations is not usually evident. Problems with selective attention are most likely to be related to response bias rather than actual sensory selection difficulties.

Attentional disturbance is the most common cognitive symptom associated with major affective disorders (R.A. Cohen et al. 1998):

1. Subjective complaints of problems with concentration and focus are among the symptoms that are considered in a diagnosis of depression.
2. Problems with reduced energetic capacity (focused attention) and sustained attention are most common. Response selection and control is often more moderately impaired. Sensory selective attention is usually less affected.
3. Attentional performance is often quite variable over time.
4. The quality of attentional impairments varies as a function of affective state. Manic patients tend to make more errors of commission and failure to inhibit responding, whereas depressed patients make more errors of omission and are likely to show low levels of arousal, with psychomotor slowing. Great effort is often required for attention.
5. Given the strong likelihood of attentional disturbance in patients with affective disorders, it is essential that depression be ruled out or factored in when one is assessing attention associated with other brain disorders.

Schizophrenia

The early researchers of schizophrenia, Kraepelin and Bleuler, reported attentional disturbances in their patients (Kraepelin 1931). They noted perseveration in thought and action, tangentiality, inability to initiate actions or sustain attention, rapid fatigue, and orientation to trivial stimuli. Bleuler (1911/1950) noted that autistically withdrawn patients had disturbances of passive attention, seemed to have little awareness of the outside world, and attended to stimuli in the environment in an almost random manner. These findings suggested to Bleuler that schizophrenia consisted of problems in both the inhibiting and the facilitating components of attention. Bleuler also concluded that these patients had a fundamental disruption of the associative organization of mental activity, which interfered with their capacity for purposeful behavior, organized thought, and discourse.

There is now general agreement that abnormal attention is a central feature of schizophrenia. Deficits across all domains of attention can be demonstrated in patients with this disorder. Filtering of irrelevant information is a major problem, as evidenced by the occurrence of hallucinations, thought insertions, and other positive symptoms. Schizophrenic patients often encounter difficulties on tests of sensory selective attention because of their susceptibility to distraction, which in turn is correlated with the presence and severity of thought disorder (Oltmanns et al. 1978; Wielgus and Harvey 1988). Slowing of reaction time is a ubiquitous feature in schizophrenic patients and may be related to distractibility caused by intrinsic factors such as auditory hallucinations and transient loss of set (Nuechterlein 1977; Nuechterlein and Dawson 1984; Schwartz et al. 1989). Performance deficits are seen on tests of divided attention when concurrent task performance is required. People with schizophrenia encounter great difficulty on tests requiring suppression of interfering information (e.g., the Stroop Test). Attentional capacity and focus, as measured by Digit Symbol Substitution, the PASAT, and other tests that require mental control, are usually impaired. Furthermore, people with schizophrenia have great difficulty with sustained attention, probably as a result of the combined interaction of all attentional problems, particularly distractibility.

Contemporary models of attention deficit in patients with schizophrenia can be broadly categorized into those that emphasize disturbances of information processing and those that focus on disturbances of arousal. Both factors appear to be important in schizophrenia. Behavioral abnormalities develop when the person with schizophrenia is confronted with excessive task demands or becomes overloaded with either internal signals or external information that taxes his or her limited available attentional capacity. This is most apparent when tasks require effortful controlled attentional processing. People with schizophrenia show better performance on tasks that are well practiced and involve automatic forms of attention (Callaway and Naghdi 1982; Neale and Oltmanns 1980). These deficits may be directly associated with disturbances of informational gating in dopaminergic brain systems.

Attention-Deficit/Hyperactivity Disorder

ADHD is characterized by difficulty paying attention to internal and external stimuli, impaired ability to organize and complete tasks, and problems controlling behaviors, emotions, and impulses (Shaffer 1994). Individuals with ADHD often do not achieve their academic, occupational, and social potential (Barkley et al. 1993; Rutter 1983; Shaywitz and Shaywitz 1987). ADHD has become one of the most widely diagnosed disorders of childhood. DSM-IV-TR distinguishes between symptoms of attentional disturbance and hyperactivity/impulsivity and provides criteria for ADHD, combined type, predominantly inattentive type, and predominantly hyperactive-impulsive type (American Psychiatric Association 2000). To meet DSM-IV-TR criteria, the symptoms must be present for at least 6 months; must cause impairment in social, occupational, or academic functioning; and must be present in two or more settings (Table 10–2).

Although attentional symptoms improve with age in people with ADHD, approximately 11%–31% of children with the disorder continue to be disabled by it in adulthood (Gittelman et al. 1985; Mannuzza et al. 1993). The diagnosis of ADHD in adults is now a common reason for neuropsychiatric evaluation, but there is not a separate category for the diagnosis of ADHD in adults. To meet criteria for ADHD in adults, some hyperactive-impulsive or inattentive symptoms must have been present and must have caused impairment before age 7.

The essential features of ADHD are inattention, impulsiveness, and hyperactivity that are developmentally inappropriate. Diagnosis of ADHD is age related, because behavioral norms change across the life span. For example, the DSM-IV-TR criteria for restlessness change from physical evidence of motor restlessness in childhood to a subjective sense of restlessness in adolescents and adults. The diagnosis of ADHD is also strongly influenced by cultural expectations of what constitutes the range of age-appropriate behavior. ADHD is most evident in cultures requiring attendance in schools for long periods of the day, during which a child must stay seated and sustain attention on highly abstract tasks with minimal ongoing reinforcement. Even in cultures as similar as the United States and Great Britain, the frequency with which this syndrome is diagnosed shows surprising variability. Rutter (1983) cites evidence that the diagnosis of hyperactivity is made nearly 50 times as often in North America as in Britain.

ADHD is more common in first- and second-degree relatives of patients with ADHD (Biederman et al. 1990; Faraone et al. 1993, 1994). Genome-wide screens have yielded a number of gene loci, and linkage analysis studies have identified several monaminergic neurotransmitter

---

TABLE 10–2. Criteria for attention-deficit/hyperactivity disorder

Inattention (six or more symptoms)

- Makes careless mistakes, has poor attention to detail
- Has difficulty sustaining attention
- Does not seem to listen
- Does not follow through or finish tasks
- Has difficulty organizing tasks
- Avoids activities that require sustained mental effort
- Loses things easily
- Is easily distracted
- Is forgetful

Hyperactivity-impulsivity (six or more symptoms)

Hyperactivity

- Fidgets, squirms
- Has difficulty remaining seated
- Runs or climbs excessively (children), experiences subjective restlessness (adults)
- Has difficulty with quiet activities
- Is "on the go," "driven by a motor"
- Talks excessively

Impulsivity

- Blurts out answers before questions are completed
- Is impatient
- Often interrupts others

Source. Adapted from American Psychiatric Association: *Diagnostic and Statistical Manual of Mental Disorders, Fourth Edition, Text Revision*, p. 92. Washington, DC, American Psychiatric Association, 2000. Copyright © 2000 American Psychiatric Association. Used with permission.

---

receptor and transporter candidate genes with mildly elevated risk, but results have been inconclusive (Faraone et al. 2005). Male relatives may be at greater risk, although results from gender studies in ADHD vary. Family members of ADHD probands also appear to have a higher incidence of comorbid psychiatric disorders, such as antisocial personality disorder, major depression, substance abuse, and anxiety disorder (Shaywitz and Shaywitz 1987).

Comorbid conditions commonly accompany ADHD in children and adults. Chang et al. (1995) assessed the presence of comorbid conditions in a retrospective chart review of 130 adults referred for evaluation of attentional disturbance and found that substance abuse, mood disorder, and learning disability were present in a large percentage of the sample. Biederman et al. (1992, 1993b) found a high incidence of conduct, mood, and anxiety disorders in children and adults with ADHD.

Structural and functional imaging studies have implicated frontal system dysfunction in persons with ADHD (Castellanos et al. 1994; Ciedd et al. 1994; Lou et al. 1984; Matochik et al. 1994; Zametkin et al. 1993). Deficits in dopaminergic and noradrenergic function have also been implicated in patients with ADHD (Kostrzewa et al. 1994; Satterfield et al. 1994). The ability of stimulants to ameliorate symptoms of ADHD lends further support to the involvement of catecholamines in this disorder. Serotonin may play a modulatory role in ADHD, particularly in relationship to symptoms of mood, aggression, and impulse control (Costall et al. 1979; Halperin et al. 1994). Functional imaging studies have also found prefrontal and anterior temporal hypometabolism in patients with secondary depression (Mayberg 1994). Dysfunction in dopaminergic systems in the nucleus accumbens appears to play a central role in substance abuse. One possible explanation for the high incidence of comorbidity between attentional symptoms and mood, impulse control, and substance abuse is that these systems share a close anatomical, neurochemical, and functional composition in the basal forebrain and anteromedial frontal lobe.

The diagnosis of ADHD can be difficult and is based primarily on subjective reports by patients and family members. It is important to obtain historical information about the attentional complaint from multiple sources (Ward et al. 1993). Situational variations in the behavioral manifestation of an attention deficit pose another diagnostic challenge. Behavior in the office and performance on cognitive tasks in a structured setting may be normal. However, the same individual may be impaired in a less structured environment with competing demands for attention.

For the most part, patients with ADHD have normal intelligence and do not exhibit major cognitive dysfunction. However, certain deficit patterns are observed on standardized tests. Poor performance on three WAIS-R subscales (Digit Span, Arithmetic, and Digit Symbol) are associated with ADHD when general verbal and visual-spatial performance are at normal or nearly normal levels (Kaufman 1979). This pattern is not unique to ADHD; other disorders that affect concentration, working memory, or processing speed also produce this profile.

Impaired sustained attention is a primary feature of ADHD. Impairments are greatest when vigilance is required to detect infrequent information, particularly when this information is not motivationally salient. Hyperactive children exhibit more errors of both omission and commission on the CPT than do children without ADHD, and they also show more rapid deterioration of task performance over time (Sykes et al. 1973). In other studies (Barkley 1977; Rapoport et al. 1978), CPT performance often improved after the administration of stimulants.

Errors of omission and commission on motor tasks requiring selective inhibition of responses (e.g., go/no-go paradigms) provide other markers for ADHD (Risser and Bowers 1993; Trommer et al. 1988). Furthermore, differences in performance between children with ADHD with and without hyperactivity may exist on this paradigm. These impairments on the go/no-go paradigm may reflect general problems with impulsivity (Barkley et al. 1992). Additional research is needed to better characterize the nature of impulsivity in persons with ADHD.

One long-standing hypothesis regarding the nature of ADHD is that the attention deficit results from susceptibility to distraction. Children with ADHD were thought to have an impairment related to the filtering of task-irrelevant stimuli. Yet children with ADHD rarely show problems with performance in the presence of distracting information on laboratory tests (Douglas and Peters 1981). Attentional filtering may not be the major problem in most cases of ADHD.

The primary symptoms of ADHD, inattentiveness and impulsiveness, cause a wide range of behaviors that vary greatly among children. Barkley (1988) has argued that this suggests a more fundamental impairment involving the use of rule-governed behavior, including the ability to use language as a discriminative stimulus for behavior control. If this is true, many of the attentional impairments of ADHD reflect difficulties in the compliance that is necessary for sustained attention in the absence of strong immediate reinforcement (Douglas 1983). Ultimately, ADHD may result from a failure of normal reinforcement in interaction with defective processes of attention and response inhibition.

CASE EXAMPLE: ADULT ADHD, CASE 1

A 38-year-old male nursing student was evaluated for complaints of difficulty paying attention. He stated that he had done poorly in school and "was ignored by the teachers and allowed to graduate from high school without doing the work." He found it difficult to pay attention to what people were saying, because his thoughts were jumping quickly from one topic to another. Sitting still to read required tremendous effort. He always had a very high energy level. He became convinced that he was a failure as a student and that he was fit only for manual labor. He also suffered from significant mood lability and heavily abused cocaine and alcohol. He reported that cocaine made him feel normal. His substance abuse habit became severe, and he admitted himself for inpatient substance abuse treatment 10 years ago. He has been drug free since that time. He has gradually resumed his education but has found that he has to work twice as hard as other students to cover the material.

Neuropsychological testing revealed his intelligence to be in the normal range, but Verbal IQ was 23 points higher than Performance IQ. Scores on tests requiring complex attention were moderately impaired. Achievement test scores revealed performance below expectations in spelling, reading, and arithmetic.

He was begun on methylphenidate, 10 mg in the morning and 10 mg at noon, with an excellent response. He became able to read for longer periods without losing his concentration or having to get up and pace. He no longer had to get up in the middle of the night to complete his assignments. He began to take tests without time limitations in a separate room and began taping lectures to review at home. His class average increased from C+ to A.

Methylphenidate was tolerated without side effects. The dose was increased to 10 mg, morning, noon, and late afternoon, to help with schoolwork in the evening. Supportive counseling has helped him improve his self-image, and he now plans to pursue graduate work in health care.

This case demonstrates a profound example of attentional disturbance that was not addressed in childhood. Subsequent academic performance and self-image were poor. This patient also showed the common comorbid features of mood lability, substance abuse, and poor academic performance. Successful treatment first required discontinuation of substance abuse. Medication, modifications to his academic environment (Table 10–3), and counseling to help with self-esteem provided significant benefits.

CASE EXAMPLE: ADULT ADHD, CASE 2

A 45-year-old woman was evaluated for difficulties paying attention and problems with short-term memory. Her son had recently been diagnosed with and treated for ADHD. She was a college graduate who throughout school had struggled with reading, processing lecture material, and keeping her work organized. She felt that she had to work twice as hard as her peers. She had no evidence of hyperactivity, mood disturbance, or substance abuse. Neuropsychological testing revealed superior intelligence with impairment of complex attention and difficulty with sustained reading and reading comprehension.

She was begun on methylphenidate, 10 mg in the morning and at noon, with a good initial response. The dose has since been increased to 20 mg in the morning and at noon, with an occasional 10-mg dose in the afternoon if she needs to work in the early evening.

This case demonstrates an example of a long-standing disturbance of attention and organization in an adult without hyperactivity, learning disability, or another psychiatric diagnosis. There appears to be a familial pattern.

Treatment with methylphenidate increased attention and organization, which led to considerable improvement in her daily functioning.

The diagnosis of ADHD should be made carefully, with special attention to the identification of comorbid conditions. In a retrospective sample (Chang et al. 1995), 50% of adults referred for evaluation of ADHD did not meet the diagnostic criteria for ADHD. Historical information about the attentional disturbance should be gathered from the patient, family, and additional sources. Adults who were referred for evaluation of ADHD and who had a history of childhood ADHD had a different pattern of cognitive performance than adults without a childhood history of ADHD. (Recommendations for the office evaluation of ADHD are provided in Table 10–4.) Neuropsychological testing can help highlight cognitive strengths and weaknesses, diagnose the presence of learning disabilities, and help distinguish attentional disturbance from an underlying memory disorder. Although cognitive testing can help document attentional disturbance, normal attentional performance on neuropsychological testing does not exclude the diagnosis of ADHD.

The first step in the treatment of ADHD is to develop a problem list in which each problem is weighted by severity. A treatment plan is then constructed that targets symptom clusters one at a time. If substance abuse is present, it must be treated before attentional symptoms can be reliably evaluated and treated. If attentional symptoms are the primary problem, then a trial of treatment with a stimulant should be initiated. If depression is the primary symptom, with secondary attentional complaints, then treatment with an antidepressant should be initiated first.

In a limited number of carefully controlled medication trials for ADHD, methylphenidate and other stimulants were superior to placebo (Elia 1993; Hechtman et al. 1984; Matochik et al. 1994; Mattes et al. 1984; Pelham et al. 1990; Rapport et al. 1994; Wender et al. 1985; Wilens and Biederman 1992). A number of medications have been approved for treatment of ADHD in children, and these medications are commonly being used to treat adults with ADHD as well. Response rates up to 70% have been reported. Responders often report feeling more composed, with improvement in symptoms of irritability, impatience, mood lability, and impulsivity in addition to improved attention, concentration, and organization.

The usual starting dosage of methylphenidate is 10 mg in the morning and 10 mg at noon. The usual dosage range is 20–90 mg/day in two to three divided doses. Most patients do well on 20–30 mg/day. The therapeutic effect lasts approximately 3–4 hours. Some patients notice a wearing-off effect with dysphoria. The medication is usually well tolerated. Jitteriness is a common side effect, and methyl-

TABLE 10–3.   Academic recommendations for patients with attention deficit disorder and learning disabilities

1. Modified test format, including open-book exams, short-answer questions, or multiple-choice evaluations, with a simplified verbal structure for the questions and answers. Having a reader available to interpret questions may be necessary.

2. Access in class to notes of another student or the instructor

3. Permission to tape lectures or workshops

4. Use of a word processor for all written assignments, including essay tests, with spelling and grammar checks

5. Untimed testing because of slow reading rate and difficulty accessing information under pressure

6. Books on tape or the assignment of a study partner who can help in getting the material from the reading assignments

7. Tutoring in coursework if the study partner is not available

8. Testing in a separate room to eliminate distractions

9. Use of a calculator and the ability to bring formulas or to have open-book exams when math is required

10. Waiver of the math requirement in academic settings if accommodations and tutoring are not successful

11. Waiver of the foreign-language requirement if accommodations and tutoring are not successful

12. Limit to one the number of courses with heavy reading requirements

Individualized tutoring is suggested to work on the following skills:

1. Basic written-language skills, including reading decoding, reading comprehension, spelling, grammar, phonetics, and punctuation

2. Advanced reading skills, including comprehension efficiency, main idea identification, and key terms scanning

3. Advanced writing skills, including syntax, use of an outline for term papers, idea development in written form, organization, and proofreading. The use of capitalization should also be addressed.

4. Study skills, including planning how to attack reading and writing assignments, memorization, scheduling, organizational strategies, and self-monitoring for comprehension

5. Test-taking skills, including how to read multiple-choice questions, organization of essay questions, strategies for deciding which questions to answer first, and how to recognize the material studied in the format of the test questions

6. Cognitive strategies to improve organization and to help overcome procrastination. Efforts to enhance concentration for listening and reading should be attempted.

phenidate should not be taken together with caffeinated beverages. Insomnia, headache, nausea, irritability, moodiness, agitation, tics, and rebound phenomena occur infrequently. For patients who have milder symptoms or those who experience a wearing-off effect, a sustained-release preparation (Ritalin SR) may be tried. This preparation tends to have a smoother onset and less of a wearing-off effect. The sustained-release form is given as a 20-mg dose in the morning and at noon. Patients and physicians need to adjust the timing and the dose of the stimulants to find the optimum regimen, particularly for individuals who work second and third shifts. Comparable effectiveness of methylphenidate sustained-release and standard preparations has been reported in patients with ADHD (Fitzpatrick et al. 1992; Lawrence et al. 1997; Pelham et al. 1990). A number of stimulants are now available in once-daily slow-release formulations, and a transdermal methylphenidate patch has been approved. Most patients take stimulants 7 days a week, but some prefer to take them only during the work or school week, and a few patients take them only as needed, before an examination or when projects require sustained attention. Dextroamphetamine and mixed-salt amphetamines are available in short-acting and sustained-release preparations and appear to have similar efficacy to methylphenidate. Pemoline is no longer used because of the risk of liver toxicity (Marotta and Roberts 1998). The U.S. Food and Drug Administration has raised concern about the risk of psychosis in children taking stimulants for ADHD and also has inserted a black box warning about increased cardiac risk in adults taking stimulants (Nissen 2006).

TABLE 10–4. Office evaluation of attention-deficit/hyperactivity disorder (ADHD)

History of attentional complaints

Duration, primary symptoms?

Are symptoms diffuse or specific to modality or setting?

Is there evidence of hyperactivity? Can they sit in class or through dinner or a movie without getting up?

Do they read for pleasure? Do they have problems reading (decoding, comprehension)? How long do they read at one time? Can they recall what they read?

Can they take effective notes in class and follow what is said?

Do they have trouble being organized? Do they misplace things?

Do they keep their room and belongings in good order?

Do they daydream? Do their thoughts jump around?

Are they forgetful? Do they feel frequently overwhelmed?

Do they have trouble completing tasks?

Do they lose interest quickly and shift from one activity to another?

Can they listen to others and keep track of conversations?

Are they easily distracted, impulsive, impatient? Can they wait in line? Are they short-tempered, irritable, and easily angered?

Do they blurt out answers and interrupt others?

Do their moods change frequently?

History from patient and informant

Developmental history; history of brain injury, tics, conduct disturbance

Academic history: highest educational level, grades at each level, best and worst subjects, resource help, special education, repetition of a grade, history of hyperactivity in school

History of depression, mood lability, or substance abuse

Family history of ADHD symptoms

Office tests

Recitation of months of the year backwards, Digit Span

Repetition of a short story

Letter cancellation task

Arithmetic problems: addition, multiplication, subtraction, division

Reading: fluency, comprehension, educational level

Test-free articulation of ideas by asking patients to describe a paragraph that they read or to answer other open-ended questions

Brief writing sample

Verbal fluency

Abstraction

Figure copying

Memory

General information

General intelligence estimation

Observation of problem-solving strategy: carefulness, consistency, and frustration and anxiety levels

Although stimulants remain the first-line treatment for ADHD, there has been a great deal of interest in the use of nonstimulant medications to treat ADHD. Patients who do not respond satisfactorily or have unacceptable side effects with one medication may do well with another drug. Methylphenidate and dextroamphetamine are controlled substances, and prescribing these agents can be cumbersome. Only a 1-month supply can be given at a time, and prescriptions cannot be renewed over the telephone. Though not approved for the treatment of ADHD, the tricyclic antidepressants that block norepinephrine reuptake (desipramine and nortriptyline) may be prescribed in doses used to treat depression. Bupropion, an antidepressant that blocks dopamine reuptake and enhances dopaminergic transmission, and venlafaxine, a mixed reuptake inhibitor, may also be helpful (Biederman et al. 1986, 1989, 1993a; Casat et al. 1989; Pataki et al. 1993; Simeon et al. 1986; Wender and Reimher 1990). Atomoxetine, a norepinephrine reuptake inhibitor, is approved for the treatment of ADHD in children and adults. Liver injury has been reported with atomoxetine. Other agents that may be tried include clonidine (an α-2 receptor agonist) and modafanil (Swanson et al. 2006). These drugs may be particularly useful in patients with a history of substance abuse who are at risk for abusing stimulant medication. There are scarce controlled data on the use of selective serotonin reuptake inhibitors in the treatment of ADHD (Barrickman et al. 1991; Jankovic 1993; Spencer et al. 1993a, 1993b; Wilens et al. 1993). Patients with ADHD and comorbid depression may require treatment with both a stimulant and an antidepressant.

Behavioral treatments for attentional disturbance can be an extremely helpful adjunct to medication. Identifying the time of day when the patient is most productive and advising him or her to concentrate on the most demanding attentional activities during that period will optimize daily performance. Academic tutoring and modifications to the academic program—such as taking untimed tests, taking tests in a separate quiet room, and taping lectures for later review—are often recommended (see Table 10–4). Limiting the number of courses and making realistic career choices will increase the likelihood of academic success. Supportive counseling and education about the illness for the patient and the family can help improve self-esteem. Coaching services that work on organizational skills can help with the development of productive new habits.

Highlights for the Clinician

The ability to pay attention forms the foundation of normal cognitive function.
Disturbances of attention are an important feature of most neuropsychiatric disorders.

This chapter highlights—

+ The *multidimensional process* of attention, broken down into its key functional components

+ *Cognitive tests* used to assess each component

+ Recent advances in understanding the *neural pathways* mediating attention in the brain

+ Advances in structural and functional *brain imaging techniques*, such as diffusion tensor imaging, functional magnetic resonance imaging, and positron emission tomography, that have fueled new understanding of neural pathways

+ *Clinical impacts* of dysregulated attention in common neurological conditions

+ The latest developments in understanding the genetic underpinnings, diagnosis, and treatment of *attention-deficit/hyperactivity disorder* in children and adults

RECOMMENDED READINGS

Biederman J: New developments in the treatment of attention deficit/hyperactivity disorder. J Clin Psychiatry 67 (suppl 8):3–6, 2006

Cohen RA: Neuropsychology of Attention. New York, Plenum, 1993

Faraone SV, Perlis RH, Doyle AE, et al: Molecular genetics of attention-deficit/hyperactivity disorder. Biol Psychiatry 57:1313–1323, 2005

Nissen SE: Perspective: ADHD drugs and cardiovascular risks. N Engl J Med 354:1445–1448, 2006

Salloway S, Malloy P, Duffy J: The Frontal Lobes and Neuropsychiatric Illness. Washington, DC, American Psychiatric Press, 2001

Sweet LH, Rao SM, Primeau M, et al: Functional magnetic resonance imaging of working memory among multiple sclerosis patients. J Neuroimaging 14:150–157, 2004

REFERENCES

Adams RD, Victor M: Principles of Neurology, 2nd Edition. New York, McGraw-Hill, 1981

Ahrens ET, Laidlaw DH, Readhead C, et al: MR microscopy of transgenic mice that spontaneously acquire experimental allergic encephalomyelitis. Magn Reson Med 40:119–132, 1998

Albert ML: A simple test of visual neglect. Neurology 23:658–664, 1973

Alexander GE, DeLong MR, Strick PL: Parallel organization of functionally segregated circuits linking basal ganglia and cortex. Annu Rev Neurosci 9:357–381, 1986

American Psychiatric Association: Diagnostic and Statistical Manual of Mental Disorders, 4th Edition, Text Revision. Washington, DC, American Psychiatric Association, 2000

Armitage SG: An analysis of certain psychological tests used for the evaluation of brain injury. Psychol Monogr 60:1–23, 1946

Arnstein A, Goldman-Rakic P: Alpha$_2$-adrenergic mechanisms in prefrontal cortex associated with cognitive decline in aged nonhuman primates. Science 230:1273–1276, 1985

Barkley RA: The effect of methylphenidate on various measures of activity level and attention in hyperkinetic children. J Abnorm Child Psychol 5:351–369, 1977

Barkley RA: Attention deficit disorder with hyperactivity, in Behavioral Assessment of Childhood Disorders. Edited by Barkley RA, Mash EJ, Terdal LG. New York, Guilford, 1988, pp 69–104

Barkley RA, DuPaul GJ, McMurray MB: Comprehensive evaluation of attention deficit disorder with and without hyperactivity as defined by research criteria. J Consult Clin Psychol 58:775–789, 1990

Barkley RA, Grodzinsky G, DuPaul GJ: Frontal lobe functions in attention deficit disorder with and without hyperactivity: a review and research report. J Abnorm Child Psychol 20:163–188, 1992

Barkley RA, Guevremont DC, Anastopoulos AD, et al: Driving-related risks and outcomes of attention deficit hyperactivity disorder in adolescents and young adults: a 3- to 5-year follow-up survey. Pediatrics 92:212–218, 1993

Barrickman L, Noyes R, Kuperman S, et al: Treatment of ADHD with fluoxetine: a preliminary trial. J Am Acad Child Adolesc Psychiatry 30:762–767, 1991

Battersby WS, Bender MB, Pollack M: Unilateral spatial agnosia (inattention) in patients with cerebral lesions. Brain 79:68–93, 1956

Baxter LR: Neuroimaging studies of obsessive compulsive disorder. Psychiatr Clin North Am 15:871–884, 1992

Baxter LR, Schwartz JM, Bergman KS, et al: Caudate glucose metabolic rate changes with both drug and behavior therapy for obsessive compulsive disorder. Arch Gen Psychiatry 49:681–689, 1992

Beauchamp MS, Petit L, Ellmore TM, et al: A parametric fMRI study of overt and covert shifts of visuospatial attention. Neuroimage 14:310–321, 2001

Beaulieu C: The basis of anisotropic water diffusion in the nervous system: a technical review. NMR Biomed 15:435–455, 2002

Bellack AS, Hersen M: Behavioral Assessment, 3rd Edition. New York, Pergamon, 1988

Benkelfat C, Nordhal TE, Semple WE, et al: Local cerebral glucose metabolic rates in obsessive compulsive disorder: patients treated with clomipramine. Arch Gen Psychiatry 47:840–848, 1990

Benton A, Hamsher K, Varney NR, et al: Contributions to Neuropsychological Assessment. New York, Oxford University Press, 1983

Biederman J, Gastfriend DR, Jellinek MS: Desipramine in the treatment of children with ADD. J Clin Psychopharmacol 6:359–363, 1986

Biederman J, Baldessarini RJ, Wright V, et al: A double-blind placebo controlled study of desipramine in the treatment of ADD: efficacy. J Am Acad Child Adolesc Psychiatry 32:199–204, 1989

Biederman J, Faraone SV, Keenan K, et al: Family genetic and psychosocial risk factors in DSM-III attention deficit disorder. J Am Acad Child Adolesc Psychiatry 29:526–533, 1990

Biederman J, Faraone SV, Keenan K, et al: Further evidence for family genetic risk factors in attention deficit hyperactivity disorder: patterns of comorbidity in probands and relatives in psychiatrically and pediatrically referred samples. Arch Gen Psychiatry 49:728–738, 1992

Biederman J, Baldessarini RJ, Wright V, et al: A double-blind placebo controlled study of desipramine in the treatment of ADD, III: lack of impact of comorbidity and family history factors on clinical response. J Am Acad Child Adolesc Psychiatry 32:199–204, 1993a

Biederman J, Faraone SV, Spencer T, et al: Patterns of psychiatric comorbidity, cognition, and psychosocial functioning in adults with attention deficit hyperactivity disorder. Am J Psychiatry 150:1792–1798, 1993b

Binkofski F, Fink GR, Geyer S, et al: Neural activity in human primary motor cortex areas 4a and 4p is modulated differentially by attention to action. J Neurophysiol 88:514–519, 2002

Bleuler E: Dementia Praecox or the Group of Schizophrenias (1911). New York, International Universities Press, 1950

Brain WR: Visual disorientation with special reference to lesions of the right cerebral hemisphere. Brain 64:224–272, 1941

Brand C: General intelligence and mental speed: their relationship and development, in Intelligence and Learning. Edited by Friedman MP, Das JP, O'Connor N. New York, Plenum, 1981, pp 589–593

Brefczynski JA, DeYoe EA: A physiological correlate of the "spotlight" of visual attention. Nat Neurosci 2:370–374, 1999

Breslow R, Kocsis J, Belkin B: Memory deficits in depressive illness. J Psychiatr Res 185–191, 1977

Broadbent DE: Perception and Communication. New York, Pergamon, 1958

Bruhn P, Parsons OA: Reaction time variability in epileptic and brain-damaged patients. Cortex 13:373–384, 1977

Bushnell MC, Goldberg ME, Robinson DL: Behavioral enhancement of visual responses in monkey cerebral cortex, I: modulation in posterior parietal cortex related to selective visual attention. J Neurophysiol 46:755–772, 1981

Byrne DC: Affect and vigilance performance in depressive illness. J Psychiatr Res 13:185–191, 1977

Callaway E, Naghdi S: An information processing model for schizophrenia. Arch Gen Psychiatry 39:339–347, 1982

Casat CD, Pleasants DZ, Schroeder DH, et al: Bupropion in children with attention deficit disorder. Psychopharmacol Bull 25:198–201, 1989

Castellanos FX, Giedd JN, Eckburg P, et al: Quantitative morphology of the caudate nucleus in attention deficit hyperactivity disorder. Am J Psychiatry 151:1791–1796, 1994

Chang K, Neeper R, Jenkins M, et al: Clinical profile of patients referred for evaluation of adult attention deficit hyperactivity disorder. J Neuropsychiatry Clin Neurosci 7:400–401, 1995

Chang L, Speck O, Miller EN, et al: Neural correlates of attention and working memory deficits in HIV patients. Neurology 57:1001–1007, 2001

Cherry EC: Some experiments on the recognition of speech, with one and with two ears. J Acoust Soc Am 26:975–979, 1953

Christensen AL: Luria's Neuropsychological Investigation, 2nd Edition. Copenhagen, Denmark, Munksgaard, 1989

Ciedd JN, Castellanos FX, Casey BJ, et al: Quantitative morphology of the corpus callosum in attention deficit hyperactivity disorder. Am J Psychiatry 151:665–669, 1994

Clemens JA, Fuller RW: Differences in the effects of amphetamine and methylphenidate on brain dopamine turnover and serum prolactin concentration in reserpine-treated rats. Life Sci 24:2077–2081, 1979

Cohen RA: Neuropsychology of Attention. New York, Plenum, 1993

Cohen RA, Fisher M: Neuropsychological correlates of fatigue associated with multiple sclerosis. J Clin Exp Neuropsychol 10:48–52, 1988

Cohen RA, Lohr I: The influence of effort on impairments of attention associated with major affective disorders (abstract). J Int Neuropsychol Soc 1:122, 1995

Cohen RA, Waters W: Psychophysiological correlates of levels and states of cognitive processing. Neuropsychologia 23:243–256, 1985

Cohen RA, McCrae V, Phillips K, et al: Neurobehavioral consequences of bilateral medial cingulotomy (abstract). Neurology 40:198, 1990

Cohen RA, Kaplan RF, Meadow ME, et al: Habituation and sensitization of the orienting response following bilateral anterior cingulotomy. Neuropsychologia 132:609–617, 1994

Cohen RA, O'Donnell BF, Meadows M-E, et al: ERP indices and neuropsychological performance as predictors of functional outcome in dementia. J Geriatr Psychiatry Neurol 8:217–225, 1995

Cohen RA, Malloy PF, Jenkins MA: Disorders of attention, in Clinical Neuropsychology: A Pocket Handbook for Assessment. Edited by Snyder PJ, Nussbaum PD. Washington, DC, American Psychological Association, 1998, pp 541–572

Cohen RM, Weingartner H, Smallberg SA, et al: Effort and cognition in depression. Arch Gen Psychiatry 39:593–597, 1982

Coles MGH, Duncan-Johnson CC: Cardiac activity and information processing: the effects of stimulus significance, and detection and response requirement. J Exp Psychol Hum Percept Perform 1:418–428, 1975

Colquhoun WP, Baddeley AD: Influence of signal probability during pretraining on vigilance decrement. J Exp Psychol 73:153–155, 1967

Conners CK: A teacher rating scale for use with children. Am J Psychiatry 126:884–888, 1969

Corbetta M, Akbudak E, Conturo TE, et al: A common network of functional areas for attention and eye movements. Neuron 21:761–773, 1998

Corcoran DW, Mullin J, Rainey MT, et al: The effects of raised signal and noise amplitude during the course of vigilance tasks, in Vigilance: Theory, Operational Performance, and Psychological Correlates. Edited by Mackie R. New York, Academic Press, 1977, pp 645–663

Costall B, Hui SC, Naylor RJ: The importance of serotonergic mechanisms for the induction of hyperactivity by amphetamine. Neuropharmacology 18:605–609, 1979

Crick F, Koch C: Towards a neurobiological theory of consciousness. Seminars in the Neurosciences 2:263–275, 1990

Culham JC, Brandt SA, Cavanagh P, et al: Cortical fMRI activation produced by attentive tracking of moving targets. J Neurophysiol 80:2657–2670, 1998

Culham JC, Cavanagh P, Kanwisher NG: Attention response functions: characterizing brain areas using fMRI activation during parametric variations of attentional load. Neuron 32:737–745, 2001

Cummings JL: Frontal-subcortical circuits and human behavior. Arch Neurol 50:873–880, 1993

Denny-Brown D, Chambers RA: The parietal lobe and behavior. Research Publication of the Association for the Research of Nervous and Mental Diseases 36:35–117, 1958

De Renzi E, Faglioni P, Previdi P: Spatial memory and hemispheric locus of lesion. Cortex 13:424–433, 1977

Desimone R, Gross CG: Visual areas in the temporal cortex of the macaque. Brain Res 178:363–380, 1979

D'Esposito M, Detre JA, Alsop DC, et al: The neural basis of the central executive system of working memory. Nature 16: 378, 279–281, 1995

Deutsch CP: Differences among epileptics and between epileptics and nonepileptics in terms of some learning and memory variables. Arch Neurol Psychiatry 70:474–482, 1953

Deutsch JA, Deutsch D: Attention: some theoretical considerations. Psychol Rev 70:80–90, 1963

Douglas VI: Attentional and cognitive problems, in Developmental Neuropsychiatry. Edited by Rutter M. New York, Guilford, 1983, pp 280–329

Douglas VI, Peters KG: Towards a clearer definition of the attention deficit of hyperactive children, in Attention and Cognitive Development. Edited by Hale GA, Lewis M. New York, Plenum, 1981, pp 173–246

Drummond SP, Gillin JC, Brown GG: Increased cerebral response during a divided attention task following sleep deprivation. J Sleep Res 10:85–92, 2001

Ebstein R, Novick O, Umansky R, et al: Dopamine D$_4$ receptor exon III polymorphism associated with the human personality trait of novelty seeking. Nat Genet 12:78–80, 1996

Elia J: Drug treatment of hyperactive children: therapeutic guidelines. Drugs 46:863–871, 1993

Faraone SV, Biederman J, Lehman BK, et al: Evidence for the independent familial transmission of attention deficit hyperactivity disorder and learning disabilities: results from a family genetic study. Am J Psychiatry 150:891–895, 1993

Faraone SV, Biederman J, Milberger S: An exploratory study of ADHD among second degree relatives of ADHD children. Biol Psychiatry 35:398–402, 1994

Faraone SV, Perlis RH, Doyle AE, et al: Molecular genetics of attention-deficit/hyperactivity disorder. Biol Psychiatry 57:1313–1323, 2005

Firth CD, Stevens M, Johnstone EC, et al: Effects of ECT and depression on various aspects of memory. Br J Psychiatry 142:610–617, 1983

Fitzpatrick PA, Klorman R, Brumaghim JT, et al: Effects of sustained release and standard preparations of methylphenidate on attention deficit disorder. J Am Acad Child Adolesc Psychiatry 31:226–234, 1992

Folkard S: Time of day and level of processing. Mem Cognit 7:247–252, 1979

Fuster JM: The Prefrontal Cortex: Anatomy, Physiology, and Neuropsychology of the Frontal Lobe. New York, Raven, 1989

Gitelman DR, Nobre AC, Parrish TB, et al: A large-scale distributed network for covert spatial attention: further anatomical delineation based on stringent behavioural and cognitive controls. Brain 122:1093–1106, 1999

Gittelman R, Mannuzza S, Shenker R, et al: Hyperactive boys almost grown up, I: psychiatric status. Arch Gen Psychiatry 42:937–947, 1985

Glowinsky H: Cognitive deficits in temporal lobe epilepsy: an investigation of memory functioning. J Nerv Ment Dis 157:129–137, 1973

Goldberg ME, Bushnell MD: Behavioral enhancement of visual response in monkey cerebral cortex, II: modulation in frontal eye fields specifically related to saccades. J Neurophysiol 46:773–787, 1981

Goldberg ME, Wurtz RH: Activity of superior colliculus in behaving monkey, I: visual receptive fields of single neurons. J Neurophysiol 35:542–559, 1972

Green DM, Swets JA: Signal Detection Theory and Psychophysics. New York, Wiley, 1966

Gronwall D: Advances in the assessment of attention and information processing after head injury, in Neurobehavioral Recovery From Head Injury. Edited by Levin HS, Grafman J, Eisenberg HM. New York, Oxford University Press, 1987, pp 355–371

Gronwall DMA, Sampson H: The Psychological Effects of Concussion. Auckland, NZ, Auckland University Press/Oxford University Press, 1974

Gronwall DMA, Wrightson P: Delayed recovery of intellectual function after minor head injury. Lancet 4:605–609, 1974

Halperin JM, Sharma V, Siever LJ, et al: Serotonergic function in aggressive and nonaggressive boys with attention deficit hyperactivity disorder. Am J Psychiatry 151:243–248, 1994

Hansch EC, Syndulko K, Cohen SN, et al: Cognition in Parkinson disease: an event-related potential perspective. Ann Neurol 11:599–607, 1982

Hansen JC, Dickstein PW, Berlin C, et al: Event-related potentials during selective attention to speech sounds. Biol Psychol 16:211–229, 1983

Hasher L, Zacks RT: Automatic and effortful processes in memory. J Exp Psychol Gen 108:356–388, 1979

Heaton RK: Wisconsin Card Sorting Test. Odessa, FL, Psychological Assessment Resources, 1985

Heaton RK, Nelson LM, Thompson DS, et al: Neuropsychological findings in relapsing/remitting and chronic/progressive multiple sclerosis. J Consult Clin Psychol 53:103–110, 1985

Hechtman L, Weiss G, Perlman T: Young adult outcome in hyperactive children who received long-term stimulant treatment. J Am Acad Child Psychiatry 23:261–269, 1984

Heilman KM, Bowers D, Coslett HB, et al: Directional hypokinesia in neglect. Neurology 35:855–860, 1985

Heilman KM, Watson RT, Valenstein E, et al: Attention: behavior and neural mechanisms. Attention 11:461–481, 1988

Heilman KM, Watson RT, Valenstein E: Neglect and related disorders, in Clinical Neuropsychology, 3rd Edition. Edited by Heilman KM, Valenstein E. New York, Oxford University Press, 1993, pp 279–336

Herath P, Klingberg T, Young J, et al: Neural correlates of dual task interference can be dissociated from those of divided attention: an fMRI study. Cereb Cortex 11:796–805, 2001

Hill D: On states of consciousness, in The Bridge Between Neurology and Psychiatry. Edited by Reynolds EH, Trimble MR. London, Churchill Livingstone, 1989, pp 56–71

Hillyard SA, Hansen JC: Attention: electrophysiological approaches, in Psychophysiology: Systems, Processes and Applications. Edited by Coles M, Donchin E, Porges S. New York, Guilford, 1986, pp 227–243

Hillyard SA, Hink RF, Schwent VL, et al: Electrical signs of selective attention in the human brain. Science 182:177–180, 1973

Hockey GRJ, Colquhoun WP: Diurnal variation in human performance: a review, in Aspects of Human Efficiency: Diurnal Rhythm and Loss of Sleep. Edited by Colquhoun WP. London, English Universities Press, 1972, pp 1–23

Hyvarinen J, Poranen A, Jokinen Y: Influence of attentive behavior on neuronal responses to vibration in primary somatosensory cortex of the monkey. J Neurophysiol 43:870–882, 1980

James W: Principles of Psychology. New York, Holt, 1890

Jancke L, Specht K, Shah JN, et al: Focused attention in a simple dichotic listening task: an fMRI experiment. Brain Res Cogn Brain Res 16:257–266, 2003

Jankovic J: Deprenyl in attention deficit associated with Tourette's syndrome. Arch Neurol 9:181–189, 1993

Jennings JR, Averill RJ, Opton ME, et al: Some parameters of heart rate change: perceptual versus motor task requirements, noxiousness, and uncertainty. Psychophysiology 7:194–212, 1980

Jerison HJ: Signal detection theory in the analysis of human vigilance. Hum Factors 9:285–288, 1967

Johnson JA, Zatorre RJ: Attention to simultaneous unrelated auditory and visual events: behavioral and neural correlates. Cereb Cortex 15:1609–1620, 2005

Jones EG, Leavitt RY: Retrograde axonal transport and demonstration of nonspecific projections to the cerebral cortex and striatum from thalamic intralaminar nuclei in the rat, cat and monkey. J Comp Neurol 154:349–378, 1974

Jones EG, Wise SP, Coulter JD: Differential thalamic relationships of sensory-motor and parietal cortical fields in monkeys. J Comp Neurol 183:833–882, 1979

Jones MR, Boltz M: Dynamic attending and responses to time. Psychol Rev 96:459–491, 1989

Jones-Gotman M, Milner B: Design fluency: the invention of nonsense drawings after focal cortical lesions. Neuropsychologia 15:61–71, 1977

Kahneman D: Attention and Effort. Englewood Cliffs, NJ, Prentice-Hall, 1973

Kahneman D, Beatty J: Pupil diameter and load on memory. Science 154:1583–1585, 1966

Kahneman D, Treisman A: Changing views of attention and automaticity, in Varieties of Attention. Edited by Parasuraman R, Davies DR. New York, Academic Press, 1984, pp 286–294

Kandel ER, Schwartz JH: Molecular biology of memory: modulation of transmitter release. Science 218:433–443, 1982

Kaplan RF, Verfaellie M, DeWitt L, et al: Effects of changes in stimulus continency on visual extinction. Neurology 40:1299–1301, 1989

Kaplan RF, Verfaellie M, Meadows ME, et al: Changing attentional demands in left hemi-spatial neglect. Arch Neurol 48:1263–1266, 1991

Kaufman AS: Intelligence Testing With the WISC-R. New York, Wiley, 1979

Kessler HR, Cohen RA, Lauer K, et al: The relationship between disability and memory dysfunction in multiple sclerosis. Int J Neurosci 62:17–34, 1992

Kim YH, Gitelman DR, Nobre AC, et al: The large-scale neural network for spatial attention displays multifunctional overlap but differential asymmetry. Neuroimage 9:269–277, 1999

Kimura D: Functional asymmetry of the brain in dichotic listening. Cortex 3:163–178, 1967

Klove H: Clinical neuropsychology, in The Medical Clinics of North America. Edited by Forster FM. New York, WB Saunders, 1963, pp 1647–1658

Kostrzewa RM, Brus R, Kalbfleisch JH, et al: Proposed animal model of attention deficit hyperactivity disorder. Brain Res Bull 34:161–167, 1994

Kraepelin E: Dementia Praecox and Paraphrenia. Edinburgh, Livingstone, 1931

LaBar KS, Gitelman DR, Parrish TB, et al: Neuroanatomic overlap of working memory and spatial attention networks: a functional MRI comparison within subjects. Neuroimage 10:695–704, 1999

Lange KW, Robbins TW, Marsden CD, et al: L-Dopa withdrawal selectively impairs performance in tests of frontal lobe function in Parkinson's disease. Psychopharmacology 107:394–404, 1992

Lawrence JD, Lawrence DB, Carson DS: Optimizing ADHD therapy with sustained-release methylphenidate. Am Fam Physician 55:1705–1709, 1997

Levin H, Kraus M: The frontal lobes and traumatic brain injury. J Neuropsychiatry Clin Neurosci 6:443–454, 1994

Levin HS, Mattis S, Ruff RM, et al: Neurobehavioral outcome of minor closed head injury: a three center study. J Neurosurgery 66:234–243, 1987

Lezak MD: Neuropsychological Assessment, 3rd Edition. New York, Oxford University Press, 1995

Lim KO, Helpern JA: Neuropsychiatric applications of DTI: a review. NMR Biomed 15:587–593, 2002

Loiseau P, Stube E, Broustet D, et al: Evaluation of memory function in a population of epileptic patients and matched controls. Acta Neurol Scand 62:58–61, 1980

Loose R, Kaufmann C, Auer DP, et al: Human prefrontal and sensory cortical activity during divided attention tasks. Hum Brain Mapp 18:249–259, 2003

Lou HC, Henriksen L, Bruhn P: Focal cerebral hypoperfusion in children with dysphasia and/or attention deficit disorder. Arch Neurol 41:825–829, 1984

Luks TL, Simpson GV: Preparatory deployment of attention to motion activates higher-order motion-processing brain regions. Neuroimage 22:1515–1522, 2004

Luria AR: Higher Cortical Functions in Man. New York, Basic Books, 1966

Makris N, Worth AJ, Sorensen AG, et al: Morphometry of in vivo human white matter association pathways with diffusion-weighted magnetic resonance imaging. Ann Neurol 42:951–962, 1997

Malone JRL, Hemsley DR: Lowered responsiveness and auditory signal detectability during depression. Psychol Med 7:717–722, 1977

Mannuzza S, Klein RG, Bessler A: Adult outcome of hyperactive boys: educational achievement, occupational rank, and psychiatric status. Arch Gen Psychiatry 50:565–576, 1993

Marotta PJ, Roberts EA: Pemoline hepatotoxicity in children. J Pediatr 132:894–897, 1998

Matochik JA, Liebenauer II, King AC, et al: Cerebral glucose metabolism in adults with attention deficit hyperactivity disorder after chronic stimulant treatment. Am J Psychiatry 151:658–664, 1994

Mattes JA, Boswell L, Oliver H: Methylphenidate effects on symptoms of attention deficit disorder in adults. Arch Gen Psychiatry 41:1059–1063, 1984

Mayberg HS: Frontal lobe dysfunction in secondary depression. J Neuropsychiatry Clin Neurosci 6:428–442, 1994

Mayer AR, Dorflinger JM, Rao SM, et al: Neural networks underlying endogenous and exogenous visual-spatial orienting. Neuroimage 23:534–541, 2004

McCormick DA: Cholinergic and noradrenergic modulation of thalamocortical processing. Trends Neurosci 12:215–221, 1989

Meck WH: Attentional bias between modalities: effect on the internal clock, memory, and decision stages used in animal time discrimination, in Timing and Time Perception. Edited by Gibbon J, Allan L. New York, Annals of the New York Academy of Sciences, New York Academy of Sciences, 1984, pp 528–541

Mega MS, Cummings JL: Frontal-subcortical circuits and neuropsychiatric disorders. J Neuropsychiatry Clin Neurosci 6:358–370, 1994

Mesulam M-M: A cortical network for directed attention and unilateral neglect. Ann Neurol 10:309–325, 1981

Mesulam M-M: Principles of Behavioral Neurology. Philadelphia, PA, FA Davis, 1985

Milner B: Interhemispheric differences in the localization of psychological processes in man. Br Med Bull 27:272–277, 1971

Mindus P, Rasmussen S, Lindquist C: Neurosurgical treatment for refractory obsessive compulsive disorder: implications for understanding frontal lobe function. J Neuropsychiatry Clin Neurosci 6:467–477, 1994

Mirsky AF: The neuropsychology of attention: elements of a complex behavior, in Integrating Theory and Practice in Clinical Neuropsychology. Edited by Perelman E. Hillsdale, NJ, Lawrence Erlbaum, 1989, pp 75–91

Mirsky AF, Primac DW, Marsan CA, et al: A comparison of the psychological test performance of patients with focal and nonfocal epilepsy. Exp Neurol 2:75–89, 1960

Modell JG, Mountz JM, Curtis GC, et al: Neurophysiological dysfunction in basal ganglia/limbic striatal and thalamocortical circuits as a pathogenetic mechanism of obsessive-compulsive disorder. J Neuropsychiatry Clin Neurosci 1:27–36, 1989

Moruzzi G, Magoun HW: Brainstem reticular formation and activation of the EEG. Electroencephalogr Clin Neurophysiol 1:455–473, 1949

Mountcastle VB, Lynch JC, Georgopoulos A, et al: Posterior parietal association cortex of the monkey: command function from operations within extrapersonal space. J Neurophysiol 38:871–908, 1975

Nauta HJ: The relationship of the basal ganglia to the limbic system, in Handbook of Clinical Neurology, Vol 5: Extrapyramidal Disorders. Edited by Vinken PJ, Bruyn GW, Klawans HL. New York, Elsevier, 1986, pp 19–29

Navon D: Attention division or attention sharing? In Attention and Performance XI. Edited by Posner MI, Marin OSM. Hillsdale, NJ, Erlbaum, 1985, pp 133–146

Neale JM, Oltmanns TF: Schizophrenia. New York, Wiley, 1980

Nehemkis AM, Lewinsohn PM: Effects of left and right cerebral lesions in the naming process. Percept Mot Skills 35:787–798, 1972

Neisser U, Becklen R: Selective looking: attending to visually specified events. Cognit Psychol 7:480–494, 1975

Nissen SE: Perspective: ADHD drugs and cardiovascular risks. N Engl J Med 354:1445–1448, 2006

Nobre AC, Coull JT, Maquet P, et al: Orienting attention to locations in perceptual versus mental representations. J Cogn Neurosci 16:363–373, 2004

Nuechterlein KH: Reaction time and attention in schizophrenia: a critical evaluation of the data and theories. Schizophr Bull 3:373–428, 1977

Nuechterlein KH, Dawson ME: Information processing and attentional functioning in the developmental course of schizophrenic disorders. Schizophr Bull 10:160–203, 1984

O'Donnell BF, Friedman S, Squires NK, et al: Active and passive P3 latency in dementia: relationship to psychometric, EEG, and CT measures. Neuropsychiatry Neuropsychol Behav Neurol 3:164–179, 1990

Oltmanns TF, Ohayon J, Neale JM: The effect of anti-psychotic medication and diagnostic criteria on distractibility in schizophrenia. J Psychiatr Res 14:81–91, 1978

Oscar-Berman M, Gade A: Electrodermal measures of arousal in humans with cortical or subcortical brain damage, in The Orienting Reflex in Humans. Edited by Kimmel H, Van Olst E, Orlebeke J. Hillsdale, NJ, Lawrence Erlbaum, 1979, pp 665–676

Owens A, James M, Leigh PN, et al: Fronto-striatal cognitive deficits at different stages of Parkinson's disease. Brain 115:1727–1751, 1992

Parasuraman R: Response bias and physiological reactivity. J Psychol 91:309–313, 1975

Parasuraman R: Sustained attention in detection and discrimination, in Varieties of Attention. Edited by Parasuraman R, Davies DR. New York, Academic Press, 1984, pp 243–289

Pardo JV, Fox PT, Raichle ME: Localization of a human system for sustained attention by positron emission topography. Nature 349:61–64, 1991

Pataki CS, Carlson GA, Kelly KL, et al: Side effects of methylphenidate and desipramine alone and in combination in children. J Am Acad Child Adolesc Psychiatry 32:1065–1072, 1993

Pavlov IP: Conditioned Reflexes. London, Oxford University Press, 1927

Peelen MV, Heslenfeld DJ, Theeuwes J: Endogenous and exogenous attention shifts are mediated by the same large-scale neural network. Neuroimage 22:822–830, 2004

Pelham WE, Greenslade KE, Vodde-Hamilton M, et al: Relative efficacy of long-acting stimulants on children with attention deficit–hyperactivity disorder: a comparison of standard methylphenidate, sustained-release methylphenidate, sustained-release dextroamphetamine, and pemoline. Pediatrics 86:226–237, 1990

Petersen SE, Fox PT, Posner MI, et al: Positron emission tomographic studies of the processing of single words. J Cogn Neurosci 1:153–170, 1989

Peterson LR, Peterson MJ: Short-term retention of individual verbal items. J Exp Psychol 58:193–198, 1959

Piccirilli M, Alessandro P, Sciarma T, et al: Attention problems in epilepsy: possible significance of the epileptogenic focus. Epilepsia 35:1091–1096, 1994

Picton T, Stuss D: Neurobiology of conscious experience. Curr Opin Neurobiol 4:256–265, 1994

Porteus SD: Porteus Maze Test: Fifty Years' Application. New York, Psychological Corporation, 1965

Posner MI: Chronometric explorations of the mind. New York, Oxford University Press, 1986

Posner MI, Boies SJ: Components of attention. Psychol Rev 78:391–408, 1971

Posner MI, Cohen Y: Facilitation and inhibition in shifts of visual attention, in Attention and Performance X. Edited by Bouma H, Bowhuis D. Hillsdale, NJ, Lawrence Erlbaum, 1984, pp 532–542

Posner MI, Walker JA, Friedrich FA, et al: How do the parietal lobes direct covert attention? Neuropsychologia 25:135–145, 1987

Pribram KH: The neurobehavioral analysis of limbic forebrain mechanisms: revision and progress report, in Advances in the Study of Behavior, Vol 2. Edited by Lehrman DS, Hinde RA, Shaw E. New York, Academic Press, 1969, pp 297–332

Pugh KR, Shaywitz, BA, Shaywitz SE, et al: Auditory selective attention: an fMRI investigation. Neuroimage 4:159–173, 1996

Rao SM: Neuropsychology of multiple sclerosis: a critical review. J Clin Exp Neuropsychol 8:503–542, 1986

Rapczak S, Verfaellie M, Fleet WS, et al: Selective attention in hemispatial neglect. Arch Neurol 46:178–182, 1989

Rapoport JL: Basal ganglia dysfunction as a proposed cause of obsessive compulsive disorder, in Psychopathology and the Brain. Edited by Carroll BJ, Barrett JE. New York, Raven, 1991, pp 77–95

Rapoport JL, Buchsbaum MS, Zahn TP, et al: Dextroamphetamine: cognitive and behavioral effects in normal prepubertal boys. Science 199:560–563, 1978

Rapport MD, Denney C, DuPaul GJ, et al: Attention deficit disorder and methylphenidate: normalization rates, clinical effectiveness and response prediction in 76 children. J Am Acad Child Adolesc Psychiatry 33:882–893, 1994

Raskin DC, Kotses H, Bever J: Autonomic indicators of orienting and defensive reflexes. J Exp Psychol 80:423–433, 1969

Rausch R, Lieb JP, Crandall PH: Neuropsychologic correlates of depth spike activity in epileptic patients. Arch Neurol 35:699–705, 1978

Risser MG, Bowers TG: Cognitive and neuropsychological characteristics of attention deficit hyperactivity disorder in children receiving stimulant medications. Percept Mot Skills 77:1023–1031, 1993

Rosen AC, Rao SM, Caffarra P, et al: Neural basis of endogenous and exogenous spatial orienting: a functional MRI study. J Cogn Neurosci 11:135–152, 1999

Rosvold HE, Mirsky AF, Sarandon I, et al: A continuous performance test of brain damage. J Consult Clin Psychol 20:343–350, 1956

Rowe J, Stephan KE, Friston K, et al: Attention to action in Parkinson's disease: impaired effective connectivity among frontal cortical regions. Brain 125:276–289, 2002

Rutter M: Issues and prospects in developmental neuropsychiatry, in Developmental Neuropsychiatry. Edited by Rutter M. New York, Guilford, 1983, pp 577–598

Salloway S: Diagnosis and treatment of patients with frontal lobe syndromes. J Neuropsychiatry Clin Neurosci 6:388–398, 1994

Salloway S, Cummings J: Subcortical disease and neuropsychiatric illness. J Neuropsychiatry Clin Neurosci 6:93–99, 1994

Salloway S, Rasmussen S, Malloy P: Resolution of long-standing obsessive compulsive disorder following left anteromedial thalamic infarction (abstract). Neurology 45 (suppl 14): A167, 1995

Sato H, Hata Y, Hagihara K, et al: Effects of cholinergic depletion on neuron activities in the cat visual cortex. J Neurophysiol 58:781–794, 1987

Satterfield JH, Schell AM, Nicholas T: Preferential neural processing of attended stimuli in attention-deficit hyperactivity disorder and normal boys. Psychophysiology 31:1–10, 1994

Scheibel AB: The problem of selective attention: a possible structural substrate, in Brain Mechanisms and Perceptual Awareness. Edited by Pompeiano O, Marsan CA. New York, Raven, 1981, pp 319 326

Schneider JS, Sun ZQ, Roeltgen DP: Effects of dopamine agonists on delayed response performance in chronic low-dose MPTP-treated monkeys. Pharmacol Biochem Behav 48:235–240, 1994

Schneider W, Shiffrin RM: Controlled and automatic human information processing, I: detection, search, and attention. Psychol Rev 84:1–66, 1977

Schwartz F, Carr AC, Munich RL, et al: Reaction time impairment in schizophrenia and affective illness: the role of attention. Biol Psychiatry 25:540–548, 1989

Shaffer D: Attention deficit hyperactivity disorder in adults. Am J Psychiatry 151:633–637, 1994

Shannon CE, Weaver W: The Mathematical Theory of Communication. Urbana, University of Illinois Press, 1949

Shaywitz SE, Shaywitz BA: Attention deficit disorder: current perspectives. Pediatr Neurol 3:129–135, 1987

Shekim WO, Bylund DB, Hodges K, et al: Platelet alpha 2–adrenergic receptor binding and the effects of d-amphetamine in boys with attention deficit hyperactivity disorder. Neuropsychobiology 29:120–124, 1994

Shenker A: The mechanism of action of drugs used to treat attention-deficit hyperactivity disorder: focus on catecholamine receptor pharmacology. Advances in Psychiatry 30:337–381, 1992

Shute CC, Lewis PR: The ascending cholinergic reticular system, neocortical, olfactory and subcortical projections. Brain 90:497–520, 1967

Siddle D, Stephenson D, Spinks JA: Elicitation and habituation of the orienting response, in Orienting and Habituation: Perspectives in Human Research. Edited by Siddle D. New York, Wiley, 1983, pp 109–182

Simeon JG, Ferguson HB, Van Wyck Fleet J: Bupropion effects in attention deficit and conduct disorders. Can J Psychiatry 31:581–585, 1986

Smith A: Symbol Digit Modalities Test Manual. Los Angeles, CA, Western Psychological Service, 1973

Smith EE, Jonides J: Working memory: a view from neuroimaging. Cognit Psychol 33:5–42, 1997

Spencer T, Biederman J, Kerman K, et al: Desipramine treatment of children with attention-deficit hyperactivity disorder and tic disorder or Tourette's syndrome. J Am Acad Child Adolesc Psychiatry 32:354–360, 1993a

Spencer T, Biederman J, Steingard R, et al: Bupropion exacerbates tics in children with attention-deficit hyperactivity disorder and Tourette's syndrome. J Am Acad Child Adolesc Psychiatry 32:205–210, 1993b

Spreen O, Strauss E: A Compendium of Neuropsychological Tests. New York, Oxford University Press, 1991

Springer SP: Dichotic listening, in Experimental Techniques in Human Neuropsychology. Edited by Hannay J. New York, Oxford University Press, 1986, pp 138–166

Squires KC, Chippendale TJ, Wrege KS, et al: Electrophysiological assessment of mental function in aging and dementia, in Aging in the 1980s. Edited by Poon LW. Washington, DC, American Psychological Association, 1980, pp 82–94

Steriade M, Glenn M: The neocortical and caudate projections of intralaminal thalamic neurons and their synaptic excitation from the thalamic reticular core. J Neurophysiol 48:352–371, 1982

Storandt M, Botwinick J, Danzinger WL, et al: Psychometric differentiation of mild senile dementia of the Alzheimer type. Arch Neurol 41:497–499, 1984

Strakowski SM, Adler CM, Holland SK, et al: A preliminary FMRI study of sustained attention in euthymic, unmedicated bipolar disorder. Neuropsychopharmacology 29:1734–1740, 2004

Stromgren LS: The influence of depression on memory. Acta Psychiatr Scand 56:109–128, 1977

Stroop JR: Studies of interference in serial verbal reactions. J Exp Psychol 18:643–662, 1935

Stuss DT: Contribution of frontal lobe injury to cognitive impairment after closed head injury: methods of assessment and recent findings, in Neurobehavioral Recovery From Head Injury. Edited by Levin HS, Grafman J, Eisenberg HM. New York, Oxford University Press, 1987, pp 166–177

Stuss DT, Benson DF: The Frontal Lobes. New York, Raven, 1986

Stuss DT, Stethem LL, Hugenholtz H, et al: Reaction time after head injury: fatigue, divided and focused attention, and consistency of performance. J Neurol Neurosurg Psychiatry 52:742–748, 1989

Sundgren PC, Dong Q, Gomez-Hassan D, et al: Diffusion tensor imaging of the brain: review of clinical applications. Neuroradiology 46:339–350, 2004

Sunshine JL, Lewin JS, Wu DH, et al: Functional MR to localize sustained visual attention activation in patients with attention deficit hyperactivity disorder: a pilot study. AJNR Am J Neuroradiol 18:633–637, 1997

Swanson JM, Greenhill LL, Lopez FA, et al: Modafinil film-coated tablets in children and adolescents with attention-deficit/hyperactivity disorder: results of a randomized, double-blind, placebo controlled, fixed-dose study followed by abrupt discontinuation. J Clin Psychiatry 67:137–147, 2006

Swedo SE, Pietrini P, Leonard HL, et al: Cerebral glucose metabolism in childhood-onset obsessive compulsive disorder: revisualization during pharmacotherapy. Arch Gen Psychiatry 49:690–694, 1992

Sweet LH, Rao SM, Primeau M, et al: Functional magnetic resonance imaging of working memory among multiple sclerosis patients. J Neuroimaging 14:150–157, 2004

Sweet LH, Paskavitz JF, O'Connor MJ, et al: FMRI correlates of the WAIS-III symbol search subtest. J Int Neuropsychol Soc 11:471–476, 2005

Sweet LH, Rao SM, Primeau M, et al: Functional magnetic resonance imaging response to increased verbal working memory demands among patients with multiple sclerosis. Hum Brain Mapp 27:28–36, 2006

Sykes DH, Douglas VI, Morgenstern G: Sustained attention in hyperactive children. J Child Psychol Psychiatry 14:213–220, 1973

Treisman AM: Strategies and models of selective attention. Psychol Rev 76:282–299, 1969

Treisman AM, Davies A: Divided attention to ear and eye, in Attention and Performance IV. Edited by Kornblum S. New York, Academic Press, 1986, pp 101–117

Treisman AM, Geffen G: Selective attention: perception or response? Q J Exp Psychol 19:1–18, 1967

Trommer BL, Hoeppner JB, Lorber R, et al: The go–no-go paradigm in attention deficit disorder. Ann Neurol 24:610–614, 1988

Tuch DS, Wedeen VJ, Dale AM, et al: Conductivity tensor mapping of the human brain using diffusion tensor MRI. Proc Natl Acad Sci U S A 98:11697–11701, 2001

Tuch DS, Reese TG, Wiegell MR, et al: High angular resolution diffusion imaging reveals intravoxel white matter fiber heterogeneity. Magn Reson Med 48:577–582, 2002

Tuch DS, Reese TG, Wiegell MR, et al: Diffusion MRI of complex neural architecture. Neuron 40:885–895, 2003

Underwood G: Attention and Memory. New York, Pergamon, 1976

Van Zomeren AH, Van Den Burg W: Residual complaints of patients 2 years after severe head injury. J Neurol Neurosurg Psychiatry 48:21–28, 1985

Van Zomeren AH, Brouwer WH, Deelman BG: Attentional deficits: the riddles of selectivity, speed and alertness, in Closed Head Injury: Psychological, Social and Family Consequences. Edited by Brooks N. New York, Oxford University Press, 1984, pp 74–107

Verfaellie M, Bowers D, Heilman KM: Attentional factors in the occurrence of stimulus-response compatibility effects. Neuropsychologia 26:435–444, 1988

Vernon PA: Speed of Information Processing and Intelligence. Norwood, NJ, Ablex, 1987

Ward MF, Wender PH, Reimherr FW: The Wender Utah Rating Scale: an aid in the retrospective diagnosis of childhood attention deficit hyperactivity disorder. Am J Psychiatry 150:885–890, 1993

Wechsler D: A standardized memory scale for clinical use. J Psychol 19:87–95, 1945

Wechsler D: Wechsler Adult Intelligence Scale, Revised. San Antonio, TX, Psychological Corporation, 1981

Wender PH, Reimher FW: Bupropion treatment of ADHD in adults. Am J Psychiatry 147:1018–1020, 1990

Wender PH, Reimherr FW, Wood D, et al: A controlled study of methylphenidate in the treatment of attention deficit disorder, residual type, in adults. Am J Psychiatry 142:547–552, 1985

Wiegell MR, Larsson HB, Wedeen VJ: Fiber crossing in human brain depicted with diffusion tensor MR imaging. Radiology 217:897–903, 2000

Wiegell MR, Tuch DS, Larsson HB, et al: Automatic segmentation of thalamic nuclei from diffusion tensor magnetic resonance imaging. Neuroimage 19:391–401, 2003

Wielgus MS, Harvey PD: Dichotic listening and recall in schizophrenia and mania. Schizophr Bull 14:689–700, 1988

Wilens TE, Biederman J: The stimulants. Psychiatr Clin North Am 15:191–222, 1992

Wilens TE, Biederman J, Geist DE, et al: Nortriptyline in the treatment of ADHD: a chart review of 58 cases. J Am Acad Child Adolesc Psychiatry 32:343–349, 1993

Wing AN, Kristofferson AB: Response delays and the timing of discrete motor responses. Perception and Psychophymology 14:5–12, 1973

Yantis S: How visual salience wins the battle for awareness. Nat Neurosci 8:975–977, 2005

Yantis S, Schwarzbach J, Serences JT, et al: Transient neural activity in human parietal cortex during spatial attention shifts. Nat Neurosci 5:995–1002, 2002

Zametkin AJ, Liebenauer M, Fitzgerald GA, et al: Brain metabolism in teenagers with attention deficit hyperactivity disorder. Arch Gen Psychiatry 50:333–340, 1993

11

NEUROPSYCHIATRIC ASPECTS OF DELIRIUM

Paula T. Trzepacz, M.D.

David J. Meagher, M.D., M.R.C.Psych.

Delirium is a commonly occurring neuropsychiatric syndrome primarily, but not exclusively, characterized by impairment in cognition, which causes a "confusional state." Delirium is a state of consciousness between normal alertness and awakeness and stupor or coma (Figure 11–1). Delirium may have a rapid, forceful onset with many symptoms, or it may be preceded by a subacute "subclinical" delirium with gradual changes over the course of a few days, such as alterations in sleep pattern or aspects of cognition. Precise clinical delineation between severe delirium and stupor is difficult when the delirium presents as hypoactive. Emergence from coma usually involves a period of delirium before normal consciousness is achieved, except in drug-induced comatose states (Ely and Dittus 2004; McNicoll et al. 2003).

Because delirium has a wide variety of underlying etiologies—identification of which is part of clinical management—it is considered a syndrome and not a unitary disorder. It may, however, represent dysfunction of a final common neural pathway that leads to its characteristic symptoms. Its broad constellation of symptoms includes not only the diffuse cognitive deficits implicit for its diagnosis but also delusions, perceptual disturbances, affective lability, language abnormalities, disordered thought processes, sleep-wake cycle disturbance, and psychomotor changes. Table 11–1 presents details of symptoms of delirium that affect nearly every neuropsychiatric do-

main, including characteristic features that help differentiate delirium from other psychiatric disorders.

Unlike symptoms of most other psychiatric disorders, delirium symptoms typically fluctuate in intensity over a 24-hour period. During this characteristic waxing and waning of symptoms, relatively lucid or quiescent periods often occur. In milder cases, such periods involve a significant diminution or even an apparent resolution of symptoms. Daily Delirium Rating Scale (DRS) ratings of postoperative patients showed patterns where symptoms diminished but reappeared consistent with either serial short episodes or diminution to subclinical levels (Rudberg et al. 1997). In addition, fluctuation in the level of symptom severity may relate to shifts between hypoactive and hyperactive periods or disruption of the sleep-wake cycle.

Much research in recent decades has focused on the elderly person with delirium. However, delirium can occur at any age, and the less mature neural pathways of children may put them at high risk. Although delirium in children is vastly understudied, descriptions indicate that symptoms are essentially identical to those in adults (Platt et al. 1994b; Prugh et al. 1980; Turkel et al. 2003, 2006).

Delirium is the accepted term to denote acute disturbances of global cognitive function, encompassing a unitary syndrome with multiple possible different etiologies, as defined in both DSM-IV/DSM-IV-TR and ICD-10 research classification systems (American Psychiatric Association

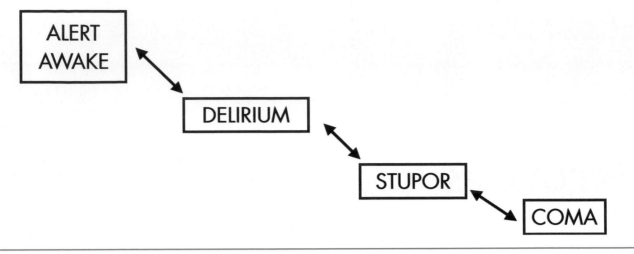

FIGURE 11–1.   Continuum of level of consciousness.

1994, 2000; World Health Organization 1992). Unfortunately, multiple synonyms, based on the etiology or setting in which delirium is encountered, persist both in the literature and between disciplines in clinical practice. Examples include *acute confusional state, intensive care unit (ICU) psychosis, hepatic encephalopathy, toxic psychosis, acute brain failure,* and *posttraumatic amnesia.* Terms such as *acute brain failure* and *acute organic brain syndrome* more accurately highlight the global nature and acute onset of cerebral cortical deficits in patients with delirium, although they lack specificity from other cognitive mental disorders. Furthermore, the term *reversible cognitive deficit* is used in geriatric literature but is poorly defined and not synonymous with delirium; it could instead represent subclinical delirium or cognitive impairment related to many other causes (e.g., pain, poor sleep, medication adverse events). Recent research shows that DSM-IV-TR delirium occurs after traumatic brain injury (Sherer et al. 2005) despite misnomers and poor recognition by nonpsychiatrists. Consistent and proper use of the term *delirium* will greatly enhance medical communication, diagnosis, and research.

DIAGNOSIS

DIAGNOSTIC CRITERIA SYSTEMS

Specific diagnostic criteria for delirium did not appear in the first two editions of the *Diagnostic and Statistical Manual of Mental Disorders* (DSM and DSM-II; American Psychiatric Association 1952, 1968) or in Research Diagnostic Criteria (RDC). Diagnostic criteria for delirium first appeared in DSM-III (American Psychiatric Association 1980). Thus, early clinical reports and research were affected by this lack of diagnostic specificity. Symptom rating scales for delirium began to appear around the time of DSM-III.

DSM was first published in 1952 and described acute and chronic brain syndromes. Most forms of delirium were encompassed within the "acute, reversible" category and were characterized by impairments of orientation, memory, all intellectual functions, and judgment, as well as lability and shallowness of affect. Other disturbances, such as hallucinations and delusions, were considered secondary to the disturbance of the sensorium. Causes of delirium were specifically noted—for example, "acute brain syndrome associated with cerebrovascular accident" (this notation of medical etiology returned in DSM-IV).

DSM-II described two organic brain syndromes, psychotic and nonpsychotic types, each with an acute or chronic delineation. DSM-II maintained the same five symptoms as DSM. DSM-III first described symptoms and diagnostic criteria for the syndrome termed *delirium.* Delirium was distinguished from dementia and other organic mental disorders; each was identified by its own explicit criteria. Some revisions were made in DSM-III-R (American Psychiatric Association 1987), especially to the major criterion involving inattention and altered consciousness.

DSM-IV (as well as its text revision, DSM-IV-TR) (see Table 11–2) has five categories of delirium; the criteria are the same for each category except the one for etiology. The categories are delirium due to 1) a general medical condition, 2) substance intoxication, 3) substance withdrawal, 4) multiple etiologies, and 5) not otherwise specified. This notation of etiology in DSM-IV is reminiscent of the first DSM.

DSM-III through DSM-IV-TR include efforts to further clarify the major criterion describing altered state of consciousness. This criterion has been considered as either inattention or "clouding of consciousness." The latter term is obfuscating because the elements of consciousness that are altered are not specified, nor is it clear

TABLE 11–1. Signs and symptoms of delirium

Diffuse cognitive deficits

Attention

Orientation (time, place, person)

Memory (short- and long-term; verbal and visual)

Visuoconstructional ability

Executive functions

Temporal course

Acute or abrupt onset

Fluctuating severity of symptoms over 24-hour period

Usually reversible

Subclinical syndrome may precede and/or follow the episode

Psychosis

Perceptual disturbances (especially visual), including illusions, hallucinations, metamorphosias

Delusions (usually paranoid and poorly formed)

Thought disorder (tangentiality, circumstantiality, loose associations)

Sleep-wake disturbance

Fragmented throughout 24-hour period

Reversal of normal cycle

Sleeplessness

Psychomotor behavior

Hyperactive

Hypoactive

Mixed

Language impairment

Word-finding difficulty/dysnomia/paraphasia

Dysgraphia

Altered semantic content

Severe forms can mimic expressive or receptive aphasia

Altered or labile affect

Any mood can occur, usually incongruent to context

Anger or increased irritability common

Hypoactive delirium often mislabeled as depression

Lability (rapid shifts) common

Unrelated to mood preceding delirium

TABLE 11–2. DSM-IV-TR criteria for diagnosis of delirium due to a general medical condition

A. Disturbance of consciousness (i.e., reduced clarity of awareness of the environment) with reduced ability to focus, sustain, or shift attention.

B. A change in cognition (such as memory deficit, disorientation, language disturbance) or the development of a perceptual disturbance that is not better accounted for by a preexisting, established, or evolving dementia.

C. The disturbance develops over a short period of time (usually hours to days) and tends to fluctuate during the course of the day.

D. There is evidence from the history, physical examination, or laboratory findings that the disturbance is caused by the direct physiological consequences of a general medical condition.

how "clouding" differs from "level" of consciousness. Attentional disturbance distinguishes delirium from dementia, for which the first criterion is memory impairment. Attentional disturbances in delirium range from general, nonspecific reduction in alertness (typically associated with nicotinic, cholinergic, histaminergic, or adrenergic actions) to decreased selective focusing or sustaining of attention (which may be related to muscarinic or cholinergic dysfunction). The contribution of attentional deficits to the altered awareness that occurs in delirium is insufficient by itself to account for other prominent symptoms—formal thought disorder, language and sleep-wake cycle disturbances, and other cognitive-perceptual deficits.

The characteristic features of the temporal course of delirium—acute onset and fluctuation of symptoms—have constituted a separate criterion in DSM-III, DSM-III-R, and DSM-IV. Temporal features assist in distinguishing delirium from most types of dementia, and most clinicians consider them to be important in making a diagnosis.

Despite the breadth of the symptoms of delirium, not all have been emphasized in the various editions of DSM. Dysexecutive symptoms (impairment of prefrontal executive cognition) are not mentioned in any DSM edition, despite the importance of prefrontal involvement in delirium (Trzepacz 1994a). Psychosis has not received much attention except in DSM-II, despite the occurrence of delusions in about one-third of patients and hallucinations in slightly more (Cutting 1987; Meagher 2005; Morita et al. 2004; Ross et al. 1991; Sirois 1988; Webster and Holroyd 2000). Characteristic features of delusions (which are usually paranoid and poorly formed) and hallucinations (often visual) have not been specified in DSM criteria, despite their usefulness to the clinician.

The World Health Organization's ICD-10 (1992) research diagnostic criteria for delirium are similar to DSM-IV-TR criteria A, C, and D. However, ICD-10 diverges from DSM-IV-TR in that cognitive dysfunction is manifested by both "(1) impairment of immediate recall and recent memory, with intact remote memory" and "(2) disorientation in time, place or person." In addition, a disturbance in sleep is present and manifested by insomnia, nocturnal worsening of symptoms, or disturbing dreams or nightmares that may continue as hallucinations or illusions when the patient is awake, which seems to indicate an etiological link between perceptual disturbances and sleep mechanisms. Despite these differences, a study of 80 delirious patients showed 100% concordance for diagnosis between DSM-III-R and ICD-10 research criteria for delirium systems (Treloar and MacDonald 1997).

Cole et al. (2003a) used DSM-III-R as the gold standard to compare the sensitivity and specificity of DSM-IV, DSM-III, and ICD-10 delirium criteria in patients with delirium only, dementia only, and comorbid delirium and dementia. The differing emphasis on "clouding of consciousness" and inattention was reflected in lower sensitivity for criteria sets in which clouding of consciousness was required, perhaps because the term *clouding of consciousness* is vague and difficult to assess. Sensitivity and specificity for DSM-IV, DSM-III, and ICD-10 criteria were 100% and 71%, 96% and 91%, and 61% and 91%, respectively. Thus, DSM-IV was found to be the most inclusive. Similarly, Laurila et al. (2003, 2004c) conducted a series of studies comparing various DSM and ICD-10 definitions of delirium and found substantial differences in rates, with only 25% of delirious patients diagnosed as such by all four schemes. Moreover, DSM-IV criteria identified almost twice as many cases of delirium compared with earlier DSM editions and ICD-10. Lesser diagnostic emphasis on disorganized thinking in DSM-IV accounts for its greater sensitivity and inclusivity (but lower specificity) in comparison to the other systems. The prognostic significance of these differences in diagnostic sensitivity between criteria sets varied little for outcome at 2 years in elderly hospital and nursing home patients. Two-year outcome in elderly hospital and nursing home patients was similar regardless of diagnostic criteria used, suggesting that DSM-IV identifies additional patients who have the poor prognosis of delirium. These studies confirm that standardized descriptions of delirium have changed during the past 25 years, potentially affecting results from studies conducted at different times.

PRODROMAL SYMPTOMS

Although delirium is usually characterized by an acute onset replete with many symptoms, it may be preceded by a subclinical delirium. Matsushima et al. (1997) prospectively studied 10 cardiac care unit patients who met DSM-III-R criteria for delirium and 10 nondelirious control subjects with an electroencephalogram (EEG). They found prodromal changes of background slowing on EEG (theta/alpha ratio) and sleep disturbance associated with changing consciousness. Duppils and Wikblad (2004) assessed a wide range of potential prodromal disturbances in elderly hip surgery patients and found that delirium was preceded by prodromal symptoms in 62% of the cases that included disorientation, calls for assistance, and anxiety in the 2 days before full delirium. De Jonghe et al. (2005) studied delirium symptoms daily with the Delirium Rating Scale—Revised-98 (DRS-R98) in elderly patients undergoing hip surgery who were involved in a study of haloperidol prophylaxis. Disorientation, short- and long-term memory disturbance, and inattention were noted in the 3 days before emergence of full delirium, whereas sleep-wake cycle disturbance, hallucinations, and thought process disorder occurred 1 day before, suggesting that cognitive impairments precede sleep-wake and psychotic symptoms. Kaneko et al. (1999) found a close correlation between development of postoperative delirium and decreased nocturnal and excessive daytime sleep. Fann et al. (2005) prospectively followed up delirium symptoms in patients undergoing stem cell transplantation and found that both psychobehavioral and cognitive disturbances predated the onset of full delirium by 4 days. The best brief tool to assess for prodromal symptoms with a high degree of predictability has not been determined. Nonspecific symptoms such as anxiety or calls for assistance may be less useful than key cognitive items.

SUBSYNDROMAL DELIRIUM

The presence of subsyndromal delirium symptoms in elderly persons appears to be associated with poorer prognosis compared with nondelirious patients and approaches that of the full syndrome. Cole et al. (2003b) prospectively studied subsyndromal delirium in 164 elderly medical patients, defined as delirium not meeting DSM-III-R criteria and the presence of one or more of four symptoms—clouding of consciousness, inattention, disorientation, and perceptual disturbances. The more symptoms present, especially on admission, the worse the prognosis, as evidenced by longer inpatient stays, poorer cognitive and functional status, and greater subsequent mortality at 12-month follow-up. Bourdel-Marchasson et al. (2004) found that subsyndromal delirium was a strong predictor (equivalent to full syndromal delirium) of postdischarge need for institutional care among elderly patients admitted to medical facilities. Marcantonio et al. (2002) found that levels of reduced independent-living status in elderly postoperative hip surgery patients with subsyndromal delirium were similar to levels in patients with mild delirium at 6-month follow-up. Moreover, a study of patients admitted to post-acute skilled nursing facilities found mortality rates (18%) in subsyndromal delirium that were lower than in full delirium (25%) but significantly higher than in nondelirious patients (5%) (Marcantonio et al. 2005). Subsyndromal illness may reflect individual neuropsychiatric symptoms that are unrelated to delirium (e.g., dementia) or an attenuated delirium in patients with lower vulnerability to delirium than in the elderly. Unfortunately, research is lacking in children and nongeriatric adults in whom frailty, diminished cognitive reserve, and dementia are not confounding issues.

MISDIAGNOSIS

Delirium frequently goes undetected in clinical practice. Between one-third and two-thirds of cases are missed across a range of therapeutic settings and by various specialists, including psychiatrists and neurologists (Johnson et al. 1992). Nonrecognition, complicated by mislabeling, represents a failure to recognize the symptoms of delirium accurately and results in poorer outcomes, including increased mortality (Kakuma et al. 2003; Rockwood et al. 1994). Poor detection also may reflect fluctuating symptom severity and breadth of symptoms, including multiple cognitive and noncognitive disturbances. Altered mental status was noted in only 16% of elderly emergency department patients with delirium (Hustey et al. 2003), and, even worse, emergency physicians did not alter management of these patients (including decisions to discharge home) when made aware of the impairments.

Misdiagnosis of delirium is more likely in patients who are older; who have sensory impairments, preexisting dementia, or a hypoactive presentation; and who are referred from surgical or intensive care settings (S.C. Armstrong et al. 1997; Inouye et al. 2001). Delirium is commonly misdiagnosed as depression by nonpsychiatrists (Farrell and Ganzini 1995; Margolis 1994; Nicholas and Lindsey 1995; Trzepacz et al. 1985). ICU populations have delirium prevalence rates ranging from 40% to 87% (Ely et al. 2001b), but delirium is unfortunately understudied and neglected either because it is "expected" to happen during severe illness or because medical resources are preferentially dedicated to managing the more immediate "life-threatening" problems. Ely et al.

(2004b) surveyed 912 physicians, nurses, respiratory therapists, and pharmacists attending international critical care meetings and found that 72% thought ventilated patients experienced delirium, 92% considered it a very serious problem, and 78% acknowledged that it was underdiagnosed; yet only 40% routinely screened for delirium, and only 16% used a specific tool for assessment.

The stereotyped image of delirium as an agitated psychotic state misrepresents most of the patients, who may not have psychotic symptoms or may have a hypoactive presentation (Meagher and Trzepacz 2000). The hypoactive presentation is less appreciated because the quiet, untroublesome patient is often presumed to have intact cognition and is more easily overlooked in the time-pressured technological environment of modern medicine. Moreover, some screening instruments are less sensitive to hypoactive presentations (P. Gagnon et al. 2000). Detection can be improved by assessing cognitive function, improving awareness of the varied presentations of delirium, and routinely using a screening tool (O'Keeffe et al. 2005; Rockwood et al. 1994). Nurses have the most contact with patients and relatives and offer the opportunity to monitor for delirium, although recognition can be affected by personal attitudes or education that reduce identification of delirium (McCarthy 2003).

DIFFERENTIAL DIAGNOSIS

Because delirium encompasses so many domains of higher cortical functions, its differential diagnosis is broad and can be mistaken for dementia, depression, primary or secondary psychosis, anxiety and somatoform disorders, and, particularly in children, behavioral disturbance (Table 11–3). Accurate diagnosis requires close attention to symptoms, temporal onset, and results of tests (e.g., cognitive, laboratory, electroencephalographic, and chart review including medication lists and anesthesia records). Given that delirium can be the presentation for serious medical illness, any patient experiencing a sudden deterioration in cognitive function should be assessed for possible delirium. Urinary tract infections in nursing home patients commonly present as delirium. Delirium occurs commonly in stroke patients (Caeiro et al. 2004a; Ferro et al. 2002) and is frequently the first indication of cerebrovascular accident (L.A. Wahlund and Bjorlin 1999).

Delirium Versus Dementia

The most difficult differential diagnosis for delirium is dementia, the other cause of generalized cognitive impairment. The broad structural damage of end-stage dementia has been likened to the severe physiologically impaired state of delirium. Lewy body dementia has a

TABLE 11–3.   Differential diagnosis of delirium

	Delirium	Dementia	Depression	Schizophrenia
Onset	Acute	Insidious[a]	Variable	Variable
Course	Fluctuating	Often progressive	Diurnal variation	Variable
Reversibility	Usually[b]	Not usually	Usually but can be recurrent	No, but has exacerbations
Level of consciousness	Impaired	Unimpaired until late stages	Generally unimpaired	Unimpaired (perplexity in acute stage)
Attention and memory	Inattention is primary with poor memory	Poor memory without marked inattention	Mild attention problems, inconsistent pattern, memory intact	Poor attention, inconsistent pattern, memory intact
Hallucinations	Usually visual; can be auditory, tactile, gustatory, olfactory	Can be visual or auditory	Usually auditory	Usually auditory
Delusions	Fleeting, fragmented, usually persecutory	Paranoid, often fixed	Complex and mood congruent	Frequent, complex, systematized, often paranoid

[a]Except for large strokes, which can be abrupt, and Lewy body dementia, which can be subacute.
[b]Can be chronic (as in paraneoplastic syndrome, central nervous system adverse events of medications, or severe brain damage).

more aggressive temporal course than Alzheimer's disease and mimics delirium with fluctuation of symptom severity, visual hallucinations, attentional impairment, alteration of consciousness, and delusions (Robinson 2002). Dementia is a potent predisposing factor for the development of delirium and is often comorbid with delirium in elderly patients.

Despite this substantial overlap, delirium and dementia can be reliably distinguished by a combination of careful history-taking for onset of characteristic symptoms and clinical investigation. Abrupt onset and fluctuating course are highly characteristic of delirium. In addition, level of consciousness and attention are markedly disturbed in delirium but remain relatively intact in uncomplicated dementia, in which memory impairment is instead the cardinal feature. Dementia patients often awaken at night, mistaking it as daytime, whereas disruption of the sleep-wake cycle, including fragmentation throughout 24 hours or even sleeplessness, is more characteristic in patients with delirium. Psychotic symptoms are more suggestive of delirium (present in approximately 50% of patients) than dementia, although Ropacki and Jeste (2005) reported psychotic symptoms in 41% of the patients with Alzheimer's disease. How-

ever, the possibility of comorbid delirium as the cause of psychosis was not well accounted for in this literature.

Only a few studies have investigated differences in symptom profile between patients with delirium and patients with dementia. O'Keeffe (1994) prospectively studied acute medically ill patients (12 in each group) with either DSM-III-diagnosed delirium, dementia, or comorbid delirium-dementia with the Delirium Assessment Scale, Brief Psychiatric Rating Scale motor item, and Mini-Mental State Examination (MMSE; Folstein et al. 1975) but was unable to distinguish delirium from dementia. In contrast, 9 of 10 DRS items—all except the cognitive item—distinguished delirious ($n = 20$) from moderately demented ($n = 9$) patients whose symptoms were diagnosed with DSM-III (Trzepacz and Dew 1995). Trzepacz et al. (2002) used the DRS-R98 and noted significant differences (after Bonferroni correction) between delirium and dementia groups (who had been blindly evaluated) for sleep-wake cycle disturbances, thought process abnormalities, motor agitation, attention, and visuospatial ability, which were more impaired in delirium, but no differences for delusions, affective lability, language, motor retardation, orientation, and short- or long-term memory. Careful assessment can distinguish groups of patients with these two disorders, but more work is needed to clarify differentiating features between delirium and dementia that can be applied to individual cases in clinical practice.

Even more challenging is distinguishing delirium from comorbid delirium-dementia. Liptzin et al. (1993) compared Delirium Symptom Inventory (DSI) items in DSM-III-R-diagnosed hospitalized elderly patients with delirium ($n=67$) and comorbid delirium-dementia ($n=58$) and found no differences for seven symptoms, although perceptual disturbances were numerically higher in the delirium-dementia group (50% vs. 28%). Trzepacz et al. (1998) compared DRS items in DSM-III-R-diagnosed delirium ($n=18$) and delirium-dementia patients ($n=43$) and found that only the DRS cognition item and the MMSE distinguished the groups (worse scores in the comorbid group). When factor analysis was done, 7 of 10 DRS items were common to both groups and loaded onto two factors: psychomotor disturbances, delusions, mood lability, sleep-wake cycle disturbances on factor 1 and temporal onset, physical disorder, and perceptual disturbances on factor 2.

Cole et al. (2002b) found only psychomotor agitation more prevalent in DSM-III-R delirium-dementia compared with delirium when the Confusion Assessment Method (CAM; Inouye et al. 1990) was used, whereas only disorganized thinking and disorientation were significantly more prevalent in delirium-dementia than in delirium when the Delirium Index was used, supporting others' findings that when individual symptoms are assessed, delirium presents similarly regardless of whether it is accompanied by dementia. Laurila et al. (2004b) compared symptom patterns in delirium with those in delirium-dementia according to an operationalized checklist of DSM and ICD criteria for delirium. Clouding of consciousness, disorganized thinking, and perceptual disturbances were especially prominent in delirium-dementia, whereas perceptual disturbances, motor abnormalities, and disorientation were most common in delirium alone. Voyer et al. (2006) compared delirium symptoms in patients with mild, moderate, and severe preexisting cognitive impairment and found similar profiles for all symptoms across groups except disorganized thinking.

Thus, it appears that when delirium and dementia are comorbid, delirium phenomenology generally overshadows that of the dementia, but when delirium and dementia are assessed as individual conditions, more symptoms can distinguish them, at least by mean scores. These research findings are consistent with the clinical rule of thumb that "altered cognition reflects delirium until proven otherwise" to prevent misattribution of delirium to dementia.

Most tools used for delirium assessment have not been validated for their ability to distinguish delirium from dementia, although three have been—the DRS (Trzepacz and Dew 1995), DRS-R98 (Trzepacz et al.

2001, 2002), and Cognitive Test for Delirium (CTD; Hart et al. 1996). Although abnormalities of the EEG are common to both delirium and dementia, diffuse slowing occurs more frequently (81% vs. 33%) in delirium and favors its diagnosis. In contrast, electroencephalographic slowing occurs later in the course of most degenerative dementias, although slowing occurs sooner with viral and prion dementias. The percentage of theta activity on quantitative EEGs allows differentiation of delirium from dementia (Jacobson and Jerrier 2000).

Delirium Versus Mood Disorders

Often the early behavior changes of delirium are mistaken for adjustment reactions to adverse events, particularly in patients who have experienced major trauma or have cancer. Hypoactive delirium is frequently mistaken for depression (Nicholas and Lindsey 1995). Farrell and Ganzini (1995) found that more than half of delirious patients referred to a consultation-liaison service for "depression" had thoughts of death, and almost one-quarter had suicidal thoughts. Although some symptoms of major depression occur in delirium (e.g., psychomotor slowing, sleep disturbances, irritability), in major depression, symptom onset tends to be less acute, and mood disturbances tend to be more sustained and typically dominate the clinical picture, with any cognitive impairments of depression resembling a mild subcortical dementia, or "depressive pseudodementia." Delirium can be precipitated by dehydration or malnutrition in severely depressed patients who are unable to maintain food or fluid intake.

The distinction of delirium from depression is particularly important because in addition to delayed treatment, use of antidepressants can aggravate delirium. Depression has been reported as a preoperative risk factor for delirium in patients undergoing surgery for abdominal aortic aneurysm (Minden et al. 2005) and a significant contributing cause of delirium in elderly patients admitted to medical facilities (L.A. Wahlund and Bjorlin 1999), but this could be a premonitory affective component of delirium. Conversely, the overactive, disinhibited profile of some delirious patients can closely mimic similar disturbances encountered in patients with agitated depression or mania. The most severe manic state ("Bell's mania") includes cognitive impairment and closely mimics delirium. Acute mania and delirium both can include emotional lability, perplexity, distractibility, inattention, jumbled speech, disinhibited behavior, and psychotic symptoms (Charlton and Kavanau 2002). However, the more widespread and profound cognitive changes of delirium, along with the etiological backdrop and differing clinical course, usually enable a firm distinction, and EEG can be diagnostic.

Delirium Versus Psychotic Disorders

Abnormalities of thought process and content and misperceptions can occur in both delirium and schizophrenia. Delusions in delirium are rarely as fixed or stereotyped as in schizophrenia, and first-rank symptoms are uncommon (Cutting 1987). Although delusions are most often persecutory, they are fragmented and can incorporate aspects of the environment that are poorly comprehended. Paranoid concerns about immediate well-being or perceived danger in the environment are common themes. Unlike in schizophrenia, hallucinations in delirium tend to be visual rather than auditory and, on occasion, olfactory, tactile, or gustatory. Tactile hallucinations (including formications) often suggest a hyperdopaminergic or hypocholinergic state. Illusions are common in delirium, and depersonalization and derealization are not uncommon, but delusional misidentification is relatively rare.

Level of consciousness, attention, and memory are generally unimpaired in schizophrenia, with the exception of the pseudodelirium that can occur as a result of marked perplexity in the acute stage of illness. Careful physical examination, coupled with EEG and/or a delirium-specific instrument, distinguishes delirium from these functional disorders or allows diagnosis of superimposed delirium in medically ill schizophrenic patients.

EPIDEMIOLOGY

INCIDENCE AND PREVALENCE

Delirium can occur at any age, although it is understudied in children and adolescents. Most epidemiological studies focus on the elderly, who are at higher risk to develop delirium than are younger adults. This is likely because of changes that occur in the brain with aging. These changes include decreased cholinergic activity, often referred to as "reduced brain reserve." The frequent occurrence of central nervous system (CNS) disorders (e.g., stroke, hypertensive and diabetic vessel changes, tumor, dementia) in the elderly further increases their vulnerability to delirium.

During the next three decades, the population of those age 60 and older will increase by 159% in less developed countries and by 59% in more developed countries (Jackson 1999). In the United States, in 1994, only 10% of elderly persons were older than 85 years. By 2050, almost 25% of elderly persons will be older than 85 years (Jackson 1999). This is particularly worrisome because dementia affects 5%–8% of those older than 65, 15%–20% of those older than 75, and 25%–50% of those older than 85 (American Psychiatric Association 1997). One would expect delirium rates to increase in parallel to the dementia prevalence rates.

Turkel et al. (2003) retrospectively applied the DRS to describe phenomenology in 84 consecutively evaluated (cross-sectional) children and adolescents (ages 6 months to 19 years) with DSM-IV delirium and found mean and median scores of 25 points, comparable to those for adults, with the only difference being fewer delusions and hallucinations in the younger children (mean age = 8 years). Turkel et al. (2006) compared the frequency of delirium symptoms between children and adults reported across many studies and, despite differences in methodologies and incidences, found delirium phenomenology essentially the same. Documentation of delirium symptoms in preverbal children or noncommunicative adults, however, is difficult. In these patients, clinicians must rely more on inference and observation of changed or unusual behaviors— for example, inferring hallucinations or recording changes in the sleep-wake cycle. Hallucinations in delirious children can be misattributed to imaginary friends (Prugh et al. 1980). When the diagnosis is uncertain, EEG shows generalized slowing that normalizes as delirium resolves in children, as in adults (Okamura et al. 2005).

Most studies of the incidence and prevalence of delirium report general hospital populations consisting of either referral samples or consecutive admissions to a given service with relatively little information about delirium rates in the general population. Community samples, however, are biased in that they do not include those at highest risk for delirium because they are hospitalized or in nursing homes. A wide range of percentages has been found in studies across different patient populations (e.g., elderly patients who have undergone hip surgery vs. liver transplant candidates vs. traumatic brain injury patients). Not all studies use sensitive and specific diagnostic and measurement techniques, possibly resulting in overestimates or underestimates of the true occurrence of delirium. Fann (2000) reviewed prospective studies and found an incidence range from 3% to 42% and a prevalence range from 5% to 44% in hospitalized patients. Up to 60% of nursing home patients older than age 65 may have delirium when assessed cross-sectionally (Sandberg et al. 1998). In addition, 10%–15% of elderly persons have delirium when admitted to a hospital, and another 10%–40% are given a diagnosis of delirium during the hospitalization. A clinical rule of thumb seems to be that, on average, approximately a fifth of general hospital patients have delirium sometime during hospitalization, with this figure increasing to 80%–90% in medical ICU and terminal cancer patients (Ely et al. 2001a; Lawlor et al. 2000a).

MORBIDITY AND MORTALITY

Delirium is associated with high rates of morbidity and mortality. It is not known whether the increased mortality rate is 1) solely attributable to the physiological perturbations resulting from the underlying medical causes of delirium, 2) attributable to indirect effects on the body related to perturbations of neuronal (or neuronal-endocrine-immunological) function during delirium, 3) attributable to damaging effects on the brain from neurochemical abnormalities associated with delirium (e.g., dysfunctional cellular metabolism or glutamatergic surges), or 4) related to consequences of delirious patients not fully cooperating with their medical care and rehabilitative programs during hospitalization. Furthermore, their behaviors can directly reduce the effectiveness of procedures meant to treat their medical problems (e.g., removing tubes and intravenous lines, climbing out of bed), as well as result in a higher incidence of serious complications (e.g., falls, infections due to hypostasis, bed sores), which adds to morbidity and possibly to further physiological injury and mortality. Gustafson et al. (1988) found more medical problems in delirious patients during hospitalization that included decubitus ulcers, feeding problems, and urinary incontinence. Saravay et al. (2004) explored the chronology of events leading to poor outcomes in elderly medical patients and found that mental disturbances preceded the occurrence of complications such as falls, intravenous line removal, uncooperative behavior, and problems with consent. Delirious patients with or without dementia were more likely to develop dehydration and pneumonia than were patients with dementia alone (Fick et al. 2005). Patients developing delirium were more than twice as likely to develop new complications (especially falls and pneumonia) that were associated with increased rehospitalization rates and reduced discharge rates when admitted to postacute treatment facilities (Marcantonio et al. 2005).

The interpretation of studies of mortality risk associated with delirium is complicated by methodological inconsistencies and shortcomings. Some studies do not compare delirium with control groups, most do not address the effects of treatment, many include comorbid dementia, many do not control for differences in severity or type of medical comorbidity, most do not address effects of advanced age as a separate risk factor, and specific delirium rating instruments are rarely used. Prospective application of DSM criteria by qualified clinicians, attention to whether the sample is incident or prevalent, identification of biases related to referral samples, and determination of whether follow-up mortality rates are cumulative to include the original sample size also vary across study designs. Finally, more research in nongeriatric age groups is greatly needed.

Given these caveats, mortality rates during index hospitalization for a delirium episode range from 4% to 65% (Cameron et al. 1987; Gustafson et al. 1988). When de-

lirium present on admission was excluded, the index mortality rate for incident cases was as low as about 1.5% (Inouye et al. 1999). Some studies found significantly elevated mortality rates for delirium compared with control subjects (Cameron et al. 1987; Jitapunkul et al. 1992; Pompeii et al. 1994; Rabins and Folstein 1982; van Hemert et al. 1994), whereas other studies did not (Forman et al. 1995; George et al. 1997; Gustafson et al. 1988; Inouye et al. 1998, 1999; Kishi et al. 1995). Many studies of longer-term follow-up of delirium mortality rates (more than 3 months after discharge) did find worse mortality rates in delirium groups, including subsyndromal delirium (Cole et al. 2003b). One study found significant differences in index mortality rate among motor subtypes, with the lowest rate (10%) in hyperalert patients compared with hypoalert patients (38%) and mixed cases (30%) (S.M. Olofsson et al. 1996). Excessive mortality in some reports was attributed to greater age (Gustafson et al. 1988; Huang et al. 1998; Kishi et al. 1995; Trzepacz et al. 1985; Weddington 1982), more serious medical problems (Cole and Primeau 1993; Jitapunkul et al. 1992; Magaziner et al. 1989; Trzepacz et al. 1985), and dementia (Cole and Primeau 1993; Gustafson et al. 1988) as well as severity of delirium symptoms (Marcantonio et al. 2002). Manos and Wu (1997) found no differences in delirium mortality rates between medical and postoperative groups after 3.5 years. Conversely, Curyto et al. (2001) found an increased mortality of 75% at 3 years for delirious compared with control (51%) elderly patients despite no differences in prehospital levels of depression, global cognitive performance, physical functioning, or medical comorbidity. Frail elderly living in nursing facilities studied for 3 months during and after an acute medical hospitalization had a high mortality rate of 18% in hospital and 46% at 3 months that was associated with severe and persistent delirium (Kelly et al. 2001). Leslie et al. (2005) found that hospitalized elderly patients with delirium had a 62% increased risk of mortality at 1-year follow-up and lost an average of 13% of a year of life compared with nondelirious control subjects. Moreover, they also noted a dose-response relation between delirium severity and mortality rate.

Inouye et al. (1998) found that delirium (diagnosed with the CAM) significantly increased mortality risk, even after they controlled for age, sex, dementia, activities of daily living (ADL) level, and Acute Physiology and Chronic Health Evaluation II (APACHE II; Knaus et al. 1985) scores in a prospective study of medically hospitalized elderly persons. Ely et al. (2004) reported that delirium in medical ICU patients was independently associated with a greater than 300% increased likelihood of dying at 6 months ($P = 0.008$), even after they corrected for numerous covariates including coma and use of psychoactive medications. McCusker et al. (2002) showed that delirium is a significant predictor of 12-month mortality for older inpatients, even after the data are adjusted for age, sex, marital status, living location, comorbidity, acute physiological severity, illness severity, dementia, and hospital service. Pitkälä and colleagues (2005) found that delirium was a predictor of mortality and institutionalization in an elderly population at both 1- and 2-year follow-up, even when level of frailty was accounted for.

Other work has found better outcomes, including reduced mortality, when delirium was actively identified and treated. In a prospective cohort study of prevalent delirium diagnosed with the CAM in emergency departments, 30 delirious and 77 nondelirious elderly patients who were discharged home instead of being admitted to the hospital were assessed at 6-month follow-up intervals until 18 months (Kakuma et al. 2003). After the investigators adjusted for age, sex, functional level, cognitive status, comorbidity, and number of medications, delirium was significantly associated with increased mortality. Those whose delirium was not detected by the emergency department staff had the highest mortality over 6 months compared with those whose delirium was detected; no mortality difference was seen between the patients whose delirium was detected and the nondelirious patients, emphasizing the importance of detection. Lundstrom et al. (2005) applied a multifactorial program focusing on more rapid recognition and treatment of delirium and enhancing relationships with informal caregivers and found reduced mortality in the delirious patients receiving treatment on this ward compared with those receiving usual care on another acute medical ward, but treatment and control groups were not randomized. Milbrandt et al. (2005) found significantly lower mortality (8%) in 989 mechanically ventilated ICU patients who had received haloperidol, although delirium was not documented as the principal reason for haloperidol use. They speculated that these differences might relate to reduced agitation, stabilization of cognitive status, or inhibition of secretion of proinflammatory cytokines by haloperidol (Moots et al. 1999). K.J. Kalisvaart et al. (2005a), in a double-blind, randomized, placebo-controlled study, noted reduced severity and duration of delirium in elderly hip surgery patients receiving prophylactic low-dose haloperidol.

Even though the mechanism is not understood, delirium is associated with an increased risk for mortality extending well beyond the index hospitalization that might be reduced by aggressive treatment of both the delirium and its comorbid medical problems, except possibly in the frailest elderly patients.

LENGTH OF STAY

Significantly increased length of stay (LOS) associated with delirium has been reported in most studies (Forman et al. 1995; Francis et al. 1990; Gustafson et al. 1988; Hales et al. 1988; Levkoff et al. 1992; Pompeii et al. 1994; R.I. Thomas et al. 1988), but not all (Cole et al. 1994; George et al. 1997; Jitapunkul et al. 1992; Rockwood 1989). A meta-analysis of eight studies (Cole and Primeau 1993) does support both numerical and statistical differences between delirium patients' and control groups' LOS. Delirium duration was associated with LOS in both the medical ICU and the hospital ($P \le 0.0001$) and was the strongest predictor of LOS, even after Ely et al. (2001a) adjusted for illness severity, age, gender, and days of opiate and narcotic use. McCusker et al. (2003b) studied elderly medical inpatients and found significantly longer LOS for incident, but not prevalent, delirium. The Academy of Psychosomatic Medicine Task Force on Mental Disorders in General Medical Practice (Saravay and Strain 1994) reviewed economic effects and outcomes of delirium in various populations and reported that comorbid delirium increased LOS 100% in general medical patients (R.I. Thomas et al. 1988), 114% in elderly patients (Schor et al. 1992), 67% in stroke patients (Cushman et al. 1998), 300% in critical care patients (Kishi et al. 1995), 27% in cardiac surgery patients, and 200%–250% in hip surgery patients (Berggren et al. 1987). They noted that delirium contributes to increased LOS via medical and behavioral mechanisms, including decreased motivation to participate in treatment and rehabilitation, medication refusal, disruptive behavior, incontinence and urinary tract infections, falls and fractures, and decubiti. Saravay et al. (2004) prospectively assessed chronology of cognitive and behavioral symptoms and found that delirium and dementia contribute to increased LOS via their consequences, such as falls, pulled intravenous lines, incontinence, restraints, and decreased cooperation. Bourgeois et al. (2006) found that any cognitive disorder increased LOS and that with increasing age, adults were less likely to have delirium without comorbid dementia. Mittal et al. (2006) compared delirious patients who were and were not referred for consultation. Those who were referred for consultation were more likely to be younger, to be hyperactive, to have greater substance abuse and less comorbid dementia, and to be recognized as delirious; no difference was found in LOS or 1-year mortality between those who were and those who were not referred.

REDUCED INDEPENDENCE

Decreased independent living status and increased rate of institutionalization during follow-up after a delirium episode were found in many studies (Cole and Primeau 1993; George et al. 1997; Inouye et al. 1998; Pitkälä et al. 2005). Reduction in ambulation and/or ADL level at follow-up was also commonly reported (Francis and Kapoor 1992; Gustafson et al. 1988; Inouye et al. 1998; Minagawa et al. 1996; Murray et al. 1993). Both full-blown delirium and subsyndromal illness have an effect in nursing home settings, where incident cases are associated with poor 6-month outcome, including behavioral decline, initiation of physical restraints, greater risk of hospitalization, and increased mortality rate (Marcantonio et al. 2005; Murphy 1999). Similarly, Pitkälä et al. (2005) identified delirium as an independent predictor of loss of independence and mortality at 2-year follow-up in a study of frail elderly patients older than 70 years. Elderly femoral neck fracture patients who had delirium on admission or postoperatively were more dependent in their ADLs at discharge and 4 months later (B. Olofsson et al. 2005). Even subsyndromal delirium is reported to increase index admission LOS and reduce postdischarge functional level and mortality after adjusting for age, sex, marital status, previous living arrangement, comorbidity, dementia status, and clinical or physiological severity of illness (Cole et al. 2003b; Marcantonio et al. 2005).

COST OF CARE

Delirium results in greater costs of care. Franco et al. (2001) found higher professional consultation, technical, and routine nursing care costs in delirious patients older than 50 years who were undergoing elective surgery; 11.4% became delirious during postoperative days 1–4. Milbrandt et al. (2004) found 39% increased cost associated with having at least one delirium episode in 183 mechanically ventilated medical ICU patients, even though analysis controlled for multiple confounds such as age, comorbidity of illness, degree of organ dysfunction, and nosocomial infection. Median ICU costs per patient were 60% greater and total hospital costs were 65% higher in delirious patients, with the cost increasing with more severe delirium. Fick et al. (2005) studied health care costs from administrative records of a managed care organization for 76,000 community-dwelling elderly patients and found that costs were twice as high for patients with delirium and especially increased for patients with delirium superimposed on dementia compared with those with either condition alone. The elevated costs were related to cerebrovascular disease, urinary tract infections, pneumonia, and dehydration and resulted in greater facility costs and more emergency department and nursing home visits.

DISTRESS AND PSYCHOLOGICAL SEQUELAE

Delirium is frequently a distressing experience for patients and their caregivers. Delirium-recovered patients may be uncomfortable discussing their delirium episodes—even to the extent of denial—because of fear that they may be "senile" or "mad" (Schofield 1997). Breitbart et al. (2002a) used the Delirium Experience Questionnaire to prospectively interview and rate 101 cancer patients with a resolved delirium episode, their spouses, and their nurses. About half (43%) recalled their episode, and recall depended on delirium severity as rated by the Memorial Delirium Assessment Scale (MDAS) (100% of patients with mild vs. 16% of patients with severe delirium recalled the episode). Mean distress levels were high for patients at 3.2 points (scored 0–4) and nurses at 3.1 but were highest for spouses at 3.8. However, among delirious patients who did not recall the episode ($n = 47$), the mean distress level was only 1.5. The experience of the delirium was frightening and stressful for all involved but for somewhat different reasons. For patients, the presence of delusions was predictive of distress level; for nurses, the presence of perceptual disturbances or a very severe delirium; and for spouses, a low Karnofsky scale level of functioning. Spouses perceived the delirium as indicating a high risk for death and loss of the loved one, contributing to bereavement. Fann et al. (2005) found that in patients undergoing hematopoietic stem cell transplantation, level of affective distress was closely linked to delirium severity, and in particular to psychosis and level of psychomotor disturbance. In nondemented elderly patients with delirium, O'Keeffe (2005) found that more than half were able to recall psychotic symptoms and that many continued to be distressed by their recollections 6 months later. Thus, delirium can have a great psychological effect on patients and those who care for them, yet it is often overlooked in the treatment care plan.

REVERSIBILITY OF A DELIRIUM EPISODE

Delirium traditionally has been distinguished from dementia by its potential for reversal and its transient neurobiological state. Bedford's (1957) study of delirium found that only 5% of the patients were still "confused" at 6-month follow-up. Full resolution of symptoms at hospital discharge of elderly patients may be the exception rather than the rule according to some (Levkoff et al. 1992; Rockwood 1993). Levkoff et al. (1992) found that only 4% of the elderly patients with delirium had complete resolution of symptoms at discharge, 20.8% at 6 weeks, and 17.7% at 6 months, but they did not exclude comorbid dementia patients. McCusker et al. (2003a) found that 12 months after diagnosis of delirium in elderly medical inpatients, inattention, disorientation, and poor memory were the most persistent individual symptoms both in those with and in those without concomitant dementia (see next section, "Persistent Cognitive Deficits").

Individual delirium symptoms can predict the episode duration. Wada and Yamaguchi (1993) found that a longer delirium (≥1 week) in elderly neuropsychiatry consults was predicted by severity of cognitive disturbance, mood lability, and sleep-wake cycle disruption. Levkoff et al. (1994) noted persistent delirium symptoms in 30% of the elderly patients hospitalized for acute care at 6-month follow-up; orientation difficulty and mood and sleep disturbances were the most common symptoms, but dementia patients were not excluded from the study. Treloar and MacDonald (1997) found that the degree of "reversibility" of an index episode of delirium was predicted by motor activity, speech and thought disturbances, and a fluctuating course.

The reversibility of delirium appears related to underlying causation and pathophysiology. Mach et al. (1995) found that full resolution of delirium was more likely with higher levels of serum anticholinergic activity, perhaps indicating that some causes of delirium, such as anticholinergic toxicity, were more reversible, although this was not specifically addressed in this study. In cancer patients, Morita et al. (2001) found that delirium caused by drugs or metabolic abnormalities such as dehydration or hypercalcemia was more reversible compared with that caused by hypoxia or global metabolic encephalopathy. Moreover, delirium was less reversible when the patient had previous episodes.

One explanation for persisting impairments may be incomplete treatment or recurring course of delirium (Meagher 2001a). The ever-increasing financial pressures to shorten hospital stays have resulted in many patients being discharged from the hospital before delirium has resolved, even though families and nursing homes are not resourced to manage delirium to its resolution. Kiely et al. (2004) studied 2,158 patients from seven Boston-area skilled nursing facilities and found that 16% had a full-blown delirium according to the CAM as well as lower MMSE and higher MDAS scores. They warned of the adverse effect of delirium persisting in subacute care settings related to loss of independent functioning. Marcantonio et al. (2005) assessed 1,248 elderly patients soon after admission to postacute facilities and found that 15% had delirium and another 51% had subsyndromal delirium.

PERSISTENT COGNITIVE DEFICITS

In the elderly, the term *persistent cognitive impairment* in the weeks or months following a delirium episode during a medical-surgical hospitalization is used, but its neuropsychological pattern and etiology are not clear and are highly confounded by difficult-to-measure comorbid pathophysiologies. Possible causes of persistent cognitive difficulties in patients who have experienced delirium are shown in Figure 11–2.

The increased diagnosis of dementia in patients who had an episode of delirium suggests a preexisting dementia heralded by the delirium. Kolbeinsson and Jonsson (1993) found that delirium was complicated by dementia at follow-up in 70% of patients. Rahkonen et al. (2000) found that when the index episode of delirium resolved, a new diagnosis of dementia was made in 27% of 51 prospectively studied community-dwelling elderly, and at 2-year follow-up, a total of 55% had a new diagnosis of dementia. Rockwood et al. (1999) reported an 18% annual incidence of dementia in patients with delirium—more than three times higher risk than in nondelirious patients when the confounding effects of comorbid illness severity and age were adjusted for. At 5-year follow-up, Parkinson's disease patients who had a delirium episode had more cognitive impairment, motor decline, and death than did nondelirious Parkinson's disease control subjects (Serrano-Dueñas and Bleda 2005).

Persistent cognitive deficits may be related to a previously undiagnosed dementia that progresses after delirium resolution. This possibility is supported by a study of undetected dementia in 252 community-dwelling older people, in whom 64% had dementia but had never been medically assessed for cognitive impairment (Sternberg et al. 2000). Koponen et al.'s (1994) 5-year longitudinal study of delirium in the elderly attributed persistence and progression of symptoms more to the underlying dementia than to the previous delirium episode. Similarly, in a cross-sectional study of consecutive psychogeriatric admissions, the only factor significantly linked to incomplete symptom resolution in delirium was the presence of preexisting cognitive impairment (Camus et al. 2000b). In nursing home patients, better cognitive function at baseline was associated with better outcome from delirium (Murphy 1999). Kasahara et al. (1996) compared delirium and dementia in young (35–45 years) and aged (older than 60 years) alcoholic patients and found similar frequency of delirium but no cases of dementia in the younger group compared with 62% of the aged group. The aged group also had more frequent and severe physical complications, hepatic injury, and cardiomyopathy, and

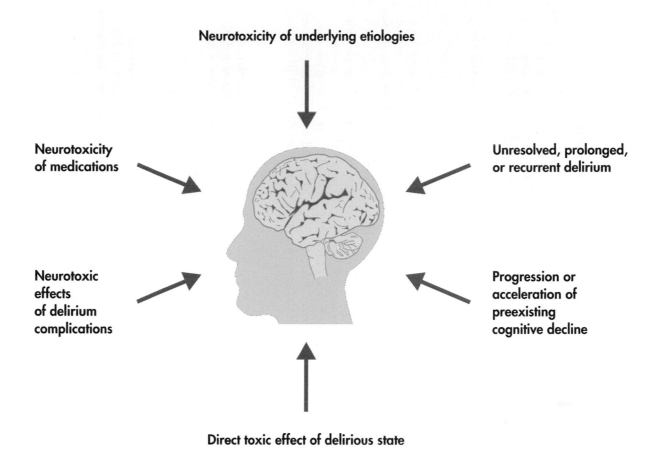

Neurotoxicity of underlying etiologies

Neurotoxicity of medications

Unresolved, prolonged, or recurrent delirium

Neurotoxic effects of delirium complications

Progression or acceleration of preexisting cognitive decline

Direct toxic effect of delirious state

FIGURE 11–2.   Possible reasons for persistent cognitive impairment in patients after an episode of delirium.

their delirium episodes were more severe, perhaps as a result of more years of exposure to toxic effects of ethanol or vulnerability due to aging. Therefore, younger adults with delirium either have better brain recovery than elders do or are at less risk for degenerative and vascular dementias that can be misattributed to delirium persistence.

Some studies attempt to account for predelirium cognitive function as a factor in postdelirium cognitive impairment (see Table 11–4). These indicate an association with the development of dementia after an episode of delirium that at least in part seems unrelated to prior cognitive function, but many important methodological issues need to be better addressed. Research is needed that uses detailed premorbid cognitive assessments and repeated neuropsychological testing designed to detect and differentiate patterns of types of dementias (Alzheimer's disease, vascular, frontal, or other dementing processes) or the medical insults experienced (e.g., hypoxia) to distinguish these from delirium-induced damage. Most of these studies (apart from Fann and Sullivan 2003) relate to older persons, but studies of longitudinal postdelirium cognitive function in younger adults who are not at risk for dementia could help

answer this question. Also, some work suggests better outcome in less severe delirium (Leslie et al. 2005; Wada and Yamaguchi 1993) and episodes of shorter duration (Liptzin and Levkoff 1992), although medical illness severity is a likely confound and covaries with delirium severity. Some (Duppils and Wikblad 2004; O'Keeffe et al. 2005; Treloar and MacDonald 1997) suggested that the rate of deterioration following a delirium episode is far in excess of that following Alzheimer's dementia, in which a reduction in MMSE score of two to three points per annum is typical (Davidson et al. 1996). Terminology problems also exist regarding when a chronic delirium becomes irreversible and whether the experience of an index episode of delirium, perhaps by virtue of a neurotoxic or kindling effect, may alter the threshold for further episodes of delirium or contribute to the progression or development of dementia.

RISK FACTORS FOR DELIRIUM

Risk factors are external or intrinsic variables that increase the likelihood of experiencing delirium and should not be confused with causes of delirium. Delirium is particularly

TABLE 11–4.   Studies of cognitive performance after an episode of delirium

Study	Population	Delirium diagnosis	Assessment of baseline cognition	Follow-up	Outcome at follow-up	Comments
Francis and Kapoor 1992	229 community-dwelling patients older than 70 undergoing medical admission; 50 developed delirium	DSM-III-R	Blessed Dementia Rating Scale Modified "telephone" MMSE	2 years	Cognitive decline much greater in delirium group (mean = 3.3 MMSE points) vs. nondelirious control group (mean = 0.6).	Delirium population was judged to be more medically morbid at admission. Only 11 patients from delirium group tested at follow-up.
Kolbeinsson and Jonsson 1993	87 emergency medical admission patients older than 70 with cognitive impairment, divided into those with DSM-III-R dementia (n = 50) and those with delirium (n = 37)	DSM-III-R	MMSE and mental status questionnaire	Up to 5 months	26 (70%) of those with delirium diagnosis at admission also fulfilled criteria for DSM-III-R dementia at discharge.	Patients divided into delirium or dementia groups at admission; whole population was significantly cognitively impaired at admission. Actual duration of follow-up was unclear, and diagnostic impressions rather than cognitive measurements were reported.
Levkoff et al. 1994	325 elderly acute hospital admission patients; 91 developed delirium	DSM-III	38 had preexisting dementia, but only new symptoms were counted toward delirium diagnosis	6 months	72 (79%) had persistent symptoms on DSI at 3 months and 62 (68%) at 6 months, with disorientation (23%) and inattention (10%) common.	Patients with preexisting dementia were included, but dementia frequency at follow-up was not reported, and cognitive symptoms were limited to DSM-III domains.
Rockwood et al. 1999	203 consecutive general medical admission patients older than 65; 38 developed delirium	DSM-IV	Canadian Study of Health and Aging dementia protocol	32.5 months	Relative risk of dementia at follow-up was 3.23 times greater in the delirium group (60%; 18.1% annual incidence) than in the nondelirium group (18.5%; 5.6% per year).	Only 16 subjects had delirium without prior dementia, and of these, only 6 were alive at final follow-up assessment.
Moller et al. 1998	1,218 patients older than 60 undergoing major surgery compared with 321 matched control subjects; 99 developed delirium postoperatively	DSM-III	MMSE score >23; various exclusion criteria such as CNS disease, history of neuropsychological testing, or receiving antidepressants or tranquilizers	3 months	Postoperative cognitive dysfunction at 3 months was significantly more common in postoperative population (10% vs. 3%), but delirium was not an identified risk factor.	Screening for delirium was conducted with orientation items of MMSE, which lacks sensitivity for delirium.

TABLE 11–4. Studies of cognitive performance after an episode of delirium (*continued*)

Study	Population	Delirium diagnosis	Assessment of baseline cognition	Follow-up	Outcome at follow-up	Comments
Rahkonen et al. 2000	51 emergency admission patients with delirium older than 65 and living at home before admission	DSM-III-R	Excluded moderate or severe dementia as per medical records and caregiver interviews	2 years	27% diagnosed with dementia at end of index delirium episode; a further 16% had dementia at 1-year follow-up and 12% at 2-year follow-up. Risk of dementia during follow-up was vastly greater (>4 times) than for age-equivalent general population.	The study included patients with mild cognitive impairment at baseline. Group with dementia at follow-up had significantly lower MMSE score at baseline.
Dolan et al. 2000	682 nondemented elderly hip fracture patients living at home before admission; 433 denoted cognitively intact preoperatively; 92 developed delirium	DSM-III-R	Judged cognitively intact if medical chart notation not suggestive of preexisting dementia, organic brain syndrome, or Alzheimer's disease	2 years	Delirium at admission was associated with poorer cognitive functioning on MMSE at 6-, 12-, 18-, and 24-month follow-up. Patients experiencing delirium were almost twice as likely to be cognitively impaired at 24 months.	Cognition was formally measured with MMSE only postoperatively. Preoperative assessment involved chart review for evidence of cognitive difficulties. Delirium group was more medically morbid and older at baseline.
McCusker et al. 2001	315 medical admissions from emergency department older than 65; 220 experienced delirium; 56 had no preexisting dementia	DSM-III-R	IQCODE and MMSE	1 year	Similar reduction in MMSE scores in patients with delirium (−3.36) and dementia (−4.99).	86% of the cases were of prevalent delirium.
Katz et al. 2001	96 elderly patients (mean age = 84 years) from two supported community residences; 12 developed delirium during a hospitalization	DSM-III-R	MMSE, Buschke Selective Reminding Test, Stroop Test, verbal vigilance	1 year	Despite similar medical morbidity and cognitive profiles at baseline, patients developing delirium experienced significantly greater reduction in MMSE scores but not in other measures of cognition at 1 year.	Small absolute numbers developing delirium resulted in underpowered study. Only severe dementia was ruled out; 40% of the sample had MMSE score of 23 or less at baseline.

TABLE 11–4. Studies of cognitive performance after an episode of delirium *(continued)*

Study	Population	Delirium diagnosis	Assessment of baseline cognition	Follow-up	Outcome at follow-up	Comments
Gruber-Baldini et al. 2003	674 patients older than 65 who were community dwelling prior to admission with hip fractures; 486 were not cognitively impaired prefracture, and 149 (31%) of these developed cognitive impairment during hospitalization	DSM-III	Preoperative cognitive function assessed by medical note review, proxy reports, and patient assessment. Patients with MMSE score<24 were considered not cognitively intact and analyzed separately.	1 year	Cognitive impairment first detected in hospital persisted in more than 40% at 1-year follow-up.	Precise nature of postoperative cognitive impairment unclear (i.e., MMSE<24 or confusion noted in case notes). Also, substantial reliance on proxy reports of MMSE for follow-up assessments.
Lundstrom et al. 2003	78 nondemented patients older than 65 undergoing surgery for femoral neck fractures	DSM-IV	Caregiver interviews and MMSE	5 years	Patients experiencing delirium were 3.5 times more likely to develop dementia over the following 5 years.	Delirium group had significantly poorer cognitive performance preoperatively.
Jackson et al. 2003	Prospective study of 275 medical ICU mechanically ventilated patients; 41 available for follow-up assessment at 6 months, of whom 34 had no evidence of preexisting cognitive impairment at baseline	DSM-III-R	Modified Blessed Dementia Rating Scale score<3	6 months	Delirium duration was longer (NS) in patients with impaired cognitive function (measured with detailed neuropsychological battery) at follow-up. Overall, delirium was not specifically associated with cognitive decline.	Very high dropout rate, resulting ultimately in small numbers. Delirium severity not assessed.
Duppils and Wikblad 2004	115 patients older than 75 years undergoing hip surgery; 32 developed delirium postoperatively	DSM-IV	Excluded patients with prevalent delirium or MMSE score<11	6 months	Patients experiencing delirium had greater cognitive decline on MMSE (mean = 2.6 points at 6-month follow-up).	Many patients had significant cognitive impairment at outset, and the group experiencing delirium was older and more morbid (less independent, more sensory impairments).

TABLE 11–4. Studies of cognitive performance after an episode of delirium (continued)

Study	Population	Delirium diagnosis	Assessment of baseline cognition	Follow-up	Outcome at follow-up	Comments
Benoit et al. 2005	102 patients undergoing elective abdominal surgery; 34 developed delirium postoperatively	DSM-IV	Scores preoperatively were within normal range for an extensive neuropsychological battery (MMSE, Wechsler Logical Memory test, Rey-Osterrieth Complex Figure, time to state months of year backward, time to print the alphabet in capital letters, Trail Making Test A and B, animal naming, delayed recall of Wechsler and Rey-Osterrieth Complex Figure tests as above)	3 months	Delirium was associated with poorer cognition at 3-month follow-up, especially regarding immediate and delayed recall on Wechsler Logical Memory test and Rey-Osterrieth Complex Figure test.	Delirium patients had poorer baseline scores, and period of follow-up was very short; raises possibility of unresolved delirium episode.
Rothenhausler et al. 2005	34 patients undergoing cardiopulmonary bypass surgery; 11 developed delirium	DSM-IV	Syndrom-Kurztest (SKT), a cognitive performance test including 9 subtests of memory and attention	1 year	30 patients were reassessed at follow-up; 6 patients (20%) had cognitive deficits at 1-year follow-up. Cognitive dysfunction at discharge and 1-year follow-up was not related to postoperative delirium.	Relatively small cohort and postoperative delirium of short duration (range = 1–7 days).
Wacker et al. 2006	572 post-elective hip or knee surgery patients; 90 were cognitively intact at baseline, of whom 31 had experienced delirium	DSM-IV	Retrospective informant-based diagnoses of cognitive function preoperatively	21 months	Relative risk of dementia was 10.5 times greater in patients with documented DSM-IV delirium in postoperative period.	Not prospective. Compared current cognitive performance in patients who had delirium with that in patients who had similar procedures but did not have documented delirium episode. Preoperative cognitive status was determined with IQCODE almost 2 years later.

Note. MMSE = Mini-Mental State Examination; DSI = Delirium Symptom Inventory; CNS = central nervous system; ICU = intensive care unit; NS = not significant.

common during hospitalization when there is a confluence of both predisposing factors—that is, vulnerabilities related to the individual, including genetics—and precipitating factors related to external stressors, medications, illness, surgery, and so on. Patient-related, illness, procedure-related, pharmacological, and environmental factors have been identified as risk factors for delirium, as illustrated in Figure 11–3. Risk factors identified for the elderly are not the same as those for ICU patients or children. Although some factors are more relevant in certain settings, age, preexisting cognitive impairment, severe comorbid illness, and medication exposure are particularly strong predictors of delirium risk across a range of populations (Inouye et al. 1999). More research is needed to identify setting and age-specific risk factors that are highly predictive and possibly modifiable as preventive strategies.

Stress-vulnerability models for the occurrence of delirium have been long recognized. Henry and Mann (1965) described "delirium readiness." More recent models of causation describe cumulative interactions between predisposing (vulnerability) factors and precipitating insults (Inouye and Charpentier 1996; O'Keeffe and Lavan 1996). Baseline risk is a more potent predictor of the likelihood of delirium: if baseline vulnerability is low, then patients are very resistant to the development of delirium despite exposure to significant precipitating factors, whereas if baseline vulnerability is high, then delirium is likely even in response to minor precipitants (Figure 11–4). Tsutsui et al. (1996), for example, found that in patients older than 80 years, delirium occurred in 52% after emergency surgery and in 20% after elective procedures, whereas no case of delirium was noted in patients younger than 50 undergoing either elective or emergency procedures. It is generally believed that the aged brain is more vulnerable to delirium, in part related to structural and degenerative changes as well as altered neurochemical flexibility. Children are also considered to be at higher risk for delirium, possibly related to developmental immaturity of brain structure and chemistry.

O'Keeffe and Lavan (1996) stratified patients into four levels of delirium risk on the basis of the presence of three factors (chronic cognitive impairment, severe illness, elevated serum urea level) and found that the risk of delirium increased as these factors accumulated. Similarly, Inouye and Charpentier (1996) developed a predictive model that included four predisposing factors (cognitive impairment, severe illness, visual impairment, and dehydration) and five precipitating factors (more than three medications added, catheterization, use of restraints, malnutrition, any iatrogenic event). These factors predicted a 17-fold variation in the relative risk of developing delirium. Subsequent work has validated this model in elderly hip surgery patients (K.J.

Kalisvaart et al. 2005b). Although the value of reducing risk factors appears self-evident, many risk factors may simply be markers of general morbidity, and therefore studies documenting preventive effects are important. Some risk factors are proxies for actual causes—in the elderly, a bladder catheter may increase risk for delirium because of infection risk or may indicate an infection that is an etiology.

Some risk factors are potentially modifiable and thus are targets for preventive interventions. Even just closer observation of patients at high risk for delirium could mean more prompt intervention in emergent delirium. In elderly hip fracture surgery patients, the presence of dehydration at the time of hospital admission predicted urinary tract infection, which predicted an increased incidence of delirium and a prolonged LOS (Kamel 2005). Medication exposure is probably the most readily modifiable risk factor for delirium, being implicated as a cause in 20%–40% of cases of delirium. Inouye et al. (1999) studied the effect of preventive measures aimed at minimizing six of the risk factors identified in their previous work with hospitalized elderly persons (Inouye et al. 1993). Standardized protocols to address cognitive impairment, sleep deprivation, immobility, visual impairment, hearing impairment, and dehydration resulted in significant reductions in the number and duration of delirium episodes. Moreover, in a subsequent study, the rate of adherence to suggested interventions was a significant predictor of improved outcome (Inouye et al. 2003). Marcantonio et al. (2001) extended this work and reported that proactive geriatric consultation with a protocol advising on 10 aspects of care reduced both incidence and severity of delirium in an elderly hip fracture population. In contrast, systematic detection of and multidisciplinary care for delirium produced minimal improvement in outcome of older medical inpatients (many with dementia) (Cole et al. 2002a). Use of preoperative psychological interventions to reduce anxiety and optimization of perioperative management with medical involvement may have a positive effect (Owens and Hutelmyer 1982; Schindler et al. 1989).

The role of baseline psychiatric status (besides dementia) as a risk factor for delirium is not well studied, although some have proposed that anxiety or depression may increase risk. The risk of delirium was increased in elderly patients who were depressed (B. Olofsson et al. 2005) and in children who were more anxious preoperatively (Kain et al. 2004).

OLD AGE

The aged brain is more vulnerable to delirium, in part related to structural and degenerative changes and reduced neurochemical flexibility. However, children are

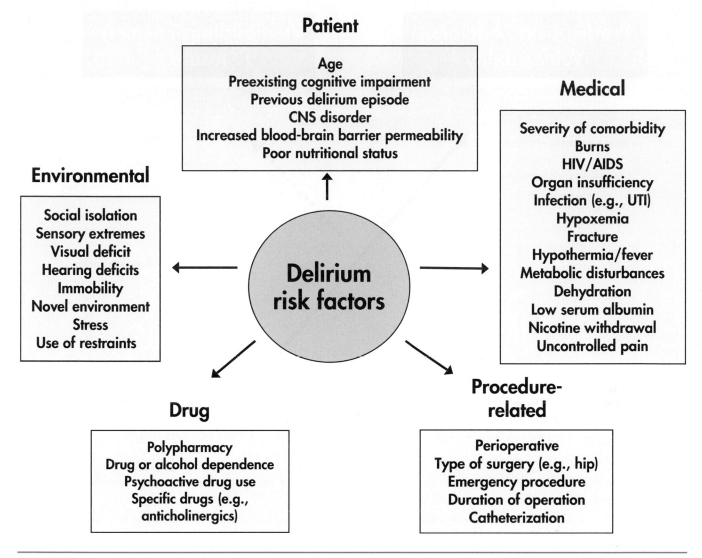

FIGURE 11–3. Risk factors for delirium. CNS=central nervous system; HIV=human immunodeficiency virus; AIDS= acquired immunodeficiency syndrome; UTI=urinary tract infection.

also considered at higher risk for delirium, possibly because of ongoing microstructural and neurochemical brain development. For example, pruning of synaptic bulbs and maturation of the cholinergic system continue into mid-adolescence, particularly in layer III of the prefrontal cortex. This layer is an associative area that interconnects with other brain association regions and is important for executive cognitive functions; this layer develops slowly throughout childhood, is especially affected by Alzheimer's neuropathological changes in the elderly, and is highly cholinergic. Perhaps immaturity or degeneration of this prefrontal cholinergic layer is relevant to vulnerability for delirium. Advanced age is also associated with a higher frequency of other risk factors such as cognitive impairment and vulnerability to drug toxicity. The elderly have diminished renal and hepatic function as well as reduced water-to-fat content ratio.

Moreover, the effects of drugs are mitigated less by counterregulatory homeostatic mechanisms (Turnheim 2003).

PREEXISTING COGNITIVE IMPAIRMENT

Up to two-thirds of the cases of delirium occur superimposed on preexisting cognitive impairment (L.A. Wahlund and Bjorlin 1999). Delirium is 2–3.5 times more common in patients with dementia than in control subjects without dementia (Erkinjuntti et al. 1986; Jitapunkul et al. 1992). Delirium risk appears to be greater in Alzheimer's disease of late onset and in vascular dementia than in other dementias, perhaps reflecting the relatively widespread neuronal disturbance associated with these conditions (Robertsson et al. 1998). Marcantonio et al. (2005) found that nondelirious elderly patients admitted

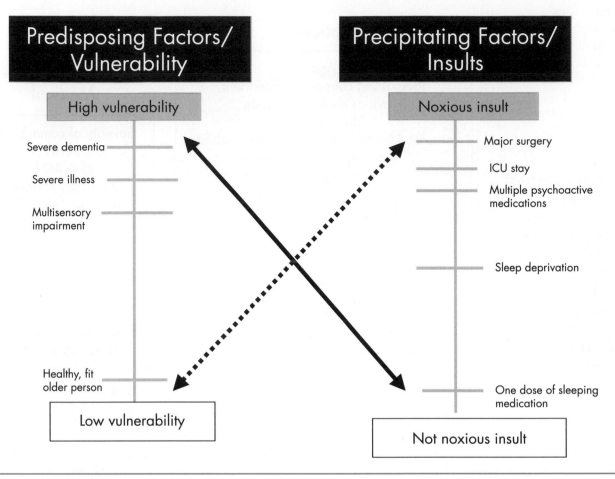

FIGURE 11-4.   Relation between an individual person's health status and the effects of insults determines the threshold for the occurrence of delirium. ICU=intensive care unit.

Source.   Adapted, with permission, from Inouye SK, Charpentier PA: "Precipitating Factors for Delirium in Hospitalized Elderly Patients: Predictive Model and Interrelationships With Baseline Vulnerability," *Journal of the American Medical Association* 275:852–857, 1996. Copyright © 1996, American Medical Association. All rights reserved.

to postacute facilities had virtually no preexisting dementia compared with those who had become delirious.

MEDICATIONS

Polypharmacy and drug intoxication or withdrawal may be the most common causes of delirium, but drug use is also a risk factor (Gaudreau et al. 2005b; Hales et al. 1988; Inouye and Charpentier 1996; Kagansky et al. 2004; Trzepacz et al. 1985). Benzodiazepines, opiates, and drugs with anticholinergic activity have a particular association with delirium (T.M. Brown 2000; Marcantonio et al. 1994). In elderly hip fracture patients, midazolam use was significantly related to delirium incidence (Santos et al. 2005). L. Han et al. (2001) studied older patients with preexisting delirium and found that exposure to anticholinergic medications worsened delirium. Many drugs (and their metabolites) can unexpectedly contribute to delirium as a result of unrecognized anticholinergic effects. Ten of the 25

most commonly prescribed drugs for the elderly had sufficient in vitro anticholinergic activity identified by radioreceptor assay to cause memory and attention impairment in elderly subjects without delirium (Tune et al. 1992). White et al. (2005) identified altered drug metabolism as a possible factor in delirium. Spectrophotometry identified reduced plasma esterase activity (including acetylcholinesterase and butyrylcholinesterase) in elderly patients with delirium compared with nondelirious control subjects and also found that mortality was associated with low plasma esterase activity at admission. It is therefore important to minimize drug exposure, especially when elderly patients are facing high-risk periods such as the perioperative phase.

NEUROLOGICAL INSULTS

Delirium can be an important presenting feature of cerebrovascular disease. L.A. Wahlund and Bjorlin (1999), in a review of elderly patients with delirium admitted to a medical facility, found that stroke without other neurological signs accounted for 14% of all cases of delirium. Ferro et al. (2002) reviewed literature relating to poststroke delirium and found that delirium can complicate the course of acute stroke in up to 48% of patients. Caeiro et al. (2004b) studied 22 delirious poststroke patients and found that delirium was more common after hemorrhagic rather than ischemic stroke and that anticholinergic medications were a particular risk factor in this population. A separate study of 218 consecutive patients with acute stroke found that delirium was more common after hemispheric than brain stem or cerebellar stroke—in particular, after right middle cerebral artery lesions—and after intracerebral rather than subarachnoid hemorrhage or cerebral infarct (Caeiro et al. 2004a). Delirium incidence was 16% in 68 consecutive cases of acute subarachnoid hemorrhage and associated with admission computed tomographic scan evidence of intraventricular bleeding, hydrocephalus, and basofrontal hematomas suggesting damage to networks subserving attention, declarative memory, and emotional expression (Caeiro et al. 2005).

Comparing parkinsonian patients with and without delirium, delirium was associated with increased risk of developing dementia, more severe motor impairment, and mortality (Serrano-Dueñas and Bleda 2005).

PAIN CONTROL MEDICATIONS

In hospitalized cancer patients, delirium risk is increased at cumulative daily doses of greater than 90 mg of morphine equivalents, greater than 15 mg of dexamethasone equivalents, and greater than 2 mg of lorazepam equivalents (Gaudreau et al. 2005a). Delirium was nine times more likely in older patients undergoing hip surgery deemed to have undertreated pain (Morrison et al. 2003), and delirium was associated with higher scores of bodily pain perioperatively (Duppils and Wikblad 2004). Similarly, Adunsky et al. (2002) found lower use of analgesia in patients developing delirium, suggesting that underuse of analgesia may be a factor in delirium genesis. Fann et al. (2005) studied the relation between delirium and pain severity with serial (thrice-weekly) assessments and found that a rise in pain severity seemed to predate delirium severity by 3 days, suggesting a possible risk factor for worsening delirium. B. Gagnon et al. (2001) identified alterations in the circadian pattern that the experience of pain typically follows in delirious patients as indicated by greater use of analgesia for breakthrough pain. Use of meperidine may be associated with an elevated risk of delirium (Adunsky et al. 2002; Morrison et al. 2003). Open-label switch from morphine to fentanyl in delirious cancer patients was associated with reduced delirium and pain severity and an escalation of opioid doses, despite the high anticholinergicity of fentanyl (Morita et al. 2005). Studies of patient-controlled analgesia have indicated that this approach to pain relief is associated with less overall opiate use, reduced delirium incidence (Tokita et al. 2001), and shorter duration of delirium when it occurs (Mann et al. 2000).

NUTRITIONAL FACTORS

Thiamine deficiency is an underappreciated cause of and/or risk factor for delirium in pediatric intensive care and oncology patients (Seear et al. 1992) and nonalcoholic elderly patients (O'Keeffe et al. 1994). Interestingly, thiamine is a cofactor necessary for adequate functioning of cholinergic neurons.

Low serum albumin is an important risk factor at any age and may signify poor nutrition, chronic disease, or liver or renal insufficiency. Hypoalbuminemia results in a greater bioavailability of many drugs that are transported in the bloodstream by albumin, and this is associated with an increased risk of side effects, including delirium (Dickson 1991; Trzepacz and Francis 1990). This increased biological drug activity occurs within the therapeutic range and is not recognized because increased levels of free drug are not reported separately in assays. Serum albumin was identified by discriminant analysis, along with Trail Making Test B and EEG dominant posterior rhythm, to sensitively distinguish delirious from nondelirious liver transplant candidates (Trzepacz et al. 1988b). Low serum albumin, along with advanced age, cognitive impairment, bone metastases, and a hematological malignancy was predictive of delirium in oncology patients (Ljubisljevic and Kelly 2003).

SMOKING AND NICOTINE WITHDRAWAL

The role of smoking in delirium risk appears complex. Benoit et al. (2005) studied risk factors for delirium in 102 patients undergoing elective abdominal surgery and found that the number of years that patients had previously smoked, but not current smoking status, was a significant predictor of delirium risk. Nicotine withdrawal has been implicated as a potential risk factor in the development of delirium, especially in heavy smokers unable to continue their habit during hospital admission. Mayer et al. (2001) and Klein et al. (2002) reported patients with presumed nicotine withdrawal–related delirium that rapidly responded to transdermal nicotine patches.

PERIOPERATIVE FACTORS

Postoperative delirium (excluding emergence from anesthesia) appears most frequently at day 3. Van der Mast (2000) proposed that surgery induces immune activation and a physical stress response. This is composed of increased limbic-hypothalamic-pituitary-adrenocortical axis activity, low triiodothyronine syndrome, and altered blood-brain barrier permeability. Increased blood-brain barrier permeability is a risk factor for delirium, as occurs in uremia. A large multicenter study (International Study of Post-Operative Cognitive Dysfunction) found age, duration of anesthesia, lower education level, second operation, postoperative infection, and respiratory complications to be predictors of postoperative cognitive impairment (Moller et al. 1998). However, this study reported little about possible pathophysiological mechanisms for impairment because delirium risk (screened for with MMSE) was not associated with hypoxemia, hypotension, or use of specific anesthetic agents or procedures. Other work has identified type of surgery (e.g., cardiothoracic), duration of operation, intraoperative complications, and emergency nature of procedure as perioperative factors associated with an elevated risk of delirium (Agnoletti et al. 2005; Bucerius et al. 2004). In postcardiotomy surgery, urgency of operation, intraoperative factors, and cerebrovascular disease were independent predictors of delirium (Bucerius et al. 2004).

Pratico and colleagues (2005) have proposed a model by which anesthetics acting on central cholinergic systems may cause postoperative delirium, but in a review of 20 randomized controlled trials that examined the role of anesthetic choice in postoperative cognitive dysfunction, Wu et al. (2004) found no evidence that general anesthetics were associated with a greater risk than regional anesthetics.

GENETIC FACTORS

Several studies have addressed the influence of genetic factors in delirium vulnerability. To date, these have focused mostly on alcohol withdrawal delirium (see Table 11–5) and suggest positive associations between the risk of delirium tremens and polymorphisms of genes for neuropeptide Y (Koehnke et al. 2002), glutamatergic kainate receptor subunit gene (Preuss et al. 2003, 2006), cannabinoid receptor (Schmidt et al. 2002), and brain-derived neurotrophic factor (BDNF) (Matsushita et al. 2004). Conversely, studies of genes for norepinephrine transporter (Samochowiec et al. 2002), dopamine β-hydroxylase (Köhnke et al. 2006), glutamate transporter (Sander et al. 2000), metabotropic glutamate receptors (Preuss et al. 2002), BDNF (Matsushita et al. 2004), and N-methyl-D-aspartate receptor subunits (Rujescu et al. 2005; Tadic et al. 2005) have not identified significant associations with delirium propensity. Studies of the dopamine transporter gene have been both positive (Gorwood et al. 2003; Wernicke et al. 2002) and negative (Köhnke et al. 2005).

A few studies addressed the role of genetic factors in the expression of delirium symptoms as well as treatment response to antipsychotics in delirium. These studies suggested that visual hallucinations during alcohol withdrawal delirium are more frequent in subjects with the A9 allele of the dopamine transporter gene (Limosin et al. 2004), cholecystokinin A receptor (Okubo et al. 2002) and promoter gene polymorphisms (Okubo et al. 2000), catechol-O-methyltransferase (COMT) polymorphisms (A. Nakamura et al. 2001), and NRH:quinone oxidoreductase 2 polymorphisms (an enzyme involved in alcohol metabolism) (Okubo et al. 2003). J.Y. Kim et al. (2005) did not find any relation between dopamine transporter gene polymorphisms and responsiveness to risperidone or haloperidol in medical-surgical patients. Pomara et al. (2004) studied the relation between the apolipoprotein E (APOE) genotype and sensitivity to anticholinergic medication exposure (trihexyphenidyl hydrochloride) in cognitively intact elderly and found that subjects with the *APOE*E4* allele experienced significantly greater cognitive impairment. On a similar note, van Munster et al. (2005) studied the *APOE* genotype in a small sample of elderly general hospital patients and were unable to find an association with delirium risk.

The temporal relation between exposure to risk factors and development of delirium has received limited study to date—the multifactorial nature of most delirium episodes suggests that various vulnerability factors may interact with changing environmental insults over time. For example, hypoalbuminemia may become more relevant to delirium on commencement of pharmacological treatment of a medical cause of delirium (e.g., respiratory infection). The dynamic relation among factors remains understudied.

ETIOLOGIES OF DELIRIUM

Delirium has a wide variety of etiologies alone or in combination. Figure 11–5 is a part of the Delirium Etiology Checklist (Paula Trzepacz, personal communication, 2006), a standardized tool used to determine etiologies within 13 categories; the etiologies can then be rated for degree of likelihood on the basis of overall clinical evaluation of a patient. These categories include primary CNS disorders, systemic disturbances that affect cerebral function, and drug or toxin exposure (including intoxication and withdrawal). Often multiple etiologies occur serially in addition to concurrently and may prolong the delirium episode. We hypothesize that delirium severity is a function of an individual's baseline delirium vulnerability, such as age or genetics, interacting with multiple overlapping or serial etiologies, as illustrated in Figure 11–6.

TABLE 11–5.   Studies of genetic factors in delirium

Study	Population	Gene	Findings
Sander et al. 1997	293 alcoholic patients	*DAT* gene	Patients with variable number tandem repeat polymorphism had increased risk of delirium.
Okubo et al. 2000	214 male alcoholic patients	CCK gene promoter region	Patients who had hallucinations were significantly more likely to possess the C allele than were control subjects.
Sander et al. 2000	166 alcoholic patients	Glutamate transporter *EAAT2* gene	No association with alcohol withdrawal delirium.
A. Nakamura et al. 2001	91 male alcoholic patients	Catechol-O-methyltransferase (COMT) gene	Frequency of visual and auditory hallucinations associated with polymorphisms in COMT gene.
Preuss et al. 2002	182 DSM-IV alcohol-dependent subjects	Metabotropic glutamate receptors 7 and 8 genes	No association with delirium tremens.
Schmidt et al. 2002	121 severe alcoholic patients	Cannabinoid receptor gene (*CNR1*)	Homozygous genotype *CNR1 1359A/A* associated with greater vulnerability to alcohol withdrawal delirium.
Okubo et al. 2002	131 male alcoholic patients	CCKA receptor gene	Significant association between polymorphism at −85 locus and hallucinations accompanying delirium tremens.
Wernicke et al. 2003	367 alcoholic patients	*R1* and *R2B* NMDA receptor genes	A allele of *R1* gene associated with delirium tremens.
Koehnke et al. 2002	216 alcoholic patients	Neuropeptide Y	Non–statistically significant elevated frequency of C allele in patients experiencing complicated withdrawal (including delirium tremens).
Samochowiec et al. 2002	157 alcoholic patients	Norepinephrine transporter gene	G1287A mutation not associated with alcohol withdrawal symptoms.
Gorwood et al. 2003	120 alcohol-dependent patients	A9 allele of dopamine transporter	Increased risk of delirium tremens.
Okubo et al. 2003	247 male alcoholic patients	NRH-quinone oxidoreductase 2 (*NQO2*) Glutathione *S*-transferase M1 (*GSTM1*) NAD(P)H-quinone oxidoreductase 1 (*NQO1*)	Polymorphism at the promoter region of the *NQO2* associated with frequency of delirium tremens and hallucinations.
Preuss et al. 2003	196 patients with DSM-IV alcohol dependence	Cannabinoid receptor gene (*CNR1*)	No association with alcohol withdrawal symptoms.

TABLE 11–5. Studies of genetic factors in delirium *(continued)*

Study	Population	Gene	Findings
Matsushita et al. 2004	377 male alcoholic patients	Brain-derived neurotrophic factor gene (*BDNF*)	Delirium tremens more frequent in patients with G196A polymorphism.
Limosin et al. 2004	64 women with alcohol withdrawal delirium	A9 allele of dopamine transporter	Increased risk of visual hallucinations (in alcohol withdrawal).
Rujescu et al. 2005	442 alcohol-dependent subjects	NMDA receptor-1 subunit (*GRIN1*)	Alcohol withdrawal seizures more frequent in patients with 2108A allele. No association with delirium tremens.
Tadic et al. 2005	377 alcoholic patients	NMDA receptor-2B subunit (*NR2B*)	No association with withdrawal-related traits.
J.Y. Kim et al. 2005	42 patients with delirium	Dopamine transporter gene	DAT polymorphisms not related to response to risperidone vs. haloperidol.
Köhnke et al. 2005	216 alcoholic patients	Dopamine transporter gene	No association between A9 allele and alcohol withdrawal symptoms.
Köhnke et al. 2006	208 alcoholic patients	Dopamine β-hydroxylase gene	DBH(*)444G/A polymorphism not associated with alcohol withdrawal symptoms.
van Munster et al. 2005	126 elderly general hospital admissions	Apolipoprotein E	No association with delirium risk.
Preuss et al. 2006	233 patients with DSM-IV alcohol dependence	Glutamatergic kainate receptor subunit (*GlurR7*) gene	Significant relation between history of delirium tremens and the Ser310 allele.

Note. NMDA = *N*-methyl-D-aspartate.

In DSM-IV-TR, delirium is coded with some regard to etiology: general medical condition, substance intoxication or withdrawal, multiple causes, or no apparent identifiable cause. For an etiology to be considered causal, 1) it should be a recognized possible cause of delirium and 2) it should be temporally related in onset and course to delirium presentation, but 3) the delirium should not be better accounted for by other factors.

Between two and six possible causes are typically identified (Breitbart et al. 1996; Francis et al. 1990; Meagher et al. 1996; O'Keeffe 1999; Trzepacz et al. 1985), with a single etiology identified in 50% or fewer of the cases (Camus et al. 2000b; Morita et al. 2001; O'Keeffe 1999; S.M. Olofsson et al. 1996; Ramirez-Bermudez et al. 2006). It is important that clinicians consider further investigation after one likely cause is determined. Multiple-etiology delir-

ium is more frequent in the elderly and those with terminal illness. For example, delirium in cancer patients can be due to the direct effect of the primary tumor or an indirect effect of metastases, metabolic problems (organ failure or electrolyte disturbance), chemotherapy, radiation and other treatments, infections, vascular complications, nutritional deficits, and paraneoplastic syndromes. This multifactorial nature has been underemphasized in research—etiological attribution is typically based on clinical impressions that are not standardized (e.g., the most likely cause identified by the referring physician) or oversimplified by documenting a single etiology for each case.

Some causes occur more frequently in particular populations. Drugs and polypharmacy commonly cause or contribute to delirium, especially in elderly patients (T.M. Brown 2000). Drug-related causes are more com-

Drug Intoxication

1❏ Alcohol   3❏ Opiate   5❏ Hallucinogenic   6❏ Prescribed drug _____
2❏ Sedative-hypnotic 4❏ Psychostimulant   7❏ Other _____
                                                          8❏ OTC _____

Drug Withdrawal

1❏ Alcohol   3❏ Prescribed drug _____
2❏ Sedative-hypnotic   4❏ Other drug _____

Metabolic/Endocrine Disturbance

1❏ Volume depletion	6❏ Uremia	12❏ Hypoalbuminemia	21❏ Hypomagnesiemia
2❏ Volume overload	7❏ Anemia	13❏ Hyperalbuminemia	22❏ Hypermagnesiemia
3❏ Acidosis	8❏ Avitaminosis _____	14❏ Bilirubinemia	23❏ Hypophosphatemia
4❏ Alkalosis	9❏ Hypervitaminosis _____	15❏ Hypocalcemia	24❏ Hypothyroidism
5❏ Hypoxia	10❏ Hypoglycemia	16❏ Hypercalcemia	25❏ Hyperthyroidism
	11❏ Hyperglycemia	17❏ Hypokalemia	26❏ Hypoparathyroidism
		18❏ Hyperkalemia	27❏ Hyperparathyroidism
		19❏ Hyponatremia	28❏ Cushing's syndrome
30❏ Other_____		20❏ Hypernatremia	29❏ Addison's disease

❏ Traumatic Brain Injury

❏ Seizures

Intracranial Infection

1❏ Meningitis   3❏ Abscess   5❏ HIV
2❏ Encephalitis   4❏ Neurosyphilis   6❏ Other _____

Systemic Infection

1❏ Bacteremia   3❏ Fungal   5❏ Viral   7❏ Urinary
2❏ Sepsis   4❏ Protozoal 6❏ Respiratory 8❏ Other _____

Intracranial Neoplasm

1❏ Primary   2❏ Metastasis   3❏ Meningeal carcinomatosis
Histology _____ Site _____

Extracranial Neoplasm

Site of primary lesion _____   ❏ Paraneoplastic syndrome

Cerebrovascular Disorder

1❏ Transient ischemic attack   3❏ Stroke   6❏ Intraparenchymal hemorrhage
2❏ Subarachnoid hemorrhage   4❏ Subdural hemorrhage 7❏ Cerebral vasculitis
                               5❏ Cerebral edema   8❏ Other _____

Organ Insufficiency

1❏ Cardiac   3❏ Hepatic   5❏ Pancreatic
2❏ Pulmonary   4❏ Renal   6❏ Other _____

Other CNS

1❏ Parkinson's disease   3❏ Multiple sclerosis   5❏ Hydrocephalus
2❏ Huntington's disease   4❏ Wilson's disease   6❏ Other _____

Other Systemic

1❏ Heatstroke   3❏ Radiation   5❏ Immunosuppressed   7❏ Fractures
2❏ Hypothermia   4❏ Postoperative state 6❏ Other_____

© Trzepacz 1999

FIGURE 11–5. Delirium Etiology Checklist worksheet. Contact author for copy of complete checklist (PTT@lilly.com).

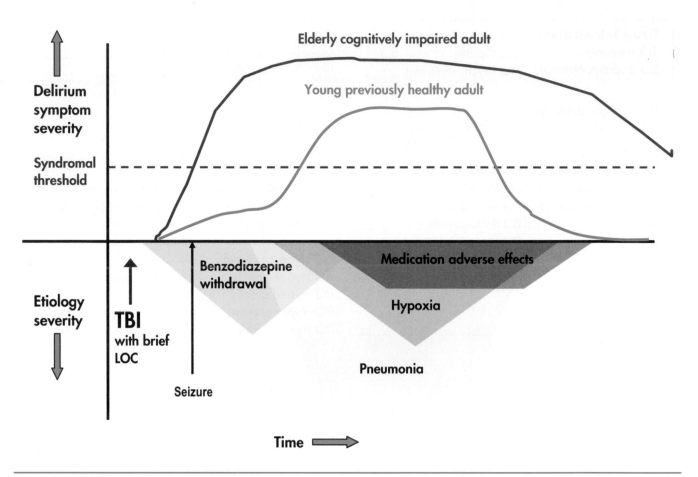

FIGURE 11–6. Delirium severity as a function of an individual's baseline delirium vulnerability interacting with multiple overlapping or serial etiologies. TBI=traumatic brain injury; LOC=loss of consciousness.

monly reported in psychiatric populations. Delirium in children and adolescents involves the same categories of etiologies as in adults, although specific causes may differ. Delirium related to illicit drugs is more common in younger populations, whereas that due to prescribed drugs and polypharmacy is more common in older populations. Cerebral hypoxia is common at age extremes, with chronic obstructive airway disease, myocardial infarction, and stroke common in older patients and hypoxia due to foreign body inhalation, drowning, and asthma more frequent in younger patients. Poisonings are also more common in children than in adults, whereas children and the elderly both have high rates of delirium related to head trauma—bicycle accidents in children and falls in the elderly.

Once the diagnosis of delirium is made, a careful and thorough, although prioritized, search for causes must be conducted. Ameliorations of specific underlying causes are important in resolving delirium, although this should not preclude treatment of the delirium itself, which can reduce symptoms even before underlying medical causes are rectified (Breitbart et al. 1996).

DELIRIUM DETECTION, SCREENING, AND ASSESSMENT

Given the high rates of missed diagnosis, there is a great need for brief screening tools that enable prompt recognition of delirium with high sensitivity even if specificity is lower. Screening tools can provide a provisional diagnosis but often have poor differential diagnostic capability. Screening tools also differ from tools that monitor severity over time and from tools that are focused on a few preclinical symptoms that are highly predictive of an episode. Validated tools for the latter two tasks do not exist yet.

Screening tools for delirium need to be convenient for use in day-to-day practice as well as suitable for use by nonpsychiatric physicians and nurses. The CAM is probably the most widely used delirium screening tool in general hospitals (Inouye et al. 1990). It is based on DSM-III-R criteria and requires the presence of three of four cardinal symptoms of delirium. It is intended for use by nonpsychiatric clinicians in hospital settings and is useful for case finding, although nurses' ratings were much less sensitive than those done by physicians (1.00 vs. 0.13) when compared with an independent physician's DSM-III-R diagnosis (Rolfson et al. 1999). One study (Rockwood 1993) suggested that lower specificity and sensitivity are a trade-off for its simplicity, although in other studies, it performed well compared with physicians' diagnoses in short-term hospital settings. It has not been well studied for its ability to distinguish delirium from dementia, depression, or other psychiatric disorders. Cole et al. (2003a) assessed the sensitivity and specificity of the full CAM in patients with DSM-III-R–diagnosed delirium, dementia, or comorbid delirium-dementia. When these investigators used a cutoff of 6 of 11 items present, they found 95% sensitivity and 83% specificity in delirium-only cases and 98% sensitivity and 76% specificity in comorbid cases; however, when they used fewer items, such as a minimum cutoff of 3 symptoms, the specificities were greatly reduced to 60% for delirium and 47% for comorbid delirium-dementia. When used to screen elderly emergency department patients for delirium based on a geriatrician's interview as compared with an observing lay person, the CAM had interrater reliability of 0.91, sensitivity of 0.86, and specificity of 1.00 (Monette et al. 2001). The CAM-ICU (Ely et al. 2001b) uses specific adjunctive tests and standardized administration to enhance reliability and validity and had 95% validity and 0.92–0.96 interrater reliability as compared with expert psychiatric DSM-IV diagnosis of delirium in two different validation studies of 150 ICU patients (Ely et al. 2001a, 2001b). However, because this population is among the highest for delirium incidence (>80%), not much variability exists to differentiate from other diagnoses.

Fanjiang and Folstein (2001) piloted a simple screening scale, the Three Item Delirium Scale, for bedside detection of delirium by medical students. It requires the presence of altered consciousness plus either cognitive impairment or hallucinations. An initial report suggested that it has high sensitivity (0.89) and specificity (1.00) compared with an attending psychiatrist diagnosis, although the medical students were not blind to patient history at the time of the ratings.

Because delirium is primarily a cognitive disorder, bedside assessment of cognition is critical to proper diagnosis. All cognitive domains are affected—orientation, attention, short- and long-term memory, visuoconstructional ability, and executive functions (the latter are poorly studied in delirium)—even though attentional deficits are most specifically emphasized in DSM. Pattern and timing of deficits assist in differential diagnosis from dementias and amnestic disorders.

Use of bedside screening tests such as the MMSE allows documentation of the presence of a cognitive disorder, although the MMSE alone is insufficient to distinguish delirium from dementia (Rolfson et al. 1999; Trzepacz et al. 1988a). The MMSE is easy for many people (ceiling effect) and has a limited breadth of items, particularly for prefrontal executive and right hemisphere functions. The emphasis on orientation, which is an unreliable indicator of delirium, is a disadvantage of the MMSE (Meagher et al. 2007). Nevertheless, O'Keeffe et al. (2005) studied 165 elderly hospital patients and found that a two-point or greater decline in the MMSE score detected CAM-diagnosed delirium with 93% sensitivity and 90% specificity, and a three-point or greater increase in the MMSE score detected delirium resolution with 77% sensitivity and 75% specificity. Serial MMSE assessments may be of some value in diagnosing and monitoring delirium, but the use of the CAM as the gold standard may not be ideal. Fayers et al. (2005) examined the predictive value for delirium of specific MMSE items in two separate large populations (elderly patients admitted to a medical facility and patients with cancer diagnoses) and found that four separate items (current year, date, backward spelling, and copying a pentagon) were accurate for identifying ICD-10 delirium, although the role of preexisting or emergent dementia was not clearly accounted for. This contrasts with studies of dementia in which orientation to time and recall of three objects provided the best discrimination for dementia of Alzheimer's type (Galasko et al. 1990; Solfrizzi et al. 2001).

The combination of a global rating of attentiveness, Digit Span Backward, and cancellation tests differentiated delirium from dementia among elderly medical inpatients, whereas the vigilance test, MMSE, and Digit Span Forward did not (O'Keeffe and Gosney 1997). However, patients were excluded from the study if their MMSE score was 10 points or less, which limits applicability to many patients with delirium and severe dementia. Trail Making Test B along with reduced serum albumin and EEG dominant posterior rhythm distinguished delirious from nondelirious liver transplant candidates with 97% sensitivity and 83% specificity (Trzepacz et al. 1988a). Fann et al. (2002) found that patients who developed delirium after stem cell transplantation had lower Trail Making Test B scores pretransplant. The Trail Making Test B may be a useful test to screen for or monitor delirium, although the patient needs to be able to write.

The Clock Drawing Test assesses constructional praxis, visuospatial ability, executive function, and verbal and semantic memory. Fisher and Flowerdew (1995) found that the Clock Drawing Test was superior to the MMSE for predicting risk of postoperative delirium in older patients. Manos (1997) found the Clock Drawing Test to be a useful screen for cognitive impairment in medically ill patients, even though it did not discriminate between delirium and dementia. K.Y. Kim et al. (2003) used the Clock Drawing Test and MMSE to plot treatment response to quetiapine in delirium and found that scores on both tests improved as delirium resolved over a 4-week period. However, Rolfson et al. (1999) found that neither the Clock Drawing Test nor the MMSE was a sensitive marker of delirium in elderly cardiac surgery patients. The Clock Drawing Test detects overall cognitive impairment in elderly medical inpatients but lacks specificity for either the severity or the presence of delirium (Adamis et al. 2005); however, it correlated reasonably with the DRS ($r = -0.60$) and MMSE ($r = 0.70$).

COGNITIVE ASSESSMENT

The CTD (Hart et al. 1996) is a bedside cognitive test designed specifically for delirious patients, who are often unable to speak or write in a medical setting. The CTD correlates highly with the MMSE ($r = 0.82$) in delirium patients and was performable in 42% of the ICU patients in whom the MMSE was not. It has two equivalent forms that correlate highly ($r = 0.90$) in dementia patients, which allows for repeated measurements. However, it correlates less well with symptom rating scales for delirium that include noncognitive symptoms—for example, the Medical College of Virginia Nurses Rating Scale for Delirium (Hart et al. 1996) ($r = -0.02$) or the DRS-R98 (Trzepacz et al. 2001) ($r = -0.62$). The CTD has many nonverbal (nondominant hemisphere) items and includes abstraction questions. R.E. Kennedy et al. (2003) tested the CTD in 65 traumatic brain injury patients in a neurorehabilitation hospital and found 72% sensitivity and 70% specificity compared with DSM-IV diagnoses of delirium.

It has been theorized that prefrontal and right hemisphere circuits are especially important in delirium neuropathophysiology (Trzepacz 1994a, 1999b, 2000). Two studies found that just a few cognitive tests (e.g., similarities and Digit Span Forward) were able to discriminate delirious from nondelirious medical patients. One assessed only right hemisphere functions—visual attention span forward and recognition memory for pictures (Hart et al. 1997)—and the other assessed prefrontal functions (Bettin et al. 1998).

DELIRIUM ASSESSMENT INSTRUMENTS

Diagnostic criteria are important in diagnosing delirium, and cognitive tests are useful to document cognitive impairment. Rating the severity of the broad range of delirium symptoms, however, requires other methods. The choice of instrument is dictated by many factors, as listed in Table 11–6. Unfortunately, the increase in the

number of instruments developed for delirium assessment has not been matched by an equivalent body of research to support their use by confirming suitability for use in different populations with well-designed psychometric studies. More than 10 instruments have been proposed to assess symptoms of delirium for screening, diagnosis, or symptom severity rating (Trzepacz 1994b). However, only a few of these have been used broadly (see descriptions below). Three instruments operationalized DSM-III criteria: the Saskatoon Delirium Checklist (Miller et al. 1988), the Organic Brain Syndrome Scale (Berggren et al. 1987), and the Delirium Assessment Scale (O'Keeffe 1994). In these, DSM-III–derived items are rated along a continuum of mild, moderate, and severe. None has been well described or validated. The Delirium Assessment Scale could not distinguish delirium from dementia patients. A more recently developed severity scale, the Confusional State Evaluation (Robertsson 1999), assessed 22 items, but 12 were determined a priori to be "key symptoms." It was not validated against control groups, and dementia patients were included in the delirium group.

TABLE 11–6. Factors relevant to choice of delirium assessment instrument

Purpose of the assessment
> Screening
>
> Diagnosis
>
> Severity
>
> Serial measurement of profile
>
> Range of symptoms measured

Assessor
> Nurse
>
> Physician
>
> Trained researcher

Ease of use
> Time available
>
> Need for training

Population to be studied and location
> Ability to cooperate with procedure
>
> Validity in different populations

Psychometric properties of the instrument
> Reliability
>
> Internal consistency
>
> Validity

The most commonly used delirium assessment tool by nurses is the NEECHAM Confusion Scale (Neelon et al. 1986). It is scored from 0 to 30 with cutoffs for levels of confusion severity and was originally validated in elderly acute medical and nursing home settings without a control group. Interrater reliability was 0.96, correlation with the MMSE was 0.81, and correlation with nurses' subjective ratings was 0.46. It has three sections—information processing, behavior, and physiological measurement. Internal consistency was between 0.73 and 0.82 (Cronbach α) in 73 elderly hip surgery patients, and factor analysis detected three factors (Johansson et al. 2002). The psychometric qualities of the NEECHAM scale also have been assessed in elderly ICU patients, indicating internal consistency (0.81) and concordance with DSM-III-R criteria (0.68) (Csokasy 1999). It has been translated into Swedish, Norwegian, Dutch, and Japanese.

The DRS (Trzepacz et al. 1988a) is a 10-item scale assessing a breadth of delirium features and can function both to clarify diagnosis and to assess symptom severity because of its hierarchical nature (Trzepacz 1999a; van der Mast 1994). It is probably the most widely used delirium rating scale and has been translated into Italian, French, Spanish, Korean, Japanese, Mandarin Chinese, Dutch, Swedish, German, Portuguese, and a language of India for international use. It is generally used by those who have some psychiatric training. The DRS has high interrater reliability and validity even compared with other psychiatric patient groups, and it distinguishes delirium from dementia. It has been modified by some researchers to a 7- or 8-item subscale for repeated measures. In one study (Treloar and MacDonald 1997), the DRS and CAM diagnosed delirium with a high level of agreement ($r = 0.81$). It has been used to assess delirium in children and adolescents (Turkel et al. 2003).

The MDAS is a 10-item severity rating scale for use after a diagnosis of delirium has been made (Breitbart et al. 1997). It was intended for repeated ratings within a 24-hour period, as occurs in treatment studies. It does not include items for temporal onset and fluctuation of symptoms, which are characteristic symptoms that help to distinguish delirium from dementia. The MDAS correlated highly with the DRS ($r = 0.88$) and the MMSE ($r = -0.91$). The Japanese version of the MDAS was validated in 37 elderly patients with delirium, dementia, mood disorder, or schizophrenia and was found to distinguish among them ($P < 0.0001$), with a mean score of 18 in the delirium group (Matsuoka et al. 2001). It correlated reasonably well with the DRS Japanese version ($r = -0.74$) and the Clinician's Global Rating of Delirium ($r = 0.67$) and less well with the MMSE ($r = 0.54$). The Italian version of the MDAS (Grassi et al. 2001) correlated well

with the DRS Italian version in a study of 105 consecutive cancer patients (66 had delirium). When the CAM was used as the diagnostic standard, the MDAS had a high specificity (94%) but low sensitivity (68%), whereas the DRS with a cutoff of 10 had high sensitivity (95%) and low specificity (68%) and with a cutoff of 12 had a sensitivity of 80% and a specificity of 76%. In this same study, the MMSE had 96% sensitivity but only 38% specificity. Factor analysis showed a three-factor structure for the DRS and a two-factor structure for the MDAS. Lawlor et al. (2000b) used the MDAS in cancer patients with DSM-IV–diagnosed delirium and found two factors: Cronbach $\alpha = 0.78$ and a correlation ($r = 0.55$) with the MMSE.

The DRS-R98 is a substantially revised version of the DRS that addresses the shortcomings of the DRS (Trzepacz et al. 2001). It allows for repeated measurements and includes separate or new items for language, thought processes, motor agitation, motor retardation, and five cognitive domains. The DRS-R98 has 16 items, with 3 diagnostic items separable from the 13-item severity subscale for serial measurements. Anchored severity descriptions for a broad range of symptoms known to occur in delirium use standard phenomenological definitions, without a priori assumptions about which symptoms occur more frequently. The total scale is used for initial evaluation of delirium to allow discrimination from other disorders. The DRS-R98 total score ($P < 0.001$) distinguished delirium from dementia, schizophrenia, depression, and other medical conditions during blind ratings, with sensitivities ranging from 91% to 100% and specificities from 85% to 100%, depending on the cutoff score chosen. It has high internal consistency (Cronbach $\alpha = 0.90$), correlates well with the DRS ($r = 0.83$) and the CTD ($r = -0.62$), and has high interrater reliability (intraclass correlation coefficient $= 0.99$). In a recent review of delirium assessment tools, Timmers and colleagues (2005) concluded that the DRS-R98 was the best overall of currently available delirium rating tools largely because of its range of symptoms and suitability for use by physicians and research assistants. Translations exist or are in progress for Spanish, Portuguese, Japanese, Korean, Greek, Danish, Dutch, German, French, Lithuanian, Norwegian, Italian, and Chinese versions. Japanese, Dutch, and Spanish (Spain) versions have been validated and published (De Rooij 2005a; Fonseca et al. 2005; Kishi et al. 2001). Colombian Spanish and Portuguese validation studies are completed but yet unpublished. A Palm Pilot version has been used for clinical research (Hill et al. 2002).

On the basis of issues such as instrument design, purpose, available translations, and breadth of use, a few of the available instruments are recommended (Table 11–7). They can be used together or separately depending on the

TABLE 11–7.   Recommended delirium assessment instruments[a]

Instrument	Type	Rater
Confusion Assessment Method (Inouye et al. 1990)	4-item diagnostic screener	Nonpsychiatric clinician
Confusion Assessment Method for ICU (Ely et al. 2001b)	4-item diagnostic screener anchored by objective tests	ICU nurses
Delirium Rating Scale[b] (Trzepacz et al. 1998)	10-item severity/diagnostic scale	Psychiatrically trained clinician
Memorial Delirium Assessment Scale (Breitbart et al. 1997)	10-item severity scale	Clinician
Delirium Rating Scale—Revised-98 (Trzepacz et al. 2001)	16-item scale (severity and diagnostic subscales)	Psychiatrically trained clinician
Cognitive Test for Delirium (Hart et al. 1996)	5 cognitive domains as bedside test	Trained technician or clinician

Note.   ICU=intensive care unit.
[a]See text for descriptions.
[b]Has been used in children.

clinical or research need. For example, a screening tool can be used for case detection, followed by a more thorough assessment for meeting DSM criteria and symptom severity.

ELECTROENCEPHALOGRAPHY

In the 1940s, Engel and Romano (1944, 1959; Romano and Engel 1944) first wrote a series of classic papers that described the relation of delirium, as measured by cognitive impairment, to electroencephalographic slowing. In their seminal work, they showed an association between abnormal electrical activity of the brain and the psychiatric symptoms of delirium; the reversibility of both conditions; the ubiquity of electroencephalographic changes for different underlying disease states; and an improvement in electroencephalography background rhythm that paralleled clinical improvement. The thalamus drives the normal awake, resting alpha rhythm, and cholinergic activity is necessary such that anticholinergic agents cause slowing of the dominant posterior rhythm. Abnormalities in evoked potentials support a role for the thalamus in delirium (Trzepacz et al. 1989).

Working with burn patients, Andreasen et al. (1977) showed that the time course of electroencephalographic slowing could precede or lag behind overt clinical symptoms of delirium, although sensitive delirium symptom ratings were not used. EEG dominant posterior rhythm, along with serum albumin and the Trail Making Test B, distinguished delirious from nondelirious cirrhosis patients in another study (Trzepacz et al. 1988b). Although generalized slowing is the typical EEG pattern for both hypoactive and hyperactive presentations of delirium and for most eti-

ologies of delirium, delirium tremens is associated with predominantly low-voltage fast activity (Kennard et al. 1945), making it an important exception. An animal model for delirium that used atropine found similar electroencephalographic slowing in rats as in humans that was associated over time with worsened cognitive function (maze performance) (Leavitt et al. 1994; Trzepacz et al. 1992).

EEG characteristics in delirium include slowing or dropout of the dominant posterior rhythm, diffuse theta or delta waves (i.e., slowing), poor organization of background rhythm, and loss of reactivity of the EEG to eye opening and closing (Jacobson and Jerrier 2000). Similarly, quantitative EEG (QEEG) in delirium shows parallel findings affecting slowing of power bands' mean frequency (see Figure 11–7) as compared with nondelirious control subjects.

Table 11–8 describes different EEG patterns that can be seen clinically in delirium. Although diffuse slowing is the most common presentation, false-negative results occur when a person's characteristic dominant posterior rhythm does not slow sufficiently to drop from the alpha to the theta range, thereby being read as normal despite the presence of abnormal slowing for that individual. (Generally, a change of more than 1 Hz from an individual's baseline is considered abnormal.) Comparison with prior baseline EEGs is often helpful to document that slowing has in fact occurred. Less commonly, but nonetheless important, an EEG may detect focal problems, such as ictal and subictal states or a previously unsuspected tumor that presents with prominent confusion. These include toxic ictal psychosis, nonconvulsive status, and complex partial status epilepticus (Drake and Coffey 1983; Trzepacz 1994a) or focal lesions (Jacobson and Jerrier 2000). New-onset complex partial seizures are un-

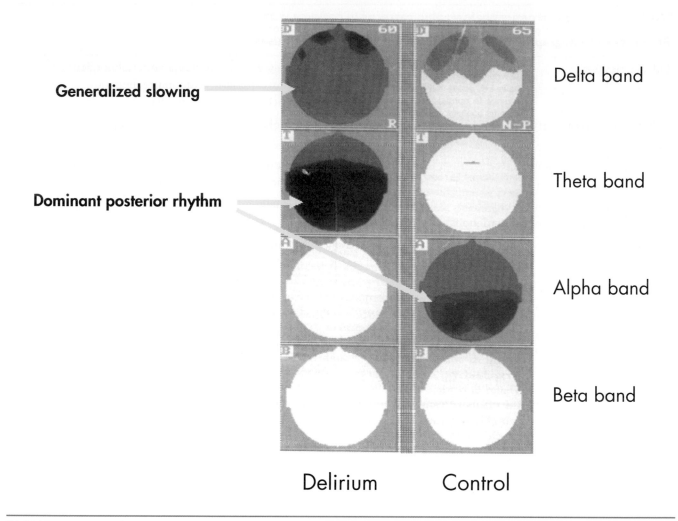

Generalized slowing

Dominant posterior rhythm

Delta band

Theta band

Alpha band

Beta band

Delirium   Control

FIGURE 11–7. Quantitative electroencephalogram (QEEG) brain map in delirium. Relative power in each of four frequency bands (higher power in darker color).

Source. Reprinted from Jacobson S, Jerrier H: "EEG in Delirium." *Seminars in Clinical Neuropsychiatry* 5:86–92, copyright 2000, with permission from Elsevier.

derappreciated in the elderly, related to ischemic damage (Sundaram and Dostrow 1995). Jacobson and Jerrier (2000) warned that it can be difficult to distinguish delirium from drowsiness and light sleep unless the technologist includes standard alerting procedures during the EEG. In most cases, EEGs are not needed to make a clinical diagnosis of delirium, instead being used when seizures are suspected or differential diagnosis is difficult, such as in schizophrenic patients with medical illness.

More recent advances in electroencephalographic technologies have expanded our knowledge. Koponen et al. (1989b) used spectral analysis of delirious elderly patients (about 75% of whom also had dementia) and found significant reductions in alpha percentage, increased theta and delta activity, and slowing of the peak and mean frequencies. All of these findings are consistent with electroencephalographic slowing. The study also found a corre-

lation between the severity of cognitive decline and the length of the patient's hospital stay and the degree of electroencephalographic slowing. Jacobson et al. (1993a) could use QEEG to distinguish delirious from nondelirious individuals with the relative power of the alpha frequency band and could distinguish delirious from demented patients according to theta activity and the relative power of the delta band. Serial EEGs of delirious patients showed associations between the relative power of the alpha band and cognitive ability, whereas in demented patients, the absolute power of the delta band was associated with cognitive changes (Jacobson et al. 1993b). QEEG could replace conventional EEG for delirium assessment in the future (Jacobson and Jerrier 2000).

Evoked potentials also may be abnormal in delirium, suggesting thalamic or subcortical involvement in the production of symptoms. Metabolic causes of delirium

TABLE 11–8.   Electroencephalographic patterns in patients with delirium

Electroencephalographic finding	Comment	Causes
Diffuse slowing	Most typical delirium pattern	Many causes, including anticholinergicity, posttraumatic brain injury, hepatic encephalopathy, hypoxia
Low-voltage fast activity	Typical of delirium tremens	Alcohol withdrawal; benzodiazepine intoxication
Spikes/polyspikes, frontocentral	Toxic ictal pattern (nonconvulsive)	Hypnosedative drug withdrawal; tricyclic and phenothiazine intoxication
Left/bilateral slowing or delta bursts; frontal intermittent rhythmic delta	Acute confusional migraine	Usually in adolescents
Epileptiform activity, frontotemporal or generalized	Status with prolonged confusional states	Nonconvulsive status and complex partial status epilepticus

precipitate abnormalities in visual, auditory, and somatosensory evoked potentials (Kullmann et al. 1995; Trzepacz et al. 1989), whereas somatosensory evoked potentials are abnormal in patients whose delirium is due to posttraumatic brain injury, suggesting damage to the medial lemniscus. In general, normalization of evoked potentials parallels clinical improvement, although evoked potentials are not routinely recorded for clinical purposes.

EEGs and evoked potentials in children with delirium show patterns similar to those in adults, with diffuse slowing on EEG and increased latencies of evoked potentials (J.A. Katz et al. 1988; Okamura et al. 2005; Prugh et al. 1980; Ruijs et al. 1993, 1994). The degree of slowing on EEGs and evoked potentials recorded serially over time in children and adolescents correlates with the severity of delirium and with recovery from delirium (Foley et al. 1981; Montgomery et al. 1991; Onofrj et al. 1991).

PHENOMENOLOGY OF DELIRIUM

Wolff and Curran's (1935) classic descriptive report of 106 consecutive "dysergastic reaction" patients is still consistent with modern-day notions of delirium symptoms. Inconsistent terminology, unclear definitions of symptoms, and underuse of standardized symptom assessment tools have hampered subsequent efforts to describe delirium phenomenology more carefully or to compare symptom incidences across studies and etiological populations (Meagher and Trzepacz 1998). Most studies are cross-sectional, so we lack an understanding of how various symptoms change over the course of an episode.

More recent longitudinal research including daily delirium ratings has focused on total scale scores and not the occurrence of individual symptoms and their pattern over time. Rudberg et al. (1997) used the DRS and DSM-III-R criteria to rate daily 432 medical-surgical patients 65 years or older at a university hospital. They found a 15% incidence of delirium ($n = 63$), in 69% of whom the delirium lasted for only a day. Mean DRS scores on day 1 were significantly higher (i.e., worse) in those whose delirium occurred for multiple days than in those whose delirium lasted 1 day, suggesting a relation between severity and duration in delirium episodes. Marcantonio et al. (2003) studied delirium symptom progression measured with nursing staff ratings of minimum data set symptoms over the first week after admission to postacute facilities. They noted that all six symptoms measured (distractibility, altered perception, disorganized speech, restlessness, lethargy, and mental fluctuation) persisted in two-thirds of patients, with symptoms worsening in 12%. Fann et al. (2005) prospectively studied patients undergoing hematopoietic stem cell transplantation with thrice-weekly assessments with the DRS and MDAS from pretransplantation to day 30 posttransplant. They found that neuropsychiatric features (psychomotor changes, sleep-wake cycle disturbance, and psychotic symptoms) dominated in the early phases but that cognitive impairment peaked a week into delirium and dominated thereafter.

Relations between symptoms also have received limited study, mainly through factor analyses of cross-sectional data (Camus et al. 2000a; Fann et al. 2005; Grassi et al. 2001; Johansson et al. 2002; Lawlor et al. 2000b; Meagher 2005; Trzepacz and Dew 1995; Trzepacz et al. 1998). Although studied on different populations, these factor analyses had some striking similarities regarding which symptoms clustered together in factors and also suggested that delirium symptoms overshadow dementia symptoms when they are comorbid.

Despite across-study inconsistencies (see Table 11–9) for symptom frequencies, certain symptoms occur more often than do others, consistent with the proposal that delirium has core symptoms irrespective of etiology (Trzepacz 1999b, 2000). The most recent data used the DRS-R98 to assess more symptoms with greater consistency than in prior studies. Only one study reported symptoms in children (Turkel et al. 2006) that differed significantly from those in adults: less frequent delusions, more fluctuation of symptoms, greater sleep-wake cycle disturbance, more affective lability, and more agitation. However, none of those adult studies used the DRS-R98, and generally symptom collection was neither well standardized nor comprehensive. In contrast, Turkel and colleagues' (2006) data in children showed frequencies more consistent with the adult DRS-R98 studies.

Figure 11–8 illustrates how multiple etiologies for delirium may "funnel" into a final common neural pathway (Trzepacz 1999b, 2000) so that the phenomenological expression becomes similar despite a breadth of different physiologies. This implies, as well, that certain brain circuits and neurotransmitter systems are more affected (Trzepacz 1994a, 1999b, 2000).

CORE SYMPTOMS

Candidates for "core" symptoms include attentional deficits, memory impairment, disorientation, sleep-wake cycle disturbance, thought process abnormalities, language disturbances, and motor alterations (see "Motor Subtypes" section below), whereas "associated" or non-core symptoms would include perceptual disturbances (illusions, hallucinations), delusions, and affective changes (Trzepacz 1999b). Analysis of DRS-R98 blinded ratings supports this separation of so-called core from associated symptoms on the basis of their relative prevalence (Trzepacz et al. 2001). The occurrence of the less frequent associated symptoms might suggest involvement of particular etiologies and their specific pathophysiologies or individual differences in brain circuitry and vulnerability. Characteristic diagnostic features of delirium, such as altered state of consciousness (called "clouding" by some) and fluctuation of symptom severity over a 24-hour period, may be epiphenomena and not symptoms per se. These may be more related to *how* the symptoms are expressed to affect the observed outward appearance of delirium.

The severity of symptoms in delirium typically fluctuates in intensity over any 24-hour period, unlike that in most other psychiatric disorders. Symptom fluctuation is thus an important indicator of delirium and emphasized in diagnostic classifications (American Psychiatric Asso-

ciation 1994, 2000; World Health Organization 1992). During this characteristic waxing and waning of symptoms, relatively lucid or quiescent periods pose challenges for accurate diagnosis and severity ratings. Some lucid periods may restore enough capacity for patients to communicate their management choices (Bostwick and Masterson 1998). The underlying reason for this fluctuation in symptom severity is not understood—it may relate to shifts between hypoactive and hyperactive periods or fragmentations of the sleep-wake cycle, including daytime rapid eye movement (REM) sleep. Alternatively, it may be similar to the diurnal fluctuation ("sundowning") that occurs in dementia, although Jagmin (1998) studied fluctuation in cognitive performance (via morning and evening assessments with the MMSE and NEECHAM scale) in elderly postoperative patients without dementia or prior cognitive impairment and found that time of day did not significantly affect development of delirium or mental status scores, suggesting that the sundowning phenomenon may be relatively specific to dementia.

Historically, delirium has been viewed by some neurologists primarily as a disturbance of attention; less importance has been attributed to its other cognitive deficits and behavioral symptoms. Attentional disturbance is the cardinal symptom required for diagnosis of delirium yet is unlikely to explain the breadth of delirium symptoms. The nondominant posterior parietal and prefrontal cortices, as well as the brain stem and anteromedial thalamus, play roles in subserving attention, but other brain regions are likely to be involved in other symptoms of delirium. Distractibility, inattention, and poor environmental awareness can be evident during interview and on formal testing. Attentional impairment was found in 100% of delirium patients in a blinded assessment with the DRS-R98 (Trzepacz et al. 2001). O'Keefe and Gosney (1997) found that attentional deficits discriminated delirium patients from either patients with dementia or elderly inpatients without psychiatric disorders when they used sensitive tests such as Digit Span Backward and Digit Cancellation Test.

Memory impairment occurs often in delirium, affecting both short- and long-term memory, although most reports have not distinguished between types of memory impairment. In delirium due to posttraumatic brain injury, procedural and declarative memory are impaired, and procedural memory improves first (Ewert et al. 1985). Patients are usually amnestic for some or all of their delirium episodes, although recent studies have highlighted that many patients can recall some of the often distressing experiences of delirium. Breitbart et al. (2002a) found that about half of their patients with resolved delirium were amnestic for their episode and that

TABLE 11–9.   Studies of delirium phenomenology

	Frequency (%) in children	Frequencies (%) from adult studies that used various classifications	Frequencies (%) from studies that used DRS-R98
Disorientation	77	43, 70, 78, 80, 88, 94, 96, 100	76, 96
Attentional deficits	100	17, 62, 100, 100, 100	97, 100
Sustained attention		89	
Shifting attention		87	
Clouded consciousness	93	58, 65, 65, 87, 91, 100	
Memory impairment (unspecified)	52	64, 90, 95, 100	
Short-term memory			88, 92
Long-term memory			89, 96
Visuospatial impairment			87, 96
Language abnormalities		41, 47, 62, 76, 93	57, 67
Disorganized thinking/thought process abnormalities		57, 64, 76, 95	54, 79
Incoherence		77	
Sleep-wake cycle disturbance	98	25, 49, 77, 95, 96	92, 97
Perceptual disturbance/hallucinations	43	24, 35, 35, 41, 45, 46, 71	50, 63
Delusions		18, 19, 25, 37, 38, 45, 68	21, 31
Affective lability/emotional disturbance	79	43, 63, 97, 97	53, 54
Apathy	68	86	
Anxiety	61	55	
Irritability	86		
Psychomotor changes (general)		38, 53, 55, 83, 88, 92, 93	
Motor agitation	69	59	62, 79
Motor retardation		71	29, 62

more severe amnesia was associated with greater severity of delirium on the MDAS, suggesting a defect in new learning during delirium (see Figure 11–9). Similarly, O'Keeffe (2005) found that about half of elderly nondemented delirious patients recalled their delirium, many of whom continued to be disturbed by their recollections 6 months later. Trzepacz et al. (2001) found a high correlation between the DRS-R98 short- and long-term memory items ($r=0.51$, $P=0.01$) in delirious patients, with attention correlating with short-term memory ($r=0.44$, $P=0.03$) but not with long-term memory. This outcome is consistent with adequate attention being a prerequisite for information to enter short-term (working) memory, followed by storage of selected data from working memory into long-term memory.

Disturbances of the sleep-wake cycle are especially common in patients with delirium. The DRS-R98 identified sleep-wake cycle disturbances in 92%–97% of delirious patients (Meagher et al. 2007; Trzepacz et al. 2001). Sleep-wake cycle disturbances may underlie fluctuations in the severity of symptoms during a 24-hour period. Sleep disturbances range from napping and nocturnal disruptions to a more severe disintegration of the normal circadian cycle. The extent to which sleep-wake cycle disturbance confounds the hyperactive-hypoactive subtyping of delirium is not known. The role of sleep disturbances in early or prodromal phases of delirium is uncertain; some have suggested that sleep disturbances may be a central feature of delirium evolution, possibly related to disturbed melatonin secretion (Charlton and Kavanau

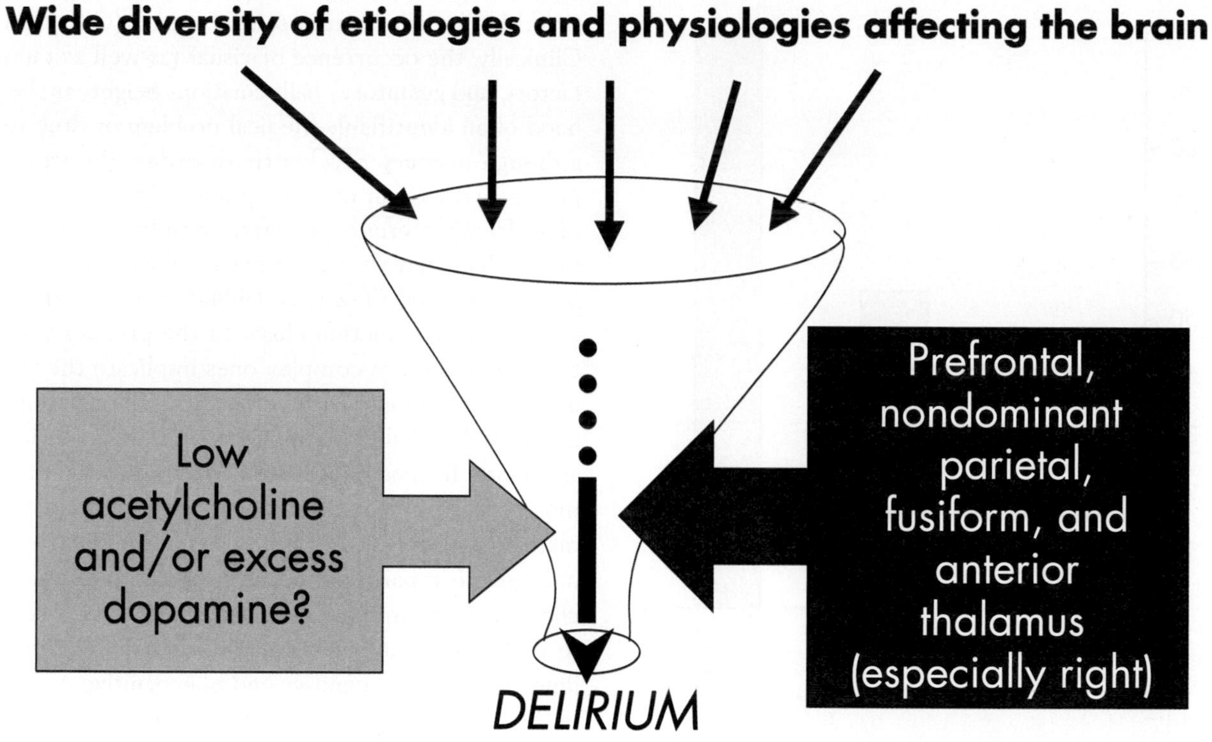

Wide diversity of etiologies and physiologies affecting the brain

Low acetylcholine and/or excess dopamine?

Prefrontal, nondominant parietal, fusiform, and anterior thalamus (especially right)

DELIRIUM

FIGURE 11–8. Delirium final common pathway.

2002; Shigeta et al. 2001). However, Harrell and Othmer (1987), in a study of postcardiotomy delirium, found that sleep disturbance mirrored reductions in MMSE scores but did not predate them. Similarly, de Jonghe et al. (2005) found that the prodromal phase of delirium was characterized principally by cognitive disturbances rather than behavioral or sleep disturbances. Disturbances in sleep pattern may be a marker for temporal course of an episode. A retrospective study measured treatment response—2 or more consecutive nights of undisturbed sleep was equated with delirium resolution (Dautzenberg et al. 2004).

Visuospatial disturbances have not been studied in detail in delirium, but Clock Drawing Test deficits and wandering behaviors indicate difficulties. Accuracy of both the overall shapes and the details of drawings is impaired, suggesting dysfunction of bilateral posterior parietal lobes and prefrontal cortex. Meagher et al. (2007) found disturbances of visuospatial function in 87% of delirious patients and noted that these were moderate or severe in 64%.

Language disturbances in delirium include dysnomia, paraphasias, impaired comprehension, dysgraphia, and word-finding difficulties. In extreme cases, language resembles a fluent dysphasia. Incoherent speech or speech disturbance is reported commonly. Dysgraphia was once believed to be specific to delirium (Chedru and Ge-

schwind 1972), but comparison of writing samples from patients with other psychiatric disorders found that dysgraphia was not specific to delirium (Patten and Lamarre 1989); rather, abnormal semantic content of language was more differentiating in delirium. The language item on the DRS-R98 did not distinguish delirium and dementia patients, but the CTD comprehension item, which incorporates language and executive function, did (Trzepacz et al. 2002).

Disorganized thinking was found in 95% of delirious patients in one study (Rockwood 1993) and was noted by Cutting (1987) to be different from schizophrenic thought processes. However, very little work has been done to characterize thought process disorder in patients with delirium, which clinically ranges from tangentiality and circumstantiality to loose associations. On the DRS-R98, 21% of delirium patients had tangentiality or circumstantiality, whereas 58% had loose associations (Trzepacz et al. 2001). Greater severity of thought process disturbances can distinguish delirium when it occurs with concomitant dementia (Laurila et al. 2004a), and thought disorder is significantly worse in delirium than in dementia (Trzepacz et al. 2002). Besides thought process abnormality, other indications of psychosis include abnormal thought content and perceptual disturbances, although these occur less often than do core symptoms (Trzepacz et al. 2001).

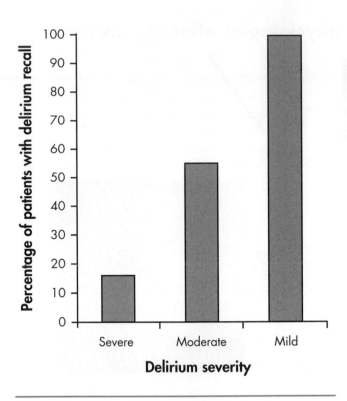

FIGURE 11–9. Ability to recall an episode of delirium worsens with more severe delirium symptoms.

Source. Reprinted from Breitbart W, Gibson C, Tremblay A: "The Delirium Experience: Delirium Recall and Delirium-Related Distress in Hospitalized Patients With Cancer, Their Spouses/Caregivers, and Their Nurses." *Psychosomatics* 43:183–194, 2002. Copyright 2002 American Psychiatric Publishing, Inc. Used with permission.

ASSOCIATED SYMPTOMS

Psychotic symptoms occur in both agitated and quiet presentations and are important determinants of the delirium experience for patients and their caregivers (Breitbart et al. 2002a). A retrospective study of 227 consecutively evaluated delirium patients found that 25.6% had delusions, 27% had visual hallucinations, 12.4% had auditory hallucinations, and 2.7% had tactile hallucinations (Webster and Holroyd 2000). O'Keeffe (2005) prospectively studied 105 elderly nondemented patients with delirium and found that 70% had delusions or misperceptions or both during delirium. Cutting (1987) noted that delusional content tended to involve delusional misidentification, imminent misadventure to others, or bizarre happenings in the patient's environment. Although psychotic symptoms are commonly equated with hyperactive presentations, recent reports emphasized their occurrence in quieter presentations (Breitbart et al. 2002a; Meagher 2005). The psychological distress associated with these symptoms often persists after resolution of the delirium episode (Morita et al. 2004; O'Keeffe 2005).

The type of perceptual disturbance and delusion distinguishes delirium from schizophrenia (Cutting 1987). Clinically, the occurrence of visual (as well as tactile, olfactory, and gustatory) hallucinations heightens the likelihood of an identifiable medical problem or drug toxicity, although primary psychiatric disorders do occasionally present with visual misperceptions. Visual hallucinations range from patterns or shapes to complex and vivid animations, which may vary according to which part of the brain is being affected (Trzepacz 1994a). Simple forms or colors suggest dysfunction closer to the primary visual cortex, whereas more complex ones implicate the temporal or fusiform regions, with peduncular hallucinations causing movielike hallucinations. Persecutory delusions that are poorly formed (not systematized) are the most common type in delirium, but other types can occur (e.g., somatic or grandiose). Delusions do not seem to be a result of cognitive impairment per se; however, the origin of psychosis in delirium remains uncertain, including its relation to underlying etiologies, patient vulnerabilities, phase of illness, and other cognitive and noncognitive components of the syndrome. Recent genetic studies of alcohol-related delirium suggested that psychosis tendency may be genetically based (see subsection "Genetic Factors" above).

Affective lability that involves unpredictable mood changes within minutes is characteristic of delirium. Mood alterations can take many forms (e.g., anxiety, fear, anger, dysphoria, elation, euphoria, apathy), with changes from one type to another without obvious relation to the context (i.e., incongruent) and outside of self-control. Mood difficulties can herald delirium as part of a prodromal phase. Hypoactive delirium is frequently mistaken for depression, whereas hyperactive delirium can mimic agitated depression or hypomania. In a study of patients referred by a consultation-liaison psychiatrist for suspected mood disorder who actually had delirium, 24% experienced suicidal thoughts, 52% had frequent thoughts of death, and 32% believed that there was no point in taking medications (Farrell and Ganzini 1995). These findings highlight the importance of careful monitoring of mental state in delirious patients. Affective lability occurred less often than did core symptoms (Meagher et al. 2007; Trzepacz et al. 2001).

MOTOR SUBTYPES

Disturbances of motor behavior are almost invariable in delirium (Camus et al. 2000b; Gupta et al. 2005; Meagher 2005) and have been considered as candidates for inclusion among its core symptoms. The varying motor presentations of delirium have been described since ancient times, when two patterns were distinguished—"phrenitis" and "lethargicus" (Lipowski 1990). Contemporary medicine recognizes three patterns: excited ("hyperactive"), lethargic ("hypoactive"), and "mixed." Often motor disturbances are characterized as psychomotor behaviors (including hyperalertness, wandering, uncooperativeness or hypersomnolence, disinterest, unawareness) that encompass nonmotor symptoms that may or may not have any specificity for delirium. Mixed presentations shift between hyper- and hypoactivity.

These motor variants are important not only because of their effect on delirium detection and management but also because of their relation to prognosis and differences in underlying etiology and pathophysiology. Delusions, hallucinations, mood lability, speech incoherence, and sleep disturbances may be somewhat more frequent in hyperactive patients (Meagher and Trzepacz 2000; Ross et al. 1991) but also occur in hypoactive patients. Neurologists have differentiated delirium such that disorientation with reduced motor activity has been called "acute confusion," whereas hyperactive disoriented patients were labeled "delirious" (Mesulam 1985; Mori and Yamadori 1987). In a study of infarctions of the right middle cerebral artery, Mori and Yamadori (1987) found that acute confusional states are disturbances of attention, resulting from frontostriatal damage, whereas acute agitated deliria are disturbances of emotion and affect resulting from injury to the middle temporal gyrus. However, these distinctions are not supported by data or neural circuitry (Trzepacz 1994a). Temporal-limbic information is linked to prefrontal cortex via the basotemporal-limbic pathways and the thalamo-frontal-striatal circuits. Thus, delirium likely relates to both frontal and temporal-limbic dysfunction.

There has been much interest in whether delirium has subtypes on the basis of various parameters such as underlying physiology, etiology, and symptom profile (Trzepacz 1994a), similar to the way heart failure is categorized. It is unclear whether subtypes even truly exist. Nonetheless, the most studied possible subtype is based on psychomotor behavior. Lipowski (1990) championed the use of the umbrella term *delirium* with secondary delineations for three motor subtypes. Lipowski's and others' definitions of motor subtypes have been subjectively described, are not standardized, and include nonmotor behavioral features such as affective changes and disturbances of speech, thinking, and perception.

Motor subtypes have similar degrees of overall cognitive impairment and electroencephalographic slowing, which are objective and diagnostic aspects of delirium (Koponen et al. 1989b; Ross et al. 1991). From a clinical perspective, the visibility of such presentations and their relevance to differential diagnosis, delirium detection, and treatment experience make their study worthwhile

(O'Keeffe 1999). In addition, studies suggest that these motorically defined subtypes differ in relation to the frequency of nonmotor symptoms (Gupta et al. 2005; Meagher et al. 2000; Sandberg et al. 1999), etiology (Gupta et al. 2005; Meagher et al. 1998; Morita et al. 2001; Ross et al. 1991), pathophysiology (Balan et al. 2003), detection rates (Inouye 1994), treatment experience (Breitbart et al. 2002b; Meagher et al. 1996; Uchiyama et al. 1996), duration of episode, and outcome (Kobayashi et al. 1992; Lam et al. 2003; Liptzin and Levkoff 1992; Liu et al. 1997; Marcantonio et al. 2002; O'Keeffe and Lavan 1999; S.M. Olofsson et al. 1996; Reyes et al. 1981; Treloar and MacDonald 1997).

However, methodological inconsistencies and variability of findings across studies make the interpretation of these findings difficult (Meagher and Trzepacz 2000; Meagher et al., in press). In particular, the definitions of motor subtypes vary considerably and include symptoms that do not directly relate to motor disturbance and have uncertain value in subtyping (e.g., affective changes, aggressive behavior, alterations in verbal output). Moreover, waxing and waning of symptom severity and sleepwake cycle abnormalities complicate our understanding of motor subtypes, as does reliance on subjective and retrospective reports of behavior over 24-hour periods. Wide variation is seen among reports of relative frequencies of motor subtypes (see Table 11–10), even when alcohol withdrawal cases are excluded. In a prospective study of delirious patients, Meagher et al. (in press) found a remarkably low level of concordance (34%) among four different methods of defining psychomotor subtypes. Preliminary work in mixed dementia-delirium patients suggests that motion analysis may be of value in distinguishing clinical subtypes (Honma et al. 1998), but studies that use objective motor activity level monitoring of delirious patients are needed to focus on and quantify motor behavior over 24-hour periods.

In many reports, up to half of patients present with a mixed motor subtype during their episode. These mixed cases may reflect different outcomes over time of multiple etiological effects on motor behavior or may be a hybrid state. More detailed longitudinal study of delirium symptoms is necessary to clarify the stability of motor subtypes. Fann et al. (2005) studied motor symptom profile in 90 patients pre–stem cell transplantation to day 30 post–stem cell transplantation and found that psychomotor disturbance (measured on the MDAS and DRS) was consistently hypoactive (in 86%) throughout a delirium episode without fluctuation. Marcantonio et al. (2003) studied delirium symptom persistence over a week in elderly patients admitted to postacute facilities and found that both lethargy and restlessness remained

TABLE 11–10.   Studies of frequency of motor subtypes in delirium

Study	Subtyping method/population	Hypo-active (%)	Hyper-active (%)	Mixed (%)	None (%)
Koponen et al. 1989c	Lipowski description Psychogeriatric admissions	13	38	49	—
Ross et al. 1991	Visual analogue scale Consultation-liaison referrals	32	68	—	—
Liptzin and Levkoff 1992	Liptzin and Levkoff criteria General hospital admissions	19	15	52	14
Kobayashi et al. 1992	Lipowski description Neuropsychiatry referrals	6	79	15	—
Platt et al. 1994a	Delirium Rating Scale psychomotor item Hospitalized AIDS patients	46	37	17	—
Uchiyama et al. 1996	Clinical observation Psychogeriatric admissions	20	80	—	—
Meagher et al. 1996	Liptzin and Levkoff criteria Consultation-liaison referrals	24	30	46	—
S.M. Olofsson et al. 1996	Clinical observation Consultation-liaison referrals with cancer	18	71	11	—
Liu et al. 1997	Liptzin and Levkoff criteria Consultation-liaison referrals	13	69	18	—
O'Keeffe and Lavan 1999	Delirium Assessment Scale score Geriatric admissions	29	21	43	7
Okamato et al. 1999	Delirium Symptom Inventory item General hospital admissions	—	73	27	—
Camus et al. 2000b	Own checklist Geriatric admissions	26	46	27	—
Sandberg et al. 1999	Own checklist Elderly patients in various settings	26	22	42	11
Lawlor et al. 2000b	Memorial Delirium Assessment Scale (MDAS) item Cancer patients	39	11	44	5
Breitbart et al. 2002a	MDAS item Cancer patients	54	47	—	—
Marcantonio et al. 2002	MDAS item Post–hip surgery patients	71	27		2
Peterson et al. 2006	Richmond Agitation and Aggression Scale Intensive care unit admissions	38	1	61	—

TABLE 11–10. Studies of frequency of motor subtypes in delirium *(continued)*

Study	Subtyping method/ population	Hypo- active (%)	Hyper- active (%)	Mixed (%)	None (%)
Balan et al. 2003	Liptzin and Levkoff criteria Geriatric admissions	32	23	45	—
Lam et al. 2003	MDAS item Palliative care admissions	70	13	17	—
Gupta et al. 2005	Delirium Rating Scale— Revised-98 motor items	16	36	48	—
De Rooij 2005a	Liptzin and Levkoff criteria Hospitalized elderly patients	35	65		—
Santos et al. 2005	Lipowski criteria Elderly postoperative patients	26	47	26	—
Fann et al. 2005	MDAS item Stem cell transplantation patients	84	3	11	2
Gaudreau et al. 2005a	MDAS item Oncology unit admissions	81	14	5	—

stable in most (95%) patients. Peterson et al. (2006) used the Richmond Agitation and Aggression Scale to have nurses rate medical ICU delirium patients three times per shift for an average of 6 days. They found very few hyperactive ($n = 4$) and mostly hypoactive ($n = 138$) or mixed ($n = 255$) subtypes; however, confounds of sedating medications were present.

To date, clinical studies have not provided convincing evidence that motor subtypes have particular etiological associations. Sites of focal cerebral lesions do not consistently associate with specific motor subtypes. Alcohol withdrawal delirium, which is generally hyperactive, is associated with increased beta electroencephalographic activity (on a background of slowing), but most other causes of delirium are typically associated with diffuse electroencephalographic slowing, regardless of motor presentation (Trzepacz 1994a). Similarly, functional neuroimaging studies of delirium indicate increased cerebral blood flow in alcohol withdrawal delirium (Hemmingsen et al. 1988), whereas other causes are associated with reductions in global or frontal cerebral blood flow irrespective of motor subtype (Trzepacz 1994a).

Disturbances of the cholinergic system have been consistently implicated in delirium. Evidence from studies in animals and nondelirious human volunteers suggests that reduced cholinergic activity is associated with relative hyperactivity, but studies measuring possible markers of CNS cholinergic function in delirium, such as

serum anticholinergic activity and cerebrospinal fluid somatostatin-like immunoreactivity, have not supported this possibility. Similarly, arguments have been made for involvement of other neurochemical systems (dopamine, serotonin, γ-aminobutyric acid [GABA], histamine) (Meagher and Trzepacz 2000).

Balan et al. (2003) showed that levels of the melatonin metabolite 6-SMT correlated closely with motor presentation during the delirium episode but normalized thereafter, with highest levels in hypoactive patients, followed by mixed motor presentation, and with lowest levels in those with hyperactivity. These findings echo those noted in studies of melatonin function and psychomotor profile in mood disorders (B. Wahlund et al. 1998). Melatonin is involved in regulation of the sleep-wake circadian cycle at the hypothalamus and has recognized hypnotic effects. It is also involved in regulation of immune response and aging, and its secretion is increased by immobilization and decreased during the daytime by light exposure. Balan et al. (2003) hypothesized that disruption of melatonin secretion is key to the emergence of delirium and that the interaction of certain extrinsic factors (e.g., abnormal light exposure in medical ICU settings) may interact with intrinsic factors to shape motor profile according to whether secretion is increased (relative hypoactivity) or decreased (relative hyperactivity).

Motor presentations of delirium may be related to different etiologies, treatment, or outcome. Delirium due to drug-related causes is most commonly hyperactive, whereas delirium due to metabolic disturbances, including hypoxia, is more frequently hypoactive in presentation (Meagher et al. 1998; Morita et al. 2001; O'Keeffe and Lavan 1999; S.M. Olofsson et al. 1996; Ross et al. 1991). Patients with a hyperactive subtype may have better outcomes after an episode of delirium, with shorter LOS, lower mortality rates, and a higher rate of full recovery (Kobayashi et al. 1992; Liptzin and Levkoff 1992; S.M. Olofsson et al. 1996). However, these differences may reflect variations in underlying causes, recognition rates, or treatment practices. Underdetection and misdiagnosis are especially common in hypoactive patients. In fact, Meagher et al. (1996) found that use of psychotropic medication and supportive environmental ward strategies were related to level of hyperactivity rather than to degree of cognitive disturbance. S.M. Olofsson et al. (1996) reported better outcome in patients with hyperactive delirium but noted that they received less haloperidol than did nonhyperactive patients. O'Keefe and Lavan (1999) reported greater use of neuroleptics and shorter hospital stays in hyperactive patients but attributed this to less severe illness at the onset of delirium and a lower incidence of hospital-acquired infections and bed sores in those who were hyperactive. Even when actively screened for earlier detection or more active investigation, hypoactive patients still may have a poorer outcome (O'Keefe and Lavan 1999). Other work has found similar outcomes in the different motor groups (Camus et al. 2000b). All work focused on implication of motor presentations of delirium may need reevaluation when motor activity monitoring redefines these categories objectively.

Treatment studies have not been designed specifically to assess response or effectiveness for different motor subtypes. In clinical practice, it is often presumed that neuroleptic agents are useful in delirium solely for sedative or antipsychotic purposes and thus more effective for hyperactive patients. However, a prospective study found comparable efficacy for haloperidol in treating both hypo- and hyperactive delirious medical patients (Platt et al. 1994a), whereas another study (Breitbart et al. 2002b) found that hypoactive symptoms were somewhat less responsive to olanzapine in an uncontrolled open trial; however, structural brain lesions may have been confounds. Uchiyama et al. (1996) found better response rates to mianserin in delirium with hyperactive motor presentation compared with hypoactive motor profile, attributed to its sedating effects. Overall, the relation between motor subtype and treatment and outcome remains unclear and confounded by methodological issues.

TREATMENT OF DELIRIUM

Delirium is an example par excellence of a disorder requiring a multifaceted biopsychosocial approach to assessment and treatment. After the diagnosis of delirium is made, the process of identifying and reversing suspected causes begins. Rapid treatment is important because of the high morbidity and mortality rates associated with delirium. Treatments include medication, environmental manipulation, and patient and family psychosocial support (American Psychiatric Association 1999). However, no drug has a U.S. Food and Drug Administration (FDA) indication for the treatment of delirium. Randomized double-blind, placebo-controlled, adequately powered efficacy trials are lacking. The American Psychiatric Association (1999) "Practice Guidelines for the Treatment of Patients With Delirium" note the need for such research, and this is ever more pertinent given the escalating range of therapeutic options available in delirium, including atypical antipsychotics, procholinergic agents, and melatonergic compounds. Most prospective drug studies use open-label designs (Table 11–11); more is published about atypical antipsychotics than about conventional neuroleptics in these studies. Whether any neuroleptic agent adequately targets all core symptoms of delirium has not been shown. Cholinergic agents hold more promise in chronic prophylactic dosing, although shorter-acting agents such as physostigmine, which offer faster onset of action in acute settings, have not been tried for non-drug-induced delirium.

PREVENTION STRATEGIES

Preoperative patient education and preparation were helpful in reducing delirium symptom rates (Chatham 1978; Owens and Hutelmyer 1982; Schindler et al. 1989; M.A. Williams et al. 1985). However, studies that used caregiver education and environmental or risk factor interventions had mixed results, with two not finding any significant effect on delirium rate (Nagley 1986; Wanich et al. 1992) and one (Rockwood et al. 1994) finding modest gains in delirium diagnosis (3%–9%) through special internal medicine house staff education efforts. In contrast, Inouye et al. (1999) studied the effect on delirium of preventive measures that minimized six of the risk factors identified in their previous work with hospitalized elderly patients. They used standardized protocols in a prospective study of 852 elderly medical inpatients to address cognitive impairment, sleep deprivation, immobility, visual impairment, hearing impairment, and dehydration, which resulted in significant reductions in the number (62 vs. 90) and duration (105 vs. 161 days) of delirium episodes relative to control subjects. Effects of adherence to the delirium risk protocol were sub-

TABLE 11–11. Prospective studies of drug treatment in delirium

Study	Agent	Population	Design	Purpose	Measure[a]	Diagnosis
Conventional antipsychotics						
Breitbart et al. 1996	Haloperidol vs. chlorpromazine vs. lorazepam	30 AIDS inpatients	Double-blind, randomized	Efficacy	DRS	DSM-III-R
K.J. Kalisvaart et al. 2005a	Haloperidol vs. placebo	430 elderly hip surgery inpatients	Double-blind, randomized	Prophylaxis (acute)	DRS-R98	DSM-IV
Kaneko et al. 1999	Intravenous haloperidol vs. intravenous placebo	78 gastrointestinal postoperative inpatients	Randomized, not blinded	Prophylaxis (acute) and rescue	Clinical assessment	DSM-III-R
Atypical antipsychotics						
Horikawa et al. 2003	Risperidone	10 consultation-liaison referrals	Open label	Efficacy	DRS	DSM-IV
Mittal et al. 2004	Risperidone	10 medical-surgical admissions	Open label	Efficacy	DRS	DSM-IV
Parellada et al. 2004	Risperidone	64 medical inpatients	Open label	Efficacy	DRS	DSM-IV
Toda et al. 2005	Risperidone	10 elderly inpatients	Open label	Efficacy	DRS	DSM-IV
C.S. Han and Kim 2004	Risperidone vs. haloperidol	28 consultation-liaison referrals	Double-blind, randomized	Efficacy	MDAS	DSM-III-R
J.Y. Kim et al. 2005	Haloperidol vs. risperidone	42 medical-surgical patients	Open label, not randomized	Efficacy	DRS-R98	DSM-IV
Sipahimalani and Masand 1998	Olanzapine vs. haloperidol	22 consultation-liaison referrals	Open label, not randomized	Efficacy	DRS	Not specified
K.S. Kim et al. 2001	Olanzapine	20 medical-surgical patients	Open label	Efficacy	DRS	DSM-IV
Breitbart et al. 2002b	Olanzapine	79 cancer inpatients	Open label	Efficacy	MDAS	DSM-IV
Hill et al. 2002	Olanzapine vs. risperidone vs. haloperidol	50 general hospital patients	Open label, not randomized	Efficacy	DRS-R98	DSM-IV
Skrobik et al. 2004	Olanzapine vs. haloperidol	103 intensive care unit patients	Randomized, not blinded	Efficacy	Delirium Index	Intensive care unit delirium screening checklist
Straker et al. 2006	Aripiprazole	14 general hospital patients	Open label	Efficacy	DRS-R98	DSM-IV

TABLE 11–11. Prospective studies of drug treatment in delirium *(continued)*

Study	Agent	Population	Design	Purpose	Measure[a]	Diagnosis
Atypical antipsychotics *(continued)*						
K. Y. Kim et al. 2003	Quetiapine	12 geriatric medical patients	Open label	Efficacy	DRS	DSM-IV
Sasaki et al. 2003	Quetiapine	12 patients	Open label	Efficacy	DRS	DSM-IV
Pae et al. 2004	Quetiapine	22 inpatients	Open label	Efficacy	DRS-R98	DSM-IV
Lee et al. 2005	Amisulpiride vs. quetiapine	40 patients	Open label, randomized	Efficacy	DRS-R98	DSM-IV
Procholinergic						
Diaz et al. 2001	Citicholine vs. placebo	81 elderly nondemented hip surgery patients	Randomized	Prophylaxis (acute)	CAM AMT	DSM-III-R
Liptzin et al. 2005	Donepezil vs. placebo	80 elderly elective hip surgery patients	Double-blind, randomized	Prophylaxis (acute)	DSI	DSM-IV
Moretti et al. 2004	Rivastigmine vs. cardioaspirin	230 elderly vascular dementia outpatients	Case-control, not randomized	Prophylaxis (chronic)	CAM Index at 2 years	DSM-IV
Other						
J. Nakamura et al. 1994	Mianserin vs. haloperidol vs. oxypertine	23 general hospital inpatients	Not specified	Efficacy	DRS	Not specified
J. Nakamura et al. 1995	Mianserin vs. haloperidol	65 consultation-liaison referrals	Open label, not randomized	Efficacy	DRS	DSM-III-R
Uchiyama et al. 1996	Mianserin	62 psychogeriatric inpatients	Open label	Efficacy	DRS	DSM-IV
J. Nakamura et al. 1997a	Mianserin vs. haloperidol	66 consultation-liaison referrals	Open label, not randomized	Efficacy	DRS	DSM-IV
J. Nakamura et al. 1997b	Mianserin suppositories	16 consultation-liaison patients	Open label	Efficacy	DRS	DSM-IV
Bayindir et al. 2000	Ondansetron	35 postcardiotomy patients	Open label	Efficacy	4-point clinical scale	Not specified
B. Gagnon et al. 2005	Methylphenidate	14 cancer patients	Open label	Efficacy	MMSE	DSM-IV

[a]Primary outcome measure.
Note. AMT = Abbreviated Mental Test; CAM = Confusion Assessment Method; DRS = Delirium Rating Scale; DRS-R98 = Delirium Rating Scale—Revised-98; MDAS = Memorial Delirium Assessment Scale; DSI = Delirium Symptom Inventory; MMSE = Mini-Mental State Examination.

sequently reported for 422 elderly patients during implementation (Inouye et al. 2003): adherence ranged from 10% for the sleep protocol to 86% for orientation. Higher levels of adherence by staff resulted in lower delirium rates up to a maximum of an 89% reduction, even after the investigators controlled for confounding variables such as medical comorbidity, functional status, and illness severity. At 6-month follow-up of 705 survivors from this intervention study of six risk factors, no differences were seen between groups for any of 10 outcome measures except for less frequent incontinence in the intervention group (Bogardus et al. 2003), suggesting that the intervention's effect was essentially during the index hospitalization without any longer-lasting benefits. When a subset of patients at high risk for delirium at baseline were compared, however, patients who received the intervention had significantly better self-rated health and functional status at follow-up.

Marcantonio et al. (2001) found that proactive geriatric consultation in patients undergoing hip surgery was associated with significantly reduced incidence and severity of delirium in the intervention group who had received a mean of 10 recommendations regarding risk factor prevention and active treatment of emergent delirium. Interestingly, more than three-quarters of these recommendations were adhered to, but with relatively less adherence to suggestions regarding analgesia, nutritional inadequacies, and correction of sensory impairments. Young and George (2003) studied the effect of introducing consensus guidelines for delirium management in general hospital settings and found that management processes improved only when the intervention was reinforced by regular teaching sessions, but these effects did not reach statistical significance.

Milisen et al. (2001) compared delirium rates in two cohorts of elderly hip surgery patients (each $n = 60$)—each before and after implementing an intervention composed of nurse education, cognitive screening, consultation by a nurse or physician geriatric/delirium specialist, and scheduled pain protocol. They found no effect on delirium incidence but, rather, a shorter delirium duration (median 1 vs. 4 days) and lower delirium severity score in the intervention group as measured by a modified (not validated) CAM. Marcantonio et al. (2001) used a different study design and randomly assigned 62 elderly hip fracture patients to either a perioperative geriatric consultation or usual care. Daily ratings on the MMSE, DSI, CAM, and MDAS indicated a lower delirium rate (32% vs. 50%) and fewer severe delirium cases (12% vs. 29%) in the consultative group. LOS was not affected, and the effect of consultation was greatest in those patients without preexisting dementia or poor ADLs, in contrast to the subgroup analysis of Bogardus et al. (2003), in which most benefit accrued at follow-up for high-risk patients.

Psychiatric consultation facilitates identification of predisposing and precipitating factors for delirium. Medication exposure, visual and hearing impairments, sleep deprivation, uncontrolled pain, dehydration, malnutrition, catheterization, and use of restraints are all factors that can be modified in the elderly, but uncertainty remains as to the precise value of multicomponent interventions that attempt to reduce the incidence and severity of delirium through modification of recognized risk factors (Bogardus et al. 2003; Cole et al. 1998; Inouye et al. 1999) or systematic detection and multidisciplinary care of identified cases (Cole et al. 2002a). Some more recent studies have suggested that proactive approaches to education of staff involved in the care of patients at high risk for delirium, risk factor reduction, systematic cognitive screening for delirium, and patient-tailored treatment of emergent delirium were associated with reduced incidence (Marcantonio et al. 2001) and severity or duration of incident delirium (Lundstrom et al. 2005; Marcantonio et al. 2001; Milisen et al. 2001) and decreased delirium-related mortality (Lundstrom et al. 2005), although such benefits may be more pronounced in patients with better baseline cognitive status (Marcantonio et al. 2001). Marcantonio et al. (2001) found that implementing suggestions about pain management, sensory impediments, and inadequate nutrition was less frequent. The effect of such interventions depends on degree of implementation, and greater adherence leads to lower delirium rates (Inouye et al. 2003). A multicomponent randomized intervention for geriatric delirium in acute medical wards resulted in no differences at 1-year follow-up for death or institutionalization but did alleviate delirium faster acutely, and cognition was improved at 6 months in the intervention group (Pitkälä et al. 2005).

PHARMACOLOGICAL PROPHYLAXIS

Cholinergic agents have engendered the most interest, consistent with the cholinergic deficiency hypothesis for delirium. Perioperative piracetam use during anesthesia was reviewed across eight studies, mostly from the 1970s, and was believed to have a positive effect on reducing postoperative delirium symptoms (Gallinat et al. 1999). Citicholine, 1.2 mg/day, given 1 day before and on each of 4 days after surgery, was assessed for acute prophylaxis of delirium in a randomized, placebo-controlled trial of 81 nondemented hip surgery patients (Diaz et al. 2001). Although no significant difference was found between groups on the Abbreviated Mental Test or the CAM, the placebo group had numerically more delirium cases (17.4% vs. 11.7%). In a retrospective review of delirium incidence in hospitalized elderly medical patients receiving various treatments over an 18-month period, Dautzenberg et al. (2004) found a lower incidence of delirium in patients who had received chronic rivastigmine treatment. A double-blind, randomized, placebo-controlled trial of donepezil given 2 weeks before and after elective orthopedic surgery in an elderly population did not find a group difference, a result that was attributed to low delirium incidence and underpowering of the study in this cognitively intact low-risk cohort (Liptzin et al. 2005). In a 24-month prophylaxis study comparing rivastigmine with cardioaspirin in elderly patients with vascular dementia, Moretti et al. (2004) found reduced occurrence of delirium (40% vs. 62%), shorter episode duration (4 vs. 7.5 days), and lower use of benzodiazepines and antipsychotics in the cholinesterase inhibitor group, supporting a role for cholinergic deficiency in delirium in these at-risk patients.

Kaneko et al. (1999) compared postoperative prophylaxis with 5 mg/day of intravenous haloperidol with intravenous saline in a randomized but not blinded trial of gastrointestinal surgery patients and found that the incidence of delirium was only 10.5% in the active drug group compared with 32.5% in the saline group ($P<0.05$). Rescue with haloperidol and flunitrazepam was allowed, however, in both groups as soon as delirium symptoms appeared, but mean doses were not reported. K.J. Kalisvaart et al. (2005a) studied 430 elderly hip surgery patients in a randomized, double-blind, acute prophylaxis study in which either haloperidol or placebo was given up to 3 days before and 3 days after surgery. Although they found a nonsignificant lower numerical difference only for delirium incidence (23% vs. 32%) with the use of haloperidol, significant differences were found for shorter delirium duration (4.4 vs. 12 days), lower DRS-R98 scores (13.6 vs. 18.2), and shorter LOS (12 vs. 23.8 days) in the active treatment group. This was the first double-blind, randomized, placebo-controlled trial of use of a neuroleptic agent for delirium, but dosing was lower than in an efficacy design.

Adjusting the types of routinely used medications can reduce iatrogenic delirium. Maldonado et al. (2004) reported an interim data analysis showing significantly reduced delirium incidence (DSM-IV and DRS) when a novel α_2-adrenergic receptor agonist—dexmedetomidine (5%)—was administered for postoperative sedation compared with propofol (54%) or fentanyl/midazolam (46%) in patients who had cardiac valve surgery. Improved pain control after hepatectomy surgery in elderly patients using patient-controlled epidural anesthesia with bupivacaine and fentanyl ($n=14$) compared with continuous epidural mepivacaine ($n=16$) was associated with lower incidences of moderate and severe delirium (36% vs. 75% and 14% vs. 50%, respectively), and antipsychotic drug use was also lower in that group (Tokita et al. 2001). Similarly, open-

label switch from morphine to fentanyl in delirious cancer patients resulted in decreased MDAS and pain scores in 13 of 20 patients on day 3, although 4 received neuroleptic rescue doses (Morita et al. 2005). Ely and Dittus (2004) encourage individual titration of sedating agents to avoid iatrogenic delirium and unresponsive states in ICU patients.

TREATMENT OF A DELIRIUM EPISODE

The principles of good ward management of delirious patients include ensuring the safety of the patient and his or her immediate surroundings (including sitters), achieving optimal levels of environmental stimulation, and minimizing the effects of any sensory impediments. The complications of delirium can be minimized by careful attention to the potential for falls and avoidance of prolonged hypostasis. The use of orienting techniques (e.g., calendars, nightlights, and reorientation by staff) and familiarizing the patient with the environment (e.g., with photographs of family members) are sometimes comforting, although it is important to remember that environmental manipulations alone do not reverse delirium (American Psychiatric Association 1999; S.D. Anderson 1995). It also has been suggested that diurnal cues from natural lighting reduce sensory deprivation and incidence of delirium (L.M. Wilson 1972), although sensory deprivation alone is insufficient to cause delirium (Francis 1993). Unfortunately, routine implementation of nursing interventions occurs primarily in response to hyperactivity and behavioral management challenges rather than in response to the core cognitive disturbances of delirium (Meagher et al. 1996).

An alternative approach is home-based care ("hospital in the home"), which results in reduced incidence and duration of delirium and substantially reduced rehabilitation costs in elderly patients undergoing physical rehabilitation (Caplan et al. 2005). The "flying delirium team" uses a nurse-led coordinated approach to multidisciplinary care (psychiatry, geriatrics, and neurology) of hospitalized patients with delirium (Lemey et al. 2005). The "Delirium Room" (Flaherty et al. 2003) is a specialized four-bed unit for management and mobilization of disturbed elderly patients without the use of restraints—a well-recognized risk factor for delirium (McCusker et al. 2001)—that involves comprehensive delirium-oriented treatment to minimize risk and aggravating factors and medication use with daily multidisciplinary reviews of progress. Preliminary investigation suggests that exposure to delirium risk factors and mortality rates are reduced in this model of care. McCaffrey and Locsin (2004) found a lower incidence of delirium in elderly postoperative patients provided with passive ("easy listening") music therapy via a bedside compact disc player, with a calming effect on the ward atmosphere.

Supportive interaction with relatives and caregivers is fundamental to good management of delirium. During implementation of a psychoeducational intervention for family caregivers of terminally ill cancer patients, P. Gagnon et al. (2002) found that few caregivers were aware of the risk of delirium or that it could be treated. The intervention was associated with significant improvements in caregiver confidence. Lundstrom et al. (2005) found reduced delirium duration and mortality in patients receiving care on a ward where staff had received training in delirium assessment and treatment, where improved caregiver-patient interaction was emphasized. Although relatives can play an integral role in efforts to support and reorient delirious patients, they can add to the burden if they are ill-informed, critical, or anxious, whereby medical staff members respond to their distress by inappropriately medicating patients. Recovered delirium patients reported that simple but firm communication, reality orientation, a visible clock, and the presence of a relative had contributed to a heightened sense of control (Schofield 1997). Clarification of the cause and meaning of symptoms combined with recognition of treatment goals can allow better management of what is a distressing experience for both patient and loved ones (Breitbart et al. 2002a; Meagher 2001b).

PHARMACOLOGICAL TREATMENT OF DELIRIUM

Current delirium pharmacotherapies are borrowed from the treatment of primary psychiatric disorders. Pharmacological treatment with a neuroleptic agent (dopamine D_2 antagonist) is the clinical standard of delirium treatment, although other agents have been tried and are described in this section (see Table 11–11). Doses need to be modified for elderly patients; however, Hally and Cooney (2005) found that these modifications were frequently overlooked for both haloperidol (62%) and lorazepam (47%) prescribing.

Benzodiazepines

Benzodiazepines are generally reserved for delirium due to ethanol or sedative-hypnotic withdrawal, for which they are first-line agents (Mayo-Smith et al. 2004). Lorazepam or clonazepam (the latter for alprazolam withdrawal) is often used. However, Klijn and van der Mast (2005) warned about overlooking other causes of delirium when patients have alcohol withdrawal and contend that haloperidol should be the first-choice treatment in these patients as well.

Some clinicians use lorazepam as an adjunctive medication with haloperidol in the most severe cases of delirium or when extra assistance with sleep is needed. Benzodiazepine

monotherapy is generally not effective for non-substance-related delirium and may exacerbate the delirium, as shown in Breitbart and colleagues' (1996) controlled blinded study. None of the survey respondents from the American Geriatrics Society would use lorazepam alone to treat severe delirium in elderly postoperative patients (Carnes et al. 2003). Anticholinergic toxicity–induced delirium and agitation were controlled and reversed with physostigmine (87% and 96%, respectively), whereas benzodiazepines controlled agitation in 24% and were ineffective in treating delirium in a retrospective report of 52 consecutive toxicology consultations (Burns et al. 2000). Additionally, patients who received physostigmine had a lower incidence of complications (7% vs. 46%) and a shorter time to recovery (median 12 vs. 24 hours) compared with patients who received benzodiazepines. Pandharipande et al. (2006) found a significant deliriogenic effect, in medical ICU patients, only for benzodiazepines when compared with other commonly used medications (propofol, morphine, and fentanyl), even though higher doses of all of these agents were used in delirious than in nondelirious ICU patients. A survey of ICU physicians found that 66% of the respondents treated delirium with haloperidol, 12% used lorazepam, and fewer than 5% used atypical antipsychotics. More than 55% administered haloperidol and lorazepam at daily doses of 10 mg or less, but some used more than 50 mg/day of either medication (Ely et al. 2004b).

Cholinergic Enhancer Drugs

The cholinergic deficiency hypothesis of delirium suggests that treatment with a cholinergic enhancer drug—generally acetylcholinesterase inhibitors—could be therapeutic. Physostigmine reverses anticholinergic delirium (Stern 1983), but its side effects (seizures) and short half-life make it unsuitable for routine clinical treatment of delirium. Tacrine also was shown to reverse central anticholinergic syndrome (Mendelson 1977), but it has not been studied formally. Three case reports found that donepezil improved delirium in postoperative state, comorbid Lewy body dementia, and comorbid alcohol dementia (Burke et al. 1999; Wengel et al. 1998, 1999). Physostigmine administered in the emergency department to patients suspected of having muscarinic toxicity resulted in reversal of delirium in 22 of 39 patients, including several in whom the cause could not be determined (Schneir et al. 2003); only 1 of the 39 patients had an adverse event (brief seizure). C.J. Kalisvaart et al. (2004) reported that three cases of prolonged delirium that was unresponsive to haloperidol or atypical antipsychotics rapidly resolved when treatment was switched to rivastigmine. (See also "Pharmacological Prophylaxis" subsection earlier in this chapter.)

Neuroleptics

Haloperidol is the neuroleptic most often chosen for the treatment of delirium. It can be administered orally, intramuscularly, or intravenously (Adams 1984, 1988; Dudley et al. 1979; Gelfand et al. 1992; Moulaert 1989; Sanders and Stern 1993; Tesar et al. 1985), although the intravenous route has not been approved by the FDA. Intravenously administered haloperidol is twice as potent as that taken orally (Gelfand et al. 1992). Bolus intravenous doses usually range from 0.5 to 20 mg, although larger doses are sometimes given. In severe, refractory cases, continuous intravenous infusions of 15–25 mg/hour (up to 1,000 mg/day) can be given (Fernandez et al. 1988; J.L. Levenson 1995; Riker et al. 1994; Stern 1994). The specific brain effects of haloperidol in alleviating delirium are not known, but positron emission tomographic scans show reduced glucose utilization in the limbic cortex, thalamus, caudate, and frontal and anterior cingulate cortices (Bartlett et al. 1994). These regions are important for behavior and cognition and have been implicated in the neuropathogenesis of delirium. Milbrandt et al. (2005) found in nearly 1,000 ICU patients that use of haloperidol was associated with reduced mortality.

Clinical use of haloperidol traditionally has been considered to be relatively safe in the seriously medically ill and does not cause as much hypotension as droperidol does (Gelfand et al. 1992; Moulaert 1989; Tesar et al. 1985). Haloperidol does not antagonize dopamine-induced increases in renal blood flow (D.H. Armstrong et al. 1986). Even when haloperidol is given intravenously at high doses in delirium, extrapyramidal symptoms (EPS) are usually not a problem except in more sensitive patients (e.g., those with HIV or Lewy body dementia) (Fernandez et al. 1989; McKeith et al. 1992; Swenson et al. 1989). A case series of five ICU patients receiving 250–500 mg/day of continuous or intermittent intravenous haloperidol had self-limited withdrawal dyskinesia following high-dose haloperidol (Riker et al. 1997). Intravenous lorazepam is sometimes combined with intravenous haloperidol in critically ill patients to lessen EPS and increase sedation.

Cases of prolonged QTc interval on electrocardiogram (ECG) and torsades de pointes tachyarrhythmia (multifocal ventricular tachycardia) have been increasingly recognized and attributed to intravenously administered haloperidol (Hatta et al. 2001; Huyse 1988; Kriwisky et al. 1990; Metzger and Friedman 1993; O'Brien et al. 1999; Perrault et al. 2000; Wilt et al. 1993; Zee-Cheng et al. 1985). The American Psychiatric Association (1999) "Practice Guidelines for the Treatment of Patients With Delirium" recommend that QTc prolongation greater than 450 ms or to greater than 25% over a previous ECG may warrant telemetry, cardiology consultation, dose re-

duction, or discontinuation. They also recommend monitoring serum magnesium and potassium in critically ill delirious patients whose QTc is 450 ms or greater because of the common use of concomitant drugs and/or electrolyte disturbances that also can prolong the QTc interval.

Empirical evidence for neuroleptic benefits in treating delirium is substantial, but efficacy trials are rare. Itil and Fink (1966) found that chlorpromazine reversed anticholinergic delirium. In a double-blind, randomized, controlled design, Breitbart et al. (1996) found that delirium in AIDS patients significantly improved with haloperidol or chlorpromazine, but not with lorazepam, but DRS and MMSE scores still did not return to normal. In addition, both hypoactive and hyperactive subtypes responded to treatment with haloperidol or chlorpromazine, and improvement was noted within hours of treatment, even before the underlying medical causes were addressed (Platt et al. 1994a).

Haloperidol use in pediatric patients with delirium is not well documented, despite its use in adult delirium and in other childhood psychiatric disorders (Teicher and Gold 1990). Its efficacy in children for delusions, hallucinations, thought disorder, aggressivity, stereotypies, hyperactivity, social withdrawal, and learning ability (Teicher and Gold 1990) suggests that it may have a potentially beneficial role in pediatric delirium. Clinical experience with haloperidol in pediatric delirium supports its beneficial effects, although no controlled studies have been done. A retrospective report of 30 children (mean age = 7 ± 1.0 years, range = 8 months to 18 years) with burn injuries supports the use of haloperidol for agitation, disorientation, hallucinations, delusions, and insomnia (R.L. Brown et al. 1996). The mean haloperidol dose was 0.47 ± 0.002 mg/kg, with a mean maximum dose in 24 hours of 0.46 mg/kg, administered intravenously, orally, and intramuscularly. Mean efficacy, as scored on a 0- to 3-point scale (3 = excellent), was 2.3 ± 0.21, but the drug was not efficacious in 17% of cases (four of five of these failures were via the oral route). EPS were not observed, and one episode of hypotension occurred with the intravenous route.

Droperidol has been used to treat acute agitation and confusion from a variety of causes, including mania and delirium (Hooper and Minter 1983; Resnick and Burton 1984; H. Thomas et al. 1992), and was superior to placebo (van Leeuwen et al. 1977). Compared with haloperidol, droperidol is more sedating, has a faster onset of action, can be used only parenterally in the United States, and is very hypotensive because of its potent α-adrenergic antagonism (Moulaert 1989). It is not recommended for use in delirium, however, because of serious cardiac safety concerns resulting from significant prolongation of the QTc interval in a dose-related manner (Lawrence and Nasraway 1997; Lischke et al. 1994; Reilly et al. 2000).

Atypical Antipsychotic Agents

Atypical antipsychotic agents differ from haloperidol and other conventional neuroleptics in a variety of neurotransmitter activities, especially serotonin. In addition to presynaptic serotonin type 2 ($5\text{-}HT_2$) receptor antagonism, it is hypothesized that loose binding at the dopamine D_2 receptor may define atypicality (Kapur and Seeman 2001). Some atypical antipsychotics are being used routinely to treat delirium, and literature on their use is accumulating—mostly case reports, retrospective case series, and a few open-label prospective trials that used standardized measures (Schwartz and Masand 2002; Torres et al. 2001). Hally and Cooney (2005) surveyed prescribing practices for delirium among general hospital medical staff and noted that risperidone was the second most frequently prescribed antipsychotic agent (38%) after haloperidol. In several patients who had a poor response to haloperidol, delirium improved after treatment was switched to an atypical antipsychotic agent (Al-Samarrai et al. 2003; Leso and Schwartz 2002; Passik and Cooper 1999). Haloperidol is avoided in posttraumatic brain injury delirium because dopamine blockade is thought to be deleterious to cognitive recovery; two traumatic brain injury patients with delirium given low-dose olanzapine showed remarkable improvement within a short time (Ovchinsky et al. 2002), suggesting a possible role for atypical antipsychotics in this population.

Because atypical antipsychotics differ in their chemical structures and are not a pharmacological class per se, they may differ in how they affect delirium. Receptor activities and adverse event profiles differ among the atypical agents, and their associated EPS, QTc prolongation, and effects on cognition are particularly relevant to any use in delirium. Ziprasidone was implicated in causing QTc prolongation in a patient with delirium (Leso and Schwartz 2002) and was temporally related to runs of torsades de pointes and QTc prolongation during rechallenge in a patient with delirium (Heinrich et al. 2006). In some case reports, risperidone, quetiapine, and olanzapine were implicated in causing delirium (Chen and Cardasis 1996; Karki and Masood 2003; Ravona-Springer et al. 1998; Samuels and Fang 2004; Sim et al. 2000).

A few reports included more than one atypical agent or compared conventional agents with atypical agents. Al-Samarrai et al. (2003) reported two cases of delirium that did not respond to either haloperidol or risperidone but settled soon after commencing quetiapine. Three elderly patients with postoperative delirium responded quickly to olanzapine up to 10 mg/day and tolerated it well, despite not responding to or having excessive sedation from either haloperidol or risperidone (Khouzam and Gazula 2001).

Hill et al. (2002) compared DRS-R98 daily ratings from 50 consecutive delirium cases treated with haloperidol, olanzapine, or risperidone and found a significant main effect of drug and time at 3 days, with olanzapine being more effective in reducing delirium severity than either haloperidol or risperidone. Skrobik et al. (2004) found similar efficacy for haloperidol and olanzapine in ICU patients, with more EPS in the haloperidol group, but standardized delirium ratings were not used and investigators were not blinded to drug. J.Y. Kim et al. (2005) used the DRS-R98 to compare haloperidol and risperidone in an open-label nonrandomized trial and found equivalent efficacy. Blinded, randomized comparator studies are clearly needed to determine whether therapeutic differences exist.

Clozapine—the first atypical antipsychotic—is clinically distinct from the others and is not recommended for delirium treatment. It is very sedating, has significant anticholinergic side effects, causes sinus tachycardia, lowers seizure threshold, and is associated with causing agranulocytosis. Clozapine treatments ($n = 391$) resulted in about an 8% incidence of delirium episodes among 315 psychiatric inpatients, and in 7 of 33 episodes it was the only drug used (Gaertner et al. 1989). The incidence and risk factors for delirium were evaluated in 139 psychiatric patients with a mean age of 41 years who were given an average daily dose of 282 ± 203 mg/day for 18.9 ± 16.4 days (Centorrino et al. 2003). Delirium was diagnosed in 10.1%, and 71.4% of those were moderate to severe; cotreatment with other centrally active antimuscarinic drugs, poor clinical outcome, older age, and longer hospitalization (by 17.5 days) were associated with delirium in these patients. Cholinergic agents can reverse clozapine-induced delirium (Schuster et al. 1977).

Risperidone in doses up to 5 mg/day has been reported to reduce delirium severity as measured by the DRS in an open-label case series (Sipahimalani and Masand 1997) and several prospective open trials (Horikawa et al. 2003; Mittal et al. 2004; Parellada et al. 2004; Toda et al. 2005). Double-blind, placebo-controlled studies (I.R. Katz et al. 1999) have reported that risperidone has dose-related EPS beginning at about 2 mg/day. The combination of risperidone and the selective serotonin reuptake inhibitor paroxetine was reported to induce delirium as part of serotonin syndrome in two elderly patients (ages 78 and 86 years) (Karki and Masood 2003). Liu et al. (2004), in a retrospective analysis, found that risperidone had efficacy similar to that of haloperidol in treating hyperactive symptoms of delirium, but patients receiving risperidone required much less anticholinergic medication for EPS.

Eleven patients with delirium taking olanzapine showed similar response on the DRS to 11 patients with delirium taking haloperidol in an open-label, nonrandomized case series, although 5 haloperidol-treated patients had EPS or excessive sedation compared with none in the olanzapine-treated group (Masand and Sipahimalani 1998). Breitbart et al. (2002b) found resolution of delirium according to the MDAS with olanzapine treatment in 79% of patients by day 3 with overall good tolerability but less responsiveness in older patients with brain damage as a result of metastases or dementia. K.S. Kim et al. (2001) found decreased DRS scores in 20 patients with delirium (mean age = 46 years) taking olanzapine, which was well tolerated without EPS. Olanzapine has a favorable EPS profile and does not appear to have a clinically significant effect on the QTc interval at therapeutic doses in schizophrenic patients (Czekalla et al. 2001). Olanzapine increases acetylcholine release measured by in vivo microdialysis in both rat prefrontal cortex (Meltzer et al. 1999) and hippocampus (Schirazi et al. 2000), consistent with procholinergic activity. J.S. Kennedy et al. (2001) theorized that presynaptic blockade by olanzapine at 5-HT_3, 5-HT_6, and muscarinic type 2 (M_2) receptors may account for this increased acetylcholine release (see discussion of ondansetron in "Agents With Serotonergic Actions" subsection later in this chapter).

Open-label studies of patients with delirium treated with quetiapine with flexible dosing suggested that it was well tolerated and associated with symptom reduction on the DRS (K.Y. Kim et al. 2003; Sasaki et al. 2003) or DRS-R98 (Pae et al. 2004). Lee et al. (2005) compared amisulpiride (mean dose = 156 mg/day) with quetiapine (mean dose = 113 mg/day) in an open-label, randomized study of delirium and found similar reductions in DRS-R98 scores, and both drugs were well tolerated.

Aripiprazole, an atypical antipsychotic with pro-dopaminergic effects related to partial agonism, was reported to be efficacious in an open-label trial in which the DRS-R98 was used and to have a low rate of adverse events (Straker et al. 2006).

Atypical agents in intramuscular formulations are therapeutic options being tried by clinicians whose medically ill patients cannot take oral medications. However, recent concerns about a possible increased risk of cerebrovascular events in elderly patients with dementia receiving chronic oral atypical antipsychotics (Brodaty et al. 2003; I.R. Katz et al. 1999) suggest a need for greater caution in their use, particularly in view of the high rate of concomitant dementia in patients with delirium. The risk of adverse cerebrovascular events is comparable for risperidone, quetiapine, and olanzapine, but the risk is elevated when they are used in patients with dementia compared with other indications (Layton et al. 2005). Other work suggests that stroke is no higher in elderly patients receiving atypical antipsychotics compared with typical antipsychotics (Herrmann et al. 2004) and that medica-

tion choice should be guided by a careful consideration of the overall risk-benefit ratio (L.S. Schneider et al. 2005).

Psychostimulants

Psychostimulants can worsen delirium—probably via increased dopaminergic activity—and their use when a depressed mood is present is contentious (J.A. Levenson 1992; P.B. Rosenberg et al. 1991). Morita et al. (2000) reported improvement of hypoactive delirium in a terminally ill cancer patient due to disseminated intravascular coagulation and multiorgan failure when methylphenidate, 10–20 mg/day, was administered, which raised the arousal level within 1 day and improved MDAS and DRS scores. They attributed the improvement to amelioration of an overstimulated GABA system. In an open-label study, B. Gagnon et al. (2005) administered 20–30 mg of methylphenidate to 14 patients with advanced metastatic cancer and hypoactive delirium; median MMSE scores improved at 1-hour postdose. Cases with psychosis were excluded.

Anticonvulsant Agents

Anticonvulsant agents such as valproic acid may have a role in some cases of delirium, and they are first-line treatments when ictal states are the cause of delirium (Bourgeois et al. 2005; A. Schneider 2005).

Agents With Serotonergic Actions

Agents with serotonergic actions may be of therapeutic value in delirium. L-Tryptophan administered thrice daily was associated with improved MMSE scores and reduced tranquilizer requirement in an uncontrolled study of 32 patients with substance-related delirium (Hebenstreit et al. 1989). Mianserin, a serotonergic tetracyclic antidepressant, has been used in Japan for delirium in elderly medical and postsurgical cohorts, administered either orally or as a suppository. Several open-label studies found reductions in the DRS scores similar to those seen with haloperidol (J. Nakamura et al. 1995, 1997a, 1997b; Uchiyama et al. 1996). Its efficacy was theorized to be related to effects on reducing agitation and improving sleep or to its weak D_2 receptor antagonism in conjunction with blockade of postsynaptic 5-HT_2, presynaptic α-adrenergic, and H_1 and H_2 histaminic receptor blockade.

A single 8-mg intravenous dose of ondansetron, a 5-HT_3 antagonist, was reported to reduce agitation in patients with delirium when a 4-point rating scale was applied prospectively in 35 postcardiotomy patients (mean age = 51 years) (Bayindir et al. 2000). Blockade of presynaptic 5-HT_3 and 5-HT_6 receptors increases release of acetylcholine, possibly the mechanism for ondansetron's apparent beneficial effects.

POSTDELIRIUM MANAGEMENT

Treatment of delirium should continue until symptoms have fully resolved, but the role of continued treatment thereafter is uncertain. Alexopoulos et al. (2004) surveyed 52 experts on the treatment of older adults and found consensus that treatment of delirium should be continued for at least a week after response before tapering and discontinuation are attempted. However, many patients experiencing delirium are discharged before full resolution of symptoms, and, unfortunately, continued monitoring and management are often not part of postdischarge planning. Problems with attention and orientation are especially persistent (McCusker et al. 2003a). Further episodes may be prevented by addressing risk factors such as medication exposure and sensory impairments. There has been little study of the psychological aftermath of delirium, but recent work suggests that approximately 50% of patients can recall the episode (Breitbart et al. 2002a; O'Keeffe 2005). Depression and posttraumatic stress disorder have been described, but most dismiss the episode once it has passed, often despite lingering concerns that the episode heralds a first step toward loss of mental faculties and independence (Schofield 1997). Other patients experience silent delirium and are ashamed or afraid to admit to symptoms. Explicit recognition and discussion of the meaning of delirium can facilitate adjustment but also can allow more detailed discussion of how best to minimize future risk. A follow-up visit can facilitate postdelirium adjustment by clarifying the transient nature of delirium symptoms in contrast to dementia (Easton and MacKenzie 1988) and by providing any ongoing medication adjustments.

NEUROPATHOPHYSIOLOGY OF DELIRIUM

Delirium is considered to result from a generalized disturbance of higher cerebral cortical processes, as reflected by diffuse slowing on the EEG and a breadth of neuropsychiatric symptoms (cognition, perception, sleep, motor, language, and thought). It is not accompanied by primary motor or sensory deficits except when related to a specific etiology (e.g., asterixis), although progressive loss of control of motor functions occurs as severity increases (e.g., difficulty with hygiene and self-feeding and incontinence) (Engel and Romano 1959). Thus, not all brain regions are equally affected in delirium. Certain regions, circuits, and neurochemistry may be integral in the neuropathogenesis of delirium (Trzepacz 1994a, 1999b, 2000). Henon et al. (1999) found that laterality of lesion location and not metabolic factors accounted for the differences in delirium incidence for superficial cortical lesions.

Even though delirium has many different etiologies, each with its own physiological effects on the body, its constellation of symptoms is largely stereotyped, with many considered "core" symptoms (Meagher et al. 2007; Trzepacz et al. 2001). Somehow this diversity of physiological perturbations translates into a common clinical expression that may well relate to dysfunction of certain neural circuits (as well as neurotransmitters)—that is, a final common neural pathway (Trzepacz 1999b, 2000). An analogy of a funnel (see Figure 11–8) can be used to represent this common neural circuitry.

NEUROANATOMICAL CONSIDERATIONS

Studies support certain neural pathways being involved in delirium. Specifically, bilateral or right prefrontal cortex, superficial right posterior parietal cortex, basal ganglia, either right or left fusiform cortex (ventromesial temporoparietal) and lingual gyrus, and right anterior thalamus appear to be particularly associated with delirium (Trzepacz 2000). In addition, the pathways linking them (thalamic-frontal-subcortical and temporolimbic-frontal/subcortical) are likely involved. This hypothesis is largely based on structural neuroimaging reports (Table 11–12), only a few of which are consecutive and prospective in design, and a limited number of functional neuroimaging studies.

Lateralization to more right-sided circuitry involvement in delirium is also supported by evidence besides lesion studies. The right prefrontal cortex cognitively processes novel situations, in contrast to the left (which processes familiar situations), and this may account for delirium patients' difficulties with comprehending new environments (E.L. Goldberg 1998). The right posterior parietal cortex subserves sustained attention and attention to the environment (Posner and Boies 1971), and both are often impaired in delirium. Bipolar patients had the highest incidence of delirium (35.5%) among 199 psychiatric inpatients (Ritchie et al. 1996), and because right-sided anterior and subcortical pathways have been implicated in mania (Blumberg et al. 1999), this suggests a predisposition to delirium possibly based on neuroanatomy. Bell's mania is a severe form of mania that causes pseudodelirium. Visual attention and visual memory tests—assessing nondominant hemisphere cognitive functions—distinguished delirious from nondelirious patients (Hart et al. 1997). Dopamine neurotransmission is lateralized such that activity is normally higher in the left prefrontal cortex (Glick et al. 1982), and this difference may become more extreme if right-sided pathways are affected in delirium.

Lesions of the right posterior parietal cortex may be present with severe delirium that overshadows sensory deficits (Boiten and Lodder 1989; Koponen et al. 1989a;

TABLE 11–12.   Lesions associated with delirium in structural neuroimaging studies

Study	Lesions associated with delirium
Mesulam et al. 1979; Price and Mesulam 1985	CVA in R posterior parietal, R prefrontal, ventromedial temporal, or occipital cortex
Horenstein et al. 1967	CVAs in fusiform and calcarine cortices
Medina et al. 1977	L or bilateral mesial temporal-occipital CVA
Medina et al. 1974	L hippocampal or fusiform CVA
Vaphiades et al. 1996	R mesial occipital, parahippocampal, and hippocampal (with visual hallucinations)
Nighoghossian et al. 1992	R subcortical CVA (with frontal deactivation)
Bogousslavsky et al. 1988	R anterior thalamus CVA on preexisting L caudate lesion (with ↓ frontal perfusion on SPECT)
Figiel et al. 1989; Martin et al. 1992	Lesions in caudate nucleus (in depressed patients treated with ECT or medications)
Figiel et al. 1991	Parkinson's disease patients (depressed and treated with ECT or medications)
Koponen et al. 1989a	R prefrontal or posterior parietal cortex CVA (many with comorbid dementia)
Dunne et al. 1986	R temporoparietal CVA
Mullaly et al. 1982	R temporal or parietal CVA
Boiten and Lodder 1989	R inferior parietal lobule CVA
Friedman 1985; Santamaria et al. 1984	R anteromedial thalamus CVA
Henon et al. 1999	R superficial CVA (prospective sample)
Caeiro et al. 2004b	CVAs in R MCA hemispheric, thalamus, and caudate

Note.   CVA = cerebrovascular accident (stroke); R = right; L = left; SPECT = single-photon emission computed tomography; ECT = electroconvulsive therapy; MCA = middle cerebral artery.

Source.   Adapted from Trzepacz PT: "Is There a Final Common Neural Pathway in Delirium? Focus on Acetylcholine and Dopamine." *Seminars in Clinical Neuropsychiatry* 5:132–148, copyright 2000, with permission from Elsevier.

Mesulam et al. 1979; Price and Mesulam 1985). Infarctions distributed in the right middle cerebral artery produce fewer localizing neurological signs when they are accompanied by agitated delirium (Schmidley and Messing 1984). Lesions of the fusiform region may be associated with an acute, agitated delirium accompanied by visual impairment (Horenstein et al. 1967; Medina et al. 1974, 1977). Despite their posterior location, lesions in this basal temporal region also may affect functions of the prefrontal cortex via temporal-limbic-frontal pathways.

The thalamus is uniquely positioned to filter, integrate, and regulate information among the brain stem, cortex, and subcortex. EEG abnormal results and somatosensory evoked potential slowing are consistent with thalamic dysfunction in delirium (see subsection "Electroencephalography" earlier in this chapter). The anterior, medial, and dorsal thalamic nuclei have important interconnections with prefrontal, subcortical, and limbic areas that are involved in cognitive and behavioral functions. Because the thalamus is extensively and reciprocally interconnected with all areas of cerebral cortex, a relatively small thalamic lesion can cause delirium. The thalamus is rich in GABAergic interneurons and glutamatergic neurons (Sherman and Kock 1990) and receives cholinergic, noradrenergic, and serotonergic afferents from brain stem nuclei. Muscarinic influences at the thalamus affect baseline electroencephalographic rhythm. Strokes in the right paramedian and anteromedial thalamus (Bogousslavsky et al. 1988; Friedman 1985; Santamaria et al. 1984) can cause delirium. Gaudreau and Gagnon (2004) have proposed a model of delirium in which both "positive" symptoms (psychosis) and "negative" symptoms (inattention) can be caused by thalamic sensory overload caused by excessive dopaminergic or glutamatergic activity and/or reduced cholinergic or GABAergic activity.

Basal ganglia lesions are also associated with delirium. Preexisting lesions of the caudate nucleus (Figiel et al. 1989; Martin et al. 1992) and Parkinson's disease (Figiel et al. 1991) increase the risk of delirium during electroconvulsive therapy and with the use of tricyclic antidepressants. From a study of delirium incidence among 175 consecutive dementia patients, Robertsson et al. (1998) concluded that subcortical damage increased delirium risk and that patients with vascular dementia were more at risk than were those with early Alzheimer's or frontotemporal dementia.

A retrospective study of 661 stroke patients found 33% to be acutely confused on presentation (Dunne et al. 1986). The 19 patients diagnosed as having delirium almost exclusively had right-sided temporoparietal cortex lesions, although another 26 patients with similar lesions were not classified as having delirium because they lacked "clouded consciousness," which likely underdiagnosed the frequency of delirium associated with such lesions. A retrospective study of 309 neurology consultations found 60 patients with acute confusional state; those with focal lesions had mostly right temporal or parietal locations (Mullaly et al. 1982).

A few prospective studies of stroke location and delirium incidence have been done. Ramirez-Bermudez et al. (2006) surveyed 202 neurological emergencies and found that delirium (incidence = 15%) was associated with lesions in the frontal and temporal lobes but did not report laterality for individual cases. When DSM-IV criteria and a DRS score of 10 or more points were used to define cases, 202 consecutive stroke patients had a 25% incidence of delirium (Henon et al. 1999). Right-sided superficial cortical lesions were more associated with delirium than were left-sided lesions ($P = 0.009$), whereas deep lesions did not show laterality. Computed tomographic scans for 69 consecutively admitted delirious (DSM-III diagnosis) elderly patients, many of whom had comorbid dementia, were compared with scans for 31 age-matched control subjects with other neurological disorders (Koponen et al. 1989a). Delirious patients had more generalized atrophy and focal changes—in particular, right hemisphere lesions in the parieto-occipital association area. On the basis of DSM-III-R criteria, 48% of 155 consecutive stroke patients were acutely confused (Gustafson et al. 1991). Among these, more patients with left-sided lesions were confused (58%) than those with right-sided lesions (38%), although the study was not designed to assess effects of laterality. Caeiro et al. (2004b) used the DRS to assess delirium prospectively in 218 consecutive acute stroke patients and a control group of 50 acute coronary syndrome patients; they found a higher incidence of delirium in the stroke patients (13%

vs. 2%). Hemispheric strokes were more associated with delirium than were brain stem or cerebellar strokes, and the most common lesions were large right MCA infarcts, and independent predictors included neglect (a nondominant cerebral dysfunction) and increased odds ratios for thalamus (1.3), caudate (6.7), and middle cerebral artery (2.4) lesion locations. Thus, many patients with strokes can become delirious through a variety of chemical or structural mechanisms—for example, glutamatergic surges and cholinergic deficiency—but most evidence supports laterality for cortical and thalamic lesions.

Findings from single photon emission computed tomography (SPECT) and positron emission tomography (PET) scans also support the relevance of the prefrontal cortex and subcortical regions in patients with delirium (Trzepacz 1994a). These tests usually show reduced flow or metabolism in the frontal cortex and either increased or decreased flow in subcortical regions. Yokota and colleagues (2003) used xenon-enhanced CT and found widespread reduction in regional cerebral blood flow (cerebral cortex, thalamus, basal ganglia) in delirious patients that returned to normal when delirium improved. Reishies et al. (2005) found altered cognition following electroconvulsive therapy that was associated with increased slow-wave activity that was most pronounced in the anterior cingulate cortex, a region important for higher cognitive functions such as error processing, working memory, verbal fluency, selective attention, and long-term memory. Dysfunction in both cortical and subcortical regions in delirium is also supported by slowing of EEG and evoked potentials (see subsection "Electroencephalography" earlier in this chapter).

NEUROTRANSMISSION

A final common neural pathway for delirium would be composed of both neuroanatomical and neurochemical dimensions. The preponderance of evidence in the literature supports a low cholinergic/excess dopaminergic state for this proposed final common neural pathway (Trzepacz 1996, 2000). Although other neurotransmitter systems are known to be involved for certain etiologies (e.g., hepatic insufficiency or alcohol withdrawal deliria), the activity of cholinergic and dopaminergic pathways can be regulated and affected by other neurotransmitters, including serotonergic, opiatergic, GABAergic, noradrenergic, and glutamatergic systems; altered metabolic states; physiological changes of inflammatory and stress responses; and glial activity. Thus, many factors can interact with the final common pathway to culminate in delirium.

Neurotransmission may be altered in many ways, including through widespread effects on oxidative metabolism. Glucose and oxygen are both critical for brain function, and their delivery is dependent on properly functioning cardiovascular and pulmonary systems. Pathways for the metabolism of glucose and production of adenosine triphosphate involve oxygen and vitamins (cofactors for enzymes) as well as substrates related to neurotransmission (e.g., amino acids and acetyl coenzyme A), so the citric acid cycle is very important for general brain metabolism and production of neurotransmitters. Seaman et al. (2006) retrospectively found that measures of oxidative stress (hemoglobin, hematocrit, and pulse oximetry) and presence of pneumonia or sepsis were worse in patients who developed delirium in an ICU than in those who did not, even though no differences in overall medical morbidity were identified with APACHE II scores. During severe illness, surgery, and trauma, ratios of plasma amino acids may affect synthesis in the brain of neurotransmitters that are associated with immune activation and adaptive metabolic changes that redirect energy consumption (van der Mast and Fekkes 2000).

Alterations in the blood-brain barrier, such as during uremia, allow penetration of molecules and drugs that would not ordinarily enter the CNS and thereby produce unwanted effects on function of the brain regions and pathways. Vascular endothelial cells and perivascular cells at the interface between peripheral blood and brain parenchyma are proposed to be involved in transmission of inflammation from periphery to brain such that signals are transmitted via activation of those parenchymal microglia, according to postmortem human brain tissue studies (Uchikado et al. 2004). This is a suggested mechanism whereby systemic inflammatory responses are relayed to the brain despite an intact blood-brain barrier and may cause delirium through release of cytokines that alter neurotransmission without overt structural damage to the brain.

Whereas some etiologies of delirium alter neurotransmission via general metabolism, others may antagonize or interfere with specific receptors and neurotransmitters. Evidence indicates both specific and widespread effects on neurotransmission in delirium. In addition to changes in major neurotransmitter systems, neurotoxic metabolites, such as quinolinic acid from tryptophan metabolism (Basile et al. 1995), and false transmitters, such as octopamine in patients with liver failure, can alter neurotransmission and also have been implicated in the neuropathogenesis of delirium. Because glia regulate neurotransmitter amounts in the synapse, glial dysfunction also may be involved.

A wide variety of medications and their metabolites have anticholinergic activity and cause delirium. Some act postsynaptically; others act presynaptically; and still others, such as norfentanyl and normeperidine, have anticholinergic metabolites (Coffman and Dilsaver 1988). Tune et al. (1992) studied and measured the anticholinergic ac-

tivity of many medications in "atropine equivalents." They identified significant anticholinergic effects in many medications usually not recognized as being anticholinergic (e.g., digoxin, nifedipine, cimetidine, and codeine). However, the assay used did not discriminate among the five muscarinic receptor subtypes, activity at which can result in opposite effects in the brain depending on location in the synapse; for example, blockade of presynaptic M_2 receptors results in an increased release of acetylcholine. Delirium induced by anticholinergic drugs is associated with generalized electroencephalographic slowing and is reversed by treatment with physostigmine or neuroleptics (Itil and Fink 1966; Stern 1983). Centrally active anticholinergic agents can cause electroencephalographic slowing and reduced verbal memory (Sloan et al. 1992).

A rat model of delirium in which a range of atropine doses was used showed similar features as human delirium: cognitive impairment, electroencephalographic slowing and increased amplitude, and hyperactivity during objective motor monitoring (Leavitt et al. 1994; Trzepacz et al. 1992) (see Figure 11–10). A different rat model in which lower atropine doses were used showed cognitive impairment, but because EEGs were not recorded, intoxication, but not delirium per se, was found (O'Hare et al. 1997).

In addition, several medical conditions have anticholinergic effects, including thiamine deficiency, hypoxia, and hypoglycemia, all of which may reduce acetylcholine by affecting the oxidative metabolism of glucose and the production of acetyl coenzyme A, the rate-limiting step for acetylcholine synthesis (Trzepacz 1994a, 1996). Consistent with these findings, glucose has been shown to enhance memory performance via a CNS muscarinic mechanism (Kopf and Baratti 1994). Parietal cortex levels of choline are reduced in chronic hepatic encephalopathy, as measured by magnetic resonance imaging (MRI) spectroscopy (Kreis et al. 1991).

Serum levels of anticholinergic activity are elevated in patients with postoperative delirium and correlate with severity of cognitive impairment (Tune et al. 1981), improving with resolution of the delirium (Mach et al. 1995). Post–electroconvulsive therapy delirium is also associated with higher serum anticholinergic levels (Mondimore et al. 1983). Higher serum anticholinergic activity levels were associated with reduced self-care ability among nursing home patients (Rovner et al. 1988). A double-blind intervention study in a nursing home showed that reduction of anticholinergic drugs improved cognitive status in those who had had elevated serum anticholinergic levels (Tollefson et al. 1991). This assay also detects substances circulating in peripheral blood that reflect inflammation and are not specific to the cholinergic system but may still have relevance to delirium.

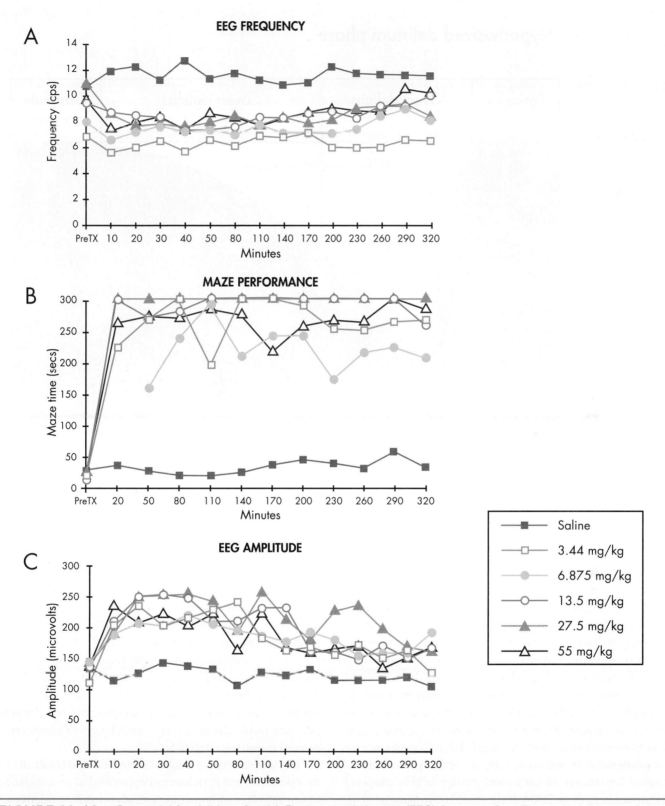

FIGURE 11–10. Rat model for delirium. *Panel A.* Electroencephalogram (EEG) frequency for saline control group and atropine dose groups at all times. *Panel B.* Maze performance for saline control group and atropine dose groups at all times. *Panel C.* EEG amplitude for saline control group and atropine dose groups at all times. PreTX=baseline; cps=cycles per second.

Source. Reprinted from Leavitt M, Trzepacz PT, Ciongoli K: "Rat Model of Delirium: Atropine Dose-Response Relationships." *Journal of Neuropsychiatry and Clinical Neurosciences* 6:279–284, 1994. Copyright 1994, American Psychiatric Press, Inc. Used with permission.

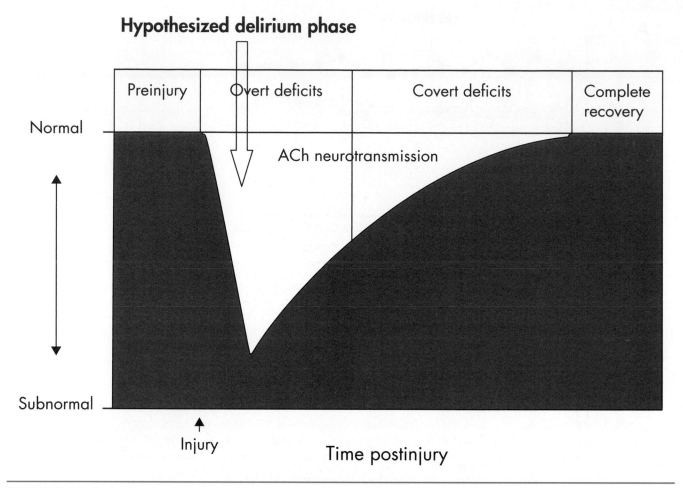

FIGURE 11–11.   Cholinergic hypofunction after traumatic brain injury. ACh = acetylcholine.

Source.   Reprinted from Dixon CE, Hamm RJ, Taft WC, et al: "Increased Anticholinergic Sensitivity Following Closed Skull Impact and Controlled Cortical Impact Traumatic Brain Injury in the Rat." *Journal of Neurotrauma* 11:275–287, 1994. Copyright 1994. Used with permission.

Age-associated changes in cholinergic function also increase delirium propensity. Alzheimer's and vascular dementias reduce cholinergic activity and are associated with increased risk for delirium. Lewy body dementia mimics delirium with its fluctuating symptom severity, confusion, hallucinations (especially visual), delusions, and electroencephalographic slowing and is associated with significant loss of cholinergic nucleus basalis neurons (Robinson 2002). Its delirium symptoms respond to donepezil (Kaufer et al. 1998). Use of cholinergic agents has been associated with reduced delirium incidence or improvement in delirium (see subsection "Pharmacological Treatment of Delirium" earlier in this chapter) (Dautzenberg et al. 2004; Diaz et al. 2001; Moretti et al. 2004), including in vascular dementia patients.

Stroke and traumatic brain injury are associated with decreased cholinergic activity—especially in the thalamus, amygdala, frontal cortex, hippocampus, and basal forebrain (Yamamoto et al. 1988)—and with increased vulnerability to antimuscarinic drugs (Dixon et al. 1994).

The low cholinergic state seems to correlate temporally with delirium following the acute event (see Figure 11–11). Thus, broad support exists for an anticholinergic mechanism from diverse mechanisms of delirium: metabolic, neurochemical, and structural.

On the contrary, cholinergic toxicity from organophosphate insecticides, nerve poisons, and tacrine (Trzepacz et al. 1996) also can cause delirium, although this is not as well described as anticholinergic delirium. Perhaps delirium results from extreme imbalances of cholinergic neurotransmitter activity levels.

Dopamine activity may be increased as a result of reduced cholinergic activity, conceptualized as an imbalance of the activities of dopamine and acetylcholine relative to each other. Hypoxia is associated with increased release of dopamine while decreasing the release of acetylcholine (Broderick and Gibson 1989). In striatum, D_2 receptor stimulation reduces acetylcholine release, whereas D_1 stimulation increases it (Ikarashi et al. 1997). Phasic dopamine release is associated with salience attribution to external stimuli, and it mediates working memory in the prefrontal cortex, which is essential for problem-solving and decision-making (Kienast and Heinz 2006). Both of these functions are important for a delirious patient trying to interact with the environment. D_1 receptors are highly involved in the modulation of working memory, and their activation follows an inverted U-shaped curve so that too little or too much D_1 agonism disrupts performance.

Delirium can occur from intoxication with dopaminergic drugs, including levodopa, dopamine, and bupropion (Ames et al. 1992), and from cocaine binges (Wetli et al. 1996). Patients with alcohol withdrawal delirium are more likely to have the A9 allele of the dopamine transporter gene compared with matched control subjects without delirium (Sander et al. 1997), suggesting a role for dopamine in delirium propensity, although subsequent reports were inconsistent (Köhnke et al. 2005). Delirium from opiates may be mediated by increased dopamine and glutamate activity in addition to decreased acetylcholine (Gibson et al. 1975). Excess dopamine levels occur during hepatic encephalopathy, presumably as a result of increased levels of tyrosine and phenylalanine in CSF (Knell et al. 1974) or changes in dopamine regulation by altered serotonin activity. Dopamine agonists (active at D_1 and D_2 receptors) have been shown to cause electroencephalographic slowing and behavioral arousal in rats (Ongini et al. 1985), findings similar to those seen in rats treated with atropine (Leavitt et al. 1994; Trzepacz et al. 1992). A rat model for delirium that used apomorphine (a direct D_1 and D_2 agonist) in a choice reaction task showed reversal of performance deficits by administration of haloperidol and aniracetam, a cholinomimetic, but not by administration of tacrine, which worsened deficits (K. Nakamura et al. 1998). The investigators concluded that cognitive deficits were mediated by a D_2 mechanism, but because EEGs were not recorded, it is not clear if this could be a delirium animal model.

Little is known about which dopamine receptor subtypes are involved in the neuropathogenesis of delirium, although those related to mesolimbic and mesofrontal dopaminergic pathways are probably involved. Antidopaminergic agents, particularly neuroleptics, can be successfully used to treat delirium, including that arising from anticholinergic causes (Itil and Fink 1966; Platt et al. 1994a). Traditional neuroleptics that are effective in treating delirium are not subtype specific; haloperidol predominantly affects D_2 receptors, although it also affects D_1, D_3, and D_4 receptors (Piercey et al. 1995). Use of selective dopamine antagonists might shed light on the mechanism underlying delirium. For example, differential effects on D_1, D_2, and D_3 receptors might underlie different motor presentations during an individual delirium episode (Trzepacz 2000). Polymorphisms in genes related to dopamine receptors

(e.g., through mutations, single nucleotide polymorphisms, and variable number tandem repeats) may mediate more subtle differences in dopamine receptor function and open the door to better understanding of delirium occurrence and risk as well as treatment through genetic studies (see Table 11–5) (Wong et al. 2000).

Norepinephrine is well known for its importance in cognition, especially with regard to attention, working memory, and executive functions. J. Nakamura et al. (1997a) described decreased plasma-free 3-methoxy-4-hydroxy-phenylglycol concentration, a norepinephrine metabolite, in association with improvement on the DRS in response to treatment, that reached levels for nondelirious control subjects but no difference in plasma-free homovanillic acid. This suggests that delirium is a hyperadrenergic state, even though plasma levels may not reflect CNS levels. Norepinephrine modulates and attenuates the effect of dopamine's disruption of normal gating; that is, suppression of irrelevant information at the nucleus accumbens. Low doses of dopamine can enhance gating, whereas higher doses disrupt it; this may be related to distractibility in delirium (Swerdlow et al. 2006).

Both increased and decreased GABA have been implicated in causing delirium. Increased GABAergic activity, in addition to reduced glutamate and increased serotonin activity, is one of several putative mechanisms implicated in hepatic encephalopathy (Mousseau and Butterworth 1994). Increased GABA activity may result from elevated ammonia levels, which increase levels of glutamate and glutamine, which are then converted into GABA (B. Anderson 1984; Schafer and Jones 1982). Consistent with this hypothesis is the improvement observed in some patients with hepatic encephalopathy who are taking flumazenil, which blocks $GABA_A$-benzodiazepine receptors. Glutamine levels have been shown to be elevated in hepatic encephalopathy, as measured by MRI spectroscopy, although the chemical relations among glutamine, GABA, and glutamate confound the meaning of this measurement (Kreis et al. 1991). Reduced GABA activity occurs in delirium during withdrawal from ethanol and from sedative-hypnotic drugs. Decreased GABA activity is also implicated in the mechanism of antibiotic delirium caused by penicillins, cephalosporins, and quinolones (Akaike et al. 1991; Mathers 1987).

Both low and excessive levels of serotonin are associated with delirium (van der Mast and Fekkes 2000). Serotonin activity may be increased in patients with hepatic encephalopathy—related to increased tryptophan uptake in the brain (Mousseau and Butterworth 1994; van der Mast and Fekkes 2000)—as well as in sepsis (Mizock et al. 1990) and serotonergic syndromes (R.J. Goldberg and Huk 1992). The precursor of serotonin, tryptophan, is also implicated in delirium. Increases in free tryptophan levels in plasma correlate with reductions in cerebral blood flow on xenon-enhanced computed tomographic scans in patients with subclinical hepatic encephalopathy (Rodriguez et al. 1987), and L-5-hydroxytryptophan induces delirium (Irwin et al. 1986). In contrast, tryptophan is decreased in patients with postcardiotomy delirium (van der Mast et al. 1994). Serotonin regulates dopamine activity in some brain regions, including the striatum and limbic system (Meltzer 1993), which may explain why neuroleptics are useful in treating serotonergic deliria.

Histamine may play a role in delirium through its effects on arousal and hypothalamic regulation of sleep-wake circadian rhythms. H_1 agonists and H_3 antagonists increase wakefulness (Monti 1993), whereas antihistamines (H_1 antagonists) reduce arousal and are associated with REM sleep (Marzanatti et al. 1989) and delirium (Tejera et al. 1994). H_1 antagonists increase catechols and serotonin levels and have anticholinergic properties (Jones et al. 1986), possibly mediating delirium. H_2 antagonists also cause delirium, possibly related to their anticholinergic properties (Picotte-Prillmayer et al. 1995), although they do not affect brain sleep centers.

Glutamate release is increased during hypoxia, and glutamatergic receptors may be activated by quinolone antibiotics (P.D. Williams and Helton 1991). Activation of glutamatergic receptors is a possible mechanism for quinolones causing delirium. Dopamine and glutamate are both neurotransmitters at the thalamus, a region potentially important in the neuropathogenesis of delirium.

Disruption of normal biological rhythms is well recognized in delirium, particularly in relation to sleep-wake cycles and other circadian cycles. Melatonin receptors exist at the suprachiasmatic nucleus of the hypothalamus. Several studies have suggested a possible relation between these disruptions and altered melatonin metabolism; tryptophan is the precursor for both melatonin and serotonin. Shigeta et al. (2001) compared melatonin secretion patterns of nondelirious and delirious patients with and without complications after major abdominal surgery. In the patients with delirium, reduced melatonin levels were not associated with complications, and markedly elevated melatonin levels resulted in complications (infection, shock, cardiac failure). Similarly, K. Olofsson et al. (2004) advocated a trial of melatonin as a treatment for delirium on the basis of observed disruption of circadian rhythm to melatonin secretion in ICU patients. Balan et al. (2003) found high levels of melatonin metabolites in the urine in delirium, especially in patients with hypoactive delirium. Lewis and Barnett (2004) proposed that administration of melatonin in delirium may restore tryptophan levels by reducing its breakdown and thereby treat not only hypoactive but also hyperactive forms by blunting activity of an alternative metabolic pathway for tryptophan that produces an abnormal metabolite that is believed to produce excitatory symptoms.

CYTOKINES AND INFLAMMATORY RESPONSE

Cytokines have been implicated as causes of inflammatory or infectious-induced delirium, and they also may have a role in sleep (Moldofsky et al. 1986). They are polypeptide hormones secreted in the CNS by glia and macrophages, whose normally low extracellular levels are increased during stress, rapid growth, inflammation, tumor, trauma, and infection (Hopkins and Rothwell 1995; Stefano et al. 1994). Although cytokines are not yet identified as neurotransmitters per se, they may influence the activities of catecholamines, indoleamines, GABA, and acetylcholine (Hopkins and Rothwell 1995) and can cause increased release and turnover of dopamine and norepinephrine (Stefano et al. 1994) and reduction of acetylcholine levels (Willard et al. 1999), thereby causing delirium. Cytokines acting as neurotoxins, as in HIV dementia, is another mechanism for causing brain dysfunction (Lipton and Gendelman 1995), although Broadhurst and Wilson (2001) have highlighted that inhibition of growth factor–mediated neuroprotective effects may be a significant mechanism by which they enhance neurodegeneration, especially in compromised CNS.

The use of interleukins in cancer patients is commonly associated with delirium (S. Rosenberg et al. 1989). Interleukin-1 (IL-1) is an endogenous pyrogen, high doses of IL-2 cause delirium, IL-6 levels predict lesion size in stroke, and tumor necrosis factor–α is a cytotoxic cytokine, whereas insulin growth factor–1 (IGF-1) is neuroprotective and inhibits cytotoxic cytokines (K. Wilson et al. 2005). K. Wilson et al. (2005) found that low premorbid IGF-1 levels predicted delirium incidence in a prospective study. De Rooij (2005b) found increased levels of IL-6, IL-8, and C-reactive protein in hospitalized elderly patients with delirium. Conversely, somatostatin and IGF-1 have been shown to improve cognitive function in preclinical and clinical studies of cognitively impaired subjects (Craft et al. 1999; Saatman et al. 1997) and may therefore have a role in prevention and treatment of delirium. Further work on the protective role of IGF-1 in patients at risk for delirium is needed.

CONCLUSION

Delirium is a common neuropsychiatric disorder affecting cognition, thinking, perception, sleep, language, and other behaviors. It is associated with increased mortality following an episode, the attribution of which to delirium itself or underlying medical problems is unclear. It affects persons of any age, although elderly patients may be particularly vulnerable, especially if they have dementia. Research in nongeriatric adults and children is sorely needed lest we risk error in applying data from elderly to younger persons. Clinical assessment of delirium can be aided through the use of diagnostic criteria and rating scales, as well as knowledge of which populations are at risk. Research could greatly benefit from consensus on using certain valid, specific, and sensitive instruments across studies. Underdetection and misdiagnosis are rampant, begging for valid, concise screening and monitoring tools.

Certain symptoms of delirium may represent "core" symptoms, whereas others may be associated symptoms that occur under various conditions, possibly more related to etiology or idiopathic features. Core symptoms may reflect dysfunction of certain brain regions and neurotransmitter systems that constitute a "final common neural pathway" that is responsible for the presentation of the syndrome of delirium. Regions implicated include prefrontal cortex, thalamus, basal ganglia, right temporoparietal cortex, and fusiform and lingual gyri. Diverse physiologies related to the wide variety of etiologies may funnel into a common neurofunctional expression for delirium via elevated brain dopaminergic and reduced cholinergic activity or a relative imbalance between these. Other neurochemical candidates include serotonin, melatonin, norepinephrine, GABA, glutamate, and cytokines, although these may interact to regulate or alter activity of acetylcholine and dopamine in key circuitry.

The clinical standard of treatment involves a dopamine antagonist medication—usually haloperidol—although, theoretically, procholinergic drugs should help. Drug treatment studies for delirium, particularly double-blind studies, are few, and no placebo-controlled, appropriately powered efficacy trials have been done. Newer agents deserve more study as well. It is important to initiate treatment even before medical causes have been rectified and for both hypoactive and hyperactive psychomotor presentations because target symptoms are probably cognition, thought, sleep, and language. That delirium is common yet inadequately detected; associated with increased morbidity, mortality, and length of hospitalization; and potentially caused by virtually anything from a textbook of medicine has been well substantiated. The travesty is the lack of a specific efficacious and well-tolerated treatment as substantiated by a regulatory approval in any country. Clearly, delirium needs to become a top priority for regulatory agencies and national research funding institutions.

Highlights for the Clinician

Characteristic	Caveats	Actions
Higher cortical dysfunction	✦ Such dysfunction produces acute, diffuse cognitive disorder with the cardinal symptom of inattention or altered consciousness and a breadth of other neuropsychiatric symptoms affecting thought, sleep-wake cycle, mood, language, motor activity, and perception.	✦ Do a cognitive assessment, because reliance on any one symptom of delirium alone might be misleading diagnostically.
Motor activity levels	✦ Hypoactive presentations are often missed or misdiagnosed as depression, whereas hyperactive presentations are noticed more because of the disruptions to nursing care.	✦ Maintain a high level of suspicion for delirium in the medically ill, especially quiet patients.
Comorbidity with dementia in older patients	✦ Dementia is a risk factor for delirium and also has overlapping symptoms, which complicates accurate diagnosis. Because of the poor prognosis for delirium and high potential for reversibility, the rule of thumb is: "It is delirium until proven otherwise."	✦ Assess for attention deficits that help diagnose delirium rather than most dementias; the latter have primary memory deficits, although Lewy body dementia masquerades as delirium.

(continued)

Highlights for the Clinician (continued)

Characteristic	Caveats	Actions
Multiple etiologies	✦ Delirium is caused by a wide variety of medical, surgical, and pharmacological conditions that need to be evaluated stepwise on an individualized basis to elucidate one or more etiologies.	✦ Identify and correct or treat each etiology as soon as possible while monitoring mental status.
Serious consequences	✦ Delirium is associated with high morbidity, long-term mortality, and increased length of stay and costs in the hospital.	✦ Take prompt action in managing the underlying causes and treating the delirium itself as a brain disorder.
Treatment	✦ Pharmacological and nonpharmacological methods are used to treat delirium such that treatment targets core neuropsychiatric symptoms (cognition, sleep, thoughts), and not just psychotic symptoms or motor presentation. No regulatory body has approved a particular medication for delirium.	✦ Consider empirical evidence from consensus and mostly open-label studies suggesting that neuroleptics may be useful (except in delirium tremens, for which benzodiazepines are preferred).

RECOMMENDED READINGS

Breitbart W, Gibson C, Tremblay A: The delirium experience: delirium recall and delirium-related distress in hospitalized patients with cancer, their spouses/caregivers, and their nurses. Psychosomatics 43:183–194, 2002

Engel GL, Romano J: Delirium, a syndrome of cerebral insufficiency. J Chronic Dis 9:260–277, 1959

Kalisvaart KJ, de Jonghe JFM, Bogaards MJ, et al: Haloperidol prophylaxis for elderly hip surgery patients at risk for delirium: a randomized, placebo-controlled study. J Am Geriatr Soc 53:1658–1666, 2005

Marcantonio ER, Flacker JM, Wright RJ, et al: Reducing delirium after hip fracture: a randomized trial. J Am Geriatr Soc 49:516–522, 2001

Meagher D: Delirium: optimizing management. BMJ 322:144–149, 2001

Trzepacz PT: Is there a final common neural pathway in delirium? Focus on acetylcholine and dopamine. Semin Clin Neuropsychiatry 5:132–148, 2000

REFERENCES

Adamis D, Morrison C, Treloar A, et al: The performance of the Clock Drawing Test in elderly medical inpatients: does it have utility in the identification of delirium? J Geriatr Psychiatry Neurol 18:129–133, 2005

Adams F: Neuropsychiatric evaluation and treatment of delirium in the critically ill cancer patient. Cancer Bull 36:156–160, 1984

Adams F: Emergency intravenous sedation of the delirious medically ill patient. J Clin Psychiatry 49(suppl):22–26, 1988

Adunsky A, Levy R, Mizrahi E, et al: Exposure to opioid analgesia in cognitively impaired and delirious elderly hip fracture patients. Arch Gerontol Geriatr 35:245–251, 2002

Agnoletti V, Ansaloni L, Catena F, et al: Postoperative delirium after elective and emergency surgery: analysis and checking of risk factors: a study protocol. BMC Surg 5:12, 2005

Akaike N, Shirasaki T, Yakushiji T: Quinolone and fenbufen interact with GABA-A receptors in dissociated hippocampal cells of rats. J Neurophysiol 66:497–504, 1991

Alexopoulos GS, Streim J, Carpenter D, et al: Using antipsychotic agents in older patients. Expert Consensus Panel for Using Antipsychotic Drugs in Older Patients. J Clin Psychiatry 65 (suppl 2):5–99, 2004

Al-Samarrai S, Dunn J, Newmark T, et al: Quetiapine for treatment-resistant delirium. Psychosomatics 44:350–351, 2003

American Psychiatric Association: Diagnostic and Statistical Manual: Mental Disorders. Washington, DC, American Psychiatric Association, 1952

American Psychiatric Association: Diagnostic and Statistical Manual of Mental Disorders, 2nd Edition. Washington, DC, American Psychiatric Association, 1968

American Psychiatric Association: Diagnostic and Statistical Manual of Mental Disorders, 3rd Edition. Washington, DC, American Psychiatric Association, 1980

American Psychiatric Association: Diagnostic and Statistical Manual of Mental Disorders, 3rd Edition, Revised. Washington, DC, American Psychiatric Association, 1987

American Psychiatric Association: Diagnostic and Statistical Manual of Mental Disorders, 4th Edition. Washington, DC, American Psychiatric Association, 1994

American Psychiatric Association: Practice guidelines for treatment of patients with Alzheimer's disease and other dementias of late life. Am J Psychiatry 154(suppl):1–39, 1997

American Psychiatric Association: Practice guidelines for the treatment of patients with delirium. Am J Psychiatry 156(suppl):1–20, 1999

American Psychiatric Association: Diagnostic and Statistical Manual of Mental Disorders, 4th Edition, Text Revision. Washington, DC, American Psychiatric Association, 2000

Ames D, Wirshing WC, Szuba MP: Organic mental disorders associated with bupropion in three patients. J Clin Psychiatry 53:53–55, 1992

Anderson B: A proposed theory for the encephalopathies of Reye's syndrome and hepatic encephalopathy. Med Hypotheses 15:415–420, 1984

Anderson SD: Treatment of elderly patients with delirium. Can Med Assoc J 152:323–324, 1995

Andreasen NJC, Hartford CE, Knott JR, et al: EEG changes associated with burn delirium. Dis Nerv Syst 38:27–31, 1977

Armstrong DH, Dasts JF, Reilly TE, et al: Effect of haloperidol on dopamine-induced increase in renal blood flow. Drug Intell Clin Pharm 20:543–546, 1986

Armstrong SC, Cozza KL, Watanabe KS: The misdiagnosis of delirium. Psychosomatics 38:433–439, 1997

Balan S, Leibovitz A, Zila SO, et al: The relation between the clinical subtypes of delirium and the urinary level of 6-SMT. J Neuropsychiatry Clin Neurosci 15:363–366, 2003

Bartlett EJ, Brodie JD, Simkowitz P, et al: Effects of haloperidol challenge on regional cerebral glucose utilization in normal human subjects. Am J Psychiatry 151:681–686, 1994

Basile AS, Saito K, Li Y, et al: The relationship between plasma and brain quinolinic acid levels and the severity of hepatic encephalopathy in animal models of fulminant hepatic failure. J Neurochem 64:2607–2614, 1995

Bayindir O, Akpinar B, Can E, et al: The use of the 5-HT$_3$ antagonist ondansetron for the treatment of post-cardiotomy delirium. J Cardiothorac Vasc Anesth 14:288–292, 2000

Bedford PD: General medical aspects of confusional states in elderly people. BMJ 2:185–188, 1957

Benoit AG, Campbell BI, Tanner JR, et al: Risk factors and prevalence of perioperative cognitive dysfunction in abdominal aneurysm patients. J Vasc Surg 42:884–890, 2005

Berggren D, Gustafson Y, Eriksson B, et al: Postoperative confusion following anesthesia in elderly patients treated for femoral neck fractures. Anesth Analg 66:497–504, 1987

Bettin KM, Maletta GJ, Dysken MW, et al: Measuring delirium severity in older general hospital inpatients without dementia: the Delirium Severity Scale. Am J Geriatr Psychiatry 6:296–307, 1998

Blumberg HP, Stern E, Ricketts S, et al: Rostral orbitofrontal prefrontal cortex dysfunction in the manic state of bipolar disorder. Am J Psychiatry 156:1986–1988, 1999

Bogardus ST Jr, Desai MM, Williams CS, et al: The effects of a targeted multicomponent delirium intervention on post-discharge outcomes for hospitalized older adults. Am J Med 114:383–390, 2003

Bogousslavsky J, Ferranzzini M, Regli F, et al: Manic delirium and frontal-like syndrome with paramedian infarction of the right thalamus. J Neurol Neurosurg Psychiatry 51:116–119, 1988

Boiten J, Lodder J: An unusual sequela of a frequently occurring neurologic disorder: delirium caused by brain infarct. Ned Tijdschr Geneeskd 133:617–620, 1989

Bostwick JM, Masterson BJ: Psychopharmacological treatment of delirium to restore mental capacity. Psychosomatics 39:112–117, 1998

Bourdel-Marchasson I, Vincent S, Germain C, et al: Delirium symptoms and low dietary intake in older inpatients are independent predictors of institutionalization: a 1-year prospective population-based study. J Gerontol A Biol Sci Med Sci 59:350–354, 2004

Bourgeois JA, Koike AK, Simmons JE, et al: Adjunctive valproic acid for delirium and/or agitation on a consultation-liaison service: a report of six cases. J Neuropsychiatry Clin Neurosci 17:232–238, 2005

Bourgeois JA, Hilty DM, Wegelin JA, et al: Cognitive disorder diagnoses in inpatient psychosomatic medicine consultations: associations with age and length of stay. Psychosomatics 47:414–420, 2006

Breitbart W, Marotta R, Platt MM, et al: A double-blind trial of haloperidol, chlorpromazine, and lorazepam in the treatment of delirium in hospitalized AIDS patients. Am J Psychiatry 153:231–237, 1996

Breitbart W, Rosenfeld B, Roth A, et al: The Memorial Delirium Assessment Scale. J Pain Symptom Manage 13:128–137, 1997

Breitbart W, Gibson C, Tremblay A: The delirium experience: delirium recall and delirium related distress in hospitalized patients with cancer, their spouses/caregivers, and their nurses. Psychosomatics 43:183–194, 2002a

Breitbart W, Tremblay A, Gibson C: An open trial of olanzapine for the treatment of delirium in hospitalized cancer patients. Psychosomatics 43:175–182, 2002b

Broadhurst C, Wilson K: Immunology of delirium: new opportunities for treatment and research. Br J Psychiatry 179:288–289, 2001

Brodaty H, Ames D, Snowdon J, et al: A randomized placebo-controlled trial of risperidone for the treatment of aggression, agitation, and psychosis of dementia. J Clin Psychiatry 64:134–143, 2003

Broderick PA, Gibson GE: Dopamine and serotonin in rat striatum during in vivo hypoxic-hypoxia. Metab Brain Dis 4:143–153, 1989

Brown RL, Henke A, Greenhalgh DG, et al: The use of haloperidol in the agitated, critically ill pediatric patient with burns. J Burn Care Rehabil 17:34–38, 1996

Brown TM: Drug-induced delirium. Semin Clin Neuropsychiatry 5:113–125, 2000

Bucerius J, Gummert JF, Borger MA, et al: Predictors of delirium after cardiac surgery delirium: effect of beating-heart (off-pump) surgery. J Thorac Cardiovasc Surg 127:57–64, 2004

Burke WJ, Roccaforte WH, Wengel SP: Treating visual hallucinations with donepezil. Am J Psychiatry 156:1117–1118, 1999

Burns MJ, Linden CH, Graudins A, et al: A comparison of physostigmine and benzodiazepines for the treatment of anticholinergic poisoning. Ann Emerg Med 35:374–381, 2000

Caeiro L, Ferro JM, Albuquerque R, et al: Delirium in the first days of acute stroke. J Neurol 251:171–178, 2004a

Caeiro L, Ferro JM, Claro MI, et al: Delirium in acute stroke: a preliminary study of the role of anticholinergic medications. Eur J Neurol 11:699–704, 2004b

Caeiro L, Menger C, Ferro JM, et al: Delirium in acute subarachnoid haemorrhage. Cerebrovasc Dis 19:31–38, 2005

Cameron DJ, Thomas RI, Mulvihill M, et al: Delirium: a test of DSM-III criteria on medical inpatients. J Am Geriatr Soc 35:1007–1010, 1987

Camus V, Burtin B, Simeone I, et al: Factor analysis supports evidence of existing hyperactive and hypoactive subtypes of delirium. Int J Geriatr Psychiatry 115:313–316, 2000a

Camus V, Gonthier R, Dubos G, et al: Etiologic and outcome profiles in hypoactive and hyperactive subtypes of delirium. J Geriatr Psychiatry Neurol 13:38–42, 2000b

Caplan GA, Coconis J, Board N, et al: Does home treatment affect delirium? A randomised controlled trial of rehabilitation of elderly and care at home or usual treatment (The REACH-OUT trial). Age Ageing 35:53–60, 2005

Carnes M, Howell T, Rosenberg M, et al: Physicians vary in approaches to the clinical assessment of delirium. J Am Geriatr Soc 51:234–239, 2003

Centorrino F, Albert MJ, Drago-Ferrante G, et al: Delirium during clozapine treatment: incidence and associated risk factors. Pharmacopsychiatry 36:156–160, 2003

Charlton BG, Kavanau JL: Delirium and psychotic symptoms: an integrative model. Med Hypotheses 58:24–27, 2002

Chatham MA: The effect of family involvement on patients' manifestations of postcardiotomy psychosis. Heart Lung 7:995–999, 1978

Chedru F, Geschwind N: Writing disturbances in acute confusional states. Neuropsychologia 10:343–353, 1972

Chen B, Cardasis W: Delirium induced by lithium and risperidone combination. Am J Psychiatry 153:1233–1234, 1996

Coffman JA, Dilsaver SC: Cholinergic mechanisms in delirium. Am J Psychiatry 145:382–383, 1988

Cole MG, Primeau FJ: Prognosis of delirium in elderly hospital patients. Can Med Assoc J 149:41–46, 1993

Cole MG, Primean FJ, Bailey RF, et al: Systematic intervention for elderly inpatients with delirium: a randomized trial. Can Med Assoc J 151:965–970, 1994

Cole MG, Primeau FJ, Elie LM: Delirium: prevention, treatment, and outcome studies. J Geriatr Psychiatry Neurol 11:126–137, 1998

Cole MG, McCusker J, Bellavance F, et al: Systematic detection and multidisciplinary care of delirium in older medical inpatients: a randomized trial. Can Med Assoc J 167:753–759, 2002a

Cole M[G], McCusker J, Dendukuri N, et al: Symptoms of delirium among elderly medical inpatients with or without dementia. J Neuropsychiatry Clin Neurosci 14:167–175, 2002b

Cole MG, Dendukuri N, McCusker J, et al: An empirical study of different diagnostic criteria for delirium among elderly medical inpatients. J Neuropsychiatry Clin Neurosci 15:200–207, 2003a

Cole M[G], McCusker J, Dendukuri N, et al: The prognostic significance of subsyndromal delirium in elderly medical inpatients. J Am Geriatr Soc 51:754–760, 2003b

Craft S, Asthana MD, Newcomer JW, et al: Enhancement of memory in Alzheimer's disease with insulin and somatostain, but not glucose. Arch Gen Psychiatry 56:1135–1140, 1999

Csokasy J: Assessment of acute confusion: use of the NEECHAM confusion scale. Appl Nurs Res 12:51–55, 1999

Curyto KJ, Johnson J, TenHave T, et al: Survival of hospitalized elderly patients with delirium: a prospective study. Am J Geriatr Psychiatry 9:141–147, 2001

Cushman LA: Secondary neuropsychiatric complications in stroke: implications for acute care. Arch Phys Med Rehabil 69:877–879, 1998

Cutting J: The phenomenology of acute organic psychosis: comparison with acute schizophrenia. Br J Psychiatry 151:324–332, 1987

Czekalla J, Beasley CM Jr, Dellva MA, et al: Analysis of the QTc interval during olanzapine treatment of patients with schizophrenia and related psychoses. J Clin Psychiatry 62:191–198, 2001

Dautzenberg PL, Mulder LJ, Olde Rikkert MG, et al: Delirium in elderly hospitalized patients: protective effects of chronic rivastigmine usage. Int J Geriatr Psychiatry 19:641–644, 2004

Davidson M, Harvey P, Welsh KA, et al: Cognitive functioning in late-life schizophrenia: a comparison of elderly schizophrenic patients and patients with Alzheimer's disease. Am J Psychiatry 153:1274–1279, 1996

de Jonghe JFM, Kalisvaart KJ, Eikelenboom P, et al: Early symptoms in the prodromal phase of delirium in elderly hipsurgery patients. Int Psychogeriatr 17 (suppl 2):148, 2005

De Rooij S: Delirium subtype identification and the validation of the Delirium Rating Scale—Revised-98 (Dutch version) in hospitalised elderly patients. Int Psychogeriatr 17 (suppl 2):262, 2005a

De Rooij S: Raised levels of interleukin-6, interleukin-8, and C-reactive protein in hospitalised elderly patients with delirium. Int Psychogeriatr 17 (suppl 2):146–157, 2005b

Diaz V, Rodriguez J, Barrientos P, et al: Use of procholinergics in the prevention of postoperative delirium in hip fracture surgery in the elderly: a randomized controlled trial. Rev Neurol 33:716–719, 2001

Dickson LR: Hypoalbuminemia in delirium. Psychosomatics 32:317–323, 1991

Dixon CE, Hamm RJ, Taft WC, et al: Increased anticholinergic sensitivity following closed skull impact and controlled cortical impact traumatic brain injury in the rat. J Neurotrauma 11:275–287, 1994

Dolan MM, Hawkes WG, Zimmerman SI, et al: Delirium on hospital admission in aged hip fracture patients: prediction of mortality and 2-year functional outcomes. J Gerontol Med Sci 55A:M527–M434, 2000

Drake ME, Coffey CE: Complex partial status epilepticus simulating psychogenic unresponsiveness. Am J Psychiatry 140:800–801, 1983

Dudley DL, Rowlett DB, Loebel PJ: Emergency use of intravenous haloperidol. Gen Hosp Psychiatry 1:240–246, 1979

Dunne JW, Leedman PJ, Edis RH: Inobvious stroke: a cause of delirium and dementia. Aust N Z J Med 16:771–778, 1986

Duppils GS, Wikblad K: Delirium: behavioural changes before and during the prodromal phase. J Clin Nurs 13:609–616, 2004

Easton C, MacKenzie F: Sensory-perceptual alterations: delirium in the intensive care unit. Heart Lung 17:229–237, 1988

Ely EW, Dittus RS: Pharmacological treatment of delirium in the intensive care unit. JAMA 292:168, 2004

Ely EW, Gautam S, Margolin R, et al: The impact of delirium in the intensive care unit on hospital length of stay. Intensive Care Med 27:1892–1900, 2001a

Ely EW, Gordan S, Francis J, et al: Evaluation of delirium in critically ill patients: validation of the Confusion Assessment Method for the intensive care unit (CAM-ICU). Crit Care Med 29:1370–1379, 2001b

Ely EW, Shintani A, Truman B, et al: Delirium as a predictor of mortality in mechanically ventilated patients in the intensive care unit. JAMA 291:1753–1762, 2004a

Ely EW, Stephens RK, Jackson JC, et al: Current opinions regarding the importance, diagnosis, and management of delirium in the intensive care unit: a survey of 912 healthcare professionals. Crit Care Med 32:106–112, 2004b

Engel GL, Romano J: Delirium, II: reversibility of electroencephalogram with experimental procedures. Arch Neurol Psychiatry 51:378–392, 1944

Engel GL, Romano J: Delirium, a syndrome of cerebral insufficiency. J Chronic Dis 9:260–277, 1959

Erkinjuntti T, Wikstrom J, Parlo J, et al: Dementia among medical inpatients: evaluation of 2000 consecutive admissions. Arch Intern Med 146:1923–1926, 1986

Ewert J, Levin HS, Watson MG, et al: Procedural memory during posttraumatic amnesia in survivors of severe closed head injury: implications for rehabilitation. Arch Neurol 46:911–916, 1985

Fanjiang G, Folstein M: The Three Item Delirium Scale. Psychosomatics 42:165–199, 2001

Fann JR: The epidemiology of delirium: a review of studies and methodological issues. Semin Clin Neuropsychiatry 5:86–92, 2000

Fann JR, Sullivan AK: Delirium in the course of cancer treatment. Semin Clin Neuropsychiatry 8:217–228, 2003

Fann JR, Roth-Roemer S, Burington BE, et al: Delirium in patients undergoing hematopoietic stem cell transplantation. Cancer 95:1971–1981, 2002

Fann JR, Alfano CM, Burington BE, et al: Clinical presentation of delirium in patients undergoing hematopoietic stem cell transplantation. Cancer 103:810–820, 2005

Farrell KR, Ganzini L: Misdiagnosing delirium as depression in medically ill elderly patients. Arch Intern Med 155:2459–2464, 1995

Fayers PM, Hjermstad MJ, Ranhoff AH, et al: Which Mini-Mental State Exam items can be used to screen for delirium and cognitive impairment? J Pain Symptom Manage 30:41–50, 2005

Fernandez F, Holmes VF, Adams F, et al: Treatment of severe, refractory agitation with a haloperidol drip. J Clin Psychiatry 49:239–241, 1988

Fernandez F, Levy JK, Mansell PWA: Management of delirium in terminally ill AIDS patients. Int J Psychiatry Med 19:165–172, 1989

Ferro JM, Caeiro L, Verdelho A: Delirium in acute stroke. Curr Opin Neurol 15:51–55, 2002

Fick DM, Kolanowski AM, Waller JL, et al: Delirium superimposed on dementia in a community-dwelling managed care population: a three-year retrospective study of occurrence, costs and utilization. J Gerontol Med Sci 60A:748–753, 2005

Figiel GS, Krishman KR, Breitner JC, et al: Radiologic correlates of antidepressant-induced delirium: the possible significance of basal ganglia lesions. J Neuropsychiatry Clin Neurosci 1:188–190, 1989

Figiel GS, Hassen MA, Zorumski C, et al: ECT-induced delirium in depressed patients with Parkinson's disease. J Neuropsychiatry Clin Neurosci 3:405–411, 1991

Fisher BW, Flowerdew G: A simple model for predicting postoperative delirium in older patients undergoing elective orthopedic surgery. J Am Geriatr Soc 43:175–178, 1995

Flaherty JH, Tariq SH, Raghavan S, et al: A model for managing delirious older inpatients. J Am Geriatr Soc 51:1031–1035, 2003

Foley CM, Polinsky MS, Gruskin AB, et al: Encephalopathy in infants and children with chronic renal disease. Arch Neurol 38:656–658, 1981

Folstein MF, Folstein SE, McHugh PR: "Mini-Mental State": a practical method for grading the cognitive state of patients for the clinician. J Psychiatr Res 12:189–198, 1975

Fonseca F, Bulbena A, Navarrete R, et al: Spanish version of the Delirium Rating Scale—Revised-98: reliability and validity. Psychosom Res 59:147–151, 2005

Forman LJ, Cavalieri TA, Galski T, et al: Occurrence and impact of suspected delirium in hospitalized elderly patients. J Am Osteopath Assoc 95:588–591, 1995

Francis J: Sensory and environmental factors in delirium. Paper presented at Delirium: Current Advancements in Diagnosis, Treatment and Research, Geriatric Research, Education, and Clinical Center (GRECC), Veterans Administration Medical Center, Minneapolis, MN, September 13–14, 1993

Francis J, Kapoor WN: Prognosis after hospital discharge of older medical patients with delirium. J Am Geriatr Soc 40:601–606, 1992

Francis J, Martin D, Kapoor WN: A prospective study of delirium in hospitalized elderly. JAMA 263:1097–1101, 1990

Franco K, Litaker D, Locala J, et al: The cost of delirium in the surgical patient. Psychosomatics 42:68–73, 2001

Friedman JH: Syndrome of diffuse encephalopathy due to nondominant thalamic infarction. Neurology 35:1524–1526, 1985

Gaertner HJ, Fischer E, Hoss J: Side effects of clozapine. Psychopharmacology 99:S97–S100, 1989

Gagnon B, Lawlor PG, Mancini IL, et al: The impact of delirium on the circadian distribution of breakthrough analgesia in advanced cancer patients. J Pain Symptom Manage 22:826–833, 2001

Gagnon B, Low G, Schreier G: Methylphenidate hydrochloride improves cognitive function in patients with advanced cancer and hypoactive delirium: a prospective clinical study. J Psychiatry Neurosci 30:100–107, 2005

Gagnon P, Allard P, Masse B, et al: Delirium in terminal cancer: a prospective study using daily screening, early diagnosis, and continuous monitoring. J Pain Symptom Manage 19:412–426, 2000

Gagnon P, Charbonneau C, Allard P, et al: Delirium in advanced cancer; a psychoeducational intervention for family caregivers. J Palliat Care 18:253–261, 2002

Galasko D, Klauber MR, Hofstetter R, et al: The MMSE in the early diagnosis of Alzheimer's disease. Arch Neurol 47:49–52, 1990

Gallinat J, Moller HJ, Hegerl U: Piracetam in anesthesia for prevention of postoperative delirium. Anasthesiol Intensivmed Notfallmed Schmerzther 34:520–527, 1999

Gaudreau JD, Gagnon P: Psychotogenic drugs and delirium pathogenesis: the central role of the thalamus. Med Hypotheses 64:471–475, 2004

Gaudreau JD, Gagnon P, Harel F, et al: Fast, systematic, and continuous delirium assessment in hospitalized patients: the Nursing Delirium Screening Scale. J Pain Symptom Manage 29:368–375, 2005a

Gaudreau JD, Gagnon P, Harel F, et al: Psychoactive medications and risk of delirium in hospitalized cancer patients. J Clin Oncol 23:6712–6728, 2005b

Gelfand SB, Indelicato J, Benjamin J: Using intravenous haloperidol to control delirium (abstract). Hosp Community Psychiatry 43:215, 1992

George J, Bleasdale S, Singleton SJ: Causes and prognosis of delirium in elderly patients admitted to a district general hospital. Age Ageing 26:423–427, 1997

Gibson GE, Jope R, Blass JP: Decreased synthesis of acetylcholine accompanying impaired oxidation of pyruvate in rat brain slices. Biochem J 26:17–23, 1975

Glick SD, Ross DA, Hough LB: Lateral asymmetry of neurotransmitters in human brain. Brain Res 234:53–63, 1982

Goldberg EL: Lateralization of frontal lobe functions and cognitive novelty. J Neuropsychiatry Clin Neurosci 6:371–378, 1998

Goldberg RJ, Huk M: Serotonergic syndrome from trazodone and buspirone (letter). Psychosomatics 33:235–236, 1992

Gorwood P, Limosin F, Batel P, et al: The A9 allele of the dopamine transporter gene is associated with delirium tremens and alcohol-withdrawal seizure. Biol Psychiatry 53:85–92, 2003

Grassi L, Caraceni A, Beltrami E, et al: Assessing delirium in cancer patients: the Italian versions of the Delirium Rating Scale and the Memorial Delirium Assessment Scale. J Pain Symptom Manage 21:59–68, 2001

Gruber-Baldini AL, Zimmerman S, Morrison RS, et al: Cognitive impairment in hip fracture patients: timing of detection and longitudinal follow-up. J Am Geriatr Soc 51:1227–1236, 2003

Gupta AK, Saravay SM, Trzepacz PT, et al: Delirium motoric subtypes (abstract). Psychosomatics 46:158, 2005

Gustafson Y, Berggren D, Brahnstrom B, et al: Acute confusional states in elderly patients treated for femoral neck fracture. J Am Geriatr Soc 36:525–530, 1988

Gustafson Y, Olsson T, Eriksson S, et al: Acute confusional state (delirium) in stroke patients. Cerebrovasc Dis 1:257–264, 1991

Hales RE, Polly S, Orman D: An evaluation of patients who received an organic mental disorder diagnosis on a psychiatric consultation-liaison service. Gen Hosp Psychiatry 11:88–94, 1988

Hally O, Cooney C: Delirium in the hospitalized elderly: an audit of NCHD prescribing practice. Ir J Psychol Med 22:133–136, 2005

Han CS, Kim YK: A double-blind trial of risperidone and haloperidol for the treatment of delirium. Psychosomatics 45:297–301, 2004

Han L, McCusker J, Cole M, et al: Use of medications with anticholinergic effect predicts clinical severity of delirium symptoms in older medical inpatients. Arch Intern Med 161:1099–1105, 2001

Harrell R, Othmer E: Postcardiotomy confusion and sleep loss. J Clin Psychiatry 48:445–446, 1987

Hart RP, Levenson JL, Sessler CN, et al: Validation of a cognitive test for delirium in medical ICU patients. Psychosomatics 37:533–546, 1996

Hart RP, Best AM, Sessler CN, et al: Abbreviated Cognitive Test for Delirium. J Psychosom Res 43:417–423, 1997

Hatta K, Takahashi T, Nakamura H, et al: The association between intravenous haloperidol and prolonged QT interval. J Clin Psychopharmacol 21:257–261, 2001

Hebenstreit GF, Fellerer K, Twerdy B, et al: L-Tryptophan in pre-delirium and delirium conditions. Infusionstherapie 16:92–96, 1989

Heinrich TW, Biblo LA, Schneider J: Torsades de pointes associated with ziprasidone. Psychosomatics 47:264–268, 2006

Hemmingsen R, Vorstrup S, Clemmesen L, et al: Cerebral blood flow during delirium tremens and related clinical states studied with xenon-133 inhalation tomography. Am J Psychiatry 145:1384–1390, 1988

Henon H, Lebert F, Durieu I, et al: Confusional state in stroke: relation to preexisting dementia, patient characteristics and outcome. Stroke 30:773–779, 1999

Henry WD, Mann AM: Diagnosis and treatment of delirium. Can Med Assoc J 93:1156–1166, 1965

Herrmann N, Mamdani M, Lanctot KL: Atypical antipsychotics and risk of cerebrovascular accidents. Am J Psychiatry 161:1113–1115, 2004

Hill EH, Blumenfield M, Orlowski B: A modification of the Trzepacz Delirium Rating Scale—Revised-98 for use on the Palm Pilot, and a presentation of data of symptom monitoring using haloperidol, olanzapine, and risperidone in the treatment of delirious hospitalized patients (abstract). Psychosomatics 43:158, 2002

Honma H, Kohsaka M, Suzuki I, et al: Motor activity rhythm in dementia with delirium. Psychiatry Clin Neurosci 52:196–198, 1998

Hooper JF, Minter G: Droperidol in the management of psychiatric emergencies. J Clin Psychopharmacol 3:262–263, 1983

Hopkins SJ, Rothwell NJ: Cytokines and the nervous system, I: expression and recognition. Trends Neurosci 18:83–88, 1995

Horenstein S, Chamberlin W, Conomy J: Infarction of the fusiform and calcarine regions: agitated delirium and hemianopia, in Translations of the American Neurological Association 1967, Vol 92. Edited by Yahr MD. New York, Springer, 1967, pp 85–89

Horikawa N, Yamazaki T, Miyamoto K, et al: Treatment for delirium with risperidone: results of a prospective open trial with 10 patients. Gen Hosp Psychiatry 25:289–292, 2003

Huang S-C, Tsai S-J, Chan C-H, et al: Characteristics and outcome of delirium in psychiatric inpatients. Psychiatry Clin Neurosci 52:47–50, 1998

Hustey FM, Meldon SW, Smith MD, et al: The effect of mental status screening on the care of elderly emergency department patients. Ann Emerg Med 41:678–684, 2003

Huyse F: Haloperidol and cardiac arrest. Lancet 2:568–569, 1988

Ikarashi Y, Takahashi A, Ishimaru H, et al: Regulation of dopamine D1 and D2 receptors on striatal acetylcholine release in rats. Brain Res Bull 43:107–115, 1997

Inouye SK: The dilemma of delirium: clinical and research controversies regarding diagnosis and evaluation of delirium in hospitalized elderly medical patients. Am J Med 7:278–288, 1994

Inouye SK, Charpentier PA: Precipitating factors for delirium in hospitalized elderly patients: predictive model and interrelationships with baseline vulnerability. JAMA 275:852–857, 1996

Inouye SK, van Dyke CH, Alessi CA, et al: Clarifying confusion: the Confusion Assessment Method. Ann Intern Med 113:941–948, 1990

Inouye SK, Viscoli CM, Horwitz RI, et al: A predictive model for delirium in hospitalized elderly medical patients based on admission characteristics. Arch Intern Med 119:474–481, 1993

Inouye SK, Rushing JT, Foreman MD, et al: Does delirium contribute to poor hospital outcome? J Gen Intern Med 13:234–242, 1998

Inouye SK, Bogardus ST, Charpentier PA, et al: A multicomponent intervention to prevent delirium in hospitalized older patients. N Engl J Med 340:669–676, 1999

Inouye SK, Foreman MD, Mion LC, et al: Nurses' recognition of delirium and its symptoms: comparison of nurse and researcher ratings. Arch Intern Med 161:2467–2473, 2001

Inouye SK, Bogardus ST Jr, Williams CS, et al: The role of adherence on the effectiveness of nonpharmacologic interventions: evidence from the delirium prevention trial. Arch Intern Med 163:958–964, 2003

Irwin M, Fuentenebro F, Marder SR, et al: L-5-Hydroxytryptophan-induced delirium. Biol Psychiatry 21:673–676, 1986

Itil T, Fink M: Anticholinergic drug-induced delirium: experimental modification, quantitative EEG, and behavioral correlations. J Nerv Ment Dis 143:492–507, 1966

Jackson JC, Hart RP, Gordon SM, et al: Six-month neuropsychological outcome of medical intensive care unit patients. Crit Care Med 31:1226–1234, 2003

Jackson SA: The epidemiology of aging, in Principles of Geriatric Medicine and Gerontology. Edited by Hazzard WR, Blass JP, Ettinger WH, et al. New York, McGraw-Hill, 1999, pp 203–226

Jacobson SA, Jerrier S: EEG in delirium. Semin Clin Neuropsychiatry 5:86–93, 2000

Jacobson SA, Leuchter AF, Walter DO: Conventional and quantitative EEG diagnosis of delirium among the elderly. J Neurol Neurosurg Psychiatry 56:153–158, 1993a

Jacobson SA, Leuchter AF, Walter DO, et al: Serial quantitative EEG among elderly subjects with delirium. Biol Psychiatry 34:135–140, 1993b

Jagmin MG: Postoperative mental status in elderly hip surgery patients. Orthop Nurs 17:32–42, 1998

Jitapunkul S, Pillay I, Ebrahim S: Delirium in newly admitted elderly patients: a prospective study. Q J Med 83:307–314, 1992

Johansson IS, Hamrin EK, Larsson G: Psychometric testing of the NEECHAM Confusion Scale among patients with hip fracture. Res Nurs Health 25:203–211, 2002

Johnson JC, Kerse NM, Gottlieb G, et al: Prospective versus retrospective methods of identifying patients with delirium. J Am Geriatr Soc 40:316–319, 1992

Jones J, Dougherty J, Cannon L: Diphenhydramine-induced toxic psychosis. Am J Emerg Med 4:369–371, 1986

Kagansky N, Rimon E, Naor S, et al: Low incidence of delirium in very old patients after surgery for hip fractures. Am J Geriatr Psychiatry 12:306–314, 2004

Kain ZN, Caldwell-Andrews AA, Maranets I, et al: Preoperative anxiety and emergence delirium and postoperative maladaptive behaviors. Anesth Analg 99:1648–1654, 2004

Kakuma R, du Fort GG, Arsenault L, et al: Delirium in older emergency department patients discharged home: effect on survival. J Am Geriatr Soc 51:443–450, 2003

Kalisvaart CJ, Boelaarts L, de Jonghe JF, et al: [Successful treatment of three elderly patients suffering from prolonged delirium using the cholinesterase inhibitor rivastigmine] (Dutch). Ned Tijdschr Geneeskd 148:1501–1504, 2004

Kalisvaart KJ, de Jonghe JF, Bogaards MJ, et al: Haloperidol prophylaxis for elderly hip-surgery patients at risk for delirium: a randomized placebo-controlled study. J Am Geriatr Soc 53:1658–1666, 2005a

Kalisvaart KJ, Vreeswijk R, de Jonghe J, et al: Risk factors and prediction of post-operative delirium in elderly hip surgery patients: implementation and validation of the Inouye risk factor model. Int Psychogeriatr 17 (suppl 2):261, 2005b

Kamel HK: The frequency and factors linked to a urinary tract infection coding in patients undergoing hip fracture surgery. J Am Med Dir Assoc 6:316–320, 2005

Kaneko T, Cai J, Ishikura T, et al: Prophylactic consecutive administration of haloperidol can reduce the occurrence of postoperative delirium in gastrointestinal surgery. Yonago Acta Med 42:179–184, 1999

Kapur S, Seeman P: Does fast dissociation from the dopamine d(2) receptor explain the action of atypical antipsychotics? A new hypothesis. Am J Psychiatry 158:360–369, 2001

Karki SD, Masood GR: Combination risperidone and SSRI-induced serotonin syndrome. Ann Pharmacother 37:388–391, 2003

Kasahara H, Karasawa A, Ariyasu T, et al: Alcohol dementia and alcohol delirium in aged alcoholics. Psychiatry Clin Neurosci 50:115–123, 1996

Katz IR, Jeste DV, Mintzer JE, et al: Comparison of risperidone and placebo for psychosis and behavioral disturbances associated with dementia: a randomized double-blind trial. J Clin Psychiatry 60:107–115, 1999

Katz IR, Curyto KJ, Tenhave T, et al: Validating the diagnosis of delirium and evaluating its association with deterioration over a one-year period. Am J Geriatr Psychiatry 9:148–159, 2001

Katz JA, Mahoney DH, Fernbach DJ: Human leukocyte alpha-interferon induced transient neurotoxicity in children. Invest New Drugs 6:115–120, 1988

Kaufer DI, Catt KE, Lopez OL, et al: Dementia with Lewy bodies: response of delirium-like features to donepezil. Neurology 51:1512–1513, 1998

Kelly KG, Zisselman M, Cutillo-Schmitter T, et al: Severity and course of delirium in medically hospitalized nursing facility residents. Am J Geriatr Psychiatry 9:72–77, 2001

Kennard MA, Bueding E, Wortis WB: Some biochemical and electroencephalographic changes in delirium tremens. Q J Stud Alcohol 6:4–14, 1945

Kennedy JS, Zagar A, Bymaster F, et al: The central cholinergic system profile of olanzapine compared with placebo in Alzheimer's disease. Int J Geriatr Psychiatry 16:S24–S32, 2001

Kennedy RE, Nakase-Thompson R, Nick TG, et al: Use of the Cognitive Test for Delirium in patients with traumatic brain injury. Psychosomatics 44:283–289, 2003

Khouzam HR, Gazula K: Clinical experience of olanzapine during the course of post operative delirium associated with psychosis in geriatric patients: a report of three cases. International Journal of Psychiatry in Clinical Practice 5:63–68, 2001

Kiely DK, Bergmann MA, Jones RN, et al: Characteristics associated with delirium persistence among newly admitted post-acute facility patients. J Gerontol A Biol Sci Med Sci 59:344–349, 2004

Kienast T, Heinz A: Dopamine and the diseased brain. CNS Neurol Disord Drug Targets 5:109–131, 2006

Kim JY, Jung IK, Han C, et al: Antipsychotics and dopamine transporter gene polymorphisms in delirium patients. Psychiatry Clin Neurosci 59:183–188, 2005

Kim KS, Pae CU, Chae JH, et al: An open pilot trial of olanzapine for delirium in the Korean population. Psychiatry Clin Neurosci 55:515–519, 2001

Kim KY, Bader GM, Kotlyar V, et al: Treatment of delirium in older adults with quetiapine. J Geriatr Psychiatry Neurol 16:29–31, 2003

Kishi Y, Iwasaki Y, Takezawa K, et al: Delirium in critical care unit patients admitted through an emergency room. Gen Hosp Psychiatry 17:371–379, 1995

Kishi Y, Hosaka T, Yoshikawa E, et al: Delirium Rating Scale—Revised (DRS-R-98), Japanese version. Seishin Igaku 43:1365–1371, 2001

Klein M, Payaslian S, Gomez J, et al: Acute confusional syndrome due to acute nicotine withdrawal. Medicina (B Aires) 62:335–336, 2002

Klijn IA, van der Mast RC: Pharmacotherapy of alcohol withdrawal delirium in patients admitted to a general hospital (comment). Arch Intern Med 165:346, 2005

Knaus WA, Draper EA, Wagner DP, et al: APACHE II: a severity of disease classification system. Crit Care Med 13:818–829, 1985

Knell AJ, Davidson AR, Williams R, et al: Dopamine and serotonin metabolism in hepatic encephalopathy. BMJ 1:549–551, 1974

Kobayashi K, Takeuchi O, Suzuki M, et al: A retrospective study on delirium type. Jpn J Psychiatry Neurol 46:911–917, 1992

Koehnke MD, Schick S, Lutz U, et al: Severity of alcohol withdrawal symptoms and the T1128C polymorphism of the neuropeptide Y gene. J Neural Transm 109:1423–1429, 2002

Köhnke MD, Batra A, Kolb W, et al: Association of the dopamine transporter gene with alcoholism. Alcohol Alcohol 40:339–342, 2005

Köhnke MD, Kolb W, Kohnke AM, et al: *DBH (*) 444G/A* polymorphism of the dopamine beta hydroxylase gene is associated with alcoholism but not with severe alcohol withdrawal symptoms. J Neural Transm 113:869–876, 2006

Kolbeinsson H, Jonsson A: Delirium and dementia in acute medical admissions of elderly patients in Iceland. Acta Psychiatr Scand 87:123–127, 1993

Kopf SR, Baratti CM: Memory-improving actions of glucose: involvement of a central cholinergic muscarinic mechanism. Behav Neural Biol 62:237–243, 1994

Koponen H, Hurri L, Stenback U, et al: Computed tomography findings in delirium. J Nerv Ment Dis 177:226–231, 1989a

Koponen H, Partanen J, Paakkonen A, et al: EEG spectral analysis in delirium. J Neurol Neurosurg Psychiatry 52:980–985, 1989b

Koponen H, Stenbach U, Mattila E, et al: Delirium among elderly persons admitted to a psychiatric hospital: clinical course during the acute stage and one year follow-up. Acta Psychiatr Scand 79:579–585, 1989c

Koponen H, Sirvio J, Lepola U, et al: A long-term follow-up study of cerebrospinal fluid acetylcholinesterase in delirium. Eur Arch Psychiatry Clin Neurosci 243:347–351, 1994

Kreis R, Farrow N, Ross BN: Localized NMR spectroscopy in patients with chronic hepatic encephalopathy: analysis of changes in cerebral glutamine, choline, and inositols. NMR Biomed 4:109–116, 1991

Kriwisky M, Perry GY, Tarchitsky, et al: Haloperidol-induced torsades de pointes. Chest 98:482–484, 1990

Kullmann F, Hollerbach S, Holstege A, et al: Subclinical hepatic encephalopathy: the diagnostic value of evoked potentials. J Hepatol 22:101–110, 1995

Lam PT, Tse CY, Lee CH: Delirium in a palliative care unit. Progress in Palliative Care 11:126–133, 2003

Laurila JV, Pitkala KH, Strandberg TE, et al: The impact of different diagnostic criteria on prevalence rates for delirium. Dement Geriatr Cogn Disord 16:156–162, 2003

Laurila JV, Pitkala KH, Strandberg TE, et al: Delirium among patients with and without dementia: does the diagnosis according to the DSM-IV differ from the previous classifications? Int J Geriatr Psychiatry 19:271–277, 2004a

Laurila JV, Pitkala KH, Strandberg TE, et al: Detection and documentation of dementia and delirium in acute geriatric wards. Gen Hosp Psychiatry 26:31–35, 2004b

Laurila JV, Pitkala KH, Strandberg TE, et al: Impact of different diagnostic criteria on prognosis of delirium: a prospective study. Dement Geriatr Cogn Disord 18:240–244, 2004c

Lawlor PG, Gagnon B, Mancini IL, et al: Occurrence, causes and outcome of delirium in patients with advanced cancer. Arch Intern Med 160:786–794, 2000a

Lawlor PG, Nekolaichuk C, Gagnon B, et al: Clinical utility, factor analysis, and further validation of the Memorial Delirium Assessment Scale in patients with advanced cancer: assessing delirium in advanced cancer. Cancer 88:2859–2867, 2000b

Lawrence KR, Nasraway SA: Conduction disturbances associated with administration of butyrophenone antipsychotics in the critically ill: a review of the literature. Pharmacotherapy 17:531–537, 1997

Layton D, Harris S, Wilton LV, et al: Comparison of incidence rates of cerebrovascular accidents and transient ischaemic attacks in observational cohort studies of patients prescribed risperidone, quetiapine or olanzapine in general practice in England including patients with dementia. J Psychopharmacol 19:473–482, 2005

Leavitt M, Trzepacz PT, Ciongoli K: Rat model of delirium: atropine dose-response relationships. J Neuropsychiatry Clin Neurosci 6:279–284, 1994

Lee KU, Won WY, Lee HK, et al: Amisulpride versus quetiapine for the treatment of delirium: a randomized, open prospective study. Int Clin Psychopharmacol 20:311–314, 2005

Lemey L, Vranken C, Simoens K, et al: The "flying delirium room": towards an adequate approach of acute delirium in a general hospital. Int Psychogeriatr 17 (suppl 2):260, 2005

Leslie DL, Zhang Y, Holford TR, et al: Premature death associated with delirium at 1-year follow-up. Arch Intern Med 165:1657–1662, 2005

Leso L, Schwartz TL: Ziprasidone treatment of delirium. Psychosomatics 43:61–62, 2002

Levenson JA: Should psychostimulants be used to treat delirious patients with depressed mood? (letter). J Clin Psychiatry 53:69, 1992

Levenson JL: High-dose intravenous haloperidol for agitated delirium following lung transplantation. Psychosomatics 36:66–68, 1995

Levkoff SE, Evans DA, Liptzin B, et al: Delirium: the occurrence and persistence of symptoms among elderly hospitalized patients. Arch Intern Med 152:334–340, 1992

Levkoff SE, Liptzin B, Evans D, et al: Progression and resolution of delirium in elderly patients hospitalized for acute care. Am J Geriatr Psychiatry 2:230–238, 1994

Lewis MC, Barnett SR: Postoperative delirium: the tryptophan dysregulation model. Med Hypotheses 63:402–406, 2004

Limosin F, Loze JY, Boni C, et al: The A9 allele of the dopamine transporter gene increases the risk of visual hallucinations during alcohol withdrawal in alcohol-dependent women. Neurosci Lett 362:91–94, 2004

Lipowski ZJ: Delirium: Acute Confusional States. New York, Oxford University Press, 1990

Lipton SA, Gendelman HE: Dementia associated with the acquired immunodeficiency syndrome. N Engl J Med 332:934–940, 1995

Liptzin B, Levkoff SE: An empirical study of delirium subtypes. Br J Psychiatry 161:843–845, 1992

Liptzin B, Levkoff SE, Gottlieb GL, et al: Delirium: background papers for DSM-IV. J Neuropsychiatry Clin Neurosci 5:154–160, 1993

Liptzin B, Laki A, Garb JL, et al: Donepezil in the prevention and treatment of post-surgical delirium. Am J Geriatr Psychiatry 13:1100–1106, 2005

Lischke V, Behne M, Doelken P, et al: Droperidol causes a dose-dependent prolongation of the QT interval. Anesth Analg 79:983–986, 1994

Liu CY, Yeh EK, Lee YC, et al: Delirium in a general hospital psychiatric consultation service. Int Med J 4:181–185, 1997

Liu CY, Juang YY, Liang HY, et al: Efficacy of risperidone in treating the hyperactive symptoms of delirium. Int Clin Psychopharmacol 19:165–168, 2004

Ljubisljevic V, Kelly B: Risk factors for development of delirium among oncology patients. Gen Hosp Psychiatry 25:345–352, 2003

Lundstrom M, Edlund A, Bucht G, et al: Dementia after delirium in patients with femoral neck fractures. J Am Geriatr Soc 51:1002–1006, 2003

Lundstrom M, Edlund A, Karlsson S, et al: A multifactorial intervention program reduces the duration of delirium, length of hospitalization, and mortality in delirious patients. J Am Geriatr Soc 53:622–628, 2005

Mach J, Dysken M, Kuskowski M, et al: Serum anticholinergic activity in hospitalized older persons with delirium: a preliminary study. J Am Geriatr Soc 43:491–495, 1995

Magaziner J, Simonsick EM, Kashner M, et al: Survival experience of aged hip fracture patients. Am J Public Health 79:274–278, 1989

Maldonado JR, van der Starre P, Wysong A, et al: Dexmedetomide: can it reduce the incidence of ICU delirium in postcardiotomy patients? Proceedings of 50th annual meeting of the Academy of Psychosomatic Medicine. Psychosomatics 45:145–175, 2004

Mann C, Pouzeratte Y, Boccara G, et al: Comparison of intravenous or epidural patient-controlled analgesia in the elderly after major abdominal surgery. Anesthesiology 92:433–441, 2000

Manos PJ: The utility of the ten-point clock test as a screen for cognitive impairment in general hospital patients. Gen Hosp Psychiatry 19:439–444, 1997

Manos PJ, Wu R: The duration of delirium in medical and postoperative patients referred for psychiatric consultation. Ann Clin Psychiatry 9:219–225, 1997

Marcantonio ER, Juarez G, Goldman L, et al: The relationship of postoperative delirium with psychoactive medications. JAMA 272:1518–1522, 1994

Marcantonio E[R], Ta T, Duthie E, et al: Delirium severity and psychomotor types: their relationship with outcomes after hip fracture repair. J Am Geriatr Soc 50:850–857, 2002

Marcantonio ER, Flacker JM, Wright RJ, et al: Reducing delirium after hip fracture: a randomized trial. J Am Geriatr Soc 49:516–22, 2001

Marcantonio ER, Simon SE, Bergmann MA, et al: Delirium symptoms in post-acute care: prevalent, persistent, and associated with poor functional recovery. J Am Geriatr Soc 51:4–9, 2003

Marcantonio ER, Kiely DK, Simon SE, et al: Outcomes of older people admitted to postacute facilities with delirium. J Am Geriatr Soc 53:963–969, 2005

Margolis RL: Nonpsychiatric house staff frequently misdiagnose psychiatric disorders in general hospitalized patients. Psychosomatics 35:485–491, 1994

Martin M, Figiel G, Mattingly G, et al: ECT-induced interictal delirium in patients with a history of a CVA. J Geriatr Psychiatry Neurol 5:149–155, 1992

Marzanatti M, Monopoli A, Trampus M, et al: Effects of nonsedating histamine H-1 antagonists on EEG activity and behavior in the cat. Pharmacol Biochem Behav 32:861–866, 1989

Masand PS, Sipahimalani A: Olanzapine in the treatment of delirium. Psychosomatics 39:422–430, 1998

Mathers DA: The GABA-A receptor: new insights from single channel recording. Synapse 1:96–101, 1987

Matsuoka Y, Miyake Y, Arakaki H, et al: Clinical utility and validation of the Japanese version of the Memorial Delirium Assessment Scale in a psychogeriatric inpatient setting. Gen Hosp Psychiatry 23:36–40, 2001

Matsushima E, Nakajima K, Moriya H, et al: A psychophysiological study of the development of delirium in coronary care units. Biol Psychiatry 41:1211–1217, 1997

Matsushita S, Kimura M, Miyakawa T, et al: Association study of brain-derived neurotrophic factor gene polymorphism and alcoholism. Alcohol Clin Exp Res 28:1609–1612, 2004

Mayer SA, Chong JY, Ridgway E, et al: Delirium from nicotine withdrawal in neuro-ICU patients. Neurology 57:551–553, 2001

Mayo-Smith MF, Beecher LH, Fischer TL, et al: Management of alcohol withdrawal delirium: an evidence-based practice guideline. Working Group on the Management of Alcohol Withdrawal Delirium, Practice Guidelines Committee, American Society of Addiction Medicine. Arch Intern Med 164:1405–1412, 2004

McCaffrey R, Locsin R: The effect of music listening on acute confusion and delirium in elders undergoing elective hip and knee surgery. J Clin Nurs 13:91–96, 2004

McCarthy MC: Detecting acute confusion in older adults: comparing clinical reasoning of nurses working in acute, long-term, and community health care environments. Res Nurs Health 26:203–212, 2003

McCusker J, Cole M, Abrahamowicz M, et al: Environmental risk factors for delirium in hospitalized older people. J Am Geriatr Soc 49:1327–1334, 2001

McCusker J, Cole M, Abrahamowicz M, et al: Delirium predicts 12-month mortality. Arch Intern Med 162:457–463, 2002

McCusker J, Cole MG, Dendukuri N, et al: The course of delirium in older medical inpatients: a prospective study. J Gen Intern Med 18:696–704, 2003a

McCusker J, Cole MG, Dendukuri N, et al: Does delirium increase hospital stay? J Am Geriatr Soc 51:1539–1546, 2003b

McKeith I, Fairbairn A, Perry R, et al: Neuroleptic sensitivity in patients with senile dementia of Lewy body type. BMJ 305:673–678, 1992

McNicoll L, Pisani MA, Zhang Y, et al: Delirium in the intensive care unit: occurrence and clinical course in older patients. J Am Geriatr Soc 51:591–598, 2003

Meagher D: Delirium episode as a sign of undetected dementia among community dwelling elderly subjects. J Neurol Neurosurg Psychiatry 70:821, 2001

Meagher D: Delirium: optimising management. BMJ 7279:144–149, 2001b

Meagher DJ: The significance of motoric symptoms and subtypes in delirium. Symposium presented at the 156th annual meeting of the American Psychiatric Association, San Francisco, CA, May 17–22, 2003

Meagher D[J]: Clearing the confusion: psychopathology, cognition, and motoric profile in 100 consecutive cases of delirium. Int Psychogeriatr 17 (suppl 2):120–121, 2005

Meagher DJ, Trzepacz PT: Delirium phenomenology illuminates pathophysiology, management and course. J Geriatr Psychiatry Neurol 11:150–157, 1998

Meagher DJ, Trzepacz PT: Motoric subtypes of delirium. Semin Clin Neuropsychiatry 5:76–86, 2000

Meagher DJ, O'Hanlon D, O'Mahony E, et al: Use of environmental strategies and psychotropic medication in the management of delirium. Br J Psychiatry 168:512–515, 1996

Meagher DJ, O'Hanlon D, O'Mahoney E, et al: Relationship between etiology and phenomenological profile in delirium. J Geriatr Psychiatry Neurol 11:146–149, 1998

Meagher DJ, O'Hanlon D, O'Mahony E, et al: Relationship between symptoms and motoric subtype of delirium. J Neuropsychiatry Clin Neurosci 12:51–56, 2000

Meagher DJ, Moran M, Raju B, et al: Phenomenology of 100 consecutive adult cases of delirium. Br J Psychiatry 190:135–141, 2007

Meagher DJ, Moran M, Raju B, et al: Motor symptoms in 100 cases of delirium vs. controls: comparison of subtyping methods. Psychosomatics (in press)

Medina JL, Rubino FA, Ross E: Agitated delirium caused by infarctions of the hippocampal formation and fusiform and lingual gyri. Neurology 24:1181–1183, 1974

Medina JL, Sudhansu C, Rubino FA: Syndrome of agitated delirium and visual impairment: a manifestation of medial temporo-occipital infarction. J Neurol Neurosurg Psychiatry 40:861–864, 1977

Meltzer HY: Serotonin-dopamine interactions and atypical antipsychotic drugs. Psychiatr Ann 23:193–200, 1993

Meltzer HY, O'Laughlin IA, Dai J, et al: Atypical antipsychotic drugs but not typical increased extracellular acetylcholine levels in rat medial prefrontal cortex in the absence of acetylcholinesterase inhibition (abstract). Abstr Soc Neurosci 25:452, 1999

Mendelson G: Pheniramine aminosalicylate overdosage: reversal of delirium and choreiform movements with tacrine treatment. Arch Neurol 34:313, 1977

Mesulam M-M: Attention, confusional states, and neglect, in Principles of Behavioral Neurology. Edited by Mesulam M-M. Philadelphia, PA, FA Davis, 1985, pp 125–168

Mesulam M-M, Waxman SG, Geschwind N, et al: Acute confusional states with right middle cerebral artery infarction. J Neurol Neurosurg Psychiatry 39:84–89, 1979

Metzger E, Friedman R: Prolongation of the corrected QT and torsades de pointes cardiac arrhythmia associated with intravenous haloperidol in the medically ill. J Clin Psychopharmacol 13:128–132, 1993

Milbrandt EB, Deppen S, Harrison PL, et al: Costs associated with delirium in mechanically ventilated patients. Crit Care Med 32:955–962, 2004

Milbrandt EB, Kersten A, Kong L, et al: Haloperidol use is associated with lower hospital mortality in mechanically ventilated patients. Crit Care Med 33:226–229, 2005

Milisen K, Foreman MD, Abraham IL, et al: A nurse-led interdisciplinary intervention program for delirium in elderly hip-fracture patients. J Am Geriatr Soc 49:523–532, 2001

Miller PS, Richardson JS, Jyu CA, et al: Association of low serum anticholinergic levels and cognitive impairment in elderly presurgical patients. Am J Psychiatry 145:342–345, 1988

Minagawa H, Uchitomi Y, Yamawaki S, et al: Psychiatric morbidity in terminally ill cancer patients: a prospective study. Cancer 78:1131–1137, 1996

Minden SL, Carbone LA, Barsky A, et al: Predictors and outcomes for delirium. Gen Hosp Psychiatry 27:209–214, 2005

Mittal D, Jimerson NA, Neely EP, et al: Risperidone in the treatment of delirium: results from a prospective open-label trial. J Clin Psychiatry 65:662–667, 2004

Mittal D, Majithia D, Kennedy R, et al: Differences in characteristics and outcome of delirium as based on referral patterns. Psychosomatics 47:367–375, 2006

Mizock BA, Sabelli HC, Dubin A, et al: Septic encephalopathy: evidence for altered phenylalanine metabolism and comparison with hepatic encephalopathy. Arch Intern Med 150:443–449, 1990

Moldofsky H, Lue FA, Eisen J, et al: The relationship of interleukin-1 and immune functions to sleep in humans. Psychosom Med 48:309–318, 1986

Moller JT, Cluitmans P, Rasmussen LS, et al: Long-term postoperative cognitive dysfunction in the elderly ISPOCD1 study. ISPOCD investigators. International Study of Post-Operative Cognitive Dysfunction. Lancet 351:857–861, 1998

Mondimore FM, Damlouji N, Folstein MF, et al: Post-ECT confusional states associated with elevated serum anticholinergic levels. Am J Psychiatry 140:930–931, 1983

Monette J, Galbaud du Fort G, Fung SH, et al: Evaluation of the Confusion Assessment Method (CAM) as a screening tool for delirium in the emergency room. Gen Hosp Psychiatry 23:20–25, 2001

Montgomery EA, Fenton GW, McClelland RJ, et al: Psychobiology of minor head injury. Psychosom Med 21:375–384, 1991

Monti JM: Involvement of histamine in the control of the waking state. Life Sci 53:1331–1338, 1993

Moots RJ, Al Saffar Z, Hutchinson D, et al: Old drug, new tricks: haloperidol inhibits secretion of proinflammatory cytokines. Ann Rheum Dis 58:585–587, 1999

Moretti R, Torre P, Antonello RM, et al: Cholinesterase inhibition as a possible therapy for delirium in vascular dementia: a controlled, open 24-month study of 246 patients. Am J Alzheimers Dis Other Demen 19:333–339, 2004

Mori E, Yamadori A: Acute confusional state and acute agitated delirium. Arch Neurol 44:1139–1143, 1987

Morita T, Otani H, Tsunoda J, et al: Successful palliation of hypoactive delirium due to multi-organ failure by oral methylphenidate. Support Care Cancer 8:134–137, 2000

Morita T, Tei Y, Tsunoda J, et al: Underlying pathologies and their associations with clinical features in terminal delirium of cancer patients. J Pain Symptom Manage 22:997–1006, 2001

Morita T, Hirai K, Sakaguchi Y, et al: Family perceived distress about delirium-related symptoms of terminally ill cancer patients. Psychosomatics 45:107–113, 2004

Morita T, Takigawa C, Onishi H, et al: Opioid rotation from morphine to fentanyl in delirious cancer patients: an open-label trial. J Pain Symptom Manage 30:96–103, 2005

Morrison RS, Magaziner J, Gilbert M, et al: Relationship between pain and opioid analgesics on the development of delirium following hip fracture. J Gerontol A Biol Sci Med Sci 58:76–81, 2003

Moulaert P: Treatment of acute nonspecific delirium with IV haloperidol in surgical intensive care patients. Acta Anaesthesiol Belg 40:183–186, 1989

Mousseau DD, Butterworth RF: Current theories on the pathogenesis of hepatic encephalopathy. Proc Soc Exp Biol Med 206:329–344, 1994

Mullaly W, Huff K, Ronthal M, et al: Frequency of acute confusional states with lesions of the right hemisphere (abstract). Ann Neurol 12:113, 1982

Murphy KM: The baseline predictors and 6-month outcomes of incident delirium in nursing home residents: a study using the minimum data set. Psychosomatics 40:164–165, 1999

Murray AM, Levkoff SE, Wetle TT, et al: Acute delirium and functional decline in the hospitalized elderly patient. J Gerontol 48:M181–M186, 1993

Nagley SJ: Predicting and preventing confusion in your patients. J Gerontol Nurs 12:27–31, 1986

Nakamura A, Inada T, Kitao Y, et al: Association between catechol-O-methyltransferase (COMT) polymorphism and severe alcoholic withdrawal symptoms in male Japanese alcoholics. Addict Biol 6:233–238, 2001

Nakamura J, Uchimura N, Yamada S, et al: Effects of mianserin hydrochloride on delirium: comparison with the effects of oxypertine and haloperidol. Nihon Shinkei Seishin Yakurigaku Zasshi 14:269–277, 1994

Nakamura J, Uchimura N, Yamada S, et al: The effect of mianserin hydrochloride on delirium. Hum Psychopharmacol 10:289–297, 1995

Nakamura J, Uchimura N, Yamada S, et al: Does plasma free-3-methoxy-4-hydroxyphenyl(ethylene)glycol increase the delirious state? A comparison of the effects of mianserin and haloperidol on delirium. Int Clin Psychopharmacol 12:147–152, 1997a

Nakamura J, Uchimura N, Yamada S, et al: Mianserin suppositories in the treatment of post-operative delirium. Hum Psychopharmacol 12:595–599, 1997b

Nakamura K, Kurasawa M, Tanaka Y: Apomorphine-induced hypoattention in rat and reversal of the choice performance impairment by aniracetam. Eur J Pharmacol 342:127–138, 1998

Neelon VJ, Champagne MT, Carlson JR, et al: The NEECHAM scale: construction, validation, and clinical testing. Nurs Res 45:324–330, 1986

Nicholas LM, Lindsey BA: Delirium presenting with symptoms of depression. Psychosomatics 36:471–479, 1995

Nighoghossian N, Trouillas P, Vighetto A, et al: Spatial delirium following a right subcortical infarct with frontal deactivation. J Neurol Neurosurg Psychiatry 55:334–335, 1992

O'Brien JM, Rockwood RP, Suh KI: Haloperidol-induced torsades de pointes. Ann Pharmacother 33:1046–1050, 1999

O'Hare E, Weldon DT, Bettin K, et al: Serum anticholinergic activity and behavior following atropine sulfate administration in the rat. Pharmacol Biochem Behav 56:151–154, 1997

Okamato Y, Matsuoka Y, Sasaki T, et al: Trazodone in the treatment of delirium. J Clin Psychopharmacol 19:280–282, 1999

Okamura A, Nakano T, Fukumoto Y, et al: Delirious behaviour in children with influenza: its clinical features and EEG findings. Brain Dev 27:271–274, 2005

O'Keeffe ST: Rating the severity of delirium: the Delirium Assessment Scale. Int J Geriatr Psychiatry 9:551–556, 1994

O'Keeffe ST: Clinical subtypes of delirium in the elderly. Dement Geriatr Cogn Disord 10:380–385, 1999

O'Keeffe S[T]: The experience of delirium in older people. Int Psychogeriatr 17 (suppl 2):120, 2005

O'Keeffe ST, Gosney MA: Assessing attentiveness in older hospitalized patients: global assessment vs. test of attention. J Am Geriatr Soc 45:470–473, 1997

O'Keeffe ST, Lavan JN: Predicting delirium in elderly patients: development and validation of a risk-stratification model. Age Ageing 25:317–321, 1996

O'Keeffe ST, Lavan JN: Clinical significance of delirium subtypes in older people. Age Ageing 28:115–119, 1999

O'Keeffe ST, Tormey WP, Glasgow R, et al: Thiamine deficiency in hospitalized elderly patients. Gerontology 40:18–24, 1994

O'Keeffe ST, Mulkerrin EC, Nayeem K, et al: Use of serial Mini-Mental State Examinations to diagnose and monitor delirium in elderly hospital patients. J Am Geriatr Soc 53:867–870, 2005

Okubo T, Harada S, Higuchi S, et al: Genetic polymorphism of the CCK gene in patients with alcohol withdrawal symptoms. Alcohol Clin Exp Res 24 (4 suppl):2–4, 2000

Okubo T, Harada S, Higuchi S, et al: Investigation of quantitative loci in the CCKAR gene with susceptibility to alcoholism. Alcohol Clin Exp Res 26 (8 suppl):2–5, 2002

Okubo T, Harada S, Higuchi S, et al: Association analyses between polymorphisms of the phase II detoxification enzymes (GSTM1, NQO1, NQO2) and alcohol withdrawal symptoms. Alcohol Clin Exp Res 27 (8 suppl):68S–71S, 2003

Olofsson B, Lundström M, Borssén B, et al: Delirium is associated with poor rehabilitation outcome in elderly patients treated for femoral neck fractures. Scand J Caring Sci 19:119–127, 2005

Olofsson K, Alling C, Lundberg D, et al: Abolished circadian rhythm of melatonin secretion in sedated and artificially ventilated intensive care patients. Acta Anaesthesiol Scand 48:679–684, 2004

Olofsson SM, Weitzner MA, Valentine AD, et al: A retrospective study of the psychiatric management and outcome of delirium in the cancer patient. Support Care Cancer 4:351–357, 1996

Ongini E, Caporali MG, Massotti M: Stimulation of dopamine D-1 receptors by SKF 38393 induces EEG desynchronization and behavioral arousal. Life Sci 37:2327–2333, 1985

Onofrj M, Curatola L, Malatesta G, et al: Reduction of P3 latency during outcome from post-traumatic amnesia. Acta Neurol Scand 83:273–279, 1991

Ovchinsky N, Pitchumoni S, Skotzko CE: Use of olanzapine for the treatment of delirium following traumatic brain injury. Psychosomatics 43:147–148, 2002

Owens JF, Hutelmyer CM: The effect of postoperative intervention on delirium in cardiac surgical patients. Nurs Res 31:60–62, 1982

Pae CU, Lee SJ, Lee CU, et al: A pilot trial of quetiapine for the treatment of patients with delirium. Hum Psychopharmacol 19:125–127, 2004

Pandharipande P, Shintani A, Peterson J, et al: Lorazepam is an independent risk factor for transitioning to delirium in intensive care unit patients. Anesthesiology 104:21–26, 2006

Parellada E, Baeza I, de Pablo J, et al: Risperidone in the treatment of patients with delirium. J Clin Psychiatry 65:348–353, 2004

Passik SD, Cooper M: Complicated delirium in a cancer patient successfully treated with olanzapine. J Pain Symptom Manage 17:219–223, 1999

Patten SB, Lamarre CJ: Dysgraphia (letter). Can J Psychiatry 34:746, 1989

Perrault LP, Denault AY, Carrier M, et al: Torsades de pointes secondary to intravenous haloperidol after coronary artery bypass graft surgery. Can J Anesth 47:251–254, 2000

Peterson JF, Pun BT, Dittus RS, et al: Delirium and its motoric subtypes: a study of 614 critically ill patients. J Am Geriatr Soc 54:479–484, 2006

Picotte-Prillmayer D, DiMaggio JR, Baile WF: H-2 blocker delirium. Psychosomatics 36:74–77, 1995

Piercey MF, Camacho-Ochoa M, Smith MW: Functional roles for dopamine-receptor subtypes. Clin Neuropharmacol 18:S34–S42, 1995

Pitkälä KH, Laurila JV, Strandberg TE, et al: Prognostic significance of delirium in frail older people. Dement Geriatr Cogn Disord 19:158–163, 2005

Platt MM, Breitbart W, Smith M, et al: Efficacy of neuroleptics for hypoactive delirium. J Neuropsychiatry Clin Neurosci 6:66–67, 1994a

Platt MM, Trautman P, Frager G, et al: Pediatric delirium: research update. Paper presented at the annual meeting of the Academy of Psychosomatic Medicine, Phoenix, AZ, November 1994b

Pomara N, Willoughby LM, Wesnes K, et al: Increased anticholinergic challenge-induced memory impairment associated with the APOE-epsilon4 allele in the elderly: a controlled pilot study. Neuropsychopharmacology 29:403–409, 2004

Pompeii P, Foreman M, Rudberg MA, et al: Delirium in hospitalized older persons: outcomes and predictors. J Am Geriatr Soc 42:809–815, 1994

Posner ML, Boies SJ: Components of attention. Psychol Rev 78:391–408, 1971

Pratico C, Quattrone D, Lucanto T, et al: Drugs of anesthesia acting on central cholinergic system may cause postoperative cognitive dysfunction and delirium. Med Hypotheses 65:972–982, 2005

Preuss UW, Koller G, Bahlmann M, et al: No association between metabotropic glutamate receptors 7 and 8 (mGlur7 and mGlur8) gene polymorphisms and withdrawal seizures and delirium tremens in alcohol-dependent individuals. Alcohol Alcohol 37:174–178, 2002

Preuss UW, Koller G, Zill P, et al: Alcoholism-related phenotypes and genetic variants of the CB1 receptor. Eur Arch Psychiatry Clin Neurosci 253:275–280, 2003

Preuss UW, Zill P, Koller G, et al: Ionotropic glutamate receptor gene GRIK3 SER310ALA functional polymorphism is related to delirium tremens in alcoholics. Pharmacogenomics J 6:34–41, 2006

Price BH, Mesulam M: Psychiatric manifestations of right hemisphere infarctions. J Nerv Ment Dis 173:610–614, 1985

Prugh DG, Wagonfeld S, Metcalf D, et al: A clinical study of delirium in children and adolescents. Psychosom Med 42:177–195, 1980

Rabins PV, Folstein MF: Delirium and dementia: diagnostic criteria and fatality rates. Br J Psychiatry 140:149–153, 1982

Rahkonen T, Luukkainen-Markkula R, Paanila S, et al: Delirium as a sign of undetected dementia among community dwelling elderly subjects: a 2 year follow up study. J Neurol Neurosurg Psychiatry 69:519–521, 2000

Ramirez-Bermudez J, Lopez-Gomez M, Sosa Ana L, et al: Frequency of delirium in a neurological emergency room. J Neuropsychiatry Clin Neurosci 18:108–112, 2006

Ravona-Springer R, Dohlberg OT, Hirschman S, et al: Delirium in elderly patients treated with risperidone: a report of three cases. J Clin Psychopharmacol 18:171–172, 1998

Reilly JG, Ayis AS, Ferrier IN, et al: QTc-interval abnormalities and psychotropic drug therapy in psychiatric patients. Lancet 355:1048–1052, 2000

Reishies FM, Neuhaus AH, Hansen ML, et al: Electrophysiological and neuropsychological analysis of a delirious state: the role of the anterior cingulate gyrus. Psychiatry Res 138:171–181, 2005

Resnick M, Burton BT: Droperidol versus haloperidol in the initial management of acutely agitated patients. J Clin Psychiatry 45:298–299, 1984

Reyes RL, Bhattacharyya AK, Heller D: Traumatic head injury: restlessness and agitation as prognosticators of physical and psychological improvement in patients. Arch Phys Med Rehabil 62:20–23, 1981

Riker RR, Fraser GL, Cox PM: Continuous infusion of haloperidol controls agitation in critically ill patients. Crit Care Med 22:433–440, 1994

Riker RR, Fraser GL, Richen P: Movement disorders associated with withdrawal from high-dose intravenous haloperidol therapy in delirious ICU patients. Chest 111:1778–1781, 1997

Ritchie J, Steiner W, Abrahamowicz M: Incidence of and risk factors for delirium among psychiatric patients. Psychiatr Serv 47:727–730, 1996

Robertsson B: Assessment scales in delirium. Dement Geriatr Cogn Disord 10:368–379, 1999

Robertsson B, Blennow K, Gottfries CG, et al: Delirium in dementia. Int J Geriatr Psychiatry 13:49–56, 1998

Robinson MJ: Probable Lewy body dementia presenting as "delirium." Psychosomatics 43:84–86, 2002

Rockwood K: Acute confusion in elderly medical patients. J Am Geriatr Soc 37:150–154, 1989

Rockwood K: The occurrence and duration of symptoms in elderly patients with delirium. J Gerontol 48:M162–M166, 1993

Rockwood K, Cosway S, Stolee P, et al: Increasing the recognition of delirium in elderly patients. J Am Geriatr Soc 42:252–256, 1994

Rockwood K, Cosway S, Carver D, et al: The risk of dementia and death after delirium. Age Ageing 28:551–556, 1999

Rodriguez G, Testa R, Celle G, et al: Reduction of cerebral blood flow in subclinical hepatic encephalopathy and its correlation with plasma-free tryptophan. J Cereb Blood Flow Metab 7:768–772, 1987

Rolfson DB, McElhaney JE, Jhangri GS, et al: Validity of the Confusion Assessment Method in detecting postoperative delirium in the elderly. Int Psychogeriatr 11:431–438, 1999

Romano J, Engel GL: Delirium, I: electroencephalographic data. Arch Neurol Psychiatry 51:356–377, 1944

Ropacki SA, Jeste DV: Epidemiology of and risk factors for psychosis of Alzheimer's disease: a review of 55 studies published from 1990 to 2003. Am J Psychiatry 162:2022–2030, 2005

Rosenberg PB, Ahmed I, Hurwitz S: Methylphenidate in depressed medically ill patients. J Clin Psychiatry 52:263–267, 1991

Rosenberg S, Loetz M, Yang J: Experience with the use of high-dose interleukin-2 in the treatment of 652 cancer patients. Ann Surg 210:474–484, 1989

Ross CA, Peyser CE, Shapiro I, et al: Delirium: phenomenologic and etiologic subtypes. Int Psychogeriatr 3:135–147, 1991

Rothenhausler HB, Grieser B, Nollert G, et al: Psychiatric and psychosocial outcome of cardiac surgery with cardiopulmonary bypass: a prospective 12-month follow-up study. Gen Hosp Psychiatry 27:182–128, 2005

Rothwell NJ, Hopkins SJ: Cytokines and the nervous system, II: actions and mechanisms of action. Trends Neurosci 18:130–136, 1995

Rovner BW, David A, Lucas-Blaustein MJ, et al: Self-care capacity and anticholinergic drug levels in nursing home patients. Am J Psychiatry 145:107–109, 1988

Rudberg MA, Pompei P, Foreman MD, et al: The natural history of delirium in older hospitalized patients: a syndrome of heterogeneity. Age Ageing 26:169–174, 1997

Ruijs MB, Keyser A, Gabreels FJ, et al: Somatosensory evoked potentials and cognitive sequelae in children with closed head injury. Neuropediatrics 24:307–312, 1993

Ruijs MB, Gabreels FJ, Thijssen HM: The utility of electroencephalography and cerebral CT in children with mild and moderately severe closed head injuries. Neuropediatrics 25:73–77, 1994

Rujescu D, Soyka M, Dahmen N, et al: GRIN1 locus may modify the susceptibility to seizures during alcohol withdrawal. Am J Med Genet B Neuropsychiatr Genet 133:85–87, 2005

Saatman KE, Contreras PC, Smith DH, et al: Insulin-like growth factor-1 improves both neurological motor and cognitive outcome following experimental brain injury. Exp Neurol 147:418–427, 1997

Samochowiec J, Kucharska-Mazur J, Kaminski R, et al: Norepinephrine transporter gene polymorphism is not associated with susceptibility to alcohol dependence. Psychiatry Res 111:229–233, 2002

Samuels S, Fang M: Olanzapine may cause delirium in geriatric patients. J Clin Psychiatry 65:582–583, 2004

Sandberg O, Gustafson Y, Brannstrom B, et al: Prevalence of dementia, delirium and psychiatric symptoms in various care settings for the elderly. Scand J Soc Med 26:56–62, 1998

Sandberg O, Gustafson Y, Brannstrom B, et al: Clinical profile of delirium in older patients. J Am Geriatr Soc 47:1300–1306, 1999

Sander T, Harms H, Podschus J, et al: Alleleic association of a dopamine transporter gene polymorphism in alcohol dependence with withdrawal seizures or delirium. Biol Psychiatry 41:299–304, 1997

Sander T, Ostapowicz A, Samochowiec J, et al: Genetic variation of the glutamate transporter *EAAT2* gene and vulnerability to alcohol dependence. Psychiatr Genet 10:103–107, 2000

Sanders KM, Stern TA: Management of delirium associated with use of the intra-aortic balloon pump. Am J Crit Care 2:371–377, 1993

Santamaria J, Blesa R, Tolosa ES: Confusional syndrome in thalamic stroke. Neurology 34:1618–1619, 1984

Santos FS, Wahlund LO, Varli F, et al: Incidence, clinical features and subtypes of delirium in elderly patients treated for hip fractures. Dement Geriatr Cogn Disord 20:231–237, 2005

Saravay SM, Strain JJ: Academy of Psychosomatic Medicine Task force on funding implications of consultation-liaison psychiatry outcome studies. Psychosomatics 35:227–232, 1994

Saravay SM, Kaplowitz M, Kurek J, et al: How do delirium and dementia increase length of stay of elderly general medical inpatients. Psychosomatics 45:235–242, 2004

Sasaki Y, Matsuyama T, Inoue S, et al: A prospective, open-label, flexible-dose study of quetiapine in the treatment of delirium. J Clin Psychiatry 64:1316–1321, 2003

Schafer DF, Jones EA: Hepatic encephalopathy and the gamma-aminobutyric acid neurotransmitter system. Lancet 1:18–20, 1982

Schindler BA, Shook J, Schwartz GM: Beneficial effects of psychiatric intervention on recovery after coronary artery bypass graft surgery. Gen Hosp Psychiatry 11:358–364, 1989

Schirazi S, Rodriguez D, Nomikos GG: Effects of typical and atypical antipsychotic drugs on acetylcholine release in the hippocampus. Abstr Soc Neurosci 26:2144, 2000

Schmidley JW, Messing RO: Agitated confusional states with right hemisphere infarctions. Stroke 5:883–885, 1984

Schmidt LG, Samochowiec J, Finckh U, et al: Association of a CB1 cannabinoid receptor gene (CNR1) polymorphism with severe alcohol dependence. Drug Alcohol Depend 65:221–224, 2002

Schneider A: Use of intravenous valproate (Depacon) in the treatment of delirium: a case series. Neurobiol Aging 25 (suppl 2):S302–S303, 2005

Schneider LS, Dagerman KS, Insel P: Risk of death with atypical antipsychotic drug treatment for dementia: meta-analysis of randomized placebo-controlled trials. JAMA 294:1934–1943, 2005

Schneir AB, Offerman SR, Ly BT, et al: Complications of diagnostic physostigmine administration to emergency department patients. Ann Emerg Med 42:14–19, 2003

Schofield I: A small exploratory study of the reaction of older people to an episode of delirium. J Adv Nurs 25:942–952, 1997

Schor JD, Levkoff SE, Lipsitz LA, et al: Risk factors for delirium in hospitalized elderly. JAMA 267:827–831, 1992

Schuster P, Gabriel E, Kufferle B, et al: Reversal by physostigmine of clozapine-induced delirium. Clin Toxicol 10:437–441, 1977

Schwartz TL, Masand PS: The role of atypical antipsychotics in the treatment of delirium. Psychosomatics 43:171–174, 2002

Seaman JS, Schillerstrom J, Carroll D, et al: Impaired oxidative metabolism precipitates delirium: a study of 101 ICU patients. Psychosomatics 47:56–61, 2006

Seear M, Lockitch G, Jacobson B, et al: Thiamine, riboflavin and pyridoxine deficiency in a population of critically ill children. J Pediatr 121:533–538, 1992

Serrano-Dueñas M, Bleda MJ: Delirium in Parkinson's disease patients: a five-year follow-up study. Parkinsonism Relat Disord 11:387–392, 2005

Sherer M, Nakas-Thompson R, Yablon SA, et al: Multidimensional assessment of acute confusion after traumatic brain injury. Arch Phys Med Rehabil 86:896–904, 2005

Sherman SM, Kock C: Thalamus, in The Synaptic Organization of the Brain, 3rd Edition. Edited by Shepherd GM. New York, Oxford University Press, 1990, pp 246–278

Shigeta H, Yasui A, Nimura Y, et al: Postoperative delirium and melatonin levels in elderly patients. Am J Surg 182:449–454, 2001

Sim FH, Brunet DG, Conacher GN: Quetiapine associated with acute mental status changes (letter). Can J Psychiatry 3:299, 2000

Sipahimalani A, Masand PS: Use of risperidone in delirium: case reports. Ann Clin Psychiatry 9:105–107, 1997

Sirois F: Delirium: 100 cases. Can J Psychiatry 33:375–378, 1988

Skrobik YK, Bergeron N, Dumont M, et al: Olanzapine vs haloperidol: treating delirium in a critical care setting. Intensive Care Med 30:444–449, 2004

Sloan EP, Fenton GW, Standage KP: Anticholinergic drug effects on quantitative EEG, visual evoked potentials, and verbal memory. Biol Psychiatry 31:600–606, 1992

Solfrizzi V, Torres F, Capursi C, et al: Analysis of individual items of MMSE in discrimination between normal and demented subjects. Arch Gerontol Geriatr 7(suppl):357–362, 2001

Stefano GB, Bilfinger TV, Fricchione GL: The immune-neuro-link and the macrophage: post-cardiotomy delirium, HIV-associated dementia and psychiatry. Prog Neurobiol 42:475–488, 1994

Stern TA: Continuous infusion of physostigmine in anticholinergic delirium: a case report. J Clin Psychiatry 44:463–464, 1983

Stern TA: Continuous infusion of haloperidol in agitated critically ill patients. Crit Care Med 22:378–379, 1994

Sternberg SA, Wolfson C, Baumgarten M: Undetected dementia in community-dwelling older people: the Canadian Study of Health and Aging. J Am Geriatr Soc 48:1430–1434, 2000

Straker DA, Shapiro PA, Muskin PR: Aripiprazole in the treatment of delirium. Psychosomatics 47:385–391, 2006

Sundaram M, Dostrow V: Epilepsy in the elderly. Neurologist 1:232–239, 1995

Swenson JR, Erman M, Labelle J, et al: Extrapyramidal reactions: neuropsychiatric mimics in patients with AIDS. Gen Hosp Psychiatry 11:248–253, 1989

Swerdlow NR, Bongiovanni MJ, Tochen L, et al: Separable noradrenergic and dopaminergic regulation of prepulse inhibition in rats: implications for predictive validity and Tourette syndrome. Psychopharmacology 186:246–254, 2006

Tadic A, Dahmen N, Szegedi A, et al: Polymorphisms in the NMDA subunit 2B are not associated with alcohol dependence and alcohol withdrawal-induced seizures and delirium tremens. Eur Arch Psychiatry Clin Neurosci 255:129–135, 2005

Teicher MH, Gold CA: Neuroleptic drugs: indications and guidelines for their rational use in children and adolescents. J Child Adolesc Psychopharmacol 1:33–56, 1990

Tejera CA, Saravay SM, Goldman E, et al: Diphenhydramine-induced delirium in elderly hospitalized patients with mild dementia. Psychosomatics 35:399–402, 1994

Tesar GE, Murray GB, Cassem NH: Use of high-dose intravenous haloperidol in the treatment of agitated cardiac patients. J Clin Psychopharmacol 5:344–347, 1985

Thomas H, Schwartz E, Petrilli R: Droperidol versus haloperidol for chemical restraint of agitated and combative patients. Ann Emerg Med 21:407–413, 1992

Thomas RI, Cameron DJ, Fahs MC: A prospective study of delirium and prolonged hospital stay. Arch Gen Psychiatry 45:937–946, 1988

Timmers JFM, Kalisvaart KJ, Schuurmans M, et al: A review of assessment scales for delirium, in Primary Prevention of Delirium in the Elderly. Edited by Kalisvaart K. Amsterdam, The Netherlands, Academisch Proefschrift, University of Amsterdam, 2005, pp 21–39

Toda H, Kusumi I, Sasaki Y, et al: Relationship between plasma concentration levels of risperidone and clinical effects in the treatment of delirium. Int Clin Psychopharmacol 20:331–333, 2005

Tokita K, Tanaka H, Kawamoto M, et al: Patient-controlled epidural analgesia with bupivacaine and fentanyl suppresses postoperative delirium following hepatectomy. Masui 50:742–746, 2001

Tollefson GD, Montagne-Clouse J, Lancaster SP: The relationship of serum anticholinergic activity to mental status performance in an elderly nursing home population. J Neuropsychiatry Clin Neurosci 3:314–319, 1991

Torres R, Mittal D, Kennedy R: Use of quetiapine in delirium: case reports. Psychosomatics 42:347–349, 2001

Treloar AJ, MacDonald AJ: Outcome of delirium, I: outcome of delirium diagnosed by DSM III-R, ICD-10 and CAMDEX and derivation of the Reversible Cognitive Dysfunction Scale among acute geriatric inpatients. Int J Geriatr Psychiatry 12:609–613, 1997

Trzepacz PT: Neuropathogenesis of delirium: a need to focus our research. Psychosomatics 35:374–391, 1994a

Trzepacz PT: A review of delirium assessment instruments. Gen Hosp Psychiatry 16:397–405, 1994b

Trzepacz PT: Anticholinergic model for delirium. Semin Clin Neuropsychiatry 1:294–303, 1996

Trzepacz PT: The Delirium Rating Scale: its use in consultation/liaison research. Psychosomatics 40:193–204, 1999a

Trzepacz PT: Update on the neuropathogenesis of delirium. Dement Geriatr Cogn Disord 10:330–334, 1999b

Trzepacz PT: Is there a final common neural pathway in delirium? Focus on acetylcholine and dopamine. Semin Clin Neuropsychiatry 5:132–148, 2000

Trzepacz PT, Dew MA: Further analyses of the Delirium Rating Scale. Gen Hosp Psychiatry 17:75–79, 1995

Trzepacz PT, Francis J: Low serum albumin and risk of delirium (letter). Am J Psychiatry 147:675, 1990

Trzepacz PT, Teague GB, Lipowski ZJ: Delirium and other organic mental disorders in a general hospital. Gen Hosp Psychiatry 7:101–106, 1985

Trzepacz PT, Baker RW, Greenhouse J: A symptom rating scale for delirium. Psychiatry Res 23:89–97, 1988a

Trzepacz PT, Brenner R, Coffman G, et al: Delirium in liver transplantation candidates: discriminant analysis of multiple test variables. Biol Psychiatry 24:3–14, 1988b

Trzepacz PT, Sclabassi R, Van Thiel D: Delirium: a subcortical mechanism? J Neuropsychiatry Clin Neurosci 1:283–290, 1989

Trzepacz PT, Leavitt M, Ciongoli K: An animal model for delirium. Psychosomatics 33:404–415, 1992

Trzepacz PT, Ho V, Mallavarapu H: Cholinergic delirium and neurotoxicity associated with tacrine for Alzheimer's dementia. Psychosomatics 37:299–301, 1996

Trzepacz PT, Mulsant BH, Dew MA, et al: Is delirium different when it occurs in dementia? A study using the Delirium Rating Scale. J Neuropsychiatry Clin Neurosci 10:199–204, 1998

Trzepacz PT, Mittal D, Torres R, et al: Validation of the Delirium Rating Scale—Revised-98: comparison to the Delirium Rating Scale and Cognitive Test for Delirium. J Neuropsychiatry Clin Neurosci 13:229–242, 2001

Trzepacz PT, Mittal D, Torres R, et al: Delirium vs dementia symptoms: Delirium Rating Scale-Revised (DRS-R-98) and Cognitive Test for Delirium (CTD) item comparisons. Psychosomatics 43:156–157, 2002

Tsutsui S, Kitamura M, Higachi H, et al: Development of postoperative delirium in relation to a room change in the general surgical unit. Surg Today 26:292–294, 1996

Tune LE, Dainloth NF, Holland A, et al: Association of postoperative delirium with raised serum levels of anticholinergic drugs. Lancet 2:651–653, 1981

Tune L[E], Carr S, Hoag E, et al: Anticholinergic effects of drugs commonly prescribed for the elderly: potential means for assessing risk of delirium. Am J Psychiatry 149:1393–1394, 1992

Turkel SB, Tavare CJ: Delirium in children and adolescents. J Neuropsychiatry Clin Neurosci 15:431–435, 2003

Turkel SB, Braslow K, Tavare CJ, et al: The delirium rating scale in children and adolescents. Psychosomatics 44:126–129, 2003

Turkel SB, Trzepacz PT, Tavare CJ: Comparison of delirium in adults and children. Psychosomatics 47:320–324, 2006

Turnheim K: When drug therapy gets old: pharmacokinetics and pharmacodynamics in the elderly. Exp Gerontol 38:843–853, 2003

Uchikado H, Akiyama H, Kondo H, et al: Activation of vascular endothelial cells and perivascular cells by systemic inflammation: an immunohistochemical study of postmortem human brain tissues. Acta Neuropathol 107:341–351, 2004

Uchiyama M, Tanaka K, Isse K, et al: Efficacy of mianserin on symptoms of delirium in the aged: an open trial study. Prog Neuropsychopharmacol Biol Psychiatry 20:651–656, 1996

van der Mast RC: Detecting and measuring the severity of delirium with the symptom rating scale for delirium, in Delirium After Cardiac Surgery. Thesis, Erasmus University Rotterdam, Benecke Consultants, Amsterdam, The Netherlands, 1994, pp 78–89

van der Mast RC, Fekkes D: Serotonin and amino acids: partners in delirium pathophysiology? Semin Clin Neuropsychiatry 5:125–131, 2000

van der Mast RC, Fekkes D, van den Broek WW, et al: Reduced cerebral tryptophan availability as a possible cause for postcardiotomy delirium (letter). Psychosomatics 35:195, 1994 van der Mast RC, Fekkes D: Serotonin and amino acids: partners in delirium pathophysiology? Semin Clin Neuropsychiatry 5:125–131, 2000

van Hemert AM, van der Mast RC, Hengeveld MW, et al: Excess mortality in general hospital patients with delirium: a 5-year follow-up study of 519 patients seen in psychiatric consultation. J Psychosom Res 38:339–346, 1994

van Leeuwen AMII, Molders J, Sterkmans P, et al: Droperidol in acutely agitated patients: a double-blind placebo-controlled study. J Nerv Ment Dis 164:280–283, 1977

Van Munster BC, Kaorevaar JC, de Rooij SE, et al: The association between delirium and APOE-epsilon 4 allele in the elderly. Int Psychogeriatrics 17 (suppl 2):149, 2005

Vaphiades MS, Celesia GG, Brigell MG: Positive spontaneous visual phenomena limited to the hemianopic field in lesions of central visual pathways. Neurology 47:408–417, 1996

Voyer P, Cole MG, McCusker J, et al: Prevalence and symptoms of delirium superimposed on dementia. Clin Nurs Res 15:46–66, 2006

Wacker P, Nunes PV, Cabrita H, et al: Post-operative delirium is associated with poor cognitive outcome and dementia. Dement Geriatr Cogn Disord 21:221–227, 2006

Wada Y, Yamaguchi N: Delirium in the elderly: relationship of clinical symptoms to outcome. Dementia 4:113–116, 1993

Wahlund B, Grahn H, Saaf J, et al: Affective disorder subtyped by psychomotor symptoms, monoamine oxidase, melatonin and cortisol: identification of patients with latent bipolar disorder. Eur Arch Psychiatry Clin Neurosci 248:215–224, 1998

Wahlund LA, Bjorlin GA: Delirium in clinical practice: experiences from a specialized delirium ward. Dement Geriatr Cogn Disord 10:389–392, 1999

Wanich CK, Sullivan-Marx EM, Gottlieb GL, et al: Functional status outcomes of a nursing intervention in hospitalized elderly. Image J Nurs Sch 24:201–207, 1992

Webster R, Holroyd S: Prevalence of psychotic symptoms in delirium. Psychosomatics 41:519–522, 2000

Weddington WW: The mortality of delirium: an underappreciated problem? Psychosomatics 23:1232–1235, 1982

Wengel SP, Roccaforte WH, Burke WJ: Donepezil improves symptoms of delirium in dementia: implications for future research. J Geriatr Psychiatry Neurol 11:159–161, 1998

Wengel SP, Burke WJ, Roccaforte WH: Donepezil for postoperative delirium associated with Alzheimer's disease. J Am Geriatr Soc 47:379–380, 1999

Wernicke C, Smolka M, Gallinat J, et al: Evidence for the importance of the human dopamine transporter gene for withdrawal symptomatology of alcoholics in a German population. Neurosci Lett 333:45–48, 2002

Wernicke C, Samochowiec J, Schmidt LG, et al: Polymorphisms in the N-methyl-D-aspartate receptor 1 and 2B subunits are associated with alcoholism-related traits. Biol Psychiatry 54:922–928, 2003

Wetli CV, Mash D, Karch SB: Cocaine-associated agitated delirium and the neuroleptic malignant syndrome. Am J Emerg Med 14:425–428, 1996

White S, Calver BL, Newsway V, et al: Enzymes of drug metabolism during delirium. Age Ageing 34:603–608, 2005

Willard LB, Hauss-Wegrzyniak B, Wenk GL: Pathological and biochemical consequences of acute and chronic neuroinflammation within the basal forebrain cholinergic system of rats. Neuroscience 88:193–200, 1999

Williams MA, Campbell EB, Raynor WJ, et al: Reducing acute confusional states in elderly patients with hip fractures. Res Nurs Health 8:329–337, 1985

Williams PD, Helton DR: The proconvulsive activity of quinolone antibiotics in an animal model. Toxicol Lett 58:23–28, 1991

Wilson K, Broadhurst C, Diver M, et al: Plasma insulin growth factor-1 and incident delirium. Int J Geriatr Psychiatry 20:154–159, 2005

Wilson LM: Intensive care delirium: the effect of outside deprivation in a windowless unit. Arch Intern Med 130:225–226, 1972

Wilt JL, Minnema AM, Johnson RF, et al: Torsades de pointes associated with the use of intravenous haloperidol. Ann Intern Med 119:391–394, 1993

Wolff HG, Curran D: Nature of delirium and allied states: the dysergastic reaction. Arch Neurol Psychiatry 33:1175–1215, 1935

Wong AHC, Buckle CE, van Tol HHM: Polymorphisms in dopamine receptors: what do they tell us? Eur J Pharmacol 410:183–203, 2000

World Health Organization: International Statistical Classification of Diseases and Related Health Problems, 10th Revision. Geneva, Switzerland, World Health Organization, 1992

Wu CL, Hsu W, Richman JM, et al: Postoperative cognitive function as an outcome of regional anesthesia and analgesia. Reg Anesth Pain Med 29:257–268, 2004

Yamamoto T, Lyeth BG, Dixon CE, et al: Changes in regional brain acetylcholine content in rats following unilateral and bilateral brainstem lesions. J Neurotrauma 5:69–79, 1988

Yokota H, Ogawa S, Kurokawa A, et al: Regional cerebral blood flow in delirious patients. Psychiatry Clin Neurosci 57:337–339, 2003

Young LJ, George J: Do guidelines improve the process and outcomes of care in delirium? Age Ageing 32:525–528, 2003

Zee-Cheng C-S, Mueller CE, Siefert CF, et al: Haloperidol and torsades de pointes (letter). Ann Intern Med 102:418, 1985

12

NEUROPSYCHIATRIC ASPECTS OF APHASIA AND RELATED DISORDERS

Mario F. Mendez, M.D., Ph.D.

David Glenn Clark, M.D.

Language is the unique human ability to communicate through symbols, whether these are in the form of spoken or written language, Braille, musical notation, or sign language. Normal human language requires the ability to access these symbols, encode and decode them, and process the strings of symbols that make up propositional communication (Hauser et al. 2002). Aphasia is the loss or impairment of language due to brain dysfunction. In aphasic patients, some or all of these language functions become disturbed, usually as a consequence of acquired brain damage in the language structures of the left hemisphere.

The aphasic syndromes disturb communication and can be severely disabling. In addition to disturbances in linguistic processing, aphasia is associated with neuropsychiatric manifestations. Aphasic patients are prone to psychiatric problems, including depression or paranoid ideation, cognitive abnormalities, and psychosocial challenges in adjusting to the effect of their disorder. These complications may cause more disability than the aphasia itself.

Despite interest in aphasia, clinicians have paid relatively little attention to the behavioral complications of aphasic syndromes. In some cases, aphasic disorders may be misinterpreted as the speech abnormalities associated with psychiatric diseases such as schizophrenia and depression.

BACKGROUND

Aphasia is a common manifestation of brain disease. The annual incidence of stroke in the United States is about 500,000, and about 20% of these stroke patients have aphasia or a related disorder (Pedersen et al. 1995). Dementia, intracranial neoplasms, traumatic brain injury, and many other neurological disorders also can produce language disturbances. Aphasia is particularly prominent in Alzheimer's disease and frontotemporal lobar degenerations, which include a specific language degeneration known as primary progressive aphasia (Clark et al. 2005).

Current approaches to aphasia stem from early work on the localization of language to discrete, interconnected areas in the left hemisphere. In 1861, Paul Broca inaugurated the modern study of aphasia with his description of a patient who had lost the ability to speak and had a focal brain injury in the frontal region. This early work established the dominance of the human left hemisphere for language function and established an anterior-posterior dichotomy of language processing. Later, Karl Wernicke and others described a group of specialized and interconnected language regions in the brain. The two major centers for this model were Broca's area in the anterior frontal region for language pro-

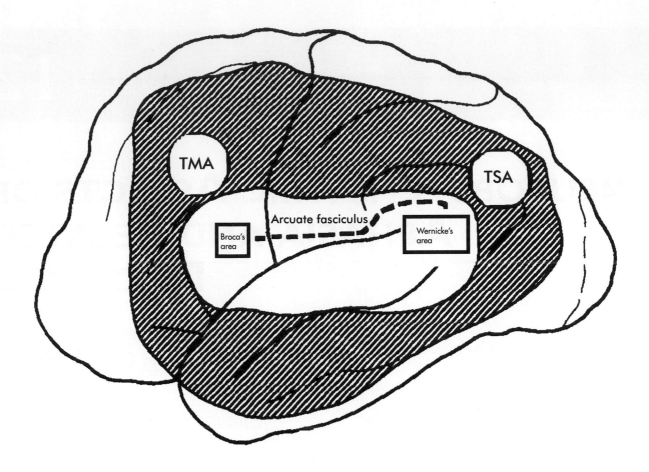

FIGURE 12–1. Lateral view of the left hemisphere indicating the perisylvian area (*central clear region*), where the major language centers are located (Catani et al. 2005). Broca's area in the frontal operculum, Wernicke's area in the superior temporal gyrus, and the arcuate fasciculus are indicated. Lesions in these corresponding structures result in Broca's aphasia, Wernicke's aphasia, and conduction aphasia, respectively. These perisylvian aphasia syndromes include disturbances in the ability to repeat spoken language. Lesions in the surrounding border zone area (*cross-hatched region*) may result in transcortical aphasia syndromes characterized by sparing of repetition. TMA = region where a lesser lesion may result in transcortical motor aphasia; TSA = region where a lesion may result in transcortical sensory aphasia.

duction and Wernicke's area in the superior temporal gyrus for language decoding. The elaboration of this model led to a view that language functions were localized in neuroanatomical regions in the left perisylvian region (Figure 12–1).

Although prominent neuroscientists and clinicians subsequently challenged this interpretation of localization of lesion studies, the original views of Broca and Wernicke were restored when Norman Geschwind (1965) reported that separation (disconnection) of cortical foci could produce distinct language impairments. Investigators have since used improved clinical and laboratory studies to confirm the clinicoanatomical syndromes formulated by the nineteenth-century French and German aphasiologists. The reborn localization concept is embodied in the Wernicke-Geschwind model of language and aphasia (Benson and Ardila 1996) (Figure 12–2).

In more recent years, many disciplines have added to our understanding of aphasia (Benson and Ardila 1996; A.R. Damasio 1992). Linguists have applied the analysis of different levels of language representation to disorders of language. These have included phonology (the sound pattern of language), morphology (the combination of language's smallest meaningful units), syntax (the structure of sentences), semantics (the relation of language to meaning), and pragmatics (nuances of articulation and discourse). Noam Chomsky's (1972) emphasis on a universal grammar suggested the existence of a common brain substrate that results in restriction of the set of possible human grammars. Such restriction is thought to underlie the speed with which children are able to acquire language. Computer scientists working in artificial intelligence have attempted to formalize the necessary and

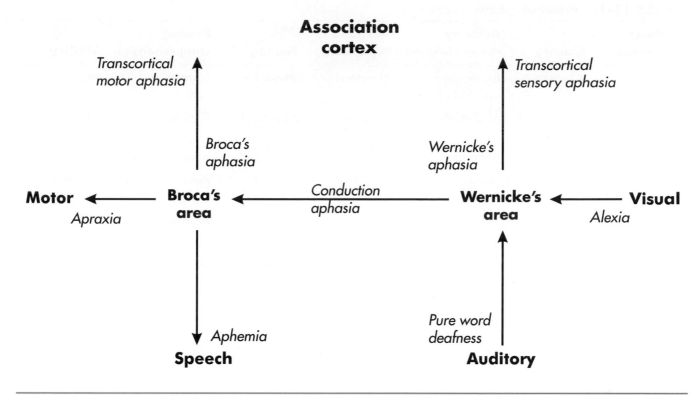

FIGURE 12–2.   Wernicke-Geschwind model. The diagram illustrates the organization of language and corresponding aphasia syndromes in the left hemisphere. The perisylvian language region receives auditory and visual input and produces speech and motor output. Disturbances in the corresponding regions are indicated in italics. Aphemia and pure word deafness are disturbances at the prelanguage and postlanguage levels, respectively. Alexia and apraxia reflect disorders of visual language input and nonspeech motor output, respectively. Language symbols must be interpreted by relating to other associations in higher association cortex. Lesions outside the perisylvian language region may result in the transcortical aphasias, sparing the direct perisylvian pathway mediating repetition.

sufficient computational abilities of human brains to account for observations that support the existence of universal grammar. Regardless of whether universal grammar is truly specialized for language or is simply a manifestation of general learning principles, evidence has accumulated that supports the role of specialized brain regions in language use. Anatomists and others have reported a larger planum temporale containing Wernicke's area in the left hemisphere in adults, in fetal brains by about 30 weeks of gestation, and in human skull imprints at least 40,000 years old. Neuropsychologists have noted greater bilaterality of language in the brains of most left-handed individuals and therefore decreased value and localization of the classic aphasia syndromes in those individuals. Finally, the recent advances in positron emission tomography, single photon emission computed tomography, and functional magnetic resonance imaging have expanded our view of the anatomical relations and functional connectivity of language organization in the brain (Muller et al. 1997).

CLASSIFICATION AND DIAGNOSIS OF APHASIA

THE LANGUAGE EXAMINATION

The syndrome classification based on the Wernicke-Geschwind model remains the core of both clinical and academic studies of aphasia. Classification of aphasia syndromes by this model requires the examination of six major language areas: 1) fluency, 2) confrontational naming, 3) auditory comprehension, 4) repetition, 5) reading (aloud and for comprehension), and 6) writing. Six additional and helpful areas of examination are 1) word-list generation, 2) automatic speech, 3) content of speech, 4) presence of language errors (paraphasias and neologisms), 5) prosody, and 6) speech mechanics. Table 12–1 presents an abridged version of this classification with the major language abnormalities associated with each syndrome (Benson and Ardila 1996; A.R. Damasio 1992; Kertesz 1979; Kirschner 1995).

TABLE 12–1.   Principal aphasia syndromes

Aphasia syndrome	Fluency	Auditory comprehension	Repetition	Naming	Reading comprehension	Writing
Broca's	Abnormal	Relatively normal	Abnormal	Abnormal	Normal or abnormal	Abnormal
Wernicke's	Normal, paraphasic	Abnormal	Abnormal	Abnormal	Abnormal	Abnormal
Global	Abnormal	Abnormal	Abnormal	Abnormal	Abnormal	Abnormal
Conduction	Normal, paraphasic	Relatively normal	Abnormal	Usually abnormal	Relatively normal	Abnormal
Transcortical motor	Abnormal	Relatively normal	Relatively normal	Abnormal	Relatively normal	Abnormal
Transcortical sensory	Normal, echolalic	Abnormal	Relatively normal	Abnormal	Abnormal	Abnormal
Anomic	Normal	Relatively normal	Normal	Abnormal	Normal or abnormal	Normal or abnormal

Fluency evaluation requires an assessment of the generation and ease of production of language. The examiner elicits language in spontaneous conversation or a structured interview, listening for several elements of potential dysfluency. These include a decrease in the number of words generated per minute (usually fewer than 50 in English); shortened phrase length (no more than a few words per phrase); a dropout of grammatical morphemes, such as prepositions, conjunctions, and inflectional suffixes (agrammatic or "telegraphic" speech); and increased effort in speech production. In addition, aphasic patients often have a dysarthric or poorly articulated verbal output with loss of the normal components of prosody or intonation. Often, their verbal output is brief and strained but succinct and informative. The patient's ability to produce automatic speech, such as counting numbers or reciting the days of the week, also reflects his or her ability to generate and produce language, but may be spared in the setting of nonfluency.

The ability to produce names is probably the most commonly impaired language function in aphasia. At the bedside, the examiner may ask the patient to name common items present in his or her environment, such as pen, watch, ring, tie, and keys. Subsequently, the examiner asks the patient to name less common items and parts of objects, such as the face of a watch, the heel of a shoe, and the cuff of a sleeve. Standardized or controlled evaluation of confrontational naming requires the patient to name pictures of objects or actions. Differences between production of nouns and verbs provide clues to lesion localization (A.R. Damasio and Tranel 1993). In the assess-

ment of naming, it is worthwhile to have the patient generate a list of words, such as animal names, in a 1-minute timed sample (normal is 12 or more). This provides a means of assessing the patient's general ability to access words without relying on visual perceptual abilities necessary for the interpretation of line drawings that are typically used for confrontational naming.

A further step in the language examination is an assessment of auditory comprehension. Comprehension may be impaired at multiple levels but may be grossly assessed by giving the patient simple commands or asking yes-or-no questions. Commands such as "close your eyes" or "open your mouth" can be escalated to more complex pointing commands such as "first touch your chin and then touch your right shoulder." The patient should be able to comprehend and follow these instructions. Should the patient fail to perform correctly, further testing may identify whether the deficit is at the level of speech sound recognition (e.g., distinguishing between words such as "bit" and "pit"), word recognition (e.g., pointing appropriately to items in response to hearing their names), or verbal working memory (e.g., dialing a telephone number correctly after it is recited). Even aphasic patients who perform well on these comprehension tasks may have difficulty integrating syntactic information. This can be assessed by comparing the patient's ability to interpret sentences with canonical and noncanonical structures. For example, these patients may have difficulty interpreting passive voice sentences (which place the object before the verb and the subject afterward), such as "The lion was killed by the tiger," despite intact ability to interpret the active voice equivalent ("The tiger killed the lion").

In addition to fluency, naming, and auditory comprehension, the examiner must evaluate repetition, reading, writing, and the presence or absence of paraphasic errors. The examiner asks the patient to repeat sentences or phrases such as "no ifs, ands, or buts" and listens for the presence of phonemic (also called *literal*) paraphasias (language errors involving the substitution of incorrect sounds in a word). The patient must read a brief written passage aloud and is then queried for his or her comprehension of the passage. A brief written sample, preferably a sentence of the patient's own composition and a dictated sentence, screens for agraphias or acquired writing disturbances. Finally, the examiner carefully assesses the patient's language output for paraphasic errors, not only phonemic but also semantic paraphasias (the substitution of an incorrect word) and neologisms (the production of "new" or made-up-sounding words, which in the setting of aphasia represent an extreme form of phonemic paraphasia) (Hillis et al. 1999).

CLINICAL APHASIA SYNDROMES

BROCA'S APHASIA

Nonfluent verbal output characterizes Broca's aphasia. Spontaneous speech is sparse, effortful, dysarthric, dysprosodic, short in phrase length, and agrammatic. Decreased fluency occurs in the presence of relatively preserved comprehension (although relational words such as "above" and "behind" may be poorly understood), abnormal repetition and naming, a disturbance in reading (particularly for relational and syntactic words), and disturbed writing. Most patients with Broca's aphasia have right-sided weakness varying from mild paresis to total hemiplegia, and some have sensory loss as well. Apraxia of the left limb and buccal-lingual apraxia are common. The neuropathology involves the left hemisphere frontal operculum containing Broca's area (Figure 12–3). If the lesion is superficial and involves only the cortex, the prognosis for improvement is good. However, if the lesion extends sufficiently deep to involve the basal ganglia and internal capsule, the language defect tends to be permanent. Evidence from neuroimaging studies implicates the anterior insula in the genesis of nonfluency, probably because of alterations of speech praxis (Peach 2004).

WERNICKE'S APHASIA

The most striking abnormality of Wernicke's aphasia is a disturbance of comprehension, which may range from a total inability to understand spoken language to a partial difficulty in decoding the spoken word. The characteristics of Wernicke's aphasia include fluent verbal output with normal word count and phrase length; no abnormal effort, articulatory problems, or prosodic difficulties; and difficulty in repetition and in word finding. The verbal output is often empty of content words and full of paraphasic substitutions and neologisms that can be considered a form of "noise" in the phonological output system. *Jargon aphasia* refers to this output when it is extreme and unintelligible, and it must be distinguished from the "word salad" of schizophrenia (Table 12–2), in which neologisms recur and are endowed with meaning by the speaker. Often no basic neurological defects are found, but a superior quadrantanopsia may be present as a result of disconnection of part of the optic radiations (Meyer's loop) from occipital cortex. The neuropathology involves the posterior superior temporal lobe of the left hemisphere (the auditory association cortex) and, in some cases, the primary auditory sensory area as well (Figure 12–4).

CONDUCTION APHASIA

Conduction aphasia features a prominent disturbance in repetition out of proportion to any other language disturbance. Patients with conduction aphasia have fluent verbal output and a preserved ability to comprehend. Paraphasias are common, particularly substitutions of phonemes, and confrontational naming is often limited by these paraphasic intrusions. Reading aloud and writing are disturbed, but reading comprehension can be entirely normal. Apraxia of both the right and the left limb is often present; this is postulated to be related to disruption of motor sequence representations ("praxicons") in the left inferior parietal lobe or to disconnection of these representations from frontal premotor cortex. Cortical sensory loss of the left hand or the left side of the face is common. Most cases of conduction aphasia have neuropathology involving the anterior inferior parietal lobe, including the supramarginal gyrus and the arcuate fasciculus (H. Damasio and Damasio 1980), but exceptions are recognized (Mendez and Benson 1985).

GLOBAL APHASIA

A severe language impairment in which all modalities—verbal fluency, comprehension, repetition, naming, reading, and writing—are impaired is known as *global aphasia*. Most patients have a right hemiparesis or hemiplegia, a right hemisensory deficit, and a right homonymous hemianopsia. Global aphasia is usually caused by a complete infarction in the territory of the middle cerebral artery. Exceptions are noted, however, including some in which global aphasia occurs without hemiparesis due to multiple emboli (usually of cardiac origin) to the left cerebral hemisphere.

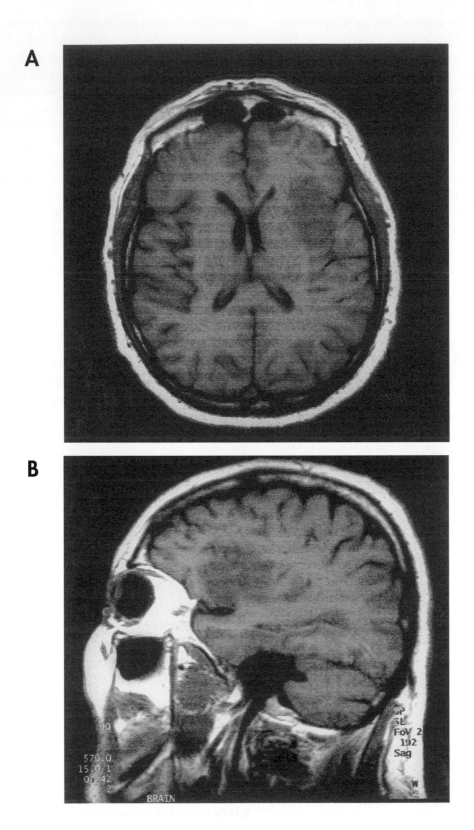

FIGURE 12–3.   Magnetic resonance images (T1 weighted) of a patient with Broca's aphasia. The horizontal (*Panel A*) and sagittal (*Panel B*) views show a stroke involving the left inferior frontal region and encompassing Broca's area.

TABLE 12–2. Comparison of language characteristics for Wernicke's aphasia, delirium, schizophrenia, and mania

	Wernicke's aphasia	Delirium	Schizophrenia	Mania
Basic language				
Fluency	Normal	Mildly abnormal	Extended	Logorrheic
Comprehension	Abnormal	Variable	Intact	Normal
Repetition	Abnormal	Mildly abnormal	Intact	Normal
Naming	Abnormal	Nonaphasic	Intact	Normal
Reading comprehension	Abnormal	Variable	Intact	Normal
Writing	Abnormal	Abnormal	Resembles spoken output	Normal
Other examination				
Word-list generation	Diminished	Abnormal	Diminished on average, bizarre	Increased
Automatic speech	Paraphasic	Normal	Normal, bizarre	Normal
Content of speech	Empty	Incoherent	Impoverished, bizarre, restricted	Grandiose
Neologisms and paraphasias	Common	Absent	Rare (stable meaning)	
Prosody	Normal	Mildly abnormal	Mildly abnormal	Mildly abnormal
Motor speech	Normal	Dysarthric and incoherent	Possible clanging	Press of speech
Associated features				
Thinking		Confused	Special productions	Rapid, flight of ideas
Awareness of deficit	Present	Partial	Absent	Absent
Neurological examination	Possibly abnormal	Possibly abnormal	Normal	Normal

TRANSCORTICAL APHASIAS

The major factor underlying transcortical aphasias is the relative preservation of the ability to repeat spoken language in the presence of other language impairments. Transcortical motor aphasia resembles Broca's aphasia in its decreased verbal fluency but differs in the normal or nearly normal ability to repeat. Patients with this disorder present the strange picture of struggling to utter words in spontaneous conversation but of easily saying the same words on repetition. Transcortical sensory aphasia resembles Wernicke's aphasia in its fluent paraphasic output and decreased comprehension but differs in the preserved ability to repeat. In its extreme version, the patient tends to have echolalia. Patients with this disorder may manifest the peculiar tendency to repeat everything that the examiner says, as if mimicking him or her. This tendency to echolalia can lead to the misdiagnosis of the aphasia as a factitious or primary psychiatric condition. These patients often complete common expressions or nursery rhymes (completion phenomenon) and may repair grammatical errors when repeating phrases.

The neuropathological lesion underlying transcortical motor aphasia is in the supplementary motor area of the left hemisphere or between that area and the frontal operculum. In cases of transcortical sensory aphasia, the lesion is generally in the left posterior superior or middle temporal gyri. The transcortical aphasia syndromes may result from watershed infarction in the anterior or posterior border zones.

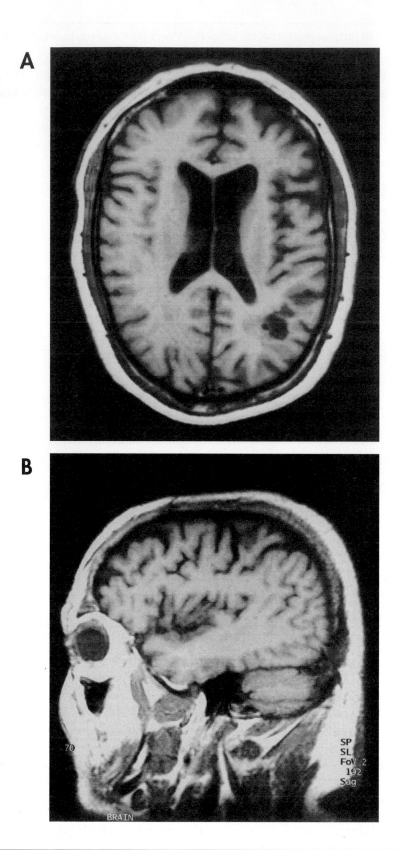

FIGURE 12–4.   Magnetic resonance images (T1 weighted) of a patient with Wernicke's aphasia. The horizontal (*Panel A*) and sagittal (*Panel B*) views show an embolic stroke involving the left temporal lobe and encompassing Wernicke's area.

The most common site of neuropathology in transcortical sensory aphasia is in the angular gyrus in the left parietal region. Mixed transcortical aphasia, also known as isolation of the speech area, is the transcortical equivalent of global aphasia. Patients with this disorder may be entirely unable to speak or to comprehend language, but they are able to repeat spoken words. The neuropathology in the mixed transcortical syndrome involves the vascular border zone or watershed areas in both the frontal and the parietal lobes. Some patients with transcortical aphasia have widespread pathology with involvement of the frontal lobes. In these cases, the echolalia is a manifestation of environmental dependency.

ANOMIC APHASIA

Anomic aphasia is a common residual effect following improvement from other types of aphasia (Maher and Raymer 2004). Although verbal output is fluent and repetition and comprehension are intact, naming to confrontation is significantly disturbed. Patients have multiple word-finding pauses, a tendency to circumlocution, and a somewhat stumbling verbal output. Many individuals with anomic aphasia also have reading and writing disturbances (alexia and agraphia). There is no specific causative location, although neuropathology often involves the left hemisphere angular gyrus. Anomic aphasia also has been reported with lesions of the left temporal pole, but some investigators have documented poor access to words within specific categories, depending on the location of the lesion within higher associative cortex (H. Damasio et al. 1996).

SUBCORTICAL APHASIA

With the advent of brain imaging, it became apparent that predominant subcortical lesions (hemorrhage or infarction) could produce acute aphasia syndromes or variable symptomatology (Nadeau and Crosson 1997). Subcortical aphasias characteristically begin with a period of mutism followed by a period of abnormal motor speech, usually hypophonia and articulatory difficulty. As recovery ensues, patients regain much of their speech but are left with paraphasic errors. Similar to the transcortical aphasias, repetition is near normal, and comprehension, naming, reading, and writing may or may not show abnormality. If the lesion is entirely subcortical, recovery usually ensues; many individuals recover totally from the aphasia but are left with residual speech impairments. Some studies suggest that basal ganglia or thalamic lesions alone are insufficient to produce permanent aphasia and that cortical involvement is necessary to produce

permanent language changes (Bhatia and Marsden 1994). Moreover, recent evidence from diffusion- and perfusion-weighted imaging suggests that such transient aphasia may occur only in the context of cortical hypoperfusion during the acute period following infarction (Hillis et al. 2004).

AMELODIA OR APROSODIA

In addition to the classic aphasia syndromes from left hemisphere damage, several related disturbances of communication result from right hemisphere lesions. The right hemisphere has a dominant role for emotional features, including emotional prosodic aspects of communication (Borod 1992). Amelodia (also called affective motor aprosodia) is a disturbance characterized by loss of melody, prosody, or emotional intonation in verbal output (Ross 1981). The individual has a flat, monotonous verbal output; inability to produce a melody when singing (expressive amusia); decreased facial grimacing; and sparse use of gestures. The result is a seemingly emotionless response easily misinterpreted as depression.

The neuropathology of amelodia involves the right frontal opercular area or its connection, the right hemisphere equivalent of Broca's area. Inasmuch as the causative lesion may be small and otherwise silent, the patient who appears depressed and is unable to produce melody deserves special consideration for neuroimaging. In addition, receptive amusias and other disorders of melody recognition are related disturbances predominantly associated with right hemisphere lesions (Hielscher 2004; Pearce 2005).

VERBAL DYSDECORUM

Verbal dysdecorum is characterized by a decreased ability to monitor and control the content of verbal output (Alexander et al. 1989). Although language itself is not defective in verbal dysdecorum, the serious psychosocial problems caused by poorly monitored output have a neurobiological source. Individuals with verbal dysdecorum speak too freely, discuss improper topics, make snide or cruel (but often true) remarks about themselves and others, argue, and are otherwise disagreeable without realizing the social consequences of their actions. Often these patients' presenting complaint is an inability to maintain friendships, and even a short exposure to such an individual identifies the problem. Verbal dysdecorum may or may not be associated with confabulation or with physical impropriety, and it must be distinguished from manic verbal output with press of speech (see Table 12–2). Current evidence suggests a right hemisphere frontal, probably lateral convexity, site of neuropathology (Alexander et al. 1989), although the disorder also may be seen in the disinhibition syndrome associated with orbitofrontal lesions and with right anterior temporal disorders. The most common causes of verbal dysdecorum are trauma, other focal lesions affecting the frontal lobes, and frontotemporal dementia.

MISCELLANEOUS DISORDERS

Several other disorders of communication may occur and are relevant to the subsequent discussion of neuropsychiatric phenomena. The alexias are language disturbances characterized by the inability to read and may or may not be accompanied by agraphia, the inability to write. Pure word deafness is a disturbance of language comprehension at the prelanguage level (see Figure 12–2). Aphemia is a disturbance of language production at the postlanguage level. Unless preserved language ability is shown in the written modality, clinicians may mistake pure word deafness, aphemia, and even auditory agnosia for the aphasia syndromes. The apraxias, or disturbances in the execution of learned motor acts, often accompany aphasias and require the interpretation of a language command prior to the execution of a motor response. Disorders of speech, or the neuromotor aspects of verbal communication, involve not only the dysarthrias and mutism but also reiterative speech disorders such as palilalia (repetition of one's own words or phrases), acquired stuttering (repetition of syllables), and logoclonia (specific repetition of the end syllables of words). In addition, the verbal output of delirium includes incoherence and nonaphasic misnaming, and clinicians must be able to distinguish the language of delirium from jargon aphasia and the language of psychiatric disorders (see Table 12–2).

Aphasia is an integral part of the multiple cognitive deficits that characterize the dementias (Kramer and Duffy 1996). Patients with Alzheimer's disease usually progress from early word-finding difficulty to a syndrome resembling transcortical sensory aphasia (albeit typically without echolalia or other phenomena, such as completion). In patients with vascular dementia, there may be a range of aphasia syndromes, given the variability in stroke location. The frontotemporal dementias, such as Pick's disease, are characterized by early verbal dysdecorum and decreased word-list generation and gradually progress to reiterative speech disturbances such as echolalia, decreased verbal output, and eventual mutism. In most other dementias, patients have decreased word-list generation and poor confrontational naming.

Asymmetric neurodegeneration of the cortex can result in a primary progressive aphasia syndrome. Autopsy usually identifies histopathological changes consistent with a frontotemporal lobar degeneration, such as Pick's bodies, "dementia lacking distinctive histology," or tau-negative, ubiquitin-positive inclusion bodies indistinguishable from those seen in amyotrophic lateral sclerosis. In about 20% of cases, the microscopic examination indicates changes of Alzheimer's disease.

Primary progressive aphasia may be fluent or nonfluent. Mesulam's criteria group all of these patients into a single progressive aphasia category, regardless of fluency. The Neary criteria, however, provide for the diagnosis of *progressive nonfluent aphasia*, a disorder characterized by the insidious onset and gradual progression of anomia, agrammatism, or phonemic paraphasias (Westbury and Bud 1997), and a fluent type termed *semantic dementia* (Hodges et al. 1992). Despite preserved speech sound, word, and sentence production in spontaneous speech, patients with semantic dementia lose the meanings of words. This manifests not only as impaired confrontational naming but also as disrupted passive naming (i.e., single word comprehension) and a failure to benefit from phonological cues. In addition to the language disorder, patients with semantic dementia may develop agnosia, or loss of knowledge, for objects and thus may be unable to recognize them or describe their use. Recent imaging studies indicate that the syndrome of progressive nonfluent aphasia is associated with left inferior frontal atrophy, whereas semantic dementia is associated with disproportionate involvement of the left anterior temporal lobe (Gorno-Tempini et al. 2004). After a period of 2 or more years of predominant language impairment, patients with these progressive aphasia syndromes usually develop impairment of other cognitive domains with an accompanying functional decline that qualifies them for the diagnosis of dementia. This dementia may bear clinical similarity to frontotemporal dementia, Alzheimer's disease, or some other dementing disease (Green et al. 1990).

Apraxia, agnosia, and Gerstmann's syndrome may accompany a language disorder and could contribute to the neuropsychiatric consequences of aphasia. Apraxia is an acquired impairment in learned motor movements not due to primarily motor or sensory deficits. The examination for apraxia involves asking the patient to perform learned movements such as waving goodbye and pantomiming brushing his or her teeth. If the patient fails a task, the examiner should demonstrate the movement and ask the patient to imitate it. Apraxia may result from damage to motor programs, disconnection of language from the areas for motor control, or the inability to understand concepts. The agnosias are disorders of recognition that may complicate aphasia. Agnosias may be visual or auditory or involve another modality, and they are often classified as either associative or apperceptive. *Associative agnosia* refers to a normal perception that is disconnected from its other associations and meanings. *Apperceptive agnosia* implies a problem with recognition because of subtle disturbances in perceptual processing. Finally, some patients may have Gerstmann's syndrome from involvement of the left angular gyrus. In addition to agraphia, these patients have right-left confusion and difficulty with finger recognition ("finger agnosia"). Another component of Gerstmann's syndrome is difficulty manipulating numbers or numerical concepts ("acalculia"). All of these cognitive disturbances can contribute to the neuropsychiatric consequences of language impairment.

NEUROPSYCHIATRIC ASPECTS OF APHASIA

Patients with aphasias or related disorders often have neuropsychiatric disturbances that may be more debilitating than the language impairment itself. Lack of awareness of these disturbances stems in part from the fact that the language disorder interferes with communication and with the psychiatric assessment of patients. The behavioral assessment of aphasic patients through their language impairment requires a great deal of skill and expertise. In the following sections, we discuss the neuropsychiatric aspects of aphasia as psychiatric aspects, cognitive aspects, and psychosocial aspects.

PSYCHIATRIC ASPECTS

Two distinct, long-term behavioral syndromes accompany aphasia syndromes. One accompanies nonfluent (anterior) aphasia, and the other appears in cases of fluent (posterior) aphasia (Benson 1973).

Anterior Aphasia Behavioral Syndrome

Persons with Broca's aphasia or transcortical motor aphasia know exactly what they wish to say, but their verbal output is restricted and barely intelligible. This inability to explain their wishes or thoughts in other than telegraphic words can cause intense frustration. These nonfluent aphasic patients may manifest their attempts to communicate with agitated gestures and expletives.

Depression is another aspect of the anterior aphasia behavioral reaction. Nonfluent aphasic patients develop intense feelings of personal worthlessness and hopelessness. Depression is considerably more common and intense in patients with anterior aphasia than in those with posterior aphasia (Robinson 1997). This is due in part to the patient's ability to recognize the disability and the frustration of not being able to express thoughts and desires, but the depression has neurobiological causes as well.

The occurrence of depression correlates with acute strokes in the left prefrontal region and surrounding areas (Robinson and Szetela 1981). The depressive reaction typically starts with feelings of futility that lead to an unwillingness to participate in self-care or in rehabilitation activities. During the depressed period, aphasic patients may sink deep within themselves; stop eating; refuse social interaction with therapists, other patients, or even family members; and manifest a strong but passive noncooperation. In rare instances, the negative reaction may become intense and explosive, a catastrophic reaction. Although the depression, frustration, and catastrophic reaction of the patient with anterior aphasia suggest a strong potential for suicide, it is rarely reported in this group.

Posterior Aphasia Behavioral Syndrome

Most patients with posterior aphasia have difficulty comprehending spoken language and remain unaware of their deficit, producing a persistent unconcern that is pathological. Because they are unable to monitor their own verbal output, they often fail to realize that they are producing an incomprehensible jargon. In fact, when tape recordings of such jargon have been made and then replayed immediately, many patients with posterior aphasia deny that it is their own speech. The persistent unawareness and unconcern in patients with posterior aphasia stand in sharp contrast to the frustrated, depressed condition in individuals with anterior aphasia.

Paranoia with agitation, another aspect of posterior aphasia behavioral syndrome, occurs when damage is limited to the posterior temporal lobe (Wernicke's aphasia). This feature is much less common in patients with transcortical sensory aphasia and is virtually unknown in those with anterior aphasia. Paranoid behavior is also universally present in the prelanguage disorder of pure word deafness. Unaware of their own comprehension disturbance, individuals with posterior aphasia or pure word deafness tend to blame their communication difficulties on others. They suggest that the person they are talking to is not speaking clearly or is not paying sufficient attention. Some of these patients come to believe that persons they observe talking together must be using a special code because their conversation cannot be understood. This reaction is similar to the paranoid reaction of acquired deafness, but the paranoia also has neurobiological causes. A paranoid reaction correlates with lesions in the left temporal lobe, suggesting that damage to this anatomical region facilitates the perception of threat.

In addition, some patients with posterior aphasia have impulsive behavior. The combination of unawareness, paranoia, and impulsiveness makes them potentially dangerous to others. Physical attacks against medical personnel, family members, or other patients can occur, particularly when the patients misinterpret the behaviors of others. Almost all aphasic patients who need custodial management because of dangerous behavior have a posterior fluent aphasia (Benson and Geschwind 1985). Moreover, compared with patients having anterior aphasia with depression, those having posterior aphasia with both paranoia and impulsiveness tend to commit suicide more often, particularly as self-awareness of their deficit occurs.

Behavior in Primary Progressive Aphasia

The clinical syndromes of primary progressive aphasia and semantic dementia are most often associated with frontotemporal lobar degeneration. In addition to aphasia, frontotemporal lobar degeneration manifests prominent neuropsychiatric abnormalities, including apathy, depression, anxiety, elation, disinhibition, eating disorders, and sleep disorders. Certain of these findings are associated with the neuroanatomical focus of the disease. For instance, sleep disturbances are more prevalent among patients with predominant temporal lobe atrophy, a finding that is associated with the syndrome of semantic dementia (Liu et al. 2004), and apathy is significantly more common in patients with predominant frontal lobe atrophy. Consequently, patients with progressive nonfluent aphasia may develop apathy with a diminution of overall verbal output. Initial anxiety and depression over their language deficit gradually give way to lack of concern or insight for their impairment. The frontal behavior changes also lead to disinhibited commentary, compulsive utterances, and reiterative speech changes. In contrast, patients with semantic dementia may become suspicious or confused over their inability to be understood. With increasing left temporal involvement, patients with semantic dementia can be plagued by complex compulsions, and with increasing right temporal involvement, they may lose all interpersonal warmth and fail to recognize emotion and prosody in speech.

Compulsive behaviors are common in all forms of frontotemporal lobar degeneration and may constitute a source of caregiver stress. Selective serotonin reuptake inhibitors may suppress these compulsions, significantly improving quality of life for the patient and caregiver.

COGNITIVE ASPECTS

Aphasic patients often present initially with delirium followed by a period of decreased insight into the existence of their language deficit. If the brain insult is sufficiently large, the patient with aphasia is lethargic or has a clouding of consciousness from the cerebral edema, diaschisis, and other acute neuropathological changes. After resolution of the initial delirium, in days to weeks, a more prolonged period ensues in which the aphasic patient fails to realize fully the alterations that have occurred. Although alert and responsive, the patient does not yet grasp the significance of the language defect. At this stage, the patient cannot participate rationally in plans for the future because of a decreased appreciation of reality. As previously discussed, some patients with posterior aphasia have a permanent impairment in awareness and concern, but for most, the insight that they are language impaired eventually dawns on them, sometimes rather acutely, and can lead directly to reactive depression.

Language facilitates thought. Among aphasic individuals, thinking processes are less efficient because of language deficits. Following Bastian, who in 1898 declared that humans think in words, many experts have emphasized the symbolic nature of cognition and have concluded that defective use of language symbols produces defective thinking. Kurt Goldstein accepted aphasia as proof that thinking was abnormal, either regressed or concrete. Furthermore, pathology of the posterior language area may be more likely than anterior damage to interfere with intellectual competency (Benson 1979).

Despite these observations, the studies of intelligence in aphasic patients have provided somewhat nebulous results (Hamsher 1981; Josse and Tzourio-Mazoyer 2004). Most aphasic patients perform poorly on standard tests of intellectual competency, sometimes in both verbal and nonverbal portions, but many retain considerable nonverbal capability. Standard IQ tests, however, emphasize language skills and thus exaggerate intellectual deficits among aphasic patients. Moreover, most intelligence studies treat aphasia as a single, unitary disturbance, failing to note that intellectual dysfunction varies considerably with the specific aphasia syndrome and the locus of neuropathology. In real life, the examiner must base a decision about the intellectual competence of an aphasic patient on observations; test results alone are not sufficient. Important information—such as retaining social graces; counting; making change; showing appropriate concern about family, business, and personal activities; finding their way about; socializing; and showing self-concern—may provide valuable indications of residual intelligence in individuals with aphasia.

PSYCHOSOCIAL ASPECTS

An important but easily overlooked factor affecting most individuals with acquired aphasia stems from the sudden, unexpected, and truly calamitous alteration of lifestyle produced by the language disorder. In many aphasic patients, the magnitude of the loss of language is overwhelming. Language is such a basic human function that, in shock value, its acute loss ranks with sudden blindness, quadriplegia, or the diagnosis of an incurable disease. Along with the sudden loss of this critical function, many of the stabilizing factors of personal existence are lost. Because of the losses incurred, aphasic patients may enter a period of bereavement, grief reaction, or reactive depression. As a rule, however, such feelings are delayed after the onset of acquired language impairment and may build over weeks, months, or even years.

The onset of aphasia disrupts previously secure patterns of interaction and communication in both social activities and employment. The changes in social status do not occur immediately, and realization of the degree of change may not occur for some time after its onset. If the language disturbance is relatively mild, the aphasic individual may retain or eventually regain his or her previous status within the family, but when the language disturbance is more severe, the spouse or another family member must assume much of the decision-making role. Aphasia can place an individual in a passive, childlike position within the family, and he or she may need help to carry out even basic everyday activities. Not infrequently, the reaction to this downgrading of family status is violent, with negative, hostile, and sometimes cruel behavior directed toward close family members. Some families are incapable of successfully managing this transition. The spouse often feels and expresses anger and hostility because of decreased income, altered social position, and numerous added responsibilities.

Physical limitations may aggravate the adjustment to the language disorder. Aphasia usually occurs in the context of stroke or other brain disorder, resulting in additional neurological impairments. Hemiparesis, balance insecurity, visual field defect, unilateral attention disorder, pain, paresthesias, epileptic seizures, the need for major medical or surgical treatments, and many other physical problems plague these patients. Among patients with aphasia, sexual maladjustment is a potential problem that can be missed by physicians and therapists. A major degree of paralysis, an inability to communicate accurately, and an underlying uncertainty of residual sexual competency can hinder healthy sexual relationships. In most instances, however, the acquired lack of sexuality is physiologically unfounded.

Legal capacity for decision making is another psychosocial consideration for aphasic patients. Many aphasic patients can manage their own affairs, whereas others are obviously unable to make decisions and deserve the protection of a conservator or a guardian. Informed medical opinion is often needed to determine whether an aphasic patient has sufficient language and comprehension to sign checks or business papers, to dispense money, to manage property or other holdings, to make a will or other testamentary documents, and so forth. A physician should evaluate and carefully record the patient's ability to comprehend both spoken and written language and to express personal decisions. Special procedures are necessary if a legal act (e.g., signing a will or entering into a contract) is to be performed by an aphasic patient. In addition to receiving added explanations, the document in question should be reviewed with the patient until both the physician and the attorney are satisfied that the patient understands its basic meaning. Such a procedure may require several sessions, and for practical reasons, the document should be kept short, simple, and as free as possible of legal jargon. An even more difficult problem arises when a physician is asked to provide retrospective testimony about an aphasic patient's legal competency, such as the question of whether a patient did or did not understand a legal document consummated after the onset of aphasia. A physician's testimony can relate only to a description of the patient's ability to understand spoken and written language and the ability to express ideas.

PROGNOSIS AND TREATMENT

Most poststroke aphasia patients recover significant language function (Ansaldo et al. 2004; Benson and Ardila 1996; Robey 1998). Patients with anomic or conduction aphasia have an excellent recovery and are often left with some more minor degree of language impairment. Many patients with initial Broca's or Wernicke's aphasia recover to anomic or conduction aphasia. The exception is patients with initial global aphasia. In general, these patients have a poor prognosis for recovery of functional language. In addition, patients with aphasia due to dementia or primary progressive aphasia continue to have a slowly progressive deterioration in their language ability, eventually complicated by deficits in other areas of cognition.

The treatment for aphasia requires a careful assessment, usually performed by a speech-language pathologist. The assessment includes evaluation with one of the commonly used aphasia tests, such as the Boston Diagnostic Aphasia Examination, the Psycholinguistic Assessment of Language Processing in Aphasia, or the Communicative Abilities of Daily Living (Lezak 1994). The therapist then formulates a therapy program based on specific goals. In addition to traditional rote repetition and rehearsal, a range of other language therapy techniques are available. These include stimulation-facilitation techniques such as melodic intonation therapy and emotional speech techniques (Benson and Ardila 1996; Reuterskiold 1991). Some techniques focus on modular treatments aimed at specific deficits, such as verbal fluency. Other techniques focus on functional improvement, caregiver interventions, manual or visual symbol systems, use of communication aids, or more recent neurocognitive and psycholinguistic approaches. Whatever the program, a significant emphasis is directed toward positive language competency, allowing few failures and rewarding all successes.

Drug treatments for language disturbances have had little success. Although bromocriptine, bupropion, and methylamphetamine have improved fluency in some nonfluent patients, more rigorous studies have failed to show significant benefits (Gupta et al. 1995; Walker-Batson et al. 2001). In addition, some aphasic patients need extensive rehabilitation measures other than speech and language therapy. These measures include physical therapy, gait training, mechanical aids such as crutches and leg braces, recreational therapy, and occupational therapy, including instruction and training in activities of daily living.

Despite the language disturbance, many forms of psychotherapy may be useful for aphasic patients, not the least of which is the support provided by family members, nursing staff, therapists, physicians, and others in contact with the patient. A positive transference almost always occurs between the patient with aphasia and the speech-language pathologist, a phenomenon that can be used therapeutically. Most language therapists, however, are not formally trained in psychotherapy, and they may become discouraged, for example, if the patient's psychiatric manifestations obviate good language rehabilitation. Moreover, the comprehension deficit of patients with posterior aphasia precludes more traditional insight-oriented psychotherapy. These barriers need to be considered and overcome. Group psychotherapy, when possible, can decrease feelings of isolation and also can provide encouragement as patients observe improvements in others. Finally, family counseling often represents a crucial factor in the successful management of an aphasic patient's neuropsychiatric problems.

Among patients with an aphasia syndrome, the early recognition of a mood disorder is critical to the treatment of depression. Awareness of the onset of depression in an aphasic patient should be immediately followed by supportive measures. Challenging therapies (e.g., language, occupational, and physical) should be halted and replaced with activities that the patient can perform successfully. The patient should not be allowed to fail, particularly at tasks that would be considered simple and mundane in normal life. Careful monitoring is needed, and suicide precautions may become necessary, particularly for patients with posterior aphasia. Physicians often use antidepressant medications, particularly for the depression of patients with anterior aphasia. Because aphasic patients are often elderly and have cardiovascular disease, selective serotonin reuptake inhibitors are usually the medications of choice. Drugs such as sertraline and paroxetine have been beneficial in relieving symptoms of depression in these patients.

In addition to antidepressants, a range of psychoactive medications can be useful in the management of aphasic patients. Benzodiazepines can help alleviate anxiety and hyperactivity, but their potential suppression of learning and memory may impede rehabilitation. Atypical antipsychotics, such as quetiapine, olanzapine, and risperidone, are useful in selected aphasic patients, especially those with posterior aphasia who have impulsive, paranoid behavior. Patients with Wernicke's aphasia and pure word deafness who are given these psychotropic medications appear to have less agitation and are more compliant with rehabilitation measures. Doses should be kept low to avoid interference with residual mental functions. When brain damage causes apathy, lethargy, and decreased drive, judicious use of a stimulant such as methylphenidate could be beneficial. Again, these drugs need to be monitored carefully because of the increased susceptibility of brain-damaged patients to potential complications.

CONCLUSION

Patients with aphasia and related disorders often have significant psychiatric, cognitive, and psychosocial complications. These changes result from their altered ability to communicate, from their compromised personal and social status, and directly from the brain lesion itself. The neuropsychiatric aspects of aphasia hamper language rehabilitation and may produce serious dysfunction. The optimal management of aphasic patients does not stop with language therapy but also requires competence in the management of the neuropsychiatric aspects of these syndromes.

Highlights for the Clinician

✦ The aphasias are disturbances of the brain's use of symbols.

✦ In addition to language impairment, the aphasias can result in devastating neuropsychiatric manifestations.

✦ The different aphasic syndromes can be organized by the Wernicke-Geschwind model of language in the brain.

✦ These syndromes are characterized by the language examination, which assesses fluency, comprehension, naming, repetition, reading, and writing.

✦ The aphasias must be distinguished from the language manifestations of delirium, schizophrenia, and mania.

✦ The anterior aphasic syndrome is characterized by frustration, depression, and a possible catastrophic reaction.

✦ The posterior aphasic syndrome is characterized by unawareness and unconcern, paranoia with agitation, and impulsive behavior.

✦ The aphasias result in multiple additional cognitive and psychosocial issues, such as major alterations in lifestyle with significant social and occupational limitations.

✦ The aphasias include a range of considerations that affect prognosis and treatment.

RECOMMENDED READINGS

Berthier ML: Poststroke aphasia: epidemiology, pathophysiology and treatment. Drugs Aging 22:163–182, 2005

Grossman M, Ash S: Primary progressive aphasia: a review. Neurocase 10:3–18, 2004

REFERENCES

Alexander MP, Benson DE, Stuss DT: Frontal lobes and language. Brain Lang 37:641–691, 1989

Ansaldo AI, Arguin M, Lecours AR: Recovery from aphasia: a longitudinal study on language recovery, lateralization patterns, and attentional resources. J Clin Exp Neuropsychol 26:621–627, 2004

Benson DF: Psychiatric aspects of aphasia. Br J Psychiatry 123:555–566, 1973

Benson DF: Aphasia, Alexia, and Agraphia. New York, Churchill Livingstone, 1979

Benson DF, Ardila A: Aphasia: A Clinical Approach. New York, Oxford University Press, 1996

Benson DF, Geschwind N: The aphasias and related disturbances, in Clinical Neurology, Vol 1. Edited by Baker AB, Joynt R. Philadelphia, PA, Harper & Row, 1985, pp 1–34

Bhatia KP, Marsden CD: The behavioural and motor consequences of focal lesions of the basal ganglia in man. Brain 117:859–876, 1994

Borod JC: Interhemispheric and intrahemispheric control of emotion: a focus on unilateral brain damage. J Consult Clin Psychol 60:339–348, 1992

Catani M, Jones DK, Ffytche DH: Perisylvian language networks of the brain. Ann Neurol 57:8–16, 2005

Chomsky N: Language and Mind, 2nd Edition. New York, Harcourt Brace Jovanovich, 1972

Clark DG, Charuvastra A, Miller BL, et al: Fluent versus nonfluent primary progressive aphasia: a comparison of clinical and functional neuroimaging features. Brain Lang 94:54–60, 2005

Damasio AR: Aphasia. N Engl J Med 326:531–539, 1992

Damasio AR, Tranel D: Nouns and verbs are retrieved with differently distributed neural systems. Proc Natl Acad Sci U S A 90:4957–4960, 1993

Damasio H, Damasio A: The anatomical basis of conduction aphasia. Brain 103:337–350, 1980

Damasio H, Grabowski TJ, Tranel D, et al: A neural basis for lexical retrieval. Nature 380:499–505, 1996

Geschwind N: Disconnexion syndromes in animals and man. Brain 88:237–294, 585–644, 1965

Gorno-Tempini ML, Dronkers NF, Rankin KP, et al: Cognition and anatomy in three variants of primary progressive aphasia. Ann Neurol 55:335–346, 2004

Green J, Morris JC, Sandson J, et al: Progressive aphasia: a precursor of global dementia? Neurology 40:423–429, 1990

Gupta SR, Mlcoch G, Scolaro C, et al: Bromocriptine treatment of nonfluent aphasia. Neurology 45:2170–2173, 1995

Hamsher K: Intelligence and aphasia, in Acquired Aphasia. Edited by Sarno MT. New York, Academic Press, 1981, pp 327–359

Hauser MD, Chomsky N, Fitch WT: The faculty of language: what is it, who has it, and how did it evolve? Science 298:1569–1579, 2002

Hielscher M: Comprehension of emotional information in patients with aphasia. Folia Phoniatr Logop 56:14–26, 2004

Hillis AE, Boatman D, Hart J, et al: Making sense out of jargon: a neurolinguistic and computational account of jargon aphasia. Neurology 53:1813–1824, 1999

Hillis AE, Barker PB, Wityk RJ, et al: Variability in subcortical aphasia is due to variable sites of cortical hypoperfusion. Brain Lang 89:524–530, 2004

Hodges JR, Patterson K, Oxbury S, et al: Semantic dementia. Brain 115:1783–1806, 1992

Josse G, Tzourio-Mazoyer N: Hemispheric specialization for language. Brain Res Brain Res Rev 44:1–12, 2004

Kertesz A: Aphasia and Associated Disorders. New York, Grune & Stratton, 1979

Kirschner HS (ed): Handbook of Neurological Speech and Language Disorders. New York, Marcel Dekker, 1995

Kramer JH, Duffy JM: Aphasia, apraxia, and agnosia in the diagnosis of dementia. Dementia 7:23–26, 1996

Lezak M: Neuropsychological Assessment, 3rd Edition. New York, Oxford University Press, 1994

Liu W, Miller BL, Kramer JH, et al: Behavioral disorders in the frontal and temporal variants of frontotemporal dementia. Neurology 62:742–748, 2004

Maher LM, Raymer AM: Management of anomia. Top Stroke Rehabil 11:10–21, 2004

Mendez MF, Benson DE: Atypical conduction aphasia: a disconnection syndrome. Arch Neurol 42:886–891, 1985

Muller R-A, Rothermel RD, Behen ME, et al: Receptive and expressive language activation for sentences. Neuroreport 8:3767–3770, 1997

Nadeau SE, Crosson B: Subcortical aphasia. Brain Lang 58:355–402, 1997

Peach RK: Acquired apraxia of speech: features, accounts, and treatment. Top Stroke Rehabil 11:49–58, 2004

Pearce JM: Selected observations on amusia. Eur Neurol 54:145–148, 2005

Pedersen PM, Jorgensen HS, Nakayama H, et al: Aphasia in acute stroke: incidence, determinants, and recovery. Ann Neurol 38:659–666, 1995

Reuterskiold C: The effects of emotionality on auditory comprehension in aphasia. Cortex 27:595–604, 1991

Robey RR: A meta-analysis of clinical outcomes in the treatment of aphasia. J Speech Lang Hear Res 41:172–187, 1998

Robinson RG: Neuropsychiatric consequences of stroke. Annu Rev Med 48:217–229, 1997

Robinson R, Szetela B: Mood change following left hemisphere brain injury. Ann Neurol 9:447–453, 1981

Ross ED: The aprosodias: functional-anatomic organization of the affective components of language in the right hemisphere. Arch Neurol 38:561–569, 1981

Walker-Batson D, Curtis S, Natarajan R, et al: A double-blind, placebo-controlled study of the use of amphetamine in the treatment of aphasia. Stroke 32:2093–2098, 2001

Westbury C, Bud D: Primary progressive aphasia: a review of 112 cases. Brain Lang 60:381–406, 1997

13

NEUROPSYCHIATRIC ASPECTS OF AGGRESSION AND IMPULSE-CONTROL DISORDERS

Eric Hollander, M.D.
Heather A. Berlin, Ph.D., M.P.H.

The concepts of impulsivity and aggression play important roles not only in clinical psychiatry but also in everyday life. *Impulsivity* is defined as the failure to resist an impulse, drive, or temptation that is harmful to oneself or others. Impulsive behavior is impetuous and lacks deliberation. An impulse may be sudden in onset and transitory, or a gradual increase in tension may reach a crescendo in an explosive expression of the impulse, resulting in violence without regard for self or others. What makes an impulse pathological is an inability to resist it and its expression in an inappropriate environment.

Aggression is any form of behavior directed toward harm or injury of another person. It constitutes a multideterminated act that often results in physical (or verbal) injury to others, self, or objects. The behavioral manifestations of aggression are characterized by heightened vigilance and enhanced readiness to attack. Aggressive acts may be classified as defensive, premeditated, or impulsive. *Impulsive aggression* refers to impulsive and aggressive behavior occurring simultaneously. Sometimes impulsivity has been confused with aggression. Pathological gambling, for example, is impulsive but does not necessarily involve aggression. Likewise, a premeditated, well-planned assassination attempt is aggressive but not neces-

sarily impulsive. Impulsive aggression correlates more clearly with biological indices of neurotransmitter function than does premeditated aggression. Often impulsivity and aggression are expressed together, as in antisocial personality disorder (ASPD).

Impulsivity and aggression may be part of the defining characteristics of many psychiatric illnesses, including personality disorders such as borderline personality disorder (BPD) and ASPD; neurological disorders characterized by disinhibited behavior; attention-deficit/hyperactivity disorder; substance and alcohol abuse; bulimia; and impulse-control disorders such as intermittent explosive disorder. Impulsivity is also a significant correlate of suicide and violent behavior.

The concepts of impulsivity and aggression are diagnostically nonspecific but may be viewed as dimensional constructs. A closer look at clinical syndromes characterized by these behaviors may also help elucidate the biological underpinnings of impulsivity and aggression.

Impulsive aggressive behaviors are severe behavioral disturbances with substantial associated morbidity and mortality. These behaviors may also lead to prolonged social, vocational, and family dysfunction; violent crimes (including murder, rape, robbery, and assault); accidents

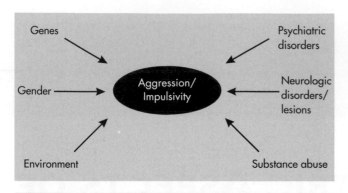

FIGURE 13–1. Factors contributing to aggression and impulsivity.

(including reckless driving); and injuries. Individuals who manifest impulsivity and aggression often become involved with the legal system and need repeated psychiatric evaluation and treatment and government financial assistance.

Clearly, the causes of impulsivity and aggression are complex and involve a combination of biological, developmental, psychosocial, and cultural factors (Figure 13–1). In this chapter, we focus on the neuropsychiatry and neurobiology of impulsivity and aggression, discuss specific disorders of impulse control, and highlight treatment strategies for managing impulsive and aggressive behavior.

EPIDEMIOLOGY

We live in a violent society. In the United States, homicide is the second leading cause of death among those 15–24 years of age. The four crimes classified as violent by the Federal Bureau of Investigation (FBI) are homicide, armed robbery, rape, and assault. Impulsivity and aggression are often the causes of crime, violence, homicide, suicide, substance abuse, and accidents and injuries. A greater percentage of the aggression in our society is associated with the young, and half of all homicides are committed by those younger than age 25. A 2000 report by the Bureau of Alcohol, Tobacco and Firearms revealed that 40.9% of crime gun possessors were 25 years of age or younger (U.S. Department of the Treasury 2002).

The highest rates of death and homicide are among young, poor, urban men. Overall, rates of death by homicide are about three times greater for men than for women. Homicide remains the leading cause of death of black men and women between ages 15 and 34. The fact that homicide is the leading cause of death for young blacks is explained partly by the low rate of natural deaths in the young in general and partly by high rates of poverty and concentration in large central cities, protecting them from the leading cause of death for young whites—motor

vehicle accidents. Much lower rates of homicide have been reported in countries such as England, Sweden, and Japan, which all have strict gun control laws.

There are more than 20,000 homicides in the United States each year, and men are three times more likely than women to be killed. In 90% of homicides, the perpetrator and victim involved are the same race, and a handgun is used in more than 50% of the murders. Alcohol use is associated with 25%–75% of homicides. Homicide often occurs in families in the context of domestic quarrels and when members have access to firearms. In domestic violence, women are more likely to attack their husbands than vice versa. The Epidemiologic Catchment Area (ECA) project suggested that the rate of family violence was increasing among both blacks and whites, particularly in the younger populations (Federal Bureau of Investigation 1991).

Aggression and impulsivity are clearly linked to violence in our society. The etiology of violence, impulsivity, and aggression is multifactorial and not fully understood. A better understanding of the biological underpinnings of violence and aggression is only a part of the remedy, and these statistics help convey the depth of the problem and the degree to which it affects our culture.

MEASUREMENTS OF IMPULSIVITY AND AGGRESSION

Direct in vitro laboratory tests of impulsivity and aggression are currently unavailable. This discussion focuses on instruments that have been specifically designed to quantify aggressive and impulsive behavior. Most studies examining the biological basis of impulsivity and aggression in humans have used either interview or self-reported assessments. Rating scales measuring aggressive or impulsive behavior have been developed, covering both personality dimensions and clinical syndromes. These rating scales have been used as tools for measuring prognosis and outcome. The scales, which can be specific or comprehensive, measure both internally experienced variables (e.g., mood) and externally observable variables (e.g., behavior).

One of the problems in measuring aggression is the potential for discrepancies between self-rating scales and observer scales. Verbal aggression is difficult to assess because it may be a function of social class and clinical status. Some patients threaten others but are not aggressive in person, whereas others store their rage and ultimately explode in anger. How a patient handles aggressive urges requires evaluation not only of what he or she says but also of past behavior. On the other hand, measurement of severe aggressive behavior (i.e., physical aggression) is often limited to observer scales because data based on the patients' own reports are likely to be biased on the basis of social desirability. Because there is social stigma attached to violent, aggressive behavior, few patients will honestly report their true behavior. In addition, patients with reduced verbal capacity or cognitive impairments (i.e., dementia) are often limited in their self-reporting. Observer scales are mainly used with moderately to severely aggressive hospitalized or institutionalized patients and are limited in distinguishing between chronic baseline aggression and exacerbations or heightened states of sporadic verbal or physical aggression.

Traditionally, before more valid and reliable instruments were developed, projective tests such as the Rorschach test or Thematic Apperception Test (TAT) were used to quantify aggression. Currently the most commonly used aggression questionnaire is the Buss-Durkee Hostility Inventory. In the subsections that follow, we summarize briefly the various strategies used to assess aggression and impulsivity in humans.

SELF-REPORT ASSESSMENTS

Buss-Durkee Hostility Inventory

The Buss-Durkee Hostility Inventory (BDHI; Buss and Durkee 1957) is the most widely used self-report assessment of aggression. It is a 75-item true/false questionnaire that measures different aspects of hostility, aggression, and danger (e.g., "I seldom strike back, even if someone hits me first: true or false"). There are eight subscales: assault, indirect hostility, irritability, negativism, resentment, suspicion, verbal hostility, and guilt. The BDHI has good test-retest reliability and good reports of positive concurrent validity.

Hostility and Direction of Hostility Questionnaire

The Hostility and Direction of Hostility Questionnaire (HDHQ; Philip 1969) is a true/false questionnaire containing 51 items derived from the Minnesota Multiphasic Personality Inventory (Hathaway and McKinley 1989). It contains five subscales, of which only one, "acting out hostility," is relevant to aggressive behavior. The HDHQ has modest to good test-retest reliability for its subscales.

Spielberger State-Trait Anger Expression Inventory

The Spielberger State-Trait Anger Expression Inventory (STAEI; Spielberger 1988) is a 44-item scale that divides behavior into state anger (i.e., current feelings) and trait anger (i.e., disposition toward angry reactions). (Sample items: "How I feel right now: I feel irritated"; "How I generally feel: I fly off the handle.") The STAEI takes about 15 minutes to complete.

Barratt Impulsiveness Scale, Version 11

The Barratt Impulsiveness Scale, version 11 (BIS-11; Patton et al. 1995) is a self-administered questionnaire of trait impulsivity with 30 items scored on a 4-point scale. The BIS-11 assesses long-term patterns of behavior; subjects are asked questions about the way they think and act without relation to any specific time period. The BIS-11 is made up of three subscales: nonplanning impulsivity (attention to details), motor impulsivity (acting without thinking), and cognitive impulsivity (future-oriented thinking and coping stability). This and previous versions of the BIS were designed primarily as research instruments to aid in the description of impulsivity in healthy individuals and to explore the role of impulsivity in psychopathology. Barratt (Barratt et al. 2005) has suggested that a Total score at or higher than 75 could indicate an impulse-control disorder, whereas a Total score in the range of 70–75 could indicate pathological impulsivity.

Massachusetts General Hospital Hairpulling Scale

The Massachusetts General Hospital (MGH) Hairpulling Scale (Keuthen et al. 1995) is a seven-item self-report questionnaire, scored on a 5-point Likert scale, that was developed to evaluate the severity of trichotillomania. This measure was modeled after the Yale-Brown Obsessive Compulsive Scale (Y-BOCS) but differs from the Y-BOCS in that it does not include questions on obsessional ideation. The MGH Hairpulling Scale assesses the urge to pull hair, the actual amount of pulling, perceived control over hair pulling, and associated distress. The scale was designed to evaluate the baseline severity of trichotillomania and to assess change in symptom severity over time. It is intended for both clinical and research settings. Because the MGH Hairpulling Scale was developed relatively recently, there are no standardized scores.

Gambling Symptom Assessment Scale

The Gambling Symptom Assessment Scale (G-SAS; Kim et al. 2001) is a 12-item self-rated scale designed to assess gambling symptom severity and change during a treatment (an outcome measure). It measures gambling urges, thoughts, and behavior. The scale was designed primarily for gamblers who have prominent gambling urges. Since almost all gamblers have urges to gamble, the scale can be applied to pathological gamblers in general, but it was not designed for those who do not have urges to gamble. Each item is scored on a 5-point scale. All items ask for an average symptom based on the past 7 days.

Kleptomania Symptom Assessment Scale

The Kleptomania Symptom Assessment Scale (K-SAS; Grant and Kim 2002) is an 11-item self-rated scale designed to measure the thoughts, urges, and behaviors associated with compulsive stealing. The scale was constructed on the basis of the observation that the thought patterns and behaviors of patients with kleptomania are similar to those of patients with substance addiction or behaviors such as compulsive gambling. The K-SAS is a modification of the G-SAS (Kim et al. 2001) and is designed to measure the change in kleptomania symptoms during treatment. Each item is scored from 0 to 4. Higher total scores reflect greater symptom severity. In two treatment samples, the mean scores ranged from 22 to 37 (Grant and Kim 2002; Grant et al. 2003).

INTERVIEW ASSESSMENTS

Life History Assessments: The Brown-Goodwin Assessment for Life History of Aggression

The Brown-Goodwin Assessment (BGA; G. Brown et al. 1979) is one of the most commonly used assessments of aggressive behavior. It is rated by a clinician on the basis of direct interview with the patient and/or review of medical records and other information about the patient (including information from informants). The BGA has 11 assessments of aggression: temper, fighting, assault, school discipline, civilian discipline, antisocial behavior not involving police, antisocial behavior involving police, military discipline, military judicial discipline, property damage, and verbal aggression.

Pathological Gambling Modification of the Yale-Brown Obsessive Compulsive Scale

The Pathological Gambling Modification of the Yale-Brown Obsessive Compulsive Scale (PG-YBOCS; DeCaria et al. 1998) was modified from the original reliable and valid Y-BOCS (Goodman et al. 1989a, 1989b). Although a relatively new measure, PG-YBOCS is one of the most widely used clinician-rated measures of PG. It consists of 10 clinician-administered questions that measure the severity of pathological gambling over a recent time interval (usually within the past 1–2 weeks). The first five questions assess urges and thoughts associated with pathological gambling, whereas the last five questions assess the behavioral component of the disorder. Both sets of questions focus on time occupied by gambling, interfer-

ence due to gambling, distress associated with gambling, resistance against gambling, and degree of control over gambling, which corresponds to DSM-IV criteria for pathological gambling (American Psychiatric Association 1994). Scores of 0 through 4 are assigned according to the severity of the response. Each set of questions is totaled separately as well as together for a total score.

South Oaks Gambling Screen— Interview or Self-Report

The South Oaks Gambling Screen (SOGS; Lesieur and Blume 1987, 1993), developed as a quantifiable structured instrument to assess pathological gambling, is a 20-item questionnaire that can be administered in either interview (by professionals and nonprofessionals) or self-report format. The SOGS may also be completed by an informant to provide a cross-check of an individual's responses. Although the SOGS questions do not correspond exactly with either DSM-III-R (American Psychiatric Association 1987) or DSM-IV criteria for pathological gambling, they assess the essential features of the disorder as defined in both DSM editions. Specifically, the SOGS assesses recurrent and maladaptive gambling behavior that disrupts personal, family, and vocational pursuits. Whereas DSM-III-R and DSM-IV also address the emotional components of gambling, the SOGS does not; rather, it focuses primarily on associated maladaptive social and financial behavior. The SOGS addresses gambling behavior across the lifetime. Past-year (Abbott and Volberg 1991) and past 6-month (Ladouceur and Sylvain 2000) versions have been developed for research. Scores are obtained by summing all positive responses. The authors identify 5 as a cutoff score for indicating probable pathological gambling, a score of 3–4 as signifying some problem, and a score of 0–2 as suggesting no problem.

Psychiatric Institute Trichotillomania Scale

The Psychiatric Institute Trichotillomania Scale (PITS; Winchel et al. 1992), developed to assess trichotillomania, is a six-item semistructured interview designed to be administered by a clinician. This measure assesses the number of hair-pulling sites, quantity of hair loss, time spent pulling and thinking about pulling, resistance to hair-pulling urges, distress regarding hair-pulling behavior and its consequences, and interference with daily activities. The PITS is designed to evaluate current symptom severity (i.e., during the past week) as well as change in symptom profile and severity over time. The measure includes a seven-item hair-pulling history interview, in which the interviewer asks questions about age at onset, course of illness, sites of hair pulling, and associated maladaptive behavior. The responses from this section are not included in the final score but are used to aid scoring of the six items that form the heart of the interview. Items are rated on an 8-point scale. Higher total scores reflect greater severity. Neither normative data nor cutoff scores are provided.

DIRECT LABORATORY ASSESSMENTS OF AGGRESSION

Direct laboratory assessments of aggression assess the extent to which a subject responds aggressively to an opponent in a simulated "game" involving the subject giving an electric shock to his or her "opponent" or another measure of aggression. The three major direct laboratory assessments are discussed below.

Buss "Aggression Machine" Paradigm

In the Buss "Aggression Machine" (BAM; Buss 1961), the experimental subject's task is to teach his or her opponent a concept by showing an example of the concept. If the opponent is correct, a feedback button notifies the experimental subject, who is instructed beforehand not to deliver a shock in this circumstance. If the opponent is incorrect, the experimental subject has to press one of 10 buttons that deliver increasing intensities of electric shock.

Taylor Competitive Reaction Time-Task

The Taylor Competitive Reaction Time-Task (TCRTT; Taylor 1987) is a modification of the BAM. In the TCRTT, the experimental subject is engaged in a reaction time-task with an opponent.

Cherek Point Subtraction Aggression Paradigm

The Cherek Point Subtraction Aggression Paradigm (PSAP; Kelly and Cherek 1993) is a modification of the TCRTT, whereby the investigator is able to set the level of preoccupation for each session.

Although these rating measurements are useful, it is helpful to consider their limitations in the evaluation of dangerousness. Assessment of release from prison or hospital depends more on subjective parameters, such as the patient's alliance or compliance with medication, than on several tests, and the patient's history is still the most important determinant in the process of risk assessment.

DIRECT LABORATORY ASSESSMENTS OF IMPULSIVITY

The advantages of laboratory measures of impulsivity include their suitability for repeated use and thus for treatment studies, and their potential for use in both animals

and humans, allowing for comparative studies of the basic biochemistry of these behaviors. For example, animal studies using paradigms that are based on reward-choice models and response disinhibition/attentional models have found evidence for a negative correlation between impulsivity and serotonin function (Evenden 1999; Puumala and Sirviö 1998). The primary disadvantages of these measures are that they do not incorporate the social aspects of impulsivity and do not measure long-term patterns of behavior.

Three broad categories of behavioral laboratory paradigms have been used to measure impulsivity: 1) punishment and/or extinction paradigms (Matthys et al. 1998), 2) reward-choice paradigms (Ainslie 1975), and 3) response disinhibition/attentional paradigms (Dougherty et al. 1999; Halperin et al. 1991). However, the construct of impulsivity is multifaceted and can be described in a variety of different ways.

Some tests measure impulsivity in terms of behavioral inhibition or the ability to suppress behavior when faced with punishment, novelty, or nonreward. This inhibition or suppression is typically measured by a go/no-go task in which behavioral inhibition is needed or an overt conflict emerges between making ("go") and refraining from ("no-go") a response based on reward, punishment, or nonreward. Another behavioral measure of impulsivity is delay of reinforcement. This approach, taken by Logue (1995) and others such as Trevor Robbins and his colleagues (e.g., Cardinal et al. 2001), considers self-control (the inverse of impulsivity) as a function of factors controlling the choice of delayed reinforcers (Logue 1988; Rachlin 1995). In other words, impulsivity is considered a problem with the ability to delay gratification. In this approach, impulsivity is usually measured as preference for a small immediate reward over a delayed larger reward.

Dickman (1993) identified two aspects of impulsivity: disinhibition and reflection-impulsivity. Syndromes of disinhibition are evidenced by, for example, an increased number of correct "go" responses in a "go/no-go" discrimination test (Newman et al. 1985). Reflection-impulsivity has been conceptualized as the cognitive processes involved in reflecting on the accuracy of available hypotheses (Kagan and Messer 1975). Operationally, the variable has been defined as a composite of two dimensions: latency to first response and accuracy of choice or total errors, which are combined in the Matching Familiar Figures Test (MFFT; Kagan et al. 1964; see also Kagan 1966), regarded as the primary (and often the only used) index of reflection-impulsivity. The MFFT is a standard, internally consistent, stable, reliable, and well-validated (Glow et al. 1981) measure of impulsivity in which participants select, from the set of highly similar pictures, the one that is exactly the same as the standard picture.

Participants were given 12 trials with 8 variants each to choose from, with a different target object for each trial. Mean time latency of the participants' first response across all trials and number of errors made before choosing the correct item were recorded. Dickman (1993) suggested reflection-impulsivity is a separate dimension, since results on the MFFT do not correlate with either self-report or other behavioral measures of impulsivity.

NEUROBIOLOGY AND NEUROPSYCHIATRY

In this section, we review neuroanatomical and neurotransmitter research that has focused on aggression and impulsivity as underlying personality or behavioral traits. Much of this work has used aggression and suicidality as indices of impulsivity. Although not all aggressive and suicidal behaviors are impulsive, these behaviors can arguably be seen as constituting a measure of the tendency to be impulsive (i.e., impulsive aggression). In addition, we discuss neuroendocrine and genetic correlates of impulsivity and aggression. Impulsivity and aggression are likely to be the result of several different independent factors interacting to modulate an individual's behavior.

NEUROLOGICAL STRUCTURES INVOLVED IN AGGRESSION

A vast body of literature exists linking specific brain structures to aggressive behavior in mammals and nonhuman primates. Clinicians have also commonly observed that patients with neurological lesions may present with symptoms of aggression (Weiger and Bear 1988). A number of investigators hypothesize that for a subgroup of chronically aggressive persons, the root of the aggressive behavior is brain damage. D.O. Lewis et al. (1982) reported that every death row inmate studied by her team had a history of head injury, often inflicted by abusive parents. Her study concluded that death row inmates constitute an especially neuropsychiatrically impaired prison population. Although the connection between physical abuse, head injury, and aggression is uncertain, many studies do show an association between physical abuse and later aggressive behavior. Clinical reports of aggressive patients with specific neurological lesions may help delineate the structures that mediate these symptoms. In patients who present with aggressive symptoms, researchers have demonstrated neurological "soft signs"—a marker of subtle neurological dysfunction (Shaffer et al. 1985). Research on the major brain structures involved in mediating aggression has focused on the hypothalamus, amygdala, and prefrontal cortex. We briefly review the relationships between impulsive aggressive behavior, and these three structures.

Hypothalamus

The hypothalamus monitors internal status and orchestrates neuroendocrine responses via sympathetic arousal. It is involved in the regulation of the sleep-wake cycle, appetite, body temperature, and sexual activity. In combination with the pituitary, it is the major regulator of the autonomic nervous system. The mesolimbic dopaminergic pathway and the ascending serotonergic, noradrenergic, and cholinergic pathways from the brain stem have terminations in the hypothalamus.

The hypothalamus plays a major role in the expression of aggression in animals (Adams 2006; Eichelman 1971; Hassanain et al. 2005; Wasman and Flynn 1962). Stimulation of the anterior hypothalamus causes predatory attacks in cats, whereas activation of the dorsomedial aspect produces aggression in which the animal ignores the presence of a rat and attacks the experimenter. Destruction of aggression-inhibitory areas, such as the ventromedial nucleus of the hypothalamus, produces permanently aggressive cats and rats (Bard 1928; Reeves and Plum 1969). After cortical ablation, stimulation of the posterior lateral hypothalamus of the cat elicits sham-rage, a posture of preparation for attack. Stimulation of the posterior lateral portion of the hypothalamus shortens the latency of the attack, whereas stimulation of the medial ventral area prolongs the latency of attack (Eichelman 1971; Wasman and Flynn 1962). Hamsters tested for offensive aggression after microinjections of arginine vasopressin (AVP) directly within the anterior hypothalamus in combination with a 5-hydroxytryptamine (5-HT; serotonin) type 1B (5-HT$_{1B}$) receptor agonist have increased aggression, whereas those injected with AVP and a serotonin type 1A (5-HT$_{1A}$) receptor agonist have a dose-dependent inhibition of AVP-affiliated offensive aggression (Ferris et al. 1999). Structural lesions of the hypothalamus in humans may be associated with unplanned and undirected aggressive symptoms that often appear unprovoked but may be in response to physical discomfort (Haugh and Markesbery 1983; Ovsiew and Yudofsky 1983; Reeves and Plum 1969).

Amygdala

The limbic system encompasses the amygdala and temporal cortex. The amygdala activates and/or suppresses the hypothalamus and modulates input from the neocortex. It also has efferents to the extrapyramidal system. The amygdala may have a role in associating sensory experience with (hypothalamically directed) affects and behaviors, including anger (Bear 1991). In a study using positron emission tomography (PET), the amygdala was shown to be more activated during the processing of visually presented linguistic threats than during the processing of neutral words (Isenberg et al. 1999).

Bilateral lesions of the amygdala tame a variety of hostile and vicious animals (Klüver and Bucy 1939), whereas irritative lesions or electrical stimulation can lead to rage outbursts. Removal of the amygdala from monkeys has been shown to result in decreased or no change in aggression (Downer 1961; Izquierdo et al. 2005). However, amygdalectomy in submissive monkeys may result in increased aggression (Dicks et al. 1969). Aggressive behavior following stimulation of the amygdala in cats varies according to their preexisting temperament (Adamac 1990). These findings suggest that the amygdala may not simply function to increase regulatory affects and behaviors, but rather it may mediate and balance their control. In monkeys, bilateral temporal lobectomy leads to hyperorality, hypersexuality, absence of fear response, increased touching, and visual agnosia (Klüver-Bucy syndrome). Bilateral temporal lobe damage in humans leads to similar symptoms, including hypersexuality and visual and auditory agnosias (Lilly et al. 1983; Trimble et al. 1997). In addition, humans exhibit placidity, apathy, bulimia, and aphasia (Isern 1987; Marlowe et al. 1975). This syndrome appears to be a disconnection between sensory information about the environment and the regulation of affects and behaviors (e.g., aggression, sex, food) that usually help the person or animal negotiate that environment.

Seizure studies of the limbic area in humans give insight into the possible neuroanatomical underpinnings of aggression. Whereas bilateral temporal lobe damage in humans may lead to Klüver-Bucy syndrome with a decrease in regulatory affects and behaviors, disorders of temporal lobe excitation may result in increased affect and aggression (Nachson 1988; Trimble and Van Elst 1999). Researchers have noted associations between aggression and temporal lobe epilepsy (TLE). Elliot (1992) found that 30% of 286 patients with intermittent violent outbursts had TLE. D.O. Lewis (1982) found psychomotor epilepsy in 18 of 97 (19%) incarcerated delinquent boys with a history of violence. Patients with TLE may demonstrate hyperemotionality and increased aggression. Interictal aggression is much more common than ictal or postictal aggression in TLE. Interictal aggression is often characterized by intense affect in response to environmental stimuli, whereas ictal and postictal aggression are spontaneous and unfocused.

In humans, reports of surgical intervention for the relief of mental or structural brain disease or epilepsy have shown that both the amygdala and other temporal lobe and limbic system structures contribute to aggression modula-

tion. Two patients who underwent bilateral amygdalotomy for intractable aggression showed a reduction in autonomic arousal in response to stressful stimuli and a decrease in aggressive outbursts (Lee et al. 1998). Limbic system tumors, infections, and blood vessel abnormalities have also been associated with violence. Although it is clear that various limbic system structures have an inhibitory or excitatory effect on aggression, the precise mechanism of the aggression pathway is still far from established.

Prefrontal Cortex

The prefrontal cortex (PFC) modulates limbic and hypothalamic activity and is associated with the social and judgment aspects of aggression. The frontal cortex coordinates timing of social cues, often before the expression of associated emotions. Lesions in this area give rise to disinhibited anger after minimal provocation, characterized by an individual showing little regard for the consequences of affect and behavior. Weiger and Bear (1988) suggest that whereas TLE patients may express deep remorse over an aggressive act, patients with prefrontal lesions often indicate indifference. Patients with violent behavior have been found to have a high frequency of prefrontal lobe lesions, and orbitofrontal cortex lesions, in particular, tend to result in antisocial behaviors (Blair 2004; Seguin 2004). In a study of Vietnam veterans with a history of penetrating head injuries, patients with ventromedial lesions had higher verbal aggression scores than control subjects and patients with lesions in other brain areas (Grafman et al. 1996). Frontal lesions may result in the sudden discharge of limbic- and/or amygdala-generated affects that are no longer modulated, processed, or inhibited by the frontal lobe. Individuals consequently respond with rage or aggression when acting on feelings that would have ordinarily been modulated. Prefrontal damage may cause aggression by a secondary process involving lack of inhibition of the limbic area. Dorsal lesions of the PFC are associated with impairment in long-term planning and increased apathy. Orbital lesion s of the PFC are associated with increases in reflexive emotional responses to environmental stimuli (Luria 1980).

The PFC is involved in the executive functions that guide behavior like planning, response modulation, and inhibition, and plays an important role in self-regulation (Ernst et al. 2003; Goudriaan et al. 2004; Jentsch and Taylor 1999; Lyvers 2000; Rogers and Robbins 2001). Numerous studies report that patients with impulsivity have neurobiological and neurocognitive deficits in executive functions related to the PFC (Berlin et al. 2004, 2005; Cheung et al. 2004; Goudriaan et al. 2004, 2005; Spinella 2004). Findings indicate that pathological gamblers have impairments in several aspects of executive functioning, including response inhibition, planning, and decision making (Cavedini et al. 2002; Goudriaan et al. 2004, 2005; Petry 2001a, 2001b; Petry and Casarella 1999; Regard et al. 2003).

PFC damage can cause disinhibition, such that behavior becomes largely guided by previously conditioned or prepotent responses that are inappropriate in the current situation (Berlin et al. 2004; Milner 1982; Robbins 1996). Specifically, damage within the orbitofrontal cortex (OFC) or prelimbic cortex of humans leads to a tendency to preferentially respond for immediate small rewards over delayed, more efficient rewards (Bechara et al. 2000; Damasio 1996). Further, studies of OFC lesions in humans have revealed an autonomic pattern of deficits (Damasio et al. 1990) and subtle executive deficits in real-world social contexts (Eslinger and Damasio 1985; Grattan et al. 1994). In accord, damage to the OFC has been associated with disinhibited or socially inappropriate behavior, misinterpretation of moods, and impulsivity (Damasio 1994; Levin et al. 1991; Rolls et al. 1994). In one study (Berlin et al. 2004), OFC lesion patients performed more impulsively on both self-report and cognitive-behavioral tests of impulsivity, reported more inappropriate behaviors, and performed worse on a stimulus-reinforcement association reversal task than patients with non-OFC prefrontal cortex lesions and neuropsychiatrically healthy control participants. Further, in another study (Berlin et al. 2005), OFC lesion patients and BPD patients performed similarly in that they were more impulsive and reported more inappropriate behaviors, BPD characteristics, anger, and less happiness than patients with non-OFC prefrontal cortex lesions and neuropsychiatrically healthy control groups. They were also less open to experience and had a faster perception of time (underproduced time) than the neuropsychiatrically healthy control participants. This implies that OFC dysfunction may contribute to some of the core characteristics of BPD, in particular impulsivity.

Orbitofrontal and ventrolateral PFC activation is thought to exhibit top-down control over limbic pathways (Drevets 1999; Herpertz et al. 2001; Morgan et al. 1993; Rauch et al. 1998) via extensive reciprocal connections with the amygdala and other limbic structures, thus playing a role in correcting and regulating emotional and behavioral responses (Drevets 1998; Hornak et al. 2003, 2004; Rolls et al. 1994). Therefore, limbic-orbitofrontal circuit dysfunction may be involved in impulsivity in at least in a subgroup of patients (Van Reekum 1993), via underactivation of prefrontal areas involved in inhibiting behavior, overstimulation of the limbic regions involved in drive, or a combination of both.

Positron emission tomography has allowed researchers to explore whether reduced serotonergic functioning occurs in specific brain regions in individuals with increased aggression and impulsivity. One imaging study showed that in contrast to control subjects, BPD patients have diminished response to serotonergic stimulation (*d,l*-fenfluramine) in areas of PFC associated with regulation of impulsive behavior, specifically the medial and orbital regions of the right prefrontal cortex, left middle and superior temporal gyri, left parietal lobe, and left caudate body (Soloff et al. 2000). Siever et al. (1999) found that impulsive aggressive patients had significantly blunted metabolic responses in orbital frontal, adjacent ventral medial, and cingulate cortex compared with control subjects. Finally, impulsive murderers have been shown to have lower left and right prefrontal functioning and higher right subcortical functioning in comparison to predatory murderers (Raine et al. 1998).

Other areas implicated in impulsivity and aggression include the midline thalamus, lateral preoptic region, mamillary bodies, hippocampus, and basal ganglia.

NEUROPHARMACOLOGY OF IMPULSIVITY AND AGGRESSION

Decreased Serotonin Function

There is significant evidence for the role of serotonergic dysregulation in impulsive aggression in both animals and humans (Table 13–1) (Åsberg et al. 1976; G. Brown et al. 1979, 1982; Ferrari et al. 2005; Sabrie 1986). This association has been shown with a variety of measures of serotonergic function. A decrease in brain serotonin is found in the brain stems of muricidal rats (i.e., aggressive rats that spontaneously kill mice introduced into their cages) and other animals made aggressive by isolation. The administration of tryptophan, a serotonin precursor, reduces or abolishes the violence (Depue and Spoont 1986). In primate studies, researchers have noted higher blood levels of serotonin and higher cerebrospinal fluid (CSF) levels of 5-hydroxyindoleacetic acid (5-HIAA) in monkeys that tend to be dominant and high-ranking in their colonies (Higley et al. 1992) and lower CSF concentration of 5-HIAA as an antecedent to greater alcohol consumption (Higley et al. 1996b).

In humans, Åsberg et al. (1976) initially noted an inverse relationship between violent/lethal suicidal behavior and CSF concentration of the serotonin metabolite 5-HIAA in depressed patients. Subsequent studies on populations in eight different countries confirmed that suicidal depressed patients have lower CSF concentration of 5-HIAA than nonsuicidal depressed patients. For example, Lidberg et al. (2000) found that homicide offenders with a history of suicide attempts had a lower CSF concentration of 5-HIAA than the remaining homicide offenders. This correlation is particularly strong in those

TABLE 13–1. Studies of serotonin with aggression and impulsivity

Study type	Study	Findings
Animal studies	Higley et al. 1996b	Lower CSF concentration of 5-HIAA in primates correlated with greater alcohol consumption
	Depue and Spoont 1986	Decreased brain 5-HT in the brain stems of aggressive rats
CSF 5-HIAA	Lidberg et al. 2000	Low 5-HIAA concentration in CSF in homicide offenders with history of suicide attempts
	Stanley et al. 2000	Low 5-HIAA concentration in CSF in aggressive population independent of suicidal behavior
	G. Brown et al. 1982	Low 5-HIAA concentration in CSF of patients with personality disorders: decrease correlated with scores on lifetime aggression scale
	G. Brown et al. 1982; Bioulac 1980; Lidberg et al. 1984; Linnoila et al. 1983	Inverse relationship between CSF levels of 5-HIAA and impulsive/violent behaviors
5-HT platelet studies	Coccaro et al. 1996	Reduced numbers of platelet 5-HT transporter sites associated with history of aggressive behavior in patients with personality disorders
	Mann et al. 1992	Increased platelet 5-HT content correlated with lifetime aggression in BPD patients
	Biegon et al. 1990; Marazziti and Conti 1991	Abnormal 5-HT levels in platelets correlated with impassivity and aggression
	Stoff et al. 1987	Decreased numbers of platelet 5-HTT sites in aggressive institutionalized subjects
	C. S. Brown et al. 1989	Platelet 5-HT uptake inversely correlated with Barratt Impulsivity Scale score in aggressive males
Serum tryptophan	C. E. Lewis 1991	Low serum ratio of tryptophan to other neutral amino acids in alcoholic persons arrested for assaultive behaviors compared with other alcoholic persons
5-HT PET studies	Siever et al. 1999	No significant increases in glucose metabolism in cingulate, orbital frontal, ventral medial frontal, and inferior parietal cortices in impulsive aggressive patients after administration of serotonergic releasing agent d,l-fenfluramine (significant increases were seen in healthy control subjects)
	New et al. 2002	No activation in the left anteromedial orbital cortex of patients with impulsive aggression in response to the serotonergic agonist m-CPP (such activation was seen in control subjects). The anterior cingulate, normally activated by m-CPP, was deactivated in patients, while the posterior cingulate gyrus was activated in patients and deactivated in controls.
	New et al. 2004b	Blunted prolactin response in impulsive aggressive men with personality disorders after administration of d,l-fenfluramine compared with healthy controls

TABLE 13–1.   Studies of serotonin with aggression and impulsivity (*continued*)

Study type	Study	Findings
	New et al. 2004a	Increases in relative metabolic rate in the orbitofrontal cortex and significant clinical improvement in impulsive aggressive BPD patients after receiving the SSRI fluoxetine
	Frankle et al. 2005	Significant reduction in 5-HTT availability in the anterior cingulate cortex of individuals with impulsive aggression compared with healthy subjects

Note.   BPD = borderline personality disorder; CSF = cerebrospinal fluid; 5-HIAA = 5-hydroxyindoleacetic acid; 5-HT = serotonin; 5-HTT = serotonin transporter; m-CPP = *m*-chlorophenylpiperazine; PET = positron emission tomography; SSRI = selective serotonin reuptake inhibitor.

with violent suicide attempts. Low CSF concentration of 5-HIAA has also been shown to be related to aggressive behavior independent of suicidal behavior in patients with Axis I disorders (Stanley et al. 2000). In addition, G. Brown et al. (1982) demonstrated a decrease in CSF concentration of 5-HIAA in patients with personality disorders and found that this decrease correlated with scores on a lifetime aggression scale. Many studies have confirmed an inverse relationship between CSF 5-HIAA level and impulsive and violent behaviors (Bioulac 1980; G. Brown et al. 1982; Lidberg et al. 1984; Linnoila et al. 1983). The individual case subjects and small populations studied include psychopathic military personnel, arsonists, murderers, violent suicidal patients, and behaviorally disrupted children and adolescents. Linnoila et al. (1983) reported reduced CSF 5-HIAA concentration in both impulsive violent offenders and impulsive arsonists compared with persons who commit premeditated violence, suggesting that it is nonpremeditated ("impulsive") aggression, specifically, that correlates with reduced central serotonin function in these individuals.

Suicidal behavior can be conceptualized as aggressive behavior directed toward the self, and studies have found that decreased brain stem levels of serotonin and 5-HIAA are consistent postmortem findings in suicide victims. Investigators have also correlated abnormal serotonin platelet studies with impulsivity and aggression (Biegon et al. 1990; Marazziti and Conti 1991). Platelets bind and transport serotonin. Decreased numbers of platelet serotonin transporter (5-HTT) sites are found in aggressive subjects with conduct disorder and in "aggressive" institutionalized psychiatric subjects (Stoff et al. 1987). In addition, an inverse correlation between platelet serotonin uptake and Barratt "Impulsivity" score has been reported in aggressive adult males (C.S. Brown et al. 1989). In children and adolescents with conduct disorder, there is a negative correlation between platelet imipramine binding

and impulsive aggression (Stoff et al. 1987). In individuals with personality disorders, platelet-titrated paroxetine binding has been shown to be inversely correlated with Life History of Aggression total score and aggression score and with the BDHI Assault score (Coccaro et al. 1996).

Researchers have noted consistently reduced imipramine binding (C.S. Brown et al. 1989) and increased platelet serotonin type 2 (5-HT$_2$) binding in suicide victims (Biegon et al. 1990). Reduced numbers of platelet 5-HTT sites are associated with life history of aggressive behavior in patients with personality disorder (Coccaro et al. 1996). The reduced imipramine binding may reflect decreased serotonin release. Increased 5-HT$_2$ binding may reflect the brain's compensatory response to a decrease in functional serotonergic neurons, with consequent upregulation of postsynaptic 5-HT$_2$ binding sites. Additional findings that suggest the role of serotonin in impulsivity and aggression include reports of low serum ratios of tryptophan to other neutral amino acids in alcoholic subjects arrested for assaultive behaviors compared with other alcoholic subjects or nonalcoholic control subjects (C.E. Lewis 1991). Type 2 alcoholism is associated with both violent behavior and serotonergic deficit (LeMarquand et al. 1994; Virkkunen and Linnoila 1990). Individuals with a family history of alcoholism may be more sensitive to impulsivity in response to low serotonin levels, because tryptophan-depleted individuals with a family history of alcoholism made more errors in a modified Taylor task than did those with no family history of alcoholism (LeMarquand et al. 1999).

Several PET studies also suggest decreased serotonin function in brain areas involved in inhibition in impulsive and aggressive patients (Frankle et al. 2005; New et al. 2002, 2004a, 2004b; Siever et al. 1999). In one study, 5-HTT (PET radiotracer ^{11}C-labeled McN 5652) availability was significantly reduced in the anterior cingulate cortex of individuals with impulsive aggression compared

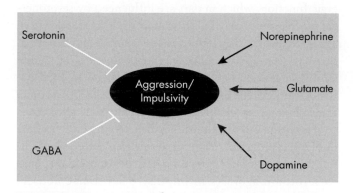

FIGURE 13-2. Neurochemistry of aggression and impulsivity. *White T-shaped lines* indicate that relative decrease in these neurotransmitters is related to increased impulsivity and aggression. *Black arrows* indicate that relative excess of these neurotransmitters is related to increased impulsivity and aggression. GABA = γ-aminobutyric acid.

with healthy controls (Frankle et al. 2005). Thus, pathological impulsive aggression may be associated with lower serotonergic innervation in the anterior cingulate cortex, an area involved in affective regulation.

Neurotransmitters other than serotonin likely influence aggressive and impulsive behavior—for example, γ-aminobutyric acid (GABA), norepinephrine, and dopamine (Oquendo and Mann 2000) (Figure 13-2). An α-amino-3-hydroxy-5-methylisoxazole-4-propionate (AMPA) receptor antagonist, NBQX, was found to increase impulsivity in rats. Normal behavior was restored by injection of a positive allosteric modulator of AMPA receptors, which indicated that the AMPA receptor, a type of glutamate receptor, is involved in the regulation of impulsivity (Nakamura et al. 2000).

One way to study the biology of impulsivity and aggression is to study the traits that cut across personality disorder diagnoses. For example, BPD and ASPD are characterized by impulsivity and aggression, behavioral dimensions that are hypothesized to have specific neurobiological correlates. Studies of patients with BPD have found increased platelet serotonin content that correlated with hostility and lifetime aggression, whereas platelet serotonin content was decreased in depressed patients (Mann et al. 1992). Platelet monoamine oxidase (MAO) has been described as a peripheral marker of cerebral MAO activity and has been found to occur at lower levels in individuals with a high level of impulsiveness—for example, in bullfighters (Carrasco et al. 1999) and bulimic patients (Carrasco et al. 2000). One study found platelet MAO levels significantly decreased in BPD patients compared with control subjects (Yehuda et al. 1989). However, another study (Soloff et al. 1991) did not find this association. These contradictory results suggest the

complexity of neuronal mechanisms in producing behavior. One point to consider is that MAO is relatively nonspecific—it is involved in the breakdown of a number of monoamines—and the activity of MAO in platelets may not reflect MAO activity in the central nervous system (CNS).

PHARMACOLOGICAL CHALLENGE STUDIES

Pharmacological challenges have confirmed a role for serotonin in impulsivity and aggression. The hypothalamic-pituitary-adrenal axis is involved in regulating the interaction between various neurotransmitters that appear, in part, to be stimulated by serotonin. Serotonin stimulation of the hypothalamus causes release of an unidentified prolactin-releasing factor (Ben-Jonathan et al. 1989) that acts on the pituitary, resulting in increased prolactin release. One way that impulsive, aggressive behavior has been linked to serotonergic abnormalities is via measurement of prolactin response to serotonin agonists. Serotonin agonists such as *m*-chlorophenylpiperazine (m-CPP) and fenfluramine stimulate serotonin release through the limbic-hypothalamic-pituitary axis and thereby increase plasma prolactin levels. This action is blocked by serotonin antagonists.

Pharmacological studies provide insight into the possible mechanisms of impulsivity and aggression. In animal studies, monkeys that have a low prolactin response to fenfluramine display more aggressive gestures when shown a slide of a threatening human being than do those with a high prolactin response (Kyes et al. 1995). Researchers have administered m-CPP and fenfluramine to impulsive and aggressive subjects, assaultive BPD and ASPD patients, and patients who attempted suicide, and found a blunted prolactin response that correlated inversely with impulsive aggression (Coccaro et al. 1997; Lopez-Ibor et al. 1990; Moss et al. 1990; New et al. 1997; O'Keane et al. 1992; Siever et al. 1999; 2002, 2004b). In patients with personality disorders, the prolactin response to these agents was inversely correlated with self-reported irritability and aggression, possibly reflecting decreased receptor sensitivity (Coccaro and Murphy 1990; Coccaro et al. 1989). This blunted prolactin response to selective and nonselective serotonergic agents may reflect multiple abnormalities at different functional levels of the serotonergic system. More recently, Siever et al. (1999) found that after receiving the serotonergic releasing agent *d,l*-fenfluramine, impulsive aggressive patients showed significantly blunted metabolic responses in orbital frontal, ventral medial, and cingulate cortex when compared with healthy controls, suggesting reduced serotonergic modulation of these regions in patients with impulsive aggression. In another study (New et al. 1997), patients with a personality disorder and history of self-mutilation or suicide had blunted prolactin and cortisol responses to *d,l*-fenfluramine compared with those with neither, and those with both had the most blunted responses to fenfluramine. Thus, a central serotonin abnormality may be associated with both self-directed violence and suicidal behavior. In a later study using PET, New et al. (2004b) also found that the prolactin response to *d,l*-fenfluramine was blunted in impulsive aggressive men with personality disorders, both with and without suicidal histories, compared with controls. This response was not seen in impulsive aggressive women with personality disorders. This study replicates previous studies in which male patients with a personality disorder and related impulsive aggression and suicide attempts showed a blunted prolactin response to fenfluramine (see New et al. 2004b).

Rinne et al. (2000) found that the cortisol and prolactin responses to an m-CPP challenge in BPD patients were significantly lower than in control subjects and were inversely correlated with frequency of physical and sexual abuse. These data suggest that severe and traumatic stress during childhood affects the serotonergic system. In another study (New et al. 2002), patients with impulsive aggression did not show activation in the left anteromedial orbital cortex in response to the serotonergic agonist m-CPP, whereas control subjects did. The anterior cingulate, normally activated by m-CPP, was deactivated in patients, while the posterior cingulate gyrus was activated in patients and deactivated in controls. The decreased activation of inhibitory regions in patients with impulsive aggression in response to a serotonergic stimulus may contribute to their difficulty in modulating aggressive impulses.

Another line of evidence for serotonergic dysregulation in impulsive aggressive BPD patients stems from the fact that serotonergic drugs have been shown to improve these symptoms. Lithium, for example, has been reported to enhance presynaptic transmission of serotonin via second messenger systems (Coccaro et al. 1991) and has been shown to produce global improvement in BPD patients (Links et al. 1990). Fluoxetine, a selective serotonin reuptake inhibitor (SSRI), has been reported to decrease impulsivity and aggression in BPD patients (Coccaro and Murphy 1990; Cornelius et al. 1989; Norden 1989). New et al. (2004a) found that impulsive aggressive patients with BPD had increases in relative metabolic rate in the orbitofrontal cortex and significant clinical improvement after receiving the SSRI fluoxetine. Thus, fluoxetine appears to have a normalizing effect on prefrontal cortex metabolism in impulsive aggressive patients. On the other hand, MAO inhibitors (MAOIs) have been shown to increase agitation and irritability in some BPD patients (Cowdry and Gardner 1988; Soloff et al. 1986). These studies support the hypothesis that increases in noradren-

ergic function, which in part are influenced by serotonergic mechanisms, may be associated with the tendency to act aggressively. Although studies are limited, the association between pharmacological enhancement of serotonin neurotransmission and reduced impulsivity in BPD patients supports the hypothesis that a decrease in serotonin transmission may underlie impulsivity in BPD patients.

However, a few studies failed to replicate the finding of blunted prolactin response in selected disorders of impulsivity and found augmented neuroendocrine response to serotonin agonists in impulsive substance abusers (Moss et al. 1990), patients with BPD (Hollander et al. 1994), and pathological gamblers. Patients with alcohol abuse (Moss et al. 1990), trichotillomania (Stein et al. 1993a, 1993b), and pathological gambling (DeCaria 1996) experienced a "high" compared with control subjects after receiving m-CPP. This high was characterized by feelings of "spaciness" and feelings of mild derealization or depersonalization and was described as similar to the highs reported when these patients were actually pulling hair (Stein 1995) or gambling (DeCaria 1996). In addition, male patients with BPD had greater increases in cortisol levels and marginally blunted prolactin responses compared with control subjects after receiving m-CPP (Hollander et al. 1994). The blunted prolactin response to serotonin agonists and the reported feeling of being high in impulsive and aggressive patients suggest aberrant serotonergic functioning in this population.

Although most of the research in impulsivity and aggression has focused on serotonergic function, there is also limited evidence for the role of norepinephrine. In fact, the serotonergic, noradrenergic, and dopaminergic systems are highly connected, and it is difficult to stimulate one without affecting the others. Animal studies support the hypothesis that the norepinephrine system has a direct effect on aggression. For example, MAOIs and tricyclic antidepressants, which increase the amount of central norepinephrine in the synaptic cleft, increase shock-induced fighting in rodents (Kantak et al. 1981). One study involving humans found that CSF concentration of 3-methoxy-4-hydroxyphenylglycol (MHPG) correlated with aggressive behavior in a sample of subjects with personality disorders (G. Brown et al. 1979). Another study found a correlation between irritability and growth hormone response to the α-noradrenergic agonist clonidine in patients with personality disorders (Coccaro et al. 1991). Norepinephrine may modulate serotonergically mediated impulsive aggression. Decreases in norepinephrine, for example, may mediate depression, suicide, and inwardly directed aggression, whereas increases in norepinephrine may mediate outwardly directed aggression and irritability (Siever and Davis 1991). Overall, however, the role of norepinephrine is less studied and is not as clear as the role of serotonin in impulsivity and aggression. Nonserotonergic medications have been useful in treating impulsivity and aggression in BPD patients. These include neuroleptics (Soloff et al. 1986), carbamazepine (Cowdry and Gardner 1988), and valproic acid (Hollander et al. 2001a; Stein et al. 1995). The reason for the effectiveness of these agents has not been established and lends support to the role of multiple neurotransmitters in the mediation of aggression and impulsivity.

GENETIC STUDIES

Genetic studies in humans and animals have not yet supported a definitive association among impulsivity, aggression, and reduced serotonergic activity, but there is evidence to suggest they are related (Meyer-Lindenberg et al. 2006; Popova 2006). The Maudsley rat study, however, was an example of genetic breeding for aggressive behavior. Two groups of rats were bred. The first group (MNR) included rats that had low measures of impulsivity and high measures of inhibition. The second group (MR) had the opposite features. The MR strains bred from the second group were significantly more impulsive and demonstrated increased aggressive behavior compared with the MNR rats (Eichelman 1971). Neurochemically, the MNR strain showed lower limbic brain serotonin levels than the MR strain (Sudak and Maas 1964).

At the synaptic level, reuptake of serotonin is accomplished by a plasma membrane carrier called *serotonin transporter*, or 5-HTT. The gene for 5-HTT has been mapped to chromosome 17 (Collier et al. 1996). Preliminary evidence for a genetic disturbance in serotonergic function that might predispose individuals to impulsive aggressive behavior includes a study of the gene for the rate-limiting enzyme for serotonin synthesis, tryptophan hydroxylase (TPH). The gene for TPH has been mapped to the short arm of chromosome 11 and is one of the major candidate genes for psychiatric and behavioral disorders. Part of the gene for TPH has been discovered to exist as two alleles, U and L, with certain genotypes (UL and LL) being associated with impulsive aggressive behavior and suicidal behavior and low CSF levels of 5-HIAA in violent offenders (Nielson et al. 1994). Persons having the TPH U allele scored significantly higher on measures of aggression than did individuals homozygous for the L allele. Also, peak prolactin response was attenuated among male subjects, but not female subjects, having any U allele relative to LL homozygotes (Manuck et al. 1999). In another study, TPH genotype was found to be associated with impulsive aggressive behaviors in male patients with personality disorders, but not in female patients

with the same disorders (New et al. 1998). Further studies are needed to clarify the role of TPH alleles in aggression and the differences between genders. The gene for the serotonin type 1B receptor (*HTR1B*) is located on chromosome 6 (Hamblin et al. 1992). A common polymorphism in the coding region of this gene is caused by a silent G to C substitution (Lappalainen et al. 1995). Some postmortem studies have reported decreased numbers of 5-HT$_{1B}$ receptors in the frontal cortex of nondepressed suicide victims (Arranz et al. 1994). The allelic variability at the *HTR1B* locus may be associated with the susceptibility to suicide attempts in patients with personality disorders. New et al. (2001) found that the G allele at the *HTR1B* locus was associated with a history of suicide attempts in white patients with personality disorders. No relationship was found between *HTR1B* genotype and self-reported impulsive aggression, but self-report measures of aggression may not accurately reflect impulsive aggressive behavior. In summary, serotonin synthesis and regulation are at least partially controlled by genetic factors that likely contribute to an individual's propensity for impulsive and aggressive behaviors.

Currently, there are no controlled family history studies of individuals with impulse-control disorders (i.e., intermittent explosive disorder, kleptomania, pyromania, pathological gambling, and trichotillomania). There are studies supporting associations between major mood disorder and alcohol and substance abuse in first-degree relatives of individuals with kleptomania and in first-degree relatives of pathological gamblers (Linden et al. 1986; Ramirez et al. 1983; Saiz et al. 1992). Other findings include associations between anxiety disorders in the families of individuals with kleptomania and violent behavior and attention-deficit/hyperactivity disorder in families of individuals with intermittent explosive disorder (McElroy et al. 1991).

Research involving monozygotic twins supports a hereditary aspect to aggressive behavior, with concordance rates for monozygotic twins being greater than those for dizygotic twins. Twin studies suggest that antisocial behavior in adult life is related more to genetic factors than to environmental factors (Cadoret et al. 1995).

Chromosomal studies have looked at the influence of chromosomal abnormalities in aggression, particularly the XYY syndrome (Bioulac et al. 1980). However, the link between XYY syndrome and violence has not been confirmed. Inborn metabolic disorders that affect the nervous system can be associated with aggressive personalities. These disorders, which diffusely affect the CNS and are inherited, include phenylketonuria, Lesch-Nyhan syndrome, Prader-Willi syndrome, Vogt's syndrome (a neuronal storage disorder), and Sanfilippo's syndrome (increased mucopolysaccharide storage).

EVIDENCE FOR THE ROLE OF THE SEROTONIN$_{1B}$ RECEPTOR IN AGGRESSION

Animal models have been used to define more clearly the role of specific serotonin receptors in impulsivity and aggression. To define the contribution of serotonin receptor subtypes to behavior, mutant mice lacking the 5-HT$_{1B}$ receptor were generated by homologous recombination. These mice did not exhibit any obvious developmental or cognitive defects. However, they were noted to be extremely aggressive and attacked intruders faster and more intensely than did wild-type mice (Hen 1994). They also had increased impulsive aggression, more rapidly acquired cocaine self-administration, and increased alcohol consumption (Brunner and Hen 1997). These findings suggest a role for the 5-HT$_{1B}$ receptors in modulating aggressive, impulsive, and addiction behavior (Hen 1994).

Findings from genetic studies involving the 5-HT$_{1B}$ receptor gene in human subjects have been equivocal. In one study, a polymorphism of the 5-HT$_{1B}$ receptor gene was linked to aggressive and impulsive behavior in alcoholic individuals (Lappalainen et al. 1998). However, Huang et al. (1999), using two common polymorphisms, found no relationship between suicide, alcoholism, or pathological aggression and 5-HT$_{1B}$ receptor–binding indices or genotype.

Hollander et al. (1992) observed that a subgroup of patients with obsessive-compulsive disorder (OCD) experienced exacerbation of obsessive symptoms following m-CPP challenge studies. m-CPP has affinity for the 5-HT$_{1A}$, 5-HT$_{2C}$, and 5-HT$_{1D}$ receptor subtypes. Patients who underwent challenge studies with MK212, a serotonin agonist with affinity for the 5-HT$_{1A}$ and 5-HT$_{2C}$ receptor subtypes but not for the 5-HT$_{1D}$ subtype, did not manifest exacerbation of obsessions and compulsions. Because there are behavioral changes in a subgroup of OCD patients after administration of m-CPP but not of MK212, and because the activity of these two agonists differs with regard to only one receptor subtype, the 5-HT$_{1D}$ receptor, there is a suggestion that this receptor may modulate obsessions, of which sexual and aggressive symptoms may be prominent.

ENDOCRINE STUDIES

Animal studies show that testosterone levels of male rhesus monkeys correlate positively with behavioral dominance and aggression. If a single male monkey is placed with other aggressive males, he becomes submissive and shows a decrease in plasma testosterone, revealing that endogenous hormone production can be affected by behavioral variables. The connection between the endocrine system and aggression and impulsivity is not clear. Some researchers have hypothesized that androgens may play a role in aggression. They suggest that the androgen insensitivity syndrome and the androgenital syndrome are examples of androgen excesses and deficiencies associated with aggressive and inhibited behavior, respectively. In one study, inmates who had committed personal crimes of sex and violence had higher testosterone levels than inmates who had committed property crimes of burglary, theft, and drugs. Inmates with higher testosterone levels also violated more rules in prison, especially rules involving overt confrontation (Dabbs et al. 1995). CSF free testosterone has been shown to be correlated with overall aggressiveness but not with measures of impulsivity (Higley et al. 1996a). Estrogens and antiandrogens have been used to reduce aggressiveness effectively in some violent sex offenders, although these agents clearly need to be better studied. Low salivary cortisol levels have been associated with persistence and early onset of aggression in school-age boys, suggesting that low hypothalamic-pituitary-adrenal axis activity correlates with aggressive activity (McBurnett et al. 2000).

NEUROPSYCHIATRIC/ NEUROPSYCHOLOGICAL STUDIES OF IMPULSIVITY AND AGGRESSION

Because aggression and impulsivity appear to be core features of both BPD and ASPD, much of the neuropsychiatric research in this area has focused on patients who meet criteria for these disorders. Researchers have suggested that impaired neuropsychiatric development could lead to personality pathology and that individuals with aggressive symptoms manifest subtle neuropsychiatric impairment. In this section, we review the neuropsychiatric and neuropsychological aspects of BPD and ASPD that give greater insight into the biological basis of impulsivity and aggression in these disorders.

Borderline Personality Disorder

BPD patients are often in a state of crisis. Their behavior is unpredictable and sometimes dangerous to self or others, and they rarely are able to achieve up to the level of their abilities. The painful nature of their lives is reflected in repetitive self-destructive acts that may include impulsive wrist slashing, self-mutilation, or suicide. There are fewer neuropsychological studies of BPD patients than of ASPD patients. BPD patients have commonly been thought, however, to have cognitive impairment on the basis of clinical observation of "ego deficits" (Kernberg 1975). BPD patients show no impairments in performance on structured psychological tests, such as the Wechsler Adult Intelligence Scale, but they have disturbed performance on unstructured projective tests such as the Rorschach (Singer 1977). Although there is limited support for cognitive impairment in BPD, these studies support the idea that cognitive capacities in BPD are vulnerable to affective disruption and that patients lack stable self-organizing strategies. Neuropsychological studies of BPD patients support the association with impairment in complex information processing. Researchers have shown that, compared with control subjects, BPD patients had deficits on tests requiring the ability to plan multiple operations, to maintain a prolonged response over time, and to perform complex auditory and visual memory tasks (Burgess 1991). In addition, BPD patients also had significant impairment on tests of visual filtering and discrimination. These neuropsychological disturbances, particularly defects of memory, have been linked to the unstable, chaotic interactions characterized by impulsivity that are often seen in BPD patients. Neuropsychological studies have shown a variety of disturbances in BPD, including deficits in recall of learned material and completion of complex cognitive tasks (Burgess 1990; O'Leary et al. 1991).

In a time production task, where BPD patients were asked to read random numbers off of a computer screen (distracter task) and to stop at variable set time intervals, patients produced less time compared with healthy controls, indicative of a faster subjective sense of time (Berlin and Rolls 2004). Further, BPD patients' faster subjective sense of time correlated with both self-report and behavioral impulsivity. BPD patients also were less conscientious, extraverted, and open to experience, as well as more impulsive (by self-report and behaviorally), emotional, and neurotic, and they reported more BPD characteristics than did controls. The results suggest that some of these core characteristics of BPD may be on a continuum with impulsivity seen in the general population and that impulsivity, in particular, may be related to time perception deficits (i.e., a faster subjective sense of time). While impulsivity was correlated with time perception across all participants, emotionality, introversion, and lack of openness to experience were not. This suggests that different symptoms of the borderline personality syndrome may be separable and, therefore, may be related to different cognitive deficits and potentially to different brain systems.

Researchers have also studied neurological soft signs in BPD patients. The term *neurological soft signs* refers to nonlocalizing abnormalities not indicative of gross neurological disease. Soft signs are associated with a wide variety of developmental disabilities and include involuntary movements, a variety of apraxias, difficulties in performing rapid alternate movements, difficulties in discerning double simultaneous stimulation, and dysgraphesthesia. The assessment of neurological soft signs appears reliable and stable.

Work on patients with personality disorders characterized by impulsivity supports an association between these disorders and increased soft signs. Gardner et al. (1987) found significantly more soft sign neurological abnormalities in BPD patients compared with control subjects. Vitiello et al. (1990) found that increased soft signs were associated with impulsive responding on cognitive tests but not with global cognitive functioning.

Our group (Stein et al. 1993a) found that patients with DSM-III-R–diagnosed BPD had significantly more left-sided soft signs than did control subjects. These left-sided soft signs correlated with lowered neuropsychological test performance of visuospatial tasks and are thus consistent with right hemisphere dysfunction. However, there was also a significant association between history of aggression and right-sided soft signs. These findings are consistent with an association between impulsive aggression and left hemisphere dysfunction.

Evidence of neuropsychiatric abnormalities in personality disorders characterized by impulsivity has a number of clinical implications. Impairment in tasks of complex information processing, which appears to be associated with increased neurological soft signs, may contribute to difficulties in building and maintaining a coherent and stable sense of self and in using past experiences to organize present behavior and to predict future consequences. Impairment on verbal functions mediated by the left hemisphere may also contribute to impaired regulation of impulsivity and aggression insofar as verbal processing facilitates mental exploration before motor enactment, allowing greater appreciation of consequences and alternatives. In view of their nonspecificity and unclear etiology, however, neurological soft signs provide only a limited view of the neuropsychiatry of impulsivity and aggression.

In the only study to date comparing precise lesion patients with BPD patients on neuropsychological tests, Berlin et al. (2005) found that OFC and BPD patients performed similarly in that they were more impulsive and reported more inappropriate behaviors, BPD characteristics, anger, and less happiness than non-OFC prefrontal cortex lesion and neurologically and psychiatrically healthy control groups. They were also less open to experience and had a faster perception of time (underproduced time) than the neurologically and psychiatrically healthy controls. This implies that OFC dysfunction may contribute to some of the core characteristics of BPD, in particular impulsivity. In fact, neuroimaging studies show differences in the prefrontal cortex in people with BPD compared with normal subjects at baseline (De la Fuente et al. 1997; Goyer et al. 1994; Lyoo et al. 1998) and in response to aversive stimuli (Herpertz et al. 2001) and neuropharmacological probes associated with impulsivity (Leyton et al.

2001; Soloff et al. 2000). More specifically, there is some evidence from brain imaging studies for OFC dysfunction in BPD (Driessen et al. 2004; Schmahl et al. 2004; Van Elst et al. 2003; Vollm et al. 2004) and specifically for hypometabolism (De la Fuente et al. 1997; Goyer et al. 1994; Soloff et al. 2000) and reduced brain volume (Lyoo et al. 1998; Van Elst et al. 2003) of the OFC.

Electroencephalographic abnormalities have been associated with impulsive aggression, although definitive results have been inconclusive. While some have found no significant differences between these groups (Archer et al. 1988; Cornelius et al. 1986), electroencephalogram (EEG) abnormalities have been reported to be more prevalent in BPD patients than in control patients with other psychiatric disorders (Andrulonis et al. 1981; Cowdry et al. 1985; Snyder and Pitts 1984). The site of the reported abnormalities varies in that slow, fast, and mixed waves have been reported in frontal, frontotemporal, and occipital brain regions (Snyder and Pitts 1984). Increased risk for head injury might exist in patients with BPD because of their impulsivity and may account for the findings of different locations of EEG abnormalities in the brain (New et al. 1995).

PET studies in subjects with BPD have repeatedly reported functional abnormalities in the frontal lobe of the brain. One PET study showed an inverse correlation of global cerebral glucose metabolic rate and aggression; this finding was specific to the BPD group compared with patients with other personality disorders. Regional metabolic glucose rates in the frontal and parietal lobes were also depressed in BPD patients (Goyer et al. 1994). Similarly, in a PET study, De la Fuente et al. (1997) reported that patients with BPD had bilateral hypometabolism in premotor and prefrontal cortical areas compared with control subjects. Further, using PET neuroimaging during a pharmacological challenge with d,l-fenfluramine, Soloff et al. (2000) found that impulsive aggression in BPD patients was associated with diminished serotonergic regulation in the PFC, including medial and orbital regions. BPD patients had reduced activity in areas of the PFC associated with regulation of impulsive behavior following serotonergic stimulation. The diminished frontal metabolism in BPD patients could cause, act in parallel with, or exacerbate impaired serotonergic function and therefore be related to their impulsivity (De la Fuente et al. 1997).

Using magnetic resonance spectroscopy, Van Elst et al. (2001) examined the brains of patients with BPD and found a significant reduction of absolute N-acetylaspartate (NAA) concentrations in the dorsolateral frontal cortex of BPD patients compared with control subjects. In the first functional magnetic resonance imaging (fMRI) study with BPD patients, Herpertz et al. (2001) found that BPD patients, but not control subjects, had an elevated blood oxygen level–dependent fMRI signal bilaterally in the amygdala and fusiform gyrus and in the left medial and right ventrolateral PFC in response to aversive emotional stimuli. They suggested that BPD subjects' perceptual cortex may be modulated through the amygdala, leading to increased attention to emotionally relevant environmental stimuli, and that the medial/ventrolateral PFC may be a gateway for distinctive sensorial information and may modulate or inhibit amygdaladriven emotional responses and thus provide top-down control of the amygdala (see also Drevets 1999; Morgan et al. 1993; Rauch et al. 1998). More fMRI studies are needed to help clarify the previous, less differentiated, PET findings of hypofrontality in patients with BPD.

The functional abnormalities reported in studies of BPD patients suggest that structural brain abnormalities might exist in BPD as well. However, neither gross inspection nor quantitative measures have revealed brain computed tomography (CT) abnormalities in BPD patients more frequently than in psychiatrically healthy controls (Lucas et al. 1989; Schulz et al. 1983; Snyder et al. 1983). However, CT technology may not be sensitive enough to detect subtle variations in structural neuroanatomy. More advanced MRI studies have found structural abnormalities in BPD patients compared with healthy controls. The first MRI study that evaluated the structural abnormalities of the brain in subjects with the sole diagnosis of BPD found that BPD patients had a smaller frontal lobe volume compared with healthy subjects (Lyoo et al. 1998). Since impulsivity, a defining feature of BPD, has been reported to be closely related to frontal lobe dysfunction in people with impulsive personality disorders (Goyer et al. 1994; Stein et al. 1993a), and people with frontal lobe structural damage have shown problems with impulse control (Damasio et al. 1990), the finding of a smaller frontal lobe in BPD patients (Lyoo et al. 1998) may provide a structural basis for understanding this psychopathology in the context of BPD. While a number of lines of research are suggestive of biological disturbances associated, in particular, with the impulsive aspect of BPD, a neuroanatomical/physiological explanation of the etiology of BPD remains to be clarified.

Antisocial Personality Disorder

ASPD is characterized by continued antisocial or criminal acts but is not synonymous with criminality. Rather, it is an inability to conform to social norms and a pervasive pattern of disregard for and violation of the rights of others. A notable finding is patients' lack of remorse for their behavior. Persons with ASPD repeatedly get into fights or are assaultive. Impulsivity in ASPD may manifest itself in a failure to show normal cautions and in increased recklessness. Impulsive behaviors may be driven by a need for excitement that expresses a disregard for the person's own safety and an intolerance for the feelings that he or she would otherwise experience. Conduct disorder is associated with ASPD later in life. Both ASPD and conduct disorder are associated with an increased use of illicit substances. Substance use and abuse is often impulsive, is frequently characterized by behavioral disinhibition, and commonly results in harm to oneself or others. The neurobiological association between certain behavioral characteristics of substance abuse, ASPD, and impulsive aggressive behavior in other contexts is beyond the scope of this chapter.

Neuropsychological testing of patients with ASPD has yielded mixed results. Using the Halstead-Reitan battery, Yeudall and Fromm-Auch (1979) studied laterality of cerebral dysfunction in various subject groups. They found impairments on variables sensitive primarily to left hemisphere dysfunction in violent criminals, alcoholic individuals with personality disorders, and adolescents with conduct disorders, but predominantly right hemisphere dysfunction in nonviolent criminals, alcoholic individuals with affective disorders, and individuals with affective personality disorders. Fedora and Fedora (1983) also found that prisoners with impulsive behaviors had evidence of left hemisphere impairment, particularly of the anterior regions.

EEGs and brain stem auditory evoked potentials of ASPD patients are not significantly different from those of control subjects (Fishbein et al. 1989). Conduct disorder in some children appears to be associated with later ASPD. Both disorders are characterized by impulsivity, aggression toward others, and violation of the rights of others. Our group has shown that patients with conduct disorder have greater neuropsychological impairment compared with control subjects (Aronowitz 1994). Conduct disorder patients have greater visuospatial, visuoperceptual, and visuoconstructional impairments compared with non–conduct-disordered patients (Aronowitz 1994). Socially appropriate behavior requires modulation of activity, self-restraint, flexibility, adaptation, and planning and anticipation of consequences. These abilities may be difficult for individuals with ASPD and conduct disorder, perhaps because of their neuropsychological deficits.

Using PET, Goyer et al. (1994) found that OFC, anterior medial frontal, and anterior temporal glucose metabolic rates were inversely associated with aggressive history in 17 patients with personality disorders (6 antisocial, 6 borderline, 2 dependent, and 3 narcissistic) compared with 43 healthy controls. In addition, using PET and replicating their earlier pilot study (Volkow and Tancredi 1987), Volkow et al. (1995) found that, compared with healthy controls ($N = 8$), 7 of 8 psychiatric patients with a history of repetitive violent behavior had significantly lower resting cerebral glucose metabolism values in the medial temporal and prefrontal cortices—regions that have been implicated in aggression and impulsivity.

Using PET during the continuous performance task, Raine et al. (1994) found that accused murderers ($n = 22$) had significantly lower glucose metabolism in both lateral and medial prefrontal cortices relative to age- and gender-matched controls ($n = 22$). On the same task, compared with age- and gender-matched controls ($n = 41$), murderers pleading not guilty by reason of insanity ($n = 41$) had reduced glucose metabolism in the prefrontal cortex, superior parietal gyrus, left angular gyrus, and corpus callosum, while abnormal metabolic asymmetries (left < right) were also found in the amygdala, thalamus, and medial temporal lobe (Raine et al. 1997). Thus, a network of abnormal cortical and subcortical brain processes may predispose people to violence. In a reanalysis of these data, Raine et al. (1998) found that the reduction in frontal activation was much more pronounced in murderers whose crimes had an affective rather than predatory basis. Affectively motivated crimes generally are considered to be more impulsive in nature than predatory murders that are, by definition, planned (Hoptman 2003). Davidson et al. (2000) suggest that impulsive violence results from a breakdown in the brain's ability to regulate negative affect. Thus, affective crimes may provide a window into the brain mechanisms underlying impulsive aggression. Finally, in a structural MRI study, ASPD ($n = 21$) patients, compared with healthy ($n = 34$), substance-dependent ($n = 26$), and psychiatric ($n = 21$) controls, showed an 11% reduction in prefrontal gray matter volume in the absence of brain lesions and a reduction in autonomic activity (skin conductance and heart rate) during a social stressor in which participants gave a videotaped speech on their faults (Raine et al. 2000). These deficits predicted group membership independent of psychosocial risk factors. This structural prefrontal deficit may underlie the lack of conscience, poor fear conditioning, low arousal, and decision-making deficits that often characterize antisocial psychopathic behavior.

Impulse-Control Disorders

The five impulse-control disorders listed in DSM-IV-TR are intermittent explosive disorder, kleptomania, pathological gambling, pyromania, and trichotillomania (American Psychiatric Association 2000). Self-mutilation and sexual impulsivity are considered impulse-control disorders not otherwise specified and include behavioral characteristics that overlap with those of a number of other DSM-IV-TR disorders.

There have been few studies examining the neurobiological underpinnings of DSM-IV-TR impulse-control disorders. Most of the studies have involved controlled pharmacotherapy studies for the treatment of impulsivity, which is discussed in the treatment section of this chapter. Pathological gamblers have higher CSF MHPG levels but similar CSF 5-HIAA levels compared with control subjects (Bergh et al. 1997). Pathological gamblers demonstrated dysregulated plasma prolactin response to intravenous clomipramine challenges (Moreno et al. 1991; Vazquez Rodriguez et al. 1991) relative to normal control subjects, indicative of serotonergic dysregulation. Our group demonstrated augmented neuroendocrine and behavioral response to m-CPP in pathological gamblers (DeCaria 1996). Some investigators have found clomipramine (Hollander et al. 1992) and fluvoxamine (Hollander et al. 1998, 2000) useful in the treatment of pathological gambling. There are also reports of the successful use of lithium in treating this disorder (Hollander et al. 2005a; Pallanti et al. 2002), as well as for kleptomania (Rocha and Rocha 1992), trichotillomania (Christenson et al. 1991), and sexual compulsions (Nishimura et al. 1997). Other mood stabilizers have been shown to be effective for impulse-control disorders—for example, divalproex sodium and topiramate for pathological gambling (Dannon et al. 2005; Pallanti et al. 2002) and tiagabine for impulse-control disorders with aggression (Kaufman et al. 2002).

Virkkunen et al. (1987) found lower CSF 5-HIAA and MHPG concentrations in persons who set fires compared with control subjects. All of the arsonists in the study met DSM-III criteria for BPD, and many demonstrated explosive behavior.

Very little neurobiological research has been done on kleptomania and trichotillomania. There is some anecdotal evidence that patients with kleptomania respond to various antidepressants, including SSRIs. Self-mutilation has been studied in patients with personality disorders, and one study showed a negative correlation between impulsive self-mutilation and the number of platelet imipramine-binding receptor sites (Stoff et al. 1987). Patients with personality disorders who exhibited self-mutilative behavior did not differ from patients with personality disorders without self-mutilative behavior in CSF 5-HIAA level or in platelet imipramine binding (Simeon et al. 1992). Case reports have noted the usefulness of lithium, SSRIs, and opiate antagonists in ameliorating self-mutilative behavior, again suggesting the heterogeneous nature of self-mutilation and the complexity of its underlying neurobiology.

TREATMENT OF IMPULSIVITY AND AGGRESSION

PHARMACOTHERAPEUTIC INTERVENTIONS

Impulsivity and aggression are behavioral characteristics that encompass a broad range of clinical problems. Studies on impulsivity and aggression have focused on a heterogeneous group of disorders with varied responses to pharmacotherapeutic interventions. In this section, we do not focus on the treatment of patients with epilepsy and patients with drug-induced aggression. These areas are reviewed elsewhere (see Chapter 16, Chapter 23, and Chapter 31).

Controlled studies suggest that a number of medications may be useful in the treatment of impulsivity and aggression. Given the evidence for decreased serotonergic function in impulsive and aggressive behaviors, many, but not all, of these medications involve direct serotonergic mechanisms. SSRIs have been shown to reduce impulsive aggressive behaviors in different psychiatric disorders. For example, fluvoxamine resulted in improvement in gambling severity in patients with pathological gambling compared with placebo in one double-blind study (Hollander et al. 2000). However, in some disorders characterized by impulsivity, SSRIs have a quick onset, but these effects may be transient and some patients may require additional augmentation with compounds such as lithium, buspirone, and anticonvulsants (Hollander and Wong 1995). The neurotransmitter effects of lithium are complex and include an effect on second-messenger systems related to the serotonergic system. Lithium has been found effective for impulsivity and aggression across different population such as prison inmates (Sheard 1971, 1975; Sheard et al. 1976, 1977; Tupin 1978; Tupin et al. 1973), children and adolescents with conduct disorders (Campbell et al. 1984, 1995; Fava 1997; Malone et al. 2000; Moll and Rothenberger 1998), deaf patients with impulsive aggression (Altshuler et al. 1977), and aggressive children (Siassi 1982).

Medications that are not serotonergically mediated, such as anticonvulsants, have also been useful in treating impulsivity and aggression across disorders (Berlin HA, Hollander E: "Mood Stabilizers for Personality Disorders and Impulsive Aggression," unpublished). Although evidence suggests that impulsivity and aggression are serotonergically mediated, a serotonergic hypothesis of impulsivity is not a definitive model. The complete role of serotonin activity and its complex interactions with other neurotransmitters and receptors in impulsivity and aggression have not yet been fully delineated.

BPD is a common clinical problem whereby researchers have used pharmacological interventions to target the characteristic symptoms of impulsivity, aggression, lability, and hostility. Fluoxetine is the best-studied SSRI for the treatment of impulsivity and aggression. A number of open trials of fluoxetine in BPD suggest its efficacy in the treatment of impulsivity and aggression in BPD. Markowitz (1990) reported that BPD patients showed significant decreases in self-injurious behavior after treatment with fluoxetine 80 mg/day for 12 weeks. Three subsequent double-blind, placebo-controlled trials of fluoxetine confirmed the findings of the open trials (Markowitz 1992). Overall, controlled studies of fluoxetine, sertraline, and fluvoxamine suggest that these medications are of benefit to patients with impulsivity and aggression in the context of BPD. More studies are needed to assess further which behaviors are associated with responsivity to an SSRI, appropriate dosage, and longitudinal efficacy of those agents.

Researchers and clinicians have used lithium, carbamazepine, valproic acid, and, more recently, gabapentin, lamotrigine, and topiramate to treat the impulsivity, aggression, and mood instability seen in patients with bipolar disorder, and they subsequently reasoned that it might stabilize these same symptoms in BPD. In a double-blind, placebo-controlled trial (Cowdry and Gardner 1988), carbamazepine decreased impulsivity in a group of BPD patients. MAOIs have not been shown to decrease the behavioral dyscontrol or impulsivity seen in BPD. Furthermore, in BPD patients, overdosing on psychotropic agents is a common form of suicide, and MAOIs are clearly dangerous in these situations.

The tricyclic antidepressants have been extensively studied for their effects on depression in BPD patients. Although they are clearly effective for depressive symptoms, tricyclic antidepressants have not been shown to be particularly helpful in decreasing aggression and impulsivity in BPD (Soloff et al. 1986). Some BPD patients actually experienced increased anger, hostility, and aggression while taking imipramine (Klein 1968) and amitriptyline (Soloff et al. 1986). There are case reports of using desipramine or clomipramine effectively to treat violent outbursts in some patients and of using amitriptyline, trazodone, or fluoxetine for aggression associated with brain injury and anoxic encephalopathy. The potential for worsening impulsive aggressive symptoms and the danger of overdose in patients who have impaired self-control may limit the use of tricyclic antidepressants.

Neuroleptics are among the most studied medications for treatment of BPD, and they have been effective in treating violence associated with psychosis. Although they are the most commonly used medications for violence and aggression related to psychosis, neuroleptics are often chronically misused as sedatives. Further, some studies with BPD patients have shown that neuroleptics were not

well tolerated and were statistically no better than placebo in the reduction of hostility, anger, and aggression (Goldberg et al. 1986; Soloff et al. 1986). However, in contrast, many studies demonstrate the efficacy of neuroleptics for the treatment of impulsivity and aggression in BPD patients (Nickel et al. 2006; Soler et al. 2005; Villeneuve and Lemelin 2005). In one 8-week open-label pilot study, BPD patients treated with olanzapine had decreased BIS-11 and BDHI scores compared with those treated with placebo (Schultz et al. 1999). Clinicians should keep in mind that neuroleptics, despite their efficacy, may result in a number of adverse side effects. They may cause tolerance to sedation and lead to increased doses and thereby increased side effects such as akathisia, extrapyramidal side effects, and anticholinergic toxicity. These specific side effects can worsen aggression in predisposed patients, particularly those with organic brain injury.

Mood stabilizers and anticonvulsants have been effective in treating impulsivity and aggression in patient populations. Our group (Stein et al. 1995) found that valproate led to significant overall improvement in 50% of a small sample of BPD patients who completed an 8-week open-label trial. Also, in a 10-week double-blind study, we found that valproate may be more effective than placebo (Hollander et al. 1998, 2001a). The medication was helpful for impulsivity, anger, and irritability, as well as for mood instability and anxiety. More recently, Hollander et al. (2003) conducted a large placebo-controlled, multicenter trial of divalproex for the treatment of impulsive aggression in Cluster B personality disorder, intermittent explosive disorder, or posttraumatic stress disorder. Entry criteria required evidence of current impulsive aggressive behavior (e.g., two or more impulsive aggressive outbursts per week on average for the previous month) and an Overt Aggression Scale—Modified (OAS-M) score of 15 or greater. Divalproex was superior to placebo in the treatment of impulsive aggression, irritability, and global severity in a large subgroup of patients with Cluster B disorders in terms of OAS-M Aggression scores. These results support previous findings of decreased impulsive aggressive behavior and irritability in BPD patients treated with divalproex (Hollander et al. 2001a), including those who failed to respond to other antiaggressive agents (i.e., SSRIs) (Kavoussi and Coccaro 1998). In the Hollander et al. (2003) study, unlike a previous pilot study in which divalproex was superior to placebo for the treatment of irritability and hostility in women with bipolar II and BPD (Frankenburg and Zanarini 2002), patients were excluded if they had bipolar I or bipolar II disorder with recent hypomania (during the past year). This suggests that the effect of divalproex in impulsive aggression may be unrelated to its effect in mania. However, the possibility that the impulsive aggression of Cluster B personality disorders has an affective component, or that there is a subclinical mood disorder in Cluster B personality disorders, cannot be excluded.

Hollander et al. (2005b) examined clinical characteristics of BPD outpatients that might predict treatment response to divalproex for impulsive aggression. In this 12-week randomized, double-blind study, divalproex was superior to placebo in reducing impulsive aggression in BPD patients. Both pretreatment trait impulsivity and state aggression symptoms, independently of one another, predicted a favorable response to divalproex relative to placebo. However, baseline affective instability did not affect differential treatment response. These data may be helpful in identifying patient subgroups (e.g., those with high levels of trait impulsivity or state aggression) or baseline characteristics of BPD that could guide future trials of mood stabilizers. These data also suggest that BPD may be characterized by independent symptom domains that are amenable to treatment (Berlin and Rolls 1994; Berlin et al. 2004, 2005).

The potential efficacy of valproate in the treatment of BPD raises the question of the neurobiological underpinnings of the core features of BPD, namely, impulsivity and aggression. A number of points are relevant. First, a link between impulsive aggression and limbic abnormality has long been postulated. Although only a small percentage of BPD patients have seizure activity, more subtle neuropsychiatric abnormalities, including increased neurological soft signs, have been found in this population. The hypothesis that valproate alters limbic dysfunction by interrupting neuronal kindling is therefore of interest. Second, there is increasing evidence that serotonergic hypofunction may play a role in the mediation of BPD symptoms. Although valproate has multiple effects on neurotransmission, it is notable that valproate increases 5-HIAA levels. Further studies and larger sample sizes for the use of valproate in the treatment of BPD are warranted. Other anticonvulsants have all been shown to be effective in treating BPD—for example, carbamazepine (Cowdry and Gardner 1988; Gardner and Cowdry 1986; De la Fuente and Lotstra 1994; Denicoff et al. 1994), topiramate (Nickel et al. 2004, 2005), gabapentin (Biancosino et al. 2002), and lamotrigine (Pinto and Akiskal 1998; Preston et al. 2004).

TREATMENT IN DEVELOPMENTALLY DISABLED PERSONS

Autistic disorder and mental retardation are often associated with impulsive outbursts, emotional lability, rage episodes, and aggression toward self and others. Treatment with fluoxetine has been found to decrease aggression, self-injury, and agitation in profoundly mentally retarded patients (Markowitz 1992). Lithium has been shown to be beneficial in a subset of children with rage, aggression, and irritability (DeLong 1978) and in mentally retarded patients with repeated, uncontrolled aggression and self-injury (Craft et al. 1987). Beta-blockers, which also bind to 5-HT$_1$-like receptors, have been found in open trials to lead to improvements in aggressive patients with neuropsychological disorders and in patients with impulsive aggression (Silver and Yudofsky 1995). Williams et al. (1982) documented the efficacy of propranolol in a diagnostically diverse population sharing the problem of rage outbursts. A series of case reports has indicated that carbamazepine treatment decreased rage outbursts and aggression in a group of patients demonstrating heterogeneous behaviors associated with aggression. In an open trial, our group reported that divalproex sodium (valproate) resulted in improvement in impulsive aggressive symptoms and affective instability in autism spectrum disorders (Hollander et al. 2001b). Further, in a double-blind, placebo-controlled trial of divalproex sodium, we (Hollander et al. 2006) found significant improvement in repetitive behaviors of autism spectrum disorders with divalproex sodium. In a multisite randomized, double-blind, placebo-controlled trial, McCracken et al. (2002) found that the atypical antipsychotic risperidone was well tolerated and efficacious for the treatment of aggression, self-injurious behavior, and tantrums in children with autistic disorder. Buspirone, a nonbenzodiazepine, nonsedating 5-HT$_{1A}$ agonist, may be effective in the treatment of patients with developmental disabilities and head injury. These findings need further controlled trials. Eltoprazine, a phenylpiperazine derivative and mixed 5-HT$_1$ agonist, has shown antiaggressive properties in animal models. Eltoprazine-like compounds may be used in future treatment strategies and as a probe to further study the basis of impulsivity and aggression (Mak et al. 1995).

Highlights for the Clinician

Measurements of impulsivity and aggression

Self-report assessments

◆ Buss-Durkee Hostility Inventory

◆ Hostility and Direction of Hostility Questionnaire

◆ Spielberger State-Trait Anger Expression Inventory

◆ Barratt Impulsiveness Scale, Version 11

◆ Massachusetts General Hospital Hairpulling Scale

◆ Gambling Symptom Assessment Scale

◆ Kleptomania Symptom Assessment Scale

Interview assessments

◆ Brown-Goodwin Assessment for Life History of Aggression

◆ Pathological Gambling Modification of the Yale-Brown Obsessive Compulsive Scale

◆ South Oaks Gambling Screen

◆ Psychiatric Institute Trichotillomania Scale

Direct laboratory assessments of aggression

◆ Buss "Aggression Machine" Paradigm

◆ Taylor Competitive Reaction Time-Task

◆ Cherek Point Subtraction Aggression Paradigm

Direct laboratory assessments of impulsivity

Advantages: Suitable for repeated use and thus for treatment studies, have potential for use in both animals and humans, and allow for comparative studies of the basic biochemistry of these impulsive behaviors

Disadvantages: Do not incorporate the social aspects of impulsivity and do not measure long-term patterns of behavior

◆ Three broad categories of behavioral laboratory paradigms have been used to measure impulsivity:

  1. Punishment and/or extinction paradigms (Matthys et al. 1998)

  2. Reward-choice paradigms (Ainslie 1975)

  3. Response disinhibition/attentional paradigms (Dougherty et al. 1999; Halperin et al. 1991).

◆ Commonly used laboratory tests: go/no-go task, Matching Familiar Figures Test

Neurobiology and neuropsychiatry

Neurological structures involved in aggression

◆ Hypothalamus

◆ Amygdala

◆ Prefrontal cortex

Neuropharmacology of impulsivity and aggression

◆ Decreased serotonin function (see Table 13–1)

(continued)

Highlights for the Clinician (continued)

Pharmacological challenge studies

◆ Studies confirm a role for serotonin in impulsivity and aggression.

◆ In general, studies show that a blunted prolactin response to serotonin agonists is related to aggressive/impulsive behavior.

Genetic studies

◆ Genetic studies in humans and animals have not yet supported a definitive association among impulsivity, aggression, and reduced serotonin activity, but there is evidence to suggest they are related.

Evidence for the role of the 5-HT$_{1B}$ receptor in aggression

◆ Animal studies suggest a role for the 5-HT$_{1B}$ receptors in modulating aggressive, impulsive, and addiction behavior.

◆ Genetic studies involving the 5-HT$_{1B}$ receptor gene in human subjects have been equivocal.

Endocrine studies

◆ Animal studies show that testosterone levels of male rhesus monkeys correlate positively with behavioral dominance and aggression.

◆ Some researchers suggest that the androgen insensitivity syndrome and the androgenital syndrome are examples of androgen excesses and deficiencies associated with aggressive and inhibited behavior, respectively.

Neuropsychiatric/neuropsychological studies of impulsivity and aggression

◆ Because aggression and impulsivity appear to be core features of both borderline personality disorder (BPD) and antisocial personality disorder (ASPD), much of the neuropsychiatric research in this area has focused on patients who meet criteria for these disorders.

◆ Researchers have suggested that impaired neuropsychiatric development could lead to personality pathology and that individuals with aggressive symptoms manifest subtle neuropsychiatric impairment.

◆ A number of lines of research (e.g., imaging, neuropsychological testing, neurological soft signs) are suggestive of biological disturbances, in particular those related to prefrontal cortex, that are associated with the impulsive and aggressive aspects of BPD and ASPD.

◆ Few studies have examined the neurobiological underpinnings of DSM-IV-TR impulse-control disorders (i.e., intermittent explosive disorder, kleptomania, pathological gambling, pyromania, and trichotillomania).

◆ Most of the studies of impulse-control disorders involve controlled pharmacotherapy studies for the treatment of impulsivity, which is discussed in the treatment section of this chapter.

Treatment of impulsivity and aggression

◆ Controlled studies suggest that a number of medications may be useful in the treatment of impulsivity and aggression.

◆ Given the evidence for decreased serotonergic function in impulsive and aggressive behaviors, many (but not all) of these medications involve direct serotonergic mechanisms. Selective serotonin reuptake inhibitors have been shown to reduce impulsive aggressive behaviors in impulsive or aggressive psychiatric disorders.

◆ Lithium has been found effective for impulsivity and aggression across different patient populations.

Highlights for the Clinician (continued)

✦ Researchers and clinicians have used lithium, carbamazepine, valproic acid, and, more recently, gabapentin, lamotrigine, and topiramate to treat the impulsivity, aggression, and mood instability in patient populations.

✦ Monoamine oxidase inhibitors (MAOIs) have not been shown to decrease the behavioral dyscontrol or impulsivity seen in BPD. Further, in BPD patients, overdosing on psychotropic agents is a common form of suicide, and MAOIs are clearly dangerous in these situations.

✦ Although they are clearly effective for depressive symptoms, tricyclic antidepressants have not been shown to be particularly helpful in decreasing aggression and impulsivity in BPD. Further, the potential for worsening impulsive, aggressive symptoms and the danger of overdose in patients who have impaired self-control may limit the use of tricyclic antidepressants.

✦ Neuroleptics are among the most studied medications for treatment of BPD, and they have been effective in treating violence associated with psychosis. However, neuroleptics are often chronically misused as sedatives and may not be well tolerated. Despite the efficacy of these agents, clinicians should keep in mind that neuroleptics may result in a number of adverse side effects.

✦ Mood stabilizers/anticonvulsants such as valproate (divalproex), carbamazepine, topiramate, gabapentin, and lamotrigine have been effective in treating impulsivity and aggression in patient populations, in particular BPD patients.

Treatment in the developmentally disabled

✦ Autistic disorder and mental retardation are often associated with impulsive outbursts, emotional lability, rage episodes, and aggression toward self and others.

✦ Various treatments have been shown to be effective in treating aggressive and impulsive symptoms (included self-harm) in these populations. These treatments include fluoxetine, lithium, β-blockers (which also bind to 5-HT_1–like receptors, such as propranolol), carbamazepine, divalproex sodium (valproate), risperidone, and buspirone (a 5-HT_{1A} agonist).

✦ Eltoprazine, a phenylpiperazine derivative and mixed 5-HT_1 agonist, has shown antiaggressive properties in animal models.

✦ Eltoprazine-like compounds may be used in future treatment strategies and as a probe to further study the basis of impulsivity and aggression.

RECOMMENDED READINGS

Coccaro E (ed): Aggression: Psychiatric Assessment and Treatment. New York, Informa Healthcare, 2003

Hollander E, Stein DJ (eds): Impulsivity and Aggression. Sussex, UK, Wiley, 1995

Hollander E, Stein DJ (eds): Clinical Manual of Impulse-Control Disorders. Washington, DC, American Psychiatric Publishing, 2006

REFERENCES

Abbott M, Volberg R: Gambling and Problem Gambling in New Zealand: Report on Phase One of the National Survey. Research Series No 12. Wellington, New Zealand, Department of Internal Affairs, 1991

Adamac R: Does the kindling model reveal anything clinically significant? Biol Psychiatry 27:249–279, 1990

Adams DB: Brain mechanisms of aggressive behavior: an updated review. Neurosci Biobehav Rev. 30:304–e18, 2006

Ainslie G: Specious reward: a behavioral theory of impulsiveness and impulse control. Psychol Bull 82:463–496, 1975

Altshuler KZ, Abdullah S, Rainer JD: Lithium and aggressive behavior in patients with early total deafness. Dis Nerv Syst 38:521–524, 1977

American Psychiatric Association: Diagnostic and Statistical Manual of Mental Disorders, 3rd Edition, Revised. Washington, DC, American Psychiatric Association, 1987

American Psychiatric Association: Diagnostic and Statistical Manual of Mental Disorders, 4th Edition. Washington, DC, American Psychiatric Association, 1994

American Psychiatric Association: Diagnostic and Statistical Manual of Mental Disorders, 4th Edition, Text Revision. Washington, DC, American Psychiatric Association, 2000

Andrulonis PA, Glueck BC, Stroebel CF, et al: Organic brain dysfunction and the borderline syndrome. Psychiatr Clin North Am 4:47–66, 1981

Archer RP, Struve FA, Ball JD, et al: EEG in borderline personality disorder. Biol Psychiatry 24:731–732, 1988

Aronowitz B: Neuropsychiatric and neuropsychological findings in conduct disorder and attention-deficit hyperactivity disorder. J Neuropsychiatry Clin Neurosci 6:245–249, 1994

Arranz B, Eriksson A, Mellerup E, et al: Brain 5-HT$_{1A}$, 5-HT$_{1D}$ and 5-HT$_2$ receptors in suicide victims. Biol Psychiatry 35:457–463, 1994

Åsberg M, Träskman L, Thorèn P: 5-HIAA in the cerebrospinal fluid: a biochemical suicide predictor? Arch Gen Psychiatry 33:1193–1197, 1976

Bard P: A diencephalic mechanism for the expression of rage with special reference to the sympathetic nervous system. Am J Psychol 84:490–515, 1928

Barratt ES, Lijffijt M, Moeller FG: When does impulsivity become pathologic? Psychiatric Times 22:23–26, 2005

Bear DM: Neurological perspectives on aggression. J Neuropsychiatry Clin Neurosci 3 (suppl 1):3–8, 1991

Bechara A, Tranel D, Damasio H: Characterization of the decision-making deficit of patients with ventromedial prefrontal cortex lesions. Brain 123:2189–2202, 2000

Ben-Jonathan N, Abbogast LA, Hyde JF: Neuroendocrine regulation of prolactin release. Prog Neurobiol 33:399–447, 1989

Bergh C, Eklund T, Sodersten P, et al: Altered dopamine function in pathological gambling. Psychol Med 27:473–475, 1997

Berlin HA, Rolls ET: Time perception, impulsivity, emotionality, and personality in self-harming borderline personality disorder patients. J Personal Disord 18:358–378, 2004

Berlin HA, Rolls ET, Kischka U: Impulsivity, time perception, emotion, and reinforcement sensitivity in patients with orbitofrontal cortex lesions. Brain 127:1108–1126, 2004

Berlin HA, Rolls ET, Iversen SD: Borderline personality disorder, impulsivity, and the orbitofrontal cortex. 162:2360–2373, 2005

Biancosino B, Facchi A, Marmai L, et al: Gabapentin treatment of impulsive-aggressive behaviour. Can J Psychiatry 47:483–484, 2002

Biegon A, Grinspoon A, Blumfeld R, et al: Increased serotonin 5-HT$_2$ receptor binding on blood platelets of suicidal men. Psychopharmacology (Berl) 100:165–167, 1990

Bioulac B, Benezech M, Renaud B, et al: Biogenic amines in 47 XYY syndrome. Biol Psychiatry 15:917–923, 1980

Blair RJ: The roles of orbital frontal cortex in the modulation of antisocial behavior. Brain Cogn 55:198–208, 2004

Brown CS, Kent TA, Bryant SG, et al: Blood platelet uptake of serotonin in episodic aggression. Psychiatry Res 27:5–12, 1989

Brown G, Goodwin F, Ballenger J, et al: Aggression in humans correlates with cerebrospinal fluid amine metabolites. Psychiatry Res 1:131–139, 1979

Brown G, Ebert M, Grayer P, et al: Aggression, suicide, and serotonin. Am J Psychiatry 139:741–746, 1982

Brunner D, Hen R: Insights into the neurobiology of impulsive behavior from serotonin receptor knockout mice. Ann NY Acad Sci 836:81–105, 1997

Burgess JW: Cognitive information processing in borderline personality disorder. Jefferson Journal of Psychiatry 3:34–49, 1990

Burgess JW: Relationship of depression and cognitive impairment to self-injury in borderline personality disorder, major depression, and schizophrenia. Psychiatry Res 38:77–87, 1991

Buss AH: The Psychology of Aggression. New York, Wiley, 1961

Buss AH, Durkee A: An inventory for assessing different kinds of hostility. J Consult Clin Psychol 21:343–349, 1957

Cadoret RJ, Yates WR, Troughton E, et al: Adoption study demonstrating two genetic pathways to drug abuse. Arch Gen Psychiatry 52:42–52, 1995

Campbell M, Small AM, Green WH, et al: Behavioral efficacy of haloperidol and lithium carbonate: a comparison in hospitalized aggressive children with conduct disorder. Arch Gen Psychiatry 41:650–656, 1984

Campbell M, Adams PB, Small AM, et al: Lithium in hospitalized aggressive children with conduct disorder: a double-blind and placebo-controlled study. J Am Acad Child Adolesc Psychiatry 34:445–453, 1995

Cardinal RN, Pennicott DR, Sugathapala CL, et al: Impulsive choice induced in rats by lesions of the nucleus accumbens core. Science 292:2499–2501, 2001

Carrasco JL, Saiz-Ruiz J, Diaz-Marsa M, et al: Low platelet monoamine oxidase activity in sensation-seeking bullfighters. CNS Spectrums 4:21–24, 1999

Carrasco JL, Diaz-Marsa M, Hollander E, et al: Decreased platelet monoamine oxidase activity in female bulimia nervosa. Eur Neuropsychopharmacol 10:113–117, 2000

Cavedini P, Riboldi G, Keller R, et al: Frontal lobe dysfunction in pathological gambling patients. Biol Psychiatry 51:334–341, 2002

Cheung AM, Mitsis EM, Halperin JM: The relationship of behavioral inhibition to executive functions in young adults. J Clin Exp Neuropsychol 26:393–404, 2004

Christenson GA, Popkin MK, Mackenzie TB, et al: Lithium treatment of chronic hair pulling. J Clin Psychiatry 52:116–120, 1991

Coccaro EF, Murphy DL (eds): Serotonin in Major Psychiatric Disorders. Washington, DC, American Psychiatric Press, 1990

Coccaro EF, Siever LJ, Klar H, et al: Serotonergic studies in affective and personality disorder patients: correlates with suicidal and impulsive aggressive behavior. Arch Gen Psychiatry 46:587–599, 1989

Coccaro EF, Lawrence T, Trestman R, et al: Growth hormone responses to intravenous clonidine challenge correlates with behavioral irritability in psychiatric patients and in healthy volunteers. Psychiatry Res 39:129–139, 1991

Coccaro EF, Kavoussi RJ, Sheline YI, et al: Impulsive aggression in personality disorders correlates with tritiated paroxetine binding in the platelet. Arch Gen Psychiatry 53:531–536, 1996

Coccaro EF, Kavoussi RJ, Cooper TB, et al: Central serotonin activity and aggression: inverse relationship with prolactin response to D-fenfluramine, but not CSF 5-HIAA concentration, in human subjects. Am J Psychiatry 154:1430–1435, 1997

Collier DA, Stober G, Li T, et al: A novel functional polymorphism within the promoter of the serotonin transporter gene: possible role in susceptibility to affective disorders. Mol Psychiatry 1:453–460, 1996

Cornelius JR, Brenner RP, Soloff PH, et al: EEG abnormalities in borderline personality disorder: specific or nonspecific. Biol Psychiatry 21:974–977, 1986

Cornelius JR, Soloff PH, George AWA, et al: An evaluation of the significance of selected neuropsychiatric abnormalities in the etiology of borderline personality disorder. J Personal Disord 3:19–25, 1989

Cowdry RW, Gardner DL: Pharmacotherapy of borderline personality disorder: alprazolam, carbamazepine, trifluoperazine, and tranylcypromine. Arch Gen Psychiatry 45:111–119, 1988

Cowdry RW, Pickar D, Davies R: Symptoms and EEG findings in the borderline syndrome. Int J Psychiatry Med 15:201–211, 1985

Craft M, Ismail IA, Krishnamurti D, et al: Lithium in the treatment of aggression in mentally handicapped patients: a double blind trial. Br J Psychiatry 150:685–689, 1987

Dabbs JM, Carr TS, Frady RL, et al: Testosterone, crime, and misbehavior among 692 male prison inmates. Pers Individ Dif 18:627–633, 1995

Damasio AR: Descartes' Error: Emotion, Reason, and the Human Brain. New York, Putnam, 1994

Damasio AR: The somatic marker hypothesis and the possible functions of the prefrontal cortex. Philos Trans R Soc Lond B Biol Sci 351:1413–1420, 1996

Damasio AR, Tranel D, Damasio H: Individuals with sociopathic behavior caused by frontal damage fail to respond autonomically to social stimuli. Behav Brain Res 41:81–94, 1990

Dannon PN, Lowengrub K, Gonopolski Y, et al: Topiramate versus fluvoxamine in the treatment of pathological gambling: a randomized, blind-rater comparison study. Clin Neuropharmacol 28:6–10, 2005

Davidson RJ, Putnam KM, Larson CL: Dysfunction in the neural circuitry of emotion regulation: a possible prelude to violence. Science 289:591–594, 2000

DeCaria CM: Diagnosis, neurobiology and treatment of pathological gambling. J Clin Psychiatry 57 (suppl 8):80–83, 1996

DeCaria CM, Hollander E, Begaz T, et al: Reliability and validity of a pathological gambling modification of the Yale-Brown Obsessive-Compulsive Scale (PG-YBOCS): preliminary findings. 12th National Conference of Problem Gambling, Las Vegas, NV, July 17–20, 1998

De la Fuente JM, Lotstra F: A trial of carbamazepine in borderline personality disorder. Eur Neuropsychopharmacol 4:479–486, 1994

De la Fuente JM, Goldman S, Stanus E, et al: Brain glucose metabolism in borderline personality disorder. J Psychiatr Res 31:531–541, 1997

DeLong GR: Lithium carbonate treatment of select behavior disorders in children suggesting manic-depressive illness. J Pediatr 93:689–694, 1978

Denicoff KD, Meglathery SB, Post RM, et al: Efficacy of carbamazepine compared with other agents: a clinical practice survey. J Clin Psychiatry 55:70–76, 1994

Depue RA, Spoont MR: Conceptualizing a serotonin trait: a behavioral dimension of constraint. Ann N York Acad Sci 487:47–62, 1986

Dickman SJ: Impulsivity and information processing, in The Impulsive Client: Theory, Research, and Treatment. Edited by McCown WG, Johnson JL, Shure MB. Washington, DC, American Psychological Association, 1993, pp 151–184

Dicks P, Meyers RE, Kling A: Uncus and amygdala lesions: effects on social behavior in the free-ranging monkey. Science 165:69–71, 1969

Dougherty DM, Bjork JM, Huckabee HC, et al: Laboratory measures of aggression and impulsivity in women with borderline personality disorder. Psychiatry Res 85:315–326, 1999

Downer JL: Changes in visual gnostic functions and emotional behavior following unilateral temporal pole damage in the "split brain" monkey. Nature 191:50–51, 1961

Drevets WC: Functional neuroimaging studies of depression: the anatomy of melancholia. Annu Rev Med 49:341–361, 1998

Drevets WC: Prefrontal cortical-amygdalar metabolism in major depression. Ann NY Acad Sci 877:614–637, 1999

Driessen M, Beblo T, Mertens M, et al: Posttraumatic stress disorder and fMRI activation patterns of traumatic memory in patients with borderline personality disorder. Biol Psychiatry 55:603–611, 2004

Eichelman B: Effect of subcortical lesions on shock-induced aggression in the rat. J Comp Physiol Psychol 74:331–339, 1971

Elliot FA: Violence: the neurological contribution: an overview. Arch Neurol 49:595–603, 1992

Ernst M, Grant SJ, London ED, et al: Decision making in adolescents with behavior disorders and adults with substance abuse. Am J Psychiatry 160:33–40, 2003

Eslinger PJ, Damasio AR: Severe disturbance of higher cognition after bilateral frontal lobe ablation: patient EVR. Neurology 35:1731–1741, 1985

Evenden JL: The pharmacology of impulsive behaviour in rats, VII: the effects of serotonergic agonists and antagonists on responding under a discrimination task using unreliable visual stimuli. Psychopharmacology (Berl) 146:422–431, 1999

Fava M: Psychopharmacologic treatment of pathologic aggression. Psychiatr Clin North Am 20:427–451, 1997

Federal Bureau of Investigation: Crime in the United States: Uniform Crime Reports, 1990. Washington, DC, U.S. Government Printing Office, 1991

Fedora O, Fedora S: Some neuropsychological and psychophysiological aspects of psychopathic and nonpsychopathic criminals, in Laterality and Psychopathology. Edited by Flor-Henry P, Gruzelier J. Amsterdam, Elsevier, 1983, pp 20–25

Ferrari PF, Palanza P, Parmigiani S, et al: Serotonin and aggressive behavior in rodents and nonhuman primates: predispositions and plasticity. Eur J Pharmacol. 526:259–273, 2005

Ferris CF, Stolberg T, Delville Y: Serotonin regulation of aggressive behavior in male golden hamsters (Mesocricetus auratus). Behav Neurosci 113:804–815, 1999

Fishbein DH, Lozovsky D, Jaffe JH: Impulsivity, aggression, and neuroendocrine responses to serotonergic stimulation in substance abusers. Biol Psychiatry 25:1049–1066, 1989

Frankenburg FR, Zanarini MC: Divalproex sodium treatment of women with borderline personality disorder and bipolar II disorder: a double-blind placebo-controlled pilot study. J Clin Psychiatry 63:442–446, 2002

Frankle WG, Lombardo I, New AS, et al: Brain serotonin transporter distribution in subjects with impulsive aggressivity: a positron emission study with [11C]McN 5652. Am J Psychiatry 162:915–923, 2005

Gardner DL, Cowdry RW: Positive effects of carbamazepine on behavioral dyscontrol in borderline personality disorder. Am J Psychiatry 143:519–522, 1986

Gardner D, Lucas PB, Cowdry RW: Soft sign neurological abnormalities in borderline personality disorder and normal control subjects. J Nerv Ment Dis 3:177–180, 1987

Glow PH, Lange RV, Glow RA, et al: The measurement of cognitive impulsiveness: psychometric properties of two automated versions of the Matching Familiar Figures Test. J Behav Assess 3:281–295, 1981

Goldberg SC, Schulz SC, Schulz PM, et al: Borderline and schizotypal personality disorders treated with low-dose thiothixene vs placebo. Arch Gen Psychiatry 43:680–686, 1986

Goodman W, Price L, Rasmussen S, et al: The Yale-Brown Obsessive Compulsive Scale, I: development, use, and reliability. Arch Gen Psychiatry 49:1006–1011, 1989a

Goodman W, Price L, Rasmussen S, et al: The Yale-Brown Obsessive Compulsive Scale, II: validity. Arch Gen Psychiatry 49:1012–1016, 1989b

Goudriaan AE, Oosterlaan J, de Beurs E, et al: Pathological gambling: a comprehensive review of biobehavioral findings. Neurosci Biobehav Rev 28:123–141, 2004

Goudriaan AE, Oosterlaan J, de Beurs E, et al: Decision making in pathological gambling: a comparison between pathological gamblers, alcohol dependents, persons with Tourette syndrome, and normal controls. Brain Res Cogn Brain Res 23:137–151, 2005

Goyer PF, Andreason PJ, Semple WE, et al: Positron emission tomography and personality disorders. Neuropsychopharmacology 10:21–28, 1994

Grafman J, Schwab K, Warden D, et al: Frontal lobe injuries, violence, and aggression: a report of the Vietnam Head Injury Study. Neurology 46:1231–1238, 1996

Grant JE, Kim SW: An open label study of naltrexone in the treatment of kleptomania. J Clin Psychiatry 63:349–356, 2002

Grant JE, Kim SW, Grosz RL: Perceived stress in kleptomania. Psychiatr Q 74:251–258, 2003

Grattan LM, Bloomer RH, Archambault FX, et al: Cognitive flexibility and empathy after frontal lobe lesion. Neuropsychiatry Neuropsychol Behav Neurol 7:251–259, 1994

Halperin JM, Wolf L, Greenblatt ER, et al: Subtype analysis of commission errors on the Continuous Performance Test. Dev Neuropsychol 7:207–217, 1991

Hamblin MW, Metcalf MA, McGuffin RW, et al: Molecular cloning and functional characterization of a human 5-HT$_{1B}$ serotonin receptor: a homologue of the rat 5-HT$_{1B}$ receptor with 5-HT$_{1D}$-like pharmacologic specificity. Biochem Biophys Res Commun 184:752–759, 1992

Hassanain M, Bhatt S, Zalcman S, et al: Potentiating role of interleukin-1beta (IL-1beta) and IL-1beta type 1 receptors in the medial hypothalamus in defensive rage behavior in the cat. Brain Res 1048:1–11, 2005

Hathaway SR, McKinley JC: Minnesota Multiphasic Personality Inventory–2. Minneapolis, University of Minnesota, 1989

Haugh RM, Markesbery WR: Hypothalamic astrocytoma: syndrome of hyperphagia, obesity, and disturbances of behavior and endocrine and autonomic function. Arch Neurol 40:560–563, 1983

Hen R: Enhanced aggressive behavior in mice lacking HT$_{1B}$ receptor. Science 265:119–123, 1994

Herpertz SC, Dietrich TM, Wenning B, et al: Evidence of abnormal amygdala functioning in borderline personality disorder: a functional MRI study. Biol Psychiatry 50:292–298, 2001

Higley JD, Mehlman PT, Taub PM, et al: Cerebrospinal fluid monoamine and adrenal correlates of aggression in free-ranging rhesus monkeys. Arch Gen Psychiatry 48:437–441, 1992

Higley JD, Mehlman PT, Poland RE, et al: CSF testosterone and 5-HIAA correlate with different types of aggressive behaviors. Biol Psychiatry 40:1067–1082, 1996a

Higley JD, Suomi SJ, Linnoila M: A nonhuman primate model of type II excessive alcohol consumption? I: low cerebrospinal fluid 5-hydroxyindoleacetic acid concentrations and diminished social competence correlate with excessive alcohol consumption. Alcohol Clin Exp Res 20:629–642, 1996b

Hollander E, Wong CM: Obsessive-compulsive spectrum disorders. J Clin Psychiatry 56 (suppl 4):3–6, 53–55, 1995

Hollander E, Frenkel M, DeCaria C, et al: Treatment of pathological gambling with clomipramine (letter). Am J Psychiatry 149:710–711, 1992

Hollander E, Stein DJ, DeCaria CM, et al: Serotonergic sensitivity in borderline personality disorder: preliminary findings. Am J Psychiatry 151:277–280, 1994

Hollander E, DeCaria CM, Mari E, et al: Short-term single-blind fluvoxamine treatment of pathological gambling. Am J Psychiatry 155:1781–1783, 1998

Hollander E, DeCaria CM, Finkell J, et al: A randomized double-blind fluvoxamine/placebo crossover trial in pathological gambling. Biol Psychiatry 47:813–817, 2000

Hollander E, Allen A, Lopez, RP, et al: A preliminary double-blind placebo controlled trial of divalproex sodium in borderline personality disorder. J Clin Psychiatry 62:199–203, 2001a

Hollander E, Dolgoff-Kaspar R, Cartwright C, et al: An open trial of divalproex sodium in autism spectrum disorders. J Clin Psychiatry 62:530–534, 2001b

Hollander E, Tracy KA, Swann AC, et al: Divalproex in the treatment of impulsive aggression: efficacy in Cluster B personality disorders. Neuropsychopharmacology 28:1186–1197, 2003

Hollander E, Pallanti S, Allen A, et al: Does sustained-release lithium reduce impulsive gambling and affective instability versus placebo in pathological gamblers with bipolar spectrum disorders? Am J Psychiatry 162:137–145, 2005a

Hollander E, Swann AC, Coccaro EF, et al: Impact of trait impulsivity and state aggression on divalproex versus placebo response in borderline personality disorder. Am J Psychiatry 162:621–624, 2005b

Hollander E, Soorya L, Wasserman S, et al: Divalproex sodium vs placebo in the treatment of repetitive behaviors in autism spectrum disorder. Int J Neuropsychopharmacol 9:209–213, 2006

Hoptman MJ: Neuroimaging studies of violence and antisocial behavior. J Psychiatr Pract 9:265–278, 2003

Hornak J, Bramham J, Rolls ET, et al: Changes in emotion after circumscribed surgical lesions of the orbitofrontal and cingulate cortices. Brain 126:1691–1712, 2003

Hornak J, O'Doherty J, Bramham J, et al: Reward-related reversal learning after surgical excisions in orbitofrontal and dorsolateral prefrontal cortex in humans. J Cogn Neurosci 16:463–478, 2004

Huang YY, Grailhe R, Arango V, et al: Relationship of psychopathology to the human serotonin$_{1B}$ genotype and receptor binding kinetics in postmortem brain tissue. Neuropsychopharmacology 21:238–246, 1999

Isenberg N, Silbersweig D, Engelien A, et al: Linguistic threat activates the human amygdala. PNAS Online 96:10456–10459, 1999

Isern R: Family violence and the Klüver-Bucy syndrome. South Med J 80:373–377, 1987

Izquierdo A, Suda RK, Murray EA: Comparison of the effects of bilateral orbital prefrontal cortex lesions and amygdala lesions on emotional responses in rhesus monkeys. J Neurosci 25:8534–8542, 2005

Jentsch JD, Taylor JR: Impulsivity resulting from frontostriatal dysfunction in drug abuse: implications for the control of behavior by reward-related stimuli. Psychopharmacology (Berl) 146:373–390, 1999

Kagan J: Reflection-impulsivity: the generality of dynamics of conceptual tempo. J Abnorm Psychol 1:17–24, 1966

Kagan J, Messer SB: Some misgivings about the Matching Familiar Figures Test as a measure of reflection-impulsivity: commentary reply. Developmental Psychology 11:244–248, 1975

Kagan J, Rosen BL, Day D, et al: Information processing in the child: significance of analytic and reflective attitudes. Psychol Monogr (Gen Appl) 78, No 578, 1964

Kantak RM, Hegstrand LR, Eichelman B: Facilitation of shock-induced fighting following intraventricular 5,7-dihydroxytryptamine and 6-hydroxydopa. Psychopharmacology (Berl) 74:157–160, 1981

Kaufman KR, Kugler SL, Sachdeo RC: Tiagabine in the management of postencephalitic epilepsy and impulse control disorder. Epilepsy Behav 3:190–194, 2002

Kavoussi RJ, Coccaro EF: Divalproex sodium for impulsive aggressive behavior in patients with personality disorder. J Clin Psychiatry 59:676–680, 1998

Kelly TH, Cherek DR: The effects of alcohol on free-operant aggressive behavior. J Stud Alcohol Suppl 11:40–52, 1993

Kernberg O: Borderline Conditions and Pathological Narcissism. New York, Jason Aronson, 1975

Keuthen NJ, O'Sullivan RL, Ricciardi JN, et al: The Massachusetts General Hospital (MGH) Hairpulling Scale, I: development and factor analyses. Psychother Psychosom 64:141–145, 1995

Kim SW, Grant JE, Adson D, et al: Double-blind naltrexone and placebo comparison study in the treatment of pathological gambling. Biol Psychiatry 49:914–921, 2001

Klein DF: Psychiatric diagnosis and a typology of clinical drug effects. Psychopharmacologia 13:359–386, 1968

Klüver H, Bucy PC: Preliminary analysis of functions of the temporal lobes in monkeys. Archives of Neurological Psychiatry 42:979–1000, 1939

Kyes RC, Botchin MB, Kaplan JR, et al: Aggression and brain serotonergic responsivity: response to slides in male macaques. Physiol Behav 57:205–208, 1995

Ladouceur R, Sylvain C: Treatment of pathological gambling: a controlled study. Anuaria de Psicologia 30:127–135, 2000

Lappalainen J, Dean M, Charbonneau L, et al: Mapping of the serotonin 5-HT$_{1D}$ autoreceptor gene on chromosome 6 and direct analysis for sequence variants. Am J Med Genet 60:157–160, 1995

Lappalainen J, Long JC, Eggert M, et al: Linkage of antisocial alcoholism to the serotonin 5-HT$_{1B}$ receptor gene in two populations. Arch Gen Psychiatry 55:989–994, 1998

Lee GP, Bechara A, Adolphs R, et al: Clinical and physiological effects of stereotaxic bilateral amygdalotomy for intractable aggression. J Neuropsychiatry Clin Neurosci 10:413–420, 1998

LeMarquand D, Pihl RO, Benkelfat C: Serotonin and alcohol intake, abuse, and dependence: clinical evidence. Biol Psychiatry 36:326–337, 1994

LeMarquand DG, Benkelfat C, Pihl RO, et al: Behavioral disinhibition induced by tryptophan depletion in nonalcoholic young men with multigenerational family histories of paternal alcoholism. Am J Psychiatry 156:1771–1779, 1999

Lesieur HR, Blume SB: The South Oaks Gambling Screen (SOGS): a new instrument for the identification of pathological gamblers. Am J Psychiatry 144:1184–1188, 1987

Lesieur HR, Blume S: Revising the South Oaks Gambling Screen in different settings. Journal of Gambling Studies 9:213–223, 1993

Levin HS, Goldstein FC, Williams DH, et al: The contribution of frontal lobe lesions to the neurobehavioral outcome of closed head injury, in Frontal Lobe Function and Dysfunction. Edited by Levin HS, Eisenberg HM, Benton LB. Oxford, UK, Oxford University Press, 1991, pp 318–338

Lewis CE: Neurochemical mechanisms of chronic antisocial behavior: a literature review. J Nerv Ment Dis 179:720–729, 1991

Lewis DO, Pincus JH, Sharok SS, et al: Psychomotor epilepsy and violence in a group of incarcerated adolescent boys. Am J Psychiatry 139:882–887, 1982

Leyton M, Okazawa H, Diksic M, et al: Brain regional alpha-[^{11}C]methyl-L-tryptophan trapping in impulsive subjects with borderline personality disorder. Am J Psychiatry 158:775–782, 2001

Lidberg L, Åsberg M, Sundqvist-Stensman UB: 5-Hydroxyindoleacetic acid levels in attempted suicides who have killed their children (letter). Lancet 2:928, 1984

Lidberg L, Belfrage H, Bertilsson L, et al: Suicide attempts and impulse control disorder are related to low cerebrospinal fluid 5-HIAA in mentally disordered violent offenders. Acta Psychiatr Scand 101:395–402, 2000

Lilly R, Cummings JL, Benson DF, et al: The human Klüver-Bucy syndrome. Neurology 33:1141–1145, 1983

Linden RD, Pope HG Jr, Jonas JM: Pathological gambling and major affective disorder: preliminary findings. J Clin Psychiatry 47:201–203, 1986

Links PS, Steiner M, Boiago I, et al: Lithium therapy for borderline patients: preliminary findings. J Clin Psychopharmacol 4:173–181, 1990

Linnoila M, Virkkunen M, Scheinin M, et al: Low cerebrospinal fluid 5-hydroxyindoleacetic acid concentration differentiates impulsive from nonimpulsive violent behavior. Life Sci 33:2609–2614, 1983

Logue AW: Research on self-control: an integrated framework. Behav Brain Sci 11:665–709, 1988

Logue AW: Self-Control. Englewood Cliffs, NJ, Prentice Hall, 1995

Lopez-Ibor JJ, Lana F, Saiz Ruiz J: Conductas autoliticas impulsivas y serotonina. Actas Luso-Espanolas de Neurologia, Psiquiatria y Ciencias Afines 18:316–325, 1990

Lucas PB, Gardner DL, Cowdry RW, et al: Cerebral structure in borderline personality disorder. Psychiatry Res 27:111–115, 1989

Luria AR: Higher Cortical Functions in Man. New York, Basic Books, 1980

Lyoo IK, Han MH, Cho DY: A brain MRI study in subjects with borderline personality disorder. J Affect Disord 50:235–243, 1998

Lyvers M: "Loss of control" in alcoholism and drug addiction: a neuroscientific interpretation. Exp Clin Psychopharmacol 8:225–249, 2000

Mak M, DeKoning P, Mos J, et al: Preclinical and clinical studies on the role of the 5-HT$_1$ receptors in aggression, in Impulsivity and Aggression. Edited by Hollander E, Stein DJ. New York, Wiley, 1995, pp 289–311

Malone RP, Delaney MA, Luebbert JF, et al: A double-blind placebo-controlled study of lithium in hospitalized aggressive children and adolescents with conduct disorder. Arch Gen Psychiatry 57:649–654, 2000

Mann JJ, McBride PA, Anderson GM, et al: Platelet and whole blood serotonin content in depressed inpatients: correlations with acute and lifetime psychopathology. Biol Psychiatry 32:243–257, 1992

Manuck SB, Flory JD, Ferrell RE, et al: Aggression and anger-related traits associated with a polymorphism of the tryptophan hydroxylase gene. Biol Psychiatry 45:603–614, 1999

Marazziti D, Conti L: Aggression, hyperactivity, and platelet IMI-binding. Acta Psychiatr Scand 84:209–211, 1991

Markowitz PI: Fluoxetine treatment of self-injurious behavior in the mentally retarded (letter). J Clin Psychopharmacol 10:299–300, 1990

Markowitz PI: Effect of fluoxetine on self-injurious behavior in the developmentally disabled: a preliminary study. J Clin Psychopharmacol 12:27–31, 1992

Marlowe WB, Mancall EL, Thomas JJ: Complete Klüver-Bucy syndrome in man. Cortex 11:53–59, 1975

Matthys W, Van Goozen SH, de Vries H, et al: The dominance of behavioural activation over behavioural inhibition in conduct disordered boys with or without attention deficit hyperactivity disorder. J Child Psychol Psychiatry 39:643–651, 1998

McBurnett K, Lahey BB, Rathouz PJ, et al: Low salivary cortisol and persistent aggression in boys referred for disruptive behavior. Arch Gen Psychiatry 57:38–43, 2000

McCracken JT, McGough J, Shah B, et al: Risperidone in children with autism and serious behavioral problems. Research Units on Pediatric Psychopharmacology Autism Network. N Engl J Med 347:314–321, 2002

McElroy SC, Hudson JI, Pope HG Jr, et al: Kleptomania: clinical characteristics and associated psychopathology. Psychol Med 21:93–108, 1991

Meyer-Lindenberg A, Buckholtz JW, Kolachana B, et al: Neural mechanisms of genetic risk for impulsivity and violence in humans. Proc Natl Acad Sci USA 103:6269–6274, 2006

Milner B: Some cognitive effects of frontal-lobe lesions in man. Philos Trans R Soc Lond B Biol Sci 298:211–226, 1982

Moll GH, Rothenberger A: [Lithium salts in child and adolescent psychiatry] Nervenarzt 69:935–943, 1998 (in German)

Moreno I, Saiz-Ruiz JY, Lopez-Ibor JJ: Serotonin and gambling dependence. Hum Psychopharmacol 6:9–12, 1991

Morgan MA, Romanski LM, LeDoux JE: Extinction of emotional learning: contribution of medial prefrontal cortex (letter). Neuroscience 163:109–113, 1993

Moss HB, Yao YK, Panzak GL: Serotonergic responsivity and behavioral dimensions in antisocial personality disorder with substance abuse. Biol Psychiatry 28:325–338, 1990

Nachson I: Hemisphere function in violent offenders, in Biological Contributions to Crime Causation. Edited by Moffitt TE, Mednick SA. Dordrecht, Germany, Martinus Nijhoff, 1988, pp 55–67

Nakamura K, Kurasawa M, Shirane M: Impulsivity and AMPA receptors: aniracetam ameliorates impulsive behavior induced by a blockade of AMPA receptors in rats. Brain Res 862:266–269, 2000

New AS, Trestman RL, Siever LJ: Borderline personality disorder, in Impulsivity and Aggression. Edited by Hollander E, Stein DJ. New York, Wiley, 1995, pp 153–173

New AS, Trestman RL, Mitropoulou V, et al: Serotonergic function and self-injurious behavior in personality disorder patients. Psychiatry Res 69:17–26, 1997

New AS, Gelernter J, Yovell Y, et al: Tryptophan hydroxylase genotype is associated with impulsive-aggression measures: a preliminary study. Am J Med Genet 81:13–17, 1998

New AS, Gelernter J, Goodman M, et al: Suicide, impulsive aggression, and HTR1B genotype. Biol Psychiatry 50:62–65, 2001

New AS, Hazlett EA, Buchsbaum MS, et al: Blunted prefrontal cortical 18fluorodeoxyglucose positron emission tomography response to meta-chlorophenylpiperazine in impulsive aggression. Arch Gen Psychiatry 59:621–629, 2002

New AS, Buchsbaum MS, Hazlett EA, et al: Fluoxetine increases relative metabolic rate in prefrontal cortex in impulsive aggression. Psychopharmacology (Berl) 176:451–458, 2004a

New AS, Trestman RF, Mitropoulou V, et al: Low prolactin response to fenfluramine in impulsive aggression. J Psychiatr Res 38:223–230, 2004b

Newman JP, Widom CS, Nathan S: Passive avoidance in syndromes of disinhibition: psychopathy and extraversion. J Pers Soc Psychol 48:1316–1327, 1985

Nickel MK, Nickel C, Mitterlehner FO, et al: Topiramate treatment of aggression in female borderline personality disorder patients: a double-blind, placebo-controlled study. J Clin Psychiatry 65:1515–1519, 2004

Nickel MK, Nickel C, Kaplan P, et al: Treatment of aggression with topiramate in male borderline patients: a double-blind, placebo-controlled study. Biol Psychiatry 57:495–499, 2005

Nickel MK, Muehlbacher M, Nickel C, et al: Aripiprazole in the treatment of patients with borderline personality disorder: a double-blind, placebo-controlled study. Am J Psychiatry 163:833–838, 2006

Nielson DA, Goldman D, Virkkunen M, et al: Suicidality and 5-hydroxyindoleacetic acid concentration associated with a tryptophan hydroxylase polymorphism. Arch Gen Psychiatry 51:34–38, 1994

Nishimura H, Suzuki M, Kasahara H, et al: Efficacy of lithium carbonate on public and compulsive masturbation: a female case with mild mental disability. Psychiatry Clin Neurosci 51:411–413, 1997

Norden MJ: Fluoxetine in borderline personality disorder. Prog Neuropsychopharmacol Biol Psychiatry 13:885–893, 1989

O'Keane V, Moloney E, O'Neill H, et al: Blunted prolactin responses to d-fenfluramine in sociopathy: evidence for subsensitivity of central serotonergic function. Br J Psychiatry 160:643–646, 1992

O'Leary KM, Brouwers P, Gardner DL, et al: Neuropsychological testing of patients with borderline personality disorder. Am J Psychiatry 148:106–111, 1991

Oquendo MA, Mann JJ: The biology of impulsivity and suicidality. Psychiatr Clin North Am 23:11–25, 2000

Ovsiew F, Yudofsky S: Aggression: a neuropsychiatric perspective, in Rage, Power, and Aggression: The Role of Affect in Motivation, Development and Adaptation. Edited by Glick RA, Roose SP. New Haven, CT, Yale University Press, 1983, pp 213–230

Pallanti S, Quercioli L, Sood E, et al: Lithium and valproate treatment of pathological gambling: a randomized single-blind study. J Clin Psychiatry 63:559–564, 2002

Patton JH, Stanford MS, Barratt ES: Factor structure of the Barratt Impulsiveness Scale. J Clin Psychol 51:768–774, 1995

Petry NM: Pathological gamblers, with and without substance use disorders, discount delayed rewards at high rates. J Abnorm Psychol 110:482–487, 2001a

Petry NM, Casarella T: Excessive discounting of delayed rewards in substance abusers with gambling problems. Drug Alcohol Depend 56:25–32, 1999

Petry NM: Substance abuse, pathological gambling, and impulsiveness. Drug Alcohol Depend 63:29–38, 2001b

Philip A: The development and use of the Hostility and Direction of Hostility Questionnaire. J Psychosom Res 13:283–287, 1969

Pinto OC, Akiskal HS: Lamotrigine as a promising approach to borderline personality: an open case series without concurrent DSM-IV major mood disorder. J Affect Disord 51:333–343, 1998

Popova NK: From genes to aggressive behavior: the role of serotonergic system. Bioessays 28:495–503, 2006

Preston GA, Marchant BK, Reimherr FW, et al: Borderline personality disorder in patients with bipolar disorder and response to lamotrigine. J Affect Disord 79:297–303, 2004

Puumala T, Sirviö J: Changes in activities of dopamine and serotonin systems in the frontal cortex underlie poor choice accuracy and impulsivity of rats in an attention task. Neuroscience 83:489–499, 1998

Rachlin H: Self-control: beyond commitment. Behav Brain Sci 18:109–159, 1995

Raine A, Buchsbaum MS, Stanley J, et al: Selective reductions in prefrontal glucose metabolism in murderers. Biol Psychiatry 36:365–373, 1994

Raine A, Buchsbaum M, LaCasse L: Brain abnormalities in murderers indicated by positron emission tomography. Biol Psychiatry 42:495–508, 1997

Raine A, Melroy JR, Bihrle S, et al: Reduced prefrontal and increased subcortical brain functioning assessed using positron emission tomography in predatory and affective murderers. Behav Sci Law 16:319–332, 1998

Raine A, Lencz T, Bihrle S, et al: Reduced prefrontal gray matter volume and reduced autonomic activity in antisocial personality disorder. Arch Gen Psychiatry 57:119–129, 2000

Ramirez LF, McCormick RA, Russo AM, et al: Patterns of substance abuse in pathological gamblers undergoing treatment. Addict Behav 8:425–428, 1983

Rauch SL, Shin LM, Whalen PJ, et al: Neuroimaging and the neuroanatomy of posttraumatic stress disorder. CNS Spectrums 3 (suppl 2):30–41, 1998

Reeves AG, Plum F: Hyperphasia, rage, and dementia accompanying a ventromedial hypothalamus neoplasm. Arch Neurol 20:616–624, 1969

Regard M, Knoch D, Guetling E, et al: Brain damage and addictive behavior: a neuropsychological and electroencephalogram investigation with pathologic gamblers. Cogn Behav Neurol 16:47–53, 2003

Rinne T, Westenberg HG, den Boer JA, et al: Serotonergic blunting to meta-chlorophenylpiperazine (m-CPP) highly correlates with sustained childhood abuse in impulsive and autoaggressive female borderline patients. Biol Psychiatry 47:548–556, 2000

Robbins TW: Dissociating executive functions of the prefrontal cortex. Philos Trans R Soc Lond B Biol Sci 351:1463–1471, 1996

Rocha FL, Rocha ME: Kleptomania, mood disorder and lithium. Arq Neuropsiquiatr 50:543–546, 1992

Rogers RD, Robbins TW: Investigating the neurocognitive deficits associated with chronic drug misuse. Curr Opin Neurobiol 11:250–257, 2001

Rolls ET, Hornak J, Wade D, et al: Emotion-related learning in patients with social and emotional changes associated with frontal lobe damage. J Neurol Neurosurg Psychiatry 57:1518–1524, 1994

Sabrie P: Reconciling the role of central serotonin neurons in human and animal behavior. Behav Brain Sci 9:319–364, 1986

Saiz J, Moreno I, Lopez-Ibor JJ: Ludopatia: estudio clínico y terapéutico-evolutivo de un grupo de jugadores patológicos. Actas Luso-Españolas de Neurologia, Psiquiatrica y Ciencias Afines 20:189–197, 1992

Schmahl CG, Vermetten E, Elzinga BM, et al: A positron emission tomography study of memories of childhood abuse in borderline personality disorder. Biol Psychiatry 55:759–765, 2004

Schultz SC, Camlin KL, Berry SA, et al: Olanzapine safety and efficacy in patients with borderline personality disorder and comorbid dysthymia. Biol Psychiatry 46:1429–1435, 1999

Schulz SC, Koller MM, Kishore PR, et al: Ventricular enlargement in teenage patients with schizophrenia spectrum disorder. Am J Psychiatry 140:1592–1595, 1983

Seguin JR: Neurocognitive elements of antisocial behavior: relevance of an orbitofrontal cortex account. Brain Cogn 55:185–197, 2004

Shaffer D, Schonfeld IS, O'Connor PA, et al: Neurological soft signs and their relationship to psychiatric disorder and intelligence in childhood and adolescence. Arch Gen Psychiatry 42:342–351, 1985

Sheard M: Effect of lithium on human aggression. Nature 230:113–114, 1971

Sheard MH: Lithium in the treatment of aggression. J Nerv Ment Dis 160:108–118, 1975

Sheard MH, Marini JL, Bridges CI, et al: The effect of lithium on impulsive aggressive behavior in man. Am J Psychiatry 133:1409–1413, 1976

Sheard MH, Marini JL, Giddings SS: The effect of lithium on luteinizing hormone and testosterone in man. Dis Nerv Syst 38:765–769, 1977

Siassi I: Lithium treatment of impulsive behavior in children. J Clin Psychiatry 43:482–484, 1982

Siever LJ, Davis KL: A psychological perspective on the personality disorders. Am J Psychiatry 148:1647–1658, 1991

Siever LJ, Buchsbaum MS, New AS, et al: d,l-Fenfluramine response in impulsive personality disorder assessed with [^{18}F]fluorodeoxyglucose positron emission tomography. Neuropsychopharmacology 20:413–423, 1999

Silver JM, Yudofsky SC: Organic mental disorder and impulsive aggression, in Impulsivity and Aggression. Edited by Hollander E, Stein D. New York, Wiley, 1995, pp 243–259

Simeon D, Stanley B, Frances A, et al: Self-mutilation in personality disorders: psychological and biological correlates. Am J Psychiatry 149:221–226, 1992

Singer MT: The borderline diagnosis and psychological tests: review and research, in Borderline Personality Disorder. Edited by Harticollis P. New York, International Universities Press, 1977, pp 193–212

Snyder S, Pitts WM Jr: Electroencephalography of DSM-III borderline personality disorder. Acta Psychiatr Scand 69:129–134, 1984

Snyder S, Pitts WM, Gustin Q: CT scans of patients with borderline personality disorder (letter). Am J Psychiatry 140:272, 1983

Soler J, Pascual JC, Campins J, et al: Double-blind, placebo-controlled study of dialectical behavior therapy plus olanzapine for borderline personality disorder. Am J Psychiatry 162:1221–1224, 2005

Soloff PH, George A, Nathan RS, et al: Progress in pharmacology of borderline disorders. Arch Gen Psychiatry 43:691–697, 1986

Soloff PH, Cornelius J, Foglia J, et al: Platelet MAO in borderline personality disorder. Biol Psychiatry 29:499–502, 1991

Soloff PH, Meltzer CC, Greer PJ, et al: A fenfluramine-activated FDG-PET study of borderline personality disorder. Biol Psychiatry 47:540–547, 2000

Spielberger CD: Anger Expression Inventory. Odessa, FL, Psychological Assessment Resources, 1988

Spinella M: Neurobehavioral correlates of impulsivity: evidence of prefrontal involvement. Int J Neurosci 114:95–104, 2004

Stanley B, Molcho A, Stanley M, et al: Association of aggressive behavior with altered serotonergic function in patients who are not suicidal. Am J Psychiatry 157:609–614, 2000

Stein DJ: Trichotillomania and obsessive-compulsive disorder. J Clin Psychiatry 56 (suppl 4):28–34, 1995

Stein DJ, Hollander E, Cohen L, et al: Neuropsychiatric impairment in impulsive personality disorders. Psychiatry Res 48:257–266, 1993a

Stein DJ, Hollander E, Liebowitz MR: Neurobiology of impulsivity and the impulse control disorders. J Neuropsychiatry Clin Neurosci 5:9–17, 1993b

Stein DJ, Simeon D, Frenkel M, et al: An open trial of valproate in borderline personality disorder. J Clin Psychiatry 56:506–510, 1995

Stoff DM, Pollack L, Vitello B, et al: Reduction of (^{3}H)-imipramine binding sites on platelets of conduct disordered children. Neuropsychopharmacology 1:55–62, 1987

Sudak HW, Maas JW: Behavioral neurochemical correlation in reactive and nonreactive strains of rats. Science 146:418–420, 1964

Taylor SP: Aggressive behavior and physiological arousal as a function of provocation and the tendency to inhibit aggression. J Pers 35:297–310, 1987

Trimble MR, Van Elst LT: On some clinical implications of the ventral striatum and the extended amygdala: investigations of aggression. Ann NY Acad Sci 877:638–644, 1999

Trimble MR, Mendez MF, Cummings JL: Neuropsychiatric symptoms from the temporolimbic lobes. J Neuropsychiatry Clin Neurosci 9:429–438, 1997

Tupin JP: Usefulness of lithium for aggressiveness. Am J Psychiatry 135:1118, 1978

Tupin JP, Smith DB, Clanon TL, et al: The long-term use of lithium in aggressive prisoners. Compr Psychiatry 14:311–317, 1973

U.S. Department of the Treasury, Bureau of Alcohol, Tobacco and Firearms: Crime Gun Trace Reports (2000) National Report. Youth Crime Gun Interdiction Initiative. Washington, DC, U.S. Department of the Treasury, 2002

Van Elst LT, Thiel T, Hesslinger B, et al: Subtle prefrontal neuropathology in a pilot magnetic resonance spectroscopy study in patients with borderline personality disorder. J Neuropsychiatry Clin Neurosci 13:511–514, 2001

Van Elst TL, Hesslinger B, Thiel T, et al: Frontolimbic brain abnormalities in patients with borderline personality disorder: a volumetric magnetic resonance imaging study. Biol Psychiatry 54:163–171, 2003

Van Reekum R: Acquired and developmental brain dysfunction in borderline personality disorder. Can J Psychiatry 38 (suppl 1):S4–S10, 1993

Vazquez Rodriguez AM, Arranz Pena MI, Lopez Ibor JJ, et al: Clomipramine test: serum level determination in three groups of psychiatric patients. J Pharm Biomed Anal 9:949–952, 1991

Villeneuve E, Lemelin S: Open-label study of atypical neuroleptic quetiapine for treatment of borderline personality disorder: impulsivity as main target. J Clin Psychiatry 66:1298–1303, 2005

Virkkunen M, Linnoila M: Serotonin in early-onset, male alcoholics with violent behavior. Ann Med 22:327–331, 1990

Virkkunen M, Nuutila A, Goodwin FK, et al: Cerebrospinal fluid monoamine metabolite levels in male arsonists. Arch Gen Psychiatry 44:241–247, 1987

Vitiello B, Stoff D, Atkins M, et al: Soft neurological signs and impulsivity in children. J Dev Behav Pediatr 11:112–115, 1990

Volkow ND, Tancredi L: Neural substrates of violent behaviour: a preliminary study with positron emission tomography. Br J Psychiatry 151:668–673, 1987

Volkow ND, Tancredi LR, Grant C, et al: Brain glucose metabolism in violent psychiatric patients: a preliminary study. Psychiatry Res 61:243–253, 1995

Vollm B, Richardson P, Stirling J, et al: Neurobiological substrates of antisocial and borderline personality disorder: preliminary results of a functional fMRI study. Crim Behav Ment Health 14:39–54, 2004

Wasman M, Flynn JP: Directed attack elicited from the hypothalamus. Arch Neurol 6:220–227, 1962

Weiger WE, Bear DM: An approach to the neurology of aggression. J Psychiatr Res 22:85–98, 1988

Williams DT, Mehl R, Yudofsky S, et al: The effect of propranolol on uncontrolled rage outbursts in children and adolescents with organic brain dysfunction. J Am Acad Child Psychiatry 21:129–135, 1982

Winchel RM, Jones JS, Molcho A, et al: The Psychiatric Institute Trichotillomania Scale (PITS). Psychopharmacol Bull 28:463–476, 1992

Yehuda R, Southwick SM, Edell WS, et al: Low platelet monoamine oxidase activity in borderline personality disorder. Psychiatry Res 30:265–273, 1989

Yeudall LT, Fromm-Auch D: Neuropsychological impairments in various psychopathological populations, in Hemisphere Asymmetries of Function in Psychopathology. Edited by Gruzelier J, Flor-Henry P. Amsterdam, Elsevier, 1979, pp 81–83

14

NEUROPSYCHIATRIC ASPECTS OF MEMORY AND AMNESIA

Yaakov Stern, Ph.D.

Harold A. Sackeim, Ph.D.

MEMORY SYSTEMS

The research and clinical understanding of memory has increased dramatically since the 1990s. Three related lines of research have demonstrated that memory is not a unitary entity and have outlined the nature of different memory "systems":

1. In experimental cognitive research with healthy individuals, comparisons of different types of tasks have dissected memory into interrelated, but discriminable, processes.
2. Studies of abilities that are differentially affected and retained in patients with discrete brain lesions have also supported the concept of distinct memory systems.
3. Functional brain imaging studies using cognitive challenge procedures with positron emission tomography (PET) or functional magnetic resonance imaging (fMRI) have contributed to the separation of memory processes and contributed to the understanding of the neural network mediating memory performance.

For some memory systems, there is relatively good evidence that they are subserved by specific areas of the brain or by specific neural networks. Other systems without clear-cut anatomical correlates have been identified experimentally on the basis of the type of information they

process or the way they operate. Thus, whether some distinct memory systems actually represent different brain systems remains to be seen. In this section, we review the different aspects of memory that have been identified. The various systems are summarized in Figure 14–1.

Most memory researchers make an initial separation of memory into two categories: 1) declarative and 2) nondeclarative (Cohen and Squire 1980; Squire 1992). *Declarative memory* describes the conscious recollection of words, scenes, faces, stories, and events. It is the type of memory assessed by traditional tests of recall and recognition, which rely on what has been called the *explicit* retrieval of information (Graf and Schacter 1985). *Nondeclarative memory* is best described in the negative—as a collection of memory processes that are not declarative. The hallmark of nondeclarative memory is evidence that some types of life experience can result in behavioral change without requiring conscious access to the experience—that is, without explicit recall. Tests of nondeclarative memory typically rely on what has been called *implicit* retrieval; these tests attempt to demonstrate that a particular type of experience has resulted in a later change in behavior. Several types of memory are subsumed under the heading of nondeclarative memory, including procedural memory, classical conditioning, simple associative learning, and priming. Another category of memory separate from the declarative-nondeclarative distinction is *working mem-*

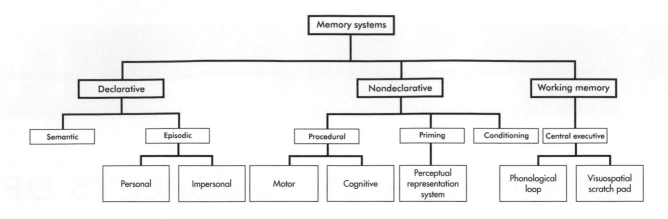

FIGURE 14–1.   An outline of the components of memory.

Source.   Adapted from Squire 1992.

ory. Working memory is viewed as an active memory buffer that can serve either as a scratch pad for newly acquired information or as a locus and mechanism for retrieving and operating on already stored information. Later discussed in this chapter are the *system* and *process* concepts of memory and the coordination of memory systems.

DECLARATIVE MEMORY

Declarative memory is the aspect of memory that is most often assessed clinically with tests of recall or recognition. It is usually subdivided into two components: semantic memory and episodic memory (Tulving 1972, 1983). *Semantic memory* refers to the acquisition of factual information about the world. Typically, semantic memories cannot be fixed as having been acquired at a specific time. For example, although people know Shakespeare is the author of *Hamlet,* few could recall when this information was first encoded. *Episodic memory* refers to the recording and conscious recollection of personal experiences. Semantic memory is required for episodic memory. However, typical recollections are more than simple facts. They include the spatial and temporal context of events as well as other associated features, such as the emotions associated with life events and the specific details that encompass life events. Episodic memory encompasses personal or autobiographical memories as well as memories of public events. Most standard clinical assessments of memory evaluate semantic memory. It is important to recognize that personal or autobiographical events may become semantic memories, losing any associated recall of spatial or temporal context. People may remember, as a fact, that they graduated from college in a particular year but have no recall of the events surrounding the graduation.

A key observation underlying the current memory taxonomy is that declarative memory is dependent on the integrity of the hippocampus and its related structures. This dependence was demonstrated most dramatically by the famous case of H.M., who underwent surgery for severe epilepsy (Milner 1959). The medial temporal region of this individual's brain, including the uncus, amygdala, anterior two-thirds of the hippocampus, and hippocampal gyrus, was removed bilaterally. After the operation, he was unable to retain new information if he was distracted for more than a few seconds from rehearsing the material. Thus, his performance on standard tests of recall was impaired, and he could not learn new vocabulary words. However, his recall of events remote from the operation was close to normal (Corkin 1984; Marslen-Wilson and Teuber 1975). Other intellectual functions, including IQ, were spared. H.M. remains densely amnesic to this day. H.M.'s case provides compelling evidence for the importance of the hippocampus and related structures to the process of memory formation and storage that supports the laying down of new declarative memories. Indeed, the strongest argument for the existence of a memory system can be made for declarative memory, which can be convincingly demonstrated to rely, at least in part, on a specific set of brain structures.

An fMRI paradigm called the *subsequent memory effect* elegantly demonstrates the brain areas involved in the encoding of episodic memories. Using this approach, Wagner et al. (1998) conducted brain scans of subjects as words were presented to them; following these encoding scans, subjects' memory for the words was assessed by a recognition test. The fMRI data were analyzed by categorizing encoding trials on the basis of whether the word was either subsequently remembered or forgotten on the postscan memory test. The event-related design permitted identification of regions that demonstrate differential activation during the encoding of words subsequently remembered and those subsequently forgotten. When the investigators compared high-confidence hits with misses, they noted greater activation in multiple left prefrontal regions and left parahippocampal and fusiform gyri for remembered words. This study demonstrates the role of the hippocampus and surrounding areas in the encoding of memories. In addition, the left prefrontal regions may serve to organize information in working memory, with this serving as input to the parahippocampal gyrus and the medial temporal memory system (see the section "Working Memory" later in this chapter for more detail).

NONDECLARATIVE MEMORY

The concept of nondeclarative memory stems from the observation that several types of memory tasks can be performed successfully even by patients who have sustained damage to the hippocampus and its associated structures (Cohen and Squire 1980), with marked deficits in declarative memory. The fact that studies of healthy control subjects have also demonstrated dissociations in task performance suggests that some tasks do not require declarative memory. Unlike declarative memory, nondeclarative memory cannot be considered a system. Rather, the term is simply a general classification for a disparate group of tasks (and presumably memory processes) whose performance is not mediated by conscious recall. Some of these tasks have been grouped into hypothetical systems, which are discussed below: procedural memory, simple conditioning and simple associative learning, and priming. One unifying feature of nondeclarative memory tasks is that they demand implicit recall, in which there is no need for conscious storage or recall of material.

Procedural Memory

The term *procedural memory* is typically applied to tasks that assess the acquisition of motor or cognitive skills. One can describe procedural memory as "knowing how," as opposed to declarative memory's "knowing that" (Cohen and Squire 1980).

A well-investigated test of procedural memory is the Tower of Hanoi task. In this task, which is based on an old puzzle, the subject is given a board with three posts. On one of the posts is a pile of disks of graduated sizes, so that each disk is smaller than the one below it. The subject's task is to move all of the disks from one post to another, following two rules: only one disk can be moved at a time, and a larger disk can never be put on top of a smaller disk. The key to solving this puzzle is to develop the optimal sequence of moves needed to move the disks. With practice, an amnesic patient can improve his or her performance on this task to the optimal level (Cohen 1984;

Cohen and Corkin 1981). When given the task again at a later date, the amnesic patient does not remember ever having performed it and needs to be taught the rules as if this were his or her first exposure. However, once the patient begins to perform the task, it is clear that the performance level is far better than at the first exposure to the task. Thus, although the individual has no episodic memory for the task or its rules, the procedures or strategies that contribute to task performance have been retained. This procedural memory is implicit and is thought to be not dependent on the perihippocampal structures.

Procedural memory has also been demonstrated for motor tasks. One example is the pursuit rotor task, in which the subject must learn to keep a stylus touching a spot on a revolving turntable. As with the more cognitively based Tower of Hanoi task, amnesic patients can learn and retain this skill (Corkin 1968). Other tests of procedural learning include mirror reading and jigsaw puzzle assembly.

The brain areas that mediate procedural memory have not been identified. However, because several studies have suggested that learning the pursuit rotor task depends on the integrity of the basal ganglia, it is possible that procedural memory for motor tasks depends on areas of the brain associated with initial task acquisition and performance (Butters et al. 1990). Similarly, it has been suggested that the brain structures that mediate the acquisition and initial performance of motor tasks also mediate procedural memory for these cognitive skills.

Simple Conditioning and Simple Associative Learning

Amnesic patients can acquire new conditioned responses. In one early study, Weiskrantz and Warrington (1979) assessed classical conditioning of the blink response in two amnesic patients. These patients retained conditioned responses for as long as 24 hours even though they did not recognize the conditioning apparatus. Other simple associative learning is also intact in amnesic patients.

Priming

Priming is another type of nondeclarative memory that requires implicit recall. Some investigators have suggested that distinct memory systems may underlie performance on priming tasks. *Priming* can be defined as the facilitated identification of perceptual objects from reduced cues as a consequence of prior exposure to those objects (Tulving and Schacter 1990).

In a typical priming task, the subject studies some material but is not told that he or she will be expected to recall it. For example, the subject may be given a list of words and asked to identify those that contain a particular letter or to make some judgment about the words (e.g., degree of pleasantness). A key feature of the subsequent retrieval task is that it is also implicit. For example, in one typical retrieval task, the subject is given the first three letters of words (i.e., word stems) and asked to generate words that begin with those stems as quickly as possible. Half of the word stems are the beginnings of words to which the subject was previously exposed, while the other half correspond to new words. In this experiment, the subject will generate words more rapidly for stems of previously studied words. This priming effect is not dependent on explicit recall and is present in amnesic patients (Graf and Schacter 1985). In addition, this priming experiment includes an explicit-recall component, usually a recognition task in which the subject is given a list of words containing both previously studied and new words. Typically the subject's ability to discriminate the "old" from the "new" words is quite poor, thus demonstrating that exposure to the words was not sufficient for retrieval in a standard explicit-recall task.

A wide range of priming paradigms has been used. The studied material has included words, shapes, and sounds. The mode of exposure of the studied list also has been extensively varied, and these studies have provided insight into the memory processes underlying priming. An important feature of the subject's initial exposure to the list is the level of processing. A distinction can be made between instructions that call attention to the perceptual features of items (e.g., their shape, constituent letters) and those that require a deeper or more conceptual level of processing (e.g., making judgments about whether words belong to specific categories). In general, the more the mode of study is perceptual in nature (a quality some researchers call "data driven"), the better the priming performance. In contrast, deeper conceptual study is more beneficial to declarative modes of recall (Blaxton 1995).

Some priming tasks benefit from deeper levels of processing. These tasks, known as *conceptual priming tasks*, require semantic processing of the task stimuli and often require responses that are conceptually or semantically related to a stimulus. For example, subjects are given the name of a category (e.g., animal) and asked to produce the first instance that comes to mind (e.g., bear). It has been argued that these conceptual priming tasks differ from standard perceptual priming and rely on semantic learning (Tulving and Schacter 1990).

The sensitivity of priming performance to perceptual manipulation, as well as the lack of reliance on hippocampal systems in priming, has led some theorists to suggest that priming is an expression of *perceptual representation systems* (PRS)—a group of domain-specific subsystems that process and represent information about the form and structure, but not the meaning or other associative properties, of words and objects (Tulving and Schacter 1990). PRS are thought to involve the brain areas responsible for the initial perception and processing of material. Schacter and colleagues have proposed three such systems: 1) visual word form (Schacter 1990), 2) auditory word form (Schacter and Church 1992), and 3) structural description (Schacter et al. 1990). The most carefully developed of these hypothesized systems is the visual word form PRS, which presumably mediates most of the visually presented verbal priming tasks. This system would include areas in the occipital cortex and elsewhere that are important for visual processing, but it would exclude both those areas involved in the semantic processing of words and those implicated in explicit recall.

Working Memory

Working memory is typically viewed as distinct from the declarative and nondeclarative memory systems. In one sense, working memory is similar to what in the past has been called *short-term memory*. It provides a repository for briefly holding on to information such as a telephone number or the name of a newly met person. It is also important in tasks that require mental manipulation of information, such as multistep arithmetic problems. However, for many theorists (e.g., Goldman-Rakic 1992), working memory also has a more important role as the "work space" where recalled information is actually used, manipulated, and related to other information, thus allowing complex cognitive processes such as comprehension, learning, and reasoning to take place.

A detailed model of working memory was proposed by Baddeley (1986). In this model, working memory is viewed not as a single memory buffer, but instead as three interrelated components comprising an attentional controller (the *central executive*) aided by two active "slave" subsystems: the articulatory or phonological loop and the visuospatial "scratch pad" or "sketch pad." The phonological loop maintains speech-based information. Without this loop, such information would fade rapidly. However, the information can be maintained for longer periods by an articulatory control process, which in effect recycles or rehearses the information. Thus, one way to remember a telephone number until it is dialed is to mentally repeat it continuously. Similar to the phonological loop, the visuospatial scratch pad briefly stores and rehearses visuospatial information. Baddeley's current version of the working memory also incorporates a fourth component, termed the *episodic buffer* (Baddeley 2000). This buffer plays a role in integrating information from subsidiary systems and from long-term memory.

Although the central executive is presumably the most important component of working memory, its role is the least well defined. One function of the central executive is to coordinate information from the separate subsystems. In one study of this function, subjects were asked to simultaneously perform pursuit-tracking and digit-span tasks, the latter of which involves remembering a newly presented string of numbers. Because these two tasks rely on the phonological loop and the visuospatial scratch pad, a subject's relative ability or inability to perform them simultaneously may reflect the capacity of the central executive. Another function attributed to the central executive is the organization and generation of new strategies for the retrieval or processing of information.

Memory Consolidation

Studies of amnesic patients—as well as of normal humans and animals treated with electroconvulsive shock or specific medications—suggest that there is a difference between how memory is stored for short and longer periods of time.

The short-term memory store has limited capacity and persists for just a few minutes without rehearsal. This level of storage is probably comparable to that described in the working memory system. The short-term memory store is thought to be based either on short-term changes in synaptic transmission or on some form of ongoing neural activity that maintains the information. Manipulations that silence neuronal activity, such as cooling or anoxia, can disrupt short-term but not long-term memories.

If memory is to persist longer, it must be transferred into a long-term memory store. Long-term memory storage can be subdivided into 1) an earlier phase that is relatively sensitive to disruption and 2) a later phase that is more insensitive to disruption. Studies in electroconvulsive therapy (ECT) support this theory (for more detail, see "Electroconvulsive Therapy and Other Brain Stimulation Treatments" later in this chapter). For example, immediately following ECT treatment course, deficits in the recall or recognition of both personal and public information learned before ECT treatment (i.e., retrograde amnesia) are common (Lisanby et al. 2000; Sackeim 1992; Sackeim et al. 1993, 2000). These deficits are greatest for events that occurred temporally closest to the treatment, typically within weeks or months (Lisanby et al. 2000; McElhiney et al. 1995; Squire 1986). Thus, whereas memory for more remote events is intact, patients may have difficulty recalling events that occurred during and several months, or in some cases a few years, before the ECT course. This observation is consistent with the idea that the more recent memories are more easily disrupted because they have not yet been stored in their final long-term memory form. In classic amnesia, the retrograde amnesia also can have a temporal gradient, with poorer recall for more recent information (Russell and Nathan 1946). The observation that ECT-caused retrograde amnesia is mostly transitory argues that the memory stores themselves are not affected by ECT, but rather the ability to retrieve these memories (Sackeim 1992).

Animal studies using agents designed to block protein or mRNA synthesis have shown that long-term memory is selectively impaired and short-term memory is unaffected (Davis and Squire 1984). In this case, the actual long-term storage of the material may be affected rather than the retrieval from long-term storage. Thus memories in the later phase of long-term storage are probably in the form of actual protein changes that alter the connections between neurons.

SYSTEM VERSUS PROCESS CONCEPTS

Some investigators have preferred to categorize memory tasks in a way that does not rely on the concept of systems. Thus, for example, the dissociations in performance between a task that requires implicit retrieval (such as priming) and a task that requires explicit retrieval (such as a word recognition test) might not be a function of the use of separate memory systems. Rather, a *process-based* view of memory would posit that these dissociations are a function of the type of processing performed on the test material at study and test. In general, to the degree that the type of processing at study is recapitulated at test, memory performance will improve (Blaxton 1995; Gabrieli 1995). Two types of processing are typically considered: 1) conceptually driven processing, which is based on the semantic meaning of stimuli; and 2) data-driven processing, which is based on the perceptual features of stimuli. Often, the study phase of priming tests is data driven, with the subject instructed to attend to some perceptual feature of the studied material. This procedure creates an advantage in a data-driven test such as the word-fragment technique sometimes used in priming tasks (see the section "Priming" earlier in this chapter) and a disadvantage in a more conceptually driven task such as word recognition. Alternatively, when material is studied at a conceptually driven level—for example, by generating synonyms to the studied words—an advantage is created in tests that also require this type of processing. Thus, the process-based approach argues that it is not necessary to posit that implicit and explicit retrieval reflect two distinct memory systems. Rather, processing matches or mismatches can be introduced into tasks requiring either type of retrieval with predictable results.

Proponents of the process-based approach most often study healthy subjects, although predictions from this approach have been supported in some studies of populations with brain damage, including left temporal lobe epilepsy and Alzheimer's disease (Blaxton 1992). However, the process-based predictions are not completely upheld in individuals with diencephalic or bilateral medial temporal amnesia (Keane et al. 1993). These patients appear to have normal priming on implicit conceptual memory tasks but are impaired on explicit conceptual tasks. This pattern supports the argument that these patients have a deficit in explicit recall, as systems theorists would predict. Most theorists now agree that systems- and process-based approaches are not mutually exclusive and that manipulations of processing type can enrich insights about the nature of memory systems.

COORDINATION OF MEMORY SYSTEMS

Although experimental manipulations and careful observation of patients with brain lesions support the concept of dissociable memory systems, it should be stressed that these systems do not usually operate independently. For example, in a healthy subject, a priming task probably does not measure implicit recall only, because performance might also be aided by explicit recall. Consequently, most experimenters design priming studies to minimize the influence of explicit recall. Other investigators, however, have developed techniques that attempt to evaluate the relative contributions of explicit (or conscious) and implicit (or unconscious) recall during the performance of a memory task (Jacoby et al. 1992).

More importantly, memory theorists have proposed models of memory that suggest how the different memory systems are normally integrated. Presented here is a simplification of one such model, proposed by Moscovitch (1994). Modules similar to the PRS (described earlier in this chapter, in the section "Priming") are responsible for the perception and encoding of information. Other associated central systems semantically encode the perceptual information. These systems operate automatically (without awareness) and may subserve implicit recall. The information from these systems can be delivered to working memory, where it can be briefly stored or processed. According to Moscovitch (1994), information in working memory that receives full conscious attention is automatically processed by the hippocampus and related structures. Storage in these structures is in the form of simple association, in which a cue in working memory will produce the associated memories from the hippocampal structures regardless of whether they are relevant. Input to the hippocampus from working memory and output from the hippocampus to working memory can be guided, organized, and evaluated by executive systems, most likely located in prefrontal cortex. In this model, "the frontal lobes are necessary for converting remembering from a stupid reflexive act triggered by a cue to an intelligent, reflective, goal-directed activity under voluntary control" (Moscovitch 1994, pp. 278–279). Acquisition and retention of skills in procedural memory tasks may be mediated by modification of the same structures that are involved in task performance, similar to the operation of PRS in priming tasks. This model integrates the reviewed declarative and nondeclarative memory systems, as well as the components of working memory, into a coordinated system and provides a framework for how these systems interact. Clearly, in the course of day-to-day activities, all of these systems must work together to allow individuals to store, recall, and use memories.

AMNESIA

Amnesia is the generic term for severe memory deficit, regardless of cause. Table 14–1 summarizes the DSM-IV-TR (American Psychiatric Association 2000) criteria for amnesia.

Four clinical characteristics are typical of most amnesic patients: anterograde amnesia, retrograde amnesia, confabulation, and intact intellectual function. *Anterograde amnesia* is the hallmark of an amnestic disorder; it refers to the inability after the onset of the disorder to acquire new information for explicit retrieval. *Retrograde amnesia* refers to difficulty in retrieving events that occurred before the onset of the amnestic disorder, often demarcated as the time of head trauma, stroke, or other injury. Retrograde amnesia is more variably present in different amnesias. When amnesic patients are asked to recall information and cannot, they may *confabulate;* that is, they may provide made-up or inaccurate information without having any apparent awareness that their responses are incorrect. Again, confabulation does not occur in all amnesias, and it is often more common in the acute stage of the neuropsychiatric illness. Finally, in the classic amnestic disorders, the patients' intellectual function remains relatively intact even though some specific secondary cognitive defects may be noted on careful neuropsychological testing.

LESIONS OF THE MEDIAL REGIONS OF THE TEMPORAL LOBES

The classic case of bilateral medial temporal lobe (MTL) ablation is the patient H.M., who was described earlier in this chapter in the section "Declarative Memory." Since

TABLE 14–1. DSM-IV-TR criteria for amnestic disorder

A. The development of memory impairment as manifested by impairment in the ability to learn new information or the inability to recall previously learned information.

B. The memory disturbance causes significant impairment in social or occupational functioning and represents a significant decline from a previous level of functioning.

C. The memory disturbance does not occur exclusively during the course of a delirium or a dementia.

D. There is evidence from the history, physical examination, or laboratory findings that the disturbance is the direct physiological consequence of a general medical condition (including physical trauma).

Source. Reprinted from American Psychiatric Association: *Diagnostic and Statistical Manual of Mental Disorders*, 4th Edition, Text Revision. Washington, DC, American Psychiatric Association, 2000. Used with permission.

his surgery, H.M. has had severe anterograde amnesia and essentially cannot recall or recognize virtually any newly learned information. He can remember events from his early childhood but has difficulty with events that occurred just before his operation, indicating a restricted retrograde amnesia. His IQ is in the normal range.

Although bilateral temporal lobectomies are rare, unilateral temporal lobectomies are commonly performed to treat intractable seizure disorders. This operation is usually effective in treating the seizure disorder, and patients may have no obvious memory deficits. However, careful testing often demonstrates subtle memory impairments: removal of the left temporal lobe commonly produces relative deficits in verbal memory, and removal of the right temporal lobe commonly produces relative deficits in remembering nonverbal information. These results indicate material-specific amnesia. A similar pattern has often been demonstrated in the acute postictal state following ECT, where unilateral treatment with electrodes on the left side produces greater persistence of postictal confusion and verbal anterograde and retrograde memory deficits, while stimulation over the right hemisphere produces greater anterograde and retrograde memory deficits for nonverbal material (Sackeim 1992). Likewise, left and right medial temporal lobe sclerosis due to epilepsy has been associated with material-specific amnesia.

WERNICKE-KORSAKOFF SYNDROME

Wernicke-Korsakoff syndrome is the prototypical example of diencephalic amnesia, given that the memory disorders seen in this condition are attributed to lesions of medial diencephalic brain structures, including the dorsomedial nucleus of the thalamus and/or the mammillary bodies (Victor et al. 1989). The syndrome is typically observed in nutritionally depleted alcoholic patients. When the diet is insufficient, neuronal injury occurs in thiamine-dependent areas of the brain and can lead to the characteristic lesions associated with this condition. In the acute phase, Wernicke's encephalopathy, patients commonly present with complaints of mental confusion, staggering gait, ocular symptoms, and polyneuropathy. The chronic phase of the disease, Korsakoff's psychosis, is characterized by both anterograde and retrograde memory deficits. The anterograde amnesia is dense, with the patient unable to recall events that are no longer in working memory. Retrograde amnesia consists of difficulty recalling past personal or public events. Recall is poorest for events that are closest to the onset of the amnesia and improves for events in the more distant past. This pattern of retrograde amnesia is called a *temporal gradient* (Albert et al. 1979). Performance on IQ tests is comparable to that of chronic alcoholic individuals without amnesia. Deficits can be demonstrated, however, on tests that require speed and visuoperceptual and spatial organization components. The neuropathology of this syndrome consists of lesions to the paraventricular regions of the thalamus, the hypothalamus, the mammillary bodies, the periaqueductal region of the midbrain, the floor of the fourth ventricle, and the superior vermis (Victor et al. 1989).

FRONTAL LOBE LESIONS AND THE ROLE OF THE FRONTAL LOBES IN MEMORY

Most of the literature investigating frontal lobe lesions has concentrated on cognitive functions other than memory. Although the frontal lobes are complex structures with many differentiated areas and functions, the consensus had long been that lesions to the frontal lobes do not produce the kinds of memory deficits that are seen in amnesia. Memory performance is affected in patients with frontal lobe lesions, but deficits have been attributed to the roles of frontal structures in the placement of information into spatial and temporal contexts and in the execution of complex mnemonic strategies (Baddeley 1986; Milner et al. 1985). Without spatial and temporal contexts, organizing information for storage or retrieval is difficult. Some patients with frontal lobe lesions have been described as not being able to remember to remember; that is, they do not spontaneously initiate the activity required to retrieve information or to identify a retrieval strategy. This view of the frontal lobes in memory loss is concordant with the model of memory systems set forth above (see the section "Coordination of Memory Systems" earlier in this chapter).

However, a recent meta-analysis of studies relating frontal lobe lesions to tests of recognition, cued recall, and free recall suggests that all three types of performance are disrupted in patients with frontal lobe lesions (Wheeler et al. 1995). In many published studies, there was a nonsignificant trend toward better performance in the control groups, with the failure to obtain statistically significant differences often attributed to a lack of statistical power. This weakness is eliminated with meta-analysis. The review found that patients with frontal lobe lesions performed more poorly on recall than on recognition tests, which again may implicate the processes involved in the organization of information and the initiation of recall as the primary reasons for the memory deficit. However, the patients also performed more poorly than control subjects on recognition tasks, which may suggest that the frontal lobes have a more primary role in episodic memory.

Nonetheless, the role of the frontal lobe in memory processes is undergoing substantial reevaluation. This stems principally from several sources of evidence. First, frontal lobe damage can result in a profound, temporally graded retrograde amnesia (Kopelman 1992; Kopelman et al. 1999; Moscovitch 1994; Shimamura 1994; Stuss and Benson 1986), in some comparisons as great as MTL pathology (Kopelman et al. 1999) and presumably due to the disruption of retrieval processes. In amnesic patients, anterograde and retrograde amnesia are often weakly associated, and there is evidence that tests of frontal lobe (executive) function covary with the magnitude of retrograde amnesia (Kopelman 1992).

Markowitsch (1995, 2000) conducted a careful analysis of the sites of injury in brain-damaged patients with preserved anterograde memory but marked retrograde amnesia. He proposed that ventrolateral (orbital) prefrontal cortex and temporopolar cortex, interconnected through the ventral branch of the uncinate fasciculus, are essential for the retrieval of declarative information from long-term memory, with the caveat that right-sided damage was especially associated with retrograde amnesia. A host of imaging studies in normal samples have shown activation of ventrolateral prefrontal cortex and anterolateral portions of the temporal cortex during episodic memory retrieval (Buckner 1996; Buckner et al. 1995, 1998a, 1998b, 1999, 2000; S. Kapur et al. 1995; Lepage et al. 2000; Shallice et al. 1994; Tulving and Markowitsch 1997; Tulving et al. 1994a, 1994b, 1999). Thus, the evidence from focal retrograde amnesia (N. Kapur 1999) and

imaging studies of normal recall or recognition of newly learned information emphasize a key contribution of the ventrolateral prefrontal cortex and the temporal pole.

More generally and surprisingly, early imaging studies of the retrieval of newly learned information had difficulty in showing MTL activation (Schachter and Wagner 1999). However, other work has suggested that there may be differential encoding and retrieval activation within the hippocampus along the rostral-caudal axis (Lepage et al. 1998). In addition, the novelty of stimuli may strongly impact the nature of MTL activation. Using fMRI in normal participants, Saykin et al. (1999) and Johnson et al. (2001) found that the processing of novel words led to activation of the left anterior hippocampus, whereas recognition of familiar words activated the left posterior parahippocampal gyrus and right dorsolateral prefrontal cortex. In particular, retrieval success was strongly associated with activation of the right dorsolateral prefrontal cortex (Johnson et al. 2001).

Overall, it is more firmly established from imaging studies that dorsal prefrontal cortical regions participate in retrieval of newly learned information. Tulving and colleagues offered the hemispheric encoding/retrieval asymmetry (HERA) model (S. Kapur et al. 1995; Nyberg et al. 1996a, 1996b, 1996c, 1998, 2000; Tulving and Markowitsch 1997, 1998; Tulving et al. 1994a, 1994b), which posits that that the left prefrontal cortex (particularly the dorsolateral prefrontal cortex) is critical to the encoding of novel information in episodic memory and retrieval from semantic memory. In contrast, the right prefrontal cortex (particularly the dorsolateral prefrontal cortex) is critical in episodic memory retrieval. HERA has been carefully critiqued (Buckner 1996; Nyberg et al. 1996a), and regions involved in encoding and retrieval have been refined. For instance, S. Kapur et al. (1995) distinguished between general retrieval attempt and successful retrieval of stored memories, or *ecphory*. Whereas the former was associated with primarily right prefrontal activation (Brodmann area [BA] 9/10/46), the latter was characterized by activation of more posterior right-sided regions (right cuneus-precuneus). Subsequently, Lepage et al. (2000) made the distinction between episodic retrieval mode (REMO) and ecphory. REMO was associated with greater right than left prefrontal cortical activation, including BA 9/10. The investigators concluded that the retrieval asymmetry in HERA is explained by the asymmetry in REMO but that the new findings did not necessitate reformulation of the encoding asymmetry aspect of HERA (left > right). In other work, Nyberg et al. (2000) used partial least squares analyses of imaging data and identified a functional network involving the right prefrontal cortex, left MTL, and left parietal regions (cuneus-precuneus) in episodic retrieval. Thus, beyond the MTL, recent work on memory retrieval of newly learned information in normal subjects has generally emphasized right-sided dorsal prefrontal (typically dorsolateral) structures, as well as ventromedial and temporopolar regions. Notably, the left dorsolateral prefrontal cortex is thought to be critical in the retrieval of semantic memories (i.e., facts about the world).

This imaging work with normal participants has focused on retrieval of (impersonal) newly learned information (e.g., word lists). Relevance to the understanding of retrograde amnesia in patients with lesions (or who have received ECT) or for the processes mediating memories of the personal past may be questionable. Only a small set of studies has examined activation patterns during recall of autobiographical memories in healthy subjects (with only case studies of patients with retrograde amnesia), and in general this literature is methodologically compromised (e.g., no control over the age of events recalled, no verification of accuracy of recall). Andreasen et al. (1995) found left dorsolateral prefrontal activation during recall of autobiographical or personal memories. As the investigators' procedure involved verbalization during scanning, they repeated the experiment with silent recall (Andreasen et al. 1999), finding activation of medial and orbital frontal cortex, anterior cingulate, left parietal regions, and left thalamus. In line with HERA, Fink et al. (1996) found that retrieval of autobiographical memories activated multiple right hemisphere regions, including dorsal prefrontal cortex (BA 6); temporomedial, temporoparietal, and temporolateral cortex; and posterior cingulate. There was also activation of MTL structures, including amygdala, hippocampus, and parahippocampus. In contrast, Conway et al. (1999) found predominantly left-sided activation (frontal BA 6/44/45) and inferior temporal lobe activation (BA 20) in response to recall of both recent and remote autobiographical memories. The investigators also detected hippocampal activation under both conditions, implying that even if remote memory storage extends beyond MTL regions, intact hippocampal function may be necessary for successful retrieval. Finally, Maguire and Mummery (1999) found evidence of left temporal pole, left medial frontal cortex (BA 10), and left hippocampal activation during retrieval of autobiographical memories. Taken together, these studies indicate that there is great uncertainty about the exact region(s) necessary for retrieval of autobiographical memories in normal participants. Furthermore, unlike the larger literature on retrieval of newly learned information, this handful of imaging studies of autobiographical memory has not explicitly examined the consequences of unsuccessful ecphory of events (i.e., amnesia). Finally, aside from Conway et al. (1999), no study has examined differential activation of recent versus remote autobiographical memories, despite the fact that most theories suggest a time-limited role for events to be stored in the MTL before permanent transfer to cortical representations (e.g., Moscovitch 1994).

ALZHEIMER'S DISEASE

Alzheimer's disease is a progressive dementing disorder that affects a wide range of intellectual functions. The hallmark of all dementias is acquired amnesia, along with deficits in other cognitive functions. Patients with Alzheimer's disease have difficulty learning new material. In addition, their memory deficit is characterized by rapid forgetting of newly acquired material (Welsh et al. 1992). In addition, as the disease progresses, there is a growing retrograde amnesia, typically manifesting a classic temporal gradient, with greatest preservation of remote memories. Recent studies suggest that the memory deficit of Alzheimer's disease is actually present years before the clinical diagnosis becomes apparent (Jacobs et al. 1995). The histopathological manifestations of Alzheimer's disease—cell loss, senile plaques, and neurofibrillary tangles—are relatively widespread but early in the disease are primarily present in the hippocampus and surrounding entorhinal cortex (Ball et al. 1985).

Twelve elders who had documented isolated memory decline over 3 years but no dementia were studied with an fMRI paradigm in which they studied pictured faces for later recall (Small et al. 1999). The subjects were dichotomized into two subgroups: four with diminished entorhinal activation (i.e., entorhinal activation at least two standard deviations below that of the normal elderly) and eight with normal entorhinal activation. The diminished entorhinal activation subgroup had diminished activation in the hippocampus proper and the subiculum compared with normal elderly. The diminished-activation subgroup may have preclinical Alzheimer's disease. The normal-activation subgroup had diminished activation restricted to the subiculum. This subgroup of subjects is unlikely to have early Alzheimer's disease but may have memory decline for some other reason.

Other imaging work suggests that some patients with early Alzheimer's disease utilize the same neural networks as matched elderly controls when performing memory tasks (Stern et al. 2000). In contrast, the investigators found that other patients with Alzheimer's disease appear to utilize different and apparently compensatory networks. The use of compensatory networks is associated with poorer memory performance and may mark a stage of disease progression in which pharmacological attempts to arrest the disease process may be less successful.

PSYCHIATRIC DISORDERS AND NORMAL AGING

The major psychiatric disorders—schizophrenia, mania, and major depression—almost invariably compromise aspects of attention and concentration (Goldberg and Gold 1995; Sackeim and Steif 1988). Because the ability to focus and sustain attention is central to the acquisition of new information in general and declarative memory in particular, deficits in acquiring new information are common among these patients. Traumatic episodes can lead to amnesia. Finally, normal aging is associated with specific declines in memory.

MOOD DISORDERS

Since the classic work of Cronholm and Ottosson (1961), it has been repeatedly demonstrated that although patients experiencing an episode of major depression or mania have a reduced capacity to learn new, unstructured information, they usually have less impairment in retaining the information that they do learn. For example, in verbal and nonverbal paired-associate tasks, depressed patients will typically recall fewer items than will matched control subjects when tested immediately after stimulus presentation, with the extent of this deficit often associated with measures of depression severity and reversal with successful treatment (Bornstein et al. 1991; Steif et al. 1986; Sternberg and Jarvik 1976). In contrast, after controlling for the amount of information learned, researchers have found that depressed patients and control subjects typically do not differ in the percentage of the material recalled after a delay. Thus, in general, depression appears to have a greater influence on the acquisition than the retention of information (D.B. Burt et al. 1995). However, memory impairments have been identified in mood disorder samples. Zakzanis et al. (1998), in a meta-analysis, found that anterograde memory tests were among the most discriminative neuropsychological measures in distinguishing patients with major depression from matched controls. In part, this finding may be due to the contribution of attentional deficits to memory performance.

This acquisition impairment is most marked for material that is unstructured and that exceeds the capacity of working memory. Healthy individuals are capable of recalling or recognizing 7 ± 2 items immediately after presentation, and this aspect of short-term memory is often assessed with digit-span tests. The evidence is mixed that digit-span performance is impaired in the major mood disorders (Breslow et al. 1980; Gass and Russell 1986; Whitehead 1973). When deficits on this measure are observed in mood disorder patients, it is generally thought that the deficits reflect not an inherent limitation in the capacity of working memory, but rather an attentional dysfunction, with difficulties in concentration leading to greater distractibility and interference effects.

Other sources support the notion that attentional dysfunction and, more generally, impaired executive skills commonly form the basis for memory deficits in mood disorders (Sackeim and Steif 1988). Calev and Erwin (1985) compared depressed patients and healthy control subjects on a verbal memory task in which the difficulty of recall and recognition was matched. Depressed patients demonstrated deficits in recall but not in recognition. This finding suggested that there were no deficits in the consolidation and storage of information, but that depressed patients had a reduced ability to organize effective retrieval strategies. Furthermore, the deficits in episodic memory seen in depressed patients are most pronounced when the material to be learned is unstructured. For example, when given a list of words to remember that are drawn from semantic categories (e.g., pants, shirt, shoe) in which the order of words is clustered by category, depressed patients are typically equivalent to healthy control subjects in recall. However, when overt clustering is not provided, patients manifest a recall deficit (Backman and Forsell 1994; Channon et al. 1993; Weingartner et al. 1981). This finding suggests that depressed patients are less likely both to spontaneously impose organization on new information and to link that information to preexisting knowledge. Consequently, the depth of encoding is more shallow, resulting in impaired learning and retrieval.

Automatic and Effortful Processing

Cognitive psychologists have distinguished between automatic and effortful processing (Hasher and Zacks 1979). Similar to the notion of nondeclarative memory, automatic operations place limited demands on attentional capacity and occur without intention or awareness. A person's learning and retaining knowledge of what he or she had for breakfast—that is, incidental learning—is an example of automatic processing. In contrast, effortful processing requires the use of limited attentional capacity, is initiated intentionally, and benefits from rehearsal. Committing to memory a long shopping list is an example of effortful processing. In general, depressed patients are more likely to manifest deficits on tasks that require effort or greater depth of processing but not on tasks that can be completed automatically (Roy-Byrne et al. 1986; Weingartner et al. 1981). Similarly, most studies that have compared implicit and explicit memory in major depression have noted deficits in the declarative (explicit) domain but not in the nondeclarative (implicit) domain (Bazin et al. 1994; Watkins et al. 1996). This overall pattern may be useful clinically in distinguishing depressed patients from those with Alzheimer's disease. Antero- grade memory deficits are expected in Alzheimer's dis- ease even when tasks call for shallow processing and min- imal effort. Furthermore, a conservative response bias is commonly observed in major depression, where recogni- tion errors tend to be false-negative errors; that is, pa- tients fail to recognize a previously learned stimulus (Cor- win et al. 1990). In contrast, patients with Alzheimer's disease are often more prone to false-positive errors, mis- identifying a novel stimulus as part of a learning set (Gain- otti and Marra 1994; Lachner and Engel 1994).

Mood-Congruence Effects

Often, depressed patients not only are impaired in their capacity for effortful learning but also manifest changes in the content of memory. In clinical interviews, it is evident that much of the recollection of depressed patients involves autobiographical events with negative emotional valence. The concept of the effects of mood congruence on memory stipulates that the efficiency of mnemonic processing is influenced by the match between an existing mood state and the affective tone of the material to be remembered (Blaney 1986; Singer and Salovey 1988). There will be greater access to those memories whose affective valence is congruent with the current mood state. For example, some evidence exists that depressed psychi- atric patients are more likely to recall experiences of fail- ure relative to experiences of success (DeMonbreun and Craighead 1977). Furthermore, this biasing of memory may extend beyond explicit, conscious recall. Watkins et al. (1996) found that whereas healthy control subjects showed greater implicit priming effects for positively emo- tionally toned words than for negative words, the opposite characterized depressed patients. The concept of mood congruence is attractive in helping to account for the apparent bias in accessibility of personal memories among depressed patients. However, in clinical samples, such mood-congruence effects have been observed mostly in memory tests for experimenter-presented material (Breslow et al. 1981). When effects have been obtained for "real-life" autobiographical memories, they have often pertained to the latency of recall (e.g., Lloyd and Lishman 1975) or to the extent of detail in the reported memories (Brittlebank et al. 1993). In addition, there is evidence that mood-congruence effects are most readily obtained when the recall of autobiographical memories is relatively unstructured (Eich et al. 1994). Typical procedures involve presentation of cue words as free-association stimuli for recalling autobiographical events. In contrast, when using procedures that required a deliberate memory search for specific classes of events, McElhiney et al. (1995) found no difference between severely depressed patients and healthy control subjects in capacity to recall negatively ver- sus positively charged autobiographical memories. If this formulation is correct, it suggests that the spontaneous trains of thought of depressed patients are biased to retrieve negative affective memories but that no abnormal- ities are seen when retrieval is guided or structured.

Impact of Episodic Frequency

There is increasing evidence that the neuropsychological impairments, and in particular memory disturbance, in mood disorder patients may not fully reverse with reso- lution of the depressive or manic episode and may inten- sify with repeated episodes. T. Burt et al. (2000) com- pared young and elderly unipolar and bipolar patients in an episode of major depression on a variety of antero- grade memory tasks. The elderly bipolar patients, even though free of psychotropic medication, had the poorest performance of all groups, suggesting a particular iatro- genic effect of a long-term history of bipolar disorder. This finding is all the more impressive because in evalua- tions of neuropsychological differences between young adults with unipolar and bipolar illness, subjects with bipolar disorder have generally fared better (Donnelly et al. 1982; Mason 1956; McKay et al. 1995; Overall et al. 1978). In a meta-analysis of 40 studies, Kindermann and Brown (1997) reported that studies that examined both bipolar and unipolar patients found greater dysfunction of moderate effect size when compared to studies exam- ining patients with unipolar depression alone. The larger differences were found for 1) figural (vs. verbal) mem- ory; 2) delayed (vs. immediate) memory; and 3) recogni- tion (vs. free and cued recall). Similarly, D. B. Burt et al. (1995) in another meta-analysis noted that recall deficits were of greater magnitude in samples that contained both bipolar and unipolar depressed patients compared with samples restricted to unipolar major depression.

Anatomical Correlates

Several studies have shown that bipolar patients in the euthymic state manifest neuropsychological deficits rela- tive to matched control subjects—but the characterization of these deficits is still unclear, with the exception possibly of impairments in verbal learning and executive function (Coffman et al. 1990; Kessing 1998; van Gorp et al. 1998) and the suggestion that greater frequency of episodes or duration of illness may be related to greater impairment. Of particular note, Shelline et al. (1999) examined euthy- mic women with a history of unipolar major depression and reported that the number of days lifetime in a depressive episode was inversely related to hippocampal volume. The interpretation offered is that excessive glucocorticoids (e.g., hypercortisolemia) during the episode have an atrophic effect on hippocampal volume. Notably, reduced hippocampal size was associated with inferior performance on a verbal memory test. Thus, there has been a major change in perspective. Memory deficits in mood disorders were largely seen as a state-dependent phenomenon, mainly attributable to attentional disturbance and difficulties with effortful processing. There is incomplete, but increasing, evidence that learning and memory abnormalities may persist during euthymia and may reflect structural brain abnormalities induced by the mood disorder episodes.

SCHIZOPHRENIA

Schizophrenia is associated with disturbances in attention, motor behavior, processing speed, abstraction, learning, and memory. Indeed, patients with schizophrenia perform poorly on a wide variety of cognitive and behavioral tasks. This generalized intellectual decline seems to be present early in the illness and, in most cases, does not appear to be subsequently progressive (Hyde et al. 1994; Nopoulos et al. 1994). Given the multiple dimensions of deficit, one goal of neuropsychological investigation has been to determine whether certain cognitive domains are especially impaired in schizophrenia. The belief has been that identifying such differential deficits may provide leads regarding the cognitive dysfunction that plays a more primary role in the disorder's pathoetiology (Blanchard and Neale 1994; Chapman and Chapman 1973). Related goals have been to determine whether subgroups of patients differ in their profiles of cognitive disability and to relate findings of cognitive impairment to functional and structural brain abnormalities (Goldberg and Gold 1995).

A major focus of research on memory impairment in schizophrenia has been to improve characterization of the deficits in working and declarative memory. In line with imaging studies of function and structure, the most characteristic neuropsychological profile in schizophrenia is compatible with deficits in systems mediated by the prefrontal and temporohippocampal cortex (M.A. Taylor and Abrams 1984), with relative sparing of language and visuospatial processing mediated by posterior cortex.

There is debate concerning whether schizophrenia's deficits in working memory and associated executive functions are less or more profound than those in verbal, declarative memory (Goldberg and Gold 1995; Saykin et al. 1994). In a large study of first-episode, never medicated patients, previously treated, medication-free patients, and healthy control subjects, Saykin et al. (1994) reported that verbal memory impairment was the most profound deficit and was present early in the course of the illness. The magnitude of impairment in this domain was extensive even after the investigators controlled for impairments in executive functions (i.e., attention-vigilance, abstraction-flexibility). Similarly, in a community-based study of 138 patients with schizophrenia, Kelly et al. (2000) found that 15% had significant global cognitive impairment, 81% had impaired memory, 25% had executive dyscontrol, and 49% had impaired verbal fluency. Elvevag et al. (2000) attempted to examine how various manipulations of paired-associate learning would interfere with the memory performance of patients with schizophrenia in a manner akin to the interference seen with patients with frontal lobe damage. The investigators concluded that the susceptibility to interference effects was not a specific problem in patients with schizophrenia but reflected a more general disturbance in memory. Verdoux and Liraud (2000) compared the memory and executive abilities of patients with schizophrenia, other schizophrenic psychoses, bipolar disorder, and major depression. Memory deficits were most discriminatory between patients with schizophrenia and those with other psychotic or mood disorders.

The verbal memory deficit seen in patients with schizophrenia is compatible with left temporohippocampal dysfunction and has been observed in patients with schizotypal personality disorder (Voglmaier et al. 2000). Related imaging research with fluorodeoxyglucose-PET in the resting state revealed that increased metabolic activity in the left inferior frontal and left midtemporal regions was associated with increased verbal memory deficits (Mozley et al. 1996). This finding was interpreted as indicating dysfunction in the circuitry subserving declarative verbal memory and, in particular, excessive activation in these regions. Compatible with these findings is a highly consistent set of observations of volume reduction in the left temporal lobe of patients with schizotypal personality disorder, first-episode schizophrenia, and chronic schizophrenia (Gur et al. 2000; McCarley et al. 1999) and reduced P300 evoked potential amplitudes over the left temporal lobe in patients with schizophrenia (O'Donnell et al. 1999; Salisbury et al. 1999). Compared to controls and patients with manic psychosis, patients with first-episode schizophrenia have smaller gray matter left planum temporale and Heschl gyrus volumes (Hirayasu et al. 2000). Patients with chronic schizophrenia may be more likely to show volume reductions in MTL structures, particularly the hippocampus (Dickey et al. 1999).

However, Gold et al. (1995) compared neuropsychological profiles in patients with schizophrenia and patients with left or right temporal lobe epilepsy. Among the epileptic patients, particularly those with left temporal lobe epilepsy, memory was selectively impaired relative to other domains, particularly attention. Among patients with schizophrenia, the magnitude of attentional and memory impairments was relatively equal. Other research has suggested that individual patients may differ in the extent to which they manifest neuropsychological impairments characteristic of frontal lobe (executive function) or temporal lobe (episodic memory) dysfunction (Harvey et al. 1995) and that impairments in each domain may have distinct clinical correlates (Sullivan et al. 1994). Indeed, in a recent study, Weickert et al. (2000) examined neuropsychological profiles in a large group of patients with chronic schizophrenia in relation to estimates of current and premorbid intellectual level. Across the subgroups, the investigators concluded that deficits in attention and executive function may be core cognitive features of the disorder, independent of variations in intelligence. In examining patients with schizophrenia, healthy siblings, and controls, Staal et al. (2000) found that executive function deficits and, to some extent, sensorimotor impairments characterized both the patients and siblings, suggesting that these cognitive abnormalities may be related to the schizophrenia genotype.

Impairments in executive function and in working memory suggest disruption of prefrontal cortical function. Compatible physiological and biochemical data have been obtained. Callicott et al. (2000) reported that during the performance of a working memory task (N-Back), patients with schizophrenia manifested abnormal activation in the dorsolateral prefrontal cortex; in patients and controls, the direct correlation between the degree of activation response and performance was opposite in direction. Furthermore, N-acetylaspartate (NAA) concentrations, measured by proton magnetic resonance spectroscopy, were lower in this region (BA 9, 46) in patients with schizophrenia compared to controls, suggesting prefrontal neuronal pathology; NAA levels predicted the fMRI response to the working memory challenge. Thus, in addition to the substantial evidence for a (verbal) declarative memory deficit in schizophrenia, it is evident that many patients also manifest deficits in working memory and other executive functions.

The nature of the declarative memory deficits in schizophrenia has been further specified. Deficits are usually more pronounced in tests of recall than in tests of recognition (Beatty et al. 1993; Calev 1984). The deficits in explicit recall have often been attributed to shallow or inefficient encoding of information, disorganized or inefficient retrieval strategies, and rapid forgetting (Goldberg and Gold 1995; McKenna et al. 1990). Notably, a growing number of studies have reported that patients with schizophrenia evidence little or no deficits in nondeclarative memory

tasks, including procedural memory (as reflected in motor skill learning) and implicit memory (as reflected in various tests of perceptual and conceptual priming) (Clare et al. 1993; Gras-Vincendon et al. 1994; Perry et al. 2000).

As indicated, schizophrenia is also associated with often profound impairments in aspects of working memory. Primate and human research has indicated that various prefrontal areas are critical to the capacity to hold information in consciousness, update past and current information based on a changing environment, and guide behavior on the basis of these representations (Goldman-Rakic 1994). Lesions in selective prefrontal areas in primates result in characteristic deficits in modality-specific aspects of working memory. Neuropsychological tests designed to sample analogous functions in humans have repeatedly shown marked deficits in patients with schizophrenia (Keefe et al. 1995; Park and Holzman 1993). Indeed, a diverse number of deficits are subsumed under the concepts of "working memory" and "executive function." The central executive is responsible for selecting stimuli for further processing (i.e., allocating attention). Deficits in this function will be reflected in increased distractibility and inability to maintain vigilance. In line with decades of research suggesting increased distractibility, Fleming et al. (1995) demonstrated that even a simple concurrent task will interfere with short-term memory performance in patients with schizophrenia. Furthermore, the central executive is responsible for shifting sets (i.e., changing strategies and behaviors when they no longer meet environmental demands). A deficit in this domain would be expressed as perseveration and as difficulty with rule learning and concept formation. Impairments in these domains are characteristic of schizophrenia, as reflected in performance deficits on the Wisconsin Card Sorting Test (Heaton et al. 1993) or the Category Test from the Halstead-Reitan Battery (Reitan and Wolfson 1985). Nonetheless, it has still not been established that dysfunction of specific prefrontal areas is responsible for the working memory deficits seen in schizophrenia. Indeed, there is preliminary evidence that patients with schizophrenia may have marked deficits in aspects of working memory that are less reliant on the prefrontal cortex. Using a remarkably simple task, Strous et al. (1995) demonstrated that patients with schizophrenia were impaired in matching two tones after a brief delay of only 300 milliseconds but were unimpaired when there was no intertone interval. This aspect of auditory sensory (echoic) memory is thought to be subserved by nonassociation cortex outside the frontal lobes (e.g., superior temporal plane). Thus, both prefrontal and nonprefrontal components of working memory may be preferentially disturbed in schizophrenia.

TABLE 14–2.   DSM-IV-TR criteria for dissociative amnesia

A. The predominant disturbance is one or more episodes of inability to recall important personal information, usually of a traumatic or stressful nature, that is too extensive to be explained by ordinary forgetfulness.

B. The disturbance does not occur exclusively during the course of Dissociative Identity Disorder, Dissociative Fugue, Posttraumatic Stress Disorder, Acute Stress Disorder, or Somatization Disorder and is not due to the direct physiological effects of a substance (e.g., a drug of abuse, a medication) or a neurological or other general medical condition (e.g., Amnestic Disorder Due to Head Trauma).

C. The symptoms cause clinically significant distress or impairment in social, occupational, or other important areas of functioning.

Source.   Reprinted from American Psychiatric Association: *Diagnostic and Statistical Manual of Mental Disorders*, 4th Edition, Text Revision. Washington, DC, American Psychiatric Association, 2000. Used with permission.

DISSOCIATIVE AMNESIA

Table 14–2 provides the DSM-IV-TR diagnostic criteria for dissociative amnesia (formerly psychogenic amnesia). Dissociative amnesia is a disorder in which memory loss is attributed to functional factors. The memory loss may be localized in time, may be selective for elements of past history, and, most rarely, may be generalized and continuous. In the generalized form, patients may have amnesia for their own identity and history.

Dissociative amnesia is rarely diagnosed. Several factors may account for its low incidence. First, even among patients who at one time received diagnoses of hysterical disorders, amnesia was a relatively uncommon symptom. Perley and Guze (1962) examined the frequency of a wide range of symptoms in a sample of patients with "hysterical neurosis" (at that time, dissociative disorders were included in this grouping). First, whereas symptoms such as dizziness, headache, fatigue, and abdominal pain occurred at high rates (all in more than 70% of patients), amnesia was found in only 8% of cases. Second, patients presenting with forms of functional amnesia typically have a number of other psychiatric disorders or manifest the amnesia after a trauma—as, for instance, may occur in combat situations. Current nosology excludes diagnosis of dissociative amnesia in many such instances. Third, a functional amnesia does not necessarily interfere with

social or occupational functioning. The most common varieties involve forgetting of isolated events. Furthermore, patients with dissociative amnesia may display indifference to their symptomatology and thus be unlikely to present for treatment.

Dissociative amnesia may be more common among females, and it is thought to occur more often in adolescents and young adults than in the elderly. Most cases show rapid recovery of memory, and therefore the disorder is usually transient. Abeles and Schilder (1935) and Herman (1938) reported on 63 cases of dissociative amnesia (the investigators also included fugue states in this categorization). In these studies, 27 subjects recovered within 24 hours, 21 within 5 days, 7 within a week, and 4 within 3 weeks or more.

Differential Diagnosis

Problems of differential diagnosis usually involve distinguishing dissociative amnesia from two other types of conditions: 1) trauma to the brain, which may produce similar syndromes; and 2) amnesia that may be malingered. (See further discussion of malingering later in this section.)

The DSM-IV grouping of dissociative disorders is an attempt to categorize disturbances of higher cognitive functions that resemble effects of neurological dysfunction but that are believed to be functional in origin. If a patient's amnesia can be related to a neurological disorder, the diagnosis of dissociative disorder is inappropriate. To date, no studies have examined the frequency with which patients with dissociative disorder diagnoses concurrently or ultimately show signs of neurological disease. However, such work in the case of hysterical conversion reactions indicates that a disturbingly large number of patients thus diagnosed manifested neurological disorders (at the time or shortly thereafter) that in some patients proved fatal (Slater and Glithero 1965; Whitlock 1967).

The difficulties of differential diagnosis of dissociative disorders can be illustrated with the syndrome of transient global amnesia (Fisher and Adams 1964; Pantoni et al. 2000). Without warning, individuals, usually middle-aged, display retrograde amnesia for events that occurred in the previous days, weeks, or years and a dense anterograde amnesia. The amnesia is typically transient, lasting from minutes to several hours. When memory returns, there is typically a progressive recall of distant events, with memory of the most recent past returning last. Retrograde amnesia may resolve before the anterograde component (N. Kapur et al. 1998). During the amnesia, the individual is usually well oriented, with perception, sense of identity, and other higher cognitive functions intact. There is typically considerable concern and upset on the part of the individual about the memory loss. An attack may strike only once or may be recurrent (Heathfield et al. 1973).

The transient nature of the amnesia and its occurrence in individuals who appear medically healthy might suggest a dissociative reaction. Heathfield et al. (1973) reported on 31 patients who were referred for transient loss of memory. Of the 31 patients, memory loss was associated with epilepsy in 6 patients, with migraine in 1 patient, and with temporal lobe encephalitis in 2 patients. Three patients received the diagnosis of dissociative (psychogenic) amnesia. The remaining 19 patients were considered as presenting the syndrome of transient global amnesia. The age of these 19 patients (13 men, 6 women) ranged from 46 to 68 years; amnestic episodes lasted from 30 minutes to 5 days; and 11 patients had only one attack during the period of study. Cerebrovascular dysfunction was suggested in 9 of the 19 patients. Heathfield et al. (1973) concluded, "It is probable that most episodes of transient global amnesia result from bilateral temporal lobe or thalamic lesions. In some of our patients there was clear evidence of ischemia in the territory of the posterior cerebral circulation, and we consider that such ischemia is the cause of this syndrome" (p. 735). However, recent investigations have suggested that etiologies based on migraine, seizures, transient cerebral arterial ischemia, or a thromboembolic pathogenesis are unlikely to account for transient global amnesia (Lauria et al. 1998; Lewis 1998). Receiving greater attention is the possibility that a blockage of venous return (as in a Valsalva maneuver) results in high venous retrograde pressure to the cerebral venous system and produces venous ischemia in the diencephalon and MTL (Lewis 1998; Sander et al. 2000). Regardless, several imaging studies, using single-photon computed tomography (SPECT), PET, or diffusion-weighted magnetic resonance imaging have reported decreased activity in MTL structures during transient global amnesia, with normalization on recovery (Jovin et al. 2000; Strupp et al. 1998; Tanabe et al. 1999).

Some general guidelines may be useful in distinguishing dissociative amnesia from the memory loss that accompanies neurological disease. Typically, the memory loss associated with head trauma, Korsakoff's psychosis, temporal lobe dysfunction, and ECT has both retrograde and anterograde components, whereas patients with dissociative amnesia will often show unaltered ability to acquire and retain new information (as also opposed to transient global amnesia). It is rare in the context of neurological disease for a patient to manifest global amnesia across the life span, and personal identity and early memories are typically preserved. Dissociative amnesia may selectively affect autobiographical memory, whereas both personal and impersonal memory are disturbed in amnesia associated with neurological insult.

Contributing to differential diagnosis is the collateral behavior of the patient and the nature of the recovery of memory. Patients who present with amnesia accompanied by clouded consciousness, disorientation, and/or mood change are likely manifesting neurological disturbance. Indifference to an amnesia concerning events that would ordinarily be associated with guilt and shame for the patient suggests a dissociative basis. Dissociative amnesia usually pertains to traumatic events, and amnesia for the ordinary events of life would suggest a neurological disturbance. Amnesia during or after a stressful experience is not, however, a reliable sign of dissociative origin (it is excluded by DSM-IV). Stress may precipitate a transient ischemic attack or an epileptic event, resulting in amnesia. Retrograde amnesia associated with known neurological insult typically also has a standard course of recovery; events in the most distant past are recovered before more recent events. In dissociative amnesia, there is usually a sudden return of memory (Nemiah 1979). Hypnotic and/or sodium amobarbital interviews may be useful to distinguish dissociative amnesia from neurological disturbance. A number of reports exist of patients who recovered memory with either procedure, and in some cases the recovery was permanent (e.g., Herman 1938). Recovery of memory with the use of hypnosis or amobarbital should not occur in cases of neurological disturbance.

Malingering

Malingering refers to deliberate and voluntary simulation of psychological or physical disorder. The assumption in a diagnosis of dissociative amnesia is that the loss of memory and its subsequent recovery are not under voluntary control. It should be noted that some clinicians with considerable exposure to amnesias of psychological origin question whether a distinction between malingering and dissociative amnesia can or should be made. Differentiating between dissociative amnesia and malingering is difficult. The degree to which malingering is successful at simulation likely depends on the sophistication of the malingering patient regarding manifestations of psychological and neurological disease. In a somewhat similar context, it should be noted that experienced hypnotists cannot reliably distinguish hypnotized subjects from individuals simulating the effects of hypnosis (Orne 1979). Since the late 1990s, psychometric instruments have been validated that appear successful in distinguishing between the malingering of anterograde amnesia and a true amnestic syndrome. The basis of this approach is to use memory tests that are subjectively experienced as difficult, but in which patients with amnesia show high performance accuracy. In contrast, individuals who are malingering generate low scores (Rees et al. 1998; Tombaugh 1996).

NORMAL AGING

Complaints about memory loss are common in the elderly, and normal aging is accompanied by characteristic decrements in memory performance (Parkin et al. 1995; West 1996). However, the decline in memory with aging is selective, affecting some cognitive processes more than others. The capacity to deliberately acquire and retain new information (declarative episodic memory) is often impaired by age 50, particularly when the material to be learned is unstructured, such as random lists of words (Albert et al. 1987). This deficit seems to reflect not a more rapid forgetting with aging, but rather the use of less-efficient encoding and retrieval strategies. In part, this deficit, as in major depression, may reflect limited attentional capacity and reduced capacity for effortful processing. Aging also exerts greater negative effects on memory for the context in which information was learned as opposed to memory for the information itself. For example, age-related changes have been demonstrated in memory for the temporal order (Parkin et al. 1995) and the source (Craik et al. 1990) of information. This pattern of memory deficits, with decrements in source memory and in the acquisition and retention of unstructured material (but not of highly structured material), is suggestive of an age-related decline in the memory processes supported by prefrontal cortex (West 1996). Indeed, the age-related impairment in source memory has been found to covary with other measures of frontal lobe function, the Wisconsin Card Sorting Test, and verbal fluency (Craik et al. 1990; Parkin et al. 1995). There is also evidence that with aging, the frontal lobe undergoes greater reductions in volume and in resting functional activity than do other brain areas (West 1996).

The literature on the effects of aging on nondeclarative memory is inconsistent. Although it appears that many of the cognitive processes that underlie these aspects of learning and memory are unaltered by age (Light and La Voie 1993), age-related deficits have been reported, particularly for priming tasks. Indeed, there is also evidence linking impaired implicit memory to age-related frontal lobe dysfunction (Winokur et al. 1996).

METAMEMORY: SUBJECTIVE EVALUATION OF MEMORY

In clinical circumstances, a psychiatrist often obtains patients' assessments of their own memory functioning, a domain referred to as *metamemory*. The perception of memory decline may be the first indication of valid incipient changes in cognitive function. A large number of studies, conducted in neurological, psychiatric, and healthy populations, have examined the relationships between self-evaluations of memory and objective test results.

The most consistent finding in this literature is that the strongest predictor of memory self-evaluation is current mood state (Bennett-Levy and Powell 1980; Coleman et al. 1996; Hinkin et al. 1996; Larrabee and Levin 1986). Almost invariably, depressed mood, whether assessed by observers or by self-report, is associated with self-evaluations of impaired cognitive function (Prudic et al. 2000). In contrast, although significant associations between objective neuropsychological and subjective cognitive evaluations have been occasionally reported (Riege 1982), for the most part such associations are either small in magnitude or nonexistent. Furthermore, when associations have been reported, they have not always been in the expected direction. Hinkin et al. (1996) found that men who were seropositive for human immunodeficiency virus type 1 (HIV-1) with a low level of memory complaints performed worse on memory testing than those with a higher level of complaints.

It is sobering that independent of neurological or psychiatric illness, human beings are generally poor judges of the quality of their memory. To some extent, this lack of association might be attributed to the limited ecological validity of standard memory-assessment batteries, which may fail to capture the type of memory failures experienced in everyday life (e.g., incidental learning and forgetting). Furthermore, it is clear that a variety of neurological and psychiatric conditions, including but not limited to Alzheimer's disease and schizophrenia, may be associated with distinct deficits in metamemory, such that patients are particularly likely to deny or be unaware of cognitive deficits. However, the fact that current mood state is a consistent predictor of memory functioning strongly implies that factors other than actual memory performance influence self-evaluations. Figure 14–2 illustrates changes on the Squire Subjective Memory Questionnaire (Squire et al. 1979) in patients with major depression who did and did not respond to ECT (Coleman et al. 1996). Both at baseline and shortly after the ECT course, patient scores on this metamemory measure were strongly associated with depression severity scores. The investigators found that although patients had characteristic anterograde and retrograde memory disturbances at the time of post-ECT metamemory evaluation, approximately 80% of patients reported improved memory functioning after ECT relative to before ECT. Although the magnitude of these memory deficits was gen-

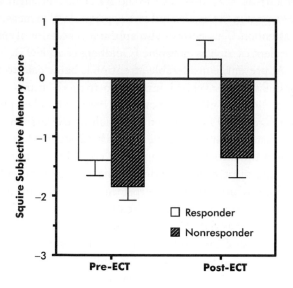

FIGURE 14–2. Scores on the Squire Subjective Memory Questionnaire in depressed patients treated with electroconvulsive therapy (ECT). A score of 0 indicates that the patient assesses memory function to be the same as it was before the episode of depressive illness, whereas a negative score indicates that the patient considers current memory function to be impaired. Before receiving ECT, patients report marked impairment, the magnitude of which covaries with the severity of depressive symptoms. Patients who respond to ECT report marked improvement even though objective tests indicate memory deficits.

Source. Adapted from Coleman et al. 1996.

erally equivalent in ECT responders and nonresponders, the improvement in the metamemory measure was particularly pronounced in patients whose depression responded to ECT.

Little consensus exists about the theoretical underpinnings of metamemory or subjective memory judgments. The field is largely driven by empirical interest in the relationship of objective memory performance to subjective complaints and, particularly, the disjunction between the two—that is, why reports of memory performance often deviate so markedly from actual performance. For example, one hypothesis proposed that an internal memory monitor reviews memory contents in an unbiased manner and forms judgments about the retrievability of these memories (Burke et al. 1991). A later view suggested that judgments about memory are highly inferential and that evaluations of the objective status of memory must be made based on sources of information other than access to a review of memory content. Other sources of information that affect subjective judgments may include retrieval fluency, the amounts of related and unrelated information activated by attempts to remem-

ber (Koriat 1993), and feelings about memory, such as the feeling of familiarity (Schwartz et al. 1997).

As a result, there are likely to be multiple dimensions to assess when evaluating subjective memory. An inclusive conceptual approach offered four dimensions: 1) memory knowledge, which involves factual knowledge about memory and its processes; 2) memory monitoring, which includes awareness of the current state of one's memory and of how one uses memory; 3) memory-related affect; and 4) memory self-efficacy, which involves a set of beliefs about one's memory, including changes in memory status (Hultsh et al. 1988). Evaluations of the psychometric properties of questionnaires developed to examine subjective assessments of memory indicated that assessments of memory capacity and change in memory status were best related to beliefs about memory which were, in turn, subject to a variety of influences, including mood and locus of control (Cavanaugh and Green 1990). In a meta-analysis of the effects of memory training on subjective memory assessment, Floyd and Scogin (1997) found that memory training and improvement in performance did not alter subjective memory assessment in normal elderly adults. Instead, techniques such as relaxation training, which may impact affect or mood, and interventions directed at altering participants' beliefs about the effects of aging on memory significantly improved subjective assessment of memory. This finding suggests that interventions that improve objective memory performance have less impact on subjective evaluations than interventions that target either affective state or beliefs about memory.

EFFECTS OF SOMATIC TREATMENTS ON LEARNING AND MEMORY

PSYCHOTROPIC AGENTS

In addition to the deleterious effects of benzodiazepines on psychomotor performance, this class of medications can produce consistent adverse effects on memory. The most characteristic deficit is diminished delayed recall for newly learned information (J.L. Taylor and Tinklenberg 1987). This deficit is most evident acutely after ingestion and is most marked 1–2 hours postingestion for diazepam and 3–4 hours postingestion for lorazepam. Despite producing this deficit in anterograde declarative memory, benzodiazepines do not appear to impair retrograde memory. Indeed, lists of words learned before benzodiazepine administration may be better recalled in the postingestion period, a phenomenon termed *retrograde facilitation.* This effect may be more pronounced at higher benzodiazepine dosages and has been interpreted as reflecting reduced retroactive interference due to diminished learning after drug ingestion. The capacity of short-term or working memory does not appear to be altered by benzodiazepine use, although the speed at which information is processed may be slowed. Contrary to tolerance to benzodiazepine's effects on psychomotor performance, which appears to persist with chronic use, tolerance to adverse acute effects of benzodiazepines on memory functions may not develop with chronic use (Gorenstein et al. 1994). There is also evidence to suggest that elderly individuals are particularly sensitive to the amnestic effects of benzodiazepines.

A wide range of medications have anticholinergic properties, including heterocyclic antidepressants (e.g., amitriptyline, imipramine, nortriptyline), neuroleptics (e.g., chlorpromazine), antiparkinsonian agents (e.g., benztropine), and sleep and cold preparations that contain antihistamines. Anticholinergic medications can produce sedation, attentional impairment, memory disturbance, and, in extreme cases, an anticholinergic delirium. There is compelling evidence that psychotropic medications that differ in anticholinergic properties also differ in their effects on learning and memory. For example, despite equivalent clinical improvement, patients with major depression will show superior performance on declarative memory measures when treated with fluoxetine relative to amitriptyline (Richardson et al. 1994). In a double-blind crossover study in patients with chronic schizophrenia, Silver and Geraisy (1995) found that biperiden (an anticholinergic medication) but not amantadine (a dopamine agonist) produced detectable deficits in both working and declarative memory. As with the benzodiazepines, vulnerability to the adverse cognitive effects of anticholinergic agents may be augmented in the elderly. There is evidence that tolerance develops to the adverse cognitive effects of anticholinergic medications, but there is no such evidence for benzodiazepines. Nonetheless, avoidance of agents with pronounced anticholinergic effects may be advisable, particularly in patients with preexisting memory impairment.

Aside from the anticholinergic properties of antidepressants or neuroleptics, there is not convincing evidence that standard antidepressants or traditional neuroleptics exert intrinsic detrimental effects on learning and memory. For example, differences among the selective serotonin reuptake inhibitors (SSRIs) in neuropsychological effects are largely attributable to differences among their anticholinergic properties. Although excessive dosages can produce sedation with traditional neuroleptic treatment, most studies of cognitive function in patients with schizophrenia—comparing patients' unmedicated states with their neuroleptic-treated states—have found no change or slight improvement in the medicated states, particularly in measures of attention. This pattern also appears to hold for atypical neuroleptics such as clozapine (Goldberg et al. 1993).

At present, considerable attention is being paid to the possibility that atypical antipsychotic medications have an ameliorative effect on cognitive deficits in schizophrenia (Purdon 1999). Currently, much of the evidence is circumstantial and tentative. At least 12 studies have examined the effects of clozapine on cognitive parameters, with the most general finding being an improvement in measures of attention and verbal fluency, with some additional evidence for improved executive function. However, as reviewed by Meltzer and McGurk (1999), effects of clozapine on working memory and on standard measures of verbal and nonverbal learning and memory are inconclusive. Somewhat similarly, risperidone appears to exert positive effects on working memory, executive function, and attention, whereas effects on standard measures of learning and memory are inconsistent. There is preliminary evidence that olanzapine may have a different profile, improving verbal learning and memory, verbal fluency, and executive function, but not attention, working memory, or visual (nonverbal) learning and memory (e.g., Purdon et al. 2000). Thus, the possibility has been raised that atypical antipsychotics differ in their effects on memory, with risperidone having stronger beneficial effects on working (short-term) memory and olanzapine exerting stronger action on verbal learning and memory.

ELECTROCONVULSIVE THERAPY AND OTHER BRAIN STIMULATION TREATMENTS

ECT is a remarkably effective treatment for specific psychiatric disorders (American Psychiatric Association 2001; Sackeim et al. 1995). However, its cognitive side effects are the major factor limiting its use. As with spontaneous seizures, in the immediate postictal period, patients may manifest transient neurological abnormalities, alterations of consciousness (disorientation, attentional dysfunction), sensorimotor abnormalities, and disturbances in higher cognitive functions, particularly learning and memory (Sackeim 1992). Technical factors in ECT administration—including electrode placement (bilateral versus unilateral), stimulus dosage, and electrical waveform—strongly determine the severity and persistence of these acute effects. Indeed, these factors determine whether patients require on average a few minutes or several hours to achieve full reorientation after seizure termination (Sackeim 1992; Sackeim et al. 1993, 2000; Weiner et al. 1986).

There is rapid recovery of cognitive function after a single treatment. However, with forms of ECT that exert more severe acute cognitive effects, recovery may be incomplete by the time of the next treatment. In such cases, deterioration may occur over the treatment course, particularly when treatments are closely spaced in time. Some patients may develop an organic mental syndrome with marked disorientation during the ECT course. With milder forms of ECT, cumulative deterioration in cognitive functions need not occur. Indeed, with specific alterations of ECT technique, cumulative *improvement* in some acute cognitive measures has been demonstrated (Sackeim 1992).

Associations between the magnitude of cognitive effects and ECT treatment parameters diminish as time from ECT progresses. Differences between bilateral and unilateral electrode placement are difficult to detect after more than a few months have elapsed since the end of the ECT course (Lisanby et al. 2000; Sackeim 1992; Sackeim et al. 1993, 2000; Weiner et al. 1986). Within days of the end of an ECT course, depressed patients manifest superior performance in most cognitive domains relative to their pretreatment baseline. On tests of intelligence, patients' scores shortly after ECT will typically be superior to those produced in the untreated depressed state (Sackeim et al. 1992). Similarly, before treatment, depressed patients usually manifest deficits in the acquisition of information, as revealed by tests of immediate recall or recognition of item lists. Within days after an ECT course, patients are typically unchanged or improved in these measures of learning, with the change in clinical state being the critical predictor of the magnitude of improvement. In contrast, patients often manifest impaired ability to retain information over a delay. This impairment reflects a double dissociation between the effects of depression and ECT on anterograde learning and memory (Steif et al. 1986). ECT introduces a new deficit in consolidation or retention, so that information that is newly learned is rapidly forgotten.

During and shortly after a course of ECT, patients also display retrograde amnesia. Deficits in the recall or recognition of both personal and public information learned before ECT are common, and there is evidence that these deficits are greatest for events that occurred temporally closest to the treatment (McElhiney et al. 1995; Squire 1986). Thus, whereas memory for more remote events is intact, patients may have difficulty recalling events that occurred during and several months to years before the ECT course. The retrograde amnesia is rarely dense, as patients typically show spottiness in memory for recent events. It has typically been thought that the amnesia is most dense for autobiographical information (Weiner 1984). However, careful analysis of the extent of amnesia for public and personal events, and the details of those events, indicates that information about the world (i.e.,

public events) is subject to greater memory loss (Lisanby et al. 2000). This finding is in contrast to the pattern often seen with MTL brain damage, in which retrograde amnesia for personal information is greater than that for impersonal or public events (Nadel and Moscovitch 1997).

As time from treatment increases, retrograde memory function improves, with a return of more distant memories (Lisanby et al. 2000; McElhiney et al. 1995). This temporally graded pattern is compatible with similar findings of the effects of repeated electroconvulsive shock in animals (Krueger et al. 1992). Both the anterograde and the retrograde amnesia are most marked for explicit or declarative memory, whereas no effects of ECT have been seen on measures of implicit or procedural memory (Squire et al. 1985). In this respect, the effects of ECT on memory are similar to those associated with MTL dysfunction. In general, there is no relation between the magnitude of ECT's adverse effects on memory and its therapeutic properties (McElhiney et al. 1995).

Within a few weeks after the end of ECT, objective evidence of persistent cognitive deficits is difficult to document. The anterograde amnesia typically resolves rapidly after ECT termination (Sackeim et al. 1993, 2000). The retrograde amnesia will often show a more gradual reduction, with substantial return of memory for events that were seemingly "forgotten" when assessed immediately after the treatment course. However, ECT can result in persistent deficits (McElhiney et al. 1995; Sackeim 2000a; Weiner et al. 1986), most likely due to a combination of retrograde and anterograde effects. Even when tested at substantial time periods after treatment, patients may manifest persistent amnesia for some events that occurred several months immediately before and after ECT. Recent work suggests that the patients most vulnerable to persistent retrograde amnesia are those with preexisting cognitive impairment and those who manifest the most prolonged disorientation immediately after seizure induction (Sobin et al. 1995). In rare cases, the extent of persistent or permanent retrograde amnesia may extend several years into the past (Sackeim 2000a).

Since the late twentieth century, other brain stimulation treatments have been developed. There have been over 20 reports on the use of *repetitive transcranial magnetic stimulation* (rTMS) in the treatment of major depression, as well as rTMS application to other neuropsychiatric conditions (George et al. 1999). This noninvasive technique involves inducing focal current flow in cortical tissue by imposing a time-varying magnetic field. When combined with functional imaging techniques, rTMS has shown remarkable promise as a method to map brain function (through transitory disruption of local activity) and brain connectivity. Although neuropsychological investigation has been limited in the standard treatment trials in neuropsychiatric disorders (usually at least 10 days of stimulation, each for 15–20 periods), initial impressions are that rTMS (either at slow or fast frequencies) is benign in cognitive effects. Of greater uncertainty, at least in the treatment of major depression, is whether nonconvulsive rTMS will have a significant clinical role. Therapeutic properties have been highly variable in effect size and there is little information on the persistence of clinical benefit (Sackeim 2000b). Using similar technology, an alternative that is being developed is the deliberate induction of seizure activity under general anesthesia with rTMS, termed *magnetic seizure therapy* (MST). Due to the greater control magnetic stimulation affords over the site of seizure initiation and electrical dosage in the brain, MST may have advantages over ECT in reducing adverse amnestic effects (Lisanby et al. 2001).

Finally, another new brain stimulation approach is the use of *vagus nerve stimulation* (VNS) in the therapy of treatment-resistant major depressive episodes. VNS is approved for treatment-resistant epilepsy. The procedure involves inserting a stimulator in the chest wall and running leads to electrodes attached to the left vagus nerve in the neck. Stimulation is continuous within a 24-hour cycle, usually involving 30 seconds of stimulation followed by a 5-minutes-off period. Intensity of the current administered is the primary variable adjusted, and it is usually varied in relation to tolerability. An initial open-label pilot study suggested that a substantial number of patients with treatment-resistant depression showed marked and sustained clinical improvement (Rush et al. 2000). Neuropsychological investigation in this sample before and after the acute VNS treatment phase did not reveal any deleterious effects. Indeed, there was improvement in a variety of neurocognitive measures, including memory, but especially executive functions, that tended to covary with the extent of clinical improvement (Sackeim et al. 2001).

Highlights for the Clinician

+ Memory is not a unitary entity. A set of "systems" has been outlined that encompasses different aspects of memory. Most memory researchers make an initial separation of memory into two categories: a) *declarative* (the type of memory assessed by traditional recall and recognition tests) and b) *nondeclarative* (including conditioning, priming, and procedural memory).

+ *Amnesia* is the generic term for severe memory deficit. Four clinical characteristics are typical of most amnesic patients: anterograde amnesia, retrograde amnesia, confabulation, and intact intellectual function.

+ Normal aging is accompanied by characteristic decrements in memory performance. However, the decline in memory with aging is selective, affecting some cognitive processes more than others. Alzheimer's disease is the most common dementia. Its hallmark, and typically earliest symptom, is amnesia.

+ The major psychiatric disorders—schizophrenia, mania, and major depression—almost invariably compromise aspects of attention and concentration. Because the ability to focus and sustain attention is central to the acquisition of new information in general and declarative memory in particular, deficits in acquiring new information are common among patients with these disorders.

+ Psychotropic agents and electroconvulsive therapy can have specific effects on memory.

RECOMMENDED READINGS

Budson AE, Price BH: Memory dysfunction. N Engl J Med 352:692–699, 2005
Tulving E, Craik F (eds): The Oxford Handbook of Memory. New York, Oxford University Press, 2000

REFERENCES

Abeles M, Schilder P: Psychogenic loss of personal identity. Arch Neurol Psychiatry 34:587–604, 1935

Albert MS, Butters N, Levin J: Temporal gradients in the retrograde amnesia of patients with alcoholic Korsakoff's disease. Arch Neurol 36:211–216, 1979
Albert MS, Duffy FH, Naeser MA: Nonlinear changes in cognition and their neurophysiologic correlates. Can J Psychol 41:141–157, 1987
American Psychiatric Association: Diagnostic and Statistical Manual of Mental Disorders, 4th Edition, Text Revision. Washington, DC, American Psychiatric Association, 2000

American Psychiatric Association: The Practice of Electroconvulsive Therapy: Recommendations for Treatment, Training and Privileging, 2nd Edition: A Task Force Report of the American Psychiatric Association. Washington, DC, American Psychiatric Association, 2001

Andreasen NC, O'Leary DS, Cizadlo T, et al: Remembering the past: two facets of episodic memory explored with positron emission tomography. Am J Psychiatry 152:1576–1585, 1995

Andreasen NC, O'Leary DS, Paradiso S, et al: The cerebellum plays a role in conscious episodic memory retrieval. Hum Brain Mapp 8:226–234, 1999

Backman L, Forsell Y: Episodic memory functioning in a community-based sample of old adults with major depression: utilization of cognitive support. J Abnorm Psychol 103:361–370, 1994

Baddeley AD: Working Memory. Oxford, UK, Oxford University Press, 1986

Baddeley AD: The episodic buffer: a new component of working memory? Trends Cogn Sci 4:417–423, 2000

Ball MJ, Fishman M, Hachinski V, et al: A new definition of Alzheimer's disease: a hippocampal dementia. Lancet 1:14–16, 1985

Bazin N, Perruchet P, De Bonis M, et al: The dissociation of explicit and implicit memory in depressed patients. Psychol Med 24:239–245, 1994

Beatty WW, Jocic Z, Monson N, et al: Memory and frontal lobe dysfunction in schizophrenia and schizoaffective disorder. J Nerv Ment Dis 181:448–453, 1993

Bennett-Levy J, Powell GE: The Subjective Memory Questionnaire (SMQ): an investigation into the self-reporting of "real-life" memory skills. Br J Soc Clin Psychol 19:177–188, 1980

Blanchard JJ, Neale JM: The neuropsychological signature of schizophrenia: generalized or differential deficit? Am J Psychiatry 151:40–48, 1994

Blaney PH: Affect and memory: a review. Psychol Bull 99:229–246, 1986

Blaxton TA: Dissociations among memory measures in memory-impaired subjects: evidence for a processing account of memory. Mem Cognit 20:549–562, 1992

Blaxton TA: A process-based view of memory. J Int Neuropsychol Soc 1:112–114, 1995

Bornstein RA, Baker GB, Douglass AB: Depression and memory in major depressive disorder. J Neuropsychiatry Clin Neurosci 3:78–80, 1991

Breslow R, Kocsis J, Belkin B: Memory deficits in depression: evidence utilizing the Wechsler Memory Scale. Percept Mot Skills 51:541–542, 1980

Breslow R, Kocsis J, Belkin B: Contribution of the depressive perspective to memory function in depression. Am J Psychiatry 138:227–230, 1981

Brittlebank AD, Scott J, Williams JM, et al: Autobiographical memory in depression: state or trait marker? Br J Psychiatry 162:118–121, 1993

Buckner RL: Beyond HERA: contributions of specific prefrontal brain areas to long-term memory retrieval. Psychon Bull Rev 3:149–158, 1996

Buckner RL, Petersen SE, Ojemann JG, et al: Functional anatomical studies of explicit and implicit memory retrieval tasks. J Neurosci 15 (pt 1):12–29, 1995

Buckner RL, Koutstaal W, Schacter DL, et al: Functional-anatomic study of episodic retrieval, II: selective averaging of event-related fMRI trials to test the retrieval success hypothesis. Neuroimage 7:163–175, 1998a

Buckner RL, Koutstaal W, Schacter DL, et al: Functional-anatomic study of episodic retrieval using fMRI, I: retrieval effort versus retrieval success. Neuroimage 7:151–162, 1998b

Buckner RL, Kelley WM, Petersen SE: Frontal cortex contributes to human memory formation. Nat Neurosci 2:311–314, 1999

Buckner RL, Koutstaal W, Schacter DL, et al: Functional MRI evidence for a role of frontal and inferior temporal cortex in amodal components of priming. Brain 123 (pt 3):620–640, 2000

Burke D, MacKay DG, Worthley JS, et al: On the tip of the tongue: What causes word findings failures in young and older adults. J Mem Lang 30:542–579, 1991

Burt DB, Zembar MJ, Niederehe G: Depression and memory impairment: a meta-analysis of the association, its pattern, and specificity. Psychol Bull 117:285–305, 1995

Burt T, Prudic J, Peyser S, et al: Learning and memory in bipolar and unipolar major depression: effects of aging. Neuropsychiatry Neuropsychol Behav Neurol 13:246–253, 2000

Butters N, Heindel WC, Salmon DP: Dissociation of implicit memory in dementia: neurological implications. Bull Psychon Soc 28:230–246, 1990

Calev A: Recall and recognition in mildly disturbed schizophrenics: the use of matched tasks. Psychol Med 14:425–429, 1984

Calev A, Erwin P: Recall and recognition in depressives: use of matched tasks. Br J Clin Psychol 24:127–128, 1985

Callicott JH, Bertolino A, Mattay VS, et al: Physiological dysfunction of the dorsolateral prefrontal cortex in schizophrenia revisited. Cereb Cortex 10:1078–1092, 2000

Cavanaugh JC, Green EE: I believe, therefore I can: self-efficacy beliefs in memory aging, in Aging and Cognition: Mental Processes, Self Awareness and Interventions. Edited by Lovelace EA. New York, Elsevier Science, 1990, pp 189–230

Channon S, Baker JE, Robertson MM: Effects of structure and clustering on recall and recognition memory in clinical depression. J Abnorm Psychol 102:323–326, 1993

Chapman LJ, Chapman JP: Disordered Thought in Schizophrenia. Englewood Cliffs, NJ, Prentice-Hall, 1973

Clare L, McKenna PJ, Mortimer AM, et al: Memory in schizophrenia: what is impaired and what is preserved? Neuropsychologia 31:1225–1241, 1993

Coffman JA, Bornstein RA, Olson SC, et al: Cognitive impairment and cerebral structure by MRI in bipolar disorder. Biol Psychiatry 27:1188–1196, 1990

Cohen NJ: Preserved learning capacity in amnesia: evidence for multiple memory systems, in The Neuropsychology of Memory. Edited by Squire LR, Butters N. New York, Guilford, 1984, pp 83–103

Cohen NJ, Corkin S: The amnesic patient H.M.: learning and retention of a cognitive skill (abstract). Society of Neuroscience Abstracts 7:235, 1981

Cohen NJ, Squire LR: Preserved learning and retention of pattern analyzing skill in amnesia: dissociation of knowing how and knowing that. Science 210:207–209, 1980

Coleman EA, Sackeim HA, Prudic J, et al: Subjective memory complaints before and after electroconvulsive therapy. Biol Psychiatry 39:346–356, 1996

Conway MA, Turk DJ, Miller SL, et al: A positron emission tomography (PET) study of autobiographical memory retrieval. Memory 7:679–702, 1999

Corkin S: Acquisition of motor skill after bilateral medial temporal lobe excision. Neuropsychologia 6:225–265, 1968

Corkin S: Lasting consequences of bilateral medial temporal lobectomy: clinical course and experimental findings in H.M. Semin Neurol 4:249–259, 1984

Corwin J, Peselow E, Feenan K, et al: Disorders of decision in affective disease: an effect of beta-adrenergic dysfunction? Biol Psychiatry 27:813–833, 1990

Craik FIM, Morris LW, Morris RG, et al: Relations between source amnesia and frontal lobe functioning in older adults. Psychol Aging 5:148–151, 1990

Cronholm B, Ottosson J-O: Memory functions in endogenous depression: before and after electroconvulsive therapy. Arch Gen Psychiatry 5:193–199, 1961

Davis H, Squire L: Protein synthesis and memory. Psychol Bull 96:518–559, 1984

DeMonbreun B, Craighead W: Selective recall of positive and neutral feedback. Cognit Ther Res 1:311–329, 1977

Dickey CC, McCarley RW, Voglmaier MM, et al: Schizotypal personality disorder and MRI abnormalities of temporal lobe gray matter. Biol Psychiatry 45:1393–1402, 1999

Donnelly EF, Murphy DL, Goodwin FK, et al: Intellectual function in primary affective disorder. Br J Psychiatry 140:633–636, 1982

Eich E, Macaulay D, Ryan L: Mood dependent memory for events of the personal past. J Exp Psychol Gen 123:201–215, 1994

Elvevag B, Egan MF, Goldberg TE: Paired-associate learning and memory interference in schizophrenia. Neuropsychologia 38:1565–1575, 2000

Fink GR, Markowitsch HJ, Reinkemeier M, et al: Cerebral representation of one's own past: neural networks involved in autobiographical memory. J Neurosci 16:4275–4282, 1996

Fisher C, Adams R: Transient global amnesia. Acta Neurol Scand 40 (suppl 9):1–83, 1964

Fleming K, Goldberg TE, Gold JM, et al: Verbal working memory dysfunction in schizophrenia: use of a Brown-Peterson paradigm. Psychiatry Res 56:155–161, 1995

Floyd M, Scogin F: Effects of memory training on the subjective memory functioning and mental health of older adults: a meta-analysis. Psychol Aging 12:150–161, 1997

Gabrieli JDE: A systematic view of human memory processes. J Int Neuropsychol Soc 1:115–118, 1995

Gainotti G, Marra C: Some aspects of memory disorders clearly distinguish dementia of the Alzheimer's type from depressive pseudo-dementia. J Clin Exp Neuropsychol 16:65–78, 1994

Gass C, Russell E: Differential impact of brain damage and depression on memory test performance. J Consult Clin Psychol 54:261–263, 1986

George MS, Lisanby SH, Sackeim HA: Transcranial magnetic stimulation: applications in psychiatry. Arch Gen Psychiatry 56:300–311, 1999

Gold JM, Blaxton TA, Hermann BP, et al: Memory and intelligence in lateralized temporal lobe epilepsy and schizophrenia. Schizophr Res 17:59–65, 1995

Goldberg TE, Gold JM: Neurocognitive deficits in schizophrenia, in Schizophrenia. Edited by Hirsch SR, Weinberger DR. Oxford, UK, Blackwell, 1995, pp 146–162

Goldberg TE, Greenberg R, Griffin S: The impact of clozapine on cognition and psychiatric symptoms in patients with schizophrenia. Br J Psychiatry 162:43–48, 1993

Goldman-Rakic PS: Working memory and the mind. Sci Am 267:110–117, 1992

Goldman-Rakic PS: Working memory dysfunction in schizophrenia. J Neuropsychiatry Clin Neurosci 6:348–357, 1994

Gorenstein C, Bernik MA, Pompeia S: Differential acute psychomotor and cognitive effects of diazepam on long-term benzodiazepine users. Int Clin Psychopharmacol 9:145–153, 1994

Graf P, Schacter DL: Implicit and explicit memory for new associations in normal and amnesic patients. J Exp Psychol Learn Mem Cogn 11:501–518, 1985

Gras-Vincendon A, Danion JM, Grange D, et al: Explicit memory, repetition priming and cognitive skill learning in schizophrenia. Schizophr Res 13:117–126, 1994

Gur RE, Turetsky BI, Cowell PE, et al: Temporolimbic volume reductions in schizophrenia. Arch Gen Psychiatry 57:769–775, 2000

Harvey PD, Powchik P, Mohs RC, et al: Memory functions in geriatric chronic schizophrenic patients: a neuropsychological study. J Neuropsychiatry Clin Neurosci 7:207–212, 1995

Hasher L, Zacks R: Automatic and effortful processes in memory. J Exp Psychol Gen 108:356–388, 1979

Heathfield K, Croft P, Swash M: The syndrome of transient global amnesia. Brain 96:729–736, 1973

Heaton R, Chelune G, Talley J, et al: Wisconsin Card Sorting Test (WCST) Manual, Revised and Expanded. Odessa, FL, Psychological Resources, 1993

Herman M: The use of intravenous Sodium Amytal in psychogenic amnesic states. Psychiatr Q 12:738–742, 1938

Hinkin CH, van Gorp WG, Satz P, et al: Actual versus self-reported cognitive dysfunction in HIV-1 infection: memory-metamemory dissociations. J Clin Exp Neuropsychol 18:431–443, 1996

Hirayasu Y, McCarley RW, Salisbury DF, et al: Planum temporale and Heschl gyrus volume reduction in schizophrenia: a magnetic resonance imaging study of first-episode patients. Arch Gen Psychiatry 57:692–699, 2000

Hultsch DF, Hertzog C, Dixon RA, et al: Memory self-knowledge in the aged, in Cognitive Development in Adulthood: Progress in Cognitive Development Research. Edited by Howe ML, Brainerd CJ. New York, Springer, 1988, pp 65–92

Hyde TM, Nawroz S, Goldberg TE, et al: Is there cognitive decline in schizophrenia? a cross-sectional study. Br J Psychiatry 164:494–500, 1994

Jacobs DM, Sano M, Dooneief G, et al: Neuropsychological detection and characterization of preclinical Alzheimer's disease. Neurology 45:957–962, 1995

Jacoby LL, Lindsay DS, Toth JP: Unconscious influences revealed: attention, awareness, and control. Am Psychol 47:802–809, 1992

Johnson SD, Saykin AJ, Flashman LA, et al: Brain activation on fMRI and verbal memory ability: functional neuroanatomic correlates of CVLT performance. J Int Neuropsychol Soc 7:55–62, 2001

Jovin TG, Vitti RA, McCluskey LF: Evolution of temporal lobe hypoperfusion in transient global amnesia: a serial single photon emission computed tomography study. J Neuroimaging 10:238–241, 2000

Kapur N: Syndromes of retrograde amnesia: a conceptual and empirical synthesis. Psychol Bul 125:800–825, 1999

Kapur N, Millar J, Abbott P, et al: Recovery of function processes in human amnesia: evidence from transient global amnesia. Neuropsychologia 36:99–107, 1998

Kapur S, Craik FI, Jones C, et al: Functional role of the prefrontal cortex in retrieval of memories: a PET study. Neuroreport 6:1880–1884, 1995

Keane MM, Gabrieli JDE, Monti LA, et al: Amnesic patients show normal priming and a normal depth-of-processing effect in a conceptually driven implicit task (abstract). Society of Neuroscience Abstracts 19:1079, 1993

Keefe RS, Roitman SE, Harvey PD, et al: A pen-and-paper human analogue of a monkey prefrontal cortex activation task: spatial working memory in patients with schizophrenia. Schizophr Res 17:25–33, 1995

Kelly C, Sharkey V, Morrison G, et al: Nithsdale Schizophrenia Surveys 20: cognitive function in a catchment-area-based population of patients with schizophrenia. Br J Psychiatry 177:348–353, 2000

Kessing LV: Cognitive impairment in the euthymic phase of affective disorder. Psychol Med 28:1027–1038, 1998

Kindermann SS, Brown GG: Depression and memory in the elderly: a meta-analysis. J Clin Exp Neuropsychol 19:625–642, 1997

Kopelman MD: The "new" and the "old": components of the anterograde and retrograde memory loss in Korsakoff and Alzheimer patients, in Neuropsychology of Memory, 2nd Edition. Edited by Squire LR, Butters N. New York, Guilford, 1992, pp 130–146

Kopelman MD, Stanhope N, Kingsley D: Retrograde amnesia in patients with diencephalic, temporal lobe or frontal lesions. Neuropsychologia 37:939–958, 1999

Korait A: How do we know that we know? the accessibility model of the feeling of knowing. Psychol Rev 100:609–639, 1993

Krueger RB, Sackeim HA, Gamzu ER: Pharmacological treatment of the cognitive side effects of ECT: a review. Psychopharmacol Bull 28:409–424, 1992

Lachner G, Engel RR: Differentiation of dementia and depression by memory tests: a meta-analysis. J Nerv Ment Dis 182:34–39, 1994

Larrabee GJ, Levin HS: Memory self-ratings and objective test performance in a normal elderly sample. J Clin Exp Neuropsychol 8:275–284, 1986

Lauria G, Gentile M, Fassetta G, et al: Transient global amnesia and transient ischemic attack: a community-based case-control study. Acta Neurol Scand 97:381–385, 1998

Lepage M, Habib R, Tulving E: Hippocampal PET activations of memory encoding and retrieval: the HIPER model. Hippocampus 8:313–322, 1998

Lepage M, Ghaffar O, Nyberg L, et al: Prefrontal cortex and episodic memory retrieval mode. Proc Natl Acad Sci U S A 97:506–511, 2000

Lewis SL: Aetiology of transient global amnesia. Lancet 352:397–399, 1998

Light LL, La Voie D: Direct and indirect measures of memory in old age, in Implicit Memory. Edited by Graf P, Masson MEJ. Hillsdale, NJ, Lawrence Erlbaum, 1993, pp 207–230

Lisanby SH, Maddox JH, Prudic J, et al: The effects of electroconvulsive therapy on memory of autobiographical and public events. Arch Gen Psychiatry 57:581–590, 2000

Lisanby SH, Schlaepfer TE, Hans-Ulrich Fisch H-U, et al: Magnetic seizure therapy of major depression. Arch Gen Psychiatry 58:303–305, 2001

Lloyd GG, Lishman WA: Effect of depression on the speed of recall of pleasant and unpleasant experiences. Psychol Med 5:173–180, 1975

Maguire EA, Mummery CJ: Differential modulation of a common memory retrieval network revealed by positron emission tomography. Hippocampus 9:54–61, 1999

Markowitsch HJ: Which brain regions are critically involved in the retrieval of old episodic memory? Brain Res Brain Res Rev 21:117–127, 1995

Markowitsch HJ: The neuroanatomy of memory, in The Oxford Handbook of Memory. Edited by Tulving E, Craik FIM. New York, Oxford University Press, 2000, pp 465–484

Marslen-Wilson WD, Teuber H: Memory for remote events in anterograde amnesia: recognition of public figures from news photographs. Neuropsychologia 13:353–364, 1975

Mason CF: Pre-illness intelligence of mental hospital patients. J Consult Psychol 20:297–300, 1956

McCarley RW, Wible CG, Frumin M, et al: MRI anatomy of schizophrenia. Biol Psychiatry 45:1099–1119, 1999

McElhiney MC, Moody BJ, Steif BL, et al: Autobiographical memory and mood: effects of electroconvulsive therapy. Neuropsychology 9:501–507, 1995

McKay AP, Tarbuck AF, Shapleske J, et al: Neuropsychological function in manic-depressive psychosis: evidence for persistent deficits in patients with chronic, severe illness. Br J Psychiatry 167:51–57, 1995

McKenna PJ, Tamlyn D, Lund CE, et al: Amnesic syndrome in schizophrenia. Psychol Med 20:967–972, 1990

Meltzer HY, McGurk SR: The effects of clozapine, risperidone, and olanzapine on cognitive function in schizophrenia. Schizophr Bull 25:233–255, 1999

Milner B: The memory defect in bilateral hippocampal lesions. Psychiatr Res Rep Am Psychiatr Assoc 11:43–58, 1959

Milner B, Petrides M, Smith ML: Frontal lobes and the temporal organization of memory. Hum Neurobiol 4:137–142, 1985

Moscovitch M: Memory and working with memory: evaluation of a component process model and comparisons with other models, in Memory Systems. Edited by Schacter D, Tulving E. Cambridge, MA, MIT Press, 1994, pp 269–310

Mozley LH, Gur RC, Gur RE, et al: Relationships between verbal memory performance and the cerebral distribution of fluorodeoxyglucose in patients with schizophrenia. Biol Psychiatry 40:443–451, 1996

Nadel L, Moscovitch M: Memory consolidation, retrograde amnesia and the hippocampal complex. Curr Opin Neurol 7:217–227, 1997

Nemiah J: Dissociative amnesia: a clinical and theoretical reconsideration, in Functional Disorders of Memory. Edited by Kihlstrom J, Evans F. Hillsdale, NJ, Lawrence Erlbaum, 1979, pp 303–323

Nopoulos P, Flashman L, Flaum M, et al: Stability of cognitive functioning early in the course of schizophrenia. Schizophr Res 14:29–37, 1994

Nyberg L, Cabeza R, Tulving E: PET Studies of encoding and retrieval: the HERA model. Psychon Bull Rev 3:135–148, 1996a

Nyberg L, McIntosh AR, Cabeza R, et al: General and specific brain regions involved in encoding and retrieval of events: what, where, and when. Proc Natl Acad Sci U S A 93:11280–11285, 1996b

Nyberg L, McIntosh AR, Houle S, et al: Activation of medial temporal structures during episodic memory retrieval. Nature 380:715–717, 1996c

Nyberg L, McIntosh AR, Tulving E: Functional brain imaging of episodic and semantic memory with positron emission tomography. J Mol Med 76:48–53, 1998

Nyberg L, Persson J, Habib R, et al: Large scale neurocognitive networks underlying episodic memory. J Cogn Neurosci 12:163–173, 2000

O'Donnell BF, McCarley RW, Potts GF, et al: Identification of neural circuits underlying P300 abnormalities in schizophrenia. Psychophysiology 36:388–398, 1999

Orne M: On the simulating subjects as a quasi-control group in hypnosis research: what, why, and how, in Hypnosis: Developments in Research and New Perspectives. Edited by Fromm E, Shor R. New York, Aldine, 1979, pp 519–565

Overall JE, Hoffmann NG, Levin H: Effects of aging, organicity, alcoholism, and functional psychopathology on WAIS subtest profiles. J Consult Clin Psychol 46:1315–1322, 1978

Pantoni L, Lamassa M, Inzitari D: Transient global amnesia: a review emphasizing pathogenic aspects. Acta Neurol Scand 102:275–283, 2000

Park S, Holzman PS: Association of working memory deficit and eye tracking dysfunction in schizophrenia. Schizophr Res 11:55–61, 1993

Parkin AJ, Walter BM, Hunkin NM: Relationships between normal aging, frontal lobe function, and memory for temporal and spatial information. Neuropsychology 9:304–312, 1995

Perley M, Guze S: Hysteria—the stability and usefulness of clinical criteria. N Engl J Med 266:421–426, 1962

Perry W, Light GA, Davis H, et al: Schizophrenia patients demonstrate a dissociation on declarative and nondeclarative memory tests. Schizophr Res 46:167–174, 2000

Prudic J, Peyser S, Sackeim HA: Subjective memory complaints: a review of patient self-assessment of memory after electroconvulsive therapy. J ECT 16:121–132, 2000

Purdon SE: Cognitive improvement in schizophrenia with novel antipsychotic medications. Schizophr Res 35(suppl):S51–S60, 1999

Purdon SE, Jones BD, Stip E, et al: Neuropsychological change in early phase schizophrenia during 12 months of treatment with olanzapine, risperidone, or haloperidol. The Canadian Collaborative Group for research in schizophrenia. Arch Gen Psychiatry 57:249–258, 2000

Rees LM, Tombaugh TN, Gansler DA, et al: Five validation experiments of the Test of Memory Malingering (TOMM). Psychol Assess 10:10–20, 1998

Reitan R, Wolfson D: The Halstead-Reitan Neuropsychological Test Battery: Theory and Clinical Interpretation. Tucson, AZ, Neuropsychology Press, 1985

Richardson JS, Keegan DL, Bowen RC, et al: Verbal learning by major depressive disorder patients during treatment with fluoxetine or amitriptyline. Int Clin Psychopharmacol 9:35–40, 1994

Riege WH: Self-report and tests of memory aging. Clin Gerontol 1:23–36, 1982

Roy-Byrne PP, Weingartner H, Bierer LM, et al: Effortful and automatic cognitive processes in depression. Arch Gen Psychiatry 43:265–267, 1986

Rush AJ, George MS, Sackeim HA, et al: Vagus nerve stimulation (VNS) for treatment-resistant depressions: a multicenter study. Biol Psychiatry 47:276–286, 2000

Russell WR, Nathan PW: Traumatic amnesia. Brain 69:280–300, 1946

Sackeim HA: The cognitive effects of electroconvulsive therapy, in Cognitive Disorders: Pathophysiology and Treatment. Edited by Moos WH, Gamzu ER, Thal LJ. New York, Marcel Dekker, 1992, pp 183–228

Sackeim HA: Memory and ECT: from polarization to reconciliation. J ECT 16:87–96, 2000a

Sackeim HA: Repetitive transcranial magnetic stimulation: what are the next steps? Biol Psychiatry 48:959–961, 2000b

Sackeim HA, Steif BL: The neuropsychology of depression and mania, in Depression and Mania. Edited by Georgotas A, Cancro R. New York, Elsevier, 1988, pp 265–289

Sackeim HA, Freeman J, McElhiney M, et al: Effects of major depression on estimates of intelligence. J Clin Exp Neuropsychol 14:268–288, 1992

Sackeim HA, Prudic J, Devanand DP, et al: Effects of stimulus intensity and electrode placement on the efficacy and cognitive effects of electroconvulsive therapy. N Engl J Med 328:839–846, 1993

Sackeim HA, Devanand DP, Nobler MS: Electroconvulsive therapy, in Psychopharmacology: The Fourth Generation of Progress. Edited by Bloom F, Kupfer D. New York, Raven, 1995, pp 1123–1142

Sackeim HA, Prudic J, Devanand DP, et al: A prospective, randomized, double-blind comparison of bilateral and right unilateral electroconvulsive therapy at different stimulus intensities. Arch Gen Psychiatry 57:425–434, 2000

Sackeim HA, Keilp JG, Rush AJ, et al: The effects of vagus nerve stimulation on cognitive performance in patients with treatment-resistant depression. Neuropsychiatry Neuropsychol Behav Neurol 14:53–62, 2001

Salisbury DF, Shenton ME, McCarley RW: P300 topography differs in schizophrenia and manic psychosis. Biol Psychiatry 45:98–106, 1999

Sander D, Winbeck K, Etgen T, et al: Disturbance of venous flow patterns in patients with transient global amnesia. Lancet 356:1982–1984, 2000

Saykin AJ, Shtasel DL, Gur RE, et al: Neuropsychological deficits in neuroleptic naive patients with first-episode schizophrenia. Arch Gen Psychiatry 51:124–131, 1994

Saykin AJ, Johnson SC, Flashman LA, et al: Functional differentiation of medial temporal and involved in processing novel and familiar words: an fMRI study. Brain 122:1963–1971, 1999

Schacter DL: Perceptual representation systems and implicit memory: towards a resolution of the multiple memory systems debate. Ann N Y Acad Sci 608:543–571, 1990

Schacter DL, Church B: Auditory priming: implicit and explicit memory for words and voices. J Exp Psychol Learn Mem Cogn 18:915–930, 1992

Schacter DL, Wagner AD: Medial temporal lobe activations in fMRI and PET studies of episodic encoding and retrieval. Hippocampus 9:7–24, 1999

Schacter DL, Cooper LA, Delaney SM: Implicit memory for unfamiliar objects depends on access to structural descriptions. J Exp Psychol Gen 119:5–24, 1990

Schwartz BL, Benjamin AS, Bjork RA: The inferential and experiential bases of metamemory. Current Directions in Psychological Science 6:132–137, 1997

Shallice T, Fletcher P, Frith CD, et al: Brain regions associated with acquisition and retrieval of verbal episodic memory. Nature 368:633–635, 1994

Shelline YI, Sanghavi M, Mintun MA, et al: Depression duration but not age predicts hippocampal volume loss in medically healthy women with recurrent major depression. J Neurosci 19:5034–5043, 1999

Shimamura AP: Memory and frontal lobe function, in The Cognitive Neurosciences. Edited by Gazzaniga MS. Cambridge, MA, MIT Press, 1994, pp 803–813

Silver H, Geraisy N: Effects of biperiden and amantadine on memory in medicated chronic schizophrenic patients: a double-blind cross-over study. Br J Psychiatry 166:241–243, 1995

Singer JA, Salovey P: Mood and memory: evaluating the network theory of affect. Clin Psychol Rev 8:211–251, 1988

Slater E, Glithero E: A follow-up of patients diagnosed as suffering from "hysteria." J Psychosom Res 9:9–13, 1965

Small SA, Perera GM, DeLaPaz R, et al: Differential regional dysfunction of the hippocampal formation among elderly with memory decline and Alzheimer's disease. Ann Neurol 45:466–472, 1999

Sobin C, Sackeim HA, Prudic J, et al: Predictors of retrograde amnesia following ECT. Am J Psychiatry 152:995–1001, 1995

Squire LR: Memory functions as affected by electroconvulsive therapy. Ann N Y Acad Sci 462:307–314, 1986

Squire LR: Declarative and nondeclarative memory: multiple brain systems supporting learning and memory. J Cogn Neurosci 99:195–231, 1992

Squire LR, Wetzel CD, Slater PC: Memory complaint after electroconvulsive therapy: assessment with a new self-rating instrument. Biol Psychiatry 14:791–801, 1979

Squire L, Shimamura A, Graf P: Independence of recognition memory and priming effects: a neuropsychological analysis. J Exp Psychol Learn Mem Cogn 11:37–44, 1985

Staal WG, Hijman R, Hulshoff Pol HE, et al: Neuropsychological dysfunctions in siblings discordant for schizophrenia. Psychiatry Res 95:227–235, 2000

Steif BL, Sackeim HA, Portnoy S, et al: Effects of depression and ECT on anterograde memory. Biol Psychiatry 21:921–930, 1986

Stern Y, Moeller JR, Anderson KE, et al: Different brain networks mediate task performance in normal aging and AD: defining compensation. Neurology 55:1291–1297, 2000

Sternberg DE, Jarvik ME: Memory function in depression: improvement with antidepressant medication. Arch Gen Psychiatry 33:219–224, 1976

Strous RD, Cowan N, Ritter W, et al: Auditory sensory (echoic) memory dysfunction in schizophrenia. Am J Psychiatry 152:1517–1519, 1995

Strupp M, Bruning R, Wu RH, et al: Diffusion-weighted MRI in transient global amnesia: elevated signal intensity in the left mesial temporal lobe in 7 of 10 patients. Ann Neurol 43:164–170, 1998

Stuss DT, Benson DF: The Frontal Lobes. New York, Raven, 1986

Sullivan EV, Shear PK, Zipursky RB, et al: A deficit profile of executive, memory, and motor functions in schizophrenia. Biol Psychiatry 36:641–653, 1994

Tanabe M, Watanabe T, Ishibashi M, et al: Hippocampal ischemia in a patient who experienced transient global amnesia after undergoing cerebral angiography: case illustration. J Neurosurg 91:347, 1999

Taylor JL, Tinklenberg JR: Cognitive impairment and benzodiazepines, in Psychopharmacology: The Third Generation of Progress. Edited by Meltzer H. New York, Raven, 1987, pp 1449–1454

Taylor MA, Abrams R: Cognitive dysfunction in schizophrenia. Am J Psychiatry 141:196–201, 1984

Tombaugh T: Test of Memory Malingering (TOMM). New York, Multi Health Systems, 1996

Tulving E: Episodic and semantic memory, in Organization of Memory. Edited by Tulving E, Donaldson W. New York, Academic Press, 1972, pp 381–403

Tulving E: Elements of Episodic Memory. Oxford, UK, Oxford University Press, 1983

Tulving E, Markowitsch HJ: Memory beyond the hippocampus. Curr Opin Neurobiol 7:209–216, 1997

Tulving E, Markowitsch HJ: Episodic and declarative memory: role of the hippocampus. Hippocampus 8:198–204, 1998

Tulving E, Schacter DL: Priming and human memory systems. Science 247:301–306, 1990

Tulving E, Kapur S, Craik FI, et al: Hemispheric encoding/retrieval asymmetry in episodic memory: positron emission tomography findings. Proc Natl Acad Sci U S A 91:2016–2020, 1994a

Tulving E, Kapur S, Markowitsch HJ, et al: Neuroanatomical correlates of retrieval in episodic memory: auditory sentence recognition. Proc Natl Acad Sci U S A 91:2012–2015, 1994b

Tulving E, Habib R, Nyberg L, et al: Positron emission tomography correlations in and beyond medial temporal lobes. Hippocampus 9:71–82, 1999

van Gorp WG, Altshuler L, Theberge DC, et al: Cognitive impairment in euthymic bipolar patients with and without prior alcohol dependence: a preliminary study. Arch Gen Psychiatry 55:41–46, 1998

Verdoux H, Liraud F: Neuropsychological function in subjects with psychotic and affective disorders: relationship to diagnostic category and duration of illness. Eur Psychiatry 15:236–243, 2000

Victor M, Adams RD, Collins GH: The Wernicke-Korsakoff Syndrome, 2nd Edition. Philadelphia, PA, FA Davis, 1989

Voglmaier MM, Seidman LJ, Niznikiewicz MA, et al: Verbal and nonverbal neuropsychological test performance in subjects with schizotypal personality disorder. Am J Psychiatry 157:787–793, 2000

Wagner AD, Schacter DL, Rotte M, et al: Building memories: remembering and forgetting of verbal experiences as predicted by brain activity. Science 281:1188–1191, 1998

Watkins PC, Vache K, Verney SP, et al: Unconscious mood-congruent memory bias in depression. J Abnorm Psychol 105:34–41, 1996

Weickert TW, Goldberg TE, Gold JM, et al: Cognitive impairments in patients with schizophrenia displaying preserved and compromised intellect. Arch Gen Psychiatry 57:907–913, 2000

Weiner RD: Does ECT cause brain damage? Behavioral Brain Science 7:1–53, 1984

Weiner RD, Rogers HJ, Davidson JR, et al: Effects of stimulus parameters on cognitive side effects. Ann N Y Acad Sci 462:315–325, 1986

Weingartner H, Cohen R, Murphy D, et al: Cognitive processes in depression. Arch Gen Psychiatry 38:42–47, 1981

Weiskrantz L, Warrington EK: Conditioning in amnesic patients. Neuropsychologia 17:187–194, 1979

Welsh KA, Butters N, Hughes JP, et al: Detection and staging of dementia in Alzheimer's disease: use of the neuropsychological measures developed for the Consortium to Establish a Registry for Alzheimer's Disease. Arch Neurol 49:448–452, 1992

West RL: An application of prefrontal cortex function theory to cognitive aging. Psychol Bull 120:272–292, 1996

Wheeler MA, Stuss DT, Tulving E: Frontal lobe damage produces episodic memory impairment. J Int Neuropsychol Soc 1:525–536, 1995

Whitehead A: Verbal learning and memory in elderly depressives. Br J Psychiatry 123:203–208, 1973

Whitlock F: The etiology of hysteria. Acta Psychiatr Scand 43:144–162, 1967

Winokur G, Moscovitch M, Stuss DT: Explicit and implicit memory in the elderly: evidence for double dissociation involving medial temporal- and frontal-lobe functions. Neuropsychology 10:57–65, 1996

Zakzanis KK, Leach L, Kaplan E: On the nature and pattern of neurocognitive function in major depressive disorder. Neuropsychiatry Neuropsychol Behav Neurol 11:111–119, 1998

Part IV

Neuropsychiatric Disorders

15

Neuropsychiatric Aspects of Traumatic Brain Injury

Jonathan M. Silver, M.D.

Robert E. Hales, M.D., M.B.A.

Stuart C. Yudofsky, M.D.

Each year in the United States, more than 2 million people sustain a traumatic brain injury (TBI); 300,000 of these persons require hospitalization, and more than 80,000 of the survivors are afflicted with the chronic sequelae of such injuries (J.F. Kraus and Sorenson 1994). In this population, psychosocial and psychological deficits are commonly the major source of disability for the victims and of stress for their families. The psychiatrist, neurologist, and neuropsychologist are often called on by other medical specialists or the families to treat these patients. In this chapter, we review the role these professionals play in the prevention, diagnosis, and treatment of the cognitive, behavioral, and emotional aspects of TBI.

EPIDEMIOLOGY

death among persons under age 35. What is often not stated is that the most common cause is injuries incurred during motor vehicle accidents. TBI accounts for 2% of all deaths and 26% of all injury deaths (Sosin et al. 1989). A conservative estimate of the annual incidence of individuals hospitalized with TBI is approximately 120 per 100,000 (J.F. Kraus and Chu 2005). There are almost

100,000 new disabilities from TBI per year (J.F. Kraus and Chu 2005). In the United States, between 2.5 million and 6.5 million individuals live with the long-term consequences of TBI (NIH Consensus Development Panel 1999). Disorders arising from traumatic injuries to the brain are more common than any other neurological disease, with the exception of headaches (Kurtzke 1984).

Those at the highest risk for brain injury are men ages 15–24 years. Alcohol use is common in brain injury; a positive blood alcohol concentration was demonstrated in 56% of one sample of victims (J.F. Kraus et al. 1989). Motor vehicle accidents account for approximately one-half of traumatic injuries; other common causes are falls (21%), assaults and violence (20%), and accidents associated with sports and recreation (3%) (although as many as 90% of injuries in this category may be unreported) (NIH Consensus Development Panel 1999). Children are highly vulnerable to accidents as passengers, to falls as pedestrians, to impact from moving objects (e.g., rocks or baseballs), and to sports injuries. In the United States, as many as 5 million children sustain head injuries each year, and of this group 200,000 are hospitalized (Raphaely et al. 1980). As a result of bicycle accidents alone, 50,000 children sustain head injuries, and 400 children die each year (U.S. Department of Health and Human Services 1989). Tragically, among infants, most head injuries are the result of child abuse (64%) (U.S. Department of Health and Human Services 1989).

The total economic cost of brain injury is staggeringly high: an estimated $37.8 billion per year for the United States alone to treat 328,000 victims of brain injury (W. Max et al. 1991). The average lifetime cost of treatment per person ranges from $600,000 to $1,875,000 (NIH Consensus Development Panel 1999). Because the victims of TBI most commonly are young adults, they may require prolonged rehabilitation.

Statistics form only a piece of the picture of the cost of TBI. Mental health professionals must deal with individuals and families who have endured these tragic events. The psychological and social disability after brain injury can be dramatic. As with patients who have many psychiatric illnesses, and in distinction to patients with neurological disorders such as stroke and Parkinson's disease, many survivors of TBI appear to be physically well (without sensorimotor impairment). In addition to the neurological consequences of TBI, the cognitive, social, and behavioral problems result in significant impairment. Studies examining the psychosocial functioning and adjustment at 1 month, 2 years, or 7 years after severe TBI have shown that patients have extreme difficulty in numerous critical areas of functioning, including work, school, familial, interpersonal, and avocational activities (Crawford 1983; McLean et al. 1984; Oddy et al. 1985; Weddell et al. 1980).

NEUROANATOMY AND PATHOPHYSIOLOGY OF TRAUMATIC BRAIN INJURY

NEUROANATOMY

The patient who sustains brain injury from trauma may incur damage through several mechanisms, which are listed in Table 15–1. Contusions affect specific areas of the brain and usually occur as the result of low-velocity injuries, such as falls. Courville (1945) examined the neuroanatomical sites of contusions and found that most injuries were in the basal and polar portions of the temporal and frontal lobes. Most of these lesions were the result of the location of bony prominences that surround the orbital, frontal, and temporal areas along the base of the skull. Coup injuries occur at the site of impact due to local tissue strain. Contrecoup injuries occur away from the site of impact during sudden deceleration and translational and angular movements of the head. Impact is not required for contrecoup injuries to occur, and they usually occur in frontal and temporal areas (Gennarelli and Graham 1998).

TABLE 15–1.   Mechanisms of neuronal damage in traumatic brain injury

Primary effects

    Contusions

    Diffuse traumatic axonal injury

Secondary effects

    Hematomas

       Epidural effects

       Subdural effects

       Intracerebral effects

    Cerebral edema

    Hydrocephalus

    Increased intracranial pressure

    Infection

    Hypoxia

    Neurotoxicity

    Inflammatory response

    Protease activation

    Calcium influx

    Excitotoxin and free radical release

    Lipid peroxidation

    Phospholipase activation

Diffuse axonal injury refers to mechanical or chemical damage to the axons in cerebral white matter that commonly occurs with lateral angular or rotational acceleration. The axon is vulnerable to injury during high-velocity accidents when there is twisting and turning of the brain around the brain stem (as can occur in "whiplash" car accidents). Axons are stretched, causing delayed (hours) disruption of the cytoskeleton and impaired axoplasm transport. This results in axoplasmic swelling and detachment, changes in membrane structure, disruption in neurofilaments, and wallerian degeneration of the distal stump of the axon (Gennarelli and Graham 2005). The disruption of axons can occur as long as 2 weeks after the injury (Gennarelli and Graham 1998). Chemically, metabolic changes occur, leading to axonal damage (discussion follows). The most vulnerable sites in the brain to axonal injury are the reticular formation, superior cerebellar peduncles, regions of the basal ganglia, hypothalamus, limbic fornices, and corpus callosum (Cassidy 1994).

Diffuse axonal injury can often but does not necessarily result in sudden loss of consciousness (LOC) and can occur in mild brain injury or *concussion* (Jane et al. 1985; Povlishock et al. 1983). Among cases of TBI without diffuse axonal injury, there is a lower incidence of skull fractures, contusions, and intracranial hematomas (Adams et al. 1982).

Subdural hematomas (acute, subacute, and chronic) and intracerebral hematomas have effects that are specific to their locations and degree of neuronal damage. In general, subdural hematomas affect arousal and cognition.

PATHOPHYSIOLOGY

After TBI, the damaged neurons have an increased demand for energy. However, a decrease in cerebral blood flow occurs, which results in a mismatch between needed and available energy supply. These injured cells are more vulnerable to hypoxia, resulting in further neuronal damage (DeKosky et al. 1998). Secondary neurotoxicity is caused by calcium influx, phospholipase activation, inflammatory response, protease activation, excitotoxin release, and lipid peroxidation that further damage axons and neuronal systems (DeKosky et al. 1998; Honig and Albers 1994). During hypoxia, free radicals and excitotoxic neurotransmitters, such as glutamate, are released and result in further neuronal damage (Becker et al. 1988; Faden et al. 1989), especially hippocampal damage to the CA1 neurons (Gennarelli and Graham 1998). Palmer et al. (1994) found that the brain concentration of aspartate, glutamate, glycine, and γ-aminobutyric acid (GABA) significantly increased in 5 patients with severe TBI. In evaluating the concentrations of glutamate in the cerebrospinal fluid (CSF) of 12 brain-injured patients, elevations were found that persisted for days after the injury (A.J. Baker et al. 1993).

Studies in animals suggest that the hippocampal formation is differentially sensitive to injury relative to other regions of the brain, that the CA1 and CA3 subfields and the dentate hilar region are most commonly affected, that such injury can occur even in the absence of hypoxia or elevated intracranial pressure (Hicks et al. 1993; Lowenstein et al. 1992; D.H. Smith et al. 1991; Toulmond et al. 1993), and that functional alterations may occur without actual neuronal cell death (Reeves et al. 1995). Furthermore, these lesions correlate with decrements in memory performance (Hamm et al. 1992; Hicks et al. 1993; Lowenstein et al. 1992; D.H. Smith et al. 1991).

Animal models of TBI, including fluid percussion models in cats and rodents and controlled angular acceleration devices in nonhuman primates, suggest that even mild TBI can result in neuronal injury with the appearance of axonal edema, separation of proximal and distal portions of the injured axons, and subsequent wallerian degeneration of the distal axonal segment (Jane et al.

1985; Povlishock and Coburn 1989). This is accompanied by disruption of axoplasmic transport and by secondary deafferentation. These changes evolve over a broad period of time—for example, from hours to weeks in the cat model (Povlishock and Coburn 1989)—perhaps providing some rationale for evolving symptoms in the days and weeks following a mild TBI. Although there is a general correlation between the length of unconsciousness and the amount of diffuse axonal injury, neuropathological changes characteristic of those seen in brain injury have been shown in cases of very mild TBI in humans, even those in whom there was no LOC (Blumbergs et al. 1994; Gennarelli et al. 1982; Oppenheimer 1968).

NEUROTRANSMITTER CHANGES AFTER TBI

Neuropsychiatric symptoms arising from penetrating and/or focal trauma are often understandable given the functions known to be subserved by the site of injury (e.g., behavioral disinhibition and aggression following bilateral orbitofrontal contusion), but the etiology of cognitive impairments following nonpenetrating (or "nonfocal") injuries is relatively less well understood. Cytotoxic processes such as calcium and magnesium dysregulation, free radical induced injury, neurotransmitter (especially glutamate and cholinergic) excitotoxicity, and diffuse axonal injury due to straining and shearing biomechanical forces may be produced by nonpenetrating injuries (see Halliday 1999 and McIntosh et al. 1999 for review). These processes functionally and structurally disrupt the neural networks subserving many critical neuropsychiatric functions (i.e., cognition, emotion, and behavior). Although TBI-induced glutamatergic disturbances are almost certainly important in the genesis of injury to areas critical to neuropsychiatric function (see Obrenovitch and Urenjak 1997 for review), there are at present no therapies available to directly ameliorate neuropsychiatric problems predicated on disturbances in this system. Several studies of neurochemical changes subsequent to TBI suggest that alterations in neurotransmitter production and/or delivery occur within these networks both acutely and chronically, and may therefore play a role in the development of neuropsychiatric problems following TBI. These studies have shown that neurotransmitter systems including norepinephrine, serotonin, dopamine, and acetylcholine are altered by TBI, although the timing of such effects following TBI is important to consider. Multiple pharmacotherapies are available to modify the function of these neurotransmitter systems and the neuropsychiatric problems arising from disturbances within them.

In this chapter, we focus on TBI-induced neurotransmitter disturbances that are both related to neuropsychiatric functioning and amenable to modification using agents presently available. These two limits will focus this portion of the discussion on disturbances in dopamine, norepinephrine, serotonin, and acetylcholine.

Catecholamines

Discrete lesions to ascending monoaminergic projections may interfere with the function of systems dependent on such afferent pathways (Morrison et al. 1979). Monoaminergic afferents course from the brain stem anteriorly, curving around the hypothalamus, the basal ganglia, and the frontal cortex, placing them in anatomical areas that are especially vulnerable to the effects of TBI.

Two studies found markedly elevated plasma norepinephrine levels after acute head injury (Clifton et al. 1981; Hamill et al. 1987). However, most of the studies in this area suggest only that acute elevations of striatal dopamine are predictive of poor recovery from TBI (Donnemiller et al. 2000; Hamill et al. 1987; Woolf et al. 1987). No human studies have demonstrated a clear relationship between in vivo markers of dopaminergic function and long-term cognitive deficits in traumatically brain-injured humans. Thus, the extent of dopaminergic and noradrenergic dysfunction in the late period following TBI remains uncertain, and the implications of such findings with respect to long-term neuropsychiatric disturbances require further study. Nonetheless, the observation of cognitive improvements (e.g., arousal, speed of processing, attention, and perhaps memory) among some persons with TBIs during treatment with agents that increase dopaminergic neurotransmission suggests that dopamine dysfunction (primary, secondary, or both) may play an important role in the genesis of cognitive impairment following TBI.

Serotonin

Serotonergic projections to the frontal cortical areas are susceptible to biomechanical injury, and both diffuse axonal injury and contusions may produce dysfunction in this neurotransmitter system. Secondary neurotoxicity that is caused by excitotoxins and lipid peroxidation may also damage the neuronal systems that mediate serotonin (Karakucuk et al. 1997) and perhaps also norepinephrine. Studies of serotonin activity after TBI are somewhat variable in their findings, although differences in the methodology (especially location of CSF sampling) appear to account for much of the difference in study findings.

This may offer some explanation for the discrepancy of findings related to CSF serotonin, norepinephrine, and dopamine metabolites following TBI in humans, in that that the site from which samples are obtained may yield substantially different findings. Consistent with this experimental observation, Vecht et al. (1975) and Bareggi et al. (1975) found that lumbar CSF 5-hydroxyindoleacetic acid (5-HIAA) was below normal in conscious patients and was normal in patients who were unconscious. Decreased CSF levels of serotonin were reported by Karakucuk et al. (1997) in 45 adults undergoing minor surgery with spinal anesthesia within 24 hours of TBI. However, Porta et al. (1975) demonstrated elevated ventricular CSF 5-HIAA levels in patients within days of severe TBI. Additionally, focal and diffuse lesions may result in differences with respect to monoaminergic alterations after TBI. For example, Van Woerkom et al. (1977) investigated patients with frontotemporal contusions and those with diffuse contusions. They documented decreased levels of 5-HIAA in patients with frontotemporal contusions but increased 5-HIAA levels in those with more diffuse contusions. In summary, the animal and human studies suggest acute increases in hemispheric serotonin levels following TBI, and suggest that such increases are associated with decreased glucose utilization. Whether or to what extent similar changes persist into the late period following TBI remains uncertain, as does the role of such changes in the genesis of neuropsychiatric symptoms following TBI.

Acetylcholine

Findings from both basic and clinical neuroscience suggest that both acute and long-term alterations in cortical cholinergic function develop following TBI. TBI appears to produce an acute increase in cholinergic neurotransmission followed by chronic reductions in neurotransmitter function and cholinergic afferents. Consistent with observations in experimental injury studies, Grossman et al. (1975) demonstrated that patients with TBI had elevated acetylcholine levels in fluid obtained from intraventricular catheters or lumbar puncture in the acute period following TBI. Dewar and Graham (1996) and Murdoch et al. (1998) demonstrated cortical cholinergic dysfunction (loss of cortical cholinergic afferents with concurrent preservation of postsynaptic muscarinic and nicotinic receptors) weeks after severe TBI. Arciniegas et al. (1999, 2000a, 2001), using the hippocampally mediated, cholinergically dependent P50 evoked waveform response to paired auditory stimuli, demonstrated electrophysiological abnormalities consistent with reduced hippocampal cholinergic function in patients with chronic symptoms of impaired auditory gating, attention, and memory in the late (>1 year) period following TBI.

NEUROPSYCHIATRIC ASSESSMENT OF TRAUMATIC BRAIN INJURY

HISTORY-TAKING

Although brain injuries subsequent to serious automobile, occupational, or sports accidents may not result in diagnostic enigmas for the psychiatrist, less severe trauma may first present as relatively subtle behavioral or affective change. Patients may fail to associate the traumatic event with subsequent symptoms. Prototypic examples include the alcoholic man who is amnestic for a fall that occurred while he was inebriated, the 10-year-old boy who falls from his bicycle and hits his head but fails to inform his parents, or the wife who was beaten by her husband but who is either fearful or ashamed to report the injury to her family physician. Confusion, intellectual changes, affective lability, or psychosis may occur directly after the trauma or as long as many years afterward. Individuals who present for emergency treatment for blunt trauma may not be adequately screened for TBI (Chambers et al. 1996). Even individuals who have identified themselves as "nondisabled" but who had experienced a blow to the head that left them at a minimum dazed and confused had symptoms and emotional distress similar to a group of individuals with known mild TBI (Gordon et al. 1998).

For all psychiatric patients, the clinician must specifically inquire whether the patient has been involved in situations that are associated with head trauma. The practitioner should ask about automobile, bicycle, or motorcycle accidents; falls; assaults; playground accidents; and participation in sports that are frequently associated with brain injury (e.g., football, soccer, rugby, and boxing). Patients must be asked whether there was any alteration in consciousness after they were injured, including feeling dazed or confused, losing consciousness, or experiencing a period of amnesia after the accident. The clinician should inquire as to whether the patients were hospitalized and whether they had posttraumatic symptoms, such as headache, dizziness, irritability, problems with concentration, and sensitivity to noise or light. Most patients will not volunteer this information without direct inquiry. Patients are usually unaware of the phenomenon of posttraumatic amnesia and may confuse posttraumatic amnesia with LOC. They assume that if they are unable to recall events, they must have been unconscious. Therefore, care must be taken to document the source of this observation (e.g., whether there were observers who witnessed the period of unconsciousness).

Because many patients are unaware of, minimize, or deny the severity of behavioral changes that occur after TBI, family members also must be asked about the effects

TABLE 15–2. Assessment of traumatic brain injury

Behavioral assessment

Structured interviews (e.g., Structured Clinical Interview for DSM-IV Diagnoses [SCID], Mini-International Neuropsychiatric Inventory [MINI])

Neurobehavioral Rating Scale (NBRS)

Positive and Negative Symptom Scale (PANSS)

Glasgow Coma Scale (GCS)

Galveston Orientation and Amnesia Test (GOAT)

Rancho Los Amigos Cognitive Scale

Rating scales for depression (Hamilton)

Rating scales for aggression (Overt Aggression Scale/ Agitated Behavior Scale)

Neuropsychiatric Inventory/Neuropsychiatric Inventory Questionnaire

Brain Injury Screening Questionnaire

Rivermead Post Concussion Symptoms Questionnaire

Brain imaging

Computed tomography (CT)

Magnetic resonance imaging (MRI) with fluid-attenuated inversion recovery (FLAIR)

Functional magnetic resonance imaging (fMRI)

Single-photon emission computed tomography (SPECT)

Regional cerebral blood flow (rCBF)

Positron emission tomography (PET)

Proton magnetic resonance spectroscopy (MRS)

Diffusion tensor imaging (DTI)

Electrophysiological assessment

Electroencephalogram (EEG), including special leads

Computerized EEG

Brain electrical activity mapping (BEAM)

Neuropsychological assessment

Attention and concentration

Premorbid intelligence

Memory

Executive functioning

Verbal capacity

Problem-solving skills

TABLE 15–3.   Glasgow Coma Scale

Eye opening

None	1. Not attributable to ocular swelling
To pain	2. Pain stimulus is applied to chest or limbs
To speech	3. Nonspecific response to speech or shout, does not imply the patient obeys command to open eyes
Spontaneous	4. Eyes are open, but this does not imply intact awareness

Motor response

No response	1. Flaccid
Extension	2. "Decerebrate." Adduction, internal rotation of shoulder, and pronation of the forearm
Abnormal flexion	3. "Decorticate." Abnormal flexion, adduction of the shoulder
Withdrawal	4. Normal flexor response; withdraws from pain stimulus with adduction of the shoulder
Localizes pain	5. Pain stimulus applied to supraocular region or fingertip causes limb to move so as to attempt to remove it
Obeys commands	6. Follows simple commands

Verbal response

No response	1. (Self-explanatory)
Incomprehensible	2. Moaning and groaning, but no recognizable words
Inappropriate	3. Intelligible speech (e.g., shouting or swearing), but no sustained or coherent conversation
Confused	4. Patient responds to questions in a conversational manner, but the responses indicate varying degrees of disorientation and confusion
Oriented	Normal orientation to time, place, and person

Source. Adapted from Teasdale and Jennett 1974.

of injury on the behavior of their relative. For example, in evaluating the social adjustment of patients years after severe brain injury, Oddy et al. (1985) compared symptoms reported by both patients and their relatives. Forty percent of relatives of 28 patients with TBI reported that their relative behaved childishly. However, this symptom was not reported by the patients themselves. Although 28% of the patients complained of problems with their vision after the injury, this difficulty was not reported by relatives. Patients overestimate their level of functioning compared with the reporting of relatives, and they report more physical than nonphysical impairment (Sherer et al. 1998).

Family members also are more aware of emotional changes than are the victims of brain injury. Whereas individuals with TBI tend to view the cognitive difficulties as being more severe than the emotional changes (Hendryx 1989), mood disorders and frustration intolerance are viewed by family members as being more disabling than cognitive disabilities (Rappaport et al. 1989).

DOCUMENTATION AND RATING OF SYMPTOMS

Symptom rating scales, electrophysiological imaging, and neuropsychiatric assessments should be used to define symptoms and signs that result from TBI (Table 15–2). The severity of injury may be determined by several parameters, including duration of unconsciousness, initial score on the Glasgow Coma Scale (GCS) (Teasdale and Jennett 1974), and degree of posttraumatic amnesia. The GCS (Table 15–3) is a 15-point scale that documents eye opening, verbal responsiveness, and motor response to stimuli and may be used to measure the depth of coma, both initially and longitudinally. The Galveston Orientation and Amnesia Test (GOAT) (Levin et al. 1979) measures the extent of posttraumatic amnesia and can be used serially to document recovery of memory (Figure 15–1). Overall cognitive and behavioral recovery may be documented using the Rancho Los Amigos Cognitive Scale (Table 15–4) (Hagen 1998).

In severe TBI, posttraumatic amnesia or LOC may persist for at least 1 week or longer or, in extreme cases, may last weeks to months. GCS scores for severe TBI are less than 10. Mild head injury is usually defined as LOC for less than 15–20 minutes, GCS score of 13–15, brief or no hospitalization, and no prominent residual neurobehavioral deficits. LOC is not required for the diagnosis of traumatic brain injury; however, there must be some evidence of alteration in consciousness, including feeling dazed or experiencing a period of posttraumatic amnesia (Committee on Head Injury Nomenclature 1966; Quality Standards Subcommittee 1997). Operationalized diagnostic criteria for mild TBI have been proposed (Table

Name_____ Date of test ___/___/___/

Age _____ Sex M F Day of the week:
  s m t w t f s

Date of birth ____/____/____/ Time A.M. P.M.

Diagnosis _____ Date of injury ___/___/___/

Galveston Orientation and Amnesia Test (GOAT) **Error points**

1. What is your name? (2) _____ ___/___/

   When were you born? (4) _____ ___/___/

   Where do you live? (4) _____ ___/___/

2. Where are you now? (5) city _____ ___/___/

   (5) hospital _____ ___/___/

   (unnecessary to state name of hospital)

3. On what date were you admitted to this hospital? (5) _____ ___/___/

   How did you get here? (5) _____ ___/___/

4. What is the first event you can remember after the injury? (5) _____ ___/___/

   Can you describe in detail (e.g., date, time, companions) the first event you can ___/___/
   recall after the injury? (5) _____

5. Can you describe the last event you recall before the accident? (5) ___/___/

   _____

   Can you describe in detail (e.g., date, time, companions) the first event you can ___/___/
   recall before the injury? (5) _____

6. What time is it now? _____ (−1 for each ¾ hour removed from correct time to ___/___/
   maximum of −5)

7. What day of the week is it? _____ (−1 for each day removed from correct one) ___/___/

   _____

8. What day of the month is it? _____ (−1 for each day removed from correct date to ___/___/
   maximum of −5) _____

9. What is the month? _____ (−5 for each month removed from correct one to ___/___/
   maximum of −15) _____

10. What is the year? _____ (−10 for each year removed from correct one to maximum ___/___/
    of −30) _____

Total error points ___/___/

Total GOAT Score (100 points minus total error points) ___/___/

FIGURE 15–1. The Galveston Orientation and Amnesia Test (GOAT).

Source. Reprinted from Levin HS, O'Donnell VM, Grossman RG: "The Galveston Orientation and Amnesia Test: A Practical Scale to Assess Cognition After Head Injury." *Journal of Nervous and Mental Disease* 167:675–684, 1979. Used with permission.

15–5) (Mild Traumatic Brain Injury Committee 1993). A specific grading scale has been developed for concussions that occur during sports: Grade 1—confusion without amnesia and no LOC; Grade 2—confusion with amnesia and no LOC; and Grade 3—LOC (Kelly 1995).

The use of structured clinical interviews and rating scales will assist the clinician in the determination of the presence of symptoms and in rating their severity. For example, the Structured Clinical Interview for DSM-IV (SCID; Spitzer et al. 1997) or the Mini-International Neu-

TABLE 15–4.   Rancho Los Amigos Cognitive Scale

I.	**No response:** Unresponsive to any stimulus
II.	**Generalized response:** Limited, inconsistent, nonpurposeful responses, often to pain only
III.	**Localized response:** Purposeful responses; may follow simple commands; may focus on presented object
IV.	**Confused, agitated:** Heightened state of activity; confusion, disorientation; aggressive behavior; unable to do self-care; unaware of present events; agitation appears related to internal confusion
V.	**Confused, inappropriate:** Nonagitated; appears alert; responds to commands; distractible; does not concentrate on task; agitated responses to external stimuli; verbally inappropriate; does not learn new information
VI.	**Confused, appropriate:** Good directed behavior, needs cueing; can relearn old skills as activities of daily living (ADLs); serious memory problems; some awareness of self and others
VII.	**Automatic, appropriate:** Appears appropriate, oriented; frequently robotlike in daily routine; minimal or absent confusion; shallow recall; increased awareness of self, interaction in environment; lacks insight into condition; decreased judgment and problem solving; lacks realistic planning for future
VIII.	**Purposeful, appropriate:** Alert, oriented; recalls and integrates past events; learns new activities and can continue without supervision; independent in home and living skills; capable of driving; defects in stress tolerance, judgment, abstract reasoning persist; may function at reduced levels in society

Source.   Reprinted with permission of the Adult Brain Injury Service of the Rancho Los Amigos Medical Center, Downey, California.

TABLE 15–5.   Definition of mild traumatic brain injury

A patient with mild traumatic brain injury is a person who has had a traumatically induced physiological disruption of brain function, as manifested by **at least** one of the following:

1. Any period of loss of consciousness;

2. Any loss of memory for events immediately before or after the accident;

3. Any alteration in mental state at the time of the accident (e.g., feeling dazed, disoriented, or confused); and

4. Focal neurological deficit(s) that may or may not be transient; but where the severity of the injury does not exceed the following: loss of consciousness of approximately 30 minutes or less; after 30 minutes, an initial Glasgow Coma Scale (GCS) score of 13–15; and posttraumatic amnesia (PTA) not greater than 24 hours.

Source.   Reprinted from Mild Traumatic Brain Injury Committee of the Head Injury Interdisciplinary Special Interest Group of the American Congress of Rehabilitation Medicine: "Definition of Mild Traumatic Brain Injury." *Journal of Head Trauma Rehabilitation* 8:86–87, 1993. Used with permission.

ropsychiatric Inventory (MINI; Sheehan et al. 1998) may be used to evaluate psychiatric diagnoses, whether or not they are associated with brain injury. Scales such as the Neurobehavioral Rating Scale (NBRS; Levin et al. 1987b) and the Positive and Negative Syndrome Scale (PANSS; S.R. Kay et al. 1987) may be used to document the presence and severity of many emotional and cognitive symptoms. The Brain Injury Screening Questionnaire (Depart-

ment of Rehabilitation Medicine 2000) or the Rivermead Post Concussion Symptoms Questionnaire (King et al. 1995) can be used to monitor the presence of multiple symptoms that often occur after TBI. The Neuropsychiatric Inventory (NPI; Cummings et al. 1994) or the abbreviated NPI Questionnaire (Kaufer et al. 2000) will enable the examiner to review symptoms with relatives or caregivers. The Overt Aggression Scale (OAS; Yudofsky et al. 1986) (Figure 15–2) and Overt Agitation Severity Scale (OASS; Yudofsky et al. 1997) can be used to document the frequency and severity of aggressive outbursts and agitation that are so commonly associated with brain injury (Silver and Yudofsky 1987, 1991). The Agitated Behavior Scale (Bogner et al. 1999) may also be helpful.

LABORATORY EVALUATION

Imaging Techniques

Brain imaging techniques are frequently used to demonstrate the location and extent of brain lesions (Belanger et al. 2007). Computed tomography (CT) is used for the acute assessment of the patient with head trauma to document hemorrhage, edema, midline shifts, herniation, fractures, and contusions. The timing of such imaging is important because this establishes a baseline day of injury

Overt Aggression Scale (OAS)

Stuart Yudofsky, M.D., Jonathan Silver, M.D., Wynn Jackson M.D., and Jean Endicott, Ph.D.

Identifying Data

Name of patient	Name of rater
Sex of patient: 1 male 2 female	Date / / (mo/da/yr) Shift: 1 night 2 day 3 evening

☐ No aggressive incident(s) (verbal or physical) against self, others, or objects during the shift (check here).

Aggressive Behavior (check all that apply)

Verbal aggression	Physical aggression against self
☐ Makes loud noises, shouts angrily	☐ Picks or scratches skin, hits self, pulls hair (with no or minor injury only)
☐ Yells mild personal insults (e.g., "You're stupid!")	☐ Bangs head, hits fist into objects, throws self onto floor or into objects (hurts self without serious injury)
☐ Curses viciously, uses foul language in anger, makes moderate threats to others or self	☐ Small cuts or bruises, minor burns
☐ Makes clear threats of violence toward others or self (I'm going to kill you.) or requests to help to control self	☐ Mutilates self, makes deep cuts, bites that bleed, internal injury, fracture, loss of consciousness, loss of teeth

Physical aggression against objects	Physical aggression against other people
☐ Slams door, scatters clothing, makes a mess	☐ Makes threatening gesture, swings at people, grabs at clothes
☐ Throws objects down, kicks furniture without breaking it, marks the wall	☐ Strikes, kicks, pushes, pulls hair (without injury to them)
☐ Breaks objects, smashes windows	☐ Attacks others, causing mild to moderate physical injury (bruises, sprain, welts)
☐ Sets fires, throws objects dangerously	☐ Attacks others, causing severe physical injury (broken bones, deep lacerations, internal injury)

Time incident began: ___ ___ : ___ ___ am/pm	Duration of incident: ___ ___ : ___ ___ (hours/minutes)

Intervention (check all that apply)

☐ None	☐ Immediate medication given by mouth	☐ Use of restraints
☐ Talking to patient	☐ Immediate medication given by injection	☐ Injury requires immediate medical treatment for patient
☐ Closer observation	☐ Isolation without seclusion (time out)	☐ Injury requires immediate treatment for other person
☐ Holding patient	☐ Seclusion	

Comments

FIGURE 15–2. The Overt Aggression Scale (OAS).

Source. Reprinted from Yudofsky SC, Silver JM, Jackson W, et al.: "The Overt Aggression Scale for the Objective Rating of Verbal and Physical Aggression." *American Journal of Psychiatry* 143:35–39, 1986. Used with permission.

scan, since lesions may be visualized months after the injury that cannot be seen during the acute phase (Bigler 2005). Thus, for a significant number of patients with severe brain injury, initial CT evaluations may not detect lesions that are observable on CT scans performed 1 and 3 months after the injury (Cope et al. 1988).

Magnetic resonance imaging (MRI) has been shown to detect clinically meaningful lesions in patients with severe brain injury when CT scans have not demonstrated anatomical bases for the degree of coma (Levin et al. 1987a; Wilberger et al. 1987). MRI is especially sensitive in detecting lesions in the frontal and temporal lobes that are not visualized by CT, and these loci are frequently related to the neuropsychiatric consequences of the injury (Levin et al. 1987a). MRI has been found to be more sensitive for the detection of contusions, shearing injury, and subdural and epidural hematomas (Orrison et al. 1994), and it has been able to document evidence of diffuse axonal injury in patients who have a normal CT scan after experiencing mild TBI (Mittl et al. 1994). When MRI is used, fluid-attenuated inversion recovery (FLAIR) is superior to T2-weighted spin-echo technique, especially in visualizing central diffuse axonal injury of the fornix and corpus callosum (Ashikaga et al. 1997). MR imaging in the chronic stage is better correlated with neuropsychiatric symptoms (Bigler 2005).Quantitative analyses of individuals with TBI have revealed multiple affected brain structures, including the frontal and temporal lobes, thalamus, hippocampus, and basal ganglia (Bigler 2005).

Functional techniques in brain imaging, such as regional cerebral blood flow (rCBF) and positron emission tomography (PET), can detect areas of abnormal function when even CT and MRI scans fail to show any abnormalities of structure (Anderson et al. 2005). Single-photon emission computed tomography (SPECT) also shows promise in documenting brain damage after TBI. Abnormalities are visualized in patients who have experienced mild TBI (Gross et al. 1996; Masdeu et al. 1994; Nedd et al. 1993) or who have chronic TBI (Nagamachi et al. 1995), even in the presence of normally appearing areas on CT scans. Abnormalities on SPECT appear to correlate with the severity of trauma (Jacobs et al. 1994). These techniques were utilized in examining a group of individuals with late whiplash syndrome (Bicik et al. 1998). Although there was significant frontopolar hypometabolism, it correlated significantly with scores on the Beck Depression Inventory (Beck et al. 1961). However, in individual cases, the reliability of the depiction of hypometabolism was low. A "normal" SPECT scan does not imply normal pathology; in addition, SPECT abnormalities after TBI have not been shown to correlate with cognitive deficits or behavioral symptoms (Anderson et al. 2005). SPECT abnormalities can also be seen in many of the concurrent problems experienced by those with TBI, including depression and substance use. Although some studies have found correlations between neuropsychological deficits and abnormalities on PET, other studies have found no relation between lesion location and deficits (Anderson et al. 2005).

Proton magnetic resonance spectroscopy (MRS), which provides information on intracellular function, has been investigated for the detection of abnormalities in TBI. N-acetyl aspartate (NAA) is associated with neuronal or axonal loss. Cech et al. (1998) examined 35 patients with TBI and found that a majority of those with mild TBI as well as severe TBI showed abnormal levels of NAA in the splenium, consistent with diffuse axonal injury. Early changes in NAA concentrations in gray matter were predictive of outcome in a group of 14 patients after TBI (S.D. Friedman et al. 1999). Ariza et al. (2004) found a correlation between performance on neuropsychological tests and NAA concentrations. Even in mild TBI, abnormalities may be found in areas that are frequent sites of diffuse axonal injury (Inglese 2005).

McAllister et al. (1999, 2001) used functional MRI (fMRI) to assess patterns of regional brain activation in response to working memory loads in a group of individuals 1 month after they had sustained mild TBI. This group demonstrated significantly increased activation during a high-load task, particularly in the right parietal and right dorsolateral frontal regions. However, there were no differences in task performance compared with the control group. This study appears to correlate with the complaints of patients who state that they have to "work harder" to recall things but in whom no deficits are found on objective testing. Other studies (Christodoulou et al. 2001; Easdon et al. 2004) suggest that there is impairment in brain structures required for appropriate responding to stimuli.

Caution must be observed in applying the findings in this literature to a clinical population. We are unable to determine the presence of abnormalities before the accident. Abnormalities on SPECT or PET have been demonstrated in individuals with no history of brain injury who have psychiatric disorders including posttraumatic stress disorder (PTSD) (Rauch et al. 1996), somatization disorder (Lazarus and Cotterell 1989), major depression (Dolan et al. 1992), and chronic alcoholism (Kuruoglu et al. 1996). When the evidence was reviewed in 1996, the American Academy of Neurology concluded that there currently was insufficient evidence for the use of SPECT to diagnose TBI, and its use in this condition should be considered investigational (Therapeutics and Technology Assessment Subcommittee 1996). With the present state of the art, functional imaging results can only be used as part of an overall evaluation to confirm findings documented elsewhere (Silver and McAllister 1997).

Electrophysiological Techniques

Electrophysiological assessment of the patient after TBI may also assist in the evaluation. Electroencephalography can detect the presence of seizures or abnormal areas of functioning. To enhance the sensitivity of this technique, the electroencephalogram (EEG) should be performed after sleep deprivation, with photic stimulation and hyperventilation and with anterotemporal and/or nasopharyngeal leads (Goodin et al. 1990). Computed interpretation of the EEG and brain electrical activity mapping (BEAM) may be useful in detecting areas of dysfunction not shown in the routine EEG (Watson et al. 1995). There is controversy regarding the usefulness of these techniques. The American Academy of Neurology and the American Clinical Neurophysiology Society have concluded that "the evidence of clinical usefulness or consistency of results [is] not considered sufficient for us to support [the] use [of quantitative electroencephalography] in diagnosis of patients with postconcussion syndrome, or minor or moderate head injury" (Nuwer 1997). However, the EEG and Clinical Neuroscience Society addressed significant concerns regarding the interpretation of this report (Thatcher et al. 1999). Their opinion is that there is significant scientific literature on the use and interpretation of quantitative electroencephalography, and that several findings have been consistent (reduced amplitude of high-frequency electroencephalography, especially in the frontal lobes, a shift toward lower increased electroencephalographic frequencies, and changes in electroencephalographic coherence) (Thatcher et al. 1999). A detailed discussion of electrophysiological techniques can be found elsewhere (Arciniegas et al. 2005).

Neuropsychological Testing

Neuropsychological assessment of the patient with TBI is essential to document cognitive and intellectual deficits and strengths. Tests are administered to assess the patient's attention, concentration, memory, verbal capacity, and executive functioning. This latter capacity is the most difficult to assess and includes problem-solving skills, abstract thinking, planning, and reasoning abilities. A valid interpretation of these tests includes assessment of the patient's preinjury intelligence and other higher levels of functioning. Because multiple factors affect the results of testing (Table 15–6), tests must be performed and interpreted by a clinician with skill and experience.

Patients' complaints may not be easily or accurately categorized as either functional (i.e., primarily due to a

TABLE 15–6. Major factors affecting neuropsychological test findings

- Original endowment
- Environment
- Motivation (effort)
- Physical health
- Psychological distress
- Psychiatric disorders
- Medications
- Qualifications and experience of neuropsychologist
- Errors in scoring
- Errors in interpretation

Source. Reprinted from Simon RI: "Ethical and Legal Issues," in *Textbook of Traumatic Brain Injury.* Edited by Silver JM, McAllister TM, Yudofsky SC. Washington, DC, American Psychiatric Publishing, 2005, pp. 583–605. Used with permission.

psychiatric disorder) or neurological (i.e., primarily caused by the brain injury). Nonetheless, outside agencies (e.g., insurance companies and lawyers) may request a neuropsychiatric evaluation to assist with this "differential." In reality, most symptoms result from the interaction of many factors, including neurological, social, emotional, educational, and vocational. Because important insurance and other reimbursement decisions may hinge on whether or not disabilities stem from brain injury, the clinician should take care that his or her impressions are based on data and are not misapplied to deprive the patient of deserved benefits. For example, mood disorders and cognitive sequelae of brain injury are often miscategorized as "mental illnesses" that are not covered by some insurance policies.

CLINICAL FEATURES

The neuropsychiatric sequelae of TBI include problems with attention and arousal, concentration, and executive functioning; intellectual changes; memory impairment; personality changes; affective disorders; anxiety disorders; psychosis; posttraumatic epilepsy; sleep disorders; aggression; and irritability. Physical problems such as headache, chronic pain, vision impairment, and dizziness complicate recovery. Key clinical features of TBI are outlined in the "Highlights for the Clinician" table at the end of this chapter. The severity of the neuropsychiatric sequelae of the brain injury is determined by multiple factors existing before, during, and after the injury (Dikmen and Machamer 1995) (Table 15–7). In general, prognosis is associated with the severity of injury. Although duration of posttraumatic amnesia correlates with subsequent cognitive recovery (Levin et al. 1982), in an analysis of 1,142 patients assessed after hospitalization for TBI, the simple presence or absence of LOC was not significantly related to performance on neuropsychological tests (Smith-Seemiller et al. 1996). There is a lack of correlation between the occurrence of LOC and neuropsychological test results in patients with mild brain injury (Lovell et al. 1999). In addition, the symptoms of injury are correlated with the type of damage sustained. For example, those with diffuse axonal injury often experience problems with arousal, attention, and slow cognitive processing. The presence of total anosmia in a group of patients with closed head injury predicted major vocational problems at least 2 years after these patients had been given medical clearance to return to work (Varney 1988). Posttraumatic anosmia may occur as a result of damage to the olfactory nerve, which is located adjacent to the orbitofrontal cortex, although there may be peripheral nerve involvement that results in anosmia. Impairment in olfactory naming and recognition frequently occurs in patients with moderate or severe brain injury and is related to frontal and temporal lobe damage (Levin et al. 1985).

In a review by Corrigan (1995), victims of TBI who were intoxicated with alcohol at the time of the injury had longer periods of hospitalization, had more complications during hospitalization, and had a lower level of functioning at the time of discharge from the hospital compared with patients with TBI who had no detectable blood alcohol level at the time of hospitalization. One factor complicating the interpretation of these data is the fact that intoxication may produce decreased responsiveness even without TBI, which can result in a GCS score that indicates greater severity of injury than is actually present. Furthermore, even a history of substance abuse is associated with increased morbidity and mortality rates.

Morbidity and mortality rates after brain injury increase with age. Elderly persons who experience TBI have longer periods of agitation and greater cognitive impairment and are more likely to develop mass lesions and permanent disability than are younger victims (Kim 2005). Individuals who have a previous brain injury do not recover as well from subsequent injuries (Carlsson et al. 1987).

The interaction between the brain injury and the psychosocial factors cannot be underestimated. Demographic factors have been found to predict cognitive dysfunction after TBI (Smith-Seemiller et al. 1996). Preexisting emotional and behavioral problems are exacerbated after injury. It also appears that having a preexisting psychiatric disorder increases the risk of TBI (Fann et al. 2002). Social conditions and support networks that existed before the injury affect the symptoms and course of recovery. In

TABLE 15–7. Factors influencing outcome after brain injury

- Severity of injury
- Type of injury
- Anosmia
- Intellectual functioning
- Psychiatric diagnosis
- Sociopathy
- Premorbid behavioral problems (children)
- Social support
- Substance use
- Neurological disorder
- Age
- Apolipoprotein E status

general, individuals with greater preinjury intelligence recover better after injury (G. Brown et al. 1981). Factors such as level of education, level of income, and socioeconomic status are positive factors in the ability to return to work after minor head injury (Rimel et al. 1981).

There have been several studies that have associated the presence of apolipoprotein E epsilon 4 allele (*APOE*E4*)with prognosis of recovery from TBI. Examining recovery in professional boxers, Jordan et al. (1997) found that the presence of *APOE*E4* was associated with chronic neurologic deficits in "high-exposure" boxers. In individuals with TBI who were admitted to a neurosurgical unit, the presence of *APOE*E4* predicted poor recovery after 6 months, even after controlling for severity of injury (Teasdale et al. 1997). Poorer recovery was also found by G. Friedman et al. (1999), Lichtman et al. (2000), and Kutner et al. (2000). However, Chamelian et al. (2004) found no relationship between recovery after mild to moderate TBI and *APOE* status. Although these results need additional confirmation, especially in those with mild TBI, they emphasize the fact that there are prognostic factors that influence recovery that we do not assess or that have not yet been determined. We must avoid "blaming the victim" or concluding that the individual does not "want" to improve (for psychological or monetary reasons) when there may be biological factors that influence recovery. Our belief is that many more biological factors will be discovered that significantly affect recovery from TBI.

PERSONALITY CHANGES

Unlike many primary psychiatric illnesses that have gradual onset, TBI often occurs suddenly and devastatingly.

Although some patients recognize that they no longer have the same abilities and potential that they had before the injury, many others with significant disabilities deny that there have been any changes. Prominent behavioral traits such as disorderliness, suspiciousness, argumentativeness, isolativeness, disruptiveness, social inappropriateness, and anxiousness often become more pronounced after brain injury.

In a study of children with head injury, G. Brown et al. (1981) found that disinhibition, social inappropriateness, restlessness, and stealing were associated with injuries in which there was LOC extending for more than 7 days. In a survey of the relatives of victims of severe TBI, McKinlay et al. (1981) found that 49% of 55 patients developed personality changes 3 months after the injury. After 5 years, 74% of these patients were reported to have changes in their personality (N. Brooks et al. 1986). More than one-third of these patients had problems of "childishness" and "talking too much" (N. Brooks et al. 1986; McKinlay et al. 1981).

Thomsen (1984) found that 80% of 40 patients with severe TBI had personality changes that persisted for 2 to 5 years, and 65% had changes lasting 10–15 years after the injury. These changes included childishness (60% and 25%, respectively), emotional lability (40% and 35%, respectively), and restlessness (25% and 38%, respectively). Approximately two-thirds of patients had less social contact, and one-half had loss of spontaneity and poverty of interests after 10–15 years.

Because of the vulnerability of the prefrontal and frontal regions of the cortex to contusions, injury to these regions is common and gives rise to changes in personality known as the frontal lobe syndrome. For the prototypic patient with frontal lobe syndrome, the cognitive functions are preserved while personality changes abound. Psychiatric disturbances associated with frontal lobe injury commonly include impaired social judgment, labile affect, uncharacteristic lewdness, inability to appreciate the effects of one's behavior or remarks on others, a loss of social graces (such as eating manners), a diminution of attention to personal appearance and hygiene, and boisterousness. Impaired judgment may take the form of diminished concern for the future, increased risk taking, unrestrained drinking of alcohol, and indiscriminate selection of food. Patients may appear shallow, indifferent, or apathetic, with a global lack of concern for the consequences of their behavior.

Certain behavioral syndromes have been related to damage to specific areas of the frontal lobe (Auerbach 1986). The orbitofrontal syndrome is associated with behavioral excesses, such as impulsivity, disinhibition, hyperactivity, distractibility, and mood lability. Injury to the dorsolateral frontal cortex may result in slowness, apathy,

and perseveration. This may be considered similar to the negative (deficit) symptoms associated with schizophrenia, wherein the patient may exhibit blunted affect, emotional withdrawal, social withdrawal, passivity, and lack of spontaneity (S.R. Kay et al. 1987). As with TBI, deficit symptoms in patients with schizophrenia are thought to result from disordered functioning of the dorsolateral frontal cortex (Berman et al. 1988). Outbursts of rage and violent behavior occur after damage to the inferior orbital surface of the frontal lobe and anterior temporal lobes.

Patients also develop changes in sexual behavior after brain injury, most commonly decreased sex drive, erectile function, and frequency of intercourse (Zasler 1994). Kleine-Levin syndrome—characterized by periodic hypersomnolence, hyperphagia, and behavioral disturbances that include hypersexuality—has also been reported to occur subsequent to brain injury (Will et al. 1988).

Although there have been studies examining personality changes after TBI, few have focused on Axis II psychopathology in individuals with TBI. In utilizing a structured clinical interview to diagnose personality disorders in 100 individuals with TBI, Hibbard et al. (2000) found that several personality disorders developed after TBI that were reflective of persistent challenges and compensatory coping strategies facing these individuals. Whereas before TBI, 24% of the sample population had personality disorders, 66% of the sample met criteria for personality disorders after TBI. The most common disorders were borderline, avoidant, paranoid, obsessive-compulsive, and narcissistic. Koponen et al. (2002), in a 30-year follow-up study of 60 patients with TBI, found that the most frequent personality disorders were paranoid, schizoid, avoidant, and organic personality disorders.

In DSM-IV-TR (American Psychiatric Association 2000), these personality changes would be diagnosed as personality change due to traumatic brain injury. Specific subtypes are provided as the most significant clinical problems (Table 15–8).

INTELLECTUAL CHANGES

Problems with intellectual functioning may be among the most subtle manifestations of brain injury. Changes can occur in the ability to attend, concentrate, remember, abstract, calculate, reason, plan, and process information (McCullagh and Feinstein 2005). Problems with arousal can take the form of inattentiveness, distractibility, and difficulty switching and dividing attention (Ponsford and Kinsella 1992). Mental sluggishness, poor concentration, and memory problems are common complaints of both patients and relatives (N. Brooks et al. 1986; McKinlay et al. 1981; Thomsen 1984). High-level cognitive functions, termed

TABLE 15–8.   DSM-IV-TR diagnostic criteria for personality change due to traumatic brain injury

A. A persistent personality disturbance that represents a change from the individual's previous characteristic personality pattern. (In children, the disturbance involves a marked deviation from normal development or a significant change in the child's usual behavior patterns lasting at least 1 year).

B. There is evidence from the history, physical examination, or laboratory findings that the disturbance is the direct physiological consequence of a general medical condition.

C. The disturbance is not better accounted for by another mental disorder (including other Mental Disorders Due to a General Medical Condition).

D. The disturbance does not occur exclusively during the course of a delirium.

E. The disturbance causes clinically significant distress or impairment in social, occupational, or other important areas of functioning.

Specify type:

> **Labile Type:**   if the predominant feature is affective lability
>
> **Disinhibited Type:**   if the predominant feature is poor impulse control as evidenced by sexual indiscretions, etc.
>
> **Aggressive Type:**   if the predominant feature is aggressive behavior
>
> **Apathetic Type:**   if the predominant feature is marked apathy and indifference
>
> **Paranoid Type:**   if the predominant feature is suspiciousness or paranoid ideation
>
> **Other Type:**   if the presentation is not characterized by any of the above subtypes
>
> **Combined Type:**   if more than one feature predominates in the clinical picture
>
> **Unspecified Type**

Source.   Reprinted from American Psychiatric Association: *Diagnostic and Statistical Manual of Mental Disorders*, 4th Edition, Text Revision. Washington, DC, American Psychiatric Association, 2000. Used with permission.

executive functions, are frequently impaired, although such impairments are difficult to detect and diagnose with cursory cognitive testing (Table 15–9) (McCullagh and Feinstein 2005). Only specific tests that mimic real-life deci-

TABLE 15–9.   Aspects of executive functions potentially impaired after traumatic brain injury

- Goal establishment, planning, and anticipation of consequences
- Initiation, sequencing, and inhibition of behavioral responses
- Generation of multiple response alternatives (in contrast to perseverative or stereotyped responses)
- Conceptual/inferential reasoning, problem solving
- Mental flexibility/ease of mental and behavioral switching
- Transcending the immediately salient aspects of a situation (in contrast to "stimulus-bound behavior" or "environmental dependency")
- Executive attentional processes
- Executive memory processes
- Self-monitoring and self-regulation, including emotional responses
- Social adaptive functioning: sensitivity to others, using social feedback, engaging in contextually appropriate social behavior

Source.   Reprinted from McCullagh S, Feinstein A: "Cognitive Changes," in *Textbook of Traumatic Brain Injury*. Edited by Silver JM, McAllister TW, Yudofsky SC. Washington, DC, American Psychiatric Publishing, 2005, pp. 321–335. Used with permission.

sion-making situations may objectively demonstrate the problems encountered in daily life (Bechara et al. 1994).

Studies suggest that among the long-term sequelae of brain trauma is Alzheimer's disease (Amaducci et al. 1986; Graves et al. 1990). Amyloid protein deposition has been found in the brains of patients who experienced severe TBI (Roberts et al. 1994; Sheriff et al. 1994). Several investigators have found this association in elderly persons who have brain injury (Mayeux et al. 1993; Van Duijn et al. 1992). Sustaining TBI reduced the time to onset of Alzheimer's disease among those who were at risk (Nemetz et al. 1999). There have been several studies that have examined the influence of *APOE* status on the risk of developing Alzheimer's disease subsequent to TBI. Mayeux et al. (1995) found that the presence of the *APOE*E4* allele combined with a history of head injury results in synergistic effect, increasing the risk from twofold with *APOE*E4* alone to a 10-fold increase in risk with *APOE*E4* and TBI. Katzman et al. (1996) determined that in their population, there was an additive effect. However, in another large family study, the influence of TBI on the development of Alzheimer's disease was greater among persons lacking *APOE*E4* (Guo et al. 2000). This connection between these disorders is logical, given the pathological features of these disorders, and must be considered when reviewing the lifelong implications of recovery from TBI (Jellinger 2004).

Children who survive head trauma often return to school with behavioral and learning problems (Mahoney et al. 1983). Children with behavioral disorders are much more likely to have a history of prior head injury (Michaud et al. 1993). In addition, children who sustained injury at or before age 2 years had significantly lower IQ scores (Michaud et al. 1993). The risk factors for the sequelae of TBI in children are controversial (J.E. Max 2005). In a study of 43 children and adolescents who had sustained TBI, J.E. Max et al. (1998b) found that preinjury family functioning was a significant predictor of psychiatric disorders after 1 year. Whereas some investigators have demonstrated neuropsychological sequelae after mild TBI when careful testing is done (Gulbrandsen 1984), others have shown that mild TBI produces virtually no clinically significant long-term deficits (Fay et al. 1993). In patients who survive moderate to severe brain injury, the degree of memory impairment often exceeds the level of intellectual dysfunction (Levin et al. 1988). The following case example illustrates a typical presentation of an adolescent with TBI presenting with behavioral and academic problems.

CASE EXAMPLE

A 17-year-old girl was referred by her father for neuropsychiatric evaluation because of many changes that were observed in her personality during the past 2 years. Whereas she had been an A student and had been involved in many extracurricular activities during her sophomore year in high school, there had been a substantial change in her behavior during the past 2 years. She was barely able to maintain a C average, was "hanging around with the bad kids," and was frequently using marijuana and alcohol. A careful history revealed that 2 years earlier, her older brother had hit her in the forehead with a rake, which stunned her, but she did not lose consciousness. Although she had had a headache after the accident, no psychiatric or neurological follow-up was pursued.

Neuropsychological testing at the time of evaluation revealed a significant decline in intellectual functioning from her "preinjury" state. Testing revealed poor concentration, attention, memory, and reasoning abilities. Academically, she was unable to "keep up" with the friends she had before her injury, and she began to socialize with a group of students with little interest in academics and began to conceptualize herself as being a rebel. When neuropsychological testing results were explained to the patient and her family as a consequence of the brain injury, she and her family were able to understand the "defensive" reaction to her changed social behavior.

PSYCHIATRIC DISORDERS

Studies that utilize standard psychiatric diagnostic criteria have found that several psychiatric disorders are common in individuals with TBI (Deb et al. 1999; Fann et al. 1995; Hibbard et al. 1998a; Jorge et al. 1993; van Reekum et al. 2000). In a group of patients referred to a brain injury rehabilitation center, Fann et al. (1995) found that 26% had current major depression, 14% had current dysthymia, 24% had current generalized anxiety disorder, and 8% had current substance abuse. There was a 12% occurrence of pre-TBI depression. Deb et al. (1999) performed a psychiatric evaluation of 196 individuals who were hospitalized after TBI. They found that a psychiatric disorder was present in 21.7% versus 16.4% of a control population of individuals hospitalized for other reasons. Compared with the control group, the individuals with TBI had a higher rate of depression (13.9% vs. 2.1%) and panic disorder (9.0% vs. 0.8%). Factors associated with these psychiatric disorders included a history of psychiatric illness, preinjury alcohol use, unfavorable outcome, lower Mini-Mental State Exam scores, and fewer years of education. Hibbard et al. (1998a) administered a structured psychiatric interview to 100 individuals with TBI. Major depression (61%), substance use disorder (28%), and PTSD (19%) were the most common psychiatric diagnoses elicited. Jorge et al. (1993) found that 26% of individuals had major depression 1 month after injury; 11% had comorbid generalized anxiety disorder.

In the New Haven portion of the National Institute of Mental Health Epidemiologic Catchment Area (ECA) program, individuals were administered standardized and validated structured interviews (Silver et al. 2001). Among 5,034 individuals interviewed, 361 admitted to a history of severe brain trauma with LOC or confusion (weighted rate of 8.5/100). When controlling for sociodemographic factors, quality-of-life indicators, and alcohol use, risk was increased for major depression, dysthymia, panic disorder, obsessive-compulsive disorder, phobic disorder, and drug abuse/dependence.

Several studies suggest that individuals who experience TBI have a higher than expected rate of preinjury psychiatric disorders. Histories of prior psychiatric disorders in individuals with TBI have varied between 17% and 44%, and pre-TBI substance use figures have ranged from 22% to 30% (Jorge et al. 1994; van Reekum et al. 1996). Fann et al. (1995) found that 50% of individuals who had sustained TBI reported a history of psychiatric problems prior to the injury. The Research and Training Center for the Community Integration of Individuals with TBI at Mt. Sinai Medical Center in New York found that in a group of 100 individuals with TBI, 51% had pre-TBI psychiatric disorders, most commonly major depression or substance use disorders, which occurred at rates more than twice those reported in community samples (Hibbard et al. 1998a). Fann et al. (2002) analyzed the HMO database of 450,000 members for the occurrence of a TBI and evidence of a psychiatric condition. They found that the relative risk for TBI was 1.3- to 4-fold higher in individuals with a preceding psychiatric diagnosis (24.2% vs. 14.3%). Interestingly, this held for all psychiatric disorders except attention-deficit/hyperactivity disorder.

AFFECTIVE CHANGES

Depression occurs frequently after TBI. There are several diagnostic issues that must be considered in the evaluation of the patient who appears depressed after TBI. Sadness is a common reaction after TBI, as patients describe "mourning" the loss of their "former selves," often a reflection of deficits in intellectual functioning and motoric abilities. Careful psychiatric evaluation is required to distinguish grief reactions, sadness, and demoralization from major depression.

Although scales such as the Hamilton Rating Scale for Depression (Hamilton 1960) or the Beck Depression Inventory (Beck et al. 1961) are useful in evaluating the severity of depression in patients with major depressive disorder, these are not substitutes for careful and thorough clinical evaluation. When the relationship between Beck Depression Inventory scores and the current diagnosis of depression was examined, high scores on the Beck Depression Inventory appeared to represent hyperreactivity to post-TBI symptoms rather than clinical depression (Sliwinski et al. 1998). Patients with depressed mood may not experience the somatic symptoms required for the diagnosis of major depressive disorder. The clinician must distinguish mood lability that occurs commonly after brain injury from major depression. Lability of mood and affect may be caused by temporal limbic and basal forebrain lesions (Ross and Stewart 1987) and has been shown to be responsive to standard pharmacological interventions of depression (discussion follows). In addition, apathy (diminished motivation) secondary to brain injury (which includes decreased motivation, decreased pursuit of pleasurable activities, or schizoid behavior) and complaints of slowness in thought and cognitive processing may resemble depression (Marin and Chakravorty 2005).

The clinician should endeavor to determine whether a patient may have been having an episode of major depression before an accident. Traumatic injury may occur as a result of the depression and suicidal ideation. Alcohol use, which frequently occurs with and complicates depressive illness, is also a known risk factor for motor vehicle accidents. One common scenario is depression leading to poor concentration, to substance abuse, and to risk taking (or even overt suicidal behavior), which together contribute to the motor vehicle accident and brain injury.

Prevalence of Depression After TBI

The prevalence of depression after brain injury has been assessed through self-report questionnaires, rating scales, and assessments by relatives. For mild TBI, estimates of depressive complaints range from 6% to 39%. For depression after severe TBI, in which patients often have concomitant cognitive impairments, reported rates of depression vary from 10% to 77%.

Robert Robinson and his colleagues have performed prospective studies of the occurrence of depression after brain injury (Federoff et al. 1992; Jorge et al. 1993). They evaluated 66 hospitalized patients who sustained acute TBI and followed the course of their mood over 1 year. Diagnoses were made using structured interviews and DSM-III-R criteria. Patients were evaluated at 1 month, 3 months, 6 months, and 1 year after injury. At each period, approximately 25% of patients fulfilled criteria for major depressive disorder. The mean duration of depression was 4.7 months, with a range of 1.5–12 months. Of the entire group of patients, 42% developed major depression during the first year after injury. The researchers also found that patients with generalized anxiety disorder and comorbid major depression have longer lasting mood problems than do those patients with depression and no anxiety (Jorge et al. 1993). More recently, this group extended their observations to another group of 91 patients (Jorge et al. 2004). During the first year after TBI, 33% developed depression, significantly more than the "other injury" control group. In those individuals, there was a high rate of comorbid anxiety (75%), aggression (56%), and reduced executive and social functioning.

In an unselected population sample, major depression was found in 11.1% of those with a history of brain injury (Silver et al. 2001). Deb et al. (1999) found 13.9% of individuals developed depression after TBI. Major depression occurred in 61% of a sample of individuals with TBI who were administered a structured psychiatric interview (Hibbard et al. 1998a). In a group of patients referred to a brain injury rehabilitation center, Fann et al. (1995) found that 26% had current major depression, and 14% had current dysthymia. Kreutzer et al. (2001) evaluated the presence of depression in 722 outpatients and found that major depression occurred in 42%. Koponen et al. (2002) followed a group of 60 patients who were injured an average of 30 years earlier and found a lifetime prevalence of depression of 26.7%. Holsinger (2002) followed a group of 520 World War II veterans with an average of 50 years since head injury. In comparison with a group of 1,198 veterans without brain injury, the lifetime prevalence of depression was 18.5 versus 13.4%, and the rate of current depression was 11.2% versus 8.5%. The risk of depression increased with the severity of TBI.

Studies consistently report increased risk of suicide subsequent to TBI (Tate et al. 1997). Data from a follow-up study (N. Brooks, personal communication, 1990) of 42 patients with severe TBI showed that 1 year after injury, 10% of those surveyed had spoken about suicide and 2% had made suicide attempts. Five years after the traumatic event, 15% of the patients had made suicide attempts. In addition, many other patients expressed hopelessness about their condition and a belief that life was not worth living. Silver et al. (2001) found that those with brain injury reported a higher frequency of suicide attempts than individuals without TBI (8.1% vs. 1.9%). This remained significant even after controlling for sociodemographic factors, quality-of-life variables, and presence of any coexisting psychiatric disorder. Mann et al. (1999) found an increased occurrence of TBI in individuals who have made suicide attempts. Simpson and Tate (2002) evaluated 172 outpatients with TBI who were in a brain injury rehabilitation unit. Hopelessness was found in 35%, suicidal ideation was found in 23%, and a suicide attempt was found in 18%. The relationship between suicidal behavior and TBI is complicated. Oquendo et al. (2004) evaluated the predictors of suicidal ideation in 340 patients with major depression. Subjects with TBI reported more aggressive behavior during childhood compared with subjects without TBI. Twenty percent of suicide attempters with TBI made their first suicide attempt prior to their brain injury. In addition, there were higher levels of aggressive behavior that antedated the TBI. It appeared that both suicidal behavior and TBI share an antecedent risk factor: aggression. Thus, it appears that the high incidence of suicide attempts in this population is caused by the combination of several factors, namely, major depression with disinhibition secondary to frontal lobe injury and preexisting risk factors such as aggressive behavior. The medical team, family, and other caregivers must work closely together, on a regular and continuing basis, to gauge suicide risk.

The incidence and severity of depression have not been found to be related to the duration of LOC (Bornstein et al. 1989; Levin and Grossman 1978), to the duration of posttraumatic amnesia (Bornstein et al. 1988), or to the presence or absence of skull fracture (Bornstein et al. 1988). However, depression may be related to the extent of neuropsychological impairment as documented by neuropsychological testing (Bornstein et al. 1989; Dikmen and Reitan 1977). Patients with post-TBI depression had a greater incidence of poor social adjustment and dissatisfaction before the injury (Federoff et al. 1992). Those who experienced an early transient depressive episode had left frontodorsolateral and left basal ganglia lesions. Depression that lasted longer than 6 months was associated with poorer social functioning and activities of daily living (Jorge et al. 1994). Analysis of MRIs revealed depression was correlated with reduced left prefrontal gray matter (Jorge et al. 2004). Fann et al. (1995) have shown that individuals with coexistent anxiety and depression had a greater severity of postconcussive symptoms and rated themselves as having a lesser degree of recovery. Satz et al. (1998) found that individuals with depressive symptoms and TBI had poorer outcome as related on the Glasgow Outcome Scale but not on neuropsychological measures. Depressed individuals with mild or moderate TBI had lower scores on working memory, processing speed, verbal memory, and executive functioning (Rapoport et al. 2005).

Mania After TBI

Manic episodes and bipolar disorder have also been reported to occur after TBI (Burstein 1993), although the occurrence is less frequent than that of depression after brain injury (Bakchine et al. 1989; Bamrah and Johnson 1991; Bracken 1987; Clark and Davison 1987; Nizamie et al. 1988). In the New Haven ECA sample, bipolar disorder occurred in 1.6% of those with brain injury, although the odds ratio was no longer significant when sociodemographic factors and quality of life were controlled (Silver et al. 2001). Predisposing factors for the development of mania after brain injury include damage to the basal region of the right temporal lobe (Starkstein et al. 1990) and right orbitofrontal cortex (Starkstein et al. 1988) in patients who have family histories of bipolar disorder.

DELIRIUM

When a psychiatrist is consulted during the period when a patient with a brain injury is emerging from coma, the usual clinical picture is one of delirium with restlessness, agitation, confusion, disorientation, delusions, and/or hallucinations. As Trzepacz and Kennedy (2005) observed, this period of recovery is often termed *posttraumatic amnesia* in the brain injury literature and is classified as Rancho Los Amigos Cognitive Scale Level IV or V (see Table 15–4). Although delirium in patients with TBI is most often the result of the effects of the injury on brain tissue chemistry, the psychiatrist should be aware that there may be other causes for the delirium (such as side effects of medication, withdrawal, or intoxication from drugs ingested before the traumatic event) and

TABLE 15–10. Causes of delirium in patients with traumatic brain injury

- Mechanical effects (acceleration or deceleration, contusion, and others)
- Cerebral edema
- Hemorrhage
- Infection
- Subdural hematoma
- Seizure
- Hypoxia (cardiopulmonary or local ischemia)
- Increased intracranial pressure
- Alcohol intoxication or withdrawal, Wernicke's encephalopathy
- Reduced hemoperfusion related to multiple trauma
- Fat embolism
- Change in pH
- Electrolyte imbalance
- Medications (barbiturates, steroids, opioids, and anticholinergics)

Source. Reprinted from Trzepacz PT, Kennedy RE: "Delirium and Posttraumatic Amnesia," in *Textbook of Traumatic Brain Injury.* Edited by Silver JM, McAllister TW, Yudofsky SC. Washington, DC, American Psychiatric Publishing, 2005, pp. 175–200. Used with permission.

environmental factors (such as sensory monotony). Table 15–10 lists common factors that can result in posttraumatic delirium.

Stuss et al. (1999) examined patients recovering from acute TBI using tests of attention and memory. Attention improved before performance on memory tasks, especially in individuals with mild TBI. The researchers concluded that the phenomenon currently termed posttraumatic amnesia is actually a confusional state and that the term *posttraumatic confusional state* should be used instead.

PSYCHOTIC DISORDERS

Psychosis can occur either immediately after brain injury or after a latency of many months of normal functioning (Corcoran et al. 2005). McAllister (1998) observed that psychotic symptoms may result from a number of different post-TBI disorders, including mania, depression, and epilepsy. The psychotic symptoms may persist despite improvement in the cognitive deficits caused by trauma (Nasrallah et al. 1981). Review of the literature published

between 1917 and 1964 (Davison and Bagley 1969) revealed that 1%–15% of schizophrenic inpatients have histories of brain injury. Violon and De Mol (1987) found that of 530 head injury patients, 3.4% developed psychosis 1–10 years after the injury. Wilcox and Nasrallah (1987) found that a group of patients diagnosed with schizophrenia had a significantly greater history of brain injury with LOC before age 10 than did patients who were diagnosed with mania or depression or patients who were hospitalized for surgery. Achte et al. (1991) reported on a sample of 2,907 war veterans in Finland who sustained brain injury. They found that 26% of these veterans had psychotic disorders. In a detailed evaluation of 100 of these veterans, the authors found that 14% had paranoid schizophrenia. In a comparison of patients who developed symptoms of schizophrenia or schizoaffective disorder subsequent to TBI, left temporal lobe abnormalities were found only in the group who developed schizophrenia (Buckley et al. 1993). The rate of schizophrenia in the group of individuals with a history of TBI in the New Haven group in the ECA study was 3.4% (Silver et al. 2001). However, after controlling for alcohol abuse and dependence, the risk for the occurrence of schizophrenia was of borderline significance.

Patients with schizophrenia may have had brain injury that remains undetected unless the clinician actively elicits a history specific for the occurrence of brain trauma. One high-risk group is homeless mentally ill individuals. To examine the relationship of TBI to schizophrenia and homelessness, Silver et al. (1993) conducted a case–control study of 100 homeless and 100 never-homeless indigent schizophrenic men, and a similar population of women. In the group of men, 55 patients had a prior TBI (36 homeless, 19 domiciled, $P < 0.01$). In the group of women, 35 had previous TBI (16 homeless, 19 domiciled, $P =$ not significant). We believe that the cognitive deficits subsequent to TBI in conjunction with psychosis increase the risk for becoming homeless; in addition, being homeless, and living in a shelter, carries a definite risk for trauma (Kass and Silver 1990).

There is evidence of an interaction between genetic predisposition to schizophrenia and TBI. Malaspina et al. (2001) analyzed data from their study of the effect of TBI on the development of schizophrenia in families with bipolar disorder or schizophrenia. They found that members of the schizophrenia pedigrees, even those without a schizophrenia diagnosis, had greater exposure to TBI compared with members of the bipolar disorder pedigrees (i.e., having genetic loading for schizophrenia increased one's risk for acquiring a TBI). Within the schizophrenia pedigrees, TBI was associated with a greater risk of schizophrenia, consistent with synergistic effects between genetic vulnerability for schizophrenia and TBI. AbdelMalik et al. (2003) compared history and severity of TBI in childhood (age

10 years or younger) and adolescence in 67 subjects with schizophrenia and 102 unaffected siblings in 23 families with familial schizophrenia with evidence of genetic linkage. The TBI was almost all of mild severity. The individuals with schizophrenia were more likely to have childhood TBI and a younger mean age at onset. The severity of TBI correlated with younger age at onset. Genetic vulnerability appears to be the greatest risk factor for the development of posttraumatic psychosis (Sachdev et al. 2001).

POSTTRAUMATIC EPILEPSY

A varying percentage of patients, depending on the location and severity of injury, will have seizures during the acute period after the trauma. Posttraumatic epilepsy, with repeated seizures and the requirement for anticonvulsant medication, occurs in approximately 12%, 2%, and 1% of patients with severe, moderate, and mild head injuries, respectively, within 5 years of the injury (Annegers et al. 1980). Risk factors for posttraumatic epilepsy include skull fractures and wounds that penetrate the brain, a history of chronic alcohol use, intracranial hemorrhage, and increased severity of injury (Yablon 1993).

Salazar et al. (1985) studied 421 Vietnam veterans who had sustained brain-penetrating injuries and found that 53% had posttraumatic epilepsy. In 18% of these patients, the first seizure occurred after 5 years; in 7%, the first seizure occurred after 10 years. In addition, 26% of the patients with epilepsy had an organic mental syndrome as defined in DSM-III. In a study of World War II veterans, patients with brain-penetrating injuries who developed posttraumatic epilepsy had a decreased life expectancy compared with patients with brain-penetrating injuries without epilepsy or compared with patients with peripheral nerve injuries (Corkin et al. 1984). Patients who develop posttraumatic epilepsy have also been shown to have more difficulties with physical and social functioning and to require more intensive rehabilitation efforts (Armstrong et al. 1990).

Posttraumatic epilepsy is associated with psychosis, especially when seizures arise from the temporal lobes. Brief episodic psychoses may occur with epilepsy; about 7% of patients with epilepsy have persistent psychoses (McKenna et al. 1985). These psychoses exhibit a number of atypical features, including confusion and rapid fluctuations in mood. Psychiatric evaluation of 101 patients with epilepsy revealed that 8% had organic delusional disorder that, at times, was difficult to differentiate symptomatically from schizophrenia (Garyfallos et al. 1988).

Anticonvulsant drugs can produce cognitive and emotional symptoms (Reynolds and Trimble 1985; Rivinus 1992; M.C. Smith and Bleck 1991). Phenytoin has more profound effects on cognition than does carbamazepine

(Gallassi et al. 1988), and negative effects on cognition have been found in patients who received phenytoin after traumatic injury (Dikmen et al. 1991). Minimal impairment in cognition was found with both valproate and carbamazepine in a group of patients with epilepsy (Prevey et al. 1996). Dikmen et al. (2000) found no adverse cognitive effects of valproate when it was administered for 12 months after TBI. The effects of phenytoin and carbamazepine in patients recovering from TBI were compared by K.R. Smith et al. (1994). They found that both phenytoin and carbamazepine had negative effects on cognitive performance, especially those that involved motor and speed performance. Although in the patient group as a whole, the effects were of questionable clinical significance, some individual patients experienced significant effects. Intellectual deterioration in children undergoing long-term treatment with phenytoin or phenobarbital also has been documented (Corbett et al. 1985). Treatment with more than one anticonvulsant (polytherapy) has been associated with increased adverse neuropsychiatric reactions (Reynolds and Trimble 1985). Of the newer anticonvulsant medications, topiramate, but not gabapentin or lamotrigine, demonstrated adverse cognitive effects in healthy young adults (Martin et al. 1999; Salinsky et al. 2005). Hoare (1984) found that the use of multiple anticonvulsant drugs to control seizures resulted in an increase in disturbed behavior in children.

Patients who have a seizure immediately after brain injury are often given an anticonvulsant drug for seizure prophylaxis. Temkin et al. (1990) showed that the administration of phenytoin soon after traumatic injury had no prophylactic effect on seizures that occurred subsequent to the first week after injury. Similarly, valproate did not demonstrate any efficacy in preventing late posttraumatic seizures (Temkin et al. 1999). It should be noted that there was a nonsignificant trend toward a higher mortality rate. Anticonvulsant medications are not recommended after 1 week of injury for prevention of posttraumatic seizures (Brain Injury Special Interest Group 1998; Brain Trauma Foundation 2000). Any patient with TBI who is treated with anticonvulsant medication requires regular reevaluations to substantiate continued clinical necessity.

ANXIETY DISORDERS

Several anxiety disorders may develop after TBI (Warden and Labatte 2005). Jorge et al. (1993) found that 11% of 66 patients with TBI developed generalized anxiety disorder in addition to major depression. Fann et al. (1995) evaluated 50 outpatients with TBI and found that 24% had generalized anxiety disorder. Deb et al. (1999) evaluated 196 individuals who were hospitalized after TBI.

Panic disorder developed in 9%. Salazar et al. (2000) evaluated 120 military members after moderate to severe TBI. At 1 year after enrollment to the study of cognitive rehabilitation, 15% met criteria for generalized anxiety disorder. Hibbard et al. (1998a) found that 18% developed PTSD, 14% developed obsessive-compulsive disorder, 11% developed panic disorder, 8% developed generalized anxiety disorder, and 6% developed phobic disorder. All of these were more frequent after TBI compared with before TBI. In analysis of data from the New Haven portion of the ECA study, Silver et al. (2001) found that of individuals with a history of brain injury during their lifetime, the incidences of anxiety disorders were 4.7% for obsessive-compulsive disorder, 11.2% for phobic disorder, and 3.2% for panic disorder. Dissociative disorders, including depersonalization (Grigsby and Kaye 1993) and dissociative identity disorder (Sandel et al. 1990), may occur. It is our clinical observation that patients with histories of prior trauma are at higher risk for developing these disorders.

Because of the potential life-threatening nature of many of the causes of TBI, including motor vehicle accidents and assaults, one would expect that these patients are at increased risk of developing PTSD. There is a 9.2% risk of developing PTSD after exposure to trauma, highest for assaultive violence (Breslau et al. 1998). PTSD and acute stress response, including symptoms of peritraumatic dissociation (Ursano et al. 1999b), are not uncommon after serious motor vehicle accidents (Koren et al. 1999; Ursano et al. 1999a).

PTSD has been found in individuals with TBI (Bryant 1996; McMillan 1996; Ohry et al. 1996; Parker and Rosenblum 1996; Rattok 1996; Silver et al. 1997). In utilizing the SCID in evaluating 100 individuals with a history of TBI, Hibbard et al. (1998a) found that 18% met criteria for PTSD. Harvey and Bryant conducted a 2-year study of 79 survivors of motor vehicle accidents who sustained mild TBI. They found that acute stress disorder developed in 14% of these patients at 1 month. After 2 years, 73% of the group with acute stress disorder developed PTSD (Harvey and Bryant 2000). Six months after severe TBI, 26 of 96 individuals (27.1%) developed PTSD (Bryant et al. 2000). Although few patients had intrusive memories (19.2%), 96.2% reported emotional reactivity. The authors suggested that traumatic experiences may be mediated at an implicit level. Similarly, in 47 subjects with moderate TBI who were amnestic for the traumatic event, Warden et al. (1995) found that no patients met the full criteria for the diagnosis of PTSD, which includes reexperiencing the event. However, 14% of patients had avoidance and arousal symptoms. Not all investigators have found that PTSD occurs with TBI. In evaluating a group of 70 patients diagnosed with PTSD or mild TBI, Sbordone and Liter (1995) found that no patients

had both disorders (although the presence of subsyndromal PTSD was not assessed). Feinstein et al. (2002) evaluated 282 outpatients with TBI and stratified them according to their duration of posttraumatic amnesia. There was no difference in levels of PTSD and distress. However, the intrusive and avoidant symptoms were greater in those with posttraumatic amnesia of less than 1 hour. Children are also susceptible to the development of PTSD after TBI. J.E. Max et al. (1998a) evaluated 50 children who were hospitalized after TBI. Although only 4% of subjects developed PTSD, 68% had one PTSD symptom after 3 months, suggesting subsyndromal PTSD despite neurogenic amnesia.

Because of the overlap among symptoms of PTSD and mild TBI, it can be difficult to ascribe specific symptoms to the brain injury or to the circumstances of the accident. In studies of patients with PTSD, memory deficits consistent with temporal lobe injury have been demonstrated (Bremner et al. 1993). Imaging studies have shown smaller hippocampal volumes with PTSD (Bremner et al. 1995, 1997). It is therefore apparent that exposure to extreme stressors results in brain dysfunction that may be similar to that found after TBI.

We present the following case as an illustration.

CASE EXAMPLE

While Mr. A was working, a machine was activated accidentally, and his head was crushed. He had full recall of the sound of his skull cracking and the sensation of blood coming down his forehead. It was several hours before he was transported to a hospital, but he never lost consciousness. His EEG revealed irregular right cerebral activity, and MRI was compatible with contusion and infarction of the right temporal parietal region.

Since the accident, Mr. A developed the full syndrome of PTSD; he experienced flashbacks, mood lability, sensitivity to noise, decreased interest, distress when looking at pictures of the accident, and problems with concentration.

SLEEP DISORDERS

It is common for individuals with TBI to complain of disrupted sleep patterns, ranging from hypersomnia to difficulty maintaining sleep (Rao et al. 2005). Fichtenberg et al. (2000) assessed 91 individuals with TBI who were admitted to an outpatient neurorehabilitation clinic. The presence of depression (as indicated by score on the Beck Depression Inventory) and mild severity of the TBI were correlated with the occurrence of insomnia. Guilleminault et al. (2000) assessed 184 patients with head trauma and hypersomnia. Abnormalities were demonstrated on the Multiple Sleep Latency Test (MSLT). Sleep-disordered breathing was common (59/184 patients). Hypersomnia must be differentiated from lack of motivation and apathy.

In addition, the contribution of pain to disruption of sleep must be considered. Although depression and sleep disorders can be related and have similarities in the sleep endocrine changes (Frieboes et al. 1999), in our experience with depressed individuals after TBI, the sleep difficulties persist after successful treatment of the mood disorder. In addition, we have seen patients who have developed sleep apnea or nocturnal myoclonus subsequent to TBI.

MILD TRAUMATIC BRAIN INJURY AND POSTCONCUSSION SYNDROME

Patients with mild TBI may present with somatic, perceptual, cognitive, and emotional symptoms that have been characterized as the postconcussion syndrome (Table 15–11). By definition, mild TBI is associated with a brief duration of LOC (less than 20 minutes) or no LOC, and posttraumatic amnesia of less than 24 hours; the patient usually does not require hospitalization after the injury (see Table 15–5). For each patient hospitalized with mild TBI, probably four to five others sustain mild TBIs but receive treatment as outpatients or perhaps get no treatment at all. The psychiatrist is often called to assess the patient years after the injury, and the patient may not associate brain-related symptoms such as depression and cognitive dysfunction with the injury. The results of laboratory tests, such as structural brain imaging studies, often do not reveal significant abnormalities. However, as discussed previously, functional imaging studies such as SPECT (Masdeu et al. 1994; Nedd et al. 1993) and computerized electroencephalography and brain stem auditory evoked potential recordings have demonstrated abnormal findings (Watson et al. 1995). Diffuse axonal injury may occur with mild TBI, as demonstrated in the pathological examination of brains from patients who have died from systemic injuries (Oppenheimer 1968), as well as in nonhuman primates (Gennarelli et al. 1982). In addition, the balance between cellular energy demand and supply can be disrupted (McAllister 2005).

Most studies of cognitive function subsequent to mild TBI suggest that patients report trouble with memory, attention, concentration, and speed of information processing, and patients can in fact be shown to have deficits in these areas shortly after their injury (1 week to 1 month) (S.J. Brown et al. 1994; McAllister 2005; McMillan and Glucksman 1987). In an evaluation of neuropsychological deficits in 53 patients who were experiencing postconcussive problems from 1 to 22 months after injury, Leininger et al. (1990) detected significantly poorer performance (P<0.05) on tests of reasoning, information processing, and verbal learning than that found in a control population. Hugenholtz et al. (1988) reported that significant atten-

TABLE 15–11. Postconcussion syndrome

Somatic symptoms
- Headache
- Dizziness
- Fatigue
- Insomnia

Cognitive symptoms
- Memory difficulties
- Impaired concentration

Perceptual symptoms
- Tinnitus
- Sensitivity to noise
- Sensitivity to light

Emotional symptoms
- Depression
- Anxiety
- Irritability

Source. Adapted from Lishman 1988.

tional and information processing impairment (P<0.01) occurred in a group of adults after mild concussion. Although there was improvement over time, the patient group continued to have abnormalities 3 months after the injury. Warden et al. (2001) found that even in previously high-functioning individuals who sustained mild concussion (West Point cadets), there was impairment in processing speed several days after the injury.

Individuals with mild TBI have an increased incidence of somatic complaints, including headache, dizziness, fatigue, sleep disturbance, and sensitivity to noise and light (S.J. Brown et al. 1994; Dikmen et al. 1986; Levin et al. 1987c; Rimel et al. 1981). In the behavioral domain, the most common problems include irritability, anxiety, and depression (Dikmen et al. 1986; Fann et al. 1995; Hibbard et al. 1998a). McAllister (2005) has opined that it may be more accurate to discuss postconcussive symptoms rather than a syndrome.

The majority of individuals with mild TBI recover quickly, with significant and progressive reduction of complaints in all three domains (cognitive, somatic, and behavioral) at 1, 3, and certainly 6 months from the injury (Bernstein 1999). Unfortunately, good recovery is not universal. A significant number of patients continue to complain of persistent difficulties 6–12 months and even longer after their injury. For example, Keshavan et al. (1981) found that 40% of their patients had significant symptoms 3 months after injury. Levin et al. (1987c), in a multicenter study, found that 3 months postinjury, 47% complained of headache, 22% of decreased energy, and 22% of dizziness. In a review of this topic, Bohnen et al. (1992) found a range of 16%–49% of patients with persistent symptoms at 6 months and 1%–50% with persistent symptoms at 1 year. Those with persistent symptoms have been found to have impaired cognitive function (Leininger et al. 1990). S.J. Brown et al. (1994) suggest that if symptoms are present at 3–6 months subsequent to injury, they tend to persist. Alves et al. (1993) prospectively assessed 587 patients with uncomplicated mild TBI for 1 year. The most frequent symptoms were headache and dizziness. The researchers found that fewer than 6% of these subjects complained of multiple symptoms consistent with postconcussion syndrome.

Therefore, there may be two groups of mild TBI patients: those who recover by 3 months and those who have persistent symptoms. It is not known whether the persistent symptoms are part of a cohesive syndrome or simply represent a collection of loosely related symptoms resulting from the vagaries of an individual injury (Alves et al. 1986). However, it is increasingly recognized that "mild" TBI and concussions that occur in sports injuries result in clinically significant neuropsychological impairment (Freeman et al. 2005).

Compensation and litigation do not appear to affect the course of recovery after "mild" brain injury (Bornstein et al. 1988), and many patients return to work despite the continuation of psychiatric symptoms (Hugenholtz et al. 1988). In fact, professional athletes who sustain mild TBI and have a negative financial incentive to stop playing have the same symptoms of postconcussion syndrome as do individuals who sustain mild TBI at work or in motor vehicle accidents. As McAllister (1994) has pointed out,

> [T]here may be times when a patient's attorney gives clear encouragement to maintain symptoms when litigation extends over a period of several years.... [However,] there is virtually no evidence at this point to suggest that it is the primary factor in the overwhelming majority of patients with mild brain injury. (p. 375)

In an extensive review of the literature, Alexander (1995) highlighted several important aspects regarding patients who develop prolonged postconcussion syndrome: 1) they are more likely to have been under stress at the time of the accident, 2) they develop depression and/or anxiety soon after the accident, 3) they have extensive social disruption after the accident, and 4) they have problems with physical symptoms such as headache and dizziness.

The treatment of patients with mild TBI involves initiating several key interventions (T. Kay 1993). In the early phase of treatment, the major goal is prevention of the postconcussion syndrome. This involves providing information and education about understanding and predicting symptoms and their resolution and actively managing a gradual process of return to functioning. Education about the postconcussion syndrome and its natural history improves prognosis (Wade et al. 1998). It is important to involve the patient's family or significant other, so that they understand the disorder and predicted recovery. After the postconcussion syndrome has developed, the clinician must develop an alliance with the patient and validate his or her experience of cognitive and emotional difficulties while not prematurely confronting emotional factors as primary. A combined treatment strategy is required that addresses the emotional problems along with cognitive problems.

As discussed in the previous section, patients with mild TBI may have vivid recollections of the traumatic event; this may contribute to the development of PTSD in addition to postconcussive symptoms. There is overlap between these two syndromes, and determining the predominant diagnosis may be difficult. In general, postconcussion symptoms should decrease within 3 months, whereas the symptoms of PTSD may not diminish until 3–6 months after the trauma. Reexperiencing the traumatic event (e.g., in flashbacks or nightmares) is characteristic of PTSD.

AGGRESSION

Individuals who have traumatic brain injury may experience irritability, agitation, and aggressive behavior (Silver et al. 2005b). These episodes range in severity from irritability to outbursts that result in damage to property or assaults on others. In severe cases, affected individuals cannot remain in the community or with their families and often are referred to long-term psychiatric or neurobehavioral facilities. Increased isolation and separation from others often occur.

In the acute recovery period, 35%–96% of patients are reported to have exhibited agitated behavior (Silver et al. 2005b). After the acute recovery phase, irritability or bad temper is common. There has been only one prospective study of the occurrence of agitation and restlessness that has been monitored by an objective rating instrument, the OAS (Brooke et al. 1992b). These authors found that of 100 patients with severe TBI (GCS score less than 8, more than 1 hour of coma, and more than 1 week of hospitalization), only 11 patients exhibited agitated behavior. Only 3 patients manifested these behaviors for more than 1 week. However, 35 patients were observed to be restless but not agitated. In a prospective sample of 100 patients admitted to a brain injury rehabilitation unit, 42% exhibited agitated behavior during at least one nursing shift (Bogner and Corrigan 1995). In follow-up periods ranging from 1 to 15 years after injury, these behaviors occurred in 31%–71% of patients who experienced severe TBI (Silver et al. 2005b). Studies of mild TBI have evaluated patients for much briefer periods of time; 1-year estimates from these studies range from 5% to 70% (Silver et al. 2005b). Tateno et al. (2003), studying an inpatient TBI population, found that aggression was associated with the presence of major depression, frontal lobe lesions, poor premorbid social functioning, and a history of alcohol and substance abuse.

Carlsson et al. (1987) examined the relationship between the number of traumatic brain injuries associated with LOC and various symptoms, and they demonstrated that irritability increases with subsequent injuries. Of the men who did not have head injuries with LOC, 21% reported irritability, whereas 31% of men with one injury with LOC and 33% of men with two or more injuries with LOC admitted to this symptom ($P < 0.0001$).

Explosive and violent behaviors have long been associated with focal brain lesions as well as with diffuse damage to the central nervous system (Anderson and Silver 1999). The current diagnostic category in DSM-IV-TR is personality change due to a general medical condition (American Psychiatric Association 2000) (see Table 15–8). Patients with aggressive behavior would be specified as aggressive type, whereas those with mood lability are specified as labile type. Characteristic behavioral features occur in many individuals who exhibit aggressive behavior after brain injury (Yudofsky et al. 1990). Typically, violence seen in these patients is *reactive* (i.e., triggered by modest or trivial stimuli). It is *nonreflective*, in that it does not involve premeditation of planning, and *nonpurposeful*, in the sense that the aggression serves no obvious long-term aims or goals. The violence is *periodic*, with brief outbursts of rage and aggression interspersed between long periods of relatively calm behavior. The aggression is *ego-dystonic*, such that the individual is often upset or embarrassed after the episode. Finally, it is generally *explosive*, occurring suddenly with no apparent buildup.

PHYSICAL PROBLEMS

Coldness

Complaints of feeling cold, without actual alteration in body temperature, are occasionally seen in patients who have sustained brain injury. This feeling can be distressing to those who experience it. Patients may wear excessive amounts of clothing and may adjust the thermostat so that other members of the family are uncomfortable. Although this is not a commonly reported symptom of TBI, Hibbard et al. (1998b) found that in a sample of 331 individuals with TBI, 27.9% complained of changes in body temperature, and 13% persistently felt cold. Eames

(1997), while conducting a study of the cognitive effects of vasopressin nasal spray in patients with TBI, reported incidentally that 13 patients had the persistent feeling of coldness, despite normal sublingual temperature. All were treated with nasal vasopressin spray for 1 month. Eleven of these patients stopped complaining of feeling cold after 1 month of treatment, and 1 other patient had improvement in the symptom, without complete relief. We describe below a series of 6 patients with brain injury whose subsequent complaints of feeling cold were treated with 1-desamino-8-D-arginine vasopressin (DDAVP) (intranasal vasopressin or desmopressin acetate).

In a pilot study, 6 patients who complained of persisting coldness after brain injury were treated with DDAVP twice daily for 1 month (Silver and Anderson 1999). Response was assessed after 1 month of treatment. DDAVP was discontinued, and reassessment was done 1 month later. Five of the 6 patients had a dramatic response to DDAVP, as soon as 1 week after initiating treatment and no longer complained of feeling cold. Response persisted even after discontinuation of treatment. Patients denied any side effects from treatment with DDAVP. The experience of persisting coldness can respond dramatically to brief treatment with intranasal DDAVP. It is striking that the beneficial effects of DDAVP persisted after the treatment period ended. DDAVP may reverse physiological effects of a relative deficit in vasopressin in the hypothalamus, caused by injury to the vasopressin precursor producing cells in the anterior hypothalamus, and corrects an internal temperature set point disrupted by the brain injury.

Other Somatic Problems

The psychiatrist treating an individual who has sustained TBI should be aware of many other somatic problems that interfere with functioning and may exacerbate emotional problems. This includes chronic pain (Zasler and Martelli 2005), headaches (including recurrence of migraines) (Ward and Levin 2005), dizziness from vestibular disorders (Richter 2005), and visual problems (Kapoor and Ciuffreda 2005). There are specific modalities (such as vestibular therapy and vision therapy) that can alleviate these problems and improve quality of ife.

THERAPEUTIC STRATEGIES

There are many useful therapeutic approaches available for people who have brain injuries. Brain-injured patients may develop neuropsychiatric symptoms based on the location of their injury, the emotional reaction to their injury, their preexisting strengths and difficulties, and their social expectations and supports. Comprehensive rehabilitation centers address many of these issues with therapeutic strategies that are developed specifically for this population (Ben-Yishay and Lakin 1989; Binder and Rattok 1989; Pollack 1989; Prigatano 1989).

Although these programs meet many of the needs of patients with TBI, comprehensive neuropsychiatric evaluation (including the daily evaluation and treatment of the patient by a psychiatrist) is rarely available. Although we propose a multifactorial, multidisciplinary, collaborative approach to treatment, for purposes of exposition we have divided treatment into psychopharmacological, behavioral, psychological, and social interventions.

PSYCHOPHARMACOLOGICAL TREATMENT

It is critical to conduct a thorough assessment of the patient before any intervention is initiated. Two issues require particular attention in the evaluation of the potential use of medication. First, the presenting complaints must be carefully assessed and defined. Second, the current treatment must be reevaluated. Although consultation may be requested to decide whether medication would be helpful, it is often the case that 1) other treatment modalities have not been properly applied, 2) there has been misdiagnosis of the problem, or 3) there has been poor communication among treating professionals. On occasion, a potentially effective medication has not been beneficial because it has been prescribed in a dose that is too low or for a period of time that is too brief. In other instances, the most appropriate pharmacological recommendation is that no medication is required and that other therapeutic modalities need to be reassessed. In reviewing the patient's current medication regimen, two key issues should be addressed: 1) the indications for all drugs prescribed and whether they are still necessary, and 2) the potential side effects of these medications. Patients who have had a severe brain trauma may be receiving many medications that result in psychiatric symptoms such as depression, mania, hallucinations, insomnia, nightmares, cognitive impairments, restlessness, paranoia, or aggression.

Few controlled clinical trials have been conducted to assess the effects of medication in patients with brain injury. Unfortunately, there are few rigorous studies that provide guidelines for tratment (Neurobehavioral Guidelines Working Group 2006). Therefore, the decision regarding which medication (if any) to prescribe is based on 1) current knowledge of the efficacy of these medications in other psychiatric disorders, 2) side-effect profiles of the medications, 3) the increased sensitivity to side effects shown by patients with brain injury, 4) analogies

from the brain injury symptoms to the recognized psychiatric syndromes (e.g., amotivational syndrome after TBI may be analogous to the deficit syndrome in schizophrenia), and 5) hypotheses regarding how the neurochemical changes after TBI may affect the proposed mechanisms of action of psychotropic medications.

There are several general guidelines that should be followed in the pharmacological treatment of the psychiatric syndromes that occur after TBI: 1) start low, go slow, 2) conduct a therapeutic trial of all medications, 3) maintain continuous reassessment of clinical condition, 4) monitor drug-drug interactions, 5) augment partial response, and 6) discontinue or lower the dose of the most recently prescribed medication if there is a worsening of the treated symptom soon after the medication had been initiated (or increased). In our experience, patients with brain injury of any type are far more sensitive to the side effects of medications than are patients who do not have brain injury. Doses of psychotropic medications must be raised and lowered in small increments over protracted periods of time, although patients ultimately may require the same doses and serum levels that are therapeutically effective for patients without brain injury.

When medications are prescribed, it is important that they be given in a manner that enhances the probability of benefit and reduces the possibility of adverse reactions. Medications often should be initiated at dosages that are lower than those usually administered to patients without brain injury. However, comparable doses to those used to treat primary psychiatric disorders may be necessary to treat TBI-related neuropsychiatric conditions effectively. Dose increments should be made gradually, to minimize side effects and enable the clinician to observe adverse consequences. It is important that such medications be given sufficient time to impart their full effects. Thus, when a decision is made to administer a medication, the patient must receive an adequate therapeutic trial of that medication in terms of dosage and duration of treatment.

Because of frequent changes in the clinical status of patients after TBI, continuous reassessment is necessary to determine whether each prescribed medication is still required. For depression following TBI, the standard guidelines for the treatment of major depression offered by the American Psychiatric Association (2000) may offer a reasonable framework within which to develop a working treatment plan, including continuation of medication for a minimum of 16–20 weeks following complete remission of depressive symptoms. For this and all other neuropsychiatric sequelae of TBI, however, no formal treatment guidelines specific to this population are available. Although there is increasingly useful literature regarding the types and doses of medications useful for the treatment of such problems, there are few if any studies regarding the optimal duration of treatment and/or the issues pertaining to treatment discontinuation and relapse risk. In general, if the patient has responded favorably to initial medication treatment for one or another neuropsychiatric problem after TBI, the clinician must use sound judgment and apply risk-benefit determinations to each specific case in deciding whether and/or when to taper and attempt to discontinue the medication following TBI. Continuous reassessment is necessary because spontaneous remission of some symptoms may occur, in which case the medication can be permanently discontinued, or a carryover effect of the medication may occur (i.e., its effects may persist after the duration of treatment), in which case a reinstatement of the medication may not be required.

When a new medication is initiated in combination with medications previously prescribed, the clinician must be vigilant for the development of drug-drug interactions. These interactions may include alteration of pharmacokinetics that result in increased half-lives and serum levels of medications, as can occur with the use of multiple anticonvulsants. Additionally, alterations of pharmacodynamics may develop during the administration of medications with additive or synergistic clinical effects (e.g., increased sedative effects when several sedating medications are administered simultaneously).

If a patient does not respond favorably to the initial medication prescribed, several alternatives are available. If there has been no response, changing to a medication with a different mechanism of action is suggested, much as is done in the treatment of depressed patients without brain injury. If there has been a partial response to the initial medication, addition of another medication may be useful. The selection of a second supplementary or augmenting medication should be based on consideration of the possible complementary or contrary mechanisms of action of such agents and on the individual and combined side-effect profiles of the initial and secondary agents and their potential pharmacokinetic and pharmacodynamic interactions.

Although individuals after TBI may experience multiple concurrent neuropsychiatric symptoms (e.g., depressed mood, irritability, poor attention, fatigue, and sleep disturbances) suggesting a single "psychiatric diagnosis" such as major depression, we have found that some of these symptoms often persist despite treatment of the apparent "diagnosis." In other words, diagnostic parsimony should be sought but may not always be the best or most accurate diagnostic approach in this population. For this reason, the neuropsychiatric approach of evaluating and monitoring individual symptoms is necessary and differs from the usual "syndromal" approach of the present conventional psychiatric paradigm. Several medications may be required to allevi-

ate several distinct symptoms following TBI, although it is prudent to initiate each treatment one at a time to determine the efficacy and side effects of each prescribed drug.

Studies of the effects of psychotropic medications in patients with TBI are few, and rigorous double-blind, placebo-controlled studies are rare (see Arciniegas et al. 2000b). The recommendations contained in this chapter represent a synthesis of the available treatment literature in TBI, the extensions of the known uses of these medications in phenotypically similar non-brain-injured psychiatric populations of patients with other types of brain injury (stroke, multiple sclerosis, etc.), and the opinions of the authors of this chapter. We recognize that the pathophysiology of these symptoms may differ in patients with TBI; thus, generalization of response to treatment seen in the context of other forms of brain dysfunction (e.g., stroke, Alzheimer's disease) to TBI may not always be valid. Where there are treatment studies in the TBI population to offer guidance regarding medication treatments, these are noted and referenced for further consideration by interested readers.

AFFECTIVE ILLNESS

Depression

Affective disorders subsequent to brain damage are common and are usually highly detrimental to a patient's rehabilitation and socialization. However, the published literature is sparse regarding the effects of antidepressant agents and/or electroconvulsive therapy (ECT) in the treatment of patients with brain damage in general and TBI in particular (Arciniegas et al. 1999; Bessette and Peterson 1992; Cassidy 1989; Saran 1985; Varney et al. 1987) (see Silver et al. 2005a for review).

Guidelines for using antidepressants for patients with TBI.   The choice of an antidepressant depends predominantly on the desired side-effect profile. Usually, antidepressants with the fewest sedative, hypotensive, and anticholinergic side effects are preferred. Thus, the selective serotonin reuptake inhibitors (SSRIs) are usually the first-line medications prescribed. Fann and colleagues performed a single-blind placebo run-in trial of sertraline in 15 patients with major depression after TBI. Two-thirds of these patients achieved a Hamilton Rating Scale for Depression score consistent with remission by 2 months (Fann et al. 2000). In addition, those patients showed improvements in psychomotor speed, recent verbal memory, recent visual memory, and general cognitive efficiency (Fann et al. 2001). In a study comparing nortriptyline and fluoxetine in poststroke depression, nortriptyline was superior in efficacy to fluoxetine, and fluoxetine demonstrated no benefit above placebo

(Robinson et al. 2000). If a heterocyclic antidepressant (HCA) is chosen, we suggest nortriptyline or desipramine and careful plasma monitoring to achieve plasma levels in the therapeutic range for the parent compound and its major metabolites (e.g., nortriptyline levels 50–100 ng/mL; desipramine levels greater than 125 ng/mL) (American Psychiatric Association Task Force 1985).

ECT remains a highly effective and underused modality for the treatment of depression overall, and ECT can be used effectively after acute or severe TBI (Kant et al. 1999; Ruedrich et al. 1983). If the patient has preexisting memory impairment, nondominant unilateral ECT should be used.

Side effects. The most common and disabling antidepressant side effects in patients with TBI are the anticholinergic effects, especially with the older HCAs. These medications may impair attention, concentration, and memory, especially in patients with brain lesions. SSRIs, venlafaxine, and bupropion all have minimal or no anticholinergic action.

In some individuals, SSRIs may result in word-finding problems or apathy. This may be due to the effects of SSRIs in decreasing dopaminergic functioning, and it may be reversible with the addition of a dopaminergic or stimulant medication.

The choice of SSRI may require similar consideration. Schmitt et al. (2001) demonstrated that healthy middle-aged adults experienced significantly greater impairments of delayed recall in a word-learning test during treatment with paroxetine 20–40 mg per day than during treatment with placebo, an effect attributed to paroxetine's nontrivial antimuscarinic properties. This study also demonstrated significant improvements in verbal fluency among healthy middle-aged adults treated with sertraline 50–100 mg when compared with treatment with placebo, an effect attributed to sertraline's dopamine reuptake inhibition. Whether similar differences in cognitive profiles distinguish between these and other SSRIs in the TBI population is not yet clear. Nonetheless, observations of distinct cognitive profiles among these agents may merit consideration when selecting an agent in this population.

The available evidence suggests that, overall, antidepressants may be associated with a greater frequency of seizures in patients with brain injury. The antidepressants maprotiline and bupropion may be associated with a higher incidence of seizures (Davidson 1989; Pinder et al. 1977). Wroblewski et al. (1990) reviewed the records of 68 patients with TBI who received HCA treatment for at least 3 months. The frequencies of seizures were compared for the 3 months before treatment, during treatment, and after treatment. Seizures occurred in 6 patients (9%) during the baseline period, in 16 (24%) during HCA treatment, and in 4 (6%) after treatment was discontinued. Fourteen patients

(19%) had seizures shortly after the initiation of HCA treatment. For 12 of these patients, no seizures occurred after HCA treatment was discontinued. Importantly, 7 of these patients were receiving anticonvulsant medication before and during HCA treatment. The occurrence of seizures was related to greater severity of brain injury. However, Zimmer et al. (1992) treated 17 patients with neurological disorders (e.g., TBI, stroke, degenerative disease) with bupropion at an average dosage of 200 mg/day. No seizures occurred in this group of patients. Other investigations have found that seizure control does not appear to worsen if psychotropic medication is introduced cautiously and if the patient is on an effective anticonvulsant regimen (Ojemann et al. 1987). Although there have been reports of seizures occurring with fluoxetine, Favale et al. (1995) demonstrated an anticonvulsant effect in patients with seizures. In our experience, few patients have experienced seizures during treatment with SSRIs and other newer antidepressants. Although antidepressants should be used with continuous monitoring in patients with severe TBI, we also believe that antidepressants can be used safely and effectively in patients with TBI.

Mania

Manic episodes that occur after TBI have been successfully treated with lithium carbonate, carbamazepine (Stewart and Nemsath 1988), valproic acid (Pope et al. 1988), clonidine (Bakchine et al. 1989), and ECT (Clark and Davison 1987). Lamotrigine and gabapentin are other options, although evidence as to efficacy, especially in individuals with TBI, is sparse. Because of the increased incidence of side effects when lithium is used in patients with brain lesions, we limit the use of lithium in patients with TBI to those with mania or with recurrent depressive illness that preceded their brain damage.

Lithium has been reported to aggravate confusion in patients with brain damage (Schiff et al. 1982), as well as to induce nausea, tremor, ataxia, and lethargy in this population. In addition, lithium may lower seizure threshold (Massey and Folger 1984). Hornstein and Seliger (1989) reported a patient with preexisting bipolar disorder who experienced a recurrence of mania after experiencing closed head injury. Before the injury, this patient's mania was controlled with lithium carbonate without side effects. However, after the brain injury, dysfunctions of attention and concentration emerged that reversed with lowering of the lithium dosage.

Lability of Mood and Affect

In contrast to mood disorders—conditions in which the baseline emotional state is pervasively disturbed over a relatively long period of time (i.e., weeks)—disorders of affect denote conditions in which the more moment-to-moment variation and regulation of emotion is disturbed. The classic disorder of affective dysregulation is pathological laughing and/or crying (PLC), also sometimes referred to as "emotional incontinence" or "pseudobulbar affect." Patients with this condition experience episodes of involuntary crying and/or laughing that may occur many times per day, are often provoked by trivial (i.e., not sentimental) stimuli, are quite stereotyped in their presentation, are uncontrollable, do not evoke a concordant subjective affective experience, and do not produce a persistent change in the prevailing mood (Poeck 1985). In this classic presentation, PLC appears to be a relatively infrequent (5.3%) consequence of TBI (Zeilig et al. 1996). Affective lability differs from PLC in that both affective expression and experience are episodically dysregulated, the inciting stimulus may be relatively minor but is often somewhat sentimental, and the episodes are somewhat more amenable to voluntary control and are less stereotyped. However, these episodes do not produce a persistent change in mood and are often sources of significant distress and embarrassment to patients that otherwise (quite correctly) report their mood as "fine" (euthymic). The prevalence of affective lability following TBI is not clear, but it is a commonly observed acute and chronic problem after TBI at all levels of severity.

Antidepressants may be used to treat the labile mood that frequently occurs with neurological disease. However, it appears that the control of lability of mood and affect may differ from that of depression, and the mechanism of action of antidepressants in treating mood lability in those with brain injuries may differ from that in the treatment of patients with "uncomplicated" depression (Lauterbach and Schweri 1991; Panzer and Mellow 1992; Ross and Rush 1981; Schiffer et al. 1985; Seliger et al. 1992; Sloan et al. 1992). Schiffer et al. (1985) conducted a double-blind crossover study with amitriptyline and placebo in 12 patients with pathological laughing and weeping secondary to multiple sclerosis. Eight patients experienced a dramatic response to amitriptyline at a maximum dose of 75 mg/day.

There have been several reports of the beneficial effects of fluoxetine for "emotional incontinence" secondary to several neurological disorders (K.W. Brown et al. 1998; Nahas et al. 1998; Panzer and Mellow 1992; Seliger et al. 1992; Sloan et al. 1992). K.W. Brown et al. (1998) treated 20 patients with poststroke emotionalism with fluoxetine in a double-blind, placebo-controlled study. The individuals receiving fluoxetine exhibited statistically and clinically significant improvement. In our experience, all SSRIs can be effective, and the dosage guidelines are similar to those used in the treatment of depression. In addition, other antidepressants, such as nortriptyline, can

also be effective for emotional lability. We emphasize that for many patients it may be necessary to administer these medications at standard antidepressant dosages to obtain full therapeutic effects, although response may occur for others within days of initiating treatment at relatively low doses. Preliminary data suggest that dextromethorphan may improve this syndrome in certain neurological disorders (B.R. Brooks et al. 2004).

COGNITIVE FUNCTION AND AROUSAL

Stimulants, such as dextroamphetamine and methylphenidate, and dopamine agonists, such as amantadine and bromocriptine, may be beneficial in treating the patient with apathy and impaired concentration to increase arousal and to diminish fatigue. These medications all act on the catecholaminergic system but in different ways. Dextroamphetamine blocks the reuptake of norepinephrine and, in higher doses, also blocks the reuptake of dopamine. Methylphenidate has a similar mechanism of action. Amantadine acts both presynaptically and postsynaptically at the dopamine receptor and may also increase cholinergic and GABAergic activity (Cowell and Cohen 1995). In addition, amantadine is an N-methyl-D-aspartate (NMDA) glutamate receptor antagonist (Weller and Kornhuber 1992). Bromocriptine is a dopamine type 1 receptor antagonist and a dopamine type 2 receptor agonist. It appears to be a dopamine agonist at midrange doses (Berg et al. 1987). Assessment of improvement in attention and arousal may be difficult (Whyte 1992), and further work needs to be conducted in this area to determine whether these medications affect outcome. Therefore, careful objective assessment with appropriate neuropsychological tests may be helpful in determining response to treatment.

Dextroamphetamine and Methylphenidate

Several reports have indicated that impairments in verbal memory and learning, attention, and behavior are alleviated with either dextroamphetamine or methylphenidate (Bleiberg et al. 1993; Evans et al. 1987; Kaelin et al. 1996; Lipper and Tuchman 1976; Weinberg et al. 1987; Weinstein and Wells 1981). C.T. Gualtieri and Evans (1988), in a double-blind, placebo-controlled crossover study, studied 15 patients with TBI who were currently functioning at a Rancho Los Amigos Scale level of VII or VIII. Patients received a 2-week treatment with placebo, methylphenidate 0.15 mg/kg of body weight twice daily, or methylphenidate 0.30 mg/kg twice daily. Of the 15 patients treated, 14 improved with active medication and had increased scores on ratings of mood and performance. The authors observed that this short-term response was not sustained over time. In a double-blind, placebo-controlled trial of the administration of methylphenidate in the subacute setting to individuals with moderate to moderately severe TBI, Plenger et al. (1996) found that attention and performance were improved at 30 days but did not differ from a control group at 90 days. Therefore, the rate, but not the extent, of recovery was improved with stimulants. Speech et al. (1993) conducted a double-blind, placebo-controlled study of the effects of methylphenidate in 10 patients with chronic TBI. They found no significant increase in measures of attention, arousal, learning, cognitive processing speed, or behavior. Mooney and Haas (1993) found that methylphenidate improved anger and other personality problems after TBI. Whyte et al. (1997) performed a randomized, placebo-controlled trial of methylphenidate on 19 patients who exhibited attentional deficits after TBI. Although there was improvement in speed of mental processing, there were no improvements noted in orienting to distractions, sustained attention, and motor speed.

When used, methylphenidate should be initiated at 5 mg twice daily and dextroamphetamine at 2.5 mg twice daily. Maximum dosage of each medication is usually 60 mg/day, administered twice daily or three times daily. However, we have seen some patients who have required higher dosages of methylphenidate to obtain a reasonable serum level of 15 mg/mL.

Sinemet and Bromocriptine

Lal et al. (1988) reported on the use of L-dopa/carbidopa (Sinemet) in the treatment of 12 patients with brain injury (including anoxic damage). With treatment, patients exhibited improved alertness and concentration; decreased fatigue, hypomania, and sialorrhea; and improved memory, mobility, posture, and speech. Dosages administered ranged from 10/100 to 25/250 four times daily. Eames (1989) suggests that bromocriptine may be useful in treating cognitive initiation problems of brain-injured patients at least 1 year after injury. He recommended starting at 2.5 mg/day and administering treatment for at least 2 months at the highest dose tolerated (up to 100 mg/day). Other investigators have found that patients with nonfluent aphasia (Gupta and Mlcoch 1992), akinetic mutism (Echiverri et al. 1988), and apathy (Catsman-Berrevoets and Harskamp 1988) have improved after treatment with bromocriptine. Parks et al. (1992) suggest that bromocriptine exerts specific effects on the frontal lobe and increases goal-directed behaviors.

Amantadine

Amantadine may be beneficial in the treatment of anergia, abulia, mutism, and anhedonia subsequent to brain injury (Chandler et al. 1988; Cowell and Cohen 1995;

T. Gualtieri et al. 1989; Nickels et al. 1994). M.F. Kraus and Maki (1997) administered amantadine 400 mg/day to six patients with TBI. Improvement was found in motivation, attention, and alertness, as well as executive function and dyscontrol. Dosages should initially be 50 mg twice daily and should be increased every week by 100 mg/day to a maximum dosage of 400 mg/day.

Tricyclic Antidepressants

Although the drugs involved are not in the category of stimulants or dopamine agonists, Reinhard et al. (1996) administered amitriptyline (1 patient) and desipramine (2 patients) and found improvement in arousal and initiation after TBI. The authors hypothesize that the improvement is from the noradrenergic effects of the HCA.

Side Effects of Medications for Impaired Concentration and Arousal

Adverse reactions to medications for impaired concentration and arousal are most often related to increases in dopamine activity. Dexedrine and methylphenidate may lead to paranoia, dysphoria, agitation, and irritability. Depression often occurs on discontinuation, so stimulants should be discontinued using a slow regimen. Interestingly, there may be a role for stimulants to increase neuronal recovery subsequent to brain injury (Crisostomo et al. 1988). Side effects of bromocriptine include sedation, nausea, psychosis, headaches, and delirium. Amantadine may cause confusion, hallucinations, edema, and hypotension; these reactions occur more often in elderly patients.

There is often concern that stimulant medications may lower seizure threshold in patients with TBI who are at increased risk for posttraumatic seizures. Wroblewski et al. (1992) reviewed their experience with methylphenidate in 30 patients with severe brain injury and seizures and examined changes in seizure frequency after initiation of methylphenidate. The number of seizures was monitored for 3 months before treatment with methylphenidate, for 3 months during treatment, and for 3 months after treatment was discontinued. The researchers found that whereas only 4 patients experienced more seizures during methylphenidate treatment, 26 had either fewer or the same number of seizures during treatment. The authors concluded that there is no significant risk in lowering seizure threshold with methylphenidate treatment in this high-risk group. Although many patients in this study were treated concomitantly with anticonvulsant medications that may have conferred some protection against the development of seizures, this does not explain why 13 patients had fewer seizures when treated with methylphenidate. In a double-blind, placebo-controlled study of the effects of methylphenidate (0.3 mg/kg twice daily) in 10 children with well-controlled seizures and attention-deficit/hyperactivity disorder, no seizures occurred during the 4 weeks of treatment either with active drug or with placebo (Feldman et al. 1989). Dextroamphetamine has been used adjunctively in the treatment of refractory seizures (S. Livingston and Pauli 1975), and bromocriptine may also have some anticonvulsant properties (Rothman et al. 1990). Amantadine may lower seizure threshold (T. Gualtieri et al. 1989). We have also observed several patients who had not experienced seizures for months before the administration of amantadine to have had a seizure weeks after it was prescribed.

PROBLEMS WITH PROCESSING MULTIPLE STIMULI

Although individuals with TBI may have difficulty with maintaining attention on single tasks, they can also have difficulty in processing multiple stimuli. This difficulty has been called an abnormality in auditory gating, and it is consistent with an abnormal response in processing auditory stimuli that are given 50 milliseconds apart (P50 response) (Arciniegas et al. 2000b). Preliminary evidence suggests that this response normalizes after treatment with donepezil 5 mg, which also results in symptomatic improvement (Arciniegas et al. 2001).

FATIGUE

Stimulants (methylphenidate and dextroamphetamine) and amantadine can diminish the profound daytime fatigue experienced by patients with TBI. Dosages utilized would be similar to those used for treatment of diminished arousal and concentration. Modafinil, a medication recently approved for the treatment of excessive daytime somnolence in patients with narcolepsy, also may have a role in treatment of post-TBI fatigue. There have been studies specifically in patients with multiple sclerosis that have shown benefit (Rammahan et al. 2000; Terzoudi et al. 2000), whereas another controlled study showed no benefit (Stankoff et al. 2005). Teitelman (2001) described his use of modafinil among 10 outpatients with nonpenetrating TBI and functionally significant excessive daytime sleepiness and in 2 patients with somnolence caused by sedating psychiatric medications. The patients included in his report were between 42 and 72 years of age, were outpatients, and were treated in an open-label fashion. Doses of modafinil ranged between 100 mg and 400 mg and were taken once each morning. Nine of these patients reported improvements in excessive daytime sleepiness, and some patients also reported

subjective improvements in attention as well as other cognitive benefits. Although this medication was generally well tolerated, this report also describes treatment intolerance due to increased "emotional instability" in 2 women with brain injury complicated by multiple other medical conditions who were receiving multiple additional medications. Dosages should start with 100 mg in the morning and can be increased to up to 600 mg/day administered in two doses (i.e., 400 mg in the morning and 200 mg in the afternoon).

COGNITION

Cholinesterase Inhibitors

TBI may produce cognitive impairments via disruption of cholinergic function (Arciniegas et al. 1999), and the relative sensitivity of TBI patients to medications with anticholinergic agents has prompted speculation that cognitively impaired TBI patients may have a relatively reduced reserve of cholinergic function. This has prompted trials of procholinergic agents, and in particular physostigmine, to treat behavioral dyscontrol and impaired cognition in TBI survivors (Eames and Sutton 1995). However, the significant peripheral effects and narrow margin of safety of physostigmine have made treatment with this agent impractical. With the advent of relatively centrally selective acetylcholinesterase inhibitors such as donepezil, the issue of cholinergic augmentation strategies in the treatment of cognitive impairment following TBI is currently being revisited, and preliminary reports suggest that donepezil may improve memory and global functioning (Kaye et al. 2003; Morey et al. 2003; Taverni et al. 1998; Whelan et al. 2000; Zhang et al. 2004). Doses of donepezil range from 5mg to 10 mg per day. A report of rivastigmine (3–12 mg/day) used in a double-blind randomized, placebo-controlled multicenter study of 154 patients suggested improvements in cognition in those individuals with the most significant memory problems (Silver et al. 2006). The most common side effects include sedation, insomnia, diarrhea, and dizziness, which are minimized by starting with the lower dosage and adjusting upward slowly. Although these adverse effects are generally transient, a few patients will be unable to tolerate the medication due to persistent severe diarrhea.

PSYCHOSIS

The psychotic ideation resulting from TBI is generally responsive to treatment with antipsychotic medications. However, side effects such as hypotension, sedation, and confusion are common. Also, brain-injured patients are particularly subject to dystonia, akathisia, and other parkinsonian side effects—even at relatively low doses of antipsychotic medications (Wolf et al. 1989). Antipsychotic medications have also been reported to impede neuronal recovery after brain injury (Feeney et al. 1982). Therefore, we advise that antipsychotics should be used sparingly during the acute phases of recovery after the injury. Of the newer "atypical" antipsychotic medications, quetiapine has the fewest extrapyramidal effects. Risperidone, olanzapine, aripiprazole, and ziprasidone may all have a role in the treatment of post-TBI psychosis, although published literature is limited. Therapeutic effect may not be evident for 3 weeks after treatment at each dosage. In general, we recommend a low-dose neuroleptic strategy for all patients with neuropsychiatric disorders. Clozapine is a novel and effective antipsychotic medication that does not produce extrapyramidal side effects. Although its use in patients with neuropsychiatric disorders has yet to be investigated fully, its side-effect profile poses many potential disadvantages. It is highly anticholinergic, produces significant sedation and hypotension, lowers seizure threshold profoundly, and is associated with a 1% risk of agranulocytosis that requires lifetime weekly monitoring of blood counts.

Among all the first-generation antipsychotic drugs, molindone and fluphenazine have consistently demonstrated the lowest potential for lowering the seizure threshold (Oliver et al. 1982). Clozapine treatment is associated with a significant dose-related incidence of seizures (ranging from 1% to 2% of patients who receive doses below 300 mg/day and 5% of patients who receive 600–900 mg/day); thus, in patients with TBI it must be used with extreme caution and for most carefully considered indications (Lieberman et al. 1989).

SLEEP

Sleep patterns of patients with brain damage are often disordered, with impaired rapid eye movement (REM) recovery and multiple nocturnal awakenings (Prigatano et al. 1982). Hypersomnia that occurs after severe missile head injury most often resolves within the first year after injury, whereas insomnia that occurs in patients with long periods of coma and diffuse injury has a more chronic course (Askenasy et al. 1989). Barbiturates and long-acting benzodiazepines should be prescribed for sedation with great caution, if at all. These drugs interfere with REM and Stage IV sleep patterns and may contribute to persistent insomnia (Buysse and Reynolds 1990). Clinicians should warn patients of the dangers of using over-the-counter preparations for sleeping and for colds because of the prominent anticholinergic side effects of these agents.

Trazodone, a sedating antidepressant medication that is devoid of anticholinergic side effects, may be used for nighttime sedation. A dose of 50 mg should be administered initially; if this is ineffective, doses up to 150 mg may be prescribed. Nonpharmacological approaches should be considered. These include minimizing daytime naps, adhering to regular sleep times, and engaging in regular physical activity during the day.

AGGRESSION AND AGITATION

Although there is no medication approved by the U.S. Food and Drug Administration (FDA) that is specifically for the treatment of aggression, medications are widely used (and commonly misused) in the management of patients with acute or chronic aggression. The reported effectiveness of these medications is highly variable, as are the reported rationales for their prescription. Some of these medications are offered in order to inhibit excessive activity in temporolimbic areas (e.g., as with anticonvulsants), to reduce "hyperactive" limbic monoaminergic neurotransmission (e.g., noradrenergic blockade with propranolol, dopaminergic blockade with haloperidol), to augment orbitofrontal and/or dorsolateral prefrontal cortical activity with monoaminergic agonists (e.g., amantadine, methylphenidate, and perhaps buspirone), or to increase serotonergic input (SSRIs). Unfortunately, there is a paucity of rigorous double-blind, placebo-controlled studies (i.e., "Level I" studies) or even prospective cohort studies (i.e., "Level II" studies) to guide clinicians in the use of pharmacological interventions. The International Brain Injury Association has assembled a task force on reviewing the literature pertaining to the neurobehavioral consequences of TBI, which is in progress. At this time, we suggest utilizing *The Expert Consensus Guideline Series: Treatment of Agitation in Older Persons With Dementia* as a framework for the assessment and management of agitation and aggression after TBI (Alexopolous et al. 1998). After appropriate assessment of possible etiologies of these behaviors, treatment is focused on the occurrence of comorbid neuropsychiatric conditions (depression, psychosis, insomnia, anxiety, delirium) (see Figure 15–3), whether the treatment is in the acute (hours to days) or chronic (weeks to months) phase, and the severity of the behavior (mild to severe). The clinician must be aware that patients may not respond to just one medication but may require combination treatment, similar to the pharmacotherapeutic treatment for refractory depression.

Chronic Aggression

If a patient continues to exhibit periods of agitation or aggression beyond several weeks, the use of specific anti-aggressive medications should be initiated to prevent these episodes from occurring. Because no medication

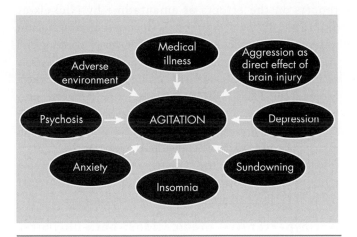

FIGURE 15–3. Factors associated with agitation in brain injury.

has been approved by the FDA for treatment of aggression, the clinician must use medications that may be antiaggressive but that have been approved for other uses (e.g., seizure disorders, depression, hypertension) (Silver and Yudofsky 1994a; Yudofsky et al. 1998).

Antipsychotic medications. If, after thorough clinical evaluation, it is determined that the aggressive episodes result from psychosis, such as paranoid delusions or command hallucinations, then antipsychotic medications will be the treatment of choice. Risperidone has been used to treat agitation in elderly patients with dementia with good results (Goldberg and Goldberg 1995). Olanzapine appears to be more sedating, and quetiapine may have fewer extrapyramidal symptoms than does risperidone. Clozapine may have greater antiaggressive effects than other antipsychotic medications (Michals et al. 1993; Ratey et al. 1993). However, the increased risk of seizures must be carefully assessed.

Antianxiety medications. Serotonin appears to be a key neurotransmitter in the modulation of aggressive behavior. In preliminary reports, buspirone, a serotonin type 1A agonist, has been reported to be effective in the management of aggression and agitation for patients with head injury, dementia, and developmental disabilities and autism (Silver and Yudofsky 1994a; Yudofsky et al. 1998). In rare instances, some patients become more aggressive when treated with buspirone. Therefore, buspirone should be initiated at low dosages (i.e., 5 mg twice daily) and increased by 5 mg every 3–5 days. Dosages of 45–60 mg/day may be required before there is improvement in aggressive behavior, although we have noted dramatic improvement within 1 week.

Clonazepam may be effective in the long-term management of aggression, although controlled, double-blind studies have not yet been conducted. Freinhar and Alvarez (1986) found that clonazepam decreased agitation in three elderly patients with organic brain syndromes. Keats and Mukherjee (1988) reported antiaggressive effects of clonazepam in a patient with schizophrenia and seizures. We use clonazepam when pronounced aggression and anxiety occur together or when aggression occurs in association with neurologically induced tics and similarly disinhibited motor behaviors. Dosages should initially be 0.5 mg twice daily and may be increased to as high as 2–4 mg twice daily, as tolerated. Sedation and ataxia are frequent side effects.

Anticonvulsive medications. The anticonvulsant carbamazepine has been demonstrated to be effective for treatment of bipolar disorders and has also been advocated for control of aggression in both epileptic and nonepileptic populations. Several open studies have indicated that carbamazepine may be effective in decreasing aggressive behavior associated with TBI dementia (Chatham-Showalter 1996), developmental disabilities, and schizophrenia and in patients with a variety of other organic brain disorders (Silver and Yudofsky 1994; Yudofsky et al. 1998). Carbamazepine can be a highly effective medication to treat aggression in the brain-injured patient, and we believe it is the drug of choice for patients who have aggressive episodes with concomitant seizures or epileptic foci. Reports also indicate that the antiaggressive response of carbamazepine can be found in patients with and without electroencephalographic abnormalities (Silver and Yudofsky 1994; Yudofsky et al. 1998). Azouvi and colleagues (1999) found that 8 of 10 patients with aggressive behavior after TBI responded to carbamazepine.

In our experience and that of others, the anticonvulsant valproic acid may also be helpful to some patients with organically induced aggression (Geracioti 1994; Giakas et al. 1990; Horne and Lindley 1995; Mattes 1992; Wroblewski et al. 1997). For patients with aggression and epilepsy whose seizures are being treated with anticonvulsant drugs such as phenytoin and phenobarbital, switching to carbamazepine or to valproic acid may treat both conditions.

Gabapentin may be beneficial for the treatment of agitation in patients with dementia (Herrmann et al. 2000; Roane et al. 2000). Dosages have ranged from 200–2400 mg/day. However, Childers and Holland (1997) report an increase in anxiety and restlessness (i.e., agitation) in two cognitively impaired TBI patients for whom gabapentin was prescribed to reduce chronic pain.

Antimanic medications. Although lithium is known to be effective in controlling aggression related to manic excitement, many studies suggest that it may also have a role in the treatment of aggression in selected nonbipolar patient populations (Yudofsky et al. 1998). Included are patients with TBI (Bellus et al. 1996; Glenn et al. 1989) as well as patients with mental retardation who exhibit self-injurious or aggressive behavior, children and adolescents with behavioral disorders, prison inmates, and patients with other organic brain syndromes.

Patients with brain injury have increased sensitivity to the neurotoxic effects of lithium (Hornstein and Seliger 1989; Moskowitz and Altshuler 1991). Because of lithium's potential for neurotoxicity and its relative lack of efficacy in many patients with aggression secondary to brain injury, we limit the use of lithium in patients whose aggression is related to manic effects or recurrent irritability related to cyclic mood disorders.

Antidepressants. The antidepressants that have been reported to control aggressive behavior are those that act preferentially (amitriptyline) or specifically (trazodone and fluoxetine) on serotonin. In open studies, Mysiw et al. (1988) and Jackson et al. (1985) reported that amitriptyline (maximum dose 150 mg/day) was effective in the treatment of patients with recent severe brain injury whose agitation had not responded to behavioral techniques. Trazodone has also been reported to be effective in the treatment of aggression that occurs with organic mental disorders (Silver and Yudofsky 1994; Yudofsky et al. 1998). Two individuals with Huntington's disease and aggressiveness were treated effectively with sertraline (Ranen et al. 1996). Thirteen patients who had irritability and aggression after TBI also exhibited improvement after treatment with sertraline (Kant et al. 1998). Fluoxetine has been reported to be effective in the treatment of aggressive behavior in a patient who sustained brain injury as well as in patients with personality disorders and depression, and adolescents with mental retardation and self-injurious behavior (Silver and Yudofsky 1994; Yudofsky et al. 1998). We have used SSRIs with considerable success in aggressive patients with brain lesions. The dosages used are similar to those for the treatment of mood lability and depression.

We have evaluated and treated many patients with emotional lability that is characterized by frequent episodes of tearfulness and irritability and the full symptomatic picture of neuroaggressive syndrome (Silver and Yudofsky 1994a). These patients—who would be diagnosed under DSM-IV with personality change, labile type, due to traumatic brain injury—have responded well to antidepressants. This is discussed above in the section on mood lability.

Stimulants. Several studies have examined the role of dopaminergic medications and stimulants in the treatment of agitation and aggression. There have been three case

reports on the effects of amantadine by Nickels et al. (1994) (2 of 3 subjects with postcoma agitation improved), Chandler et al. (1988) (2 cases of agitation and aggression in the postacute stage improved), and Nickels et al. (1994) (2 of 3 subjects with severe agitation improved). Mooney and Haas (1993) conducted a randomized, pretest–posttest, placebo-controlled, single-blind study of the effect of methylphenidate 30 mg/day for 6 weeks on brain injury–related anger in 38 individuals with "serious" TBIs 6 months or more after their injuries. Although those taking methylphenidate had a lower level of anger after treatment, they also had greater levels of pretreatment anger.

Antihypertensive medications: beta-blockers. Since the first report of the use of β-adrenergic receptor blockers in the treatment of acute aggression in 1977, more than 25 articles have appeared in the neurologic and psychiatric literature reporting experience in using β-blockers with more than 200 patients with aggression (Yudofsky et al. 1987). Most of these patients had been unsuccessfully treated with antipsychotics, minor tranquilizers, lithium, and/or anticonvulsants before being treated with β-blockers. The β-blockers that have been investigated in controlled prospective studies include propranolol (a lipid-soluble, nonselective receptor antagonist), nadolol (a water-soluble, nonselective receptor antagonist), and pindolol (a lipid-soluble, nonselective β receptor antagonist with partial sympathomimetic activity). A growing body of preliminary evidence suggests that β-adrenergic receptor blockers are effective agents for the treatment of aggressive and violent behaviors, particularly those related to organic brain syndrome. The effectiveness of propranolol in reducing agitation has been demonstrated during the initial hospitalization after TBI (Brooke et al. 1992a). Guidelines for the use of propranolol are listed in Table 15–12. When a patient requires the use of a once-a-day medication because of compliance difficulties, long-acting propranolol (i.e., Inderal LA) or nadolol (Corgard) can be used. When patients develop bradycardia that prevents prescribing therapeutic dosages of propranolol, pindolol (Visken) can be substituted, using one-tenth the dosage of propranolol. The intrinsic sympathomimetic activity of pindolol stimulates the β receptor and restricts the development of bradycardia.

The major side effects of β-blockers when used to treat aggression are lowering of blood pressure and pulse rate. Because peripheral β receptors are fully blocked with dosages of 300–400 mg/day, further decreases in these vital signs usually do not occur even when doses are increased to much higher levels. Despite reports of depression with the use of β-blockers, controlled trials and our experience indicate that it is a rare occurrence. Because the use of pro-

TABLE 15–12.   Clinical use of propranolol

1. Conduct a thorough medical evaluation.

2. Exclude patients with the following disorders: bronchial asthma, chronic obstructive pulmonary disease, insulin-dependent diabetes mellitus, congestive heart failure, persistent angina, significant peripheral vascular disease, hyperthyroidism.

3. Avoid sudden discontinuation of propranolol (particularly in patients with hypertension).

4. Begin with a single test dose of 20 mg/day in patients for whom there are clinical concerns with hypotension or bradycardia. Increase dose of propranolol by 20 mg/day every 3 days.

5. Initiate propranolol on a 20-mg-three-times-daily schedule for patients without cardiovascular or cardiopulmonary disorder.

6. Increase the dosage of propranolol by 60 mg/day every 3 days.

7. Increase medication unless the pulse rate is reduced below 50 beats/minute or systolic blood pressure is less than 90 mm Hg.

8. Do not administer medication if severe dizziness, ataxia, or wheezing occurs. Reduce or discontinue propranolol if such symptoms persist.

9. Increase dose to 12 mg/kg of body weight or until aggressive behavior is under control.

10. Doses greater than 800 mg are not usually required to control aggressive behavior.

11. Maintain the patient on the highest dose of propranolol for at least 8 weeks before concluding that the patient is not responding to the medication. Some patients, however, may respond rapidly to propranolol.

12. Use concurrent medications with caution. Monitor plasma levels of all antipsychotic and anticonvulsive medications.

Source.   Reprinted from Silver JM, Yudofsky SC: "Pharmacologic Treatment of Aggression." *Psychiatric Annals* 17:397–407, 1987. Used with permission.

pranolol is associated with significant increases in plasma levels of thioridazine, which has an absolute dosage ceiling of 800 mg/day, the combination of these two medications should be avoided whenever possible.

Table 15–13 summarizes our recommendations for the use of various classes of medication in the treatment of

TABLE 15–13.   Pharmacotherapy of agitation

Acute agitation/severe aggression

  Antipsychotic drugs

  Benzodiazepines

Chronic agitation

  Atypical antipsychotics

  Anticonvulsants (VPA, CBZ, ?gabapentin)

  Serotonergic antidepressants (SSRI, trazodone)

  Buspirone

  β-Blockers

Note.   CBZ=carbamazepine; SSRI=selective serotonin reuptake inhibitor; VPA=valproic acid.

chronic aggressive disorders associated with TBI. Acute aggression may be treated by using the sedative properties of neuroleptics or benzodiazepines. In treating aggression, the clinician, when possible, should diagnose and treat underlying disorders and should use, when possible, antiaggressive agents specific for those disorders. When there is partial response after a therapeutic trial with a specific medication, adjunctive treatment with a medication with a different mechanism of action should be instituted. For example, a patient with partial response to β-blockers can have additional improvement with the addition of an anticonvulsant.

Acute Aggression and Agitation

In the treatment of agitation and of acute or severe episodes of aggressive behavior, medications that are sedating may be indicated. However, because these drugs are not specific in their ability to inhibit aggressive behavior, there may be detrimental effects on arousal and cognitive function. Therefore, the use of sedation-producing medications must be time limited to avoid the emergence of seriously disabling side effects ranging from oversedation to tardive dyskinesia.

After the diagnosis and treatment of underlying causes of aggression and the evaluation and documentation of aggressive behaviors (such as with the OAS; see Figure 15–2), the use of pharmacological interventions can be considered in two categories: 1) the use of the sedating effects of medications, as required in acute situations, so that the patient does not harm him/herself or others; and 2) the use of nonsedating antiaggressive medications for the treatment of chronic aggression (Silver and Yudofsky 1994; Yudofsky et al. 1995).

Antipsychotic drugs.   Antipsychotics are the most commonly used medications in the treatment of aggression. Although these agents are appropriate and effective when aggression is derivative of active psychosis, the use of neuroleptic agents to treat chronic aggression, especially that secondary to organic brain injury, is often ineffective and entails significant risks that the patient will develop serious complications. Usually, it is the sedative side effects rather than the antipsychotic properties of antipsychotics that are used (i.e., misused) to "treat" (i.e., mask) the aggression. Often, patients develop tolerance to the sedative effects of the neuroleptics and therefore require increasing doses. As a result, extrapyramidal and anticholinergic-related side effects occur. Paradoxically (and frequently), because of the development of akathisia, the patient may become more agitated and restless as the dose of neuroleptic is increased, especially when a high-potency antipsychotic such as haloperidol is administered. The akathisia is often mistaken for increased irritability and agitation, and a vicious cycle of increasing neuroleptics and worsening akathisia occurs.

Studies of injury to motor neurons in animals provide some evidence that haloperidol impedes recovery. This effect was seen only when animals actively participated in a behavioral task and not when the animals were restrained after drug administration (Feeney et al. 1982). It is possible that the effect on decreasing dopamine and inhibiting neuronal function, which may be the mechanism of action to treat aggression, may have other detrimental effects on recovery. Whether this finding is generalizable to recovery in brain injury remains unclear. However, the finding raises important potential risk-benefit issues that must be considered before antipsychotic drugs are used to treat aggressive behavior in patients with neuronal damage.

In patients with brain injury and acute aggression, we recommend starting a neuroleptic such as risperidone at low doses of 0.5 mg orally, with repeated administration every hour until control of aggression is achieved. If after several administrations of risperidone the patient's aggressive behavior does not improve, the hourly dose may be increased until the patient is so sedated that he or she no longer exhibits agitation or violence. Once the patient is not aggressive for 48 hours, the daily dosage should be decreased gradually (i.e., by 25%/day) to ascertain whether aggressive behavior reemerges. In this case, consideration should then be made about whether it is best to increase the dose of risperidone and/or to initiate treatment with a more specific antiaggressive drug.

Sedatives and hypnotics.   There is an inconsistent body of literature on the effects of the benzodiazepines in the treatment of aggression. The sedative properties of benzodiazepines are especially helpful in the management of acute agitation and aggression. Most likely, this is due to the effect of benzodiazepines on increasing the inhibitory neurotransmitter GABA. Paradoxically, several studies report increased hostility and aggression as well as the induction of rage in patients treated with benzodiazepines. However, these reports are balanced by the observation that this phenomenon is rare (Dietch and Jennings 1988). Benzodiazepines can produce amnesia, and preexisting memory dysfunction can be exacerbated by the use of benzodiazepines. Brain-injured patients may also experience increased problems with coordination and balance with benzodiazepine use.

For treatment of acute aggression, lorazepam 1–2 mg may be administered every hour by either oral or intramuscular route until sedation is achieved (Silver and Yudofsky 1994). Intramuscular lorazepam has been suggested as an effective medication in the emergency treatment of the violent patient (Bick and Hannah 1986). Intravenous lorazepam is also effective, although the onset of action is similar when administered intramuscularly. Caution must be taken with intravenous administration, and it should be injected in doses less than 1 mg/minute to avoid laryngospasm. As with neuroleptics, gradual tapering of lorazepam may be attempted when the patient has been in control for 48 hours. If aggressive behavior recurs, medications for the treatment of chronic aggression may be initiated. Lorazepam in 1- or 2-mg doses, administered either orally or by injection, may be administered, if necessary, in combination with a neuroleptic medication (haloperidol, 2–5 mg). Other sedating medications such as paraldehyde, chloral hydrate, or diphenhydramine may be preferable to sedative antipsychotic agents.

CONCERNS REGARDING PHARMACOTHERAPY

There has been a bias held by patients, families, and, often, treatment centers against the use of medications for the treatment of neuropsychiatric disorders in patients with brain injury. This issue is important because the psychiatrist is often faced with resistance from patients, families, and staff about the use of medications. The bias against the use of psychiatric medications may have several sources, including the stigma associated with mental illness and psychiatry as well as the patient's previous suboptimal experience with psychotropic medications. The stigma may be related to the view that psychiatric symptoms are a sign of weakness, indolence, or even moral decline. We have suggested that the neuropsychiatric paradigm that uses a "medical model," reducing the misleading demarcation between "brain" and "mind" and emphasizing neurobiological effects (without negating emotional and psychological factors), is our strongest weapon against stigma (Yudofsky and Hales 1989). It is helpful to tell patients that their symptoms may be due to alterations in neurotransmitter function that may be treated with centrally active medications.

Unfortunately, for patients with TBI, a common experience with the use of psychotropic medications has indeed often been a negative one. Neuroleptics are widely misused as a general "tranquilizer" to sedate patients agitated after TBI, with resulting impairment in alertness, cognition, and initiation and the production, over time, of severe extrapyramidal side effects. For example, we evaluated in consultation one patient who had been treated with low-dose fluphenazine to control agitated behavior. One month later, the staff and family complained that she was "underaroused." On our examination, the patient had severe cogwheel rigidity that had not been diagnosed previously. One hour after administration of benztropine 1 mg, she was "active" again.

Another fear about medication is that it will interfere with a "natural healing process" that occurs after TBI. Evidence obtained from animal models suggests that certain drugs may interfere with recovery after neuronal injury. Feeney et al. (1982) studied the effect of dextroamphetamine on recovery from hemiplegia after ablation of the sensorimotor cortex in rats. The researchers found that dextroamphetamine accelerated the rate of recovery and that this effect was blocked by haloperidol. In addition, haloperidol, when administered alone, resulted in delayed recovery. Importantly, recovery was affected only when the animal was allowed to move during drug administration. This implies that haloperidol delays a process during active rehabilitation rather than interfering with spontaneous recovery. In another model, Hovda and Fenney (1984) found that haloperidol blocked the positive effect of dextroamphetamine on recovery of depth perception after visual cortex injury. It has been suggested that the mechanism of action of haloperidol in delaying recovery is through effects as an α-adrenergic antagonist (Sutton et al. 1987). Clonidine, an α-agonist, and prazosin, an α_1-antagonist, reinstate deficits after sensorimotor cortex ablation (Sutton and Feeney 1987), an effect not seen with propranolol (Boyeson and Feeney 1984). Other studies have demonstrated that clonidine has deleterious effects on recovery (Feeney and Westerberg 1990; L.B. Goldstein and Davis 1990). It should be noted that these experimental methods in animals do not produce the same neuropathological findings as contusions or diffuse axonal injury in humans and therefore may not apply to many patients with TBI. These results also suggest that patients must be in active rehabilitation during drug administration for these effects to occur.

In animal studies that involve the neurotransmitter GABA, increase in GABA function has been associated with greater neuromotor deficits and poorer recovery (Boyeson 1991). Increased production of GABA associated with benzodiazepine administration may result in greater glutamate neurotoxicity (Simantov 1990). Diazepam has been found to block recovery of sensory deficits after rat neocortex ablation (Schallert et al. 1986).

The studies cited above relating the use of psychotropic medications to impaired neuronal recovery after laboratory-induced brain injury have all used animal models. In reviewing the medical records of 100 patients who were admitted to the hospital after head injury, L.B. Goldstein (1995) reported that only 14% were taking medications at the time of injury. However, during hospitalization, 72% of the patients received one or a combination of the drugs that animal studies suggest may impair recovery (neuroleptics and other central dopamine receptor antagonists, benzodiazepines, phenytoin, and phenobarbital).

There have been no carefully controlled clinical trials of this important issue in humans. Interestingly, when the medical records of recovering stroke patients were reviewed, the use of antihypertensive medications or haloperidol was associated with poorer recovery (Porch et al. 1985). Goldstein and Davis (1988) found that phenytoin, benzodiazepines, dopamine receptor antagonists, clonidine, and prazosin prescribed for patients who had experienced ischemic strokes were each associated with poorer sensorimotor function and lower measures of activities of daily living than in patients who did not receive those drugs.

BEHAVIORAL AND COGNITIVE TREATMENTS

Behavioral treatments are important in the care of patients who have sustained TBI. These programs require careful design and execution by a staff well versed in behavioral techniques. Behavioral methods can be used in response to aggressive outbursts and other maladaptive social behaviors (Corrigan and Bach 2005). One study (Eames and Wood 1985) found that behavior modification was 75% effective in dealing with disturbed behavior after severe brain injury.

After brain injury, patients may need specific cognitive strategies to assist with impairments in memory and concentration (Cicerone et al. 2005; Gordon and Hibbard 2005). As opposed to earlier beliefs that cognitive therapy should "exercise" the brain to develop skills that have been damaged, current therapies involve teaching the patient new strategies to compensate for lost or impaired functions. Salazar et al. (2000) for the Defense and Veterans Head Injury Program (DVHIP) Study Group compared an intensive 8-week in-hospital cognitive rehabilitation program to a limited home program. Both groups improved, but there was no significant difference between the two treatments. (For more information on cognitive treatments, see Chapter 33 of this book.) We emphasize that for most patients, treatment strategies are synergistic. For example, the use of β-adrenergic receptor antagonists to treat agitation and aggression may enhance a patient's ability to benefit from behavioral and cognitive treatments.

PSYCHOLOGICAL AND SOCIAL INTERVENTIONS

In the broadest terms, psychological issues involving patients who incur brain injury revolve around four major themes: 1) psychopathology that preceded the injury, 2) psychological responses to the traumatic event, 3) psychological reactions to deficits brought about by brain injury, and 4) psychological issues related to potential recurrence of brain injury.

Preexisting psychiatric illnesses are most frequently intensified with brain injury. Therefore, the angry, obsessive patient or the patient with chronic depression will exhibit a worsening of these symptoms after brain injury. Specific coping mechanisms that were used before the injury may no longer be possible because of the cognitive deficits caused by the neurological disease. Therefore, patients need to learn new methods of adaptation to stress. In addition, as mentioned above, the social, economic, educational, and vocational status of the patient (and how these are affected by brain lesions) influences the patient's response to the injury.

The events surrounding brain injury often have far-reaching experiential and symbolic significance for the patient. Such issues as guilt, punishment, magical wishes, and fears crystallize about the nidus of a traumatic event. For example, a patient who sustains brain injury during a car accident may view his injury as punishment for long-standing violent impulses toward an aggressive father. In such cases, reassurance and homilies about his lack of responsibility for the accident are usually less productive than psychological exploration.

A patient's reactions to being disabled by brain damage have realistic as well as symbolic significance. When intense effort is required for a patient to form a word or to move a limb, frustration may be expressed as anger, depression, anxiety, or fear. Particularly in cases in which brain injury results in permanent impairment, a psychiatrist may experience countertransferential discomfort that results in failure to discuss directly with the patient and his or her family the implications of resultant disabilities and limitations. Gratuitous optimism, collaboration with denial of the patient, and facile solutions to complex problems are rarely effective and can erode the therapeutic alliance and ongoing treatment. Tyerman and Humphrey (1984) assessed 25 patients with severe brain injury for changes in self-concept. Patients viewed themselves as markedly changed after their injury but believed that they would regain preexisting capacities within a year. The authors concluded that these unrealistic expectations may hamper rehabilitation and adjustment of both the patient and his or her relatives. By gently and persistently directing the patient's attention to the reality of the disabilities, the psychiatrist may help the patient begin the process of acceptance and adjustment to the impairment. Clinical judgment will help the psychiatrist in deciding whether and when explorations of the symbolic significance of the patient's brain injury should be pursued. The persistence of anxiety, guilt, and fear beyond the normative stages of adjustment and rehabilitation may indicate that psychodynamic approaches are required (Drubach et al. 1994; Pollack 2005).

Families of patients with neurological disorders are under severe stress. The relative with a brain injury may be unable to fulfill his or her previous role or function as parent or spouse, thus significantly affecting the other family members (Cavallo and Kay 2005). Oddy et al. (1978) evaluated 54 relatives of patients with brain injury within 1, 6, and 12 months of the traumatic event. Approximately 40% of the relatives showed depressive symptoms within 1 month of the event; 25% of the relatives showed significant physical or psychological illness within 6–12 months of the brain damage. Mood disturbances, especially anxiety, depression, and social role dysfunction, are also seen within this time (Kreutzer et al. 1994; Linn et al. 1994; M.G. Livingston et al. 1985a, 1985b). Family members may experience increased substance use, unemployment, and decreased financial status over time (K.M. Hall et al. 1994). By treating the psychological responses of relatives to the brain injury, the clinician can foster a supportive and therapeutic atmosphere for the patient as well as significantly help the relative. In one study (Leach et al. 1994), teaching the family how to implement problem-solving techniques and behavioral coping strategies resulted in lower levels of depression in the person who sustained the injury.

For both patients and their families, severe TBI results in multifaceted losses, including the loss of dreams about and expectations for the future. The psychiatrist may be of enormous benefit in treating the family and patient by providing support, insight, and other points of view. A patient from a high-achieving family who lost his ability to do theoretical physics told one of us (S.C.Y.), "If I can't go to graduate school in physics at Princeton like my brother and my cousin, I am worthless."

Educational and supportive treatment of families can be therapeutic when used together with appropriate social skills training. Patient advocacy groups, such as the National Brain Injury Foundation, can provide important peer support for families. Many patients require clear, almost concrete statements describing their behaviors because insight and judgment may be impaired.

It is a distressing fact that brain injury can and often does recur. With repeated injury, there is an increase in the incidence of neuropsychiatric and emotional symptoms (Carlsson et al. 1987). Patients' fears and anxieties about recurrence of injury are more than simply efforts at magical control over terrifying conditions. Therapeutic emphasis should be placed on actions and activities that will aid in preventing recurrence, including compliance with appropriate medications and abstinence from alcohol and other substances of abuse.

PREVENTION

MOTOR VEHICLE ACCIDENTS

The proper use of seat belts with upper-torso restraints is 45% effective in preventing fatalities, 50% effective in preventing moderate to critical injuries, and 10% effective in preventing minor injuries when used by drivers and passengers (U.S. Department of Transportation 1984). This translates to 12,000–15,000 lives saved per year (National Safety Council 1986). Orsay et al. (1988) noted that victims of motor vehicle accidents who wore seat belts had a 60.1% reduction in injury severity. Without specific legislation, car restraints are used infrequently. Many brain injuries occur in side impacts, when the heads of occupants collide with the structural column between the windshield and the side window. More than 7,000 motor vehicle–related deaths are caused by side impacts, nearly half of which are due to brain trauma (Jagger 1992). In 2003, there were 44,800 motor vehicle accident–related fatalities (National Safety Council 2006). There were 2.2 million disabling injuries from motor vehicle accidents in 1998 (National Safety Council 1999).

The use of safety belts has prevented a significant number of deaths and injuries (Centers for Disease Control 1992; Kaplan and Cowley 1991). Driver and passenger air bags have decreased the number and severity of injuries, although they have not been as effective in controlling severe injuries of the lower extremities (Kuner et al. 1996).

Alcohol dependence is a highly prevalent and destructive illness. In addition, alcohol abuse is a common concomitant of affective and characterological disorders. Alcohol intoxication is frequently found in the patient who has suffered brain injury, whether from violence, falls, or motor vehicle accidents (Brismar et al. 1983). In the United States, the proportion of alcohol involvement in motor vehicle fatalities has been decreasing over the past several years. Whereas during the week, 24% of fatally injured drivers had blood alcohol concentration (BAC) at or above 0.087%, on weekends, the proportion increases to 45% (Insurance Institute for Highway Safety 2005a). Alcohol-related deaths have been decreased by a combination of "zero tolerance" laws and laws lowering the allowable BAC for impaired driving from 0.10% to 0.08% (Insurance Institute for Highway Safety 2005a).

Drivers in fatal accidents have a more frequent history of alcohol use, previous accidents, moving traffic violations, psychopathology, stress, paranoid thinking, and depression. They often have less control of hostility and anger, with a decreased tolerance for tension, and a history of increased risk taking (Tsuang et al. 1985). Cigarette smoking, alcohol use, obesity, and physical inactivity were found to be associated with nonuse of seat belts (Goldbaum et al. 1986). Therefore, we strongly advocate that in all psychiatric and other medical histories a detailed inquiry about alcohol use, seat belt use, and driving patterns be present. Examples of driving patterns, accident records, violations, driving while intoxicated, speeding patterns, car maintenance, presence of distractions such as children and animals, and hazardous driving conditions should be included in a complete driving record. The use of illicit substances and medications that may induce sedation, such as antihistamines, antihypertensive agents, anticonvulsants, minor tranquilizers, and antidepressants, should also be assessed and documented. Psychiatric patients are at greater risk for motor vehicle accidents because they often have several of these characteristics (Noyes 1985).

Clearly, motorcycle riding, with or without helmets, and using bicycles for commuting purposes are associated with head injuries, even when safety precautions are taken and when driving regulations are observed. In 2005, there were 4,439 motorcyclist deaths (Insurance Institute for Highway Safety 2005c). It has been estimated that for every motorcycle-related death, there are another 37 injuries and many more that remain unreported to the police (S.P. Baker et al. 1987). Helmets can reduce the risk of on-highway motorcycle fatalities by about 37% and are 67% effective in preventing brain injuries (Insurance Institute for Highway Safety 2005c). Death rates from TBI are twice as high in states with weak or nonexistent helmet laws, compared with rates in states with helmet laws that apply to all riders (Sosin et al. 1989). Fewer than half of the states mandate all riders to wear helmets. In 2005, there were 782 bicyclists killed in crashes with motor vehicles, a number that has been decreasing over the years (Insurance Institute for Highway Safety 2005b). Virtually all of those riders were not wearing helmets (Insurance Institute for Highway Safety 2005b). Every year, 1,300 cyclists are killed in the United States (Centers for Disease Control 1988). The use of bicycle helmets can significantly decrease the morbidity and mortality resulting from bicycle-related head injuries (Thompson et al. 1989). However, only 16 states have mandatory helmet laws, and even these apply only to riders under age 18.

Significant preventive measures to reduce head trauma include counseling a patient about risk taking; the treatment of alcoholism and depression; the judicious prescription of medications and full explanations of sedation, cognitive impairment, and other potentially dangerous side effects; and public information activities on topics such as the proper use of seat belts, the dangers of drinking and driving, and automobile safety measures.

PREVENTION OF BRAIN INJURY IN CHILDREN

Beyond nurturance, children rely on their parents or guardians for guidance and protection. Each year in the United States more than 1,500 children under age 13 die as motor vehicle passengers; more than 90% of these children were not using car seat restraints (Insurance Institute for Highway Safety 2005d). Child safety seats have been found to be 80%–90% effective in the prevention of injuries to children (National Safety Council 1985). In a sample of 494 children younger than 4 years old who had suffered motor vehicle accident trauma (Agran et al. 1985), 70% had been unrestrained, 12% were restrained with seat belts, and 22% were restrained in child safety seats. In general, restrained children tended to sustain less serious injuries than the unrestrained children.

Children younger than 4 years old who are not restrained in safety seats are 11 times more likely to be killed in motor vehicle accidents (National Safety Council 1985). It is not safe for the child to sit on the lap of the parent, with or without restraints, because the adult's weight can crush the child during an accident. Young children traveling with drivers who themselves are not wearing seat belts are four times as likely to be left unrestrained (National Safety Council 1985). Legislation in Britain mandating the use of child safety seats has had a significant effect on decreasing fatal and serious injuries to children (Avery and Hayes 1985). In the United States, all 50 states and the District of Columbia have mandatory laws for child safety seats (National Safety Council 1985). Children who ride on bicycle-mounted child seats are highly subject to injuries to the head and face and should wear bicycle helmets. Alcohol use by adults is frequently a factor in child injuries and fatalities (Li 2000). In the majority of drinking driver–related child passenger deaths, the child was an unrestrained passenger (Quinlan et al. 2000).

Children are often involved in sports that carry the risk of brain injury. Sports such as boxing, gymnastics, diving, soccer, football, basketball, and hockey are associated with considerable risk of TBI. It has been estimated that 300,000 cases of TBI occur during sports or recreation (Centers for Disease Control and Prevention 1997). For children ages 10–14 years, sports and recreational activities account for 43% of TBI (J.F. Kraus and Nourjah 1988). J.W. Powell and Barber-Foss (1999) found that 3.9% of 17,815 high school athletes had sustained a mild TBI. Mild brain injury is not uncommon in football and can result in persistent symptoms and disabilities (Gerberich et al. 1983). An estimated 20% of high school football players sustain concussion during a single football season, with some reporting symptoms persisting as long as 6–9 months after the end of the season (Gerberich et al. 1983). Soccer may involve the use of the head with sudden twists to strike the ball that may also result in neuropsychiatric abnormalities (Tysvaer et al. 1989).

The clinician must always be alert to the possibility that parents may be neglectful, may use poor judgment, and may even be directly violent in their treatment of children. Unfortunately, it is not uncommon for head trauma to result from overt child abuse on the part of parents, other adults, and peers. We must always be alert to such possibilities in our patients, and when these problems are discovered, we must take direct actions to address them. We encourage direct counseling of parents who do not consistently use infant and child car seats for their children.

CONCLUSION

Invariably, brain injury leads to emotional damage in the patient and in the family. In this chapter, we have reviewed the most frequently occurring psychiatric symptoms that are associated with TBI. We have emphasized how the informed psychiatrist is not only effective but essential in both the prevention of brain injury and, when it occurs, the treatment of its sequelae. In addition to increased efforts devoted to the prevention of brain injury, we advocate a multidisciplinary and multidimensional approach to the assessment and treatment of neuropsychiatric aspects of brain injury.

Highlights for the Clinician

Key clinical features of TBI

Epidemiology

+ There are 100,000 new disabilities from adult traumatic brain injury (TBI) each year.

+ Between 2.5 million and 6.5 million adults live with long-term consequences of TBI.

+ Five million children sustain TBI each year, 200,000 of whom are hospitalized.

Neurotransmitter changes after TBI

+ Catecholamines

  • Discrete lesions to ascending monoaminergic projections may interfere with the function of systems dependent on such afferent pathways.

  • Levels tend to increase acutely after TBI, and increased levels—especially of dopamine—may portend increased neuropsychiatric deficits.

+ Serotonin

  • Serotonergic projections to the frontal cortical areas are susceptible to biomechanical injury, and both diffuse axonal injury and contusions may produce dysfunction in this neurotransmitter system.

  • Excitotoxins and lipid peroxidation may also damage serotonergic neuronal systems.

  • Studies of serotonergic activity after acute and chronic TBI have variable findings.

+ Acetylcholine

  • Findings from both basic and clinical neuroscience suggest that both acute and long-term alterations in cortical cholinergic function develop following TBI.

  • TBI appears to produce an acute increase in cholinergic neurotransmission followed by chronic reductions in neurotransmitter function and cholinergic afferents.

Neuropsychiatric assessment of patients with TBI

+ History-taking: Although brain injuries subsequent to serious automobile, occupational, or sports accidents may not result in diagnostic enigmas for the psychiatrist, less severe trauma may first present as relatively subtle behavioral or affective change.

+ Documentation and rating of symptoms: Table 15–2 summarizes the systematic assessment of neuropsychiatric function following TBI.

+ Laboratory evaluation

  • Computed tomography (CT) for acute assessment of the patient with head trauma documents hemorrhage, edema, midline shifts, herniation, fractures, and contusions.

  • Magnetic resonance imaging (MRI) is used with patients with severe brain injury when CT scans have not demonstrated anatomical bases for the degree of coma.

  • MRI is especially sensitive in detecting lesions in the frontal and temporal lobes that are not visualized by CT.

  • Functional techniques in brain imaging, such as regional cerebral blood flow (rCBF) and positron emission tomography (PET), can detect areas of abnormal function, when even CT and MRI scans fail to show any abnormalities of structure.

  • Single-photon emission computed tomography (SPECT) also shows promise in documenting brain damage after TBI.

  • Electrophysiological techniques for assessment after TBI may also assist in the evaluation.

(continued)

Highlights for the Clinician (continued)

Neuropsychiatric sequelae of TBI

✦ Personality changes: Frontal lobe syndrome subsequent to TBI is associated with profound changes in relatedness and social functioning.

✦ Intellectual changes: Problems with intellectual functioning may be among the most subtle manifestations of brain injury. Changes encompass dysfunctions in the ability to attend, concentrate, remember, use abstractions and logic, calculate, reason, and remember and process information.

✦ Psychiatric disorders

• Mood and affect: Depression and increased risk of suicide occur frequently after TBI.

• Mania: Mania is more frequently associated with damage to basal region of right temporal lobe and in patients with family histories of bipolar disorder.

• Delirium: Delirium can be related to direct effects of injury on brain tissue, side effects of medication, drug withdrawal or intoxication, and/or environmental factors.

• Posttraumatic epilepsy: A varying percentage of patients, depending on the location and severity of injury, will have seizures during the acute period after the trauma.

• Anxiety disorders: Generalized anxiety disorder, panic disorder, obsessive-compulsive disorder, posttraumatic stress disorder, and phobic disorder may develop after TBI.

• Sleep disorders: It is common for individuals with TBI to complain of disrupted sleep patterns, ranging from hypersomnia to difficulty maintaining sleep.

RECOMMENDED READING

Silver JM, McAllister TW, Yudofsky SC (eds): Textbook of Traumatic Brain Injury. Washington, DC, American Psychiatric Publishing, 2005

REFERENCES

AbdelMalik P, Husted J, Chow EW, et al: Childhood head injury and expression of schizophrenia in multiply affected families. Arch Gen Psychiatry 60:231–236, 2003

Achte K, Jarho L, Kyykka T, et al: Paranoid disorders following war brain damage: preliminary report. Psychopathology 24:309–315, 1991

Adams JH, Graham DI, Murray LS, et al: Diffuse axonal injury due to nonmissile head injury in humans: an analysis of 45 cases. Ann Neurol 12:557–563, 1982

Agran PF, Dunkie DE, Winn DG: Motor vehicle accident trauma and restraint usage patterns in children less than 4 years of age. Pediatrics 76:382–386, 1985

Alexander MP: Mild traumatic brain injury: pathophysiology, natural history, and clinical management. Neurology 45:1253–1260, 1995

Alexopoulos GS, Silver JM, Kahn DA, et al: The Expert Consensus Guideline Series: Treatment of Agitation in Older Persons with Dementia. Postgrad Med (A Special Report). April 1998

Alves WM, Coloban ART, O'Leary TJ, et al: Understanding posttraumatic symptoms after minor head injury. J Head Trauma Rehabil 1:1–12, 1986

Alves W, Macciocchi SN, Barth JT: Postconcussive symptoms after uncomplicated mild head injury. J Head Trauma Rehabil 8:48–59, 1993

Amaducci LA, Fratiglioni L, Rocca WA, et al: Risk factors for clinically diagnosed Alzheimer's disease: a case control study of an Italian population. Neurology 36:922–931, 1986

American Psychiatric Association: Diagnostic and Statistical Manual of Mental Disorders, 4th Edition. Washington, DC, American Psychiatric Association, 1994

American Psychiatric Association: Diagnostic and Statistical Manual of Mental Disorders, 4th Edition, Text Revision. Washington, DC, American Psychiatric Association, 2000

American Psychiatric Association Task Force on the Use of Laboratory Tests in Psychiatry: Tricyclic antidepressants: blood level measurements and clinical outcome: an APA Task Force report. Am J Psychiatry 142:155–162, 1985

Anderson KE, Silver JM: Neurological and mental diseases and violence, in Medical Management of the Violent Patient: Clinical Assessment and Therapy. Edited by Tardiff K. New York, Marcel Dekker, 1999, pp 87–124

Anderson KE, Taber KH, Hurley RA: Functional imaging, in Textbook of Traumatic Brain Injury. Edited by Silver JM, McAllister TM, Yudofsky SC. Washington, DC, American Psychiatric Publishing, 2005, pp 107–134

Annegers JF, Grabow JD, Groover RV, et al: Seizures after head trauma: a population study. Neurology 30:683–689, 1980

Arciniegas D, Adler L, Topkoff J, et al: Attention and memory dysfunction after traumatic brain injury: cholinergic mechanisms, sensory gating, and a hypothesis for further investigation. Brain Inj 13:1–13, 1999

Arciniegas D, Olincy A, Topkoff J, et al: Impaired auditory gating and P50 nonsuppression following traumatic brain injury. J Neuropsychiatry Clin Neurosci 12:77–85, 2000a

Arciniegas DB, Topkoff J, Silver JM: Neuropsychiatric aspects of traumatic brain injury. Curr Treat Options Neurol 2:169–186, 2000b

Arciniegas DB, Topkoff JL, Anderson CA, et al: Normalization of P50 physiology by donepezil hydrochloride in traumatic brain injury patients (abstract). J Neuropsychiatry Clin Neurosci 13:140, 2001

Arciniegas DB, Anderson CA, Rojas DC: Electrophysiological techniques, in Textbook of Traumatic Brain Injury. Edited by Silver JM, McAllister TM, Yudofsky SC. Washington, DC, American Psychiatric Publishing, 2005, pp 135–158

Armstrong KK, Sahgal V, Bloch R, et al: Rehabilitation outcomes in patients with posttraumatic epilepsy. Arch Phys Med Rehabil 71:156–160, 1990

Ariza M, Junque C, Mataro M, et al: Neuropsychological correlates of basal ganglia and medial temporal lobe NAA/Cho reductions in traumatic brain injury. Arch Neurol 61:541–544, 2004

Ashikaga R, Araki Y, Ishida O: MRI of head injury using FLAIR. Neuroradiology 39:239–242, 1997

Askenasy JJM, Winkler I, Grushkiewicz J, et al: The natural history of sleep disturbances in severe missile head injury. J Neurol Rehabil 3:93–96, 1989

Auerbach SH: Neuroanatomical correlates of attention and memory disorders in traumatic brain injury: an application of neurobehavioral subtypes. J Head Trauma Rehabil 1:1–12, 1986

Avery JG, Hayes HRM: Death and injury to children in cars: Britain. BMJ 291:515, 1985

Azouvi P, Jokic C, Attal N, et al: Carbamazepine in agitation and aggressive behaviour following severe closed head injury: results of an open trial. Brain Inj 13:797–804, 1999

Bakchine S, Lacomblez L, Benoit N, et al: Manic-like state after bilateral orbitofrontal and right temporoparietal injury: efficacy of clonidine. Neurology 39:777–781, 1989

Baker AJ, Moulton RJ, MacMillan VH, et al: Excitatory amino acids in cerebrospinal fluid following traumatic brain injury in humans. J Neurosurg 79:369–372, 1993

Baker SP, Whitfield RA, O'Neill B: Geographic variations in mortality from motor vehicle crashes. N Engl J Med 316:1384–1387, 1987

Bamrah JS, Johnson J: Bipolar affective disorder following head injury. Br J Psychiatry 158:117–119, 1991

Bareggi SR, Porta M, Selenati A, et al: Homovanillic acid and 5-hydroxyindole-acetic acid in the CSF of patients after a severe head injury, I: lumbar CSF concentration in chronic brain post-traumatic syndromes. Eur Neurol 13:528–544, 1975

Bechara A, Damasio AR, Damasio H, et al: Insensitivity to future consequences following damage to human prefrontal cortex. Cognition 50:7–15, 1994

Beck AT, Ward CH, Mendelson M, et al: An inventory for measuring depression. Arch Gen Psychiatry 4:561–571, 1961

Becker DP, Verity MA, Povlishock J, et al: Brain cellular injury and recover: horizons for improving medical therapies in stroke and trauma. West J Med 148:670–684, 1988

Belanger HG, Vanderploeg RD, Curtiss G, et al: Recent neuroimaging techniques in mild traumatic brain injury. J Neuropsychiatry Clin Neurosci 19:5–20, 2007

Bellus SB, Stewart D, Vergo JG, et al: The use of lithium in the treatment of aggressive behaviours with two brain-injured individuals in a state psychiatric hospital. Brain Inj 10:849–860, 1996

Ben-Yishay Y, Lakin P: Structured group treatment for brain-injury survivors, in Neuropsychological Treatment After Brain Injury. Edited by Ellis DW, Christensen A-L. Boston, MA, Kluwer Academic, 1989, pp 271–295

Berg MJ, Ebert B, Willis DK, et al: Parkinsonism—drug treatment: part I. Drug Intell Clin Pharm 21:10–21, 1987

Berman KF, Illowsky BP, Weinberger DR: Physiological dysfunction of dorsolateral prefrontal cortex in schizophrenia, IV: further evidence for regional and behavioral specificity. Arch Gen Psychiatry 45:616–622, 1988

Bernstein DM: Recovery from head injury. Brain Inj 13:151–172, 1999

Bessette RF, Peterson LG: Fluoxetine and organic mood syndrome. Psychosomatics 33:224–225, 1992

Bicik I, Radanov BP, Schafer N, et al: PET with 18-fluorodeoxyglucose and hexamethylpropylene amine oxime SPECT in late whiplash syndrome. Neurology 51:345–350, 1998

Bick PA, Hannah AL: Intramuscular lorazepam to restrain violent patients. Lancet 1:206–207, 1986

Bigler ED: Structural imaging, in Textbook of Traumatic Brain Injury. Edited by Silver JM, McAllister TM, Yudofsky SC. Washington, DC, American Psychiatric Publishing, 2005, pp 79–106

Binder LM, Rattok J: Assessment of the postconcussive syndrome after mild head trauma, in Assessment of the Behavioral Consequences of Head Trauma. Edited by Lezak MD. New York, Alan R Liss, 1989, pp 37–48

Bleiberg J, Garmoe W, Cederquist J, et al: Effects of Dexedrine on performance consistency following brain injury: a double-blind placebo crossover case study. Neuropsychiatry Neuropsychol Behav Neurol 6:245–248, 1993

Blumbergs PC, Scott G, Manavis J, et al: Staining of amyloid precursor protein to study axonal damage in mild head injury. Lancet 344:1055–1056, 1994

Bogner JA, Corrigan JD: Epidemiology of agitation following brain injury. NeuroRehabilitation 5:293–297, 1995

Bogner JA, Corrigan JD, Strange M, et al: Reliability of the Agitated Behavior Scale. J Head Trauma Rehabil 14:91–96, 1999

Bohnen N, Twijnstra A, Jolles J: Post-traumatic and emotional symptoms in different subgroups of patients with mild head injury. Brain Inj 6:481–487, 1992

Bornstein RA, Miller HB, van Schoor T: Emotional adjustment in compensated head injury patients. Neurosurgery 23:622–627, 1988

Bornstein RA, Miller HB, van Schoor JT: Neuropsychological deficit and emotional disturbance in head-injured patients. J Neurosurg 70:509–513, 1989

Boyeson MG: Neurochemical alterations after brain injury: clinical implications for pharmacologic rehabilitation. Neurorehabilitation 1:33–43, 1991

Boyeson MG, Feeney DM: The role of norepinephrine in recovery from brain injury. Abstr Soc Neurosci 10:68, 1984

Bracken P: Mania following head injury. Br J Psychiatry 150:690–692, 1987

Brain Injury Special Interest Group of the American Academy of Physical Medicine and Rehabilitation: Practice parameter: antiepileptic drug treatment of posttraumatic seizures. Arch Phys Med Rehabil 79:594–597, 1998

Brain Trauma Foundation: Role of antiseizure prophylaxis following head injury. The American Association of Neurological Surgeons. The Joint Section on Neurotrauma and Critical Care. J Neurotrauma 17:549–553, 2000

Bremner JD, Scott TM, Delaney RC, et al: Deficits in short-term memory in posttraumatic stress disorder. Am J Psychiatry 150:1015–1019, 1993

Bremner JD, Randall P, Scott TM, et al: MRI-based measurement of hippocampal volume in patients with combat-related posttraumatic stress disorder. Am J Psychiatry 152:973–981, 1995

Bremner JD, Randall P, Vermetten E, et al: Magnetic resonance imaging–based measurement of hippocampal volume in posttraumatic stress disorder related to childhood physical and sexual abuse: a preliminary report. Biol Psychiatry 41:23–32, 1997

Breslau N, Kessler RC, Chilcoat HD, et al: Trauma and posttraumatic stress disorder in the community: the 1996 Detroit Area Survey of Trauma. Arch Gen Psychiatry 55:626–632, 1998

Brismar B, Engstrom A, Rydberg U: Head injury and intoxication: a diagnostic and therapeutic dilemma. Acta Chir Scand 149:11–14, 1983

Brooke MM, Patterson DR, Questad KA, et al: The treatment of agitation during initial hospitalization after traumatic brain injury. Arch Phys Med Rehabil 73:917–921, 1992a

Brooke MM, Questad KA, Patterson DR, et al: Agitation and restlessness after closed head injury: a prospective study of 100 consecutive admissions. Arch Phys Med Rehabil 73:320–323, 1992b

Brooks BR, Thisted RA, Appel SH, et al: Treatment of pseudobulbar affect in ALS with dextromethorphan/quinidine: a randomized trial. ALS Study Group. Neurology 63:1364–1370, 2004

Brooks N: Personal communication, reported in Eames P, Haffey WJ, Cope DN: Treatment of behavioral disorders, in Rehabilitation of the Adult and Child with Traumatic Brain Injury, 2nd Edition. Edited by Rosenthal M, Griffith ER, Bond MR, et al. Philadelphia, PA, FA Davis, 1990, pp 410–432

Brooks N, Campsie L, Symington C, et al: The five year outcome of severe blunt head injury: a relative's view. J Neurol Neurosurg Psychiatry 49:764–770, 1986

Brown G, Chadwick O, Shaffer D, et al: A prospective study of children with head injuries, III: psychiatric sequelae. Psychol Med 11:63–78, 1981

Brown KW, Sloan RL, Pentland B: Fluoxetine as a treatment for post-stroke emotionalism. Acta Psychiatr Scand 98:455–458, 1998

Brown SJ, Fann JR, Grant I: Postconcussional disorder: time to acknowledge a common source of neurobehavioral morbidity. J Neuropsychiatry Clin Neurosci 6:15–22, 1994

Bryant RA: Posttraumatic stress disorder, flashbacks, and pseudomemories in closed head injury. J Trauma Stress 9:621–629, 1996

Bryant RA, Marosszeky JE, Crooks J, et al: Posttraumatic stress disorder after severe traumatic brain injury. Am J Psychiatry 157:629–631, 2000

Buckley P, Stack JP, Madigan C, et al: Magnetic resonance imaging of schizophrenia-like psychoses associated with cerebral trauma: clinicopathological correlates. Am J Psychiatry 150:146–148, 1993

Burstein A: Bipolar and pure mania disorders precipitated by head trauma. Psychosomatics 34:194–195, 1993

Buysse DJ, Reynolds CF III: Insomnia, in Handbook of Sleep Disorders. Edited by Thorpy MJ. New York, Marcel Dekker, 1990, pp 373–434

Carlsson GS, Svardsudd K, Welin L: Long-term effects of head injuries sustained during life in three male populations. J Neurosurg 67:197–205, 1987

Cassidy JW: Fluoxetine: a new serotonergically active antidepressant. J Head Trauma Rehabil 4:67–69, 1989

Cassidy JW: Neuropathology, in Neuropsychiatry of Traumatic Brain Injury. Edited by Silver JM, Yudofsky SC, Hales RE. Washington, DC, American Psychiatric Press, 1994, pp 43–80

Catsman-Berrevoets CE, Harskamp FV: Compulsive pre-sleep behavior and apathy due to bilateral thalamic stroke: response to bromocriptine. Neurology 38:647–649, 1988

Cavallo MM, Kay T: The family system, in Textbook of Traumatic Brain Injury. Edited by Silver JM, McAllister, Yudofsky SC. Washington, DC, American Psychiatric Publishing, 2005, pp 533–558

Cech KM, Hills EC, Sandel ME, et al: Proton magnetic resonance spectroscopy for detection of axonal injury in the splenium of the corpus callosum of brain-injured patients. J Neurosurg 88:795–801, 1998

Centers for Disease Control: Bicycle-related injuries: data from the National Electronic Injury Surveillance System. MMWR Morb Mortal Wkly Rep 36:269–271, 1988

Centers for Disease Control: Increased safety-belt use: United States, 1991. MMWR Morb Mortal Wkly Rep 41:421–423, 1992

Centers for Disease Control and Prevention: Sports-related recurrent brain injuries—United States. MMWR Morb Mortal Wkly Rep 46:224–227, 1997

Chambers J, Cohen SS, Hemminger L, et al: Mild traumatic brain injuries in low-risk trauma patients. J Trauma 41:976–979, 1996

Chandler MC, Barnhill JL, Gualtieri CT: Amantadine for the agitated head-injury patient. Brain Inj 2:309–311, 1988

Chamelian L, Reis M, Feinstein A: Six-month recovery from mild to moderate traumatic brain injury: the role of APOE-epsilon4 allele. Brain 127:2621–2628, 2004

Chatham-Showalter PE: Carbamazepine for combativeness in acute traumatic brain injury. J Neuropsychiatry Clin Neurosci 8:96–99, 1996

Childers MK, Holland D: Psychomotor agitation following gabapentin use in brain injury. Brain Inj 11:537–540, 1997

Christodoulou C, DeLuca J, Ricker JH, et al: Functional magnetic resonance imaging of working memory impairment after traumatic brain injury. J Neurol Neurosurg Psychiatry 71:161–168, 2001

Cicerone KD, Dahlberg C, Malec JF, et al: Evidence-based cognitive rehabilitation: updated review of the literature from 1998 through 2002. Arch Phys Med Rehabil 86:1681–1692, 2005

Clark AF, Davison K: Mania following head injury: a report of two cases and a review of the literature. Br J Psychiatry 150:841–844, 1987

Clifton GL, Ziegler MG, Grossman RG: Circulating catecholamines and sympathetic activity after head injury. Neurosurgery 8:10–14, 1981

Committee on Head Injury Nomenclature: Report of the Ad Hoc Committee to study head injury nomenclature: proceedings of the Congress of Neurological Surgeons in 1964. Clin Neurosurg 12:386–394, 1966

Cope DN, Date ES, Mar EY: Serial computerized tomographic evaluations in traumatic head injury. Arch Phys Med Rehabil 69:483–486, 1988

Corbett JA, Trimble MR, Nichol TC: Behavioral and cognitive impairments in children with epilepsy: the long-term effects of anticonvulsant therapy. J Am Acad Child Psychiatry 24:17–23, 1985

Corcoran C, McAllister TW, Malaspina D: Psychotic disorders, in Textbook of Traumatic Brain Injury. Edited by Silver JM, McAllister, Yudofsky SC. Washington, DC, American Psychiatric Publishing, 2005, pp 213–229

Corkin S, Sullivan EV, Carr A: Prognostic factors for life expectancy after penetrating head injury. Arch Neurol 41:975–977, 1984

Corrigan JD: Substance abuse as a mediating factor in outcome from traumatic brain injury. Arch Phys Med Rehabil 76:302–309, 1995

Corrigan PW, Bach PA: Behavioral treatment, in Textbook of Traumatic Brain Injury. Edited by Silver JM, McAllister TW, Yudofsky SC. Washington, DC, American Psychiatric Publishing, 2005, pp 661–678

Courville CB: Pathology of the Nervous System, 2nd Edition. Mountain View, CA, Pacific Press Publications, 1945

Cowell LC, Cohen RF: Amantadine: a potential adjuvant therapy following traumatic brain injury. J Head Trauma Rehabil 10:91–94, 1995

Crawford C: Social problems after severe head injury. N Z Med J 96:972–974, 1983

Crisostomo EA, Duncan PW, Propst M, et al: Evidence that amphetamine with physical therapy promotes recovery of motor function in stroke patients. Ann Neurol 23:94–97, 1988

Cummings JL, Mega M, Gray K, et al: The Neuropsychiatric Inventory: comprehensive assessment of psychopathology in dementia. Neurology 44:2308–2314, 1994

Davidson J: Seizures and bupropion: a review. J Clin Psychiatry 50:256–261, 1989

Davison K, Bagley CR: Schizophrenic-like psychoses associated with organic disorders of the central nervous system: a review of the literature, in Current Problems in Neuropsychiatry: Schizophrenia, Epilepsy, the Temporal Lobe. Edited by Herrington RN. Br J Psychiatry (special publication no 4), 1969, pp 113–184

Deb S, Lyons I, Koutzoukis C, et al: Rate of psychiatric illness 1 year after traumatic brain injury. Am J Psychiatry 156:374–378, 1999

DeKosky ST, Kochanek PM, Clark RS, et al: Secondary injury after head trauma: subacute and long-term mechanisms. Semin Clin Neuropsychiatry 3:176–185, 1998

Department of Rehabilitation Medicine: Brain Injury Screening Questionnaire 2000 (BISQ): Research and Training Center on Community Integration of Individuals With Traumatic Brain Injury. New York, Department of Rehabilitation Medicine, The Mount Sinai Center, 2000

Dewar D, Graham DI: Depletion of choline acetyltransferase but preservation of M1 and M2 muscarinic receptor binding sites in temporal cortex following head injury: a preliminary human postmortem study. J Neurotrauma 13:181–187, 1996

Dietch JT, Jennings RK: Aggressive dyscontrol in patients treated with benzodiazepines. J Clin Psychiatry 49:184–189, 1988

Dikmen S, Machamer JE: Neurobehavioral outcomes and their determinants. J Head Trauma Rehabil 10:74–86, 1995

Dikmen S, Reitan RM: Emotional sequelae of head injury. Ann Neurol 2:492–494, 1977

Dikmen S, McLean A, Temkin N: Neuropsychological and psychosocial consequences of minor head injury. J Neurol Neurosurg Psychiatry 49:1227–1232, 1986

Dikmen SS, Temkin NR, Miller B, et al: Neurobehavioral effects of phenytoin prophylaxis of posttraumatic seizures. JAMA 265:1271–1277, 1991

Dikmen SS, Machamer JE, Win HR, et al: Neuropsychological effects of valproate in traumatic brain injury: a randomized trial. Neurology 54:895–902, 2000

Dolan RJ, Bench CJ, Brown RG, et al: Regional cerebral blood flow abnormalities in depressed patients with cognitive impairment. J Neurol Neurosurg Psychiatry 55:768–773, 1992

Donnemiller E, Brenneis C, Wissel J, et al: Impaired dopaminergic neurotransmission in patients with traumatic brain injury: a SPECT study using 123I-beta-CIT and 123I-IBZM. Eur J Nucl Med 27:1410–1414, 2000

Drubach D, McAlaster R, Hartman P: The use of a psychoanalytic framework in the rehabilitation of patients with traumatic brain injury. Am J Psychoanal 54:255–263, 1994

Easdon C, Levine B, O'Connor C, et al: Neural activity associated with response inhibition following traumatic brain injury: an event-related fMRI investigation. Brain Cogn 54:136–138, 2004

Eames P: The use of Sinemet and bromocriptine. Brain Inj 3:319–320, 1989

Eames P: Feeling cold: an unusual brain injury symptom and its treatment with vasopressin. J Neurol Neurosurg Psychiatry 62:198–199, 1997

Eames P, Sutton A: Protracted post-traumatic confusional state treated with physostigmine. Brain Inj 9:729–734, 1995

Eames P, Wood R: Rehabilitation after severe brain injury: a follow-up study of a behavior modification approach. J Neurol Neurosurg Psychiatry 48:613–619, 1985

Echiverri HC, Tatum WO, Merens TA, et al: Akinetic mutism: pharmacologic probe of the dopaminergic mesencephalofrontal activating system. Pediatr Neurol 4:228–230, 1988

Evans RW, Gualtieri CT, Patterson D: Treatment of chronic closed head injury with psychostimulant drugs: a controlled case study and an appropriate evaluation procedure. J Nerv Ment Dis 175:106–110, 1987

Faden AI, Demediuk P, Panter S, et al: The role of excitatory amino acids and NMDA receptors in traumatic brain injury. Science 244:798–800, 1989

Fann JR, Katon WJ, Uomoto JM, et al: Psychiatric disorders and functional disability in outpatients with traumatic brain injuries. Am J Psychiatry 152:1493–1499, 1995

Fann JR, Uomoto JM, Katon WJ: Sertraline in the treatment of major depression following mild traumatic brain injury. J Neuropsychiatry Clin Neurosci 12:226–232, 2000

Fann JR, Uomoto JM, Katon WJ: Cognitive improvement with treatment of depression following mild traumatic brain injury. Psychosomatics 42:48–54, 2001

Fann JR, Leonetti A, Jaffe K, et al: Psychiatric illness and subsequent traumatic brain injury: a case control study. J Neurol Neurosurg Psychiatry 72:615–620, 2002

Favale E, Rubino V, Mainaardi P, et al: Anticonvulsant effect of fluoxetine in humans. Neurology 45:1926–1927, 1995

Fay GC, Jaffe KM, Polissar NL, et al: Mild pediatric brain injury: a cohort study. Arch Phys Med Rehabil 74:895–901, 1993

Federoff PJ, Starkstein SE, Forrester AW, et al: Depression in patients with acute traumatic brain injury. Am J Psychiatry 149:918–923, 1992

Feeney DM, Westerberg VS: Norepinephrine and brain damage: alpha noradrenergic pharmacology alters functional recovery after cortical trauma. Can J Psychol 44:233–252, 1990

Feeney DM, Gonzalez A, Law WA: Amphetamine, haloperidol, and experience interact to affect rate of recovery after motor cortex injury. Science 217:855–857, 1982

Feinstein A, Hershkop S, Ouchterlony D, et al: Posttraumatic amnesia and recall of a traumatic event following traumatic brain injury. J Neuropsychiatry Clin Neurosci 14:25–30, 2002

Feldman H, Crumrine P, Handen BL, et al: Methylphenidate in children with seizures and attention-deficit disorder. Am J Dis Child 143:1081–1086, 1989

Fichtenberg NL, Millis SR, Mann NR, et al: Factors associated with insomnia among post-acute traumatic brain injury survivors. Brain Inj 14:659–667, 2000

Freeman JR, Barth JT, Broshek DK, et al: Sports injuries, in Textbook of Traumatic Brain Injury. Edited by Silver JM, McAllister, Yudofsky SC. Washington, DC, American Psychiatric Publishing, 2005, pp 453–476

Freinhar JP, Alvarez WA: Clonazepam treatment of organic brain syndromes in three elderly patients. J Clin Psychiatry 47:525–526, 1986

Frieboes R-M, Muller U, Murck H, et al: Nocturnal hormone secretion and the sleep EEG in patients several months after traumatic brain injury. J Neuropsychiatry Clin Neurosci 11:354–360, 1999

Friedman G, Froom P, Sazbon ML, et al: Apolipoprotein E-epsilon4 genotype predicts a poor outcome in survivors of traumatic brain injury. Neurology 52:244–248, 1999

Friedman SD, Brooks WM, Jung RE, et al: Quantitative proton MRS predicts outcome after traumatic brain injury. Neurology 52:1384–1391, 1999

Gallassi R, Morreale A, Lorusso S, et al: Carbamazepine and phenytoin: comparison of cognitive effects in epileptic patients during monotherapy and withdrawal. Arch Neurol 45:892–894, 1988

Garyfallos G, Manos N, Adamopoulou A: Psychopathology and personality characteristics of epileptic patients: epilepsy, psychopathology and personality. Acta Psychiatr Scand 78:87–95, 1988

Gennarelli TA, Graham DI: Neuropathology of the head injuries. Semin Clin Neuropsychiatry 3:160–175, 1998

Gennarelli TA, Graham DI: Neuropathology, in Textbook of Traumatic Brain Injury. Edited by Silver JM, McAllister TM, Yudofsky SC. Washington, DC, American Psychiatric Publishing, 2005, pp 27–50

Gennarelli TA, Thibault LE, Adams JH, et al: Diffuse axonal injury and traumatic coma in the primate. Ann Neurol 12:564–574, 1982

Geracioti TD: Valproic acid treatment of episodic explosiveness related to brain injury. J Clin Psychiatry 55:416–417, 1994

Gerberich SG, Priest JD, Boen JR, et al: Concussion incidences and severity in secondary school varsity football players. Am J Public Health 73:1370–1375, 1983

Giakas WJ, Seibyl JP, Mazure CM: Valproate in the treatment of temper outbursts (letter). J Clin Psychiatry 51:525, 1990

Glenn MB, Wroblewski B, Parziale J, et al: Lithium carbonate for aggressive behavior or affective instability in ten brain-injured patients. Am J Phys Med Rehabil 68:221–226, 1989

Goldbaum GM, Remington PL, Powell KE, et al: Failure to use seat belts in the United States: the 1981–1983 behavioral risk factor surveys. JAMA 255:2459–2462, 1986

Goldberg RJ, Goldberg JS: Low-dose risperidone for dementia related disturbed behavior in nursing home. Paper presented at the annual meeting of the American Psychiatric Association, Miami, FL, May 20–25, 1995

Goldstein LB: Prescribing of potentially harmful drugs to patients admitted to hospital after head injury. J Neurol Neurosurg Psychiatry 58:753–755, 1995

Goldstein LB, Davis JN: Physician prescribing patterns following hospital admission for ischemic cerebrovascular disease. Neurology 38:1806–1809, 1988

Goldstein LB, Davis JN: Clonidine impairs recovery of beamwalking after a sensorimotor cortex lesion in the rat. Brain Res 508:305–309, 1990

Goodin DS, Aminoff MJ, Laxer KD: Detection of epileptiform activity by different noninvasive EEG methods in complex partial epilepsy. Ann Neurol 27:330–334, 1990

Gordon WA, Hibbard MR: Cognitive rehabilitation, in Textbook of Traumatic Brain Injury. Edited by Silver JM, McAllister, Yudofsky SC. Washington, DC, American Psychiatric Publishing, 2005, pp 655–660

Gordon WA, Brown M, Sliwinski M, et al: The enigma of "hidden" traumatic brain injury. J Head Trauma Rehabil 13:1–18, 1998

Graves AB, White E, Koepsell TD, et al: The association between head trauma and Alzheimer's disease. Am J Epidemiol 131:491–501, 1990

Grigsby J, Kaye K: Incidence and correlates of depersonalization following head trauma. Brain Inj 7:507–513, 1993

Gross H, Kling A, Henry G, et al: Local cerebral glucose metabolism in patients with long-term behavioral and cognitive deficits following mild traumatic brain injury. J Neuropsychiatry Clin Neurosci 8:324–334, 1996

Grossman R, Beyer C, Kelly P, et al: Acetylcholine and related enzymes in human ventricular and subarachnoid fluids following brain injury, in Proceedings of the 5th Annual Meeting for Neuroscience 76:506, 1975

Gualtieri CT, Evans RW: Stimulant treatment for the neurobehavioural sequelae of traumatic brain injury. Brain Inj 2:273–290, 1988

Gualtieri T, Chandler M, Coons TB, et al: Amantadine: a new clinical profile for traumatic brain injury. Clin Neuropharmacol 12:258–270, 1989

Guilleminault C, Yuen KM, Gulevich MG, et al: Hypersomnia after head-neck trauma: a medicolegal dilemma. Neurology 54:653–659, 2000

Gulbrandsen GB: Neuropsychological sequelae of light head injuries in older children 6 months after trauma. J Clin Neuropsychol 6:257–268, 1984

Guo Z, Cupples LA, Kurz A, et al: Head injury and the risk of AD in the MIRAGE study. Neurology 54:1316–1323, 2000

Gupta SR, Mlcoch AG: Bromocriptine treatment of nonfluent aphasia. Arch Phys Med Rehabil 73:373–376, 1992

Hagen C: The Rancho Levels of Cognitive Function, 3rd Edition. Downey, CA, Rancho Los Amigos Medical Center, 1998

Hall KM, Karzmark P, Stevens M, et al: Family stressors in traumatic brain injury: a two-year follow-up. Arch Phys Med Rehabil 75:876–884, 1994

Halliday AL: Pathophysiology, in Traumatic Brain Injury. Edited by Marion DW. New York, Thieme Medical Publishers, 1999, pp 29–38

Hamill RW, Woolf PD, McDonald JV, et al: Catecholamines predict outcome in traumatic brain injury. Ann Neurol 21:438–443, 1987

Hamilton M: A rating scale for depression. J Neurol Neurosurg Psychiatry 23:56–62, 1960

Hamm RJ, Dixon CE, Gbadebo DM, et al: Cognitive deficits following traumatic brain produced by controlled cortical impact. J Neurotrauma 9:11–20, 1992

Harvey AG, Bryant RA: Two-year prospective evaluation of the relationship between acute stress disorder and posttraumatic stress disorder following mild traumatic brain injury. Am J Psychiatry 15:626–628, 2000

Hendryx PM: Psychosocial changes perceived by closed-head-injured adults and their families. Arch Phys Med Rehabil 70:526–530, 1989

Herrmann N, Lanctot K, Myszak M: Effectiveness of gabapentin for the treatment of behavioral disorders in dementia. J Clin Psychopharmacol 20:90–93, 2000

Hibbard MR, Uysal S, Kepler K, et al: Axis I psychopathology in individuals with traumatic brain injury. J Head Trauma Rehabil 13:24–39, 1998a

Hibbard MR, Uysal S, Sliwinski M, et al: Undiagnosed health issues in individuals with traumatic brain injury living in the community. J Head Trauma Rehabil 13:47–57, 1998b

Hibbard MR, Bogdany J, Uysal S, et al: Axis II psychopathology in individuals with traumatic brain injury. Brain Inj 14:45–61, 2000

Hicks RR, Smith DH, Lowenstein DH, et al: Mild experimental brain injury in the rat induces cognitive deficits associated with regional neuronal loss in the hippocampus. J Neurotrauma 10:405–414, 1993

Hoare P: The development of psychiatric disorder among schoolchildren with epilepsy. Dev Med Child Neurol 26:3–13, 1984

Holsinger T, Steffens DC, Phillips C, et al: Head injury in early adulthood and the lifetime risk of depression. Arch Gen Psychiatry 59:17–22, 2002

Honig LS, Albers GW: Neuropharmacological treatment for acute brain injury, in Neuropsychiatry of Traumatic Brain Injury. Edited by Silver JM, Yudofsky SC, Hales RE. Washington, DC, American Psychiatric Press, 1994, pp 771–804

Horne M, Lindley SE: Divalproex sodium in the treatment of aggressive behavior and dysphoria in patients with organic brain syndromes. J Clin Psychiatry 56:430–431, 1995

Hornstein A, Seliger G: Cognitive side effects of lithium in closed head injury (letter). J Neuropsychiatry Clin Neurosci 1:446–447, 1989

Hovda DA, Fenney DM: Amphetamine with experience promotes recovery of locomotor function after unilateral frontal cortex injury in the cat. Brain Res 298:358–361, 1984

Hugenholtz H, Stuss DT, Stethem LL, et al: How long does it take to recover from a mild concussion? Neurosurgery 22:853–858, 1988

Inglese M, Makani S, Johnson G, et al: Diffuse axonal injury in mild traumatic brain injury. J Neurosurg 103:298–303, 2005

Insurance Institute for Highway Safety, Highway Loss Data Institute: Fatality facts: alcohol. Washington, DC, Insurance Institute for Highway Safety, Highway Loss Data Institute, 2005a. Available at: http://www.iihs.org/research/fatality_facts/alcohol.html. Accessed January 10, 2007.

Insurance Institute for Highway Safety, Highway Loss Data Institute: Fatality facts: bicycles. Washington, DC, Insurance Institute for Highway Safety, Highway Loss Data Institute, 2005b. Available at: http://www.iihs.org/research/fatality_facts/bicycles.html. Accessed January 10, 2007.

Insurance Institute for Highway Safety, Highway Loss Data Institute: Fatality facts: motorcycles. Washington, DC, Insurance Institute for Highway Safety, Highway Loss Data Institute, 2005c. Available at: http://www.iihs.org/research/fatality_facts/motorcycles.html. Accessed January 10, 2007.

Insurance Institute for Highway Safety, Highway Loss Data Institute: Fatality facts: children. Washington, DC, Insurance Institute for Highway Safety, Highway Loss Data Institute, 2005d. Available at: http://www.iihs.org/research/fatality_facts/children.html. Accessed January 10, 2007.

Jackson RD, Corrigan JD, Arnett JA: Amitriptyline for agitation in head injury. Arch Phys Med Rehabil 66:180–181, 1985

Jacobs A, Put E, Ingels M, et al: Prospective evaluation of technetium-99m-HMPAO SPECT in mild and moderate traumatic brain injury. J Nucl Med 35:942–947, 1994

Jagger J: Prevention of brain trauma by legislation, regulation, and improved technology: a focus on motor vehicles. J Neurotrauma 9 (suppl):S313–S316, 1992

Jane JA, Steward O, Gennarelli T: Axonal degeneration induced by experimental noninvasive minor injury. J Neurosurg 62:96–100, 1985

Jellinger KA: Head injury and dementia. Curr Opin Neurol 17:719–723, 2004

Jordan BD, Relkin NR, Ravdin LD, et al: Apolipoprotein E epsilon4 associated with chronic traumatic brain injury in boxing. JAMA 278:136–140, 1997

Jorge RE, Robinson RG, Starkstein SE, et al: Depression and anxiety following traumatic brain injury. J Neuropsychiatry Clin Neurosci 5:369–374, 1993

Jorge RE, Robinson RG, Starkstein SE, et al: Influence of major depression on 1-year outcome in patients with traumatic brain injury. J Neurosurg 81:726–733, 1994

Jorge RE, Robinson RG, Moser D, et al: Major depression following traumatic brain injury. Arch Gen Psychiatry 61:42–50, 2004

Kaelin DL, Cifu DX, Matthies B: Methylphenidate effect on attention deficit in the acutely brain-injured adult. Arch Phys Med Rehabil 77:6–9, 1996

Kant R, Smith-Seemiller L, Zeiler D: Treatment of aggression and irritability after head injury. Brain Inj 12:661–666, 1998

Kant R, Coffey CE, Bogyi AM: Safety and efficacy of ECT in patients with head injury: a case series. J Neuropsychiatry Clin Neurosci 11:32–37, 1999

Kaplan BH, Cowley RA: Seatbelt effectiveness and cost of noncompliance among drivers admitted to a trauma center. Am J Emerg Med 9:4–10, 1991

Kapoor N, Ciuffreda KJ: Vision problems, in Textbook of Traumatic Brain Injury. Edited by Silver JM, McAllister, Yudofsky SC. Washington, DC, American Psychiatric Publishing, 2005, pp 405–417

Karakucuk EI, Pasaoglu H, Pasaoglu A, et al: Endogenous neuropeptides in patients with acute traumatic head injury, II: changes in the levels of cerebrospinal fluid substance P, serotonin and lipid peroxidation products in patients with head trauma. Neuropeptides 31:259–263, 1997

Kass F, Silver JM: Neuropsychiatry and the homeless. J Neuropsychiatry Clin Neurosci 2:15–19, 1990

Katzman R, Galasko DR, Saitoh T, et al: Apolipoprotein-epsilon4 and head trauma: synergistic or additive risks? Neurology 46:889–891, 1996

Kaufer DI, Cummings JL, Ketchel P, et al: Validation of the NPI-Q, a brief clinical form of the Neuropsychiatric Inventory. J Neuropsychiatry Clin Neurosci 12:233–239, 2000

Kay SR, Fiszbein A, Opler LA: The Positive and Negative Syndrome Scale (PANSS) for schizophrenia. Schizophr Bull 13:261–276, 1987

Kay T: Neuropsychological treatment of mild traumatic brain injury. J Head Trauma Rehabil 8:74–85, 1993

Kaye NS, Townsend JB 3rd, Ivins R: An open-label trial of donepezil (Aricept) in the treatment of persons with mild traumatic brain injury. J Neuropsychiatry Clin Neurosci 15:383–384, 2003

Keats MM, Mukherjee S: Antiaggressive effect of adjunctive clonazepam in schizophrenia associated with seizure disorder. J Clin Psychiatry 49:117–118, 1988

Kelly JP: Concussion, in Current Therapy in Sports Medicine, 3rd Edition. Edited by Torg JS, Shephard RJ. Philadelphia, PA, CV Mosby, 1995, pp 21–24

Keshavan MS, Channabasavanna SM, Narahana Reddy GN: Post-traumatic psychiatric disturbances: patterns and predictors of outcome. Br J Psychiatry 138:157–160, 1981

Kim E: Elderly, in Textbook of Traumatic Brain Injury. Edited by Silver JM, McAllister TM, Yudofsky SC. Washington, DC, American Psychiatric Publishing, 2005, pp 495–508

King NS, Crawford S, Wenden FJ, et al: The Rivermead Post Concussion Symptoms Questionnaire: a measure of symptoms commonly experienced after head injury and its reliability. J Neurol 242:587–592, 1995

Koponen S, Taiminen T, Portin R, et al: Axis I and II psychiatric disorders after traumatic brain injury: a 30 year follow-up study. Am J Psychiatry 159:1315–1321, 2002

Koren D, Arnon I, Klein E: Acute stress response and posttraumatic stress disorder in traffic victims: a one-year prospective, follow-up study. Am J Psychiatry 156:367–373, 1999

Kraus JF, Chu LD: Epidemiology, in Textbook of Traumatic Brain Injury. Edited by Silver JM, McAllister TM, Yudofsky SC. Washington, DC, American Psychiatric Publishing, 2005, pp 3–26

Kraus MF, Maki PM: Effect of amantadine hydrochloride on symptoms of frontal lobe dysfunction in brain injury: case studies and review. J Neuropsychiatry Clin Neurosci 9:222–230, 1997

Kraus JF, Nourjah P: The epidemiology of mild, uncomplicated brain injury. J Trauma 28:1637–1643, 1988

Kraus JF, Sorenson SB: Epidemiology, in Neuropsychiatry of Traumatic Brain Injury. Edited by Silver JM, Yudofsky SC, Hales RE. Washington, DC, American Psychiatric Press, 1994, pp 3–41

Kraus JF, Morgenstern H, Fife D, et al: Blood alcohol tests, prevalence of involvement, and outcomes following brain injury. Am J Public Health 79:294–299, 1989

Kreutzer JS, Gervasio AH, Camplair PS: Primary caregivers' psychological status and family functioning after traumatic brain injury. Brain Inj 8:197–210, 1994

Kreutzer JS, Seel RT, Gourley E: The prevalence and symptom rates of depression after traumatic brain injury: a comprehensive examination. Brain Inj 15:563–576, 2001

Kuner EH, Schlickewei W, Oltmanns D: Injury reduction by the airbag in accidents. Injury 27:185–188, 1996

Kurtzke JF: Neuroepidemiology. Ann Neurol 16:265–277, 1984

Kuruoglu AC, Arikan Z, Vural G, et al: Single photon emission computerized tomography in chronic alcoholism: antisocial personality disorder may be associated with decreased frontal perfusion. Br J Psychiatry 169:348–354, 1996

Kutner KC, Erlanger DM, Tsai J, et al: Lower cognitive performance of older football players possessing apolipoprotein E e4. Neurosurgery 47:651–657, 2000

Lal S, Merbitz CP, Grip JC: Modification of function in head-injured patients with Sinemet. Brain Inj 2:225–233, 1988

Lauterbach EC, Schweri MM: Amelioration of pseudobulbar affect by fluoxetine: possible alteration of dopamine-related pathophysiology by a selective serotonin reuptake inhibitor. J Clin Psychopharmacol 11:392–393, 1991

Lazarus A, Cotterell KP: SPECT scan reveals abnormality in somatization disorder patient. J Clin Psychiatry 50:475–476, 1989

Leach LR, Frank RG, Bouman DE, et al: Family functioning, social support and depression after traumatic brain injury. Brain Inj 8:599–606, 1994

Leininger BE, Gramling SE, Farrell AD, et al: Neuropsychological deficits in symptomatic minor head injury patients after concussion and mild concussion. J Neurol Neurosurg Psychiatry 53:293–296, 1990

Levin HS, Grossman RG: Behavioral sequelae of closed head injury: a quantitative study. Arch Neurol 35:720–727, 1978

Levin HS, O'Donnell VM, Grossman RG: The Galveston Orientation and Amnesia Test: a practical scale to assess cognition after head injury. J Nerv Ment Dis 167:675–684, 1979

Levin HS, Benton AL, Grossman RG: Neurobehavioral Consequences of Closed Head Injury. New York, Oxford University Press, 1982

Levin HS, High WM, Eisenberg HM: Impairment of olfactory recognition after closed head injury. Brain 108:579–591, 1985

Levin HS, Amparo E, Eisenberg HM, et al: Magnetic resonance imaging and computerized tomography in relation to the neurobehavioral sequelae of mild and moderate head injuries. J Neurosurg 66:706–713, 1987a

Levin HS, High WM, Goethe KE, et al: The Neurobehavioral Rating Scale: assessment of the behavioral sequelae of head injury by the clinician. J Neurol Neurosurg Psychiatry 50:183–193, 1987b

Levin HS, Mattis S, Ruff RM, et al: Neurobehavioral outcome following minor head injury: a three-center study. J Neurosurg 66:234–243, 1987c

Levin HS, Goldstein FC, High WM Jr, et al: Disproportionately severe memory deficit in relation to normal intellectual functioning after closed head injury. J Neurol Neurosurg Psychiatry 51:1294–1301, 1988

Li G: Child injuries and fatalities from alcohol-related motor vehicle crashes: call for a zero-tolerance policy. JAMA 283:2291–2292, 2000

Lichtman SW, Seliger G, Tycko B, et al: Apolipoprotein E and functional recovery from brain injury following postacute rehabilitation. Neurology 55:1536–1539, 2000

Lieberman JA, Kane JM, Johns CA: Clozapine: guidelines for clinical management. J Clin Psychiatry 50:329–338, 1989

Linn RT, Allen K, Willer BS: Affective symptoms in the chronic stage of traumatic brain injury: a study of married couples. Brain Inj 8:135–147, 1994

Lipper S, Tuchman MM: Treatment of chronic post-traumatic organic brain syndrome with dextroamphetamine: first reported case. J Nerv Ment Dis 162:266–371, 1976

Livingston MG, Brooks DN, Bond MR: Patient outcome in the year following severe head injury and relatives' psychiatric and social functioning. J Neurol Neurosurg Psychiatry 48:876–881, 1985a

Livingston MG, Brooks DN, Bond MR: Three months after severe head injury: psychiatric and social impact on relatives. J Neurol Neurosurg Psychiatry 48:870–875, 1985b

Livingston S, Pauli LL: Dextroamphetamine for epilepsy. JAMA 233:278–279, 1975

Lovell MR, Iverson GL, Collins MW, et al: Does loss of consciousness predict neuropsychological decrements after concussion? Clin J Sport Med 9:193–198, 1999

Lowenstein DH, Thomas MJ, Smith DH, et al: Selective vulnerability of dentate hilar neurons following traumatic brain injury: a potential mechanistic link between head trauma and disorders of the hippocampus. J Neurosci 12:4846–4853, 1992

Mahoney WJ, D'Souza BJ, Haller JA, et al: Long-term outcome of children with severe head trauma and prolonged coma. Pediatrics 71:754–762, 1983

Malaspina D, Goetz RR, Friedman JH, et al: Traumatic brain injury and schizophrenia in members of schizophrenia and bipolar disorder pedigrees. Am J Psychiatry 36:1278–1285, 2001

Mann JJ, Waternaux C, Haas GL, et al: Toward a clinical model of suicidal behavior in psychiatric patients. Am J Psychiatry 156:181–189, 1999

Marin RS, Chakravorty S: Disorders of diminished motivation, in Textbook of Traumatic Brain Injury. Edited by Silver JM, McAllister TM, Yudofsky SC. Washington, DC, American Psychiatric Publishing, 2005, pp 337–352

Martin R, Kuzniecky R, Ho S, et al: Cognitive effects of topiramate, gabapentin, and lamotrigine in healthy young adults. Neurology 52:321–327, 1999

Masdeu JC, Van Heertum RL, Kleiman A, et al: Early single-photon emission computed tomography in mild head trauma: a controlled study. J Neuroimaging 4:177–181, 1994

Massey EW, Folger WN: Seizures activated by therapeutic levels of lithium carbonate. South Med J 77:1173–1175, 1984

Mattes JA: Valproic acid for nonaffective aggression in the mentally retarded. J Nerv Ment Dis 180:601–602, 1992

Max JE: Children and adolescents, in Textbook of Traumatic Brain Injury. Edited by Silver JM, McAllister TM, Yudofsky SC. Washington, DC, American Psychiatric Publishing, 2005, pp 477–494

Max JE, Castillo CS, Robin DA, et al: Posttraumatic stress symptomatology after childhood traumatic brain injury. J Nerv Ment Dis 186:589–596, 1998a

Max JE, Robin DA, Lindgren SD, et al: Traumatic brain injury in children and adolescents: psychiatric disorders at one year. J Neuropsychiatry Clin Neurosci 10:290–297, 1998b

Max W, MacKenzie E, Rice D: Head injuries: costs and consequences. J Head Trauma Rehabil 6:76–91, 1991

Mayeux R, Ottman R, Tang MX, et al: Genetic susceptibility and head injury as risk factors for Alzheimer's disease among community-dwelling elderly persons and their first-degree relatives. Ann Neurol 33:494–501, 1993

Mayeux R, Ottman R, Maestre G, et al: Synergistic effects of traumatic head injury and apolipoprotein-epsilon 4 in patients with Alzheimer's disease. Neurology 45:555–557, 1995

McAllister TW: Mild traumatic brain injury and the postconcussive syndrome, in Neuropsychiatry of Traumatic Brain Injury. Edited by Silver JM, Yudofsky SC, Hales RE. Washington, DC, American Psychiatric Press, 1994, pp 357–392

McAllister TW: Traumatic brain injury and psychosis: what is the connection? Semin Clin Neuropsychiatry 3:211–223, 1998

McAllister TW: Mild brain injury and the postconcussion syndrome, in Textbook of Traumatic Brain Injury. Edited by Silver JM, McAllister, Yudofsky SC. Washington, DC, American Psychiatric Publishing, 2005, pp 279–308

McAllister TW, Saykin AJ, Flashman LA, et al: Brain activation during working memory 1 month after mild traumatic brain injury: a functional MRI study. Neurology 53:1300–1308, 1999

McAllister TW, Sparling MB, Flashman LA, et al: Differential working memory load effects after mild traumatic brain injury. Neuroimage 14:1004–1012, 2001

McCullagh S, Feinstein A: Cognitive changes, in Textbook of Traumatic Brain Injury. Edited by Silver JM, McAllister TM, Yudofsky SC. Washington, DC, American Psychiatric Publishing, 2005, pp 321–335

McIntosh TK, Juhler M, Raghupathi R, et al: Secondary brain injury: neurochemical and cellular mediators, in Traumatic Brain Injury. Edited by Marion DW. New York, Thieme Medical Publishers, 1999, pp 39–54

McKenna PJ, Kane JM, Parrish K: Psychotic syndromes in epilepsy. Am J Psychiatry 142:895–904, 1985

McKinlay WW, Brooks DN, Bond MR, et al: The short-term outcome of severe blunt head injury as reported by the relatives of the injured person. J Neurol Neurosurg Psychiatry 44:527–533, 1981

McLean A Jr, Dikmen S, Temkin N, et al: Psychosocial functioning at 1 month after head injury. Neurosurgery 14:393–399, 1984

McMillan TM: Post-traumatic stress disorder following minor and severe closed head injury: 10 single cases. Brain Inj 10:749–758, 1996

McMillan TM, Glucksman EE: The neuropsychology of moderate head injury. J Neurol Neurosurg Psychiatry 50:393–397, 1987

Michals ML, Crismon ML, Roberts S, et al: Clozapine response and adverse effects in nine brain-injured patients. J Clin Psychopharmacol 13:198–203, 1993

Michaud LJ, Rivara FP, Jaffe KM, et al: Traumatic brain injury as a risk factor for behavioral disorders in children. Arch Phys Med Rehabil 74:368–375, 1993

Mild Traumatic Brain Injury Committee of the Head Injury Interdisciplinary Special Interest Group of the American Congress of Rehabilitation Medicine: Definition of mild traumatic brain injury. J Head Trauma Rehabil 8:86–87, 1993

Mittl RL, Grossman RI, Hiehle JF, et al: Prevalence of MR evidence of diffuse axonal injury in patients with mild head injury and normal head CT findings. AJNR Am J Neuroradiol 15:1583–1589, 1994

Mooney GF, Haas LJ: Effect of methylphenidate on brain injury–related anger. Arch Phys Med Rehabil 74:153–160, 1993

Morey CE, Cilo M, Berry J, et al: The effect of Aricept in persons with persistent memory disorder following traumatic brain injury: a pilot study. Brain Inj 17:809–816, 2003

Morrison JH, Molliver ME, Grzanna R: Noradrenergic innervation of cerebral cortex: widespread effects of local cortical lesions. Science 205:313–316, 1979

Moskowitz AS, Altshuler L: Increased sensitivity to lithium-induced neurotoxicity after stroke: a case report. J Clin Psychopharmacol 11:272–273, 1991

Murdoch I, Perry EK, Court JA, et al: Cortical cholinergic dysfunction after human head injury. J Neurotrauma 15:295–305, 1998

Mysiw WJ, Jackson RD, Corrigan JD: Amitriptyline for post-traumatic agitation. Am J Phys Med Rehabil 67:29–33, 1988

Nagamachi S, Nichikawa T, Ono S, et al: A comparative study of 123I-IMP SPET and CT in the investigation of chronic-stage head trauma patients. Nucl Med Commun 16:17–25, 1995

Nahas Z, Arlinghaus KA, Kotrla KJ, et al: Rapid response of emotional incontinence to selective serotonin reuptake inhibitors. J Neuropsychiatry Clin Neurosci 10:453–455, 1998

Nasrallah HA, Fowler RC, Judd LL: Schizophrenia-like illness following head injury. Psychosomatics 22:359–361, 1981

National Safety Council: Accident Facts. Chicago, IL, National Safety Council, 1985

National Safety Council: Accident Facts. Chicago, IL, National Safety Council, 1986

National Safety Council: Accident Facts. Chicago, IL, National Safety Council, 1999

National Safety Council: Report on Injuries in America. 2006. Available at: http://www.nsc.org/library/report_injury_usa.htm.Accessed January 15, 2007.

Nedd K, Sfakianakis G, Ganz W, et al: 99mTc-HMPAO SPECT of the brain in mild to moderate traumatic brain injury patients: compared with CT: a prospective study. Brain Inj 7:469–479, 1993

Nemetz PN, Leibson C, Naessens JM, et al: Traumatic brain injury and time to onset of Alzheimer's disease: a population-based study. Am J Epidemiol 149:32–40, 1999

Neurobehavioral Guidelines Working Group; Warden DL, Gordon B, McAllister TW, et al: Guidelines for the pharmacologic treatment of neurobehavioral sequelae of traumatic brain injury. J Neurotrama 23:1468–1501, 2006

NIH Consensus Development Panel on Rehabilitation of Persons With Traumatic Brain Injury: Rehabilitation of persons with traumatic brain injury. JAMA 282:974–983, 1999

Nickels JL, Schneider WN, Dombovy ML, et al: Clinical use of amantadine in brain injury rehabilitation. Brain Inj 8:709–718, 1994

Nizamie SH, Nizamie A, Borde M, et al: Mania following head injury: case reports and neuropsychological findings. Acta Psychiatr Scand 77:637–639, 1988

Noyes R Jr: Motor vehicle accidents related to psychiatric impairment. Psychosomatics 26:569–580, 1985

Nuwer MR: Assessment of digital EEG, quantitative EEG and EEG brain mapping: report of the American Academy of Neurology and the American Clinical Neurophysiology Society. Neurology 49:277–292, 1997

Obrenovitch TP, Urenjak J: Is high extracellular glutamate the key to excitotoxicity in traumatic brain injury? J Neurotrauma 14:677–698, 1997

Oddy M, Humphrey M, Uttley D: Stresses upon the relatives of head-injured patients. Br J Psychiatry 133:507–513, 1978

Oddy M, Coughlan T, Tyerman A, et al: Social adjustment after closed head injury: a further follow-up seven years after injury. J Neurol Neurosurg Psychiatry 48:564–568, 1985

Ohry A, Rattok J, Solomon Z: Post-traumatic stress disorder in brain injury patients. Brain Inj 10:687–695, 1996

Ojemann LM, Baugh-Bookman C, Dudley DL: Effect of psychotropic medications on seizure control in patients with epilepsy. Neurology 37:1525–1527, 1987

Oliver AP, Luchins DJ, Wyatt RJ: Neuroleptic-induced seizures: an in vitro technique for assessing relative risk. Arch Gen Psychiatry 39:206–209, 1982

Oppenheimer DR: Microscopic lesions in the brain following head injury. J Neurol Neurosurg Psychiatry 31:299–306, 1968

Oquendo MA, Friedman JH, Grunebaum MF, et al: Mild traumatic brain injury and suicidal behavior in major depression. J Nerv Ment Dis 192:430–434, 2004

Orrison WW, Gentry LR, Stimac GK, et al: Blinded comparison of cranial CT and MR in closed head injury evaluation. AJNR Am J Neuroradiol 15:351–356, 1994

Orsay EM, Turnbull TL, Dunne M, et al: Prospective study of the effect of safety belts on morbidity and health care costs in motor-vehicle accidents. JAMA 260:3598–3603, 1988

Palmer AM, Marion DW, Botscheller ML, et al: Increased transmitter amino acid concentration in human ventricular CSF after brain trauma. Neuroreport 30:153–156, 1994

Panzer MJ, Mellow AM: Antidepressant treatment of pathologic laughing or crying in elderly stroke patients. J Geriatr Psychiatry Neurol 4:195–199, 1992

Parker RS, Rosenblum A: IQ loss and emotional dysfunctions after mild head injury in a motor vehicle accident. J Clin Psychol 52:32–43, 1996

Parks RW, Crockett DJ, Manji HK, et al: Assessment of bromocriptine intervention for the treatment of frontal lobe syndrome: a case study. J Neuropsychiatry Clin Neurosci 4:109–110, 1992

Pinder RM, Brogden RN, Speight TM, et al: Maprotiline: a review of its pharmacological properties and therapeutic efficacy in mental states. Drugs 13:321–352, 1977

Plenger PM, Dixon CE, Castillo RM, et al: Subacute methylphenidate treatment for moderate to moderately severe traumatic brain injury: a preliminary double-blind placebo-controlled study. Arch Phys Med Rehabil 77:536–540, 1996

Poeck K: Pathological laughter and crying, in Handbook of Clinical Neurology, Vol. 45: Clinical Neuropsychology, No 1. Edited by Fredericks JAM. Amsterdam, Elsevier, 1985, pp 219–225

Pollack IW: Traumatic brain injury and the rehabilitation process: a psychiatric perspective, in Neuropsychological Treatment After Brain Injury. Edited by Ellis D, Christensen A-L. Boston, MA, Kluwer Academic, 1989, pp 105–127

Pollack IW: Psychotherapy, in Textbook of Traumatic Brain Injury. Edited by Silver JM, McAllister, Yudofsky SC. Washington, DC, American Psychiatric Publishing, 2005, pp 641–654

Ponsford J, Kinsella G: Attention deficits following closed head injury. J Clin Exp Neuropsychol 14:822–838, 1992

Pope HG Jr, McElroy SL, Satlin A, et al: Head injury, bipolar disorder, and response to valproate. Compr Psychiatry 29:34–38, 1988

Porch B, Wyckes J, Feeney DM: Haloperidol, thiazides and some antihypertensives slow recovery from aphasia. Abstr Soc Neurosci 11:52, 1985

Porta M, Bareggi SR, Collice M, et al: Homovanillic acid and 5-hydroxyindole-acetic acid in the CSF of patients after a severe head injury, II: ventricular CSF concentrations in acute brain post-traumatic syndromes. Eur Neurol 13:545–554, 1975

Povlishock JT, Coburn TH: Morphopathological change associated with mild head injury, in Mild Head Injury. Edited by Levin HS, Eisenberg HM, Benton AL. New York, Oxford University Press, 1989, pp 37–53

Povlishock JT, Becker DP, Cheng CLY, et al: Axonal change in minor head injury. J Neuropathol Exp Neurol 42:225–242, 1983

Powell JW, Barber-Foss KD: Traumatic brain injury in high school athletes. JAMA 282:958–963, 1999

Prevey ML, Delany RC, Cramer JA, et al: Effect of valproate on cognitive functioning: comparison with carbamazepine. Arch Neurol 53:1008–1016, 1996

Prigatano GP: Work, love, and play after brain injury. Bull Menninger Clin 53:414–431, 1989

Prigatano GP, Stahl ML, Orr WC, et al: Sleep and dreaming disturbances in closed head injury patients. J Neurol Neurosurg Psychiatry 45:78–80, 1982

Quality Standards Subcommittee of the American Academy of Neurology: Practice parameter. Neurobiology (Bp) 48:1–5, 1997

Quinlan KP, Brewer RD, Sleet DA, et al: Characteristics of child passenger deaths and injuries involving drinking drivers. JAMA 283:2249–2252, 2000

Rammahan KW, Rosenberg JH, Pollak CP, et al: Modafinil: efficacy for the treatment of fatigue in patients with multiple sclerosis (abstract). Neurology 54 (suppl 3):A24, 2000

Ranen NG, Lipsey JR, Treisman G, et al: Sertraline in the treatment of severe aggressiveness in Huntington's disease. J Neuropsychiatry Clin Neurosci 8:338–340, 1996

Rao V, Rollings P, Spiro J: Fatigue and sleep problems, in Textbook of Traumatic Brain Injury. Edited by Silver JM, McAllister, Yudofsky SC. Washington, DC, American Psychiatric Publishing, 2005, pp 369–384

Raphaely RC, Swedlow DB, Downes JJ, et al: Management of severe pediatric head trauma. Pediatr Clin North Am 27:715–727, 1980

Rapoport MJ, McCullagh S, Shammi P, et al: Cognitive impairment associated with major depression following mild and moderate traumatic brain injury. J Neuropsychiatry Clin Neurosci 17:61–65, 2005

Rappaport M, Herrero-Backe C, Rappaport ML, et al: Head injury outcome up to ten years later. Arch Phys Med Rehabil 70:885–892, 1989

Ratey JJ, Leveroni C, Kilmer D, et al: The effects of clozapine on severely aggressive psychiatric inpatients in a state hospital. J Clin Psychiatry 54:219–223, 1993

Rattok J: Do patients with mild brain injuries have posttraumatic stress disorder, too? J Head Trauma Rehabil 11:95–97, 1996

Rauch SL, van Der Kolk BA, Fisler RE, et al: A symptom provocation study of posttraumatic stress disorder using positron emission tomography and script-driven imagery. Arch Gen Psychiatry 53:380–387, 1996

Reeves TM, Lyeth BG, Povlishock JT: Long-term potentiation deficits and excitability changes following traumatic brain injury. Exp Brain Res 106:248–256, 1995

Reinhard DL, Whyte J, Sandel ME: Improved arousal and initiation following tricyclic antidepressant use in severe brain injury. Arch Phys Med Rehabil 77:80–83, 1996

Reynolds EH, Trimble MR: Adverse neuropsychiatric effects of anticonvulsant drugs. Drugs 29:570–581, 1985

Richter EF III: Balance problems and dizziness, in Textbook of Traumatic Brain Injury. Edited by Silver JM, McAllister, Yudofsky SC. Washington, DC, American Psychiatric Publishing, 2005, pp 393–404

Rimel RW, Giordani B, Barht JT, et al: Disability caused by minor head injury. Neurosurgery 9:221–228, 1981

Rivinus TM: Psychiatric effects of the anticonvulsant regimens. J Clin Psychopharmacol 2:165–192, 1992

Roane DM, Feinberg TE, Meckler L, et al: Treatment of dementia-associated agitation with gabapentin. J Neuropsychiatry Clin Neurosci 12:40–43, 2000

Roberts GW, Gentleman SM, Lynch A, et al: Beta amyloid protein depositions in the brain after severe head injury: implications for the pathogenesis of Alzheimer's disease. J Neurol Neurosurg Psychiatry 57:419–423, 1994

Robinson RG, Schultz SK, Castillo C, et al: Nortriptyline versus fluoxetine in the treatment of depression and in short-term recovery after stroke: a placebo-controlled, double-blind study. Am J Psychiatry 157:351–359, 2000

Ross ED, Rush AJ: Diagnosis and neuroanatomical correlates of depression in brain-damaged patients: implications for a neurology of depression. Arch Gen Psychiatry 38:1344–1354, 1981

Ross ED, Stewart RS: Pathological display of affect in patients with depression and right frontal brain damage. An alternative mechanism. J Nerv Ment Dis 176:165–172, 1987

Rothman KJ, Funch DP, Dreyr NA: Bromocriptine and puerperal seizures. Epidemiology 1:232–238, 1990

Ruedrich I, Chu CC, Moore SI: ECT for major depression in a patient with acute brain trauma. Am J Psychiatry 140:928–929, 1983

Sachdev P, Smith JS, Cathcart S: Schizophrenia-like psychosis following traumatic brain injury: a chart-based descriptive and case-control study. Psychol Med 31:231–239, 2001

Salazar AM, Jabbari B, Vance SC, et al: Epilepsy after penetrating head injury, I: clinical correlates: a report of the Vietnam head injury study. Neurology 35:1406–1414, 1985

Salazar AM, Warden DL, Schwab K, et al: Cognitive rehabilitation for traumatic brain injury: a randomized trial. Defense and Veterans Head Injury Program (DVHIP) Study Group. JAMA 283:3075–3081, 2000

Salinsky MC, Storzbach D, Spenceer DC, et al: Effects of topiramate and gabapentin on cognitive abilities in healthy volunteers. Neurology 64:792–798, 2005

Sandel ME, Weiss B, Ivker B: Multiple personality disorder: diagnosis after a traumatic brain injury. Arch Phys Med Rehabil 71:523–535, 1990

Saran AS: Depression after minor closed head injury: role of dexamethasone suppression test and antidepressants. J Clin Psychiatry 46:335–338, 1985

Satz P, Forney DL, Zaucha K, et al: Depression, cognition, and functional correlates of recovery outcome after traumatic brain injury. Brain Inj 12:537–553, 1998

Sbordone RJ, Liter JC: Mild traumatic brain injury does not produce post-traumatic stress disorder. Brain Inj 9:405–412, 1995

Schallert T, Hernandez TD, Barth TM: Recovery of function after brain damage: severe and chronic disruption by diazepam. Brain Res 379:104–111, 1986

Schiff HB, Sabin TD, Geller A, et al: Lithium in aggressive behavior. Am J Psychiatry 139:1346–1348, 1982

Schiffer RB, Herndon RM, Rudick RA: Treatment of pathologic laughing and weeping with amitriptyline. N Engl J Med 312:1480–1482, 1985

Schmitt JA, Kruizinga MJ, Reidel WJ: Non-serotonergic pharmacological profiles and associated cognitive effects of serotonin reuptake inhibitors. J Psychopharmacol 15:173–179, 2001

Seliger GM, Hornstein A, Flax J, et al: Fluoxetine improves emotional incontinence. Brain Inj 6:267–270, 1992

Sheehan DV, Lecrubier Y, Sheehan KH, et al: The Mini-International Neuropsychiatric Interview (MINI): the development and validation of a structured diagnostic psychiatric interview for DSM-IV and ICD-10. J Clin Psychiatry 59 (suppl 20):22–33; quiz 34–57, 1998

Sherer M, Boake C, Levin E, et al: Characteristics of impaired awareness after traumatic brain injury. J Int Neuropsychol Soc 4:380–387, 1998

Sheriff FE, Bridges LR, Sivaloganaathan S: Early detection of axonal injury after human head trauma using immunocytochemistry for beta-amyloid precursor protein. Acta Neuropathol (Berl) 87:55–62, 1994

Silver JM, Anderson KA: Vasopressin treats the persistent feeling of coldness after brain injury. J Neuropsychiatry Clin Neurosci 11:248–252, 1999

Silver JM, McAllister TW: Forensic issues in the neuropsychiatric evaluation of the patient with mild traumatic brain injury. J Neuropsychiatry Clin Neurosci 9:102–113, 1997

Silver JM, Yudofsky SC: Pharmacologic treatment of aggression. Psychiatr Ann 17:397–407, 1987

Silver JM, Yudofsky SC: The Overt Aggression Scale: overview and clinical guidelines. J Neuropsychiatry Clin Neurosci 3:S22–S29, 1991

Silver JM, Yudofsky SC: Aggressive disorders, in Neuropsychiatry of Traumatic Brain Injury. Edited by Silver JM, Yudofsky SC, Hales RE. Washington, DC, American Psychiatric Press, 1994, pp 313–356

Silver JM, Caton CM, Shrout PE, et al: Traumatic brain injury and schizophrenia. Paper presented at the annual meeting of the American Psychiatric Association, San Francisco, CA, May 22–27, 1993

Silver JM, Rattok J, Anderson K: Post-traumatic stress disorder and traumatic brain injury. Neurocase 3:151–157, 1997

Silver JM, Weissman M, Kramer R, et al: Association between severe head injuries and psychiatric disorders: findings from the New Haven NIMH Epidemiologic Catchment Area Study. Brain Inj 15:935–945, 2001

Silver JM, Arciniegas DA, Yudofsky SC: Psychopharmacology, in Textbook of Traumatic Brain Injury. Edited by Silver JM, McAllister TM, Yudofsky SC. Washington, DC, American Psychiatric Publishing, 2005a, pp 609–640

Silver JM, Yudofsky SC, Anderson KE: Aggressive disorders, in Textbook of Traumatic Brain Injury. Edited by Silver JM, McAllister TM, Yudofsky SC. Washington, DC, American Psychiatric Publishing, 2005b, pp 259–278

Silver JM, Koumaras B, Chen M, et al: The effects of rivastigmine on cognitive function in patients with traumatic brain injury. Neurology 67:748–755, 2006

Simantov R: Gamma-aminobutyric acid (GABA) enhances glutamate cytotoxicity in a cerebellar cell line. Brain Res Bull 24:711–715, 1990

Simpson G, Tate R: Suicidality after traumatic brain injury: demographic, injury and clinical correlates. Psychol Med 32:687–697, 2002

Sliwinski M, Gordon WA, Bogdany J: The Beck Depression Inventory: is it a suitable measure of depression for individuals with traumatic brain injury? J Head Trauma Rehabil 13:40–46, 1998

Sloan RL, Brown KW, Pentland B: Fluoxetine as a treatment for emotional lability after brain injury. Brain Inj 6:315–319, 1992

Smith DH, Okiyama K, Thomas MJ, et al: Evaluation of memory dysfunction following experimental brain injury using the Morris water maze. J Neurotrauma 8:259–269, 1991

Smith KR, Goulding PM, Wilderman D, et al: Neurobehavioral effects of phenytoin and carbamazepine in patients recovering from brain trauma: a comparative study. Arch Neurol 51:653–660, 1994

Smith MC, Bleck TP: Convulsive disorders: toxicity of anticonvulsants. Clin Neuropharmacol 14:97–115, 1991

Smith-Seemiller L, Lovell MR, Smith SS: Cognitive dysfunction after closed head injury: contributions of demographics, injury severity and other factors. Appl Neuropsychol 3:41–47, 1996

Sosin DM, Sacks JJ, Smith SM: Head injury-associated deaths in the United States from 1979–1986. JAMA 262:2251–2255, 1989

Speech TJ, Rao SM, Osmon DC, et al: A double-blind controlled study of methylphenidate treatment in closed head injury. Brain Inj 7:333–338, 1993

Spitzer RL, Williams JBW, Gibbon M, et al: Structured Clinical Interview for DSM-IV (SCID) User's Guide. Washington, DC, American Psychiatric Press, 1997

Stankoff B, Waubant E, Confavreux C, et al: Modafinil for fatigue in MS: a randomized placebo-controlled double-blind study. French Modafinil Study Group. Neurology 64:1139–1143, 2005

Starkstein SE, Boston JD, Robinson RG: Mechanisms of mania after brain injury: 12 case reports and review of the literature. J Nerv Ment Dis 176:87–100, 1988

Starkstein SE, Mayberg HS, Berthier ML, et al: Mania after brain injury: neuroradiological and metabolic findings. Ann Neurol 27:652–659, 1990

Stewart JT, Nemsath RH: Bipolar illness following traumatic brain injury: treatment with lithium and carbamazepine. J Clin Psychiatry 49:74–75, 1988

Stuss DT, Binns MA, Carruth FG, et al: The acute period of recovery from traumatic brain injury: posttraumatic amnesia or posttraumatic confusional state? J Neurosurg 90:635–643, 1999

Sutton RL, Feeney DM: Yohimbine accelerates recovery and clonidine and prazosin reinstate deficits after recovery in rats with sensorimotor cortex ablation. Abstr Soc Neurosci 13:913, 1987

Sutton RL, Weaver MS, Feeney DM: Drug-induced modifications of behavioral recovery following cortical trauma. J Head Trauma Rehabil 2:50–58, 1987

Tate R, Simpson G, Flanagan S, et al: Completed suicide after traumatic brain injury. J Head Trauma Rehabil 12:16–20, 1997

Tateno A, Jorge RE, Robinson RG. Clinical correlates of aggressive behavior after traumatic brain injury. J Neuropsychiatry Clin Neurosci 15:155–160, 2003

Taverni JP, Seliger G, Lichtman SW: Donepezil mediated memory improvement in traumatic brain injury during post acute rehabilitation. Brain Inj 12:77–80, 1998

Teasdale G, Jennett B: Assessment of coma and impaired consciousness: a practical scale. Lancet 2:81–84, 1974

Teasdale GM, Nicoll JAR, Murray G, et al: Association of apolipoprotein E polymorphism with outcome after head injury. Lancet 350:1069–1071, 1997

Teitelman E: Off-label uses of modafinil. Am J Psychiatry 158:1431, 2001

Temkin NR, Dikmen SS, Wilensky AJ, et al: A randomized, double-blind study of phenytoin for the prevention of post-traumatic seizures. N Engl J Med 323:497–502, 1990

Temkin NR, Dikmen SS, Anderson GD, et al: Valproate therapy for prevention of posttraumatic seizures: a randomized trial. J Neurosurg 91:593–600, 1999

Terzoudi M, Gavrielidou P, Heilakos G, et al: Fatigue in multiple sclerosis: evaluation of a new pharmacological approach (abstract). Neurology 54 (suppl 3):A61–A62, 2000

Thatcher RW, Moore N, John ER, et al: QEEG and traumatic brain injury: rebuttal of the American Academy of Neurology 1997 Report by the EEG and Clinical Neuroscience Society. Clin Electroencephalogr 30:94–98, 1999

Therapeutics and Technology Assessment Subcommittee of the American Academy of Neurology: Assessment of brain SPECT. Neurology 46:278–285, 1996

Thompson RS, Rivara FP, Thompson DC: A case-control study of the effectiveness of bicycle safety helmets. N Engl J Med 320:1361–1367, 1989

Thomsen IV: Late outcome of very severe blunt head trauma: a 10–15 year second follow-up. J Neurol Neurosurg Psychiatry 47:260–268, 1984

Toulmond S, Duval D, Serrano A, et al: Biochemical and histological alterations induced by fluid percussion brain injury in the rat. Brain Res 620:24–31, 1993

Trzepacz PT, Kennedy RE: Delirium and posttraumatic amnesia, in Textbook of Traumatic Brain Injury. Edited by Silver JM, McAllister TM, Yudofsky SC. Washington, DC, American Psychiatric Publishing, 2005, pp 175–200

Tsuang MT, Boor M, Fleming JA: Psychiatric aspects of traffic accidents. Am J Psychiatry 142:538–546, 1985

Tyerman A, Humphrey M: Changes in self-concept following severe head injury. Int J Rehabil Res 7:11–23, 1984

Tysvaer AT, Storli O, Bachen NI: Soccer injuries to the brain. Acta Neurol Scand 80:151–156, 1989

Ursano RJ, Fullerton CS, Epstein RS, et al: Acute and chronic posttraumatic stress disorder in motor vehicle accident victims. Am J Psychiatry 156:589–595, 1999a

Ursano RJ, Fullerton CS, Epstein RS, et al: Peritraumatic dissociation and posttraumatic stress disorder following motor vehicle accidents. Am J Psychiatry 156:1808–1810, 1999b

U.S. Department of Health and Human Services: Interagency Head Injury Task Force Report. Washington, DC, U.S. Department of Health and Human Services, 1989

U.S. Department of Transportation: Final regulatory impact assessment on amendments to Federal Motor Vehicle Safety Standard 208, Front Seat Occupant Protection (DOT Publ No HS-806-572). Washington, DC, U.S. Department of Transportation, 1984

Van Duijn CM, Tanja TA, Haaxma R, et al: Head trauma and the risk of Alzheimer's disease. Am J Epidemiol 135:775–782, 1992

van Reekum R, Bolago I, Finlayson MA, et al: Psychiatric disorders after traumatic brain injury. Brain Inj 10:319–327, 1996

van Reekum R, Cohen T, Wong J: Can traumatic brain injury cause psychiatric disorders? J Neuropsychiatry Clin Neurosci 12:316–327, 2000

Van Woerkom TCAM, Teelken AW, Minderhoud JM: Difference in neurotransmitter metabolism in frontotemporal-lobe contusion and diffuse cerebral contusion. Lancet 1:812–813, 1977

Varney NR: Prognostic significance of anosmia in patients with closed-head trauma. J Clin Exp Neuropsychol 10:250–254, 1988

Varney NR, Martzke JS, Roberts RJ: Major depression in patients with closed head injury. Neuropsychology 1:7–9, 1987

Vecht CJ, Van Woerkom TCAM, Teelken AW, et al: Homovanillic acid and 5-hydroxyindoleacetic acid cerebrospinal fluid levels. Arch Neurol 32:792–797, 1975

Violon A, De Mol J: Psychological sequelae after head trauma in adults. Acta Neurochir (Wien) 85:96–102, 1987

Wade DT, King NS, Crawford S, et al: Routine follow up after head injury: a second randomised clinical trial. J Neurol Neurosurg Psychiatry 65:177–183, 1998

Ward TM, Levin M: Headaches, in Textbook of Traumatic Brain Injury. Edited by Silver JM, McAllister, Yudofsky SC. Washington, DC, American Psychiatric Publishing, 2005, pp 385–391

Warden DL, Labbate LA: Posttraumatic stress disorder and other anxiety disorders, in Textbook of Traumatic Brain Injury. Edited by Silver JM, McAllister, Yudofsky SC. Washington, DC, American Psychiatric Publishing, 2005, pp 231–243

Warden DL, Labbate LA, Salazar AM, et al: PTSD symptoms in moderate traumatic brain injury. Paper presented at the annual meeting of the American Psychiatric Association, Miami Beach, FL, May 20–25, 1995

Warden D, Bleiberg J, Cameron KL, et al: Persistent prolongation of simple reaction time in sports concussion. Neurology 57:524–526, 2001

Watson MR, Fenton GW, McClelland RJ, et al: The postconcussional state: neurophysiological aspects. Br J Psychiatry 167:514–521, 1995

Weddell R, Oddy M, Jenkins D: Social adjustment after rehabilitation: a two year follow-up of patients with severe head injury. Psychol Med 10:257–263, 1980

Weinberg RM, Auerbach SH, Moore S: Pharmacologic treatment of cognitive deficits: a case study. Brain Inj 1:57–59, 1987

Weinstein GS, Wells CE: Case studies in neuropsychiatry: posttraumatic psychiatric dysfunction—diagnosis and treatment. J Clin Psychiatry 42:120–122, 1981

Weller M, Kornhuber J: A rationale for NMDA receptor antagonist therapy of the neuroleptic malignant syndrome. Med Hypotheses 38:329–333, 1992

Whelan FJ, Walker MS, Schulz SK: Donepezil in the treatment of cognitive dysfunction associated with traumatic brain injury. Ann Clin Psychiatry 12:131–135, 2000

Whyte J: Neurologic disorders of attention and arousal: assessment and treatment. Arch Phys Med Rehabil 73:1094–1103, 1992

Whyte J, Hart T, Schuster K, et al: Effects of methylphenidate on attentional function after traumatic brain injury: a randomized placebo-controlled trial. Am J Phys Med Rehabil 76:440–450, 1997

Wilberger JE, Deeb A, Rothfus W: Magnetic resonance imaging in cases of severe head injury. Neurosurgery 20:571–576, 1987

Wilcox JA, Nasrallah HA: Childhood head trauma and psychosis. Psychiatry Res 21:303–306, 1987

Will RG, Young JPR, Thomas DJ: Klein-Levin syndrome: report of two cases with onset of symptoms precipitated by head trauma. Br J Psychiatry 152:410–412, 1988

Wolf B, Grohmann R, Schmidt LG, et al: Psychiatric admissions due to adverse drug reactions. Compr Psychiatry 30:534–545, 1989

Woolf PD, Hamill RW, Lee LA, et al: The predictive value of catecholamines in assessing outcome in traumatic brain injury. J Neurosurg 66:875–882, 1987

Wroblewski BA, McColgan K, Smith K, et al: The incidence of seizures during tricyclic antidepressant drug treatment in a brain-injured population. J Clin Psychopharmacol 10:124–128, 1990

Wroblewski BA, Leary JM, Phelan AM, et al: Methylphenidate and seizure frequency in brain-injured patients with seizure disorders. J Clin Psychiatry 53:86–89, 1992

Wroblewski BA, Joseph AB, Kupfer J, et al: Effectiveness of valproic acid on destructive and aggressive behaviours in patients with acquired brain injury. Brain Inj 11:37–47, 1997

Yablon SA: Posttraumatic seizures. Arch Phys Med Rehabil 74:983–1001, 1993

Yudofsky SC, Hales RE: The reemergence of neuropsychiatry: definition and direction. J Neuropsychiatry Clin Neurosci 1:1–6, 1989

Yudofsky SC, Silver JM, Jackson W, et al: The Overt Aggression Scale for the objective rating of verbal and physical aggression. Am J Psychiatry 143:35–39, 1986

Yudofsky SC, Silver JM, Schneider SE: Pharmacologic treatment of aggression. Psychiatric Annals 17:397–407, 1987

Yudofsky SC, Silver JM, Hales RE: Pharmacologic management of aggression in the elderly. J Clin Psychiatry 51 (suppl 10):22–28, 1990

Yudofsky SC, Silver JM, Hales RE: Psychopharmacology of aggression, in American Psychiatric Press Textbook of Psychopharmacology. Edited by Schatzberg AF, Nemeroff CB. Washington, DC, American Psychiatric Press, 1995, pp 735–751

Yudofsky SC, Kopecky HJ, Kunik ME, et al: The Overt Agitation Severity Scale for the objective rating of agitation. J Neuropsychiatry Clin Neuroscience 9:541–548, 1997

Yudofsky SC, Silver JM, Hales RE: Treatment of agitation and aggression, in Textbook of Psychopharmacology, 2nd Edition. Edited by Schatzberg AF, Nemeroff CB. Washington, DC, American Psychiatric Press, 1998, pp 881–900

Zasler N: Sexual dysfunction, in Neuropsychiatry of Traumatic Brain Injury. Edited by Silver JM, Yudofsky SC, Hales RE. Washington, DC, American Psychiatric Press, 1994, pp 443–470

Zasler ND, Martelli MF, Nicholson K: Chronic pain, in Textbook of Traumatic Brain Injury. Edited by Silver JM, McAllister, Yudofsky SC. Washington, DC, American Psychiatric Publishing, 2005, pp 419–433

Zeilig G, Drubach DA, Katz-Zeilig M, Karatinos J: Pathological laughter and crying in patients with closed traumatic brain injury. Brain Inj 10:591–597, 1996

Zhang L, Plotkin RC, Wang G, et al: Cholinergic augmentation with donepezil enhances recovery in short-term memory and sustained attention after traumatic brain injury. Arch Phys Med Rehabil 85:1050–1055, 2004

Zimmer B, Garber HJ, Price TRP, et al: Bupropion use in patients at risk for seizures. Paper presented at the annual meeting of the American Psychiatric Association, Washington, DC, May 2–7, 1992

16

NEUROPSYCHIATRIC ASPECTS OF SEIZURE DISORDERS

H. Florence Kim, M.D.

Stuart C. Yudofsky, M.D.

Robert E. Hales, M.D.

Gary J. Tucker, M.D.

Before the development of the electroencephalogram (EEG) by Dr. Hans Berger in the 1930s, all seizure disorders were classified with mental disorders (Berger 1929–1938). Indeed, a strong link between epilepsy and psychiatry has been known for more than a century. In the late nineteenth century, the noted neuropsychiatrist Emil Kraepelin (1922/1968) described three types of psychoses: dementia praecox, manic-depressive illness, and psychosis associated with epilepsy. Until recently, the conception that epilepsy is a mental disorder was held in many countries.

Epilepsy represents one of the more interesting aspects of brain-behavior relations. Epilepsy is not only an important medical condition but also an important part of the differential diagnosis of behavior disorders. Epilepsy—and its ability to cause behavioral symptoms without overt classical seizures—is an important natural model of behavioral disturbance.

The behavioral symptoms associated with either insults to the central nervous system (CNS) or diseases of the CNS are actually very few; consequently, a wide variety of etiologies can cause the same symptoms (Table 16–1). Epilepsy can cause both chronic and episodic behavior disorders. However, as with all disturbances of the CNS, when clear evidence of pathology is found, either by EEG or by imaging, the possible etiological diagnosis of behavioral disturbance is enhanced. Unfortunately, with various epileptic conditions, clear laboratory diagnostic evidence is often not present, and the hypothesis about etiology is based solely on the clinical picture.

SEIZURE DISORDERS

SEIZURES AND EPILEPSY

Epilepsy is a term applied to a broad group of disorders. The defining feature of any of the epilepsies is the seizure. A seizure can have almost protean manifestations, and it is usually defined as having all or parts of the following: an impairment of consciousness, involuntary movements, behavior changes, and altered perceptual experiences (Table 16–2).

The diagnosis of epilepsy is made only when a person has recurrent seizures. A seizure involves paroxysmal cerebral neuronal firing, which may or may not produce disturbed consciousness and perceptual or motor alterations. The classic image of a seizure is that of the *grand mal* or generalized tonic-clonic seizure. These seizures usually involve relatively short (10–30 seconds) tonic movements, with marked extension and flexion of mus-

TABLE 16–1.　Primary symptoms and dysfunctions of central nervous system disturbances

Cognitive

　Affect modulation

　Intellectual function

　Judgment

　Memory

　Orientation

Behavioral

　Anxiety

　Arousal

　Mood

　Motor

　Personality traits

Perceptions

　Auditory

　Kinesthetic pain

　Olfactory

　Taste

　Visual

TABLE 16–2.　International League Against Epilepsy (ILAE) proposed diagnostic scheme

Axis I: Ictal phenomenology describing the ictal events

Axis II: Seizure type

　Specify from ILAE List of Epileptic Seizures. Identify localization within the brain or precipitating stimuli when appropriate.

Axis III: Epileptic syndrome

　Specify from ILAE List of Epilepsy Syndromes. Specify only when syndromic diagnosis is possible.

Axis IV: Etiology

　Specify genetic defects or specific pathologies from ILAE Classification of Diseases Frequently Associated With Epileptic Seizures or Epilepsy Syndromes. Specify only when etiology is known.

Axis V: Impairment classification derived from World Health Organization (optional)

Source. Adapted from International League Against Epilepsy Commission Report: A proposed diagnostic scheme for people with epileptic seizures and with epilepsy: report of the ILAE Task Force on Classification and Terminology. *Epilepsia* 42:796–803, 2001b. Used with permission.

cles, without shaking. A longer phase (15–60 seconds) involving clonic movements, manifesting as rhythmic muscle group shaking, follows the tonic phase. Tonic phase movements may be associated with laryngeal stridor manifested as a high-pitched screaming sound. Urinary, and occasionally fecal, incontinence may occur as a result of sphincteric relaxation, and the seizures are almost invariably followed by headache, sleepiness, and confusion. Seizures preceded by perceptual, autonomic, affective, or cognitive alterations (aura) usually indicate a focal onset with secondary generalization. There are many types of seizures that vary markedly from the above description (Chadwick 1993; Engel 1992).

CLASSIFICATION OF SEIZURES

The classification of seizures and epilepsy is constantly evolving. It has shifted away from terms such as *grand mal* to an attempt to correlate clinical seizure type with electroencephalographic ictal (i.e., during the seizure) and interictal (i.e., between seizures) changes. The most recent classification of epileptic seizures by the International League Against Epilepsy (ILAE) in 2001 has moved away from previous phenomenological descriptions to the creation of a list of seizure types that repre-

sent diagnostic entities on the basis of common pathophysiology and anatomy (International League Against Epilepsy Commission Report 2001a).

In place of a fixed classification, a diagnostic scheme consisting of five levels or axes to provide a standardized description of epilepsy is now recommended by the International League Against Epilepsy Commission Report (2001b) (see Table 16–2). Axis I is a description of the ictal event according to the International League Against Epilepsy Commission Report's (2001a) standardized *Glossary of Descriptive Terminology for Ictal Semiology.* This description will not reference etiology, anatomy, or mechanisms. Axis II consists of the epileptic seizure type, diagnostic entities denoting therapeutic, prognostic, and etiological mechanisms. If anatomical localization is possible, it should be specified here. Reflex seizures, or seizures precipitated by sensory stimuli, should specify precipitating factors on this axis as well. Selected seizure types are listed in Table 16–3. These seizure types are separated into self-limited and continuous seizures and further divided into generalized and focal seizures. Axis III is the epileptic syndrome, a constellation of signs and symptoms that define an epileptic condition. It is not necessary to specify a syndromic diagnosis, if one is not known. Selected epileptic syndrome diagnoses are listed in Table 16–4. Axis IV lists the etiology if known, such as

TABLE 16–3. International League Against Epilepsy epileptic seizure types

Self-limited seizure types

  Generalized seizures

    Tonic-clonic seizures

    Clonic seizures

    Absence seizures

    Tonic seizures

    Spasms

    Myoclonic seizures

    Atonic seizures

  Focal seizures

    Focal sensory seizures

    Focal motor seizures

    Gelastic seizures

    Hemiclonic seizures

    Secondarily generalized seizures

Continuous seizure types

  Generalized status epilepticus

  Focal status epilepticus

Precipitating stimuli for reflex seizures

  Visual stimuli, thinking, music, eating, praxis, somatosensory, proprioceptive, reading, hot water, startle

Source. Adapted from International League Against Epilepsy Commission Report: "Glossary of Descriptive Terminology for Ictal Semiology: Report of the ILAE Task Force on Classification and Terminology." *Epilepsia* 42:1212–1218, 2001a. Used with permission.

TABLE 16–4. International League Against Epilepsy selected epilepsy syndromes

Benign familial neonatal seizures

Benign infantile seizures

Lennox-Gastaut syndrome

Landau-Kleffner syndrome

Childhood absence epilepsy

Reflex epilepsies

Familial temporal lobe epilepsies

Conditions with epileptic seizures that do not require a diagnosis of epilepsy

  Benign neonatal seizures

  Febrile seizures

  Reflex seizures

  Alcohol withdrawal seizures

  Drug or other chemically induced seizures

  Immediate and early posttraumatic seizures

  Single seizures or isolated seizure clusters

Source. Adapted from International League Against Epilepsy Commission Report: "Glossary of Descriptive Terminology for Ictal Semiology: Report of the ILAE Task Force on Classification and Terminology." *Epilepsia* 42:1212–1218, 2001a. Used with permission.

a specific disease or a genetic or pathological abnormality. Axis V is a classification of impairment associated with the epileptic condition and is considered optional.

Generalized Seizures

Generalized seizures (or generalized attacks) are epileptic seizures that manifest immediately and spread bilaterally through the cerebral cortex. They are generalized in that subcortical fibers may be involved, and there is simultaneous spread throughout the cerebral cortex. No preceding motor or perceptual experiences occur, and there is almost invariably total loss of consciousness.

Focal (Partial) Seizures

In *focal seizures* (or partial or localization-related seizures), epileptic firing starts in a specific focus in the brain (usually the cerebral cortex). This evokes a physiological experience that stimulating that focus would produce.

When such seizures involve no alteration in consciousness, they are called *simple partial seizures* (previously called *elementary partial seizures*). When there is a defect in consciousness (i.e., confusion, dizziness), they are called *complex partial seizures* (CPSs). Some authors further subdivide CPSs into type 1 (temporal lobe) and type 2 (extratemporal). It is important to note that 40% of all patients with epilepsy will have CPSs (International League Against Epilepsy Commission 1985). The terms *simple* and *complex partial seizures* are no longer recommended for use in classification of specific seizure types as in the past but may still be used as descriptive terms.

Tonic-Clonic Seizures

Tonic-clonic seizures (or grand mal seizures) are the most common form of generalized seizure. They manifest as total loss of consciousness with a tetanic muscular phase, usually several seconds (tonic), followed by a phase of repetitive jerking, usually 1–2 minutes (clonic). These seizures may be generalized from the start or begin as partial seizures and secondarily generalize.

Partial seizures secondarily generalized are seizures that start as partial seizures. This phase may or may not be remembered. They then spread bilaterally throughout the cerebral cortex, producing secondary generalization. This terminology is different from a previous classification that spoke of secondary generalized epilepsy, which referred to a kind of epilepsy generalized from the start, with features of a diffuse cerebral pathology.

Absence Seizures

Typical *absence seizures* (or *petit mal* seizures) are a common seizure type that occurs primarily in children. These are generalized from the start, with loss of consciousness for a few seconds without any motor phase. Typical electroencephalographic findings are bilateral and synchronous and have spike waves of 3–4 Hz.

Status Epilepticus

Status epilepticus is a continuous seizure state that involves two or more seizures superimposed on each other without total recovery of consciousness and is a true medical emergency. Generalized status epilepticus can be convulsive, consisting of tonic-clonic seizures, or nonconvulsive. The nonconvulsive form of generalized status epilepticus is defined as behavioral or cognitive changes from baseline such as confusion, stupor, or coma, accompanied by continuous or near-continuous seizure activity on EEG. Several other forms of status epilepticus exist, including absence status epilepticus and focal status epilepticus types, when consciousness may be preserved, and the diagnosis is often made by EEG (Novak et al. 1971).

CAUSES OF EPILEPSY

The idiopathic or genetic epilepsies, in which no CNS pathology is evident, are usually childhood syndromes. In patients older than 30, the onset of epilepsy or recurrent seizures is usually associated with CNS pathology, and a search must be made for the cause of the seizures. When CNS pathology is present, these syndromes are usually described as symptomatic or secondary seizure disorders, or epilepsy. Conditions such as head injury, encephalitis, birth trauma, or hyperpyrexia represent rather static and permanent lesions that can cause epilepsy or seizures. Conditions that can be progressive and that change over time include medication overdose or withdrawal, tumor, infections, metabolic disease (e.g., hypoglycemia and uremia), and endocrine diseases. Alzheimer's disease and other dementias, multiple sclerosis, cerebral arteriopathy, and other degenerative or infiltrative conditions can all lead to a progressive and changing picture of seizures.

Seizures can also be a reaction to various medical or physiological stresses. This fact is particularly evident at both ends of the age spectrum. For example, febrile conditions are more likely to cause seizures in young people and older people. The tendency to have seizures is related to an inherited predisposition for variations in the seizure threshold because not all young or older patients with the same fever will have a seizure.

TEMPORAL LOBE EPILEPSY

In this chapter, we use the term *temporal lobe epilepsy*, which is no longer recognized by the ILAE, but we emphasize that the term is used in the descriptive sense, implying both complex and simple partial seizures, including psychomotor automatisms and tonic-clonic seizures that may originate from the temporal lobe. Many such phenomena interpreted as having originated in the temporal lobe may, in fact, be extratemporal.

Although the term *temporal lobe epilepsy* has formally become an anachronism, in practice it is still commonly used in the absence of an adequate alternative. The phenomena of temporal lobe epilepsy are *not* synonymous with those of its proposed nonanatomical replacement, CPSs, because CPSs are restricted to patients who have focal firing with defects of consciousness.

In practice, many patients with temporal lobe epilepsy have no defect of consciousness and have simple partial seizures (e.g., olfactory hallucinations), which may derive from the temporal lobes. In addition, they may have simple partial seizures with psychic symptomatology (e.g., cognitive alterations, such as flashbacks or déjà vu experiences occurring in clear consciousness). Temporal lobe epilepsy may also manifest with the *temporal lobe absence* or behavioral arrest that is associated with a brief loss of consciousness of 10–30 seconds. These episodes may be associated with minor automatisms (e.g., chewing movements) and at times with "drop attacks" (the falling associated with loss of muscle tone). Patients with temporal lobe epilepsy often appear to be staring and after the episode may be aware that they had a loss of consciousness. They may experience postictal features such as headache and sleepiness. Thus, the temporal lobe absence differs from petit mal because the latter is a shorter episode, without muscle movements and postictal features (Fenton 1986).

Temporal lobe epilepsy also may manifest with psychomotor automatisms alone, which are no longer regarded as a form of CPS. Psychomotor automatisms may involve a psychic (cognitive-affective, somatosensory, or perceptual) phase followed by a motor phase. The psychic phase may be very brief and not recognized by the patient, who may be amnestic for it. It may be associated with many perceptual alterations, such as an auditory buzz or hum, complex verbalizations, or aphasias. Visual abnormalities include diplopia, misperceptions of movement, and changes in perceived object size or shape. Other alter-

TABLE 16–5. Behavioral symptoms often associated with seizures, particularly temporal lobe epilepsy

Hallucinations: all sensory modalities

Illusions

Déjà vu

Jamais vu

Depersonalization

Repetitive thoughts and nightmares

Flashbacks and visual distortions

Epigastric sensations

Automatisms

Affective and mood changes

Catatonia

Cataplexy

Amnestic episodes

ations may include illusions, tactile distortions, olfactory phenomena (e.g., generally unpleasant, burning, or rotting smells), gustatory phenomena (e.g., metallic tastes), and somatosensory autonomic symptoms (e.g., piloerection, gastric sensations, or nausea). Flashbacks and alterations of consciousness (*jamais vu*, depersonalization, derealization, and déjà vu) may occur. These are followed by automatisms of various degrees of complexity. There may be simple buttoning or unbuttoning or masticatory movements, more complex "wandering" fugue states, furor-type anger (which is very rare), or speech automatisms (which are far more common than is recognized).

The features of temporal lobe epilepsy are varied and protean (Bear 1986; Blumer 1975). Table 16–5 describes some of the symptoms that have often been associated with temporal lobe disturbances.

EPIDEMIOLOGY OF SEIZURE DISORDERS

As can be seen from the variety of seizures and syndromes that constitute epilepsy, it is often difficult to get a clear idea of the epidemiology. The prevalence of epilepsy is believed to be 5–40 per 1,000 people. The incidence is estimated to be 40–70 per 100,000 people per year in industrialized countries and more than twice as high in developing countries. Worldwide, 50 million people are affected by epilepsy, with 2.4 million new cases occurring every year (GCAE Secretariat 2003). The incidence of epilepsy is highest in young children, decreases in adults, and peaks again in the elderly (Dekker 2002). Shovron

and Reynolds (1986) presented convincing data that most patients developing seizures enter long-term remission. Annegers et al. (1979) indicated that of 475 patients, 76% experienced at least one seizure-free period for 5 or more years. Seventy percent of the patients were in continual remission 20 years after the diagnosis. Another community survey by Goodridge and Shovron (1983) reported that 122 patients from a sample of 6,000 had at least one epileptic seizure (excluding febrile seizures), and 70% of these patients, after 15 years following the initial diagnosis, were in long-term remission. The earlier the remission of seizures after onset, the more likely it was that the patient would have a permanent remission. Those whose seizures continued beyond 2 years were more likely to have seizures at the end of the longitudinal study. A study by Sillanpaa et al. (1995) confirmed these findings. Many of the patients in remission were able to be withdrawn completely from medication. Consequently, the image of epilepsy as a chronic condition is not necessarily a valid one; however, in a condition that consists of so many different manifestations and causes, it is often difficult to generalize beyond the individual case. Unfortunately, no good long-term studies of the behavioral disturbances associated with seizure disorders have been done. It would be of some interest, considering the high remission rate of epilepsy, to see if the behavior also ceased.

PSYCHOSOCIAL FACETS OF EPILEPSY

The epileptic patient encounters major psychosocial stressors. First is the stress of having a chronic illness. Studies comparing the epileptic patient with groups of patients with other chronic illnesses, such as rheumatic heart disease, diabetes mellitus, and cancer, have concluded that each of these conditions has its own special stressors (Dodrill and Batzel 1986). However, when comparing any of these populations with patients with organic brain disease, specific problems arise because damage to the CNS, in and of itself, leads to unique consequences (Szatmari 1985).

A special difficulty of the epileptic patient is the often paroxysmal (or episodic) element to the illness. Between episodes, the person with epilepsy may be functioning normally. Substantial covert stress leads the person with epilepsy to be afraid of performing normal social activities, such as dating during adolescence. The fear of a seizure is greater than the occurrence. In addition, the witnessing of an actual tonic-clonic seizure is a frightening experience for many members of the general population, and much folklore is associated with seizures (Temkin 1979). Consequently, conceptions of epilepsy may be distorted thereafter, and even an isolated seizure may have grave consequences on interpersonal relationships.

Within American culture, persons with epilepsy are, at times, perceived as an inferior minority group. In some preliterate subcultures, an epileptic seizure is often regarded as a type of communication with ancestors or with higher beings, and epileptic individuals may be perceived as having special powers. Many of them become shamans or witch doctors and are highly respected members of their culture (Temkin 1979). Also, the disorders create limitations on the patient's activities (i.e., epileptic individuals cannot operate complex machinery, work in jobs that expose them to dangers, swim alone, or, in some instances, even bathe autonomously). The consequences of not being allowed to drive are a major obstacle in our society, particularly in rural areas. These functional limitations can be considerable, particularly because they are often disregarded by the patient (e.g., driving), which may create additional guilt, moral and ethical consequences, and legal complications. Frequently, in families with epileptic members, abnormal relationships develop that may lead to increased dependency or isolation. Patterns of dependency can be difficult to dislodge, and it is sometimes easier to remain ill than to become seizure-free and healthy. The epileptic patient needs to learn to develop independence and a sense of self-care and to create constructive relationships that promote health. The degree of influence that apparent psychological factors may have on the course of epilepsy should not be underestimated (Hoare 1984; Stevens 1988; Ziegler 1982).

DIAGNOSIS

The diagnosis of epilepsy is basically a clinical one, much as is the diagnosis of schizophrenia. Although an EEG can often be confirmatory, 20% of patients with epilepsy will have normal EEG findings, and 2% of patients without epilepsy will have spike and wave formations (Engel 1992). The best diagnostic test for seizures is the observation of the patient or the report of someone who has observed the patient having a seizure. Thus, the history taken from the patient and the family is crucial. Key factors important in the history of these patients are the age at onset of seizures, any history of illness or trauma to the nervous system that could cause seizures, a family history of epilepsy, and some idea of whether the condition is progressive or static. Attempts should be made to determine whether the seizures are idiopathic or secondary. Certainly, these descriptions are most helpful in the diagnosis of major motor seizures or generalized seizures. They are also useful in attempting to determine the relation between the seizures and various behavioral disturbances. Because the seizure focus can reside in any location in the brain, as well as affecting various circuits

within the brain, the number of behavioral symptoms associated with seizures is considerable (see Table 16–5).

Laboratory

Finding an elevated prolactin level is the only major laboratory test used in the diagnostic workup of seizures. A hormone secreted by the anterior pituitary gland, serum prolactin is released by epileptic activity spreading from the temporal lobe to the hypothalamic-pituitary axis (Bauer 1996). After a seizure, usually within 15–20 minutes after a generalized tonic-clonic seizure, an abrupt rise in prolactin levels occurs. As a rule, the prolactin level decreases to normal within 60 minutes; therefore, blood should be drawn 15–20 minutes after the seizure. These levels are typically three to four times the patient's baseline prolactin level. This response of prolactin is seen more often in major motor seizures and less frequently in CPSs. Widespread activation of the temporal lobe structures, however, is often associated with increasing prolactin levels. In a recent study of 200 consecutive patients seen in the emergency department setting with a diagnosis of seizure followed by syncope, the sensitivity of serum prolactin level was 42%, specificity was 82%, positive predictive value was 74%, negative predictive value was 54%, and overall diagnostic accuracy was 60% (Vukmir 2004). Furthermore, elevated prolactin levels have not been helpful in differentiating true seizures from nonepileptic or pseudoseizures (Shukla et al. 2004; Willert et al. 2004). Some data indicate that repeated seizures and shorter seizure-free periods decrease the prolactin response (Malkowicz et al. 1995). Prolactin levels also may be elevated by neuroleptic use. Thus, elevated serum prolactin levels may be helpful as a confirmatory test for suspected seizure but not as a singular diagnostic test.

Imaging

Structural imaging techniques such as magnetic resonance imaging (MRI) and computed tomography (CT) scans are crucial for the evaluation of symptomatic epilepsies. Both structural and functional imaging modalities are also useful for localization of seizure foci to evaluate candidates for surgical intervention. Functional imaging such as single-photon emission computed tomography (SPECT) and positron emission tomography (PET) has been valuable in evaluating ictal events and blood flow to focal lesions during a seizure. However, postictal and interictal evaluations are much less informative. SPECT studies are very reliable for localizing ictal events. PET is somewhat better in the detection of interictal temporal lobe hypermetabolism (Ho et al. 1995). Undoubtedly, as these instruments become more sensitive, their use will increase in the clinical evaluation of seizure disorders.

EEG

The EEG is one of the most important tests in the evaluation of seizures, suspected seizures, or episodic behavioral disturbances. In this day of major advances in imaging, the EEG is also frequently overlooked, and often when it is used, it is misinterpreted. The paroxysmal interictal EEG with spikes and wave complexes can confirm the clinical diagnosis of a seizure disorder. It can, when positive, differentiate between seizure types (e.g., absence seizures from generalized seizures) and indicate the possibility of a structural lesion when there are focal findings in the EEG. However, a normal EEG result cannot eliminate the possibility of a seizure disorder being present in a particular patient. The EEG is a reflection of surface activity in the cortex and may not reflect seizure activity deep in the brain. Most clinicians, when confronted with a behavior disorder that does not fit the usual clinical picture of a schizophrenic psychosis (particularly if the disorder is episodic), will obtain an EEG. If the EEG result is negative, the clinicians may then be deterred from further pursuing the idea that this episodic behavior may represent a seizure disorder. It is important to remember that the diagnosis of epilepsy (as with schizophrenia) is a clinical one and that although the EEG can confirm the diagnosis, it cannot exclude it. Even with elaborate recordings (24-hour EEGs) and concomitant videotaping, a seizure disorder cannot always be diagnosed.

Special techniques have been used to help with EEG diagnosis. Nasopharyngeal electrodes are one commonly used technique. However, the increased yield with nasopharyngeal electrodes is not substantial—some studies indicate less than 10% detection (Bickford 1979). In contrast, the yield with sphenoidal electrodes is greatly increased (Ebersole and Leroy 1983). Unfortunately, placement of sphenoidal electrodes requires time and expertise, which are not readily available.

One suggestion has been the placement of electrodes on the buccal skin surface in the area of the submandibular notch. It appears that these placements may entirely eclipse the use of nasopharyngeal electrodes because they are almost as effective at picking up foci as sphenoidal placements are (Sadler and Goodwin 1986). Much more definitive, however, is the use of cerebral cortical placements during neurosurgery procedures. These may show firing (e.g., in patients with temporal lobe epilepsy and psychosis) in the region of the hippocampus (Heath 1982). The improvement in signal detection gained from the direct placement of intracranial electrodes underscores the insensitivity of the scalp electrode placement commonly used in surface EEGs.

Several methods are used for evoking electroencephalographic abnormalities. One very common method is the use of sleep records. In this method, the yield of actual ictal-related events is not substantially increased. However, the potential for detecting a particular focus or focal abnormality may increase because of the extra synchronization that may occur. Phases of sleep may differ in threshold for inducing seizures (i.e., less potentiality for seizures), and during such phases, focal abnormalities may be more evident (Brodsky et al. 1983). This fact explains the apparent paradox of the use, for many years, of barbiturates such as secobarbital sodium in sleep records.

The preferred means of evaluating brain wave activity during sleep is the natural induction of sleep. However, in a laboratory situation, this is often not practical, and at times (e.g., overnight) the patient is sleep deprived so that no medication need be given. Such a practice is a good one but is not applicable to the psychiatric patient who is generally disturbed enough to require a sedative. The alternative is the administration of chloral hydrate, 1–3 g, as premedication before the sleep record. The chloral hydrate has little effect on the EEG and does not prevent the demonstration of focal abnormalities. Overall, a sleep electroencephalographic record increases the chances of detecting a focal abnormality, such as a temporal lobe focus, approximately fourfold. For example, Gibbs and Gibbs (1952) found only 20% interseizure waking electroencephalographic abnormalities in temporal lobe epilepsy; this figure went up to 80% in sleep records in a nonhomogeneous neurological population. A study by Cendes et al. (2000) reported that when the EEG showed lateralization, hippocampal atrophy was also evident on the MRI. Thus, in those suspected of having temporal lobe epilepsy, the lateralized EEG was very helpful in making the diagnosis.

Certain medications should be particularly avoided when obtaining electroencephalographic studies. The first are those in the benzodiazepine group, which may have, by virtue of their strong antiepileptic effects, profound effects in normalizing the EEG. Because effects on receptor activity may last weeks, even with the short-acting benzodiazepines, the yield of demonstrating abnormal activity after administration of benzodiazepines may decrease substantially. The second medication to avoid for sleep is L-tryptophan. Adamec and Stark (1983) found that L-tryptophan has some effect in raising the seizure threshold during electroconvulsive therapy (ECT). Some psychotropic medications, such as neuroleptics, the tricyclic and heterocyclic antidepressants, and the benzodiazepines (Pincus and Tucker 1985), also may increase synchronization of the EEG (leading to a seizure-like pattern). One report (Ryback and Gardner 1991) described a small series in which procaine activation of the EEG was useful in identifying patients with episodic behavior disorders responsive to anticonvulsants.

Recent advances in electroencephalographic technology may ultimately change the whole perspective of its use in psychiatry Evoked potentials and quantitative EEG are promising research tools that have yet to show specific clinical utility in the diagnosis and treatment of neuropsychiatric disorders.

DIFFERENTIAL DIAGNOSIS OF BEHAVIORAL SYMPTOMS ASSOCIATED WITH EPILEPSY

A range of medical conditions must be distinguished from seizures: panic disorder, hyperventilation, hypoglycemia, various transient cerebral ischemias, migraine, narcolepsy, malingering, and conversion reactions. The defining characteristics of temporal lobe epilepsy are typically subjective experiences or feelings, automatisms, and, more rarely, catatonia or cataplexy. Because the symptoms are usually related to a focal electrical discharge in the brain, they are generally consistent and few in number. Although the list of possible symptoms may be quite large (see Table 16–5), each patient will have a limited number of specific symptoms—for example, auditory hallucinations (usually voices), repetitive sounds, or visual hallucinations and misperceptions that are of a consistent type that includes a visual disturbance. The automatisms, as related previously, are simple (e.g., chewing, swallowing, pursing of the lips, looking around, smiling, grimacing, crying). Other types of automatisms are attempting to sit up, examining or fumbling with objects, and buttoning or unbuttoning clothes. Complex, goal-directed behavior is unusual during these episodes. Aggressive behavior is also rare. The only time the patient will sometimes become aggressive is when an attempt is made to restrain or prevent ambulation (Rodin 1973). Typical attacks usually consist of a cessation of activity, followed by automatism and impairment of consciousness. The entire episode usually lasts from 10 seconds to as long as 30 minutes. The motor phenomena and postural changes, such as catatonia, are rarer (Fenton 1986; Kirubakaran et al. 1987).

The profile of patients who present primarily with behavioral symptoms is usually of episodic "brief" disturbances lasting for variable periods of time (hours to days). Historically, the patient often states that such episodes have occurred mainly once a month or once every 3 months. The patient seeks psychiatric attention when the frequency of the episodes increases to daily or several times per day with resultant impairment of functioning. Critical factors helpful in the diagnosis of temporal lobe epilepsy are shown in Table 16–6.

TABLE 16–6. Factors helpful in the diagnosis of temporal lobe epilepsy

Does the patient describe typical subjective alterations?

Has the patient been observed performing characteristic automatisms?

Was the patient confused during the episode?

Is the patient's memory for events that occurred impaired?

Did the patient experience postictal depression?

Has the patient had other lapses during which he or she engaged in nearly identical behavior?

A final term that requires clarification does not refer to epileptic seizures at all. The term *pseudoseizure* is used synonymously with *nonepileptic seizure* or *conversion reaction*. The differentiation of this condition from true seizures is at times extremely difficult (Table 16–7), often complicated by the fact that the person who is suspected of having "seizures," primarily related to psychological reasons, often has a history of true seizures. Devinsky and Gordon (1998) noted that nonepileptic seizures often can follow epileptic seizures. They postulated that the epileptic seizure, particularly the CPS, leads to possible loss of inhibition of impulses and emotions. The patients with nonepileptic seizures differ from seizure disorder patients in that they may have significantly more stress, more negative life events, and a history of child abuse, and they often have more somatic symptoms and awareness of their bodies (Arnold and Privitera 1996; Tojek et al. 2000). Most of the nonepileptic seizure patients have somatoform disorders, particularly conversion, rather than dissociative disorders. Interestingly, the patients with nonepileptic seizures who did not fit the criteria for conversion had a high incidence of anxiety and psychotic disorders (Alper et al. 1995; Kuyk et al. 1999). A significant number of patients with nonepileptic seizures also have concomitant mood and anxiety disorders. Therefore, combination treatment with psychotropic medications such as selective serotonin reuptake inhibitors (SSRIs), benzodiazepines, and atypical antipsychotics and individual psychotherapy can be extremely helpful in decreasing the frequency and morbidity associated with nonepileptic seizures (M. Thomas and Jankovic 2004).

However, patients will at times have episodes that are extremely difficult to interpret. These episodes may be very short-lived, lasting seconds or minutes, but on occasion can last for days. Such patients behave out of character and usually show a profound lability of affect, with disturbances ranging from depression to mania. The patients may

TABLE 16–7.   General features of nonepileptic seizures ("pseudoseizures")

Setting

Environmental gain (audience usually present)

Seldom sleep related

Often triggered (e.g., by stress)

Suggestive profile on Minnesota Multiphasic Personality Inventory (Hathaway and McKinley 1989)

Attack

Atypical movements, often bizarre or purposeful

Seldom results in injury

Often starts and ends gradually

Out-of-phase movements of extremities

Side-to-side movements

Examination

Restraint accentuates the seizure

Inattention decreases over time

Plantar flexor reflexes

Reflexes intact (corneal, pupillary, and blink)

Consciousness preserved

Autonomic system uninvolved

Autonomically intact

After attack

No postictal features (lethargy, tiredness, abnormal electroencephalogram findings)

Prolactin normal (after 30 minutes)

No or little amnesia

Memory exists (hypnosis or amobarbital sodium)

appear to be markedly thought disordered, delusional, or hallucinating. Very often, these episodes are repetitive and of the same quality each time. These patients may have behavioral alterations perceived as characterological disorders. Clinically, these nonepileptic seizures often occur in young women and consist of significant amounts of staring, shaking, blacking out without falling, and stiffening without loss of consciousness (Devinsky et al. 1996). Pelvic thrusting can occur in many types of seizures and is not alone diagnostic of nonepileptic seizures (Geyer et al. 2000).

In such episodes, EEGs or 24-hour monitoring may not provide any additional information. However, if the patients have temporal spikes, even if they do not correlate

with video monitoring, they may respond to anticonvulsant medication. But in most cases, the patient will be left with the label of having nonepileptic seizures. Twenty percent of intractable seizures remain as nonepileptic seizures (Krumholz 1999). Kanner et al. (1999) studied 45 patients with the diagnosis of nonepileptic seizures. Interestingly, 29% of the patients stopped having seizures after being told that the seizures were psychogenic. Twenty-seven percent had only brief recurrences, and the seizures persisted in 44%. The patients in whom the seizures persisted often had psychiatric diagnoses of recurrent affective disorder, dissociative disorders, or personality disorders. However, an abnormal MRI finding predicted the recurrence of seizures with 75% accuracy, which may indicate some covert biological basis for the nonepileptic seizure.

Frontal lobe epilepsy can also present with bizarre behavioral symptoms and can be confused with nonepileptic seizures. Laskowitz et al. (1995) noted that the symptoms often appear as spells with an aura of panic symptoms, with weird vocalizations and with bilateral limb movements but no periods of postictal tiredness and no confusion; also, no oral or alimentary movements occur. These spells last about 60–70 seconds. Fortunately, most of these seizures are symptomatic of a CNS lesion, and usually the correct diagnosis is made with the EEG or imaging studies. P. Thomas et al. (1999) described a form of nonconvulsive status epilepticus of frontal origin. These patients often presented with a mood disturbance similar to hypomania, subtle cognitive impairments, some disinhibition, and some indifference.

ETIOLOGICAL LINKS OF SEIZURES TO PSYCHOPATHOLOGY

The increased incidence of psychopathology and seizure disorders is clear and evident, but the exact etiology of this increased incidence is unclear. There have been two major theories historically. One is an affinity theory, best exemplified by the classic articles of Slater et al. (1963), which described a group of patients with epilepsy and psychosis. An opposing theory was first postulated by Von Meduna (1937), who observed (incorrectly) that the schizophrenic patients under his care had few epileptic conditions (Fink 1984). He then hypothesized that the induction of a seizure in a psychotic patient might be therapeutic. Landolt (1958) observed a group of patients whose EEG results seemed to normalize during a psychotic episode. This has been called "forced normalization," and Pakalinis et al. (1987) observed seven patients who had this pattern. This inverse relation between seizures and behavioral disturbances has been noted by many clinicians. For example, it is not uncommon for a patient with epilepsy to have a marked decrease in seizures for a prolonged time and then later to have an increase in behavioral disturbances. After a seizure, the behavior seems to normalize again. Although these observations are clinically and statistically apparent (Schiffer 1987), their exact etiological importance to all patients with epilepsy and behavioral disturbance is unclear. The relation between psychopathology and seizures is not clear and is complicated by whether the behavioral disturbance is a preictal event, an ictal event, or a postictal event. Many hypothesize the existence of subictal electrical events in the brain that are pathological, leading to disturbances of CNS function that manifest as behavioral disturbance. *Kindling*, a pathophysiological event, is the sequence whereby repetitive subthreshold electrical or chemical stimuli to specific brain areas eventually induce a seizure or a behavioral disturbance that persists. This process has been hypothesized as one of the possible causes of psychopathology. However, kindling remains only a tantalizing hypothesis, and it has never been demonstrated in humans (Adamec and Stark 1983).

Other hypotheses about the cause of the psychopathology have been that seizures create a type of organic brain syndrome related to some underlying diffuse process or are caused by active focal damage (Pincus and Tucker 1985). Toxicity of the medicines used to treat seizure disorders also has been implicated, and although most anticonvulsant drugs cause significant cognitive impairment, they do not seem to be associated with the development of major psychopathology (Dodrill and Troupin 1991; Meador et al. 1993; Moehle et al. 1984; Trimble 1988). Overmedication with anticonvulsant medications before the availability of blood level monitoring was a likely cause of confusion and behavioral disturbance in some of these patients; however, with present-day monitoring, these disturbances occur much less frequently.

TEMPORAL LOBE SPECIFICITY AND PSYCHOPATHOLOGY

A major question about the behavior changes in epilepsy is whether behavioral disturbances occur more commonly in patients with temporal lobe epilepsy specifically or whether the behavioral disturbances are related to seizure disorders in general.

This issue is complex, with many confounding variables. For example, more complicated patients gravitate toward university hospitals, where studies are usually undertaken. In the hospital study by Currie et al. (1970) in London, 25% of the 2,664 patients seen in a university hospital clinic had a history of psychiatric hospitalization, whereas only 5%–9% of 678 patients in a private clinic in

the same city had a similar history of psychiatric hospitalization. Another confounding variable is the age at onset of psychomotor epilepsy, which is similar to that of schizophrenia. Moreover, three-quarters of patients with psychomotor seizures or CPSs are older than 16 years at the onset of the seizure disorder (Stevens 1988).

The vast majority of patients with seizure disorders will have temporal lobe foci on electroencephalographic examination at some point during their illness. Kristensen and Sindrup (1978) compared CPS patients with psychosis with CPS patients without psychosis and could find little difference in the two groups with regard to age at onset, laterality of focus, and interval between epilepsy onset and time of examination. The patients with psychosis had significantly more neurological signs, spike EEGs, a history of brain damage, and no family history of seizure disorders, suggesting that these patients may have had other associated organic brain syndromes. The increased incidence of psychosocial problems in these groups may further confound the relation to behavioral disturbances.

Additionally, patients with CPSs and secondary generalization are often more difficult to keep seizure-free than are those with generalized seizures. Consequently, they are often taking high doses of anticonvulsants and/or anticonvulsant polytherapy. Their greater number of seizures and the frequent evidence of associated organic brain syndromes further confound the relation to behavioral disturbance.

The confounding variables include increased seizures, increased amounts of anticonvulsants, and increased numbers of different types of seizures. The temporal lobe constitutes 40% of the cerebral cortex (Stevens 1988). These factors could differentially be perceived as important causal, predisposing, or incidental features. However, patients with temporal lobe epilepsy have increased difficulties with seizure control and medication, and this may be related to the more primitive embryological structure of the archipallium. The relative degree of encephalization in this area is less than that in other areas of the brain. This primitive structure could predispose to psychopathology.

Despite these confounding factors and limited available data, it appears that patients with temporal lobe epilepsy and other focal epilepsies are at greater risk for developing psychiatric disorders than are patients with primary generalized seizure disorders. A study of 88 epilepsy outpatients found psychiatric disorders in 60% of the temporal lobe epilepsy patients and 54% of the patients with other focal epilepsies, compared with 37% of the patients with primary generalized epilepsy (Edeh and Toone 1987). Poor response to treatment is also related to increased psychiatric comorbidity. Patients with treatment-refractory epilepsy quite often have temporal lobe epilepsy. In one study, patients awaiting temporal lobectomy had a lifetime prevalence of psychiatric disorders of 75% (Glosser et al. 2000). Thus, epilepsy patients most at risk for developing psychiatric comorbidity are those with localization-related epilepsies and a chronic, treatment-resistant course (Blumer et al. 1995; Cockerell et al. 1996; Fiordelli et al. 1993; Glosser et al. 2000).

COMORBID PSYCHIATRIC SYNDROMES

The relation of psychopathology and seizure disorders is difficult to establish. Most of the studies rest at the level of case report, and even large-scale studies usually deal with populations that have come to psychiatric attention rather than community-based samples (Popkin and Tucker 1994). The following question constantly arises: Are we dealing with behavior associated with a seizure disorder, or is the behavior associated with another underlying disease of the CNS that can cause seizures? Comparison of symptoms between patients with seizure disorders and those with other disturbances of the CNS indicates a considerable overlap. For example, symptoms of impulsiveness and irritability, emotional lability, paranoia, changes in sexual behavior, regression, and poor sleep have been noted in patients with seizure disorders, head trauma, and tumors and in patients with abnormal EEG results as the only finding. Therefore, at the symptom level, we are frequently dealing with general symptoms related to damage of the CNS and not specific to any one condition or region of the brain. The symptoms can be episodic changes in mood, irritability or impulsiveness, psychosis, anxiety disorders, or confusional syndromes. The other major types of symptoms usually seen with CNS dysfunction are related to more insidious disorders, such as dementia, depression, various motor diseases, or distinctive personality changes such as those seen after head trauma (Popkin and Tucker 1994). Consequently, when we talk about psychopathology associated with seizure disorders, we see a wide range of syndromes. The etiologies of these syndromes may be related to the seizure specifically or to the underlying damage to the CNS. The various symptom patterns may be related to individual genetic predispositions, environmental influences, or genetic-environmental interactions.

The temporal relation of mood or psychotic symptoms to seizure episodes is also important and thus has been classified into peri-ictal, ictal, postictal, and interictal episodes. The term *peri-ictal* (or premonitory) refers to psychiatric symptoms immediately before and after the seizure. These symptoms may last hours to days and may resolve when the seizure itself occurs. *Ictal* symptoms are affective or psy-

chotic symptoms that occur during the seizure itself. *Postictal* psychiatric symptoms begin shortly after the cessation of seizure activity. And *interictal* refers to chronic psychiatric symptoms that appear during seizure-free periods. This classification is important in that each type appears to follow a differing constellation and severity of symptoms and thus may require different treatment approaches.

PSYCHOSIS

It is clear that *all* of the symptoms described in schizophrenic patients can occur in patients with seizure disorders (Toone et al. 1982). The classic study by Slater et al. (1963) conducted at Maudsley Hospital in London evaluated patients hospitalized for psychosis who had seizure disorders. These patients had all the symptoms associated with schizophrenia. A community sample studied by Matsuura et al. (2004) showed that 50% of the patients with epilepsy and psychosis met diagnostic criteria for schizophrenia by standardized rating scales. However, the question of definition remains. There are similarities in the cognitive deficits noted in both epileptic patients and schizophrenic patients. Mellers et al. (2000) used neuropsychological testing to compare a group of patients with epilepsy and psychosis, epilepsy alone, and schizophrenia with a group of neuropsychologically healthy control subjects. Patients with psychosis and epilepsy had almost identical neuropsychological test patterns. Often, what patients with seizure disorders and behavior problems describe is a single complaint such as auditory hallucinations or a solitary perceptual change. The patients with these single symptoms are frequently classified by clinicians as psychotic. Conversely, psychiatric patients with several symptoms are sometimes dubiously labeled as epileptic based on a history of a seizure disorder, a solitary seizure, seizures associated with alcohol or other substance withdrawal, or vaguely described and poorly characterized "blackouts." Such cases are difficult to interpret, but there seems to be no denying the relation of seizures to psychopathology. Kanner et al. (1996) studied patients admitted to a video electroencephalographic monitoring unit for evaluation of their seizures. As part of the evaluation, all anticonvulsants were stopped. The researchers found that of the 140 patients admitted to the unit, there was a 7.8% incidence of postictal psychiatric events; 6.4% were psychotic and 1.4% were nonpsychotic. The psychotic events were mostly depressive, hypomanic, or delusional, and all seemed to take place in a confused state. These episodes responded to psychotropic medication and lasted about 69 hours on average. A similar finding was noted by Ketter et al. (1994), who described increased anxiety and depressive symptoms in

38% of 32 patients withdrawn from their anticonvulsant medications in order to enter a controlled trial.

Seizure disorders and schizophrenia have many empirical similarities that also make the differential diagnosis difficult. Both disorders are also phenomenologically based constructs presenting primarily as behavioral disturbances, and often no specific pathological changes are evident in either of these conditions. Furthermore, the peak age at onset is similar. Both disorders may occur in early to late adolescence, although epilepsy often presents in childhood and may occur at any age. The neurotransmitter dopamine is somehow related in both conditions because dopamine antagonists are antipsychotic and mildly epileptogenic. Dopamine agonists are psychotogenic and mildly antiepileptic (Trimble 1977). Perhaps most significant is that both conditions require a team approach to rehabilitate patients. However, they do differ in that many seizure disorders go into complete remission, whereas most schizophrenic disorders do not. The family history can be of help in that the genetic frequencies are similar for both conditions, with 10%–13% of the offspring of parents with either schizophrenia or epilepsy having the same condition (Metrakos and Metrakos 1961), but this leaves most cases without a family history of either condition.

Despite more than 100 publications in the scientific literature dealing with core issues of epilepsy in relation to psychosis, the cause of the increased psychopathology in epileptic conditions remains unclear, and a precise clinical picture has not been established (Diehl 1989; McKenna et al. 1985; Neppe 1986). Ey (1954), Gibbs and Gibbs (1952), Gudmundsson (1966), Krohn (1961), Lindsay et al. (1979), Qin et al. (2005), Sachdev (1998), and Sengoku et al. (1983) have all described a clear association between these two conditions. These diverse studies come from several different countries and range from national surveys of unselected populations to studies of patients in outpatient clinics as well as psychiatric hospital populations. These studies suggest that the incidence of psychosis in relation to epilepsy ranges from 4% (Trimble 1977) to 27% (average, about 7%) (Dongier 1959–1960).

Clinically, there seem to be three psychotic presentations that one sees with seizure disorders. One is an episodic course that is usually related to seizure activity, manifested by perceptual changes, alterations in consciousness, and poor memory for the events. Peri-ictal, ictal, and postictal psychoses often follow this episodic course. A chronic interictal psychotic condition also occurs in which the pa-

tient may have simple auditory hallucinations, paranoia, or other perceptual changes, and this condition closely resembles schizophrenia. The third type is simply a variation in which the patient usually has some type of persistent experience of depersonalization or visual distortion that, for lack of a better name, is usually labeled as psychotic. The latter is probably a variant of the chronic psychotic state.

Peri-ictal psychoses develop during seizure activity. Duration of symptoms can be days to weeks, and consciousness may be impaired (Trimble et al. 2000). Ictal psychoses usually occur in patients with generalized nonconvulsive status or complex partial status epilepticus, manifesting as altered consciousness, confusion, or even delusions and hallucinations. Psychotic symptoms may last hours to days, and EEG findings are consistent with status epilepticus (Gaitatzis et al. 2004). Postictal psychoses, also episodic in nature, will often appear after a lucid period following prolonged seizures or an increase in seizure frequency. Hallucinations or delusions may be prominent and may or may not be accompanied by impaired consciousness. Symptoms may resolve spontaneously in days, even without treatment with neuroleptics, although sometimes postictal psychoses may develop into a chronic psychotic condition (Gaitatzis et al. 2004). Interictal psychoses occur during seizure-free periods and do not appear to be directly related to seizure activity. In fact, a form of interictal psychosis may occur that is related to remission of seizures that is often referred to as *forced normalization*. These psychoses may consist of delusions and hallucinations but are distinct from primary psychotic disorders such as schizophrenia because of less deterioration of premorbid affect and personality, fewer negative symptoms, and less severe psychotic episodes (Toone et al. 1982).

Although Slater et al. (1963) postulated a long period between the onset of seizures and subsequent psychosis, it is not uncommon for a clinician to treat a patient for "schizophrenia" who is often completely unresponsive to antipsychotic medications. During the course of this treatment, the patient has a grand mal seizure. An EEG is then obtained that confirms the diagnosis of epilepsy.[1] The patient is then given anticonvulsant medication, and a marked decrease in the "psychotic" symptoms occurs.

In retrospect, patients with a seizure disorder and psychosis, such as the one noted earlier, have subtly different clinical characteristics than the typical schizophrenic patient. Patients with a seizure disorder and psychosis often talk about their symptoms in almost a detached manner.

---

[1]It is important to note that although neuroleptics may lower the seizure threshold, they do not usually cause seizures in patients who are not predisposed to them. Among inpatients taking psychotropic medication, seizures were infrequent, occurring in 0.03% of psychiatric inpatients (Popli et al. 1995).

TABLE 16–8. Diagnostic clues indicating psychosis may be due to lesion of the central nervous system or seizures

Presentation that does not meet DSM-IV-TR criteria

Good premorbid social history

Abrupt change in personality, mood, or ability to function

Rapid fluctuations in mental status

Unresponsiveness to usual biological or psychological interventions

Some might say the patients view the symptoms as ego-dystonic—the symptoms are not part of them, as though something was imposed on them such as a physical illness. Second, most of these patients seem quite intact even when experiencing the symptoms, particularly so between episodes. Their mental status examinations seem to show no evidence of other schizophrenic symptoms. During the episode, what is often seen is a confusional state and an alteration in consciousness rather than an inability to communicate. It is not uncommon to talk to one of these patients on the telephone, have a fairly normal conversation, and then, at the end, ask if the hallucinations are still present. These patients will note that the hallucinations are still occurring on a frequent basis. Additionally, many of these patients have good premorbid social histories. What they and their families describe is an abrupt change in personality, mood, or ability to function. It is important to remain suspicious of altered perceptual experiences that do not completely meet DSM-IV-TR (American Psychiatric Association 2000) criteria for schizophrenia and to reevaluate patients whose symptoms do not respond to antipsychotic medication (Table 16–8).

Possibly Related Seizure Disorders

An interesting area of speculation involves the concept of so-called atypical psychosis. Clinicians have often noted that the distinctions made by classification systems are more distinct in theory than in practice. Consequently, although some cases are clear and are unambiguously labeled as either schizophrenia or mood disorder, a large group of patients does not fit neatly into either category. These patients are frequently given diagnoses of schizoaffective disorder or atypical psychosis. In an excellent review, Procci (1976) noted that the atypical psychotic patients usually have an acute onset, more frequent remissions, good premorbid functioning (often with symptoms of schizophrenia), affective symptoms, and confusion and agitation.

Monroe (1982) extended this concept by delineating a group he called "episodic psychotics," and he related this to a limbic ictal disorder that was unresponsive to antidepressants and neuroleptics. He noted that these patients' psychoses were of a precipitous onset, with intense affects, and had an intermittent course characterized by symptom-free intervals. He postulated that this represented some type of limbic seizure disorder. As an extension of these studies, Tucker et al. (1986) described a series of patients who had documented temporal lobe dysfunction on EEGs with symptomatology very similar to that in the group described by Procci (1976) and the episodic psychosis described by Monroe (1982). All of the patients described had spell-type episodes. They also experienced marked mood lability, often with suicidal ideation and suicide attempts, as well as psychotic phenomena and cognitive changes. All patients returned to normal baseline with symptom-free intervals. It is extremely important that many of these conditions occur in a state of clear consciousness and do not necessarily present with either a clouding of consciousness or symptoms of disorientation.

Such studies of patients with possible temporolimbic dysfunction have been continued from other sources (Wells and Duneau 1980), including chronically ill nonepileptic psychiatric patients who have electroencephalographic temporal lobe foci, violent patients who have refractory schizophrenia (Hakola and Laulumaa 1982), patients who have borderline personality disorder (Cowdry and Gardner 1988), and patients who become dysphoric when taking neuroleptics and have abnormal EEG findings (Brodsky et al. 1983). Although many of these patients' conditions respond to carbamazepine in particular, it should not be seen as a panacea. If carbamazepine is used inappropriately, some patients appear to deteriorate, and response to anticonvulsants does not imply the presence of seizure disorder.

Treatment of Psychotic Conditions

The major treatment of the episodic psychotic conditions is usually the appropriate use of anticonvulsant medications. The treatment of chronic conditions involves both anticonvulsant and antipsychotic medications. In general, the use of medication in these patients is difficult in that very small doses of any medication often cause an increase in symptoms that diminishes over time. Consequently, very small doses and infrequent changes seem to be the major guidelines in treating these conditions. Although all of the neuroleptics can lower the seizure threshold, the rate of seizures with atypical antipsychotic agents is quite low, and their use is increasing in patients with seizures and psychosis, despite lack of controlled clinical trials as to their efficacy in treating seizure-related psychosis. Of the traditional neuroleptics, haloperidol, fluphenazine, molindone, pimozide, and trifluoperazine seem to lower the seizure threshold the least. The propensity for clozapine to lower the seizure threshold is quite well known, so it is only used in patients whose symptoms do not respond to all other antipsychotic medications. Furthermore, the use of clozapine and carbamazepine is contraindicated because of the risk of agranulocytosis.

With anticonvulsant drugs, it is best to adjust their doses as far as possible to the top range of the therapeutic window. However, in cases of forced normalization or psychoses related to seizure remission, a moderate reduction of antiepileptic medications can be helpful. Because all of the anticonvulsants can cause cognitive side effects, it is important to distinguish between toxicity from the drugs and a worsening in behavior (Armon et al. 1996; Hamer et al. 2000; Martin et al. 1999; Meador et al. 1995). Vigabatrin has been reported to have a side-effect profile that shows a 2.5% incidence of psychotic symptoms and a 17.1% incidence of affective symptoms (Levinson and Devinsky 1999).

ANXIETY DISORDERS

The correspondence between seizure disorders and anxiety disorders is a fascinating topic, and the substantial overlapping of symptoms often makes differentiation between these classes of disorders complex. Either type of syndrome can be confused with the other, and the same class of medications (benzodiazepines) helps to reduce the symptoms and subsequent impairment of both types. Panic disorder and CPSs are each included in the differential diagnosis of the other. Although many symptoms overlap, evidence of neurophysiological linkage between anxiety and seizure disorder remains tenuous, except that both involve underlying limbic dysfunction (Fontaine et al. 1990). This connection appears to be more relevant between partial seizure and CPS than other seizure disorders, and it has been speculated that a subgroup of patients exists who have panic disorder that has a pathophysiological relation to epilepsy (Dantendorfer et al. 1995). This relation is not surprising given that modulation of fear is associated with the temporal lobes; others have hypothesized relations between the parietal and the frontal lobe neural circuits and panic attacks (Alemayehu et al. 1995; McNamara and Fogel 1990).

Despite few studies of the relation between anxiety and epilepsy disorders, the available evidence suggests that the prevalence of anxiety disorders is high in both outpatient and hospitalized epilepsy patients. Estimates of anxiety disorders in outpatient and hospitalized epilepsy patients are between 14% and 25%, much higher than those in the general population (Edeh and Toone 1987; Gureje 1991; Jacoby et al. 1996; Perini et al. 1996).

TABLE 16–9.   Anxiety disorder symptoms that overlap with those of seizure disorder

Panic disorder

Fear

Depersonalization

Derealization

Déjà vu

Jamais vu

Misperceptions

Illusions

Dizziness

Paresthesias

Chills or hot flashes

Obsessive-compulsive disorder

Obsessions, forced or intrusive

Posttraumatic stress disorder

Recurrent memories or distressing recollections

Flashback-like episodes

Irritability

Difficulty concentrating

Agoraphobia

Fear of recurrent episodes that leads to restriction of activities

The relation between posttraumatic stress disorder, obsessive-compulsive disorder, generalized anxiety, social phobia, and simple phobias has not been articulated. As is the case with panic disorder, there are overlapping symptoms. Table 16–9 lists many of the symptoms that overlap between CPS and anxiety disorders.

Roth and Harper (1962) have pointed out some of the similarities between epilepsy and anxiety disorders. Both are episodic disorders with sudden onset without a precipitating event; both sometimes present with dissociative symptoms: depersonalization, derealization, and déjà vu; both often present with abnormal perceptual and emotional disturbances, such as intense fear and terror; and both have associated physical symptoms. Significant clinical differences between panic disorder and CPS help to differentiate the two: In panic disorders, consciousness is usually preserved, olfactory hallucinations are unusual, the patient has a positive family history, electroencephalographic results are usually normal, and many patients do not respond well to anticonvulsants (Handal et al. 1995). Individuals with CPS generally do not have agoraphobia, they may have automatisms, their attacks are generally shorter, they often have abnormal brain scans, and antidepressants may worsen the course of their illness (Roth and Harper 1962). Patients with refractory anxiety, in particular panic disorder, and patients who have atypical responses to psychotropic medications should be reevaluated for a seizure disorder. A pilot study by Weilburg et al. (1995) found that in patients with atypical panic attacks, ambulatory electroencephalographic monitoring helped to identify an underlying seizure disorder. Electroencephalographic changes occurred in 33% of the subjects ($n=15$), and among subjects with "captured" panic attacks, 45% showed focal paroxysmal electroencephalographic changes. Two of these five subjects previously had a normal routine EEG.

Treatment of Comorbid Anxiety

Patients with seizure disorders and comorbid anxiety disorder should receive treatment for their anxiety. No controlled clinical trials of the efficacy of treatment of anxiety disorders have been done in epilepsy patients. However, clinical experience indicates that SSRIs, first-line treatments for primary anxiety disorders such as generalized anxiety disorder, panic disorder, and obsessive-compulsive disorder, are also helpful in the treatment of anxiety disorders in epilepsy patients. SSRIs can cause potential interactions with hepatically metabolized antiepileptic medications because they can inhibit various cytochrome P450 enzymes. Benzodiazepines such as clonazepam and alprazolam also can be helpful in the treatment of anxiety disorders in epilepsy patients, although the clinician must be aware of side effects of sedation, impaired cognition, psychomotor slowing, tolerance, addiction, and withdrawal-related seizures. Psychotherapeutic approaches such as cognitive-behavioral therapy, behavioral modification, short-term symptom-focused therapies, and psychoeducation may be helpful as well, but few data exist as to their treatment efficacy.

MOOD DISORDERS

CNS disorders and chronic medical illnesses are frequently associated with increased incidence of mood disorders (Silver et al. 1990); however, there seems to be a distinct relation between mood disorders and epilepsy. Suicide is of special concern because its prevalence is greater in patients with epilepsy than in the general population (Gehlert 1994; Nilsson et al. 2002). Suicide is the cause of death in 10% of all patients with epilepsy, compared with 1% in the general population (Jones et al. 2003).

Patients with uncontrolled seizures have a prevalence of depression up to 10 times greater than in the general population and up to 5 times greater than in patients with controlled seizures (Harden and Goldstein 2002; Hermann et al. 2000; Lambert and Robertson 1999). Patients with epilepsy appear to have higher rates of depression and more severe depression than do patients with other chronic illnesses such as asthma and diabetes mellitus. Furthermore, health care utilization in depressed epilepsy patients is significantly higher than in nondepressed epilepsy patients. Depressed epilepsy patients had twice as many emergency department and nonpsychiatric office visits as did their nondepressed counterparts (Cramer et al. 2004).

Little is known about the prevalence of other mood disorders such as mania and dysthymia in patients with seizure disorders. It is also unknown whether vulnerability to depression is increased as a result of type, frequency, or age at onset of seizures. Several studies have identified a link between left-sided epileptogenic lesions and depression, although a conclusive link has yet to be established (Mendez et al. 1994; Schmitz et al. 1999; Victoroff et al. 1994). Partial seizures, male gender, and depressive symptoms also have been associated with a left epileptogenic focus (Altshuler et al. 1990; Septien et al. 1993; Strauss et al. 1992). Blumer et al. (1995) evaluated 97 patients admitted to a neurodiagnostic electroencephalographic/video monitoring unit and noted that 34% had atypical depression and 22% had nonepileptic seizures. He defined eight key symptoms that he thought were characteristic of the affective disorders of these patients: depressed mood, anergy, irritability, euphoria, pain, insomnia, fear, and anxiety. These patients also had a history of suicide attempts and hallucinations. Blumer and colleagues (1995) believed that this was an epilepsy-specific syndrome, but again many of these symptoms are associated with many types of insult to the CNS. Altshuler et al. (1999) did a 10-year follow-up of 49 patients who had undergone surgery for refractory temporal lobe seizures. The incidence of affective disorder in these patients was quite high: 45% had a lifetime history of depression, 77% had a prior history of depression, 10% developed depression for the first time after surgery, and 50% showed complete remission of their depression after surgery. Forty-seven percent had no recurrence of their depression after surgery. This study certainly implicates the temporal lobes as an anatomical area of some interest in mood disorder.

Several features of depression in epilepsy require special consideration before one diagnoses a comorbid mood disorder. Sometimes it can be difficult to distinguish affective symptoms from symptoms related to the seizure disorder or the underlying pathology. Peri-ictal depression or premonitory dysphoria may occur before or after the seizure, lasting hours to days. Depressive or dysphoric symptoms of this type may stop when the seizure occurs or may continue for days after the seizure. It is unknown whether these affective symptoms are subclinical symptoms of the seizure itself. Ictal depressive symptoms occur during the seizure and are characterized by sudden onset of symptoms without precipitating factors and can even manifest as impulsive suicidality (Prueter and Norra 2005). Postictal depressive episodes occur after seizure activity resolves and may last for up to 2 weeks. The most common type of depression in epilepsy is interictal depression, which may manifest as major depressive or dysthymic episodes. Interictal depression does not fit DSM-IV-TR classification well because it tends to have a chronic course and atypical mood symptoms of pain, mixed phases of euphoria and dysphoria, and short intervals without affective symptoms (Kanner 2003).

In evaluating depression in a patient with epilepsy, it is very important to examine the medications the patient is taking. Anticonvulsants have been identified as causal agents of depression and cognitive impairments; phenobarbital, the anticonvulsant vigabatrin, and multiple combinations of anticonvulsants appear to contribute to mood disturbance (Bauer and Elger 1995; Brent et al. 1990; Levinson and Devinsky 1999; Mendez et al. 1993). Other anticonvulsants have minimal effect, and some, such as carbamazepine and lamotrigine, may have beneficial effects on mood.

Treatment of Comorbid Mood Disorders

Data on the treatment of depression in seizure patients are extremely limited. In general, preictal and ictal depressive symptoms may not require antidepressant treatment because these episodes are often self-limited, and improved seizure control will reduce their occurrence (Lambert and Robertson 1999). However, postictal and interictal depressions require treatment with antidepressant medication.

When depression does occur, the clinician should determine whether the patient has had a recent change in antiepileptic medication regimen. If the patient recently discontinued an antiepileptic medication with mood-stabilizing medications, the medication should be restarted. Or if the patient is taking an antiepileptic medication with known depressogenic effects, it should be replaced, if possible, by one with mood-stabilizing effects such as carbamazepine, valproate, or lamotrigine. For patients with a bipolar diathesis or suspected mood lability, monotherapy with carbamazepine or valproic acid (or now lamotrigine) may suffice to prevent episodes, decrease severity of symptoms, and minimize overall decompensation.

All antidepressants, including the SSRI antidepressants, are proconvulsive, although the incidence of seizures in healthy individuals is low (Alldredge 1999). Despite few controlled clinical data on the efficacy of SSRI antidepressants in the treatment of mood disorders in epilepsy patients, SSRIs are generally recommended as first-line treat-

ments (Kanner and Nieto 1999). Citalopram and sertraline are often used because of their minimal interactions with antiepileptic medications. It is important to start any medication with smaller doses than are conventionally given for primary psychiatric disorders, with gradual dose increases over time. Regular monitoring of interval EEGs and antiepileptic medication levels is recommended. Of the older antidepressant medications, most of the tricyclic antidepressants are known to lower the seizure threshold. This is particularly true of amitriptyline, maprotiline, and clomipramine. Bupropion is also very likely to cause seizures. However, doxepin, trazodone, and the monoamine oxidase inhibitors have less of a tendency to lower the seizure threshold (Rosenstein 1993). Most of the seizures reported with any of these medications are dose related; therefore, blood level monitoring in these patients can be quite useful.

In most cases, treating the depression often improves seizure control. In an open study evaluating the use of fluoxetine as an adjunctive medication in patients with CPSs, 6 of 17 patients showed a dramatic improvement, and the others had a 30% reduction in their seizure frequency over 14 months (Favale et al. 1995). To date, no evidence shows that any one particular antidepressant is more effective than another, and the choice should be made on clinical grounds. Epileptic patients with refractory or severe depression and even mania should be considered for ECT because it is not contraindicated in people with epilepsy. ECT raises the seizure threshold by more than 50% (Sackeim 1999). However, controlled clinical trials with ECT are lacking in epilepsy patients as well (Zwil and Pelchat 1994).

The role of psychotherapeutic approaches seems intuitively beneficial, but few empirical studies have evaluated this topic. Several studies have suggested that psychological interventions help children and adults with seizure disorders to comply with medications, accept and manage the illness, cope with stressful events, and develop improved self-esteem (Fenwick 1994; Mathers 1992; Regan et al. 1993). A study by Gillham (1990) reported that psychological intervention with education to improve coping skills could be helpful in reducing seizure frequency and psychological symptoms (as well as depressive symptoms) in patients with refractory seizures.

Vagus nerve stimulation (VNS) is a well-tolerated, efficacious treatment for refractory epilepsy. More than 15,000 patients worldwide receive VNS treatment (Ben-Menachem 2002). Its efficacy in the treatment of mood disorders is not conclusively established, although results from open, long-term studies of treatment-resistant depression are promising. It has not been studied systematically in epilepsy patients with concomitant mood disorders, although this may be a promising treatment option in the future. Repetitive transcranial magnetic stimulation (rTMS) is currently being investigated as a treatment for epilepsy and mood disorders but is not recommended for clinical use at this time.

BEHAVIORAL AND PERSONALITY DISTURBANCES

The literature and clinical experience clearly point to an association between seizure disorders and behavioral disturbances, particularly in patients who have had a chronic course (Neppe and Tucker 1988). Evidence for personality pathology with seizure disorders is sparse because of methodological constraints, but many case reports cite personality disturbance (Blumer 1999; Blumer et al. 1995). Hermann and Riel (1981) underscored the issues that have perpetuated misunderstanding of the relation between personality and seizures. Methods of measuring personality pathology and comparisons among epilepsy and control groups have not been uniform. No longitudinal studies have assessed behavior and personality before the onset of a seizure disorder. Most of our knowledge in this area comes from cross-sectional case–control studies, case reports, and tertiary centers that treat the most severe cases. As a result, it is difficult to extricate the relation between personality formation and the course of a seizure disorder. Several factors, such as stigma of the illness, adverse social factors, level of social support, cultural acceptability, consequences of the illness on psychosocial adaptation, and interpersonal relationships, play an important role in shaping patterns of behavior and have a significant effect on the integrity of personality development. Factors that may assume a role in the pathogenesis of personality and behavioral disturbance are the age at onset of the seizure disorder, the type of seizure disorder, the location and the laterality, the frequency of the seizures, the etiology, the presence of a structural lesion, the presence of another medical illness or behavioral dysfunction, and the ongoing administration of anticonvulsants.

It is unlikely that an epileptic personality exists (Dam and Dam 1986; Devinsky and Najjar 1999), and only a tenuous link is found between any formal DSM-IV-TR personality disorders and seizure disorders. Some have suggested that neurological dysfunction, including epilepsy, may play a role in the development of symptoms in subtypes of borderline personality disorder (Andrulonis et al. 1982; Gunderson and Zanarini 1989). Maladaptive personality characteristics and specific personality profiles have been described—a preoccupation with philosophical and moral concerns; a belief in a personal destiny; dependency; and traits such as humorlessness (circumstantiality), hypergraphia, hyposexuality, religiosity, viscosity, and paranoia (Bear and Fedio 1977; Hermann and Riel 1981; Waxman and Geschwind 1975)—

but large-scale studies do not confirm these case reports or even that a specific personality type is associated with seizure disorders (Mungus 1982; Rodin and Schmaltz 1984; Stark-Adamec et al. 1985; Stevens 1975).

An increase in episodic and impulsive aggression also has been associated with seizure disorders, particularly CPS (Blake et al. 1995; Mann 1995). Following the postictal period, uncooperative and aggressive behavior may occur when a confused patient is restrained or may occur in a patient who develops a postictal paranoid psychosis (Rodin 1973). Aggressive behavior during a seizure is very unusual, and aggressive activity is usually carried out in a disordered, uncoordinated, and nondirected way (Fenwick 1986). The relation between aggression and seizure disorders traditionally has been controversial because of methodological concerns. The prevalence of interictal aggression is increased in some seizure disorders, CPS, and generalized seizure disorders but may be an epiphenomenon of epilepsy. This probably can be accounted for by other factors associated with violence and aggression: exposure to violence as a child, male sex, low IQ, low socioeconomic status, adverse social factors, focal or diffuse neurological lesions, refractory seizures, cognitive impairment, history of institutionalization, and drug use (Devinsky and Vazquez 1993).

The manner in which a particular seizure disorder promotes psychopathic behavioral syndromes is not well understood. Auras have been hypothesized as manifestations of an underlying mechanism that contributes to the development of personality disturbance (Mendez et al. 1993). Evidence indicates that patients with chronic seizure disorders develop brain neuropathology, and histological studies of the temporal lobes in CPS show neuronal loss (Sloviter and Tamminga 1995).

Devinsky and Vazquez (1993) emphasized the diversity of symptoms, behaviors, and profiles and that the most important characteristic of patients with a seizure disorder is the tendency for extremes of behavior to be accentuated in numerous manners. Not all of the symptoms and consequences of a seizure disorder are debilitating, and some may even play a positive role. It is the maladaptive consequences and dysfunctional traits that should be of paramount importance in treatment.

COGNITIVE DISORDERS

Cognitive function in patients with epilepsy is highly variable, often related to the pathogenesis or etiology of the seizure disorder, anatomical localization of seizure foci, and severity and clinical course of the disorder. Results from several studies suggested that cognitive deficits may be apparent at disease onset. In one study, newly diagnosed patients with temporal lobe epilepsy had verbal memory deficits compared with control subjects, whereas another study of newly diagnosed mixed epilepsy patients found deficits in memory, attention, mental flexibility, and visuomotor tasks (Aikia et al. 2001; Pulliainen et al. 2000). Thus, epilepsy patients may have cognitive impairment at the outset, and these deficits are modulated by the long-term course of the disease (Elger et al. 2004). No controlled, long-term studies of idiopathic generalized tonic-clonic seizures and absence seizures are available, so the long-term effects on cognition are unknown. Temporal lobe epilepsy, a focal or localization-related epilepsy, is often associated with memory impairment. Left-sided temporal lobe epilepsy is often characterized by verbal memory deficits because of the language-dominant hemisphere being affected. However, right-sided temporal lobe epilepsy is not necessarily characterized by nonverbal memory impairment.

Generalized tonic-clonic seizures are more likely to cause cognitive impairment than are focal seizures. And status epilepticus, whether convulsive or nonconvulsive, can lead to severe and persistent amnesia (Dietl et al. 2004; Oxbury et al. 1997). However, the long-term cognitive effects of status epilepticus have not been comprehensively studied (Dodrill and Wilensky 1990).

Thus, it appears that cognitive function is compromised at disease onset in adult epilepsy patients and that cognitive function is fairly stable early in the disease course. Further cognitive impairment is modulated by clinical course of the disease, with seizure remission resulting in arrest or even reversal of cognitive decline. However, the long-term cognitive outcome of epilepsy patients is largely unknown (Elger et al. 2004).

OVERALL GUIDELINES FOR TREATMENT OF COMORBID PSYCHIATRIC SYNDROMES

With any chronic illness, basic principles should be applied in developing a treatment plan. Seizure disorders are no exception, and guidelines for treatment are summarized in Table 16–10. A thorough assessment of premorbid functioning, past episodes, previous trials and responses, duration of the current episode, and level of impairment and psychosocial dysfunction facilitates proper intervention and guides subsequent management. Patients with seizure disorders vary greatly in their degree of functioning and coping with life's vicissitudes. Careful attention to ongoing interpersonal and psychosocial impairment, stigmatization, and the effects of the illness on self-esteem and behavior will aid in strengthening the therapeutic alliance and promote psychoeducational and psychopharmacological interventions. Given that

insults to the CNS produce only a limited amount of symptom expression, the mood, anxiety, psychotic, cognitive, and behavioral symptoms and signs associated with seizure disorders do not fit neatly into the DSM-IV-TR psychiatric categories (Tucker 1996). The protean nature of the manifestations of various types of seizure disorders may make diagnostic confirmation difficult, especially if no electroencephalographic abnormalities are seen or if, after neurological consultation, the clinician has reservations about the diagnosis. Under such conditions, the neuropsychiatrist may elect to treat patients with a suspected seizure disorder empirically. These patients, and some patients with refractory psychiatric illness, may find benefit with the addition of an anticonvulsant (Post et al. 1985). In a few patients with concomitant psychiatric illness, anticonvulsant monotherapy for the seizure disorder may suffice. The degree of seizure control is not associated with an increase in the number of anticonvulsants (Neppe et al. 1988). Patients taking anticonvulsants should have serum blood levels checked at the first indication of incipient or worsening psychiatric symptoms or signs. Increase in the dosage of an anticonvulsant may be all that is necessary to diminish symptoms and prevent decompensation. Conversely, patients with complex medication regimens may realize symptom improvement after dosage reduction (Trimble and Thompson 1983).

Most patients will require treatment of psychiatric syndromes. Individual, group, family, or couples therapies can provide specific syndrome-focused treatments. Psychotherapeutic approaches have many advantages. They avoid drug interactions, circumvent the tendency of psychotropic medications to alter seizure thresholds, and can teach patients behavior and coping skills that may have a positive effect on symptoms and dysfunction.

Many patients will require pharmacotherapy, either combined with psychotherapeutic approaches or alone. Patients with temporal lobe epilepsy have a wide variety of mood, anxiety, dissociative, psychotic, and behavioral disturbances that frequently resemble psychiatric disorders. Discriminating the symptoms of previous seizures from target psychiatric symptoms will ensure a greater likelihood of response to medication.

Although we recommend an aggressive approach for the treatment of comorbid psychiatric syndromes, we are judicious with the dosing of psychotropics and prefer gradual increases. Clinical experience shows that many patients with seizure disorders seem to respond to smaller doses. Given the concern about anticonvulsant and psychotropic drug interactions, such an approach is warranted. Anytime a new drug is added, it is mandatory for the clinician to be aware of potential drug interactions.

TABLE 16–10. Basic principles of treating patients with a seizure disorder and concomitant psychiatric symptoms

1. Perform a thorough assessment of biopsychosocial factors that aggravate neuropsychiatric symptoms.

2. Evaluate the need for adjustment of the anticonvulsant.

3. Consider psychotherapeutic approaches (individual, group, family) that are specific for the syndrome or that target behaviors or stressors.

4. Preferably—but not always—use anticonvulsant monotherapy.

5. Optimize the addition of psychotropic medication by targeting specific psychiatric symptoms.

6. Start with smaller than usual dose and wait until symptoms stabilize (often weeks) before changing doses.

7. Anticipate interactions between anticonvulsant and psychotropic medications.

8. Collaborate with other caregivers.

Many anticonvulsants will lower the serum drug level of psychotropics through enzyme induction (Perucca et al. 1985), and psychotropics may increase the levels of anticonvulsants secondary to increased P450 hepatic enzyme competition (Cloyd et al. 1986). For patients receiving tricyclic antidepressants, monitoring of serum levels is recommended, and avoiding elevated blood levels may prevent seizure promotion (Preskorn and Fast 1992). Initially, anticonvulsant blood levels should be monitored weekly and then monthly, after the addition of a psychotropic. After a few months, serum levels can be checked less frequently. Thereafter, any changes in the dosage of medications require reexamination of serum blood levels.

Finally, the importance of coordinating care with other professionals and health care providers cannot be overemphasized. It behooves the psychiatrist to work with a neurologist (if available) to develop a long-term strategy. Often, psychiatrists will assume the role of supervising all treatment planning (Schoenenberger et al. 1995).

SPECIFIC ASPECTS OF ANTICONVULSANT USE

It is important to recognize that in many of the patients who have suspected seizure disorders, the psychiatrist will be left to manage the anticonvulsants. Often, even when the patient has a documented seizure disorder and the major persistent symptoms are behavioral, the psychiatrist will also be managing these medications alone. Until the psychiatrist is comfortable with these medications, collaboration with a neurologist is not only helpful but also a good learning technique. However, as valproic acid and carbamazepine have become more common in the treatment of bipolar illness, the basic principles are known to most psychiatrists (McElroy et al. 1988; Neppe et al. 1988).

PHARMACOKINETIC INTERACTIONS

Anticonvulsant administration is particularly important and particularly difficult by virtue of enzyme induction and inhibition occurring in the liver. This enzyme induction tends to affect predominantly the P450 cytochrome enzyme system in the liver. This implies that both the metabolism of anticonvulsants (particularly carbamazepine) and the metabolism of other lipid-soluble compounds are accelerated (Alldredge 1999; Post et al. 1985). However, some of the new anticonvulsants—oxcarbazepine, gabapentin, and vigabatrin—have few drug interactions (Dichter and Brodie 1996).

Of the major anticonvulsants, phenobarbital, phenytoin, carbamazepine, lamotrigine, topiramate, and tiagabine have potent drug interactions. Table 16–11 indicates what is known about some interactions and shows the complexity of these drug interactions (Bertilsson 1978; Birkhimer et al. 1985; Bramhall and Levine 1988; Dichter and Brodie 1996; Dorn 1986; Jann et al. 1985; Kidron et al. 1985; Shukla et al. 1984; Zimmerman 1986).

Phenobarbital

Phenobarbital is the most potent of the enzyme inducers; when it is used in combination, levels of other anticonvulsants are commonly reduced because of the extensive enzyme induction. In addition, phenobarbital causes psychological depression, has the potential for addiction (although this is generally low among patients receiving phenobarbital for seizures), and is potentially lethal in overdose. Indeed, it was the major cause of death due to overdose during the 1950s. It also produces a cognitive impairment, which may explain the rigidity of personality that was at times seen in patients with seizure disorders taking phenobarbital.

We see little role for barbiturates in the outpatient management of seizure disorders today; their only place is with patients who are already taking them and who do not have significant side effects. In our experience, most patients have side effects such as CNS depression, psychological depression, or cognitive impairments of one kind or another. It is extremely difficult to taper off barbiturates without producing an epileptic seizure in the patients.

TABLE 16–11. Known interactions between carbamazepine and other drugs

Drugs that increase carbamazepine level

Isoniazid

Valproic acid (increased free carbamazepine in vitro)

Carbamazepine epoxide only

Troleandomycin

Propoxyphene

Erythromycin

Nicotinamide

Cimetidine

Viloxazine

Drugs that decrease carbamazepine level

Phenobarbital

Phenytoin

Primidone and phenobarbital

Carbamazepine itself (autoinduction)

Alcohol (chronic use)

Cigarettes

Conditions caused by carbamazepine

Pregnancy test failure

Escape from dexamethasone suppression

Oral contraceptive failure

Substances whose effects are decreased by carbamazepine

Vitamin D, calcium, and folate; causes possible hyponatremia

Clonazepam

Dicumarol

Doxycycline

Phenytoin

Sodium valproate

Theophylline

Ethosuximide

Haloperidol

Isoniazid

Note. Because enzyme induction is the mechanism in most of these interactions, it can be hypothesized that similar effects occur with phenytoin, phenobarbital, and primidone.

Phenytoin

Although not as problematic as phenobarbital, diphenyl-hydantoin sodium (or phenytoin) is now less popular than it was and has limited use in the neuropsychiatric patient, despite being an outstanding anticonvulsant in controlling generalized tonic-clonic and some partial seizures. Its problem, like phenobarbital's, is its side-effect profile (Pulliainen and Jokelainen 1994). Mild cognitive impairment occurs, particularly in higher doses. Because phenytoin has a small therapeutic range, patients can easily become drug toxic, and (ironically) one of the side effects of significant toxicity is seizures. Additionally, it can make petit mal seizures worse. Gum hyperplasia is a particular problem with the long-term use of phenytoin, producing an appearance that can, at times, be unsightly (Trimble 1979, 1988). Phenytoin is a potent enzyme inducer but is weaker than phenobarbital.

Carbamazepine

There has been an increasing trend to use carbamazepine rather than phenytoin because it has fewer side effects, may have some psychotropic properties, and has proven value in severe disorders and bipolar illness. It is as effective as phenytoin in both generalized tonic-clonic seizures and partial seizures and thus is the drug of choice for such conditions. It is ineffective in petit mal absences, for which sodium valproate or ethosuximide is generally used.

A possible further role for carbamazepine is its use in treating nonresponsive psychotic patients or atypical psychotic patients with any electroencephalographic temporal lobe abnormalities, with episodic hostility, or with affective lability (Blumer et al. 1988; Cowdry and Gardner 1988; Neppe et al. 1991).

Carbamazepine and the other anticonvulsants involved in enzyme induction can cause many unanticipated side effects (Cloyd et al. 1986) (e.g., patients taking oral contraceptives may have their steroid levels lowered, patients may become vitamin D deficient, folic acid may be depleted). Finally, a slight elevation in hepatic enzyme levels such as glutamyl transferase commonly occurs; this does not imply that the anticonvulsant drugs should be stopped.

Early on, patients taking neuroleptics who are given carbamazepine may have more side effects as a consequence of raised levels from competition at enzyme system pathways. Because of induction by the neuroleptic, the levels of all anticonvulsants can be higher. Consequently, the necessary doses of anticonvulsant for monotherapy are lower when the anticonvulsant is given in conjunction with psychotropic agents, partly because of competition and partly because the additive pharmacodynamics produce sedation.

In addition to the phenomenon of induction of hepatic enzymes, a second phenomenon of deinduction of hepatic enzyme systems occurs (Neppe and Kaplan 1988). It is probable that patients going off anticonvulsant medication will experience a reverse process whereby the rate of liver metabolism will decrease, with the consequence that there may be an accumulation of psychotropic agents.

Valproate

Sodium valproate is particularly useful in combined tonic-clonic and petit mal seizures. It also appears to be effective against CPSs.

Valproate does not induce enzymes but metabolically competes; thus, theoretically, it raises levels of psychotropics and has its own level raised. It is safe, relatively nontoxic, and generally well tolerated. The major concern with its use is potentially fatal, primarily rare hepatotoxicity in young children, particularly when they are taking other anticonvulsants (McElroy et al. 1988).

New Antiepileptic Drugs

There are many new antiepileptic drugs: gabapentin, felbamate, oxcarbazepine, tiagabine, topiramate, vigabatrin, levetiracetam, and lamotrigine. Most of these drugs for which the actions are known affect either the inhibitory γ-aminobutyric acid system (gabapentin, tiagabine, vigabatrin) or the excitatory glutaminergic system (felbamate, lamotrigine). Many of these have been well studied throughout the world and in the United States, and all have various mild to serious side effects (Table 16–12) (Dichter and Brodie 1996; Ketter et al. 1999). Gabapentin, lamotrigine, and topiramate have been increasingly used in psychiatry for bipolar disorder and anxiety disorders and may have uses for similar disorders in seizure disorder patients (Ghaemi and Gaughan 2000; Ketter et al. 1999).

CONCLUSION

Psychopathology occurs in only a minority of persons with epilepsy. Attempted etiological explanations such as kindling, lateralization, localization, and biochemical changes are all, therefore, explanations for a small proportion of the epileptic population. Medications used to treat seizure disorders often do not alleviate behavior changes, and at times agents such as neuroleptics and antidepressants help behavior change but not seizure disturbances. The exact etiology of these conditions remains to be determined. Clinical judgment in the individual case remains the essential standard of care in the absence of solid evidence for specific indications and protocols for the use of anticonvulsant/psychotropic combinations in specific populations.

TABLE 16–12. Selected clinical aspects of the newer anticonvulsants

Felbamate[a,b]

Irritability, insomnia, stimulant effects

Aplastic anemia, hepatitis

Gabapentin

Weight gain

Few drug interactions

Anxiolytic

Lamotrigine[a,b]

No weight gain

Occasional tourettism

Rash

Does not induce P450 system

Can increase neurotoxicity of carbamazepine

Levetiracetam

Increased incidence of depression and behavioral disturbance

Oxcarbazepine

Few drug interactions (not affected by enzyme inducers)

Induces 3A family of P450 system weakly

Hyponatremia

Tiagabine

Confusion, fatigue

Does not induce P450 system

Topiramate[a]

Hyperammonemic encephalopathy when combined with valproate

Cognitive impairments

Weak effect on P450 system

Vigabatrin[a]

Increased incidence of depression and psychosis

Weight gain

Possible retinal damage

No drug interactions

[a]Can affect phenytoin, carbamazepine, or phenobarbital levels.
[b]Valproate decreases levels of this compound.

Highlights for the Clinician

✦ Diagnosis of a seizure disorder is a clinical diagnosis.

✦ An EEG may be confirmatory, but 20% of patients with epilepsy will have a normal EEG result.

✦ Structural and functional neuroimaging modalities can be helpful in the localization of seizure foci.

✦ Seizure disorders and the medications used to treat them are both associated with chronic and episodic neuropsychiatric symptoms.

✦ Mood or psychotic symptoms related to seizure episodes are classified temporally into peri-ictal, ictal, postictal, and interictal episodes and differ in terms of intensity and duration.

✦ Treatment of neuropsychiatric symptoms in epilepsy patients can be complex:

- The clinician should administer very small doses of psychotropic medications with infrequent changes.

- Psychotherapy in addition to pharmacotherapy can be helpful.

- Anticonvulsant and psychotropic medications often have significant drug interactions.

- A multidisciplinary treatment team, including neurologist, psychiatrist, psychotherapist, and social worker, can provide optimal treatment for epilepsy patients.

RECOMMENDED READING

Trimble M, Schmitz B (eds): The Neuropsychiatry of Epilepsy. Cambridge, UK, Cambridge University Press, 2002

REFERENCES

Adamec RE, Stark AC: Limbic kindling and animal behavior: implications for human psychopathology associated with complex partial seizures. Biol Psychiatry 18:269–293, 1983

Adams PF, Benson V: Current estimates from the National Health Interview Survey, 1989. Vital Health Stat 10 (176):1–221, 1990

Aikia M, Salmenpera T, Partanen K, et al: Verbal memory in newly diagnosed patients and patients with chronic left temporal lobe epilepsy. Epilepsy Behav 2:20–27, 2001

Alemayehu S, Bergey GK, Barry E, et al: Panic attacks as ictal manifestations of parietal lobe seizures. Epilepsia 36:824–830, 1995

Alldredge BK: Seizure risk associated with psychotropic drugs: clinical and pharmacokinetic considerations. Neurology 53 (suppl 2):S68–S75, 1999

Alper K, Devinsky O, Perrine K, et al: Psychiatric classification of nonconversion nonepileptic seizures. Arch Neurol 52:199–201, 1995

Altshuler LL, Devinsky O, Post RM, et al: Depression, anxiety, and temporal lobe epilepsy: laterality of focus and symptoms. Arch Neurol 47:284–288, 1990

Altshuler LL, Rausch R, Delrahim S, et al: Temporal lobe epilepsy, temporal lobectomy, major depression. J Neuropsychiatry Clin Neurosci 11:436–443, 1999

American Psychiatric Association: Diagnostic and Statistical Manual of Mental Disorders, 4th Edition, Text Revision. Washington, DC, American Psychiatric Association, 2000

Andrulonis PA, Glueck BC, Stroebel CF, et al: Borderline personality subcategories. J Nerv Ment Dis 170:670–679, 1982

Annegers JF, Hauser WA, Elveback LR: Remission of seizures and relapse in patients with epilepsy. Epilepsia 10:729–737, 1979

Armon C, Shin M, Miller P, et al: Reversible parkinsonism and cognitive impairment with chronic valproate use. Neurology 47:626–635, 1996

Arnold LM, Privitera MD: Psychopathology and trauma in epileptic and psychogenic seizure patients. Psychosomatics 37:438–443, 1996

Bauer J: Epilepsy and prolactin in adults: a clinical review. Epilepsy Res 24:1–7, 1996

Bauer J, Elger CE: Anticonvulsive drug therapy: historical and current aspects. Nervenarzt 66:403–411, 1995

Bear DM: Behavioural changes in temporal lobe epilepsy: conflict, confusion challenge, in Aspects of Epilepsy and Psychiatry. Edited by Trimble ME, Bolwig TG. London, England, Wiley, 1986, pp 19–29

Bear DM, Fedio P: Quantitative analysis of interictal behavior in temporal lobe epilepsy. Arch Neurol 34:454–467, 1977

Ben-Menachem E: Vagus-nerve stimulation for the treatment of epilepsy. Lancet Neurol 1:477–482, 2002

Berger H: Ueber das Elektrenkephalogramm des Menschen. Archives of Psychiatry I–XIV:87–108, 1929–1938

Bertilsson L: Clinical pharmacokinetics of carbamazepine. Clin Pharmacokinet 3:128–143, 1978

Bickford RG: Activation procedures and special electrodes, in Current Practice of Unusual Electroencephalography. Edited by Kass D, Daly DD. New York, Raven, 1979, pp 269–306

Birkhimer LJ, Curtis JL, Jann MW: Use of carbamazepine in psychiatric disorders. Clin Pharm 4:425–434, 1985

Blake P, Pincus J, Buckner C: Neurologic abnormalities in murderers. Neurology 45:1641–1647, 1995

Blumer D: Temporal lobe epilepsy and its psychiatric significance, in Psychiatric Aspects of Neurological Disease. Edited by Benson FD, Blumer D. New York, Grune & Stratton, 1975, pp 171–198

Blumer D: Evidence supporting the temporal lobe epilepsy personality syndrome: Neurology 53 (suppl 2):S9–S12, 1999

Blumer D, Heilbronn M, Himmelhoch J: Indications for carbamazepine in mental illness: atypical psychiatric disorder or temporal lobe syndrome? Compr Psychiatry 29:108–122, 1988

Blumer D, Montouris G, Hermann B: Psychiatric morbidity in seizure patients on a neurodiagnostic monitoring unit. J Neuropsychiatry Clin Neurosci 7:445–456, 1995

Bramhall D, Levine M: Possible interaction of ranitidine with phenytoin. Drug Intell Clin Pharm 22:979–980, 1988

Brent DA, Crumrine PK, Varma R, et al: Phenobarbital treatment and major depressive disorder in children with epilepsy: a naturalistic follow-up. Pediatrics 85:1086–1091, 1990

Brodsky L, Zuniga JS, Casenas ER, et al: Refractory anxiety: a masked epileptiform disorder? Psychiatr J Univ Ott 8:42–45, 1983

Cendes F, Li LM, Watson C, et al: Is ictal recording mandatory in temporal lobe epilepsy? Arch Neurol 57:497–500, 2000

Chadwick D: Seizures, epilepsy, and other episodic disorders, in Brain's Diseases of the Nervous System, 10th Edition. Edited by Walton J. London, England, Oxford University Press, 1993, pp 697–733

Cloyd JC, Levy RH, Wedlund RH: Relationship between carbamazepine concentration and extent of enzyme autoinduction (abstract). Epilepsia 27:592, 1986

Cockerell OC, Moriarty J, Trimble M, et al: Acute psychological disorders in patients with epilepsy: a nationwide study. Epilepsy Res 25:119–131, 1996

Cowdry R, Gardner DL: Pharmacotherapy of borderline personality disorder. Arch Gen Psychiatry 45:111–119, 1988

Cramer JA, Blum D, Fanning K, et al: The impact of comorbid depression on health resource utilization in a community sample of people with epilepsy. Epilepsy Behav 5:337–342, 2004

Currie S, Heathfield RWG, Henson RA, et al: Clinical course and prognosis of temporal lobe epilepsy: a survey of 666 patients. Brain 94:173–190, 1970

Dam M, Dam AM: Is there an epileptic personality? In Aspects of Epilepsy and Psychiatry. Edited by Trimble MR, Bolwig TG. New York, Wiley, 1986, pp 9–18

Dantendorfer K, Amering M, Baischer W, et al: Is there a pathophysiological and therapeutic link between panic disorder and epilepsy? Acta Psychiatr Scand 91:430–432, 1995

Dekker PA: Epilepsy: A Manual for Medical and Clinical Officers in Africa. Geneva, World Health Organization, 2002

Devinsky O, Gordon E: Epileptic seizures progressing into nonepileptic conversion seizures. Neurology 51:1293–1296, 1998

Devinsky O, Najjar S: Evidence against the existence of a temporal lobe epilepsy personality syndrome. Neurology 53 (suppl 2):S12–S25, 1999

Devinsky O, Vazquez B: Behavioral changes associated with epilepsy. Neurol Clin 11:127–149, 1993

Devinsky O, Sanchez-Villasenor F, Vazquez B, et al: Clinical profile of patients with epileptic and nonepileptic seizures. Neurology 46:1530–1533, 1996

Dichter M, Brodie M: New antiepileptic drugs. N Engl J Med 334:1583–1590, 1996

Diehl LW: Schizophrenic syndromes in epilepsies. Psychopathology 22:65–140, 1989

Dietl T, Urbach H, Helmstaedter C, et al: Persistent severe amnesia due to seizure recurrence after unilateral temporal lobectomy. Epilepsy Behav 6:394–400, 2004

Dodrill CB, Batzel LW: Interictal behavioral features of patients with epilepsy. Epilepsia 27 (suppl 2):S64–S76, 1986

Dodrill CB, Troupin AS: Neuropsychological effects of carbamazepine and phenytoin. Neurology 41:141–143, 1991

Dodrill CB, Wilensky AJ: Intellectual impairment as an outcome of status epilepticus. Neurology 40 (suppl 2):23–27, 1990

Dongier S: Statistical study of clinical and electroencephalographic manifestations of 536 psychotic episodes occurring in 516 epileptics between clinical seizures. Epilepsia 1:117–142, 1959–1960

Dorn JM: A case of phenytoin toxicity possibly precipitated by trazodone. J Clin Psychiatry 47:89–90, 1986

Ebersole JS, Leroy RJ: Evaluation of ambulatory EEG monitoring. Neurology 33:853–860, 1983

Edeh J, Toone B: Relationship between interictal psychopathology and the type of epilepsy: results of a survey in general practice. Br J Psychiatry 151:95–101, 1987

Elger CE, Helmstaedter C, Kurthen M: Chronic epilepsy and cognition. Lancet Neurol 3:663–672, 2004

Engel J: The epilepsies, in Cecil's Textbook of Medicine, 19th Edition. Edited by Wyngoorden J, Smith L, Bennet C. Philadelphia, PA, WB Saunders, 1992, pp 2202–2213

Ey H: Etudes psychiatriques. Paris, Desclee de Brouwer, 1954

Favale E, Rubino P, Mainardi P, et al: Anticonvulsant effect of fluoxetine in humans. Neurology 45:1926–1927, 1995

Fenton GW: The EEG, epilepsy and psychiatry, in What Is Epilepsy? Edited by Trimble MR, Reynolds EH. Edinburgh, UK, Churchill Livingstone, 1986, pp 139–160

Fenwick P: In dyscontrol epilepsy, in What Is Epilepsy? Edited by Trimble MR, Reynolds EH. Edinburgh, UK, Churchill Livingstone, 1986, pp 161–182

Fenwick P: The behavioral treatment of epilepsy generation and inhibition of seizures. Neurol Clin 12:175–202, 1994

Fink M: Meduna and the origins of convulsive therapy. Am J Psychiatry 141:1034–1041, 1984

Fiordelli E, Beghi E, Bogliun G, et al: Epilepsy and psychiatric disturbance: a cross-sectional study. Br J Psychiatry 163:446–450, 1993

Fontaine R, Breton G, D'ery R, et al: Temporal lobe abnormalities in panic disorder: an MRI study. Biol Psychiatry 27:304–310, 1990

Gaitatzis A, Trimble MR, Sander JW: The psychiatric comorbidity of epilepsy. Acta Neurol Scand 110:207–220, 2004

GCAE Secretariat: Epilepsy: Out of the Shadows. ILAE/IBE/WHO Global Campaign Against Epilepsy. Heemstede, The Netherlands, World Health Organization, 2003

Gehlert S: Perceptions of control in adults with epilepsy. Epilepsia 35:81–88, 1994

Geyer J, Payne T, Drury I: The value of pelvic thrusting in the diagnosis of seizures and pseudoseizures. Neurology 54:227–229, 2000

Ghaemi S, Gaughan S: Novel anticonvulsants: a new generation of mood stabilizers. Harv Rev Psychiatry 8:1–7, 2000

Gibbs FA, Gibbs EL: Atlas of Electroencephalography. Cambridge, MA, Addison-Wesley, 1952

Gillham RA: Refractory epilepsy: an evaluation of psychological methods in outpatient management. Epilepsia 31:427–432, 1990

Glosser G, Zwil AS, Glosser DS, et al: Psychiatric aspects of temporal lobe epilepsy before and after anterior temporal lobectomy. J Neurol Neurosurg Psychiatry 68:53–58, 2000

Goodridge DMG, Shovron SD: Epileptic seizures in a population of 6000. BMJ 287:641–644, 1983

Gudmundsson G: Epilepsy in Iceland. Acta Neurol Scand 43 (suppl 25):1–124, 1966

Gunderson JG, Zanarini MC: Pathogenesis of borderline personality, in American Psychiatric Press Review of Psychiatry, Vol 8. Edited by Tasman A, Hales RE, Frances AJ. Washington, DC, American Psychiatric Press, 1989, pp 25–48

Gureje O: Interictal psychopathology in epilepsy: prevalence and pattern in a Nigerian clinic. Br J Psychiatry 158:700–705, 1991

Hakola HP, Laulumaa VA: Carbamazepine in treatment of violent schizophrenics (letter). Lancet 1:1358, 1982

Hamer H, Knake S, Schomburg M, et al: Valproate induced hyperammonemic encephalopathy in the presence of topiramate. Neurology 54:230–232, 2000

Handal N, Masand P, Weilburg J: Panic disorder and complex partial seizures: a truly complex relationship. Psychosomatics 36:498–502, 1995

Harden CL, Goldstein MA. Mood disorders in patients with epilepsy: epidemiology and management. CNS Drugs 16:291–302, 2002

Hathaway SR, McKinley JC: Minnesota Multiphasic Personality Inventory—2. Minneapolis, University of Minnesota, 1989

Heath RG: Psychosis and epilepsy: similarities and differences in the anatomic-physiologic substrate. Advances in Biological Psychiatry 8:106–116, 1982

Hermann BP, Riel P: Interictal personality and behavioral traits in temporal lobe and generalized epilepsy. Cortex 17:125–128, 1981

Hermann BP, Seidenberg M, Bell B: Psychiatric comorbidity in chronic epilepsy: identification, consequences, and treatment of major depression. Epilepsia 41 (suppl 2):S31–S41, 2000

Ho S, Berkovic S, Berlangieri S, et al: Comparison of ictal SPECT and interictal PET in the presurgical evaluation of TLE. Ann Neurol 37:738–745, 1995

Hoare P: Does illness foster dependency? Dev Med Child Neurol 26:20–24, 1984

International League Against Epilepsy Commission: Proposal for classification of epilepsies and epileptic syndromes. Epilepsia 26:268–278, 1985

International League Against Epilepsy Commission Report: Glossary of descriptive terminology for ictal semiology: report of the ILAE task force on classification and terminology. Epilepsia 42:1212–1218, 2001a

International League Against Epilepsy Commission Report: A proposed diagnostic scheme for people with epileptic seizures and with epilepsy: report of the ILAE Task Force on Classification and Terminology. Epilepsia 42:796–803, 2001b

Jacoby A, Baker GA, Steen N, et al: The clinical course of epilepsy and its psychosocial correlates: findings from a UK community study. Epilepsia 37:148–161, 1996

Jann MW, Ereshefsky L, Saklad SR, et al: Effects of carbamazepine on plasma haloperidol levels. J Clin Psychopharmacol 5:106–109, 1985

Jones JE, Hermann BP, Barry JJ, et al: Rates and risk factors for suicide, suicidal ideation, and suicide attempts in chronic epilepsy. Epilepsy Behav 4:S31–S38, 2003

Kanner A, Stagno S, Kotagal P, et al: Postictal psychiatric events during prolonged video-EEG monitoring studies. Arch Neurol 53:258–263, 1996

Kanner AM: Depression in epilepsy: a frequently neglected multifaceted disorder. Epilepsy Behav 4:S11–S19, 2003

Kanner AM, Nieto JC: Depressive disorders in epilepsy. Neurology 53 (5 suppl 2):S26–S32, 1999

Kanner A, Parra J, Frey M, et al: Psychiatric and neurologic predictors of psychogenic seizure outcome. Neurology 53:933–938, 1999

Ketter T, Malow B, Flamini R, et al: Anticonvulsant withdrawal emergent psychopathology. Neurology 44:55–61, 1994

Ketter T, Post R, Theodore W: Positive and negative psychiatric effects of antiepileptic drugs in patients with seizure disorders. Neurology 53 (suppl 2):S53–S67, 1999

Kidron R, Averbuch I, Klein E, et al: Carbamazepine-induced reduction of blood levels of haloperidol in chronic schizophrenia. Biol Psychiatry 20:219–222, 1985

Kirubakaran V, Sen S, Wilkinson C: Catatonic stupor: unusual manifestation of TLE. Psychiatr J Univ Ott 12:244–246, 1987

Kraepelin E: Lecture VI: epileptic insanity (1922), in Lectures in Clinical Psychiatry. Translated by Johnstone T. New York, Hafner, 1968, pp 48–57

Kristensen O, Sindrup EH: Psychomotor epilepsy and psychosis, II: electroencephalographic findings. Acta Neurol Scand 57:370–379, 1978

Krohn W: A study of epilepsy in northern Norway: its frequency and character. Acta Psychiatr Scand Suppl 36:215–225, 1961

Krumholz A: Nonepileptic seizures: diagnosis and management. Neurology 53 (suppl 2):S76–S83, 1999

Kuyk J, Spinhoven P, Boas W, et al: Dissociation in temporal lobe epilepsy and pseudo-epileptic seizure patients. J Nerv Ment Dis 187:713–720, 1999

Lambert MV, Robertson MM: Depression in epilepsy: etiology, phenomenology, and treatment. Epilepsia 40 (suppl 10):S21–S47, 1999

Landolt H: Serial encephalographic investigations during psychotic episodes in epileptic patients and during schizophrenic attacks, in Lectures on Epilepsy. Edited by Lorentz de Haas AM. London, England, Elsevier, 1958, pp 91–133

Laskowitz D, Sperling M, French J, et al: The syndrome of frontal lobe epilepsy. Neurology 45:780–787, 1995

Levinson D, Devinsky O: Psychiatric events during vigabatrin therapy. Neurology 53:1503–1511, 1999

Lindsay J, Ounstead C, Richards P: Long-term outcome in children with temporal lobe seizures, III: psychiatric aspects in childhood and adult life. Dev Med Child Neurol 21:630–636, 1979

Malkowicz D, Legido A, Jackel R, et al: Prolactin secretion following repetitive seizures. Neurology 45:448–452, 1995

Mann JJ: Violence and aggression, in Psychopharmacology: The Fourth Generation of Progress. Edited by Bloom FE, Kupfer DJ. New York, Raven, 1995, pp 1919–1928

Martin R, Kuzniecky R, Ho S, et al: Cognitive effects of topiramate, gabapentin, and lamotrigine in healthy young adults. Neurology 52:321–327, 1999

Mathers CB: Group therapy in the management of epilepsy. Br J Med Psychol 65:279–287, 1992

Matsuura M, Adachi N, Oana Y, et al: A polydiagnostic and dimensional comparison of epileptic psychoses and schizophrenia spectrum disorders. Schizophr Res 69:189–201, 2004

McElroy S, Keck P, Pope H, et al: Valproate in primary psychiatric disorders, in Use of Anticonvulsants in Psychiatry. Edited by McElroy S, Pope H. Clifton, NJ, Oxford Health Care, 1988, pp 25–42

McKenna PJ, Kane JM, Parrish K: Psychotic syndromes in epilepsy. Am J Psychiatry 142:895–904, 1985

McNamara ME, Fogel BS: Anticonvulsant-responsive panic attacks with temporal lobe EEG abnormalities. J Neuropsychiatry Clin Neurosci 2:193–196, 1990

Meador KJ, Loring DW, Abney OL, et al: Effects of carbamazepine and phenytoin on EEG and memory in healthy adults. Epilepsia 34:153–157, 1993

Meador KJ, Loring D, Moore E, et al: Comparative effects of phenobarbital, phenytoin, and valproate in healthy adults. Neurology 45:1494–1499, 1995

Mellers J, Toone B, Lishman A: A neuropsychological comparison of schizophrenia and schizophrenia-like psychosis of epilepsy. Psychol Med 30:325–335, 2000

Mendez MF, Doss RC, Taylor JL, et al: Depression in epilepsy: relationship to seizures and anticonvulsant therapy. J Nerv Ment Dis 181:444–447, 1993

Mendez MF, Taylor JL, Doss RC, et al: Depression in secondary epilepsy: relation to lesion laterality. J Neurol Neurosurg Psychiatry 57:232–233, 1994

Metrakos K, Metrakos JD: Genetics of convulsive disorders, II: genetics and encephalographic studies in centrencephalic epilepsy. Neurology 11:454–483, 1961

Moehle KA, Bolter JF, Long CJ: The relationship between neuropsychological functioning and psychopathology in temporal lobe epileptic patients. Epilepsia 25:418–422, 1984

Monroe RR: Limbic ictus and atypical psychoses. J Nerv Ment Dis 170:711–716, 1982

Mungus D: Interictal behavior abnormality in temporal lobe epilepsy. Arch Gen Psychiatry 39:108–111, 1982

Neppe VM: Epileptic psychosis: a heterogeneous condition (letter). Epilepsia 27:634, 1986

Neppe VM, Kaplan C: Short-term treatment of atypical spells with carbamazepine. Clin Neuropharmacol 11:287–289, 1988

Neppe VM, Tucker GJ: Modern perspectives on epilepsy in relation to psychiatry: behavioral disturbances of epilepsy. Hosp Community Psychiatry 39:389–396, 1988

Neppe VM, Tucker GJ, Wilensky AJ: Fundamentals of carbamazepine use in neuropsychiatry. J Clin Psychiatry 49 (suppl 4):4–6, 1988

Neppe VM, Bowman B, Sawchuk KSLJ: Carbamazepine for atypical psychosis with episodic hostility: a preliminary study. J Nerv Ment Dis 179:339–340, 1991

Nilsson L, Ahlbom A, Farahmand BY, et al. Risk factors for suicide in epilepsy: a case control study. Epilepsia 43:664–651, 2002

Novak J, Corke P, Fairley N: "Petit mal status" in adults. Dis Nerv Syst 32:245–248, 1971

Oxbury S, Oxbury J, Renowden S, et al: Severe amnesia: an unusual late complication after temporal lobectomy. Neuropsychologia 35:975–988, 1997

Pakalinis A, Drake M, Kellum J: Forced normalization: acute psychosis after seizure control in seven patients. Arch Neurol 44:289–292, 1987

Perini GI, Tosin C, Curraro C, et al: Interictal mood and personality disorders in temporal lobe epilepsy and juvenile myoclonic epilepsy. J Neurol Neurosurg Psychiatry 61:601–605, 1996

Perucca E, Manzo L, Crema A: Pharmacokinetic interactions between antiepileptic and psychotropic drugs, in The Psychopharmacology of Epilepsy. Edited by Trimble M. Chichester, UK, Wiley, 1985, pp 95–105

Pincus JH, Tucker GJ: Behavioral Neurology, 3rd Edition. New York, Oxford University Press, 1985

Popkin M, Tucker GJ: Mental disorders due to a general medical condition and substance-induced disorders: mood, anxiety, psychotic, catatonic, and personality disorders, in DSM-IV Source Book. Edited by Widiger T, Frances J, Pincus HA, et al. Washington, DC, American Psychiatric Press, 1994, pp 243–276

Popli A, Kando J, Pillay S, et al: Occurrence of seizures related to psychotropic medication among psychiatric inpatients. Psychiatr Serv 46:486–488, 1995

Post RM, Uhde TW, Joffe RT, et al: Anticonvulsant drugs in psychiatric illness: new treatment alternatives and theoretical implications, in The Psychopharmacology of Epilepsy. Edited by Trimble MR. Chichester, UK, Wiley, 1985, pp 141–171

Preskorn SH, Fast GA: Tricyclic antidepressant-induced seizures and plasma drug concentration. J Clin Psychiatry 53:160–162, 1992

Procci WR: Schizo-affective psychosis: fact or fiction? A survey of the literature. Arch Gen Psychiatry 33:1167–1178, 1976

Prueter C, Norra C: Mood disorders and their treatment in patients with epilepsy. J Neuropsychiatry Clin Neurosci 17:20–28, 2005

Pulliainen V, Jokelainen M: Effects of phenytoin and carbamazepine on cognitive functions in newly diagnosed epileptic patients. Acta Neurol Scand 89:81–86, 1994

Pulliainen V, Kuikka P, Jokelainen M: Motor and cognitive functions in newly diagnosed adult seizure patients before antiepileptic medication. Acta Neurol Scand 101:73–78, 2000

Qin P, Xu H, Laursen TM: Risk for schizophrenia and schizophrenia-like psychosis among patients with epilepsy: population based cohort study. BMJ 331:23–28, 2005

Regan KJ, Banks GK, Beran RG: Therapeutic recreation programmes for children with epilepsy. Seizure 2:195–200, 1993

Rodin EA: Psychomotor epilepsy and aggressive behavior. Arch Gen Psychiatry 28:210–213, 1973

Rodin EA, Schmaltz S: The Bear-Fedio Personality Inventory and temporal lobe epilepsy. Neurology 34:591–596, 1984

Rosenstein DL, Nelson JC, Jacobs SC, et al: Seizures associated with antidepressants: a review. J Clin Psychiatry 54:289–299, 1993

Roth M, Harper M: Temporal lobe epilepsy and the phobic anxiety-depersonalization syndrome, II: practical and theoretical considerations. Compr Psychiatry 3:215–226, 1962

Ryback R, Gardner E: Limbic system dysrhythmia: a diagnostic EEG procedure utilizing procaine activation. J Neuropsychiatry Clin Neurosci 3:321–329, 1991

Sachdev P: Schizophrenia-like psychosis and epilepsy: the status of the association. Am J Psychiatry 155:325–336, 1998

Sackeim HA: The anticonvulsant hypothesis of the mechanisms of action of ECT: current status. J ECT 15:5–26, 1999

Sadler M, Goodwin J: The sensitivity of various electrodes in the detection of epilepsy from potential patients with partial complex seizures (letter). Epilepsia 27:627, 1986

Schiffer R: Epilepsy, psychosis, and forced normalization (editorial). Arch Neurol 44:253, 1987

Schmitz B, Robertson MM, Trimble MR: Depression and schizophrenia in epilepsy: social and biological risk factors. Epilepsy Res 35:59–68, 1999

Schoenenberger R, Tonasijevic M, Jha A, et al: Appropriateness of antiepileptic drug level monitoring. JAMA 274:1622–1626, 1995

Sengoku A, Yagi K, Seino M, et al: Risks of occurrence of psychoses in relation to the types of epilepsies and epileptic seizures. Folia Psychiatr Neurol Jpn 37:221–225, 1983

Septien L, Giroud M, Didi-Roy R, et al: Depression and partial epilepsy: relevance of laterality of the epileptic focus. Neurol Res 15:136–138, 1993

Shovron SD, Reynolds EH: The nature of epilepsy: evidence from studies of epidemiology, temporal patterns of seizures, prognosis and treatment, in What Is Epilepsy? Edited by Trimble MR, Reynolds EH. Edinburgh, UK, Churchill Livingstone, 1986, pp 36–45

Shukla G, Bhatia M, Vivekanandhan S: Serum prolactin levels for differentiation of nonepileptic versus true seizures: limited utility. Epilepsy Behav 5:517–521, 2004

Shukla S, Godwin CD, Long LE, et al: Lithium-carbamazepine neurotoxicity and risk factors. Am J Psychiatry 141:1604–1606, 1984

Sillanpaa M, Camfield P, Camfield C: Predicting long-term outcome of childhood epilepsy in Nova Scotia, Canada and Turku, Finland. Arch Neurol 52:589–592, 1995

Silver JM, Hales RE, Yudofsky SC: Psychopharmacology of depression in neurologic disorders. J Clin Psychiatry 51:33–39, 1990

Slater E, Beard AW, Glithero E: The schizophrenia-like psychoses of epilepsy. Br J Psychiatry 109:95–150, 1963

Sloviter RS, Tamminga CA: Cortex, VII: the hippocampus in epilepsy (letter). Am J Psychiatry 152:659, 1995

Stark-Adamec C, Adamec RE, Graham JM, et al: Complexities in the complex partial seizures personality controversy. Psychiatr J Univ Ott 10:231–236, 1985

Stevens JR: Interictal clinical manifestations of complex partial seizures, in Advances in Neurology. Edited by Penry JK, Daly DD. New York, Raven, 1975, pp 85–107

Stevens JR: Psychiatric aspects of epilepsy. J Clin Psychiatry 49 (suppl 4):49–57, 1988

Strauss E, Wada J, Moll A: Depression in male and female subjects with complex partial seizures. Arch Neurol 49:391–392, 1992

Szatmari P: Some methodologic criteria for studies in developmental neuropsychiatry. Psychiatr Dev 3:153–170, 1985

Temkin O: The Falling Sickness, 2nd Edition. Baltimore, MD, Johns Hopkins University Press, 1979

Thomas M, Jankovic J: Psychogenic movement disorders: diagnosis and management. CNS Drugs 18:437–452, 2004

Thomas P, Zifkin B, Migneco O, et al: Nonconvulsive status epilepticus of frontal origin. Neurology 52:1174–1183, 1999

Tojek TM, Lumley M, Barkley G, et al: Stress and other psychosocial characteristics of patients with psychogenic nonepileptic seizures. Psychosomatics 41:221–226, 2000

Toone BK, Garralda ME, Ron MA: The psychoses of epilepsy and the functional psychoses: a clinical and phenomenological comparison. Br J Psychiatry 141:256–261, 1982

Trimble MR: The relationship between epilepsy and schizophrenia: a biochemical hypothesis. Biol Psychiatry 12:299–304, 1977

Trimble MR: The effects of anticonvulsant drugs on cognitive abilities. Pharmacol Ther 4:677–685, 1979

Trimble MR: Cognitive hazards of seizure disorders. Epilepsia 29 (suppl 1):S19–S24, 1988

Trimble MR, Thompson PJ: Anticonvulsant drugs, cognitive impairment, and behavior. Epilepsia 24 (suppl):S55–S63, 1983

Trimble MR, Ring HA, Schmitz B: Epilepsy, in Synopsis of Neuropsychiatry. Edited by Fogel BS, Schiffer RB, Rao SM. Philadelphia, PA, Lippincott Williams & Wilkins, 2000, pp 469–489

Tucker GJ: Current diagnostic issues in neuropsychiatry, in Neuropsychiatry. Edited by Fogel BS, Schiffer RB. Baltimore, MD, Williams & Wilkins, 1996, pp 1009–1014

Tucker GJ, Price TP, Johnson VB, et al: Phenomenology of temporal lobe dysfunction: a link to atypical psychosis—a series of cases. J Nerv Ment Dis 174:348–356, 1986

Victoroff JI, Benson F, Grafton ST, et al: Depression in complex partial seizures. Arch Neurol 51:155–163, 1994

Von Meduna L: Die Konvulsionstherapie der Schizophrenia. Halle, Germany, Marhold, 1937

Vukmir RB: Does serum prolactin indicate the presence of seizure in the emergency department patient? J Neurol 251:736–739, 2004

Waxman SG, Geschwind N: The interictal behavior syndrome of temporal lobe epilepsy. Arch Gen Psychiatry 32:1580–1586, 1975

Weilburg JB, Schacter S, Worth J, et al: EEG abnormalities in patients with atypical panic attacks. J Clin Psychiatry 56:358–362, 1995

Wells C, Duneau GW: Neurology for Psychiatrists. Philadelphia, PA, FA Davis, 1980

Willert C, Spitzer C, Kusserow S, et al: Serum neuron-specific enolase, prolactin, and creatine kinase after epileptic and psychogenic non-epileptic seizures. Acta Neurol Scand 109:318–323, 2004

Ziegler R: Epilepsy: individual illness, human prediscontent and family dilemma. Fam Relat 31:435–444, 1982

Zimmerman AW: Hormones and epilepsy. Neurol Clin 4:853–861, 1986

Zwil AS, Pelchat RJ: ECT in the treatment of patients with neurological and somatic disease. Int J Psychiatry Med 24:1–29, 1994

17

NEUROPSYCHIATRIC ASPECTS OF SLEEP AND SLEEP DISORDERS

Max Hirshkowitz, Ph.D.

Amir Sharafkhaneh, M.D.

As a scientific field, sleep was first studied by psychiatrists, neurologists, and psychologists. More recently, sleep research has attracted the attention of internists, pulmonologists, cardiologists, and pediatricians. This growing interdisciplinary interest has allowed sleep medicine to emerge as a subspecialty in its own right. Human sleep, however, is a very broad topic. We therefore restrict this chapter's scope to eight main topics, beginning with a general overview and background concerning the study of human sleep. This is followed by a review of the physiology of normal human sleep that includes a description of the stages of sleep, their characteristics, their correlates, and their pattern. A description of the basic underlying mechanisms that regulate sleep follows, and sleep in patients with psychiatric conditions is considered. Clinical sleep medicine topics begin with an overview of sleep disorders classification systems and continue with characterization of the most common sleep disorders presenting as insomnia, hypersomnia, and parasomnia.

The most fundamental concept for understanding sleep is that sleep is a brain process. Furthermore, it is not one process. There are several different types of sleep, each having distinctly different neuronal generators, regulatory mechanisms, and electroencephalographic correlates. Moreover, some of the sleep processes involve cortical activation. Thus, at times sleep is active rather than passive (Chase 1972; Kleitman 1972).

When considering basic states of neurological organization, sleep versus wakefulness usually marks the first conceptual division. Hans Berger (1930), the grandfather of electroencephalography, used his string galvanometer to make the first human electroencephalographic recordings during sleep. He described the disappearance of the alpha rhythm when his subject fell asleep. Cessation of alpha rhythm in an individual with closed eyes who is not engaged in mental activity (for example, solving arithmetic equations) is essentially the definition still used today for defining sleep onset.

The first continuous overnight electroencephalographic recordings in humans were published by Loomis et al. (1937). Using the tracings from their giant 8-foot-long drum polygraph, they developed a sleep stage classification system (stages A, B, C, D, and E) and graphically illustrated sleep stages in a manner remarkably similar to that currently used. They defined sleep stages according to sleep electroencephalogram (EEG) frequency bands, including beta activity (>13 Hz), sleep spindles (bursts of 12–14 Hz), alpha rhythm (8–13 Hz, sometimes slower), theta rhythm (4–7 Hz, more common in adolescents than adults), sawtooth theta waves (4–7 Hz, with notched appearance), delta rhythm (<4 Hz), and slow waves (≤ 2 Hz).

The next major milestone was Eugene Aserinsky's discovery (while a graduate student working with Nathaniel Kleitman) of periodic electro-oculographic activity episodes during sleep. These activity episodes occurred approximately every 90–120 minutes. At first the electro-oculographic activation was thought to be a recording artifact, but continued research verified that actual eye movements were occurring. At first called jerky eye movements (JEMs), the phenomenon was renamed rapid eye movement (REM) sleep, reportedly by William C. Dement (a medical student at that time). Subsequent studies revealed that individuals awakened from REM sleep reported dreaming on 20 of the 27 instances (Aserinsky and Kleitman 1953).

The discovery of a connection between REM sleep and dreaming generated tremendous excitement in the psychiatric community. Freud had characterized dreams as "the royal road to the unconscious" (Freud 1900/1953). The sleep EEG–electro-oculogram (EOG) recording technique held promise as an objective way to explore the mysteries of the unconscious mind. Hundreds of studies attempted to exploit this paradigm; however, no unified "dream theory" emerged. Many of the concepts forwarded by Freud were verified (for example, daytime residue), whereas others were not. Modern theoretical framework varies widely. The neurophysiologically grounded "activation-synthesis hypothesis" casts dreams as epiphenomena arising from the cortex making its best attempt to interpret random subcortical activation. By contrast, the cognitive theories consider dreaming an extension of daytime thought, albeit governed by a different grammar and looser rules (Foulkes 1982; Hobson and McCarley 1977).

In the late 1950s, Michel Jouvet introduced the concept that REM sleep was a third state of consciousness and not just another component of the basic rest activity cycle (BRAC) (Jouvet et al. 1959). He observed postural changes in the cat associated with different states of sleep, and using electromyographic recordings he found muscle atonia accompanying REM sleep in normal animals. This discovery of "functional paralysis" using electromyographic recording was the final step toward development of what is now standard recording practice. The final transition step that helped launch modern sleep research was the development and publication of *A Manual of Standardized Terminology, Techniques and Scoring System for Sleep Stages of Human Subjects*. This manual was the result of efforts by leading sleep researchers throughout the world. An ad hoc standardization committee was formed, chaired by Allan Rechtschaffen and Anthony Kales (1968), and the stages of sleep were defined. The project's success derives, in no small measure, from the chairmen's insistence on consensus. The "R&K system," as it is often called, remains *the* system for recording and classifying sleep stages in humans. It provided a common language for sleep researchers and clinicians.

PHYSIOLOGY OF NORMAL HUMAN SLEEP

THE STAGES OF SLEEP

In humans, sleep stages are differentiated on the basis of activity occurring in central (C3 or C4) and occipital (O3 or O4) EEGs, right and left eye EOGs (recorded from the outer canthi), and submental electromyograms (EMGs). Traditional sleep recordings were paper polygraphic tracings usually made at a chart speed of 10 mm/second. The resulting polysomnogram (PSG) represented each 30 seconds of recording (1 epoch) as one polygraph page. It is for this reason that standard practice was designed to classify each 30-second epoch as either awake or as one or another of the stages of sleep. The practice of epoch classification according to sleep stage continues even though computerized polygraph systems allow page resizing and temporal resolution alteration (Rechtschaffen and Kales 1968).

Stage W (also called wakefulness or Stage 0) is characterized by EEG containing predominantly alpha activity and/or low voltage, mixed frequency activity. Muscle activity is fairly high, and both rapid and slow eye movements may occur. Sleep-onset epoch is determined when the duration of alpha activity decreases to less than 50% of an epoch and/or a vertex wave, a K complex, a sleep spindle, or delta activity occurs. The K complex is a high-voltage biphasic slow or sharply contoured wave that begins with a negative component and is followed by a positive component. The sleep spindle is a burst of 11.5–16 Hz waves with a duration greater than 0.5 second. If a sleep spindle or K complex occurs and high-amplitude (75µ V or greater) delta electroencephalographic activity occupies less than 20% of an epoch, Stage II is scored. If there is 20%–50% delta activity, Stage III is designated, and if there is more than 50% delta activity, the epoch is classified as sleep Stage IV. Stage I is an intermediate non-alpha state that has low voltage, mixed-frequency electroencephalographic activity that is a deltaless, spindleless stage that does not have K complexes. Rapid eye movements and muscle atonia accompanying Stage I EEG define REM sleep. Sawtooth theta is another common electroencephalographic feature of REM sleep. Table 17–1 shows the electroencephalographic, electro-oculographic, and electromyographic characteristics for the different sleep stages, and Figure 17–1 shows an example of each stage.

Stages I, II, III, and IV are sometimes collectively referred to as non-REM (NREM) sleep. Stages III and IV are often combined and called slow-wave sleep. NREM and REM sleep differ for a wide variety of physiological measures (Table 17–2).

TABLE 17–1. Sleep stage electroencephalographic, electro-oculographic, and electromyographic characteristics

Stage	Electroencephalographic characteristics	EOG	Electromyographic muscle activity
I	Low voltage, mixed frequency	Slow	Decreased from awake
II	Sleep spindles and K complexes	None	Decreased from awake
III	Sleep spindles and slow waves	None	Decreased from awake
IV	Mostly slow waves	None	Decreased from awake
REM	Low voltage, mixed frequency	Rapid	Nearly absent

Note. EOG = electro-oculogram.

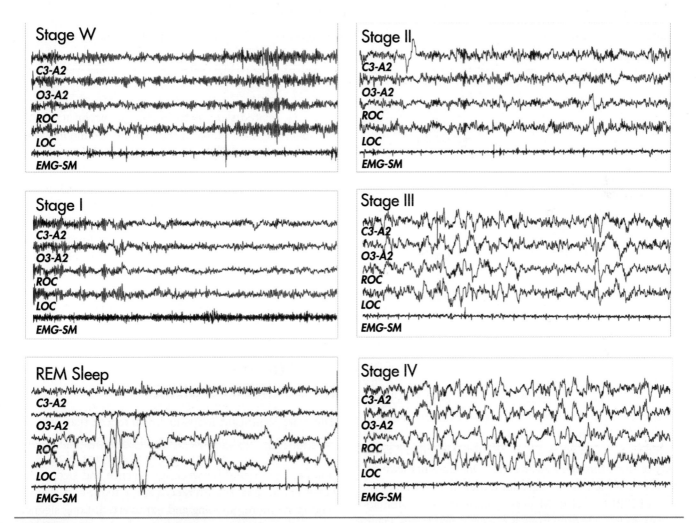

FIGURE 17–1. Polysomnographic recordings of the stages of sleep.

NORMAL SLEEP PATTERN: GENERALIZATIONS

In a good sleeper, 5% or less of total time in bed should be spent awake. Sleep onset should be swift (less than 15 minutes) and nocturnal awakenings brief. Under normal circumstances, Stage II sleep comprises approximately half of a night's sleep in a healthy young adult. About one-quarter is REM sleep, and the remainder is distributed between slow-wave sleep and Stage I. Figure 17–2 shows the nightly percentages for each stage. Sleeping for the first time in a new environment (for example, a sleep laboratory) is usually associated with delayed sleep onset, general disruption, and decreased REM and/or slow-wave sleep

TABLE 17–2.   Comparison of NREM and REM sleep activity

Physiological measure	NREM sleep	REM sleep
Heart and breathing rate	Regular, slow	Variable
Oxygen consumption	Low	High
Cerebral blood flow	Low	High
Penile blood flow (erections)	Absent	Present
Vaginal blood flow and uterine activity	Low	Increased
Breathing response to O_2	Similar to awake	Similar to awake
Breathing response to CO_2	Similar to awake	Depressed
Electrodermal activity	Present, active	Absent
Temperature regulation	Homeothermic	Poikilothermic
Mental activity	Thoughtlike	Dreamlike

Note.   NREM = non–rapid eye movement; REM = rapid eye movement.

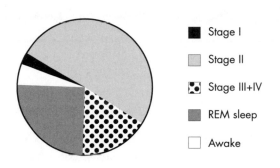

Stage I
Stage II
Stage III+IV
REM sleep
Awake

FIGURE 17–2.   Sleep stage percentages in a healthy young adult.

percentages. This adaptation-related phenomenon is termed the *first-night effect*. Nonetheless, age-specific normative values have been derived empirically for both first and succeeding nights. Such data are useful for clinical sleep assessments (Hirshkowitz et al. 1992; Roffwarg et al. 1966; R.L. Williams et al. 1974).

Sleep architecture refers to the progression and continuity of sleep through a given night. One does not have single blocks of each sleep stage, but rather there is a repeating cycle of NREM and REM sleep. There are also systematic alterations in cycle properties as the night progresses. Figure 17–3 shows a typical night with normal sleep architecture in a healthy young adult. The following five generalizations can be made about sleep architecture: 1) sleep is entered through NREM sleep; 2) NREM and REM sleep alternate approximately every 90 minutes; 3) slow-wave sleep predominates in the first third of the night; 4) REM sleep predominates in the last third of the night; and 5) REM sleep occurs in 4–6 discrete episodes each night, with episodes generally being longer later in the sleep period.

Aging-related sleep pattern changes occur across the life span; the most global is the gradual decline in overall total sleep time. REM sleep percentage (of total sleep time) decreases from birth to adolescence and then stabilizes at 20%–25%; however, some additional decline may occur after age 65 years. By contrast, slow-wave sleep begins to decline after adolescence and continues that trend with age, disappearing completely in some elderly individuals. Aging, especially after middle age, is associated with greater wakefulness intermixed with sleep (fragmentation) and increased incidence of sleep-related breathing and movement disorders. Figure 17–4 shows changes in sleep stage composition from adulthood to old age.

MECHANISMS REGULATING SLEEP

There are significant individual differences that produce variation in normal human sleep. Some of us are naturally long sleepers, whereas others are short sleepers. No correlation has been found between intelligence and sleep need; however, personality differences are noted. Short sleepers tend to be more outgoing and extraverted. Long sleepers tend to be more introverted and possibly creative (Hartmann et al. 1972). There are three basic factors involved in the general coordination of sleep and wakefulness: 1) autonomic nervous system balance, 2) homeostatic sleep drive, and 3) circadian rhythms (Hirshkowitz et al. 1997).

AUTONOMIC NERVOUS SYSTEM BALANCE

In general, sleep depends on decreasing sympathetic activation and increasing parasympathetic balance. Consequently,

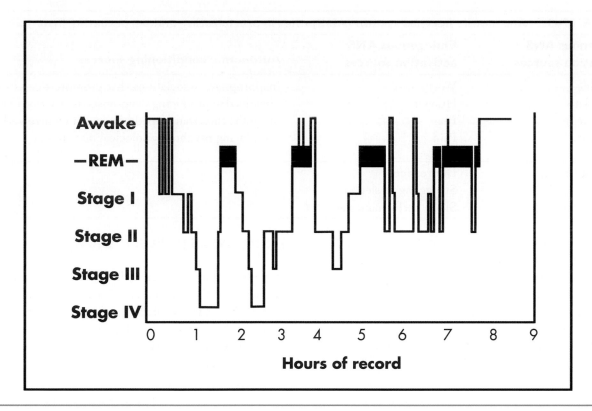

FIGURE 17–3. Sleep stage histogram for a healthy young adult.

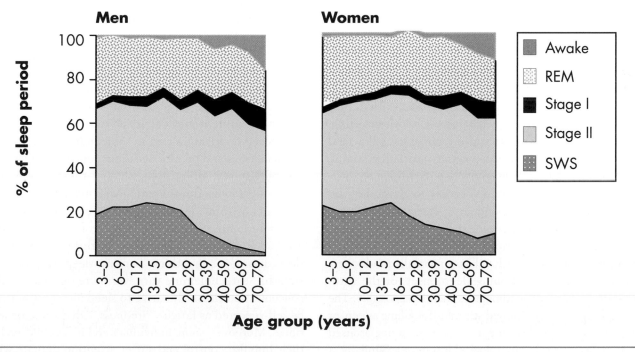

FIGURE 17–4. Sleep macroarchitecture (stages) as a function of age. SWS=slow-wave sleep.

TABLE 17–3.   Autonomic nervous system (ANS) roles in precipitating and perpetuating insomnia

Exogenous ANS activation sources	Endogenous ANS activation sources	Autonomic conditioning sources
Caffeine	Worry	Inappropriate associations that promote sleep can be
Chocolate	Hunger	involved in producing sleep-onset association disorder
Nicotine	Fear	Stimulus cues that impede sleep can be involved in
Exercise	Pain	producing psychophysiological insomnia
Heat	Anxiety	
Unfamiliar sounds	Depression	
Noise	Struggling to sleep	
Bright light	Sleep performance anxiety	

activities and influences that increase sympathetic outflow have the potential to disturb sleep. It does not matter whether the cause of sympathetic arousal is exogenous or endogenous. That is, ingesting stimulants before bedtime (exogenous) and anxious rumination when trying to sleep (endogenous) work via the same autonomic mechanism. Table 17–3 shows some common exogenous and endogenous sources of arousal that can cause sleep disruption. Sometimes an exogenous stimulus can trigger and be amplified by an internal source of arousal. For example, an unfamiliar noise in the house can provoke an anxiety or fear response that will prevent an individual from falling asleep.

Another property of autonomic arousal is that it commences rapidly but dissipates slowly. Thus, if one gets "worked up" about an issue right before bedtime, it is unrealistic to expect the arousal to cease immediately because one retires for the night. Rituals are often helpful during the presleep period to promote progressive relaxation and gradual reorientation away from daytime stressors and toward nocturnal tranquility. In children who sleep well, elaborate presleep rituals are common. Such rituals may include bedtime stories, a light snack, teeth brushing, prayers, and having a favorite stuffed animal toy, pillow, and blanket. The latter act as sleep-onset association stimuli and likely also play a role in respondent conditioning.

Autonomic activities are susceptible to classical conditioning (also known as respondent or Pavlovian conditioning). The great Russian physiologist Pavlov was able to condition a dog to salivate by ringing a bell that had been paired with presenting food (which will automatically produce canine salivation). Conditioning sleep onset, or the autonomic properties surrounding it, is therefore possible. The bed can become a conditioned stimulus for falling asleep, or in some cases it can become a cue for becoming aroused and alert (as in psychophysiological insomnia). Similarly, if a parent becomes the infant's conditioned stimulus for sleep onset, the parent may find him- or herself having to rock the baby back to sleep at any and all times of the night.

HOMEOSTATIC SLEEP DRIVE

In general, the longer an individual remains awake, the sleepier he or she becomes. Such are the dynamics of sleep debt. Homeostatic regulation of sleepiness is similar to that for thirst, hunger, and sex. These motivated states direct behavior to perform action to reduce drive. The hypothalamus is implicated in all of these physiological drive states. If one attempts continuous, uninterrupted prolonged wakefulness, sleep eventually becomes irresistible.

Sleep deprivation studies explore changes resultant from stretching the homeostatic mechanism beyond its normal limits. Such studies ultimately hope to gain insight into the role or function of sleep by examining deficits produced by its loss. Sleep deprivation can be total, partial, or stage specific. Sleep loss not only increases sleepiness, it adversely affects a variety of coping mechanisms. Sleep-deprived individuals become irritable and easily frustrated. As sleep deprivation continues, attention becomes impaired and performance lapses occur on tasks that challenge the ability to remain vigilant. Psychomotor impairment may occur and mood suffers. Longer-term sleep deprivation can, in some individuals, produce hallucinations and on rare occasions seizures. Psychological stability and affect diminish, and there may be episodes of paranoia, disorientation, and mood swings. After 72 hours of total sleep deprivation, executive function may deteriorate. Similar failure in "frontal lobe" abilities is found in patients whose sleep is disturbed long term by sleep-disordered breathing. Because sleep deprivation is stressful, catecholamine turnover increases and cortisol concentration rises. The drive to sleep increases but may be self-reported as fatigue, tiredness, exhaustion, or weariness. Moreover, some individuals and most children lose their impulse control and suffer attention deficits when sleepy (Binks et al. 1999; Dinges 1992; Horne 1988).

However, in your own experience you may have noticed that during an extended wakeful vigil, sleepiness waxes and wanes. Sometimes after staying up all night, the chronobiological self-abuser will note a surge of energy at daybreak. This indicates the presence of another sleep-wake factor: the circadian rhythm.

CIRCADIAN RHYTHMS

An approximate daylong or 24-hour rhythm is called a circadian rhythm (from the Latin *circa*, around, plus *dias*, day). There are many circadian rhythms; however, the one that regulates the sleep-wake cycle is superimposed on the homeostatic mechanisms. The biological clock believed to regulate the sleep-wake circadian rhythm is located in the suprachiasmatic nucleus (SCN). SCN firing patterns oscillate in concert and persist even in isole preparations (in vitro). Because the daily core body temperature cycle is entrained to this sleep-wake oscillator, the temperature cycle is commonly used as a marker of circadian rhythm. In general, 1) when temperature is at its peak, there is maximum alertness; 2) when temperature starts to fall, drowsiness ensues; 3) when temperature reaches nadir, sleepiness can be overwhelming; 4) as temperature starts to rise, sleepiness decreases and alertness increases; and 5) when temperature reaches maximal level, the cycle begins again. Lack of synchrony between scheduled bedtime and the sleepiness biological rhythm could mean less than optimal sleep and/or less than optimal daytime alertness (some degree of daytime drowsiness) (Aschoff 1965; Borbely and Achermann 1992; Moore-Ede et al. 1982).

SLEEP IN PATIENTS WITH PSYCHIATRIC CONDITIONS

Thirty-five percent of patients seen in sleep disorders centers with a chief complaint of insomnia had a psychiatric disorder (Coleman et al. 1982). Half of these patients had a major depressive disorder (MDD). Moreover, 90% of patients with MDD have insomnia (Reynolds and Kupfer 1987). Insomnia is a risk factor (or marker) for depression on 3-year follow-up, conferring an odds ratio of 3.95 compared with individuals without insomnia (Breslau et al. 1996). It has been also been suggested that treating insomnia may help prevent mental disorders, especially depression (Ford and Kamerow 1989). Sleep disturbances in MDD, as defined by electroencephalographic criteria, include 1) generalized sleep disturbance (increase sleep latency, increased nocturnal awakenings, and early morning awakenings), 2) slow-wave sleep decrease in the first NREM-REM cycle with delta activity shifts to the second NREM period, 3) latency to REM sleep shortened, 4) REM sleep occurring earlier in the night, and 5) REM

density increase (especially early in the night). Selective REM sleep deprivation alleviates depression. Furthermore, this antidepressant action can persist several days or more. Interestingly, most antidepressant medication suppresses REM sleep (including selective serotonin reuptake inhibitors [SSRIs], tricyclic antidepressants, and monoamine oxidase inhibitors). Arecoline (a cholinergic agonist) infusion will induce REM sleep in depressed patients, and scopolamine withdrawal mimics depression in normal subjects (including electroencephalographic sleep changes). These data support the cholinergic-aminergic imbalance theory of major depression. Although it still holds that any drug capable of suppressing REM sleep has potential antidepressant properties, a couple of newer antidepressants do not suppress REM sleep (i.e., bupropion and nefazodone). Thus, a piece is missing from the theory. Restated, REM suppression is sufficient but not necessary for antidepressant action (Benca et al. 1992; Ford and Kamerow 1989; Hirshkowitz, in press; Vogel et al. 1980).

Patients with *mania* and *hypomania* seldom complain of sleep problems even though they sleep only a short time (2–4 hours per night), have very prolonged latency to sleep, and sometimes have reduced slow-wave sleep. Patients with *schizophrenia* have no consistent electroencephalographic sleep changes except that they do not have REM sleep rebound in response to REM sleep deprivation. The only other consistent finding is that patients with schizophrenia frequently deny having slept even though sleep appears normal on the EEG-EOG-EMG. Patients with *anxiety* and *personality* disorders often have sleep-onset and sleep-maintenance insomnia (Culebras 1996; Joseph et al. 1989; Zarcone 1989).

SLEEP DISORDERS OVERVIEW AND CLASSIFICATION SYSTEMS

The seriousness of sleep disorders and their contribution to diminished quality of life are poorly recognized. Although individuals afflicted with sleep problems may desperately seek help, often they are met with indifference on the part of health care providers. Medical education for sleep disorders is inadequate, amounting usually to an hour or two in the curriculum. This level of ignorance—coupled with an attitude jaded by a sleepless, overworked internship or residency—leaves many practitioners with little empathy for those with sleep disorders. It is easy to forget that sleep disorders can be life-threatening either directly (e.g., obstructive sleep apnea) or indirectly as a result of sleep-related accidents.

Several classifications systems have been developed to categorize sleep disorders, including the *International*

Classification of Disease (ICD), the *Diagnostic and Statistical Manual of Mental Disorders* (DSM), and the *International Classification of Sleep Disorders* (ICSD). The most complete nosology is ICSD, which is now in its second edition (ICSD-2). The major differences between ICSD-1 and ICSD-2 are 1) ICSD-2 is not an axial system, 2) ICSD-2 does not list diagnostic procedures, 3) the terms *intrinsic* and *extrinsic* have been eliminated as categories for dyssomnias, 4) secondary sleep disorders are not included, and 5) ICSD-2 lists only one set of diagnostic criteria (rather than minimal and full) and does not list severity criteria. ICSD-2 is organized into eight sections: 1) insomnias, 2) sleep-related breathing disorders, 3) hypersomnias of central origin not due to circadian rhythm sleep disorder, sleep-related breathing disorder, or other cause of disturbed nocturnal sleep, 4) circadian rhythm sleep disorder, 5) parasomnias, 6) sleep-related movement disorders, 7) isolated symptoms, apparently normal variants, and unresolved issues, and 8) other sleep disorders. Table 17–4 outlines ICSD-2 (American Academy of Sleep Medicine 2005).

For instructional purposes, however, it is useful to consider sleep disorders categorized according to presenting complaint; that is, insomnia (disorders of initiating or maintaining sleep), hypersomnia (disorders of excessive sleepiness), and parasomnias (disorders of arousal [things that go bump in the night]). The national cooperative study (Coleman et al. 1982) of patients (*N* = 5,000) seen in accredited sleep disorders centers found 31% of patients had insomnias, 51% had hypersomnias, and 15% had parasomnias. Additionally, 3% of patients had disorders of the sleep-wake schedule (circadian dysrhythmia).

INSOMNIA

According to DSM-IV-TR (American Psychiatric Association 2000), insomnia is difficulty initiating sleep, difficulty maintaining sleep, or having nonrestorative sleep for 1 month or more. The insomnia or resulting sleepiness must cause clinically significant impairment or distress. To be considered primary insomnia, the etiology of the insomnia must not be rooted in psychiatric conditions, parasomnias, substance use or abuse, sleep-disordered breathing, or circadian rhythm disorders. However, insomnia usually has multiple and overlapping causes, and ruling in the assorted contributors is more helpful clinically for devising a treatment plan than ruling out factors for the sake of diagnostic purity.

Essentially, insomnia can exist a) as a specific condition or b) as a symptom. Insomnia can accompany a wide variety of sleep, medical, and psychiatric disorders.

When possible, the goal is to treat the cause(s); however, in many cases symptomatic relief is desirable while therapeutic modalities progress. Descriptively, insomnia is sometimes categorized in terms of how it affects sleep (e.g., sleep-onset insomnia, sleep maintenance insomnia, or early morning awakening). It is also classified according to its duration (e.g., transient, short-term, and long-term). Approximately a third of the American population has several serious bouts of insomnia yearly, and in 9% insomnia is a chronic condition. Individuals with chronic insomnia have more than twice as many motor vehicle accidents as the general population, but only 5% of those with chronic insomnia will see a health care provider to seek help for sleeplessness. Nonetheless, more than 40% of individuals with chronic insomnia will self-medicate with over-the-counter drugs, alcohol, or both (Gallup Organization 1991; Mellinger et al. 1985).

Spielman et al. (1987a) conceptualized insomnia in terms of the dynamic model depicted in Figure 17–5. In this model, an individual's generalized threshold for sleeplessness acts in conjunction with three factors: 1) predisposition, 2) precipitating event, and 3) perpetuating factors. In the preclinical state, every person falls within some range from being a very *sound sleeper* to a *light sleeper*. A light sleeper may have a lower sleeplessness threshold such that even minor changes in routine or mildly disquieting daytime events will trigger insomnia. The sound sleeper may be conceptualized has having a high threshold for sleeplessness and thus has no difficulty sleeping even in novel or environmentally adverse conditions. Nonetheless, a precipitating factor may usher in an episode of insomnia regardless of the individual trait disposition for sound or light sleep. Precipitating factors can vary widely. Examples include job stress, relocation, anxiety about taking an examination, undergoing a tax audit, being sued, developing a medical condition, changing medications, becoming separated or divorced, or having a grief reaction. Over time, the impact of most of these factors will wane and one would expect the sleeplessness to follow suit; however, the insomnia often persists. The persistence of sleeplessness, notwithstanding diminution of the original cause's influence (for example, having taken the examination and passed), is considered resultant from perpetuating factors. Examples of perpetuating factors would include chronically using alcohol as a sleep aid, developing habits that are inconsistent with good quality sleep (e.g., watching television in bed), or having a grief reaction evolve into depression. In some cases, the bed and bedroom become conditioned stimuli for wakefulness, and psychophysiological insomnia is the perpetuating factor.

TABLE 17–4. Outline of the International Classification of Sleep Disorders, second edition

I. Insomnia
1. Adjustment insomnia
2. Psychophysiological insomnia
3. Paradoxical insomnia
4. Idiopathic insomnia
5. Insomnia due to mental disorder
6. Inadequate sleep hygiene
7. Behavioral insomnia of childhood
8. Insomnia due to drug or substance
9. Insomnia due to medical condition
10. Insomnia not due to substance or known physiological condition, unspecified (nonorganic insomnia, NOS)
11. Physiological (organic) insomnia, unspecified

II. Sleep-related breathing disorders
A. Central sleep apnea syndromes
1. Primary central sleep apnea
2. Central sleep apnea due to Cheyne-Stokes breathing pattern
3. Central sleep apnea due to high-altitude periodic breathing
4. Central sleep apnea due to medical condition not Cheyne-Stokes
5. Central sleep apnea due to drug or substance
6. Primary sleep apnea of infancy
B. Obstructive sleep apnea syndrome
7. Obstructive sleep apnea, adult
8. Obstructive sleep apnea, pediatric
C. Sleep-related hypoventilation/hypoxemic syndrome
9. Sleep-related nonobstructive alveolar hypoventilation, idiopathic
10. Congenital central alveolar hypoventilation syndrome
D. Sleep-related hypoventilation/hypoxemia due to medical condition
11. Sleep-related hypoventilation/hypoxemia due to pulmonary parenchymal or vascular pathology
12. Sleep-related hypoventilation/hypoxemia due to lower airway obstruction
13. Sleep-related hypoventilation/hypoxemia due to neuromuscular and chest wall disorders
E. Other sleep-related breathing disorder
14. Sleep apnea/sleep-related breathing disorder, unspecified

III. Hypersomnia of central origin not due to a circadian rhythm sleep disorder, sleep-related breathing disorder, or other cause of disturbed nocturnal sleep
1. Narcolepsy with cataplexy
2. Narcolepsy without cataplexy
3. Narcolepsy due to medical condition
4. Narcolepsy, unspecified
5. Recurrent hypersomnia
   Kleine-Levin syndrome
   Menstrual-related hypersomnia
6. Idiopathic hypersomnia with long sleep time
7. Idiopathic hypersomnia without long sleep time
8. Behaviorally induced insufficient sleep syndrome
9. Hypersomnia due to medical condition
10. Hypersomnia due to drug or substance
11. Hypersomnia not due to substance or known physiological condition (nonorganic hypersomnia, NOS)
12. Physiological (organic) hypersomnia, unspecified (organic hypersomnia, NOS)

IV. Circadian rhythm sleep disorders
1. Circadian rhythm sleep disorder, delayed sleep phase type
2. Circadian rhythm sleep disorder, advanced sleep phase type
3. Circadian rhythm sleep disorder, irregular sleep-wake type
4. Circadian rhythm sleep disorder, free-running type
5. Circadian rhythm sleep disorder, jet lag type (jet lag disorder)
6. Circadian rhythm sleep disorder, shift work type (shift work disorder)
7. Circadian rhythm sleep disorder due to medical condition
8. Other circadian rhythm sleep disorder
9. Other circadian rhythm sleep disorder due to drug or substance

V. Parasomnias
A. Disorders of arousal (from NREM sleep)
1. Confusional arousals
2. Sleepwalking
3. Sleep terrors
B. Parasomnias usually associated with REM sleep
4. REM sleep behavior disorder (including parasomnia overlap disorder and status dissociatus)
5. Recurrent isolated sleep paralysis
6. Nightmare disorder
C. Other parasomnias
7. Sleep-related dissociative disorder
8. Sleep enuresis
9. Sleep-related groaning (catathrenia)
10. Exploding head syndrome
11. Sleep-related hallucinations
12. Sleep-related eating disorder
13. Parasomnia, unspecified
14. Parasomnia due to drug or substance
15. Parasomnia due to medical condition

VI. Sleep-related movement disorders
1. Restless legs syndrome
2. Periodic limb movement disorder
3. Sleep-related leg cramps
4. Sleep-related bruxism
5. Sleep-related rhythmic movement
6. Sleep-related movement disorder, unspecified
7. Sleep-related movement disorder due to drug or substance
8. Sleep-related movement disorder due to medical condition

VII. Isolated symptoms, apparently normal variants, and unresolved issues
1. Long sleeper
2. Short sleeper
3. Snoring
4. Sleep talking
5. Sleep starts (hypnic jerks)
6. Benign sleep myoclonus of infancy
7. Hypnagogic foot tremor and alternating leg muscle activation during sleep
8. Propriospinal cyclones at sleep onset
9. Executive fragmentary myoclonus

VIII. Other sleep disorders
1. Other physiological (organic) sleep disorders
2. Other sleep disorder not due to substance or known physiological conditions
3. Environmental sleep disorder

Note. NOS = not otherwise specified.
Source. Adapted from American Academy of Sleep Medicine 2005.

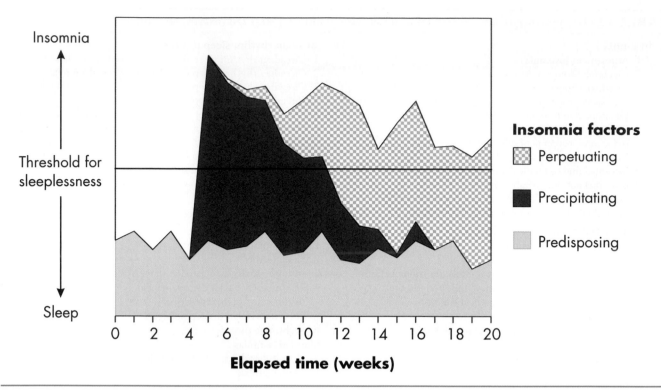

FIGURE 17–5. Spielman's dynamic model of insomnia.

Source. Adapted from Spielman et al. 1987a.

According to the multicenter cooperative study (Coleman et al. 1982), the most common types of insomnia (primary diagnosis) in patients seen at sleep disorders centers were psychiatric disorders, psychophysiological insomnia, drug and alcohol dependence, periodic limb movement disorder or restless legs syndrome, sleep-state misperception, and sleep-disordered breathing (Figure 17–6A). In the following paragraphs, each of these conditions will be reviewed along with several other important etiologies for insomnia that are less frequently seen at sleep centers; that is, inadequate sleep hygiene, idiopathic insomnia, and circadian rhythm dyssomnia.

PSYCHOPHYSIOLOGICAL INSOMNIA

Psychophysiological insomnia often occurs in combination with stress and anxiety disorders, delayed sleep phase syndrome, and hypnotic drug use and withdrawal. The patient with psychophysiological insomnia has developed a conditioned arousal associated with the thought of sleeping. Objects related to sleep (e.g., the bed, the bedroom) likewise have become conditioned stimuli that evoke insomnia. Daytime adaptation is usually good. Work and relationships are satisfying; however, there can be extreme tiredness, and the individual can become desperate. By contrast, daytime adaptation in patients with psychiatrically related insomnia is often impaired. Other

psychophysiological insomnia features include 1) excessive worry about not being able to sleep, 2) trying too hard to sleep, 3) rumination or inability to clear one's mind while trying to sleep, 4) increased muscle tension when getting into bed, 5) other somatic manifestations of anxiety, 6) ability to fall asleep when not trying to (e.g., watching television), and 7) sleeping better away from own bedroom (including the sleep laboratory). In one sense, the individual has developed a performance anxiety concerning the ability to sleep, and autonomic nervous system conditioning reinforces the situation. Stimulus control therapy is well suited for treating psychophysiological insomnia (see the section "Behavioral Treatment: Cognitive-Behavioral Therapy," below) (American Sleep Disorders Association 1997; Hauri and Fisher 1986).

DRUG AND ALCOHOL DEPENDENCE

Use of alcohol and hypnotic drugs initially promotes sleep onset because of the sedating properties of these substances. The problem is that the sleep, although apparently greater in quantity, is poorer in quality. Alcohol may relax a tense person and thereby decrease his or her latency to sleep. Sleep later in the night, however, is fragmented by arousals. As tolerance develops to the alcohol, greater amounts are needed to sustain the effects. Furthermore, during withdrawal or after tolerance has devel-

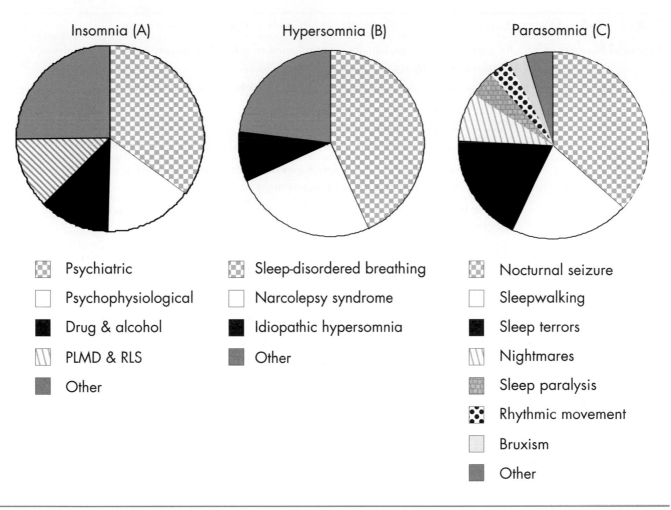

FIGURE 17–6. Proportions for the most common insomnias *(A)*, hypersomnias *(B)*, and parasomnias *(C)* seen in sleep disorders centers. PLMD = periodic limb movement disorder; RLS = restless legs syndrome.

Source. Adapted from Coleman et al. 1982.

oped, the sleep disturbance can rebound to a level more severe than the initial problem. If sleep is considered a behavior and this behavior is dependent on the use of alcohol, then by definition this is a form of alcoholism. Interestingly, one of the earliest effective hypnotic drugs was chloral hydrate, which may be considered essentially alcohol in pill form (because it is metabolized to alcohol).

Barbiturates and, later, benzodiazepines represented the most commonly used prescription medications for insomnia during the twentieth century. Both have potential for abuse and dependency, especially those that produce euphoria. Except in rare cases, sedative-hypnotic medicines are not recommended for long-term use. Benzodiazepines that alter sleep architecture and produce rebound insomnia on withdrawal tend to be habit-forming and can act as a perpetuating factor for insomnia. Abnormally increased electroencephalographic beta and sleep spindle activity commonly developed with long-term or high-dose benzodiazepines ingestion (for further discus-

sion, see "Drug Treatments," below) (American Sleep Disorders Association 1997; Hirshkowitz, in press).

RESTLESS LEGS SYNDROME AND PERIODIC LIMB MOVEMENT DISORDER

Restless legs syndrome (RLS) is characterized by the irresistible urge to move the legs when at rest or while trying to fall asleep. Patients often report crawling feelings in their legs. Moving the legs or walking around helps alleviate the discomfort. Thus, as the individual is lying in bed and relaxing, he or she is disturbed by these sensations. The individual then moves the legs and again tries to fall asleep. This cycle sometimes continues for hours and results in profound insomnia. A National Institutes of Health workshop has established criteria for the diagnosis of RLS (Table 17–5) (Walters et al. 2003). Uremia, neuropathies, and iron and folic acid deficiency anemias can produce secondary RLS. RLS is also reported in association with fibromy

TABLE 17–5.   International study group diagnostic criteria for restless legs syndrome

Essential features	An urge to move legs, usually accomplished or caused by uncontrollable or unpleasant sensations in the legs
	The urge to move or unpleasant sensations that begin or worsen during periods of rest or inactivity such as lying or sitting
	The urge to move or unpleasant sensations that are partially or totally relieved by movement such as walking or stretching, at least as long as the activity continues
	The urge to move or unpleasant sensations that are worse in the evening or night than during the day or occur only in the evening or night
Common features	Positive family history: 3–5 times higher prevalence of restless legs syndrome among first-degree relatives
	Response to dopaminergic therapy
	Periodic leg movements during sleep or wakefulness
	Clinical course: middle-age onset and usually with progressive course
	Sleep disturbance resulting in sleep-onset insomnia or daytime sleepiness
	No abnormality in primary form of the syndrome

algia, rheumatoid arthritis, diabetes, thyroid diseases, and chronic obstructive pulmonary disease (Montplaisir 2005). A detailed history and physical examination are an important part of the RLS workup. In addition, ferritin level should be checked in every patient with symptoms consistent with RLS. Nonpharmacological treatments of RLS include avoiding alcohol close to bedtime, massaging the affected parts, taking hot baths, applying a hot or cold bag to the area, and exercising in moderation. Pharmacologically, the dopaminergic agonists pramipexole and ropinirole are the treatments of choice and have evidence-based support. However, other agents sometimes used include dopamine precursors (e.g., levodopa), benzodiazepines, opiates, and antiepileptic drugs (e.g., gabapentin).

Another type of leg movement disorder associated with insomnia is periodic limb movement disorder (PLMD) (previously called *nocturnal myoclonus*). PLMD involves brief, stereotypic, repetitive, nonepileptiform movements of the limbs, usually the legs. It occurs primarily in NREM sleep and involves an extension of the big toe. A partial flexion of the ankle, knee, and hip may also occur. These movements range from 0.5 to 5 seconds in duration and occur every 20–40 seconds. The leg movements are frequently associated with brief arousals from sleep and as a result can (but do not always) disturb sleep architecture. The prevalence of PLMD increases with aging and can occur in association with folate deficiency, renal disease, anemia, and the use of antidepressants (American Sleep Disorders Association 1997; Ekbom 1960; Lugaresi et al. 1986; Walters 1995; Walters et al. 1991). Pharmacotherapy for PLMD associated with RLS is the same as that for

RLS. There has yet to be a clinical trial of pharmacotherapy for other forms of PLMD. However, benzodiazepines, especially clonazepam, and opiates have been shown to improve sleep in patients with PLMD (Montplaisir 2003).

PARADOXICAL INSOMNIA (FORMERLY SLEEP-STATE MISPERCEPTION)

Most individuals are under the mistaken impression that mental activity necessarily ceases during sleep. One might arrive at this conclusion because of the inability to recall anything between retiring to bed and arising in the morning. However, this confuses the amnesic property of sleep with lack of mentation. Most people readily acknowledge dreaming and understand that dreams constitute mental activity. Nonetheless, under normal circumstances sleep and unconsciousness are coupled; however, they can dissociate. Anxiety can provoke sleep-state misperception, and ruminative worry about not sleeping adds fuel to the fire. Thus, if one lies in bed attempting to sleep and has ruminative thoughts, it is perceived as insomnia even if brain physiology indicates sleep (American Sleep Disorders Association 1997; Carskadon et al. 1976).

This type of insomnia has previously been called pseudoinsomnia or insomnia without objective findings. Both of these appellations imply invalidation of the complaint and place the clinician at odds with the patient. However, one study reported increased metabolic rate and maximum oxygen uptake in patients with sleep-state misperception compared with normal control subjects (Bonnet and Arand 1997). Often a psychoeducational approach that attempts to explain the dissociability between physiological brain correlates of sleep and perception of sleep is more helpful. Furthermore, the ruminations (which seem so urgent at the time but lose their importance or may not even be remembered in the morning) may actually be a useful marker of sleep onset. If individuals can interpret the rumination as an indicator that they *are* asleep and it belays their worrying about not being able to sleep, the sleep-state misperception often diminishes or disappears.

SLEEP-DISORDERED BREATHING

Sleep-related breathing disorders are more commonly associated with excessive daytime sleepiness than insomnia. In some individuals, particularly if the breathing disorder is mild or at an early stage of development, the predominant complaint will be insomnia. Similarly, in obstructive forms of sleep apnea, sleep disruption results from awakenings that return ventilation to voluntary control and thus allow breathing to resume. These recurrent awakenings produce (sometimes severe) sleep maintenance insomnia. Further discussion of sleep-disordered breathing follows in the section on conditions associated with hypersomnolence.

IDIOPATHIC INSOMNIA

Patients with idiopathic insomnia have a lifelong inability to obtain adequate sleep. The insomnia must predate any psychiatric condition, and other etiologies—including psychophysiological insomnia, environmental sleep disturbances, and practices that would constitute poor sleep hygiene—must be ruled out or treated. If the insomnia persists, then it is assumed that there is a defect in the neurological mechanisms that govern the sleep-wake system. That is, the sleep homeostatic process is dysfunctional. Sleep restriction therapy may provide some benefit and will also give the clinician a clue to the limits of the patient's homeostatic process. Sleep restriction is a technique by which homeostatic drive is maximized by sleep schedule compression (see the section "Behavioral Treatment: Cognitive-Behavioral Therapy," below). Unfortunately, patients with idiopathic insomnia never slept well and will likely never have normal sleep. Although it is controversial, long-term pharmacotherapeutic intervention with this group may be required.

CIRCADIAN RHYTHM DYSSOMNIAS

In an optimal schedule, hours in bed must coincide with the sleepy phase of the circadian cycle. *Advanced sleep phase* is when the circadian rhythm cycle is shifted earlier. Therefore, the sleepiness cycle is advanced with respect

to clock time. Individuals with advanced sleep phase are drowsy in the evening, want to retire to bed earlier, awaken earlier, and are more alert in the early morning. Individuals with this pattern of advanced sleep phase are sometimes called "larks" (sometimes called "surgeons" in the medical center). By contrast, the biological clock may run slow or be shifted later than the desired schedule. This produces a *phase delay* in the sleepiness-alertness cycle. Individuals with delayed sleep phase are more alert in the evening and early nighttime, stay up later, and are more tired in the morning. These individuals are referred to as "owls" (Moore-Ede 1982; Zammit 1997).

Under the extreme condition of time isolation, most adults exhibit features of delayed sleep phase. In the absence of time cues, the sleep-wake cycle will drift later and later on each successive day. Furthermore, there can be a dissociation of the sleep-wake and temperature rhythms. Under normal circumstances, however, the biological clock is reset each day by bright light, social cues, stimulants, and activity. In cases where these factors are unable to reentrain the circadian rhythm, the advanced sleep phase and delayed sleep phase disorders of the sleep-wake cycle may occur associated with complaints of early morning awakening insomnia and sleep-onset insomnia, respectively. In the past, chronotherapy was used to reentrain the circadian rhythm; however, it has largely been replaced by bright light therapy (see next section) (Czeisler et al. 1989).

INSOMNIA TREATMENT OPTIONS

Behavioral Treatment: Cognitive-Behavioral Therapy

Behavioral treatment of insomnia is now widely recognized as an important and effective modality. The 2005 National Institutes of Health State-of-the-Science Conferences on Insomnia strongly advocated for increasing use of behavioral therapy. Cognitive-behavioral therapy (CBT), which combines patient-appropriate behavioral therapies with cognitive and psychoeducational approaches, has been found to be both effective and durable. The individual components of CBT are described below and include cognitive therapy, universal sleep hygiene, relaxation training, stimulus control therapy, sleep restriction therapy, and bright light therapy.

Cognitive therapy. Psychoeducational training can be extremely helpful because individuals with insomnia often have unusual notions about their condition. The therapist must first help an individual develop realistic expectations about his or her sleep and a timetable for expected improvement. The patient's beliefs are critically important, especially with respect to dysfunctional thinking, performance anxiety, cortical arousal, sleep misperception, automaticity, and attention. There must be awareness that the therapy will take time and involves active participation. If the patient identifies him- or herself as an "insomniac"—that is, if having insomnia is part of his or her identity and/or personality structure—this must be addressed and dispelled if one is to make progress.

Universal sleep hygiene. Many individuals with insomnia, regardless of the underlying cause, make things worse with poor sleep hygiene. Essentially, they have developed bad habits with respect to sleep. These habits may operate through autonomic, homeostatic, or circadian mechanisms. When these habits are a primary etiology, inadequate sleep hygiene can be diagnosed. Universal sleep hygiene essentially involves recommending that the individual promote sleep-enhancing habits and avoid sleep-destroying behaviors. Table 17–6 lists some recommendations to improve sleep hygiene. In applying this approach, the clinician should review the patient's day-to-day habits and obtain an appreciation of the sleep environment. From the assortment of potentially sleep-impeding activities, the clinician must judiciously choose one or two items (three at the most) to initially address. The reason for limiting the scope is that most of these directives amount to asking the patient to change an element of his or her lifestyle. Such changes are difficult at best, and therapy that overloads a person is doomed to fail. Continued follow-up with monitoring progress is essential. As goals are achieved, additional sleep hygiene issues can be addressed. Often a few simple alterations can produce dramatic results. In addition, improving sleep hygiene usually enhances sleep even when the insomnia is clearly psychiatric or physical. Presumably, adopting good sleep hygienic practices optimizes sleep, and for most people there is room for improvement (Lacks and Rotert 1986; Morgan and Closs 1999b).

Relaxation training. This type of behavioral therapy takes many forms, including progressive relaxation, breathing exercises (or yoga), biofeedback, and guided visualization. The goal of relaxation training is twofold. Primarily, it provides a systematic technique for reducing tension and stress. Thus, it acts through the autonomic mechanisms that can enhance or impede sleep. Additionally, however, it provides a distraction such that the individual thinks about something other than his or her inability to sleep. The therapy must be properly performed and overlearned before it is applied. Many individuals immediately reject relaxation therapy when it is suggested on the basis that they have tried it and it did not work. Questioning typically reveals that they pur-

TABLE 17–6. Sleep hygiene recommendations
Maintain a regular sleep-wake schedule
Get a steady daily amount of exercise
Avoid chronic use of alcohol or over-the-counter drugs as sleep aids
Do not try to fall asleep; let sleep come
Insulate the bedroom against loud noises
Make sure the bedroom is not excessively warm
A *light* snack before bedtime may be helpful
Do not eat a heavy meal close to bedtime
Avoid caffeine or chocolate in the evening
Quit smoking or avoid smoking near bedtime

chased a self-help tape and listened to it when in bed unable to sleep. Such an approach indeed does not work. Whatever the approach, be it using biofeedback or listening to an instructional tape, the technique must first be mastered. Practicing during the daytime, sometimes for weeks, is needed so that the individual can immediately move through the technique and become relaxed. Trying to learn a method while struggling to sleep must be avoided because it creates an adverse conditioning paradigm. Moreover, if the person starts to fall asleep, he will arouse himself to finish the exercise. The clinician should monitor the progress during training to ensure the technique is performed correctly and to judge when it is time for it to be applied in the sleepless bed. Finally, relaxation techniques are readily combined with other behavioral therapies (Espie et al. 1989; Lichstein and Riedel 1994).

Stimulus control therapy. For individuals with psychophysiological insomnia, stimulus control directly addresses the underlying autonomic conditioning. Secondarily it arranges homeostatic and circadian factors so that they will work in concert with attempts to recondition sleep onset. Stimulus control therapy directives attempt to enhance stimulus cues for sleeping and diminish bedroom stimulus associations with sleeplessness. The instructions are simple; however, following them consistently and keeping sleep diaries are the keys to success. The first rule is to go to bed only when sleepy. Second, use the bed only for sleeping. That is, in bed one should not eat, read, talk on the telephone, watch television, do paperwork, write letters, exercise, argue with one's spouse, or worry about things that happened in the past or are expected to happen in the future. If one is unable to sleep, rule three instructs getting up, going to another room, and doing something nonarousing until one becomes sleepy. One should not watch the clock, and in fact should hide it from view so as not to know the time when nocturnal arousals occur. Nonetheless, if it feels as if more than a few minutes have passed, getting out of bed avoids increasing frustration with the inability to sleep. Ultimately, the goal is to associate the bed and bedroom with rapid sleep onset. Rule three should be repeated as often as needed. A diary should be kept indicating how many times getting out of bed was necessary. This information can be correlated with specific daytime events to promote insight into the precipitating factors for the individual's insomnia. In addition, it will serve as a memory aid because results may not be seen for the first few weeks. Having such a record can show that bouts of insomnia are diminishing in both frequency and severity. This provides reinforcement and hope when a sudden sleeplessness recurrence prompts a patient to become discouraged and want to try something else. The final stimulus control therapy instructions address circadian and homeostatic factors to increase sleep pressure. Patients are instructed to awaken at the same time every morning, regardless of bedtime, total sleep time, or day of week, and to totally avoid napping (Bootzin 1972, 1977).

Sleep restriction therapy. This therapy is designed to enhance sleep through the homeostatic mechanism. In cases in which the patient spends a diminished percentage of his or her time in bed actually sleeping, sleep restriction therapy attempts to compress the sleep episode and enhance sleep drive. The initial step is to have a patient keep a diary of bedtimes, arising times, and amount of time actually sleeping. From this, the total sleep time can be estimated. Sometimes, patients will spend an inordinate amount of time in bed in an attempt to increase their sleep time, only to find their sleep becoming more and more fragmented. We have seen patients spending 11 hours in bed in order to attain a reported 6 hours of sleep. The second step in sleep restriction therapy is to compress the sleep schedule to the reported sleep time. Thus, in a patient reporting 6 hours of sleep in an 11-hour total bedtime, we set arising time at 6 hours after retiring time. It should be noted that restricting bedtime schedule to less than 4 hours per night is not advised. In addition, patients must be advised that they will likely be very sleepy the next day and must exercise extreme care, especially when performing potentially dangerous actions (e.g., driving). Sleep at other times during the day must be avoided, except in elderly persons, who may take a 30-minute nap. Each night, the amount of time spent asleep is reported and the clinician calculates sleep efficiency (the ratio of total sleep time to total bed time). If the patient attains a 5-night moving average sleep efficiency of 0.85 or greater,

time in bed is increased by 15 minutes (some clinicians use a 3-night average). In this manner, time awake in bed is controlled while time asleep gradually and steadily increases. Moreover, when the sleep efficiency plateaus, the clinician has an empirical estimate of the patient's homeostatic drive limit and can better judge if idiopathic insomnia is present. Nonetheless, greater sleep consolidation is achieved, and the patient spends less time lying in bed becoming frustrated by inability to sleep (Morin et al. 1994; Spielman et al. 1987b).

Bright light therapy. Bright light appears to be the critical factor in controlling the biological clock. With precise timing of bright light exposure, the biological clock phase advanced, phase delayed, or even stopped and reset. The use of bright light exposure to overcome desynchrony between environmental and biological clocks produced by rapid time zone change (jet lag), shift work, and space travel is an exciting frontier in sleep research. In general, bright light in the evening will delay the sleep phase and bright light in the morning will advance the sleep phase. Thus, the phase-delayed "owl" who stays up cruising the Internet until 2:00 A.M. with his or her face less than a meter from a 19-inch video monitor is probably further phase delaying the sleep-wake cycle. What the phase-delaying "owl" needs is to avoid bright light in the evening and replace it with bright light in the early morning (Czeisler et al. 1989; Zammit 1997).

Drug Treatments

Specific drug therapies have been applied for periodic limb movement disorder and restless legs syndrome. Currently, the most popular pharmacotherapy is with the dopaminergic agents pramipexole and ropinirole. These drugs can affect blood pressure and produce rebound movement disorders upon discontinuation. Dopamine agonists are contraindicated in patients who are taking monoamine oxidase inhibitors, who have a history of melanoma, or who have narrow-angle glaucoma. However, clonazepam and narcotics (propoxyphene, codeine, hydrocodone) are in common use (notwithstanding their addiction liability and high abuse potential) and are quite effective (Chockroverty 2000).

It should go without saying that antidepressants are indicated if depression is comorbid. Most antidepressants, however, alter sleep architecture and exacerbate the leg movement disorders. Tricyclic antidepressants and SSRIs (especially clomipramine and amitriptyline) suppress REM sleep. Amitriptyline, doxepin, and trazodone have strong sedative properties. Most tricyclics increase slow-wave sleep, whereas serotonin reuptake inhibitors generally decrease or do not change slow-wave activity. Monoamine oxidase inhibitors are powerful REM sleep suppressors and also diminish slow-wave sleep. By contrast, nefazodone and bupropion are not associated with decreased REM sleep (Hirshkowitz, in press).

The more general, nonspecific drug therapy approach to insomnia involves using sedative-hypnotic medications. The profile for an ideal hypnotic is shown in Table 17–7. Sleep-promoting substances (e.g., opium and alcohol) have been used since antiquity, but in the 1860s chloral hydrate was formulated as a sleeping pill. In essence it represented alcohol in pill form, and it gained widespread acceptance. At the turn of the last century, barbiturates became available. As strong partial γ-aminobutyric acid (GABA) agonists, barbiturates were very effective at producing sedation and immediately became popular, notwithstanding their toxic liability. Most of the barbiturates have a large REM sleep suppression and a smaller slow-wave sleep suppression effect. Sleep latency decreases, sleep efficiency increases, and there are fewer awakenings after sleep onset. The toxic liability, however, spurred further development, and in the 1960s a new class of GABA partial agonists, the benzodiazepines, largely replaced barbiturates for treating insomnia. Their wide dose safety range, minimum side effects, and milder abstinence syndrome on withdrawal made benzodiazepines far more attractive than previously available medications. Perhaps the most clinically salient advantage of benzodiazepines compared with barbiturates was the increased dose-range margin of safety (that is, a much wider effective dose to lethal dose ratio [ED:LD]). The safety range for toxicity is critically important because of the incidence of patients with MDD who present with a complaint of insomnia. Barbiturates have a long legacy of lethality. Nonetheless, even with benzodiazepines, long-term use is considered problematic. Pharmaceutical companies developed a wide variety of benzodiazepines, differing in speed of onset, half-life, and presence or absence of active metabolites (see Table 17–8). Benzodiazepines are very effective at decreasing sleep latency, increasing sleep efficiency, and decreasing awakenings after sleep onset; however, they also alter sleep macroarchitecture with slow-wave sleep and, to a lesser extent, REM sleep suppression. Sleep microarchitecture is also altered in that benzodiazepines can powerfully increase sleep spindle activity. Longer-acting benzodiazepines (especially those with active metabolites) often have carryover effects (hangover) in terms of both residual sedation and diminished psychomotor performance. The efficacy of shorter-acting benzodiazepines is marred by early morning rebound and withdrawal rebound insomnia.

Pharmaceutical development continued, and a class of more specific benzodiazepine receptor agonists was developed: cyclopyrrolones (zopiclone) and imadazopyri-

TABLE 17–7. Profile for an ideal hypnotic

Desired effect	Parameter
Increase	Sleep efficiency
	Total sleep time
Decrease	Latency to sleep onset
	Wake after sleep onset time
	Number of awakenings
Remain unchanged	Sleep macroarchitecture (stages)
	Sleep microarchitecture
Avoid producing	Carryover—hangover
	Early morning rebound insomnia
	Withdrawal rebound insomnia
	Psychomotor impairment
	Cognitive impairment
	Dependency

dine (zolpidem) in the 1980s and pyrazolopyrimidine (zaleplon) in the 1990s. These further pharmacological strides have been made because the newer medications target specific GABA receptor subtypes. These hypnotics now dominate the market. These drugs are effective hypnotics and appear to produce fewer rebound problems. The newer drugs tend to have very rapid onset, be short acting, and have little or no effect on sleep macroarchitecture. Zolpidem and zaleplon are also associated with fewer side effects, most notably the lack of residual sedation (due to their short half-lives and lack of active metabolites). Amnesia, however, persists as a side effect (less in zaleplon than zolpidem, but present in both). There is evidence that memory effects may be related to sleep induction (inasmuch as sleep itself produces amnesia). Consequently, it may not be possible to entirely eliminate amnesia as an undesirable effect of sleep-promoting substances (Morgan and Closs 1999a; Shneerson 2000).

Current Recommendations

Short-term insomnia treatment recommendations include several areas of intervention. First, it is important to review and address any behaviors or habits that are counterproductive to a good night's sleep by initiating a sleep hygiene program. Next, if other factors are identified as contributory to perpetuating sleeplessness (for example, psychophysiological insomnia), they should be treated aggressively. If pharmacotherapy is intended, an effective dose of a short-acting sedative-hypnotic should be used. Finally, treatment course should usually be less than 3 weeks in duration, and intermittent dosing is preferred.

TABLE 17–8. Pharmacokinetics of drugs approved for treating insomnia

Generic name	Brand name	Manufacturer	Dose (mg)	Onset time (minutes)	Half-life (hours)	Active metabolite
Benzodiazepine hypnotics						
Triazolam	Halcion	Upjohn	0.125–0.25	15–30	1.5–5.4	None
Estazolam	Prosom	Abbot	1–2	15–30	10–24	None
Temazepam	Restoril	Sandoz	7.5–30	45–120	10–20	None
Quazepam	Doral	Baker-Cummins	7.5–15	20–45	15–70	N-desalkyl-flurazepam
Flurazepam	Dalmane	Roche	15–30	30–60	47–100	N-desalkyl-flurazepam
Benzodiazepine receptor agonist hypnotics						
Zolpidem	Ambien	Sanofi-Aventis	5–10	30	1.4–4.5	None
Zolpidem MR	Ambien CR	Sanofi-Aventis	6.25 and 12.5	30	2.5–3.0	None
Zaleplon	Sonata	King	10–20	30–60	1–2	None
Zopiclone	Imovane	Aventis	3.75–7.5	30–60	5–6	None
Eszopiclone	Lunesta	Sepracor	1–3	30–60	6+	None

Treatment is more difficult for chronic insomnia. First, any underlying conditions, if present, that predispose the individual to sleeplessness must be identified and treated. For example, if an underlying depression exists, treating only the insomnia is ill-advised. Similarly, any perpetuating factors (e.g., inadequate sleep hygiene, ongoing use of alcohol, conditioned insomnia) should be a main therapeutic target. In chronic insomnia it is important to improve sleep behaviorally as much as possible even if other treatments are planned. Thus, combined behavioral, psychological, and pharmacological treatment can be used concurrently. In chronic insomnias resulting from RLS and PLMD, sedative-hypnotic, dopaminergic, and opioid medications have been used successfully. If a vitamin or mineral deficiency is found, its cause should be determined and nutritional supplementation should commence. For primary insomnia, when selecting medication the clinician should consider the etiology of insomnia and pharmacokinetic factors (duration of action, half-life, and whether or not metabolites are psychoactive). In insomnias from causes other than RLS and PLMD, a time-limited and intermittent dosing is usually preferred. Nonetheless, there will be patients who require continuing pharmacotherapy.

Clinicians should be cautious when prescribing hypnotic medications for patients who are elderly; who have a history of heavy snoring; who have renal, hepatic, or pulmonary disease; or who are using concomitant psychoactive medication (especially depressants). Cautious use is also warranted when prescribing sedating drugs for patients who use alcohol regularly, have suicidal tendencies, or work in hazardous occupations. If a person needs to be able to become alert rapidly during his or her usual sleep period (for example, a physician on call), sedative-hypnotics are generally contraindicated unless they are ultra-short-acting. Sedative-hypnotic medications are clearly contraindicated in patients who are pregnant, have sleep-disordered breathing, or use alcohol to excess.

HYPERSOMNIA

Excessive sleepiness is a serious, debilitating, potentially life-threatening, noncommunicable condition. It affects not only the afflicted individuals but also their family, coworkers, and the public at large. Sleepiness can be a consequence of insufficient sleep, disrupted sleep, or nonrestorative sleep. The sleep debt produced by insufficient sleep is cumulative. If one reduces sleep duration by 1–2 hours per night and continues this regimen for a week, sleepiness will reach pathological levels. When sleep debt is added to sleep disruption or nonrestorative sleep, there is increasing risk that an individual will lapse unexpectedly into sleep. Sleep onset in such circumstances characteristically occurs without warning. Sleepiness can be episodic and occur as irresistible sleep attacks, can occur in the morning as sleep drunkenness, or can be chronic. *Fatigue*, *tiredness*, and *sleepiness* are terms that are used by most people synonymously; however, one can be tired but not sleepy, sleepy but not tired, or sleepy and tired.

Sleepiness adversely affects attention, concentration, memory, and higher-order cognitive processes. Serious results of sleepiness include failure at school, loss of employment, motor vehicle accidents, and industrial disasters. The transportation industry—including trucking, rail, shipping, and aviation—is particularly susceptible to sleep-related accidents (National Commission on Sleep Disorders Research 1993). Determinants of daytime sleepiness include insufficient sleep, drug use, aging, circadian phase, and sleep disorders. Although *insufficient sleep syndrome* is a diagnostic entity, most individuals are aware of the cause; therefore, medical help is seldom sought. Disregard for the sleep-wake schedule has reached nearly epidemic proportions in some segments of the population, especially teenagers and young professionals. Insufficient sleep is an insidious killer of otherwise healthy individuals in its role as the underlying cause of countless vehicular accidents. Alcohol ingestion, sedentary situations, a warm room, or a heavy meal unmasks and worsens sleepiness, sometimes making it difficult to maintain concentration or remain alert (Dinges and Kribbs 1991; Horne 1991; Lubin 1967; H.L. Williams et al. 1959).

There are many sleep disorders associated with excessive daytime sleepiness; however, sleep-disordered breathing is by far the most common dyssomnia seen in sleep disorders centers. In the cooperative study by Coleman et al. (1982), sleep apnea syndromes accounted for 43.2% of sleepy patients. More recent statistics estimate that sleep-disordered breathing accounts for 67.8% of all patients seen in sleep disorders centers (Punjabi et al. 2000). The two next most common sleep disorders producing hypersomnia are narcolepsy and idiopathic hypersomnia (see Figure 17–6B). Other disorders of excessive sleepiness include recurrent hypersomnia (Kleine-Levin syndrome) and posttraumatic hypersomnia (resultant from brain or brain stem injury).

SLEEP-DISORDERED BREATHING

Sleep-disordered breathing includes disorders ranging from upper-airway resistance syndrome to severe obstructive sleep apnea. An episode of sleep apnea is defined as a cessation of breathing for 10 seconds or more during sleep. A reduction in breathing is termed a *hypopnea*. These sleep-related breathing impairments are most often caused by airway obstruction; however, sometimes respiratory reduction results from central (brain stem) changes in ventilatory control, metabolic factors, or heart failure. We classify each sleep-disordered breathing event as either *central, obstructive, or mixed*. Central apnea or hypopnea is the absence of breathing due to lack of respiratory effort. In obstructive events, respiratory effort continues but airflow stops due to

reduced or loss of airway patency. Mixed apnea or hypopnea episodes contain components of both, often beginning as a central apnea and progressing to an obstructive apnea.

Sleep-disordered breathing events may be accompanied by oxygen desaturation and cardiac arrhythmias. Clinical features associated with obstructive sleep apnea (the most common form of sleep-disordered breathing) include 1) excessive daytime sleepiness, 2) loud snoring with frequent awakenings, 3) awakening with choking and/or gasping for breath, 4) morning dry mouth, and 5) witnessed apnea. Predisposing factors include 1) male gender, 2) middle age, 3) obesity, 4) micrognathia or retrognathia and nasal pharyngeal abnormalities, and 5) hypothyroidism and acromegaly. Other features and comorbidities include sleep choking, morning headaches, nocturnal sweating, sleepwalking, sleep talking, nocturia, enuresis, impotence, memory impairment, depression, anxiety, hearing loss, automatic behaviors, hypertension, congestive heart failure, coronary artery disease, stroke, polycythemia, and right-sided heart failure (Robinson and Guilleminault 1999; Sharafkhaneh et al. 2004, 2005).

Treatment

Many treatments are available for sleep-disordered breathing, including weight loss, positive airway pressure therapy, use of oral appliances, and surgery. Weight loss is difficult to achieve and maintain; therefore, it is recommended but not relied on (Fairbanks et al. 1987; Loube et al. 1999; Sanders 2000; Thorpy and Ledereich 1990).

Continuous positive airway pressure.   Currently, the most popular therapy is positive airway pressure. Positive airway pressure comes in three varieties: continuous, bilevel, and auto-adjusting. Continuous positive airway pressure (CPAP) is the most common and represents the preferred treatment. It delivers fan-generated flow at a set pressure to the nares usually via a nasal mask. In so doing it creates a "pneumatic splint" and thereby maintains airway patency. It is highly effective in most patients; however, it requires nightly utilization. Patients who have more severe sleep-disordered breathing or who are sleepier at baseline are the most compliant with this therapy. It is important that the proper pressure be selected. If pressure is too low, then airway obstructions continue; if pressure is too high, sleep is disturbed. Pressures are usually adjusted during a sleep study. Often a rebound in REM and/or slow-wave sleep will occur when an effective pressure is reached. Sleep normalization is impressive. Sleep-disordered breathing is marked by frequent brief arousals. These arousals are needed to return ventilatory control to the voluntary system so that breathing will resume after airway closure. Once airway patency is achieved, these constant sleep disruptions disappear, permitting the first good night of sleep the patient has had in possibly decades.

Bilevel and self-adjusting positive airway pressure.
Some patients have difficulty exhaling against the constant pressure of CPAP. In such cases, a variant of CPAP called bilevel positive airway pressure (bilevel PAP) can be used. Bilevel PAP allows differential setting of inspiratory and expiratory pressures and is sometimes also used as a nasal ventilatory assist for central sleep apnea. Bilevel inspiratory pressure is always set higher than expiratory pressure. This setting helps to keep the upper airway patent during inspiration while it prevents complete collapse of upper airway during expiration. Another variant of CPAP is self-adjusting CPAP, or AutoCPAP. In Auto-CPAP devices, a sensor tries to detect sleep-disordered breathing events and compensate by changing airflow pressure. In developing AutoCPAP, it was hypothesized that lower pressure will be needed to overcome airway obstruction, and thus with lower pressure, utilization will improve. However, a meta-analysis concluded that utilization did not differ significantly when AutoCPAP was compared with CPAP, despite a mean decrease in overnight pressure of 2 cm H_2O (Ayas et al. 2004).

Oral appliances.
For patients who cannot tolerate positive airway pressure, other options include oral appliances or surgery. Oral appliances were developed to treat snoring and have also been found to be sometimes effective for upper airway resistance syndrome and mild to moderate obstructive sleep apnea. Most appliances in current use either manipulate the position of the mandible or retain the tongue, or both. Breathing, although improved, may not reach satisfactory levels; therefore, follow-up sleep studies are needed. A recent review of literature showed that in comparison to CPAP, oral appliances were less effective but were used more often by the patients, and in many studies they were preferred by patients over CPAP (Ferguson et al. 2006).

Surgery.
The earliest surgical intervention for severe obstructive sleep apnea was tracheostomy. There was little doubt that tracheostomy succeeded in creating an airway. Although it is no longer a preferred treatment, it remains a standard against which newer therapies are judged. The next generation of surgical intervention was uvulopalatopharyngoplasty (UPPP). Initial results indicated that this modification of soft palate was effective. More recent studies have tempered the initial enthusiasm. Clinically significant improvement is attained with UPPP in approximately 50% of patients with sleep apnea. The soft palate surgeries are also sometimes performed using a

laser. Nonetheless, predicting success is difficult, and complications may occur. Another surgical intervention includes maxillomandibular advancement. This procedure seems particularly effective in retrognathic patients or in patients with cephalometrics revealing compromised posterior airway space. Finally, the most recent anatomical alteration performed for sleep-disordered breathing, called somnoplasty, uses radiofrequency ablation.

Other treatments.
Position-dependent sleep-disordered breathing, although rare, is sometimes encountered. Typically, breathing will be impaired when the patient sleeps supine. In such cases, tennis balls sewn onto or placed into pockets on the back of the nightshirt may prevent the patient from sleeping on his or her back. Finally, it would be a great advantage if a medication to treat sleep apnea were discovered. Methoxyprogesterone acetate was once thought to be helpful but is seldom used now. Similarly, tricyclic antidepressants (e.g., protriptyline) may decrease apnea severity by increasing upper airway tone and/or reducing REM sleep (the sleep stage in which worse sleep-disordered breathing usually occurs). Theophylline also reportedly reduces sleep-disordered breathing; however, further study is needed. Recent trials failed to show clinically significant effects of atrial overdrive pacing in the treatment of obstructive sleep apnea (Sharafkhaneh et al. 2006). However, the role of biventricular pacing in patients with congestive heart failure and central sleep apnea is not known. Stimulants such as modafinil may effectively alleviate sleepiness symptoms in patients with obstructive sleep apnea who have residual sleepiness despite adequate CPAP utilization.

NARCOLEPSY

Narcolepsy results from a hypocretin deficit. It is characterized by a tetrad of symptoms: 1) excessive daytime sleepiness, 2) cataplexy, 3) sleep paralysis, and 4) hypnagogic hallucinations. Patients with narcolepsy often have an abnormal sleep architecture in which REM sleep occurs soon after sleep onset both at night and during daytime naps. This, in connection with the symptom tetrad, makes narcolepsy appear to be a REM sleep intrusion syndrome, presumably resulting from dysfunction of REM sleep generator gating mechanisms. The features of the tetrad match REM sleep characteristics. The sleep paralysis is similar to the muscle atonia that occurs during REM sleep. The hypnagogic hallucinations are vivid "dreams" that occur while the patient is still conscious or partially conscious. However, not all patients have the full constellation of symptoms. Narcolepsy is estimated to afflict 10–60 individuals per 10,000. Symptoms commonly appear in the second decade of life. Strong emotions usually act as the "trigger" for cataplexy. Common emotional triggers include laughter and anger. Severity of cataplexy ranges widely from transient weakness in knees to total paralysis while the patient is fully conscious. Episodes may last from several seconds to minutes. Usually, the patient is unable to speak and may fall to the floor. Nocturnal sleep is often fragmented, and there can be considerable sleep disturbance (Aldrich 1996; Fry 1998; American Sleep Disorders Association 1994).

It has become apparent that the hypocretin system plays a critical role in narcolepsy. In a canine model of narcolepsy, mutations of hypocretin receptor 2 were identified that resulted in receptor malfunction (Lin et al. 1999). In cases of human narcolepsy with *HLA-DQB1*0602* positive (the genetic marker for narcolepsy), levels of hypocretin-1 are undetectable in cerebrospinal fluid (Ripley et al. 2001). Strong association between narcolepsy and specific human leukocyte antigen suggests an autoimmune process that damages hypocretin-containing cells in the central nervous system (Mignot 2005).

Narcolepsy is diagnosed with an overnight sleep study, followed by a multiple sleep latency test (MSLT). The overnight sleep study helps rule out sleep-disordered breathing, PLMD, or other identifiable pathophysiologies that could be responsible for the sleepiness and other symptoms. The MSLT is a series of four to six 20-minute nap opportunities provided at 2-hour intervals on the day after the sleep study, commencing 2 hours from morning arising. On the clinical version of MSLT, if a patient falls asleep within the 20-minute limit, he or she is allowed to sleep for an additional 15 minutes. The MSLT provides two categories of important diagnostic data. First, it objectively documents sleepiness. If the mean latency to sleep across all nap sessions is 5 minutes or less, then sleepiness is considered pathological. A mean sleep latency in the 6- to 10-minute range is borderline. The MSLT also measures REM sleep coordination and pressure. If REM sleep occurs on two or more naps in a symptomatic patient, then the diagnosis is confirmed. Alternatively, a sleep-onset REM period on the previous night's sleep study and one MSLT nap with REM sleep also confirm the diagnosis. Current standard of practice and regulations in many states require diagnostic validation of narcolepsy with the MSLT if stimulants are used for treatment (Carskadon et al. 1986). Decreased levels of hypocretin-1 in cerebrospinal fluid (below 110 pg/mL) are especially predictive in patients with definite cataplexy (99% specificity, 87% sensitivity). However, in narcoleptic patients with cataplexy, the sensitivity is very low (16%), whereas specificity remains high (Mignot et al. 2002).

TREATMENT

In general, the ancillary symptoms of narcolepsy (cataplexy, sleep paralysis, and hypnagogia) are treated with REM-suppressing medications. For years, tricyclic antidepressants (especially imipramine and protriptyline) were widely used. In the past decade, however, the use of SSRIs has become commonplace for controlling daytime cataplexy. In patients in whom cataplexy is not well controlled with tricyclics or SSRIs, effective control is achieved with γ-hydroxybutyrate (sodium oxybate) (U.S. Xyrem Multicenter Study Group 2004). Sodium oxybate controls cataplexy even in patients with whom all other medications have failed. There is also evidence that sodium oxybate consolidates sleep, increases slow-wave activity, and improves daytime alertness.

The excessive daytime sleepiness associated with narcolepsy presents a greater challenge than treating cataplexy. Nonpharmacological therapy of narcolepsy includes avoiding alcohol and heavy meals, regularization and extension of sleep time, and scheduled naps during the day. Stimulant medications are used palliatively to provide symptom relief. Until recently, methylphenidate was the usual first-line treatment, followed by amphetamines if methylphenidate was ineffective. Pemoline was used with some success but was withdrawn from the U.S. market after increasing reports of serious adverse events. The introduction of modafinil, a nonstimulant somnolytic, provides clinicians with an alternative option for treating sleepiness in narcolepsy. Modafinil's benign side-effect profile makes it more attractive for long-term use than traditional stimulants. Other strategies to help offset the loss of effectiveness of these medications in combating sleepiness include having the patient take prophylactic naps to replace a scheduled stimulant dose. Periodic withdrawals of medication, so-called drug holidays, are also used when sleepiness increases to uncontrollable levels notwithstanding increased dosing. The abstinence period usually restores efficacy of the drug when it is readministered.

IDIOPATHIC HYPERSOMNIA

Idiopathic hypersomnia is another disorder of excessive sleepiness; however, patients do not have the ancillary symptoms associated with narcolepsy. Unlike in narcolepsy, sleep is usually well preserved, and sleep efficiency remains high even with very extended sleep schedules (12 hours or more). Furthermore, the patient readily falls asleep if given an opportunity to nap the following day. The proportion of slow-wave sleep is often increased; however, the electroencephalographic sleep pattern is essentially the same as that found in healthy individuals who are sleep deprived. Unlike a sleep-deprived individual, however, the sleep pattern continues in this profile even after several nights of extended sleep. As the name indicates, the etiology of idiopathic hypersomnia is not known; however, a central nervous system cause is presumed. Three general categories have been developed to attempt classification in hopes of furthering our understanding of whether this is one dyssomnia or a collection of several disorders. *Subgroup 1* includes individuals who are human lymphocyte antigen (HLA) Cw2 positive, have autonomic nervous system dysfunctions, and have other affected family members. *Subgroup 2* includes patients who are status postviral infection (e.g., Guillain-Barré syndrome [ascending polyneuropathy], mononucleosis, and atypical viral pneumonia). *Subgroup 3* patients do not have other affected family members and have not had viral infections (i.e., truly idiopathic hypersomnia). Age at onset is characteristically between ages 15 and 30 years, and the dyssomnia becomes a lifelong problem. In addition to the prolonged, undisturbed, and unrefreshing sleep, idiopathic hypersomnia is associated with long nonrefreshing naps, difficulty awakening, sleep drunkenness, and automatic behaviors with amnesia. Other symptoms suggesting autonomic nervous system dysfunction, including migraine-like headaches, fainting spells, syncope, orthostatic hypotension, and Raynaud's-type phenomena with cold hands and feet, are typical (Aldrich 1996; Guilleminault and Pelayo 2000).

TREATMENT

The sleepiness is treated palliatively in a similar fashion to the approach used in narcolepsy. Stimulants are usually less effective than in narcolepsy, however, and prophylactic napping does not seem to be as beneficial. Modafinil has not been tested in patients with idiopathic hypersomnia. However, in pivotal clinical trials in the United States, modafinil was equally effective for patients with and without cataplexy who were diagnosed with narcolepsy.

PARASOMNIAS

Parasomnias are sometimes referred to as disorders of partial arousal. In general, the parasomnias are a large and diverse collection of sleep disorders characterized by physiological or behavioral phenomena that occur during or that are potentiated by sleep. One conceptual framework posits many parasomnias as overlap or intrusion of one basic sleep-wake state into another (Figure 17–7). Wakefulness, NREM sleep, and REM sleep can be characterized as the three basic states that differ in their neurological organization. In the awake state, both the body and brain are active,

whereas in NREM sleep, both the body and brain are inactive. REM sleep involves an inactive body (atonic, in fact) and an active brain (capable of creating elaborate dream fantasies). Regional cerebral blood flow studies have confirmed increased brain activation during REM sleep. It certainly appears that in some parasomnias there are state boundary violations. For example, all of the arousal disorders (confusional arousals, sleepwalking, and sleep terrors) involve momentary or partial wakeful behaviors suddenly occurring in NREM (slow-wave) sleep. Similarly, isolated sleep paralysis is the persistence of REM sleep atonia into the wakefulness transition, whereas REM sleep behavior disorder is the failure of the mechanism creating paralytic atonia such that individuals literally act out their dreams (American Sleep Disorders Association 1997).

Significant parasomnia can occur frequently or rarely. The clinical significance of a parasomnia has more to do with the medical consequences or the distress than with how often it occurs. REM sleep behavior disorder that occurs infrequently but during which the patient is seriously injured while enacting a dream constitutes a more urgent scenario than weekly bruxism. Similarly, monthly recurrent nightmares that provoke severe insomnia and fear of sleeping can be more distressing than night terrors of the same frequency (at least to the patient). The irregularities of occurrence of most parasomnias make them difficult to document in the sleep laboratory. Sleep studies, however, are often conducted to make a differential diagnosis and ensure that the unusual behavior is not secondary to seizure, sleep-disordered breathing, or another sleep disorder.

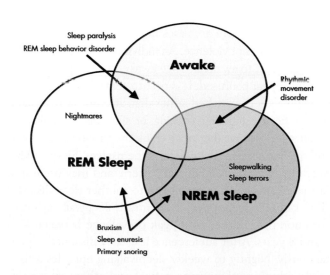

FIGURE 17–7. The relationship of common parasomnias to REM sleep, NREM sleep, and the awake state.

The nosological classification for parasomnias has evolved over the years, and the system used in the multicenter cooperative study differed from today's nosology. Figure 17–6C shows recalculated percentages of occurrence of different parasomnias among patients seen at sleep disorders centers using the cooperative study data (Coleman et al. 1982). According to this study, the most commonly encountered parasomnias are secondary to nocturnal seizure activity (33.7%). After that, the most common conditions currently classified as parasomnias include sleepwalking, sleep terrors, sleep-related enuresis, nightmares, familial sleep paralysis, head banging (rhythmic movement disorder), bruxism, and other parasomnias.

SLEEPWALKING

Sleepwalking in its classic form is, as the name implies, a condition in which an individual arises from bed and ambulates without awakening. Sleepwalking individuals can engage in a variety of complex behaviors while unconscious. Sometimes called somnambulism, sleepwalking usually occurs during slow-wave sleep and lies in the middle of a parasomnia continuum that ranges from confused arousal to sleep terror. Sleepwalks characteristically begin toward the end of the first or second slow-wave sleep episodes. Sleep deprivation and interruption of slow-wave sleep appear to exacerbate, or even provoke, sleepwalking in susceptible individuals. Sleepwalking episodes may range from sitting up and attempting to walk to conducting an involved sequence of semipurposeful actions. The sleepwalker often can successfully interact with the environment (for example, avoiding tripping over objects in his path). However, the sleepwalker will often interact with the environment inappropriately, which sometimes results in injury (for example, stepping out of an upstairs window or walking into the roadway). There are cases in which sleepwalkers have committed acts of violence. An individual who is sleepwalking is difficult to awaken. Once awake, the sleepwalker will usually appear confused. It is best to gently attempt to lead a sleepwalker back to bed rather than attempting to awaken him or her by grabbing, shaking, or shouting. In their confused state, sleepwalkers may think they are being attacked and may react violently to defend themselves. Sleepwalking in adults is rare, has a familial pattern, and may occur as a primary parasomnia or secondary to another sleep disorder (for example, sleep apnea). By contrast, sleepwalking is very common in children, with peak prevalence between ages 4 and 8 years. After adolescence it usually disappears spontaneously. Nightly to weekly sleepwalking episodes associated with physical injury to patient and others are considered severe (American Sleep Disorders Association 1997; Kales et al. 1966, 1980b).

SLEEP TERRORS

A sleep terror (sometimes called pavor nocturnus, incubus, or night terror) is characterized by a sudden arousal with intense fearfulness. It may begin with a piercing scream or cry. Autonomic and behavioral correlates of fright typically mark the experience. An individual experiencing a sleep terror usually sits up in bed, is unresponsive to stimuli, and, if awakened, is confused or disoriented. Vocalizations may occur, but the individual usually is incoherent. Notwithstanding the intensity of these events, amnesia for the episodes usually occurs. Like sleepwalking, these episodes usually arise from slow-wave sleep. Fever and withdrawal from central nervous system depressants can potentiate sleep terror episodes. Unlike nightmares in which an elaborate dream sequence unfolds, sleep terrors may be devoid of images or contain only fragments of very brief but frighteningly vivid, though sometimes static, images. A familial pattern has been reported. Like other slow-wave sleep parasomnias, sleep terrors can be provoked or exacerbated by sleep deprivation. Psychopathology is seldom associated with sleep terrors in children; however, a history of traumatic experiences or frank psychiatric problems is often comorbid in adults with this disorder. Frequency ranges from less than once per month to almost nightly occurrence (with injury to patient or others) (American Sleep Disorders Association 1997; Fisher et al. 1973; Hartmann 1988).

SLEEP ENURESIS

Sleep enuresis is a disorder in which the individual urinates during sleep while in bed. Bedwetting, as it is commonly called, has primary and secondary forms. In children, primary sleep enuresis is the continuance of bedwetting since infancy. Secondary enuresis refers to relapse after toilet training was complete and there was a period where the child remained dry. Usually, after toilet training bedwetting spontaneously resolves before age 6 years. Prevalence progressively declines from 30% at age 4 years to 10% at age 6 to 5% at age 10 and 3% at age 12. If a parent had primary enuresis, it increases the likelihood that the children will be enuretic. A single recessive gene is suspected. Secondary enuresis in children may occur with the birth of a sibling and represent a "cry for attention." Secondary enuresis can also be associated with nocturnal seizures, sleep deprivation, and urological anomalies. In adults, sleep enuresis is occasionally seen in patients with sleep-disordered breathing. In most cases, embarrassment is the most serious consequence. Nonetheless, if sleep enuresis is not addressed, it may leave psychosocial scars. A variety of medications have also been used to treat sleep enuresis, including imipramine, oxybutynin chloride, and synthetic vasopressin. Behavioral treatments, including bladder training, conditioning devices (bell and pad), and fluid restriction, reportedly have good success when properly administered. Other treatments include psychotherapy, motivational strategies, and hypnotherapy. Frequency ranges from nightly to monthly, and severity ranges from mild embarrassment to severe shame and guilt (Nino-Murcia and Keenan 1987; Scharf et al. 1987).

NIGHTMARES

Nightmares are frightening or terrifying dreams. Sometimes called dream anxiety attacks, they produce sympathetic activation and ultimately awaken the dreamer. Nightmares occur in REM sleep and usually evolve from a long, complicated dream that becomes increasingly frightening. When the person is aroused to wakefulness, the dream content is typically remembered (in contrast to sleep terrors). Some nightmares are recurrent, and—reportedly when occurring in association with posttraumatic stress disorder—they may be recollections of actual events. Common in children ages 3–6 years (prevalence estimates range from 10%–50%), nightmares are rare in adults (1% or less). Frequent and distressing nightmares are sometimes responsible for insomnia because the individual is afraid to sleep. In Freudian terms, the nightmare is an example of the failure of dream process that defuses the emotional content of the dream by disguising it symbolically, thus preserving sleep. Most patients who experience nightmares are free from psychiatric conditions. Nonetheless, individuals at risk for nightmares include those with schizotypal personality, borderline personality disorder, schizoid personality disorder, and schizophrenia. Hartmann (1984) posits that nightmares are more common in individuals with "thin boundaries," who are open and trusting and who often have creative or artistic inclinations. Having thin boundaries makes these individuals more vulnerable; furthermore, they may be at risk for schizophrenia. Traumatic events are known to induce nightmares, sometimes immediately but at other times delayed. The nightmares can persist for many years. Several medications, including levodopa and β-adrenergic blockers, and withdrawal from REM-suppressant medications are known to sometimes provoke nightmares. Finally, drug and/or alcohol abuse is associated with nightmares (Ermin 1987; Hartmann 1984, 1998; Kales et al. 1980a).

Frequently occurring nightmares often produce a "fear of sleeping" type of insomnia. In turn, the insomnia may provoke sleep deprivation, which is known to exacerbate nightmares. In this manner, a vicious cycle is created.

Treatment using behavioral techniques can be helpful. Universal sleep hygiene, stimulus control therapy, lucid dream therapy, and cognitive therapy reportedly improve sleep and reduce nightmares. In patients with nightmares related to posttraumatic stress disorder, nefazodone (an atypical antidepressant) and prazocin (an α-adrenergic antagonist) reportedly provides therapeutic benefit. Benzodiazepines may also be helpful; however, systematic controlled trials are lacking (Hirshkowitz and Moore 2000).

SLEEP PARALYSIS

Sleep paralysis is, as the name implies, an inability to make voluntary movements during sleep. It becomes a parasomnia when it occurs at sleep onset or on awakening, a time when the individual is partially conscious and aware of his or her surroundings. This inability to move can be extremely distressing, especially when it is coupled with the feeling that there is an intruder in the house or when hypnagogic hallucinations are occurring. Sleep paralysis is one of the tetrad of symptoms associated with narcolepsy; however, it is known to occur (with or without hypnagogia) in individuals who have neither cataplexy nor excessive daytime sleepiness. Although sometimes frightening, sleep paralysis is a feature of normal REM sleep briefly intruding into wakefulness. The paralysis may last from one to several minutes. It is interesting that the occurrence of sleep paralysis with hypnagogia may account for a variety of experiences where the sleeper is confronted or attacked by some sort of creature. The common description is that a "presence" is felt to be near; the individual is paralyzed; and the creature talks, attacks, or sits on the sleeper's chest and then vanishes. Whether it is called incubus, "Old Hag," vampire, ghost oppression (*kanashibari*), witch riding, or alien encounter, elements common to sleep paralysis are seen. Irregular sleep, sleep deprivation, psychological stress, and shift work are thought to increase the likelihood of sleep paralysis occurring. Occasional sleep paralysis occurs in 7%–8% of young adults. Estimates of at least one lifetime experience of sleep paralysis range from 25% to 50%. Improving sleep hygiene and ensuring sufficient sleep are first-line therapies. Sometimes, if the individual voluntarily makes very rapid eye movements or is touched by another person, the episode will terminate (Broughton 1982; Ness 1978; Wing et al. 1994).

RHYTHMIC MOVEMENT DISORDER

More commonly known as head banging, rhythmic movement disorder is characterized by stereotypic, repetitive movements that most often occur at the transition from wakefulness to sleep. Large muscle groups produced a movement that is rhythmic, most commonly involving the head and neck. The majority of infants will sometimes move rhythmically at sleep onset; however, prevalence drops from 66% to 8% by age 4 years. Estimates indicate a 4-to-1 male-to-female ratio. One theory posits that the infant or child is creating vestibular stimulation, which has a soothing effect and helps promote sleep (like the rocking of a cradle). Other names for rhythmic movement disorder include *jactatio capitis nocturna*, head banging, head rolling, body rocking, and *rhythmie du sommeil*. Onset after adolescence is rare. In most cases, rhythmic movement disorder is benign; however, it is sometimes associated with drug abuse and withdrawal. The movements can cause injury, and this is the manner by which this parasomnia becomes a serious condition. Particularly with head banging, precautions must be taken to avoid injury (using padding and wearing a helmet if necessary). When the condition occurs in an adult, a full neurological evaluation is important to determine if the movements are secondary to seizures or other central nervous system dysfunction (Thorpy 1990).

SLEEP BRUXISM

Sleep bruxism is a parasomnia in which individuals grind or clench their teeth during sleep. Sleep bruxism can produce abnormal wear on the teeth, damage teeth, provoke tooth and jaw pain, and/or make loud, unpleasant sounds that disturb the bed partner. Sometimes atypical facial pain and headache also result. It is estimated that more than 85% of the population will have sleep bruxism at some time during their lives; however, it is clinically significant in only about 5%. Sleep bruxism can occur in any stage of sleep but appears to be most common at transition to sleep, during Stage II, and during REM sleep. Some evidence indicates that teeth grinding during REM sleep is more commonly associated with dental wear or damage. Sleep bruxism does not appear to be exacerbated by dental malocclusion but rather worsens during periods of stress. Researchers studying sleep bruxism find that many patients seem to have less frequent teeth grinding when sleeping in the laboratory; therefore, repeated study may be needed to document the disorder. By contrast, bruxism frequently appears on polysomnographic recordings made for other purposes. Sleep bruxism can occur secondary to sleep-related breathing disorders, use of monoaminergic stimulants (e.g., amphetamine, cocaine), alcohol ingestion, and treatment with SSRIs. Differential diagnosis should rule out nocturnal seizure. Sleep bruxism can occur infrequently (monthly), regularly (weekly), or frequently (nightly).

Severity is judged on the basis of dental injury, consequent pain, and sleep disruption. Usual treatment involves having the patient wear an oral appliance to protect the teeth during sleep. There are two basic types of appliances used. The soft one (mouth guard) is typically used in the short term, whereas the hard acrylic one (bite splint) is used for a longer term and requires regular follow-up. Relaxation, biofeedback, hypnosis, physical therapy, and stress management are also used to treat sleep bruxism. A variety of drug therapies (benzodiazepines, muscle relaxants, dopaminergic agonists, and propranolol) have been tried; however, outcome data are not available (Rugh and Harlan 1988; Ware and Rugh 1988).

REM SLEEP BEHAVIOR DISORDER

REM sleep behavior disorder involves a failure of the atonia mechanism (sleep paralysis) during stage REM sleep. The result is that the patient literally enacts his or her dreams. Under normal circumstances, the dreamer is immobilized by REM-related hypopolarization of alpha and gamma motor neurons. Without this paralysis or with intermittent atonia, punching, kicking, leaping, and running from bed occur during attempted dream enactment. The activity has been correlated with dream imagery, but unlike during sleepwalking, the individual seems unaware of the actual environment. Although complex behaviors can be performed, the individual is acting on the dream sensorium. Thus, a sleepwalker may calmly go to a bedroom window, open it, and step out. By contrast, a person with REM sleep behavior disorder would more likely dive through the window thinking it is a dream-visualized lake. Patients and bed partners frequently sustain injury, sometimes serious (e.g., lacerations, fractures). Animal research ascribes REM sleep atonia to peri–locus coeruleus exerting an excitatory influence on the medulla (reticularis magnocellularis nucleus), which in turn paralyzes spinal motor neurons. Cats with pontine tegmental lesions perform a variety of behaviors during REM sleep. Neurological examinations of patients with REM sleep behavior disorder suggest diffuse lesions of the hemispheres, bilateral thalamic abnormalities, or primary brain stem lesions. Biperiden, tricyclic antidepressants, monoamine oxidase inhibitors, caffeine, venlafaxine, selegiline, and serotonin agonists can precipitate or exacerbate REM behavior disorder. In addition, REM behavior disorder may occur during withdrawal from alcohol, meprobamate, pentazocine, and nitrazepam. A variety of neurological conditions, including Parkinson's disease, dementia, progressive supranuclear palsy, Shy-Drager syndrome, and narcolepsy, have been associated with this parasomnia. Other conditions that may provoke a secondary REM sleep behavior disorder include sleep-disordered breathing, posttraumatic stress disorder, and nocturnal seizures. REM sleep behavior disorder is rare. Severity ranges from a mild form in which nonviolent episodes occur less than once a month to a severe form in which injury-associated episodes occur more than once a week (Schenck et al. 1986, 1989).

Highlights for the Clinician

Phenomenology of sleep

✦ Sleep is not one phenomenon. There are several types of sleep, each with its own characteristics, functions, and regulatory mechanisms.

✦ What the different types of sleep share is that each represents an important brain process. In a broad sense, sleep is a brain process.

Regulation of sleep

✦ Sleep is regulated by the autonomic nervous system, homeostatic processes, and the sleep-wake circadian rhythm.

✦ Misalignment of these factors, or situations in which one or more of these underlying mechanisms go awry, gives rise to sleep disorders.

Sleep disorders

Sleep disorders present as:

✦ Difficulty initiating and/or maintaining sleep (insomnia), **or**

✦ Difficulty maintaining or inability to maintain alertness (hypersomnia or excessive daytime sleepiness), **or**

✦ Strange, unusual, or inappropriate behaviors occurring in and around sleep (parasomnias, or things that go bump in the night [e.g., nightmares, sleepwalking, REM sleep behavior disorder])

Treatment of insomnia

✦ Effective treatment of insomnia involves behavioral, cognitive, and/or pharmacological therapy.

✦ Cognitive-behavioral therapy is a reliable alternative to the use of sleep-promoting substances.

Sleep apnea

✦ Sleep apnea is a common sleep disorder characterized by cessation or significantly restricted breathing during sleep.

✦ Sleep apnea can arise from airway occlusion (obstructive type) or from loss of respiratory drive (central type).

✦ Positive airway pressure therapy is safe and effective and is the treatment most often prescribed. Various other treatment options exist.

Sleep medicine

✦ Sleep medicine has become a recognized clinical subspecialty in recent years and is now an important part of mainstream medicine.

RECOMMENDED READINGS

Avidan A, Zee P: Handbook of Sleep Medicine. Baltimore, MD, Lippincott Williams & Wilkins, 2006
Glovinsky P, Spielman A: The Insomnia Answer. New York, The Penguin Group, 2006

REFERENCES

Aldrich M: The clinical spectrum of narcolepsy and idiopathic hypersomnia. Neurology 46:393–401, 1996
American Academy of Sleep Medicine: The International Classification of Sleep Disorders, 2nd Edition: Diagnostic and Coding Manual. Westchester, IL, American Academy of Sleep Medicine, 2005

American Psychiatric Association: Diagnostic and Statistical Manual of Mental Disorders, 4th Edition, Text Revision. Washington, DC, American Psychiatric Association, 2000

American Sleep Disorders Association: Practice parameters for the use of stimulants in the treatment of narcolepsy. Sleep 17:348–351, 1994

American Sleep Disorders Association: The International Classification of Sleep Disorders, Revised: Diagnostic and Coding Manual. Rochester, MN, American Sleep Disorders Association, 1997

Aschoff J: Circadian rhythms in man. Science 148:1427–1432, 1965

Aserinsky E, Kleitman N: Regularly occurring periods of eye motility, and concomitant phenomena. Science 118:273–274, 1953

Ayas NT, Patel SR, Malhotra A, et al: Auto-titrating versus standard continuous positive airway pressure for the treatment of obstructive sleep apnea: results of a meta-analysis. Sleep 27:249–253, 2004

Benca RM, Obermeyer WH, Thisted RA, et al: Sleep and psychiatric disorders: a meta-analysis. Arch Gen Psychiatry 49:651–668, 1992

Berger H: Ueber das elektroenkephalogramm des menschen. J Psychol Neurol 40:160–179, 1930

Binks GP, Waters FW, Hurry M: Short-term total sleep deprivations does not selectively impair higher cortical functioning. Sleep 22:328–334, 1999

Bonnet MH, Arand DL: Physiological activation in patients with sleep state misperception. Psychosom Med 59:533–540, 1997

Bootzin RR: A stimulus control treatment for insomnia. Proceedings of the American Psychological Association 4:395–396, 1972

Bootzin RR: Effects of self-control procedures for insomnia, in Behavioral Self-Management: Strategies, Techniques, and Outcomes. Edited by Stuart RB. New York, Brunner/Mazel, 1977, pp 176–195

Borbely AA, Achermann P: Concepts and models of sleep regulation: an overview. J Sleep Res 1:63–79, 1992

Breslau N, Roth T, Rosenthal L, et al: Sleep disturbance and psychiatric disorders: a longitudinal epidemiological study of young adults. Biol Psychiatry 39:411–418, 1996

Broughton RJ: Neurology and dreaming. Psychiatr J Univ Ott 7:101–110, 1982

Carskadon M, Dement WC, Mitler M, et al: Sleep report versus sleep laboratory findings in 122 drug free subjects with the complaint of chronic insomnia. Am J Psychiatry 133:1382–1388, 1976

Carskadon MA, Dement WC, Mitler MM, et al: Guidelines for the Multiple Sleep Latency Test (MSLT): a standard measure of sleepiness. Sleep 9:519–524, 1986

Chase MH (ed): The Sleeping Brain. Los Angeles, CA, Brain Information Service/Brain Research Institute, UCLA, 1972

Chockroverty S: Clinical Companion to Sleep Disorders Medicine, 2nd Edition. Boston, MA, Butterworth-Heinemann, 2000

Coleman RM, Roffwarg HP, Kennedy SJ, et al: Sleep-wake disorders based on a polysomnographic diagnosis: a national cooperative study. JAMA 247:997–1003, 1982

Culebras A: Sleep disorders associated with psychiatric, medical, and neurologic disorders, in Clinical Handbook of Sleep Disorders. Boston, MA, Butterworth-Heinemann, 1996, pp 233–281

Czeisler CA, Kronauer RE, Allan JS, et al: Bright light induction of strong (type 0) resetting of the human circadian pacemaker. Science 244:1328–1333, 1989

Dinges D: Proving the limits of functional capability: the effects of sleep loss on short-duration tasks, in Sleep, Arousal, and Performance. Edited by Broughton RJ, Ogilvie RD. Boston, MA, Birkhauser, 1992, pp 177–188

Dinges DF, Kribbs NB: Performing while sleepy: effects of experimentally induced sleepiness, in Sleep, Sleepiness, and Performance. Edited by Monk TM. Chichester, England, Wiley, 1991, pp 97–128

Ekbom KA: Restless legs syndrome: Neurology 10:868–873, 1960

Ermin MK: Dream anxiety attacks (nightmares). Psychiatr Clin North Am 10:667–674, 1987

Espie CA, Lindsay WR, Brooks DN, et al: A controlled comparative investigation of psychological treatments for chronic sleep-onset insomnia. Behav Res Ther 27:79–88, 1989

Fairbanks DNF, Fujita S, Ikematsu T, et al: Snoring and Obstructive Sleep Apnea. New York, Raven, 1987

Ferguson KA, Cartwright R, Rogers R, et al: Oral appliances for snoring and obstructive sleep apnea: a review. Sleep 29:244–262, 2006

Fisher C, Kahn E, Edwards A: A psychophysiological study of nightmares and night terrors, I: psychophysiological aspects of the stage 4 terror. J Nerv Ment Dis 157:75–98, 1973

Ford DE, Kamerow DB: Epidemiologic study of sleep disturbances and psychiatric disorders: an opportunity for prevention? JAMA 262:1479–1484, 1989

Foulkes D: A cognitive-psychological model of REM dream production. Sleep 5:169–187, 1982

Freud S: The interpretation of dreams (1900), in Standard Edition of the Complete Psychological Works of Sigmund Freud, Vols 4 and 5. Translated and edited by Strachey J. London, Hogarth Press, 1953, pp 1–715

Fry JM: Treatment modalities for narcolepsy. Neurology 50 (suppl 1):S43–S48, 1998

Gallup Organization: Sleep in America. Princeton, NJ, Gallup, 1991

Guilleminault C, Pelayo R: Idiopathic central nervous system hypersomnia, in Principles and Practice of Sleep Medicine. Edited by Kryger MH, Roth T, Dement WC. Philadelphia, PA, WB Saunders, 2000, pp 687–692

Hartmann E: The Nightmare: The Psychology and Biology of Terrifying Dreams. Basic Books, New York, 1984

Hartmann E: Two case reports: night terrors with sleep-walking a potentially lethal disorder. J Nerv Ment Dis 171:503–550, 1988

Hartmann E: Dreams and Nightmares. New York, Plenum, 1998

Hartmann E, Baekeland R, Zwilling G: Psychological differences between long and short sleepers. Arch Gen Psychiatry 26:463–468, 1972

Hauri PJ, Fisher J: Persistent psychophysiological (learned) insomnia. Sleep 2:38–53, 1986

Hirshkowitz M: Clinical pharmacology of sleep, in Sleep Disorders Medicine, 3rd Edition. Edited by Chokroverty S. Boston, MA, Butterworth-Heinmenann (in press)

Hirshkowitz M, Moore CA: Nightmares, in Encyclopedia of Stress, Vol 3. Edited by Fink G. San Diego, CA, Academic Press, 2000, pp 49–53

Hirshkowitz M, Moore CA, Hamilton CR, et al: Polysomnography of adults and elderly: sleep architecture, respiration, and leg movements. J Clin Neurophysiol 9:56–63, 1992

Hirshkowitz M, Moore CA, Minhoto G: The basics of sleep, in Understanding Sleep: The Evaluation and Treatment of Sleep Disorders. Edited by Pressman MR, Orr WC. Washington, DC, American Psychological Association, 1997, pp 11–34

Hobson JA, McCarley R: The brain as a dream stage generator: an activation-synthesis hypothesis of the dream process. Am J Psychiatry 134:1335–1348, 1977

Horne J: Why We Sleep. Oxford, England, Oxford University Press, 1988

Horne J: Dimensions to sleepiness, in Sleep, Sleepiness, and Performance. Edited by Monk TM. Chichester, England, Wiley, 1991, pp 169–196

Joseph KC, Dube D, Sitaram N: Sleep electroencephalographic characteristics of anxiety disorders, in Principles and Practice of Sleep Medicine. Edited by Kryger MH, Roth T, Dement WC. Philadelphia, PA, WB Saunders, 1989, pp 424–425

Jouvet M, Michel F, Courjon J: [On a stage of rapid cerebral electrical activity in the course of physiological sleep.] C R Seances Soc Biol Fil 153:1024–1028, 1959

Kales A, Jacobson A, Paulson MJ, et al: Somnambulism: psychophysiological correlates, I: all-night EEG studies. Arch Gen Psychiatry 14:586–594, 1966

Kales A, Soldatos C, Caldwell A, et al: Nightmares: clinical characteristics and personality patterns. Am J Psychiatry 137:1197–1201, 1980a

Kales A, Soldatos CR, Caldwell AB, et al: Sleepwalking. Arch Gen Psychiatry 37:1406–1410, 1980b

Kleitman N: Sleep and Wakefulness, 2nd Edition. Chicago, IL, University of Chicago, 1972

Lacks P, Rotert M: Knowledge and practice of sleep hygiene techniques in insomniacs and good sleepers. Behav Res Ther 24:365–368, 1986

Lichstein KL, Riedel BW: Behavioral assessment and treatment of insomnia: a review with an emphasis on clinical application. Behav Ther 25:659–688, 1994

Lin L, Faraco J, Li R, et al: The sleep disorder canine narcolepsy is caused by a mutation in the hypocretin (orexin) receptor 2 gene. Cell 98:365–376, 1999

Loomis AL, Harvey N, Hobart GA: Cerebral states during sleep, as studied by human brain potentials. J Exp Psychol 21:127–144, 1937

Loube DI, Gay PC, Strohl KP, et al: Indications for positive airway pressure treatment of adult obstructive sleep apnea patients: a consensus statement. Chest 115:863–866, 1999

Lubin A: Performance under sleep loss and fatigue, in Sleep and Altered States of Consciousness. Edited by Kety SS, Evarts EV, Williams HL. Baltimore, MD, Williams & Wilkins, 1967, pp 506–513

Lugaresi E, Cirgnotta F, Coccagna G, et al: Nocturnal myoclonus and restless legs syndrome. Adv Neurol 43:295–306, 1986

Mellinger GD, Balter MB, Uhlenhuth EH: Insomnia and its treatment: prevalence and correlates. Arch Gen Psychiatry 42:225–232, 1985

Mignot E: Narcolepsy: Pharmacology, pathophysiology, and genetics, in Principal and Practice of Sleep Medicine. Edited by Kryger M, Roth T, Dement WC. Philadelphia, PA, WB Saunders, 2005, pp 761–779

Mignot E, Lammers GJ, Ripley B, et al: The role of cerebrospinal fluid hypocretin measurement in the diagnosis of narcolepsy and other hypersomnias. Arch Neurol 59:1553–1562, 2002

Montplaisir J: Periodic limb movement in sleep, in Sleep and Movement Disorders. Edited by Chokroverty S, Hening WA, Walters AS. Philadelphia, PA, Butterworth-Heinemann, 2003, pp 300–311

Montplaisir J: Restless leg syndrome and periodic limb movement during sleep, in Principle and Practice of Sleep Medicine. Edited by Kryger M, Roth T, Dement WC. Philadelphia, PA, WB Saunders, 2005, pp 839–852

Moore-Ede MC, Sulzman FM, Fuller CA: The Clocks That Time Us. Cambridge, MA, Harvard University Press, 1982

Morgan K, Closs SJ: Hypnotic drugs in the treatment of insomnia, in Sleep Management in Nursing Practice. Edinburgh, Scotland, Churchill Livingstone, 1999a, pp 143–159

Morgan K, Closs SJ: Sleep hygiene, in Sleep Management in Nursing Practice. Edinburgh, Scotland, Churchill Livingstone, 1999b, pp 95–104

Morin CM, Culbert JP, Schwartz SM: Nonpharmacological interventions for insomnia: a meta-analysis of treatment efficacy. Am J Psychiatry 151:1172–11780, 1994

National Commission on Sleep Disorders Research: Wake Up America: A National Sleep Alert, Vol 1: Executive Summary and Executive Report, Report of the National Commission on Sleep Disorders Research. National Institutes of Health. Washington, DC, U.S. Government Printing Office, 1993

Ness RC: The old hag phenomenon as sleep paralysis: a biocultural interpretation. Cult Med Psychiatry 2:15–39, 1978

Nino-Murcia G, Keenan SA: Enuresis and sleep, in Sleep and Its Disorders in Children. Edited by Guilleminault C. New York, Raven, 1987, pp 253–267

Punjabi NM, Welch D, Strohl K: Sleep disorders in regional sleep centers: a national cooperative study. Sleep 23:471–480, 2000

Rechtschaffen A, Kales A (eds): A manual of standardized terminology, techniques and scoring system for sleep stages of human subjects (NIH Publ No 204). Washington, DC, U.S. Government Printing Office, 1968

Reynolds CF, Kupfer DJ: Sleep research in affective illness: state of the art circa 1987. Sleep 10:199–215, 1987

Ripley B, Overeem S, Fujiki N, et al: CSF hypocretin/orexin levels in narcolepsy and other neurological conditions. Neurology 57:2253–2258, 2001

Robinson A, Guilleminault C: Obstructive sleep apnea syndrome, in Sleep Disorders Medicine. Edited by Chokroverty S. Boston, MA, Butterworth-Heinemann, 1999, pp 331–354

Roffwarg HP, Muzio JN, Dement WC: Ontogenetic development of the human sleep-dream cycle. Science 152:604–619, 1966

Rugh JD, Harlan J: Nocturnal bruxism and temporomandibular disorders. Adv Neurol 49:329–341, 1988

Sanders MH: Medical therapy for obstructive sleep apnea-hypopnea syndrome, in Principles and Practice of Sleep Medicine. Edited by Kryger MH, Roth T, Dement WC. Philadelphia, PA, WB Saunders, 2000, pp 879–893

Scharf MB, Pravda MF, Jennings SW, et al: Childhood enuresis: a comprehensive treatment program. Psychiatr Clin North Am 10:655–674, 1987

Schenck CH, Bundlie SR, Ettinger MG, et al: Chronic behavioral disorders of human REM sleep: a new category of parasomnia. Sleep 9:293–308, 1986

Schenck CH, Hurwitz TD, Bundlie SR, et al: Sleep-related injury in 100 adult patients: a polysomnographic and clinical report. Am J Psychiatry 146:1166–1173, 1989

Sharafkhaneh A, Richardson P, Hirshkowitz M: Sleep apnea in a high risk population: a study of Veterans Health Administration beneficiaries. Sleep Med 5:345–350, 2004

Sharafkhaneh A, Giray N, Richardson P, et al: Association of psychiatric disorders and sleep apnea in a large cohort. Sleep 28:1405–1411, 2005

Sharafkhaneh A, Sharafkhaneh H, Bredikus A, et al: Effect of atrial overdrive pacing on obstructive sleep apnea in patients with systolic heart failure. Sleep Med 8:31–36, 2006

Shneerson JM: Handbook of Sleep Medicine. Oxford, England, Blackwell Scientific, 2000

Spielman AJ, Caruso LS, Glovinsky PB: A behavioral perspective on insomnia treatment. Psychiatr Clin North Am 10:541–553, 1987a

Spielman AJ, Saskin P, Thorpy MJ: Treatment of chronic insomnia by restriction of time in bed. Sleep 10:45–65, 1987b

Thorpy MJ: Rhythmic movement disorder, in Handbook of Sleep Disorders. Edited by Thorpy MJ. New York, Marcel Dekker, 1990, pp 609–629

Thorpy MJ, Ledereich PS: Medical treatment of obstructive sleep apnea, in Handbook of Sleep Disorders. Edited by Thorpy MJ. New York, Marcel Dekker, 1990, pp 285–309

U.S. Xyrem Multicenter Study Group: Sodium oxybate demonstrates long-term efficacy for the treatment of cataplexy in patients with narcolepsy. Sleep Med 5:119–123, 2004

Vogel GW, Vogel F, McAbee RS, et al: Improvement of depression by REM sleep deprivation. Arch Gen Psychiatry 37:247–253, 1980

Walters AS: Toward a better definition of the restless legs syndrome. The International Restless Legs Syndrome Study Group. Mov Disord 10:634–642, 1995

Walters AS, Hening W, Rubinstein, et al: A clinical and polysomnographic comparison of neuroleptic-induced akathisia and the idiopathic restless legs syndrome. Sleep 14:339–345, 1991

Walters AS, LeBrocq C, Dhar A, et al: Validation of the International Restless Legs Syndrome Study Group rating scale for restless legs syndrome. Sleep Med 4:121–132, 2003

Ware JC, Rugh JD: Destructive bruxism: sleep stage relationship. Sleep 11:172–181, 1988

Williams HL, Lubin A, Goodnow JJ: Impaired performance and acute sleep loss. Psychol Monogr 73 (part 14):1–26, 1959

Williams RL, Karacan I, Hursch CJ: EEG of Human Sleep: Clinical Applications. New York, Wiley, 1974

Wing YK, Lee ST, Chen CN: Sleep paralysis in Chinese: ghost oppression phenomenon in Hong Kong. Sleep 17:609–613, 1994

Zammit GK: Delayed sleep phase syndrome and related conditions, in Understanding Sleep: The Evaluation and Treatment of Sleep Disorders. Edited by Pressman MR, Orr WC. Washington, DC, American Psychological Association, 1997, pp 229–248

Zarcone V: Sleep abnormalities in schizophrenia, in Principles and Practice of Sleep Medicine. Edited by Kryger MH, Roth T, Dement WC. Philadelphia, PA, WB Saunders, 1989, pp 422–423

18

NEUROPSYCHIATRIC ASPECTS OF CEREBROVASCULAR DISORDERS

Robert G. Robinson, M.D.

Sergio E. Starkstein, M.D., Ph.D.

Cerebral vascular disease includes a wide range of disorders, from atherosclerotic narrowing of cerebral blood vessels to transitory or permanent brain infarction to hemorrhagic phenomena caused by weakness of the vascular wall. In this chapter, however, we focus on neuropsychiatric disorders associated with stroke. *Stroke* is defined as a sudden loss of blood supply to the brain leading to permanent tissue damage and with clinical symptoms lasting for more than 24 hours.

Stroke is the most common serious neurological disorder in the world and is the leading cause of long-term disability. Stroke accounts for half of all the acute hospitalizations for neurological disease. According to the American Heart Association, there are 700,000 strokes annually and 5.5 million survivors of stroke in the United States, with 10% of individuals over age 75 years being stroke survivors (Thom et al. 2006).

Although the annual incidence of stroke declined linearly from about 1945 to 1975, several studies have reported increased incidence of stroke in the 1980s and 1990s. For example, Pessah-Rasmussen (2003) reported the age-standardized incidence of stroke in Malmö, Sweden, was 647 per 100,000 person-years for men and 400 for women. The annual incidence increased by 3.1% in men and 2.9% in women between 1989 and 1998. There is general agreement, however, that stroke-related mortality has declined in the past 20–30 years. Pessah-Rasmussen (2003) found no change in mortality rate

among men from 1989 to 1998, but among women mortality dropped from 12.3% in 1989 to 2.0% in 1998 (odds ratio [OR] –0.89, 95% confidence interval [CI] 0.8–0.95). This declining mortality has led to an increased prevalence of stroke survivors. In the United States, estimated survivors were 1.5 million in 1973 and 2.4 million in 1991 (American Heart Association 1997), and currently there are 5.5 million (Thom et al. 2006).

The neuropsychiatric complications of cerebrovascular disease include a wide range of emotional and cognitive disturbances. In this chapter we present the latest research on many of the emotional disorders associated with stroke. The chapter is organized into three sections: the historical development of concepts in neuropsychiatry related to cerebrovascular disease, the classification of types of cerebrovascular disease, and the description and classification of clinical psychiatric disorders associated with cerebrovascular disease.

HISTORICAL PERSPECTIVE

Meyer (1904) warned that new discoveries of cerebral localization in the early 1900s, such as language function, led to an overhasty identification of centers and functions. He identified several disorders such as delirium, dementia, and aphasia that were the direct result of brain injury. In keeping with his view of the biopsychosocial causes of most mental "reactions," however, he saw manic-depressive illness and paranoiac conditions as arising from a combination of head injury (specifically citing left frontal lobe and cortical convexities) along with a family history of psychiatric disorder and premorbid personal psychiatric disorders. Bleuler (1951) noted that after stroke, "melancholic moods lasting for months and sometimes longer appear frequently" (p. 230). Kraepelin (1976) recognized an association between manic-depressive insanity and cerebrovascular disease. He stated that the diagnosis of states of depression may offer difficulties, especially when arteriosclerosis is involved. Cerebrovascular disorder may be an accompanying phenomenon of manic-depressive disease or may itself engender states of depression.

In contrast to mood and delusional disorders seen in patients with or without brain injury, Goldstein (1939) described an emotional disorder thought to be uniquely associated with brain disease. This disorder, which he termed *catastrophic reaction*, is an emotional outburst characterized by various degrees of anger, frustration, depression, tearfulness, refusal, shouting, swearing, and sometimes aggressive behavior. Goldstein ascribed this reaction to the inability of the subject to cope when faced with a serious defect in physical or cognitive functions. In his extensive studies of brain injuries in war, Goldstein (1942) described two symptom clusters: those related directly to physical damage of a circumscribed area of the brain and those—as with the catastrophic reaction—related secondarily to the subject's psychological response to injury. (Catastrophic reaction is also discussed in this chapter under "Neuropsychiatric Syndromes Associated With Cerebrovascular Disease.")

A second emotional abnormality, also thought to be characteristic of brain injury, was the indifference reaction. Babinski (1914) noted that patients with right hemisphere disease often displayed the symptoms of anosognosia, euphoria, and indifference. The indifference reaction, associated with right hemisphere lesions, consisted of symptoms of indifference toward failures, lack of interest in family and friends, enjoyment of foolish jokes, and minimization of physical difficulties (Denny-Brown et al. 1952; Hecaen et al. 1951).

A third emotional disorder that has been historically associated with brain injury such as cerebral infarction is pathological laughter or crying. Ironside (1956) described the clinical manifestations of a particular type of pathological emotional disorder he termed *pseudobulbar affect*. This disorder was associated with bilateral, often multiple, lesions affecting the corticobulbar pathways above the pons. These upper motor neuron lesions produced dysphagia, dysarthria, and paralysis of the voluntary facial muscles as well as emotional displays that were characteristically unrelated to their inner emotional state. Crying, for example, occurred spontaneously or after some seemingly minor provo-

cation. This phenomenon has also been termed *emotional incontinence, emotional lability,* and *pathological emotionalism.* (This disorder is also discussed under "Neuropsychiatric Syndromes Associated With Cerebrovascular Disease.")

The first systematic study to contrast the emotional reactions of patients with right- and left hemisphere brain damage (caused by a variety of etiologies) was done by Gainotti (1972). He reported that catastrophic reactions were more frequent among 80 patients with left hemisphere brain damage, particularly in those with aphasia, than were indifference reactions, which occurred more frequently among 80 patients with right hemisphere brain damage. Indifference reactions were also associated with neglect of the opposite half of the body and space. Gainotti agreed with Goldstein's (1942) explanation of catastrophic reaction as the desperate reaction of the subject confronted with severe physical disability. Indifference reaction, on the other hand, was not as easy to understand. Gainotti suggested that denial of illness and disorganization of the nonverbal type of synthesis may have been responsible for this emotional symptom.

Studies in which the emotional symptoms specifically associated with cerebrovascular disease were examined began to appear in the early 1960s. Fisher (1961) described depression associated with cerebrovascular disease as reactive and understandable because "the brain is the most cherished organ of humanity" (p. 379). Thus, depression was viewed as a natural emotional response to a decrease in self-esteem from a life-threatening injury and the resulting disability and dependence.

Systematic studies, however, led other investigators, impressed by the frequency of association between brain injury and emotional disorders, to hypothesize more direct causal links. In a study of 100 elderly patients with affective disorder, Post (1962) stated that the high frequency of brain ischemia associated with first episodes of depressive disorder suggested that the causes for atherosclerosis and depression may be linked. Folstein et al. (1977) compared 20 stroke patients with 10 orthopedic patients and found that although the functional disability in both groups was comparable, more of the stroke patients were depressed. These authors concluded that "mood disorder was a more specific complication of stroke than simply a response to motor disability" (p. 1018).

CLASSIFICATION OF CEREBROVASCULAR DISEASE

Although there are many ways to classify the wide range of disorders that constitute cerebrovascular disease from the perspective of its neuropsychiatric complications, probably the most pragmatic way of classifying this disease is to examine the means by which parenchymal changes in the brain occur. The first of these, ischemia, may occur either with or without infarction of parenchyma and includes transient ischemic attacks (TIAs), atherosclerotic thrombosis, cerebral embolism, and hemorrhage. The last of these, hemorrhage, may cause either direct parenchymal damage by extravasation of blood into the surrounding brain tissue, as in intracerebral hemorrhage (ICH), or indirect damage by hemorrhage into the ventricles, subarachnoid space, extradural area, or subdural area. These changes result in a common mode of expression, defined by Adams and Victor (1985) as a sudden, convulsive, focal neurological deficit, or stroke.

To expand slightly on this categorization (i.e., the means by which parenchymal changes occur), there are four major categories of cerebrovascular disease. These include 1) atherosclerotic thrombosis, 2) cerebral embolism, 3) lacunae, and 4) intracranial hemorrhage. In various studies of the incidence of cerebrovascular disease (e.g., Wolf et al. 1977), the ratio of infarcts to hemorrhages has been shown to be about 5:1. Atherosclerotic thrombosis and cerebral embolism each accounts for approximately one-third of all incidents of stroke.

ATHEROSCLEROTIC THROMBOSIS

Atherosclerotic thrombosis is often the result of a dynamic interaction between hypertension and the atherosclerotic deposition of hyaline-lipid material in the walls of peripheral, coronary, and cerebral arteries. Risk factors in the development of atherosclerosis include hyperlipidemia, diabetes mellitus, hypertension, and cigarette smoking. Atheromatous plaques tend to propagate at the branchings and curves of the internal carotid artery or the carotid sinus, in the cervical part of the vertebral arteries and their junction to form the basilar artery, in the posterior cerebral arteries as they wind around the midbrain, and in the anterior cerebral arteries as they curve over the corpus callosum. These plaques may lead to stenosis of one or more of these cerebral arteries or to complete occlusion. TIAs, defined as periods of transient focal ischemia associated with reversible neurological deficits, almost always indicate that a thrombotic process is occurring. Only rarely is embolism or ICH preceded by transient neurological deficits. Thrombosis of virtually any cerebral or cerebellar artery can be associated with TIAs.

TIAs, therefore, although not listed among the main causes of stroke, may precede, accompany, or follow the development of stroke or may occur by themselves without leading to complete occlusion of a cerebral or cere-

bellar artery. Most commonly, TIAs have a duration of from 2 to 15 minutes, with a range from a few seconds to 24 hours. Whereas the neurological examination between successive episodes of this thrombotic process is entirely normal, the permanent neurological deficits of atherosclerotic thrombosis indicate that infarction has occurred. The progression of events leading to the completed thrombotic stroke, however, can be quite variable.

CEREBRAL EMBOLISM

Cerebral embolism, which like atherosclerotic thrombosis accounts for approximately one-third of all strokes, is usually caused by a fragment breaking away from a thrombus within the heart and traveling up the carotid artery. Less often, the source of the embolism may be from an atheromatous plaque within the lumen of the carotid sinus or from the distal end of a thrombus within the internal carotid artery, or it may represent a fat, tumor, or air embolus within the internal carotid artery. The possible causes of thrombus formation within the heart include cardiac arrhythmias, congenital heart disease, infectious processes (e.g., syphilitic heart disease, rheumatic valvular disease, or endocarditis), valve prostheses, postsurgical complications, or myocardial infarction with mural thrombus.

Of all the types of stroke, those due to cerebral embolism develop most rapidly. In general, there are no warning episodes; embolism can occur at any time. A large embolus may occlude the internal carotid artery or the stem of the middle cerebral artery, producing a severe hemiplegia. More often, however, the embolus is smaller and passes into one of the branches of the middle cerebral artery. This may produce infarction distal to the site of the arterial occlusion, which is characterized by a pattern of neurological deficits consistent with that of vascular distribution, or may result in a transient neurological deficit that resolves as the embolus fragments and travels into smaller, more distal arteries.

LACUNAE

Lacunae, which account for nearly one-fifth of strokes, are the result of occlusion of small penetrating cerebral arteries. They are infarcts that may be so small as to produce no recognizable deficits or, depending on their location, may be associated with pure motor or sensory deficits. Lacunae are strongly associated with both atherosclerosis and hypertension, suggesting that lacunar infarction is the result of the extension of the atherosclerotic process into small-diameter vessels.

INTRACEREBRAL HEMORRHAGE

ICH is the fourth most frequent cause of stroke. The main causes of ICH that present as acute stroke include hypertension, rupture of saccular aneurysms or arteriovenous malformations (AVMs), a variety of hemorrhagic disorders of assorted etiologies, and trauma. Primary (hypertensive) ICH occurs within the brain tissue when the extravasation of blood forms a roughly circular or oval-shaped mass that disrupts and displaces the parenchyma. Adjacent tissue is compressed, and seepage into the ventricular system usually occurs, producing bloody spinal fluid in more than 90% of patients.

ICHs can range in size from massive bleeds of several centimeters in diameter to petechial hemorrhages of a millimeter or less, most commonly occurring within the putamen, in the adjacent internal capsule, or in various portions of the white matter underlying the cortex. Hemorrhages of the thalamus, cerebellar hemispheres, or pons are also common. Severe headache is generally considered to be a constant accompaniment of ICH, but this occurs in only about 50% of cases. The prognosis for ICH is grave: 70%–75% of patients die within 30 days (Adams and Victor 1985).

ANEURYSMS AND ARTERIOVENOUS MALFORMATIONS

Ruptured aneurysms and AVMs are the next most common type of cerebrovascular disease after thrombosis, embolism, lacunae, and ICH. Aneurysms are usually located at arterial bifurcations and are presumed to result from developmental defects in the formation of the arterial wall. Rupture occurs when the intima bulges outward and eventually breaks through the adventitia. AVMs consist of a tangle of dilated vessels that form an abnormal communication between the arterial and venous systems. They are developmental abnormalities consisting of embryonic patterns of blood vessels. Most AVMs are clinically silent but ultimately bleed. Hemorrhage from aneurysms or AVMs may occur within the subarachnoid space, leading to an identifiable presentation as a bleeding vessel anomaly, or may occur within the parenchyma, leading to hemiplegia or death.

SUBDURAL AND EPIDURAL HEMATOMAS

Although it could be contended that subdural hematomas (SDHs) and epidural hematomas do not represent forms of cerebrovascular disease, their behavior as vascular space–occupying lesions that produce many of the signs and symptoms of stroke nonetheless warrants a brief description here.

Chronic SDHs are frequently (60%), but not exclusively, caused by head trauma, followed by a gradual progression of signs and symptoms during the subsequent days to weeks. Traumatic chronic SDH may be caused by tears of bridging veins in the subdural space. Nontraumatic causes include ruptured aneurysms or AVMs of the pial surface or rapid deceleration injuries. The most common symptom of chronic SDH is headache that has a variety of neuropsychiatric manifestations paralleling the gradual increase in intracranial pressure. These manifestations include confusion, inattention, apathy, memory loss, drowsiness, and coma. Chronic SDH is also one of the many conditions in the differential diagnosis of treatable causes of dementia. Fluctuations in the level of consciousness predominate over any focal or lateralizing signs, which may include hemiparesis, hemianopsia, cranial nerve abnormalities, aphasia, or seizures. If left unchecked, chronic SDH may continue to expand or may reabsorb spontaneously.

OTHER TYPES OF CEREBROVASCULAR DISEASE

Another cause of cerebrovascular disease is fibromuscular dysplasia, which leads to narrowed arterial segments caused by degeneration of elastic tissue, disruption and loss of the arterial muscular coat, and an increase in fibrous tissue. Inflammatory diseases of the arterial system can also lead to stroke. These diseases include meningovascular syphilis, pyogenic or tuberculous meningitis, temporal arteritis, and systemic lupus erythematosus.

It appears obvious that examining the many causes and types of cerebrovascular disease in relation to specific neuropsychiatric disorders is a formidable task. In studies comparing traumatic brain injury with thromboembolic stroke, or hemorrhagic with ischemic infarcts, it has been found that the associated moods share many characteristics, depending on the size and location of the lesion and the time that has elapsed since the injury (Robinson and Szetela 1981). As indicated previously, however, the type or pattern of neuronal damage may be different, depending on the cause of the cerebrovascular disease, and resultant neuropsychiatric disorders must be systematically examined.

NEUROPSYCHIATRIC SYNDROMES ASSOCIATED WITH CEREBROVASCULAR DISEASE

A number of emotional disorders, many of which are discussed in this section, have been associated with cerebrovascular disease (Table 18–1). The neuropsychiatric disorder that has received the greatest amount of investigation, however, is poststroke depression (PSD).

TABLE 18–1. Clinical syndromes associated with cerebrovascular disease

Syndrome	Prevalence	Clinical symptoms	Associated lesion location
Major depression	20%	Depressed mood, diurnal mood variation, loss of energy, anxiety, restlessness, worry, weight loss, decreased appetite, early morning awakening, delayed sleep onset, social withdrawal, and irritability	Left front lobe and left basal ganglia during the acute period after stroke
Minor depression	19%	Depressed mood, anxiety, restlessness, worry, diurnal mood variation, hopelessness, loss of energy, delayed sleep onset, early morning awakening, social withdrawal, weight loss, and decreased appetite	Left posterior parietal and occipital regions during the acute poststroke period
Mania	Unknown, rare	Elevated mood, increased energy, increased appetite, decreased sleep, feeling of well-being, pressured speech, flight of ideas, and grandiose thoughts	Right basotemporal or right orbitofrontal lesions
Bipolar mood disorder	Unknown, rare	Symptoms of major depression alternating with mania	Right basal ganglia or right thalamic lesions
Anxiety disorder	27%	Symptoms of major depression plus intense worry and anxious foreboding in addition to depression, associated light-headedness or palpitations and muscle tension or restlessness, and difficulty concentrating or falling asleep	Left cortical lesions, usually dorsolateral frontal lobe
Psychotic disorder	Unknown, rare	Hallucinations or delusions	Right temporoparietal-occipital junction
Apathy			
Without depression	11%	Loss of drive, motivation, interest, low energy, and unconcern	Posterior internal capsule
With depression	11%		
Pathological laughing and crying	20%	Frequent, usually brief, laughing and/or crying; crying not caused by sadness or out of proportion to it; and social withdrawal secondary to emotional outbursts	Frequently, bilateral hemispheric lesions; can occur with almost any lesion location
Anosognosia	24%	Denial of impairment related to motor function, sensory perception, visual perception, or other modality with an apparent lack of concern	Right hemisphere and enlarged ventricles
Catastrophic reaction	19%	Anxiety reaction, tears, aggressive behavior, swearing, displacement, refusal, renouncement, and compensatory boasting	Left anterior-subcortical
Aprosodias			
Motor	Unknown	Poor expression of emotional prosody and gesturing, good prosodic comprehension and gesturing, and denial of feelings of depression	Right hemisphere: posterior inferior frontal lobe and basal ganglia
Sensory	32%	Good expression of emotional prosody and gesturing, poor prosodic comprehension and gesturing, and difficulty empathizing with others	Right hemisphere: posterior inferior parietal lobe and posterior superior temporal lobe

POSTSTROKE DEPRESSION

Diagnosis

Although strict diagnostic criteria have not been used in some studies of emotional disorders associated with cerebrovascular disease (Andersen et al. 1993), most studies have used structured interviews and diagnostic criteria defined by DSM-IV-TR (American Psychiatric Association 2000) or Research Diagnostic Criteria (Aben et al. 2002; Cassidy et al. 2004; Morris et al. 1990). Poststroke major depression is now categorized in DSM-IV-TR (American Psychiatric Association 2000) as "mood disorder due to stroke with major depressive-like episode" (pp 404–405). For patients with less severe forms of depression, there are "research criteria" in DSM-IV for minor depression (i.e., subsyndromal major depression; depression or anhedonia with at least one but fewer than four additional symptoms of major depression) or, alternatively, a diagnosis of mood disorder due to stroke with depressive features (i.e., depressed mood but criteria for major depression not met).

Investigators of depression associated with physical illness have debated the most appropriate method for diagnosis of depression when some symptoms (e.g., sleep or appetite disturbance) could result from the physical illness. Cohen-Cole and Stoudemire (1987) reported that four approaches have been used to assess depression in the physically ill. These approaches are the "inclusive approach," in which depressive diagnostic symptoms are counted regardless of whether they may be related to physical illness (Rifkin et al. 1985); the "etiological approach," in which a symptom is counted only if the diagnostician feels that it is not caused by the physical illness (Rapp and Vrana 1989); the "substitutive approach" of Endicott (1984), in which other psychological symptoms of depression replace the vegetative symptoms; and the "exclusive approach," in which symptoms are removed from the diagnostic criteria if they are not found to be more frequent in depressed than nondepressed patients (Bukberg et al. 1984).

Paradiso et al. (1997) and Spalletta et al. (2005) have examined the specificity of these symptoms in the diagnosis of PSD during the first 2 years following stroke. In the Paradiso study, 142 patients were followed up for examination at 3, 6, 12, or 24 months following stroke. Of these 142 patients, 60 (42%) reported the presence of a depressed mood (depressed group) while they were in the hospital, and the remaining 82 patients (58%) were nondepressed. There were no significant differences in the background characteristics between the depressed and nondepressed groups except that the depressed group was significantly younger ($P=0.006$) and had a significantly higher frequency of personal history of psychiatric disorder ($P=0.04$).

The frequency of vegetative symptoms in the hospital and at each of the follow-up visits is shown in Figure 18–1. Throughout the 2-year follow-up, depressed patients showed a higher frequency of both vegetative and psychological symptoms compared with the nondepressed patients. The only symptoms that were not more frequent in the depressed than in the nondepressed patients were weight loss and early awakening at the initial evaluation; weight loss and early morning awakening at 6 months; weight loss, early morning awakening, anxious foreboding, and loss of libido at 1 year; and weight loss and loss of libido at 2 years. Among the psychological symptoms, the depressed patients had a higher frequency of most psychological symptoms throughout the 2-year follow-up. The only psychological symptoms that were not significantly more frequent in the depressed than in the nondepressed group were suicide plans, simple ideas of reference, and pathological guilt at 3 months; pathological guilt at 6 months; pathological guilt, suicide plans, guilty ideas of reference, and irritability at 1 year; and pathological guilt and self-depreciation at 2 years.

Spalletta et al. (2005) examined 200 first-ever stroke patients within 3 months of stroke. All symptoms of major depression were significantly different in their frequencies among major, minor, and nondepressed patients except feelings of guilt. The effect of using each of the proposed alternative diagnostic methods for PSD using DSM-IV criteria was examined by Paradiso et al. (1997). The symptoms were obtained using the inclusive approach (i.e., symptoms that the patients acknowledged were included as positive even if there was some suspicion that the symptom may have been related to the physical illness). Thus, the initial diagnoses were based on the inclusive criteria. During the in-hospital evaluation, 26 patients (18%) met DSM-IV diagnostic criteria for major depression. Modified DSM-IV diagnostic criteria required five or more specific symptoms (i.e., we excluded weight loss and early morning awakening from DSM-IV diagnostic criteria because they were not significantly more frequent in the depressed than in the nondepressed patients). Of 26 patients with major depression, 3 were excluded. Compared with diagnoses based solely on the existence of five or more specific symptoms for the diagnosis of DSM-IV major depression, diagnoses based on unmodified symptoms (i.e., early awakening and weight loss included) had a specificity of 98% and a sensitivity of 100%.

Modified DSM-IV criteria are then used to examine the substitutive approach (i.e., all vegetative symptoms were eliminated and the presence of four psychological symptoms plus depressed mood was required for the diagnosis of major depression). Using this approach, none

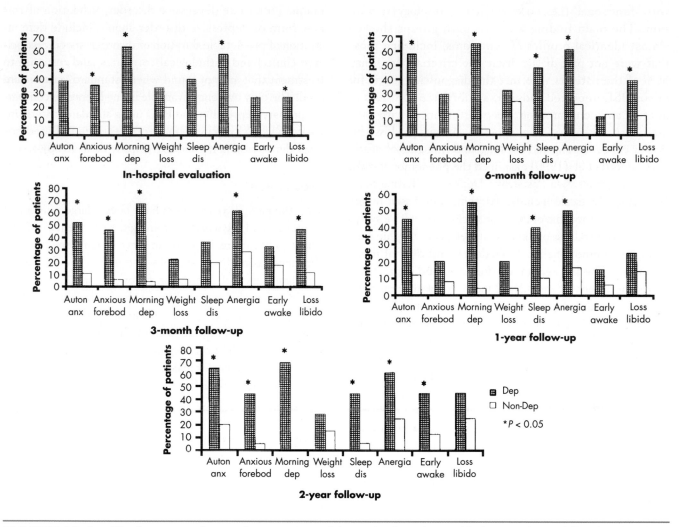

FIGURE 18–1. The frequency of vegetative symptoms of depression in patients with depressed mood (Dep) and without depressed mood (Non-Dep) following stroke. Symptom frequency is shown over the 2-year follow-up. Morning depression (i.e., diurnal mood variation) and anergia were associated with depression through the entire 2-year period. Loss of libido was only seen early in the follow-up, whereas early morning awakening was only seen late in the follow-up. These findings suggest changes over time in both the effects of chronic medical illness and the phenomenology of depression following stroke. Auton anx=autonomic anxiety; Anxious forebod=anxious foreboding; Morning dep=morning depression; Sleep dis=sleep disturbance; Early awake=early morning awakening; Loss libido=loss of libido.

Source. Reprinted from Robinson RG: *The Clinical Neuropsychiatry of Stroke, 2nd Edition.* Cambridge, UK, Cambridge University Press, 2006, p. 70 (data taken from Paradiso et al. 1997). Used with permission.

of the original 26 patients with major depression was excluded. There were, in addition, four patients who presented with four or more specific symptoms of major depression but denied the presence of a depressed mood. These cases may represent "masked" depression.

Similar results were found at 3, 6, 12, and 24 months' follow-up. The sensitivity of unmodified DSM-IV criteria was consistently 100% with a specificity that ranged from 95% to 98% compared with criteria using only specific symptoms. Thus, one could reasonably conclude that modifying DSM-IV criteria because of the existence of an acute stroke is unnecessary.

These findings also suggest that the nature of PSD may be changing over time. Since the symptoms that were specific to depression changed over time, this may reflect an alteration in the underling etiology of PSD associated with early-onset depression compared with the late or chronic poststroke period (see Figure 18–1).

Phenomenology

Lipsey et al. (1986) examined the frequency of depressive symptoms in a group of 43 patients with major PSD compared with that in a group of 43 age-matched patients with "functional" (i.e., no known brain pathology) depression. The main finding was that both groups showed almost identical profiles of symptoms, including those that were not part of the diagnostic criteria. More than 50% of the patients who met the diagnostic criteria for major PSD reported sadness, anxiety, tension, loss of interest and concentration, sleep disturbances with early morning awakening, loss of appetite with weight loss, difficulty concentrating and thinking, and thoughts of death.

Gainotti et al. (1999) examined the phenomenology of PSD using their own Poststroke Depression Rating Scale (PSDRS). The scale includes 10 items: depressed mood, guilt feelings, thoughts of death or suicide, vegetative symptoms, apathy and loss of interest, anxiety, catastrophic reactions, hyperemotionalism, anhedonia, and diurnal mood variations. The last section on diurnal mood variations is scored between +2 and −2, +2 indicating a motivated depression associated with situational stresses, handicaps, or disabilities, and −2 indicating a lack of associated motivation, with depression being more prominent in the early morning. This scale was used to compare patients with poststroke major depression less than 2 months ($n = 58$), 2–4 months ($n = 52$), and greater than 4 months ($n = 43$) after stroke with 30 patients admitted to the psychiatric hospital with a diagnosis of endogenous major depression. Although statistical adjustment controlling for the large number of comparisons was not provided, the data were interpreted to indicate that poststroke patients with endogenous depression had higher scores on suicide and anhedonia, while those with PSD only had higher scores on catastrophic reactions, hyperemotionalism, and diurnal mood variation, which indicates an association with disability.

These authors asserted that failure to assess these aspects of depression (included in the PSDRS) indicates methodological errors in the assessment of depression by Robinson's group (Gianotti et al. 1999). There are, however, clearly established criteria for the diagnosis of major depression as validated through numerous studies supporting DSM-IV-TR (American Psychiatric Association 2000). Catastrophic reactions, hyperemotionalism, and diurnal variations are idiosyncratic criteria for the diagnosis of depression, arbitrarily added to the diagnostic criteria to show differences with primary depression. As is shown later in this chapter, catastrophic reaction and hyperemotionalism are commonly seen in patients with stroke and are often associated with depression. Both catastrophic reactions and hyperemotionalism, however, occur in patients without depression, indicating that these conditions are comorbid in nature and are not symptoms that are integral to the diagnosis of depression. The addition of symptoms to the widely accepted criteria for depression must be validated as defining a specific population of patients with a unique poststroke depressive disorder. Validation of this new form of depressive disorder should include demonstration of predictable duration of disorder, specific associated clinical and pathological correlates, and response to treatment that are not found when "standard" criteria are used. The only evidence available in the literature comparing primary depression and PSD using standard criteria indicates a very close correspondence between PSD and primary depression in the elderly (Lipsey et al. 1986).

Prevalence

Over the past 10 years, there have been a large number of studies around the world examining the prevalence of PSD. These publications indicate an increasing interest among clinicians caring for poststroke patients in the frequency and significance of depression following stroke. The findings of many of these studies are shown in Table 18–2. In general, these studies have found similar rates of major and minor depression among patients hospitalized for acute stroke, in rehabilitation hospitals, and in outpatient clinics. The mean frequency of major depression among patients in acute and rehabilitation hospitals was 22% for major depression and 20% for minor depression. Among patients studied in community settings, however, the mean prevalence of major depression was 14% and minor depression was 9%. Thus, PSD is common both among patients who are receiving treatment for stroke and among community samples. The higher rates of depression among patients who were receiving treatment for stroke are probably related to the greater severity of stroke seen in treatment settings compared with community settings, in which many patients have no physical or intellectual impairment.

Duration

A series of 142 acute stroke patients was prospectively studied in a 2-year longitudinal study of PSD (Robinson 2006). At the time of the initial in-hospital evaluation, 19% of the patients had the DSM-IV-TR symptom cluster of major depression, whereas 25% had the symptom cluster of minor depression. Of those with major depression, 47% still had major depression at the 6-month follow-up evaluation, whereas only 11% of the original group still had major depression at 1-year follow-up, and none were still depressed at 2 years (Figure 18–2). In contrast, however, patients with minor depression had a less favorable prognosis; more than 50% of the patients with in-hospital minor depression continued to have major or minor depression throughout the 2-year follow-up. In addition, about 30% of patients who were not depressed in the hospital became depressed after discharge. Thus, the natural course of major depression appeared to be

TABLE 18–2. Prevalence studies of poststroke depression

Study	Patient population	N	Criteria	% Major	% Minor	Total%
Finset et al. 1989	Rehab hospital	42	Cutoff score			36
Morris et al. 1990	Rehab hospital	99	CIDI, DSM-III	14	21	35
Schubert et al. 1992	Rehab hospital	18	DSM-III-R	28	44	72
Gainotti et al. 1999	Rehab hospital	153	DSM-III-R	31	NR	31+
Schwartz et al. 1993	Rehab hospital	91	DSM-III	40		40[a]
Cassidy et al. 2004	Rehab hospital	91	DSM-IV	20	NR	20
Spalletta et al. 2005	Rehab hospital	200	SCID, DSM IV	25	31	56
Feibel et al. 1982	Outpatient (6 months)	91	Nursing evaluation			26
Robinson and Price 1982	Outpatient (6 months–10 years)	103	Cutoff score			29
Collin et al. 1987	Outpatient	111	Cutoff score			42
Astrom et al. 1993a, 1993b	Outpatient					
	(3 months)	73	DSM-III	31	NR	31[a]
	(1 year)	73	DSM-III	16	NR	16[a]
	(2 years)	57	DSM-III	19	NR	19[a]
	(3 years)	49	DSM-III	29	NR	29[a]
Castillo et al. 1995	Outpatient					33
	(3 months)	77	PSE, DSM-III	20	13	
	(6 months)	80	PSE, DSM-III	21	21	42
	(1 year)	70	PSE, DSM-III	11	16	27
	(2 years)	67	PSE, DSM-III	18	17	35
Pohjasvaara 1998	Outpatient	277	DSM-III-R	26	14	40
Dennis et al. 2000	Outpatient (6 months)	309	Cutoff score			38
Herrmann et al. 1998	Outpatient					
	(3 months)	150	Cutoff score			27
	(1 year)	136				22
Kotila et al. 1998	Outpatient					
	(3 months)	321	Cutoff score			47
	(1 year)	311				48
Wade et al. 1987	Community	379	Cutoff score			30
House et al. 1991	Community	89	PSE, DSM-III	11	12	23
Burvill et al. 1995	Community	294	PSE, DSM-III	15	8	23
Ebrahim et al. 1987	Acute hospital	149	Cutoff score			23
Fedoroff et al. 1991	Acute hospital	205	PSE, DSM-III	22	19	41
Castillo et al. 1995	Acute hospital	291	PSE, DSM-III	20	18	38
Starkstein et al. 1992	Acute hospital	80	PSE, DSM-III	16	13	29
Astrom et al. 1993a, 1993b	Acute hospital	80	DSM-III	25	NR	25[a]
Herrmann et al. 1993	Acute hospital	21	RDC	24	14	38
Andersen et al. 1994a	Acute hospital or outpatient	285	Ham-D cutoff	10	11	21
Aben et al. 2002	Acute hospital	190	SCID, DSM-IV	23	16	39
			Mean	20	21	34[a]

Note. CIDI = Composite International Diagnostic Interview; DSM-III = *Diagnostic and Statistical Manual of Mental Disorders, 3rd Edition;* DSM-III-R = *Diagnostic and Statistical Manual of Mental Disorders, 3rd Edition, Revised;* DSM-IV = *Diagnostic and Statistical Manual of Mental Disorders, 4th Edition;* Ham-D = Hamilton Rating Scale for Depression; NR = not reported; PSE = Present State Examination; RDC = Research Diagnostic Criteria; SADS = Schedule for Affective Disorders and Schizophrenia; SCID = Structured Clinical Interview for DSM-IV.
[a]Because depression was not included, these values may be low.

Source. Reprinted from Robinson RG: *The Clinical Neuropsychiatry of Stroke, 2nd Edition.* Cambridge, UK, Cambridge University Press, 2006. Used with permission.

between 6 months and 1 year, whereas the duration of minor depression was more variable, and in many cases the patients appeared to be chronically depressed.

Morris et al. (1990) found that among a group of 99 patients in a stroke rehabilitation hospital in Australia, those with major depression had a duration of major depression of 40 weeks, whereas those with adjustment disorders (minor depression) had a duration of depression of only 12 weeks. These findings confirm that major depression has a duration of approximately 9 months to 1 year but suggest that less severe depressive disorders may be more variable in their duration. Astrom et al. (1993a) found that, among 80 patients with acute stroke, 27 (34%) developed major depression in the hospital or at 3-month follow-up. Of these patients with major depression, 15 (60%) had recovered by 1-year follow-up, but by 3-year follow-up, only 1 more patient had recovered. This finding indicates that there may be a minority of patients with either major or minor depression who develop prolonged PSD.

The percentage of patients with major depression who had recovered by 1-year follow-up is shown in Figure 18–2. Although all studies found that the majority of depressions were less than 1 year in duration, the mean frequency of major depression that was persistent beyond 1 year was 26%.

The available data suggest that PSD is not transient but is usually a long-standing disorder with a natural course of approximately 9–10 months for most major cases of depression. Depression lasting more than 2 years, however, does occur in some patients with major or minor depression. Lesion location and severity of associated impairments may influence the longitudinal evolution of PSD.

Two factors have been identified that can influence the natural course of PSD. One factor is treatment of depression with antidepressant medications (discussed below). The second factor is lesion location. Starkstein et al. (1988c) compared two groups of depressed patients: one group ($n=6$) had spontaneously recovered from depression by 6 months after stroke, whereas the other group ($n=10$) remained depressed at this point. There were no significant between-group differences in important demographic variables, such as age, sex, and education, and both groups had similar levels of social functioning and degrees of cognitive dysfunction. There were, however, two significant between-group differences. One was lesion location: the recovered group had a higher frequency of subcortical and cerebellar–brain stem lesions; the nonrecovered group had a higher frequency of cortical lesions ($P<0.01$). Impairments in activities of daily living (ADL) were also significantly different between the two groups: the nonrecovered group had significantly more severe impairments in ADL in hospital than did the recovered group ($P<0.01$).

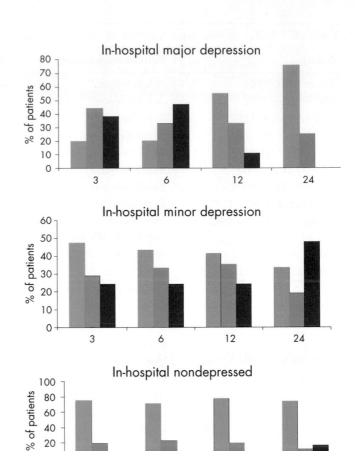

FIGURE 18–2. Diagnostic outcome at 3, 6, 12, and 24 months follow-up for 142 patients based on their in-hospital diagnoses of DSM-IV major depression ($n=27$), DSM-IV minor depression ($n=36$), or no mood disorder ($n=79$). Among the patients with in-hospital major depression (*top panel*), note the increase in the nondepressed group at 12 and 24 months. This is not seen in the minor depression patients (*middle panel*). About 25% of the initially nondepressed patients were found to have a depression diagnosis at follow-up.

Source. Reprinted from Robinson RG: *The Clinical Neuropsychiatry of Stroke*, 2nd Edition. Cambridge, UK, Cambridge University Press, 2006. Used with permission.

The available data suggest that PSD is not transient but is usually a long-standing disorder with a natural course of approximately 9–10 months for most major cases of depression. Depression lasting more than 2 years, however, does occur in some patients with major or minor depression. Lesion location and severity of associated impairments may influence the longitudinal evolution of PSD.

Relationship to Lesion Variables

Relationship between depressive disorder and lesion location has been perhaps the most controversial area of research in the field of poststroke mood disorder. Although establishing an association between specific clinical symptoms and lesion location is one of the fundamental goals of clinical practice in neurology, this has rarely been the case with psychiatric disorders. Cognitive impairment, speech impairment, and the extent and severity of motor or sensory impairment are all symptoms of stroke that are commonly used by clinicians to localize lesions to particular brain regions. There is, however, no known neuropathology consistently associated with primary mood disorders (i.e., mood disorders without known brain injury) or secondary mood disorders (i.e., mood disorders associated with a physical illness). The idea that there may be a neuropathology associated with a development of major depression has led to both surprise and skepticism.

The first study to report a significant correlation of clinical to pathological variables in PSD was an investigation by Robinson and Szetela (1981) of 29 patients with left hemisphere brain injury secondary to stroke ($n = 18$) or to traumatic brain injury ($n = 11$). Based on localization of the lesion by computed tomography (CT), there was a significant inverse correlation between the severity of depression and the distance of the anterior border of the lesion from the frontal pole ($r = 0.76$). This surprising finding led to a number of subsequent examinations of this phenomenon in other populations. Robinson et al. (1984) found a significant correlation in 10 patients with left frontal acute stroke who were right-handed and had no known risk factors for depression ($r = 0.92$; $P < 0.05$). A meta-analysis by Narushima et al. (2003) found eight independent studies of severity of depression and proximity of the stroke lesion to the right or left frontal pole done within the first 6 months following stroke. In total, 163 patients had an overall correlation coefficient of –0.53 using fixed and –0.59 using random model assumptions ($P < 0.001$). In the right hemisphere, however, a total of 106 patients had nonsignificant correlations between severity of depression and distance of the lesions from the right frontal pole ($r = -0.20$, fixed model; $r = -0.23$, random model) (Narushima et al. 2003).

In addition, however, lesion location also influences the frequency of depression. In a study of 45 patients who were on average 2–3 weeks poststroke with single lesions restricted to either cortical or subcortical structures in the left or right hemisphere, Starkstein et al. (1987b) found that 44% of patients with left cortical lesions were depressed, whereas 39% of patients with left subcortical lesions, 11% of patients with right cortical lesions, and 14%

of patients with right subcortical lesions were depressed. When patients were further divided into those with anterior and those with posterior lesions, 5 of 5 patients with left cortical lesions involving the frontal lobe had depression compared with 2 of 11 patients with left cortical posterior lesions. Moreover, 4 of the 6 patients with left subcortical anterior lesions had depression compared with 1 of 7 patients with left subcortical posterior lesions.

In a subsequent study, Starkstein et al. (1988a) examined the relationship between lesions of specific subcortical nuclei and depression. Basal ganglia (caudate and/or putamen) lesions produced major PSD in 7 of 8 patients with left-sided lesions, as compared with only 1 of 7 patients with right-sided lesions and 0 of 10 with thalamic lesions ($P < 0.001$).

Although Astrom et al. (1993a) also found that among patients with acute stroke, 12 of 14 with left anterior lesions had major depression, compared with only 2 of 7 patients with left posterior lesions ($P = 0.017$) and 2 of 23 with right hemisphere lesions ($P < 0.001$), numerous studies have failed to replicate these findings (Gainotti et al. 1999). A meta-analysis by Carson et al. (2000) concluded that there was "no support for the hypothesis that the risk of depression after stroke is affected by the location of the brain lesion." Shimoda and Robinson (1999), however, examined the relationship between lesion location and time since stroke using a longitudinally studied patient population. The study examined 60 patients with single lesions involving either the right or left middle cerebral artery distribution that was visible on CT scan and who had follow-up at 3 or 6 months (short-term follow-up) and at 12 or 24 months (long-term follow-up). There were no statistically significant differences between the patients with right and left hemisphere lesions in their age, gender, race, marital status, or other background characteristics. The frequency of depression in patients during the initial evaluation at approximately 2 weeks poststroke was significantly higher for both major and minor depression among patients with left hemisphere stroke compared with patients with right hemisphere stroke ($P = 0.0006$). At 3- to 6-month and at 1- to 2-year follow-up, however, there were no significant differences between right and left hemisphere lesion groups in the frequency of major or minor depression.

Based on the finding that PSD and lesion location were dependent on time since stroke, Robinson (2003) conducted a meta-analysis of studies conducted within 2 months following stroke, comparing the frequency of major depression among patients with left anterior versus left posterior lesions and left anterior versus right anterior lesions (Table 18–3). There were 128 patients in the left anterior–left posterior comparison, with a fixed model OR of 2.29 (95% CI 1.6–3.4, $P < 0.001$) and random model

TABLE 18–3.   Meta-analysis of the relationship of depression to lesion location

Study	N	L ant.	L post.	RR	95% CI	P	N	L ant.	R ant.	RR	95% CI	P
Astrom et al. 1993b	21	12/14	2/7	2.62[*]	1.20–8.63	0.017	25	12/13	2/12	5.54[*]	1.55–19.82	0.000
Morris 1996	20	9/10	3/10	3.00[*]	1.14–7.91	0.006	29	9/14	3/15	3.21[*]	1.08–9.51	0.016
Robinson et al. 1984	18	6/7	4/11	2.36[*]	1.02–5.45	0.040	16	6/6	4/10	2.27[*]	1.09–4.75	0.028
Robinson et al. 1986b	15	6/7	2/8	2.35[*]	1.16–9.54	0.019	11	6/6	2/5	2.23	0.85–5.87	0.46
House 1990	13	1/1	7/12	1.3	0.52–3.28	0.642	15	1/1	7/14	1.50	0.58–3.87	0.506
Hermann 1995	17	7/7	3/10	2.95[*]	1.21–7.13	0.007	NA	NA	NA	NA	NA	NA
Gainotti et al. 1999	22	1/4	8/18	0.56	0.95–3.32	0.474	16	1/4	8/12	0.38	0.07–2.15	0.146
Fixed combined	128	42/50	29/76	2.29[*]	1.6–3.4	0.000	112	35/44	26/68	2.18[*]	1.4–3.3	0.000
Random combined	126	42/50	29/76	2.29[*]	1.5–3.4	0.000	112	35/44	26/68	2.16[*]	1.3–3.6	0.004

Note.   Major depression was significantly more frequent following left anterior (L ant.) lesions than right anterior (R ant.) or left posterior (L post.) lesions. CI = confidence interval; RR = relative risk.

[*]$P < 0.05$.

Source.   Reprinted from Robinson RG: "The Controversy Over Post-Stroke Depression and Lesion Location." *Psychiatric Times* 20:39–40, 2003. Used with permission.

OR of 2.29 (95% CI 1.5–3.4, $P < 0.001$). Similarly, the comparison of left and right anterior lesions had an OR of 2.18 (fixed model: 95% CI 1.4–3.3, $P < 0.001$) and 2.16 (random model: 95% CI 1.3–3.6, $P < 0.004$), respectively.

This study suggests that the failure of other investigators to replicate the association of left anterior lesion location with increased frequency of depression may in most cases be related to time since stroke. The lateralized effect of left anterior lesions on both major and minor depression is a phenomenon of the acute poststroke period when the patients are less than 2 months poststroke. The most recent review by Bhogal al. (2004) concluded that the association between left hemisphere lesion location and PSD was dependent on whether the patients were inpatients or community patients (OR 1.36, 95% CI 1.05–1.76, $P < 0.05$) or acute versus chronic patients (OR acute 2.14, 95% CI 1.5–3.04, $P < 0.05$).

Although it is uncertain why this temporal dynamic occurs in the relationship between severity of depression and lesion location, it suggests that if physiological changes such as depletion of biogenic amines occur in patients with left

anterior lesions that lead to depression, these changes are hemisphere specific for only a few weeks. By 3 months after stroke, similar alternative mechanisms occur in patients with right frontal lesions that lead to correlations of depression severity with proximity of the lesion to the frontal pole.

Premorbid Risk Factors

The studies just reviewed indicate that although a significant proportion of patients with left anterior or right posterior lesions develop PSD, not every patient with a lesion in these locations developed a depressive mood. This observation raises the question of why clinical variability occurs and why some but not all patients with lesions in these locations develop depression.

Starkstein et al. (1988b) examined these questions by comparing 13 patients with major PSD with 13 stroke patients without depression, all of whom had lesions of the same size and location. Eleven pairs of patients had left hemisphere lesions; two pairs had right hemisphere lesions. Damage was cortical in 10 pairs and subcortical in 3 pairs. The groups did not differ on important demographic variables, such as age, sex, socioeconomic status, or education. They also did not differ on family or personal history of psychiatric disorders or neurological deficits. Patients with major PSD, however, had significantly more subcortical atrophy ($P < 0.05$), as measured both by the ratio of third ventricle to brain (i.e., the area of the third ventricle divided by the area of the brain at the same level) and by the ratio of lateral ventricle to brain (i.e., the area of the body of the lateral ventricle contralateral to the brain lesion divided by the brain area at the same level). It is likely that the subcortical atrophy preceded the stroke. Thus, a mild degree of subcortical atrophy may be a premorbid risk factor that increases the risk of developing major depression following a stroke.

In a study of patients with right hemisphere lesions, Starkstein et al. (1989b) found that patients who developed major depression after the occurrence of a right hemisphere lesion had a significantly higher frequency of family history of psychiatric disorders than did either nondepressed patients with right hemisphere lesions or patients with major depression following the occurrence of left hemisphere lesions. This finding suggests that a genetic predisposition for depression may play an important role after the occurrence of right hemisphere lesions. Eastwood et al. (1989) and Morris et al. (1990) have also reported that depressed patients were more likely than nondepressed patients to have either a personal or family history of psychiatric disorders.

In summary, lesion location is not the only factor that influences the development of PSD. Subcortical atrophy that probably precedes the stroke and a family or personal history of affective disorders also seems to play an important role. The most consistently identified risk factor for depression, however, is severity of functional physical impairment.

Relationship to Physical Impairment

Numerous investigators have reported a significant association between depression and functional physical impairment (i.e., ADL). Of 18 studies involving 3,281 patients, 15 (83%) found a statistically significant relationship between PSD and severity of impairment in ADLs. This association, however, might be construed as the severe functional impairment producing depression or, alternatively, the severity of depression influencing the severity of functional impairment. Studies, in fact, support both interpretations.

Sinyor et al. (1986) reported that although nondepressed stroke patients showed either a slight increase or no change in functional status over time, depressed patients had significant decreases in function during the first month after stroke ($P < 0.05$). In another study, Parikh et al. (1990) compared a consecutive series of 63 stroke patients who had major or minor depression with nondepressed stroke

patients during a 2-year follow-up. Although both groups had similar impairments in ADL during the time they were in hospital, the depressed patients had significantly less improvement by 2-year follow-up than did the nondepressed patients. This finding held true after the authors controlled for important variables such as the type and extent of in-hospital and rehabilitation treatment, the size and location of the lesion, the patients' demographic characteristics, the nature of the stroke, the occurrence of another stroke during the follow-up period, and the patients' medical history. Similar results were reported by Pohjasvaara et al. (2001), who found that among 256 patients, depression at 3 months was associated with Ranken scale >2 (i.e., poor physical outcome) ratings at 15 months (OR –2.5, 95% CI 1.6–3.8). A recent review by Hackett and Anderson (2005) reported that 9 of 11 studies that assessed physical disability found that it was significantly associated with depression.

Narushima and Robinson (2003) compared 34 patients who received antidepressant treatment with either nortriptyline (100 mg/day) or fluoxetine (40 mg/day) for 12 weeks beginning 19–25 days after stroke with 28 patients who received the same antidepressant treatment but began at 140 ($\pm$ 28 SD) days poststroke. There were no significant differences between groups in the potentially confounding factors of age, education, lesion volume, lesion location, or amount of rehabilitation services. During the period from 6 to 24 months following stroke, with the two groups matched for time since stroke, there was a significant group by time interaction using either intention to treat or efficacy analysis (Figure 18–3). The early-treatment group continued to show gradual recovery in ADLs over 2 years, whereas the late-treatment group showed gradual deterioration between the 12- and 24-months' follow-up. A logistic regression analysis examining the effects of diagnosis (depressed or nondepressed), medication (fluoxetine or nortriptyline), presence of severe motor impairment (NIH stroke scale rating), presence of prior psychiatric history, use of antidepressants beyond the 12-week study period, and use of early versus late antidepressant treatment showed that only the use of early versus late antidepressants predicted ADL scores at 2-year follow-up (Narushima and Robinson 2003).

Relationship to Cognitive Impairment

Numerous investigators have reported that elderly patients with functional major depression have intellectual deficits that improve with treatment of depression (Wells 1979). This issue was first examined in patients with PSD by Robinson et al. (1986a). Patients with major depression after a left hemisphere infarct were found to have significantly lower (more impaired) scores on the Mini-Mental State Examination (MMSE) (Folstein et al. 1975) than did a

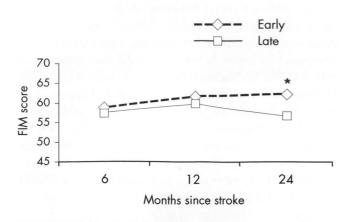

FIGURE 18–3.   Recovery in activities of daily living as measured by the Functional Independence Measure (FIM) over 2 years of follow-up. All patients were treated for 12 weeks in a double-blind study with fluoxetine or nortriptyline. Patients who received treatment within 1 month poststroke (mean 2 weeks, "Early") improved significantly more than those who received treatment after the first month poststroke (mean 12 weeks, "Late"). FIM scores were measured at the same times following stroke to control for group differences in time since stroke when the 3-month treatment was given. *Intention to treat, *P*=0.02. Efficacy, *P*=0.02.

Source.   Reprinted from Robinson RG: *The Clinical Neuropsychiatry of Stroke, 2nd Edition.* Cambridge, UK, Cambridge University Press, 2006. Used with permission.

comparable group of nondepressed patients. Both the size of patients' lesions and their depression scores correlated independently with severity of cognitive impairment.

In a second study (Starkstein et al. 1988b), stroke patients with and without major depression were matched for lesion location and volume. Of 13 patients with major PSD, 10 had an MMSE score lower than that of their matched control subjects, 2 had the same score, and only 1 patient had a higher score ($P<0.001$). Thus, even when patients were matched for lesion size and location, depressed patients were more cognitively impaired.

In a follow-up study, Bolla-Wilson et al. (1989) administered a comprehensive neuropsychological battery and found that patients with major depression and left hemisphere lesions had significantly greater cognitive impairments than did nondepressed patients with comparable left hemisphere lesions ($P<0.05$). These cognitive deficits involved tasks of temporal orientation, language, and executive motor and frontal lobe functions. On the other hand, among patients with right hemisphere lesions, patients with major depression did not differ from nondepressed patients on any of the measures of cognitive impairment.

Spalleta et al. (2002) examined 153 patients with first-ever stroke lesions of the left ($n=87$) or right ($n=66$)

hemisphere who were less than 1 year poststroke. Patients with left hemisphere lesions and major depression ($n=30$) showed significantly more impairment on the MMSE than nondepressed patients with left hemisphere lesions ($n=27$) (MMSE scores: 12.3 ± 9 [SD], major depression; 18.9 ± 8.5 [SD], nondepressed; $P<0.001$) (Figure 18–4).

Treatment studies of PSD have consistently failed to show an improvement in cognitive function even when poststroke mood disorders responded to antidepressant therapy (Andersen et al. 1996). Kimura et al. (2000) examined this issue in a study comparing nortriptyline and placebo using a double-blind treatment methodology among patients with major ($n=33$) or minor ($n=14$) PSD. Although the groups showed no significant differences in the change in MMSE scores from beginning to end of the treatment study, when patients were divided into those who responded to treatment (i.e., greater than 50% decline in Hamilton Rating Scale for Depression [Ham-D] [Hamilton 1960] score and no longer meeting depression diagnosis criteria) and those who did not respond, there was a significantly greater improvement in MMSE among patients who responded to treatment ($n=24$) compared with patients who did not respond to treatment ($n=23$) (Figure 18–5). The responding group included 16 patients treated with nortriptyline and 8 treated with placebo, whereas the nonresponder group included 5 patients treated with nortriptyline and 18 treated with placebo. There were no significant differences between the two groups in baseline Ham-D scores, demographic characteristics, stroke characteristics, or neurological findings. A repeated-measures analysis of variance (ANOVA) demonstrated a significant group by time interaction ($P=0.005$), and planned post hoc comparisons demonstrated that the responders had significantly less impaired MMSE scores than did the nonresponders, at nortriptyline doses of 75 mg ($P=0.036$) and 100 mg ($P=0.024$). If only nortriptyline-treated patients were used in the treatment response group compared with all placebo-treated patients in the treatment failure group, there was still a significant group by time interaction ($P=0.036$), which indicates that the failure to demonstrate cognitive improvement in prior studies was not the result of nortriptyline drug effects such as sedation or impaired attention due to anticholinergic effects. When the effect of major versus minor depression was examined, patients with major depression who responded to treatment ($n=15$) showed significantly greater improvement in MMSE scores than patients with major depression who did not respond ($n=18$) ($P=0.0087$). Among patients with minor depression (9 responders and 5 nonresponders), repeated-measures ANOVA of MMSE scores showed no significant group by time interaction.

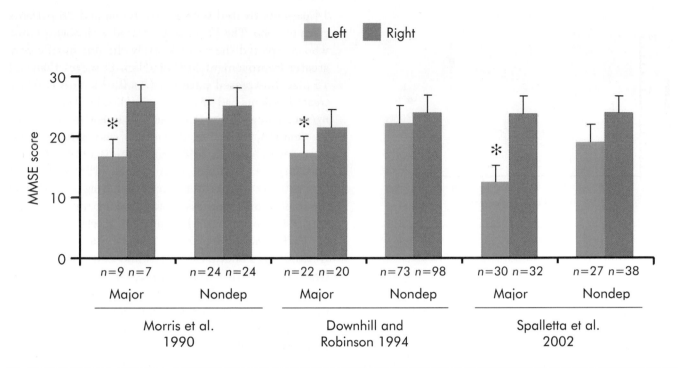

FIGURE 18–4. Mini-Mental State Examination (MMSE) scores following acute stroke in three studies among patients with major or no mood disturbance grouped according to the hemisphere of ischemia. In all three studies, there was a significant difference between patients with major depression (Major) after left hemisphere stroke and nondepressed (Nondep) patients with similar lesions. Major depression after right hemisphere lesions did not lead to the same phenomenon. Error bars represent the standard deviation divided by the square root of N.

*$P=0.001$.

Source.   Reprinted from Robinson RG: *The Clinical Neuropsychiatry of Stroke, 2nd Edition.* Cambridge, UK, Cambridge University Press, 2006. Used with permission.

The fact that earlier treatment studies did not show a significant effect of treatment of depression on cognitive function was the result of effect size. When nortriptyline-treated patients (some of whom responded to treatment and some of whom did not) were compared with placebo-treated patients (some of whom responded to treatment and some of whom did not), the effect size was only 0.16. When patients were divided into those who responded and those who did not respond, the effect size increased to 0.96, thus allowing a significant difference to be demonstrated with a much smaller group size.

Mechanism of Poststroke Depression

Although the cause of PSD remains unknown, one of the mechanisms that has been hypothesized to play an etiological role is dysfunction of the biogenic amine system. The noradrenergic and serotonergic cell bodies are located in the brain stem and send ascending projections through the median forebrain bundle to the frontal cortex. The ascending axons then arc posteriorly and run longitudinally through the deep layers of the cortex,

arborizing and sending terminal projections into the superficial cortical layers (Morrison et al. 1979). Lesions that disrupt these pathways in the frontal cortex or the basal ganglia may affect many downstream fibers. On the basis of these neuroanatomical facts and the clinical findings that the severity of depression correlates with the proximity of the lesion to the frontal pole, Robinson et al. (1984) suggested that PSD may be the consequence of depletions of norepinephrine and/or serotonin produced by lesions in the frontal lobe or basal ganglia.

In support of this hypothesis, a lateralized biochemical response to ischemia in human subjects was reported by Mayberg et al. (1988). Patients with stroke lesions in the right hemisphere had significantly higher ratios of ipsilateral to contralateral spiperone binding (presumably serotonin type 2 receptor binding) in noninjured temporal and parietal cortex than patients with comparable left hemisphere strokes. Patients with left hemisphere lesions, on the other hand, showed a significant inverse correlation between the amount of spiperone binding in the left temporal cortex and depression scores (i.e., higher depression scores were associated with lower serotonin receptor binding).

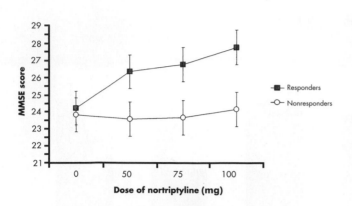

FIGURE 18–5.   Change of Mini-Mental State Examination scores (MMSE) in patients with poststroke major depression during a double-blind treatment study of nortriptyline versus placebo. Treatment responders (*n* = 15) showed significantly greater improvement in cognitive function than nonresponders (*n* = 18) (*P* = 0.0087). Error bars represent standard error of the mean (SE).

Source.   Reprinted from Kimura M, Robinson RG, Kosier T: "Treatment of Cognitive Impairment After Poststroke Depression." *Stroke* 31:1482–1486, 2000. Used with permission.

Thus, a greater depletion of biogenic amines in patients with right hemisphere lesions than in those with left hemisphere lesions could lead to a compensatory upregulation of receptors that might protect against depression. On the other hand, patients with left hemisphere lesions may have moderate depletions of biogenic amines but without a compensatory upregulation of serotonin receptors and, therefore, a dysfunction of biogenic amine systems in the left hemisphere. This dysfunction may ultimately lead to the clinical manifestations of depression.

A recent hypothesis by Spalletta et al. (2006) suggested that proinflammatory cytokines due to ischemic brain damage may lead to PSD. Stroke is known to produce cytokine release such as intracellular anthocyanin 1 (AN1) or interleukin 1, beta (IL1B), which have been found to be elevated in deceased individuals over age 60 years who had a history of major depression compared with control subjects. Cytokines might then activate the enzyme indole-2,3 dioxygenase (IDO) that catabolizes tryptophan, leading to decreased levels of serotonin (Capuron and Dantzer 2003). Thus, depletion of serotonin may trigger depressions following stroke.

Treatment of Poststroke Depression

At the present time, there are eight placebo-controlled, randomized, double-blind treatment studies on the efficacy of single-antidepressant treatment of PSD (Table 18–4). In the first study, Lipsey et al. (1984) examined

14 patients treated with nortriptyline and 20 patients given placebo. The 11 patients treated with nortriptyline who completed the 6-week study showed significantly greater improvement in their Ham-D scores than did 15 placebo-treated patients (*P* < 0.01). Successfully treated patients had serum nortriptyline levels of 50–150 ng/mL. Three patients experienced side effects (including delirium, confusion, drowsiness, and agitation) that were severe enough to require the discontinuation of nortriptyline. Similarly, Reding et al. (1986) reported that patients with PSD (defined as having an abnormal dexamethasone suppression test) taking trazodone had greater improvement in Barthel ADL scores (Granger et al. 1979) than did placebo-treated control subjects (*P* < 0.05). In another double-blind controlled trial in which the selective serotonin reuptake inhibitor (SSRI) citalopram was used, Ham-D scores were significantly more improved over 6 weeks in patients receiving active treatment (*n* = 27) than in the placebo group (*n* = 32) (Andersen et al. 1994a). At both 3 and 6 weeks, the group receiving active treatment had significantly lower Ham-D scores than did the group receiving placebo. This study established for the first time the efficacy of an SSRI in the treatment of PSD.

In another study, Robinson et al. (2000) compared depressed patients treated with fluoxetine (*n* = 23), nortriptyline (*n* = 16), or placebo (*n* = 17) in a double-blind, randomized treatment design. Patients were enrolled if they had a diagnosis of either major or minor PSD and had no contraindication to the use of fluoxetine or nortriptyline such as intracerebral hemorrhage (fluoxetine) or cardiac induction abnormalities (nortriptyline). Patients in the fluoxetine group were treated with 10-mg doses for the first 3 weeks, 20 mg for weeks 4–6, 30 mg for weeks 6–9, and 40 mg for weeks 9–12. The patients in the nortriptyline group were given 25 mg for the first week, 50 mg for weeks 2 and 3, 75 mg for weeks 3–6, and 100 mg for weeks 6–12. Patients treated with placebo were given identical capsules in the same number used for the actively treated patients. Intention-to-treat analysis demonstrated a significant time by treatment interaction with patients treated with nortriptyline showing a significantly greater decline in Ham-D scores than either the placebo-treated or fluoxetine-treated patients at 12 weeks of treatment. Intention-to-treat response rates were 10 of 16 (62%) for nortriptyline, 2 of 23 (9%) for fluoxetine, and 4 of 17 (24%) for placebo. There were no significant differences between the fluoxetine and the placebo groups (Figure 18–6).

A more recent study by Rampello et al. (2005) compared reboxetine and placebo in PDS with psychomotor retardation. Of 16 patients given reboxetine (4 mg/day),

TABLE 18–4.   Treatment studies of poststroke depression

Study	N	Medication (n) (max dose)	Duration	Evaluation method	Results	Response rate	Completion rate
Double-blind placebo-controlled studies							
Lipsey et al. 1984	34	Nortriptyline (14) (100 mg), placebo (20)	6 weeks	Ham-D, ZDS	Nortriptyline > placebo intention to treat and efficacy	100% nortriptyline, 33% placebo	11 of 14 nortriptyline, 15 of 20 placebo
Reding et al. 1986	27	Trazodone (7) (200 mg), placebo (9)	32 ± 6 days	ZDS	Trazodone > placebo on Barthel ADL scores for patients with abnormal DST	NR	NR
Andersen 1994b	66	Citalopram (33) (20 mg, 10 mg >65 years), placebo (33)	6 weeks	Ham-D, MES	Intention-to-treat response rates: citalopram > placebo	61% citalopram, 29% placebo	26 of 33 citalopram, 31 of 33 placebo
Grade et al. 1998	21	Methylphenidate (10) (30 mg), placebo (11)	3 weeks	Ham-D	Intention-to-treat response rates: methylphenidate > placebo	NR	9 of 10 methylphenidate, 10 of 11 placebo
Wiart et al. 2000	31	Fluoxetine (16) (20 mg), placebo (15)	6 weeks	MADRS	Intention-to-treat response rates: fluoxetine > placebo	62% fluoxetine, 33% placebo	14 of 16 fluoxetine, 15 of 15 placebo
Robinson et al. 2000	56	Fluoxetine (23) (40 mg), nortriptyline (16) (100 mg), placebo (17)	12 weeks	Ham-D	Intention-to-treat response rates: nortriptyline > placebo = fluoxetine = placebo	14% fluoxetine, 77% nortriptyline, 31% placebo	14 of 23 fluoxetine, 13 of 16 nortriptyline, 13 of 17 placebo
Fruehwald et al. 2003	54	Fluoxetine (28) (20 mg), placebo (26)	12 weeks	BDI, Ham-D	Ham-D > 15 fluoxetine = placebo Ham-D scores	69% fluoxetine Ham-D < 13, 75% placebo	26 of 28 fluoxetine, 24 of 26 placebo
Rampello et al. 2005	31	Reboxetine (16) (4 mg), placebo (15)	16 weeks	BDI, Ham-D	Reboxetine > placebo for PSD patients with retardation	NR	NR
Double-blind studies without placebo control							
Miyai et al. 2000	24	Desipramine (13) (100 mg), trazodone (6) (100 mg), fluoxetine (5) (20 mg)	4 weeks	Ham-D	Desipramine = trazodone = fluoxetine, no placebo comparison	NR	8 of 13 desipramine, 6 of 6 trazodone, 4 of 5 fluoxetine
Lauritzen et al. 1994	20	Imipramine (mean 75 mg) and mianserin (mean 25 mg); desipramine (mean 66 mg) and mianserin (mean 27 mg)	6 weeks	Ham-D, MES	Intention-to-treat response rates: imipramine+mianserin > desipramine and mianserin on MES but not Ham-D	Ham-D no different than MES, 81% imipramine + mianserin, 13% desipramine + mianserin	8 of 10 imipramine + mianserin, 5 of 10 desipramine + mianserin

Note.   ADL=activities of daily living; BDI=Beck Depression Inventory; DSI=dexamethasone suppression test; Ham-D=Hamilton Rating Scale for Depression; MADRS=Montgomery-Åsberg Depression Rating Scale; MES=Melancholia Scale; NR=not reported; PSD=poststroke depression; ZDS=Zung Self-Rating Depression Scale.

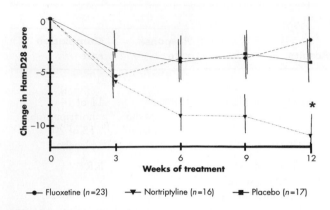

FIGURE 18–6. Intention-to-treat analysis. Change in (28-item) Hamilton Rating Scale for Depression score over 12 weeks of treatment for all patients who were entered in the study. Error bars represent the standard deviation divided by the square root of N.

*P<0.05 compared with fluoxetine or placebo.

Source. Reprinted from Robinson RG, Schultz SK, Castillo C, et al: "Nortriptyline Versus Fluoxetine in the Treatment of Depression and in Short Term Recovery After Stroke: A Placebo Controlled, Double-Blind Study." *American Journal of Psychiatry* 157:351–359, 2000. Used with permission.

there was a significantly greater decline in Ham-D and Beck Depression Inventory (BDI) (Beck et al. 1961) scores (mean ± SD: Ham-D, 24.1 ± 1.5 to 9.3 ± 2.1; BDI, 20.6 ± 2.2 to 8.1 ± 3.4) compared with placebo over the 16-week trial (Ham-D, 24.0 ± 1.3 to 22.7 ± 2.4; BDI, 19.9 ± 1.5 to 18.4 ± 3.3). The number of completers and the relative frequencies of response and remission, however, were not given.

Based on the available data, if there are no contraindications to nortriptyline such as heart block, cardiac arrhythmia, narrow-angle glaucoma, sedation, or orthostatic hypotension, nortriptyline remains the first-line treatment for PSD. Doses of nortriptyline should be increased slowly and blood levels should be monitored with a goal of achieving serum concentrations between 50 and 150 ng/mL. If there are contraindications to the use of nortriptyline, citalopram (20 mg under age 66 years, 10 mg age 66 years and over) or reboxetine (2 mg bid) would be alternate choices. Electroconvulsive therapy has also been reported to be effective for treating PSD (Murray et al. 1986). It causes few side effects and no neurological deterioration. Psychostimulants have also been reported in open-label trials to be effective for the treatment of PSD. Finally, psychological treatment using cognitive-behavioral therapy (CBT) in 123 stroke patients has been found by Lincoln et al. (2003) to be no more effective than an attention placebo treatment (*n*=39, CBT completers; *n*=43, placebo completers).

Psychosocial Adjustment

Psychosocial adjustment after stroke is an important issue to consider. Thompson et al. (1989) examined 40 stroke patients and their caregivers at an average of 9 months after the occurrence of stroke. They found that a lack of meaningfulness in life and overprotection by the caregiver were independent predictors of depression. Kotila et al. (1998) examined depression after stroke as part of the Finnstroke study. This study examined the effect of active rehabilitation programs after discharge together with support and social activities on the frequency of depression among patients and caregivers at 3 months and 1 year after stroke. At both 3 months and 1 year, the frequency of depression was significantly lower among patients receiving active outpatient treatment than among patients without active rehabilitation programs (41% vs. 54% at 3 months and 42% vs. 55% at 1 year). Although there were no significant differences between districts with and without active programs in the rate of depression among caregivers at 3 months, at 12 months there were significantly more severely depressed caregivers in districts without active programs (*P*=0.036). Greater severity of impairment as measured by the Rankin Scale (Rankin 1957) was also associated with increased depression among caregivers at 3 months after stroke.

POSTSTROKE MANIA

Although poststroke mania occurs much less frequently than depression (we have observed only 3 cases among a consecutive series of more than 300 stroke patients), manic syndromes are sometimes associated with stroke. Among 366 patients with bipolar disorder, Cassidy and Carroll (2002) found that late-onset mania (i.e., after age 47 years) was significantly associated with risk factors for vascular disease.

Phenomenology of Secondary Mania

Starkstein et al. (1988a) examined a series of 12 consecutive patients who met DSM-III criteria for an organic affective syndrome, manic type. These patients, who developed mania after a stroke, traumatic brain injury, or tumors, were compared with patients with functional (i.e., no known neuropathology) mania (Starkstein et al. 1987a). Both groups of patients showed similar frequencies of elation, pressured speech, flight of ideas, grandiose thoughts, insomnia, hallucinations, and paranoid delusions. Thus, the symptoms of mania that occurred after brain damage (secondary mania) appeared to be the same as those found in patients with mania without brain damage (primary mania).

Lesion Location

Several studies of patients with brain damage have found that patients who develop secondary mania have a significantly greater frequency of lesions in the right hemisphere than patients with depression or no mood disturbance. The right hemisphere lesions that lead to mania tend to be in specific right hemisphere structures that have connections to the limbic system. The right basotemporal cortex appears to be particularly important, because direct lesions as well as distant hypometabolic effects (diaschisis) of this cortical region are frequently associated with secondary mania.

Cummings and Mendez (1984) reported on two patients who developed mania after right thalamic stroke lesions. After a review of the literature, these authors suggested a specific association between secondary mania and lesions in the limbic system or in limbic-related areas of the right hemisphere.

Robinson and colleagues (1988) reported on 17 patients with secondary mania. Most had right hemisphere lesions involving either cortical limbic areas, such as the orbitofrontal cortex and the basotemporal cortex, or subcortical nuclei, such as the head of the caudate or the thalamus. The frequency of right hemisphere lesions was significantly greater than in patients with major depression, who tended to have left frontal or basal ganglia lesions.

These findings have been replicated in another study of eight patients with secondary mania (Starkstein et al. 1990b). All eight patients had right hemisphere lesions (seven unilateral and one bilateral injury). Lesions were either cortical (basotemporal cortex in four patients and orbitofrontal cortex in one patient) or subcortical (frontal white matter, head of the caudate nucleus, and anterior limb of the internal capsule in three patients, respectively). Positron emission tomography scans with (^{18}F)fluorodeoxyglucose were carried out in the three patients with purely subcortical lesions. They all showed a focal hypometabolic deficit in the right basotemporal cortex.

Risk Factors

Not every patient with a lesion in limbic areas of the right hemisphere will develop secondary mania. Therefore, there must be risk factors for this disorder.

In one study (Robinson et al. 1988), patients with secondary mania were compared with patients with secondary major depression. Results indicated that patients with secondary mania had a significantly higher frequency of positive family history of mood disorders than did depressed patients or patients with no mood disturbance ($P<0.05$). Therefore, it appears that genetic predisposition to mood disorders may constitute a risk factor for mania.

In another study (Starkstein et al. 1987a), patients with secondary mania were compared with patients with no mood disturbance who were matched for size, location, and etiology of brain lesion. The groups were also compared with patients with primary mania and control subjects. No significant between-group differences were found in either demographic variables or neurological evaluation. Patients with secondary mania, however, had a significantly greater degree of subcortical atrophy, as measured by bifrontal-to-brain ratio and third ventricular–to-brain ratio ($P<0.001$). Moreover, of the patients who developed secondary mania, those with a positive family history of psychiatric disorders had significantly less atrophy than those without such a family history ($P<0.05$), suggesting that genetic predisposition to affective disorders and brain atrophy may be independent risk factors.

The relatively rare occurrence of mania after stroke suggests that there are premorbid risk factors that have an impact on the expression of this disorder. Studies thus far have identified two such factors. One is a genetic vulnerability for affective disorder, and the other is a mild degree of subcortical atrophy. The subcortical atrophy probably preceded the stroke, but its cause remains unknown.

Mechanism of Secondary Mania

Several studies have demonstrated that the amygdala (located in the medial portion of the temporal lobe) has an important role in the production of instinctive reactions and the association between stimulus and emotional response (Adolphs et al. 1995; Drevets and Charney 2005). The amygdala receives its main afferents from the basal diencephalon (which in turn receives psychosensory and psychomotor information from the reticular formation) and the temporopolar and basolateral cortices (which receive main afferents from heteromodal association areas) (Beck 1949; Crosby et al. 1962). The basotemporal cortex receives afferents from association cortical areas and the orbitofrontal cortex and sends efferent projections to the entorhinal cortex, hippocampus, and amygdala. By virtue of these connections, the basotemporal cortex may represent a cortical link between sensory afferents and instinctive reactions.

The orbitofrontal cortex may be subdivided into two regions: a posterior one, which is restricted to limbic functions and should be considered part of the limbic system, and an anterior one, which exerts tonic inhibitory control over the amygdala by means of its connection through the uncinate fasciculus with the basotemporal cortex (Nauta 1971). Thus, the uncinate fasciculus and the basotemporal cortex may mediate connections between psychomotor and volitional processes, generated in the frontal lobe, and vital processes and instinctive behaviors, generated in the amygdala (Starkstein et al. 1988a).

A case report by Starkstein et al. (1989a) suggested that the mechanism of secondary mania is not related to the release of transcallosal inhibitory fibers (i.e., the release of left limbic areas from tonic inhibition due to a right hemisphere lesion). A patient who developed secondary mania after bleeding from a right basotemporal arteriovenous malformation underwent a Wada test before the therapeutic embolization of the malformation. Injection of amobarbital in the left carotid artery did not abolish the manic symptoms (which would be expected if the "release" theory were correct).

Although the mechanism of secondary mania remains unknown, both lesion studies and metabolic studies suggest that the right basotemporal cortex may play an important role. A combination of biogenic amine system dysfunction and release of tonic inhibitory input into the basotemporal cortex and lateral limbic system may lead to the production of mania.

Treatment of Secondary Mania

Although no systematic treatment studies of secondary mania have been conducted, one report suggested several potentially useful treatment modalities. Bakchine et al. (1989) carried out a double-blind, placebo-controlled treatment study in a single patient with secondary mania. Clonidine (0.6 mg/day) rapidly reversed the manic symptoms, whereas carbamazepine (1,200 mg/day) was associated with no mood changes and levodopa (375 mg/day) was associated with an increase in manic symptoms. In other treatment studies, however, the anticonvulsants valproic acid and carbamazepine as well as neuroleptics and lithium therapy have been reported to be useful in treating secondary mania (Starkstein et al. 1991). None of these treatments, however, have been evaluated in double-blind, placebo-controlled studies.

POSTSTROKE BIPOLAR DISORDER

Although some patients have one or more manic episodes after brain injury, other manic patients also have depression after brain injury. In an effort to examine the crucial factors in determining which patients have bipolar as opposed to unipolar disorder, Starkstein et al. (1991) examined 19 patients with the diagnosis of secondary mania. The bipolar (manic-depressive) group consisted of patients who, after the occurrence of the brain lesion, met DSM-III-R criteria for organic mood syndrome, mania, followed or preceded by organic mood syndrome, depressed. The unipolar-mania group consisted of patients who met the criteria for mania described previously (i.e., DSM-III-R

organic mood syndrome, mania), not followed or preceded by depression. All patients had CT scan evidence of vascular, neoplastic, or traumatic brain lesion and no history of other neurological, toxic, or metabolic conditions.

Patients in the bipolar group were found to have significantly greater intellectual impairment as measured by MMSE scores ($P < 0.05$). Almost half of the patients in the bipolar group had recurrent episodes of depression, whereas approximately one-fourth of patients in both the unipolar and bipolar groups had recurrent episodes of mania.

Of the 7 patients with bipolar disorder, 6 had lesions restricted to the right hemisphere, which involved the head of the caudate nucleus (2 patients); the thalamus (3 patients); and the head of the caudate nucleus, the dorsolateral frontal cortex, and the basotemporal cortex (1 patient). The remaining patient developed bipolar illness after surgical removal of a pituitary adenoma. In contrast to the primarily subcortical lesions in the bipolar group, 8 of 12 patients in the unipolar-mania group had lesions restricted to the right hemisphere, which involved the basotemporal cortex (6 patients), orbitofrontal cortex (1 patient), and head of the caudate nucleus (1 patient). The remaining 4 patients had bilateral lesions involving the orbitofrontal cortex (3 patients) and the orbitofrontal white matter (1 patient).

This study suggests that a prior episode of depression may have occurred in about one-third of patients with secondary mania. Patients with bipolar disorder tend to have subcortical lesions (mainly involving the right head of the caudate or the right thalamus), whereas patients with pure mania tend to show a higher frequency of cortical lesions (particularly in the right orbitofrontal and right basotemporal cortices). Finally, bipolar patients tend to have greater cognitive impairment than do patients with unipolar mania, which may either reflect differences in lesion location or suggest that the presence of a previous episode of depression may produce residual cognitive effects.

How might subcortical lesions produce bipolar disorder? Subcortical lesions have been reported to produce hypometabolic effects in widespread regions, including contralateral brain areas (i.e., crossed-hemisphere and crossed-cerebellar diaschisis) (Pappata et al. 1987). Thus, it is possible that subcortical lesions may have induced metabolic changes in left frontocortical regions, which (as noted previously) are associated with depression. Mania may develop at a later stage, when these metabolic changes become restricted to the orbitofrontal and/or basotemporal cortices of the right hemisphere.

POSTSTROKE ANXIETY DISORDER

Studies of patients with functional depression (i.e., of no known neuropathology) have demonstrated that it is important to distinguish depression associated with significant anxiety symptoms (i.e., agitated depressions) from depression without these symptoms (i.e., retarded depressions) because their cause and course may be different (Stavrakaki and Vargo 1986). This finding raises questions not only about the frequency and correlates of anxiety in stroke victims, but also about the nature of the relationship between anxiety and depression among patients with brain injury.

Starkstein et al. (1990a) examined a consecutive series of patients with acute stroke lesions for the presence of both anxiety and depressive symptoms. Slightly modified DSM-III criteria for generalized anxiety disorder (GAD) (i.e., excluding 6-month duration criteria) were used for the diagnosis of anxiety disorder. The presence of anxious foreboding and excessive worry was required, as were one or more symptoms of motor tension (i.e., muscle tension, restlessness, and easy fatigability), one or more symptoms of autonomic hyperactivity, and one or more symptoms of vigilance and scanning (i.e., feelings of being keyed up or on edge, difficulty concentrating because of anxiety, trouble falling or staying asleep, and irritability). Of a consecutive series of 98 patients with first-episode acute stroke lesions, only 6 met the criteria for GAD in the absence of any other mood disorder. On the other hand, 23 of 47 patients with major depression also met the criteria for GAD. Patients were then divided into those with anxiety only ($n=6$), anxiety and depression ($n=23$), depression only ($n=24$), and no mood disorder ($n=45$).

The only significant between-group difference in demographic variables was the presence of a higher frequency of alcoholism in patients with anxiety only. Examination of patients with positive CT scans revealed that anxious-depressed patients had a significantly higher frequency of cortical lesions (16 of 19 patients) than did either the depression-only group (7 of 15 patients) or the control group (13 of 27 patients). On the other hand, the depression-only group showed a significantly higher frequency of subcortical lesions than did the anxious-depressed group.

Castillo et al. (1993, 1995) found that 78 patients (27%) of a group of 288 patients hospitalized with an acute stroke met DSM-III-R criteria for GAD (excluding the 6-month duration criteria). Most patients with GAD also had major or minor depression (i.e., 58 of 78 patients with GAD also had depression). Depression plus anxiety was associated with left cortical lesions, whereas anxiety alone was associated with right hemisphere lesions. In a 2-year follow-up in a subgroup of 142 of these 288 patients, it was found that 32 (23%) developed GAD after the initial in-hospital evaluation (i.e., between 3 and 24 months after stroke). Early-onset but not late-onset GAD was associated with a history of psychiatric disorder, including alcohol abuse, and early-onset anxiety had a mean

duration of 1.5 months, whereas delayed-onset GAD had a mean duration of 3 months (Castillo et al. 1995).

Astrom (1996) examined 71 acute stroke patients for anxiety disorder and followed these patients over 3 years. The strongest correlates of GAD were the absence of social contacts outside the family and dependence of patients on others to perform their primary ADL. These factors were significantly more common in the GAD compared with the non-GAD population at 3 months, 1 year, 2 years, and 3 years after stroke. At 3-year follow-up, however, GAD was associated with both cortical atrophy (7 of 7 GAD patients had cortical atrophy vs. 19 of 39 non-GAD patients) and greater subcortical atrophy (as measured by frontal horn ratios on CT scan, $P=0.03$).

Leppavuori et al. (2003) found among 277 outpatients 21% with a DSM-IV diagnosis of GAD 4 months after stroke. The majority of those diagnosed (i.e., 17%) were comorbid with depression, whereas the remaining cases (i.e., 4%) had GAD without comorbid disorder. The correlates of anxiety based on logistic regression included prior history of epilepsy, comorbid depression, and use of anxiolytic drugs. The onset of GAD after stroke was associated with psychosocial function, history of migraine, and anterior circulation stroke. Morrison et al. (2005) found that anxiety after stroke remained stable in prevalence over 3 years and that the existence of poststroke anxiety at 3 years was significantly associated with prior anxiety and female gender.

Shimoda and Robinson (1998) examined the effect of GAD on outcome in patients with stroke. A group of 142 patients examined during hospitalization for acute stroke and followed for 2 years were diagnosed with GAD ($n=9$), major depressive disorder alone ($n=10$), both GAD and major depression ($n=10$), or neither GAD nor depression ($n=36$). An examination of the effect of GAD and major depression at the time of the initial hospital evaluation on recovery in ADL at short-term follow-up (3–6 months) demonstrated a significant effect of major depression but no significant effect of GAD and no interaction. At long-term follow-up (1–2 years), however, there was a significant interaction between major depression and GAD to inhibit recovery in ADL.

Similarly, an analysis of social functioning at short-term follow-up showed significant main effects of both major depression and GAD but no interaction (Shimoda and Robinson 1998). At long-term follow-up there were significant interactions between GAD and time as well as between major depression, GAD, and time. These findings indicate that patients with GAD were more impaired in their social functioning over the entire 2-year follow-up period and that patients with major depression plus GAD had the most severe impairment in social functioning of any group. Perhaps the most significant finding from this study, however, was that major depressive disorder and anxiety disorder diagnosed at the time of the initial in-hospital evaluation had a greater effect on impairment in ADL at 1-year and 2-year follow-up than major depression alone, anxiety disorder alone, or no mood or anxiety disturbance. These findings suggest that anxiety disorder is an important variable affecting long-term prognosis after stroke.

Another interesting finding from this study was that patients with major depression plus GAD had depressions that were significant longer in duration and greater in severity than patients with major depression alone.

A recent treatment study has examined the effect of nortriptyline on GAD that is comorbid with PSD (Kimura and Robinson 2003). The study included 29 patients who met criteria for GAD (17 with comorbid major depression, 10 with minor depression, and 2 with no depression). Analysis of the 27 GAD patients with comorbid depression used an intention-to-treat analysis that included 4 patients who dropped out of the study. There were no significant differences between nortriptyline and the placebo-treated patients in background characteristics including age, education, and time since stroke. There were also no significant differences between actively treated and placebo-treated patients in their neurological findings or the nature of the stroke lesion. In the group treated with nortriptyline, 54% of the patients had right hemisphere lesion; 64% of the placebo group had similar lesions. Motor impairments were present in 77% of the nortriptyline-treated patients and in 86% of the placebo-treated patients. Aphasia was found in 23% of the nortriptyline-treated patients and in 14% of the placebo patients. Because some patients in the study had been treated for 6 weeks whereas others had been treated for 12 weeks, they were combined based on the dose of nortriptyline that they were receiving.

A repeated-measures ANOVA of Hamilton Anxiety Scale (Ham-A) (Hamilton 1959) scores using an intention-to-treat analysis demonstrated a significant group by time interaction ($P=0.002$) (i.e., the nortriptyline group improved more quickly than the placebo group) (Figure 18–7). Planned comparisons revealed that the nortriptyline group was significantly more improved than the placebo group at nortriptyline doses of 50 mg, 75 mg, and 100 mg. Nine of 13 (69%) in the nortriptyline-treated group had a greater than 50% reduction in Ham-A scores, whereas only 3 of 14 placebo-treated patients (21%) had a similar reduction ($P=0.017$). When patients were divided into those with GAD plus major depression ($n=6$ treated with nortriptyline, $n=11$ treated with placebo) and those with GAD plus minor depression, there were too few patients with minor depression treated with placebo ($n=3$) to analyze the data on the patients with minor depression. How-

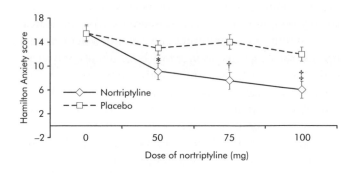

FIGURE 18–7. Mean Hamilton Anxiety Scale scores among patients with generalized anxiety disorder and comorbid depression after stroke following treatment with nortriptyline and placebo. The nortriptyline group ($n=13$) showed significantly greater improvement in anxiety symptoms than the placebo group ($n=14$) ($P=0.002$). Error bars represent standard error of the mean (SE).
$*P<0.05$; $†P<0.01$; $‡P<0.02$.

Source. Reprinted from Kimura M, Robinson RG: "Treatment of Poststroke Generalized Anxiety Disorder Comorbid With Poststroke Depression: Merged Analysis of Nortriptyline Trials." *American Journal of Geriatric Psychiatry* 11:320–327, 2003. Used with permission.

ever, repeated-measures ANOVA of Ham-A scores for the patients with major depression showed a significant group by time interaction ($P=0.022$). The patients treated with nortriptyline improved significantly more quickly than patients treated with placebo. To determine whether depression and anxiety symptoms were responding independently, the rate of change in symptom severity was compared between a Ham-A and a Ham-D measurement. At 50 mg of nortriptyline (i.e., 2–3 weeks), there was a 39% improvement in Ham-A scores and only a 14% improvement in Ham-D scores ($P=0.03$). This suggests that anxiety symptoms were responding more rapidly than depressive symptoms with nortriptyline therapy. This was the first study using double-blind, placebo-controlled methodology to demonstrate that GAD following stroke can be effectively treated with the tricyclic antidepressant nortriptyline.

POSTSTROKE PSYCHOSIS

The phenomenon of hallucinations and delusions in patients who have experienced stroke has been called agitated delirium, acute atypical psychosis, peduncular hallucinosis, release hallucinations, and acute organic psychosis. In a study of acute organic psychosis occurring after stroke lesions, Rabins et al. (1991) found a very low prevalence of psychosis among stroke patients (only 5 in more than 300 consecutive admissions). All 5 of these patients, however, had right hemisphere lesions, primarily involving frontoparietal regions. When compared with 5 age-matched patients with cerebrovascular lesions in similar locations but no psychosis, patients with secondary psychosis had significantly greater subcortical atrophy, as manifested by significantly larger areas of both the frontal horn of the lateral ventricle and the body of the lateral ventricle (measured on the side contralateral to the brain lesion). Several investigators have also reported a high frequency of seizures among patients with secondary psychosis (Levine and Finkelstein 1982). These seizures usually started after the occurrence of the brain lesion but before the onset of psychosis. The study by Rabins et al. (1991) found seizures in 3 of 5 patients with poststroke psychosis, compared with 0 of 5 poststroke, nonpsychiatric control subjects.

It has been hypothesized that three factors may be important in the mechanism of organic hallucinations, namely 1) a right hemisphere lesion involving the temporoparietal cortex, 2) seizures, and/or 3) subcortical brain atrophy (Starkstein et al. 1992).

Secondary psychosis is a rare finding in patients with brain injury and is frequently associated with lesions involving the temporoparietal junction in the right hemisphere as well as subcortical atrophy or seizure disorder. Treatment has been primarily pharmacological, with either neuroleptics or antiseizure drugs. The mechanism resulting in hallucinations and delusions has not been determined.

APATHY

Apathy is the absence or lack of motivation as manifested by decreased motor function, cognitive function, emotional feeling, and interest and has been reported frequently among patients with brain injury. Using the Apathy Scale, Starkstein et al. (1993a) examined a consecutive series of 80 patients with single-stroke lesions and no significant impairment in comprehension. Of 80 patients, 9 (11%) showed apathy as their only psychiatric disorder, whereas another 11% had both apathy and depression. The only demographic correlate of apathy was age, as apathetic patients (with or without depression) were significantly older than nonapathetic patients. In addition, apathetic patients showed significantly more severe deficits in ADL, and a significant interaction was noted between depression and apathy on ADL scores, with the greatest impairment found in patients who were both apathetic and depressed.

Patients with apathy (without depression) showed a significantly higher frequency of lesions involving the posterior limb of the internal capsule than did patients without apathy (Starkstein et al. 1993a). Lesions in the internal globus pallidus and the posterior limb of the internal capsule have been reported to produce behavioral changes, such as motor neglect, psychic akinesia, and akinetic mutism (Helgason et al. 1988). The ansa lenticularis is one of the main internal pallidal outputs, and it ends in the pedunculopontine nucleus after going through the posterior limb of the internal capsule (Nauta 1989). In rodents, this pathway has a prominent role in goal-oriented behavior (Bechara and van der Kooy 1989), and dysfunction of this system may explain the presence of apathy in patients with lesions of the posterior limb of the internal capsule. Angelelli et al. (2004), in a study of 124 poststroke patients, found apathy in 27%, depression in 61%, and irritability in 33%. Ghika-Schmidt and Bogousslavsky (2000) studied 12 patients with anterior thalamic infarcts. Within a few months' follow-up, the persisting abnormalities included memory dysfunction and apathy. Kobayashi and coworkers, using xenon inhalation, showed that patients with poststroke apathy had decreased blood flow bilaterally in the frontal lobes (Okada et al. 1997) and impaired frontal lobe function (i.e., impaired fluency and prolonged latency of novelty P3 response to auditory stimuli on electroencephalogram) (Yamagata et al. 2004).

CATASTROPHIC REACTION

As described under "Historical Perspective" earlier in this chapter, *catastrophic reaction* is a term coined by Goldstein (1939) to describe the "inability of the organism to cope when faced with physical or cognitive deficits." Catastrophic reaction is expressed by anxiety, tears, aggressive behavior, swearing, displacement, refusal, renouncement, and sometimes compensatory boasting. Starkstein et al. (1993b) assessed a consecutive series of 62 patients using the Catastrophic Reaction Scale, which was developed to assess the existence and severity of catastrophic reactions. The Catastrophic Reaction Scale has been demonstrated to be a reliable instrument in the measurement of symptoms of catastrophic reaction.

Catastrophic reactions occurred in 12 of 62 (19%) consecutive patients with acute stroke lesions (Starkstein et al. 1993b). Three major findings emerged from this study. First, patients with catastrophic reactions were found to have a significantly higher frequency of familial and personal history of psychiatric disorders (mostly depression) than were patients without catastrophic reactions. Second, catastrophic reaction was not significantly more frequent among aphasic (33%) than nonaphasic (66%) patients. This finding does not support the contention that catastrophic reactions are an understandable psychological response of "frustrated" aphasic patients (Gainotti 1972). Third, 9 of the 12 patients with catastrophic reaction also had major depression, 2 had minor depression, and only 1 was not depressed. On the other hand, among the 50 patients without catastrophic reactions, 7 had major depression, 6 had minor depression, and 37 were not depressed. Thus, catastrophic reaction was significantly associated with major depression, but it does not support the proposal by Gainotti et al. (1999) that the catastrophic reaction is an integral part of PSD. It is rather a comorbid condition that occurs in some but not all patients with PSD or that may characterize a subgroup of PSD.

In addition to this association with depression, patients with catastrophic reaction had a significantly higher frequency of lesions involving the basal ganglia (Starkstein et al. 1993b). When 10 depressed patients with catastrophic reaction were compared with 10 depressed patients without catastrophic reaction, the group with catastrophic reaction showed significantly more anterior lesions, which were mostly located in subcortical regions (i.e., 8 of 9 depressed patients with catastrophic reaction had subcortical lesions, and 3 of 9 depressed patients without catastrophic reaction had subcortical lesions) ($P=0.01$).

One may conclude from the evidence presented above that catastrophic reaction may have a neurophysiological underpinning, rather than being just a behavioral response of patients confronted with their limitations. Catastrophic reactions seem to be associated with a specific type of poststroke major depression (i.e., major depressions associated with anterior subcortical lesions). Although anterior brain lesions (both cortical and subcortical) have been associated with PSD, subcortical damage has usually been hypothesized to underlie the "release" of emotional display by removing inhibitory input to the limbic areas of the cortex (Ross and Stewart 1987).

Catastrophic reaction occurs in about 20% of stroke patients (Starkstein et al. 1993b) and is associated with a family or personal history of psychiatric disorders. Catastrophic reaction is significantly associated with major depression and may be mediated by a release of emotional display produced by anterior subcortical lesions. Thus, catastrophic reaction may or may not represent an independent clinical syndrome. Catastrophic reaction may be a behavioral symptom of a subgroup of depressions provoked by anterior subcortical damage.

PATHOLOGICAL EMOTIONS

Emotional lability is a common complication of stroke lesions. It is characterized by sudden, easily provoked episodes of crying that, although frequent, generally occur in appropriate situations and are accompanied by a congruent mood change. Pathological laughing and crying is a more severe form of emotional lability and is characterized by episodes of laughing and/or crying that are not appropriate to the context. They may appear spontaneously or may be elicited by nonemotional events and do not correspond to underlying emotional feelings. These disorders have also been termed *emotional incontinence, pathologic emotions,* and *involuntary emotional expression disorder.*

Robinson et al. (1993) examined the clinical correlates and treatment of emotional lability (including pathological laughter and crying) in 28 patients with either acute or chronic stroke. A Pathological Laughter and Crying Scale (PLACS) (Robinson et al. 1993) was developed to assess the existence and severity of emotional lability. The reliability and validity of this instrument were assessed in 18 patients receiving treatment for emotional lability and 54 other patients who had experienced acute stroke. Moreover, PLACS scores did not correlate with Ham-D scores, MMSE scores, or ADL scores, indicating that the PLACS was assessing a factor other than the ones being measured by these instruments. Tang et al. (2004) found a prevalence rate of 17.9% among 127 patients with acute stroke. Logistic regression showed that pathological emotions were associated with a history of depression and cortical infarction.

A double-blind treatment trial of nortriptyline versus placebo was conducted. The doses of nortriptyline were 25 mg for 1 week, 50 mg for 2 weeks, 70 mg for 1 week, and 100 mg for the last 2 weeks of the study. One patient dropped out during the study, 2 patients withdrew before initiation of the study, and 28 completed the 6-week protocol. Patients receiving nortriptyline showed significant improvements in PLACS scores compared with the placebo-treated patients. These differences became statistically significant at 4 and 6 weeks. Although a significant improvement in depression scores was also observed, improvements in PLACS scores were significant for both depressed and nondepressed patients with pathological laughing and crying, indicating that treatment response was not simply related to an improvement in depression (Robinson et al. 1993).

Anderson et al. (1993) also conducted a double-blind study using the SSRI citalopram to treat pathological crying. This study evaluated 16 patients using a crossover design. Three of the patients were dropped from the study—1 given placebo because of a generalized seizure on day 28, and 2 others who are also taking placebo because of a lack of response to treatment after the first week. Patients were given 1 week as a baseline, 3 weeks of treatment, and 1 week of washout, followed by 1 week as a second baseline, and then 3 weeks of the crossover treatment. The number of crying episodes per day was recorded daily by patients in their journals as the measure of treatment efficacy. Their response to treatment is shown in Figure 18–8. Although the Robinson et al. (1993) study used PLACS scores to measure outcome, the two studies were compared by examining the per-

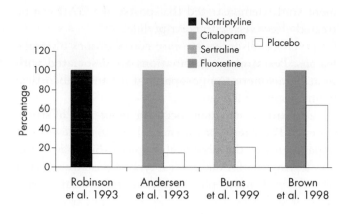

FIGURE 18–8. Comparison of double-blind treatment studies using nortriptyline, citalopram, sertraline, or fluoxetine in patients with pathological crying. Percentage of patients with >50% reduction in severity score or crying episodes. The mean pooled data response rates were 96% for active medication and 27.5% for placebo. These findings suggest that all of these medications are effective in the treatment of post-stroke pathological crying.

Source. Reprinted from Robinson RG: *The Clinical Neuropsychiatry of Stroke, 2nd Edition.* Cambridge, UK, Cambridge University Press, 2006. Used with permission.

centage reduction in baseline measure following treatment. All 13 of the patients treated with citalopram in the Anderson study responded by reduction in the number of crying episodes by at least 50%, and 2 of the patients also responded while receiving placebo. None of the patients had major depression at the start of the Anderson study, but their mean Ham-D scores decreased from 8.9 to 5.3 during the 3 weeks of treatment with citalopram ($P = 0.005$). The response to citalopram was nearly immediate, with patients reporting a 50% or greater reduction in the frequency of crying episodes during the first week of treatment; 8 patients reported response within 24 hours, 3 patients within 3 days, and only 4 patients took more than a week to respond.

There have now been four double-blind treatment studies of pathological emotion, and both fluoxetine (Brown et al. 1998) and sertraline (Burns et al. 1999) have been shown to significantly reduce the frequency of crying episodes (see Figure 18–8). These findings have supported the conclusion that SSRI antidepressant medications are rapidly effective in reducing the number of crying episodes in patients with poststroke pathological emotions.

APROSODY

Ross and Mesulam (1979) have described aprosody as abnormalities in the affective components of language,

encompassing prosody and emotional gesturing. Prosody can be defined as the "variation of pitch, rhythm, and stress of pronunciation that bestows certain semantic and emotional meaning to speech" (Ross and Mesulam 1979, p. 144).

Motor aprosody consists of marked difficulty in spontaneous use of emotional inflection in language (e.g., an absence of normal prosodic variations in speech) or emotional gesturing, whereas comprehension of emotional inflection or gesturing remains intact. Sensory aprosody, on the other hand, is manifested by intact spontaneous emotional inflection in language and gesturing, whereas comprehension of emotional inflection or gesturing is markedly impaired. In a manner analogous to the organization of propositional language in the left hemisphere, expression and comprehension of emotional inflection have been associated respectively with frontal and temporoparietal regions of the right hemisphere (Ross and Mesulam 1979).

Starkstein et al. (1994) examined prosody comprehension in 59 patients with acute stroke lesions. With the use of tapes expressing verbal emotion and photos of emotional facial expression, impaired comprehension of emotion was found in a mild form in 10 patients (17%) and in a severe form in 19 (32%). Severe aprosody was associated with the following three clinical variables: 1) neglect for tactile stimulation, 2) lesions of the right hemisphere, including the basal ganglia and temporoparietal cortex, and 3) significantly larger third ventricle–to–brain ratio. Although Ross and Rush (1981) suggested that patients with sensory aprosody might not be able to recognize their own depressed mood, major depression was found in 2 of 19 patients (11%) with severe aprosody and in 7 of 30 (23%) without aprosody (not significant).

Impairment in the ability to comprehend emotion was found in about one-third of patients. It was strongly associated with right hemisphere lesions, subcortical atrophy, and neglect but did not preclude patients from recognizing their own depression.

CONCLUSION

There are numerous emotional and behavioral disorders that occur after cerebrovascular lesions (see "Highlights for the Clinican" at the end of the chapter). Depression occurs in about 40% of stroke patients, with approximately equal distributions of major depression and minor depression. Major depression is significantly associated with left frontal and left basal ganglia lesions during the acute stroke period and may be successfully treated with nortriptyline or citalopram. Treatment of depression has also been shown to improve poststroke cognitive function.

Mania is a rare complication of stroke and is strongly associated with right hemisphere damage involving the orbitofrontal cortex, basal temporal cortex, thalamus, or basal ganglia. Risk factors for mania include a family history of psychiatric disorders and subcortical atrophy. Bipolar disorders are associated with subcortical lesions of the right hemisphere, whereas right cortical lesions lead to mania without depression.

Generalized anxiety disorder, which is present in about 27% of stroke patients, is associated with depression in the majority of cases. Among the few patients with poststroke anxiety and no depression, there is a high frequency of alcoholism and lesions of the right hemisphere. Apathy is present in about 20% of stroke patients. It is associated with older age, more severe deficits in ADL, and a significantly higher frequency of lesions involving the posterior limb of the internal capsule. A treatment study demonstrated that poststroke GAD can be treated effectively with nortriptyline.

Psychotic disorders are rare complications of stroke lesions. Poststroke hallucinations are associated with right hemisphere temporoparietal lesions, subcortical brain atrophy, and seizures.

Catastrophic reactions occur in about 20% of stroke patients. These reactions are not related to the severity of impairments or the presence of aphasia but may represent a symptom for one clinical type of poststroke major depression. Catastrophic reactions are associated with anterior subcortical lesions and may result from a "release" of emotional display in a subgroup of depressed patients. Pathological laughing and crying is another common complication of stroke lesions that may sometimes coexist with depression and may be successfully treated with nortriptyline, citalopram, fluoxetine, or sertraline.

Highlights for the Clinician

Poststroke depression

- Has repeatedly been shown to impair recovery in activities of daily living (ADL) over 2 years.

- Impairs cognitive recovery over 2 years.

- Eight double-blind treatment studies showed benefits of antidepressants on depression and/or cognitive recovery.

- Successful antidepressant treatment beginning within the first 2 months poststroke improved recovery in ADL significantly more than late treatment or nonresponse to treatment.

Poststroke anxiety disorder

- In combination with major depression, anxiety disorder has an additive effect on delaying recovery in ADL and social functioning over 2 years.

- One double-blind trial showed that antidepressants with an antianxiety component can significantly reduce poststroke anxiety symptoms.

Pathological laughing and crying

- Estimated prevalence across all studies was 15%.

- Four double-blind treatment trials showed superiority of antidepressant treatment over placebo.

Apathy, denial of illness, catastrophic reactions, impaired emotional comprehension (aprosody)

- All of these disorders occur in approximately 20% or more of stroke patients and can impede both recovery and treatment efforts.

RECOMMENDED READINGS

Robinson RG: The Clinical Neuropsychiatry of Stroke, 2nd Edition. Cambridge, UK, Cambridge University Press, 2006

Whyte EM, Mulsant BH: Poststroke depression: epidemiology, pathophysiology and biological treatment. Biol Psychiatry 52:253–264, 2002

REFERENCES

Aben I, Verhey F, Lousberg R, et al: Validity of the Beck Depression Inventory, Hospital Anxiety and Depression Scale, SCL-90, and Hamilton Depression Rating Scale as screening instruments for depression in stroke patients. Psychosomatics 43:386–393, 2002

Adams RD, Victor M: Principles of Neurology. New York, McGraw-Hill, 1985

Adolphs R, Tranel D, Damasio H, et al: Fear and the human amygdala. J Neurosci 15:5879–5891, 1995

American Heart Association: Heart and Stroke Facts: 1996 Statistical Supplement. Dallas, TX, American Heart Association, 1997

American Psychiatric Association: Diagnostic and Statistical Manual of Mental Disorders, 4th Edition, Text Revision. Washington, DC, American Psychiatric Press, 2000

Andersen G, Vestergaard K, Riis J: Citalopram for post-stroke pathological crying. Lancet 342:837–839, 1993

Andersen G, Vestergaard K, Lauritzen L: Effective treatment of poststroke depression with the selective serotonin reuptake inhibitor citalopram. Stroke 25:1099–1104, 1994a

Andersen G, Vestergaard K, Riis JO, et al: Incidence of post-stroke depression during the first year in a large unselected stroke population determined using a valid standardized rating scale. Acta Psychiatr Scand 90:190–195, 1994b

Andersen G, Vestergaard K, Riis JO, et al: Dementia of depression or depression of dementia in stroke? Acta Psychiatr Scand 94:272–278, 1996

Angelelli P, Paolucci S, Bivona Y, et al: Development of neuro-psychiatric symptoms in poststroke patients: a cross-sectional study. Acta Psychiatr Scand 110:55–63, 2004

Astrom M: Generalized anxiety disorder in stroke patients: a 3-year longitudinal study. Stroke 27:270–275, 1996

Astrom M, Adolfsson R, Asplund K: Major depression in stroke patients: a 3-year longitudinal study. Stroke 24:976–982, 1993a

Astrom M, Olsson T, Asplund K: Different linkage of depression to hypercortisolism early versus late after stroke: a 3-year longitudinal study. Stroke 24:52–57, 1993b

Babinski J: [Contribution to the study of mental disturbance in organic cerebral hemiplegia (anosognosia).] Rev Neurol (Paris) 27:845–848, 1914

Bakchine S, Lacomblez L, Benoit N, et al: Manic-like state after orbitofrontal and right temporoparietal injury: efficacy of clonidine. Neurology 39:778–781, 1989

Bechara A, van der Kooy D: The tegmental pedunculopontine nucleus: a brain-stem output of the limbic system critical for the conditioned place preferences produced by morphine and amphetamine. J Neurosci 9:3400–3409, 1989

Beck AT, Ward CH, Mendelson M, et al: An inventory for measuring depression. Arch Gen Psychiatry 4:561–571, 1961

Beck E: A cytoarchitectural investigation into the boundaries of cortical areas 13 and 14 in the human brain. J Anat 83:145–147, 1949

Bhogal SK, Teasell R, Foley N, et al: Lesion location and post-stroke depression: systematic review of the methodological limitations in the literature. Stroke 35:794–802, 2004

Bleuler EP: Textbook of Psychiatry. New York, Macmillan, 1951

Bolla-Wilson K, Robinson RG, Starkstein SE, et al: Lateralization of dementia of depression in stroke patients. Am J Psychiatry 146:627–634, 1989

Brown KW, Sloan RL, Pentland B: Fluoxetine as a treatment for post-stroke emotionalism. Acta Psychiatr Scand 98:455–458, 1998

Bukberg J, Penman D, Holland JC: Depression in hospitalized cancer patients. Psychosom Med 46:199–212, 1984

Burns A, Russell E, Stratton-Powell H, et al: Sertraline in stroke-associated lability of mood. Int J Geriatr Psychiatry 14:681–685, 1999

Burvill PW, Johnson GA, Jamrozik KD, et al: Prevalence of depression after stroke: the Perth Community Stroke Study. Br J Psychiatry 166:320–327, 1995

Capuron L, Dantzer R: Cytokines and depression: the need for a new paradigm. Brain Behav Immun 17 (suppl 1):S119–S124, 2003

Carson AJ, MacHale S, Allen K, et al: Depression after stroke and lesion location: a systematic review. Lancet 356:122–126, 2000

Cassidy F, Carroll BJ: Vascular risk factors in late onset mania. Psychol Med 32:359–362, 2002

Cassidy E, O'Connor R, O'Keane V: Prevalence of post-stroke depression in an Irish sample and its relationship with disability and outcome following inpatient rehabilitation. Disabil Rehabil 26:71–77, 2004

Castillo CS, Starkstein SE, Fedoroff JP, et al: Generalized anxiety disorder after stroke. J Nerv Ment Dis 181:100–106, 1993

Castillo CS, Schultz SK, Robinson RG: Clinical correlates of early onset and late-onset poststroke generalized anxiety. Am J Psychiatry 152:1174–1179, 1995

Cohen-Cole SA, Stoudemire A: Major depression and physical illness: special considerations in diagnosis and biologic treatment. Psychiatr Clin North Am 10:1–17, 1987

Collin J, Tinson D, Lincoln NB: Depression after stroke. Clin Rehabil 1:27–32, 1987

Crosby E, Humphrey T, Laner E: Correlative Anatomy of the Nervous System. New York, Macmillan, 1962

Cummings JL, Mendez MF: Secondary mania with focal cerebrovascular lesions. Am J Psychiatry 141:1084–1087, 1984

Dennis M, O'Rourke S, Lewis S, et al: Emotional outcomes after stroke: factors associated with poor outcome. J Neurol Neurosurg Psychiatry 68:47–52, 2000

Denny-Brown D, Meyer JS, Horenstein S: The significance of perceptual rivalry resulting from parietal lesions. Brain 75:434–471, 1952

Downhill JE Jr, Robinson RG: Longitudinal assessment of depression and cognitive impairment following stroke. J Nerv Ment Dis 182:425–431, 1994

Drevets WC, Charney DS: Anxiety disorders: neuroimaging, in Comprehensive Textbook of Psychiatry, 8th Edition. Edited by Sadock BJ, Sadock VA. Philadelphia, PA, Lippincott Williams & Wilkins, 2005, pp 1749–1750

Eastwood MR, Rifat SL, Nobbs H, et al: Mood disorder following cerebrovascular accident. Br J Psychiatry 154:195–200, 1989

Ebrahim S, Barer D, Nouri F: Affective illness after stroke. Br J Psychiatry 151:52–56, 1987

Endicott J: Measurement of depression in patients with cancer. Cancer 53 (suppl):2243–2248, 1984

Fedoroff JP, Lipsey JR, Starkstein SE, et al: Phenomenological comparisons of major depression following stroke, myocardial infarction or spinal cord lesions. J Affect Disord 22:83–89, 1991

Feibel JH, Springer CJ: Depression and failure to resume social activities after stroke. Arch Phys Med Rehabil 63:276–277, 1982

Finset A, Goffeng L, Landro NI, et al: Depressed mood and intra-hemispheric location of lesion in right hemisphere stroke patients. Scand J Rehabil Med 21:1–6, 1989

Fisher SH: Psychiatric considerations of cerebral vascular disease. Am J Cardiol 7:379–385, 1961

Folstein MF, Folstein SE, McHugh PR: Mini-Mental State: a practical method for grading the cognitive state of patients for the clinician. J Psychiatr Res 12:189–198, 1975

Folstein MF, Maiberger R, McHugh PR: Mood disorder as a specific complication of stroke. J Neurol Neurosurg Psychiatry 40:1018–1020, 1977

Fruehwald S, Gatterbauer E, Rehak P, et al: Early fluoxetine treatment of post-stroke depression: a three-month double-blind placebo-controlled study with an open-label long-term follow up. J Neurol 250:347–351, 2003

Gainotti G: Emotional behavior and hemispheric side of the brain. Cortex 8:41–55, 1972

Gainotti G, Azzoni A, Marra C: Frequency, phenomenology and anatomical-clinical correlates of major post-stroke depression. Br J Psychiatry 175:163–167, 1999

Ghika-Schmid F, Bogousslavsky J: The acute behavioral syndrome of anterior thalamic infarction: prospective study of 12 cases. Ann Neurol 48:220–227, 2000

Goldstein K: The Organism: A Holistic Approach to Biology Derived From Pathological Data in Man. New York, American Books, 1939

Goldstein K: After Effects of Brain Injuries in War. New York, Grune & Stratton, 1942

Grade C, Redford B, Chrostowski J, et al: Methylphenidate in early poststroke recovery: a double-blind, placebo-controlled study. Arch Phys Med Rehabil 79:1047–1050, 1998

Granger CV, Denis LS, Peters NC, et al: Stroke rehabilitation: analysis of repeated Barthel Index measures. Arch Phys Med Rehabil 60:14–17, 1979

Hackett ML, Anderson CS: Predictors of depression after stroke: a systematic review of observational studies. Stroke 36:2296–301, 2005

Hamilton M: The assessment of anxiety states by rating. Br J Med Psychol 32:50–55, 1959

Hamilton MA: A rating scale for depression. J Neurol Neurosurg Psychiatry 23:56–62, 1960

Hecaen H, deAjuriaguerra J, Massonet J: [Visuo-constructive disorders due to right parieto-occipital lesion; role of vestibular disturbance.] Encephale 40:122–179, 1951

Helgason C, Wilbur A, Weiss A, et al: Acute pseudobulbar mutism due to discrete bilateral capsular infarction in the territory of the anterior choroidal artery. Brain 111 (part 3):507–524, 1988

Herrmann M, Bartels C, Wallesch CW: Depression in acute and chronic aphasia: symptoms, pathoanatomical-clinical correlations and functional implications. J Neurol Neurosurg Psychiatry 56:672–678, 1993

Herrmann M, Bartels C, Schumacher M, et al: Poststroke depression: is there a pathoanatomic correlate for depression in the postacute stage of stroke? Stroke 26:850–856, 1995

Herrmann N, Black SE, Lawrence J, et al: The Sunnybrook Stroke Study: a prospective study of depressive symptoms and functional outcome. Stroke 29:618–624, 1998

House A, Dennis M, Warlow C, et al: Mood disorders after stroke and their relation to lesion location: a CT scan study. Brain 113:1113–1130, 1990

House A, Dennis M, Mogridge L, et al: Mood disorders in the year after first stroke. Br J Psychiatry 158:83–92, 1991

Ironside R: Disorders of laughter due to brain lesions. Brain 79:589–609, 1956

Kimura M, Robinson RG: Treatment of poststroke generalized anxiety disorder comorbid with poststroke depression: merged analysis of nortriptyline trials. Am J Geriatr Psychiatry 11:320–327, 2003

Kimura M, Robinson RG, Kosier T: Treatment of cognitive impairment after poststroke depression. Stroke 31:1482–1486, 2000

Kotila M, Numminen H, Waltimo O, et al: Depression after stroke: results of the FINNSTROKE study. Stroke 29:368–372, 1998

Kraepelin E: Manic Depressive Insanity and Paranoia (1921). Translated by Barclay RM. Edited by Robertson GM. New York, Arno Press, 1976

Lauritzen L, Bendsen BB, Vilmar T, et al: Post-stroke depression: combined treatment with imipramine or desipramine and mianserin: a controlled clinical study. Psychopharmacology 114:119–122, 1994

Leppavuori A, Pohjasvaara T, Vataja R, et al: Generalized anxiety disorders three to four months after ischemic stroke. Cerebrovasc Dis 16:257–264, 2003

Levine DN, Finklestein S: Delayed psychosis after right temporoparietal stroke or trauma: relation to epilepsy. Neurology 32:267–273, 1982

Lincoln NB, Flannaghan T: Cognitive behavioral psychotherapy for depression following stroke: a randomized controlled trial. Stroke 34:111–115, 2003

Lipsey JR, Robinson RG, Pearlson GD, et al: Nortriptyline treatment of post-stroke depression: a double-blind study. Lancet 1:297–300, 1984

Lipsey JR, Spencer WC, Rabins PV, et al: Phenomenological comparison of functional and post-stroke depression. Am J Psychiatry 143:527–529, 1986

Mayberg HS, Robinson RG, Wong DF, et al: PET imaging of cortical S_2-serotonin receptors after stroke: lateralized changes and relationship to depression. Am J Psychiatry 145:937–943, 1988

Meyer A: The anatomical facts and clinical varieties of traumatic insanity. American Journal of Insanity 60:373–442, 1904

Miyai I, Suzuki T, Kang J, et al: Improved functional outcome in patients with hemorrhagic stroke in putamen and thalamus compared with those with stroke restricted to the putamen or thalamus. Stroke 31:1365–1369, 2000

Morris PLP, Robinson RG, Raphael B: Prevalence and course of depressive disorders in hospitalized stroke patients. Int J Psychiatry Med 20:349–364, 1990

Morris PLP, Robinson RG, Raphael B, et al: Lesion location and post-stroke depression. J Neuropsychiatry Clin Neurosci 8:399–403, 1996

Morrison JH, Molliver ME, Grzanna R: Noradrenergic innervation of the cerebral cortex: widespread effects of local cortical lesions. Science 205:313–316, 1979

Morrison V, Pollard B, Johnston M, et al: Anxiety and depression 3 years following stroke: demographic, clinical, and psychological predictors. J Psychosom Res 59:209–213, 2005

Murray GB, Shea V, Conn DK: Electroconvulsive therapy for post-stroke depression. J Clin Psychiatry 47:258–260, 1986

Narushima K, Robinson RG: The effect of early versus late antidepressant treatment on physical impairment associated with poststroke depression: is there a time-related therapeutic window? J Nerv Ment Dis 191:645–652, 2003

Narushima K, Kosier JT, Robinson RG: A reappraisal of post-stroke depression, intra and inter-hemispheric lesion location using meta-analysis. J Neuropsychiatry Clin Neurosci 15:422–430, 2003

Nauta WJH: The problem of the frontal lobe: a reinterpretation. J Psychiatr Res 8:167–187, 1971

Nauta WJH: Reciprocal links of the corpus striatum with the cerebral cortex and the limbic system: a common substrate for movement and thought? In Neurology and Psychiatry: A Meeting of Minds. Edited by Mueller J. Basel, Switzerland, Karger, 1989, pp 43–63

Okada K, Kobayashi S, Yamagata S, et al: Poststroke apathy and regional cerebral blood flow. Stroke 28:2437–2441, 1997

Pappata S, Tran Dinh S, Baron JC, et al: Remote metabolic effects of cerebrovascular lesions: magnetic resonance and positron tomography imaging. Neuroradiology 29:1–6, 1987

Paradiso S, Ohkubo T, Robinson RG: Vegetative and psychological symptoms associated with depressed mood over the first two years after stroke. Int J Psychiatry Med 27:137–157, 1997

Parikh RM, Robinson RG, Lipsey JR, et al: The impact of post-stroke depression on recovery in activities of daily living over two year follow-up. Arch Neurol 47:785–789, 1990

Pessah-Rasmussen H, Engstrom G, Jerntorp I, et al: Increasing stroke incidence and decreasing case fatality, 1989–1998: a study from the Stroke Register in Malmö, Sweden. Stroke 34:913–918, 2003

Pohjasvaara T, Leppavuori A, Siira I, et al: Frequency and clinical determinants of poststroke depression. Stroke 29:2311–2317, 1998

Pohjasvaara T, Vataja R, Leppavuori A, et al: Depression is an independent predictor of poor long-term functional outcome post-stroke. Eur J Neurol 8:315–319, 2001

Post F: The Significance of Affective Symptoms in Old Age: A Follow-Up Study of 100 Patients, Maudsley Monograph No. 1. New York, Oxford University Press, 1962

Rabins PV, Starkstein SE, Robinson RG: Risk factors for developing atypical (schizophreniform) psychosis following stroke. J Neuropsychiatry Clin Neurosci 3:6–9, 1991

Rankin J: Cerebral vascular accidents in patients over the age of 60, III: diagnosis and treatment. Scott Med J 2:254–268, 1957

Rampello L, Alvano A, Chiechio S, et al: An evaluation of efficacy and safety of reboxetine in elderly patients affected by "retarded" post-stroke depression: a random, placebo-controlled study. Arch Gerontol Geriatr 40:275–285, 2005

Rapp SR, Vrana S: Substituting nonsomatic for somatic symptoms in the diagnosis of depression in elderly male medical patients. Am J Psychiatry 146:1197–1200, 1989

Reding MJ, Orto LA, Winter SW, et al: Antidepressant therapy after stroke: a double-blind trial. Arch Neurol 43:763–765, 1986

Rifkin A, Reardon G, Siris S, et al: Trimipramine in physical illness with depression. J Clin Psychiatry 46:4–8, 1985

Robinson RG: The controversy over post-stroke depression and lesion location. Psychiatric Times 20:39–40, 2003

Robinson RG: The Clinical Neuropsychiatry of Stroke, 2nd Edition. Cambridge, UK, Cambridge University Press, 2006

Robinson RG, Price TR: Post-stroke depressive disorders: a follow-up study of 103 patients. Stroke 13:635–641, 1982

Robinson RG, Szetela B: Mood change following left hemispheric brain injury. Ann Neurol 9:447–453, 1981

Robinson RG, Kubos KL, Starr LB, et al: Mood disorders in stroke patients: importance of location of lesion. Brain 107:81–93, 1984

Robinson RG, Bolla-Wilson K, Kaplan E, et al: Depression influences intellectual impairment in stroke patients. Br J Psychiatry 148:541–547, 1986a

Robinson RG, Lipsey JR, Rao K, et al: Two-year longitudinal study of post-stroke mood disorders: comparison of acute-onset with delayed-onset depression. Am J Psychiatry 143:1238–1244, 1986b

Robinson RG, Boston JD, Starkstein SE, et al: Comparison of mania with depression following brain injury: causal factors. Am J Psychiatry 145:172–178, 1988

Robinson RG, Parikh RM, Lipsey JR, et al: Pathological laughing and crying following stroke: validation of a measurement scale and a double-blind treatment study. Am J Psychiatry 150:286–293, 1993

Robinson RG, Schultz SK, Castillo C, et al: Nortriptyline versus fluoxetine in the treatment of depression and in short term recovery after stroke: a placebo controlled, double-blind study. Am J Psychiatry 157:351–359, 2000

Ross ED, Mesulam MM.: Dominant language functions of the right hemisphere? Prosody and emotional gesturing. Arch Neurol 36:144–148, 1979

Ross ED, Rush AJ: Diagnosis and neuroanatomical correlates of depression in brain-damaged patients: implications for a neurology of depression. Arch Gen Psychiatry 38:1344–1354, 1981

Ross ED, Stewart RS: Pathological display of affect in patients with depression and right frontal brain damage. J Nerv Ment Dis 175:165–172, 1987

Schubert DS, Burns R, Paras W, et al: Increase of medical hospital length of stay by depression in stroke and amputation patients: a pilot study. Psychother Psychosom 57:61–66, 1992

Schwartz JA, Speed NM, Brunberg JA, et al: Depression in stroke rehabilitation. Biol Psychiatry 33:694–699, 1993

Shimoda K, Robinson RG: Effect of anxiety disorder in impairment and recovery from stroke. J Neuropsychiatry Clin Neurosci 10:34–40, 1998

Shimoda K, Robinson RG: The relationship between post-stroke depression and lesion location in long-term follow-up. Biol Psychiatry 45:187–192, 1999

Sinyor D, Amato P, Kaloupek P: Post-stroke depression: relationship to functional impairment, coping strategies, and rehabilitation outcome. Stroke 17:112–117, 1986

Spalletta G, Guida G, De Angelis D, et al: Predictors of cognitive level and depression severity are different in patients with left and right hemispheric stroke within the first year of illness. J Neurol 249:1541–1551, 2002

Spalletta G, Ripa A, Caltagirone C: Symptom profile of DSM-IV major and minor depressive disorders in first-ever stroke patients. Am J Geriatr Psychiatry 13:108–115, 2005

Spalletta G, Bossù P, Ciaramella A, et al: The etiology of post-stroke depression: a review of the literature and a new hypothesis involving inflammatory cytokines. Mol Psychiatry 11:984–991, 2006

Starkstein SE, Pearlson GD, Boston J, et al: Mania after brain injury: a controlled study of causative factors. Arch Neurol 44:1069–1073, 1987a

Starkstein SE, Robinson RG, Price TR: Comparison of cortical and subcortical lesions in the production of post-stroke mood disorders. Brain 110:1045–1059, 1987b

Starkstein SE, Boston JD, Robinson RG: Mechanisms of mania after brain injury: 12 case reports and review of the literature. J Nerv Ment Dis 176:87–100, 1988a

Starkstein SE, Robinson RG, Price TR: Comparison of patients with and without post-stroke major depression matched for size and location of lesion. Arch Gen Psychiatry 45:247–252, 1988b

Starkstein SE, Robinson RG, Price TR: Comparison of spontaneously recovered versus non-recovered patients with post-stroke depression. Stroke 19:1491–1496, 1988c

Starkstein SE, Berthier PL, Lylyk A, et al: Emotional behavior after a WADA test in a patient with secondary mania. J Neuropsychiatry Clin Neurosci 1:408–412, 1989a

Starkstein SE, Robinson RG, Honig MA, et al: Mood changes after right hemisphere lesion. Br J Psychiatry 155:79–85, 1989b

Starkstein SE, Cohen BS, Fedoroff P, et al: Relationship between anxiety disorders and depressive disorders in patients with cerebrovascular injury. Arch Gen Psychiatry 47:246–251, 1990a

Starkstein SE, Mayberg HS, Berthier ML, et al: Mania after brain injury: neuroradiological and metabolic findings. Ann Neurol 27:652–659, 1990b

Starkstein SE, Fedoroff JP, Berthier MD, et al: Manic depressive and pure manic states after brain lesions. Biol Psychiatry 29:149–158, 1991

Starkstein SE, Robinson RG, Berthier ML: Post-stroke hallucinatory delusional syndromes. Neuropsychiatry Neuropsychol Behav Neurol 5:114–118, 1992

Starkstein SE, Fedoroff JP, Price TR, et al: Apathy following cerebrovascular lesions. Stroke 24:1625–1630, 1993a

Starkstein SE, Fedoroff JP, Price TR, et al: Catastrophic reaction after cerebrovascular ledions: frequency, correlates, and validation of a scale. J Neurol Neurosurg Psychiatry 5:189–194, 1993b

Starkstein SE, Federoff JP, Price TR, et al: Neuropsychological and neuroradiologic correlates of emotional prosody comprehension. Neurology 44:515–522, 1994

Stavrakaki C, Vargo B: The relationship of anxiety and depression: a review of the literature. Br J Psychiatry 149:7–16, 1986

Tang WK, Chan SS, Chiu HF, et al: Emotional incontinence in Chinese stroke patients: diagnosis, frequency, and clinical and radiological correlates. J Neurol 251:865–869, 2004

Thom T, Haase N, Rosamond W, et al: Heart disease and stroke statistics—2006 update: a report from the American Heart Association Statistics Committee and Stroke Statistics Subcommittee. Circulation 113:e85–e151, 2006

Thompson SC, Sobolew-Shobin A, Graham MA, et al: Psychosocial adjustment following stroke. Soc Sci Med 28:239–247, 1989

Wade DT, Legh-Smith J, Hewer RA: Depressed mood after stroke: a community study of its frequency. Br J Psychiatry 151:200–205, 1987

Wells CE: Pseudodementia. Am J Psychiatry 136:895–900, 1979

Wiart L, Petit H, Joseph PA, et al: Fluoxetine in early poststroke depression: a double-blind placebo-controlled study. Stroke 31:1829–1832, 2000

Wolf PA, Dawber TR, Thomas HE, et al: Epidemiology of stroke, in Advances in Neurology. Edited by Thompson RA, Green R. New York, Raven, 1977, pp 5–19

Yamagata S, Yamaguchi S, Kobayashi S: Impaired novelty processing in apathy after subcortical stroke. Stroke 35:1935–1940, 2004

19

NEUROPSYCHIATRIC ASPECTS OF BRAIN TUMORS

Trevor R.P. Price, M.D.

Kenneth L. Goetz, M.D.

Mark R. Lovell, Ph.D.

Tumors involving the central nervous system (CNS) are common. The annual incidence of primary brain tumors is 9.0 per 100,000 and that of metastatic brain tumors is 8.3 per 100,000. Evidence suggests that the overall incidence of brain tumors and the proportion of brain tumors that are malignant have been increasing over the past two decades in industrialized countries (Jukich et al. 2001; Olney et al. 1996). Brain tumors are second only to stroke as the leading cause of death from neurological diseases (Radhakrishnan et al. 1994).

Brain tumors are typically classified according to whether they are primary or metastatic, as well as according to location and histological cell type. Most primary tumors are either gliomas or meningiomas; gliomas are found more frequently (Table 19–1). The most common metastatic lesions are from lung and breast primary lesions (Table 19–2). Seventy percent of all tumors are supratentorial, with distribution by lobe as indicated in Figure 19–1. This distribution is influenced to some degree by tumor histology (Figure 19–2).

Age is also a determining factor for the frequency of various cell types. In children, astrocytomas are the most commonly seen CNS tumors, followed by medulloblastomas (Radhakrishnan et al. 1994). Gliomas are more often seen in the middle-aged population, and meningio-

TABLE 19–1. Relative frequencies of common histological types of brain tumors

Tumor type	Frequency (%)
Primary	
Gliomas	40–55
Astrocytomas	10–15
Glioblastomas	20–25
Others	10–15
Meningiomas	10–20
Pituitary adenomas	10
Neurilemmomas (mainly acoustic neuromas)	5–8
Medulloblastomas and pinealomas	5
Miscellaneous primary tumors	5
Metastatic	15–25

Source. Reprinted from Lohr JB, Cadet JL: "Neuropsychiatric Aspects of Brain Tumors," in *The American Psychiatric Press Textbook of Neuropsychiatry.* Edited by Talbott JA, Hales RE, Yudofsky SC. Washington, DC, American Psychiatric Press, 1987, p. 356. Used with permission.

TABLE 19–2.   Relative frequencies of metastatic brain tumors by site of the primary lesion

Tumor	Frequency (%)
Lung	35–45
Breast	10–20
Kidney	5–10
Gastrointestinal tract	5–10
Melanoma	2–5
Others (including thyroid, pancreas, ovary, uterus, prostate, testes, bladder, and sarcoma)	25–30

Source.   Reprinted from Lohr JB, Cadet JL: "Neuropsychiatric Aspects of Brain Tumors," in *The American Psychiatric Press Textbook of Neuropsychiatry.* Edited by Talbott JA, Hales RE, Yudofsky SC. Washington, DC, American Psychiatric Press, 1987, p. 356. Used with permission.

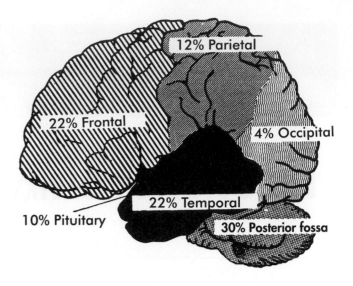

FIGURE 19–1.   Relative frequency of intracranial brain tumors according to location in the adult.

Source.   Reprinted from Lohr JB, Cadet JL: "Neuropsychiatric Aspects of Brain Tumors," in *The American Psychiatric Press Textbook of Neuropsychiatry.* Edited by Talbott JA, Hales RE, Yudofsky SC. Washington, DC, American Psychiatric Press, 1987, p. 355. Used with permission.

mas increase in incidence in the elderly (Radhakrishnan et al. 1994). Furthermore, metastatic disease is more frequent in the elderly and occurs with higher incidence than primary brain tumors.

It has been reported that primary brain tumors are up to 10 times more common among psychiatric patients than in psychiatrically healthy control subjects and that mental changes and behavioral symptoms, including confusion and various other neuropsychiatric symptoms, are more frequent early indicators of primary brain tumors than are classic physical manifestations such as headaches, seizures, and focal neurological signs (Kocher et al. 1984).

Although the various tumor classifications may eventually turn out to be important in understanding the occurrence of neuropsychiatric symptoms associated with brain tumors, no large-scale, detailed studies have yet carefully examined correlations between clinical phenomenology and various tumor parameters. Our knowledge of the neuropsychiatric and neuropsychological aspects of brain tumors is based on a relatively small number of clinical case reports and larger, uncontrolled case series from the older neurological and neurosurgical literature. Much of the discussion that follows draws on this database.

FREQUENCY OF NEUROPSYCHIATRIC SYMPTOMS IN PATIENTS WITH BRAIN TUMORS

Unfortunately, and surprisingly, few recent studies have examined the frequency of psychiatric symptoms in patients with brain tumors. This is probably because of modern imaging and neurosurgical techniques, which make early diagnosis and treatment commonplace but also prevent the opportunity to study the behavioral consequences of tumors. The studies that are available tend to be large autopsy studies, predominantly from the first half of the twentieth century.

For example, Keschner et al. (1938) noted psychiatric symptoms in 413 (78%) of 530 patients with brain tumors, and Schlesinger (1950) found behavior changes in 301 (51%) of his series of 591 patients. Although tumor-associated, complex neuropsychiatric symptoms may occur along with focal neurological signs and symptoms, often they may be the first clinical indication of a tumor, as was the case in 18% of the patients examined by Keschner et al. (1938). This, of course, also suggests that with appropriate diagnosis, 82% of this population would have had medical or surgical intervention before the advent of behavioral symptoms. On the contrary, in a study of 4 patients with intracranial tumors, Ko and Kok (1989) noted that 3 patients had initially presented to psychiatrists for diagnosis and treatment. Another more recent analysis of a group of patients with meningiomas indicated that 21% of the sample had initially presented with psychiatric symptoms in the absence of neurological signs or symptoms (Gupta and Kumar 2004). Taken together, these studies underscore the continuing need for primary care physicians and psychiatrists to be alert to

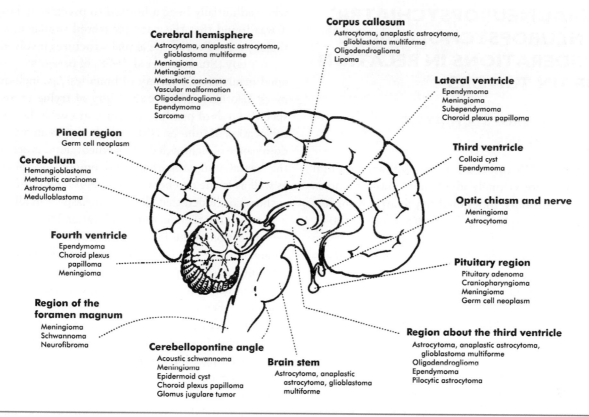

Cerebral hemisphere
Astrocytoma, anaplastic astrocytoma,
glioblastoma multiforme
Meningioma
Metingioma
Metastatic carcinoma
Vascular malformation
Oligodendroglioma
Ependymoma
Sarcoma

Corpus callosum
Astrocytoma, anaplastic astrocytoma,
glioblastoma multiforme
Oligodendroglioma
Lipoma

Lateral ventricle
Ependymoma
Meningioma
Subependymoma
Choroid plexus papilloma

Pineal region
Germ cell neoplasm

Cerebellum
Hemangioblastoma
Metastatic carcinoma
Astrocytoma
Medulloblastoma

Third ventricle
Colloid cyst
Ependymoma

Optic chiasm and nerve
Meningioma
Astrocytoma

Fourth ventricle
Ependymoma
Choroid plexus
papilloma
Meningioma

Pituitary region
Pituitary adenoma
Craniopharyngioma
Meningioma
Germ cell neoplasm

**Region of the
foramen magnum**
Meningioma
Schwannoma
Neurofibroma

Region about the third ventricle
Astrocytoma, anaplastic astrocytoma,
glioblastoma multiforme
Oligodendroglioma
Ependymoma
Pilocytic astrocytoma

Cerebellopontine angle
Acoustic schwannoma
Meningioma
Epidermoid cyst
Choroid plexus papilloma
Glomus jugulare tumor

Brain stem
Astrocytoma, anaplastic
astrocytoma, glioblastoma
multiforme

FIGURE 19–2. Topographical distribution of intracranial tumors in the adult.

Source. Reprinted from Burger PC, Scheithauer BW, Vogel FS: *Surgical Pathology of the Nervous System and Its Coverings,* 3rd Edition. New York, Churchill Livingstone, 1991. Copyright Elsevier 1991. Used with permission.

the presence of neurological abnormalities in patients who present with psychiatric and behavioral symptoms.

Minski (1933) studied 58 patients with cerebral tumors and, in addition to reporting that the psychiatric symptomatology of 25 of these patients simulated "functional psychoses," noted that 19 actually attributed the onset of their behavioral symptoms to various stresses, including financial worries and the deaths of relatives. This underscores the difficulty that clinicians face in making an appropriate diagnosis early in the course of disease. It may be impossible on purely clinical grounds to determine the organic basis of the patient's complaints until progression of the tumor has resulted in the emergence of more typical and unmistakable neurological signs and symptoms.

Despite the high prevalence of psychiatric symptoms in patients with brain tumors, the prevalence of intracranial tumors in psychiatric patients, compiled from autopsy data from mental hospitals, is only about 3%. This rate is similar to that found in autopsy series in general hospitals (Galasko et al. 1988). In a study by J.K.A. Roberts and Lishman (1984), only 1 of 323 psychiatric patients who had computed tomography (CT) scans done as part of the diagnostic evaluation was found to have a tumor. Hollister and Boutros (1991) evaluated CT or

magnetic resonance imaging (MRI) studies performed on 337 psychiatric patients. Only 2 patients were found to have brain tumors, and both had significant neurological findings on physical examination. Other studies suggest that the risk of an occult neoplasm in patients presenting with purely psychiatric complaints may be as low as 0.1% (Hobbs 1963; Remington and Robert 1962).

Two large autopsy studies (Klotz 1957; Selecki 1965) of psychiatric patients have suggested that approximately half of all tumors go undiagnosed before postmortem examination. However, these studies did not necessarily establish that brain pathology was not suspected in patients who turned out to have unrecognized brain tumors at postmortem examination or that these tumors were necessarily responsible for any or all of the psychiatric and behavioral symptoms the patients had experienced during their lifetimes. Of interest is another autopsy study, by Percy et al. (1972), which reported that before the advent of modern imaging techniques, 37% of brain tumors in an unselected population were first diagnosed at autopsy. Most of these patients were asymptomatic during their lifetimes. Undoubtedly, sophisticated brain imaging, which was unavailable at the time these series were done, would have diminished the likelihood of missing a tumor.

GENERAL NEUROPSYCHIATRIC AND NEUROPSYCHOLOGICAL CONSIDERATIONS IN RELATION TO BRAIN TUMORS

GENERAL NEUROPSYCHIATRIC CONSIDERATIONS

Patients with CNS tumors can present with mental symptoms that are virtually identical to those found in patients with primary functional psychiatric disorders (Jarquin-Valdivia 2004; Madhusoodanan et al. 2004). These symptoms run the gamut from major depression and schizophrenia to personality disorders and conversion disorders. Over the years, many clinicians and researchers have hypothesized the existence of a predictable relation between tumor location and neuropsychiatric phenomenology. Some studies have supported the generally held belief that depression is more common in frontal lobe tumors and psychosis is more common with temporal lobe neoplasms (Filley and Kleinschmidt-DeMasters 1995; Wellisch et al. 2002). Most of the older, autopsy-related studies did not strongly support this hypothesis and often concluded that observed behavior changes were of no localizing value (Keschner et al. 1938; Selecki 1965). Unfortunately, these studies were performed with little understanding of localizing phenomena, and we now are better able to recognize the role of anatomical location in determining psychiatric and neuropsychological symptomatology. Nevertheless, the nature and severity of psychiatric dysfunction accompanying tumors are determined by several other factors that are of as great or even greater importance than anatomical location. The reason that this is the case may be that neuroanatomical substrates of particular behaviors tend not to be localized to single lobes or specific anatomical locations.

The best examples of these nonlocalized substrates are behaviors mediated by tumors involving the limbic system, which includes the temporal lobes and portions of the frontal lobes, the hypothalamus, and the midbrain. Tumors affecting any of these structures may produce similar psychopathology. Furthermore, even lesions outside the limbic system may produce similar behavior changes, attributable to limbic release or disinhibition, through diaschisis or disconnection syndromes (see subsection "General Neuropsychological Considerations" later in this chapter). Limbic tumors often have been associated with depression, affective flattening, apathy, agitation, assaultive behavior, and even a variety of psychotic symptoms. In one study (Malamud 1967) of patients with tumors in or near limbic system structures who had initially been admitted to psychiatric hospitals, it was found that the patients shared similar psychopathology regardless of the actual structures involved.

A study (Starkstein et al. 1988) of patients who developed mania after a variety of brain lesions, including tumors, also illustrates the difficulty of trying to associate specific kinds of psychiatric symptoms with the anatomical location of tumors. Although there was an overall predominance of right-sided involvement, lesions occurred in the frontal, temporoparietal, and temporo-occipital lobes, as well as in the cerebellum, thalamus, and pituitary. The authors concluded that the unifying aspect in all of these lesions was not their anatomical location but rather the interconnection of the involved structures with the orbitofrontal cortex. This finding underscores the need for formulating more sophisticated localization models in which both neuroanatomical location and connectivity are considered as they relate to focal brain lesions.

Other factors also may influence presenting symptoms and thereby diminish the localizing value of a particular behavior change. Increased intracranial pressure is a nonspecific consequence of CNS tumors in general and has been implicated in behavior changes such as apathy, depression, irritability, agitation, and changes in consciousness. In one study of lesions involving the occipital lobes, it was concluded that most observed mental changes were due to increases in intracranial pressure rather than to effects of the tumors themselves (Allen 1930).

Another factor is the patient's premorbid level of functioning, which often has a significant effect on the nature of the clinical presentation. Tumors often cause an exaggeration of the individual's previous predominant character traits and coping styles. The behavior changes associated with a brain tumor usually represent a complex combination of the patient's premorbid psychiatric status, tumor-associated mental symptoms, and adaptive or maladaptive responses to the psychological stress of having been diagnosed with a brain tumor.

It has been noted that rapidly growing tumors are more commonly associated with severe, acute psychiatric symptoms, such as agitation or psychosis, as well as with more obvious cognitive dysfunctions. Patients with slow-growing tumors are more likely to present with vague personality changes, apathy, or depression, often without associated cognitive changes (Lishman 1987). Multiple tumor foci also tend to produce behavioral symptoms with greater frequency than do single lesions.

The relation between tumor type and neuropsychiatric symptoms is also complex. Several large studies (Frazier 1935; Keschner et al. 1938) have shown no association between histological type of tumor and associated behavior changes. Early reports suggested that meningiomas produced neuropsychiatric symptoms more often than other tumors did (McIntyre and McIntyre 1942). Davison and Bagley (1969) reviewed the literature on numerous patients with psychosis secondary to brain tumors and found no significant predominance of one tumor type over another. This should not be surprising, given the variability of tumor classification systems used by different pathologists (Reitan and Wolfson 1985). Schirmer and Bock (1984) found no differences in symptoms between primary brain tumors and intracranial metastases. Lishman (1987), however, suggested that gliomas may be more likely than benign tumors to produce behavior changes, possibly because of the rapidity of growth or the multiplicity of tumor sites that may be involved. One study found more anxiety and depression in patients with meningiomas than with any other tumor type (Pringle et al. 1999). Patton and Sheppard (1956) noted a greater incidence of meningiomas among psychiatric patients than among general hospital patients, whereas gliomas were equally common in both groups. Perhaps this is because meningiomas have a greater predilection to occur in proximity to the frontal lobes, where lesions are often associated with behavior changes. Furthermore, because of their location and slow growth, meningiomas often produce few focal signs and less obvious symptoms and therefore are associated with an increased likelihood that the patient will first present to a psychiatrist. For the most part, however, tumor type seems to be less important than other factors in determining the presence and nature of neuropsychiatric symptoms.

In general, the factors that most significantly influence symptom formation appear to be the extent of tumor involvement, the rapidity of its growth, and its propensity to cause increased intracranial pressure. In addition, the patient's premorbid psychiatric history, level of functioning, and characteristic psychological coping mechanisms may play a significant contributing role in determining the nature of a patient's particular symptoms. Lesion location may often, in fact, play a relatively minor role.

Nonetheless, many physicians still tend to search for certain neuropsychiatric syndromes that are characteristic of lesions located in specific neuroanatomical regions. One reason for this may be that much of what we now know about tumors and their associated psychopathology is based on retrospective, uncontrolled single case reports and clinical series. These studies often describe the nature of the symptoms associated with mass lesions occurring in particular locations rather than prospectively comparing the relative frequencies of behavior changes associated with tumors occurring in various regions of the brain. One older study (Keschner et al. 1936) examined the comparative types of psychiatric symptoms in pa-

tients with tumors of the frontal and temporal lobes and found few differences (Figure 19–3). Of course, this should not be very surprising, given the intimate anatomical interconnections between these two brain regions. Nonetheless, many of the earlier autopsy studies have supported the conclusion that the types of behavior changes observed with brain tumors tend to be similar, regardless of the specific anatomical brain region involved (Keschner et al. 1936; Schlesinger 1950; Selecki 1965).

Overall, then, lesion location is probably not the most important factor in determining the occurrence of specific types of neuropsychiatric symptoms. However, there have been some reports that brain lesions in certain locations may be associated with increased frequency of psychiatric symptoms. For example, although Keschner et al. (1936) found no overall difference in the types of behavioral symptoms associated with tumors of the frontal and temporal lobes, they did find that, to a small degree, complex visual and auditory hallucinations were more common among patients with tumors of the temporal lobe and that "facetiousness" was more frequently found among those with tumors of the frontal lobe. Behavior changes are twice as likely to occur among patients with supratentorial tumors than among those with infratentorial tumors (Keschner et al. 1938). Likewise, mental changes tended to be early symptoms in 18% of the patients with supratentorial tumors but in only 5% of those with infratentorial tumors. Psychiatric disturbances also were found to be more common among patients with tumors of the frontal and temporal lobes than in those with tumors of the parietal or occipital lobes.

Psychotic symptoms tend to be particularly frequent among patients with tumors of the temporal lobes and pituitary gland and much less common among those with occipital and cerebellar tumors, although this finding seems to depend on the particular study being reviewed (Davison and Bagley 1969). This underscores one of the major difficulties in comparing clinical series, especially when they were conducted during different time periods. Most of the available literature antedates the development of our current diagnostic system for classifying psychiatric clinical phenomenology, and therefore significant nosological and methodological problems result when one attempts to compare the conclusions of such older series either with each other or with more recent studies.

Despite these limitations, the literature taken as a whole seems to support a higher frequency of behavior changes among patients with lesions of the frontal and temporal lobes, as well as those with lesions involving deep midline structures. Similarly, bilateral tumors and those with multifocal involvement appear to be more frequently associated with neuropsychiatric symptoms.

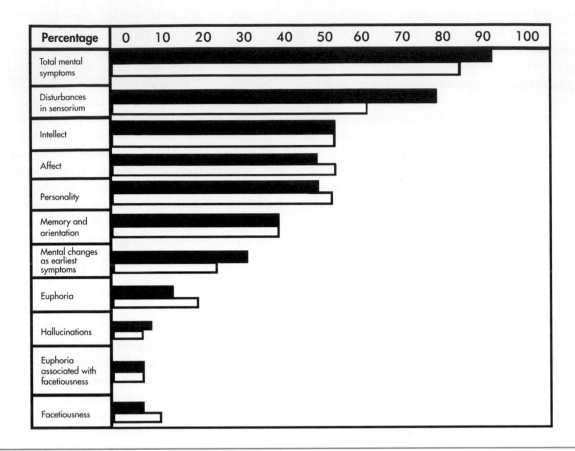

FIGURE 19–3. Comparison of incidence of mental symptoms in 110 patients with tumors of the temporal lobe (*solid bars*) and in 64 patients with tumors of the frontal lobe (*open bars*).

Source. Reprinted from Keschner M, Bender MB, Strauss I: "Mental Symptoms in Cases of Tumor of the Temporal Lobe." *Archives of Neurology and Psychiatry* 35:572–596, 1936. Copyright 1936, American Medical Association. Used with permission.

GENERAL NEUROPSYCHOLOGICAL CONSIDERATIONS

Neuropsychological testing is often useful in patients with CNS neoplasms. Although neuropsychological testing was initially used to provide diagnostic information about the location and nature of brain tumors, the current widespread availability of CT and MRI, and the consequent greater capacity for precise anatomical localization, has lessened the use of neuropsychological testing for diagnostic purposes. Currently, neuropsychological testing is most often used to determine the extent of cognitive dysfunction associated with a tumor, to provide a preoperative baseline measure of cognitive or memory functioning, or to monitor the efficacy and progress of cognitive rehabilitation efforts after treatment.

The histological type and rate of growth of a tumor may affect the nature and severity of cognitive symptoms. For example, rapidly growing, invasive tumors, such as glioblastoma multiforme, have long been thought to cause obvious cognitive dysfunction, whereas slower-growing,

noninvasive tumors, such as meningiomas, have not as frequently been associated with obvious cognitive changes or with focal neurological deficits at all (Reitan and Wolfson 1985). However, a more recent, well-controlled study did not find significant differences between patients with glioblastomas and those without glioblastomas on a battery of neuropsychological tests (Scheibel et al. 1996). In patients with slower-growing tumors, the degree to which cognitive deficits will become clinically apparent is substantially affected by the individual's level of intelligence and adaptive functioning before the development of the tumor. Thus, patients with higher premorbid IQs tend to have greater cognitive and intellectual reserves, as well as a broader range of coping and adaptive skills, which allow them to compensate for and conceal emerging cognitive impairments more successfully for longer periods. In addition, younger patients may be less likely than older patients to manifest cognitive and behavioral deficits (Bigler 1984).

In addition to the diffuse disruption of cognitive functioning secondary to these tumor-associated phenomena, other factors may result in cognitive deficits that do not reflect the anatomical location of the tumor. Specific patterns of deficits may be linked to anatomical location (Scheibel et al. 1996), and the tumor also may produce disruption of brain function in nonadjacent regions. According to Lezak (1995), several types of "distance effects" may be important in determining the types of deficits found on neuropsychological testing. First, diaschisis refers to impairment of neuronal activity in a functionally related but distant region of the brain (von Monakow 1914). Second, disconnection of a given region of the brain from a more distant region by a structural lesion can also affect the cognitive expression of the symptom. This has been dramatically demonstrated in patients who have undergone surgical sectioning of the corpus callosum as treatment for intractable seizures.

Despite its methodological and nosological limitations, the large body of descriptive literature addressing neuropsychiatric and neuropsychological symptoms associated with brain tumors over the past several decades has clearly documented that a broad array of behavior and cognitive changes may result from tumors of the brain. Thus, it underscores the need for psychiatrists to consider the possibility of an underlying brain tumor when initially evaluating any psychiatric patient. It also helps the psychiatrist in better understanding, evaluating, and treating patients with known brain tumors who have neuropsychiatric and neuropsychological symptoms. Finally, despite the generally weak association between lesion location and specific psychiatric, behavioral, and cognitive symptomatology, the literature does describe selected constellations of neuropsychiatric symptoms that are seen more frequently in patients with tumors involving certain brain regions. Thus, Hahn et al. (2003) reported that on a battery of standardized neuropsychological tests, patients with left hemisphere tumors had significantly more depressive symptoms and reported more problems with memory, inattentiveness, distractibility, and verbal fluency. Recognition of the localizing value of these associations may lead the clinician to consider organic pathology more strongly in certain patients and perhaps to pursue more vigorously the diagnosis of a previously unsuspected brain tumor.

SPECIFIC NEUROPSYCHIATRIC AND NEUROPSYCHOLOGICAL SYMPTOMS AND BRAIN TUMOR LOCATION

In the discussion that follows, we review the range of neuropsychiatric and neuropsychological signs and symptoms that have been observed to co-occur preferentially with brain tumors involving various anatomical structures, including the frontal, temporal, parietal, and occipital lobes; the diencephalon; the corpus callosum; the pituitary; and the posterior fossa.

TUMORS OF THE FRONTAL LOBE

Neuropsychiatric and Behavioral Manifestations

Tumors of the frontal lobes are frequently associated with behavioral symptoms. One study reported mental changes in as many as 90% of cases (Strauss and Keschner 1935). Of these patients, 43% manifested such changes early in the course of their illness. This is not surprising when one considers that higher-level executive and cognitive functions are mediated by this region of the cortex. Rather than being homogeneous and unidimensional in their functions, the frontal lobes are made up of a variety of functionally distinct subregions. These areas are involved in several related and unrelated tasks, such as the mediation of problem-solving behavior, the regulation of attentional processes, the temporal organization of behavior, and the modulation of affective states (McAllister and Price 1987).

Injuries to the frontal lobes have been associated with three kinds of clinical syndromes (Cummings 1993). The orbitofrontal syndrome is characterized by changes in personality. These patients typically present with irritability and lability. Cognitively, patients with this syndrome often have poor judgment and a lack of insight into their behavior. These patients have sometimes been referred to as *pseudopsychopathic* (McAllister and Price 1987).

Conversely, patients with injury to the frontal convexities, the so-called dorsolateral prefrontal syndrome, often present with apathy, indifference, and psychomotor retardation. Cognitively, such patients have difficulty initiating or persisting in behavioral activities and have problems with sustained attention and/or sequencing, and they may show perseverative behavior (Goldberg 1986). These deficits may not be especially apparent on standard intellectual or neuropsychological assessments, but they usually become apparent with more specific tests of executive functioning, such as the Wisconsin Card Sorting Test (Goldberg 1986; Heaton 1985). Patients with this syndrome have been referred to as being *pseudodepressed* because the apathy, aspontaneity, and abulia with which they often present resemble the classic symptoms of major depression (McAllister and Price 1987).

Finally, an anterior cingulate syndrome has been described. Patients with this syndrome may be akinetic with mutism and an inability to respond to commands.

Despite the occurrence of these three syndromes as relatively distinct entities compared with other types of disorders of the frontal lobe, most patients with tumors of the frontal lobe present with a combination of symptoms. This is probably due in part to the fact that tumors of the frontal lobe are rarely confined to a single subregion of the frontal lobe and may be causing effects on other areas, both directly and indirectly via pressure effects and edema, as well as by diaschisis and disconnection. It is therefore difficult to find clear descriptions of these three syndromes in pure form when reviewing the literature on neoplasms of the frontal lobe. Psychiatric symptoms also appear to be more common in patients with lesions of the anterior frontal lobe than in those with lesions of the posterior frontal lobe, suggesting that tumor location on the anteroposterior gradient within the frontal lobe may play a significant role in determining clinical presentation (Gautier-Smith 1970).

Psychiatric and behavioral presentations of frontal lobe tumors can be quite variable. Anxiety has been described and has been noted to increase with tumor progression (Kaplan and Miner 1997). Affective symptoms are common and can include depression, irritability, apathy, and euphoria. Often psychomotor retardation with aspontaneity, hypokinesia, or akinesia is present. In one study of 25 patients with frontal lobe tumors (Direkze et al. 1971), 5 (20%) had initially presented to psychiatric units with what appeared to be mood disturbances. In their study of 85 patients, Strauss and Keschner (1935) reported affective symptoms in 63%, of whom 30% presented with euphoria and 4% presented with hypomania. Although these authors found no correlation between clinical presentations and laterality of lesions, Belyi (1987) noted a tendency for patients with right frontal lesions to present with euphoria, whereas those with left frontal lesions tended to present with akinesia, abulia, and depressed affect. Another study reported psychiatric symptoms only in patients with right frontal as opposed to left frontal meningiomas (Lampl et al. 1995). A study by Burns and Swerdlow (2003) reported pedophilia and constructional apraxia signs and symptoms occurring in association with a right orbitofrontal tumor.

Changes in personality have been found in as many as 70% of patients with frontal lobe tumors (Strauss and Keschner 1935). These changes, which have been described as "characteristic" of frontal lobe disease (Pincus and Tucker 1978), include irresponsibility, childishness, facetiousness, disinhibition, and indifference toward others, as well as inappropriate sexual behavior. The term *witzelsucht* has been used to describe the tendency of patients with frontal lobe lesions to make light of everything. This humorous bent often has an angry, sarcastic, cutting quality to it. Although these behaviors are consistent with descriptions of the characteristic features of or-

bitofrontal syndrome, it should be noted that similar "frontal lobe" personality changes have been described in patients with temporal lobe and diencephalic lesions, probably as a result of the rich, reciprocal interconnections that link the temporal, limbic, and frontal regions.

Psychotic symptoms occur with some regularity in patients with frontal lobe tumors. Strauss and Keschner (1935) reported a 10% incidence of both delusions and hallucinations in their series. Other psychotic symptoms reported in patients with frontal lobe tumors have included paranoid ideation and ideas of reference. Typically, delusions secondary to intracranial tumors are less complex than those that occur as part of the delusional systems of schizophrenic patients. Likewise, simple rather than complex hallucinations and visual rather than auditory hallucinations tend to occur in patients with brain tumors.

Hypersomnolence also has been reported in these patients (Frazier 1935). A careful psychiatric assessment and evaluation of mental status may be needed to clearly differentiate this symptom from the lethargy and fatigue often encountered in patients with major depression. The presence of leg weakness, gait abnormalities, or urinary incontinence with psychiatric and behavioral symptoms should strongly indicate the need for a thorough search for frontal lobe pathology.

Neuropsychological Manifestations

Cognitively, patients with tumors of the frontal region of the brain, and of the prefrontal area in particular, often present with significant behavior changes in the absence of obvious intellectual decline or focal neurological dysfunction. In such patients, previously acquired cognitive skills are often preserved, and performance on formal intelligence testing may be quite adequate. More sophisticated neuropsychological assessment of executive functioning, however, often detects profound deficits in the individual's ability to organize, initiate, and direct personal behavior (Lezak 1995; Teuber 1972). Deficits in executive functioning, which disrupt the very core of an individual's drive, initiative, and integration as well as the ability to carry out critical higher cognitive functions, are often the most devastating and disabling types of cognitive dysfunction encountered in neurological, neurosurgical, and psychiatric patients.

Tumors of the frontal lobes also can result in significant deficits in attentional processes. In addition, tumors of the posterior frontal lobe can lead to expressive (Broca's) aphasia, when the lesion is localized to the dominant hemisphere (Benson 1979), or aprosody, when it is localized to the anterior nondominant hemisphere (Ross 1988).

TUMORS OF THE TEMPORAL LOBE

Neuropsychiatric and Behavioral Manifestations

In any discussion of the psychiatric and behavioral symptoms associated with tumors of the temporal lobe, it is important to distinguish between seizure-associated and non-seizure-associated symptoms and, within the former category, ictal and interictal phenomena. Ictal phenomena are discussed by Kim et al. in Chapter 16 of this book. In this section, we confine our discussion to non-seizure-associated and interictal symptoms due to temporal lobe tumors.

Patients with temporal lobe tumors have been noted to have a high frequency of schizophrenia-like illnesses. Malamud (1967) reported that 6 (55%) of 11 patients with temporal lobe tumors initially presented with a diagnosis of schizophrenia. Selecki (1965) reported that an initial diagnosis of schizophrenia had been made in 2 of his 9 patients with temporal lobe tumors, and he reported auditory hallucinations in 5. More recently, G.W. Roberts et al. (1990) reported that gangliogliomas, neoplastic hamartomatous lesions that preferentially involve the left medial temporal lobes, are frequently found in patients with delayed-onset, schizophrenia-like psychoses associated with chronic temporal lobe epilepsy.

Again, it must be borne in mind that many of these studies were published before the advent of DSM-IV diagnostic criteria (American Psychiatric Association 1994) and that therefore clinicians may have had a tendency to overdiagnose schizophrenia. In fact, many of the case descriptions of Malamud (1967) do not indicate that the patients had clear evidence of psychotic symptoms such as delusions, hallucinations, or formal thought disorder. Patients with temporal lobe dysfunction due to tumors or other causes often present with psychotic symptoms that are somewhat atypical for classic schizophrenia. These symptoms include episodic mood swings with suicidal ideation or attempts and visual, olfactory, and tactile hallucinations, as well as the auditory hallucinations more typically seen in schizophrenic patients (Tucker et al. 1986). Patients with schizophrenia-like psychoses due to temporal lobe disease often report having "spells" or dreamlike episodes, as well as "staring" behavior or "dazed feelings" (Tucker et al. 1986). Unlike schizophrenic patients with notably flat or inappropriate affect and a markedly diminished capacity to interact with and relate appropriately to others, patients with psychoses associated with temporal lobe disease often manifest broad-range and appropriate affect and interact with and relate to others in a relatively normal fashion. Supporting the association between psychotic symptomatology and temporal lobe tumors is the work of Davison and Bagley (1969), who reviewed 77 psychotic patients with known brain neoplasms and found that tumors of the temporal lobes were most frequent.

Other studies, however, have not confirmed the apparent high frequency of psychotic syndromes in patients with temporal lobe tumors. Keschner et al. (1936) studied 110 such patients and found that only 2 had complex hallucinations. In another study (Mulder and Daly 1952), only 4 (4%) of 100 patients with temporal lobe tumors had psychotic symptoms. Strobos (1953) noted complex auditory hallucinations in only 1 (1%) of his 62 patients with temporal lobe tumors. He found complex visual hallucinations in 5 (8%) and simple olfactory or gustatory hallucinations in 19 (31%), although these almost invariably immediately preceded the onset of seizures.

Regardless of how often specific psychotic symptoms may occur with temporal lobe tumors, these lesions are commonly associated with behavioral disturbances. Neuropsychiatric symptoms associated with temporal lobe tumors tend to be similar to those seen in patients with frontal lobe tumors and may include depressed mood with apathy and irritability or euphoric, expansive mood with hypomania or mania. As noted previously, this probably results from the complex interconnections among the frontal lobes, temporal lobes, and related structures within the limbic system.

Personality change has been described in more than 50% of patients with temporal lobe tumors and may be an early symptom thereof (Keschner et al. 1936). Research by Bear and Fedio (1977) suggests that characteristic interictal personality traits occur in patients with temporal lobe epilepsy and, furthermore, that the presence or absence of certain traits depends on whether the seizure focus is in the right or the left temporal lobe. More recent studies (Mungas 1982; Rodin and Schmaltz 1984), however, failed to confirm these initial findings. Thus, there do not appear to be specific interictal personality traits that are characteristic of temporal lobe lesions. Often patients present with an intensification of premorbid character traits or with symptoms similar to those seen in conjunction with frontal lobe tumors. Personality changes caused by brain tumors, including affective lability, episodic behavioral dyscontrol, intermittent anger, irritability, euphoria, and facetiousness, are also commonly seen (Lishman 1987).

Anxiety symptoms appear to be quite commonly associated with temporal lobe tumors. Mulder and Daly (1952) noted anxiety in 36 (36%) of their 100 patients. Two cases of panic attacks in patients with right temporal lobe tumors have been reported (Drubach and Kelly 1989; Ghadirian et al. 1986), although the number of cases is obviously too small to draw any conclusions about the influence of laterality on the appearance of such phenomena. However, these case reports are consistent with work by Reiman et al. (1986) showing abnormally low ratios of left-to-right parahippocampal blood flow in patients with panic disorder who were vulnerable to lactate-induced panic. The authors suggested that this asymmetry could be secondary to increases in neuronal activity, anatomical asymmetry, or an increase in blood-brain barrier permeability in the right parahippocampal region. Such mechanisms also could occur in conjunction with temporal lobe tumors.

Neuropsychological Manifestations

Tumors of the temporal lobes can also result in neuropsychological and cognitive deficits. First, verbal or nonverbal memory functioning may be affected, depending on the cerebral hemisphere involved. Dysfunction of the dominant temporal lobe is often associated with deficits in the ability to learn and remember verbal information, whereas that of the nondominant temporal lobe is often associated with deficits in acquiring and retaining nonverbal (i.e., visuospatial) information (Bauer et al. 1993; Butters and Milotis 1979). Tumors of the dominant temporal lobe also may result in receptive (Wernicke's) aphasia, whereas tumors of the nondominant lobe may lead to disruption of the discrimination of nonspeech sounds (Spreen et al. 1965).

Because of the high incidence of seizure disorders in patients with tumors of the temporal lobes (Strobos 1953), cognitive dysfunction in such patients may result directly from seizure activity; indirectly from dysfunction in other areas of the brain through diaschisis or disconnection; or from the administration of certain anticonvulsants, especially when they are used in high doses, for long periods, or as part of multidrug regimens.

TUMORS OF THE PARIETAL LOBE

Neuropsychiatric and Behavioral Manifestations

In general, tumors of the parietal lobe are less likely to cause behavior changes than are tumors in other locations; they are relatively "silent" with respect to psychiatric symptoms (Critchley 1964). This has been well documented in large comparative studies of psychiatric and behavioral phenomenology as a function of the anatomical location of various brain tumors. Schlesinger (1950) found affective symptoms in only 5 (16%) of 31 patients with parietal lobe tumors. The affective symptoms in these patients were predominantly depression and apa-

thy, rather than euphoria or mania, a finding consistent with the previous report of Keschner et al. (1938). Case studies also have reported depression in a woman with a left parietal lesion (Madhusoodanan et al. 2004) and mania in patients with right parietal tumors (Khouzam et al. 1994; Salazar-Calderon Perriggo et al. 1993).

Psychotic symptoms also appear to be less common in patients with parietal lobe tumors than in those with other types of lesions. Selecki (1965), however, reported episodes of "paranoid psychosis" in 2 of the 7 patients with parietal lobe tumors in his series. Cotard's syndrome, involving the denial of one's own existence, has been reported in a patient with a left parietal astrocytoma (Bhatia 1993).

Neuropsychological Manifestations

Of greater significance than the psychiatric and behavioral symptoms associated with parietal lobe tumors are the complex sensory and motor abnormalities that may accompany them. In general, parietal lobe tumors are more likely to lead to cognitive than to psychiatric symptoms. Depending on the location of a neoplasm within the parietal lobes, a variety of neuropsychological abnormalities may be observed.

Tumors of the anterior parietal lobes may result in abnormalities of sensory perception in the contralateral hand. Inability of the individual to perceive objects placed in the hand (astereognosis) is common and may have localizing value to the contralateral parietal cortex. Difficulty in recognizing shapes, letters, and numbers drawn on the hand (agraphesthesia) is common and may aid in localizing neoplasms to the parietal lobes. Apraxias also may be present. Parietal lobe tumors may interfere with the ability to decipher visuospatial information, particularly when they are localized to the nondominant hemisphere (Warrington and Rabin 1970).

Tumors of the dominant parietal lobe may lead to dysgraphia, acalculia, finger agnosia, and right-left confusion (Gerstmann's syndrome) and often affect reading and spelling. Individuals with parietal lobe tumors often present with a marked lack of awareness or even frank denial of their neurological and neuropsychiatric difficulties, even in the face of rather obvious dysfunctions, such as hemiparesis. Such phenomena are referred to as *anosognosia* or *neglect syndromes*. Because of the often bizarre neurological complaints and atypical symptoms that may accompany parietal lobe tumors, patients with these lesions are often thought to have psychiatric problems and often initially receive misdiagnoses of either a conversion disorder or some other type of somatization disorder (Jones and Barklage 1990).

TUMORS OF THE OCCIPITAL LOBE

Neuropsychiatric and Behavioral Manifestations

Patients with tumors of the occipital lobe also may present with psychiatric symptoms, but like patients with tumors involving the parietal lobes, they have been reported to be less likely to do so than those with tumors of the frontal or temporal lobes (Keschner et al. 1938). In 1930, Allen found psychiatric symptoms in 55% of a large series ($N = 40$) of patients with occipital lobe tumors. In 17% of these patients, behavioral symptoms had been the presenting complaint. The most characteristic finding was visual hallucinations, which were present in 25% of the patients. These hallucinations tended to be simple and unformed and were frequently merely flashes of light. Only 2 patients had complex visual hallucinations.

Other symptoms that have been observed in patients with occipital lobe tumors include agitation, irritability, suspiciousness, and fatigue, although Allen (1930) believed that many of these symptoms (other than the visual hallucinations) were nonspecific effects of increased intracranial pressure. Keschner et al. (1938) observed affective symptoms in 5 (45%) of 11 patients with occipital lobe tumors. Three (27%) of these patients were dysphoric, and 2 (18%) presented with euphoria or facetiousness.

Neuropsychological Manifestations

Tumors of the occipital lobes may cause significant and characteristic difficulties in cognitive and perceptual functions. A typical finding in patients with occipital lobe neoplasms is homonymous hemianopsia, the loss of one-half of the visual field in each eye. Inability to recognize items visually (visual agnosia) also may be seen (Lezak 1995). Inability to recognize familiar faces, a condition known as *prosopagnosia*, also may accompany neoplastic lesions in the occipital lobes, particularly when they are bilateral (Meadows 1974).

DIENCEPHALIC TUMORS

Neuropsychiatric and Behavioral Manifestations

Tumors of the diencephalon (thalamus, hypothalamus, and the structures surrounding the third ventricle) typically involve regions that are part of or closely contiguous to the limbic system. These lesions also interrupt the various cortical-striatal-pallidal-thalamic-cortical loops, which affect many frontal lobe functions (Alexander and Crutcher 1990). It is therefore not surprising that these lesions are often associated with psychiatric and behavioral disturbances. For example, Malamud (1967) reported diagnoses of schizophrenia in 4 of 7 patients with tumors involving structures near the third ventricle. Cairns and Mosberg (1951) reported "emotional instability" and psychosis in patients with colloid cysts of the third ventricle. Burkle and Lipowski (1978) also reported depression, affective flattening, and withdrawal in a patient with a colloid cyst of the third ventricle. Personality changes similar to those seen in patients with frontal lobe disease (Gutmann et al. 1990), akinetic mutism (Cairns et al. 1941), catatonia (Neuman et al. 1996), and obsessive-compulsive disorder (Gamazo-Garran et al. 2002) have all been reported in patients with diencephalic or deep midline tumors.

Hypothalamic tumors have been associated with disorders of eating behavior, including hyperphagia (Coffey 1989), and with symptoms indistinguishable from those of anorexia nervosa (Lin et al. 2003). Chipkevitch (1994) reported on 21 cases in the literature in which patients with brain lesions presented with symptoms consistent with a diagnosis of anorexia nervosa. Eleven (52%) of these patients had tumors of the hypothalamus. In 8 of these patients, surgical resection or radiation treatment led to improvement in the symptoms of anorexia. Patients with lesions of the hypothalamus also can present with hypersomnia and daytime somnolence.

Neuropsychological Manifestations

Neoplasms originating in subcortical brain regions often have their most dramatic effects on memory. These lesions often result in significant impairment in the retrieval of learned material, whereas other aspects of neuropsychological functioning may appear to be relatively intact on initial evaluation (Lishman 1987). However, detailed neuropsychological evaluation of a patient with a subcortical tumor may identify a pattern of "subcortical dementia" characterized by a general slowing of thought processes, forgetfulness, apathy, abulia, and depression and an impaired ability to manipulate acquired knowledge (Cummings 1990). Tumors in this area also may lead indirectly to more diffuse, generalized cognitive dysfunction by interfering with the normal circulation of cerebrospinal fluid (CSF), causing hydrocephalus.

TUMORS OF THE CORPUS CALLOSUM

Tumors of the corpus callosum have been associated with behavioral symptoms in as many as 90% of patients (Selecki 1964). Such symptoms appear to be most common in patients with tumors of the genu and splenium (Schlesinger 1950), probably because of involvement of adjacent structures (i.e., the frontal lobes and deep midline and limbic structures). Although a broad array of behavior changes, including psychosis and personality changes, have been reported, affective symptoms appear to be particularly common with tumors involving this area. In one study, patients with corpus callosum tumors were compared with patients with other types of tumors. Significantly more depression was found in the group with tumors of the corpus callosum (Nasrallah and McChesney 1981). One of these patients had received a trial of tricyclic antidepressants (TCAs) for a presumed primary affective disorder before emerging neurological symptoms led to the correct diagnosis. Tanaghow et al. (1989) also described a patient with a corpus callosum tumor without focal neurological findings who had initially presented with atypical features of depression and prominent cognitive deficits.

PITUITARY TUMORS

Patients with pituitary tumors often present with behavior changes resulting from upward extension of the tumor to other structures, particularly those in the diencephalon. This is a common occurrence in patients with craniopharyngiomas, who sometimes present with disorders of sleep or temperature regulation, clinical phenomena that are ordinarily more common with tumors of the hypothalamus. Anorexia nervosa syndromes also have been reported in patients with craniopharyngiomas (Chipkevitch 1994).

Tumors of the pituitary also can result in endocrine disturbances, which can cause neuropsychiatric symptoms. Basophilic adenomas are commonly associated with Cushing's syndrome, which is likewise often associated with affective lability, depression, or psychotic symptoms. Patients with acidophilic adenomas often present with acromegaly, which has been associated, although infrequently, with both anxiety and depression (Avery 1973).

As with brain tumors involving other anatomical locations, the entire spectrum of psychiatric symptoms, from depression and apathy (Weitzner et al. 2005) to paranoia, has been reported to occur in patients with pituitary tumors. One review of 5 patients with pituitary lesions reported delusions and hallucinations in 3 (60%) (White and Cobb 1955). In a study by Russell and Pennybacker (1961), 8 (33%) of 24 patients had severe mental disturbances that dominated their clinical picture, and 3 (13%) had initially presented to psychiatric hospitals for diagnosis and treatment. The broad spectrum of psychiatric and behavioral symptoms associated with pituitary tumors probably reflects the direct and indirect involvement of diencephalic and hypothalamic structures, as well as the effects of various endocrine dysfunctions.

TUMORS OF THE POSTERIOR FOSSA

Patients with infratentorial tumors present with psychiatric symptoms less often than do those with other types of tumors. The wide variety of behavioral symptoms that may occur in patients with such tumors again underscores the difficulty of localizing lesions on the basis of the typology of associated psychiatric symptoms. Although they are less common overall, all of the psychiatric and behavioral disturbances that have been described in patients with supratentorial tumors also have been reported in patients with infratentorial and posterior fossa lesions.

In one series, psychiatric and behavioral symptoms were found in 76% of the patients with lesions of the posterior fossa and included paranoid delusions and affective disorders (Wilson and Rupp 1946). Pollack et al. (1996) also reported affective disorders, psychosis, personality change, and somatization in their small series. Cases of mania also have been noted (e.g., Greenberg and Brown 1985). Tumors of the posterior fossa have been reported to be associated with irritability, apathy, hypersomnolence, and auditory hallucinations (Cairns 1950). Visual hallucinations have been reported in conjunction with tumors compressing the midbrain (Dunn and Weisberg 1983; Nadvi and van Dellen 1994), and manic or mixed states have been described in 3 adults with acoustic neuroma (Kalayam et al. 1994). Overanxious disorder of childhood with school phobia was reported in a 12-year-old boy with a fourth-ventricle tumor (Blackman and Wheler 1987). The anxiety symptoms were alleviated by surgical removal of the tumor. Overall, however, no convincing correlation has been established between tumors involving particular anatomical structures within the posterior fossa and the occurrence of specific psychiatric or behavioral symptomatology.

LATERALITY OF BRAIN TUMORS AND CLINICAL MANIFESTATIONS

Despite the fact that many older studies reported no consistent differences in the psychiatric and behavioral symptoms associated with left- and right-sided tumors, more recent studies have raised questions about this. The importance of cerebral hemispheric lateralization was elegantly demonstrated by Robinson et al. (1984) in their work with stroke patients. This work found an increased frequency of depression in patients with left anterior lesions and a tendency toward inappropriate cheerfulness in patients with right anterior lesions. Although few reports have specifically addressed these findings in cohorts of patients with brain tumors, studies reviewing cases of mania secondary to mixed CNS lesions, including tumors, have found a preponderance of right hemisphere lesions (Cummings and Mendez 1984; Jamieson and Wells 1979; Starkstein et al. 1988). A study of unilateral frontal tumors (Belyi 1987) reported that left-sided lesions were commonly associated with akinesia and depression, whereas right-sided lesions were more often associated with euphoria and underestimation of the seriousness of their illnesses by the patients in the study. Pringle et al. (1999) also reported a higher incidence of psychiatric disturbances overall in women with left-sided lesions. Anxiety, on the other hand, may be more common with right hemisphere tumors (Mainio et al. 2003).

These studies suggest that lesion laterality may be a more important factor in symptom formation than had previously been thought. In addition, overall, the available literature suggests the need to reevaluate tumor location and its implications for neuropsychiatric and neuropsychological symptomatology from a different, more topographical perspective. Investigators should consider not only specific regional anatomical localization but also factors such as laterality, anterior/posterior and cortical/subcortical location, and afferent and efferent projections between the region directly involved with the tumor and distant anatomical regions. More important, such a perspective will provide a more clinically relevant, although necessarily more complex, theoretical framework from which to approach the study of psychopathological symptoms and syndromes associated with brain tumors. Future studies of brain tumor–associated psychopathology patterned after the work of Robinson et al. (1984) should further enhance our understanding not only of these secondary psychiatric and behavioral symptoms and syndromes but also of the anatomical substrates of many primary psychiatric disorders.

CLINICAL DIAGNOSIS

GENERAL CLINICAL CHARACTERISTICS OF BRAIN TUMORS

For clinicians, especially psychiatrists, prompt and accurate diagnosis of brain tumors rests on awareness of the many clinical manifestations they may produce. A high index of suspicion and willingness to pursue vigorously the appropriate specialty consultations and diagnostic studies are critical to early diagnosis.

The most characteristic clinical feature of CNS tumors is the progressive appearance of focal neurological signs and symptoms in addition to neuropsychiatric symptoms. These are actually more frequent than the neurological signs and symptoms in early brain tumors and may include changes in personality and affect, altered sensorium, and cognitive and memory dysfunction. The specific constellation of clinical phenomena encountered and how rapidly they progress depend on the type, size, location, and rate of growth of the tumor; whether it is benign or malignant; and, if the latter, how aggressive it is and whether there is associated cerebral edema, increased intracranial pressure, and hydrocephalus.

Typical neurological signs and symptoms associated with brain tumors include headaches (25%–35%), nausea and vomiting (33%), seizures (20%–50%), papilledema, and visual changes, including field cuts and diplopia. Focal motor and sensory changes are of considerable value in localizing the tumor (Table 19–3).

WHEN TO SUSPECT A BRAIN TUMOR IN A PSYCHIATRIC PATIENT

Although recognition of brain tumors in patients presenting with characteristic focal neurological signs and symptoms should not ordinarily be problematic, it may be quite difficult to diagnose a brain tumor promptly and accurately in a patient presenting with predominantly psychiatric and behavioral symptoms. However, the occurrence of one or more of the following five signs and symptoms in a known psychiatric patient or in a patient presenting for the first time with psychiatric symptoms should heighten the clinician's index of suspicion regarding the possibility of a brain tumor:

1. Seizures, especially if of new onset in an adult and if focal or partial, with or without secondary generalization; seizures may be the initial neurological manifestation of a tumor in as many as 50% of cases
2. Headaches, especially if of new onset; generalized and dull (i.e., nonspecific); of increasing severity and/or frequency; or positional, nocturnal, or present immediately on awakening
3. Nausea and vomiting, especially in conjunction with headaches
4. Sensory changes: visual changes such as loss or diminution of vision, visual field defects, or diplopia; auditory changes such as tinnitus or hearing loss, especially when unilateral; and vertigo
5. Other focal neurological signs and symptoms, such as localized weakness, localized sensory loss, paresthesias or dysesthesias, ataxia, and incoordination

The clinician should bear in mind that nausea and vomiting, visual field defects, papilledema, and other focal neurological signs and symptoms often are not seen early in the course of many brain tumors. These signs may not be seen until very late, especially with "silent" tumors, such as meningiomas or slow-growing astrocytomas, and other kinds of tumors occurring in relatively "silent" locations (see subsection "Physical and Neurological Examinations" later in this chapter).

TABLE 19–3.   Neurological and neuropsychological findings with localizing value

Brain region	Neurological and neuropsychological findings
Frontal lobes	
Prefrontal	Contralateral grasp reflex, executive functioning deficits (inability to formulate goals, to plan, and to effectively carry out these plans), decreased oral fluency (dominant hemisphere), decreased design fluency (nondominant hemisphere), motor perseveration or impersistence, and inability to hold set
Posterior	Contralateral hemiparesis; decreased motor strength, speed, and coordination; and Broca's aphasia
Temporal lobes	Partial complex seizures, contralateral homonymous inferior quadrantanopsia, Wernicke's aphasia, decreased learning and retention of verbal material (dominant hemisphere), decreased learning and retention of nonverbal material (nondominant hemisphere), amusia (nondominant hemisphere), and auditory agnosia
Parietal lobes	Partial sensory seizures, agraphesthesia, astereognosis, anosognosia, Gerstmann's syndrome (acalculia, agraphia, finger agnosia, and right-left confusion), ideomotor and ideational apraxia, constructional apraxia, agraphia with alexia, dressing apraxia, prosopagnosia, and visuospatial problems
Occipital lobes	Partial sensory seizures with visual phenomena, homonymous hemianopsia, alexia, agraphia, prosopagnosia, color agnosia, and constructional apraxia
Corpus callosum	Callosal apraxia
Thalamus	Contralateral hemisensory loss and pain
Basal ganglia	Contralateral choreoathetosis, dystonia, rigidity, motor perseveration, and parkinsonian tremor
Pituitary	Bitemporal hemianopia, optic atrophy, hypopituitarism, and hypothalamus and diabetes insipidus
Pineal	Loss of upward gaze (Parinaud's syndrome)
Cerebellum	Ipsilateral hypotonia, ataxia, dysmetria, intention tremor, and nystagmus toward side of tumor
Brain stem	
Midbrain	Pupillary and extraocular muscle abnormalities and contralateral hemiparesis
Pons	Sixth and seventh nerve involvement (diplopia and ipsilateral facial paralysis)

Source.   Reprinted from Lohr JB, Cadet JL: "Neuropsychiatric Aspects of Brain Tumors," in *The American Psychiatric Press Textbook of Neuropsychiatry.* Edited by Talbott JA, Hales RE, Yudofsky SC. Washington, DC, American Psychiatric Press, 1987, p. 354. Used with permission.

DIAGNOSTIC EVALUATION

A comprehensive, careful, and detailed history of the nature and time course of both psychiatric and neurological signs and symptoms is the cornerstone of diagnosis. This should be supplemented by careful physical and neurological examinations, appropriate brain imaging and electrodiagnostic studies, and bedside neurocognitive assessment, including the Mini-Mental State Examination (MMSE), as well as formal neuropsychological testing.

Physical and Neurological Examinations

All psychiatric patients, and particularly those in whom the psychiatrist is considering a brain tumor in the differential diagnosis, should have full and careful physical, neurologi-

cal, and mental status examinations. Patients with brain tumors often manifest focal neurological findings as well as abnormalities in cognitive functioning on careful bedside neurocognitive testing. Table 19–3 highlights some of the more important and common localizing neurological findings that are found in association with brain tumors in various locations. It is important to be aware that even despite repeated careful clinical examinations, some brain tumors may not become clinically apparent until relatively late in their course. Such tumors often involve the anterior frontal lobes, corpus callosum, nondominant parietal and temporal lobes, and posterior fossa, the so-called silent regions. Thus, in patients with negative clinical examinations for focal neurological findings, other diagnostic studies are essential to rule out conclusively the presence of a tumor.

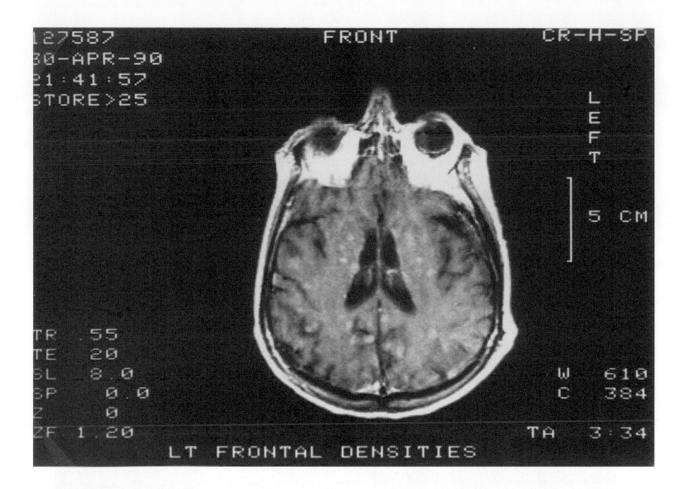

FIGURE 19–4.   Diffuse metastatic disease (small cell carcinoma of the lung) in a 66-year-old man, as seen with magnetic resonance imaging. A computed tomography scan had not shown any metastatic lesions.

Source.   Image courtesy of Dr. A. Goldberg, Department of Radiology, Allegheny General Hospital, Pittsburgh, Pennsylvania.

CT Scans

In the 1970s, the CT scan largely replaced plain skull films, radioisotope brain scans, electroencephalography, echoencephalography, and pneumoencephalography in the diagnosis of brain tumors because it provided far greater resolution of anatomical brain structures and was much more able to identify small soft-tissue mass lesions. The capacity of the CT scan to detect neoplasms has been further enhanced by the concomitant use of intravenous iodinated contrast materials, such as iohexol, that highlight tumors when they are present. CT scans can also suggest the presence of tumors by showing calcifications, cerebral edema, obstructive hydrocephalus, a shift in midline structures, or other abnormal changes in the ventricular system. Although they are extremely useful, CT scans may not identify very small tumors, tumors in the posterior fossa, tumors that are isodense with respect to brain tissue and/or CSF, and tumors diffusely involving the meninges (i.e., carcinomatosis).

MRI Scans

In general, MRI is superior to CT scanning in the diagnosis of brain tumors and other soft-tissue lesions in the brain because of its higher degree of resolution and resultant greater ability to detect very small lesions (Figures 19–4 and 19–5). In addition, MRI does not involve exposure to radiation. Its chief drawbacks are its cost and its inability to detect calcified lesions. It also cannot be used in patients in whom ferrometallic foreign objects are present. Enhancement of MRI with gadolinium further increases its diagnostic sensitivity (Figure 19–6).

Cisternography

CT cisternography, a radiographic technique for evaluating the ventricular system, subarachnoid spaces, and basilar cisterns, may be helpful in the differential diagnosis of intraventricular tumors as well as tumor-associated hydrocephalus. This technique has largely replaced pneumoencephalography, an older air-contrast imaging tech-

A

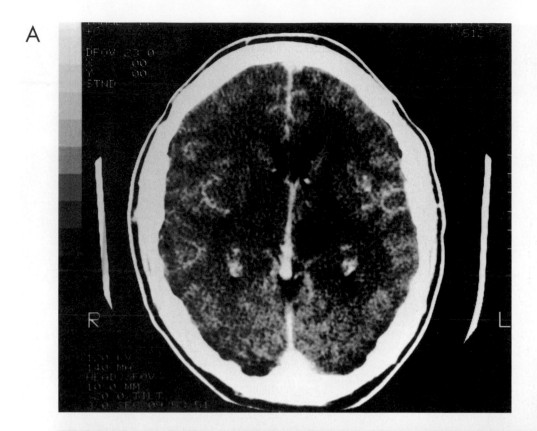

B

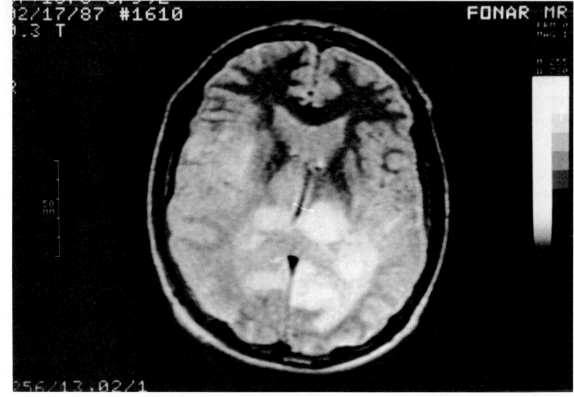

FIGURE 19–5. Brain images of a 50-year-old man with a multicentric glioma. *Panel A.* A computed tomography scan shows no evidence of tumor. *Panel B.* In a magnetic resonance imaging scan, the tumor is clearly evident.

Source. Images courtesy of Dr. A. Goldberg, Department of Radiology, Allegheny General Hospital, Pittsburgh, Pennsylvania.

A

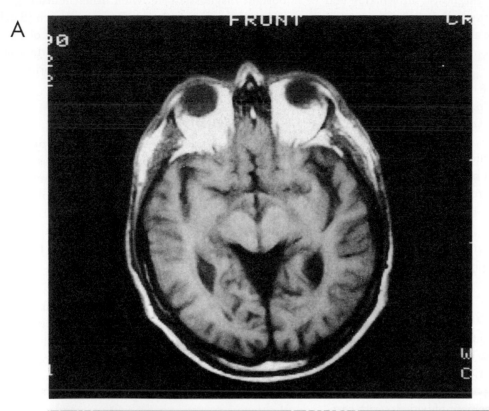

B

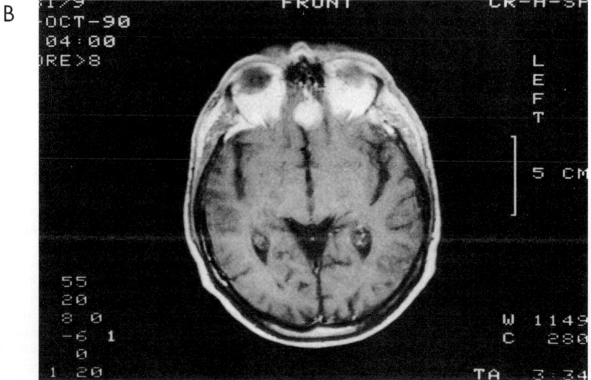

FIGURE 19–6.   Brain images of a 70-year-old man with a meningioma. *Panel A.* This tumor was not evidenced on an unenhanced magnetic resonance imaging (MRI) scan. *Panel B.* The tumor was seen clearly with a gadolinium-enhanced MRI scan.

Source.   Images courtesy of Dr. A. Goldberg, Department of Radiology, Allegheny General Hospital, Pittsburgh, Pennsylvania.

nique that provided limited diagnostic information and was poorly tolerated by patients because of associated severe headaches and nausea and vomiting.

Skull Films

Although plain skull films are no longer routinely used in the diagnosis of brain tumors, tomographs of the sella turcica may be helpful in the diagnosis of pituitary tumors, craniopharyngiomas, and the so-called empty sella syndrome. Plain skull films also may be helpful in the diagnosis of bone (skull) metastases, but bone scans are generally superior in this regard.

Cerebral Angiography

In some cases, cerebral angiography may be important in delineating the vascular supply to a brain tumor before surgery.

Neuropsychological Testing

As mentioned previously, neuropsychological testing was often used in the diagnosis and localization of brain tumors before the advent of CT and MRI. Although it is no longer used for these purposes, it still plays an important role in the overall management of patients with cerebral tumors. It can be very helpful in determining the extent of tumor-associated cognitive dysfunction and in providing baseline, preoperative, and preradiation measures of cognitive functioning. It also may be helpful in assessing the efficacy of surgery with respect to improvements in tumor-associated, preoperative, and preradiation cognitive and neuropsychological dysfunction. It is also helpful in documenting postoperative and postradiation cognitive changes and monitoring the effectiveness of rehabilitative efforts with respect to them.

Lumbar Puncture

Given the range of more sensitive, specific, and less invasive diagnostic studies currently available, lumbar puncture is now used less frequently than in the past in the diagnosis of brain tumors. Brain tumors may be associated with elevated CSF protein and increased intracranial pressure, but these findings are diagnostically nonspecific, and in the presence of the latter, herniation is a potential danger after a lumbar puncture. Therefore, before proceeding with a lumbar puncture in a patient with a brain tumor, the clinician should carefully examine the eyegrounds for indications of papilledema, and a CT or an MRI scan should be done to rule out increased intracranial pressure. With certain types of neoplastic diseases of the CNS, such as meningeal carcinomatosis and leukemia, however, lumbar puncture may play an

important diagnostic role when other neurodiagnostic studies have been unrevealing. Recent research (Batabyal et al. 2003) has suggested that measurement of carcinoembryonic antigen in the CSF may be important in the differential diagnosis and management of primary and metastatic brain tumors.

Electroencephalography

Electroencephalograms in patients with brain tumors may show nonspecific electrical abnormalities, such as spikes and slow waves, either diffuse or focal and paroxysmal or continuous. Frequently, however, the electroencephalogram is normal in such patients. It is not a very specific or sensitive test and thus is not very helpful in differentiating brain tumors from other localized structural cerebral lesions.

Other Testing

Obtaining a chest radiograph is important in evaluating brain tumors because often they may be metastatic from primary lung neoplasms. Single-photon emission computed tomography (SPECT), positron emission tomography (PET), and brain electrical activity mapping (BEAM) are newer quantitative, computer-based techniques for evaluating various aspects of brain structure and metabolic and neurophysiological functioning. At present, none of these techniques appears to have major advantages over the more standard approaches discussed previously in the routine diagnostic evaluation of brain tumors, but this may change as experience with them accumulates. SPECT may have some utility in differentiating tumor recurrence from radiation necrosis in brain tumor patients who have received radiation therapy (Figures 19–7 and 19–8) or in differentiating CNS lymphoma from toxoplasma encephalitis in AIDS patients (Ruiz et al. 1994). And PET scanning may improve diagnostic accuracy and help in the evaluation of the presence of residential or recurrent tumor tissue following initial treatments (Wong et al. 2002).

Magnetoencephalography (MEG), another recently developed technology in the assessment of brain function, relies on measurement of magnetic fields to localize neuronal cells producing abnormal electrical activity. MEG is more precise than electroencephalography in localizing sources of abnormal electrical activity in the brain and has the potential additional advantage of being able to be used sequentially in assessing brain activity over time without radiation exposure. The role MEG may play in the evaluation of brain tumors is unclear at present, but it may prove useful in the assessment of tumor-associated diaschisis and disconnection syndromes (Bartolomei et al. 2006).

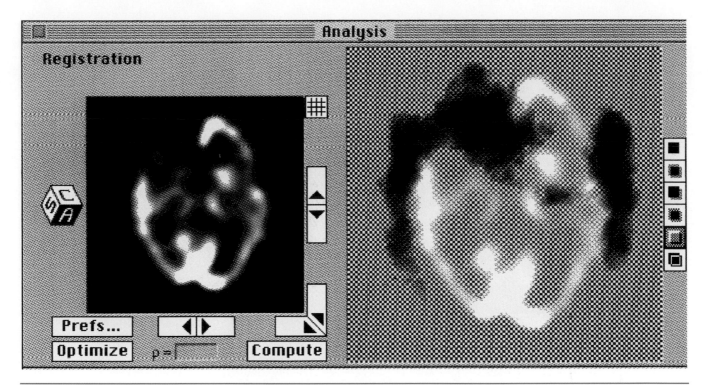

FIGURE 19–7. Single-photon emission computed tomography scans of a patient with recurrent glioblastoma. [^{99m}Tc]Hexamethylpropylene amine oxime (HMPAO) scan (*left*) indicates decreased tracer uptake in the right frontal area. Superimposed thallium scan (*right*) shows increased tracer uptake in the same area, indicating recurrent tumor.

Source. Images courtesy of Dr. M. Adatepe, Department of Nuclear Medicine, Allegheny General Hospital, Pittsburgh, Pennsylvania.

TREATMENT OF PSYCHIATRIC AND BEHAVIORAL SYMPTOMS ASSOCIATED WITH CEREBRAL TUMORS

GENERAL CONSIDERATIONS

Psychiatric and behavioral symptoms may be completely relieved after removal of the cerebral tumor with which they are associated. When this does not happen, as is often the case, decreasing the size or interfering with the growth of the tumor through surgery, chemotherapy, or radiation therapy (alone, sequentially, or in combination) may significantly ameliorate the severity of associated behavioral symptoms. Improvement in cognitive and behavioral symptoms may be rapid and dramatic with treatments that diminish increased intracranial pressure or relieve hydrocephalus associated with brain tumors.

In cases in which neuropsychiatric or behavioral symptoms persist or worsen after optimal surgical and nonsurgical interventions, psychopharmacological, psychotherapeutic, and psychosocial interventions become a major treatment focus. The persistence of such psychiatric, behavioral, and neurocognitive symptoms should lead the

neurosurgeon or neurologist to seek psychiatric consultation because these symptoms are distressing, cause functional impairment and disability, and have a very negative effect on the patient's overall quality of life (Weitzner 1999). At this juncture, the psychiatrist or neuropsychiatrist can offer the greatest assistance by providing supportive psychotherapeutic interventions to the patient and family and recommending effective somatic treatments for specific psychiatric symptoms to the patient's physician.

The interventions of the consulting psychiatrist—who works closely with the attending neurosurgeon—may significantly enhance the patient's level of functioning and overall quality of life (Fox 1998). Ameliorating the disabling dysphoria and anergia of severe depression, alleviating the distress caused by overwhelming anxiety, or simply providing consistent supportive contacts to fearful patients and their families may make an enormous difference to all concerned. Often such interventions also lead to improved treatment outcome through increased patient motivation and improved treatment compliance, which may substantially enhance the efficacy of the neurosurgeon's clinical management of the patient's brain tumor.

Although patients with cerebral tumors often have psychiatric and behavioral symptoms, only a portion of these

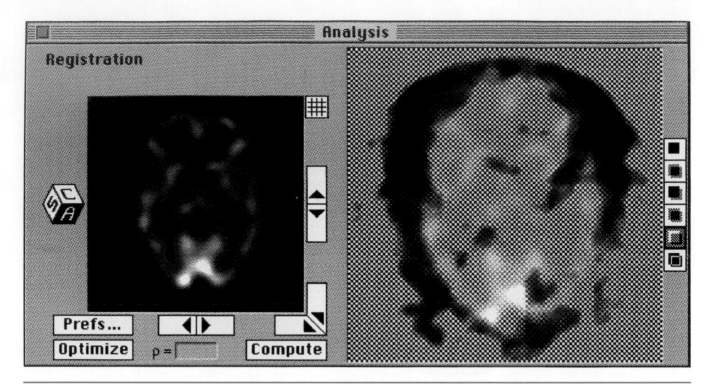

FIGURE 19–8.   Single-photon emission computed tomography scans of a patient after radiation of a left occipital tumor. Decreased uptake on [^{99m}Tc]hexamethylpropylene amine oxime (HMPAO) scan (*left*) combined with decreased uptake on superimposed thallium scan (*right*) suggests an area of postradiation necrosis rather than recurrent tumor.

Source.   Images courtesy of Dr. M. Adatepe, Department of Nuclear Medicine, Allegheny General Hospital, Pittsburgh, Pennsylvania.

are due to a mental disorder directly related to the tumor. Patients may also have persistent or recurrent symptoms of mood or anxiety disorders that were present premorbidly and were uncovered or exacerbated by the stress of having to live with a brain tumor. Anxiety and depressive symptoms may arise de novo in any brain tumor patient, with or without a history of a psychiatric disorder, as a result of psychological reactions to the stress of the initial diagnosis of a brain tumor; concerns about how it will be treated; fears about the potential adverse effects of surgery, radiation therapy, and chemotherapy; and worries about long-term prognosis. Other psychiatric symptoms may emerge later in reaction to the difficulties of adjusting to functional disabilities or distressing life changes that may result from the tumor itself or from the side effects and complications of the various therapeutic interventions brought to bear on it. It is important for the consulting psychiatrist to differentiate as precisely as possible among symptoms that are specifically tumor related (i.e., symptoms due to an organic mental syndrome), those that result from preexisting primary psychiatric disorders, and those that are predominantly reactive in nature and secondary to psychological stresses. Optimal pharmacological and psychotherapeutic interventions, individually or in combination, depend on which of these are the primary cause of the patient's symptoms.

PHARMACOLOGICAL MANAGEMENT OF PATIENTS WITH PRIMARY PSYCHIATRIC DISORDERS WHO DEVELOP BRAIN TUMORS

The psychopharmacological management of patients with preexisting primary psychiatric illnesses that persist or recur in the context of the diagnosis and treatment of cerebral tumors should follow the same general therapeutic principles that apply to tumor-free patients with similar disorders. Psychiatric and behavioral symptoms due to brain tumors may often respond to administration of appropriate psychopharmacological agents (Binder 1983). However, it is important for the psychiatrist to be cognizant of the potential need to make downward adjustments in medication dose and to use drugs that are less likely to cause delirium in patients with brain tumors, as a result of the increased susceptibility of these patients to many of the side effects of psychotropic medications. This is especially true of patients who are in the immediate postoperative period or are receiving chemotherapy or radiation therapy. Lithium, low-potency antipsychotic drugs, tertiary amine TCAs, and antiparkinsonian agents all have significant dose-related deliriogenic potential when given individually, and this is even more true when they are given in combination with each other or other potentially deliriogenic agents. Thus, these agents should be used with care in known psychiatric patients with brain tumors. It may be necessary to substitute an atypical second-generation antipsychotic, carbamazepine, valproic acid, lamotrigine, oxcarbazepine, gabapentin, or a benzodiazepine, such as lorazepam or clonazepam, for lithium in patients with mania; a newer-generation heterocyclic or secondary amine TCA, a selective serotonin reuptake inhibitor (SSRI), or one of the newer, novel-structured antidepressants for tertiary amine TCAs in patients with depression; or one of the atypical antipsychotics for old-line, standard neuroleptics in patients with schizophrenia.

Another significant concern is the potential for precipitating seizures when using these drugs, especially in patients with brain tumors in whom seizures are more likely to occur anyway. Neuroleptics, antidepressants, and lithium all can lower seizure threshold, although to varying degrees. Although the available data are inconclusive, standard neuroleptics such as molindone and fluphenazine, and possibly haloperidol (Mendez et al. 1984), are among the older antipsychotic drugs that are believed to carry the smallest risk for seizures, whereas low-potency agents such as chlorpromazine and clozapine are associated with an increased frequency of seizures (Stoudemire et al. 1993). In general, the newer atypical antipsychotics, as a class, are believed to have a lower likelihood of precipitating seizures and thus offer an important therapeutic advantage over the old-line antipsychotics. Among the antidepressants, maprotiline and bupropion appear to have the greatest seizure-inducing potential (Dubovsky 1992). Clinical and animal studies report variable effects of TCAs on seizure threshold (Edwards et al. 1986), and the evidence is unclear as to which antidepressants carry the smallest overall risk, although the SSRIs in general have been reported to have a low likelihood of precipitating seizures. In acutely manic patients with brain tumors, for whom lithium—which lowers seizure threshold and may therefore induce seizures (Massey and Folger 1984)—might otherwise be the drug of choice, carbamazepine, valproic acid, oxcarbazepine, lorazepam, clonazepam, and gabapentin—all of which have anticonvulsant properties—may be preferable alternatives.

The psychiatrist should also bear in mind that patients with brain tumors who have psychiatric disorders and are also taking anticonvulsants for a known seizure diathesis should be monitored carefully for the adequacy of anticonvulsant blood levels and should have their anticonvulsant dose increased or decreased as appropriate when psychotropic agents are given. Certain of these medications have epileptogenic effects, as well as the potential for decreasing or increasing anticonvulsant blood levels through drug-drug interactions resulting from competitive serum protein binding and/or from alterations in hepatic antiepileptic drug metabolism involving the cytochrome P450 system—which may be enhanced or inhibited, potentially leading to recrudescence of previously controlled seizures or the development of signs of anticonvulsant toxicity, respectively. A similar caution may apply to concomitant administration of anticonvulsant medications and chemotherapeutic agents that are being used in the treatment of inoperable brain tumors (Vecht et al. 2003).

PSYCHOTHERAPEUTIC MANAGEMENT OF SYNDROMES ASSOCIATED WITH BRAIN TUMORS

Supportive psychotherapy geared to the patient's current overall functional status, psychosocial situation, interpersonal and family relationships, cognitive capacities, and emotional needs is a very important element in the treatment of any brain tumor patient. The often-devastating psychological stress of initially receiving a brain tumor diagnosis and then having to undergo various invasive, painful, and potentially debilitating diagnostic studies and subsequent treatments for it can trigger both the recurrence of preexisting primary psychiatric disorders and the de novo appearance in the patient of reactive psychiatric symptoms resulting from the multiple stressors associated with the illness and its treatment. Likewise, the diagnosis and treatment of a brain tumor in a loved one is enormously stressful for families. Under any clinical scenario, supportive psychotherapy for patients and supportive psychoeducation and therapeutic interventions for their families are likely to be well received and very helpful for both and should play a major role in overall clinical management.

Ideally, supportive psychotherapy for both the patient and the family or significant others should focus primarily on concrete, reality-based cognitive and psychoeducational issues relating to diagnosis, treatment, and prognosis of the patient's brain tumor. Psychotherapeutic interactions with patients should be geared to the patient's cognitive capacities, which may be diminished by the tumor itself or by one or more of the therapeutic interventions given for it. Over time, the focus of psychotherapy often shifts to the effect of the illness on the patient's emotional and functional status, its effect on the family, the real and imagined challenges of coping with actual or anticipated functional disabilities, and the difficult processes of dealing with anticipatory grief related to potential losses and eventual death. Not surprisingly, patients with brain tumors worry a great deal about additional decrements in their cognitive and intellectual functioning, physical disability and incapacity, and, ultimately, death. Patients vary widely in their capacity to adjust to and cope with the potentially devastating consequences of brain tumors, and the success of their adjustment and adaptation greatly depends on the flexibility of their premorbid coping abilities. Some patients may appear to be little affected, whereas others may experience severe and even overwhelming symptoms of anxiety and depression. These latter patients may experience greater difficulty continuing to function optimally in their usual work and family roles and need more aggressive psychotherapeutic and psychopharmacological interventions.

Coping by brain tumor patients through the use of the defense mechanism of denial is common and may often be adaptive and effective in helping them to cope with their fears and anxieties, especially in the early stages of what may well turn out to be a life-threatening illness. On the other hand, maladaptive denial may result in the failure of patients and/or their families to comply with optimal treatment recommendations or deal appropriately and in a timely fashion with important legal, personal, family, and other reality-based issues and obligations that need to be addressed while the patient is still able. When denial is producing such maladaptive effects, the clinician may, in a sensitive and supportive manner, need to directly confront and encourage the patient and family to begin to address painful yet inevitable issues such as increasing disability, growing incapacity, and even impending death and how to best deal with these issues and then be available to them on a continuing basis as they begin to do so.

Although there are no clear-cut, generally accepted guidelines for the optimal nature and timing of discussions of prognosis with brain tumor patients, most clinicians believe that patients and families should be given realistic prognostic information in a time frame that will allow them the opportunity to make timely and well-considered decisions and appropriate plans. Such prognostic information should, of course, be conveyed by the physician in as sensitive and supportive a fashion as possible, with ample opportunity provided for questions from and detailed discussion with the patient and family. This is another juncture where the involvement of the consulting psychiatrist may be important in helping the patient and family to process unpleasant but essential clinical information in a helpful and constructive way.

Some patients who have been completely cured of a brain tumor may still manifest significant psychiatric symptoms, including anxiety, fear, and depression. They, like other patients with brain tumors, may also benefit from psychiatric treatment. Unless the psychiatric symptoms are causing functional disability, are severe and distressing, persist over an extended time, or evolve into an autonomous psychiatric syndrome, psychotherapy rather than pharmacotherapy is generally the preferred treatment approach for such patients. Short-term, symptomatically targeted pharmacotherapy can, at times, be a useful adjunct in certain cases, even if the major ongoing treatment emphasis is on psychotherapy.

It should be kept in mind that psychodynamically focused, insight-oriented psychotherapy, which is usually used in primary psychiatric syndromes when psychodynamic factors are playing a major role and which generally requires intact higher-level cognitive and abstracting capacities, may be relatively contraindicated in psychiatrically ill brain tumor patients. Such patients may have a significant degree of neurocognitive impairment in addition to their psychiatric and behavioral symptoms as a result of the effects of the tumor itself or of the various neurosurgical, chemotherapeutic, or radiotherapeutic interventions they may have undergone in attempts to cure or palliate it. When such cognitive impairment is present, psychodynamically oriented therapies are unlikely to be beneficial, and they also may cause substantial frustration and acute psychic distress as patients are confronted with psychological tasks and cognitive demands that they are unable to meet because of their brain dysfunction. In general, and in contradistinction to the more traditional, relatively passive role of the psychiatrist in insight-oriented psychotherapy, more concretely focused, "here-and-now" problem-solving psychotherapeutic approaches based on a cognitive-behavioral orientation with the psychiatrist assuming an active, supportive, and educational role in verbal interactions with the patient are likely to be most beneficial.

SOMATIC TREATMENT OF MENTAL DISORDERS DUE TO BRAIN TUMORS

The psychopharmacological treatment of organic mental symptoms and syndromes caused by cerebral tumors, whether characterized by psychotic, affective, anxiety, or neurocognitive disturbances, follows the same general principles as the drug treatment of phenomenologically similar symptoms due to primary psychiatric illnesses. In treating secondary psychiatric symptoms pharmacologically in patients with brain tumors, some important caveats must be borne in mind. As previously alluded to, patients with psychiatric symptoms that are a direct consequence of a brain tumor, like other patients with identifiable brain pathology, frequently respond favorably to medications but will frequently tolerate them only in significantly lower doses. Thus, side-effect profiles of psychotropic drugs being considered for the treatment of brain tumor patients must be very carefully evaluated, especially with regard to sedative, extrapyramidal, deliriogenic, and epileptogenic effects and potential drug interactions. The latter four of these are especially important for the clinician to keep in mind because they can result in substantial, and largely avoidable, additional clinical morbidity.

DRUG TREATMENT OF PSYCHOTIC DISORDERS DUE TO BRAIN TUMORS

Standard, first-generation antipsychotic medications may be beneficial in treating the hallucinations, delusions, and thought content and process disturbances that may accompany tumor-associated psychotic syndromes. High-potency antipsychotics, which have fewer nonneurological side effects than do the low-potency antipsychotics, are generally preferable if one of the standard neuroleptics is to be used. However, the former more often cause extrapyramidal symptoms, which may be more severe and persistent in patients with brain tumors. In patients with "organic" psychotic disorders, the therapeutically effective dose of an antipsychotic is often lower than that required for the treatment of primary "functional" psychoses. Thus, as little as 1–5 mg, rather than 10–20 mg, of haloperidol per day (or equivalent doses with other antipsychotics) may be effective. Currently there is little controlled research on the efficacy of the newer atypical antipsychotics in the treatment of psychotic symptoms in brain tumor patients, but they have been anecdotally reported to be effective in other psychotic syndromes associated with neurological disorders and have, as a result of their low side-effect profile, generally been well tolerated. Thus, they may well turn out to be the treatment of choice in brain tumor patients with psychotic symptoms. As per the general rule with the use of other psychotropics in patients with brain tumors, when initiating treatment with antipsychotics, one should "start low and go slowly." This is especially true in elderly patients, in whom effective antipsychotic doses may be lower than they are in younger patients because of aging-related pharmacokinetic and pharmacodynamic factors.

Antiparkinsonian agents, such as benztropine, trihexyphenidyl, and orphenadrine, are effective in the treatment of extrapyramidal side effects resulting from the use of neuroleptics in patients with brain tumors. However, in such patients, these agents have a greater likelihood of causing or contributing to the occurrence of anticholinergic delirium when they are used in conjunction with low-potency neuroleptics and/or tertiary amine TCAs. Thus, their use generally should be avoided unless there is a clear-cut clinical indication, and the dose should be minimized when they are used. Diphenhydramine or amantadine for dystonic and parkinsonian symptoms and benzodiazepines or β-blockers for akathisia can be effective alternatives and have less potential for causing delirium.

TREATMENT OF MOOD DISORDERS DUE TO BRAIN TUMORS

Antidepressant medications are often effective in the treatment of mood disorders with predominantly depressive features in patients with brain tumors. Standard TCAs are useful, although currently the SSRIs, newer-generation heterocyclic antidepressants, or secondary amine TCAs are often used preferentially because of their lower anticholinergic activity and sedating effects and greater overall patient acceptance, which results in improved treatment compliance. The SSRIs are therapeutically effective and do not cause delirium, have a favorable side-effect profile, and, despite their relatively high cost, often may be effective in such patients. In recent years, methylphenidate has been shown to be effective (Masand et al. 1991) and to have a rapid onset of action (Woods et al. 1986) in patients with secondary depression related to medical and neurological disorders, including brain tumors. Because methylphenidate is generally well tolerated and does not lower the seizure threshold, its use as an antidepressant in brain tumor patients is increasing. It also may have several other important therapeutic effects and thus may be a highly beneficial adjuvant to brain tumor therapy in some patients. In 30 patients with malignant gliomas with progressive neurobehavioral deficits resulting from their tumors and the radiation therapy and chemotherapy they had received for them, Meyers et al. (1998) showed that methylphenidate in as low a dosage as 10 mg twice a day had multiple significant beneficial effects. These included significant improvement in cognitive function, improved gait, increased stamina and motivation, and, in one case, improved bladder control, all of which occurred despite evidence of progressive neurological changes on MRI during the time that the subjects were receiving methylphenidate treatment. Untoward effects reported were minimal; seizure frequency did not increase, and many patients who were taking glucocorticoids were able to have their doses reduced.

Future research should focus on the relative advantages and disadvantages of alternatives such as the extended-release forms of methylphenidate, the short- and long-acting forms of dexmethylphenidate, dextroamphetamine salts, and dextroamphetamine, as well as non-amphetamine-based CNS activators such as atomoxetine and modafinil, in the treatment of psychiatric, behavioral, and neurocognitive comorbid disorders that occur in patients with brain tumors.

Monoamine oxidase inhibitors may be effective when other antidepressants are not. They do not ordinarily pose an undue risk in patients with brain tumors, but, of course, the clinician must bear in mind that the cognitive impairment that often occurs in such patients may interfere with their ability to maintain a tyramine-free diet, thereby increasing the risk associated with the use of these drugs.

If single antidepressant medication regimens are ineffective, various combinations may work. When pharmacological treatments have failed, electroconvulsive therapy should be given serious consideration. Previously, brain tumors were thought to be an absolute contraindication to electroconvulsive therapy, especially when the tumor was associated with increased intracranial pressure. Some studies (Starkstein and Migliorelli 1993; Zwil et al. 1990), however, have reported several cases of refractory depression associated with brain tumors without associated evidence of increased intracranial pressure that have been treated successfully and safely with electroconvulsive therapy when appropriate precautions have been taken.

Mood disorders with manic features due to brain tumors, although relatively rare, generally respond to lithium in the usual therapeutic range of 0.8–1.4 mEq/L. For patients in whom seizures have been a part of the clinical picture, however, carbamazepine, valproate, oxcarbazepine, lorazepam, clonazepam, gabapentin, and—in cases in which drug therapy has been ineffective—electroconvulsive therapy are preferable alternatives because they do not have the epileptogenic potential of lithium and, in fact, have anticonvulsant properties of their own.

Newer treatment approaches, including vagal nerve stimulation and transcranial magnetic stimulation, have shown promise in early clinical trials with a variety of mood disorders, including depression that has been refractory to other treatments, mania (Berman et al. 2000; Grisaru et al. 1998; Rush et al. 2000), and psychotic symptoms (Hoffman et al. 1999). Clarification of their future role in the treatment of brain tumor patients with depression and other neuropsychiatric syndromes awaits further research.

TREATMENT OF ANXIETY DISORDERS DUE TO BRAIN TUMORS

Anxiety symptoms caused either directly or indirectly by brain tumors should not be treated with neuroleptics unless psychotic features are present, for the reasons noted previously and because neuroleptics are generally not effective in patients with nonpsychotic anxiety symptoms and often cause dysphoria in nonpsychotic patients. The benzodiazepines, on the contrary, are often effective and have the added benefit of possessing anticonvulsant properties. Thus, they are frequently used. However, benzodiazepines, particularly the long-acting varieties, may induce delirium in patients with organic brain disease, including brain tumors, when used in high doses and

in older age groups. This argues for the preferential use of short-acting agents in lower doses, especially in older patients. Other disadvantages of benzodiazepines include their abuse potential and their occasional propensity (especially with the varieties that have long half-lives) to cause seemingly paradoxical reactions, characterized by increased arousal and agitation. Buspirone, which is free of these potentially negative effects, should be considered an alternative to the benzodiazepines. Its main drawbacks are its delayed onset and only modest degree of anxiolytic action. Hydroxyzine, SSRIs, or low doses of tertiary amine TCAs, such as doxepin or amitriptyline, also may have beneficial anxiolytic effects in some patients. Finally, panic attacks associated with temporal lobe tumors may respond to carbamazepine, valproate, or primidone, as well as to the usual antidepressant and antianxiety drugs.

TREATMENT OF DELIRIUM ASSOCIATED WITH BRAIN TUMORS

Delirium in patients with brain tumors may be associated with a wide variety of psychiatric and behavioral symptoms in addition to the characteristic cognitive impairments. Hallucinations (especially visual) and delusions are common in delirious patients and often respond to symptomatic treatment with low doses of haloperidol, other high-potency neuroleptics, or one of the new atypical antipsychotics while the underlying causes of the delirium are being sought and treated.

TREATMENT OF PERSONALITY CHANGES DUE TO BRAIN TUMORS

Mood lability may be associated with personality changes due to a brain tumor and may respond to lithium, carbamazepine, or other mood stabilizers. Some patients with frontal lobe syndromes associated with tumors may respond to carbamazepine, as do some patients with temporal lobe tumors who may present with associated interictal aggression and violent behavior. Patients with brain tumors who have impulse dyscontrol and rageful, explosive episodes, like patients with intermittent explosive disorders due to other medical and neurological conditions, may respond to empirical therapeutic trials of anticonvulsants, such as carbamazepine, valproic acid, or phenytoin; psychotropics, including lithium; high-potency neuroleptics; and stimulants or β-blockers.

COGNITIVE REHABILITATION

In addition to psychopharmacological and psychotherapeutic treatments, cognitive, occupational, and vocational rehabilitative interventions can be very helpful for patients whose tumors, or the treatments they have received for them, have produced behavioral, cognitive, or functional sequelae. Such sequelae can be identified and quantified by comparing preoperative with postoperative test results on the Halstead-Reitan Neuropsychological Test Battery or other comprehensive neuropsychological test batteries and various functional assessment tools. Serial testing at intervals during the patient's postoperative rehabilitation allows for objective documentation of neuropsychological and functional deficits and allows for objective monitoring of improvement or deterioration over time. Thus, in general, neuropsychological and functional assessments should be a standard part of the pretreatment evaluation and posttreatment follow-up of patients receiving treatment for brain tumors.

Cognitive, occupational, and vocational rehabilitative strategies can be developed that will seek to address deficits in intellectual, language, visuospatial, memory, and neurocognitive functioning, as well as vocational functioning and ability to carry out activities of daily living resulting from a brain tumor. In addition, behavioral techniques have been successfully applied to problematic behaviors resulting from insults to the brain. Such interventions may be used alone or in conjunction with other therapies. For a more detailed discussion of these various approaches, see "Cognitive Rehabilitation and Behavior Therapy for Patients With Neuropsychiatric Disorders," Chapter 33 of this book.

NEUROPSYCHIATRIC CONSEQUENCES OF TREATMENTS OF BRAIN TUMORS

Several psychiatric and behavioral symptoms, as well as neurocognitive deficits, may result from surgical, pharmacological, and radiation treatments of brain tumors and their complications. Unavoidable intraoperative injury to normal brain tissue in the vicinity of a brain tumor during the course of resection or debulking may result in the postoperative appearance of new or exacerbated behavioral or neurocognitive symptoms, depending on the location and connectivity of the tissues involved. The same is true of other perioperative and postoperative complications, such as infections and bleeding. Chemotherapy of brain tumors may cause transient delirium and neurocognitive dysfunction as well as other neurological complications, and the administration of steroids for secondary phenomena such as cerebral edema and increased intracranial pressure may result in the appearance of psychotic symptoms or manic, depressive, or mixed manic and depressive affective syndromes. Radiation therapy directed at brain tumors may result in immediate or delayed sequelae—neurocognitive, endocrine (in the form of late-onset hypothalamic-pituitary

dysfunction) (Agha et al. 2005), and behavioral—due to radiation-induced damage to white matter and other structures. These sequelae may be either transient (Hylton et al. 1987) or permanent (Al-Mefty et al. 1990; Burger et al. 1979) and vary considerably in severity from completely reversible changes, presumably related to edema, to widespread, permanent changes due to parenchymal necrosis. In the most severe cases, which are fortunately quite rare, progressive dementia and eventual coma and death may occur.

CONCLUSION

Brain tumors often are associated with, and frequently present, a broad range of psychiatric, behavioral, and neurocognitive symptoms. The differential diagnosis of any patient who has acute or progressive changes in behavior, personality, or cognitive function should include a brain tumor, especially if any focal neurological signs and symptoms are present. In addition to assessment of psychiatric and behavioral symptoms, a full neuropsychiatric evaluation should include physical, neurological, and mental status examinations (e.g., MMSE); appropriate brain imaging and other neurodiagnostic studies; and formal neuropsychological testing, particularly when there is any question of neurocognitive dysfunction on bedside testing with the MMSE.

The nature, frequency, and severity of psychiatric symptoms observed in patients with brain tumors depend on the combined effects of several clinical factors, including the type, location, size, rate of growth, and malignancy of the tumor. In general, behavioral symptoms associated with smaller, slower-growing, less aggressive tumors are most likely to be misdiagnosed as psychiatric in origin, particularly when they occur in "silent" regions of the brain, which do not give rise to focal neurological signs or symptoms.

Although tumors of the frontal lobe, temporal lobe, and diencephalon appear to be most commonly associated with psychiatric and behavioral symptoms, the variation in symptoms that may occur with each of these types of tumors is exceedingly broad. In general, the relation between particular neuropsychiatric symptoms and specific anatomical locations of the brain tumors that are causing them is not very consistent.

Optimal treatment of tumor-associated psychiatric, neuropsychiatric, and neuropsychological dysfunctions should be multifaceted and is dependent on the coordinated interventions of a multidisciplinary treatment team. The psychopharmacological treatment of psychiatric and behavioral syndromes should follow the same general principles as those for corresponding primary psychiatric disorders. However, the choice of drugs and/or dosages may require modification because many of the psychotropic agents can induce seizures or delirium, and patients with brain tumors are more vulnerable to these and other side effects of psychotropic medications.

Adjunctive supportive psychotherapy for both the patient and the family is very important, as are psychosocial and psychoeducational interventions tailored to their specific needs. Such psychotherapeutic and psychosocial interventions must be carefully integrated with psychopharmacological; neurocognitive, physical, occupational, and vocational rehabilitative; and behavioral treatment approaches as clinically indicated. In turn, all of these must be coordinated with the neurosurgeon's ongoing treatment interventions to optimize the patient's overall medical and surgical management. With well-planned integration and coordination of these multiple complementary therapeutic approaches, both the quantity and the quality of the patient's life may be substantially enhanced.

Highlights for the Clinician

- ✦ Psychiatric, behavioral, and neurocognitive symptoms and syndromes are frequently associated with brain tumors.

- ✦ The types of such disturbances occurring in association with brain tumors are quite varied.

- ✦ Psychiatric, behavioral, and neurocognitive symptoms associated with cerebral tumors may mimic a wide variety of primary psychiatric disorders.

- ✦ Such symptoms and syndromes may be the first indication of a previously unsuspected, underlying brain tumor.

- ✦ The possibility that a brain tumor may be causing such symptoms should always be considered in new-onset psychiatric or neurocognitive symptomatology, especially if accompanied by any neurological signs and symptoms or atypical clinical or treatment response features.

- ✦ Brain tumors may exacerbate the clinical effect of preexisting primary psychiatric illness.

- ✦ Careful neurological examination, state-of-the-art imaging studies and sophisticated scanning techniques, electrophysiological tests, and neuropsychological testing can all be quite helpful in the evaluation of a possible underlying brain tumor.

- ✦ The causes of specific types of brain tumor–associated behavioral symptomatology appear to be multiple and are believed to include anatomical location and laterality, histological type, size, and aggressiveness of the tumor in conjunction with associated factors such as cerebral edema and intracranial pressure.

- ✦ Tumor-associated psychiatric and behavioral symptoms, like those associated with primary psychiatric disorders, often respond favorably to appropriate psychopharmacological, psychotherapeutic, and psychoeducational interventions with patients and their families.

- ✦ Brain tumor patients with psychiatric and behavioral symptoms, like other patients with CNS disorders with such symptoms, often tolerate and respond to lower doses of psychopharmacological agents than are required for and tolerated by patients with similar symptoms caused by primary psychiatric illnesses.

- ✦ Psychiatrists can make valuable contributions to the overall clinical management of brain tumor patients with psychiatric, behavioral, and neurocognitive symptomatology and can help to optimize the patient's sense of well-being and overall quality of life.

RECOMMENDED READINGS

Cummings J: Clinical Neuropsychiatry. Orlando, FL, Grune & Stratton, 1985

Feinberg T, Frank M (eds): Behavioral Neurology and Neuropsychology. New York, McGraw-Hill, 1997

Jobe TH, Gaviria M: Clinical Neuropsychiatry. Oxford, UK, Blackwell Science, 1997

Kandel E, Schwartz J, Jessel T: Principles of Neural Science, 4th Edition. New York, McGraw-Hill, 2000

Lishman A, Malden MA: Organic Psychiatry: The Psychological Consequences of Cerebral Disorders, 3rd Edition. Oxford, UK, Blackwell Science, 1998

Mesulam M: Principles of Behavioral Neurology. Philadelphia, PA, FA Davis, 1986

Strub R, Black FW: Neurobehavioral Disorders: A Clinical Approach. Philadelphia, PA, FA Davis, 1988

REFERENCES

Agha A, Shenlock M, Brennan S, et al: Hypothalamic-pituitary dysfunction after irradiation of nonpituitary brain tumors in adults. J Clin Endocrinol Metab 90:6355–6360, 2005

Alexander GE, Crutcher MD: Functional architecture of basal ganglia circuits: neural substrates of parallel processing. Trends Neurosci 13:266–271, 1990

Allen IM: A clinical study of tumors involving the occipital lobe. Brain 53:196–243, 1930

Al-Mefty O, Kersh JE, Routh A, et al: The long-term side effects of radiation therapy for benign brain tumors in adults. J Neurosurg 73:502–512, 1990

American Psychiatric Association: Diagnostic and Statistical Manual of Mental Disorders, 4th Edition. Washington, DC, American Psychiatric Association, 1994

Avery TL: A case of acromegaly and gigantism with depression. Br J Psychiatry 122:599–600, 1973

Batabyal SK, Ghosh B, Sengupta S, et al: Cerebrospinal fluid and serum carcinoembryonic antigen in brain tumors. Neoplasma 50:377–379, 2003

Bartolomei F, Bosma I, Klein M, et al: How do brain tumors alter functional connectivity? A magnetoencephalography study. Ann Neurol 59:128–138, 2006

Bauer RM, Tobias B, Valenstein E: Amnesic disorders, in Clinical Neuropsychology, 3rd Edition. Edited by Heilman KM, Valenstein E. New York, Oxford University Press, 1993, pp 523–578

Bear DM, Fedio P: Quantitative analysis of interictal behavior in temporal lobe epilepsy. Arch Neurol 34:454–467, 1977

Belyi BI: Mental impairment in unilateral frontal tumors: role of the laterality of the lesion. Int J Neurosci 32:799–810, 1987

Benson DF: Aphasia, Alexia, and Agraphia. New York, Churchill Livingstone, 1979

Berman RM, Narasimhan M, Sanacora G, et al: A randomized clinical trial of repetitive transcranial magnetic stimulation in the treatment of major depression. Biol Psychiatry 47:332–337, 2000

Bhatia MS: Cotard's syndrome in parietal lobe tumor. Indian Pediatr 30:1019–1021, 1993

Bigler ED: Diagnostic Clinical Neuropsychology. Austin, University of Texas Press, 1984

Binder RL: Neurologically silent brain tumors in psychiatric hospital admissions: three cases and a review. J Clin Psychiatry 44:94–97, 1983

Blackman M, Wheler GH: A case of mistaken identity: a fourth ventricular tumor presenting as school phobia in a 12 year old boy. Can J Psychiatry 32:584–587, 1987

Burger PC, Mahaley MS, Dudka L, et al: The morphologic effects of radiation administered therapeutically for intracranial gliomas. Cancer 44:1256–1272, 1979

Burkle FM, Lipowski ZJ: Colloid cyst of the third ventricle presenting as psychiatric disorder. Am J Psychiatry 135:373–374, 1978

Burns JM, Swerdlow RH: Right orbitofrontal tumor with pedophilia symptom and constructional apraxia sign. Arch Neurol 60:437–440, 2003

Butters N, Milotis P: Amnestic disorders, in Clinical Neuropsychology. Edited by Heilman KM, Valenstein E. New York, Oxford University Press, 1979, pp 403–439

Cairns H: Mental disorders with tumors of the pons. Folia Psychiatrica Neurologica Neurochirurgica 53:193–203, 1950

Cairns H, Mosberg WH: Colloid cysts of the third ventricle. Surg Gynecol Obstet 92:545–570, 1951

Cairns H, Oldfield RC, Pennybacker JB, et al: Akinetic mutism with an epidermoid cyst of the 3rd ventricle. Brain 64:273–290, 1941

Chipkevitch E: Brain tumors and anorexia nervosa syndrome. Brain Dev 16:175–179, 1994

Coffey RJ: Hypothalamic and basal forebrain germinoma presenting with amnesia and hyperphagia. Surg Neurol 31:228–233, 1989

Critchley M: Psychiatric symptoms and parietal disease: differential diagnosis. Proc R Soc Med 57:422–428, 1964

Cummings JL: Subcortical Dementia. New York, Oxford University Press, 1990

Cummings JL: Frontal-subcortical circuits and human behavior. Arch Neurol 50:873–880, 1993

Cummings JL, Mendez MF: Secondary mania with focal cerebrovascular lesions. Am J Psychiatry 141:1084–1087, 1984

Davison K, Bagley CR: Schizophrenia-like psychoses associated with organic disorders of the central nervous system: a review of the literature, in Current Problems in Neuropsychiatry: Schizophrenia, Epilepsy, the Temporal Lobe (British Journal of Psychiatry Special Publication No 4). Edited by Harrington RN. London, Headley Brothers, 1969, pp 126–130

Direkze M, Bayliss SG, Cutting JC: Primary tumours of the frontal lobe. Br J Clin Pract 25:207–213, 1971

Drubach DA, Kelly MP: Panic disorder associated with a right paralimbic lesion. Neuropsychiatry Neuropsychol Behav Neurol 2:282–289, 1989

Dubovsky SL: Psychopharmacological treatment in neuropsychiatry, in The American Psychiatric Press Textbook of Neuropsychiatry. Edited by Yudofsky SC, Hales RE. Washington, DC, American Psychiatric Press, 1992, pp 663–701

Dunn DW, Weisberg LA: Peduncular hallucinations caused by brainstem compression. Neurology 33:1360–1361, 1983

Edwards JG, Long SK, Sedgwick EM: Antidepressants and convulsive seizures: clinical, electroencephalographic, and pharmacologic aspects. Clin Neuropharmacol 9:329–360, 1986

Filley CM, Kleinschmidt-DeMasters BK: Neurobehavioral presentations of brain neoplasms. West J Med 163:19–25, 1995

Fox S: Use of a quality of life instrument to improve assessment of brain tumor patients in an outpatient setting. J Neurosci Nurs 30:322–325, 1998

Frazier CH: Tumor involving the frontal lobe alone: a symptomatic survey of 105 verified cases. Arch Neurol Psychiatry 35:525–571, 1935

Galasko D, Kwo-On-Yuen PF, Thal L: Intracranial mass lesions associated with late-onset psychosis and depression. Psychiatr Clin North Am 11:151–166, 1988

Gamazo-Garran P, Soutullo CA, Ortuna F: Obsessive-compulsive disorder secondary to brain dysgerminoma in an adolescent boy: a positron emission tomography case report. J Child Adolesc Psychopharmacol 12:259–263, 2002

Gautier-Smith P: Parasagittal and Falx Meningiomas. London, Butterworth, 1970

Ghadirian AM, Gauthier S, Bertrand S: Anxiety attacks in a patient with a right temporal lobe meningioma. J Clin Psychiatry 47:270–271, 1986

Goldberg E: Varieties of perseverations: comparison of two taxonomies. J Clin Exp Neuropsychol 6:710–726, 1986

Greenberg DB, Brown GL: Mania resulting from brain stem tumor: single case study. J Nerv Ment Dis 173:434–436, 1985

Grisaru N, Chudakov B, Yaroslavsky Y, et al: Transcranial magnetic stimulation in mania: a controlled study. Am J Psychiatry 155:1608–1610, 1998

Gupta RK, Kumar R: Benign brain tumours and psychiatric morbidity: a 5-year retrospective data analysis. Aust N Z J Psychiatry 38:316–319, 2004

Gutmann DH, Grossman RI, Mollman JE: Personality changes associated with thalamic infiltration. J Neurooncol 8:263–267, 1990

Hahn CA, Dunn RH, Logue PE, et al: Prospective study of neuropsychologic testing and quality-of-life assessment of adults with primary malignant brain tumors. Int J Radiat Oncol Biol Phys 55:992–999, 2003

Heaton RK: Wisconsin Card Sorting Test. Odessa, FL, Psychological Assessment Resources, 1985

Hobbs GE: Brain tumours simulating psychiatric disorder. Can Med Assoc J 88:186–188, 1963

Hoffman RE, Boutros NN, Berman RM, et al: Transcranial magnetic stimulation of left temporoparietal cortex in three patients reporting hallucinated "voices." Biol Psychiatry 46:130–132, 1999

Hollister LE, Boutros N: Clinical use of CT and MR scans in psychiatric patients. J Psychiatry Neurosci 16:194–198, 1991

Hylton PD, Reichman OH, Palutsis R: Monitoring of transient central nervous system postirradiation effects by 133-xenon inhalation regional cerebral blood flow measurements. Neurosurgery 21:843–848, 1987

Jamieson RC, Wells CE: Manic psychosis in a patient with multiple metastatic brain tumors. J Clin Psychiatry 40:280–283, 1979

Jarquin-Valdivia AA: Psychiatric symptoms and brain tumors: a brief historical overview. Arch Neurol 61:1800–1804, 2004

Jones JB, Barklage NE: Conversion disorder: camouflage for brain lesions in two cases. Arch Intern Med 150:1343–1345, 1990

Jukich PJ, McCarthy BJ, Surawicz TS, et al: Trends in incidence of primary brain tumors in the United States, 1985–1994. Neuro-oncol 3:141–151, 2001

Kalayam B, Young RC, Tsuboyama GK: Mood disorders associated with acoustic neuromas. Int J Psychiatry Med 24:31–43, 1994

Kaplan CP, Miner ME: Anxiety and depression in elderly patients receiving treatment for cerebral tumours. Brain Inj 11:129–135, 1997

Keschner M, Bender MB, Strauss I: Mental symptoms in cases of tumor of the temporal lobe. Arch Neurol Psychiatry 35:572–596, 1936

Keschner M, Bender MB, Strauss I: Mental symptoms associated with brain tumor: a study of 530 verified cases. JAMA 110:714–718, 1938

Khouzam HR, Emery PE, Reaves B: Secondary mania in late life. J Am Geriatr Soc 42:85–87, 1994

Klotz M: Incidence of brain tumors in patients hospitalized for chronic mental disorders. Psychiatr Q 31:669–680, 1957

Ko SM, Kok LP: Cerebral tumours presenting with psychiatric symptoms. Singapore Med J 30:282–284, 1989

Kocher R, Linder M, Stula D: [Primary brain tumors in psychiatry.] Schweiz Arch Neurol Neurochir Psychiatr 135:217–227, 1984

Lampl Y, Barak Y, Achiron A, et al: Intracranial meningiomas: correlation of peritumoral edema and psychiatric disturbances. Psychiatry Res 58:177–180, 1995

Lezak MD: Neuropsychological Assessment, 3rd Edition. New York, Oxford University Press, 1995

Lin L, Lioa SC, Lee YJ, et al: Brain tumor presenting as anorexia nervosa in a 19-year-old man. J Formos Med Assoc 102:737–740, 2003

Lishman WA: Organic Psychiatry: The Psychological Consequences of Cerebral Disorder. New York, Oxford University Press, 1987

Madhusoodanan S, Danan D, Brenner R, et al: Brain tumor and psychiatric manifestations: a case report and brief review. Ann Clin Psychiatry 16:111–113, 2004

Mainio A, Hakko H, Niemala A, et al: The effect of brain tumour laterality on anxiety levels among neurosurgical patients. J Neurol Neurosurg Psychiatry 74:1278–1282, 2003

Malamud N: Psychiatric disorder with intracranial tumors of limbic system. Arch Neurol 17:113–123, 1967

Masand P, Murray GB, Pickett P: Psychostimulants in poststroke depression. J Neuropsychiatry Clin Neurosci 3:23–27, 1991

Massey EW, Folger WN: Seizures activated by therapeutic levels of lithium carbonate. South Med J 77:1173–1175, 1984

McAllister TW, Price TRP: Aspects of the behavior of psychiatric inpatients with frontal lobe damage: some implications for diagnosis and treatment. Compr Psychiatry 28:14–21, 1987

McIntyre HD, McIntyre AP: The problem of brain tumor in psychiatric diagnosis. Am J Psychiatry 98:720–726, 1942

Meadows JC: The anatomical basis of prosopagnosia. J Neurol Neurosurg Psychiatry 37:489–501, 1974

Mendez MF, Cummings JL, Benson DF: Epilepsy: psychiatric aspects and use of psychotropics. Psychosomatics 25:883–894, 1984

Meyers CA, Weitzner MA, Valentine AD, et al: Methylphenidate therapy improves cognition, mood, and function of brain tumor patients. J Clin Oncol 16:2522–2527, 1998

Minski L: The mental symptoms associated with 58 cases of cerebral tumor. J Neurol Psychopathol 13:330–343, 1933

Mulder DW, Daly D: Psychiatric symptoms associated with lesions of temporal lobe. JAMA 150:173–176, 1952

Mungas D: Interictal behavior abnormality in temporal lobe epilepsy: a specific syndrome or non-specific psychopathology? Arch Gen Psychiatry 39:108–111, 1982

Nadvi SS, van Dellen JR: Transient peduncular hallucinations secondary to brain stem compression by a medulloblastoma. Surg Neurol 41:250–252, 1994

Nasrallah HA, McChesney CM: Psychopathology of corpus callosum tumors. Biol Psychiatry 16:663–669, 1981

Neuman E, Rancurel G, Lecrubier Y, et al: Schizophreniform catatonia in 6 cases secondary to hydrocephalus with subthalamic mesencephalic tumor associated with hypodopaminergia. Neuropsychobiology 34:76–81, 1996

Olney JW, Farber NB, Spitznagel E, et al: Increasing brain tumor rates: is there a link to aspartame? J Neuropathol Exp Neurol 55:1115–1123, 1996

Patton RB, Sheppard JA: Intracranial tumors found at autopsy in mental patients. Am J Psychiatry 113:319–324, 1956

Percy AK, Elveback LR, Okazaki H, et al: Neoplasms of the central nervous system: epidemiologic considerations. Neurology 22:40–48, 1972

Pincus JH, Tucker GJ: Behavioral Neurology, 2nd Edition. New York, Oxford University Press, 1978

Pollack L, Klein C, Rabey JM, et al: Posterior fossa lesions associated with neuropsychiatric symptomatology. Int J Neurosci 87:119–126, 1996

Pringle AM, Taylor R, Whittle IR: Anxiety and depression in patients with an intracranial neoplasm before and after tumor surgery. Br J Neurosurg 13:46–51, 1999

Radhakrishnan K, Bohnen NI, Kurland LT: Epidemiology of brain tumors, in Brain Tumors: A Comprehensive Text. Edited by Morantz RA, Walsh JW. New York, Marcel Dekker, 1994, pp 1–18

Reiman EM, Raichle ME, Robins E, et al: The application of positron-emission tomography to the study of panic disorder. Am J Psychiatry 143:469–477, 1986

Reitan RM, Wolfson D: Neuroanatomy and Neuropathology for Neuropsychologists. Tucson, AZ, Neuropsychology Press, 1985, pp 167–192

Remington FB, Robert SL: Why patients with brain tumors come to a psychiatric hospital: a thirty-year survey. Am J Psychiatry 119:256–257, 1962

Roberts GW, Done DJ, Bruton C, et al: A "mock up" of schizophrenia: temporal lobe epilepsy and schizophrenia-like psychosis. Biol Psychiatry 28:127–143, 1990

Roberts JKA, Lishman WA: The use of CAT head scanner in clinical psychiatry. Br J Psychiatry 145:152–158, 1984

Robinson RG, Kubos KL, Starr LB, et al: Mood disorders in stroke patients: importance of location of lesion. Brain 107:81–93, 1984

Rodin E, Schmaltz S: The Bear-Fedio personality inventory and temporal lobe epilepsy. Neurology 34:591–596, 1984

Ross E: Prosody and brain lateralization: fact vs. fancy or is it all just semantics? Arch Neurol 45:338–339, 1988

Ruiz A, Ganz WI, Donovan Post J, et al: Use of thallium-201 brain SPECT to differentiate cerebral lymphoma from toxoplasma encephalitis in AIDS patients. AJNR Am J Neuroradiol 15:1885–1894, 1994

Rush AJ, George MS, Sackheim HA, et al: Vagus nerve stimulation (VNS) for refractory depressions: a multicenter study. Biol Psychiatry 47:276–286, 2000

Russell RW, Pennybacker JB: Craniopharyngioma in the elderly. J Neurol Neurosurg Psychiatry 24:1–13, 1961

Salazar-Calderon Perriggo VH, Oommen KJ, Sobonya RE: Silent solitary right parietal chondroma resulting in secondary mania. Clin Neuropathol 12:325–329, 1993

Scheibel RS, Meyers CA, Levin VA: Cognitive dysfunction following surgery for intracerebral glioma: influence of histopathology, lesion location, and treatment. J Neurooncol 30:61–67, 1996

Schirmer M, Bock WJ: The primary symptoms of intracranial metastases, in Advances in Neurosurgery, Vol 12. Edited by Piotrowski W, Brock M, Klinger M. Berlin, Germany, Springer Verlag, 1984, pp 25–29

Schlesinger B: Mental changes in intracranial tumors and related problems. Confinia Neurologica 10:225–263, 1950

Selecki BR: Cerebral mid-line tumours involving the corpus callosum among mental hospital patients. Med J Aust 2:954–960, 1964

Selecki BR: Intracranial space-occupying lesions among patients admitted to mental hospitals. Med J Aust 1:383–390, 1965

Spreen O, Benton A, Fincham R: Auditory agnosia without aphasia. Arch Neurol 13:84–92, 1965

Starkstein SE, Migliorelli R: ECT in a patient with a frontal craniotomy and residual meningioma. J Neuropsychiatry Clin Neurosci 5:428–430, 1993

Starkstein SE, Boston JD, Robinson RG: Mechanisms of mania after brain injury: 12 case reports and review of the literature. J Nerv Ment Dis 176:87–100, 1988

Stoudemire A, Fogel BS, Gulley LR, et al: Psychopharmacology in the medical patient, in Psychiatric Care of the Medical Patient. Edited by Stoudemire A, Fogel BS. New York, Oxford University Press, 1993, pp 155–206

Strauss I, Keschner M: Mental symptoms in cases of tumor of the frontal lobe. Arch Neurol Psychiatry 33:986–1005, 1935

Strobos RRJ: Tumors of the temporal lobe. Neurology 3:752–760, 1953

Tanaghow A, Lewis J, Jones GH: Anterior tumour of the corpus callosum with atypical depression. Br J Psychiatry 155:854–856, 1989

Teuber HL: Unity and diversity of frontal lobe functions. Acta Neurobiol Exp 32:615–656, 1972

Tucker GJ, Price TRP, Johnson VB, et al: Phenomenology of temporal lobe dysfunction: a link to atypical psychosis: a series of cases. J Nerv Ment Dis 174:348–356, 1986

Vecht CJ, Wagner GL, Wilms EB: Treating seizures in patients with brain tumors: drug interactions between antiepileptic and chemotherapeutic agents. Semin Oncol 30 (6 suppl 19):49–52, 2003

von Monakow C: Die Lokalisation im Grossheim und der Abbav der Funktion durch Kortikale Herde. Weisbaden, JF Bergmann, 1914

Warrington EK, Rabin P: Perceptual matching in patients with cerebral lesions. Neuropsychologia 8:475–487, 1970

Weitzner MA: Psychosocial and neuropsychiatric aspects of patients with primary brain tumors. Cancer Invest 17:285–291, 1999

Weitzner MA, Kanfer S, Booth-Jones M: Apathy and pituitary disease: it has nothing to do with depression. J Neuropsychiatry Clin Neurosci 17:159–166, 2005

Wellisch DK, Kaleita TA, Freeman D, et al: Predicting major depression in brain tumor patients. Psychooncology 11:230–238, 2002

White J, Cobb S: Psychological changes associated with giant pituitary neoplasms. Arch Neurol Psychiatry 74:383–396, 1955

Wilson G, Rupp C: Mental symptoms associated with extramedullary posterior fossa tumors. Trans Am Neurol Assoc 71:104–107, 1946

Wong TZ, van der Westhuizen GJ, Coleman RE: Positron emission tomography imaging of brain tumors. Neuroimaging Clin N Am 12:615–626, 2002

Woods SW, Tesar GE, Murray GB, et al: Psychostimulant treatment of depressive disorders secondary to medical illness. J Clin Psychiatry 47:12–15, 1986

Zwil AS, Bowring MA, Price TR, et al: Prospective electroconvulsive therapy in the presence of intracranial tumor. Convuls Ther 6:299–307, 1990

20

NEUROPSYCHIATRIC ASPECTS OF HUMAN IMMUNODEFICIENCY VIRUS INFECTION OF THE CENTRAL NERVOUS SYSTEM

Francisco Fernandez, M.D.

Jun Tan, M.D., Ph.D.

Human immunodeficiency virus (HIV) infection has become a major health and social issue of this era. It contributed to the first known decrease in average life expectancy in the United States (Kranczer 1995). Because of its complex nature, HIV may well continue to defy complete cure for some time to come. HIV not only devastates an individual's constitutional health but also attacks the central and peripheral nervous systems and causes a range of neurological syndromes and organic mental disorders with sometimes insidious courses. Our aim is to outline the neuropathology and neurobehavioral symptomatology associated with HIV infection and delineate the challenging and perplexing range of possible neuropsychiatric complications that clinicians may encounter. We discuss treatment of the various neuropsychiatric entities in relation to the special characteristics and needs of this medically ill population.

HIV: MEDICAL FACTORS

Since initial reports of the acquired immunodeficiency syndrome (AIDS) (Gottlieb et al. 1981) and the discovery that the syndrome and related illnesses were associated with a specific virus—HIV (Barre-Sinoussi et al. 1983; Gallo et al. 1983; J.A. Levy et al. 1984)—researchers have noted that infections can result from several high-risk situations. These risk factors include a venereal mode of transmission in which the virus borne on body fluids enters the bloodstream through breaks in mucous membranes; intravenous drug use with shared needles; and administration of blood transfusions, blood products, or blood factor concentrates infected with the virus. Infants are infected perinatally and through infected breast milk during lactation. Current terminology designates transmission patterns into two types: 1) the "horizontal" pattern, which includes body fluid contact through sexual activity, intravenous drug administration, and administration of blood products; and 2) the "vertical" pattern, by which infants are infected as just described.

Efforts to control this viral infection by pharmacological treatments have advanced remarkably since the onset of the pandemic. Unfortunately, there is no cure at this time, and attempts to develop vaccines for this organism have met with a confounding complexity of genetic features. HIV, a lentivirus and a retrovirus, possesses the capacity for amazing diversity and mutation. During the process of transcription of the double-stranded ribonucleic acid genome into deoxyribonucleic acid (DNA), two basic types of this highly genetically diverse virus have been identified: HIV-1 and HIV-2, both of which are thought to have originated in Africa (Clavel et al. 1986; Markovitz 1993; Miyazaki 1995; Rolfe 1994). There is increasing information that the main virus was zoonotic, with early infections arising from contact with chimpanzees. HIV-1 is more associated with the AIDS epidemic in Central and East Africa (Clavel et al. 1986), whereas HIV-2 is epidemic in West Africa but rare outside of that continent (Clavel et al. 1986; Markovitz 1993; Marlink et al. 1994; Miyazaki 1995; Rolfe 1994).

Through advances in genomic sequencing, several subtypes (referred to as *clades*) of HIV-1 (10, specified as A through J) and HIV-2 (5, indicated by A through E), and an atypical form of HIV-1 termed O for "outlier," have been identified. Moreover, each clade has several strains. Epidemiologically, the subtypes of HIV-1 were found to have rather specific geographic distributions (Brodine et al. 1997; Louwagie et al. 1993). HIV-1 clades A, C, and D are the most prevalent in Africa, whereas clade E is the modal virus in Southeast Asia, and clade C occurs most frequently in India and China (Brodine et al. 1997). Clade B is the predominant virus in North and South America and Europe (Brodine et al. 1997). It is not yet known if there are types that have a special affinity for the central nervous system (CNS), but it is known that there are mutations in a particular sequence of the viral envelope protein that more readily enter the brain. This virus possesses an amazing capacity for further diversity in that one individual, once infected, can produce myriad subspecies (Diaz et al. 1997). This is partially because during the reverse transcription process, the DNA genome that has just been produced is not proofread. This can result in a thousand-fold higher rate of nucleotide substitutions than may occur with herpesvirus DNA genomes (Brodine et al. 1997).

Both transmission modes apply to both HIV types (Miyazaki 1995), but evidence indicates that HIV-2 has a wider range of pathogenicity (Gao et al. 1994; Marlink et al. 1994). However, neurotropism is considered to be equivalent (Rolfe 1994). HIV-1 has been most investigated in research and clinical reports with regard to the pathology of AIDS and is the focus of this chapter wherever HIV is referenced.

According to the Centers for Disease Control and Prevention (2003) *HIV/AIDS Surveillance Report* through 2003, approximately 950,000 persons in the United States were living with HIV and were largely asymptomatic. An-

other estimated 920,000 (approximately 750,000 cases in males and 170,000 cases in females) had a diagnosis of AIDS (Centers for Disease Control and Prevention 2003). Worldwide, 38 million people are living with HIV. U.S. surveillance reports from 2000 to 2003 indicated that the overall annual rate of diagnosis of HIV/AIDS remained stable over this period, with an increase of 3% in the annual rates of males and a decrease of 3.7% in the annual rates of females (Centers for Disease Control and Prevention 2004). Of these HIV cases, epidemiological studies provide estimates that during the course of the infection, up to 30% may be expected to develop HIV-1–associated dementia (HAD; Heaton et al. 1995; Janssen et al. 1991, 1992), the most severe phase of HIV-1–associated cognitive/motor complex (Janssen et al. 1991). In the very young (younger than age 15 years) and in the elderly (age 75 or older), 13% and 19%, respectively, may have encephalopathy (Janssen et al. 1992; Mitsuyasu 1989). The appearance of this complication is ominous; the median survival duration after this diagnosis is about 6 months (McArthur et al. 1993, 2005).

The virus may have a long period of asymptomatic activity or dormancy, intracellularly, before symptoms of immune, neuromuscular, and CNS decline manifest (Bernad 1991; Brew et al. 1988; Hollander 1991; Koralnik et al. 1990; J.A. Levy 1993; Mitsuyasu 1989; Rowen and Carne 1991). This latency may last for 5–7 years before severe constitutional symptoms appear; however, cases of cognitive and psychiatric manifestations have been reported to occur even before the onset of AIDS case–defining criteria such as opportunistic infections, characteristic malignancies, or neurological syndromes (Beckett et al. 1987; Maccario and Scharre 1987; Navia and Price 1987).

CNS PATHOLOGY RESULTING DIRECTLY FROM HIV

AIDS is the term denoting the ultimate stage of systemic infection with HIV. However, before the realization that the disease was caused by a virus, clinicians noted that patients complained of cognitive and mood disorders. After researchers proposed a viral etiology of AIDS and AIDS-related disorders, investigations found that HIV not only is the agent of immune compromise but also may be neurotropic and neuropathogenic. The most common CNS complication is cognitive impairment of sufficient severity to warrant the diagnosis of a dementia. According to the Centers for Disease Control (1987), this dementia status is independently a diagnostic, case-defining criterion for the status of fully developed AIDS.

Cognitive disorders were originally believed to affect only a small proportion of HIV-infected individuals.

Studies have now reported that the prevalence and severity of cognitive impairment increase as the disease progresses (Heaton et al. 1995).

At the outset of the HIV epidemic, severe cognitive decline was thought to be a part of the end stage of HIV infection, associated only with AIDS. At that point, patients had opportunistic infections in addition to the effects of HIV brain infection; this combination could cause gross impairment. This severe cognitive disorder was often found to be composed of a combination of disturbances in cognitive functioning, motor behavior, and affective functioning, and this triad was termed *AIDS dementia complex* by Price and colleagues (Brew et al. 1988). Investigators also found that HIV itself produced an encephalitis or encephalopathy, which was variously termed *subacute encephalitis*, *HIV encephalopathy*, or *AIDS encephalopathy*. More recently, a behaviorally based set of criteria to distinguish levels of neurological and neurobehavioral impairment has been proposed by the American Academy of Neurology (AAN; see "Neurobehavioral Assessment of HIV Infection of the CNS" later in this chapter), which has termed these conditions *HIV-1-associated cognitive/motor complex* (Janssen et al. 1991). These criteria mainly distinguish motor impairments from mild cognitive deficits (HIV-1-associated minor cognitive/motor disorder) from the actual dementia (HAD), which is a profound state of disability.

Direct brain infection by HIV, therefore, is now widely believed to be the likely cause of related cognitive and other neurobehavioral disorders (Janssen et al. 1991). The evidence for this theory includes detection of HIV-1 in CNS 14 days after initial infection (Davis et al. 1992), presence of viral nucleic acid in the brains of some patients with this disorder, direct HIV isolation from the brain and cerebrospinal fluid (CSF) (Chiodi et al. 1992), electron microscopic findings of viral particles within infiltrating macrophages (Schindelmeiser and Gullotta 1991), and detection of viral antigens within the brains of infected individuals (Pumarola-Sune et al. 1987). The studies that showed direct brain infection by HIV provide a clear rationale for attempting to treat HIV-related cognitive disorder with an antiviral drug (see section "Treatment of HIV Infection of the CNS" later in this chapter). In addition, because the CNS in HIV infection can be regarded as a possible reservoir or sanctuary for the virus, antiviral drugs that can penetrate the blood-brain barrier and the blood-CSF barrier are clearly necessary.

With respect to how HIV gains entry to the CNS, Gyorkey and colleagues (1987), after reviewing autopsy material, postulated early in the history of the epidemic that this virus may enter the brain substance by passing through endothelial gaps in brain capillaries. A non-$CD4^+$-dependent HIV infection of brain capillary endothelial cells also has been identified (Moses et al. 1993). Investigators also have proposed that the virus gains entry to the brain parenchyma via infiltration of infected macrophage leukocytes, the so-called Trojan Horse effect (Dickson et al. 1991; Schindelmeiser and Gullotta 1991; Vazeux 1991). Regardless of the mode of entry, the virus attaches via its coat glycoprotein gp120 to binding sites (most notably, $CD4^+$ receptors) on brain microglial cells (J.A. Levy 1993; S.A. Lipton and Gendleman 1995). Hill and colleagues (1987) have detailed numerous brain sites where the virus seems to have an affinity. These areas are rich with $CD4^+$ receptors and include basal ganglia and temporolimbic structures. This localization of receptors may relate to the typical neurobehavioral symptoms associated with HAD (Hill et al. 1987; Ruscetti et al. 1988).

Much of the knowledge of central neuropathology associated with HIV infection has come from the pioneering work of Price and colleagues (Brew et al. 1988; Navia et al. 1986a, 1986b) and Wiley and colleagues (Masliah et al. 1992, 1995; Wiley et al. 1991), who have extensively reviewed autopsy material of patients with fully developed AIDS, and from subsequent histological examinations that have further delineated regional involvement. Gross examination of the brain indicates that the white matter, subcortical structures, and vacuolar myelopathy of the spinal cord are commonly involved (Brew et al. 1988). Also, at this stage, extensive atrophy, most notably reflected in increased ventricular size (as opposed to widened sulcal spaces), is found. Although neurons are thought not to be the direct target of the virus (yet some investigators have found regional neuronal loss in HIV-1 brain infection [Ketzler et al. 1990; Weis et al. 1993]), they sustain neurotoxic effects. Frequently involved subcortical gray matter structures include basal ganglia, thalamus, and temporolimbic structures. The cerebral cortex is often spared; however, some investigators have noted extensive cortical changes (Ciardi et al. 1990; Everall et al. 1991; Ketzler et al. 1990; Masliah et al. 1992; Navia et al. 1986a; Wiley et al. 1991). Wiley and colleagues applied sensitive quantitative methods to the histological analysis of cerebral cortex and found up to a 40% loss of cortical dendritic area (Masliah et al. 1992). In this analysis, the severity of cortical damage was found to be correlated with level of HIV gp41 immunoreactivity (Masliah et al. 1992).

This CNS neuropathology often results in cognitive changes, from mild memory decline and cognitive slowing to a profound dementia (Everall et al. 1993; Grafe et al. 1990). In addition, Price and colleagues noted in their series of findings that HIV-1 could be recovered mainly from brains of patients with the most severe form of dementia in which multinucleated giant cell creation had occurred

(Brew et al. 1988). However, dementia also has developed in individuals in whom the virus could not be recovered from the CNS, either directly or by hybridization methods.

Once the virus has entered the CNS, a complex cascade of events can occur to cause neural injury, which is thought to result in the various neurobehavioral syndromes (S.A. Lipton and Gendleman 1995). S.A. Lipton and Gendleman (1995) have detailed what is currently known about these events. First, in the process of binding to a CD4$^+$ receptor–containing cell, HIV gp120 irreversibly binds to a calcium channel and increases intracellular free calcium (Giulian et al. 1990; Stefano et al. 1993). HIV gp120 also induces the cell to increase neurotoxin production (S.A. Lipton and Gendleman 1995) and may alter brain glucose metabolism, which could lead to brain dysfunction (Kaiser et al. 1990; S.A. Lipton and Gendleman 1995). Second, after the virus enters the cell and incorporates its genome into the host's genome, it can induce the infected macrophage to release more injurious compounds in the presence of other stimulators, such as other CNS infectious by-products and cytokines produced in response to infections by other immunologically active cells. S.A. Lipton and Gendleman (1995) described these compounds to include glutamate-like substances such as quinolinic acid; free radicals such as superoxide anions; other cytokines such as tumor necrosis factor-α, interleukin-1-β, and interferon-γ; and eicosanoids such as arachidonic acid. Additionally, gp120 and certain fragment peptides are powerful activators of N-methyl-D-aspartate (NMDA) receptors of the CNS, the mechanism associated with neuroexcitotoxicity (Gemignani et al. 2000). These are all thought to cause neurocellular injury by several mechanisms, including increased intracellular calcium and increased concentrations of the toxic inorganic compound nitric oxide.

Another process—apoptosis, or programmed cell destruction—was proposed as an additional factor in the destruction of CD4$^+$ cells in HIV disease, for both lymphocytes and neural tissues. Apoptosis is the genetically determined cell death (Bellamy et al. 1995; Silvestris et al. 1995; Steller 1995) that is thought to maintain homeostasis in the body by eliminating excess and worn-out cells. One protein thought to participate in this process is FAS (Lynch et al. 1995; Silvestris et al. 1995), and this genetically driven action has been shown to culminate in disruption of the cell's nucleus by activation of endonucleases (Silvestris et al. 1995). The process of homeostasis is thought to go awry in cancer, AIDS, and neurodegenerative diseases (Bellamy et al. 1995; Steller 1995; Thompson 1995). Certain immune factors, such as tumor necrosis factor-α, can trigger apoptosis (Talley et al. 1995).

In the case of HIV infection, several virus-related proteins can trigger apoptosis. Gp120 also has been reported to induce apoptosis (Maccarrone et al. 2000). Tumor necrosis factor-α can be produced by HIV-related gp120 binding to macrophages, which may lead to this process (Sekigawa et al. 1995). Apoptosis also has been shown to be induced peripherally by the HIV-related Tat protein (Li et al. 1995). This cell-destroying mechanism can be inhibited, and knowledge of how to effect this inhibition can be applied to clinical AIDS treatment. Certain immunosuppressive compounds such as FK506 (Sekigawa et al. 1995) and glucocorticoids (Lu et al. 1995) have inhibited apoptosis, as have growth factors (Li et al. 1995), soluble CD4 (Maldarelli et al. 1995), N-acetylcysteine (Talley et al. 1995), and didanosine (preinfection only) (Corbeil and Richman 1995), but not zidovudine (Maldarelli et al. 1995). However, inhibiting apoptosis can present further difficulties because it has been shown that it can enhance viral production and lead to high levels of persistent viral infection (Antoni et al. 1995).

HIV-related apoptosis apparently also can affect the CNS in HIV encephalitis (Petito and Roberts 1995; Talley et al. 1995). Apoptosis was considered to be operational in the demise of neurons and astrocytes as determined by characteristic morphology and immunohistochemical labeling of cell fragments. The stimulatory mechanism for this CNS apoptosis was thought to be a viral product or component or tumor necrosis factor, the latter supported by an in vitro study in which tumor necrosis factor-α caused apoptosis in neuroblastoma cell culture (Talley et al. 1995). Thus, this naturally regulated process may be dysregulated by the complex actions of viral infection and its by-products, which may become a major contributor to the various ways that the CNS is impaired in HIV infection.

Investigators who have searched for a biochemical marker that would correlate with or predict the level of the neurobehavioral disturbance in HAD have found that levels of β$_2$-microglobulin, eicosanoids, prostaglandin E$_2$, and neopterin are promising assays at this time (Brew et al. 1992; Elovaara et al. 1989; Griffin et al. 1994; Harrison and Skidmore 1990; Karlsen et al. 1991). These levels correlated highly with degree of dementia.

Additional work on the neuropathology of excitotoxins (Cotton 1990; Heyes et al. 1991, 1992; Kieburtz et al. 1991a; S.A. Lipton 1992; S.A. Lipton and Gendleman 1995; Sardar et al. 1995; Schwarcz et al. 1983; Walker et al. 1989), the role of NMDA receptor physiology and dysregulation (Kieburtz et al. 1991a; S.A. Lipton 1992; S.A. Lipton and Gendleman 1995), and the specific neurotoxicity of quinolinic acid, a metabolite of tryptophan (Kieburtz et al. 1991a; S.A. Lipton and Gendleman 1995; Schwarcz et al. 1983), is also contributing to the explanation of how neuronal tissue is injured by remote metabolic effects of HIV infection. Quinolinic acid levels have been found to be highly correlated with levels of β_2-microglobulin and neopterin (Heyes et al. 1992; Kieburtz et al. 1991a) and with cognitive impairment (Heyes et al. 1991).

The preceding discussion clearly shows that inflammation plays an important role in the pathology of HAD. The inflammatory changes are probably initially the result of the transmigration of HIV-1-infected cells across the blood-brain barrier and include microglial activation as well as increased cytokine production and activity (Asensio and Campbell 1999). Many studies have suggested or assumed that such inflammation arises mainly from the interaction of microglia with these viral proteins, such as Tat and gp120 (McManus et al. 2000; Minghetti et al. 2004). Interestingly, D'Aversa et al. (2005) has recently shown that viral proteins also up-regulate key surface receptors, such as CD40, a type I transmembrane glycoprotein, on microglia. In a previous study, D'Aversa and colleagues (2002) found a significantly increased number of CD40-positive microglia in HIV encephalitic brain. Additionally, they showed that treatment of these cultured microglia with interferon-γ and CD40L greatly produces several cytokines that may be neurotoxic (D'Aversa et al. 2002; Tan et al. 1999). Thus, disruption of the CD40-CD40L interaction might implicate this pathway as a therapeutic target for HAD (D'Aversa et al. 2002).

CNS NEUROPATHOLOGY DUE TO OPPORTUNISTIC INFECTIONS AND NEOPLASIA

As mentioned earlier in this chapter, when severe neurological disease, opportunistic infections, or malignancies such as Kaposi's sarcoma and HIV-related lymphomas arise, the patient's condition meets criteria for full-blown AIDS. This may occur at any time, although immune compromise is usually reflected by the clinical and laboratory markers—namely, fewer than 200 CD4$^+$ cells/mm^3. Additionally, syphilis and tuberculosis are increasingly found as coinfections in patients with AIDS. These disorders must be considered in the differential diagnosis of CNS infection. These opportunistic infections and malignancies may contribute to severe neurological disorders or overwhelming dementia (Bedri et al. 1983; Belman et al. 1986; Brew et al. 1988; Budka 1989; Filley et al. 1988; Gonzales and David 1988; Gray et al. 1988; Ho et al. 1987; Lantos et al. 1989; Petito 1988). Thus, it is important to investigate and treat aggressively the cause of the neurological problem in order to postpone mortality and to seek to restore normal neurobehavioral function. Bredesen and colleagues (1988) reviewed common CNS infections, as well as neoplasia and other infection- or

treatment-induced complications. This range of CNS involvement is listed in Table 20–1 (Bredesen et al. 1988).

Toxoplasma gondii is perhaps the most common opportunistic infection in AIDS and may present as a focal or diffuse cognitive or affective disturbance. Clinically, toxoplasmosis symptoms include malaise, confusion, lethargy, headache, fever, and focal deficits. The authors have seen a case of cerebral toxoplasmosis (Figure 20–1), which initially presented as a presumed postpartum depression. This affective disorder was refractory to antidepressant treatment. Later, the patient developed hemiballismus. A neurodiagnostic evaluation, including computed tomographic imaging, subsequently identified CNS toxoplasmosis.

The results of serological testing are of limited diagnostic value. Neuroimaging may have normal findings, but a typical presentation of toxoplasmal involvement is a ring-enhancing lesion near the subcortical gray matter structures (Jarvik et al. 1988; Kelly and Brant-Zawadzki 1983; Whelan et al. 1983). Multiple lesions are common on magnetic resonance imaging (MRI), with toxoplasmal foci on T2 scans represented as areas of heightened signal intensity (Bredesen et al. 1988). Thallium-201 single-photon emission computed tomography (SPECT) can be helpful in distinguishing cerebral toxoplasmosis (negative uptake) from lymphoma (increased uptake). Definitive diagnosis for toxoplasmosis is determined by biopsy.

Cryptococcus neoformans, the other common AIDS-related intracranial infection, presents principally as a meningitis, with headache (R.B. Lipton et al. 1991), altered mental status, nuchal rigidity, fever, and nausea and vomiting. Definitive diagnosis is based on analysis of CSF.

Other viral infections producing personality and behavior changes and cognitive impairment, with and without sensorimotor impairments, that have been reported frequently in the CNS include progressive multifocal leukoencephalopathy (PML; Bedri et al. 1983; Berger et al. 1987; Fong and Toma 1995; J.K. Miller et al. 1982; Portegies et al. 1991) due to a papovavirus (Jacob-Creutzfeldt virus [JCV]); cytomegalovirus (CMV); herpes simplex virus (HSV); and varicella zoster virus (VZV). The prognosis for PML remains grave; however, combination treatment with cytarabine and zidovudine appears promising for not only extending life but also producing remission (Portegies et al. 1991). New treatments aimed at inhibiting JCV replication are expected to improve patient survival (Berger and Concha 1995; Kerr et al. 1993).

CMV is commonly seen in the CNS of AIDS patients and may produce encephalitis, retinitis, and peripheral neuropathies and demyelination (Bredesen et al. 1988; Masdeu et al. 1988). Treatment of CMV infection is currently limited to chronic administration of ganciclovir (dihydroxypropoxymethyl guanine; DHPG), foscarnet

TABLE 20–1.   CNS conditions associated with AIDS and HIV infection

HIV-associated disorders

HIV-1-associated cognitive/motor complex

HIV-1-associated dementia

HIV-1-associated minor cognitive/motor disorder

HIV-1-associated myelopathy

Opportunistic viral infections

Cytomegalovirus

Herpes simplex virus, types 1 and 2

Herpes varicella zoster virus

Papovavirus (progressive multifocal leukoencephalopathy)

Adenovirus type 2

Other opportunistic infections of the CNS

Toxoplasma gondii

Cryptococcus neoformans

Candida albicans

Aspergillus fumigatus

Coccidioides immitis

Mucormycosis

Rhizopus species

Acremonium alabamensis

Histoplasma capsulatum

Mycobacterium tuberculosis

Mycobacterium avium-intracellulare

Listeria monocytogenes

Nocardia asteroides

Neoplasms

Primary CNS lymphoma

Metastatic lymphoma

Metastatic Kaposi's sarcoma

Cerebrovascular pathology

Infarction

Hemorrhage

Vasculitis

Adverse effects of treatments for HIV and AIDS-related disorders

Note.   CNS = central nervous system; AIDS = acquired immunodeficiency syndrome; HIV = human immunodeficiency virus.

Source.   Adapted from Bredesen DE, Levy RM, Rosenblum ML: "The Neurology of Human Immunodeficiency Virus Infection." *Quarterly Journal of Medicine* 68:665–677, 1988. Copyright 1988 Oxford University Press. Used with permission.

(Reddy et al. 1992; Studies of the Ocular Complications of AIDS Research Group 1994), or, more problematically, cidofovir (Akler et al. 1998; Lalezari et al. 1998). It also has been found that the protease inhibitors and highly active antiretroviral therapy (HAART), used systemically for general HIV treatment, help control the retinitis (Macdonald et al. 1998; Reed et al. 1997).

HSV infections may manifest in temporal lobe encephalitis or encephalomyelitis in immune-deficient patients. The severity of the infection seems to correlate with the level of immune dysfunction (Bredesen et al. 1988). Progression to a chronic mental disorder due to a general medical condition with amnestic features is a danger. The usual emergency treatment for suspected HSV encephalitis—intravenous acyclovir—would apply in these cases.

VZV can reactivate in AIDS patients, causing a range of peripheral and cranial nerve inflammatory responses, encephalitis, myelitis, and inflammations of brain vasculature (Beilke 1989; Bredesen et al. 1988; Scaravilli et al. 1989; Vinters et al. 1988). Diagnosis of VZV in the CNS is associated with elevated VZV antibody titers in the CSF (Bredesen et al. 1988). VZV is treated with intravenous acyclovir or vidarabine.

Mycobacterial (especially tuberculosis) and fungal infections also occur in the brain see (see Table 20–1). Diagnosis is aided through biopsy. Tuberculous meningitis is the most frequent extrapulmonary manifestation in HIV-1 infection. Aggressive treatment for longer periods is required to avoid relapses.

Syphilis occurs as a concurrent CNS infection, and its diagnosis is problematic. It can be asymptomatic, and other causes of meningitis can obscure the picture. Cases with a negative CSF Venereal Disease Research Laboratory result have been reported (Musher et al. 1990), and the fluorescent treponemal antibody absorption test (FTA-ABS) also has not been conclusive. Other newer techniques such as polymerase chain reaction for the nucleic material of the treponema may lead to better differentiation (DeBiasi and Tyler 1999). Treatment of syphilis is with intravenous aqueous crystalline penicillin G, followed by intramuscular penicillin G benzathine.

Non-Hodgkin's lymphoma is commonly seen as a primary CNS tumor in AIDS patients (Bredesen et al. 1988). Patients with lymphoma usually present with altered mental status, hemiparesis, aphasia, seizures, or other focal symptoms. One patient in our emergency department presented with a manic episode. He had no history of affective disorder. At first, he was given a diagnosis of toxoplasmosis, but he ultimately received an accurate diagnosis of CNS lymphoma (Figure 20–2). A diagnostic investigation, including computed tomo-

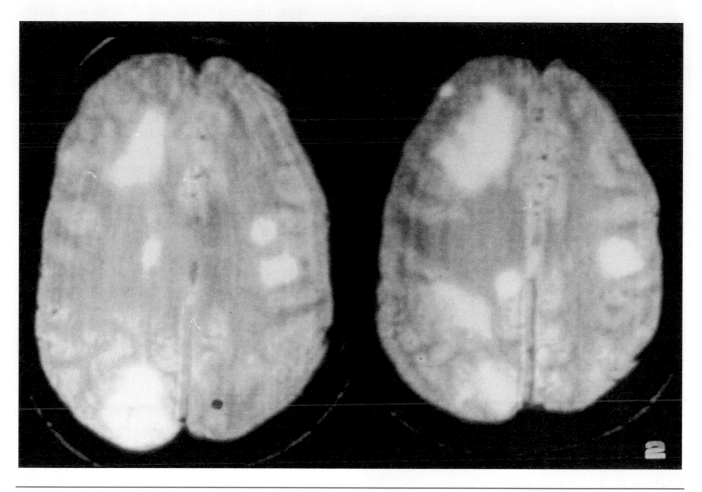

FIGURE 20–1.   Magnetic resonance imaging scan of a 35-year-old woman presenting with severe postpartum depression and history of long-term intravenous drug use. The patient's symptoms were refractory to antidepressant pharmacotherapy, and she was being evaluated for electroconvulsive therapy. Multiple foci of cerebral toxoplasmosis, confirmed by cerebrospinal fluid titer, are seen as bright patches, with the largest in the left frontal and occipital areas.

graphic imaging, detected a right frontal ring-enhancing lesion in this patient. Diagnosis of lymphoma is confirmed with the aid of neuroimaging, biopsy, and/or recovery of malignant cells from the CSF. The prognosis for survival ranges from less than 6 months to 1 year or more.

Cerebrovascular problems (Beilke 1989; Bredesen et al. 1988; Engstrom et al. 1989; Frank et al. 1989; Scaravilli et al. 1989; Snider et al. 1983; Vinters et al. 1988) commonly occur in AIDS patients. These problems may result from viral (e.g., varicella zoster virus; Frank et al. 1989) or bacterial/treponemal (Brightbill et al. 1995) vasculitis. Also, cerebral infarcts may result from emboli secondary to nonbacterial thrombotic endocarditis (Bredesen et al. 1988). Other causes of cerebrovascular problems include vasculotoxic responses to treatment of systemic infections and malignancies. Behaviorally, a multi-infarct state may be reflected as a stepwise decline in cognitive functioning and must be differentiated from the more protracted progressive viral encephalopathic process.

Thus, clinicians must rapidly assess patients presenting with focal neurocognitive findings, which may be the result of potentially treatable infections, to forestall more serious global mental status decline or death.

DIRECT ASSESSMENT OF CNS INJURY IN HIV DISEASE

NEUROIMAGING FINDINGS

Imaging, by both computed tomography (CT) and MRI, has proved helpful in showing injury by the virus and other pathological processes in the brain (Bishburg et al. 1989; Dooneief et al. 1992; Flowers et al. 1990; Freund-Levi et al. 1989; Jarvik et al. 1988; Kelly and Brant-Zawadzki 1983; H. S. Levin et al. 1990; Post et al. 1991; Whelan et al. 1983). Aside from either method being able to show atrophy, as reflected by increased ventricular size and sulcal size, both can help to define pathological entities such

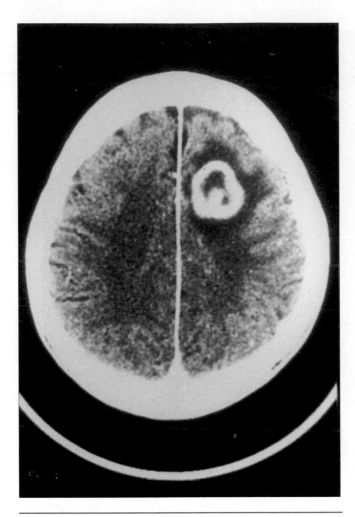

FIGURE 20–2.   Computed tomography scan of a 21-year-old man presenting in an emergency department with a first episode of mania.

Imaging reflecting functioning of the nervous system, such as positron emission tomography (PET) (Brunetti et al. 1989; Hinkin et al. 1995), SPECT (Kuni et al. 1991; Masdeu et al. 1991; Sacktor et al. 1995a), magnetic resonance spectroscopy (MRS) (Deicken et al. 1991; Jarvik et al. 1993; Menon et al. 1990), functional MRI (Navia and Gonzalez 1997), and regional cerebral blood flow (rCBF) (Schielke et al. 1990), has shown regional functional abnormalities in HIV. These imaging modalities have established themselves as sensitive to different aspects of functioning: PET reflects metabolism; SPECT, functional MRI, and rCBF reflect brain perfusion; and MRS reflects biochemical function and dysfunction.

In one study (Brunetti et al. 1989), PET-detected subcortical hypermetabolism in basal ganglia and thalamus was seen early in the course of CNS disease, followed by regional and then general hypometabolism as the disease progressed. PET scanning also has proved to be helpful in ascertaining the therapeutic effects of antiviral treatment. PET scanning noted reversal of focal cortical abnormalities of glucose metabolism after the AIDS dementia complex was treated with zidovudine (Brunetti et al. 1989). In other patients without abnormalities at baseline, glucose metabolism increased after zidovudine treatment. Improved brain glucose utilization was correlated with neurological functional improvement. As mentioned earlier in this chapter, CNS glucose utilization was found to be, in part, dysregulated by a glycoprotein associated with the HIV viral coat (Kaiser et al. 1990); thus, reduction in viral activity could be associated with this increased glucose metabolism.

SPECT scanning has been improved to provide more qualitative and quantitative reflection of brain cortical and subcortical perfusion. One study (Sacktor et al. 1995b), however, was not able to correlate focal perfusion deficits with neuropsychological deficits; only motor function impairment correlated with global perfusion deficits.

MRS presented functional evidence of neuronal loss in HIV-infected patients who had normal structure on MRI (Menon et al. 1990) and identified decreased brain adenosine triphosphate and phosphocreatine concentrations in the white matter of HIV-positive neuropsychiatric patients (Deicken et al. 1991). MRS with a quantitation of choline-to-creatine signals ratio has been suggested to characterize neuronal dysfunction. This ratio was determined to increase with cellular membrane turnover (Chong et al. 1993). The N-acetylaspartate–to–creatine ratio (Barker et al. 1995; Chong et al. 1993; Tracey et al. 1996) and phosphocreatine (Deicken et al. 1991) concentration also were found to decrease in relation to neuronal dysfunction. Studies report an increase in choline (probably reflecting a reactive astrocytosis) and reductions in N-acetylaspartate (probably reflecting neuronal injury). These findings have been correlated with

as ring-enhancing lesions and some aspects of white matter involvement. MRI is superior to CT in showing areas of focal high-signal intensities in subcortical white and gray matter by the T2-weighted signal (Dooneief et al. 1992). T1 relaxation times have been examined and have not indicated structural differences between older HIV-infected patients and control subjects or temporal changes in these older patients as their disease progressed (Freund-Levi et al. 1989). MRI also has not proven useful in depicting structural correlates of neurologically asymptomatic HIV infection (Post et al. 1991). MRI, however, has disclosed neurostructural changes in medically symptomatic but neurologically asymptomatic HIV-positive patients. Jernigan et al. (1993) found volumetric reductions in cerebral gray and white matter in these patients. Most recently, MRI that uses diffusion tensor imaging (DTI) to study white matter abnormalities such as white matter pallor has been found useful in distinguishing between HIV-1-infected patients and noninfected control subjects.

severity of cognitive changes, severity of dementia, CD4 cell count, and both plasma and CSF viral load (Chang et al. 1999). With antiretroviral treatment, these MRS changes can normalize over time (Chang et al. 2001). Proton MRS may be a useful way to follow up patients from the neurologically asymptomatic stage through HIV-1-associated minor cognitive/motor disorder and HAD (Cecil and Lenkinski 1998). It may provide an early marker of neuronal dysfunction before irreversible damage to the CNS occurs.

CEREBROSPINAL FLUID FINDINGS

The CSF of HIV-infected patients who have fever with or without altered mental status or with complaints about mental functioning should be evaluated quickly for signs of opportunistic infection such as toxoplasmosis, cryptococcal infection, HSV, varicella zoster virus, and CMV so that appropriate anti-infective treatment can be initiated before CNS damage occurs (Buffet et al. 1991). Specific signs of HIV infection that are reflected in CSF values include HIV virions, immunoglobulin G (IgG—in abnormally large quantities), HIV-specific antibody, mononuclear cells, neopterin, β_2-microglobulin, and oligoclonal bands (Brew et al. 1992; Buffet et al. 1991; Carrieri et al. 1992; Chiodi et al. 1992; Heyes et al. 1991; Larsson et al. 1991; Lolli et al. 1990; Marshall et al. 1988, 1991; McArthur et al. 1992; Portegies et al. 1989; Reboul et al. 1989; Shaskan et al. 1992; Tartaglione et al. 1991). The amount of intrathecal virus and antibody, however, has not been found to correlate with severity of neurological or cognitive symptomatology (Reboul et al. 1989). IgG production was found to increase throughout duration of infection (1-year sampling), regardless of CD4$^+$ cell count, in neurologically healthy patients (Marshall et al. 1991). The concentration of CSF β_2-microglobulin is highly correlated with both dementia severity (Brew et al. 1992; McArthur et al. 1992) and level of systemic disease (asymptomatic seropositivity to fully developed AIDS). CSF β_2-microglobulin has shown some specificity in differentiating HAD from multiple sclerosis and other CNS disorders (Carrieri et al. 1992) with regard to absolute levels and CSF-to-serum ratios. Additionally, it can reflect positive symptomatic zidovudine therapy (Brew et al. 1992) (although the amount of virus in the CSF may not be reduced with treatment [Tartaglione et al. 1991]).

Merrill (1992) has suggested that the presence of cytokines, namely interleukin-1, tumor necrosis factor-α, interleukin-6, and transforming growth factor-β, may be associated with both pro- and anti-inflammatory events in the CNS. He compared differences in myelin damage in multiple sclerosis and HIV infection of the CNS: in multiple sclerosis, effector cell–mediated lesion production, destruction

of oligodendrocytes, and demyelination occur; in HIV, virus-induced toxin production via macrophages and microglia, which can produce myelin pallor, occurs. This syndrome may cause neural dysfunction throughout the brain without frank destruction of myelin, which would be reflected in an increase in CSF levels of myelin basic protein (Marshall et al. 1988, 1991). Others have reported that demyelination occurs in HIV disease (e.g., Greenberg 1995). HIV has been associated with a demyelinating chronic inflammatory peripheral polyneuropathy that presents as Guillain-Barré syndrome (Cornblath et al. 1987; Dalakas and Pezeshkpour 1988), but debate continues as to whether it also may be centrally demyelinating (Gray and Lescs 1993; Merrill 1987; Power et al. 1993; Vago et al. 1993).

Analysis of neurotransmitter metabolites in CSF, specifically those of noradrenaline and dopamine, failed to detect significantly different levels of 3-methoxy-4-hydroxyphenylglycol (MHPG) between HIV-infected patients and noninfected, healthy volunteers (Larsson et al. 1991). However, CSF levels of homovanillic acid (HVA) were lower by almost half in HIV-infected patients than in noninfected volunteers and lowest in patients with AIDS; no direct relation was found between HVA levels and severity of dementia. The level of quinolinic acid, an excitotoxin and an NMDA receptor agonist (see earlier discussion in the section "CNS Pathology Resulting Directly From HIV"), is related to severity of dementia and clinical status (Heyes et al. 1991). In patients with early-stage disease, quinolinic acid levels were twice those of non-HIV-infected subjects, and more than 20 times normal levels were detected in patients with severe dementia or CNS AIDS involvement (opportunistic infection or CNS neoplasms) (Heyes et al. 1991). More recently, CSF quinolinic acid levels were found to correlate with regional brain atrophy as quantified by MRI, whereas CSF β_2-microglobulin levels were not (Heyes et al. 2001). The significance of these levels of an excitotoxin in the CNS continues to be investigated with regard to pathogenesis and pathophysiology of cognitive disorders.

A relation between endorsed depressive or anxious symptoms and CSF immune function markers has been found in HIV-positive U.S. Air Force personnel (Praus et al. 1990). These investigators found significant correlations between CSF nucleated cell counts or protein levels and Hamilton Rating Scale for Depression scores greater than 10 and between CSF nucleated cell counts or absolute CD4a cell counts and Hamilton Anxiety Scale scores greater than 10.

Measurements of HIV RNA in the CSF are not routinely done on a clinical basis. However, the available literature strongly suggests correlation of concentrations of CSF HIV RNA with the severity of neurological and neuropsychological deficits in untreated patients (Brew et al. 1997; McArthur et al. 1997). With antiretroviral treatment, these deficits are attenuated or reversed (Marra et al. 2003; McArthur et al. 2004).

ELECTROPHYSIOLOGICAL FINDINGS

Electrophysiological examination of HIV-infected patients with cognitive and neurological complaints is helpful in establishing an organic basis for these conditions and has detected neural dysfunction before other behavioral markers could (Goodin et al. 1990; Goodwin et al. 1990; Ollo et al. 1990, 1991; Tinuper et al. 1990). Both electroencephalogram (EEG) and specific evoked potentials have been used in this regard. HIV infection may cause a convulsive disorder (Parisi et al. 1991), but most studies have shown that, groupwise, the percentage of patients with abnormal EEG findings increases as the systemic disease progresses and that slowing of dominant frequencies is unusual. In Centers for Disease Control group II (asymptomatic) patients, 25% were found to have abnormal EEG results, with frontotemporal theta slowing as the predominant finding (Elovaara et al. 1991; Parisi et al. 1989). In Centers for Disease Control group III (persistent generalized lymphadenopathy) patients, 30% had a variety of abnormalities somewhat evenly divided among frontotemporal theta slowing, diffuse theta slowing, and frontotemporal delta slowing (Parisi et al. 1989). Thus, these significant electrophysiological disturbances occurred in pre-AIDS groups. Others (Gabuzda et al. 1988) have found even higher percentages of abnormalities in more physically symptomatic patients. Of the patients with pre-AIDS, 35% had mildly to severely abnormal findings, whereas 65% of the patients with AIDS had mildly to severely abnormal EEG activity. Across both these diagnostic groups, intermittent or continuous symmetric theta or delta slowing was characteristic.

Sleep-related EEG findings also have reflected effects of HIV on the CNS. Sleep is often disturbed in patients with HIV disease (Darko et al. 1995), and polysomnography has been used to investigate patients' complaints of dyssomnia. These studies have uncovered gross disturbances in sleep architecture (Itil et al. 1990; Norman et al. 1990; Wiegand et al. 1991a, 1991b). The viral infection may play a central role in these disorders, and medication effects such as those of zidovudine also must be included in the analysis of sleep disturbances due to HIV disease.

Evoked potential studies were able to detect abnormalities in neurologically and physically asymptomatic HIV-seropositive patients (Goodin et al. 1990; Goodwin et al. 1990; Smith et al. 1988). Brain-stem auditory and somatosensory evoked potentials from tibial nerve stimulation and oculomotor activity recordings showed signif-

TABLE 20–2. HIV-1-associated minor cognitive/motor disorder: American Academy of Neurology criteria

The patient must have all of the following:

A. Cognitive/motor/behavioral dysfunctions: at least two of the following (acquired and present for at least 1 month):

Impaired attention/concentration

Mental slowing

Impaired memory

Slowed movements

Incoordination

Personality change, irritability, or emotional lability

These cognitive/motor dysfunctions must be documented by neurological examination or neuropsychological testing.

B. The dysfunction in cognitive/motor/behavioral abilities must cause mild impairment of work-related activities or activities of daily living.

C. The level of disturbance does not meet the criteria for HIV-1-associated dementia complex or HIV-1-associated myelopathy.

D. There must be no evidence of another etiology, such as CNS opportunistic infection or malignancy or severe systemic illness (documented by history, physical examination, and laboratory and radiological investigations), or effects related to alcohol/substance use, acute or chronic substance withdrawal, adjustment disorder, or other psychiatric disorders.

Note. HIV=human immunodeficiency virus; CNS=central nervous system.
Source. Adapted from Janssen RS, Cornblath DR, Epstein LG, and the Working Group of the American Academy of Neurology AIDS Task Force: "Nomenclature and Research Case Definitions for Neurologic Manifestations of Human Immunodeficiency Virus-Type 1 (HIV-1) Infection." *Neurology* 41:778–785, 1991. Used with permission.

icant delays in latencies of response compared with those of control subjects. These authors concluded that evoked potentials may represent an early direct indication of neurological involvement in HIV disease, before overt symptomatology occurs.

Quantitative EEG results in patients with HIV disease have more consistently shown the evolution of electrophysiological abnormalities across the HIV disease spectrum. One correlation study with PET confirmed the clinical conceptualization of HAD as a subcortical dementia (Newton et al. 1993, 1994). Quantitative EEG also may be useful to monitor progress in patients taking various antiretroviral therapies (Baldeweg et al. 1995). It seems reasonable to use quantitative EEG adjunctively to adequately detect and monitor HIV-associated cognitive changes and their treatment.

NEUROBEHAVIORAL ASSESSMENT OF HIV INFECTION OF THE CNS

Dementia is generally regarded as an acquired intellectual impairment characterized by persistent deficits in multiple areas, including memory, language, cognition, visuospatial skills, personality, and emotional functioning (Cummings and Benson 1983). HAD has been portrayed as a subcortical type of dementia affecting subcortical and frontostriatal brain processes (Brew et al. 1988). However, because other CNS cortical areas have been identified as being affected (Ciardi et al. 1990; Everall et al. 1991; Grant et al. 1987; Ketzler et al. 1990; Masliah et al. 1992; Navia et al. 1986a; Wiley et al. 1991), a strict definition of HIV-related cognitive impairment as a subcortical disorder has been questioned (Poutiainen et al. 1991). Dementia's persistent cognitive impairment differentiates it from another common HIV-related mental disorder due to a general medical condition—delirium. The symptoms most frequently described and most closely associated with subcortical disorders such as Parkinson's disease and progressive supranuclear palsy, as well as multiple sclerosis, are found in HIV infection of the CNS. The description of HAD as a subcortical process suggests that neuropsychological tests that reflect memory registration, storage, and retrieval; psychomotor speed; information processing rate; and fine motor function are important in a neuropsychological battery for assessment of HIV-related cognitive impairment (Butters et al. 1990). Other traditionally cortical syndromes, such as aphasia, agnosia, apraxia, and other sensory-perceptual functions, also can be present but usually not until later in the course of the disease and perhaps as a result of some focal opportunistic infection or neoplastic invasion of the CNS.

The earliest level of cognitive impairment is a subclinical cognitive inefficiency that can range in severity from a decrement in previous level of functioning in attention, speed of information processing, memory, abstraction, and fine motor skills to formal test-defined deficits in some of these domains. Disturbances in these functions may have no observable effects on activities of daily living or functional performance. These changes occur in more

TABLE 20–3. Early signs and symptoms of HIV-related neurobehavioral impairment

Cognitive	Affective/behavioral
Memory impairment (especially with verbal, rote, or episodic)	Apathy
	Depressed mood
	Anxiety
Concentration or attention disturbance	Mild agitation
Language comprehension problems	Mild disinhibition
Conceptualization difficulties	Hallucinations or misperceptions
Problem-solving difficulties	
Visuospatial constructional deficits	
Motor slowing or impairment in coordination	
Mental tracking difficulties	
Mild frontal lobe–type symptoms	
Handwriting and fine motor control difficulties	

Note. HIV = human immunodeficiency virus.
Source. Adapted from Brew BJ, Sidtis JJ, Petito CK, et al: "The Neurologic Complications of AIDS and Human Immunodeficiency Virus Infection," in *Advances in Contemporary Neurology.* Edited by Plum F. Philadelphia, PA, FA Davis, 1988, pp. 1–49.

than 20% of asymptomatic HIV-1-infected individuals (Wilkie et al. 1990a), but the proportion of patients having these problems doubles with advanced disease (Heaton et al. 1995). More severe impairment interfering minimally with functional status is now defined by the AAN as HIV-1-associated minor cognitive/motor disorder (Table 20–2). Prevalence of HIV-1-associated minor cognitive/motor disorder is unknown, but estimates suggest that 20%–30% of asymptomatic HIV-1-infected individuals may meet formal AAN criteria for this disorder (Goodkin 2001). Indications of early HIV-1-associated minor cognitive/motor disorder may be mild and, as such, are frequently attributed to the systemic illness or a psychosocial reaction to HIV infection. However, even under the influence of an early organic process that affects cognition, many patients will be cognizant of their own mental and physical sluggishness and personality changes, and affective symptoms may occur concomitantly.

Fully developed HAD is commonly associated with significant declines in functional status. Table 20–3 shows

TABLE 20–4.   Late signs and symptoms of HIV-related neurobehavioral impairment

Cognitive	Affective/behavioral
Severe dementia affecting multiple cognitive areas	Severe behavioral disinhibition
Aphasia and/or mutism	Manic symptoms
Severe frontal lobe symptoms	Delusions
Severe psychomotor slowing	Severe hallucinations
Intense distractibility	Severe agitation
Disorientation	Paranoid ideation
	Severe depression with or without suicidality

Note.   HIV = human immunodeficiency virus.
Source.   Adapted from Brew BJ, Sidtis JJ, Petito CK, et al: "The Neurologic Complications of AIDS and Human Immunodeficiency Virus Infection," in *Advances in Contemporary Neurology.* Edited by Plum F. Philadelphia, PA, FA Davis, 1988, pp. 1–49.

signs and symptoms of both cognitive and psychiatric disturbances commonly encountered early in the course of HAD (Brew et al. 1988), and Table 20–4 shows signs and symptoms of cognitive and psychiatric difficulties encountered late in the course of HAD (Brew et al. 1988). The course of HAD can steadily worsen with the development of moderate to severe cognitive deficits, confusion, psychomotor slowing, and seizures. Patients may appear mute and catatonic. Socially inappropriate behavior; psychosis; mania; marked motor abnormalities such as ataxia, spasticity, and hyperreflexia; and incontinence of bladder and bowel can occur.

A meta-analysis of 41 primary studies of neuropsychological test performance (8,616 total participants) found that, overall, disease progression was accompanied by increasingly larger effect sizes between control (seronegative), asymptomatic, symptomatic, and AIDS subjects, respectively (Reger et al. 2002). Differences between the asymptomatic and control (seronegative) groups were present but small (<0.2 SD), whereas larger effect sizes were noted between the symptomatic and the AIDS groups compared with the control subjects. In later stages of the disease, motor deficits were most prominent, with deficits also present in problem solving and other executive functions, rate of information processing, expressive language, memory, and, to a lesser degree, attention and concentration. The progression of cognitive decline followed a frontal-subcortical pattern initially, with the areas of greatest deficit early in the disease (motor and executive functions) being those sub-

served by these brain regions and neural circuits. In later stages of the disease, abilities such as memory and visuospatial skills, which are less dependent on frontal-subcortical circuitry, also declined. Notably, a high degree of variability was seen among the studies included in this quantitative review. One factor suggested by the authors relates to test specificity; to the extent that some instruments measure more than one discrete domain of cognitive functioning, results of analyses that used these instruments varied. Another issue was the method of categorization of individuals by disease stages and failure to consistently account for the wide range of psychosocial variables that may affect test performance, such as demographic characteristics including age and education, the presence of mood disorders, and differences in medical comorbidity and substance use history.

Results of an 8-year longitudinal study in which the participants underwent neuropsychological evaluation at 6-month intervals were largely consistent with those of the previously described meta-analysis, also indicating a decline in cognitive function with HIV disease progression (Baldewicz et al. 2004). Of the five functional domains assessed (fine motor speed, attention, verbal memory, executive functioning, and information processing speed), fine motor speed and information processing speed showed the most significant decline over time, and this decline became increasingly prominent as individuals developed AIDS-defining illnesses.

Clinicians must seriously evaluate the patient's complaints, such as memory problems, mental slowing, and difficulty with attention and concentration, however, at any stage of the disease. Dysphoria due to the seriousness of the illness or induced by medications or affective disturbances could theoretically cause cognitive difficulties (e.g., pseudodementia of depression) (Cummings and Benson 1983), but several studies (Kovner et al. 1989; Pace et al. 1992; Syndulko et al. 1990) have reported that cognitive dysfunction is not correlated with mood disorder, and the level of cognitive impairment surpasses that expected by distraction from affective causes. Because of the possibility of early cognitive involvement, efforts have been devoted to construction of a neuropsychological battery of tests that would be sensitive to the earliest signs of HIV effects on cognition (Butters et al. 1990; Franzblau et al. 1991; Gibbs et al. 1990; Hart et al. 1990; Heaton et al. 1995; Jacobs et al. 1992; Klusman et al. 1991; Lunn et al. 1991; Marotta and Perry 1989; E.N. Miller et al. 1991; Perry et al. 1989; Van Gorp et al. 1989a; Wilkie et al. 1990a).

The cardinal signs of HIV-related cognitive impairment remain consistent by many reports (Butters et al. 1990; Collier et al. 1992; Dunlop et al. 1992; Fernandez et al. 1989a; Franzblau et al. 1991; Gibbs et al. 1990;

Hart et al. 1990; Jacobs et al. 1992; Janssen et al. 1988; Kaemingk and Kaszniak 1989; Karlsen et al. 1992; Klusman et al. 1991; Krikorian and Wrobel 1991; Lunn et al. 1991; Marotta and Perry 1989; Martin et al. 1992; E.N. Miller et al. 1991; Morgan et al. 1988; Nance et al. 1990; Pajeau and Roman 1991; Perry 1990; Perry et al. 1989; Riedel et al. 1992; Rubinow et al. 1988; Ryan et al. 1992; Skoraszewski et al. 1991; Stern et al. 1991; Tross et al. 1988; Van Gorp et al. 1989a, 1989b, 1991; Wilkie et al. 1990a, 1990b) and include problems with verbal memory, difficulties with attention and concentration, slowing of information processing, slowed psychomotor speed, and impairment of cognitive flexibility; in some cases, the nonverbal abilities of problem solving, visuospatial integration and construction, and nonverbal memory are impaired (Butters et al. 1990). Studies have shown that psychomotor tasks, such as the Digit Symbol and Block Design tests of the Wechsler Adult Intelligence Scale and the Trail Making Test Part B from the Halstead-Reitan Neuropsychological Test Battery, and memory tasks, such as the delayed Visual Reproduction subtest from the Wechsler Memory Scale and the delayed recall of the Rey-Osterrieth Complex Figure, were most affected in the early stages of cognitive impairment associated with HIV (Van Gorp et al. 1989a). We and others have found that tasks detecting psychomotor and neuromotor disturbances in HIV-related neural dysfunction such as visuomotor reaction time (Dunlop et al. 1992; Karlsen et al. 1992; Nance et al. 1990) and fine motor dexterity as measured by pegboard activities are also sensitive measures for the early detection of impairment. Such motor speed tasks may be more vulnerable to the effects of HIV than is central processing speed. One investigation (Martin et al. 1992) implied that graphomotor and manual slowing may be a major component of impairment on psychomotor tasks. When a memory search or reaction time paradigm was used, speed of memory search in HIV-positive patients did not differ significantly from that in control subjects. This task did not test speed of movement but rather a cognitive reaction latency.

Other areas of cognitive function usually assessed by neuropsychological batteries include aphasia, apraxia, and other complex language-associated functioning; verbal abstract reasoning and problem solving; and perceptual functioning of the different sensory modalities. These assessments, however, have not been universally sensitive for the early detection of HIV-related CNS dysfunction. Any impairment found in these areas of intellectual functioning may be associated with a more focal attack on the nervous system, such as an HIV-related opportunistic infection that forms a focal abscess or an HIV-related tumor. However, neuropsychological evaluations encompassing a broad

TABLE 20–5.   HIV neuropsychological screening battery

Attention and memory

   Wechsler Adult Intelligence Scale—Revised, Digit Span subtest

   Rey Auditory-Verbal Learning Test

Language/speech and speed of cognitive production

   Controlled Oral Word Association Test (from Benton Multilingual Aphasia Examination)

Executive/psychomotor

   Symbol Digit Modalities Test

   Trail Making Test, Parts A and B

   Grooved Pegboard

Note. HIV = human immunodeficiency virus.
Source. Reproduced with permission of authors and publisher from Selnes OA, Jacobson L, Machado AM, Becker JT, Wesch J, Miller EN, Visscher B, and McArthur JC: "Normative Data for a Brief Neuropsychological Screening Battery." *Perceptual and Motor Skills* 73:539–550. © Perceptual and Motor Skills 1991.

range of cognitive areas (Butters et al. 1990), as are effectively implemented with other clinical entities such as head trauma or other dementias, would seem to yield adequate information about focality of involvement in the later stages of HIV disease. These cognitive areas should be considered in research, as well as clinical investigations, so as to span all functions that might be attacked by the disease's neurotropism and not incur the chance of a false-negative finding (Kovner et al. 1989; Van Gorp et al. 1991). If the patient's lack of stamina or other situation precludes an extensive battery, a comprehensive but briefer battery consisting of the tests listed in Table 20–5 (Selnes et al. 1991), or tests that address similar functions (Butters et al. 1990), can assess the critical areas of cognitive functioning to detect HIV involvement at an early stage.

The ability of HIV-related cognitive dysfunction to disrupt the capacity to work and perform activities of daily living was formerly thought to occur only at the end of the infection's cycle during fully developed AIDS. However, because early cognitive impairment may occur before the diagnosis of AIDS, a means of measuring cognitive functioning was needed to define cognitive disabilities at earlier stages of infection. Early in the epidemic, investigators attempted to characterize functional impairment with a scale validated for Alzheimer's disease. This instrument, the Global Deterioration Scale of Reisberg and colleagues (1982), has been criticized as not linearly characterizing the cognitive and functional decline of Alzheimer's disease

(Eisdorfer et al. 1991), but it appears to be useful as a clinical tool for rating cognitive impairment as it affects everyday functioning in HIV-infected individuals before neuropsychological quantification of specific deficits. This scale can be used for investigational purposes to compare the cognitive impairment associated with HIV with that of other dementias (Fernandez and Levy 1990). It is also useful for rating functional level as required (but no scale has been specifically mandated) by the AAN's nomenclature for degree of impairment to determine HAD.

Another scale that has been proposed to discriminate patients with HIV infection and dementia from patients with HIV infection but not dementia is the HIV Dementia Scale (HDS; Power et al. 1995). It appears to be more sensitive than the Mini-Mental State Examination to the HIV-related subcortical effects of CNS infection. The HDS has been criticized because portions of the scale are difficult to administer by nonneurologically trained individuals. For example, it requires saccadic eye movement examination, for which no standardized scoring exists. However, even if this component is deleted, the HDS retains the ability to discriminate grossly among mild-moderate and moderate-severe dementia (Skolasky et al. 1998).

In the largest study of its kind to date, 267 HIV-positive individuals received comprehensive evaluations of neuropsychological functioning, medical status, and assessment of functional abilities, including laboratory measures of a variety of instrumental activities of daily living (Heaton et al. 2004). A comparison of group test performance found that individuals classified as having abnormal neuropsychological functioning, requiring at least mild impairment in two or more cognitive domains, performed significantly worse on laboratory measures of daily functional abilities. The domains most strongly correlated with failure on the functional measures included abstraction and executive functioning, learning, attention and working memory, and verbal abilities. This suggests that neuropsychological impairment is related to functional deficits, further emphasizing the importance of objective cognitive assessment in addition to measures of cognitive complaints and other self-report measures.

TREATMENT OF HIV INFECTION OF THE CNS

PRIMARY THERAPY: ANTIVIRALS

For a detailed review of the primary and secondary salvage therapeutic strategies for the treatment of HIV/AIDS, the reader is referred to the federal guidelines for the use of antiretroviral therapies in adults and children (Panel on Clinical Practices for Treatment of HIV Infection 2005).

No specific guidelines exist for treating cognitive impairment and HAD. However, available studies suggest that the main thrust of treatment should be to produce virological suppression of both plasma and CNS compartments.

Studies have found that zidovudine is a potent inhibitor of human retrovirus replication in vitro and is effective in reducing morbidity by decreasing the number of serious complications in patients with AIDS as well as in asymptomatic patients (Fischl et al. 1987; Groopman 1991a, 1991b; Merigan 1991; Moore et al. 1991). Preliminary observations from several studies also suggest that zidovudine therapy can attenuate the symptomatic course of the dementia and neurological disease in some patients (Arendt et al. 1991; Hollweg et al. 1991; Riccio et al. 1990; Schmitt et al. 1988; Yarchoan et al. 1987). Experimental data show that the compound penetrates the brain at a level at which one-half can be recovered from CSF (Wong et al. 1992). Therefore, findings such as those of Sidtis and colleagues (1993) that report improved cognitive functioning in patients who receive high levels of zidovudine—up to 2,000 mg/day—are consistent with this brain parenchymal bioavailability characteristic. Additionally, doses may need to be high to maintain therapeutic levels of zidovudine in the CNS because investigators have found that zidovudine is cleared from the brain through an active transport process (Stahle et al. 1993; Wang and Sawchuk 1995; Wong et al. 1993). Clinicians should keep this finding in mind when calculating the maintenance dose of zidovudine in the patient with subjective complaints consistent with HIV-1-associated minor cognitive/motor disorder or HAD.

Human data regarding the pharmacology and toxicology of zidovudine indicate that with careful clinical monitoring and appropriate dose modification, it is a safe drug to use in neurologically impaired patients (Yarchoan et al. 1987). The principal toxicity of zidovudine is hematological, with a decrease in the red blood cell, neutrophil, and, less commonly, platelet counts. Of these, neutrophil depression has proved to be the major limiting toxicity because anemia can be treated with transfusion. Most hematological side effects of zidovudine usually emerge after 6 weeks or more of therapy and, in many cases, require dose reduction or discontinuation. Typically, resuming treatment with zidovudine at a lower dose can be effective once hematopoietic toxicity has resolved. Furthermore, some studies suggest that a reduced or low-normal vitamin B_{12} level may be associated with a greater risk for neutrophil depression (Richman et al. 1987). Other minor side effects of zidovudine include myalgias, headache, insomnia, nausea, and depersonalization and derealization. Mania has been reported (Maxwell et al. 1988; Wright et al. 1989), and delirium also has been reported (Fernandez 1988). Macrocytosis is the only consistent laboratory index, excluding the previously described hematological changes. The only significant drug-drug interaction reported occurs with acetaminophen. Concurrent treatment with acetaminophen may result in an increased frequency of neutropenia. Theoretically, drugs that are hepatically cleared and disturb the process of glucuronidation also have the potential to cause neutropenia. Thus, zidovudine should be used cautiously, with regular hematological monitoring. A single report exists of a patient who developed severe neurotoxicity and died (Hagler and Frame 1986); however, confirmatory studies of mortality risk from zidovudine are lacking.

Other antivirals such as zalcitabine (ddC) (Dickover et al. 1991; Neuzil 1994), didanosine (ddI) (Connolly et al. 1991; Neuzil 1994), lamivudine (3TC) (van Leeuwen et al. 1995), and stavudine (d4T) (Murray et al. 1995; Neuzil 1994) are now being used in the control of HIV replication and, as such, may play a role in reducing the viral load available to the CNS via circulatory spread. These drugs, however, do not penetrate the blood-brain barrier as well as zidovudine does. Additionally, the protease inhibitors that prevent maturation of HIV particles (Neuzil 1994) are also showing promise alone and in combination therapy with the reverse transcriptase agents (HAART) (Greenlee and Rose 2000). Significant improvement in both cognitive (Tozzi et al. 1999) and motor (Sacktor et al. 2001) abilities on neuropsychological testing has been reported. Thus, antiviral therapy currently provides an important direct intervention for cognitive and emotional effects of HIV infection of the CNS.

What is not known is what particular combinations of antiretrovirals have the best penetration of the blood-brain barrier and provide the best parenchymal prophylaxis. Agents other than zidovudine theorized to do so include stavudine, abacavir, lamivudine, efavirenz, nevirapine, and indinavir. Some advocate the use of these agents that are known to penetrate the brain better on the assumption that these might better treat HIV infection of the CNS (Cysique et al. 2004; Sacktor et al. 2001). However, this approach remains controversial at this time.

ADJUNCTIVE THERAPY: ADDITIONAL BIOLOGICAL AND PHARMACOLOGICAL INTERVENTIONS

Peptide T (Bridge et al. 1991; Buzy et al. 1992; Julander et al. 1990; Rosen et al. 1992) has been the subject of controversy in the treatment of HIV infection of the CNS. It differs from the other antivirals in that instead of inhibiting reverse transcriptase activity, it blocks the binding of gp120 to CD4+ receptors, which, as mentioned

earlier in this chapter, appears to be the incipient pathophysiological mechanism for neurovirulence. Therefore, peptide T may serve as a primary intervention for HIV systemic and CNS proliferation. It appears to be less toxic than other antivirals, and one study (Rosen et al. 1992) reported reversal of neurobehavioral impairment.

Because of the observation that gp120 may be associated with neuronal cell injury by altering cellular calcium flux (S.A. Lipton 1991; S.A. Lipton and Gendleman 1995; Stefano et al. 1993), a remedy was suggested to counteract this calcium-induced injury. S.A. Lipton (1991) suggested that certain calcium channel blockers (e.g., flunarizine) were protective against gp120 toxicity in vitro. Nimodipine (30–60 mg orally 4–6 times daily) also was found to be protective and is being used to regulate neuron-injuring intracellular calcium increments (Dreyer et al. 1990). One calcium channel blocker cannot be readily substituted for another; verapamil and diltiazem were not as effective as nimodipine or did not help. In fact, in another study, verapamil enhanced HIV-1 replication in lymphoid cells (Harbison et al. 1991).

In addition, new agents are being tested that provide a rational approach to the treatment of the elements of neuronal injury outlined earlier—cytokines, NMDA, and calcium flux. Pentoxifylline (400 mg orally three times a day) has been tested to counter tumor necrosis factor-α, although troublesome side effects such as hallucinations have been reported (Dezube et al. 1993). NMDA receptor blockers are being evaluated to block the excitotoxin quinolinic acid from instituting the damage of increased intracellular calcium (American Psychiatric Association 1994). Memantine (10–30 mg/day orally; usual dose, 20 mg/day), an antiparkinsonian drug, binds to the NMDA receptor and also blocks gp120 toxicity (Kornhuber et al. 1991). Vitamin E (typically 1,600 IU/day orally; may require up to 3,000 IU/day) and N-acetylcysteine (9,600 mg/day orally) (Dröge 1993), well-known antioxidants, are apparently directed toward free radicals. Vitamin B_6 (25–50 mg/day orally for nonclinical deficiency; 50–200 mg/day orally for clinical deficiency, but observe for toxicity, manifesting as a neuropathic syndrome, at doses from 50 to 2,000 mg/day) is a cofactor in the metabolism of tryptophan into serotonin. Vitamin B_6 has been used to enhance the production of serotonin in preference to an alternative production of quinolinic acid (Shor-Posner et al. 1994). Vitamin B_{12} deficiency has been reported in a proportion of HIV-infected patients and can lead to "excess" cognitive disability; vitamin supplementation has been shown to improve cognition (Beach et al. 1992). Dosages for treatment of a clinical deficiency begin with 100 mg/day intramuscularly for a week, then twice a week for 1–2 months (or for 6 months if neurological symptoms are present), and then 1,000 mg intramuscularly every month indefinitely (American Psychiatric Association 1994). Unfortunately, the results of these and other trials have not demonstrated significant effects on either neuropsychological testing or neurobehavioral recovery (McArthur et al. 2005).

Microglia-associated chronic brain inflammation is the common final pathway in most neurodegenerative diseases, including HAD. Nicotine binding at microglial nicotinic acetylcholine receptors has shown anti-inflammatory properties (Shytle et al. 2004). In this study, Shytle et al. (2004) showed that nicotine and acetylcholine pretreatment inhibited lipopolysaccharide-induced tumor necrosis factor-α and nitric oxide productions in primary cultured microglia. In addition, in nicotine precultured neurons, binding at the α_7-nicotinic acetylcholine receptors provides neuroprotection from the excitatory amino acid glutamate as well as other inflammatory factors (Kaneko et al. 1997). Galantamine is a potent allosteric potentiating ligand of nicotinic acetylcholine receptors (Samochocki et al. 2003; Santos et al. 2002) and cholinesterase inhibitors (Shytle et al. 2004). Galantamine upregulates agonist responses of nicotinic acetylcholine receptors at concentrations of 0.1 to 1 μM, whereas concentrations greater than 10 μM result in nicotinic acetylcholine receptor inhibition. In vivo studies have shown that galantamine, acting as an allosteric potentiating ligand on presynaptic and tonically active nicotinic acetylcholine receptors, potentiates glutaminergic or γ-aminobutyric acid (GABA)-ergic transmission, whereas the non–allosteric potentiating ligand cholinesterase inhibitors lack this therapeutic effect on synaptic transmission (Santos et al. 2002). Our recent study showed that nicotine in the presence of galantamine synergistically attenuates HIV-1 gp120/interferon-γ-induced microglial activation, as evidenced by decreased tumor necrosis factor-α and nitric oxide releases (Giunta et al. 2004). This finding suggests a novel therapeutic combination to treat or prevent the onset of HAD through this modulation of the microglia inflammation mechanism.

Epigallocatechin gallate (EGCG), the major component of green tea, has been reported to have neuroprotective properties (Mandel et al. 2004). Recently, several studies have shown that EGCG has a protective effect against HIV-1 infection (Fassina et al. 2002; Kawai et al. 2003; Yamaguchi et al. 2002). Most important, Kawai and colleagues (2003) reported that EGCG directly binds to the CD4 receptor and interferes with HIV-1 gp120 binding at the target cell surface. Most recently, we have shown that EGCG treatment of primary neurons from normal mice reduced Janus associated kinase 1 (Jak1) and signal transducer and activator of transcrip-

tion 1 (Stat1) activation associated with HAD-like neuronal injury mediated by interferon-γ and/or HIV-1 viral proteins gp120 and Tat, as evidenced by decreased lactate dehydrogenase release and increased ratio of Bcl-xL to Bax protein. In addition, primary neurons derived from Stat1-deficient mice were largely resistant to HAD-like neuronal damage. In accord with these findings, EGCG also attenuated HAD-like neuronal damage in mice (Giunta et al. 2006). Taken together, these data suggest that blocking *Jak/Stat1* activation with green tea–derived EGCG possibly represents a novel therapeutic approach for the prevention and treatment of HAD.

ADJUVANT THERAPY: PSYCHOPHARMACOLOGICAL ENHANCEMENT OF FUNCTION

Adjuvant therapy in the form of psychostimulant treatment (see also subsection "Depression in HIV Disease" later in this chapter) can help improve functioning in cognitive domains. Early data indicated that methylphenidate, used to treat affective disorders in HIV-infected patients, significantly improved verbal rote memory and rate of cognitive tracking and mental set shifting (Fernandez et al. 1988a, 1988c). On average, this amounted to elevating associated scores on neuropsychological instruments into the normal range. Subsequent investigations (Angrist et al. 1991; White et al. 1992) have confirmed this effect. Possible support for the efficacy of psychostimulants may come from their enhancement of dopaminergic functioning in neural populations that subtend attention or concentration, memory retrieval, and speed of cognitive processing (Fernandez and Levy 1990).

BEHAVIORAL METHODS IN THE TREATMENT OF COGNITIVE DISORDER

Adaptive functioning can be improved with behavioral methods of cognitive rehabilitation currently used in patients with brain trauma, stroke, and Alzheimer's disease (Boccellari 1990; Boccellari and Zeifert 1994; J.K. Levy and Fernandez 1993, 1995). Memory compensation techniques, such as keeping notebooks and using cueing signs and timer signals, and home environmental manipulation, such as labeling contents of cabinets and making daily activity checklists, can optimize day-to-day functioning (J.K. Levy and Fernandez 1993, 1995). These techniques provide a structure to cognitive functioning that allows many patients to retain some control over their daily activities and extend active participation in their medical regimens.

MANIFESTATIONS OF SPECIFIC HIV-RELATED NEUROPSYCHIATRIC DISORDERS AND THEIR TREATMENT

The range of HIV-related neuropsychiatric disorders includes most of the major mental disorders listed in DSM-IV-TR (American Psychiatric Association 2000), including major depressive disorder, manic episode, psychotic disorder, delusional disorder, paranoid personality disorder, and anxiety disorder (Atkinson et al. 1988; Perry 1990; Perry and Marotta 1987). The most common psychiatric effects in HIV disease, in DSM-IV-TR terminology, are those "due to general medical conditions," such as delirium and psychosis (Fernandez et al. 1989b; Harris et al. 1991; Jones et al. 1987; Maccario and Scharre 1987; Wolcott et al. 1985); dementia; mood disorder, including depression (Fernandez et al. 1995b; Hintz et al. 1990; Markowitz et al. 1994) and mania (Kieburtz et al. 1991b; McGowan et al. 1991); and stress and distress syndromes such as anxiety disorders (Fernandez 1989). Personality disorder and delusional disorder also may be seen, depending on specific focal effects of the infection.

DELIRIUM AND PSYCHOSIS IN HIV DISEASE

Of all the mental disorders due to a medical condition, delirium is the most prevalent and most frequently undiagnosed; as many as 30% of hospitalized medical-surgical patients have an undetected delirium (Guze and Daengsurisri 1967; Knights and Folstein 1977). Pre-HAART, delirium was diagnosed in between 11% and 65% of patients. In the post-HAART era, delirium is reported in 20% of patients (O'Dowd and McKegney 1990). The prompt detection of delirium is crucial because of potential reversibility and, thus, diminished morbidity and mortality.

Although delirium reflects diffuse cerebral cellular metabolic dysfunction (Lipowski 1987), a prodromal phase often occurs during which patients complain of difficulty in thinking, restlessness, irritability, or insomnia interrupted with short periods of sleep containing vivid nightmares. The clinician must be alert to these symptoms and search for the causes of the delirious process. A brief mental status examination during the prodromal phase should focus on arousal, attention, short-term memory, and orientation. Diurnal variations (i.e., symptoms that are worse at night than during the day) are common. Along with cognitive deficits, abnormal involuntary movements such as tremor, picking at clothing, multifocal myoclonus, and asterixis are seen in delirium.

Timely pharmacological intervention may help to suppress the delirium symptoms; however, in our study, complete reversal of delirium occurred in only 37% of the patients with AIDS (Fernandez et al. 1989b). The use of high-potency neuroleptics to control delirium has found increasing acceptance (Adams 1988; Adams et al. 1986; Ayd 1978; Fernandez and Levy 1991; Fernandez et al. 1989a, 1989b; Tesar et al. 1985). Oral or intramuscular haloperidol has been an effective treatment of delirium without any serious adverse effects.

Breitbart and colleagues (1996a) performed a double-blind prospective trial comparing haloperidol, chlorpromazine, and lorazepam in the treatment of patients with AIDS and delirium. A mean dose as low as 2.8 mg of haloperidol or 50 mg of chlorpromazine resulted in improvement in delirious symptoms within the first 24 hours of treatment, with minimal extrapyramidal side effects. Lorazepam alone was not shown to be effective in this study; however, in combination with an intravenous neuroleptic, it has been shown to be of benefit.

The safety and efficacy of intravenous haloperidol treatment for delirium, either alone or in combination with lorazepam or additionally with hydromorphone for agitated patients with delirium, have been observed (Adams et al. 1986; Fernandez et al. 1989a; Tesar et al. 1985). Investigators have even reported that a continuous intravenous infusion of haloperidol can be used to achieve full control in refractory cases of delirium associated with agitation (Fernandez et al. 1988b). Although the administration of intravenous haloperidol is still considered investigational and not approved by the U.S. Food and Drug Administration (FDA), the relative rarity of treatment-related adverse effects (Huyse and Van Schijndel 1988; Konikoff et al. 1984) must be weighed against the dangers of delirium. Neuroleptic malignant syndrome is perhaps the most ominous potential adverse effect (Breitbart et al. 1988); however, in our experience, this syndrome is rare in this population. The rarity of this complication may stem from the intravenous route of administration. The possible protective influence of lorazepam, when coadministered with haloperidol, against the extrapyramidal side effects of haloperidol must be delineated with further controlled trials. Intravenous haloperidol can be approved for compassionate use if the clinician obtains permission through an institutional review process.

The ideal dose of any therapeutic medication is the smallest dose that achieves the desired clinical effects. We have found that HIV-positive patients are often more sensitive to neuroleptics and may require lower doses than do other medically ill patients with delirium (Fernandez et al. 1989b). Doses of intravenous medications, however, may need to be increased to high levels, provided that careful observation is maintained, to achieve effective and immediate control of severe agitation, which is essential to the individual's continued well-being as well as that of other patients and staff. Adverse effects of haloperidol in HIV-infected patients are mainly extrapyramidal and are significantly more frequent if the patient has another coexisting mental disorder due to a general medical condition (Fernandez et al. 1989b). However, we found that this therapy did not aggravate concurrent seizure disorders or cause adverse cardiovascular effects in patients who were not hypovolemic, hypokalemic, or hypomagnesmic.

New onset of psychosis in HIV-infected patients also has been reported (Edelstein and Knight 1987; Harris et al. 1991; Jones et al. 1987; Maccario and Scharre 1987). In one patient, schizophreniform conditions occurred before HIV seropositivity was identified (Maccario and Scharre 1987). In another study, dopamine supplementation in a patient with a parkinsonian syndrome ascribed to the effects of HIV induced psychosis that was reversible at the cost of relapse of the movement disorder (Edelstein and Knight 1987). Treatment with neuroleptics with the above-mentioned cautions has been beneficial.

Newer agents are entering the armamentarium to treat delirium and psychotic disorders. Risperidone (Singh et al. 1997) at various doses has been used with success to target psychotic symptoms. Olanzapine (Sockalingam et al. 2005) also may be used, but its affinity for the cytochrome P450 3A4 isoenzyme system may be problematic for patients taking specific protease inhibitors. Quetiapine, ziprasidone, and aripiprazole also may be tried, but there is little experience to date with these agents (Stolar et al. 2005).

DEPRESSION IN HIV DISEASE

Disturbances of mood, primarily depressive (Atkinson et al. 1988; Fernandez et al. 1989a, 1995b; Grant 1990; Hintz et al. 1990; Levine et al. 1990; Maj et al. 1991; Rabkin and Harrison 1990; Rabkin et al. 1991) but also manic and hypomanic episodes (Holmes and Fricchone 1989; Kieburtz et al. 1991b; McGowan et al. 1991), are found in HIV disease. The diagnosis of HIV-related mood disturbances is complex and requires that the clinician consider the interaction of organic and nonorganic factors. This consideration may produce the most timely and effective intervention. From the outset of this discussion, we emphasize that depression in HIV has heterogeneous etiologies; depression should not be considered a *normal* phenomenon of HIV infection.

The prevalence of mood disorders in HIV-infected patients, especially during the asymptomatic stage, has been an issue of investigation since the first patients presented with these affective symptoms. Atkinson and col-

leagues (1988) found a high lifetime prevalence of depression in HIV-infected homosexual men (30.3%), but the patients often had a mood disorder diagnosis before the development of HIV infection. Perkins and colleagues (1994), however, found that HIV-infected and non-HIV-infected homosexual men had similar high lifetime and current diagnoses of depression (29% vs. 45% and 8% vs. 3%, respectively). These rates were higher than those in the general population but were not related to stage of infection because the HIV-positive and HIV-negative subjects had similar proportions. Additionally, current depression was not related to neuropsychological test performance. The major risk factor for current depression in both groups was a history of depression.

The most malignant aspect of depression, of course, is suicide. Suicidal ideation may present throughout the course of the spectrum of illnesses, even from the apprehension regarding antibody testing (Perry et al. 1990). The physician's role is to assess the process accurately, particularly in cases of severe depression (Frierson and Lippthann 1988; Hall and Stevens 1988; Marzuk et al. 1988; Perry et al. 1990). The natural instinct of self-preservation, even that found with the diagnosis of HIV infection, vies with the serious consideration of the concept of rational suicide (Brown et al. 1986; Siegel 1986). The relative risk of suicide is very high. Marzuk and colleagues (1988) found that the relative risk of suicide in men with AIDS living in New York City was 36.3 times that for men without an AIDS diagnosis and 66.2 times that of the general population. Research has indicated that terminally ill patients who complete suicide had evidence of stress-impaired decision making or had been clinically depressed before the suicide (Brown et al. 1986). Breitbart and colleagues (1996b), in a survey of 370 ambulatory HIV-infected patients, found that 55% considered physician-assisted suicide for themselves; however, this wish was strongly related to high scores on instruments assessing psychological distress, such as with depression, hopelessness, and general psychological distress. The investigators reported that interest in physician-assisted suicide was not related to severity of pain, functional impairment associated with pain, other physical symptomatology, or extent of HIV disease. Therefore, because HIV-infected persons also may have this stress- or distress-related impairment of judgment, in addition to any judgment difficulties associated with cognitive impairment, the therapist must react assertively to any evidence of suicidal ideation. This reaction would include an accurate diagnostic assessment and a treatment plan that includes constant observation by someone who can provide interpersonal support until the condition can be stabilized. Although pharmacotherapy provides the most rapid intervention for symptom remission, specific guidelines for drug selection are conspicuously absent.

Anecdotal and clinical research observations (Fernandez et al. 1989b) have attested that the CNS of HIV-infected patients is susceptible to increased sensitivity to and intensity of medication side effects (Brown et al. 1986; Holmes and Fricchone 1989). The low-anticholinergic tricyclic antidepressants may be useful for treating depression in HIV-infected patients because these drugs have less risk than do the highly anticholinergic tricyclics of exacerbating cognitive deficits or causing a delirious process and also are not as apt as the highly anticholinergic tricyclics to dry the mucous membranes excessively (an important consideration in this population because of their susceptibility to candidiasis). The choice of a particular tricyclic antidepressant should be guided by its specific action and side effects (Richelson 1988) in relation to the patient's depressive symptoms and concomitant medical condition (Fernandez and Levy 1991). The therapeutic dose of a tricyclic antidepressant may be much lower (10–75 mg) for an HIV-infected patient with neuropsychiatric impairment than for a noninfected person.

Other antidepressants such as fluoxetine (Judd et al. 1995; Levine et al. 1990) and bupropion (Golden et al. 1988a, 1988b), monoamine oxidase inhibitors (Fernandez and Levy 1991), trazodone (Roccatagliata et al. 1977), clomipramine (Feravelli et al. 1983; Pollock et al. 1985), maprotiline (Drago et al. 1983), paroxetine (Elliott et al. 1998), sertraline (Ferrando et al. 1997), and psychostimulants such as methylphenidate and dextroamphetamine (Fernandez et al. 1988a, 1988c, 1995b; Holmes et al. 1989; Walling and Pfefferbaum 1991; White et al. 1992) also may be useful in the management of depression in HIV-infected patients.

Whenever possible, antidepressant agents that have significant affinity for cytochrome P450 2D6 and 3A4 should be avoided. Venlafaxine (Fernandez et al. 1995a) is a dual-action antidepressant (reuptake inhibitor of both serotonin and norepinephrine) (Hollister 1994). In addition to its effectiveness as an antidepressive agent, we have noticed a qualitative energizing or stimulant-like effect. This agent has been associated with increased diastolic blood pressure; however, this effect occurs particularly with the immediate-release type and only at the highest doses. It has a favorable pharmacokinetic and cytochrome P450 profile. However, reports of reduced indinavir levels (G.M. Levin 2001) and possible reduced antiretroviral efficacy must be considered. Duloxetine is another dual-action antidepressant (Nelson et al. 2005); however, no reports in HIV-related depression are available.

Citalopram and escitalopram have intermediate affinities and favorable pharmacokinetic profiles and should be considered as first-line selective serotonin reuptake inhibitors in the management of HIV-related depression (Currier et al. 2004; Stolar et al. 2005). Likewise, mirtazapine has a favorable profile with respect to concomitant use with antiretroviral therapy. Mirtazapine may be particularly useful in patients with HIV-1 infection with severe dyssomnia associated with weight loss (Stolar et al. 2005). Neutropenia and agranulocytosis are not as severe as once thought and should not interfere with effective treatment (Stolar et al. 2005).

Bupropion has both noradrenergic and dopaminergic effects and has been used effectively in HIV/AIDS patients with depression (Currier 2003; Maldonado et al. 2000). It has been associated with seizures and should be used cautiously in patients with neurological disease or avoided altogether (Maldonado et al. 2000).

Nefazodone is a serotonin receptor antagonist and serotonin reuptake inhibitor that works at the serotonin type 2 receptor site and is similar to trazodone in structure. It also is a minor noradrenergic reuptake inhibitor. Along with nefazodone's effectiveness in significant depressive illness, it appears not to potentiate the depressant effects of alcohol (Frewer and Lader 1993). Because of its affinity for cytochrome P450 and its propensity for hepatoxicity, nefazodone should be avoided in the treatment of depression in HIV/AIDS (Stolar et al. 2005).

The psychostimulants seem to be especially effective in HIV-infected patients who have cognitive impairment or depression and dementia (Fernandez and Levy 1991; Fernandez et al. 1988a, 1988c; Holmes et al. 1989). In HIV-infected patients without cognitive impairment, treatment with methylphenidate was associated with a remission of depressive symptoms that was statistically indistinguishable from that achieved with the tricyclic desipramine (Fernandez et al. 1995b). In this study, scores on depression inventories were not significantly different between patients taking the two medications, and the time frame to reduction of symptoms was overlapping. For methylphenidate, the usual dosage is 5–20 mg taken on awakening in the morning, at midmorning, and again in early afternoon to avoid disturbing nighttime sleep (Fernandez et al. 1989a). Amelioration of secondary, subclinical depression in a double-blind clinical trial comparing methylphenidate and pemoline in the treatment of significant fatigue has been reported, with relatively few side effects (Breitbart et al. 2001).

In general, all nontricyclic antidepressant agents are effective and lack significant anticholinergic, histaminergic, adrenergic, and cardiac side effects. However, most do inhibit the biochemical activity of drugs that metabolize the isoenzyme cytochrome P450 2D6 or 3A4. Thus, antidepressants should be chosen after careful review of their pharmacology. Citalopram, escitalopram, venlafaxine, and mirtazapine are the weakest 2D6 and 3A isoenzyme inhibitors (Greenblatt et al. 1998). Clinicians may use these agents with low affinity for the 2D6 and 3A isoenzyme system in HIV-related depression while carefully monitoring the coadministration of both prescribed and over-the-counter medications.

Hypogonadism with associated changes in libido, diminished appetite, fatigue, and loss of lean body mass can be present in a significant number of men with HIV/AIDS and can present as depression. Hormone replacement therapy with testosterone has been reported to be effective in men (Rabkin et al. 2004) and women (K. Miller et al. 1998). Hormone replacement in neurobehaviorally impaired patients may be disinhibitory and may cause irritability, rage, and violent behavior; therefore, such therapy should be used with caution.

Depressed HIV-infected patients with psychotic symptoms or an organic mood disturbance, or for whom pharmacological treatment has failed, may benefit from electroconvulsive therapy. This modality may be tried after very careful review of its use in patients with complex medical illness (Kessing et al. 1994; Weiner 1983); however, electroconvulsive therapy may increase confusion in some encephalopathic HIV-infected patients (Schaerf et al. 1989).

MANIA IN HIV DISEASE

Acute mania has been reported in patients with HIV disease and may be the result of premorbid bipolar disorder; brain lesions from HIV, opportunistic infections, or AIDS-related neoplasms; or medications (Kieburtz et al. 1991b; Maxwell et al. 1988; McGowan et al. 1991; O'Dowd and McKegney 1988; Wright et al. 1989). Mania is not as common as depression in this population, but it presents as a sign more suspicious of organic involvement. It may also be the behavioral manifestation of a right frontal lobe tumor or focus of infection. Zidovudine has been reported to induce mania in susceptible individuals (Hagler and Frame 1986; Kieburtz et al. 1991b; Maxwell et al. 1988; O'Dowd and McKegney 1988).

Treatment of manic disorder in HIV-infected patients is similar to that in non-HIV-infected patients: cautious rapid tranquilization by neuroleptics (being on guard for the potential for seizure induction) followed by lithium treatment. Lithium has been found useful in the treatment of secondary mania due to zidovudine (O'Dowd and McKegney 1988). Close monitoring of levels and blood chemistry is essential for avoidance of toxicity in debilitated patients or those with the wasting syndrome. It is especially critical when infectious complications occur, such as with cryptosporidial infection or other causes of severe diarrhea, or with other severe fluid losses. Even when doses are used to maintain therapeutic serum concentrations of 0.5–1.0 mEq/L, patients with advanced disease cannot tolerate treatment with lithium.

The anticonvulsant valproate also has been approved as a treatment for mania (McElroy et al. 1992). It may be tried cautiously in patients whose renal or electrolyte status makes lithium problematic. The efficacy of valproate provides support to the theory that, in some cases, manic symptomatology may be the reflection of complex partial seizures or temporal lobe dysrhythmias (Gillig et al. 1988). Halman and colleagues (1993) found that valproate worked better against manic symptoms when an MRI showed structural abnormalities in the brain, which corroborates the hypothesis that structural abnormalities may be related to the bases of these dysrhythmias. Electrodiagnostic evaluation of de novo presentations of mania in HIV-infected patients also may be helpful in clarifying this etiology. One should note that there is a single report of valproic acid decreasing intracellular concentration of glutathione and stimulating HIV (Melton et al. 1997). We have retrospectively evaluated our valproate-treated patients' medical records and have not found any increases in viral load to suggest that this is a clinically relevant concern. However, psychiatrists must be prepared to deal with the fear associated with this report in both their patients and their colleagues (as well as with possible hepatotoxicity in patients).

At this time, no clinical reports are available on the efficacy of newer antiepileptic agents such as gabapentin, lamotrigine, and topiramate in HIV-related mania. Of these, lamotrigine is the only FDA-approved medication for maintenance therapy in bipolar affective disorder and therefore may be equally effective in HIV-related mania. It is safe to use in the context of HIV (Simpson et al. 2003). Given the limitations cited on the use of mood stabilizers, the use of the atypical antipsychotic agents (see subsection "Delirium and Psychosis in HIV Disease" earlier in this chapter) for HIV-related mania may be preferable (Stolar et al. 2005).

ANXIETY AND INSOMNIA IN HIV DISEASE

The stresses associated with antibody testing, diagnosis, and treatment of HIV infection obviously elicit symptoms of anxiety (Fernandez 1989; Forstein 1984; Holland and Tross 1985; Nichols 1983, 1985; Perry et al. 1992; Sonnex et al. 1987), especially for those individuals predisposed to anxiety disorders. An initial intervention of supportive care may be offered through reassurance from friends, family, and medical support staff (Perry et al. 1992). In addition to this support, the use of anxiolytic agents may help the patient to function better in all aspects of daily living, including participation in the medical treatment he or she is receiving.

The systemic effects of HIV-spectrum illnesses may trigger an anxiety disorder. For example, anxiety may arise in conjunction with prophylactic treatment by sulfamethoxazole and trimethoprim for *Pneumocystis carinii* pneumonia. Pulmonary insufficiency during pneumonia, leading to hypoxemia, also may trigger highly anxious states. CNS infections and neoplastic lesions may elicit anxiety states. Again, comprehensive neurodiagnostic investigation helps in the differential diagnosis.

Anxiolytic medication is selected on the basis of the nature and severity of the situation. Neuroleptics are often effective for the treatment of debilitating anxiety, which may approach irrational, overwhelming panic. However, the appearance of extrapyramidal side effects should be monitored closely, especially with patients in the advanced stages of HIV disease (Breitbart et al. 1988; Fernandez et al. 1989b). The automatic use of benzodiazepines as anxiolytics is risky in cases of severe anxiety or restlessness because these compounds may further compromise the patient's coping capacity and may have a disinhibiting effect.

On the contrary, the anxiety and insomnia (ranging from mild to severe) that may result from treatment with zidovudine or steroids, or be secondary to the effects of HIV on the CNS, may be helped with brief periods of pharmacotherapy with short- to intermediate-acting benzodiazepines such as lorazepam and oxazepam (Fernandez 1988). Alprazolam for anxiety and triazolam and estazolam for insomnia should be avoided in patients receiving HAART because their affinity for the cytochrome P450 3A4 subenzyme system has been reported to cause drug-drug interactions specifically with the protease inhibitors. Chronic use of benzodiazepines may be warranted in some patients. If so, we advocate use of clonazepam tablets or wafers. If tolerance develops in these patients, 50–200 mg of trazodone at bedtime may be combined with or substituted for the benzodiazepine. Although the β-blocker propranolol is often useful for healthy individuals who are anxious or phobic, its propensity to result in hypotensive episodes, particularly in patients who may have undiagnosed HIV-related dysautonomia (Lin-Greenberger and Taneja-Uppal 1987), makes it undesirable for general use in persons with HIV disease. Antihistamines, such as hydroxyzine, have low efficacy for anxiolysis unless the anxiety is accompanied by specific respiratory problems.

Early studies of the effectiveness of the nonbenzodiazepine anxiolytic buspirone (Kastenholz and Crismon 1984) in HIV-infected patients indicate its value when the immediate attenuation of acute or situational anxiety or phobias is not essential. Buspirone's anxiolytic effects are not accompanied by excessive sedation or potential for dependence; however, several weeks of regular administration are often required to achieve optimal results. Batki (1990) found that buspirone can be effective in treating anxiety disorders in substance-abusing patients who are at risk for misuse or excess sedation from benzodiazepines. Buspirone should be prescribed with caution for HIV-infected patients with CNS impairment, and its use should be monitored closely because buspirone-related dyskinesias (Strauss 1988) and myoclonus may be more easily elicited in neurologically compromised HIV-infected patients than in noninfected, neurologically intact patients with anxiety. Cases of possible buspirone-related mania have been reported (McDaniel et al. 1990; Price and Bielefeld 1989), and use of this agent in an HIV-positive patient was reported to induce confusion and psychosis with delusions (Nazzareno and Yeragani 1988).

Nonbenzodiazepines in use for insomnia include zolpidem, zaleplon, and eszopiclone (Sharma et al. 2005). Zolpidem is a nonbenzodiazepine sedative-hypnotic, and it is the most prescribed agent in HIV-related insomnia. Zolpidem is primarily a substrate of cytochrome P450 3A4. Clinically significant interactions may occur with concurrent use of cytochrome P450 3A4 inhibitors and inducers such as ritonavir, delavirdine, and nevirapine. Zaleplon is a short-acting nonbenzodiazepine sedative-hypnotic. Zaleplon is primarily metabolized by aldehyde oxidase to form 5-oxo-zaleplon. To a lesser extent, zaleplon is metabolized by the hepatic isoenzyme cytochrome P450 3A4, and all its metabolites are inactive. However, antiretroviral protease inhibitors may increase the levels of zaleplon. Although clinical data do not exist, and this interaction is not expected to require routine zaleplon dosage adjustment, one should remain vigilant for possible problems. Eszopiclone is a nonbenzodiazepine hypnotic agent that is a pyrrolopyrazine derivative of the cyclopyrrolone class. Eszopiclone is metabolized by cytochrome P450 3A4 and 2E1 via demethylation and oxidation. Inhibitors of cytochrome P450 3A4, like the protease inhibitors, will result in an increase in the levels of eszopiclone. Clinical experience with eszopiclone in patients with HIV-related insomnia is limited.

CONCLUSION

The neuropsychiatric complications of HIV infection and AIDS are a perplexing assortment of neurological, neurocognitive, and affective/behavioral effects that may arise at any time during the course of the illness. Thus, all neuropsychiatrists should maintain a high index of suspicion of even the most subtle of behavioral symptoms in previously asymptomatic persons because several means of investigation (e.g., electrophysiological, neuropsychological) have disclosed that neurological involvement may occur early in the course of the disease. As the AIDS epidemic continues, these symptoms may arise in individuals other than those in the initial high-risk categories, and a careful history of possible exposure must be included in any workup of unusual cognitive, neurological, or neuropsychiatric symptoms fitting the pattern described in this chapter. If the etiology is found to be HIV related, then prompt aggressive treatment of the conditions, perhaps with innovative measures, is warranted, to maintain as optimal a quality of life as can be promoted, for as long as possible.

Highlights for the Clinician

- ✦ HIV-1 is a retrovirus that produces profound CD4 depletion leading to immunodeficiency and death.
- ✦ Infection of the central nervous system directly affects brain tissue, producing distinct neurobehavioral disorders.
- ✦ Secondary CNS dysfunction is produced by chronic immune activation by HIV-1 infection, leading to macrophage and glial cell activation that results in overproduction of inflammatory cytokines and chemokines.
- ✦ These proinflammatory cytokines and chemokines are related to the pathogenesis of cognitive disorders and dementia in HIV/AIDS.
- ✦ Cognitive, mood, and psychotic disorders are the most common clinical neuropsychiatric disorders associated with HIV infection.
- ✦ HIV-related neuropsychiatric disorders are diagnoses of exclusion.
- ✦ Although therapeutic interventions are readily available, their efficacy has not been widely studied.

RECOMMENDED READINGS

Fernandez F, Ruiz P (eds): Psychiatric Aspects of HIV/AIDS. Philadelphia, PA, Lippincott Williams & Wilkins, 2006
McArthur JC, Brew B, Nath A: Neurological complications of HIV infection. Lancet Neurol 4:543–555, 2005

REFERENCES

Adams F: Emergency intravenous sedation of the delirious medically ill patient. J Clin Psychiatry 49(suppl):22–26, 1988
Adams F, Fernandez F, Andersson BS: Emergency pharmacotherapy and delirium in the critically ill cancer patient: intravenous combination drug approach. Psychosomatics 27 (suppl 1):33–37, 1986
Akler ME, Johnson DW, Burman WJ, et al: Anterior uveitis and hypotony after intravenous cidofovir for the treatment of cytomegalovirus retinitis. Ophthalmology 105:651–657, 1998
American Psychiatric Association: AIDS Training Curriculum: HIV-Related Neuropsychiatric Complications and Treatments. Washington, DC, American Psychiatric Association, 1994
American Psychiatric Association: Diagnostic and Statistical Manual of Mental Disorders, 4th Edition, Text Revision. Washington, DC, American Psychiatric Association, 2000

Angrist B, D'Hollosy M, Sanfilipo M, et al: Central nervous system stimulants as symptomatic treatments for AIDS-related neuropsychiatric impairment. J Clin Psychopharmacol 12:268–272, 1991
Antoni BA, Sabbatini P, Rabson AB, et al: Inhibition of apoptosis in human immunodeficiency virus–infected cells enhances virus production and facilitates persistent infection. J Virol 69:2384–2392, 1995
Arendt G, Hefter H, Buesher L, et al: Improvement of motor performance of HIV-positive patients under AZT therapy. Neurology 42:891–895, 1991
Asensio VC, Campbell IL: Chemokines in the CNS: plurifunctional mediators in diverse states. Trends Neurosci 22:504–512, 1999
Atkinson JH, Grant I, Kennedy CJ, et al: Prevalence of psychiatric disorders among men infected with human immunodeficiency virus: a controlled study. Arch Gen Psychiatry 45:859–864, 1988
Ayd FF Jr: Haloperidol: twenty years' clinical experience. J Clin Psychiatry 39:807–814, 1978
Baldeweg T, Riccio M, Gruzelier J, et al: Neurophysiological evaluation of zidovudine in asymptomatic HIV-1 infection: a longitudinal placebo-controlled study. J Neurol Sci 132:162–169, 1995
Baldewicz TT, Leserman J, Silva SG, et al: Changes in neuropsychological functioning with progression of HIV-1 infection: results of an 8-year longitudinal investigation. AIDS Behav 8:345–355, 2004

Barker PB, Lee RR, McArthur JC: AIDS dementia complex: evaluation with proton MR spectroscopic imaging. Radiology 195:58–64, 1995

Barre-Sinoussi F, Chermann JC, Rey F, et al: Isolation of a T-lymphotropic retrovirus from a patient at risk for acquired immune deficiency syndrome (AIDS). Science 220:868–871, 1983

Batki SA: Buspirone in drug users with AIDS or AIDS related complex. J Clin Psychopharmacol 10(suppl):1115–1155, 1990

Beach RS, Morgan R, Wilkie F, et al: Plasma vitamin B_{12} level as a potential cofactor in studies of human immunodeficiency virus type 1–related cognitive changes. Arch Neurol 49:501–506, 1992

Beckett A, Summergrad P, Manschreck T, et al: Symptomatic HIV infection of the CNS in a patient without clinical evidence of immune deficiency. Am J Psychiatry 144:1342–1344, 1987

Bedri J, Weinstein W, DeGregoria P, et al: Progressive multifocal leukoencephalopathy in acquired immunodeficiency syndrome. N Engl J Med 309:492–493, 1983

Beilke MA: Vascular endothelium in immunology and infectious disease. Rev Infect Dis 11:273–283, 1989

Bellamy CO, Malcomson RD, Harrison DJ, et al: Cell death in health and disease: the biology and regulation of apoptosis. Semin Cancer Biol 6:3–16, 1995

Belman AL, Lantos G, Horoupian D, et al: AIDS: calcification of the basal ganglia in infants and children. Neurology 36:1192–1199, 1986

Berger JR, Concha M: Progressive multifocal leukoencephalopathy: the evolution of a disease once considered rare. J Neurovirol 1:5 18, 1995

Berger JR, Kaszovitz B, Post MJ, et al: Progressive multifocal leukoencephalopathy associated with human immunodeficiency virus infection: a review of the literature with a report of sixteen cases. Ann Intern Med 107:78–87, 1987

Bernad PG: The neurological and electroencephalographic changes in AIDS. Clin Electroencephalogr 22:65–70, 1991

Bishburg E, Eng RHK, Slim J, et al: Brain lesions in patients with acquired immunodeficiency syndrome. Arch Intern Med 149:941–943, 1989

Boccellari A: Living with and caring for the individual with AIDS dementia complex, in Caregiver Education Series on AIDS Dementia Complex Training Manual. San Francisco, CA, Family Survival Project, 1990

Boccellari A, Zeifert P: Management of neurobehavioral impairment in HIV-1 infection. Psychiatr Clin North Am 17:183–203, 1994

Bredesen DE, Levy RM, Rosenblum ML: The neurology of human immunodeficiency virus infection. Q J Med 68:665–677, 1988

Breitbart W, Marotta RF, Call P: AIDS and neuroleptic malignant syndrome. Lancet 2:1488–1489, 1988

Breitbart W, Marotta RF, Platt MM, et al: A double-blind trial of haloperidol, chlorpromazine, and lorazepam in the treatment of delirium in hospitalized AIDS patients. Am J Psychiatry 153:231–237, 1996a

Breitbart W, Rosenfeld BD, Passik SD: Interest in physician-assisted suicide among ambulatory HIV-infected patients. Am J Psychiatry 153:238–242, 1996b

Breitbart W, Rosenfeld B, Kaim M, et al: A randomized, double-blind, placebo controlled trial of psychostimulants for the treatment of fatigue in ambulatory patients with human immunodeficiency virus disease. Arch Intern Med 161:411–420, 2001

Brew BJ, Sidtis JJ, Petito CK, et al: The neurologic complications of AIDS and human immunodeficiency virus infection, in Advances in Contemporary Neurology. Edited by Plum F. Philadelphia, PA, FA Davis, 1988, pp 1–49

Brew BJ, Bhalla RB, Paul M, et al: Cerebrospinal fluid β2 microglobulin in patients infected with AIDS dementia complex: an expanded series including response to zidovudine treatment. AIDS 6:461–465, 1992

Brew BJ, Pemberton L, Cunningham P, et al: Levels of human immunodeficiency virus type 1RNA in cerebrospinal fluid correlate with AIDS dementia stage. J Infect Dis 175:963–966, 1997

Bridge TP, Heseltine PN, Parker ES, et al: Results of extended peptide T administration in AIDS and ARC patients. Psychopharmacol Bull 27:237–245, 1991

Brightbill TC, Ihmeidan IH, Post MJ, et al: Neurosyphilis in HIV-positive and HIV-negative patients: neuroimaging findings. AJNR Am J Neuroradiol 16:703–711, 1995

Brodine SK, Mascola JR, McCutchan FE: Genotypic variation and molecular epidemiology of HIV. Infect Med 14:739–748, 1997

Brown JH, Henteleff P, Barakat S, et al: Is it normal for terminally ill patients to desire death? Am J Psychiatry 143:208–211, 1986

Brunetti A, Berg G, DiChiro G, et al: Reversal of brain metabolic abnormalities following treatment of AIDS dementia complex with 3′-azido-2′,3′-dideoxythymidine (AZT, zidovudine): a PET-FDG study. J Nucl Med 30:581–590, 1989

Budka H: Human immunodeficiency virus (HIV)-induced disease of the central nervous system: pathology and implications for pathogenesis. Acta Neuropathol 77:225–236, 1989

Buffet R, Agut H, Chieze F, et al: Virological markers in the cerebrospinal fluid from HIV-1 infected individuals. AIDS 5:1419–1424, 1991

Butters N, Grant I, Haxby J, et al: Assessment of AIDS-related cognitive changes: recommendations of the NIMH workshop on neuropsychological assessment approaches. J Clin Exp Neuropsychol 12:963–978, 1990

Buzy J, Brenneman DE, Pert CB, et al: Potent gp120-like neurotoxic activity in the cerebrospinal fluid of HIV-infected individuals is blocked by peptide T. Brain Res 598:10–18, 1992

Carrieri PB, Indaco A, Maiorino A, et al: Cerebrospinal fluid beta-2-microglobulin in multiple sclerosis and AIDS dementia complex. Neurol Res 14:282–283, 1992

Cecil KM, Lenkinski RE: Proton MR spectroscopy in inflammatory and infectious brain disorders. Neuroimaging Clin N Am 8:863–880, 1998

Centers for Disease Control: Revision of the CDC surveillance case definition for acquired immunodeficiency syndrome. MMWR Morb Mortal Wkly Rep 36 (suppl 1S):3S–15S, 1987

Centers for Disease Control and Prevention: HIV/AIDS Surveillance Report. Atlanta, GA, Centers for Disease Control and Prevention, 2003

Centers for Disease Control and Prevention: Diagnoses of HIV/AIDS—32 states, 2000–2003. MMWR Morb Mortal Wkly Rep 53:1106–1110, 2004

Chang L, Ernst T, Leonido-Yee M, et al: Cerebral metabolic abnormalities correlate with clinical severity of HIV-1 cognitive motor complex. Neurology 52:100–108, 1999

Chang L, Witt M, Eric M, et al: Cerebral metabolite changes during the first nine months after HAART (abstract). Neurology 26:474, 2001

Chiodi F, Keys B, Albert J, et al: Human immunodeficiency virus type 1 is present in the cerebrospinal fluid of a majority of infected individuals. J Clin Microbiol 30:1768–1771, 1992

Chong WK, Sweeney B, Wilkinson ID, et al: Proton spectroscopy of the brain in HIV infection: correlation with clinical, immunologic, and MR imaging findings. Neuroradiology 188:119–124, 1993

Ciardi A, Sindair E, Scaravilli F, et al: The involvement of the cerebral cortex in human immunodeficiency virus encephalopathy: a morphological and immunohistochemical study. Acta Neuropathol 81:51–59, 1990

Clavel F, Guyader M, Guetard D, et al: Molecular cloning and polymorphism of the human immune deficiency virus type 2. Nature 324(6098):691–695, 1986

Collier AC, Marra C, Coombs RW, et al: Central nervous system manifestations in human immunodeficiency virus infection without AIDS. J Acquir Immune Defic Syndr 5:229–241, 1992

Connolly KJ, Allan JD, Fitch H, et al: Phase I study of 2′-3′-dideoxyinosine administered orally twice daily to patients with AIDS or AIDS-related complex and hematologic intolerance to zidovudine. Am J Med 91:471–478, 1991

Corbeil J, Richman DD: Productive infection and subsequent interaction of CD4-gp120 at the cellular membrane is required for HIV-induced apoptosis of CD4+ T cells. J Gen Virol 76 (pt 3):681–690, 1995

Cornblath DR, McArthur JC, Kennedy PG, et al: Inflammatory demyelinating peripheral neuropathies associated with human T-cell lymphotropic virus type III infection. Ann Neurol 21:32–40, 1987

Cotton P: AIDS dementia may be linked to metabolite of tryptophan. JAMA 264:305–306, 1990

Cummings JL, Benson DF: Dementia: A Clinical Approach. Boston, MA, Butterworths, 1983

Currier MB: A prospective trial of sustained release bupropion for depression in HIV seropositive and AIDS patients. Psychosomatics 44:120–125, 2003

Currier MB, Molina G, Kato M: Citalopram treatment of major depressive disorder in Hispanic HIV and AIDS patients: a prospective study. Psychosomatics 45:210–216, 2004

Cysique LA, Maruff P, Brew BJ: Antiretroviral therapy in HIV infection: are neurologically active drugs important? Arch Neurol 61:1699–1704, 2004

Dalakas MC, Pezeshkpour GH: Neuromuscular diseases associated with human immunodeficiency virus infection. Ann Neurol 23(suppl):S38–S48, 1988

Darko DF, Miller JC, Gallen C, et al: Sleep encephalogram delta-frequency amplitude, night plasma levels of tumor necrosis factor α and human immunodeficiency virus infection. Proc Natl Acad Sci U S A 92:12080–12084, 1995

Davis LE, Hjelle BL, Miller VE, et al: Early viral brain invasion in iatrogenic human immunodeficiency virus infection. Neurology 42:1736–1739, 1992

D'Aversa TG, Weidenheim KM, Berman JW: CD40-CD40L interactions induce chemokine expression by human microglia: implications for human immunodeficiency virus encephalitis and multiple sclerosis. Am J Pathol 160:559–567, 2002

D'Aversa TG, Eugenin EA, Berman JW: NeuroAIDS: contributions of the human immunodeficiency virus-1 proteins tat and gp120 as well as CD40 to microglial activation. J Neurosci Res 81:436–446, 2005

DeBiasi R, Tyler KL: Polymerase chain reaction in the diagnosis and management of central nervous system infections. Arch Neurol 56:1215–1219, 1999

Deicken RF, Hubesch B, Jensen PC, et al: Alterations in brain phosphate metabolite concentrations in patients with human immunodeficiency virus infection. Arch Neurol 48:203–209, 1991

Dezube BJ, Pardee AB, Chapman B, et al: Pentoxifylline decreases tumor necrosis factor expression and serum triglycerides in people with AIDS. J Acquir Immune Defic Syndr 6:787–794, 1993

Diaz RS, de Oliveira CF, Mayer A, et al: Evidence of enhanced v3 region diversity and recombination in a dually infected transfusion recipient (abstract), in Program and Abstracts of the 4th Conference on Retroviruses and Opportunistic Infections, Washington, DC, January 22–26, 1997

Dickover RE, Donovan RM, Goldstein E, et al: Decreases in unintegrated HIV DNA are associated with antiretroviral therapy in AIDS patients. J Acquir Immune Defic Syndr 5:31–36, 1991

Dickson DW, Mattiace LA, Kurc K, et al: Biology of disease: microglia in human disease, with an emphasis on acquired immune deficiency syndrome. Lab Invest 64:135–156, 1991

Dooneief G, Bello J, Todak G, et al: A prospective controlled study of magnetic resonance imaging of the brain in gay men and parenteral drug users with human immunodeficiency virus infection. Arch Neurol 49:38–43, 1992

Drago F, Motta A, Grossi E: Intravenous maprotiline in severe and resistant primary depression: a double-blind comparison with clomipramine. J Int Med Res 11:78–84, 1983

Dreyer EB, Kaiser PK, Offermann JT, et al: HIV-1 coat protein neurotoxicity prevented by calcium channel antagonists. Science 248:364–367, 1990

Dröge W: Cysteine and glutathione deficiency in AIDS patients: a rationale for the treatment with N-acctyl-cysteine. Pharmacology 46:61–65, 1993

Dunlop O, Bjørklund RA, Abedelnoor M, et al: Five different tests of reaction time evaluated in HIV seropositive men. Acta Neurol Scand 8:260–266, 1992

Edelstein H, Knight RT: Severe parkinsonism in two AIDS patients taking a prochlorperazine (letter). Lancet 2:314–342, 1987

Eisdorfer C, Cohen D, Paveza GJ, et al: An empirical evaluation of the Global Deterioration Scale for staging Alzheimer's disease. Am J Psychiatry 149:190–194, 1991

Elliott AJ, Uldall KK, Bergam K, et al: Randomized placebo-controlled trial of paroxetine versus imipramine on depressed HIV-positive outpatients. Am J Psychiatry 155:367–372, 1998

Elovaara I, Iivanianen M, Portiainer E, et al: CSF and serum β2-microglobulin in HIV infection related to neurological dysfunction. Acta Neurol Scand 79:81–87, 1989

Elovaara I, Saar P, Valle S-L, et al: EEG in early HIV-1 infection is characterized by anterior dysrhythmicity of low maximal amplitude. Clin Electroencephalogr 22:131–140, 1991

Engstrom JW, Lowenstein DH, Bredesen DE: Cerebral infarctions and transient neurologic deficits associated with acquired immunodeficiency syndrome. Am J Med 86:528–532, 1989

Everall I, Luthert PJ, Lantos PL: Neuronal loss in the frontal cortex in HIV infection. Lancet 337:1119–1121, 1991

Everall I, Luthert PJ, Lantos PL: A review of neuronal damage in human immunodeficiency virus infection: its assessment, possible mechanism and relationship to dementia. J Neuropathol Exp Neurol 52:561–566, 1993

Fassina G, Buffa A, Benelli R, et al: Polyphenolic antioxidant (-)-epigallocatechin-3-gallate from green tea as a candidate anti-HIV agent. AIDS 16:939–941, 2002

Feravelli C, Broadhurst AD, Ambonetti A, et al: Double blind trial with oral versus intravenous clomipramine in primary depression. Biol Psychiatry 18:695–706, 1983

Fernandez F: Psychiatric complications in HIV-related illnesses, in American Psychiatric Association AIDS Primer. Washington, DC, American Psychiatric Press, 1988

Fernandez F: Anxiety and the neuropsychiatry of AIDS. J Clin Psychiatry 50(suppl):9–14, 1989

Fernandez F, Levy JK: Adjuvant treatment of HIV dementia with psychostimulants, in Behavioral Aspects of AIDS and Other Sexually Transmitted Diseases. Edited by Ostrow D. New York, Plenum, 1990, pp 279–286

Fernandez F, Levy JK: Psychopharmacotherapy of psychiatric syndromes in asymptomatic and symptomatic HIV infection. Psychiatr Med 9:377–393, 1991

Fernandez F, Adams F, Levy JK, et al: Cognitive impairment due to AIDS-related complex and its response to psychostimulants. Psychosomatics 29:38–46, 1988a

Fernandez F, Holmes VF, Adams F, et al: Treatment of severe, refractory agitation with a haloperidol drip. J Clin Psychiatry 49:239–241, 1988b

Fernandez F, Levy JK, Galizzi H: Response of HIV-related depression to psychostimulants: case reports. Hosp Community Psychiatry 39:628–631, 1988c

Fernandez F, Holmes VF, Levy JK, et al: Consultation-liaison psychiatry and HIV-related disorders. Hosp Community Psychiatry 40:146–153, 1989a

Fernandez F, Levy JK, Mansell PWA: Management of delirium in terminally ill AIDS patients. Int J Psychiatry Med 19:165–172, 1989b

Fernandez F, Levy JK, Lachar BL, et al: The management of depression and anxiety in the elderly. J Clin Psychiatry 56 (suppl 2):20–29, 1995a

Fernandez F, Levy JK, Sampley HR, et al: Effects of methylphenidate in HIV-related depression: a comparative trial with desipramine. Int J Psychiatry Med 25:53–67, 1995b

Ferrando SJ, Goldman JD, Charness WE: Selective serotonin reuptake inhibitor treatment of depression in symptomatic HIV infection and AIDS: improvements in affective and somatic symptoms. Gen Hosp Psychiatry 19:89–97, 1997

Filley CM, Franklin GM, Heaton RK, et al: White matter dementia: clinical disorders and implications. Neuropsychiatry Neuropsychol Behav Neurol 1:239–254, 1988

Fischl MA, Richman DD, Grieco MH, et al: The efficacy of azidothymidine (AZT) in the treatment of patients with AIDS and AIDS-related complex: a double-blind, placebo-controlled study. N Engl J Med 317:185–191, 1987

Flowers CH, Mafee MF, Crowell R, et al: Encephalopathy in AIDS patients: evaluation with MR imaging. AJNR Am J Neuroradiol 11:1235–1245, 1990

Fong IW, Toma E: The natural history of progressive multifocal leukoencephalopathy in patients with AIDS. Clin Infect Dis 20:1305–1310, 1995

Forstein M: The psychosocial impact of the acquired immunodeficiency syndrome. Semin Oncol 11:77–82, 1984

Frank Y, Lin W, Kahn E, et al: Multiple ischemic infarcts in a child with AIDS, varicella zoster infection, and cerebral vasculitis. Pediatr Neurol 5:64–67, 1989

Franzblau A, Letz R, Hershman D, et al: Quantitative neurologic and neurobehavioral testing of persons infected with human immunodeficiency virus type 1. Arch Neurol 48:263–268, 1991

Freund-Levi Y, Saaf J, Wahlund L-O, et al: Ultra low field brain MRI in HIV transfusion infected patients. Magn Reson Imaging 7:225–230, 1989

Frewer LJ, Lader M: The effects of nefazodone, imipramine, and placebo, alone and combined with alcohol, in normal subjects. Int Clin Psychopharmacol 8:13–20, 1993

Frierson RL, Lippthann SB: Suicide and AIDS. Psychosomatics 29:226–231, 1988

Gabuzda DA, Levy SR, Chiappa KH: Electroencephalography in AIDS and AIDS-related complex. Clin Electroencephalogr 19:1–6, 1988

Gallo RC, Sarin PS, Gelmann EP, et al: Isolation of human T-cell leukemia virus in acquired immune deficiency syndrome. Science 220:865–867, 1983

Gao F, Yue L, Robertson DL, et al: Genetic diversity of human immunodeficiency virus type 2: evidence for distinct sequence subtypes with differences in virus biology. J Virol 68:743–747, 1994

Gemignani A, Paudice P, Pittaluga A, et al: The HIV-1 coat protein gp120 and some of its fragments potently activate native cerebral NMDA receptors mediating neuropeptide release. Eur J Neurosci 12:2839–2846, 2000

Gibbs A, Andrewes DG, Szmukler G, et al: Early HIV-related neuropsychological impairment: relationship to stage of viral infection. J Clin Exp Neuropsychol 12:766–780, 1990

Gillig P, Sackellares JC, Greenberg HS: Right hemisphere partial complex seizures: mania, hallucinations, and speech disturbances during ictal events. Epilepsia 29:26–29, 1988

Giulian D, Vaca K, Noonan CA: Secretion of neurotoxins by mononuclear phagocytes infected with HIV-1. Science 250:1593–1595, 1990

Giunta B, Ehrhart J, Townsend K, et al: Galantamine and nicotine have a synergistic effect on inhibition of microglial activation induced by HIV-1 gp120. Brain Res Bull 64:165–170, 2004

Giunta B, Obregon D, Hou H, et al: Green tea derived EGCG modulates AIDS dementia-like neuronal damage via inhibition of STAT1 activation. Brain Res 1123:216–225, 2006

Golden RN, De Vane CL, Laizure SC, et al: Bupropion in depression, II: the role of metabolites in clinical outcome. Arch Gen Psychiatry 45:145–149, 1988a

Golden RN, Rudorfer MV, Sherer MA, et al: Bupropion in depression, I: biochemical effects and clinical responses. Arch Gen Psychiatry 45:139–143, 1988b

Gonzales MF, David RL: Neuropathology of acquired immunodeficiency syndrome. Neuropathol Appl Neurobiol 14:345–363, 1988

Goodin DS, Aminoff MJ, Chernoff DN, et al: Long latency event-related potentials in patients infected with human immunodeficiency virus. Ann Neurol 27:414–419, 1990

Goodkin K, Baldewicz TT, Wilkie FL, et al: Cognitive-motor impairment and disorder in HIV-1 infection. Psychiatr Ann 31:37–44, 2001

Goodwin GM, Chiswick A, Egan V, et al: The Edinburgh cohort of HIV-positive drug users: auditory event-related potentials show progressive slowing in patients with Centers for Disease Control stage IV disease. AIDS 4:1243–1250, 1990

Gottlieb MS, Schroff R, Schanker RM, et al: Pneumocystis carinii pneumonia and mucosal candidiasis in previously healthy homosexual men: evidence of a new acquired cellular immunodeficiency. N Engl J Med 305:1425–1431, 1981

Grafe MR, Press GA, Berthoty DP, et al: Abnormalities of the brain in AIDS patients: correlation of postmortem MR findings with neuropathology. AJNR Am J Neuroradiol 11:905–913, 1990

Grant I: The neuropsychiatry of human immunodeficiency virus. Semin Neurol 10:267–275, 1990

Grant I, Atkinson JH, Hesselink JR, et al: Evidence for early central nervous system involvement in the immunodeficiency syndrome (AIDS) and other human immunodeficiency virus (HIV) infections: studied with neuropsychological testing and magnetic resonance imaging. Ann Intern Med 107:828–836, 1987

Gray F, Lescs MC: HIV-related demyelinating disease. Eur J Med 2:89–96, 1993

Gray F, Gherard R, Keohane C, et al: Pathology of the central nervous system in 40 cases of acquired immune deficiency syndrome (AIDS). Neuropathol Appl Neurobiol 14:365–380, 1988

Greenberg SJ: Human retroviruses and demyelinating diseases. Neurol Clin 13:75–97, 1995

Greenblatt DJ, VonMolke LL, Harmatz JS, et al: Drug interactions with newer antidepressants: role of human cytochromes P450. J Clin Psychiatry 59 (suppl 15):19–27, 1998

Greenlee JE, Rose JW: Controversies in neurological infectious diseases. Semin Neurol 20:375–386, 2000

Griffin DE, Wesselingh SL, McArthur JC: Elevated central nervous system prostaglandins in human immunodeficiency virus–associated dementia. Ann Neurol 35:592–597, 1994

Groopman JE: Antiretroviral therapy and immunomodulators in patients with AIDS. Am J Med 90 (suppl 4A):18S–21S, 1991a

Groopman JE: Treatment of AIDS with combinations of antiretroviral agents. Am J Med 90 (suppl 4A):27S–30S, 1991b

Guze SB, Daengsurisri S: Organic brain syndromes' prognostic significance in general medical patients. Arch Gen Psychiatry 17:365–366, 1967

Gyorkey F, Melnick JL, Gyorkey P: Human immunodeficiency virus in brain biopsies of patients with AIDS and progressive encephalopathy. J Infect Dis 155:870–876, 1987

Hagler DN, Frame PT: Azidothymidine neurotoxicity. Lancet 2:1392–1393, 1986

Hall JM, Stevens PE: AIDS: a guide to suicide assessment. Arch Psychiatr Nurs 1:115–120, 1988

Halman MH, Worth JL, Sanders KM, et al: Anticonvulsant use in the treatment of manic syndromes in patients with HIV1 infection. J Neuropsychiatry Clin Neurosci 5:430–434, 1993

Harbison MA, Kim S, Gillis JM, et al: Effect of the calcium channel blocker verapamil on human immunodeficiency virus type 1 replication in lymphoid cells. J Infect Dis 164:43–60, 1991

Harris MJ, Jeste DV, Gleghorn A, et al: New-onset psychosis in HIV-infected patients. J Clin Psychiatry 52:369–376, 1991

Harrison NA, Skidmore SJ: Neopterin and beta-2 microglobulin levels in asymptomatic HIV infection: the predictive value of combining markers. J Med Virol 32:128–133, 1990

Hart RP, Wade JB, Klinger RL, et al: Slowed information processing as an early cognitive change associated with AIDS and ARC (abstract). J Clin Exp Neuropsychol 12:72, 1990

Heaton RK, Grant I, Butters N, et al: The HNRC 500: neuropsychology of HIV infection at different disease stages. J Int Neuropsychol Soc 1:231–251, 1995

Heaton RK, Marcotte TD, Rivera Mindt M, et al: The impact of HIV-associated neuropsychological impairment on everyday functioning. J Int Neuropsychol Soc 10:317–331, 2004

Heyes MP, Brew BJ, Martin A, et al: Quinolinic acid in cerebrospinal fluid and serum in HIV-1 infection: relationship to clinical neurological status. Ann Neurol 29:202–209, 1991

Heyes MP, Brew BJ, Saito K, et al: Inter-relationships between quinolinic acid, neuroactive kynurenines, neopterin and β2-microglobulin in cerebrospinal fluid and HIV-1-infected patients. J Neuroimmunol 40:71–80, 1992

Heyes MP, Ellis RJ, Ryan L, et al: Elevated cerebrospinal fluid quinolinic acid levels are associated with region-specific cerebral volume loss in HIV infection. Brain 124 (pt 5):1033–1042, 2001

Hill JM, Farrar WL, Pert CB: Autoradiographic localization of T4 antigen, the HIV receptor, in human brain. Int J Neurosci 32:687–693, 1987

Hinkin CH, van Gorp WG, Mandelkern MA, et al: Cerebral metabolic change in patients with AIDS: report of a six-month follow-up using positron-emission tomography. J Neuropsychiatry Clin Neurosci 7:1880–1887, 1995

Hintz S, Kuck J, Peterkin JJ, et al: Depression in the context of human immunodeficiency virus infection: implications for treatment. J Clin Psychiatry 51:497–501, 1990

Ho DD, Pomerantz RJ, Kaplan JC: Pathogenesis of infection with human immunodeficiency virus. N Engl J Med 317:278–286, 1987

Holland JC, Tross S: The psychosocial and neuropsychiatric sequelae of the acquired immunodeficiency syndrome. Ann Intern Med 103:760–764, 1985

Hollander H: Neurologic and psychiatric manifestations of HIV disease. J Gen Intern Med 6 (Jan/Feb suppl):S24–S31, 1991

Hollister LE: New psychotherapeutic drugs. J Clin Psychopharmacol 14:50–63, 1994

Hollweg M, Riedel R-R, Goebel F-D, et al: Remarkable improvement of neuropsychiatric symptoms in HIV-infected patients after AZT therapy. Klinische Wochenschrift 69:409–412, 1991

Holmes VF, Fricchone GL: Hypomania in an AIDS patient receiving amitriptyline for neuropathic pain (clinical/scientific note). Neurology 39:305, 1989

Holmes VF, Fernandez F, Levy JK: Psychostimulant response in AIDS-related complex patients. J Clin Psychiatry 50:5–8, 1989

Huyse F, Van Schijndel RS: Haloperidol and cardiac arrest. Lancet 2:568–569, 1988

Itil TM, Ferracuti S, Freedman AM, et al: Computer-analyzed EEG (CEEG) and dynamic brain mapping in AIDS and HIV related syndrome: a pilot study. Clin Electroencephalogr 21:140–144, 1990

Jacobs D, Peavy G, Velin R, et al: Verbal memory in asymptomatic HIV-infection: evidence of subcortical dysfunction in a subgroup of patients (abstract). J Clin Exp Neuropsychol 14:101, 1992

Janssen RS, Saykin AJ, Kaplan JE, et al: Neurological complications of human immunodeficiency virus infection in patients with lymphadenopathy syndrome. Ann Neurol 23:49–55, 1988

Janssen RS, Cornblath DR, Epstein LG, and the Working Group of the American Academy of Neurology AIDS Task Force: Nomenclature and research case definitions for neurologic manifestations of human immunodeficiency virus-type 1 (HIV-1) infection. Neurology 41:778–785, 1991

Janssen RS, Nwanyanwu OC, Selik PM, et al: Epidemiology of human immunodeficiency virus encephalopathy in the United States. Neurology 42:1472–1476, 1992

Jarvik JG, Hesselink JR, Kennedy C, et al: Acquired immunodeficiency syndrome: magnetic resonance patterns of brain involvement with pathologic correlation. Arch Neurol 45:731–736, 1988

Jarvik JG, Lenkinski RE, Grossman RI, et al: Proton MR spectroscopy of HIV-infected patients: characterization of abnormalities with imaging and clinical correlation. Radiology 186:739–744, 1993

Jernigan TL, Archibald S, Hesselink JR, et al: Magnetic resonance imaging morphometric analysis of cerebral volume loss in human immunodeficiency virus: the HNRC group. Arch Neurol 50:250–255, 1993

Jones GH, Kelly CL, Davies JA: HIV and onset of schizophrenia (letter). Lancet 1:982, 1987

Judd FK, Mijch AM, Cockram A: Fluoxetine treatment of depressed patients with HIV-infection. Aust N Z J Psychiatry 29:433–436, 1995

Julander I, Alexius B, Britton S, et al: Treatment of HIV-1 infected patients with peptide T. Antivir Chem Chemother 1:349–354, 1990

Kaemingk KL, Kaszniak AW: Neuropsychological aspects of human immunodeficiency virus infection. Clin Neuropsychol 3:309–326, 1989

Kaiser PK, Offerman JT, Lipton SA: Neuronal injury due to HIV-1 envelope protein is blocked by anti gp120 antibodies but not by anti-CD4 antibodies. Neurology 40:1757–1761, 1990

Kaneko S, Maeda T, Kume T, et al: Nicotine protects cultured cortical neurons against glutamate-induced cytotoxicity via alpha7-neuronal receptors and neuronal CNS receptors. Brain Res 765:135–140, 1997

Karlsen NR, Reinvang I, Frøland SS: Serum level of neopterin, CD8+ cell count, and neuropsychological function in HIV-infected patients (abstract). J Clin Exp Neuropsychol 14:101, 1991

Karlsen NR, Reinvang I, Froland SS: Slowed reaction time in asymptomatic HIV-positive patients. Acta Neurol Scand 86:242–246, 1992

Kastenholz KV, Crismon ML: Buspirone, a novel nonbenzodiazepine anxiolytic. Clin Pharmacol Ther 3:600–607, 1984

Kawai K, Tsuno NH, Kitayama J, et al: Epigallocatechin gallate, the main component of tea polyphenol, binds to CD4 and interferes with gp120 binding. J Allergy Clin Immunol 112:951–957, 2003

Kelly WM, Brant-Zawadzki M: Acquired immunodeficiency syndrome: neuroradiologic findings. Radiology 149:485–491, 1983

Kerr DA, Chang CF, Gordon J, et al: Inhibition of human neurotropic virus (JCV) DNA replication in glial cells by camptothecin. Virology 196:612–618, 1993

Kessing L, LaBianca JH, Bolwig TG: HIV-induced stupor treated with ECT. Convuls Ther 10:232–235, 1994

Ketzler S, Weis S, Haug H, et al: Loss of neurons in the frontal cortex in AIDS patients. Acta Neuropathol (Berl) 80:92–94, 1990

Kieburtz KD, Epstein LG, Gelbard HA, et al: Excitotoxicity and dopaminergic dysfunction in the acquired immunodeficiency syndrome dementia complex: therapeutic implications. Arch Neurol 48:1281–1284, 1991a

Kieburtz K, Zettelmaier AE, Ketonen L, et al: Manic syndrome in AIDS. Am J Psychiatry 148:1068–1070, 1991b

Klusman LE, Moulton JM, Hornbostel LK, et al: Neuropsychological abnormalities in asymptomatic HIV seropositive military personnel. J Neuropsychiatry Clin Neurosci 3:422–428, 1991

Knights EB, Folstein MF: Unsuspected emotional and cognitive disturbance in medical patients. Ann Intern Med 87:723–724, 1977

Konikoff F, Kuritzky A, Jerushalmi Y, et al: Neuroleptic malignant syndrome induced by a single injection of haloperidol. BMJ 289:1228–1229, 1984

Koralnik IJ, Beaumanoir A, Hausler R, et al: A controlled study of early neurologic abnormalities in men with asymptomatic human immunodeficiency virus infection. N Engl J Med 323:864–870, 1990

Kornhuber J, Bormann J, Hubers M, et al: Effects of 1-aminoadamantanes at the MK-801-binding site of the NMDA-receptor-gated ion channel: a human postmortem brain study. Eur J Pharmacol 206:297–300, 1991

Kovner R, Perecman E, Lazar W, et al: Relation of personality and attentional factors to cognitive deficits in human immunodeficiency virus–infected subjects. Arch Neurol 46:274–277, 1989

Kranczer S: U.S. longevity unchanged. Stat Bull Metrop Insur Co 76:12–20, 1995

Krikorian R, Wrobel AJ: Cognitive impairment in HIV infection. AIDS 5:1501–1507, 1991

Kuni CC, Phame FS, Meier MJ, et al: Quantitative I-123-IMP brain SPECT and neuropsychological testing in AIDS dementia. Clin Nucl Med 16:174–177, 1991

Lalezari JP, Holland GN, Kramer F, et al: Randomized, controlled study of the safety and efficacy of intravenous cidofovir for the treatment of relapsing cytomegalovirus retinitis in patients with AIDS. J Acquir Immune Defic Syndr Hum Retrovirol 17:339–344, 1998

Lantos PL, McLaughlin JE, Scholtz CL, et al: Neuropathology of the brain in HIV infection. Lancet 1:309–311, 1989

Larsson M, Hagbreg L, Forsman A, et al: Cerebrospinal fluid catecholamine metabolites in HIV-infected patients. J Neurosci Res 28:406–409, 1991

Levin GM: A pharmacokinetic drug-drug interaction study of venlafaxine and indinavir. Psychopharmcol Bull 35:62–71, 2001

Levin HS, Williams DH, Borucki MJ, et al: Magnetic resonance imaging and neuropsychological findings in human immunodeficiency virus infection. J Acquir Immune Defic Syndr 3:757–762, 1990

Levine S, Anderson D, Bystritsky A, et al: A report of eight HIV-seropositive patients with major depression responding to fluoxetine. J Acquir Immune Defic Syndr 3:1074–1077, 1990

Levy JA: Pathogenesis of human immunodeficiency virus infection. Microbiol Rev 57:183–289, 1993

Levy JA, Hoffman AD, Kramer SM, et al: Isolation of lymphocytopathic retroviruses from San Francisco patients with AIDS. Science 225:840–842, 1984

Levy JK, Fernandez F: Memory rehabilitation in HIV encephalopathy. Clin Neuropathol 12 (suppl 1):S27–S28, 1993

Levy JK, Fernandez F: Effects of methylphenidate on HIV-related memory impairment (NR404). Paper presented at the 148th annual meeting of the American Psychiatric Association, Miami, FL, May 20–25, 1995, p 164

Li CJ, Friedman DJ, Wang C, et al: Induction of apoptosis in uninfected lymphocytes by HIV-1 Tat protein. Science 268:429–431, 1995

Lin-Greenberger A, Taneja-Uppal N: Dysautonomia and infection with the human immunodeficiency virus (letter). Ann Intern Med 106:167, 1987

Lipowski ZJ: Delirium (acute confusional states). JAMA 258:1789–1792, 1987

Lipton RB, Ferairu ER, Weiss G, et al: Headache in HIV-1-related disorders. Headache 31:518–522, 1991

Lipton SA: Calcium channel antagonists and human immunodeficiency virus coat protein-mediated neuronal injury. Ann Neurol 30:110–114, 1991

Lipton SA: Models of neuronal injury in AIDS: another role for the NMDA receptor. Trends Neurosci 15:75–79, 1992

Lipton SA, Gendleman HE: Dementia associated with the acquired immunodeficiency syndrome. N Engl J Med 332:934–940, 1995

Lolli F, Colao MG, De Maio E, et al: Intrathecal synthesis of anti-HIV antibodies in AIDS patients. J Neurol Sci 99:281–289, 1990

Louwagie J, McCutchan FE, Peeters M, et al: Phylogenetic analysis of gag genes from 70 international HIV-1 isolates provides evidence for multiple genotypes. AIDS 7:769–780, 1993

Lu W, Salerno-Goncalves R, Yuan J, et al: Glucocorticoids rescue CD4+ T lymphocytes from activation-induced apoptosis triggered by HIV-1: implications for pathogenesis and therapy. AIDS 9:35–42, 1995

Lunn S, Skydzbjerg M, Schulsinger H, et al: A preliminary report on the neuropsychologic sequelae of human immunodeficiency virus. Arch Gen Psychiatry 48:139–142, 1991

Lynch DH, Ramsdell F, Alderson MR: Fas and FasL in the homeostatic regulation of immune responses. Immunol Today 16:569–574, 1995

Maccario M, Scharre DW: HIV and acute onset of psychosis (letter). Lancet 2:342, 1987

Maccarrone M, Bari M, Corasaniti MT, et al: HIV-1 coat glycoprotein gp 120 induces apoptosis in rat brain neocortex by deranging the arachidonate cascade in favor of prostanoids. J Neurochem 75:196–203, 2000

Macdonald JC, Torriani FJ, Morse LS, et al: Lack of reactivation of cytomegalovirus (CMV) retinitis after stopping CMV maintenance therapy in AIDS patients with sustained elevations in CD4 T cells in response to highly active antiretroviral therapy. J Infect Dis 177:1182–1187, 1998

Maj M, Janssen R, Satz P, et al: The World Health Organization's cross-cultural study on neuropsychiatric aspects of infection with the human immunodeficiency virus 1 (HIV-1): preparation and pilot phase. Br J Psychiatry 159:351–356, 1991

Maldarelli F, Sato H, Berthold E, et al: Rapid induction of apoptosis by cell-to-cell transmission of human immunodeficiency virus type 1. J Virol 69:6457–6465, 1995

Maldonado JL, Fernandez F, Levy JK: Acquired immunodeficiency syndrome, in Psychiatric Management of Neurological Disease. Edited by Lauterbach EC. Washington, DC, American Psychiatric Press, 2000, pp 271–295

Mandel S, Weinreb O, Amit T, et al: Cell signaling pathways in the neuroprotective actions of the green tea polyphenol (-)-epigallocatechin-3-gallate: implications for neurodegenerative diseases. J Neurochem 88:1555–1569, 2004 [published erratum in: J Neurochem 89:527, 2004]

Markovitz DM: Infection with the human immunodeficiency virus type 2 (review). Ann Intern Med 118:211–218, 1993

Markowitz JC, Rabkin JG, Perry SW: Treating depression in HIV-positive patients. AIDS 8:403–412, 1994

Marlink R, Kanki P, Thior I, et al: Reduced rate of disease development after HIV-2 infection as compared to HIV-1. Science 265:1587–1590, 1994

Marotta R, Perry S: Early neuropsychological dysfunction caused by human immunodeficiency virus. J Neuropsychiatry Clin Neurosci 1:225–235, 1989

Marra CM, Lockhart D, Zunt JR, et al: Changes in CSF and plasma HIV-1 RNA and cognition after starting potent antiretroviral therapy. Neurology 60:1388–1390, 2003

Marshall DW, Brey RL, Cahill WT, et al: Spectrum of cerebrospinal fluid findings in various stages of human immunodeficiency virus infection. Arch Neurol 45:954–958, 1988

Marshall DW, Brey RL, Butzin CA, et al: CSF changes in a longitudinal study of 124 neurologically normal HIV-1-infected U.S. Air Force personnel. J Acquir Immune Defic Syndr 4:777–781, 1991

Martin EM, Robertson LC, Sorensen DJ, et al: Speed of memory scanning is not affected in early HIV-1 infection (abstract). J Clin Exp Neuropsychol 14:102, 1992

Marzuk PM, Tierney H, Tardiff K, et al: Increased risk of suicide in persons with AIDS. JAMA 259:1333–1337, 1988

Masdeu JC, Small CB, Weiss L, et al: Multifocal cytomegalovirus encephalitis in AIDS. Ann Neurol 23:97–99, 1988

Masdeu JC, Yudd A, Van Herrtum RL, et al: Single-photon-emission computed tomography in human immunodeficiency virus encephalopathy: a preliminary report. J Nucl Med 32:1471–1475, 1991

Masliah E, Achim CL, Ge N, et al: Spectrum of human immunodeficiency virus–associated neocortical damage. Ann Neurol 32:321–329, 1992

Masliah E, Ge N, Achim CL, et al: Differential vulnerability of calbindin-immunoreactive neurons in HIV encephalitis. J Neuropathol Exp Neurol 54:350–357, 1995

Maxwell S, Scheftner WA, Kessler HA, et al: Manic syndrome associated with zidovudine treatment. JAMA 259:3406–3407, 1988

McArthur JC, Nance-Sproson TE, Griffin DE, et al: The diagnostic utility of elevation in cerebral spinal fluid β2-microglobulin in HIV-1 dementia. Neurology 42:1707–1712, 1992

McArthur JC, Hoover DR, Bacellar H, et al: Dementia in AIDS patients: incidence and risk factors. Neurology 43:2245–2253, 1993

McArthur JC, McClernon DR, Cronin MF, et al: Relationship between human immunodeficiency virus-associated demential and viral load in cerebrospinal fluid and brain. Ann Neurol 42:689–698, 1997

McArthur JC, McDermott MP, McClernon D, et al: Attenuated central nervous system infection in advanced HIV/AIDS with combination antiretroviral therapy. Arch Neurol 61:1687–1696, 2004

McArthur JC, Brew BJ, Nath A: Neurological complications of HIV infection. Lancet Neruol 4:543–555, 2005

McDaniel SJ, Niran PT, Magnuson JV: Possible induction of mania by buspirone. Am J Psychiatry 147:125–126, 1990

McElroy SL, Keck PE, Pope HG, et al: Valproate in the treatment of bipolar disorder: literature review and clinical guidelines. J Clin Psychopharmacol 12 (suppl 1):42S–52S, 1992

McGowan I, Potter M, George RJD, et al: HIV encephalopathy presenting as hypomania. Genitourin Med 67:420–424, 1991

McManus CM, Weidenheim K, Woodman SE, et al: Chemokine and chemokine-receptor expression in human glial elements: induction by the HIV protein, Tat, and chemokine autoregulation. Am J Pathol 156:1441–1453, 2000

Melton ST, Kirkwood CK, Ghanemi SN: Pharmacotherapy of HIV dementia. Ann Pharmacother 31:457–473, 1997

Menon DK, Baudouin CJ, Tomlinson D, et al: Proton MR spectroscopy and imaging of the brain in AIDS: evidence of neuronal loss in regions that appear normal with imaging. J Comput Assist Tomogr 14:882–885, 1990

Merigan TC: Treatment of AIDS with combinations of antiretroviral agents. Am J Med 90 (suppl 4A):8S–17S, 1991

Merrill JE: Macroglia: neural cells responsive to lymphokines and growth factors. Immunol Today 8:146–150, 1987

Merrill JE: Proinflammatory and antiinflammatory cytokines in multiple sclerosis and central nervous system acquired immunodeficiency syndrome. J Immunother Emphasis Tumor Immunol 12:167–170, 1992

Miller EN, Satz P, Visscher B: Computerized and conventional neuropsychological assessment of HIV-1-infected homosexual men. Neurology 41:1608–1616, 1991

Miller JK, Barrett RE, Britton CB, et al: Progressive multifocal leukoencephalopathy in a male homosexual with T-cell immune deficiency. N Engl J Med 307:1436–1438, 1982

Miller K, Corcoran C, Armstrong C, et al: Transdermal testosterone administration in women with acquired immunodeficiency syndrome wasting: a pilot study. J Clin Endocrinol Metab 83:2717–2725, 1998

Minghetti L, Visentin S, Patrizio M, et al: Multiple actions of the human immunodeficiency virus type-1 Tat protein on microglial cell functions. Neurochem Res 29:965–978, 2004

Mitsuyasu RT: Medical aspects of HIV spectrum disease. Psychiatr Med 7:5–22, 1989

Miyazaki M: Epidemiological characteristics of human immunodeficiency virus type-2 infection in Africa (editorial and review). Int J STD AIDS 6:75–80, 1995

Moore RD, Hidalgo J, Sugland BW, et al: Zidovudine and the natural history of the acquired immunodeficiency syndrome. N Engl J Med 324:1412–1416, 1991

Morgan MK, Clark ME, Hartman WL: AIDS-related dementias: a case report of rapid cognitive decline. J Clin Psychol 44:1024–1028, 1988

Moses A, Bloom FE, Pauza CD, et al: Human immunodeficiency virus infection of human brain capillary endothelial cells occurs via a CD4/galactosylceramide-independent mechanism. Proc Natl Acad Sci U S A 90:10474–10478, 1993

Murray HW, Squires KE, Weiss W, et al: Stavudine in patients with AIDS and AIDS-related complex: AIDS Clinical Trials Group 089. J Infect Dis 171 (suppl 2):S123–S130, 1995

Musher DM, Hamill RJ, Baughn RE: Effects of human immunodeficiency virus (HIV) infection on the course of syphilis and on the response to treatment. Ann Intern Med 113:872–881, 1990

Nance M, Pirozzolo FJ, Levy JK, et al: Simple and choice reaction time in HIV-seronegative, HIV-seropositive and AIDS patients. Abstracts of the 6th International Conference on AIDS, Vol 2. San Francisco, CA, June 22, 1990, p 173

Navia BA, Gonzalez RG: Functional imaging of the AIDS dementia complex and the metabolic pathology of the HIV-1-infected brain. Neuroimaging Clin North Am 7:431–445, 1997

Navia BA, Price RW: The acquired immunodeficiency syndrome dementia complex as the presenting or sole manifestation of human immunodeficiency virus infection. Arch Neurol 44:65–69, 1987

Navia BA, Cho E-S, Petito CK, et al: The AIDS dementia complex, II: neuropathology. Ann Neurol 19:525–535, 1986a

Navia BA, Jordan BD, Price RW: The AIDS dementia complex, I: clinical features. Ann Neurol 19:517–524, 1986b

Nazzareno EL, Yeragani VK: Buspirone induced hypomania: a case report (letter). J Clin Psychopharmacol 8:226, 1988

Nelson JC, Wohlreich MM, Mallinckrodt CH, et al: Duloxetine for the treatment of major depression in older adults. Am J Geriatr Psychiatry 13:227–235, 2005

Neuzil KM: Pharmacologic therapy for human immunodeficiency virus infection: a review. Am J Med Sci 307:368–373, 1994

Newton TF, Leuchter AF, Walter DO, et al: EEG coherence in men with AIDS: association with subcortical metabolic activity. J Neuropsychiatry Clin Neurosci 5:316–321, 1993

Newton TF, Leuchter AF, Miller EN, et al: Quantitative EEG in patients with AIDS and asymptomatic HIV infection. Clin Electroencephalogr 25:18–25, 1994

Nichols SE: Psychiatric aspects of AIDS. Psychosomatics 24:1083–1089, 1983

Nichols SE: Psychosocial reactions of persons with the acquired immunodeficiency syndrome. Ann Intern Med 103:765–767, 1985

Norman SE, Chediak AD, Kiel M, et al: Sleep disturbances in HIV-infected homosexual men. AIDS 4:175–178, 1990

O'Dowd MA, McKegney FP: Manic syndrome associated with zidovudine. JAMA 260:3587–3588, 1988

O'Dowd MA, McKegney FP: AIDS patients compared to others seen in psychiatric consultation. Gen Hosp Psychiatry 12:50–55, 1990

Ollo C, Litman R, Rubinow D, et al: Neuropsychological correlates of smooth pursuit eye movements in HIV disease (abstract). J Clin Neuropsychol 12:73, 1990

Ollo C, Johnson R Jr, Grafman J: Signs of cognitive change in HIV disease: an event-related brain potential study. Neurology 41:209–215, 1991

Pace PL, Fama R, Bornstein RA: Depression and neuropsychological performance in asymptomatic HIV infection (abstract). J Clin Exp Neuropsychol 14:101, 1992

Pajeau AK, Roman GC: HIV encephalopathy and dementia. Psychiatr Clin North Am 15:455–466, 1991

Panel on Clinical Practices for Treatment of HIV Infection: Guidelines for the Use of Antiretroviral Agents in HIV-Infected Adults and Adolescents. Washington, DC, U.S. Department of Health and Human Services, 2005

Parisi A, Strosselli M, DiPerri G, et al: Electroencephalography in the early diagnosis of HIV-related subacute encephalitis: analysis of 185 patients. Clin Electroencephogr 20:1–5, 1989

Parisi A, Strosselli M, Pan A, et al: HIV-related encephalitis presenting as convulsant disease. Clin Electroencephalogr 22:1–4, 1991

Perkins DO, Stern RA, Golden RN, et al: Mood disorders in HIV infection: prevalence and risk factors in a nonepicenter of the AIDS epidemic. Am J Psychiatry 151:233–236, 1994

Perry SW: Organic mental disorders caused by HIV: update on early diagnosis and treatment. Am J Psychiatry 147:696–710, 1990

Perry S, Marotta RF: AIDS dementia: a review of the literature. Alzheimer Dis Assoc Disord 1:221–235, 1987

Perry S, Belsky-Barr D, Barr WB, et al: Neuropsychological function in physically asymptomatic, HIV-seropositive men. J Neuropsychiatry Clin Neurosci 3:296–302, 1989

Perry S, Jacobsberg L, Fishman B: Suicidal ideation of HIV testing. JAMA 263:679–682, 1990

Perry S, Fishman B, Jacobsberg L, et al: Relationships over 1 year between lymphocyte subsets and psychosocial variables among adults with infection by human immunodeficiency virus. Arch Gen Psychiatry 49:396–401, 1992

Petito CK: Review of central nervous system pathology in human immunodeficiency virus infection. Ann Neurol 23(suppl):S54–S57, 1988

Petito CK, Roberts B: Evidence of apoptotic cell death in HIV encephalitis. Am J Pathol 146:1121–1130, 1995

Pollock GB, Perel JM, Shostak M: Rapid achievement of antidepressant effect with intravenous clomipramine (letter). N Engl J Med 312:1130, 1985

Portegies P, Epstein LG, Hung STA, et al: Human immunodeficiency virus type 1 antigen in cerebrospinal fluid: correlation with clinical neurologic status. Arch Neurol 46:261–264, 1989

Portegies P, Algra PR, Hollak CEM, et al: Response to cytarabine in progressive multifocal leucoencephalopathy in AIDS (letter). Lancet 337:680–681, 1991

Post MJD, Berger JR, Quencer RM: Asymptomatic and neurologically symptomatic HIV-seropositive individuals: prospective evaluation with cranial MR imaging. Radiology 178:131–139, 1991

Poutiainen E, Haltia M, Elovaara I, et al: Dementia associated with human immunodeficiency virus: subcortical or cortical? Acta Psychiatr Scand 83:297–301, 1991

Power C, Kong PA, Crawford TO, et al: Cerebral white matter changes in acquired immunodeficiency syndrome dementia: alterations of the blood-brain barrier. Ann Neurol 34:339–350, 1993

Power C, Selnes OA, Grim JA, et al: HIV Dementia Scale: a rapid screening test. J Acquir Immune Defic Syndr Hum Retrovirol 8:273–278, 1995

Praus DJ, Brown GR, Rundell JR, et al: Associations between cerebrospinal fluid parameters and high degrees of anxiety or depression in United States Air Force personnel infected with human immunodeficiency virus. J Nerv Ment Dis 178:392–395, 1990

Price WA, Bielefeld M: Buspirone induced mania. J Clin Psychopharmacol 9:150–151, 1989

Pumarola-Sune T, Navia BA, Cordon-Cardo C, et al: HIV antigen in the brains of patients with the AIDS dementia complex. Ann Neurol 21:490–496, 1987

Rabkin JG, Harrison WM: Effect of imipramine on depression and immune status in a sample of men with HIV infection. Am J Psychiatry 147:495–497, 1990

Rabkin JG, Williams JBW, Remien RH, et al: Depression, distress, lymphocyte subsets, and human immunodeficiency virus symptoms on two occasions in HIV-positive homosexual men. Arch Gen Psychiatry 48:111–119, 1991

Rabkin JG, Wagner JG, McElhiney MC, et al: Testosterone versus fluoxetine for depression and fatigue in HIV/AIDS patients: a placebo controlled trial. J Clin Psychopharmacol 24:379–385, 2004

Reboul J, Schuller E, Pialoux G, et al: Immunoglobulins and complement components in 37 patients infected by HIV-1 virus: comparison of general (systemic) and intrathecal immunity. J Neurol Sci 89:243–252, 1989

Reddy MM, Grieco MH, McKinley GF, et al: Effect of foscarnet therapy on human immunodeficiency virus p24 antigen levels in AIDS patients with cytomegalovirus retinitis. J Infect Dis 166:607–610, 1992

Reed JB, Schwab IR, Gordon J, et al: Regression of cytomegalovirus retinitis associated with protease inhibitor treatment in patients with AIDS. Am J Ophthalmol 124:199–205, 1997

Reger M, Welsh R, Razani J, et al: A meta-analysis of the neuropsychological sequelae of HIV infection. J Int Neuropsychol Soc 8:410–424, 2002

Reisberg B, Ferris SH, de Leon MJ, et al: The Global Deterioration Scale (GDS): an instrument for the assessment of primary degenerative dementia (PDD). Am J Psychiatry 139:1136–1139, 1982

Riccio M, Burgess A, Hawkins D, et al: Neuropsychological and psychiatric changes following treatment of ARC patients with zidovudine. Int J STD AIDS 1:435–437, 1990

Richelson E: Synaptic pharmacology of antidepressants: an update. McLean Hospital Journal 13:67–88, 1988

Richman DD, Fischl MA, Grieco MH, et al: The toxicity of azidothymidine (AZT) in the treatment of patients with AIDS and AIDS-related complex: a double-blind, placebo-controlled trial. N Engl J Med 317:192–197, 1987

Riedel R-R, Helmstaedter C, Bulau P, et al: Early signs of cognitive deficits among human immunodeficiency virus–positive hemophiliacs. Acta Psychiatr Scand 85:321–326, 1992

Roccatagliata G, Abbruzzese G, Albano C, et al: Trazodone by intravenous infusion in depressions secondary to organic disease. Int Pharmacopsychiatry 12:72–79, 1977

Rolfe M: HIV-2 and its neurological manifestations (review). S Afr Med J 84:503–505, 1994

Rosen MI, Bridge TP, O'Malley SS, et al: Peptide T treatment of cognitive impairment in HIV-positive intravenous drug users. Am J Addict 1:332–338, 1992

Rowen D, Carne CA: Neurological manifestation of HIV infection. Int J STD AIDS 2:79–90, 1991

Rubinow DR, Berrettini CH, Brouwers P, et al: Neuropsychiatric consequences of AIDS. Ann Neurol 23(suppl):S24–S26, 1988

Ruscetti F, Farrar WL, Hill JM, et al: Visualization of human helper T lymphocyte differentiation antigen in primate brain. Peptides 9 (suppl 1):97–104, 1988

Ryan JJ, Paolo AM, Skrade M: Rey auditory verbal learning test performance of a federal corrections sample with acquired immunodeficiency syndrome. Int J Neurosci 64:177–181, 1992

Sacktor N, Prohovnik I, Van Heertum RL, et al: Cerebral single-photon emission computed tomography abnormalities in human immunodeficiency virus type 1–infected gay men without cognitive impairment. Arch Neurol 52:607–611, 1995a

Sacktor N, Van Heertum RL, Dooneief G, et al: A comparison of cerebral SPECT abnormalities in HIV-positive homosexual men with and without cognitive impairment. Arch Neurol 52:1170–1173, 1995b

Sacktor N, Tarwater PM, Skolasky RL, et al: CSF antiretroviral drug penetrance and the treatment of HIV-associated psychomotor slowing. Neurology 57:542–544, 2001

Samochocki M, Hoffle A, Fehrenbacher A, et al: Galantamine is an allosterically potentiating ligand of neuronal nicotinic but not of muscarinic acetylcholine receptors. J Pharmacol Exp Ther 305:1024–1036, 2003

Santos MD, Alkondon M, Pereira EF, et al: The nicotinic allosteric potentiating ligand galantamine facilitates synaptic transmission in the mammalian central nervous system. Mol Pharmacol 61:1222–1234, 2002

Sardar AM, Bell JE, Reynolds GP: Increased concentrations of the neurotoxin 3-hydroxykynurenine in the frontal cortex of HIV-1-positive patients. J Neurochem 64:932–935, 1995

Scaravilli F, Daniel SE, Harcourt-Webster N, et al: Chronic basal meningitis and vasculitis in acquired immunodeficiency syndrome: a possible role for human immunodeficiency virus. Arch Pathol Lab Med 113:192–195, 1989

Schaerf FW, Miller RS, Lipsey JR, et al: ECT for major depression in four patients infected with human immunodeficiency virus. Am J Psychiatry 146:782–784, 1989

Schielke E, Tatsch K, Pfister HW, et al: Reduced cerebral blood flow in early stages of human immunodeficiency virus infection. Arch Neurol 47:1342–1345, 1990

Schindelmeiser J, Gullotta F: HIV-p24-antigen-bearing macrophages are only present in brains of HIV-seropositive patients with AIDS-encephalopathy. Clin Neuropathol 10:109–111, 1991

Schmitt FA, Bigley JW, McKinnis R, et al: Neuropsychological outcome of zidovudine (AZT) treatment of patients with AIDS and AIDS-related complex. N Engl J Med 319:1573–1578, 1988

Schwarcz R, Whetsell WO, Mangano RM: Quinolinic acid: an endogenous metabolite that produces axon-sparing lesions in the rat brain. Science 219:316–318, 1983

Sekigawa I, Koshino K, Hishikawa T, et al: Inhibitory effect of the immunosuppressant FK506 on apoptotic cell death induced by HIV-1-gp120. J Clin Immunol 15:312–317, 1995

Selnes O, Jacobson L, Machado AM, et al: Normative data for a brief neuropsychological screening battery. Percept Mot Skills 73:539–550, 1991

Sharma SM, McDaniel JS, Sheehan NL: General principles of pharmacotherapy for the patient with HIV infection, in HIV and Psychiatry: A Training and Resource Manual. Edited by Citron K, Brouillete MJ, Beckett A. Cambridge, UK, Cambridge University Press, 2005, pp 56–87

Shaskan EG, Brew BJ, Rosenblum M, et al: Increased neopterin levels in brains of patients with human immunodeficiency virus type 1 infection. J Neurochem 59:1541–1546, 1992

Shor-Posner G, Feaster D, Blaney NT, et al: Impact of vitamin B6 status on psychological distress in a longitudinal study of HIV-1 infection. Int J Psychiatry Med 24:209–222, 1994

Shytle RD, Mori T, Townsend K, et al: Cholinergic modulation of microglial activation by alpha 7 nicotinic receptors. J Neurochem 89:337–343, 2004

Sidtis JJ, Gatsonis C, Price RW, et al: Zidovudine treatment of the AIDS dementia complex: results of a placebo-controlled trial: AIDS Clinical Trials Group. Ann Neurol 33:343–349, 1993

Siegel K: Psychosocial aspects of rational suicide. Am J Psychother 40:405–417, 1986

Silvestris F, Ribatti D, Nico B, et al: Apoptosi, o morte cellulare programmata: meccanismi regolatori e fisiopatologia [Apoptosis or programmed cell death: regulatory and pathophysiological mechanisms]. Ann Ital Med Int 10:7–13, 1995

Simpson DM, McArthur JC, Olney R, et al: Lamotrigine for HIV-associated painful sensory neuropathy: a placebo-controlled trial. Neurology 60:1508–1514, 2003

Singh AN, Golledge H, Catalan J: Treatment of HIV related psychotic disorders with risperidone a series of 21 cases. J Psychosom Res 42:489–493, 1997

Skolasky RL, Esposito DR, Selnes OA, et al: Modified HIV Dementia Scale: accurate staging of HIV-associated dementia: neuroscience of HIV infection (abstract). J Neurovirol 4(suppl): 366, 1998

Skoraszewski MJ, Ball JD, Mikulka P: Neuropsychological functioning of HIV-infected males. J Clin Exp Neuropsychol 13:278–290, 1991

Smith T, Jakobsen J, Gaub J, et al: Clinical and electrophysiological studies of human immunodeficiency virus–seropositive men without AIDS. Ann Neurol 23:295–297, 1988

Snider ND, Simpson DM, Nielsen S, et al: Neurological complications of acquired immune deficiency syndrome: analysis of 50 patients. Ann Neurol 14:403–418, 1983

Sockalingam S, Parekh N, Bogoch II, et al: Delirium in the postoperative cardiac patient: a review. J Card Surg 20:560–567, 2005

Sonnex C, Petherick A, Adler MW, et al: HIV infection increase in public awareness and anxiety. BMJ 295:193–195, 1987

Stahle L, Guzenda E, Ljungdahl-Stahle E: Pharmacokinetics and extracellular distribution to blood, brain, and muscle of alovudine (3′) and zidovudine in the rat studied by microdialysis. J Acquir Immune Defic Syndr 6:435–439, 1993

Stefano GB, Smith EM, Cadet P, et al: HIV gp120 alteration of DAMA and IL-1 alpha induced chemotaxic responses in human and invertebrate immunocytes. J Neuroimmunol 43:177–184, 1993

Steller H: Mechanisms and genes of cellular suicide. Science 267:1445–1449, 1995

Stern Y, Marder K, Bell K, et al: Multidisciplinary baseline assessment of homosexual men with and without human immunodeficiency virus infection, III: neurologic and neuropsychologic findings. Arch Gen Psychiatry 48:131–138, 1991

Stolar A, Catalano G, Hakala SM, et al: Mood disorders and psychosis in HIV, in HIV and Psychiatry: A Training and Resource Manual. Edited by Citron K, Brouillete MJ, Beckett A. Cambridge, UK, Cambridge University Press, 2005, pp 88–109

Strauss A: Oral dyskinesia associated with buspirone use in an elderly woman. J Clin Psychiatry 49:322–323, 1988

Studies of the Ocular Complications of AIDS Research Group (SOCA), in Collaboration With the AIDS Clinical Trials Group: Foscarnet-ganciclovir cytomegalovirus retinitis trial 4: visual outcomes. Ophthalmology 101:1250–1261, 1994

Syndulko K, Singer E, Fahychandon B, et al: Relationship of self-rated depression and neuropsychological changes in HIV-1 neurological dysfunction (abstract). J Clin Exp Neuropsychol 12:72, 1990

Talley AK, Dewhurst S, Perry SW, et al: Tumor necrosis factor alpha-induced apoptosis in human neuronal cells: protection by the antioxidant N-acetylcysteine and the genes bcl-2 and crmA. Mol Cell Biol 15:2359–2366, 1995

Tan J, Town T, Paris D, et al: Microglial activation resulting from CD40-CD40L interaction after beta-amyloid stimulation. Science 286:2352–2355, 1999

Tartaglione TA, Collier AC, Coombs RW, et al: Acquired immunodeficiency syndrome, cerebrospinal fluid findings in patients before and during long-term oral zidovudine therapy. Arch Neurol 48:695–699, 1991

Tesar GE, Murray GB, Cassem NH: Use of high-dose intravenous haloperidol in the treatment of agitated cardiac patients. J Clin Psychopharmacol 5:344–347, 1985

Thompson CB: Apoptosis in the pathogenesis and treatment of disease. Science 267:1456–1462, 1995

Tinuper P, de Carolis P, Galeotti M, et al: Electroencephalogram and HIV infection: a prospective study in 100 patients. Clin Electroencephalogr 21:145–150, 1990

Tozzi V, Balestra P, Galgani S, et al: Positive and sustained effects of highly active antiretroviral therapy on HIV-1 associated neurocognitive impairment. AIDS 13:1889–1897, 1999

Tracey I, Carr CA, Guimares AR, et al: Brain choline-containing compounds are elevated in HIV-positive patients before the onset of AIDS dementia complex: a proton magnetic resonance spectroscopic study. Neurology 46:783–788, 1996

Tross S, Price RW, Navia B, et al: Neuropsychological characterization of the AIDS dementia complex: a preliminary report. AIDS 2:81–88, 1988

Vago L, Castagna A, Lazzarin A, et al: Reduced frequency of HIV-induced brain lesions in AIDS patients treated with zidovudine. J Acquir Immune Defic Syndr 6:42–45, 1993

Van Gorp WG, Miller E, Satz P, et al: Neuropsychological performance in HIV-1 immunocompromised patients (abstract). J Clin Exp Neuropsychol 11:35, 1989a

Van Gorp WG, Mitrushina M, Cummings JL, et al: Normal aging and the subcortical encephalopathy of AIDS: a neuropsychological comparison. Neuropsychiatry Neuropsychol Behav Neurol 2:5–20, 1989b

Van Gorp WG, Satz P, Hinkin C, et al: Metacognition in HIV-1 seropositive asymptomatic individuals: self-ratings versus objective neuropsychological performance. J Clin Exp Neuropsychol 13:812–819, 1991

van Leeuwen R, Katlama C, Kitchen V, et al: Evaluation of safety and efficacy of 3TC (Lamivudine) in patients with asymptomatic or mildly symptomatic human immunodeficiency virus infection: a phase I/II study. J Infect Dis 171:1166–1171, 1995

Vazeux R: AIDS encephalopathy and tropism of HIV for brain monocytes/macrophages and microglial cells. Pathobiology 59:214–218, 1991

Vinters HV, Guerra WG, Eppolito L, et al: Necrotizing vasculitis of the nervous system in a patient with AIDS-related complex. Neuropathol Appl Neurobiol 14:417–424, 1988

Walker DG, Itagaki J, Berry K, et al: Examination of brains of AIDS cases for human immunodeficiency virus and human cytomegalovirus nucleic acids. J Neurol Neurosurg Psychiatry 52:583–590, 1989

Walling VR, Pfefferbaum B: Methylphenidate: its use in a depressed adolescent with AIDS. AIDS Patient Care 5:4–5, 1991

Wang Y, Sawchuk RJ: Zidovudine transport in the rabbit brain during intravenous and intracerebroventricular infusion. J Pharm Sci 84:871–876, 1995

Weiner RD: ECT in the physically ill. J Psychiatr Treat Eval 5:457–462, 1983

Weis S, Haug H, Budka H: Neuronal damage in the cerebral cortex of AIDS brains: a morphometric study. Acta Neuropathol (Berl) 85:185–189, 1993

Whelan MA, Kricheff II, Handler M, et al: Acquired immunodeficiency syndrome: cerebral computed tomographic manifestations. Radiology 149:477–484, 1983

White JC, Christensen JF, Singer CM: Methylphenidate as a treatment for depression in acquired immunodeficiency syndrome: an n-of-1 trial. J Clin Psychiatry 53:153–156, 1992

Wiegand M, Möller AA, Schreiber W, et al: Alterations of nocturnal sleep in patients with HIV infection. Acta Neurol Scand 83:141–142, 1991a

Wiegand M, Möller AA, Schreiber W, et al: Nocturnal sleep EEG in patients with HIV infection. Eur Arch Psychiatry Clin Neurosci 240:153–158, 1991b

Wiley CA, Masliah E, Morey M, et al: Neocortical damage during HIV infection. Ann Neurol 29:651–657, 1991

Wilkie FL, Eisdorfer C, Morgan R, et al: Cognition in early human immunodeficiency virus infection. Arch Neurol 47:433–440, 1990a

Wilkie F, Guterman A, Morgan R, et al: Cognition and electrophysiologic measures in early HIV infection (abstract). J Clin Exp Neuropsychol 12:48, 1990b

Wolcott DL, Fawzy FI, Pasnau RO: Acquired immune deficiency syndrome (AIDS) and consultation-liaison psychiatry. Gen Hosp Psychiatry 7:280–293, 1985

Wong SL, Wang Y, Sawchuk RJ: Analysis of zidovudine distribution to specific regions in rabbit brain using microdialysis. Pharm Res 9:332–338, 1992

Wong SL, Van Bell K, Sawchuk RJ: Distributional transport kinetics of zidovudine between plasma and brain extracellular fluid/cerebrospinal fluid in the rabbit: investigation of the inhibitory effect of probenecid utilizing microdialysis. J Pharmacol Exp Ther 264:899–909, 1993

Wright JM, Sachdev PS, Perkins RJ, et al: Zidovudine related mania. Med J Aust 150:339–341, 1989

Yamaguchi K, Honda M, Ikigai H, et al: Inhibitory effects of (-)-epigallocatechin gallate on the life cycle of human immunodeficiency virus type 1 (HIV-1). Antiviral Res 53:19–34, 2002

Yarchoan R, Berg G, Brouwers P, et al: Response of human immunodeficiency virus associated neurological disease to 3′-azido-3′-deoxythymidine. Lancet 1:132–135, 1987

21

NEUROPSYCHIATRIC ASPECTS OF ENDOCRINE DISORDERS

Monica Kelly Cowles, M.D., M.S.

Elizabeth B. Boswell, M.D.

Theodore J. Anfinson, M.D.

Charles B. Nemeroff, M.D., Ph.D.

The relationship between endocrine disturbances and psychiatric symptomatology has been recognized for centuries. Indeed, it was these clinical observations and early controlled studies that in part spawned the now established field of psychoneuroendocrinology. The epidemiology and phenomenology of psychiatric syndromes in the most common endocrine disorders (i.e., diabetes mellitus, thyroid, adrenal, and parathyroid disorders, and hyperprolactinemia) are reviewed as they occur in this chapter. Underlying pathophysiology is discussed when there is data available, but overall it is sparse. The cardinal signs and symptoms of each disorder are presented together with the psychiatric findings to assist clinicians in reviewing the context in which the psychiatric symptoms present.

The case literature was reviewed with scrutiny, with particular emphasis on determination of the qualitative nature of the psychiatric symptoms in a given case, the temporal relationship between onset of psychiatric symptoms and underlying endocrine disturbance, and the response to treatment. The methodology is similar to that utilized by Whybrow and Hurwitz (1976) in their classic review of the subject. Rigorous prospective studies that utilize structured interviews are highlighted.

DIABETES MELLITUS

The Centers for Disease Control and Prevention (2007) state that "the number of Americans with diabetes more than doubled (from 5.8 million to 14.7 million)" between 1980 and 2004. In 2002, about 1.3 million adults between 18 and 79 years of age were diagnosed with diabetes. It is well documented that patients with diabetes are at increased risk for comorbid psychiatric disorders. For example, patients with diabetes are at two to three times the risk for depression as the general population, yielding a rapidly expanding patient population diagnosed with both diseases (Anderson et al. 2001; Carnethon et al. 2003).

CARDINAL FEATURES OF THE DISORDER

Diabetes mellitus is a group of metabolic diseases, including type I, type II, and gestational diabetes, all of which are characterized by hyperglycemia. Defects in insulin secretion or insulin action, or a combination of the two, differentiate the disease processes and ultimate choice of treatment modalities. Acute and long-term complications of this illness are profound. Life-threatening consequences of uncontrolled hyperglycemia include ketoacidosis and the nonketotic hyperosmolar syndrome. Chronic hyperglycemia affects multiple organ systems and can lead to retinopathy, nephropathy, and peripheral neuropathy, as well as macrovascular compromise. Diabetic patients are at increased risk for a number of comorbid medical disorders, most notably coronary artery disease and stroke.

The presenting symptoms of hyperglycemia are polyuria, polydipsia, weight loss sometimes in the presence of polyphagia, and blurred vision. The majority of patients with type I or insulin-dependent diabetes mellitus (IDDM) present by age 30 years and are generally quite thin. This form of diabetes results from a cellular-mediated autoimmune destruction of the β-cells of the pancreas. These patients are insulin deficient and require insulin to prevent weight loss, ketoacidosis, or death. In contrast, type II or non-insulin-dependent diabetes mellitus (NIDDM) is often asymptomatic, being detected only through blood screening. The age at onset of NIDDM is typically after age 40 years, although presentations may occur earlier in obese patients or in Native Americans, African Americans, or persons of Mexican descent (Sherwin 1996). These patients demonstrate insulin resistance and may exhibit some level of impaired insulin secretion as well.

The American Diabetes Association continues to redefine criteria for the diagnosis of diabetes mellitus (American Diabetes Association 2005). Demonstration of a high random glucose level (>200 mg/dL) in the presence of symptoms of diabetes, an elevated fasting plasma glucose level (>126 mg/dL), or a 2-hour postload elevation of serum glucose level (>200 mg/dL) following a 75-g oral glucose loading dose is required for diagnosis. To confirm the diagnosis, repeat testing should be performed on a different day.

PSYCHIATRIC SYMPTOMS IN DIABETES MELLITUS

There is considerable literature exploring the link between psychiatric illness and diabetes. Weyerer et al. (1989) reported in their community study of 1,536 subjects that the prevalence of psychiatric disorders was higher in patients with diabetes (43.1%) and other chronic medical conditions (50.7%) compared with control subjects (26.2%). In a 10-year prospective study, Northam et al. (2004) identified a random group of 41 adolescents between the ages of 11 and 18 with newly diagnosed type I diabetes. They underwent diagnostic interviews, completed child behavior checklists, and were monitored for metabolic control over a 10-year period. At initial interview 37% received a DSM-IV diagnosis that included mood, anxiety, eating, and behavior disorders. Ten years after disease onset, those with preexisting psychiatric morbidity were more

likely to have a history of poor metabolic control. This result highlights the need for early intervention in this at-risk group and warrants further study. Although depressive disorders accounted for the significant difference noted between diabetic patients and control subjects in these studies, there is also data available on the comorbidity of diabetes and cognitive disorders and anxiety disorders.

Cognitive Disorders

There are many large cross-sectional and prospective studies that have revealed significant cognitive deficits in patients with both IDDM and NIDDM. These deficits range from cognitive impairment and decline among all ages to vascular dementia and Alzheimer's disease in older populations. Further, Yaffe et al. (2004) showed that patients with an impaired fasting glucose, but not yet fulfilling criteria for diabetes, exhibit cognitive impairment when compared with control subjects. In their evaluation of over 7,000 postmenopausal women, impaired fasting glucose led to cognitive decline intermediate to that experienced by control subjects versus those with diabetes, suggesting a causal relationship between diabetes and cognitive decline.

In the following discussion, various studies addressing this area of research are reviewed. Unless indicated otherwise the term *diabetes* or *diabetes mellitus* includes both IDDM and NIDDM. Given the recognition in the last decade of the increasing incidence of NIDDM, many of the more recent studies focus on this subtype. However, when studies have been limited to either IDDM or NIDDM, the findings have confirmed cognitive impairment in both.

IDDM is characterized by both chronic hyperglycemia and intermittent episodes of hypoglycemia resulting from insulin therapy aimed at strict glycemic control. In contrast, NIDDM is characterized solely by chronic hyperglycemia, the deleterious effects of which are clearly seen after prolonged exposure. The consequence of chronic hyperglycemia with respect to cognition is similar among both IDDM and NIDDM subjects. However, several other questions arise specific to IDDM. There continues to be concern that children and adolescents diagnosed with IDDM are at higher risk for more immediate cognitive impairment. The pathogenesis of this impairment remains under investigation, but it has been postulated to be largely caused by episodes of hypoglycemia. There is not, however, universal agreement on this issue.

Among patients with IDDM, several factors emerge consistently as important variables in the development of cognitive impairment, including age at onset, absenteeism from school, poor metabolic control, and episodes of hypoglycemia (Ryan 1988). Children with the onset of IDDM before age 4 years were compared with children with later-onset IDDM and sibling control subjects. Children with early-onset IDDM scored lower on visuospatial tasks and had more hypoglycemic seizures than did the other diabetic patients and sibling control subjects (Rovet et al. 1987). This was confirmed in a more recent study by Northam et al. (2001) in which 90 children with IDDM were followed over 6 years and compared with a community control group. The children with diabetes "performed more poorly than control subjects on measures of intelligence, attention, processing speed, long-term memory, and executive skills. Attention, processing speed, and executive skills were particularly affected in children with onset of disease before 4 years of age, whereas severe hypoglycemia was associated with lower verbal and full-scale intelligence quotient scores" (p. 1541).

In a larger study of adolescents, patients with IDDM developing before age 5 years learned new information less efficiently and remembered less of that information over a 30-minute retention interval. More errors also were noted on visuospatial tasks, in addition to slower motor performance and lower scores of general intelligence. Moreover, 24% of early-onset IDDM patients were judged to be clinically significantly impaired, compared with 6% of either the later-onset IDDM patients or nondiabetic control subjects (Ryan et al. 1985).

Hypoglycemia acutely impairs cognition, but the impairment is corrected upon return to a euglycemic state. In a study of 16 male subjects with IDDM (mean age: 28 years) who were exposed to a controlled reduction in blood glucose level via insulin infusion and recovery with intravenous glucose, subjective symptoms were recorded in addition to performance on a variety of neuropsychological tests (serial 7s, categorization, trail making, digit span, story recall, finger tapping). No patients showed symptoms when their blood glucose level fell to 52.3 mg/dL, and 25% of patients showed no symptoms with a blood glucose level of 32.4 mg/dL. In contrast, neuropsychological test results showed a decremental decline correlating with subnormal serum glucose levels and improvement with recovery (Pramming et al. 1986).

The long-term effects of hypoglycemia on cognition remain controversial. Several studies, both cross-sectional and prospective with evaluation periods up to a decade, have shown that recurrent severe hypoglycemic episodes do not have an impact on cognition in adolescents diagnosed with IDDM (Austin and Dearyl 1999; Diabetes Control and Complications Trial Research Group 1996; Ferguson et al. 2003b; Reichard et al. 1996). However, numerous studies have obtained discrepant findings. A comparison of children with IDDM to healthy control children revealed that episodes of hypoglycemia (ranging from severe to asymptomatic) in the diabetic children were correlated with a detrimental impact on abstract reasoning, memory skills, and auditory-verbal functioning (Golden et al. 1989; Hannonen et al. 2003; Hershey et al. 2003). Additionally, for patients diagnosed with IDDM after adolescence, repeated severe hypoglycemic episodes have been shown to detrimentally affect cognition (Langan et al. 1991; Lincoln et al. 1996; Sachon et al. 1992; Wredling et al. 1990). Interestingly brain magnetic resonance imaging (MRI) of a small group of adult IDDM patients revealed a correlation between cortical atrophy and exposure to recurrent severe hypoglycemia (Perros et al. 1997). Howorka et al. (2000) compared the electroencephalographic (EEG) patterns of 13 IDDM patients with a history of recurrent hypoglycemia with those of 14 IDDM patients without a history of recurrent hypoglycemia. The patients with a history of recurrent hypoglycemia showed decreased brain vigilance by EEG compared with the patients without the hypoglycemic history.

These findings are important because of emphasis on tight metabolic control resulting from the Diabetes Control and Complications Trial (Diabetes Control and Complications Trial Research Group 1993). With tighter metabolic control, the risk of hypoglycemia increases, and clinicians must be aware of the neurobehavioral risks of even mild hypoglycemia.

Regarding the long-term effects of diabetes, there is evidence to support that the mere presence of diabetes imparts a risk of cognitive impairment. Gregg et al. (2000) followed a cohort of 9,679 community-dwelling white women age 65 years and older for 3–6 years. The presence of diabetes correlated with diminished cognitive performance based on measures of concentration, language, memory, perceptual organization, visual scanning, sequential abilities, and executive function both at baseline and at end of the study. After controlling for many variables including age, education, depression, and stroke, patients with diabetes were 1.6 times more likely to experience major cognitive decline (the greatest 10th percentile decline in score for each of the three cognitive function tests) than their nondiabetic counterparts. Furthermore, the presence of diabetes for greater than 15 years considerably increased the risk of major cognitive decline. Another study composed of almost 11,000 individuals, ages 47 to 70 years, followed patients over a 6-year period. Again, the presence of diabetes at baseline was associated with significant cognitive decline at follow-up. Moreover, this finding persisted when the analysis was restricted to a youngest-age subset of patients (47–57 years) (Knopman et al. 2001).

Poor metabolic control apparently worsens the deleterious effects of diabetes on cognition. Early studies that first established a relationship between poor metabolic control and impaired neuropsychological performance relied on end-organ complications of diabetes as a marker for poor control (Rennick et al. 1968; Skenazy and Bigler 1984). Subsequent studies have utilized measurement of glycosylated hemoglobin (HgA1c) as a more precise determinant of longitudinal metabolic control.

Two investigations of older NIDDM patients have revealed an association between poor metabolic control and neuropsychological impairment. In the first study (Perlmuter et al. 1984), 140 NIDDM patients (ages 55–74 years) were compared with 38 nondiabetic control subjects using a serial learning task. Diabetic patients learned and recalled fewer words and required more study trials than did control subjects. These deficits correlated with elevations in HgA1c concentration and the severity of peripheral neuropathy (Perlmuter et al. 1984). In a later study (Reaven et al. 1990), 29 elderly patients with NIDDM (mean age: 69.8 years) exhibited more impairment on measures of verbal learning, abstract reasoning, and complex psychomotor functioning compared with 30 nondiabetic control subjects. In addition, the magnitude of the neuropsychological impairment correlated with the magnitude of metabolic dyscontrol as measured by HgA1c determination (Reaven et al. 1990).

Furthermore, structural and functional central nervous system (CNS) abnormalities have been observed after long-term poor metabolic control (which includes both chronic hyperglycemia and episodic hypoglycemia) and are likely associated with the progression of cognitive deficits. In addition to the previously summarized work by Howorka et al. (2000), two earlier investigations support their findings in that EEG abnormalities were noted to occur more frequently in children with IDDM who had recurrent severe hypoglycemia (Halonen et al. 1983; Haumont et al. 1979). With respect to diabetic patients with chronic hyperglycemia, a computed tomography (CT) study comparing 12 drug-treated NIDDM patients with 13 diet-treated NIDDM patients and 59 nondiabetic control subjects showed greater temporal lobe atrophy in the drug-treated groups (Soininen et al. 1992). This atrophy was negatively correlated with the level of fasting serum glucose. In another study, Brismar et al. (2002) obtained EEG recordings in 49 adults with IDDM and in 51 control subjects. In this study, all of the patients with diabetes had good glycemic control as evidenced by hemoglobin A1c (HbA1c) measurement. The diabetic patients revealed a focal decrease in temporal lobe fast activity. Taken together, these data suggest that the temporal lobe is especially vulnerable in patients with diabetes, and this may ultimately underlie the observed cognitive impairment.

Several biological mechanisms may contribute to the impaired cognitive performance of patients with diabetes mellitus and impaired fasting glucose. The prototypical diabetic complications, including renal disease, stroke, hypertension, hyperlipidemia, and ischemic heart disease, all likely contribute to cognitive decline. These complications are largely secondary to metabolic dyscontrol, such as ketoacidosis, hyperosmolar states, chronic hyperglycemia, recurrent mild hypoglycemia, and hypoglycemic seizures (Richardson 1990).

As mentioned previously, diabetes has also been associated with an increased incidence of dementia. In a longitudinal study of 1,262 randomly selected elderly subjects, patients were followed over an average of 4.3 years (Luchsinger et al. 2001). Those with diabetes but without dementia at baseline had an adjusted relative risk of stroke-associated dementia of 3.4. Further analysis of the data suggested that the presence of diabetes among black and Hispanic populations placed them at even higher risk for the development of stroke-associated dementia.

Many studies have identified a relationship between diabetes and dementia. This includes both vascular dementia and Alzheimer's disease, although interestingly the mechanisms appear to differ. Vascular dementia is largely a consequence of indirect neuronal damage via cerebral microvascular and macrovascular atherosclerotic disease. With regard to Alzheimer's disease, however, there is emerging genetic and biological evidence to support a possible common pathway leading to the development of both NIDDM and Alzheimer's disease (Bertram et al. 2000; Ghosh et al. 2000; Wiltshire et al. 2001). Farris et al. (2003) established that insulin-degrading enzyme catabolizes β-amyloid. Hypofunction of this enzyme may be the common link between the "recently recognized association between hyperinsulinemia, diabetes, and Alzheimer's disease" (p. 4162).

The epsilon 4 allele of the apolipoprotein E gene (APOE*E4) has also been associated with increased incidence of both impaired cognition and Alzheimer's disease in patients with IDDM and NIDDM. In a cross-sectional study of 96 male and female subjects with IDDM, women with the APOE*E4 allele scored significantly lower on tests of intellectual performance and frontal lobe and executive functions (Ferguson et al. 2003a). In a population of 5,888 Medicare-eligible individuals, those with the APOE*E4 allele and a diagnosis of diabetes were at substantially higher risk of cognitive decline than those without the allele, regardless of sex (Haan et al. 1999). In the Ferguson et al. (2003a) study, there appeared to be an age-related component suggesting that perhaps females with the APOE*E4 allele experience cognitive decline earlier than their male counterparts. Finally, the Honolulu-Asia Aging Study, in a cohort of 2,574 Japanese-American men with NIDDM, confirmed the strong association between diabetes and Alzheimer's disease in those with the APOE*E4 allele (Peila et al. 2002).

Hypoglycemia

Because of the importance of insulin-induced hypoglycemia as a putative risk factor for the development of cognitive impairment in diabetes, a brief discussion of the phenomenology of hypoglycemia is warranted.

Traditionally, the signs and symptoms of hypoglycemia are divided into autonomic and neuroglycopenic groups. The autonomic signs and symptoms include diaphoresis, palpitations, tremor, and hunger, whereas the neuroglycopenic symptoms include confusion, lethargy, speech and behavioral changes, and incoordination. Some authors have prospectively validated this construct with the inclusion of nausea and headache in a separately validated "malaise" category (Deary et al. 1993).

In a study of 125 prospective emergency room visits for symptomatic hypoglycemia, 65 patients had obtundation, stupor, or coma; 38 had confusional or bizarre behavior; 10 were dizzy or tremulous; 9 had seizures; and 3 had sudden hemiparesis (Malouf and Brust 1985). The most common underlying medical conditions were diabetes, alcoholism, or sepsis, alone or in combination. Other associated conditions included fasting, cancer, gastroenteritis, insulin abuse, and hypothyroidism. The overall mortality rate was 11%, and focal neurological sequelae were present in 4 patients (Malouf and Brust 1985). In a retrospective study of 51 patients admitted to the emergency room for acute hypoglycemia (Hart and Frier 1998), 80% were diabetic patients being treated with insulin. The other patients had hypoglycemia induced by excessive consumption of alcohol or deliberate self-poisoning with insulin. Hart and Frier (1998) noted increased rates of psychiatric illness and chronic alcoholism in the population studied.

Reactive hypoglycemia is a relatively rare, meal-induced hypoglycemic disorder occurring in patients with diabetes mellitus, gastrointestinal disease, and hormonal deficiency states, such as adrenal insufficiency or hypothyroidism. In these states, hyperinsulinemia is responsible for the hypoglycemia. Idiopathic postprandial hypoglycemia is a controversial entity with uncertain validity. It should be emphasized that the vast majority of patients who have adrenergic symptoms have diagnoses other than hypoglycemia to account for their symptoms, with panic, conversion, and somatization disorders accounting for many of the psychiatric cases (Hofeldt 1989).

Factitious hypoglycemia due to exogenous insulin administration is relatively uncommon but is suggested by the presence of elevated insulin antibodies, hypoglycemia, and low C peptide levels (Horwitz 1989; Scarlett et al. 1977). C peptide is secreted as a portion of endogenous proinsulin and is not a part of commercially prepared insulin.

Mood Disorders

As noted previously, depressive disorders accounted for the increased prevalence of psychiatric diagnoses in a community sample comparing diabetic patients with community members who did not have a medical illness (Weyerer et al. 1989). In a review of 20 studies of depression in patients with diabetes mellitus, Gavard et al. (1993) noted that prevalence rates of major depression varied from 8.5% to 27.3% in 9 controlled studies and varied from 11.0% to 19.9% in 11 uncontrolled studies. Studies utilizing symptom subscales revealed depressive symptom rates ranging from 21.8% to 60.0% in controlled studies and from 10.0% to 28.0% in uncontrolled studies. Gavard et al. (1993) cited numerous methodological problems that likely account for the wide variance in prevalence rates. Carney's (1998) review of studies of the prevalence rate of depression in diabetes emphasized that depression in diabetes is no more prevalent than depression in other chronic disease states.

A meta-analytic review of the literature through January 2000 yielded similar results (Anderson et al. 2002). In this review 42 studies met inclusion criteria with a combined sample size of 21,351. With respect to the inclusion criteria, studies were included that evaluated major depressive disorder (MDD) in addition to minor and subsyndromal depression given that each of these has been shown to be associated with adverse effects on social and physical functioning. Of the studies included, 48% were controlled, of which 15% were limited to evaluating IDDM, 40% to evaluating NIDDM, and 45% to evaluating a combination of the two. Of the uncontrolled studies, 27% included IDDM, 23% NIDDM, and 50% a combination of the two. The rates of depression in patients with IDDM versus NIDDM were statistically similar in those studies in which depression was determined by diagnostic interview or self-report scales. As in the general population, females had an increased prevalence rate of depression in comparison with males. Based on aggregate estimates, the point prevalence for major depression was 11%, the point prevalence for elevated depressive symptoms was 31%, and the lifetime prevalence was 28.5%. Taken together the data suggested that the presence of diabetes doubled the odds ratio for depression. Furthermore, as many as one in three diabetic patients reported depressive symptoms of sufficient severity to result in impaired functioning and quality of life. These results are of paramount importance in view of the finding that successful treatment of depression has been shown to improve glycemic control (Lustman et al. 1997b, 1998, 2000b), and yet two out of every three cases of depression in diabetes are left untreated by primary care physicians (Lustman and Harper 1987). Finally, a meta-analysis by de Groot et al. (2001) that included 27 studies published between 1975 and 1999 demonstrated a "significant and consistent association of diabetes complications and depressive symptoms" (p. 619). The literature certainly supports the view that depressive symptoms are common in diabetes and that careful clinical assessment is indicated.

Given the existence of a relationship between depression and diabetes, the point of interest then becomes the direction of causality, namely, does the presence of diabetes render one more susceptible to depression or vice versa? The most harmonious explanation is a bidirectional relationship. The stressor of being diagnosed and living with a chronic and debilitating illness has long been believed to precipitate the onset of depressive symptoms. However, in the last decade substantial evidence has also emerged that supports the hypothesis that depression is a risk factor for the onset and exacerbation of many illnesses including diabetes. In a study of native Hawaiians with NIDDM, Grandinetti et al. (2000) found a significant association between depressive symptoms and elevated HbA1c that remained after adjusting for age, body mass index, education, and gender and after excluding participants who reported a history of diabetes. A meta-analytic literature review of 25 years (1975–1999) supports this finding as well (Lustman et al. 2000a). Grandinetti et al. (2000) suggest that the relationship of depression to diabetes may in fact be more pathophysiological in nature rather than merely a psychological reaction to the disease. Lustman et al. (2005) concur based on their recent analysis as to the effect of self-care and depression-related hyperglycemia in IDDM. Depressive symptoms were associated with elevated HbA1c, with minimal effect secondary to the quality of self-care among depressed diabetic patients.

In the Rancho Bernardo Study, a cohort of 971 men and women over age 50 years completed an oral glucose tolerance test and the Beck Depression Inventory (BDI) at initial evaluation and at 8-year follow-up (Palinkas et al. 2004). A BDI score greater than 11 at visit one was associated with an increased prevalence of NIDDM at visit two. After adjusting for age, sex, body mass index, and exercise level, the odds of diagnosis of NIDDM at visit two, given a visit-one BDI greater than 11, was 2.5. These results are consistent with two previously published longitudinal studies (Eaton et al. 1996; Kawakami et al. 1999) suggesting that at least in older adults, depressive symptoms are a risk factor for the onset of NIDDM.

Another perspective was provided by Carnethon et al. (2003), who utilized data from the National Health and Nutrition Examination survey to evaluate over 6,000 patients followed from 1971 to 1992 who endorsed varying degrees of depressive symptoms (high, intermediate, and low) but did not have diabetes. Over that period 6% developed diabetes. It was found that those who initially endorsed high depressive symptoms had a relative risk of developing diabetes of 2.5 compared with those with low depressive symptom scores. Those with more severe depressive symptoms were also found to be less physically active, had a higher body mass index, and were more likely to be cigarette smokers. Further analysis revealed that within the more severe depressive symptom subset, those most at risk were patients with low levels of education (which has been correlated with lower socioeconomic status). This subset had threefold the risk of developing diabetes as those with low symptom scores.

Recently, Egede (2005) demonstrated that the coexistence of other chronic medical conditions, in addition to diabetes, places the patient at increasingly higher risk for depression. Data from almost 1,800 adults obtained from the 1999 National Health Interview Survey were evaluated, and the chronic medical conditions included were the following: hypertension, coronary artery disease, chronic arthritis, stroke, chronic obstructive pulmonary disease, and end-stage renal disease. The odds of major depression in the presence of diabetes plus one other medical condition was 1.31, whereas the odds increased to 2.09 and 4.09 for two and three or more other medical conditions, respectively.

Multiple biological mechanisms may contribute to the relationship between depression and diabetes. These include activation of inflammatory processes and the hypothalamic-pituitary-adrenal (HPA) axis as well as abnormalities in glucose metabolism, which have been observed in both nondiabetic and diabetic depressed patients (Lewis et al. 1983; Okamura et al. 2000). There is a well-defined metabolic syndrome associated with NIDDM, including insulin resistance, abdominal obesity, hypertension, and dyslipidemia. Recent advances in understanding the systemic effects of depression have led to the conclusion that depression leads to exacerbations of, and possibly direct contributions to, this syndrome. In addition, depressed patients have been shown to express elevated levels of several inflammatory markers, including interleukin-1, interleukin-6, tumor necrosis factor-α, and C-reactive protein (Carnethon et al. 2003; Musselman et al. 2001). Interestingly two independent population studies have revealed that elevated inflammatory markers are also associated with the development of diabetes (Ford 2002; Schmidt et al. 1999). These results, taken together, suggest a likely pathophysiological link between comorbid diabetes and depression.

Phenomenologically, depression associated with diabetes is very similar to primary MDD. In a study by Lustman et al. (1992a), the BDI was administered to a sample of 41 diabetic patients who fulfilled DSM-III-R (American Psychiatric Association 1987) criteria for depression, 68 depressed patients without medical illness, and 58 nondepressed diabetic patients; the prevalence and severity of symptoms were similar between diabetic depressed patients and patients with primary MDD.

Historically, the validity of diagnosing depression in the medically ill given the overlap of "sickness symptoms" such as fatigue, sleep disturbance, and decreased energy has been vigorously debated. Ample evidence now exists to put this issue to rest. Lustman et al. (1986) evaluated the prevalence of depression in a sample of 114 patients with diabetes mellitus and compared the prevalence rates with and without inclusion of symptoms that may be attributable to the underlying diabetes. They noted that when the symptoms of weight loss, fatigue, hypersomnia, psychomotor retardation, and decreased libido were excluded, due to their association with diabetes, the rate of depression changed from 36% to 32.5% (Lustman et al. 1986). Other authors have also noted a modest change in prevalence rates when an inclusive versus an etiological approach is used for diagnosis of depression and have advocated an inclusive approach in the clinical care of patients (Cohen-Cole et al. 1993).

Other aspects of depression associated with diabetes also resemble primary MDD, including a female predominance (Lustman et al. 1986; Robinson et al. 1988) and a higher likelihood of a positive family history of depression when comparing depressed diabetic patients with nondepressed diabetic patients (Lustman et al. 1987). Lustman et al. (1997a) noted that the BDI is an effective screening test for major depression in diabetic patients.

Depression comorbid with IDDM differs from depression comorbid with NIDDM in two respects: 1) the mean age at onset of depression is 22.1 years in IDDM patients and 28.6 years in NIDDM patients; and 2) in patients with NIDDM, the depressive symptoms appear to precede the development of diabetes, whereas in patients with IDDM, the diabetes precedes that of the depressive phenomenology (Lustman et al. 1988).

The presence of major depression has a negative impact on participation in diabetes treatment as measured by attendance at a weight-loss program for obese patients with NIDDM (Marcus et al. 1992). In addition, the presence of depression correlates with the worsened glycemic control in patients with IDDM (de Groot et al. 1999; Lustman et al. 1992b; Sachs et al. 1991). Winokur et al. (1988) administered a 5-hour oral glucose tolerance test (GTT) to 28 patients with depression and 21 nondepressed volunteers and found that depressed patients demonstrated significantly higher basal glucose levels and higher cumulative glucose responses after the GTT and showed larger cumulative insulin responses after the GTT than control subjects. These findings indicated the presence of a functional state of insulin resistance during major depressive illness in some patients. Poor glycemic control is well documented to be associated with complications of diabetes (Klein et al. 1988); therefore, the depressed diabetic patient may be at risk for later diabetic complications. Higher BDI scores were found in patients with diabetic complications compared with those without complications or nondiabetic control subjects (Leedom et al. 1991; Tun et al. 1990). In a 10-year prospective study, depression was found to be one of three factors independently associated with the onset of diabetic retinopathy in 24 children with IDDM (Kovacs et al. 1997). Likewise, S.T. Cohen et al. (1997) studied 49 patients with IDDM and found that patients with a history of psychiatric illness had significantly worse retinopathy than did patients without psychiatric illness. Other studies, however, failed to show a relationship between complications of diabetes and psychiatric illness (Lustman et al. 1988; Popkin et al. 1988).

It is important to keep in mind the often malevolent course of depression in diabetic patients. Once depression has been treated effectively, remission of symptoms is sustained only 10% of the time over the course of the next 5 years (Lustman et al. 1997c). Furthermore, relapses occur at a rate of approximately one per year (Lustman et al. 1988). These findings are not meant to suggest that treatment of depression in the diabetic population is not effective. Rates of successful treatment of depression in diabetic individuals actually approach those in the general population (Lustman and Clouse 2002). These data do support the notion that optimal treatment of depression in this population requires a multimodal approach, including pharmacotherapy, psychotherapy, and lifelong follow-up.

The psychopharmacological treatment of depression in diabetic patients requires some discussion because of the different effects of various classes of antidepressants on appetite, body weight, glucose control, cognition, cholinergic receptors, and sexual function and because of their propensity to exacerbate autonomic neuropathy–mediated orthostatic hypotension (Goodnick et al. 1995; Lustman et al. 1992b). Regarding the issues of appetite, weight, and glucose control, monoamine oxidase inhibitors (MAOIs) tend to exacerbate hypoglycemia and are associated with significant weight gain. Similarly trazodone is also associated with weight gain and postural hypotension, and thus it should be avoided. Cognitive interactions between the underlying illness and the selected medication need to be considered as well. Medications with anticholinergic or sedating properties are associated with greater cognitive impairment and can interfere with the daily management of diabetes (Lustman et al. 1992b). Furthermore, the impaired cognition often seen in diabetic patients may render compliance with an MAOI diet unattainable (Goodnick et al. 1995). In addition to the adverse effects on cognition associated with anticholinergic medications, the decrease in bowel motility caused by such agents may worsen underlying diabetes-related gastroparesis or constipation (Lustman et al. 1992b).

The use of tricyclic antidepressants (TCAs) in the diabetic population remains controversial. Though they are certainly effective in the treatment of depression, their side-effect profile includes increased appetite, body weight, and blood glucose, all of which are particularly problematic in the diabetic population. An additional long-standing concern is the lethality of TCAs in overdose. Extreme care must be taken in prescribing these medications, especially in light of elevated rates of suicide in this patient population. TCAs are contraindicated in patients with cardiovascular disease, a very common comorbidity in diabetic patients.

Having established that extreme caution is required when prescribing TCAs, the treatment of pain associated with diabetic neuropathy is one particular condition in which controlled studies have shown TCAs to be more effective than selective serotonin reuptake inhibitors (SSRIs) or placebo (Max et al. 1991, 1992). In this same patient population, paroxetine was also found to be effective but less so than imipramine (Sindrup et al. 1990). There is also evidence for the efficacy of serotonin/norepinephrine reuptake inhibitors (SNRIs), including duloxetine, venlafaxine, and milnacipran, in a variety of pain states ranging from diabetic neuropathy to fibromyalgia (Rao 2002). However, there are current concerns regarding adverse cardiovascular effects associated with venlafaxine (Davidson et al. 2005). Further studies are warranted in this area.

Surprisingly, there are few controlled studies available with respect to treatment of comorbid depression and diabetes. Lustman et al. (1997c), in a double-blind, placebo-controlled trial of nortriptyline, demonstrated efficacy of TCAs similar to that observed in nondiabetic patients, although treatment with nortriptyline was associated with a negative effect on glycemic control. A subsequent study by the same group reported on the results of a double-blind, placebo-controlled trial evaluating the efficacy and safety of fluoxetine in a similar patient population (Lustman et al. 2000b). Antidepressant efficacy was again comparable to that observed in nondiabetic patients, but in contrast to the nortriptyline study, there was an improvement in glycemic control. This is in keeping with the previous observation by Goodnick et al. (1995) that SSRIs are associated with modest reductions in serum glucose and have little effect on appetite.

Because of the combined effects of demonstrated efficacy, safety, improved glucose control, and minimal cognitive and anticholinergic effects, SSRIs should be selected as the first-line antidepressants of choice in treating the diabetic patient. Jimenez and Goodnick (1999) further advocate for sertraline as the first-line treatment of depression in diabetes, given its modest effect on the cytochrome P450 system and its apparent positive impact on cognition. Although the side-effect profile of these medications is quite favorable, it is important to note that SSRIs can often exert adverse effects on sexual function, which may exacerbate sexual dysfunction associated with preexisting diabetic neuropathy.

Table 21–1 summarizes the effects of antidepressants used in treating the diabetic patient. In addition to psychopharmacological treatment of depression, Lustman et al. (1998) reported that cognitive-behavioral therapy and supportive diabetes education are an efficacious treatment for major depression in patients with NIDDM.

Mania is a distinctly uncommon finding in diabetic patients. Wells et al. (1988) noted that the prevalence of mania in medically ill patients was no higher than in members of the general population, whereas the tertiary referral population evaluated by Lustman et al. (1986) revealed three cases of mania in 114 patients.

Anxiety Disorders

According to data from the National Comorbidity Survey, anxiety disorders are the most prevalent psychiatric illness, affecting one of every four respondents in their lifetime and 17% of respondents within the previous 12 months (Kessler et al. 1994). Anxiety disorders include generalized anxiety disorder (GAD), panic disorder, obsessive-compulsive disorder (OCD), posttraumatic stress disorder (PTSD), agoraphobia, specific phobia, and social phobia. GAD is among the most prevalent of these, affecting over 3% of the general population in the preceding 12 months, with a lifetime prevalence of 5% (Wittchen et al. 1994, 2001).

Given their prevalence in the general population, one would expect a similar or greater representation in the medically ill, which is indeed the case. In fact, in a meta-analytic review of anxiety in adults with diabetes, which included 18 studies and a combined population of 4,076, the prevalence of GAD was 14%, and anxiety symptoms were experienced by 40% of those in the population studied (Grigsby et al. 2002). Another meta-analysis by the same group reviewed the effect of poor glycemic control and exacerbation of symptoms of anxiety (Anderson et al. 2002). Although further studies are necessary, there

TABLE 21–1. Effects of antidepressant medications in diabetes mellitus

Medication type	Effects
Monoamine oxidase inhibitors	Associated with acute hypoglycemic episodes. Associated with long-term weight gain. May cause cognitive disturbances. Dietary restrictions may complicate the diabetic diet.
Tricyclic antidepressants	Increased noradrenergic (and dopaminergic) tone may block insulin release and result in higher blood glucose. Long-term use leads to weight gain, carbohydrate craving, and increased insulin requirements. May cause impaired memory and concentration. May help with chronic pain associated with diabetic neuropathy.
Selective serotonin reuptake inhibitors	Shown to decrease insulin requirements in some studies. May decrease body weight. Has fewer anticholinergic, orthostatic, hypotensive, and cardiovascular side effects. Paroxetine, sertraline, and citalopram have been found helpful in neuropathic pain.
Serotonin/norepinephrine reuptake inhibitors	Shown to be effective in diabetic neuropathic pain.
Bupropion, mirtazapine	Little known. Mirtazapine should be avoided due to possible weight gain.

Source. Adapted from Carney 1998; Goodnick et al. 1995; Jimenez and Goodnick 1999.

was a trend identified suggesting that anxiety disorders are associated with hyperglycemia in diabetic patients.

There is a minimal amount of literature specifically addressing the treatment of anxiety disorders in patients with diabetes mellitus. The current standard of care for pharmacological treatment in the general population includes the use of anxiolytics (such as benzodiazepines and azapirones), SSRIs, and SNRIs. Evidence supports using an SSRI as the first-line drug of choice (Davidson et al. 2004). When prescribing SSRIs for the treatment of an anxiety disorder, it is recommended to begin at very low doses to minimize exacerbation of existing symptoms and to then slowly titrate the dose upward. Anxiety disorders in general tend to require higher maintenance doses than affective disorders.

HYPOTHYROIDISM

CARDINAL FEATURES OF THE DISORDER

The classic symptoms of hypothyroidism include weight gain, lethargy, cold intolerance, slow and hoarse speech, constipation, cognitive slowing, depression, and decreased energy and libido. Signs of hypothyroidism include weight gain, hypothermia, bradycardia, thickening of the nails and hair, dryness of the skin, thickening of the tongue and facial skin, and a delayed relaxation phase of deep tendon reflexes. Detectable changes in thyroid size vary depending on the etiology of the syndrome. Diagnosis depends on the demonstration of decreased circulating thyroid hormone. Because more than 90% of patients with hypothy-

roidism have primary hypothyroidism as the underlying cause, measurement of a thyroid-stimulating hormone (TSH) level is considered the most useful screening test (Klee and Hay 1986); patients with primary hypothyroidism exhibit elevated TSH concentrations.

PSYCHIATRIC SYMPTOMS IN HYPOTHYROIDISM

Patients with hypothyroidism frequently exhibit cognitive, affective, psychotic, and anxiety symptoms. Early reports emphasized the psychotic and cognitive manifestations of hypothyroidism, whereas subsequent research has attempted to enhance our understanding of the phenomenology of psychiatric symptoms in hypothyroidism through the use of more sophisticated assessment tools. Psychiatric symptoms are often the first manifestation of thyroid disturbance (Logothetis 1963; Pitts and Guze 1961; Pomeranze and King 1966). This literature is summarized in Table 21–2. Figure 21–1 shows the relative prevalence of psychiatric symptoms in patients with hypothyroidism, both in the case literature and in unselected case series.

Cognitive Disorders

Disturbances in cognition are the most commonly reported psychiatric symptom in hypothyroidism, occurring in 46.3% of unselected cases and 48.2% of psychiatrically ill hypothyroid patients (see Figure 21–1). The severity of the disturbance varies from mild subjective cognitive slowing to severe delirium and encephalopathy. In the clas

TABLE 21–2.   Psychiatric symptoms in hypothyroidism

Study	N	Cognitive	Psychosis	Depression	Mania	Anxiety
Selected hypothyroid cases						
Asher 1949	14	12	9	5		
Miller 1952	2					
Wiesel 1952	1		1	1		
Jonas 1952	1			1		
Pitts and Guze 1961	3	3	2	3		1
Logothetis 1963	4	4	3	2		
Tonks 1964	18	5	7	6		
Libow and Durell 1965	1		1	1		
Pomeranze and King 1966	1			1		
Ward and Rastall 1967	1	1				
Treadway et al. 1967	1	1	1	1		
Hall et al. 1982	4		1	3	1	1
Stowell and Barnhill 2005	1				1	
Unselected hypothyroid populations						
Crown 1949	4	4				
Reitan 1953	15	15				
Schon et al. 1962	24	24				
Jellinek 1962	56	6	Noted	Noted	Noted	Noted
Easson 1966	19	1	11	2		
Whybrow et al. 1969	7	6	1	5		1
Jain 1972	30	8	3	13		10

Note.   Numbers in columns reflect numbers of patients exhibiting specific symptom or syndrome.

sic monograph on "myxoedema madness," Asher (1949) noted that 12 of 14 patients had evidence of cognitive impairment. This finding has been replicated repeatedly in hypothyroid patients with and without psychiatric symptoms (see Table 21–2). In one of the first studies to objectively measure the severity of cognitive disturbance, Whybrow et al. (1969) noted that hypothyroid patients had significantly impaired performance on the Trail Making and Porteus Maze tests compared with hyperthyroid patients. Significant improvement was noted with treatment. Delirium is the most severe manifestation of hypothyroidism. In a study of 56 patients with hypothyroidism and neurological symptoms, Jellinek (1962) noted that 6 of these patients had severe disturbances in their level of consciousness, being either stuporous or comatose, whereas 10 patients had clinical evidence of seizure disor-

ders. The pathophysiology of delirium in hypothyroidism is probably multifactorial, with hypoxia, hypercarbia, hyponatremia, panhypopituitarism, seizures, and autoimmune mechanisms (i.e., antithyroid antibodies) having been described (Jellinek 1962; Royce 1971; Shaw et al. 1991). Bunevicius et al. (1999) compared the effects of treatment with thyroxine (T_4) alone with those of T_4 plus triiodothyronine (T_3) in 33 patients with hypothyroidism, measuring biochemical, physiological, and psychological parameters. They found that partial substitution of T_3 for T_4 resulted in lower BDI scores and higher scores on neuropsychological tasks than in patients with T_4-only supplementation for hypothyroidism. This study suggests a specific effect of T_3 (which is normally derived from T_4 in the thyroid and other tissues including the brain and secreted by the thyroid as well) on mood and cognition.

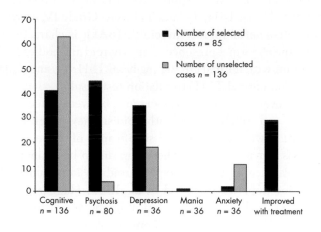

FIGURE 21–1. Psychiatric symptoms in hypothyroidism. Numbers under bars indicate the number of patients in whom the symptom was sought in unselected cases.

Source. Adapted from the case literature in Table 21–2.

It has been suspected that the severity of psychiatric symptoms often correlates with the severity of hypothyroidism. In one of the few studies to provide data in support of this hypothesis, Jain (1972) prospectively evaluated 30 hypothyroid patients; 8 were noted to have cognitive difficulties, and the severity of cognitive dysfunction increased with the magnitude of hypothyroidism. Prinz et al. (1999) found a positive relationship between total T_4 and overall cognition in healthy, euthyroid older men (mean age: 72 years).

Preliminary imaging studies confirm hypothyroid-associated changes in brain activity and regional cerebral blood flow (rCBF). In one study, Constant et al. (2001) used positron emission tomography (PET) with oxygen 15–labeled water and fluorine 18–labeled fluorodeoxyglucose as the tracers. Investigators were able to correlate rCBF and cerebral glucose uptake, two measures of regional brain activity, with the mental state in 10 patients. All subjects entered the study with diagnosed thyroid carcinoma and were scheduled for thyroidectomy (which is the indicated treatment). Patients were scanned in a euthyroid state at baseline and then in the hypothyroid state after thyroidectomy. The second scan was obtained 4–5 weeks postsurgery when patients were severely hypothyroid. At the time of the second scan, the patients were significantly more depressed, anxious, and psychomotorically slowed. The PET scans during the hypothyroid state revealed a global reduction in brain activity compared with the euthyroid state. These results are distinct from the regional CNS changes usually observed in patients with primary depression. However, there are several potential explanations for these observations in-

cluding the very severe hypothyroidism, the relatively short duration of symptoms, and the patient selection bias (i.e., all subjects had a malignancy).

In another study, 10 mildly hypothyroid patients and 10 healthy control subjects underwent MRI, single-photon emission computed tomography (SPECT), and psychometric testing (Krausz et al. 2004). A normal MRI was required of all patients for study entry. In the hypothyroid population, SPECT scans were obtained both in the hypothyroid state and again in a euthyroid state (within 4–43 days after plasma TSH concentrations had normalized). A significant reduction in rCBF was observed in the patient population, which persisted after TSH normalization. Areas of the brain that exhibited a reduction in rCBF included the right primary motor cortex, posterior cingulate, fusiform gyri, insula, and right parieto-occipital cortex, all of which may contribute to cognitive and emotional changes observed in the hypothyroid population.

Mood Disorders

Depression is the second most frequent psychiatric syndrome to occur in unselected hypothyroid patients. Although the overwhelming majority of psychiatrically ill hypothyroid patients have depressive symptoms, about 50% of unselected hypothyroid patients fulfill categorical diagnosis for a mood disorder (see Figure 21–1). Mania and hypomania are quite uncommon, occurring in only three cases in the literature (Hall et al. 1982; Mahendran 1999; Stowell and Barnhill 2005).

Table 21–2 summarizes the literature concerning the prevalence of depression in hypothyroidism; however, certain studies deserve specific mention. Whybrow et al. (1969) noted that five of seven hypothyroid patients appeared clinically depressed, one with psychotic depression. Compared with hyperthyroid patients, the hypothyroid group had higher depressive scores as measured by the Minnesota Multiphasic Personality Inventory, the Clyde Mood Scale, and the Brief Psychiatric Rating Scale. In contrast to the data regarding cognitive dysfunction, Jain (1972) could find no relationship between the severity of depression as measured by Hamilton Rating Scale for Depression (Ham-D) and BDI severity scores and the severity of hypothyroidism.

Investigators have long recognized the association between depression and hypothyroidism, and many hypotheses have been postulated as to the biological basis of this relationship. There is an emerging database that supports an underlying autoimmune process (Carta et al. 2004; Fountoulakis et al. 2004) in addition to contributions from alterations in the HPA and the hypothalamic-pituitary-thyroid (HPT) axis (see section "Hypothalamic-

Pituitary-Thyroid Axis and Depression" later in this chapter). Recent evidence suggests a genetic link as well. Polymorphisms in the Xq13 thyroid receptor coactivator named *HOPA* appear to be associated with an increased susceptibility for major depression (Philibert et al. 2002). This same gene participates in thyroid hormone signal transduction and may provide a link to the long-observed association between depression and thyroid dysfunction.

Anxiety

Anxiety occurs in approximately 30% of unselected hypothyroid patients. No correlation between the severity of anxiety as measured by the Hamilton Anxiety Scale and the severity of hypothyroidism was noted in a sample of 30 hypothyroid patients (Jain 1972). Our understanding of the phenomenology of anxiety in hypothyroidism is limited by a paucity of data. Clinical experience suggests that it is often accompanied by significant depressive symptoms and is more generalized.

Psychosis

Although psychosis is the most common symptom in the case literature on hypothyroidism (52.9%), it represents only 5% of the psychiatric morbidity in unselected samples. This disparity likely reflects a reporting bias because of the dramatic nature of psychotic symptoms. The psychotic symptoms may occur comorbidly with depression or independent of a significant affective disturbance. Paranoid delusions and auditory and visual hallucinations have been described as well. No systematic assessment of thought disorder symptoms in patients with hypothyroidism is available.

GRADES OF HYPOTHYROIDISM AND THE CONCEPT OF SUBCLINICAL HYPOTHYROIDISM

Because our ability to precisely measure thyroid function has become increasingly more sophisticated, a spectrum of disturbance in thyroid function has now been identified. Grade I (overt) or classic primary hypothyroidism is defined by low levels of circulating thyroid hormones, T_3 and T_4, and an elevated TSH concentration accompanied by clinical symptoms. Grade II hypothyroidism is defined by elevated TSH levels with normal plasma levels of thyroid hormones. An exaggerated TSH response to thyrotropin-releasing hormone (TRH) is seen in both grade I and grade II hypothyroidism, presumably due to a lack of thyroid hormone feedback. The term *subclinical hypothyroidism* generally refers to grade II hypothyroidism. Grade III hypothyroidism is characterized by an

exaggerated TSH response to TRH in the presence of normal basal TSH, T_3, and T_4 levels. Grade IV, or symptomless autoimmune thyroiditis (SAT), is characterized by the abnormal presence of antithyroid antibodies in the serum with normal circulating basal TSH, T_3, and T_4 levels and normal TRH stimulation test results.

Several interesting associations between affective illness and subclinical hypothyroidism have been identified; however, the clinical significance of these associations remains unclear. There appears to be an increased prevalence of grade II hypothyroidism in patients with major depression (Gold et al. 1981; Haggerty et al. 1993). Furthermore, subclinical hypothyroidism may be a risk factor for the development of major depression. Haggerty et al. (1993) compared the lifetime history of major depression in 16 depressed patients with grade II hypothyroidism with 15 depressed patients with normal thyroid function. The lifetime history of major depression was 56% in the patients with grade II hypothyroidism and 20% in control subjects. Ham-D scores did not differ between the groups (Haggerty et al. 1993).

Several studies have suggested that depressed patients with grade II hypothyroidism respond poorly to antidepressant treatment (Joffe and Levitt 1992; Prange et al. 1988; Targum et al. 1984). In a study of 139 patients with major depression, patients who had subclinical hypothyroidism responded less favorably to treatment with TCAs than the euthyroid group (Joffe and Levitt 1992). There are reports that grade II hypothyroidism is associated with rapid cycling among patients with affective illness, although there are discrepant reports as well (Bauer and Whybrow 1988; Cowdry et al. 1983; Joffe et al. 1988; Wehr et al. 1988). Pop et al. (1998) found that an elevated level of thyroid peroxidase antibodies, a measure of SAT, was significantly associated with later development of depression in perimenopausal women.

There is controversy as to whether thyroid hormone replacement therapy is indicated in subclinical (grade II) hypothyroidism. In a study of 33 patients with grade II hypothyroidism, 8 of 14 patients (57%) receiving levothyroxine and 3 of 12 patients (25%) receiving placebo reported symptomatic improvement, and improvement in left ventricular performance was noted in a subset of the patients treated with levothyroxine (Cooper et al. 1984). In a discussion of 2 patients with psychiatric symptoms and grade II hypothyroidism, clinical improvement in mood and psychotic symptoms was noted after treatment with levothyroxine, antidepressants, and antipsychotics, but no improvement in cognitive symptoms was seen (Haggerty et al. 1986). However, Baldini et al. (1997) evaluated affective and cognitive dysfunction in patients with euthyroidism and subclinical hypothyroidism and found that a significant decrease in logical memory was present in the subclinical hypothyroid group but not the euthyroid group. Treatment with levothyroxine significantly improved memory performance in the subclinical hypothyroid group. In one review, Smallridge (2000) noted that thyroid replacement therapy is recommended for patients with a TSH level of 10 mIU/L or higher and that replacement therapy is generally helpful for psychiatric symptoms associated with subclinical hypothyroidism.

HYPERTHYROIDISM

CARDINAL FEATURES OF THE DISORDER

The cardinal symptoms of hyperthyroidism vary, but the most common manifestations include diaphoresis, heat intolerance, fatigue, dyspnea, palpitations, weakness (especially in proximal muscles), anxiety, weight loss despite an increased appetite, hyperdefecation, and visual complaints. Signs of hyperthyroidism include noticeable anxiety and increased psychomotor activity; tachycardia, often with atrial fibrillation; bounding peripheral pulses; moist and warm skin; thinning of the individual hair shafts, as well as alopecia; tremor and hyperreflexia; and eye findings ranging from simple retraction of the upper lid with lid lag to overt exophthalmos with impairment of extraocular movement. The thyroid gland is usually enlarged, with the most notable exceptions in the elderly and in those with substernal thyroid tissue.

PSYCHIATRIC SYMPTOMS IN HYPERTHYROIDISM

Although many authors have emphasized the ubiquitous presence of psychiatric symptoms in patients with hyperthyroidism, scrutiny of the literature suggests that serious psychopathology occurs in only a minority of patients. During the acute phase of hyperthyroidism, patients can experience numerous symptoms that overlap with those occurring in psychiatric illness such as sleep disturbance, fatigue, decreased concentration, weight loss, and irritability. Recognition of this symptom overlap led investigators to attempt to delineate a relationship between the illnesses. Initially this effort yielded little and resulted in the hypothesis that coexisting hyperthyroidism and psychiatric illness are just that, comorbid but unrelated. In the last decade, however, much evidence has accrued to the contrary, supporting more than a coincident occurrence.

An interesting approach was utilized in a recent study using data from an existing Danish registry (Thomsen et al. 2005). Patient records were evaluated from 1977 to 1999, and cohorts were selected based on an index hospitalization of hyperthyroidism (experimental group), nontoxic goiter, or osteoarthritis (the later two being the control groups). The sample consisted of 183,647 patients. An index hospitalization of hyperthyroidism was associated with an increased risk of later hospitalization with an affective disorder, with the greatest risk occurring in the first 6 months after index hospitalization.

In acute hyperthyroidism, depression, anxiety, and cognitive changes are most commonly seen, and manic and psychotic manifestations are encountered less frequently. Table 21–3 summarizes the case literature and studies involving unselected hyperthyroid patients, and Figure 21–2 compares the prevalence of psychiatric symptoms in these two groups.

Cognitive Disorders

Cognitive changes associated with thyrotoxicosis range from subtle defects in attention and concentration to overt delirium. The prevalence of cognitive disturbance in thyrotoxicosis is 7.4%, considerably less than that observed in hypothyroidism. Robbins and Vinson (1960) noted frequent errors in simple conceptual tasks and an increased time for problem solving in patients with hyperthyroidism. Trzepacz et al. (1988) noted mild deficits in complex attention, immediate memory, and higher-level problem solving.

The data are mixed as to whether the severity of cognitive impairment correlates with the severity of hyperthyroidism. Alvarez et al. (1983) noted significant impairment in concentration and attention as measured by the Tolouse-Pierson Concentration Attention test in 27 patients with untreated Graves' disease compared with healthy control subjects. These deficits in attention and concentration did not correlate with the severity of hyperthyroidism. In contrast, MacCrimmon et al. (1979) noted that the severity of hyperthyroidism correlated with the severity of concentration and memory impairment. In addition, successful treatment of hyperthyroidism resulted in test scores that were indistinguishable from those of healthy control subjects.

Mood Disorders

Major depression is the most common psychiatric manifestation of hyperthyroidism, occurring in approximately 28% of unselected patients (see Figure 21–2). Furthermore, the mood symptoms may precede the development of physical signs and symptoms in some patients. In the largest sample in the literature, Sonino et al. (1993) noted that major depression occurred in 23% of 70 patients with Graves' disease. They also noted that depression occurred in the prodromal phase in 14% of these patients. Other

TABLE 21–3.   Psychiatric symptoms in hyperthyroidism

| | | Type of psychiatric disturbance | | | | |
Study	N	Cognitive	Psychosis	Depression	Mania	Anxiety
Selected hyperthyroid cases						
Bursten 1961	10	3	10	1	1	
Taylor 1975	1		1	1		
Katerndahl and Vande Creek 1983	1			1		1
Unselected hyperthyroid populations						
Lidz and Whitehorn 1949	15			9		
Mandelbrote and Wittkower 1955	25			Noted		Noted
Kleinschmidt et al. 1956	17		2	Noted		Noted
Robbins and Vinson 1960	10	1	1			1
Wilson et al. 1962	26	14		15	2	6
Artunkal and Togrol 1964	20					
Hermann and Quarton 1965	24	Noted	1			Noted
Whybrow et al. 1969	10	4	2	2		2
F.B. Thomas et al. 1970	9			6		
MacCrimmon et al. 1979	19					
Rockey and Griep 1980	14			1		11
Kathol and Delahunt 1986	33			10		20
Trzepacz et al. 1988	13			9	3	8

Note.   Numbers in columns reflect numbers of patients exhibiting specific symptom or syndrome.

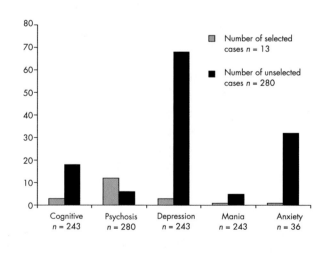

FIGURE 21–2.   Psychiatric symptoms in hyperthyroidism. Numbers under bars indicate the number of patients in whom the symptom was sought in unselected cases.

Source.   Adapted from the case literature in Table 21–3.

investigators (Wilson et al. 1962) reported that 24 of 26 patients (92%) with hyperthyroidism noted mood changes and neurovegetative symptoms involving sleep, appetite, libido, and psychomotor activity before the physical signs and symptoms of hyperthyroidism occurred. None of these patients required psychiatric treatment after euthyroidism was achieved.

In the first study to use modern operational criteria for psychiatric disorders in hyperthyroid patients, Kathol and Delahunt (1986) noted that 10 of 32 patients (31%) with untreated hyperthyroidism fulfilled DSM-III (American Psychiatric Association 1980) criteria for major depression. The severity of hyperthyroidism did not appear to predict the prevalence of depression. Trzepacz et al. (1988) noted that 9 of 13 (69%) untreated Graves' disease patients fulfilled criteria for major depression using Research Diagnostic Criteria (RDC) and the Schedule for Affective Disorders and Schizophrenia. The finding of weight loss in the presence of a voracious appetite represented a striking phenomenological difference from patients with typical major depression.

Apathetic thyrotoxicosis also has been reported and is usually seen in elderly patients with a longer duration of symptoms and more dramatic weight loss. Typically, elderly patients have apathy, depression, an increased prevalence of cardiovascular events, and a decreased prevalence of ocular manifestations. F.B. Thomas et al. (1970) found that 6 of 9 patients (67%) with apathetic thyrotoxicosis had features of mental depression; however, specific depression criteria were not described.

Mania or hypomania secondary to hyperthyroidism is distinctly uncommon, occurring in only 2.1% of unselected cases. Wilson et al. (1962) noted that 2 patients described elation as the predominant mood, and 1 patient was considered manic. Trzepacz et al. (1988) noted that 3 of 13 untreated Graves' disease patients were hypomanic. One patient with mania has been described following initiation of thyroid hormone replacement, but review of the longitudinal course of the patient's disorder suggests that the patient likely had preexisting bipolar disorder (Josephson and MacKenzie 1979).

Anxiety

Although anxiety is cited as one of the cardinal features of hyperthyroidism, it appeared in only 13% of unselected patients in whom anxiety symptoms were sought (see Figure 21–2). Anxiety due to hyperthyroidism generally has an insidious onset, often preceding overt physical signs of the disorder (Dietch 1981). Others have noted that the anxiety associated with thyrotoxicosis was indistinguishable from that observed in primary anxiety disorders (Greer et al. 1973). MacCrimmon et al. (1979) noted that more than one-half of 19 patients with untreated hyperthyroidism and psychiatric symptoms reported nervousness, jumpiness, restlessness, tension, irritability, and anxiety.

Two studies have applied operational anxiety criteria to untreated Graves' disease patients. Using RDC, Trzepacz et al. (1988) revealed that 8 of 13 patients (62%) had generalized anxiety disorder 4 of 13 (31%) met criteria for panic disorder, and 1 (8%) had agoraphobia. Kathol and Delahunt (1986) noted that 15 of 32 patients (47%) with untreated Graves' disease fulfilled DSM-III criteria for GAD. Both groups noted that the severity of anxiety correlated with the severity of hyperthyroidism and that most patients with anxiety had concurrent major depression.

Psychosis

Psychosis is an uncommon manifestation of thyrotoxicosis, occurring in 2.1% of unselected patients. Earlier estimates of prevalence ranged from 15% to 25% (Clower et al. 1969). However, review of the symptoms reported in these patients indicates that many of them would be classified as having affective disorders. Clower et al. (1969) described only 3 patients with comorbid thyrotoxicosis and psychosis in a series of 228 patients with elevated protein-bound iodine (PBI) determinations; the number of patients with elevated PBI who actually had hyperthyroidism was not noted. Bursten (1961) described 10 psychotic patients with thyrotoxicosis and noted paranoid, delusional, and hallucinatory phenomena similar to those seen in schizophreniform illnesses. Two case reports noted findings of mania with psychotic features (Irwin et al. 1997) and psychosis (Bewsher et al. 1971) following the rapid normalization of thyroid function in patients with severe, prolonged, untreated Graves' disease.

A study by Fahrenfort et al. (2000) noted that many patients with hyperthyroidism continued to have psychiatric symptoms, including depression, anxiety, fatigue, and functional impairment even after 12 months of normalization of the thyroid. The researchers advocated longer-term psychiatric follow-up of psychiatrically symptomatic hyperthyroid patients.

HASHIMOTO'S ENCEPHALITIS

Hashimoto's encephalitis is an unusual clinical syndrome that warrants separate discussion. Since 1974, several cases have been reported of a severe encephalopathic state associated with the presence of high titers of antithyroid antibodies. Most importantly, in the literature, only 3 of 13 patients (23%) were overtly hypothyroid. Ten patients (77%) were considered biochemically euthyroid when the neuropsychiatric syndrome developed (Shaw et al. 1991; Shein et al. 1986; Thrush and Boddie 1974). It is unclear whether circulating antithyroid antibodies are directly responsible for the neuropsychiatric symptoms or whether they represent a nonspecific phenomenon of immune activation. Some patients may improve after treatment with corticosteroids (van Oostrom et al. 1999).

HYPOTHALAMIC-PITUITARY-THYROID AXIS AND DEPRESSION

Affective symptoms have long been identified in thyroid disease, leading many investigators to search for the role of thyroid axis abnormalities in affective disorders. Thyroid hormone supplementation has been found to increase the rapidity of action of TCA agents (Prange et al. 1969) and was equally as effective as lithium in producing a response in depressed patients who did not respond to TCAs (Joffe et al. 1993). However, two recent large-scale controlled studies have revealed no effect of T_3 augmentation in the efficacy of SSRIs (Appelhof et al. 2004; P.T. Ninan, C.B. Nemeroff, unpublished observations, July 2005). Thus, the precise relationship between the HPT axis and affective disorders remains unclear. The complexities involved in this relationship are 1) symptoms of depression occur in both hypothyroidism and hyperthyroidism; 2) most depressed patients have HPT axis functions within the normal range (Esposito et al. 1997; Joffe and Sokolov 1994); 3) elevated levels of TRH have been reported in cerebrospinal fluid of patients with major depression (Banki et al. 1988; Kirkegaard et al. 1979); 4) 25% of patients with MDD exhibit a blunted TSH response to exogenously administered TRH (Prange et al. 1972), whereas 15% of depressed patients show an exaggerated response (Extein et al. 1981); 5) there is a higher prevalence rate of SAT in depressed patients (Gold et al. 1982; Nemeroff et al. 1985); and 6) functioning of the HPT axis can be influenced by a variety of states such as systemic or chronic illness, chronic physiological stress, nutritional status, circadian rhythms, and cognitive processes (Esposito et al. 1997). These findings preclude a simple understanding of HPT axis dysfunction in depression and emphasize the fact that considerably more research is needed in this area.

CUSHING'S SYNDROME AND DISEASE

CARDINAL FEATURES OF THE DISORDER

The most common signs and symptoms of Cushing's syndrome are centripetal obesity, hirsutism, menstrual irregularities, decreased libido, impotence, hypertension, proximal weakness, red to purple striae, acne, and easy bruisability. Osteopenia and glucose intolerance also may occur. Cushing's syndrome is classified as either adrenocorticotropic hormone (ACTH) dependent or ACTH independent. Most cases of Cushing's syndrome are due to high-dose corticosteroid administration, with adrenal carcinoma and ectopic ACTH production occurring less frequently. The term *Cushing's disease* is reserved for cases of hypercortisolism due to ACTH hypersecretion from a pituitary adenoma. Laboratory diagnosis of Cushing's syndrome depends on demonstration of either elevated urinary cortisol concentration or an abnormal dexamethasone suppression test (DST). Adrenal carcinoma, ectopic ACTH production, and Cushing's disease can be further differentiated by measuring plasma ACTH concentration, administering a high-dose DST, and performing CT or MRI of the abdomen and head.

Simmons et al. (2000) compared MRI and CT scans of the brain in 63 patients with Cushing's disease with age- and sex-matched control subjects. The "patients with Cushing's disease showed significant premature (cerebral) atrophy when compared to controls" (p. 72), further solidifying previous evidence that elevated cortisol levels cause catabolic changes most notably to soft tissues and bone. A more complete understanding is emerging regarding the systemic effects of elevated cortisol on the central nervous system.

PSYCHIATRIC SYMPTOMS IN CUSHING'S SYNDROME

Psychiatric symptoms occurring in Cushing's syndrome have been well documented in the literature (Spillane 1951; Whybrow and Hurwitz 1976; Zeiger et al. 1993). In 1913, Harvey Cushing noted psychiatric disturbance, particularly depression, in his first description of the illness that bears his name (Cushing 1932). In the decades since Cushing's observations, substantial progress has been made toward identifying the mechanisms by which excess corticosteroids affect mood, anxiety, and cognition.

Mood and Anxiety Disorders

Mood disorders, especially unipolar depression, are by far the most frequently reported psychiatric manifestations of Cushing's syndrome. Before 1980, depression was frequently noted in Cushing's syndrome, but most studies were retrospective and did not use diagnostic criteria. Whybrow and Hurwitz (1976) reviewed the literature and found that 35% of patients with Cushing's syndrome reported depressive symptoms, compared with 3.7% who reported mania. Delirium was noted in 16.2% and psychosis in 9.3% of patients. In addition, suicide attempts (Gotch 1994; Haskett 1985; Starkman et al. 1981) and completed suicides (Jeffcoate et al. 1979; Zeiger et al. 1993) have been reported during the course of Cushing's syndrome. Several investigators have used structured interviews and diagnostic criteria to scrutinize affective illness in this population. Haskett (1985) applied RDC to 30 patients with Cushing's syndrome and noted that 16 (53%) fulfilled criteria for unipolar depression and 9 (30%) met criteria for bipolar disorder. Other studies have suggested prevalence rates of depressive symptoms in Cushing's syndrome as high as 62%–94% (Kelly et al. 1996; Mazet et al. 1981; Starkman et al. 1981).

Some evidence suggests that mixed anxiety and depressive symptoms may be the most common psychiatric manifestation of Cushing's syndrome (Loosen et al. 1992; Mazet et al. 1981). Starkman et al. (1981) noted anxiety symptoms in 63% of 35 patients with Cushing's syndrome. Using the Structured Clinical Interview for DSM-III-R (SCID), Loosen et al. (1992) compared 20 patients with Cushing's disease with 20 patients with

MDD and noted that GAD was the most common psychiatric diagnosis (79%) in Cushing's disease patients. Major depression was present in 68% and panic disorder in 53%. Only one Cushing's disease patient with major depression had no syndromal comorbid anxiety diagnosis. Other investigators also have noted prominent irritability and emotional lability in depressed patients with Cushing's syndrome (Haskett 1985; Starkman et al. 1981). It is likely that reporting and investigator bias has resulted in an underappreciation of the presence of mixed anxiety and depressed states in Cushing's syndrome. Figure 21–3 illustrates the effect of reporting bias on the relative prevalence of psychiatric symptoms in Cushing's syndrome. Depression associated with Cushing's disease also may differ from primary major depression in that symptoms are often more intermittent in the former (Haskett 1985; Loosen et al. 1992; Starkman et al. 1981).

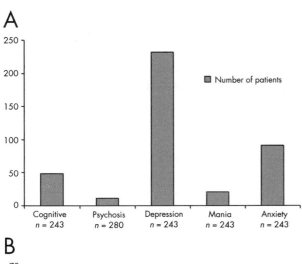

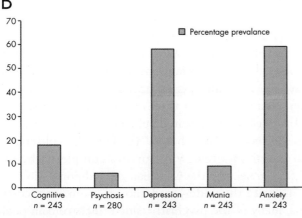

FIGURE 21–3. Psychiatric symptoms in Cushing's syndrome: the influence of publication bias on relative prevalence phenomenology. *Panel A.* All cases of psychiatric disturbances in Cushing's syndrome. *Panel B.* Relative prevalence of major psychiatric symptoms in cases of Cushing's syndrome using broad clinical or structured interview.

Several authors have noted that depressive symptoms occur early in the disorder. Sonino et al. (1993) noted that prodromal depressive symptoms occurred in 27% of 66 patients with Cushing's syndrome. Some evidence suggests that patients with antecedent psychiatric symptoms have a less favorable psychiatric outcome after treatment of the endocrinopathy (Jeffcoate et al. 1979).

Treating Cushing's syndrome—with metyrapone, adrenalectomy, or pituitary irradiation or resection—has been shown to improve the mood disorder in most patients. Sonino et al. (1993) noted that 70% of depressed Cushing's syndrome patients improved with reductions in serum cortisol. In a series of 34 patients with Cushing's syndrome, 8 of 9 depressed patients with hypercortisolism (89%) responded to bilateral adrenalectomy with improvement in their depressive symptoms (Zeiger et al. 1993). Kelly et al. (1983) reported a reduction in Ham-D scores in 26 patients with Cushing's syndrome after successful treatment. Furthermore, improvement may be related to the severity of the symptoms. In a study of 38 patients with Cushing's syndrome, 8 of 9 moderately to severely depressed patients (89%) responded to reduced plasma cortisol with an improvement in depressive symptoms compared with 6 of 13 mildly depressed patients (46%) (Jeffcoate et al. 1979). The most compelling data have arguably been provided by Starkman et al. (1986b), who noted that improvement in symptoms correlated with reduced circulating cortisol level.

Secondary mania and hypomania are relatively infrequent findings in Cushing's syndrome. Hypomania was noted in 3 (9%) and mania in 1 (3%) of 35 patients by Starkman et al. (1981). Mazet et al. (1981) noted manic symptoms in 7 of 50 patients with Cushing's syndrome (14%). Haskett (1985) used the Schedule for Affective Disorders and Schizophrenia—Lifetime Version and reported the highest prevalence rate (30%) in the literature of bipolar illness in Cushing's syndrome.

Psychosis and Cognitive Disorders

Psychosis and overt delirium have rarely been reported in patients with Cushing's disease. Psychotic symptoms in Cushing's syndrome are usually associated with affective syndromes (S.I. Cohen 1980; Haskett 1985). A case of delirium secondary to a mixed adrenal tumor secreting estrogen and cortisol in a 14-year-old boy has been reported (Ghazi et al. 1994).

Until recently, cognitive impairment in Cushing's syndrome had been relatively infrequently reported, and when documented, it had been mild. In a questionnaire study of 62 patients with Cushing's syndrome, subjective complaints of concentration and memory impairment were reported in 20 of the 41 patients (49%) who returned the questionnaire (Gotch 1994). Whelan et al. (1980) administered the Michigan Neuropsychological Test Battery to 35 patients with Cushing's syndrome. They divided the patients into four groups: group 1 (13 patients) had normal or equivocal neuropsychological findings, group 2 (10 patients) had mild or infrequent deficits, group 3 (8 patients) had moderate or frequent deficits, and group 4 (4 patients) had marked and frequent deficits in neuropsychological testing. Deficits in nonverbal visual ideation and spatial-construction abilities were more common than problems with language and verbal reasoning. In addition, impaired manual dexterity as measured by the Purdue Pegboard was noted in 46% of patients.

Of late, attention has been focused on specific areas of the brain such as the hippocampus, which plays a critical role in learning and memory and is a major target of glucocorticoids. In a series of studies from 1981 through 2003, Starkman et al. (1981, 1985, 1986a, 1986b, 1992, 1999, 2001, 2003) have explored the neuropsychiatric effects of elevated cortisol, especially with respect to cognition. In their 1992 study, 12 patients with Cushing's syndrome underwent neuropsychological testing with the Wechsler Memory Scale, the Wechsler Adult Intelligence Scale—Revised, and the Trail Making Test parts A and B. Volumetric measurements of the hippocampal formations were determined through MRI, and serum cortisol was measured. Verbal memory and verbal recall were positively associated with hippocampal volume, whereas age, educational level, and performance on the Trail Making Tests parts A and B and on full-scale IQ tests was not significantly correlated with hippocampal volume. Furthermore, the loss of hippocampal volume was negatively correlated with serum cortisol concentrations (Starkman et al. 1992).

Newcomer et al. (1994) then demonstrated that 4 days of dexamethasone administration results in impaired verbal declarative memory performance in normal healthy adult volunteers. It was then hypothesized that this effect may be mediated by site-specific glucocorticoid effects on hippocampal neurons (Bardgett et al. 1994). Brunetti et al. (1998) analyzed PET scans in 13 patients with Cushing's disease and compared them with 13 age-matched healthy control subjects. Patients with Cushing's disease had significant reduction in cerebral glucose metabolism, which the investigators theorized might contribute to the cognitive and psychiatric symptoms in patients with Cushing's disease.

After establishing a correlation among elevated cortisol levels, reduced hippocampal formation volume (HFV), and memory dysfunction before treatment of Cushing's syndrome, Starkman et al. (1999) then demonstrated that HFV increased after cortisol levels returned to normal concentrations. These results support the hy-

pothesis that the hippocampus is particularly sensitive to cortisol. In addition to several smaller studies (Forget et al. 2000; Mauri et al. 1993; Starkman et al. 1986a), a controlled study by Starkman et al. (2001) further confirmed that prior to treatment the hypercortisolemia of Cushing's disease negatively affects multiple cognitive tasks, particularly verbal learning and other verbal functions.

Finally, in their most recent study (Starkman et al. 2003), 24 patients with Cushing's disease were studied before and after treatment. In a finding consistent with previous results, patients before treatment exhibited volumetric hippocampal loss and deficits in verbal learning. After treatment, with a return to a eucortisolemic state, the patients exhibited increases in HFV with associated improvement of a specific verbal learning task. This task, the Selective Reminding Test, which requires learning unrelated words, is hypothesized to be particularly dependent on hippocampal function.

EXOGENOUS CORTICOSTEROID ADMINISTRATION

Psychiatric complications of corticosteroids were recognized shortly after they were introduced into clinical practice in the 1950s (Clark et al. 1953). Nearly all corticosteroid preparations have been implicated, including ACTH (which stimulates cortisol release), cortisone, prednisone, prednisolone, methylprednisolone, and inhaled beclomethasone (Hayreh and Watson 1970; Ling et al. 1981; Perry et al. 1984; Rosenberg et al. 1976). Psychiatric symptoms are predominantly affective, although cognitive changes, psychosis, delirium, and anxiety also have been reported (Belanoff et al. 2001b; Brown et al 2002; Campbell 1987; D'Orban 1989; Hall et al. 1979; Ling et al. 1981; Perry et al. 1984; Silva and Tolstunov 1995) (Figure 21–4). With respect to corticosteroid-associated affective symptoms, Patten (2000) estimated that the "12-month period prevalence of major depression was approximately three times as high in corticosteroid treated vs. nontreated subjects irrespective of age, gender, and perceived health" (p. 447). This observation was based on a review of surveys completed by over 73,000 subjects in the Canadian general population.

Despite the widespread clinical use of corticosteroids, many of the psychiatric side effects remain poorly characterized. Consequently, treatment options have been largely based on clinical experience and case reports rather than large controlled trials. There are tremendous methodological problems in designing the appropriate prospective study due to several factors. These include the urgency in which high-dose steroids must be initially prescribed and the need for immediate access to trained psychiatric interviewers to administer baseline rating scales. In addition, many of the conditions that respond to high-dose steroids, such as lupus and multiple sclerosis, are themselves associated with psychopathology. To minimize this effect, it is important to select an appropriate disease state when choosing a study population.

Many groups are now in the early stages of addressing these issues. Both Naber et al. (1996) and Wolkowitz et al. (1990) found that although depressive symptoms exist, manic symptoms predominate in patients undergoing short courses of steroid treatment. Naber's patient population was limited to patients with primary uveitis, whereas those in the Wolkowitz study were healthy volunteers. Based in part on these results, E.S. Brown et al. (2002) sought to address several pertinent questions, including a confirmation of whether mood changes are associated with brief courses of corticosteroid therapy at modest doses and what risk factors may exist to predict the onset of mood symptoms in patients taking corticosteroids. Thirty-two outpatients were enrolled in the study and monitored for mood changes during prednisone bursts (initial dose > 40 mg/day with treatment for at least 7 days) prescribed for treatment of preexisting asthma. Consistent with previous findings, psychiatric symptoms were primarily manic, and patients with preexisting depression tended to show improvement in their depressive symptoms. Interestingly, although not statistically significant because of the small number of participants, patients with PTSD reported exacerbations of depressive symptoms, with the three largest increases in Ham-D scores coming from patients with PTSD.

In another study, E.S. Brown et al. (2004b) addressed effects of long-term corticosteroid therapy. Seventeen patients with asthma or rheumatic disease on steroid therapy (≥10 mg/day for ≥6 months) and 15 control subjects completed multiple mood and cognitive screens in addition to functional MRI (fMRI) and proton magnetic resonance spectroscopy of the brain. The researchers found that patients receiving corticosteroid therapy had smaller hippocampal volumes and declarative memory deficits than control subjects, both of which are consistent with findings in patients with Cushing's disease.

Clinical experience suggests a correlation between severity of symptoms and corticosteroid dose, but controlled data are lacking. However, the prevalence of psychiatric disturbances associated with corticosteroid administration appears to be a dose-related phenomenon. In a prospective study of 718 hospitalized patients receiving prednisone, 1.3% had psychiatric reactions at a dosage less than or equal to 40 mg/day. This rate increased to 4.6% at dosages of 41 to 80 mg/day, and to 18.4% at dosages of 80 mg/day or more (Boston Collab-

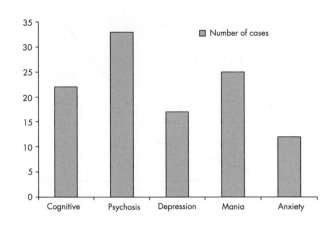

FIGURE 21–4. Psychiatric symptoms with corticosteroid administration: findings from the case literature.

Source. Adapted from Hall et al. 1979 and Perry et al. 1984.

orative Drug Surveillance Program 1972) (Figure 21–5). In a prospective evaluation of 32 asthmatic children, high-dose prednisone (mean dosage: 61.4 mg/day) was associated with more depression and anxiety symptoms and decreased verbal memory compared with low-dose prednisone (7 mg/day) (Bender et al. 1991).

Glucocorticoids regulate production and release of hypothalamic corticotropin-releasing hormone (CRH) and ACTH, modulate neurotransmitter activity, and are active in the plasticity and circuitry of many brain regions. It is therefore not surprising that the effects of glucocorticoid excess can be profound. Delineating their complex role in CNS function has been an active area of research for many decades. For example, observations of the clinical impact of excess glucocorticoids on memory, coupled with an emerging understanding of how memories are formed, have led to detailed investigation on the cellular effects of glucocorticoids. It appears that glucocorticoids are active in many processes within the brain including the mediation of neuron survival and death, dendritic branching, synapse formation, operation of various second messenger systems, and suppression of myelin content (Belanoff et al. 2001b).

Although the data are limited, a variety of strategies have been employed to prevent steroid-induced psychiatric disturbances, including administering divided doses, enteric-coated preparations (Glynne-Jones and Vernon 1986), lithium (Falk et al. 1979; Siegal 1978), valproic acid (Abbas and Styra 1994), lamotrigine (E.S. Brown et al. 2003), and olanzapine (E.S. Brown et al. 2004a). TCAs have been shown to exacerbate symptoms and are therefore not a treatment option (Hall et al. 1979).

There have been only two controlled studies to date evaluating the efficacy of pharmacotherapy in the treat-

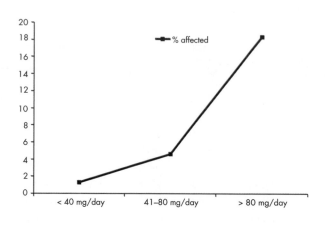

FIGURE 21–5. Prevalence of corticosteroid-related psychiatric disturbances: relationship to dosage.

Source. Adapted from Boston Collaborative Drug Surveillance Program 1972.

ment of corticosteroid-induced psychiatric symptoms. The first was the previously cited trial by Falk et al. (1979), reporting that lithium pretreatment may prevent mood disturbance due to corticosteroid treatment. The second, and much more recent, was a placebo-controlled trial evaluating the efficacy of phenytoin in the prevention of both mood and memory disturbances secondary to prescription corticosteroid therapy (E.S. Brown et al. 2005). Phenytoin was indeed found to be effective at preventing manic symptoms but interestingly did not prevent impairment of declarative memory.

ADDISON'S DISEASE (ADRENAL INSUFFICIENCY)

CARDINAL FEATURES OF THE DISORDER

The symptoms of adrenal insufficiency are best understood in terms of chronic and acute symptoms. Chronic adrenal insufficiency is manifested by fatigue, malaise, weakness, weight loss, anorexia, hyperpigmentation, hypotension, nausea, and vomiting. Hyponatremia, hyperkalemia, metabolic acidosis, anemia, and eosinophilia are often present on laboratory testing. Acute adrenal insufficiency is manifested by more profound gastrointestinal symptoms, including pain—which may mimic acute abdomen—fever, and shock.

PSYCHIATRIC SYMPTOMS IN ADRENAL INSUFFICIENCY

In contrast to many of the endocrinopathies discussed in this chapter, psychiatric symptoms are relatively uncommon in adrenal insufficiency. Addison's (1868) initial description of the disorder noted evidence of impaired

cognition. In a review of 25 cases of Addison's disease, 16 patients (64%) were noted to have disturbances in cognition (Engel and Margolin 1941). A review of these cases revealed 2 patients (13%) with delirium, 1 (6%) with psychotic symptoms, and 5 (31%) with depressive symptoms (Whybrow and Hurwitz 1976). Three other cases are present in the literature, with anxiety and depressive symptoms dominating the clinical picture (Thompson 1973; Varadaraj and Cooper 1986).

An unusual case of ACTH deficiency accompanied by delirium has been described. Mineralocorticoid functioning in the patient was normal, although he manifested severe orthostatic hypotension. The delirium resolved after administration of replacement doses of cortisone acetate (Fang and Jaspan 1989).

HYPOTHALAMIC-PITUITARY-ADRENAL AXIS AND DEPRESSION

Observations of mood disturbance, both in patients with Cushing's syndrome and in those given exogenous steroids, led many investigators to consider the role of cortisol in patients with primary mood disorders. Hypercortisolemia has since been widely documented in patients with major depression (Nemeroff et al. 1984; Ritchie et al. 1990; Rosenbaum et al. 1983; Young et al. 1994). In 1965, Bunney and Fawcett measured 24-hour urine 17-hydroxycorticosteroid levels in 143 depressed patients. Patients who later had severe or completed suicide attempts had the highest levels. Elevated cortisol levels return to normal after recovery from depression (Sachar et al. 1970). Hypercortisolemia appears to represent a state as opposed to a trait marker for depression (Gillespie and Nemeroff 2005; Musselman and Nemeroff 1996). Kiraly et al. (1997) theorized that hypercortisolemia is a treatable factor in a subset of affective and psychotic disorders and that the geriatric population may be more vulnerable to the neurotoxic effects of cortisol. Murphy et al. (1991) studied 10 patients with treatment-resistant depression and found that treatment with a steroid-suppressive agent resulted in significant improvement in 6 patients. Belanoff et al. (2001a, 2002) have reported improvement in psychotic symptoms in patients with psychotic depression after treatment with the glucocorticoid receptor antagonist mifepristone.

As previously discussed, hypercortisolemia in patients with Cushing's disease is associated with hippocampal alterations and deficits in verbal learning and memory. In a similar fashion, this relationship has been hypothesized to exist in patients with depression (Bremner 2002). Many

MRI studies support this hypothesis in that patients with depression have been shown to have smaller hippocampal volumes (Bremner et al. 2000; Sheline et al. 2002; Steffens et al. 2000; Vakili et al 2000). Bremner et al. (2004) then conducted a double-blind, placebo-controlled study to "assess the effects of dexamethasone on verbal declarative memory function in patients with major depression" (p. 812). Fifty-two subjects, 28 with MDD and 24 without MDD, were randomized to receive placebo or dexamethasone. Declarative memory was then assessed with paragraph recall at baseline and day 3. As expected, the nondepressed group on placebo showed memory improvement from day 1 to day 3 consistent with practice effect, whereas the nondepressed group taking dexamethasone showed no change in memory. In contrast, the MDD group taking dexamethasone showed improvement from day 1 to day 3, whereas those taking placebo did not. These findings are consistent with that seen in patients with Cushing's disease. At the other end of the spectrum, Newcomer et al. (1999) demonstrated a decrease in memory performance in healthy volunteers induced by stress-level cortisol administration. Hypercortisolemia, regardless of the etiology, alters declarative memory function. This is likely mediated, at least in part, through direct glucocorticoid effects on the hippocampus.

There is a growing body of literature relating stressful life events to activation of the HPA axis. Using Paykel's Interview for Recent Life Events, Sonino et al. (1988) investigated the presence of stressful life events in 30 consecutive patients with Cushing's syndrome and 30 control subjects. Patients with Cushing's syndrome had significantly more stressful life events. In a larger study in 1993, Sonino et al. noted that patients with the pituitary-dependent form of the disease had a higher number of total negative life events before onset of the disease compared with patients with pituitary-independent Cushing's syndrome. Heim et al. (2000) investigated whether early life stress resulted in a sensitization of the HPA axis later in life in a study involving women without histories of childhood abuse and women with histories of childhood abuse. Women with a history of childhood abuse exhibited increased pituitary-adrenal and autonomic responses to stress compared with the control group of women who experienced no childhood abuse. These investigators proposed that HPA axis and autonomic nervous system hyperreactivity, presumably due to hypersecretion of corticotropin-releasing factor, may be a persistent consequence of childhood abuse and contribute to the vulnerability to psychopathological conditions in adulthood. Because the early studies of HPA axis include assessments of early life stress, it is unclear how significant this factor is in the hypercortisolemia and HPA axis hyperactivity observed in depressed patients.

Carroll et al. (1968) reported nonsuppression of plasma hydroxycorticosteroid levels after administration of dexamethasone in depressed patients. DST nonsuppression has been highly correlated with depression severity, such as psychotic depression (Evans and Nemeroff 1983). Persistent DST nonsuppression may be associated with early relapse or a poorer prognosis (Arana et al. 1985).

Increased levels of CRH have been repeatedly reported in cerebrospinal fluid in depressed patients (Arato et al. 1986; Nemeroff et al. 1984; Risch et al. 1992). In addition, pituitary gland enlargement (Krishnan et al. 1991) and adrenal gland enlargement (Amsterdam et al. 1987; Nemeroff et al. 1992) have also been reported in depressed patients. CRH receptor antagonists are being actively studied as a potential novel class of antidepressants and antianxiety agents.

PHEOCHROMOCYTOMA

CARDINAL FEATURES OF THE DISORDER

Common signs in pheochromocytoma include sustained or paroxysmal hypertension, orthostatic hypotension, hyperhidrosis, hypertensive retinopathy, pallor (very rarely flushing), Raynaud's phenomenon, and livedo reticularis. Prominent symptoms include headache, diaphoresis, palpitations, tremulousness, abdominal or chest pain, nausea, vomiting, and weakness (Manger et al. 1985). In a study of 2,585 hypertensive patients, the symptom triad of headache, palpitations, and diaphoresis was predictive of a diagnosis of pheochromocytoma, with a sensitivity of 93.8%, a specificity of 90.9%, and an exclusion value of 99.9%. The absence of this triad of symptoms reduced the likelihood of pheochromocytoma to less than 1 in 1,000 (Plouin et al. 1981). Diagnosis depends on demonstration of elevated circulating catecholamines, after which localization of the tumor is undertaken (Manger et al. 1985).

PSYCHIATRIC SYMPTOMS IN PHEOCHROMOCYTOMA

Anxiety is the most frequent psychiatric symptom in pheochromocytoma, having been described in 22%–44% of patients with this tumor (Modlin et al. 1979; J.E. Thomas et al. 1966). When other symptoms such as diaphoresis and palpitations are included in this evaluation, the prevalence increases to 86% (Modlin et al. 1979). Although anxiety symptoms are frequently encountered in patients with pheochromocytoma, full syndromal states resembling panic disorder or GAD are relatively uncommon. In a study of 17 patients with pheochromocytoma, only 1 patient fulfilled criteria for possible panic disorder, 2 for GAD, and 2 for major depressive episode. None of the patients experienced the apprehension and fear characteristic of panic attacks, and none had agoraphobia (Starkman et al. 1985). Given the relative rarity of the syndrome even in hypertensive populations, evaluation for pheochromocytoma should probably be reserved for those patients whose anxiety symptoms are accompanied by headache, palpitations, significant blood pressure abnormalities, and diaphoresis.

HYPERPROLACTINEMIA

CARDINAL FEATURES OF THE DISORDER

The primary consequence of hyperprolactinemia is the presence of gonadal dysfunction. Amenorrhea and galactorrhea are the primary manifestations in females, whereas impotence is the primary symptom in males, although gynecomastia and galactorrhea can occur. Diagnosis requires demonstration of an elevated serum prolactin level (>25 ng/mL). Drug-induced causes of hyperprolactinemia (e.g., typical antipsychotics) need to be considered in the differential diagnosis, along with hyperprolactinemia due to other endocrinopathies or due to hepatic or renal disease. Idiopathic hyperprolactinemia and pituitary adenomas constitute the remainder of cases. MRI of the sella is the preferred modality for pituitary imaging. Treatment involves administration of dopamine agonists or surgical resection.

PSYCHIATRIC SYMPTOMS IN HYPERPROLACTINEMIA

Compared with other endocrinopathies, the assessment of the prevalence of psychiatric symptoms and syndromes in patients with hyperprolactinemia has received little attention. To date, no evidence-based assessment of hyperprolactinemic patients has been conducted.

Most of the literature regarding psychiatric manifestations of hyperprolactinemia is focused on symptoms such as aggression and hostility. Data from laboratory animals reveal high levels of aggression in lactating mammals in association with high prolactin levels (Erskine et al. 1978). In humans, the first studies suggesting a relationship between prolactin levels and hostility involved patients with premenstrual syndrome (Steiner et al. 1984). In another investigation, Kellner et al. (1984) used the Kellner Symptom Questionnaire (SQ) to compare hyperprolactinemic patients with family practice patient control subjects, psychiatric patient control subjects, and nonpatient employees. The SQ is a 92-item self-report scale concerning emotional symptoms and statements of well-being. Four scales are contained within the questionnaire concerning depression, anxiety, somatization, and anger-hostility. Hyperprolactinemic patients differed from family practice control subjects and nonpatient employees in the anger-hostility domain of the SQ (Kellner et al. 1984). In another study (Mastrogiacomo et al. 1983), 10 postpartum patients were compared with 10 hyperprolactinemic patients and 10 employee control subjects. Hostility scores were higher in the postpartum group than in either the control subjects or patients with hyperprolactinemia. Depression scores were higher in the hyperprolactinemic patients than in both the postpartum and control subjects (Mastrogiacomo et al. 1983). Hostility and anger are nonspecific symptoms, occurring as a manifestation of normal behavior and noted in increased frequency in a variety of disease states. Although an attempt was made to correlate hostility and depression scales of the SQ, no attempt was made in these studies to evaluate the relationship between hostility and psychiatric diagnostic entities as currently defined.

Bromocriptine, a dopamine agonist used in treating hyperprolactinemia, has been demonstrated to reduce depression, anxiety, and anger-hostility, based on the SQ scales; this improvement in symptoms correlated with a reduced serum prolactin level (Buckman and Kellner 1982). In a double-blind crossover study, six patients with hyperprolactinemia were given bromocriptine, and significant reductions in Ham-D scores were noted (Koppelman et al. 1987). Furthermore, bromocriptine has been demonstrated to have antidepressant properties in primary affectively ill patients (Theohar et al. 1982), as have other dopamine agonists such as pramipexole. All of these data taken together suggest that hyperprolactinemia may contribute to affective symptoms, although the precise relationship between hyperprolactinemia and specific diagnostic syndromes remains to be defined. In a case report, Soygur et al. (1997) described a patient with organic delusional syndrome induced by hyperprolactinemia. The patient's case was notable for the worsening of psychiatric symptoms under bromocriptine therapy and a worsening of her prolactin levels with conventional neuroleptic therapy. The atypical neuroleptic melperone successfully treated her psychotic symptoms without affecting prolactin levels.

HYPERPARATHYROIDISM

CARDINAL FEATURES OF THE DISORDER

The ability to diagnose primary hyperparathyroidism has changed dramatically over the last several decades, primarily because of automated screening laboratory panels (Heath 1991). Most patients today either are asymptomatic or have vague, nonspecific complaints. Fatigue, malaise, weakness, and cognitive complaints are common. Other manifestations include nephrolithiasis, proximal weakness of the lower extremities, chondrocalcinosis, and band keratopathy. Subperiosteal bone resorption and osteitis fibrosa cystica are rarely seen today. Most cases are caused by a solitary adenoma, with hyperplasia of multiple glands being the second most common etiology, usually in the setting of one of the multiple endocrine neoplasia syndromes. Diagnosis depends on demonstration of elevated circulating parathyroid hormone.

PSYCHIATRIC SYMPTOMS IN HYPERPARATHYROIDISM

A variety of psychiatric disturbances have been associated with hyperparathyroidism, including mood, anxiety, psychotic, and cognitive disorders. Most of the literature consists of case reports and small case series; prospective studies have been undertaken more recently. Okamoto et al. (1997) provided a comprehensive review of the literature on the relation of primary hyperparathyroidism to mild hypercalcemia and psychiatric disturbances. Table 21–4 summarizes the case literature. Alarcon and Franceschini (1984) reviewed the early literature and noted that affective and cognitive changes were the predominant symptoms and that most of the patients were elderly women.

In a retrospective series of 33 patients with primary hyperparathyroidism, Karpati and Frame (1964) noted that 14 patients had only psychiatric symptoms, with anxiety symptoms being most common, whereas 4 patients had both depression and cognitive symptoms. Petersen (1968) prospectively evaluated 54 patients with hyperparathyroidism and noted that more than 50% had psychiatric symptoms. Furthermore, he noted that the severity of psychiatric symptoms correlated with the degree of elevated serum calcium.

Review of the case literature reveals that most patients improve with correction of serum calcium. In a prospective study of 18 patients scheduled for hyperparathyroidectomy, Solomon et al. (1994) noted that preoperative symptoms of psychological distress as measured by the Symptom Checklist-90—Revised (SCL-90-R) improved within 1 month after removal of the parathyroid adenoma. In another prospective series of 34 patients with hyperparathyroidism, a detailed neurobehavioral assessment was performed in addition to a psychiatric interview (G.G. Brown et al. 1987). Only 29% of patients with hyperparathyroidism were neurobehaviorally asymptomatic; 32% had signs of affective disorder, and 39% had evidence of cognitive impairment. In addition, the serum calcium increased with progression from the

asymptomatic (mean: 10.9 mg/dL) to the affectively ill (11.3 mg/dL) and cognitively impaired groups (12.2 mg/dL). Despite the correlation between psychiatric syndromes and serum calcium, no improvement occurred with correction of the serum calcium in the series by G.G. Brown et al. (1987). However, Joborn et al. (1988) described a case–control study measuring psychiatric symptom severity before and after parathyroidectomy and found a significant reduction in the Comprehensive Psychopathological Rating Scale 1–1.5 years after surgery. Figure 21–6 illustrates the relationship between serum calcium and the nature of the psychiatric disturbance.

HYPOPARATHYROIDISM

CARDINAL FEATURES OF THE DISORDER

Hypoparathyroidism most commonly occurs as an idiopathic variant and in surgical patients after thyroidectomy. Its most prominent feature is evidence of neuromuscular irritability, ranging from paresthesias to muscle cramps, carpopedal spasm, laryngospasm, and seizures. However, deep tendon reflexes are often decreased or absent. Ocular findings include cataracts and, more rarely, papilledema. Skin changes include alopecia; transverse nail growth; dry, scaling, pigmented skin; and a propensity to develop candidal infections (Juan 1979).

PSYCHIATRIC SYMPTOMS IN HYPOPARATHYROIDISM

Phenomenology

Numerous psychiatric symptoms have been reported in hypoparathyroidism, including irritability and affective, anxiety, psychotic, and cognitive disorders. Cognitive disorders are the most frequently encountered syndromes. Researchers have emphasized the importance of recognizing anxiety features of hypoparathyroidism (Carlson 1986; Lawlor 1988).

The literature on psychiatric manifestations of hypoparathyroidism continues to be dominated by the exhaustive study by Denko and Kaelbling (1962). They reviewed 268 cases of hypoparathyroidism selected for psychiatric symptoms and compared them with 58 cases of pseudohypoparathyroidism and 11 cases of pseudopseudohypoparathyroidism. Among patients with hypoparathyroidism, these investigators noted severe intellectual impairment in 56 patients, organic brain syndromes in 47, psychotic symptoms in 29, and neurotic symptoms in 32. Fifty-seven patients were considered to have undiagnosable psychiatric illness, yet scrutiny of the data reveals that several of these patients had affective and anxiety symptoms.

TABLE 21–4.   Psychiatric symptoms in hyperparathyroidism: case reports

Study	Age/sex	Symptoms	Serum Ca^{2+} (mg/dL)	Improved with treatment
Fitz and Hallman 1952	55/M	Psychosis	14	Yes
	52/M	Delirium	19	Yes
Nielsen 1955	47/F	Mood symptoms	13	Yes
Bogdonoff 1956	58/F	Depression/anxiety	15.4	
W.C. Thomas 1958	69/F	Delirium	18.3	
Lehrer and Levitt 1960	62/F	Delirium	13.3	No (died)
Reinfrank 1961	38/M	Depression	11.1	Yes
Agras and Oliveau 1964	64/F	Psychotic depression	15	Yes
Karpati and Frame 1964	40/F	Depression	12.8	Yes
	64/F	Depression/anxiety	11.6	Yes
	?/F	Delirium	12.2	Yes
	43/F	Anxiety/obsessive-compulsive symptoms	11.6	Yes
Reilly and Wilson 1965	34/M	Psychosis	11.6	Yes
	62/F	Delirium	12.2	Yes
	67/F	Anxiety/depression	13.8	Yes
Jacobs and Merritt 1966	63/F	Delirium	21.2	Yes
Noble 1974	53/F	Depression	14.2	No
Gatewood et al. 1975	63/M	Delirium	11.9	Yes
Rosenblatt and Faillace 1977	30/M	Psychosis	12.9	Yes
Alarcon and Franceschini 1984	53/F	Psychosis	13	Yes
Kleinfeld et al. 1984	67/F	Psychosis	13.2	Yes
Borer and Bhanot 1985	45/F	Depression/delirium	12.3	Yes
Oztunc et al. 1986	45/M	Delirium	12.4	No (suicide 4 months later)
G.G. Brown et al. 1987	49/F	Depression/anxiety	11.4	No
	60/F	Depression/anxiety	11.2	No
	73/F	Anxiety	10.9	No
	59/F	Psychosis/cognitive changes	12.5	No
R.S. Brown et al. 1987	68/M	Psychosis	12.3	Yes
Hayabara et al. 1987	68/F	Psychosis	11	Yes
	60/F	Delirium	15	Yes
Thurling 1987	52/F	Psychosis	14.8	Yes
Watson and Marx 2002	63/M	Psychosis	11.1	Yes

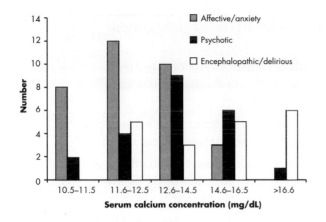

FIGURE 21–6. Psychiatric symptoms in hyperparathyroidism: phenomenological association with changes in serum calcium.

Source. Adapted from Peterson et al. 1968, updated to include case data from Table 21–4.

Several differences emerged between patients with surgical hypoparathyroidism and those with the idiopathic form. Although the overall prevalence of cognitive dysfunction was approximately 50% in both groups, isolated intellectual dysfunction was more uncommon in patients with surgical hypoparathyroidism (3.7% versus 19.0%), and delirium was much more prevalent in the surgical patients (29.2% versus 17.2%). Depressive, psychotic, and anxiety symptoms were more common in the surgical group than in the patients with idiopathic hypoparathyroidism. Depressive symptoms were present in 13.2% of surgical patients, compared with 4.9% of the idiopathic group. Psychotic symptoms were present in 19.8% of surgical patients, compared with 6.2% of the patients with idiopathic hypoparathyroidism. Anxiety symptoms were noted in 17.9% of surgical cases, whereas 11.7% of idiopathic cases were characterized by anxiety. Interestingly, manic symptoms were equally represented in both groups, being present in 4.3% of idiopathic hypoparathyroid patients and 4.7% of surgical patients. These results are summarized in Figure 21–7.

Improvement With Treatment

The overwhelming majority of the patients in the Denko and Kaelbling (1962) series improved in their psychiatric symptoms with treatment of the underlying hypoparathyroidism. Seventy-four percent of the idiopathic hypoparathyroidism patients improved, compared with 79% of the surgical patients. Residual symptoms were noted in many of the patients. Other investigators have noted

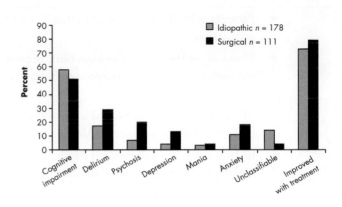

FIGURE 21–7. Psychiatric symptoms in hypoparathyroidism.

Source. Adapted from Denko and Kaelbling 1962.

improved symptoms with correction of serum calcium concentration (Carlson 1986; Gertner et al. 1976; Hossain 1970; Lawlor 1988).

CONCLUSION

The foregoing review represents a clinically oriented discussion of the prevalence and phenomenology of psychiatric symptoms in endocrine disease. It remains unknown whether the associated psychiatric disturbances are directly the result of primary metabolic derangement in each endocrine disorder or are due to some heretofore unknown factors. The pathophysiological mechanisms involved in the development of psychiatric symptoms in endocrine disturbances undoubtedly vary with the particular endocrine disorder. Therefore, an understanding of the phenomenology of these relationships is also critical to developing hypotheses concerning the precise mechanisms by which endocrine disorders can produce psychiatric symptoms.

It appears that the severity of the endocrine disturbance is often correlated with the prevalence or severity of psychiatric symptoms, although this is not always the case. In addition, it is important to note that serious psychiatric syndromes are often present in only a minority of patients. Potential risk factors (e.g., genetic predisposition) for the development of psychiatric symptoms in endocrine disease need to be identified as well. Continued neuroendocrine studies with these patients will be important to enhance our understanding of the pathophysiology of their psychiatric symptoms.

Highlights for the Clinician

- Patients with **diabetes** are at two to three times the risk for depression of the general population.

- There is evidence that the long-term presence of diabetes imparts a risk of cognitive impairment. Furthermore, poor metabolic control appears to worsen the deleterious effects of diabetes on cognition.

- Many studies have identified a relationship between diabetes and dementia. This includes both vascular dementia and Alzheimer's disease, though the mechanisms appear to differ.

- In patients with diabetes and depression, once the depression has been treated effectively, remission of symptoms is sustained only 10% of the time over the course of the following 5 years. Furthermore, relapses occur at a rate of approximately once a year.

- Patients with **hypothyroidism** frequently exhibit cognitive, affective, psychotic, and anxiety symptoms.

- Disturbances in cognition are the most commonly reported psychiatric symptom in hypothyroidism, occurring in 46.3% of unselected cases and 48.2% of psychiatrically ill hypothyroid patients.

- Depression is the second most frequent psychiatric syndrome to occur in unselected hypothyroid patients.

- Although many authors have emphasized the ubiquitous presence of psychiatric symptoms in patients with **hyperthyroidism,** scrutiny of the literature suggests that serious psychopathology occurs in only a minority of patients.

- Major depression is the most common psychiatric manifestation of hyperthyroidism, occurring in approximately 28% of unselected patients.

- Whybrow and Hurwitz (1976) reviewed the literature and found that 35.0% of patients with **Cushing's syndrome** reported depressive symptoms, compared with 3.7% who reported mania. Delirium was noted in 16.2% and psychosis in 9.3% of patients.

- Depressive symptoms resolve in 70% of Cushing's syndrome patients with correction in serum cortisol.

- In patients with Cushing's syndrome, there is a correlation between elevated cortisol levels, reduced hippocampal formation volume (HFV), multiple cognitive tasks (particularly verbal learning), and memory dysfunction. After treatment of Cushing's syndrome, it has been demonstrated that HFV increased after cortisol levels returned to normal concentrations.

- **Exogenous corticosteroid administration** imparts approximately three times the 12-month period prevalence of major depression seen in nontreated subjects, regardless of age, gender, and perceived health.

- **Hypercortisolemia** appears to represent a state as opposed to a trait marker for depression.

- A growing body of literature relates **stressful life events** to activation of the hypothalamic-pituitary-adrenal (HPA) axis. Investigators propose that HPA axis and autonomic nervous system hyperreactivity, presumably due to hypersecretion of corticotropin-releasing factor, may be a persistent consequence of childhood abuse and contribute to a vulnerability to psychopathological conditions in adulthood.

RECOMMENDED READINGS

Egede LE: Effect of comorbid chronic diseases on prevalence and odds of depression in adults with diabetes. Psychosom Med 67:46–51, 2005

Gillespie CF, Nemeroff CB: Hypercortisolemia and depression. Psychosom Med 67 (suppl 1):S26–S28, 2005

Patten SB: Exogenous corticosteroids and major depression in the general population. J Psychosom Res 49:447–449, 2000

REFERENCES

Abbas A, Styra R: Valproate prophylaxis against steroid-induced psychosis. Can J Psychiatry 39:188–189, 1994

Addison T: Disease of the supra-renal capsules, in Collection of the Published Writings of the Late Thomas Addison. London, UK, New Sydenham Society, 1868, pp 209–239

Agras S, Oliveau DC: Primary hyperparathyroidism and psychosis. Can Med Assoc J 91:1366–1367, 1964

Alarcon RD, Franceschini JA: Hyperparathyroidism and paranoid psychosis: case report and review of the literature. Br J Psychiatry 145:477–486, 1984

Alvarez MA, Gomez A, Alvarez E, et al: Short communication attention disturbance in Graves' disease. Psychoneuroendocrinology 8:451–454, 1983

American Diabetes Association: Diagnosis and classification of diabetes mellitus. Diabetes Care 28:S37–S42, 2005

American Psychiatric Association: Diagnostic and Statistical Manual of Mental Disorders, 3rd Edition. Washington, DC, American Psychiatric Association, 1980

American Psychiatric Association: Diagnostic and Statistical Manual of Mental Disorders, 3rd Edition, Revised. Washington, DC, American Psychiatric Association, 1987

Amsterdam JD, Marinelli DL, Arger P, et al: Assessment of adrenal gland volume by computed tomography in depressed patients and healthy volunteers. Psychiatry Res 21:189–197, 1987

Anderson RJ, Freedland KE, Clouse RE, et al: The prevalence of comorbid depression in adults with diabetes. Diabetes Care 24:1069–1078, 2001

Anderson RJ, Grigsby AB, Freedland KE, et al: Anxiety and poor glycemic control: a meta-analytic review of the literature. Int J Psychiatry Med 32:235–247, 2002

Appelhof BC, Brouwer JP, van Dyck R, et al: Triiodothyronine addition to paroxetine in the treatment of major depressive disorder. J Clin Endocrinol Metab 89:6271–6276, 2004

Arana GW, Baldessarini RJ, Ornsteen M: The dexamethasone suppression test for diagnosis and prognosis in psychiatry. Arch Gen Psychiatry 42:1193–1204, 1985

Arato M, Banki CM, Nemeroff CB: Hypothalamic-pituitary-adrenal axis and suicide. Ann N Y Acad Sci 487:263–270, 1986

Artunkal S, Togrol B: Psychological studies in hyperthyroidism. Brain Thyroid Relationships 92–114, 1964

Asher R: Myxoedematous madness. BMJ 2:555–562, 1949

Austin EJ, Deary IJ: Effects of repeated hypoglycemia on cognitive function: a psychometrically validated reanalysis of the Diabetes Control and Complications Trial data. Diabetes Care 22:1273–1277, 1999

Baldini IM, Vita A, Mauri MC, et al: Psychopathological and cognitive features in subclinical hypothyroidism. Prog Neuropsychopharmacol Biol Psychiatry 21:925–935, 1997

Banki CM, Bissette G, Arato M, et al: Elevation of immunoreactive CSF TRH in depressed patients. Am J Psychiatry 145:1526–1531, 1988

Bardgett ME, Taylor GT, Csernansky JG, et al: Chronic corticosterone treatment impairs spontaneous alternation behavior in rats. Behav Neural Biol 61:186–190, 1994

Bauer MS, Whybrow PC: Thyroid hormones and the central nervous system in affective illness: interactions that may have clinical significance. Integr Psychiatry 6:75–100, 1988

Belanoff JK, Flores BH, Kalezhan M, et al: Rapid reversal of psychotic depression using mifepristone. J Clin Psychopharmacol 21:516–521, 2001a

Belanoff JK, Gross K, Yager A, et al: Corticosteroids and cognition. J Psychiatr Res 35:127–145, 2001b

Belanoff JK, Rothschild AJ, Cassidy F, et al: An open label trial of C-1073 (mifepristone) for psychotic major depression. Biol Psychiatry 52:386–392, 2002

Bender BG, Lerner JA, Poland JE: Association between corticosteroids and psychologic change in hospitalized asthmatic children. Ann Allergy 66:414–419, 1991

Bertram L, Blacker D, Mullin K, et al: Evidence for genetic linkage of Alzheimer's disease to chromosome 10q. Science 290:2302–2303, 2000

Bewsher PD, Gardiner AQ, Hedley AJ, et al: Psychosis after acute alteration of thyroid status. Psychol Med 1:260–262, 1971

Bogdonoff MD: Hyperparathyroidism. Am J Med 21:583–595, 1956

Borer MS, Bhanot VK: Hyperparathyroidism: neuropsychiatric manifestations. Psychosomatics 26:597–601, 1985

Boston Collaborative Drug Surveillance Program: Acute adverse reactions to prednisone in relation to dosage. Clin Pharmacol Ther 13:694–698, 1972

Bremner JD: Structural changes in the brain in depression and relationship to symptom recurrence. CNS Spectr 7:129–139, 2002

Bremner JD, Narayan M, Anderson ER, et al: Hippocampal volume reduction in major depression. Am J Psychiatry 157:115–188, 2000

Bremner JD, Vythilingam M, Vermetten E, et al: Effects of glucocorticoids on declarative memory function in major depression. Biol Psychiatry 55:811–815, 2004

Brismar T, Hyllienmark, Ekberg K, et al: Loss of temporal lobe beta power in young adults with type 1 diabetes mellitus. Neuroreport 13:2469–2473, 2002

Brown ES, Suppes T, Khan DA, et al: Mood changes during prednisone bursts in outpatients with asthma. J Clin Psychopharmacol 22:55–61, 2002

Brown ES, Frol A, Bobadilla L, et al: Effect of lamotrigine on mood and cognition in patients receiving chronic exogenous corticosteroids. Psychosomatics 44:204–208, 2003

Brown ES, Chamberlain W, Dhanani N, et al: An open-label trial of olanzapine for corticosteroid-induced mood symptoms. J Affect Disord 83:277–281, 2004a

Brown ES, Woolston DJ, Frol A, et al: Hippocampal volume, spectroscopy, cognition, and mood in patients receiving corticosteroid therapy. Biol Psychiatry 55:538–545, 2004b

Brown ES, Stuard G, Liggin JDM, et al: Effect of phenytoin on mood and declarative memory during prescription corticosteroid therapy. Biol Psychiatry 57:543–548, 2005

Brown GG, Preisman RC, Kleerkoper M: Neurobehavioral symptoms in mild primary hyperparathyroidism: related to hypercalcemia but not improved by parathyroidectomy. Henry Ford Hosp Med J 35:211–215, 1987

Brown RS, Fischman A, Showalter CR: Primary hyperparathyroidism, hypercalcemia, paranoid delusions, homicide and attempted murder. J Forensic Sci 32:1460–1463, 1987

Brunetti A, Fulham MJ, Aloj L, et al: Decreased brain glucose utilization in patients with Cushing's disease. J Nucl Med 39:786–790, 1998

Buckman MT, Kellner R: Reduction of distress in hyperprolactinemia with bromocriptine. Am J Psychiatry 142:242–244, 1982

Bunevicius R, Kazanavicius G, Zalinkevicius R, et al: Effects of thyroxine as compared with thyroxine plus triiodothyronine in patients with hypothyroidism. N Engl J Med 340:424–429, 1999

Bunney WE, Fawcett SA: Possibility of a biochemical test for suicide potential. Arch Gen Psychiatry 13:232–239, 1965

Bursten B: Psychosis associated with thyrotoxicosis. Arch Gen Psychiatry 4:267–273, 1961

Campbell IA: Aggressive psychosis in AIDS patient on high-dose steroids. Lancet 2:750–751, 1987

Carlson RJ: Longitudinal observations of two cases of organic anxiety syndrome. Psychosomatics 27:529–531, 1986

Carnethon MR, Kinder LS, Fair JM, et al: Symptoms of depression as a risk factor for incident diabetes: findings from the National Health and Nutrition Examination epidemiologic follow-up study. Am J Epidemiol 158:416–423, 2003

Carney C: Diabetes mellitus and major depressive disorder: an overview of prevalence, complications, and treatment. Depress Anxiety 7:149–157, 1998

Carroll BJ, Martin FI, Davis B: Pituitary-adrenal function in depression. Lancet 1:1373–1374, 1968

Carta MG, Loviselli A, Hardoy MC, et al: The link between thyroid autoimmunity (antithyroid peroxidase autoantibodies) with anxiety and mood disorders in the community: a field of interest for public health in the future. BMC Psychiatry 4:25, 2004

Centers for Disease Control and Prevention: National Center for Chronic Disease Prevention and Health Promotion. Diabetes Public Health Resource. Available at: http://www.cdc.gov/diabetes/statistics/prev/national/figpersons.htm. Accessed February 28, 2007.

Clark LD, Quarton GC, Cobb S, et al: Further observations on mental disturbances associated with cortisone and ACTH therapy. N Engl J Med 249:178–183, 1953

Clower CG, Young AJ, Kepas D: Psychotic states resulting from disorders of thyroid function. Johns Hopkins Med J 124:305–310, 1969

Cohen SI: Cushing's syndrome: a psychiatric study of 29 patients. Br J Psychiatry 136:120–124, 1980

Cohen ST, Welch G, Jacobson AM, et al: The association of lifetime psychiatric illness and increased retinopathy in patients with type I diabetes mellitus. Psychosomatics 38:98–108, 1997

Cohen-Cole S, Brown FW, McDaniel JS: Assessment of depression and grief reactions in the medically ill, in Psychiatric Care of the Medical Patient. Edited by Stoudemire A, Fogel BS. New York, Oxford University Press, 1993, pp 53–70

Constant EL, De Volder AG, Ivanoiu A, et al: Cerebral blood flow and glucose metabolism in hypothyroidism: a positron emission tomography study. J Clin Endocrinol Metab 86:3864–3870, 2001

Cooper DS, Halpern R, Wood LC, et al: L-Thyroxine therapy in subclinical hypothyroidism: a double-blind placebo controlled trial. Ann Intern Med 101:18–24, 1984

Cowdry RW, Wehr TA, Ziz AP, et al: Thyroid abnormalities associated with rapid-cycling bipolar illness. Arch Gen Psychiatry 40:414–420, 1983

Crown S: Notes on an experimental study of intellectual deterioration. BMJ 2:684–685, 1949

Cushing H: The basophil adenomas of the pituitary body and their clinical manifestations (pituitary basophilism). Bull Johns Hopkins Hosp 50:137–195, 1932

Davidson JRT, Connor KM: Treatment of anxiety disorders, in The American Psychiatric Publishing Textbook of Psychopharmacology, 3rd Edition. Edited by Schatzberg AF, Nemeroff CB. Arlington, VA, American Psychiatric Publishing 2004, pp 913–934

Davidson J, Watkins L, Owens MJ, et al: Effects of paroxetine and venlafaxine-XR on heart rate variability in depression. J Clin Psychopharmacol 25:1–5, 2005

Deary IJ, Hepburn DA, MacLeod KM, et al: Partitioning the symptoms of hypoglycemia using multi-sample confirmatory factor analysis. Diabetologia 36:771–777, 1993

de Groot M, Jacobson AM, Samson JA, et al: Glycemic control and major depression in patients with type 1 and type 2 diabetes mellitus. J Psychosom Res 46:425–435, 1999

de Groot M, Anderson R, Freedland KE, et al: Association of depression and diabetes complications: a meta-analysis. Psychosom Med 63:619–630, 2001

Denko J, Kaelbling R: The psychiatric aspects of hypoparathyroidism. Acta Psychiatr Scand Suppl 164:1–70, 1962

Diabetes Control and Complications Trial Research Group: The effect of intensive treatment of diabetes on the development and progression of long-term complications in insulin-dependent diabetes mellitus. N Engl J Med 329:977–986, 1993

Diabetes Control and Complications Trial Research Group: Effects of intensive diabetes therapy on neuropsychological function in adults in the Diabetes Control and Complications Trial. Ann Intern Med 124:379–388, 1996

Dietch JT: Diagnosis of organic anxiety disorders. Psychosomatics 22:661–669, 1981

D'Orban PT: Steroid-induced psychosis (letter). Lancet 2:684, 1989

Easson WM: Myxedema with psychosis. Arch Gen Psychiatry 14:277–283, 1966

Eaton WW, Armenian H, Gallo J, et al: Depression and risk for onset of type II diabetes: a prospective population-based study. Diabetes Care 19:1097–1102, 1996

Egede LE: Effect of comorbid chronic diseases on prevalence and odds of depression in adults with diabetes. Psychosom Med 67:46–51, 2005

Engel GL, Margolin SG: Neuropsychiatric disturbances in Addison's disease and the role of impaired carbohydrate metabolism in production of abnormal cerebral function. Arch Neurol Psychiatry 45:881–884, 1941

Erskine MS, Barfield JR, Goldman BD: Intraspecific fighting during late pregnancy and lactation in rats and effects of litter removal. Behav Neural Biol 23:206–213, 1978

Esposito S, Prange AJ, Golden RN: The thyroid axis and mood disorders: overview and future prospects. Psychopharmacol Bull 33:205–217, 1997

Evans D, Nemeroff CB: Use of dexamethasone suppression test using DSM-III criteria on an inpatient psychiatric unit. Biol Psychiatry 18:505–511, 1983

Extein I, Pottash ALC, Gold MS: The thyrotropin-releasing hormone test in the diagnosis of unipolar depression. Psychiatry Res 5:311–316, 1981

Fahrenfort JJ, Wilterdink AM, van der Veen EA: Long-term residual complaints and psychosocial sequelae after remission of hyperthyroidism. Psychoneuroendocrinology 25:201–211, 2000

Falk WE, Mahnke MW, Pozkanzer DC: Lithium prophylaxis of corticotropin-induced psychosis. JAMA 241:1011–1012, 1979

Fang VS, Jaspan JB: Delirium and neuromuscular symptoms in an elderly man with isolated corticotroph-deficiency syndrome completely reversed with glucocorticoid replacement. J Clin Endocrinol Metab 69:1073–1077, 1989

Farris W, Mansourian S, Chang Y, et al: Insulin-degrading enzyme regulates the levels of insulin, amyloid β-protein, and the β-amyloid precursor protein intracellular domain in vivo. Proc Natl Acad Sci U S A 100:4162–4167, 2003

Ferguson SC, Blane A, Perros P, et al: Cognitive ability and brain structure in type 1 diabetes: relation to microangiopathy and preceding severe hypoglycemia. Diabetes 52:149–156, 2003a

Ferguson SC, Deary IJ, Evans JC, et al: Apolipoprotein-E influences aspects of intellectual ability in type 1 diabetes. Diabetes 52:145–148, 2003b

Fitz TE, Hallman BL: Mental changes associated with hyperparathyroidism. Arch Intern Med 89:547–551, 1952

Ford ES: Leukocyte count, erythrocyte sedimentation rate, and diabetes incidence in a national sample of US adults. Am J Epidemiol 155:57–64, 2002

Forget H, Lacroix A, Somma M, et al: Cognitive decline in patients with Cushing's syndrome. J Int Neuropsychol Soc 6:20–29, 2000

Fountoulakis KN, Iacovides A, Grammaticos P, et al: Thyroid function in clinical subtypes of major depression: an exploratory study. BMC Psychiatry 4:6, 2004

Gatewood JW, Organ CH, Mead BT: Mental changes associated with hyperparathyroidism. Am J Psychiatry 132:129–132, 1975

Gavard JA, Lustman PJ, Clouse RE: Prevalence of depression in adults with diabetes: an epidemiological evaluation. Diabetes Care 16:1167–1178, 1993

Gertner JM, Hodsman AB, Neuberger JN: 1-Alpha-hydroxycalciferol in the treatment of hypocalcaemic psychosis. Clin Endocrinol (Oxf) 5:539–543, 1976

Ghazi AAM, Mofid D, Rahimi F, et al: Oestrogen and cortisol producing adrenal tumor. Arch Dis Child 71:358–359, 1994

Ghosh S, Watanabe RM, Valle TT, et al: The Finland-United States investigation of non-insulin-dependent diabetes mellitus genetics (FUSION) study, I: an autosomal genome scan for genes that predispose to type 2 diabetes. Am J Hum Genet 67:1174–1185, 2000

Gillespie CF, Nemeroff CB: Hypercortisolemia and depression. Psychosom Med 67 (suppl 1):526–528, 2005

Glynne-Jones R, Vernon CC: Is steroid psychosis preventable by divided doses (letter)? Lancet 2:1404, 1986

Gold MS, Pottash ALC, Extein I: Hypothyroidism and depression: evidence from complete thyroid function evaluation. JAMA 245:1919–1922, 1981

Gold MS, Pottash ALC, Extein I: "Symptomless" autoimmune thyroiditis in depression. Psychiatry Res 6:261–269, 1982

Golden MP, Ingersoll GM, Brack CJ, et al: Longitudinal relationship of asymptomatic hypoglycemia to cognitive function in IDDM. Diabetes Care 12:89–93, 1989

Goodnick PJ, Henry JH, Buki VMV: Treatment of depression in patients with diabetes. J Clin Psychiatry 56:128–136, 1995

Gotch PM: Cushing's syndrome from the patient's perspective. Endocrinol Metab Clin North Am 23:607–617, 1994

Grandinetti A, Kaholokula JK, Crabbe KM, et al: Relationship between depressive symptoms and diabetes among native Hawaiians. Psychoneuroendocrinology 25:239–246, 2000

Greer S, Ramsay I, Bagley C: Neurotoxic and thyrotoxic anxiety: clinical, psychological and physiological measurements. Br J Psychiatry 122:549–554, 1973

Gregg EW, Yaffe K, Cauley JA, et al: Is diabetes associated with cognitive impairment and cognitive decline among older women? Study of Osteoporotic Fractures Research Group. Arch Intern Med 160:174–180, 2000

Grigsby AB, Anderson RJ, Freedland KE, et al: Prevalence of anxiety in adults with diabetes: a systematic review. J Psychosom Res 53:1053–1060, 2002

Haan MN, Shemanski L, Jagust WJ, et al: The role of APOE epsilon4 in modulating effects of other risk factors for cognitive decline in elderly persons. JAMA 282:40–46, 1999

Haggerty JJ, Evans DL, Prange AJ: Organic brain syndrome associated with marginal hypothyroidism. Am J Psychiatry 143:785–786, 1986

Haggerty JJ, Stern RA, Mason GA, et al: Subclinical hypothyroidism: a modifiable risk factor for depression? Am J Psychiatry 150:508–510, 1993

Hall RCW, Popkin MK, Stickney SK, et al: Presentation of the steroid psychosis. J Nerv Ment Dis 167:229–236, 1979

Hall RCW, Popkin MK, DeVaul R, et al: Psychiatric manifestations of Hashimoto's thyroiditis. Psychosomatics 23:337–342, 1982

Halonen H, Hiekkala H, Huupponen T, et al: A follow-up EEG study in diabetic children. Ann Clin Res 15:167–172, 1983

Hannonen R, Tupola S, Ahonen T, et al: Neurocognitive functioning in children with type-1 diabetes with and without episodes of severe hypoglycaemia. Dev Med Child Neurol 45:262–268, 2003

Hart SP, Frier BM: Causes, management and morbidity of acute hypoglycaemia in adults requiring hospital admission. QJM 91:505–510, 1998

Haskett RF: Diagnostic categorization of psychiatric disturbance in Cushing's syndrome. Am J Psychiatry 142:911–916, 1985

Haumont D, Dorchy H, Pelc S: EEG abnormalities in diabetic children: influence of hypoglycemia and vascular complications. Clin Pediatr (Phila) 18:750–753, 1979

Hayabara T, Hashimoto K, Izumi H, et al: Neuropsychiatric disorders in primary hyperparathyroidism. Jpn J Psychiatry Neurol 41:33–40, 1987

Hayreh SS, Watson PG: Prednisolone-21-stearoylglycolate in scleritis. Br J Ophthalmol 54:394–398, 1970

Heath H III: Clinical spectrum of primary hyperparathyroidism: evolution with changes in medical practice and technology. J Bone Miner Res 6 (suppl 2):S63–S70, 1991

Heim C, Newport D, Heit S, et al: Pituitary-adrenal and autonomic responses to stress in women after sexual and physical abuse in childhood. JAMA 284:592–597, 2000

Hermann HT, Quarton GC: Psychological changes and psychogenesis in thyroid hormone disorders. J Clin Endocrinol Metab 25:327–338, 1965

Hershey T, Lillie R, Sadler M, et al: Severe hypoglycemia and long-term spatial memory in children with type 1 diabetes mellitus: a retrospective study. J Int Neuropsychol Soc 9:740–750, 2003

Hofeldt FD: Reactive hypoglycemia. Endocrinol Metab Clin North Am 18:185–201, 1989

Horwitz DL: Factitious and artifactual hypoglycemia. Endocrinol Metab Clin North Am 18:203–210, 1989

Hossain M: Neurologic and psychiatric manifestations in idiopathic hypoparathyroidism: response to treatment. J Neurol Neurosurg Psychiatry 33:153–156, 1970

Howorka K, Pumprla J, Saletu B, et al: Decrease of vigilance assessed by EEG-mapping in type I diabetic patients with history of recurrent severe hypoglycaemia. Psychoneuroendocrinology 25:85–105, 2000

Irwin R, Ellis PM, Delahunt J: Psychosis following acute alteration of thyroid status. Aust N Z J Psychiatry 31:762–764, 1997

Jacobs JK, Merritt CR: Magnesium deficiency in hyperparathyroidism: case report of toxic psychosis. Ann Surg 162:260–262, 1966

Jain VK: A psychiatric study of hypothyroidism. Psychiatrica Clinica 5:121–130, 1972

Jeffcoate WJ, Silverstone JT, Edwards CRW, et al: Psychiatric manifestations of Cushing's syndrome: response to lowering of plasma cortisol. QJM 191:465–472, 1979

Jellinek EH: Fits, faints, coma, and dementia in myxoedema. Lancet 2:1010–1012, 1962

Jimenez IM, Goodnick P: Depression in patients with diabetes mellitus. Dir Psychiatry 19:231–248, 1999

Joborn C, Hetta J, Rastad J, et al: Psychiatric symptoms and cerebrospinal fluid monoamine metabolites in primary hyperparathyroidism. Biol Psychiatry 23:149–158, 1988

Joffe RT, Levitt AJ: Major depression and subclinical hypothyroidism. Psychoneuroendocrinology 17:215–221, 1992

Joffe RT, Sokolov STH: Thyroid hormones, the brain, and affective disorders. Crit Rev Neurobiol 8:45–63, 1994

Joffe RT, Kutcher S, MacDonald C: Thyroid function and bipolar affective disorder. Psychiatry Res 25:117–121, 1988

Joffe RT, Singer W, Levitt AJ, et al: A placebo-controlled comparison of lithium and triiodothyronine augmentation of tricyclic antidepressants in unipolar refractory depression. Arch Gen Psychiatry 50:387–394, 1993

Jonas AD: Hypothyroidism and neurotic depression. Am Pract Dig Treat 3:103–105, 1952

Josephson AM, MacKenzie TB: Appearance of manic psychosis following rapid normalization of thyroid status. Am J Psychiatry 136:846–847, 1979

Juan D: Hypocalcemia: differential diagnosis and mechanisms. Arch Intern Med 139:1166–1171, 1979

Karpati G, Frame B: Neuropsychiatric disorders in primary hyperparathyroidism. Arch Neurol 10:387–397, 1964

Katerndahl DA, Vande Creek L: Hyperthyroidism and panic attacks. Psychosomatics 24:491–496, 1983

Kathol RG, Delahunt JW: The relationship of anxiety and depression to symptoms of hyperthyroidism using operational criteria. Gen Hosp Psychiatry 8:23–28, 1986

Kawakami N, Takatsuka N, Shimizu H, et al: Depressive symptoms and occurrence of type 2 diabetes among Japanese men. Diabetes Care 22:1071–1076, 1999

Kellner R, Buckman MT, Fava M, et al: Prolactin, aggression, and hostility: a discussion of recent studies. Psychiatr Dev 2:131–138, 1984

Kelly WF, Checkley SA, Bender DA, et al: Cushing's syndrome and depression: a prospective study of 26 patients. Br J Psychiatry 142:16–19, 1983

Kelly WF, Kelly MJ, Faragher B: A prospective study of psychiatric and psychological aspects of Cushing's syndrome. Clin Endocrinol (Oxf) 45:715–720, 1996

Kessler RC, McGonagle KA, Zhao S, et al: Lifetime and 12-month prevalence of DSM-III-R psychiatric disorders in the United States: results from the National Comorbidity Survey. Arch Gen Psychiatry 51:8–19, 1994

Kiraly SF, Ancill RJ, Dimitrova G: The relationship of endogenous cortisol to psychiatric disorder: a review. Can J Psychiatry 42:415–420, 1997

Kirkegaard CJ, Faber J, Hummer L, et al: Increased levels of TRH in cerebrospinal fluid from patients with endogenous depression. Psychoneuroendocrinology 4:227–235, 1979

Klee GC, Hay ID: Assessment of sensitive thyrotropin assays for an expanded role in thyroid function testing: proposed criteria for analytic performance and clinical utility. J Clin Endocrinol Metab 64:461–471, 1986

Klein R, Klein BE, Moss SE, et al: Glycosylated hemoglobin predicts the incidence and progression of diabetic retinopathy. JAMA 260:2864–2871, 1988

Kleinfeld M, Peter S, Gilbert GM: Delirium as the predominant manifestation of hyperparathyroidism: reversal after parathyroidectomy. J Am Geriatr Soc 32:689–690, 1984

Kleinschmidt HJ, Waxenberg SE, Cuker R: Psychophysiology and psychiatric management of thyrotoxicosis: a two year follow-up study. J Mt Sinai Hosp N Y 23:131–153, 1956

Knopman D, Boland LL, Mosley T, et al: Cardiovascular risk factors and cognitive decline in middle-aged adults. Neurology 56:42–48, 2001

Koppelman MCS, Parry BL, Hamilton JA, et al: Effect of bromocriptine on affect and libido in hyperprolactinemia. Am J Psychiatry 144:1037–1041, 1987

Kovacs M, Obrosky DS, Goldstone D, et al: Major depressive disorder in youth with IDDM: a controlled prospective study of course and outcome. Diabetes Care 20:45–51, 1997

Krausz Y, Freedman N, Lester H, et al: Regional cerebral blood flow in patients with mild hypothyroidism. J Nucl Med 45:1712–1715, 2004

Krishnan KRR, Doraiswamy PM, Lurie SN, et al: Pituitary size in depression. J Clin Endocrinol Metab 72:256–259, 1991

Langan SJ, Deary IJ, Hepburn DA, et al: Cumulative cognitive impairment following recurrent severe hypoglycaemia in adult patients with insulin-treated diabetes mellitus. Diabetalogia 34:337–344, 1991

Lawlor BA: Hypocalcemia, hypoparathyroidism, and organic anxiety syndrome. J Clin Psychiatry 49:317–318, 1988

Leedom L, Meehan WP, Procci W, et al: Symptoms of depression in patients with type II diabetes mellitus. Psychosomatics 32:280–286, 1991

Lehrer G, Levitt M: Neuropsychiatric presentation of hypercalcemia. J Mt Sinai Hosp N Y 27:10–18, 1960

Lewis DA, Kathol RG, Sherman BM, et al: Differentiation of depressive subtypes by insulin insensitivity in the recovered phase. Arch Gen Psychiatry 40:167–170, 1983

Libow LS, Durell J: Clinical studies on the relationship between psychosis and the regulation of thyroid gland activity. Psychosom Med 27:369–376, 1965

Lidz T, Whitehorn JC: Psychiatric problems in a thyroid clinic. JAMA 139:698–701, 1949

Lincoln NB, Faleiro RM, Kelly C, et al: Effect of long-term glycemic control on cognitive function. Diabetes Care 19:656–658, 1996

Ling MH, Perry PJ, Tsuang MT: Side effects of corticosteroid therapy: psychiatric aspects. Arch Gen Psychiatry 38:741–747, 1981

Logothetis J: Psychotic behavior as the initial indicator of adult myxedema. J Nerv Ment Dis 136:561–568, 1963

Loosen PT, Chambliss R, DeBold CR, et al: Psychiatric phenomenology in Cushing's disease. Pharmacopsychiatry 25:192–198, 1992

Luchsinger JA, Tang M, Stern Y, et al: Diabetes mellitus and risk of Alzheimer's disease and dementia with stroke in a multiethnic cohort. Am J Epidemiol 154:635–641, 2001

Lustman PJ, Clouse RE: Treatment of depression in diabetes: impact on mood and medical outcomes. J Psychosom Res 53:917–924, 2002

Lustman PJ, Harper GW: Nonpsychiatric physicians' identification and treatment of depression in patients with diabetes. Compr Psychiatry 28:22–27, 1987

Lustman PJ, Harper GW, Griffith LS, et al: Use of the Diagnostic Interview Schedule in patients with diabetes mellitus. J Nerv Ment Dis 174:743–746, 1986

Lustman PJ, Clouse RE, Carney RM, et al: Characteristics of depression in adults with diabetes, in Proceedings of the National Institute of Mental Health Conference on Mental Disorders in the General Health Care Setting, Vol 1. Seattle, WA, 1987, pp 127–129

Lustman PJ, Griffith LS, Clouse RE: Depression in adults with diabetes: results of a 5-year follow-up study. Diabetes Care 11:605–612, 1988

Lustman PJ, Freedland KE, Carney RM, et al: Similarity of depression in diabetic and psychiatric patients. Psychosom Med 54:602–611, 1992a

Lustman PJ, Griffith LS, Gavard JA, et al: Depression in adults with diabetes. Diabetes Care 15:1631–1639, 1992b

Lustman PJ, Clouse RE, Griffith LS, et al: Screening for depression in diabetes using the Beck Depression Inventory. Psychosom Med 59:24–31, 1997a

Lustman PJ, Griffith LS, Clouse RE, et al: Effects of nortriptyline on depression and glucose regulation in diabetes: results of a double-blind, placebo-controlled trial. Psychosom Med 59:241–250, 1997b

Lustman PJ, Griffith LS, Freedland KE, et al: The course of major depression in diabetes. Gen Hosp Psychiatry 19:138–143, 1997c

Lustman PJ, Griffith LS, Freedland KE, et al: Cognitive behavior therapy for depression in type 2 diabetes mellitus: a randomized, controlled trial. Ann Intern Med 129:613–621, 1998

Lustman PJ, Anderson RJ, Freedland KE, et al: Depression and poor glycemic control. Diabetes Care 23:934–942, 2000a

Lustman PJ, Freedland KE, Griffith LS, et al: Fluoxetine for depression in diabetes: a randomized double-blind placebo-controlled trial. Diabetes Care 23:618–623, 2000b

Lustman PJ, Clouse RE, Ciechanowski PS, et al: Depression-related hyperglycemia in type 1 diabetes: a mediational approach. Psychosom Med 67:195–199, 2005

MacCrimmon DJ, Wallace JE, Goldberg WM, et al: Emotional disturbance and cognitive deficits in hyperthyroidism. Psychosom Med 41:331–340, 1979

Mahendran R: Hypomania in a patient with congenital familial hypothyroidism and mild mental retardation. Singapore Med J 40:425–427, 1999

Malouf R, Brust JCM: Hypoglycemia: causes, neurological manifestations, and outcome. Ann Neurol 17:421–430, 1985

Mandelbrote BM, Wittkower ED: Emotional factors in Graves' disease. Psychosom Med 17:109–123, 1955

Manger WM, Gifford RW Jr, Hoffman BB: Pheochromocytoma: a clinical and experimental overview. Curr Probl Cancer 9:1–85, 1985

Marcus MD, Winey RR, Guare J, et al: Lifetime prevalence of major depression and its effect on treatment outcome in obese type II diabetic patients. Diabetes Care 15:253–255, 1992

Mastrogiacomo I, Fava M, Fava G, et al: Postpartum hostility and prolactin. Int J Psychiatry Med 12:289–294, 1983

Mauri M, Sinforiani E, Bono G, et al: Memory impairment in Cushing's disease. Acta Neurol Scand 87:52–55, 1993

Max MB, Kishore-Kumar R, Schafer SC, et al: Efficacy of desipramine in painful diabetic neuropathy: a placebo-controlled trial. Pain 45:3–9, 1991

Max MB, Lynch SA, Muir J, et al: Effects of desipramine, amitriptyline, and fluoxetine on pain in diabetic neuropathy. N Engl J Med 326:1250–1256, 1992

Mazet P, Simon D, Luton J-P, et al: [Psychic symptoms and personality of 50 patients with Cushing's syndrome]. Nouvelle Presse Med 10:2565–2570, 1981

Miller R: Mental symptoms from myxedema. J Lab Clin Med 40:267–270, 1952

Modlin IM, Farndon JR, Shepherd A, et al: Phaeochromocytomas in 72 patients: clinical and diagnostic features, treatment and long-term results. Br J Surg 66:456–465, 1979

Murphy BE, Dhar V, Ghadirian AM, et al: Response to steroid suppression in major depression resistant to antidepressant therapy. J Clin Psychopharmacol 11:121–126, 1991

Musselman DL, Nemeroff CB: Depression and endocrine disorders: focus on the thyroid and adrenal system. Br J Psychiatry (suppl 30):123–128, 1996

Musselman DL, Miller AH, Porter MR, et al: Higher than normal plasma interleukin-6 concentrations in cancer patients with depression: preliminary findings. Am J Psychiatry 158:1252–1257, 2001

Naber D, Sand P, Heigl B: Psychopathological and neuropsychological effects of 8-days' corticosteroid treatment: a prospective study. Psychoneuroendocrinology 21:25–31, 1996

Nemeroff CB, Widerlov E, Bissette G, et al: Elevated concentrations of CSF corticotropin-releasing factor–like immunoreactivity in depressed patients. Science 226:1342–1344, 1984

Nemeroff CB, Simon JS, Haggerty JJ, et al: Antithyroid antibodies in depressed patients. Am J Psychiatry 142:840–843, 1985

Nemeroff CB, Krishnan KKR, Reed D, et al: Adrenal gland enlargement in major depression: a computed tomographic study. Arch Gen Psychiatry 49:384–387, 1992

Newcomer JW, Craft S, Hershey T, et al: Glucocorticoid-induced impairment in declarative memory performance in adult humans. J Neurosci 14:2047–2053, 1994

Newcomer JW, Selke G, Melson AK, et al: Decreased memory performance in healthy humans induced by stress-level cortisol treatment. Arch Gen Psychiatry 56:527–533, 1999

Nielsen H: Familial occurrence, gastro-intestinal symptoms and mental disturbances in hyperparathyroidism. Acta Med Scand 15:359–366, 1955

Noble P: Depressive illness and hyperparathyroidism. Proc R Soc Med 67:1066–1067, 1974

Northam EA, Anderson PJ, Jacobs R, et al: Neuropsychological profiles of children with type 1 diabetes 6 years after disease onset. Diabetes Care 24:1541–1546, 2001

Northam EA, Matthews LK, Anderson PJ, et al: Psychiatric morbidity and health outcome in type 1 diabetes: perspectives from a prospective longitudinal study. Diabet Med 22:152–157, 2004

Okamoto T, Gerstein HC, Obara T: Psychiatric symptoms, bone density and non-specific symptoms in patients with mild hypercalcemia due to primary hyperparathyroidism: a systematic overview of the literature. Endocr J 44:367–374, 1997

Okamura F, Tashiro A, Utumi A, et al: Insulin resistance in patients with depression and its changes during the clinical course of depression: minimal model analysis. Metabolism 49:1255–1260, 2000

Oztunc A, Guscott RG, Soni J, et al: Psychosis resulting in suicide in a patient with primary hyperparathyroidism. Can J Psychiatry 31:342–343, 1986

Palinkas LA, Lee PP, Barrett-Connor E: A prospective study of type 2 diabetes and depressive symptoms in the elderly: The Rancho Bernardo Study. Diabet Med 21:1185–1191, 2004

Patten SB: Exogenous corticosteroids and major depression in the general population. J Psychosom Res 49:447–449, 2000

Peila R, Rodriguez BL, Launer LJ: Type 2 diabetes, APOE gene, and the risk for dementia and related pathologies: The Honolulu-Asia Aging Study. Diabetes 51:1256–1262, 2002

Perlmuter LC, Hakami MK, Hodgson-Harrington C, et al: Decreased cognitive function in aging non–insulin-dependent patients. Am J Med 77:1043–1048, 1984

Perros P, Deary IJ, Sellar RJ, et al: Brain abnormalities demonstrated by magnetic resonance imaging in adult IDDM patients with and without a history of recurrent severe hypoglycemia. Diabetes Care 20:1013–1018, 1997

Perry PJ, Tsuang MT, Hwang MH: Prednisolone psychosis: clinical observations. Drug Intell Clin Pharm 18:603–609, 1984

Petersen P: Psychiatric disorders in primary hyperparathyroidism. J Clin Endocrinol Metab 28:1491–1495, 1968

Philibert R, Caspers K, Langbehn D, et al: The association of a HOPA polymorphism with major depression and phobia. Compr Psychiatry 43:404–410, 2002

Pitts FN, Guze SB: Psychiatric disorders and myxedema. Am J Psychiatry 118:142–147, 1961

Plouin PF, Degoulet P, Tugaye A, et al: [Screening for phaeochromocytoma : in which hypertensive patients? A semiological study of 2585 patients, including 11 with phaeochromocytoma]. Nouv Presse Med 10:869–872, 1981

Pomeranze J, King E: Psychosis as first sign of thyroid dysfunction. Geriatrics 21:211–212, 1966

Pop VJ, Maartens LH, Leusink G, et al: Are autoimmune thyroid dysfunction and depression related? J Clin Endocrinol Metab 83:3194–3197, 1998

Popkin MK, Callies AL, Lentz RD, et al: Prevalence of major depression, simple phobia, and other psychiatric disorders in patients with longstanding type I diabetes mellitus. Arch Gen Psychiatry 45:64–68, 1988

Pramming S, Thorsteinsson B, Theilgaard A, et al: Cognitive function during hypoglycemia in type I diabetes mellitus. BMJ 292:647–650, 1986

Prange AJ, Wilson IC, Rabon AM, et al: Enhancement of imipramine antidepressant activity by thyroid hormone. Am J Psychiatry 126:457–469, 1969

Prange AJ, Lara PP, Wilson IC, et al: Effects of thyrotropin-releasing hormone in depression. Lancet 2:999–1002, 1972

Prange AJ, Haggerty JJ, Rice J, et al: Marginal hypothyroidism in mental illness: preliminary assessments of prevalence and significance. Proceedings of the 16th Congress of International Neuropharmacology Conference, Munich, West Germany, August 1988

Prinz PN, Vitaliano PP, Moe KE, et al: Thyroid hormones: positive relationships with cognition in healthy, euthyroid older men. J Gerontol A Biol Sci Med Sci 54:M111–M116, 1999

Rao SG: The neuropharmacology of centrally acting analgesic medications in fibromyalgia. Rheum Dis Clin North Am 28:235–259, 2002

Reaven GM, Thompson LW, Nahum D, et al: Relationship between hyperglycemia and cognitive function in older NIDDM patients. Diabetes Care 13:16–21, 1990

Reichard P, Pihl M, Rosenqvist U, et al: Complications in IDDM are caused by elevated blood glucose level: the Stockholm Diabetes Intervention Study (SDIS) at 10-year follow up. Diabetologia 39:1483–1488, 1996

Reilly EL, Wilson WP: Mental symptoms in hyperparathyroidism: a report of three cases. Dis Nerv Syst 26:361–363, 1965

Reinfrank RF: Primary hyperparathyroidism with depression. Arch Intern Med 108:162–166, 1961

Reitan RM: Intellectual functions in myxedema. Arch Neurol Psychiatry 69:436–449, 1953

Rennick PM, Wilder RM, Sargent J, et al: Retinopathy as an indicator of cognitive-perceptual-motor impairment in diabetic adults (summary), in Proceedings of the 76th Annual Convention of the American Psychological Association, San Francisco, CA, August 1968, pp 473–474

Richardson JT: Cognitive function in diabetes mellitus. Neurosci Biobehav Rev 14:385–388, 1990

Risch SC, Lewine RJ, Kalin NH, et al: Limbic-hypothalamic-pituitary-adrenal axis activity and ventricular-to-brain ratio studies in affective illness and schizophrenia. Neuropsychopharmacology 6:95–100, 1992

Ritchie JC, Belkin BM, Krishnan KR, et al: Plasma dexamethasone concentrations and the dexamethasone suppression test. Biol Psychiatry 27:159–173, 1990

Robbins LR, Vinson DB: Objective psychological assessment of the thyrotoxic patient and the response to treatment: preliminary report. J Clin Endocrinol 20:120–129, 1960

Robinson N, Fuller JH, Edmeades SP: Depression and diabetes. Diabet Med 5:268–274, 1988

Rockey PH, Griep RJ: Behavioral dysfunction in hyperthyroidism. Arch Intern Med 140:1194–1197, 1980

Rosenbaum AH, Maruta T, Schatzberg AF, et al: Toward a biochemical classification of depressive disorders, VII: urinary free cortisol and urinary MHPG in depression. Am J Psychiatry 140:314–317, 1983

Rosenberg FR, Sander S, Nelson CT: Pemphigus: a 20-year review of 107 patients treated with corticosteroids. Arch Dermatol 112:962–970, 1976

Rosenblatt S, Faillace LA: Psychiatric manifestations of hyperparathyroidism. Tex Med 73:59–60, 1977

Rovet JF, Ehrlich RM, Hoppe M: Intellectual deficits associated with early onset of insulin-dependent diabetes mellitus in children. Diabetes Care 10:510–515, 1987

Royce PC: Severely impaired consciousness in myxedema: a review. Am J Med Sci 261:46–50, 1971

Ryan CM: Neurobehavioral complications of type-I diabetes: examination of possible risk factors. Diabetes Care 11:86–93, 1988

Ryan CM, Vega A, Drash A: Cognitive deficits in adolescents who developed diabetes early in life. Pediatrics 75:921–927, 1985

Sachar E, Hellman L, Fukushima D, et al: Cortisol production in depressive illness. Arch Gen Psychiatry 23:289–298, 1970

Sachon C, Grimaldi A, Digy JP, et al: Cognitive function, insulin-dependent diabetes and hypoglycaemia. J Intern Med 231:471–475, 1992

Sachs G, Spiess K, Moser G, et al: Glycosylated hemoglobin and diabetes: self-monitoring (compliance) in depressed and non-depressed type I diabetes patients. Psychother Psychosom Med Psychol 41:306–312, 1991

Scarlett JA, Mako ME, Rubenstein AH, et al: Factitious hypoglycemia: diagnosis by measurement of serum C-peptide immunoreactivity and insulin-binding antibodies. N Engl J Med 297:1029–1032, 1977

Schmidt MI, Duncan BB, Sharrett AR, et al: Markers of inflammation and prediction of diabetes mellitus in adults (Atherosclerosis Risk in Communities study): a cohort study. Lancet 353:1649–1652, 1999

Schon M, Sutherland AM, Rawson RW: Hormones and neuroses: the psychological effects of thyroid deficiency, in Proceedings of the 3rd World Congress of Psychiatry. Toronto, University of Toronto Press, 1962, pp 835–839

Shaw PJ, Walls TJ, Newman PK, et al: Hashimoto's encephalopathy: a steroid-responsive disorder associated with high anti-thyroid antibody titers: report of 5 cases. Neurology 41:228–233, 1991

Shein M, Apter A, Dickerman Z, et al: Encephalopathy in compensated Hashimoto thyroiditis: a clinical expression of autoimmune cerebral vasculitis. Brain Dev 8:60–64, 1986

Sheline YI, Mittler BL, Mintun MA: The hippocampus and depression. Eur Psychiatry 17 (suppl 3):300–305, 2002

Sherwin RS: Diabetes mellitus, in Cecil Textbook of Medicine, 20th Edition. Edited by Bennett JC, Plum F. Philadelphia, PA, WB Saunders, 1996, pp 1258–1277

Siegal FP: Lithium for steroid-induced psychosis. N Engl J Med 299:155–156, 1978

Silva RG, Tolstunov L: Steroid-induced psychosis: report of a case. J Oral Maxillofac Surg 53:183–186, 1995

Simmons NE, Do HM, Lipper MH, et al: Cerebral atrophy in Cushing's disease. Surg Neurol 53:72–76, 2000

Sindrup SH, Gram LF, Brosen K, et al: The selective serotonin reuptake inhibitor paroxetine is effective in the treatment of diabetic neuropathy symptoms. Pain 42:135–144, 1990

Skenazy JA, Bigler ED: Neuropsychological findings in diabetes mellitus. J Clin Psychol 40:246–258, 1984

Smallridge RC: Disclosing subclinical thyroid disease. Postgrad Med 107:143–152, 2000

Soininen H, Puranen M, Helkala E-L, et al: Diabetes mellitus and brain atrophy: a computerized tomography study in an elderly population. Neurobiol Aging 13:717–721, 1992

Solomon BL, Schaaf M, Smallridge RC: Psychologic symptoms before and after parathyroid surgery. Am J Med 96:101–106, 1994

Sonino N, Fava GA, Boscaro M: A role for life events in the pathogenesis of Cushing's disease. Clin Endocrinol (Oxf) 38:261–264, 1988

Sonino N, Fava G, Belluardo P, et al: Course of depression in Cushing's syndrome: response to treatment and comparison with Graves' disease. Horm Res 39:202–206, 1993

Soygur H, Palaoglu O, Altinors N, et al: Melperone treatment in an organic delusional syndrome induced by hyperprolactinemia: a case report. Eur Neuropsychopharmacol 7:161–163, 1997

Spillane JD: Nervous and mental disorders in Cushing's syndrome. Brain 74:72–94, 1951

Starkman MN, Schteingart DE, Schork MA: Depressed mood and other psychiatric manifestations of Cushing's syndrome: relationship to hormone levels. Psychosom Med 43:3–18, 1981

Starkman MN, Zelnick TC, Nesse RM, et al: Anxiety in patients with pheochromocytomas. Arch Intern Med 145:248–252, 1985

Starkman MN, Schteingart DE, Schork MA: Correlation of bedside cognitive and neuropsychological tests in patients with Cushing's syndrome. Psychosomatics 27:508–511, 1986a

Starkman MN, Schteingart DE, Schork MA: Cushing's syndrome after treatment: changes in cortisol and ACTH levels, and amelioration of the depressive syndrome. Psychiatry Res 19:177–188, 1986b

Starkman MN, Gebarski SS, Berent S, et al: Hippocampal formation volume, memory dysfunction, and cortisol levels in patient's with Cushing's syndrome. Biol Psychiatry 32:756–765, 1992

Starkman MN, Giordani B, Gebarski SS, et al: Decrease in cortisol reverses human hippocampal atrophy following treatment of Cushing's disease. Biol Psychiatry 46:1595–1602, 1999

Starkman MN, Giordani B, Berent S, et al: Elevated cortisol levels in Cushing's disease are associated with cognitive decrements. Psychosom Med 63:985–993, 2001

Starkman MN, Giordani B, Gebarski SS, et al: Improvement in learning associated with increase in hippocampal formation volume. Biol Psychiatry 53:233–238, 2003

Steffens DC, Byrum CE, McQuoid DR, et al: Hippocampal volume in geriatric depression. Biol Psychiatry 48:301–309, 2000

Steiner M, Haskett RF, Carroll BJ, et al: Plasma prolactin and severe premenstrual tension. Psychoneuroendocrinology 9:29–35, 1984

Stowell CP, Barnhill JW: Acute mania in the setting of severe hypothyroidism. Psychosomatics 46:259–261, 2005

Targum SD, Greenberg RD, Harmon RL, et al: Thyroid hormone and the TRH stimulation test in refractory depression. J Clin Psychiatry 45:345–346, 1984

Taylor JW: Depression in thyrotoxicosis. Am J Psychiatry 132:552–553, 1975

Theohar C, Fischer-Cornellssen K, Brosch H, et al: A comparative, multi-center trial between bromocriptine and amitriptyline in the treatment of endogenous depression. Arzneimittelforschung 32:783–787, 1982

Thomas FB, Mazzaferri EL, Skillman TG: Apathetic thyrotoxicosis: a distinctive clinical and laboratory entity. Ann Intern Med 72:679–685, 1970

Thomas JE, Rooke ED, Kuale WF: The neurologist's experience with pheochromocytoma: a review of 100 cases. JAMA 197:754–758, 1966

Thomas WC: Hypercalcemic crisis due to hyperparathyroidism. Am J Med 24:229–239, 1958

Thompson WF: Psychiatric aspects of Addison's disease: report of a case. Med Ann Dist Columbia 42:62–64, 1973

Thomsen AF, Kvist TK, Andersen PK, et al: Increased risk of affective disorder following hospitalization with hyperthyroidism: a register-based study. Eur J Endocrinol 152:535–543, 2005

Thrush DC, Boddie HG: Episodic encephalopathy associated with thyroid disorders. J Neurol Neurosurg Psychiatry 37:696–700, 1974

Thurling ML: Primary hyperparathyroidism in a schizophrenic woman. Can J Psychiatry 32:785–787, 1987

Tonks CM: Mental illness in hypothyroid patients. Br J Psychiatry 110:706–710, 1964

Treadway CR, Prange AJ, Doehne EF, et al: Myxedema psychosis: clinical and biochemical changes during recovery. J Psychiatr Res 5:289–296, 1967

Trzepacz P, McCue M, Klein I, et al: A psychiatric and neuropsychological study of patients with untreated Graves' disease. Gen Hosp Psychiatry 10:49–55, 1988

Tun PA, Nathan DM, Pulmuter LC: Cognitive and affective disorders in elderly diabetics. Clin Geriatr Med 6:731–746, 1990

Vakili K, Pillay SS, Lafer B, et al: Hippocampal volume in primary unipolar major depression: a magnetic resonance imaging study. Biol Psychiatry 47:1087–1090, 2000

van Oostrom JC, Schaafsma A, Haaxma R: Variable manifestations of Hashimoto's encephalopathy. Ned Tijdschr Geneeskd 143:25, 1319–1322, 1999

Varadaraj R, Cooper AJ: Addison's disease presenting with psychiatric symptoms (letter). Am J Psychiatry 143:553–554, 1986

Ward DJ, Rastall ML: Prognosis in "myxoedematous madness." Br J Psychiatry 113:149–151, 1967

Watson LC, Marx CE: New onset of neuropsychiatric symptoms in the elderly: possible primary hyperparathyroidism. Psychosomatics 43:413–417, 2002

Wehr T, Sack D, Rosenthal N, et al: Rapid cycling affective disorder: contributing factors in treatment response in 51 patients. Am J Psychiatry 145:179–184, 1988

Wells KB, Golding JM, Burnam MA: Psychiatric disorder in a sample of the general population with and without chronic medical conditions. Am J Psychiatry 145:976–981, 1988

Weyerer S, Hewer W, Pfeifer-Kurda M, et al: Psychiatric disorders and diabetes: results from a community study. J Psychosom Res 33:633–640, 1989

Whelan TB, Schteingart DE, Starkman MN, et al: Neuropsychological deficits in Cushing's syndrome. J Nerv Ment Dis 168:753–757, 1980

Whybrow PC, Hurwitz T: Psychological disturbances associated with endocrine disease and hormone therapy, in Hormones, Behavior, and Psychopathology. Edited by Sachar EJ. New York, Raven, 1976, pp 125–143

Whybrow PC, Prange AJ, Treadway CR: Mental changes accompanying thyroid gland dysfunction. Arch Gen Psychiatry 20:48–63, 1969

Wiesel C: Psychosis with myxedema. J Ky Med Assoc 50:395–397, 1952

Wilson WP, Johnson JE, Smith RB: Affective change in thyrotoxicosis and experimental hypermetabolism. Recent Adv Biol Psychiatry 4:234–243, 1962

Wiltshire S, Hattersley AT, Hitman GA, et al: A genomewide scan for loci predisposing to type 2 diabetes in a UK population (the Diabetes UK Warren 2 Repository): analysis of 573 pedigrees provides independent replication of a susceptibility locus on chromosome 1q. Am J Hum Genet 69:553–569, 2001

Winokur A, Maislin G, Phillips J, et al: Insulin resistance after oral glucose tolerance testing in patients with major depression. Am J Psychiatry 145:325–330, 1988

Wittchen HU, Zhao S, Kessler RC, et al: DSM-III-R generalized anxiety disorder in the National Comorbidity Survey. Arch Gen Psychiatry 51:355–364, 1994

Wittchen HU, Hoyer J: Generalized anxiety disorder: nature and course. J Clin Psychiatry 62 (suppl 11):15–19, 2001

Wolkowitz OM, Rubinow D, Doran AR, et al: Prednisone effects on neurochemistry and behavior: preliminary findings. Arch Gen Psychiatry 47:963–968, 1990

Wredling R, Levander S, Adamson U, et al: Permanent neuropsychological impairment after recurrent episodes of severe hypoglycaemia in man. Diabetologia 33:152–157, 1990

Yaffe K, Blackwell T, Kanaya AM, et al: Diabetes, impaired fasting glucose, and development of cognitive impairment in older women. Neurology 63:658–663, 2004

Young EA, Haskett RF, Grunhaus L, et al: Increased evening activation of the hypothalamic-pituitary-adrenal axis in depressed patients. Arch Gen Psychiatry 51:701–707, 1994

Zeiger MA, Fraker DL, Pass HI, et al: Effective reversibility of the signs and symptoms of hypercortisolism by bilateral adrenalectomy. Surgery 114:1138–1143, 1993

22

NEUROPSYCHIATRIC ASPECTS OF POISONS AND TOXINS

Shreenath V. Doctor, M.D., Ph.D.

All substances are poisons; there is none which is not a poison. The right dose differentiates a poison and a remedy.

Paracelsus, sixteenth century

A *poison* is defined in this chapter as a material or substance that is capable of producing a harmful response in a biological life form, seriously injuring function that, if critical, results in the death of the organism. *Toxins* are further categorized as poisons produced by various animal, plant, fungal, and microbial species to which humans are either intentionally or unintentionally exposed. *Neurotoxic agents* are poisons or toxins that specifically produce an adverse change in the structure and/or function of the nervous system. Exposure to poisons and toxins, particularly neurotoxic agents, often cause neuropsychiatric manifestations. Several different classes of chemical poisons producing neuropsychiatric sequelae are shown in Table 22–1.

Short-term or long-term exposure to neurotoxic chemical agents can result in various neuropsychiatric manifestations, such as those shown in Tables 22–2 through 22–5.

Exposures to neurotoxic agents may occur from the air, water, food, environmental surfaces, soil, microbes, fungi, plants, and animals or by envenomation via bites and stings. In our industrialized society, the number of new chemicals produced every year is estimated to be in the thousands, and each has the potential for neuropsychiatric sequelae. The multitude of adverse effects of the numerous inorganic and organic chemicals present in our environment makes the subject of this chapter a broad topic area. I discuss poisons and toxins that have prominent neuropsychiatric sequelae in humans and provide information, if available, on their exposure, absorption, mechanisms of action, diagnosis, and treatment of their effects. Included are biocides, chemicals deliberately placed in our environment to selectively injure or kill microbes, plants, animals, and other forms of life. Intoxications due to medications are beyond the scope of this chapter.

TABLE 22–1.   Selected poisons producing neuropsychiatric sequelae

Gases	Metals	Organic solvents	Pesticides
Carbon monoxide	Alkyltins	Acetone	Carbamates
Ethylene oxide	Aluminum	Carbon disulfide	Organochlorines
	Arsenic	Ethylbenzene	Organophosphates
	Bismuth	Methanol	Pyrethroids
	Copper	Methyl-*n*-butyl ketone	
	Lead	Methyl chloride	
	Manganese	Styrene	
	Mercury	Toluene	
	Thallium	Trichloroethylene	
	Zinc	Xylene	

Source.   Adapted from Bleecker 1994.

METALS AND ORGANOMETALS

Organometallic compounds are composed of a heavy metal atom with valence sites attached to a hydrocarbon or organic moiety. Organometals are more lipid soluble than the inorganic forms and easily cross the blood-brain barrier. As a result, exposure at smaller doses to organolead, organotin, or organomercury compounds can produce neurotoxicity and neuropsychiatric symptoms of greater severity than their respective heavy metal moiety.

ALUMINUM

Constituting 5% of the earth's crust, aluminum is mined and refined for use in electrical wiring, thermal insulation, paint, bricks, mufflers, and household and industrial utensils. Sources of household exposure include processed food such as pickles, aluminum-containing deodorants, oral antidiarrheal and antacid agents, and phosphate-binding gels. Other medical sources of aluminum exposure include aluminum-contaminated dialysis solutions, total parenteral nutrition solutions, and human serum albumin used in plasmapheresis. Table 22–6 lists additional sources of aluminum exposure.

The normal diet contains 3–5 mg/day of aluminum. The total body burden is approximately 30 mg. Patients taking antacids or phosphate-binding therapy may ingest enough to be in a positive balance of 200–300 mg/day (Schonwald 2004a). Aluminum is poorly absorbed through the gastrointestinal tract; however, depending on the intraluminal speciation, quantity, competing or complexing substances, and intraluminal pH (Van der Voet 1992a, 1992b), absorption can range from approximately 0.0005% to 24% in humans (Wilhelm et al. 1990). Transport in the blood occurs in association with high-molecular-weight transferrin as well as low-molecular-weight phosphate, citrate, and hydroxide (Harris 1992). Transport across the blood-brain barrier is also variable, similar to intestinal absorption.

Neuropsychiatric Manifestations

Neurotoxicity from aluminum occurs almost exclusively in persons who are unable to excrete dietary aluminum. Patients with chronic renal failure receiving long-term dialysis develop a disease known as dialysis encephalopathy (Alfrey and Froment 1990; D.N.S. Kerr et al. 1992), characterized by gradual development of personality changes and visual and auditory hallucinations leading to paranoid and suicidal behavior. A combination of dysarthria, dyspraxia, and dysphasia—considered the early-onset symptoms of the disease—can occur both during and immediately after dialysis. Myoclonic jerks, usually occurring in the facial region and upper limbs, are often present with speech disturbances. Focal motor and generalized tonic-clonic seizures can also occur with a high incidence. Dementia, the most consistent feature of dialysis encephalopathy, manifests gradually as disturbances of concentration, attention, orientation, and memory. In later stages, confusion and gross signs of dementia are noted. Finally, the patient may become immobile, mute, and obtunded, with death ensuing 6–9 months after onset. Electroencephalographic abnormalities, such as paroxysms of high-voltage delta activity with spike and wave discharges, may precede the clinical symptoms by many months (Schonwald 2004a).

After focal accumulations of the metal were observed in the central cores of senile plaques and in neurons bear-

TABLE 22–2. Neuropsychiatric sequelae associated with metal exposure

Metal	Neuropsychiatric symptoms
Alkyltin (trimethyltin)	Depression, rage, loss of libido and motivation, sleep disturbance, forgetfulness, personality deterioration
Aluminum	Personality change; fatigue; impaired memory, attention, and executive motor functions
Arsenic	Impaired verbal memory, agitation, drowsiness, confusion, emotional lability, stupor, delirium, psychosis resembling paranoid schizophrenia
Bismuth	Depression, anxiety, irritability, tremulousness, confusion, dysarthria
Copper	Schizophrenia-like symptoms; personality changes; irritability; dysarthria; impaired cognition, memory, and abstract reasoning
Gold	Depression, hallucinations
Lead	
Inorganic	
Children	Lethargy; hyperactivity; impaired intellect, reaction time, perceptual motor performance, memory, reading, spelling, auditory processing, and attention
Adults	Depression; apathy; confusion; fatigue; tension; restlessness; anger; decreases in visual intelligence, general intelligence, memory, psychomotor speed, rate of learning, attention, and visuoconstruction
Organic	Euphoria; psychosis; hallucinations; restlessness; nightmares; delirium; impaired concentration, memory, and abstract reasoning
Manganese	Somnolence, asthenia, anorexia, impaired speech, insomnia, hallucinations, excitement, aggression, mania, dementia, frontal lobe dysfunction, emotional lability, Parkinson-like symptoms, impaired judgment and memory
Mercury	
Inorganic	Irritability; avoidance; shyness; depression; lassitude; fatigue; agitation; decreases in visual memory, reaction time, motor speech, and learning
Organic (methylmercury)	Incoordination, mood lability, dementia
Thallium	Emotional lability, anxiety and hysteriform behavior, dyssomnia, headache, tremor, ataxia, polyneuritis, peripheral sensory and motor neuropathy
Zinc	Irritability

Source. Adapted from Bleecker 1994; and Bolla and Roca 1994.

ing neurofibrillary tangles, investigators suggested that aluminum might have a role in the etiology of Alzheimer's disease (D.P. Perl and Brody 1980). Neurofibrillary tangles, senile plaques, and granulovacuolar degeneration are the diagnostic hallmarks of Alzheimer's disease. However, no causal relation between aluminum and this neurological disorder has yet been elucidated.

As in Alzheimer's disease, focal accumulations of aluminum have been detected in patients with endemic amyotrophic lateral sclerosis and parkinsonian dementia, which has a high incidence of occurrence among the Chamorro population of Guam and nearby islands in the South Pacific (Garruto 1991). Epidemiological evidence suggests a link between these endemic illnesses in the Guamanian population and the prevalence of high aluminum and low calcium levels in the soil of the area.

Mechanisms of Action

The hallmarks of neurotoxicity of aluminum in experimental animal models are aberrations of cytoskeletal proteins (Bugiani and Ghetti 1990). Neurofilaments and neurofibrillary tangles form in these experimental encephalopathies; however, the symptomatology and pathology are different from those seen in subjects with Alzheimer's disease, dialysis encephalopathy, or the parkinsonian dementia/amyotrophic lateral sclerosis com-

TABLE 22–3.   Neuropsychiatric sequelae associated with solvent exposure

Solvent	Neuropsychiatric symptoms
Carbon disulfide	Psychosis; depression; personality change; insomnia; retarded speech; impaired hand-eye coordination, motor speed, energy level, psychomotor performance, reaction time, vigilance, visuomotor functions, and construction
Carbon tetrachloride	Lethargy, confusion
Ethylbenzene	Headache, irritability, fatigue
Ethylene glycol	Fatigue, personality change, depression
Methanol	Visual toxicity with diminution of pupillary light reflex, loss of visual acuity and papilledema, parkinsonian syndrome with reduced emotions, hypophonia, masked facies, tremor, rigidity, bradykinesia
Methyl chloride	Somnolence; confusion; euphoria; personality change; depression; emotional lability; impaired psychomotor speed, vigilance, reaction time, and hand-eye coordination
Methyl-*n*-butyl ketone	Peripheral neuropathy
Styrene	Depression; fatigue; dizziness; impaired memory, concentration, vigilance, reaction time, psychomotor speed, and visual construction
Toluene	
Short-term exposure	Initial excitation with depression at higher concentrations, fatigue, confusion, anxiety, increased reaction time, and impaired concentration
Long-term exposure	Exhilaration; euphoria; disinhibition; impaired performance IQ, memory, motor control, and attention; flattened affect; apathy; dementia
Trichloroethylene	Headaches; dizziness; fatigue; diplopia; anxiety; lability; insomnia; impaired concentration, manual dexterity, reaction time, memory, and visuospatial accuracy
Xylene	Confusion; impaired reaction time, attention, and concentration

Source.   Adapted from Bleecker 1994 and Bolla and Roca 1994.

TABLE 22–4.   Neuropsychiatric sequelae associated with gas exposure

Gas	Neuropsychiatric symptoms
Carbon monoxide	Impaired cognitive efficiency and flexibility and verbal and visual memory, disorientation, irritability, distractibility, masklike facies, dementia, amnesia
Ethylene oxide	Polyneuropathy, diminished intelligence, impaired verbal and visual memory and auditory and visual attention
Formaldehyde	Light-headedness, dizziness, impaired concentration and memory, mood alteration
Hydrogen sulfide	Headaches; dizziness; light-headedness; nervousness; fatigue; sleep disturbances; extremity weakness; spasms; convulsions; delirium; impaired cognition, memory, and psychomotor and perceptual abilities
Nitrous oxide	Polyneuropathy, confusion, visual hallucinations and delusions, episodic crying and agitation, sexual misbehavior, mild ataxia, impaired attention

Source.   Adapted from Bleecker 1994 and Bolla and Roca 1994.

TABLE 22–5. Neuropsychiatric sequelae associated with pesticide exposure

Pesticide	Neuropsychiatric symptoms
Carbamates (e.g., carbaril)	Headache, nausea, giddiness, blurred vision, weakness, increased sweating, vomiting, miosis, delayed neuropathy
Organophosphates (e.g., chlorpyrifos)	
Mild	Weakness, headache, dizziness, nausea, salivation, lacrimation, miosis, moderate bronchial spasm
Moderate	Abrupt weakness, visual disturbances, excessive salivation, sweating, vomiting, diarrhea, bradycardia, hypertonia, tremor of hands and head, impaired gait, miosis, chest pain, cyanosis of mucous membranes
Severe	Abrupt tremor, generalized convulsions, psychiatric disturbance, intense cyanosis, death from respiratory or cardiac failure
Organochlorines (e.g., kepone)	Nervousness, tremor, ataxia, weight loss, headache, disorientation, confusion, auditory and visual hallucinations, irritability, memory loss

Source. Adapted from Bleecker 1994 and Bolla and Roca 1994.

TABLE 22–6. Sources of aluminum exposure

Agricultural pesticides

Aluminum pots and pans

Antacids

Antiperspirants

Astringents

Buffered aspirin

Catalyst in manufacture of chemicals

Clarifying oils and fats

Cosmetics and soaps

Explosives and fireworks

Fireproofing and waterproofing cloth

Flocculent for sewage/water purification

Food additives

Food stored in aluminum foil

Fumigation

Mordant in dyeing

Paper and pulp industry

Soil conditioner to increase acidity for plants

Tanning leather

Waterproofing concrete

Source. Adapted from Schonwald 2004a.

plex of Guam. Binding of aluminum to nuclear and cytosolic phosphates and the resultant derangement of nuclear and second-messenger processes have been hypothesized in a cascade model (Lukiw and McLachlan 1993). The primary target cell in the central nervous system is the astroglia, which internalizes aluminum amino acid complexes, which results in apoptosis (Aremu and Meshitsuka 2005). Aluminum is known to inhibit glutamate dehydrogenase; the resultant disruption of glutamate neurotransmission is also implicated in the neurotoxicity of aluminum (S.J. Yang et al. 2003). Aluminum causes an inhibition of rat cerebral synaptosomal sodium/potassium adenosine triphosphatase (Na^+/K^+-ATPase) as a result of a reduction in the activity of isozymes containing the α_1, α_2, and α_3 subunits of Na^+/K^+-ATPase. The inhibition of synaptosomal Na^+/K^+-ATPase preceded major damage in plasma membrane integrity and energy supply, as indicated by the analysis of lactate dehydrogenase leakage and endogenous adenine nucleotides (Silva et al. 2005).

Diagnosis

After oral or parenteral exposure, the diagnosis of aluminum neurotoxicity is established by characteristic electroencephalographic changes, clinical abnormalities, and concentration in plasma or serum (Alfrey and Froment 1990). The electroencephalogram (EEG) is distinguished from that of other metabolic encephalopathies by the normal background frequency and characteristic mild slowing of the dominant rhythm, including bursts of predominantly anterior high-voltage delta waves with intermittent spike activity. Clinical abnormalities include

TABLE 22–7.   Serum aluminum concentrations associated with neurotoxicity

Plasma concentration (μg/L)	Effect
<10	None
10–60	Increased body burden; objective changes in neurophysiological and neuropsychological measures
61–100	Subtle mental changes such as directional disorientation and personality changes
101–200	Impairment in memory, abstract reasoning, and depression in addition to above effects
>200	Cognitive deficits, incoordination, intention tremor, loss of balance, and myoclonic jerks. Continued exposure can result in paranoid and suicidal ideation, auditory and visual hallucinations, memory loss, dementia, convulsions, coma, and death.

Source.   Adapted from Alfrey and Froment 1990 and from Ellenhorn 1997.

intermittent speech disturbances, mutism, asterixis, myoclonic jerks, seizures, personality changes, and dementia. In healthy control subjects, the normal concentration of aluminum is less than 10 mg/L of plasma or serum. Table 22–7 lists plasma or serum aluminum levels and their correlation with clinical effects.

Treatment

Preventive measures are more effective than treatment of aluminum exposure and are carried out by preventing accumulation of a "body burden," or exchangeable pool of aluminum. Because aluminum readily crosses the dialyzing membrane, levels of aluminum in the dialysis medium need to be kept at a minimum (<10 mg/L). Oral aluminum compounds should be administered in quantities as low as possible, and plasma aluminum should be checked on a regular basis to confirm the absence of any accumulation (De Wolff and Van der Voet 1986). The progressive and fatal course of aluminum encephalopathy can be treated and reversed by chelation and removal with deferoxamine, with repeated administration over a period of several months (Alfrey and Froment 1990). The prophylactic effect of melatonin as an antioxidant in aluminum encephalopathy recently has been suggested (Abd-Elghaffar et al. 2005).

ARSENIC

Industry continues to be the major source of arsenic compounds. Arsenic trioxide is obtained mainly from copper smelting, a process that continues to be a source of arsenic exposure. In the past, inorganic arsenic was used as a constituent in pharmaceutical preparations for the treatment of anemia, rheumatism, psoriasis, and syphilis, and even today, arsenic is a constituent of several preparations such as Korean herbal remedies (Mitchell-Heggs

et al. 1990) and in some homeopathic preparations (H. D. Kerr and Saryan 1986). Arsenic is used in the manufacture of agricultural agents, such as insecticides and rodenticides, and is applied in wood preservatives. Other applications of arsenic include marine paints and pigments, glassware, and food additives to promote growth in farm animals. Arsine gas (AsH_3) aids in the production of microchips in the semiconductor industry (Caravati et al. 2004; Ellenhorn 1997). Table 22–8 provides an overview of the various sources of arsenic exposure.

The biodistribution of arsenic is dependent on the duration of exposure and the chemical species. After absorption, rapid localization in erythrocytes and leukocytes is noted. Arsenic is also detected in the liver, kidney, heart, and lung and is retained in bone and teeth. Smaller amounts are found in nerve and muscle tissue. Although penetration of the blood-brain barrier is minimal, arsenic readily crosses the placenta and may produce fetal damage (Klaassen 2001a).

Neuropsychiatric Manifestations

Most patients develop a dose-dependent onset of toxicity, with latency of weeks to months for neurological and neuropsychiatric symptoms. General manifestations include malaise, weakness, anorexia, weight loss, metallic taste, and cardiac irregularities. Neurological and neuropsychiatric symptoms include headache, confusion, dysesthesia, sensory and motor peripheral neuropathy in a stocking-and-glove distribution, muscular weakness of the extremities, muscle atrophy, ataxia, spasms, muscular twitching, and seizures. Long-term exposure may result in mild dementia, peripheral neuropathies, visual disturbances, photophobia, conjunctivitis, and other ocular effects (Caravati et al. 2004; Hall and Robertson 1990). Ingestion of high doses of inorganic arsenic compounds leads to dramatic gastrointestinal manifestations.

TABLE 22–8. Sources of arsenic exposure

Arsenic trioxide (Trisenox)

Cattle and sheep dips

Some ceramic glazes

Some Chinese proprietary medicines

Clarifier in glass industry

Desiccants and defoliants

Folk herbal medicines from India and China

Mining release into air, water, and soil

Moonshine

Museum artifacts preserved with arsenic

Pesticides

Pigments

Python-brand "black snakes" Chinese fireworks

Residential herbicides

Rodenticides

Seafood and seaweed

Semiconductors (gallium arsenide)

Smelting of nonferrous metals

Wood preservative (copper arsenide) for wood decks

Source. Adapted from Caravati 2004.

Intense nausea and vomiting precede diarrhea. The stool may be watery and may contain blood. A burning sensation in the throat and esophagus may occur, and a garlic-like odor may be noted from the breath. Arsenic also causes damage to blood vessel and vascular linings, resulting in fluid leakage into interstitial spaces. This may lead to depletion of intravascular volume and shock.

Mechanisms of Action

Arsenate, the pentavalent form of arsenic, is considerably less toxic than the trivalent arsenite and is commonly found in nature. Arsenate, for the most part, is converted by cellular reduction with glutathione and methylation to arsenite (Caravati 2004). In the tissues, arsenite exerts toxic effects by two mechanisms. First, it may interact with biological micromolecules by combining with sulf-hydryl groups. Enzyme systems such as the pyruvate and succinate pathways are especially sensitive to arsenite. Second, a loss of high-energy phosphate bonds may occur as arsenic anions substitute for phosphate and disrupt oxidative phosphorylation. Thus, arsenic is able to exert cytotoxicity by inhibiting oxidative phosphorylation by two separate mechanisms (Winship 1984).

Diagnosis

Diagnosis of arsenic poisoning requires laboratory support because no signs of acute or chronic arsenic poisoning are specific. When symptoms lead to a differential diagnosis that includes arsenic poisoning, a request for arsenic analysis should be made to a laboratory specializing in the analysis of trace elements. The most sensitive and expensive method is neutron activation analysis (Lauwerys et al. 1979). The human sample of choice for arsenic analysis is urine for establishing recent exposure and hair for establishing information on long-term exposure.

Treatment

Patients should be hospitalized for stabilization following acute poisoning and receive intravenous isotonic fluid replacement for fluid loss. Blood pressure and cardiac monitoring are necessary for assessment of hypotension and cardiac dysrhythmias. At present, the antidote of choice in the treatment of arsenic poisoning is meso-2,3,-dimercapto-succinic acid (DMSA) or 2,3,-dimercapto-1-propane-sulfonic acid (DMPS). Both drugs have been shown to be more effective in the treatment of experimental arsenic poisoning than British anti-lewisite (BAL or dimercaprol) (Aposhian et al. 1984), the classic antidote for arsenic poisoning. BAL should no longer be used because it has been shown to increase arsenic content in the brain, probably by forming a lipophilic complex that readily passes the blood-brain barrier (Aposhian et al. 1984; Kreppel et al. 1990).

LEAD

Lead is the sixth most ubiquitous metal on our planet, and its use by humans was extensive in early recorded history. Plumbism, or lead poisoning, was probably the first disease recognized as an occupational hazard, by Nikander around 150 B.C. (Major 1945). Exposure occurs through air, water, and food. The elimination of lead in gasoline has dramatically reduced levels of lead in the air in the United States. Even now, after its removal from gasoline and paints, lead continues to be an environmental hazard with varied sources of exposure in a multitude of industries (Table 22–9). Although lead can be absorbed through the lungs, skin, and digestive tract, the main route of exposure is oral. The daily intake of lead is 5–15 µg/day throughout all age groups. Adults usually absorb about 15%–20% of intake; children usually absorb about 45%.

Neuropsychiatric Manifestations

Clinical symptoms of lead poisoning in adults appear when blood levels reach approximately 40 µg/dL. The most common presentation is a chronic encephalopathy affecting mood and cognitive function. Headaches,

TABLE 22–9.   Sources of lead exposure

Ammunition production

Battery production

Brass works

Bronze works

Cable making/splicing

Chemical operations

Glassworks

Jewelry production

Lead smelting

Metal casting

Metal refining

Paint production

Pigment production

Pipe cutting

Pottery manufacturing

Printing

Soldering

Stained-glass manufacturing

Welding

Source.   Adapted from Ellenhorn 1997.

fatigue, bradyphrenia, and anxiety are usually the heralding symptoms, along with sleep disturbances, insomnia, and early-morning awakening. Irritability, anorexia, nervousness, myalgia, pallor, and loss of libido are common. Patients at this stage usually recover following cessation of exposure and chelation therapy (Dart et al. 2004; Ellenhorn 1997). Chronic lead exposure in 256 adult lead smelter workers was shown to result in significant impairments in encoding, storage, and retrieval of memory (Bleecker et al. 2005). Acute encephalopathy occurs with a blood lead level greater than 150 µg/dL. As blood levels increase, headaches and tremor may follow, as well as attacks of abdominal pain alternating with diarrhea. Persistent headaches, vomiting, ataxia, and generalized or focal seizures that are refractory to medication characterize acute lead encephalopathy. The patient may appear obtunded and confused, with intermittent episodes of stupor alternating with lucid intervals. If the condition remains unrecognized, death may ensue (Bruyn and De Wolff 1994). In children, compared with adults, clinical signs and symptoms of lead toxicity can occur at blood lead levels as low as 10–15 µg/dL (Dart et al. 2004).

Mechanisms of Action

Lead is a heavy metal affecting several biochemical processes, which may explain the diverse symptoms of lead poisoning. Neuropathology findings indicated that lead targeted large motor axons producing axonal degeneration and segmental demyelination (Dart et al. 2004). Lead interferes with the function of erythrocytes, kidneys, the peripheral and central nervous system, and the intestinal tract. Lead produces diffuse effects as it complexes ligands, particularly sulfhydryl groups, at active sites of enzyme systems throughout the body (Ellenhorn 1997). Lead has an affinity for sulfhydryl groups and is toxic to zinc- and calcium-ion-dependent enzyme systems. The cytoplasmic enzyme Δ-aminolevulinic acid dehydratase (ALA-D) and ferrochetalase, a mitochondrial enzyme, are both involved in heme synthesis and are both inhibited by lead. Lead interferes with deoxyribonucleic acid (DNA) transcription factors by binding to cysteine sites. Lead interfering with calcium-dependent protein kinase C (PKC) (Godwin 2001) disrupts many cellular events such as regulation of cell growth, learning, and memory.

Evidence is accumulating on the effects of lead on brain glutamatergic synapses. Specifically, the N-methyl-D-aspartate type of excitatory amino acid receptor (NMDAR) is the direct target for lead in the brain. In animal models of lead neurotoxicity, disruption of the ontogenetically defined pattern of NMDAR subunit expression and NMDAR-mediated calcium signaling in glutamatergic synapses is a principal mechanism for induced learning and memory deficits (Toscano and Guilarte 2005). In the central nervous system, areas of neuronal damage are evident in the hippocampal CA1 and CA3 regions. Moderate lead exposure elicits a neurotrophic effect in cerebral cortical precursor cells in culture by markedly reducing apoptosis. As a result, cell survival and process development are affected, potentially altering cortical arrangement (Davidovics and Cicco-Bloom 2005).

Diagnosis

The diagnosis of lead poisoning requires eliciting a history of exposure and detecting the presence of lead in urine and blood samples. Magnetic resonance imaging (MRI) scans show widespread calcification, particularly in the cerebellar hemispheres, basal ganglia, and thalamus, and increased signal intensity of T2-weighted images of the periventricular white matter, basal ganglia, hypothalamus, and pons (Petsas et al. 1992).

Treatment

The most common detoxification method available for lead poisoning is chelation therapy. At present, the least toxic of the chelating agents are DMSA and DMPS (Aposhian and Aposhian 1990). Recommended dosages of these compounds are 30 mg/kg three times a day for 5 days. Elimination of lead in urine should be monitored before, during, and after treatment to evaluate the effectiveness of treatment. In recent studies in animals, curcumin, the major constituent of turmeric and a potent natural antioxidant, has been shown to chelate lead and provide neuroprotection by significantly attenuating the potential damage to the hippocampal CA1 and CA3 regions (Daniel et al. 2004). The use of N-acetylcysteine on lead-exposed neural cells indicates protection from the oxidative stress of lead (Aykin-Burns et al. 2005).

MANGANESE

Manganese is an essential trace element that is widely distributed in the earth's crust primarily as pyrolusite, a mineral form of manganese dioxide. Manganese is used in the production of dry-cell batteries, metal alloys, fungicides, germicides, antiseptics, glass, matches, fireworks, fertilizers, animal feeds, paints, varnish, welding rods, and antiknock gasoline additives. Manganese is also used in textile bleaching and leather tanning. Exposure is usually by inhalation or the oral route. Intestinal absorption is estimated at 3% (Mena 1980).

After its absorption through the intestinal wall, manganese is carried through the bloodstream bound to a β_1-globulin in plasma. Manganese crosses the blood-brain barrier with iron (Aschner and Aschner 1990). Murphy et al. (1991) reported that entry into the brain is through a saturable transport mechanism, primarily across the cerebral capillary-glial network.

Neuropsychiatric Manifestations

Manganese exposure causes selective toxicity to the nigrostriatal dopaminergic system, resulting in a parkinsonian-like neurological condition known as *manganism*. The early stages of manganese intoxication are characterized by mood changes, emotional lability, auditory and visual hallucinations, and neuropsychological impairment referred to as *manganese psychosis*. Continuing long-term exposure may cause progression to a second stage, a parkinsonian disorder that includes gait disturbance, speech disorder, slowing and clumsiness of movements, and postural imbalance. In the third stage, signs of dystonia may appear, including an awkward, high-stepping gait, tremor, and chorea (Feldman 1994).

Neurological symptoms have been attributed to manganese fumes generated during welding. Welding without proper protection was associated with syndromes of parkinsonism, multifocal myoclonus, mild cognitive impair-

ment, and vestibular-auditory dysfunction. Individual susceptibility and progression to further stages of intoxication are probably related to preexisting states of deficiency of other divalent cations, such as calcium and iron, and preexisting illnesses, such as hepatic cirrhosis, alcoholism, and chronic infections (Mena 1980). The presence of other metallotoxins may also contribute to the severity of toxicity by a given exposure (Shukla and Singhal 1984).

Mechanisms of Action

Manganese can form the powerfully oxidizing species Mn^{3+}, which can oxidize catecholamines by transfer of one electron to semiquinones and orthoquinones, generating superoxide and hydroxyl radicals as well as hydrogen peroxide (Graham 1984; Normandin and Hazell 2002). Oxidative stress on the cell increases with the depletion of protective enzymes, such as superoxide dismutase, catalase, and glutathione peroxidase, and substrates, such as reduced glutathione. Manganese has a saturable transport system across the blood-brain barrier (Murphy et al. 1991). A divalent metal transporter protein (DMT-1) is thought to be the transporter of manganese into astrocytes and subsequently responsible for the brain accumulation of manganese (Erikson and Aschner 2006). Oxidative stress on the cell in dopamine-containing neurons increases with the formation of neurotoxins such as 6-hydroxydopamine (Garner and Nachtman 1989). Cell death occurs when continued oxidative stress damages the hydroxy radicals of critical neuronal membrane sites and results in the peroxidation of cell membrane lipids (Segura-Aguilar and Lind 1989). Manganese poisoning results in damage to neuromelanin cells in the substantia nigra and locus coeruleus as well as loss of cells in the caudate nucleus, pallidum, putamen, and thalamus. Caspases are enzymes that signal a damaged or worn-out cell to undergo programmed cell death or apoptosis. Recent results suggest that the mitochondrial-dependent caspase-3, an enzyme that contributes to DNA fragmentation and induces proteolytic activation of PKCΔ, plays a critical role in manganese-induced apoptotic cell death and neurotoxicity (Kitazawa et al. 2005).

Diagnosis

Correlations between blood manganese and intoxication are rather poor (Chandra et al. 1974). Similarly, urinary manganese concentration does not correlate with changes in clinical neurological status; however, urinary manganese does indicate recent exposure (Cook et al. 1974; Roels et al. 1987). In addition to a good clinical history, the most promising techniques for differentiation of Parkinson's disease from parkinsonism secondary to a neurotoxin are MRI

TABLE 22–10. Sources of mercury exposure

Antiseptics	Jewelry
Bactericides and fungicides	Laundry and diaper services
Barometers	Manometers
Batteries	Mercury vapor lamps
Carbon brush production	Paints and dyes
Caustic soda production	Paper and paper pulp manufacturing
Ceramics	Photography
Chemical laboratory workers	Pressure gauges
Chloralkali production	Semiconductor solar cells
Dentistry	Silver and gold extraction
Direct current meters	Silvering in mirrors
Electroplating	Tannery workers
Embalming preparations	Tattooing materials
Fingerprint detectors	Taxidermists
Fluorescent, neon, and mercury arc lamps	Thermometers
Infrared detectors	Ultrasonic amplifiers
Ink manufacturing	Vinyl chloride production
Insecticide manufacturing	Wood preservatives

Source. Adapted from Yip L, Dart R, Sullivan J: "Mercury," in *Clinical Environmental Health and Toxic Exposures,* 2nd edition. Edited by Sullivan JB, Krieger CR. Philadelphia, PA, Lippincott Williams & Wilkins, 2001, pp 867–878.

and positron emission tomography (PET) (Wolters et al. 1989). In patients with Parkinson's disease, MRI and PET scans show selective abnormalities and decreased dopamine-binding sites, respectively, in the area of the substantia nigra. Neurological symptoms have been attributed to manganese fumes generated during welding. Recent studies have associated welding and parkinsonism. Welding without proper protection was associated with syndromes of parkinsonism, multifocal myoclonus, mild cognitive impairment, and vestibular-auditory dysfunction. Also noted was an MRI T1 hyperintensity in the basal ganglia of the workers suggestive of manganese neurotoxicity. An increased MRI T1 signal in the basal ganglia is a biological marker of manganese accumulation (Josephs et al. 2005). The clinical history should include the symptoms, age at onset, identification and proof of exposure, and nature of response to levodopa therapy. The presence of Lewy bodies indicates Parkinson's disease. In addition, more selective and severe degeneration of the substantia nigra postmortem would indicate primary Parkinson's disease.

Treatment

Preventive measures that decrease body burden are most effective in the treatment of manganese exposure. Chelation therapy with calcium disodium ethylenediaminetetraacetic acid (EDTA) may be used to hasten elimination (Cook et al. 1974) but has limited success when given in the presence of existing neurological damage

(Wynter 1962). A lack of response to levodopa therapy in relieving the persistent extrapyramidal effects of manganese poisoning suggests damage that is more widespread. Moreover, the use of levodopa therapy may actually add to the neurotoxicity by increasing the production of free radicals (Parenti et al. 1988).

MERCURY

The general population is exposed to mercury primarily by inhalation and fish consumption. Mercury enters the atmosphere from the mining of cinnabar (HgS), smelting of the ore, and burning of coal. Levels in the atmosphere range from 4 to 50 ng/m^3. Levels in coastal and surface waters average 6 ng/L and 50 ng/L, respectively. Currently, mercury is used in the manufacture of electric meters, batteries, and industrial control instruments; in the production of chloralkali and fungicidal paints; and as catalysts (Dart and Sullivan 2004; Wide 1986). Additional sources and industries in which exposure can occur are listed in Table 22–10. Occupational use of mercury is declining. The groups that are most likely to be exposed are health care providers, dentists, dental technicians, electrical equipment technicians, and miners.

Neuropsychiatric Manifestations

Mercury in elemental form is a liquid and is poorly absorbed through the gastrointestinal tract. However, mercury vaporizes easily and is well absorbed by inhalation, with a predilection for the central nervous system. Organic mercury, particularly methylmercury, is lipid soluble and is absorbed well through the gastrointestinal tract, crosses the blood-brain barrier, and has substantial neurotoxic effects.

A urinary mercury concentration of 30–50 µg/L may result in subclinical neuropsychiatric effects, and at 50–100 µg/L, a subclinical tremor is noted. Overt neuropsychiatric disturbances are noted at a urine mercury concentration of 100 µg/L or greater, and an overt tremor is noted at 200 µg/L or greater (Dart and Sullivan 2004). Exposure to inhaled elemental mercury vapor is associated with symptoms such as insomnia; nervousness; mild tremor; headache; emotional lability; fatigue; decreased sexual drive; depression; and impaired cognition, judgment, and coordination (Louria 1988). Chronic low-level toxicity from inhalation of mercury vapor includes a syndrome known as *erythrism*, consisting of irritability; pathological shyness; and impairment of memory, attention span, and intellect (Landrigan 1982). Ngim et al. (1995) reported that dentists, occupationally exposed to elemental mercury vapor, had significant deficits in motor speed, visual scanning, concentration, memory, and coordination (Dart and Sullivan 2004).

Most of the information on the toxicity of organomercury compounds is derived from information on exposures to methylmercury. Because of the lipid solubility of methylmercury, the most toxic of the short-chain alkylmercury compounds, absorption is almost complete, with subsequent slow dealkylation in tissues to mercury. The classic triad of methylmercury poisoning includes dysarthria, ataxia, and constricted visual fields (Hunter et al. 1940). Methylmercury produces insidious early symptoms such as paresthesia, followed by motor incoordination, loss of position sense, dysarthria, hearing deficits, muscle rigidity, or spasticity with hyperreflexia. Neuropsychiatric symptoms reported include headache, sleep disturbances, dizziness, irritability, emotional instability, mania, and depression (Elhassani 1983). Methylmercury is a cumulative poison with similar clinical presentations resultant from both acute and chronic exposures. Symptoms may not manifest, even with acute intoxication, for several weeks to several months. Worsening of symptoms may continue for up to 10 years, during which the condition may be frequently misdiagnosed (Dart and Sullivan 2004).

Mechanisms of Action

Mercury has a high affinity for sulfhydryl groups, leading to inhibition of various enzymes such as choline acetyltransferase. Mercury also binds to membrane proteins, causing disruption of transport processes (Elhassani 1983). Methylmercury intoxication causes a disturbance in mitochondrial energy metabolism in skeletal muscle and apoptosis in cerebellum. Methylmercury-mediated oxidative stress plays an important role in the in vivo pathological process of intoxication (Usuki et al. 2001). During methylmercury-induced neurotoxicity, degeneration of the granule cell layer in the cerebellum occurs, which leads to deficits in motor function. Methylmercury appears to act preferentially on cerebellar granule cells by an increased spontaneous release of glutamate, which, coupled with methylmercury's ability to impair glutamate uptake by astrocytes, would cause calcium-mediated cell death (Atchinson 2005).

Diagnosis

Physical examination, history of exposure, and determination of blood, urine, hair, and food levels of mercury will help confirm the diagnosis of mercury poisoning. The normal concentration of mercury is less than 2 µg/dL in the blood and less than 10 µg/L in urine. Abdominal radiography may show radiopaque inorganic mercury; however, a negative radiograph does not exclude the presence of mercury. Electromyography and nerve conduction studies may be helpful in identifying peripheral nerve abnormalities in chronically exposed workers. To rule out corrosive effects on the gastrointestinal tract following ingestion, endoscopy is recommended.

Treatment

After acute ingestion of inorganic and organic mercury, treatment consists of inducing emesis or performing gastric lavage, in addition to administering activated charcoal. The use of BAL and its derivatives, as well as penicillamine, has been shown to be helpful in the treatment of poisoning with elemental and inorganic mercury. However, these agents have minimal effect in patients with organic mercury intoxication. BAL is actually contraindicated in the treatment of methylmercury poisoning because it has been shown to increase methylmercury levels in laboratory animals (Klaassen 2001a). Polymeric vinyl resins may be more effective than penicillamine in removing the organic mercury compounds from the body (Klaassen 2001a). In patients with renal impairment secondary to acute inorganic mercury poisoning, hemodialysis may be very helpful. Conventional hemodialysis in the treatment of organic mercury intoxication is of little value; however, the use of L-cysteine has been effective in complexing methylmercury into a form that is more dialyzable (Klaassen 2001a). Mercury is sequestered in lysosomal dense bodies in neurons and is known to persist in the brain for long periods (Cavanagh 1988). In the central and peripheral nervous systems, the damage caused by mercury poisoning appears to be permanent. Elhassani

(1983) reported that the administration of neostigmine improved motor strength in patients with methylmercury intoxication. More recently, an antioxidant—Trolox (6-hydroxy-2,5,7,8-tetramethylchroman-2-carboxylic acid), a water-soluble vitamin E analogue—was reported to have in vivo effectiveness against the induced cellular toxicity following methylmercury exposure (Usuki et al. 2001).

ORGANOTINS

Organotin compounds are a group of biologically active organometallics increasingly used as biocides, preservatives, catalysts, and polymer stabilizers. Figure 22–1 shows the three-dimensional structure of the various trialkyltin compounds. The trimethyltin and triethyltin compounds are absorbed via the gastrointestinal tract and skin and are the most neurotoxic of the organotin compounds, whereas the organotins with larger alkyl groups appear less neurotoxic. Tributyltin is used as a molluscacide and is incorporated into marine paints.

Neuropsychiatric Manifestations

Trimethyltin has been implicated in cases of occupational poisoning in the chemical industry (Ross et al. 1981). After exposure due to spillage, 22 chemical plant workers were noted to develop symptoms of depression, including forgetfulness, fatigue and weakness, loss of libido, headaches, sleep disturbance, and loss of motivation. In another case, 6 chemical factory workers (Ross et al. 1981) who had been exposed for multiple short periods over a 3-day period developed headache, tinnitus, deafness, impaired memory, disorientation, aggressiveness, psychosis, syncope, and loss of consciousness. The severity of symptoms correlated with urinary tin concentrations. Electroencephalographic findings included right-sided frontal temporal delta waves and, in one case, focal spikes in the temporal region. Fortemps et al. (1978) had previously described memory dysfunction, anorexia, insomnia, headache, disorientation that progressed to acute mental confusion, and seizures. In the early 1950s, a preparation with diethyltin iodide (Stalinon), containing the contaminant triethyltin, was responsible for the poisoning of several hundred people (Rouzaud and Lutier 1954). Increased intracranial pressure and seizures, common clinical findings in subjects exposed to trimethyltin, were present in the individuals poisoned with the contaminated diethyltin iodide.

Mechanisms of Action

Neuropathological examination of mice treated with trimethyltin detected damage to the hippocampus, primarily a loss of pyramidal cells in the CA1 and CA3 regions (Dyer et al. 1982), as well as some alteration in the pyriform cor-

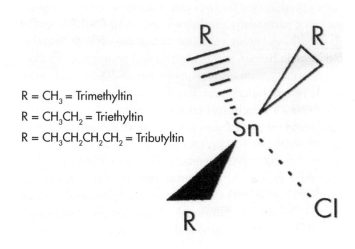

R = CH$_3$ = Trimethyltin
R = CH$_3$CH$_2$ = Triethyltin
R = CH$_3$CH$_2$CH$_2$CH$_2$ = Tributyltin

FIGURE 22–1. Chemical structures of trialkyltin compounds.

tex, amygdala, and neocortex (A.W. Brown et al. 1979). Triethyltin appears to have a different neuronal target than trimethyltin does in rats. White matter edema of the brain and spinal cord, intramyelinic vacuolation, and myelin splitting are found in subjects poisoned with triethyltin (Magee et al. 1957). Organotins inhibit oxidative phosphorylation in vitro and in vivo, inhibit production of adenosine triphosphatases, and thus can act as ionophores (Selwyn 1976). Trimethyltin can inhibit the uptake of neurotransmitters into mouse forebrain synaptosomes in vitro and in vivo (Doctor et al. 1982), as well as protein synthesis in the cortex and hippocampus of treated mice (Costa and Sulaiman 1986). Although the exact mechanism of neurotoxicity is unclear, recent studies suggested that interleukin-1α and interleukin-1β expressed in reactive astrocytes participated in trimethyltin neurotoxicity via type II glucocorticoid receptors. These changes coincided with trimethyltin-induced neuronal death in CA3 pyramidal cells of the hippocampus (Liu et al. 2005).

Diagnosis and Treatment

Diagnosis of organotin poisoning is based on a history of exposure together with clinical symptoms. Supportive care is the mainstay of treatment.

GASES

CARBON MONOXIDE

Carbon monoxide (CO) poisoning continues to be a significant cause of death throughout the world. In the United States, approximately 3,500 deaths occur each year because of CO intoxication. It occurs less frequently in developed countries today as a result of changes in combustion systems and heating fuels. The most common source of CO poisoning is the incomplete combustion of carbon-based fuels and inadequate ventilation during the operation of machinery using internal combustion engines. Space heaters, oil or gas burners, tobacco smoke, blast furnaces, and building fires are other sources of the gas (Bleecker 1994).

Neuropsychiatric Manifestations

Very low concentrations (0.01%) of CO in the air can cause a slight headache. At concentrations of 0.05%, 0.1%, and 0.2%, CO can cause severe headaches, dizziness, tachycardia, tachypnea, and coma (Dart 2004b; Ellenhorn 1997). Inhalation of 1% CO is usually fatal within 30–45 minutes. Very low concentrations of carboxyhemoglobin can produce impairment of visual, auditory, and temporal discriminations (Beard and Grandstaff 1970). Headache, nausea, and vomiting, as well as dizziness and disorientation to time, place, and person, follow acute intoxication. The patient also may experience arousal, lethargy, and, at times, coma. Generalized muscular hypertonia and spasticity may occur. Seizures also may be a presenting feature.

Neurological examination of a CO-intoxicated patient finds "lead-pipe" rigidity (i.e., an even resistance) without cogwheeling (i.e., a rhythmically interrupted or ratchetlike resistance). Parkinsonism, generalized dystonia, tremor, tics, and chorea also have been reported. Patients also may have a delayed clinical picture of neuropsychiatric symptoms (Dart 2004b; Ellenhorn 1997). Patients may recover from a short-term exposure after several days, during which initial neuropsychiatric symptoms may have already disappeared. After a period averaging 2–4 weeks, a sudden deterioration may develop consisting of amnestic disturbances, disorientation, signs of dementia, hypokinesia, bizarre and occasionally psychotic behavior, urinary incontinence, personality changes, apathy, emotional instability, anxiety, and autonomic dysregulation (Min 1986). Patients also may experience diarrhea, vomiting, periodic nausea, fever, and palpitations. Table 22–11 lists the delayed neuropsychiatric sequelae after CO intoxication.

Mechanisms of Action

CO combines with hemoglobin in the blood to form carboxyhemoglobin. Hemoglobin in its carboxyhemoglobin form cannot bind with oxygen and cannot oxygenate the tissues. The intrinsic affinity of hemoglobin for CO is 200 times greater than that for oxygen and accounts for the potency and lethality of CO via carboxyhemoglobin.

Factors involved in determining the toxicity of CO include the concentration of the gas in the air, duration of exposure, respiratory minute volume, cardiac output, hematocrit, oxygen demand of tissues, and preexisting

TABLE 22–11. Neuropsychiatric symptoms in delayed syndrome associated with carbon monoxide intoxication

Symptom	Number (%) of patients (N=86)
Psychiatric	
Apathy	86 (100)
Disorientation	86 (100)
Amnesia	86 (100)
Hypokinesia	82 (95)
Mutism	82 (95)
Irritability, distractibility	78 (91)
Apraxia	65 (76)
Bizarre behaviors	60 (70)
Stereotyped behavior	35 (41)
Confabulation	26 (30)
Insomnia	16 (19)
Depressed mood	13 (15)
Delusions	10 (12)
Echolalia	2 (2)
Elated mood	2 (2)
Neurological	
Urinary and fecal incontinence	80 (93)
Gait disturbance	78 (91)
Glabella sign	78 (91)
Grasp reflex	75 (87)
Increased muscle tone	74 (86)
Retropulsion	62 (72)
Increased deep tendon reflexes	19 (22)
Flaccid paralysis	16 (19)
Tremor	12 (14)
Dysarthria	8 (9)

Source. Adapted from Ellenhorn 1997 and Min 1986.

cerebrovascular disease. Children are inherently more sensitive than adults are to the effects of CO because of increased metabolic activity (Klaassen 2001b).

Poisoning with CO causes an increase in intracranial pressure because of transudation across capillaries of the brain. Pathological changes in the brain observed in postmortem examination include congestion, edema, petechiae, hemorrhagic focal necrosis, and perivascular infarcts. The characteristic pathology of CO toxicity is bilateral necrosis of the globus pallidus. The hippocampus, cerebral cortex, cerebellum, and substantia nigra are also vulnerable to CO toxicity (Ginsberg 1985).

Diagnosis

The clinical features of CO poisoning approximately correlate with carboxyhemoglobin levels. Laboratory tests usually are not helpful in establishing the diagnosis. Abnormal electroencephalographic findings such as low-voltage waves and diffuse slowing are common and can reflect the progression of hypoxic encephalopathy. However, EEGs have much less predictive value because patients with markedly abnormal EEG findings may show complete recovery (Dart 2004b; Ellenhorn 1997). Horowitz et al. (1987), reporting MRI findings in two patients, described areas of high signal intensity in the globus pallidus.

Treatment

Control of airway, support of breathing, a high oxygen concentration, and cardiac monitoring should be initiated in a patient with CO toxicity. Supplemental oxygen is continued until the carboxyhemoglobin level is significantly reduced (Dart 2004b; Ellenhorn 1997). Dextroamphetamine, a potent dopaminergic agent, has been used for treating the neuropsychiatric symptoms of CO poisoning. This agent shortens cognitive and motor recovery time and shows therapeutic benefit within the first 10 days of use (Smallwood and Murray 1999).

ETHYLENE OXIDE

Ethylene oxide is an intermediary agent used in the production of antifreeze, polyester fibers and bottles, photographic films, glycol ethers, and nonionic surface-active agents. Health care workers are exposed through its use as a sterilant for heat-sensitive materials in central supply units.

Neuropsychiatric Manifestations

High levels of exposure to ethylene oxide result in acute encephalopathy and peripheral neuropathy (Gross 1979). Ethylene oxide has been reported to produce persistent neurological and neuropsychological impairment after long-term low-level exposure (Crystal et al. 1988). Impairments in visual and verbal memory and decrements in auditory and visual attention were noted in individuals after exposure. Central processing of visual and verbal information was also slowed.

Mechanisms of Action

Ethylene oxide is a highly reactive gas that produces a primary axonal neuropathy and mild Schwann's cell changes. It also affects myelinated fibers (Kuzuhara et al. 1983).

Diagnosis

A history of exposure to ethylene oxide is of prime importance in establishing the diagnosis. Tests found to be helpful are the P300 evoked potential amplitude and psychomotor speed tests. Workers exposed to ethylene oxide had lower P300 amplitude, hypoactive reflexes, and poor performance on tests measuring psychomotor speed (Metter and Bleecker 1994).

Treatment

At present, no treatment is known for ethylene oxide poisoning. Symptoms improve when an exposed individual is removed from the environment containing the gas, and long-term improvement is noticeably present when ethylene oxide exposure ceases altogether (Gross 1979).

SOLVENTS

Hydrocarbon solvents have been used for many years as therapeutic agents for anesthesia, in the chemical industry to dissolve chemicals, as refrigerant agents, as typewriter correction fluid, and as cleaning agents. Workers are exposed primarily through inhalation and dermal exposure. Abuse of solvents occurs commonly through sniffing of glue or paint.

NEUROPSYCHIATRIC MANIFESTATIONS

Long-term exposure to solvents often results in subjective complaints of headache, dizziness, fatigue, malaise, weakness, memory impairment, and anxiety. Table 22–3 lists some of the neuropsychiatric manifestations of solvent exposure. Exposed individuals also may have emotional lability, irritability, sexual dysfunction, difficulties in concentration and problem solving, and general intellectual slowing, as well as sensory and motor neuropathies after long-term exposure (Bleecker 1994). An association exists between exposure to solvents and lower neurobehavioral performance, with significant neurobehavioral deficits among children exposed to solvents in comparison with working children not exposed to solvents and nonworking schoolchildren. Memory and motor dexterity appear to be particularly affected in solvent-exposed working children (Saddik et al. 2005). Solvent toxicity also may cause cardiac effects such as dysrhythmias, which result from the abuse of freons and other fluorinated hydrocarbons as well as industrial exposure in the manufacture of aliphatic and aromatic solvents.

Trichloroethylene is well known for causing peripheral neuropathy, particularly of the trigeminal nerve, an effect known as *tic douloureux*. Chlorinated hydrocarbon solvents are likely to cause hepatocellular damage, and periodic measurements of enzymes may be a useful technique to detect overexposure (Dart 2004b; Ellenhorn 1997).

n-Hexane is an industrial solvent known to cause peripheral neuropathy, the major manifestation of its toxicity. Although used primarily as a glue and solvent for adhesives, it can also be found in gasoline. *n*-Hexane neuropathy has been described, and its metabolite methyl-*n*-butylketone-2-5-hexanedione is known to be a reactive intermediate agent that inhibits the glycolytic pathway of metabolism, resulting in peripheral neuropathy. Although most of the solvents produce consistent neuropsychiatric sequelae with short-term exposure, certain solvents, such as *n*-hexane, produce peripheral neuropathies due to metabolites produced by the liver and structural differences of the original solvent (Dart 2004b).

DIAGNOSIS AND TREATMENT

A history of exposure, cognitive impairment as shown on a neuropsychological test battery, and the presence of clinical symptoms are helpful in establishing the diagnosis of solvent toxicity. At present, few treatments exist for solvent-induced neurotoxicity. Symptoms decrease when the patient is removed from the offending agent. Treatment primarily involves minimizing future exposure. Monitoring of levels in the workplace is helpful.

PESTICIDES

Pesticides are unique among environmental chemicals in that they are placed deliberately into the environment to injure or kill animal, plant, or microbial life. The well-known classes of pesticides are the organochlorines, pyrethroids, organophosphates, and carbamates. Table 22–5 lists the neuropsychiatric sequelae of exposure to various classes of pesticides.

ORGANOCHLORINE

Figure 22–2 depicts the chemical structures of representative organochlorine pesticides. The organochlorine insecticides chlordane and chlordecone (Kepone) are not biodegradable and accumulate in the environment; therefore, they are no longer used. Chlordane was primarily used in the past for termite and fire ant control. At present, the Environmental Protection Agency prohibits the delivery, sale, and use of chlordane in the United States. A National Cancer Institute study found that it causes hepatocellular carcinoma in mice (Bleecker 1994).

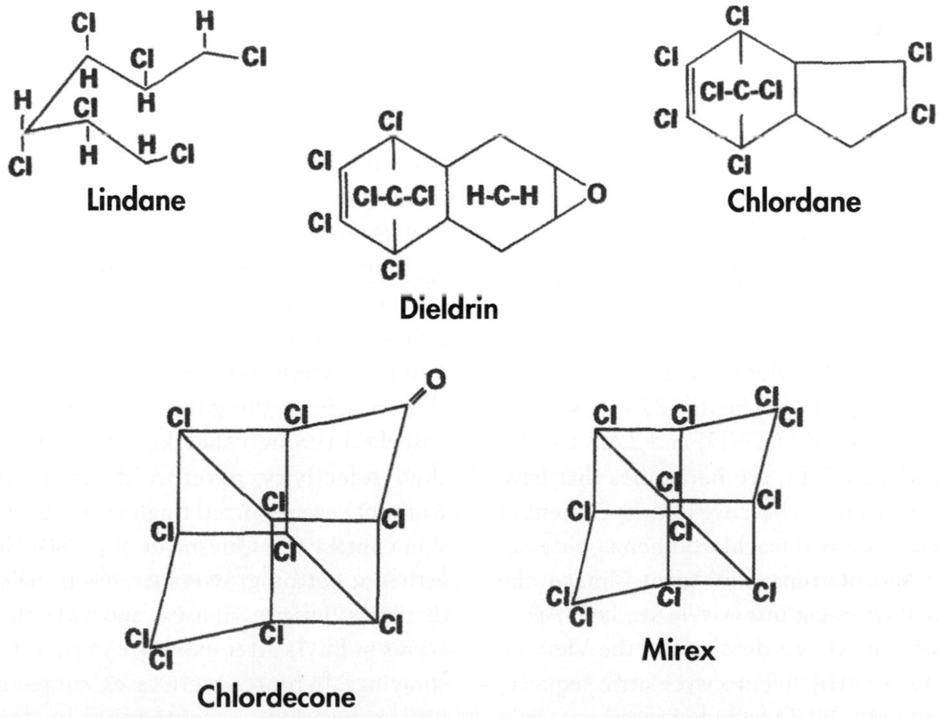

FIGURE 22–2. Chemical structures of representative organochlorine pesticides.

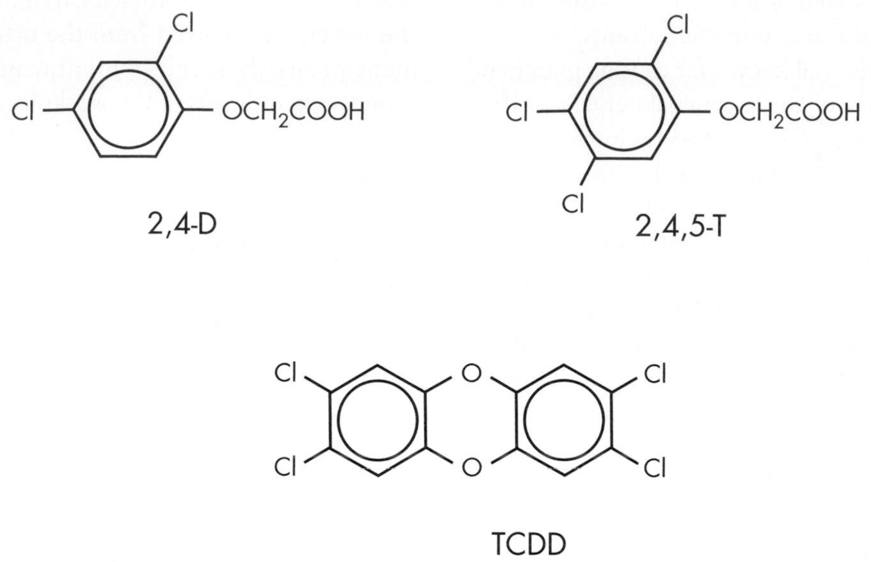

FIGURE 22–3.   Chemical structures of 2,4-dichlorophenoxyacetic acid (2,4-D), 2,4,5-trichlorophenoxyacetic acid (2,4,5-T), and 2,3,7,8-tetrachlorodibenzo-p-dioxin (TCDD).

The neuropsychiatric sequelae of long-term exposure to chlordane include early symptoms of fatigue, nausea, anorexia, and circumoral numbness. After a delay of 1 month, myoclonic jerks have been observed. After a longer time, cramps, seizures, and tremors occur. Cramps have been noted to be severe enough to produce vertebral fractures (Curley and Gerrettson 1969; Stranger and Kerridge 1968).

Chlordecone, an organochlorine pesticide, was used in the past primarily for the extermination of ants and roaches. In August 1974, the Environmental Protection Agency banned the delivery, sale, and use of chlordecone. The main route of chlordecone poisoning is by dermal or oral exposure due to careless use. Neuropsychiatric manifestations include nervousness, tremor, ataxia, weight loss, opsoclonus, and headaches. Changes in mental status, in addition to startle myoclonus, disorientation, confusion, and auditory and visual hallucinations, occur in many poisoned individuals (Taylor et al. 1978).

Chlorophenoxy compounds (Figure 22–3), such as 2,4-dichlorophenoxyacetic acid (2,4-D) and 2,4,5-trichlorophenoxyacetic acid (2,4,5-T), are herbicides that have received considerable attention because of their content of the extremely toxic 2,3,7,8-tetrachlorodibenzo-p-dioxin (TCDD or dioxin), a contaminant in Agent Orange, the toxicity of which is now being intensively studied. Agent Orange is an herbicide used as a defoliant in the Vietnam War (Roberts 1991a, 1991b). Neuropsychiatric sequelae of acute intoxication with 2,4-D include paresthesia, pain in the extremities, decreased vibration sense, reversible flaccid paralysis, and peripheral neuropathy (Food and Agriculture Organization/World Health Organization 1975). Acute intoxication with 2,4,5-T produces weakness in the muscles of mastication and swallowing, lethargy, anorexia, weakness in the lower extremities, and fatigue (Food and Agriculture Organization/World Health Organization 1975). Organochlorine pesticides remain in the environment and persist in tissues of humans and even animals in remote regions of the earth (Kannan et al. 2005).

PYRETHROIDS

Pyrethroids are recently developed, economical synthetic pesticides that have greater selective toxicity against insects than do carbamates or organophosphates. These synthetic insecticides are derived from an older class of botanical insecticides known as *pyrethrins*, a mixture of six insecticidal esters derived from desiccated chrysanthemum or pyrethrum flowers. The pyrethroids are readily absorbed from the gut and respiratory tract and poorly absorbed through the skin (Proudfoot 2005). Despite their selectivity, pyrethroids are neurotoxic; exposed workers have reported tingling and burning of the face on skin contact (Le Quesne et al. 1980). In addition to paresthesia, cotton growers experienced severe headaches, dizziness, fatigue, nausea, anorexia, and transient alterations in EEGs after exposure to pyrethroids from several sprayings. In more severe cases, subjects developed tremors, convulsions accompanied by fasciculations, and repetitive discharges on electromyograms (He et al.

TABLE 22–12. Representative commercially available organophosphate and carbamate insecticides and comparison of their relative toxicities by LD_{50}[a] on a rat lethality model

Organophosphates

High toxicity ($LD_{50} < 50$ mg/kg)	Moderate to low toxicity ($LD_{50} = 50$ to $>1,000$ mg/kg)
Azinphos-methyl (Guthion)	Acephate (Orthene)
Bomyl (Swat)	Bensulide (Betasan)
Carbophenothion (Trithion)	Chlorpyrifos (Dursban, Lorsban)
Chlorfenvinphos (Birlane)	Cythioate (Proban)
Chlormephos (Dotan)	Diazinon (Basudin, Spectracide)
Coumaphos (Co-ral)	Dichlorvos (DDVP, Vapona)
Demeton (Systox)	Dimethoate (Cygon)
Dialifor (Torak)	Ethion (Nialate)
Dicrotophos (Bidrin)	Fenitrothion (Accothion)
Disulfoton (Diasyston)	Fenthion (Baytex, Entex)
Fenamiphos (Nemacur)	Formothion (Anthio)
Fenophosphon (Agritox)	Propetamphos (Safrotin)
Isofluorophate mephosfolan (Cytrolane)	Pyrazophos (Afugan, Curamil)
Isophenfos (Amaze, Oftanol)	Quinalphos (Bayrusil)
Parathion-methyl (Penncap-M)	Sulprofos (Bolstar)
Phosphamidon (Dimecron)	Thiometon (Ekatin)
Prothoate (Fac)	Triazophos (Hostathion)
Sulfotepp (Bladafum)	Tribufos (Butonate)
Tetraethylpyrophosphate (Bladan, TEPP)	Trichlorfon (Tugon)

Carbamates

High toxicity ($LD_{50} < 50$ mg/kg)	Moderate to low toxicity ($LD_{50} = 50$ to >200 mg/kg)
Aldicarb (Temik)	Bufencarb (Bux)
Aldoxycarb (Standak)	Carbaril (Sevin)
Carbofuran (Furadan)	Pirimicarb (Pirimor)
Dimetilan (Snip)	Carbosulfan
Dioxacarb (Eleocron, Famid)	Thiodicarb (Larvin)
Propoxur (Baygon)	Trimethacarb (Broot)

[a]The LD_{50} is the dose of pesticide administered that kills 50% of test animals exposed. The LD_{50} is used to compare the relative toxicities of chemicals.

Source. Adapted from Erdman 2004.

1984). Ocular exposures have resulted in corneal erosion (Proudfoot 2005). Tetramethrin, a synthetic pyrethroid insecticide, was used globally for agriculture, but now environmental exposure is of greater concern because it exerted endocrine-disrupting effects in experimental animals through antiestrogenic action (Kim et al. 2005).

Pyrethroids act on the membrane level, particularly on sodium channels, resulting in a period of increased neuronal excitability followed by reduced excitability on submaximal stimulus (Le Quesne et al. 1980). Vitamin E, a biological antioxidant that may stabilize membranes, is recommended for preventing dysesthesias secondary to dermal exposure (Flannigan et al. 1984). Mephenesin is also an effective compound that provides some protection against pyrethroid neurotoxicity (Bradbury et al. 1983).

ORGANOPHOSPHATE AND CARBAMATE COMPOUNDS

In contrast to the organochlorine pesticides, which tend to accumulate in the environment, the organophosphate and carbamate pesticides (which constitute the largest group of pesticides) degrade rapidly. The organophosphate and carbamate pesticides include approximately 60–100 individual compounds used throughout the world, more than 40 of which are currently in commercial use in the United States (Table 22–12). Figures 22–4 and 22–5 illustrate representative chemical structures of common and widely used organophosphate and carbamate pesticides, respectively, that can produce neuropsychiatric symptoms.

As discussed later in this chapter, there has been a renewed interest in organophosphate compounds as a result of production and deployment of nerve agents by hostile military forces in the past few years. An increase in terrorism and concern that these lethal agents would be used on civilian populations in the United States have led to civil disaster preparations that included the training of physicians and other medical personnel to identify and treat organophosphate toxicity.

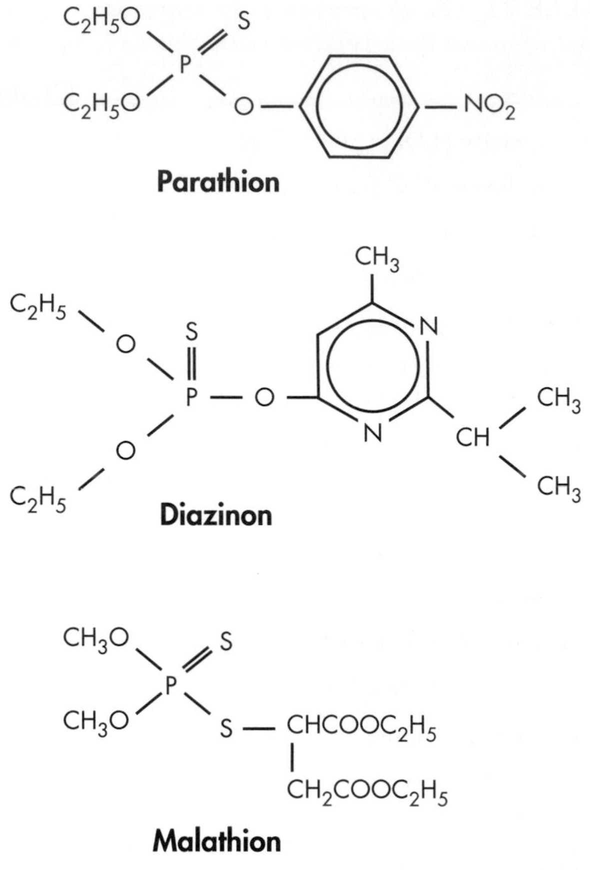

Neuropsychiatric Manifestations

Neuropsychiatric effects of exposure to organophosphates include anxiety, restlessness, apprehension, tension, labile mood, insomnia, and headache. Increasing levels of exposure may result in tremors, nightmares, increased dreaming, apathy, withdrawal, and depression. On further exposure, drowsiness, confusion, slurred speech, ataxia, generalized weakness, and coma predominate.

The onset of action of organophosphates is dependent on the type of organophosphate and the route of exposure. The onset may be quite sudden after inhalation or massive ingestion or delayed by as long as 12–48 hours following dermal exposure. Organophosphates, which are highly lipophilic, produce mild initial symptoms followed by severe cholinergic symptoms 48 hours later (Erdman 2004; Ellenhorn 1997).

The organophosphates produce chronic and delayed effects, including polyneuropathies and neurobehavioral alterations. Sensorimotor peripheral neuropathies may occur 8–14 days after exposure and do not necessarily follow acute cholinergic symptoms (Barret and Oehme 1985). The peripheral neuropathy associated with long-term exposure to organophosphates is a component of organophosphate-induced delayed neurotoxicity. Organophosphate-induced

FIGURE 22–4.   Chemical structures of organophosphate pesticides parathion, diazinon, and malathion.

delayed neurotoxicity may occur as early as 2 weeks following an exposure, and symptoms may begin with cramping in the calves and numbness and tingling in the feet, followed by progressive weakness in the lower extremities. Eventually, bilateral foot drop and equilibrium are also disturbed. In addition to triorthocresyl phosphate, mipafox and leptophos are known to cause organophosphate-induced delayed neurotoxicity, from which recovery is poor (Bidstrup et al. 1953). Long-term neuropsychiatric and neurobehavioral symptoms of organophosphate exposure include fatigue, anxiety, depression, restlessness and irritability, drowsiness, lability, confusion, and occasionally frank psychosis. These symptoms are usually subtle and mild, begin within days to weeks after the exposure, and resolve spontaneously over the course of several months to a year (Erdman 2004). A few cases may be long lasting and may persist for longer than a year. Memory and concentration deficits may cause a decline in work performance (Lerman et al. 1984).

Mechanisms of Action

Organophosphate and carbamate compounds inhibit the enzyme acetylcholinesterase, an essential enzyme for

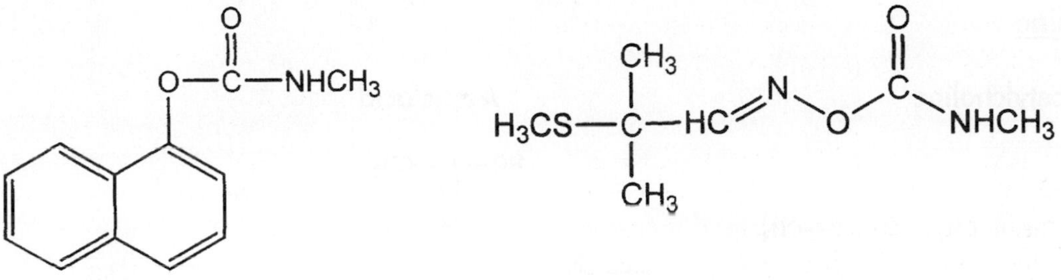

Aldicarb (Temik)   **Carbaril (Sevin)**

FIGURE 22–5. Chemical structures of representative carbamate pesticides.

normal nervous system function, by binding with the serine hydroxyl group in the active site of the enzyme (Figure 22–6). A resultant increase in acetylcholine concentration, particularly in the central nervous system, is responsible for many of the symptoms produced by exposure to organophosphates.

Diagnosis

The diagnosis of organophosphate toxicity is primarily by a history of exposure to pesticides, as well as signs and symptoms of excessive cholinergic activity. To help confirm the diagnosis, organophosphates usually have garlic-like odor, which may emanate from the patient or from the container from which the poison was dispensed. Red blood cell cholinesterase is the preferred marker for organophosphate toxicity because it is the same enzyme found in nervous tissue. Decreased acetylcholinesterase activity, in conjunction with a history of exposure, usually confirms the diagnosis. Short-term exposure may decrease acetylcholinesterase activity to 50% of baseline. There may be a return to normal activity after several weeks (Ellenhorn 1997; Erdman 2004).

Treatment

After exposure to organophosphates, the primary concern is stabilization of vital signs, followed by decontamination. Decontamination procedures include removing all contaminated clothing and thoroughly washing all exposed skin surfaces. Atropine is administered because it noncompetitively antagonizes both muscarinic and nicotinic receptors, thereby blocking the effect of excess acetylcholine (Erdman 2004). In addition to atropine, pralidoxime, an oxime and acetylcholinesterase reactivator, is useful in both organophosphate pesticide and nerve agent poisoning. The side effects of pralidoxime usually occur in only a small group of patients and include excitement, confusion, tachycardia, headache, and blurred vision possibly caused by central anticholinergic toxicity (Erdman 2004; Goetz 1985).

TOXINS

Neurotoxins occurring naturally from marine, microbial, plant, and animal species have led to many episodes of poisoning in humans. Clinical observations of these episodes of poisoning and their resulting sequelae have led to the study of these toxic compounds in model systems. Some of these naturally occurring neurotoxins have become significant tools in studying the pathogenesis of neurodegeneration within the central nervous system as well as the etiology of resultant neuropsychiatric manifestations. Because the neuropsychiatric sequelae of neurotoxins are currently a matter of interest, the subject can be only partially covered in this chapter. Rather, I focus on a few selective compounds with mechanisms and neuropsychiatric sequelae that seem to be of major relevance. For a complete review of the general toxicology of marine, microbial, fungal, plant, and animal toxins, the interested reader should refer to the work of Dart (2004b).

MARINE TOXINS

Domoic Acid

Domoic acid is a heat-stable, potent excitatory tricarboxylic amino acid found in high concentrations in cultured blue mussels (*Mytilus edulis*). It is structurally related to glutamic and kainic acid (D.J. Wu and Li 2005). It is formed by *Nitzchia pungens*, a phytoplanktonic diatom that is bioconcentrated in the blue mussel. In November 1987, at least 150 individuals in Canada had acute symptoms of intoxication after consuming cultured blue mussels; 19 individuals required hospitalization and 4 died (Jeffery et al. 2004).

The neuropsychiatric consequences of domoic acid intoxication include altered states of arousal, such as coma, abdominal paralysis, limbic seizures, and myoclonus; chronic impairment of memory; atrophy of distal musculature; and motor weakness (T.M. Perl et al. 1990;

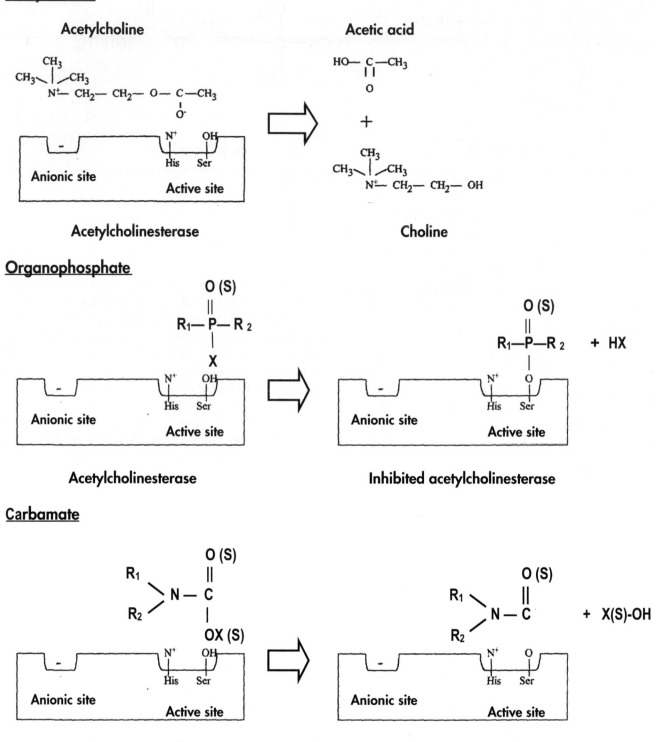

FIGURE 22–6. Interaction between an organophosphate or carbamate ester with the serine hydroxyl group in the active site of the enzyme acetylcholinesterase. The inhibited enzyme undergoes dephosphorylation or decarbamoylation when bound to an organophosphate and carbamate, respectively, and forms, as a result, free enzyme. R_1 and R_2 = alkyl or aryl groups; X = leaving group (varies with pesticide); (S) = sulfur moiety.

Teitelbaum et al. 1990). These symptoms usually were not accompanied by sensory deficits (Teitelbaum et al. 1990). Elderly persons appeared to be more affected than younger patients were.

PET studies carried out in 4 subjects 2–3 months after intoxication found decreased glucose metabolism in the mesial temporal lobe, which correlated well with the patients' memory scores. Neuropathological studies in 4 patients also showed a marked loss of neurons in the hippocampus and amygdaloid nucleus, as well as lesions in the septal area, secondary olfactory area, claustrum, dorsal medial nucleus of the thalamus, and insular and subfrontal cortex. The pattern of neurotoxic injury, particularly hippocampal damage, seems to be similar to the abnormalities induced experimentally by the excitotoxin kainate in the same structures of rodents (Chandrasekaran et al. 2004; Teitelbaum et al. 1990). In monkeys, excitatory damage from domoic acid administration is predominantly observed in the hypothalamus, hippocampus, and area postrema (Perez-Mendes et al. 2005; Tryphonas et al. 1990), a pattern similar to that of neuronal degeneration produced by kainate. Impairment of the blood-brain barrier integrity within the piriform cortex accompanied the onset of domoic acid neurotoxicity (Scallet et al. 2005). Domoic acid induces late neuronal death and caspase-3-like activity in cortical and hippocampal cells in culture (Erin and Billingsley 2004). Domoic acid appears to induce a pattern of acute neuropsychiatric change and permanent neurological deficits that resemble changes induced experimentally by kainate.

Tetrodotoxin

Puffer fish poisoning or tetrodotoxin intoxication is usually caused by improper preparation of the fish, which causes gastroenteritis and severe neurological manifestations. Tetrodotoxin-producing bacteria are in the ovaries, liver, intestines, and gallbladder of the puffer fish. Tetrodotoxin-producing bacteria have been isolated, and thus far, 19 Bacillus species have been identified (Z. Wu et al. 2005). Analysis of puffer fish tissue extracts by a fluorometric tetrodotoxin analyzer reported the presence of three tetrodotoxin derivatives besides tetrodotoxin. The toxic derivatives were isolated and identified as tetrodonic acid, 4-epitetrodotoxin, and anhydrotetrodotoxin (Nakamura and Yasumoto 1985). The highest concentrations of the toxins are in the cytosolic fraction of the liver homogenates of the puffer fish (Nagashima et al. 1999).

Tetrodotoxin is one of the most toxic of the natural toxins. Tetrodotoxin prevents the flow of sodium ions by blocking the channel through which sodium ions flow, producing neuronal conduction abnormalities in both motor and sensory nerves. The neuropsychiatric manifestations of tetrodotoxin after oral ingestion include weakness, ataxia, paresthesia in the face spreading to the extremities, nausea, diarrhea, pallor, and sweating. Intoxication may begin with oral paresthesia, sometimes with gastroenteric symptoms, that progresses to generalized paresthesia and motor paralysis of the extremities. In subacute poisoning, recovery is usually complete in 24 hours. In acute poisoning, hypoactive reflexes, gross muscular incoordination, aphonia, dysphagia, and respiratory distress in severe cases may occur, but consciousness is preserved. Unusual features of poisoning reported include hypertension, pinpoint pupils, bronchorrhea, and a facial flush (C.C. Yang et al. 1996). The last stages of the illness are characterized by mental impairment and respiratory paralysis. Rapid onset of symptoms and greater severity are associated with poorer prognosis (Ellenhorn 1997). Patients should receive symptomatic and supportive treatment and care, including gastric lavage and intravenous fluid. Intubation and mechanical ventilation should be considered if paralysis progresses quickly (Kanchanapongkul 2001; Stommel and Watters 2004).

MICROBIAL TOXINS

Botulinum Toxin

Botulinum toxin produced by *Clostridium botulinum* is the most potent natural poison known. Of the seven immunologically distinct types of botulinum toxin, types A, B, and E are the causes of most human cases of poisoning. Epidemiological analysis of cases of botulism has shown that 60% of cases are caused by type A toxin, 30% by type B, and 10% by type E, usually associated with ingestion of contaminated seafood. The bacterial spores may be found during the home canning process and tend to be resistant to heat. They may survive at temperatures greater than 120°C. The exotoxin is heat labile and can be inactivated at 85°C, in contrast to the heat-resistant spores (Dunbar 1990).

Neuropsychiatric manifestations of botulinum toxin appear within 12–36 hours after ingestion of contaminated food. The patient initially develops bulbar symptoms, including diplopia, ptosis, dysarthria, and dysphagia. These symptoms are followed by a descending pattern of weakness affecting first the upper and then the lower limbs (Cherington 1974, 1990). In severe cases, respiratory paralysis occurs, requiring assisted ventilation. Mild forms of botulism are characterized by bulbar findings and subtle weakness of muscles of the limbs that may mimic myasthenia gravis. A striking response to intravenous anticholinesterase agents is noted (Ryan and Cherington 1971). The pattern of descending weakness is a clinical hallmark of botulism and distinguishes it from the classic form of Guillain-Barré syndrome, which usually presents with an ascending pattern of weakness. Patients should receive symptomatic and supportive treatment and care, including assisted ventilation and, if indicated, intubation and mechanical ventilation.

Tetanus Toxin

Tetanospasmin, or tetanus toxin, is a soluble-protein exotoxin produced by the bacterium *Clostridium tetani*. Tetanus is a syndrome of autonomic dysfunction, neuromuscular junction blockade, muscle stiffness, and spasms caused by tetanospasmin. Although tetanus is rare in countries with immunization programs, an estimated 800,000 newborns die from neonatal tetanus every year. At present, tetanus is the second leading cause of death from diseases included in the expanded immunization program of the World Health Organization (WHO) (Traverso et al. 1991; World Health Organization 1988).

In most cases, the incubation period for tetanus after the introduction of organisms into a wound is 3–14 days, with an average of 7 days (Habermann 1978). Neuropsychiatric manifestations include backache, stiff neck, leg pains, spasms, dysphagia, abdominal cramps, vertigo, and facial weakness resembling Bell's palsy. The most common presentation is trismus due to the spasm of masseter muscles. The initial symptoms are usually followed by generalized rigidity as well as spasms with painful tonic contractions of both agonist and antagonist muscles. Superimposed on the baseline rigidity are proximal spasms that can be so severe that they resemble a generalized seizure or intense decorticate posturing, referred to as *tetanic seizures* (Weinstein 1973). Patients often remain conscious during these episodes (Bleck 1991). Treatment of tetanus involves wound care, antitoxin therapy and immunization, management of rigidity and spasms, and treatment of the autonomic derangements.

PLANT TOXINS

Exposure to poisonous plants is a common occurrence. Fortunately, most commonly encountered plants produce either no toxicity or mild to moderate toxicity consisting of gastroenteritis. A few plants produce serious neuropsychiatric effects. These include oleander and foxglove, which cause digitalis-type toxicity; water hemlock herbal remedies that have convulsant properties; and jequirity pea and castor beans, which contain the neurotoxic polypeptides abrin and ricin, respectively, both potent inhibitors of ribosomal function known to produce multiorgan failure and death (Balint 2004; Ellenhorn 1997).

Diagnosis of plant toxicity involves identification of the plant, which is often difficult. Because individual sus-

ceptibility varies, prediction of toxicity is also difficult. Further complicating management is the lack of antidotes to most plant toxins (Caravati et al. 2004). Table 22–13 lists psychoactive substances with neuropsychiatric effects found in herbal preparations. Table 22–14 lists the major plants that produce the neuropsychiatric symptoms of hallucinations and their active ingredients. Table 22–15 lists the major plants abused recreationally for their ability to alter the sensorium.

FUNGAL TOXINS

Fungi are ubiquitous in the environment, and greater than 50,000 fungal species exist. Mushrooms or macrofungi make mushroom poisons, whereas molds or microfungi produce multiple complex heterocyclic compounds that are medicinally useful as well as highly toxic secondary products known as *mycotoxins*.

Macrofungi

Mushrooms are used in religious rites, are consumed recreationally, and may be ingested accidentally by children and amateur mushroom hunters who collected, cooked, and ate what was misidentified as a delectable species (Bennett and Klich 2003; Sudakin 2004). Mushrooms fall into two classes: those with delayed toxic response after ingestion and those with an immediate effect. Mushrooms producing a delayed response seldom affect the nervous system. Mushrooms that produce poisons that predominantly affect the central nervous system generally produce an immediate response such as hallucinations. Mushrooms in the genus *Psilocybe* contain the indolealkylamine hallucinogen psilocybin and its dephosphorylated congener psilocin (Figure 22–7).

Psilocin is about one and a half times more potent than psilocybin. Neuropsychiatric manifestations of mushroom toxins may be observed 20–30 minutes after ingestion. Visual hypersensitivity usually leads to illusions and hallucinations. Dysphoria, hyperreflexia, drowsiness, and euphoria also may occur. The individual may experience flushing of the face, tachycardia, hyperthermia, and hypertension. Dangerous complications may be suicidality and trauma secondary to reckless behavior under the influence of the substance, and psychiatric symptoms may persist long after immediate effects have abated (Benjamin 1979). No specific therapy exists for psilocybin intoxication. Anxiety may be treated with benzodiazepines (Ellenhorn 1997; Schonwald 2004b; Sudakin 2004), and anticholinergic effects may be reversed with physostigmine (Van Poorten et al. 1982). Multifocal cerebral demyelination has been reported after mushroom abuse (Spengos et al. 2000).

TABLE 22–13. Psychoactive substances used in herbal preparations

Ingredient	Scientific name	Active ingredients	Use	Effects
Bufo toad secretions	*Bufo* species	Bufotenin	Secretions smoked or ingested as hallucinogen	Hallucinogen
California poppy	*Eschscholtzia californica*	Isoquinoline alkaloids	Smoked as marijuana substitute	Probably none
Catnip	*Nepeta cataria*	Nepetalactone	Smoked or tea as marijuana substitute	Euphoriant
Cinnamon	*Cinnamomum camphora*	Unknown	Smoked with marijuana	Mild stimulant
Coca leaves	*Erythroxylum coca*	Cocaine	Chewed as stimulant	Stimulant
Cola nut	*Cola* species	Caffeine	Smoked, tea, or capsules as stimulant	Stimulant
Cuarana	*Paullinia cupana*	Caffeine	Capsules or tea as stimulant	Stimulant
Damiana	*Turnera diffusa*	Unknown	Smoked as marijuana substitute	Mild stimulant
Hemlock	*Conium maculatum*	Coniine	Tea or ingested as sedative	Sedative, cholinergic effects
Hops	*Humulus lupulus*	Humulene, myrcene, 3-caryophylline, farnesene	Smoked or tea as sedative and marijuana substitute	Mild sedative
Iboga	*Tabernanthe iboga*	Indole alkaloids	Tea or chewed as hallucinogen	Hallucinogen
Juniper	*Juniper macropoda*	Unknown	Smoked as hallucinogen	Hallucinogen
Kava	*Piper methysticum*	Kava lactones	Smoked or tea as marijuana substitute	Hallucinogen
Khat	*Catha edulis*	Cathine, cathinone	Tea, chewed	Stimulant
Lobelia	*Lobelia inflate*	Lobeline	Smoked or tea as marijuana substitute	Mild euphoriant
Mandrake	*Mandragora officinarum*	Scopolamine, hyoscyamine	Tea as hallucinogen	Anticholinergic effects
Maté tea	*Ilex paraguensis*	Caffeine	Tea as stimulant	Stimulant
Mormon tea	*Ephedra nevadensis*	Ephedra	Tea as stimulant	Stimulant
Morning glory	*Ipomoea violacea, Ipomoea purpurea, Ipomoea corymbosa*	Lysergic acid hydroxyethylamide	Seeds crushed and ingested as hallucinogen	Hallucinogen
Nutmeg	*Myristica fragrans*	Myristicene, volatile oils	Tea as hallucinogen	Hallucinogen
Passion flower	*Passiflora incarnata*	Harmine alkaloids	Smoked, tea, or capsules as marijuana substitute	Mild stimulant

TABLE 22–13.   Psychoactive substances used in herbal preparations *(continued)*

Ingredient	Scientific name	Active ingredients	Use	Effects
Periwinkle	*Catharanthus roseus*	Indole alkaloids	Smoked or tea as euphoriant	Hallucinogen
Peyote	*Lophophora williamsii*	Mescaline	Chewed or tea as hallucinogen	Hallucinogen
Prickly poppy	*Argemone mexicana*	Protopine, berberine, isoquinolines	Smoked as euphoriant	Analgesic
Scotch broom	*Cytisus* species	Sparteine	Smoked as marijuana substitute	Mild euphoriant
Snakeroot	*Rauwolfia serpentine*	Reserpine	Smoked or tea as tobacco substitute	Sedative
Thorn-apple	*Datura stramonium*	Atropine, scopolamine	Smoked or tea as tobacco substitute or hallucinogen	Anticholinergic effects
Tobacco	*Nicotiana* species	Nicotine	Smoked as tobacco	Strong stimulant
Valerian	*Valeriana officinalis*	Valepotriates, volatile oils	Tea or capsules as sedative	Sedative
Wild lettuce	*Lactuca sativa*	Unknown	Smoked as opioid substitute	Possibly analgesic, sedative
Wormwood	*Artemisia absinthium*	Thujone	Smoked or tea as relaxant	Sedative
Yohimbine	*Corynanthe johimbe*	Yohimbine	Smoked or tea as stimulant	Mild hallucinogen

Source.   Adapted from DeWitt RC, Dart RC: "Herbal and Indigenous Remedies," in *Medical Toxicology.* Edited by Dart RC. Philadelphia, PA, Lippincott Williams & Wilkins, 2004, pp 1741–1747; Siegel RK: "Herbal Intoxication." *Journal of the American Medical Association* 236:474–476, 1976.

Microfungi

Molds or microfungi, in addition to mycotoxins, produce medicinally useful antibiotics that include penicillin, cephalosporin, erythromycin, griseofulvin, and neomycin. Molds also produce the potent immunosuppressants cyclosporine and tacrolimus used for organ transplantation and coumadin used commonly as an anticoagulant and antithrombotic agent. Also derived from mold are the structurally complex ergot alkaloids (Figure 22–8), such as ergotamine, lysergic acid diethylamide, and bromocriptine.

Chemically synthesized analogues of specific less toxic and nonhallucinogenic ergot alkaloids continue to be medically useful in uterine stimulation, to inhibit prolactin production, to control postpartum hemorrhage, to treat migraine headaches and Parkinson's disease, and to stimulate cerebral and peripheral metabolism (Bennett and Klich 2003).

Molds or microfungi produce three types of illness: allergy, toxicity, and infection. Consistent with the objective of this chapter, only the toxic effects of microfungi are covered. The toxic effects of mold or microfungi are caused by mycotoxins. Mycotoxins, produced by filamentous fungi, are low-molecular-weight secondary metabolites not critical to fungal cell processes that are extremely toxic in low concentrations. These metabolites are chemically heterogeneous yet grouped together solely because of their ability to cause disease and death in humans and other vertebrates (Bennett and Klich 2003). Mycotoxins seem to give mold a competitive advantage in the biological struggle over other mold species, bacteria, and other organisms competing for the same ecological niche. Approximately 400 known mycotoxins exist, of which only a dozen groups of mycotoxins are well known. Exposure to mycotoxins can occur through ingestion, inhalation, and

TABLE 22–14. Major hallucinogenic plants and their active components

Plant	Family	Active component
Cannabis sativa	Cannabinaceae	Tetrahydrocannabinol
Lophophora williamsii	Cactaceae	Mescaline
Piptadenia species	Leguminosae	Substituted tryptamines
Mimosa species	Leguminosae	Substituted tryptamines
Virola species	Myristicaceae	Substituted tryptamines
Banisteriopsis species	Malpighiaceae	Harmaline, harmine
Peganum harmala	Zygophyllaceae	Harmaline, harmine
Tabernanthe iboga	Apocynaceae	Ibogaine
Ipomoea violacea	Convolvulaceae	D-Lysergic acid amide, D-isolysergic acid amide
Turbina corymbosa	Convolvulaceae	D-Lysergic acid amide, D-isolysergic acid amide
Datura species	Solanaceae	Scopolamine
Methysticodendron amesianum	Solanaceae	Scopolamine
Amanita muscaria	Agaricaceae	Pantherine, ibotenic acid
Psilocybe mexicana	Agaricaceae	Psilocybin

Source. Adapted from Farnsworth 1986.

dermal exposure of viable or nonviable mold spores, spore fragments, and mycelia. Mycotoxins are lipid soluble and readily absorbed by the intestinal lining, airways, and skin. The public has an increased awareness of and interest in mycotoxins because of both their presence in water-damaged homes and buildings in which mold is present and their production and deliberate use by terrorists.

Commonly found mycotoxins include aflatoxins, which are very potent carcinogens, and hepatotoxins produced by the *Aspergillus* species; ochratoxins, which are nephrotoxic and carcinogenic, produced by several species of *Aspergillus* and *Penicillium;* sterigmatocystin, which is immunosuppressive and a liver carcinogen, produced by species of *Aspergillus*, particularly *Aspergillus versicolor;* and trichothecenes, which are produced primarily by species of *Stachybotrys* and *Fusarium*. Physicians have recently become more aware of the effects of mycotoxins. In 1994, attention focused on a cluster of 10 cases of infants with acute idiopathic pulmonary hemorrhage and hemosiderosis. A case–control study comparing those 10 infants with 30 age-matched control infants from the same area of Cleveland, Ohio, reported that the infants with acute pulmonary hemorrhage resided in homes with water damage and resultant mold infestation. Because of the rapid growth of the lungs in an infant, the effects of inhaled mycotoxins in infants were severe (Kilburn 2003a). As a result, the American Academy of Pediatrics currently recommends that physicians ask parents about mold exposure.

Mycotoxins appear in water-damaged homes and buildings because intrusion of water into houses, offices, and buildings leads to the growth of mold. Building materials, including wood and wood products, insulation materials, carpet, fabric and upholstery, drywall, and cellulose substrates (including paper and paper products, cardboard, ceiling tiles, and wallpaper), are suitable nutrient sources for fungal growth. Health symptoms associated with mold infestation or water damage in a building involve multiple organs such as upper and lower respiratory tracts, gastrointestinal tract, urinary tract, circulatory system, and the central and peripheral nervous systems. Studies have shown adverse effects on the nervous system in humans exposed to mold in buildings with water damage. Mycotoxins, which are prominent neurotoxins or produce neuropsychiatric effects, include the ergot alkaloids, trichothecenes, fumonisins, patulin, and tremorgens (Figure 22–9).

Neuropsychiatric manifestations. The neuropsychiatric manifestations of mycotoxins were first noted in the Middle Ages, when outbreaks of ergotism were caused by eating wheat or rye contaminated with the mold *Claviceps purpurea*, which produced ergot alkaloids and hallucinogens such as lysergic acid diethylamide, resulting in the deaths of thousands of people in Europe. Human ergotism manifests in a disorder characterized by mania, hallucinations, delusions, severe peripheral paresthesias,

TABLE 22–15.   Plants of abuse

Plant	Part used	Toxic agent
Argyreia nervosa	Seed	Ergoline hallucinogens
Atropa belladonna	Seed	Tropane alkaloids
Banisteriopsis species	Various	Harmaline (hallucinogen)
Cola nitida	Seed	Caffeine
Datura species	Seed	Tropane alkaloids
Hyoscyamus niger	Whole plant	Tropane alkaloids
Ilex paraguariensis	Leaf	Caffeine
Lophophora	—	—
Mandragora officinarum	Whole plant	Tropane alkaloids
Methysticodendron amesianum	Stem/leaf	Tropane alkaloids
Mimosa hostilis	Root	Phenylamine hallucinogens
Olmedioperebea sclerophylla	Fruit	Unknown hallucinogen
Passiflora incarnate	Stem/leaf	Harmaline (hallucinogen)
Peganum harmala	Seed	Harmaline (hallucinogen)
Piper methysticum	Root	Methysticin/kawain
Piptadenia colubrina	Seed	Phenylamine hallucinogens
Piptadenia excelsa	Seed	Phenylamine hallucinogens
Piptadenia macrocarpa	Seed	Phenylamine hallucinogens
Piptadenia peregrina	Seed/bark	Phenylamine hallucinogens
Salvia divinorum	Leaf	Unknown hallucinogen
Sophora secundiflora	Seed	Cytosine (stimulant)
Tabernanthe iboga	Root	Ibogaine (hallucinogen)
Trichocereus pachanoi	Cactus	Mescaline
Virola calophylla	Bark	Phenylamine hallucinogens

Source.   Adapted from Spoerke DG, Hall AH: "Plants and Mushrooms of Abuse." *Emergency Medicine Clinics of North America* 8:579–593, 1990.

convulsions, violent muscle spasms, vomiting, diarrhea, abdominal pain, coronary vasoconstriction, peripheral vasoconstriction, and gangrene (Bennett and Klich 2003).

Indoor molds present following water damage include *Penicillium*, *Aspergillus*, *Cladosporium*, *Alternaria*, *Stachybotrys*, and *Fusarium* species. Each is capable of producing varying amounts of mycotoxins, including the neurotoxic ergot alkaloids, trichothecenes, and tremorgens. However, the health effects of an exposure to building-related mold are difficult to assess because the exposures are inevitably from multiple species, each producing multiple mycotoxins, and consequently, health effects of exposure are termed a *mixed-mold mycotoxicosis* (Gray et al. 2003).

A significant body of literature exists regarding the neuropsychiatric and neuropsychological effects of mixed-mold exposure in the form of independent case series. Independent studies of more than 1,600 patients with ill effects associated with fungal exposure were presented at the 21st Annual Symposium on Man and His Environment in Dallas, Texas, in 2003. Two case series of 48 and 150 mold-exposed patients found significant fatigue and weakness in 70% and 100% of patients, respectively, and neurocognitive dysfunction, including memory loss, irritability, anxiety, and depression, in more than 40% of the patients in both series. Classic manifestations of neurotoxicity, including numbness, tingling, and tremor, were observed in a significant number of the patients (Lieberman 2003; Rea et al. 2003).

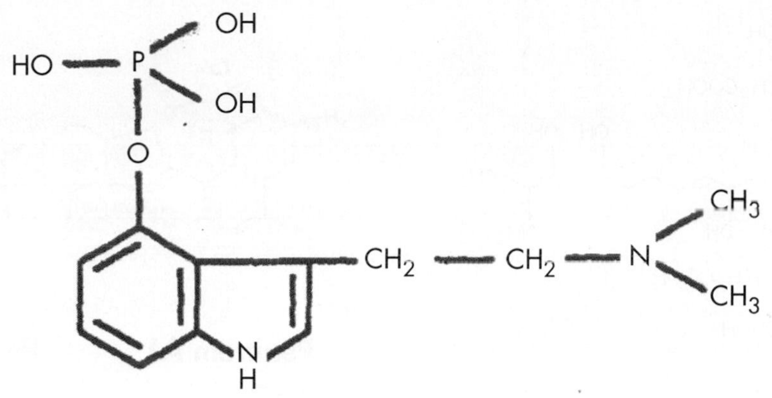

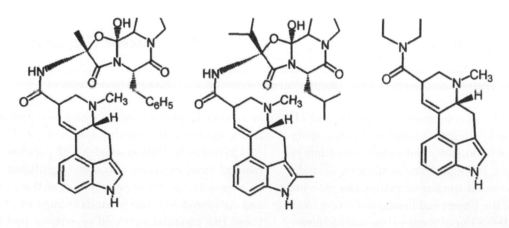

Psilocybin

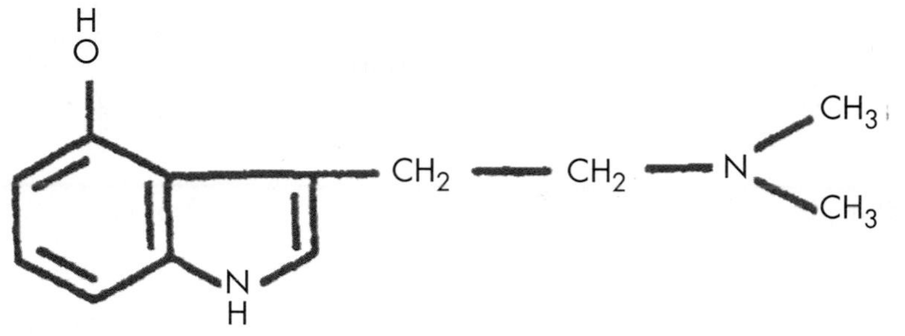

Psilocin

FIGURE 22–7.　Chemical structures of psilocybin and psilocin.

Ergotamine　　　**2-Bromo-α-ergocryptine**　　　**Lysergic acid diethylamide**

FIGURE 22–8.　Chemical structures of pharmacologically active ergot alkaloids derived from mold.

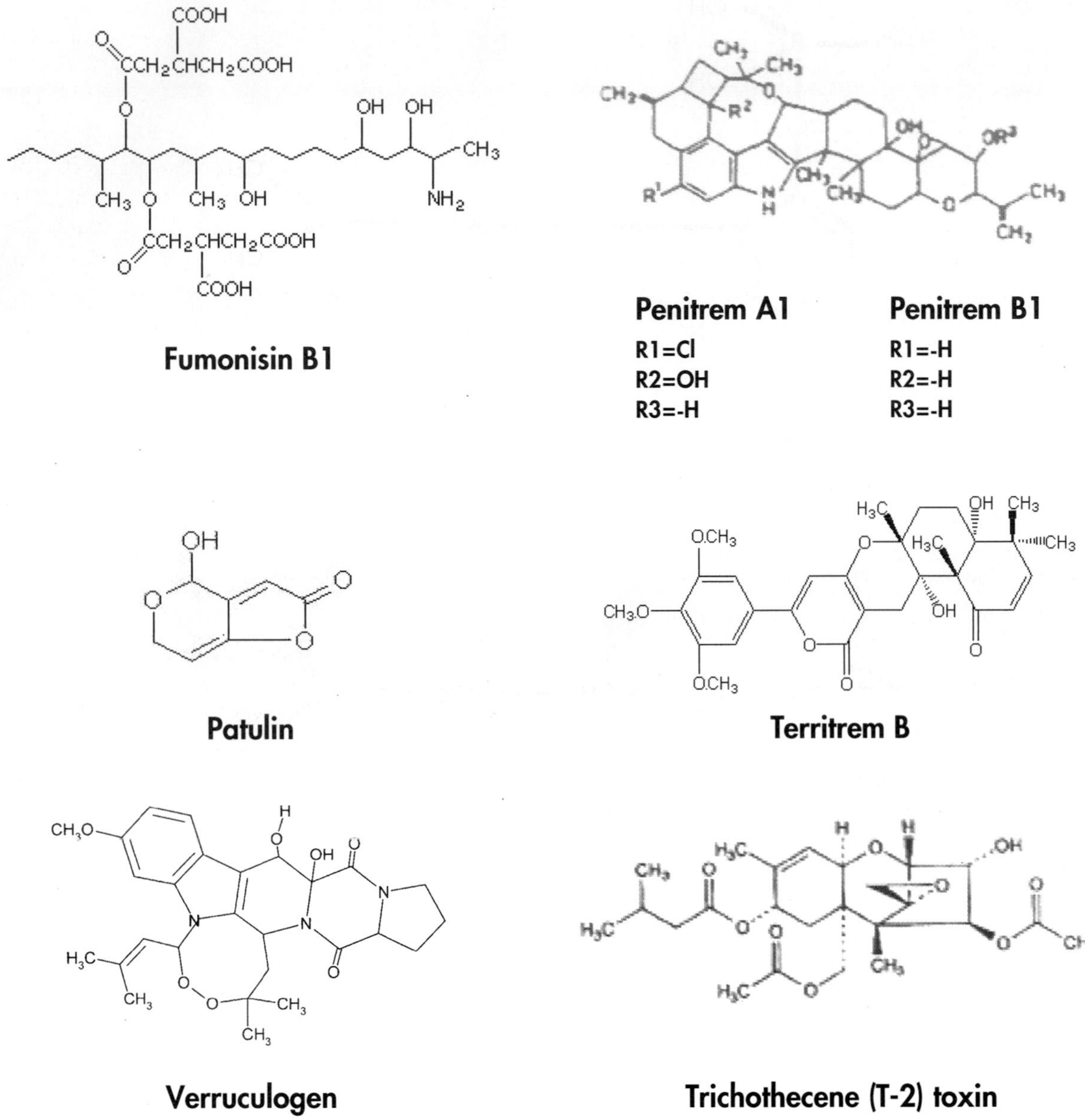

FIGURE 22–9.   Chemical structures of some representative mycotoxins with reported neurotoxicity.

A study by Campbell and colleagues (2003) evaluated 119 mixed-mold-exposed patients who had multiorgan symptoms and peripheral neuropathy. Subjective complaints included severe fatigue, decreased muscle strength, sleep disturbances, numbness and tingling of extremities with and without tremors of the fingers and hands, and severe headache. Objectively, 99 (83%) of these individuals had abnormal nerve conduction velocities in association with autoantibodies against nine neural antigens, whereas the remaining 20 (17%) had normal test results (Campbell et al. 2004). A study of 43 mixed-mold-exposed patients found that they performed significantly worse (P<0.0001) than 202 control subjects on many neuropsychiatric tests, including balance

sway speed, blinking reflex, color perception, reaction times, and left grip strength (Gray et al. 2003).

Quantitative EEG studies in 182 patients with documented mold exposure also noted significant differences in brain waves, with hypoactivation of the frontal cortex and narrowed frequency bands (Crago et al. 2003). In these 182 patients, increased severity of mold exposure, by either increased duration of exposure, increased density of spores in air, or presence of a more toxigenic species, was significantly associated with more abnormal quantitative EEG results as well as worse scores on concentration, motor skills, and verbal skills tests (Crago et al. 2003). Triple-headed single photon emission computed tomography (SPECT) brain scans identified neurotoxic patterns in 26 of 30 (87%) mold-exposed patients (Simon and Rea 2003). Assessment of the autonomic nervous function in 60 mixed-mold-exposed patients by iriscorder found that 95% had abnormal autonomic responses of the pupil compared with the population reference range. Visual contrast sensitivity studies had significantly abnormal results in indoor mold–exposed patients (Rea et al. 2003).

Additional studies have reported that compared with the general population reference range, mold-exposed patients perform significantly worse on tests of attention, balance, reaction time, verbal recall, concentration, memory, and finger tapping (Didricksen 2003; Gordon et al. 1999; Kilburn 2003a, 2003b). Studies of children and adults who were exposed to indoor molds found significantly more neurophysiological abnormalities than in control subjects, including abnormal EEG findings and abnormal brain stem, visual, and somatosensory evoked potentials (Anyanwu et al. 2003a, 2003b; Baldo et al. 2002; Campbell et al. 2003).

Lieberman (2003) presented a case series of 12 patients who developed tremors following documented heavy mixed-indoor-mold exposure. Numerous articles have reported domestic dogs developing tremors following ingestion of moldy food (Boysen et al. 2002; Naude et al. 2002). Tremorgens are mycotoxins that contain an indole moiety, presumably derived from tryptophan, and that produce tremors or seizures in animals consuming toxic amounts of contaminated foodstuffs (Peterson et al. 1982). Molds of the genera *Penicillium* and *Aspergillus* produce most of the tremorgenic mycotoxins. At least five groups of tremorgens exist, including the penitrems, verruculogens, paspalitrems, fumitremorgins, and tryptoquivaline group. The more common tremorgens—penitrems and verruculogens—grow in moldy refrigerated foods, cottage cheese, and cream cheese as well as moldy peanuts and grain.

Mechanisms of action. Verruculogens increase the spontaneous release of glutamate and aspartate by 1,300% and 1,200%, respectively, but not that of γ-aminobutyric acid (GABA) from cerebrocortical synaptosomes in sheep (Bradford et al. 1990). The stimulus for the release appears to be subcortical (Peterson et al. 1982). Territrem B, produced by the common fungus *Aspergillus terreus*, can, like an organophosphate pesticide, irreversibly bind to and inhibit the enzyme acetylcholinesterase (Chen et al. 1999). Similarly, the potent tremorgenic mycotoxin fumitremorgin A produces violent clonic-tonic convulsions, nystagmus, miosis, bradycardia, and arrhythmia consistent with excessive cholinergic stimulation (Nishiyama and Kuga 1986). Fumonisins and fumonisin analogues disrupt formation of complex sphingolipids through inhibition of ceramide synthase, with resultant apoptosis (Desai et al.

2002) and disruption of folate transport, which can potentially result in human neural tube defects (Marasas et al. 2004). Paxilline, a tremorgenic alkaloid mycotoxin produced by *Penicillium paxilline*, is a reversible inhibitor of cerebellar inositol 1,4,5-triphosphate receptor that decreases the extent of inositol 1,4,5-triphosphate–induced calcium release (Longland et al. 2000).

Penitrem A, produced by the common *Penicillium* and *Aspergillus* genera, can cause severe generalized tremors and ataxia that persist for up to 48 hours, and it affects the cerebellar region: initial exposure to penitrem A results in a three- to fourfold increase in cerebellar cortical blood flow. Mitochondrial swelling occurs in cerebellar stellate and basket cells. Purkinje's cells develop intense cytoplasmic condensation with eosinophilia that resembles "ischemic cell change," whereas many other Purkinje's cells show marked watery swelling. Astrocytes swell from hypertrophy of organelles, and discrete foci of necrosis appear in the granule cell layer, while permeability of overlying meningeal vessels becomes evident. All changes are more severe in vermis and paravermis, with no morphological changes in other brain regions. The affinities of penitrem A for high-conductance calcium-dependent potassium channels and for GABA receptors and resultant excitotoxity appear to be important underlying factors for these changes (Cavanagh et al. 1998). Penitrem A increased the spontaneous release of endogenous glutamate, GABA, and aspartate by 213%, 455%, and 277%, respectively, from cerebrocortical synaptosomes. In neurons, penitrem A increased the resting potential, end-plate potential, duration of depolarization, and presynaptic transmitter release (Norris et al. 1980).

Diagnosis. It is important to elicit a patient's history of exposure to mold whether in the workplace or at home. A neuropsychiatrist should evaluate patients exposed to mixed mold carefully, particularly if neurocognitive symptoms and neuropsychiatric symptoms arise after indoor exposure to high levels of mixed mold. For patients who have had substantial exposure to mold, a battery of tests has been developed that includes visual contrast sensitivity and pupillometry to assist in determining autonomic nervous system functioning. The evaluation should include a neuropsychiatric examination and a comprehensive metabolic panel that includes electrolytes, blood glucose, liver and kidney function tests, immune tests for autoantibodies, antibodies to the mold or mycotoxin, complement, gamma globulins, and lymphocyte panels. EEG and brain imaging such as MRI and SPECT are helpful tools in determination of neurological injury. Presence of mycotoxins or metabolites in the urine usually confirms the diagnosis (Curtis et al. 2004).

Treatment. The most important facet of treatment involves preventing any further exposure of the patient to mold. The potent toxicity of these agents warrants prudent prevention of exposures when levels of mold species indoors exceed outdoor levels by any significant amount.

ANIMAL TOXINS

Animals capable of secreting a poison by biting or stinging are termed *venomous*. Animals referred to as *poisonous* are organisms whose tissues, in part or in entirety, are toxic. Venoms are complex mixtures of enzymes and proteins (Table 22–16) with various components that are neurotoxins, myotoxins, hemostatic system toxins, hemorrhagins, nephrotoxins, cardiotoxins, and necrotoxins (Ellenhorn 1997; Russell 1983; White 2004a). Venomous snakes cause more than 30,000 deaths worldwide each year. Most deaths caused by snakebites in the United States are due to rattlesnake bites. Of the five families of venomous snakes, only Elapidae, or elapids, which include cobras, mambas, sea snakes, kraits, and death adders, and Viperidae, or vipers, which include Russell's viper and pit vipers, produce significant neurotoxic symptoms (White 2004b, 2004c). Effects of bites from these snakes include flaccid neurotoxic paralysis that is usually the result of neuromuscular junction pre- and postsynaptic neurotoxins, which act systemically rather than locally, affecting voluntary and respiratory muscle. Flaccid paralysis is progressive and may take from 1 to 12 hours to become evident. The paralysis of the cranial nerves is often seen first, with partial ptosis, followed by complete ophthalmoplegia, loss of facial tone, dysarthria, and dysphagia. The pupils may become dilated and unresponsive to light, followed by progressive weakness of the limbs and bulbar function. The accessory muscles of respiration may become more prominent, and the patient may become more agitated or drowsy as hypoxia ensues. The diaphragm is frequently the last muscle affected and, even so, may not be fully affected for 24 hours. Without timely intubation and ventilation to secure the airway, complete respiratory paralysis and death follow (White 2004a).

Treatment of venomous snakebites includes diagnosis and history surrounding the incident involving the bite. Diagnostic tests should include urine output, complete blood count, electrolytes and renal function, creatine kinase and liver function tests, and coagulation studies. Optimal management for major envenomation with respiratory support may require treatment in an intensive care unit. Medical management includes administration of antivenoms, local wound care, supportive measures, administration of antibiotics, and tetanus prophylaxis (Ellenhorn 1997; Nelson 1989; White 2004a).

TABLE 22–16. Composition of snake venoms

Acetylcholinesterase

L-Amino acid oxidase

Arginine ester hydrolase

Collagenase

DNase

Hyaluronidase

Lactate dehydrogenase

Nicotinamide adenine dinucleotide (NAD)-nucleotidase

5´-Nucleotidase

Phosphodiesterase

Phospholipase A_2 (A)

Phospholipase B

Phospholipase C

Phosphomonoesterase

Proteolytic enzymes

RNase

Thrombinlike enzyme

Source. Adapted from Ellenhorn MJ: *Ellenhorn's Medical Toxicology: Diagnosis and Treatment of Human Poisoning.* Baltimore, MD, Williams & Wilkins, 1997; Russell FE: *Snake Venom Poisoning.* Great Neck, NY, Scholium International, 1983.

CHEMICAL WARFARE AGENTS

Around the world, terrorism has become a stark reality. News reports steadily remind us of groups of terrorists that are intent on harming or killing civilians or noncombatants for fanatical causes. Terrorist attacks in the United States including those of September 11, 2001, on the World Trade Center and the Pentagon, attacks in more than 250 other countries, and, most recently, chlorine gas attacks in Iraq in 2007 have led the United States into an era of awareness and resolve to prepare for future attacks. With certainty that terrorism will continue, the use of chemical agents and toxins purposefully to induce fear in, injure, or kill both civilian and military personnel has become a realistic concern.

NERVE AGENTS

Nerve agents are particularly potent organophosphates used for chemical warfare (Figure 22–10). Nerve agents encompass a variety of compounds that have the capacity to inactivate the enzyme acetylcholinesterase. The Germans developed the G agents, tabun (GA), sarin (GB), soman (GD), and cyclosarin (GF) during World War II. These volatile compounds pose mainly an inhalation hazard. In searching for organophosphorus pesticides, German chemist Gerhard Schrader developed anticholinesterase nerve agents with extremely lethal potency with the first nerve agent, tabun. Schrader further developed sarin in 1937, followed by soman in 1944. In 1952, Great Britain developed the first V agent, VX. VX is approximately 10 times more toxic than sarin and is persistent in remaining on surfaces for long periods. The consistency of V agents is oily; therefore, they pose mainly a contact hazard. Full-scale production of nerve agents ceased in Britain and the United States in 1959 and 1969, respectively. However, during and following the Cold War, the United States stockpiled tens of thousands of tons of sarin and VX loaded in weapons. The former Soviet Union held captured German reserves of nerve agents and continued production of tabun and soman. In 1981, the United States began to produce components for binary weapons in which precursors of nerve agents are stored in separate chambers of the artillery shells or warheads and mixed on firing to form the lethal nerve agents. In 1990, following the fall of the Soviet Union, the U.S. Army began to destroy the decades-old stockpiles of weapons containing sarin, soman, and VX.

In June 1994, terrorists of the Aum Shinrikyo cult deployed the nerve agent sarin against civilian populations in the Japanese city of Matsumoto, which resulted in the deaths of 7 individuals and hospitalization of an additional 274 people. In March 1995, the same cult deployed the nerve agent sarin against commuters in the subways in the center of Tokyo, Japan, which resulted in the deaths of 12 civilians and treatment of more than 5,000 civilians for acute symptoms (Inoue 2003). The Hussein regime in Iraq used chemical weapons on civilian populations in their own country by launching chemical attacks against approximately 40 Kurdish villages during the period from 1987 to 1988 (U.S. Department of State 2003). Iraq also used the nerve agent tabun against Iran in the Iran-Iraq War in the 1980s. During Operation Desert Storm in the Persian Gulf, in late January and February 1991, coalition forces, including those of the United States, conducted aerial bombing that damaged two chemical munitions facilities in the central part of Iraq in which approximately 3 metric tons of sarin and 17 metric tons of cyclosarin were stored. The large release of the nerve agents and prevailing winds resulted in likely low-level exposure to coalition troops. Smoke, combustion products from oil well fires, and heavy concentrations of hydrocarbons present in the air made distinguishing the effects of the nerve agents difficult.

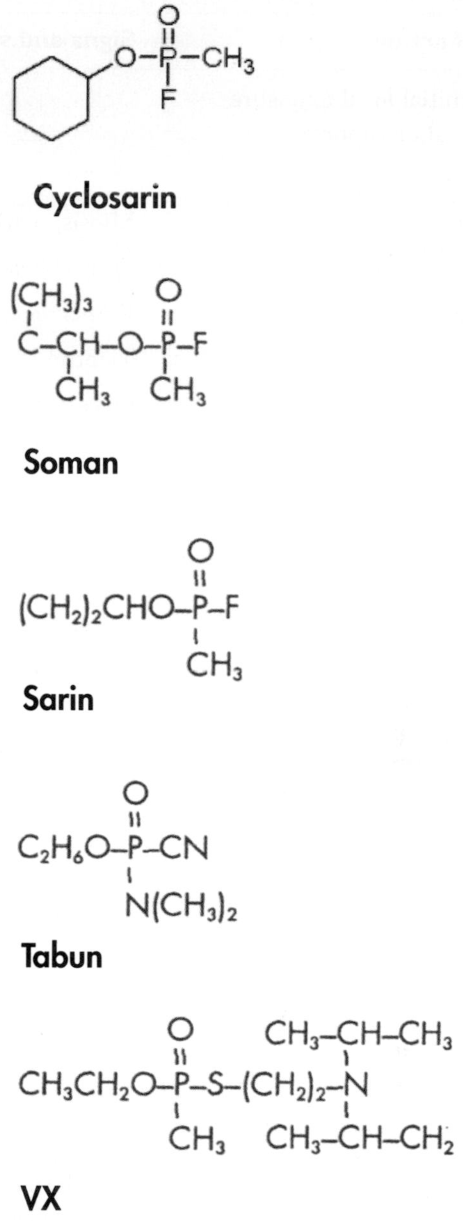

FIGURE 22–10. Chemical structures of nerve agents cyclosarin (GF), soman (GD), sarin (GB), tabun (GA), and VX.

Neuropsychiatric Manifestations

Nerve agents act on the human nervous system as their primary target organ and produce neuropsychiatric symptoms as listed in Table 22–17.

After inhalation, onset is extremely rapid because of the high vascularity of the lungs. The lungs are also important primary target organs. After dermal exposure, in the case of the G or volatile agents, systemic effects may be delayed for minutes to as long as several hours for VX. Onset of symptoms also depends on the area of skin exposed because absorption is greatest in the thinner areas of the skin.

TABLE 22–17. Signs and symptoms of nerve agent poisoning

Site of action	Signs and symptoms
After initial local exposure (dermal or vapor)	
Muscarinic	
Pupils	Miosis, marked, usually maximal (pinpoint), sometimes unequal
Ciliary body	Frontal headache, eye pain on focusing, blurring of vision
Nasal mucous membranes	Rhinorrhea, hyperemia
Bronchial tree	Tightness in chest, bronchoconstriction, increased secretion, cough
Gastrointestinal	Occasional nausea and vomiting
After systemic absorption (depending on dose)	
Muscarinic	
Bronchial tree	Tightness in chest, with prolonged wheezing expiration suggestive of bronchoconstriction or increased secretion, dyspnea, pain in chest, increased bronchial secretion, cough, cyanosis, pulmonary edema
Gastrointestinal	Anorexia, nausea, vomiting, abdominal cramps, epigastric and substernal tightness (cardiospasm) with "heartburn" and eructation, diarrhea, tenesmus, involuntary defecation
Sweat glands	Increased sweating
Salivary glands	Increased salivation
Lacrimal glands	Increased lacrimation
Heart	Bradycardia
Pupil	Miosis, occasionally unequal, later maximal miosis (pinpoint)
Ciliary body	Blurring of vision, headache
Bladder	Frequency, involuntary micturition
Nicotinic	
Striated muscle	Easy fatigue, mild weakness, muscular twitching, fasciculations, cramps, generalized weakness, flaccid paralysis (including muscles of respiration) with dyspnea and cyanosis
Sympathetic ganglia	Pallor, transitory elevation of blood pressure followed by hypotension
Central nervous system	*Immediate (acute) effects:* generalized weakness; depression of respiratory and circulatory centers with dyspnea, cyanosis, and hypotension; convulsions, loss of consciousness; coma
	Delayed (chronic) effects: giddiness, tension, anxiety, jitteriness, restlessness, emotional lability, excessive dreaming, insomnia, nightmares, headaches, tremor, withdrawal and depression, bursts of slow waves of elevated voltage on electroencephalogram (especially on hyperventilation), drowsiness, difficulty concentrating, slowness of recall, confusion, slurred speech, ataxia

Source. Adapted from Army FM8–285, Navy NAVMED P5041, and Air Force AFM160–11 Field Manual: *The Treatment of Chemical Agent Casualties and Conventional Military Chemical Injuries.* Washington, DC, Departments of the Army, Navy, and Air Force, February 28, 1990.

Low doses of nerve agents cause a range of characteristic symptoms, including increased saliva production, running nose, watery eyes, sweating, pupillary constriction, deteriorated short-range vision, feeling of pain when focusing on nearby objects, and headache. Gastrointestinal symptoms include salivation, nausea, cramping, diarrhea, and vomiting. Respiratory symptoms imclude bronchoconstriction and profuse secretion of mucus, resulting in coughing and difficulty in respiration. In addition to the previously mentioned symptoms, moderate doses of nerve agents may cause muscular weakness, convulsions, or local tremors. Higher doses of nerve agents produce convulsions, loss of consciousness, and central nervous system–mediated paralysis of the respiratory muscles. Consequently, death is often the result of suffocation (Keyes 1994).

Following the initial exposure, humans may be susceptible to lower doses of nerve agents. Acetylcholinesterase activity in humans recovers at about 10% a day following exposure to intermediate to high levels of sarin (M.A. Brown and Brix 1998). The initial outcome of nerve agent poisoning is the result of acute cholinergic effects that occur in the minutes and hours following exposure. These effects may lead to death or recovery in the days or weeks following the exposure. Following recovery in patients who had survived exposure to nerve agents, neuropsychological tests showed subtle changes in intellectual functioning, academic skills, abstraction and flexibility of thinking, and simple motor skills involving speed and coordination, as well as sleep disturbances, EEG changes, and depression. Symptoms may last for months or years after recovery from the initial cholinergic effects (Steenland 1996). A cross-sectional sleep survey of 163 victims conducted 10 years after injury with sarin on Tokyo subway trains yielded a significantly higher prevalence of poor sleep, difficulty falling asleep, intermittent awakening, early-morning awakening, a feeling of light overnight sleep, and frank insomnia compared with a control group (Kawada et al. 2005). The Centers for Disease Control and Prevention cited accidental exposures of workers and civilians during stockpile destruction as being associated with delayed peripheral neuropathy and electroencephalographic changes as well as birth defects.

Exposure to certain organophosphate nerve agents and pesticides also produces a delayed-onset distal sensorimotor polyneuropathy known as *organophosphate-induced delayed neuropathy* (Bidstrup et al. 1953; M.A. Brown and Brix 1998; Morgan and Penovich 1978). Organophosphate-induced delayed neuropathy typically appears 7–14 days after exposure to acute cholinergic poisoning but less than 4 weeks after exposure. Symptoms of organophosphate-induced delayed neuropathy include numbness, tingling, fatigue, lack of muscular coordination, muscle weakness and cramplike pain in the calf muscles, and paralysis in the lower limbs; if severe, the upper limbs also are affected. It is hypothesized that the cause of organophosphate-induced delayed neuropathy is the inhibition and subsequent "aging" or irreversible modification of an enzyme called neurotoxic esterase or neuropathy target esterase rather than the inhibition and aging of acetylcholinesterase (Bertoncin et al. 1985; Jokanovic et al. 2002).

Mechanisms of Action

Nerve agents bind and inhibit acetylcholinesterase much more potently than do organophosphate and carbamate insecticides. Acetylcholinesterase converts acetylcholine into acetic acid and choline, which subsequently undergoes reuptake into the presynaptic cell and regenerates acetylcholine. Nerve agents bind to the active site of acetylcholinesterase, rendering it incapable of deactivating acetylcholine. Acetylcholine can continue to interact with the receptor, resulting in persistent and uncontrolled stimulation of two types of peripheral postsynaptic receptors, nicotinic receptors at the skeletal muscle and autonomic ganglia and muscarinic receptors found mainly in the postganglionic parasympathetic fibers. This interaction leads to activation of the acetylcholine receptor and signal transmission in the postsynaptic side of the cleft and the resulting symptoms of excess cholinergic stimulation. In the initial step, the enzyme becomes temporarily inactivated. Some degree of reactivation of the acetylcholinesterase enzyme occurs in this initial phase, but the process is slow. The initial binding of the organophosphate nerve agent to the enzyme is reversible. However, with the more toxic organophosphate pesticides or lethal organophosphate nerve agents, the acetylcholinesterase-organophosphate nerve agent complex can undergo "aging" when the acetylcholinesterase-organophosphate complex dealkylates itself to form an irreversibly inhibited enzyme, as shown in Figure 22–11 (Dunn and Sidell 1989).

Organophosphate nerve agents have varying half-lives until the "aged" acetylcholinesterase complex is produced (M.A. Brown and Brix 1998; Sidell 1992). Recovery from organophosphate nerve agents is slow because of the need to regenerate acetylcholinesterase after the existing acetylcholinesterase is permanently inactivated. Table 22–18 lists the typical aging half-lives for the different nerve agents, after which the ability to reactivate the enzyme diminishes. Following accidental exposure to soman, symptoms such as pupil dilation can linger for weeks, as shown in Figure 22–12 (Sidell 1974).

The rapid increase in acetylcholine concentration in the central and peripheral nervous systems is responsible for many of the lethal symptoms produced by exposure to

Step 1. Formation of a reversible enzyme-inhibitor complex.

$$\text{AChE-OH} \quad + \quad R_1O\text{-}P\text{-}X \quad \longleftrightarrow \quad \text{AChE-OH} \approx R_1O\text{-}P\text{-}X$$

Active serine group
on acetylcholinesterase

Organophosphate
nerve agent

Reversible acetylcholinesterase-
organophosphate complex

Step 2. Phosphorylation and inactivation of the enzyme molecule.

$$\text{AChE-OH} \approx R_1O\text{-}P\text{-}X \quad \longrightarrow \quad \text{AChE-O-P-}R_1 \quad + \quad HX$$

Reversible acetylcholinesterase-
organophosphate complex

Inactivated acetylcholinesterase

Step 3. "Aging" reaction with formation of monophosphoric acid residue bound enzyme.

$$\text{AChE-O-P-}OR_1 \quad \longrightarrow \quad \text{AChE-O-P-OH} \quad + \quad R_1O$$

Inactivated acetylcholinesterase

"Aged" or irreversible inhibited
acetylcholinesterase by covalent binding

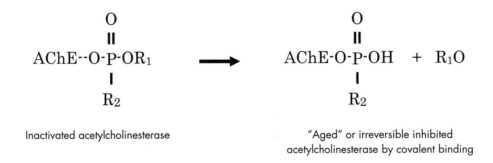

FIGURE 22–11.   The "aging" reaction between organophosphorus pesticides or nerve agents and acetylcholinesterase occurs in a three-step process. The "aging" reaction forms an enzyme-modified nerve agent that is more stable, covalently bound, and resistant to reactivation by oximes or similar antidotes. AChE-OH=active serine group of the enzyme acetylcholinesterase; R_1 and R_2=alkyl groups; X=sulfur (V nerve agents) or fluorine or cyanide (G nerve agents).

TABLE 22–18. Aging of the nerve agent acetylcholinesterase complex

Agent	Aging half-life
Tabun (GA)	46 hours
Sarin (GB)	5.2–12 hours
VX	>12 days
Soman (GD)	40 seconds to 10 minutes
Paraxon	2.1–5.4 days

Source. Adapted from Dunn and Sidell 1989.

nerve agents. Although most clinical signs and symptoms are related to excessive stimulation at the cholinergic nicotinic and muscarinic receptors, some central nervous system effects may not be mediated by cholinergic receptors. In particular, some effects occur on glutamate NMDA and GABA receptors, which may contribute to nerve agent–mediated seizures and CNS neuropathology.

Diagnosis

In the event of exposure to nerve agents, occupational history may aid in making the diagnosis. Military personnel and laboratory personnel are at risk for exposures to the nerve agents. In case of a terrorist attack, the diagnosis should be suspected when patients present with symptoms of cholinergic excess as listed in Table 22–17. The clinical sign that provides rapid confirmation of symptoms of cholinergic excess is the prominent miosis of the pupils as shown in Figure 22–12.

Treatment

After exposure to nerve agents, the primary concern is treatment and stabilization of vital signs, followed by decontamination.

Treatment requires the drugs atropine, pralidoxime or another acetylcholinesterase reactivator, and diazepam administered as soon as possible or, if warning is available, even 30 minutes to 1 hour prior to the attack. Atropine noncompetitively antagonizes both muscarinic and nicotinic receptors, thereby blocking the effect of excess acetylcholine (Dart 2004a; Holstege et al. 1997). Administration of oximes, shown in Figure 22–13—pralidoxime, obidoxime, or the Hagedorn oxime HI-6—can reactivate acetylcholinesterase if administered prior to the process of "aging" (Worek et al. 1998).

Diazepam prevents convulsions that can result in permanent neurological deficits or death. Because of the brief time between exposure and the onset of symptoms, self-administered autoinjectors are used immediately following exposure to deliver the nerve gas antidotes intramuscularly.

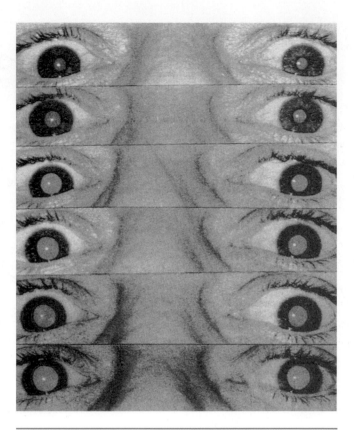

FIGURE 22–12. Prolonged miosis after accidental exposure to soman. As with other volatile nerve agents, miosis tends to be predominant and prolonged. This series of photographs was taken by Dr. Frederick Sidell to show the long duration of miosis after soman exposure. These photographs were taken over a 62-day period in which the patient was maximally dark-adapted, and then a flash photograph was taken of the pupil faster than its ability to constrict.

Source. Reprinted from Sidell FR: "Soman and Sarin: Clinical Manifestations and Treatment of Accidental Poisoning by Organophosphates." *Clinical Toxicology* 7:1–17, 1974.

In the event that advance warning is given, pretreatments are available; however, the drugs take approximately 30 minutes to be effective. The maximum protective effect occurs after 2 hours; thereafter, the effectiveness declines. The active ingredient of the preventive antidote is pyridostigmine, which is taken in the form of a tablet. Pyridostigmine is a reversible acetylcholinesterase inhibitor and thus prevents the irreversible inhibition of acetylcholinesterase by organophosphate agents through competitive binding. The usual dose is low and provides an approximate 25% inhibition of acetylcholinesterase. As a result of the reversible inhibition, pyridostigmine-bound acetylcholinesterase converts back to active acetylcholinesterase, and as a result, the synapse will continue to function. Research has shown that as little as 1%–2% active enzyme is necessary for the synapse to function. However, pyri-

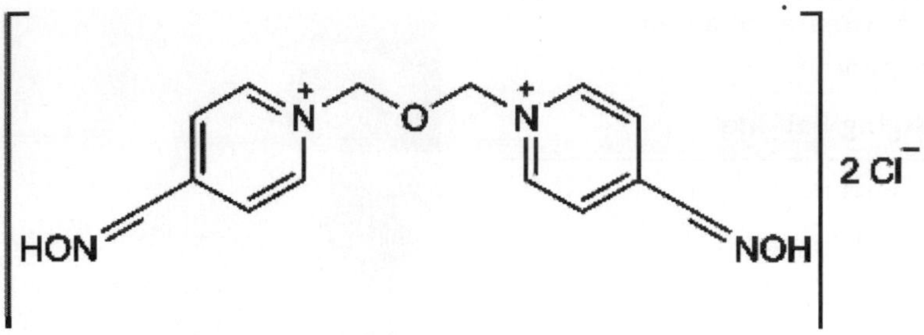

FIGURE 22–13.   Oxime acetylcholinesterase reactivators obidoxime chloride, pralidoxime (2-PAM), and Hagedorn oxime (HI-6).

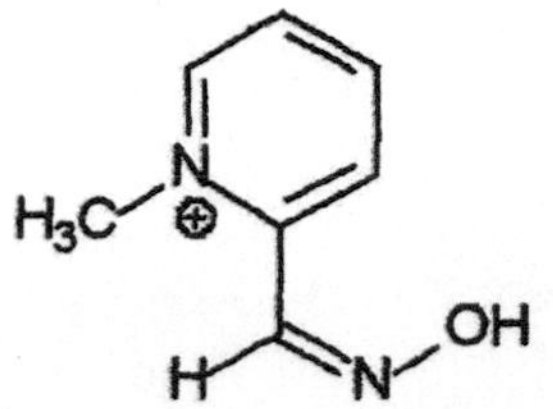

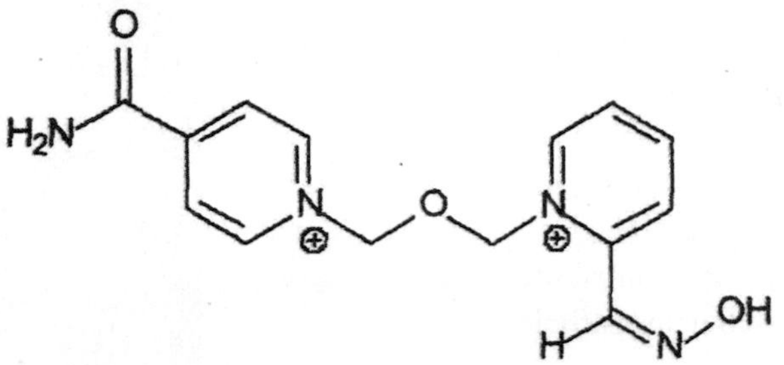

dostigmine does not cross the blood-brain barrier (Lallement et al. 2002). As a result, it will protect only the peripheral nervous system. In addition to pyridostigmine, a diazepam tablet is a pretreatment. Diazepam acts on the central nervous system, unlike pyridostigmine, as an anticonvulsive. In addition to strengthening the effects of other nerve agent antidotes, diazepam protects against permanent brain damage from seizures associated with exposure to high concentrations of organophosphate agents (Lallement et al. 1997). The physician may give the victim atropine in addition to a dose of diazepam. Research has shown that the effects of diazepam and atropine decrease after about 10–20 minutes of seizures and that overstimulation of NMDA receptors may be responsible for the seizures and the brain damage that follows. GK-11, a noncompetitive NMDA receptor antagonist, has shown promise in providing supplemental anticonvulsive and neuroprotective effects to conventional treatments (Lallement et al. 1998).

ADDITIONAL POISONS AND TOXINS USED AS CHEMICAL WEAPONS

In addition to the organophosphate nerve agents, chemical weapons include mycotoxins, staphylococcal entero-

toxin B, epsilon toxin produced by *Clostridium perfringens* types B and D, botulinum toxin, ricin, and benzilate (Marks 2004). The ability to obtain precursors and to manufacture nerve agents and toxins is relatively easy when compared with manufacturing other weapons of mass destruction, particularly nuclear weapons.

Considerable evidence indicates that Iraqi scientists developed, manufactured, and stockpiled nerve agents, mycotoxins, and bacterial and plant toxins as part of their bioweapons program in the 1980s. Approximately 2,300 liters of concentrated aflatoxin from toxigenic strains of *Aspergillus flavus* and *Aspergillus parasiticus* filled warheads on missiles. Despite the lethal effects of aflatoxins being neither apparent nor immediate on a battlefield, use of chemical weapons evokes fear and horror even before visible effects of the toxin. Unlike aflatoxins, trichothecene mycotoxins act immediately on contact, and an exposure to a few milligrams of T-2 toxin, a trichothecene toxin, can be lethal. In addition, considerable evidence exists that Iraqi scientists developed and stockpiled several thousand liters of botulinum toxin, the most potent natural poison, produced by *Clostridium botulinum*. In Fallujah, Iraq, a castor oil production facility produced powdered ricin, a potent inhibitor of protein syn-

TABLE 22–19. Comparative lethality and molecular weight of neurotoxic substances used as chemical weapons in a laboratory mice model

Agent	LD_{50}[a] (μg/kg)	Molecular weight	Source
Botulinum toxin type A1	0.001	150,000	Bacteria (*Clostridium botulinum*)
Abrin	0.04	65,000	Plant (jequirity beans, seeds of *Abrus precatorius*)
Ricin	3	64,000	Plant (castor bean, seeds of *Ricinus communis*)
Saxitoxin	10	299	Marine dinoflagellate
VX	15	267	Chemical nerve agent
Cyclosarin (GF)	16	180	Chemical nerve agent
Soman (GD)	64	182	Chemical nerve agent
Sarin (GB)	100	140	Chemical nerve agent
Anatoxin-a	375	500	Blue-green algae toxin
T-2 toxin	1,210	466	Fungal toxin (*Fusarium* species)

[a]The LD_{50} value is the dose in units of micrograms per kilogram of body weight that produces death in half (50%) of the mice tested. The LD_{50} (LD = lethal dose) is a standardized measure for expressing and comparing the toxicity of chemicals. *Source.* Adapted from Sidell 1992.

thesis and lethal in minute amounts, from castor bean oil (U.S. Central Intelligence Agency 2002). Ricin, the toxic protein of the castor oil, inhibits mammalian ribosomal protein production and subsequently affects every major organ influenced, particularly the liver, kidneys, lymph nodes, and lungs. It causes hyperpyrexia and interacts with the electrolyte and hormone metabolism. After the intoxication, a relatively symptomless "silent period" occurs, followed by a progressive multisystem failure including a hemolytic uremic syndrome, which consists of thrombotic microangiopathy, hemolytic anemia, thrombocytopenia, acute renal failure, and death. No specific therapy is available; therefore, treatment is primarily supportive (Balint 2004; Korcheva et al. 2005). To help the reader to appreciate the relative lethality of these agents, Table 22–19 shows the comparative toxicity of various agents that have potential for use as chemical weapons.

ASSESSMENT OF TOXIC EXPOSURE

The Poison Severity Score is a useful guide for communicating to a poison control center the severity of neurotoxic symptoms following acute exposure (Ellenhorn 1997). In cases of suspected toxic exposure, obtaining a thorough history and performing a clinical examination are essential. Sources such as a family member who knows the patient well may provide information about behavior or personality changes and changes in cognitive status that may interfere with an accurate history. A history should

include determining the patient's symptoms and the manner of onset of symptoms, identifying the poison, and establishing the duration and severity of exposure for any identified poisons. A careful review of symptoms by each system of the body is important. For unknown poisons, information about the patient's home location, proximity to nearby industry, occupation, source of drinking water, dietary habits and recent changes in diet, insect bites, herbal remedies, travel, hobbies, and medications may help identify the poison and route of exposure.

Laboratory studies include a complete blood count and differential, electrolytes, comprehensive metabolic function, endocrine function, and urinalysis. Because toxins may act as endocrine disruptors or toxins, a history and clinical examination for symptoms of both endocrine deficiency and excess are important.

Following a history, clinical examination, and laboratory testing, in the case of a known poison, the evaluation should focus on the target organ(s) affected. However, if the poison is unknown, qualitative analysis of blood and urine for heavy metals and screens of the blood, urine, and fat for organic and other toxins may help identify the poison. Quantitative analysis of the poison and, if applicable, metabolites in body tissues may indicate the severity of exposure, establish the time elapsed since exposure, correlate levels of the poison with severity of symptoms, and aid in monitoring elimination of the poison. Several types of testing are indicated because solvents, pesticides, metals, drugs, and plant and animal toxins may affect varied aspects of central nervous system functioning. Electroencephalography may be invaluable in certain cases in determining encephalopathic states induced by toxins. The use of quantitative EEG further increases the sensitivity of detection. Neural conduction studies can identify neuropathies as well as demyelination caused by peripheral neurotoxins. The use of computed tomography and MRI, volumetric if indicated, is helpful in identifying and localizing structural abnormalities secondary to toxin exposure. The use of SPECT and functional MRI might be helpful in studying metabolic derangements secondary to neurotoxin exposure (Simon et al. 2003). PET scans are useful as a tool to quantitate neurological effects occurring following neurotoxin exposure (Prockop 1995). Because toxic chemicals cause immune suppression either by direct effects or because of sleep disruption, components of cellular and humoral immunity are important to evaluate. A polysomnogram or sleep study can be invaluable because neurotoxins can disrupt normal sleep architecture, cause sleep disorders, and affect circadian rhythms. The presence of neural antibodies can indicate the presence of an autoimmune response. Evaluations of sensory evoked potentials are tools for identifying deficits in various sensory modalities.

Neuropsychological assessment also may be helpful. Several tests are available to assess the level of neuropsychological impairment (Hartman 1988). Ideally, workers in the chemical industry have had preexposure neuropsychological testing as part of the preemployment physical examination. Annual physical examinations and laboratory studies conducted on chemical workers should include, at a minimum, relevant tests that evaluate for the toxicity specific to the particular chemicals to which that worker is exposed.

DEVELOPMENTAL EFFECTS

The neuropsychiatric manifestations of toxin exposure discussed in this chapter are primarily those reported for adults. In experimental animals, the age of the exposed animal influences the degrees of neurological damage from neurotoxins such as metals, and the highest risks occur during the fetal and perinatal periods. The developing nervous system of the fetus, child, and early adolescent undergoes the critical cellular events of cell division, migration and differentiation, formation of synapses, pruning of synapses, myelinization, and apoptosis, during which exposure to a toxic substance may cause damage. In general, young children are at greater risk for injury than are adults subsequent to an exposure to neurotoxins. The full extent of the damage would be difficult to determine because of the long latent periods between relevant environmental exposures and emergence of evidence of impairments. On the other end of the life cycle, elderly adults have a greater susceptibility to neurotoxins because compensatory mechanisms are impaired as a result of the process of neuronal aging, with loss of neurons and supporting cells, cell death, and loss of neuronal "plasticity." The study of neurotoxins and their use as research tools continues to be important because they aid in the understanding of the pathophysiology of both psychiatric and neurological illness.

Highlights for the Clinician

Exposure to poisons and toxins can be acute or chronic and can occur through the respiratory tract via inhalation, through the skin by dermal contact or bite and envenomation, and through the digestive tract via oral ingestion, including through eating or smoking with contaminated hands or in contaminated work areas.

1. Obtain a history

In a neuropsychiatric interview of a patient, a thorough history should include questions to determine whether an exposure to poisons or toxins plays a role in the patient's illness. Family members who know the patient well may be a source of information regarding behavior or personality changes as well as changes in cognitive status that may interfere with an accurate history. In the event of a suspected poison or toxin, information obtained should include the following:

✦ Ask about the patient's occupation and that of other household members; description and duration of employment; and exposure to hazards such as pesticides, solvents, chemicals, fumes, fibers, radiation, metals, and biological agents. Ask about use of protective equipment at work such as a respirator, gloves, or safety glasses. Obtain a list of previous jobs, including full-time, part-time, and summer jobs, and military experience.

Highlights for the Clinician (continued)

- ◆ Ask if the patient smokes or eats at his or her worksite with contaminated hands or in contaminated work areas.

- ◆ Ask if anyone in the family worked with hazardous materials that they may have brought home.

- ◆ Ask if the patient has a hobby with exposure to hazardous materials such as paints, ceramics, solvents, resins, glue, adhesives, cements, or metals. Ask if the patient does repairs on his or her own or another automobile.

- ◆ Ask about pesticide use in the patient's garden and home or on a pet, safe storage of the pesticides, and removal of pesticide residue by thoroughly washing fruits and vegetables.

- ◆ Ask whether the patient has ever lived near a facility that contaminated the surrounding area such as a plant, dump, smelter, or mine.

- ◆ Ask whether the patient has changed residence because of a health problem.

- ◆ Ask whether the source of the patient's drinking water is a private well, the city water supply, or a grocery store.

- ◆ Ask what year the patient's home was built and if the home had any recent or previous water damage or flooding, underwent any recent remodeling, or received new carpet or furniture. Inquire as to the presence of an air conditioner or purifier, oil or gas central heating, gas or electric stove, wood stove, fireplace, or humidifier.

- ◆ Obtain any previous records, including laboratory testing, neuroimaging, neurophysiological and neuropsychological testing, and consultations, for comparison. Most workers in this industry have had preemployment physical examinations, laboratory studies, and an electrocardiogram.

2. Characterize symptoms

- ◆ Inquire about the timing of the patient's symptoms having any relation to work hours or to environmental activities listed above.

- ◆ Determine whether any other household members or nearby neighbors had similar symptoms.

- ◆ Determine whether anyone else at work had the same or similar problems.

- ◆ Ask whether the patient uses tobacco or drinks alcohol. Ask whether the patient takes any medications, including prescription, herbal, or homeopathic remedies.

3. Evaluate the patient

- ◆ Perform a physical examination of all systems following a thorough review of symptoms by each body system. Annual physical examinations and laboratory studies conducted on chemical workers should include, at a minimum, relevant tests that evaluate for the toxicity specific to the particular chemicals to which a worker is exposed.

- ◆ Obtain laboratory or basic clinical studies, including a complete blood count, platelet count and differential, comprehensive metabolic function including electrolytes, liver and kidney function, endocrine function, urinalysis, and electrocardiogram.

- ◆ Analyze blood and urine for heavy metals, and screen the blood, urine, and fat for organics. This analysis may be of limited value; however, in conjunction with other testing, it may help categorize the toxin.

- ◆ Complete neuropsychological testing to assess the level of neuropsychological impairment and to monitor any changes (if previous testing is available). Ideally, workers in the chemical industry have had preexposure neuropsychological testing as part of the preemployment physical examination.

(continued)

Highlights for the Clinician (*continued*)

✦ Use electroencephalography, which may be invaluable in certain cases in determining encephalopathic states induced by toxins. The use of quantitative electroencephalography further increases the sensitivity of detection.

✦ Perform nerve conduction studies to identify neuropathies and demyelination caused by peripheral neurotoxins.

✦ Use computed tomography and magnetic resonance imaging (MRI), volumetric if indicated, to help identify and localize structural abnormalities secondary to toxin exposure.

✦ Use single-photon emission computed tomography and/or functional MRI to study metabolic derangements secondary to neurotoxin exposure.

✦ Perform positron emission tomography scans to quantitate neurological effects occurring following neurotoxin exposure.

A team approach is encouraged in the identification of the offending agent and management of the patient, in the form of consultations with a regional poison control center, medical toxicologist, industrial medicine specialist, and other medical specialties.

RECOMMENDED READINGS

Dart RC: Medical Toxicology. Philadelphia, PA, Lippincott Williams & Wilkins, 2004

Ellenhorn MJ: Ellenhorn's Medical Toxicology: Diagnosis and Treatment of Human Poisoning. Baltimore, MD, Williams & Wilkins, 1997

Rea WJ, Didriksen N, Simon TR, et al: Effects of toxic exposure to molds and mycotoxins in building-related illnesses. Arch Environ Health 58:399–405, 2003

REFERENCES

Abd-Elghaffar SK, El-Sokkary GH, Sharkawy AA: Aluminum-induced neurotoxicity and oxidative damage in rabbits: protective effect of melatonin. Neuro Endocrinol Lett 26:609–616, 2005

Alfrey AC, Froment DC: Dialysis encephalopathy, in Aluminum and Renal Failure. Edited by DeBroe ME, Coburn JW. Dordrecht, The Netherlands, Kluwer, 1990, pp 249–257

Anyanwu E, Campbell AW, Jones J, et al: The neurological significance of abnormal natural killer cell activity in chronic toxigenic mold exposures. ScientificWorldJournal 3:1128–1137, 2003a

Anyanwu EC, Campbell AW, Vojdani A: Neurophysiological effects of chronic indoor environmental toxic mold exposure on children. ScientificWorldJournal 3:281–290, 2003b

Aposhian HV, Aposhian MM: Meso-2,3-dimercaptosuccinic acid: chemical, pharmacological and toxicological properties of an orally effective metal chelating agent. Annu Rev Pharmacol Toxicol 30:279–306, 1990

Aposhian HV, Carter DE, Hoover TD, et al: DMSA, DMPS, and DMPA—as arsenic antidotes. Fundam Appl Toxicol 4 (2 pt 2):S58–70, 1984

Aremu DA, Meshitsuka S: Accumulation of aluminum by primary cultured astrocytes from aluminum amino acid complex and its apoptotic effect. Brain Res 1031:284–296, 2005

Army FM8–285, Navy NAVMED P5041, and Air Force AFM160–11 Field Manual: The Treatment of Chemical Agent Casualties and Conventional Military Chemical Injuries. Washington, DC, Departments of the Army, Navy, and Air Force, February 28, 1990

Aschner M, Aschner JL: Manganese transport across the blood-brain barrier: relationship to iron homeostasis. Brain Res Bull 24:857–860, 1990

Atchinson WD: Is chemical neurotransmission altered specifically during methylmercury-induced cerebellar dysfunction? Trends Pharmacol Sci 26:549–557, 2005

Aykin-Burns N, Franklin EA, Ercal N: Effects of N-acetylcysteine on lead-exposed PC-12 cells. Arch Environ Contam Toxicol 49:119–123, 2005

Baldo JV, Ahmad L, Ruff R: Neuropsychological performance of patients following mold exposure. Appl Neuropsychol 9:193–202, 2002

Balint GS: [Ricin—2004] (in Hungarian). Orv Hetil 145:2379–2381, 2004

Barret DS, Oehme FW: A review of organophosphate ester induced delayed neurotoxicity. Vet Hum Toxicol 27:22–37, 1985

Beard RR, Grandstaff N: Carbon monoxide exposure and cerebral function. Ann N Y Acad Sci 174:385–395, 1970

Benjamin C: Persistent psychiatric symptoms after eating psilocybin mushrooms. BMJ 1:1319–1320, 1979

Bennett JW, Klich M: Mycotoxins. Clin Microbiol Rev 16:497–516, 2003

Bertoncin D, Russolo A, Caroldi S, et al: Neuropathy target esterase in human lymphocytes. Arch Environ Health 40:139–144, 1985

Bidstrup PL, Bonnell JA, Beckett AG: Paralysis following poisoning by a new organic phosphorus insecticide (mipafox): report on two cases. BMJ 1:1068–1072, 1953

Bleck TP: Tetanus: pathophysiology, management, and prophylaxis. Disease-a-Month 37:547–603, 1991

Bleecker M: Clinical presentation of selected neurotoxic compounds, in Occupational Neurology and Clinical Neurotoxicology. Edited by Bleecker ML, Hansen J. Baltimore, MD, Williams & Wilkins, 1994, pp 207–233

Bleecker ML, Ford DP, Lindgren KN, et al: Differential effects of lead exposure on components of verbal memory. Occup Environ Med 62:181–187, 2005

Bolla KI, Roca R: Neuropsychiatric sequelae of occupational exposure to neurotoxins, in Occupational Neurology and Clinical Neurotoxicology. Edited by Bleecker ML, Hansen JA. Baltimore, MD, Williams & Wilkins, 1994, pp 133–159

Boysen SR, Rozanski EA, Chan DL, et al: Tremorgenic mycotoxicosis in four dogs from a single household. J Am Vet Med Assoc 221:1420, 1441–1444, 2002

Bradbury JE, Forshaw PJ, Gray AJ, et al: The action of mephenesin and other agents on the effects produced by two neurotoxic pyrethroids in the intact and spinal rat. Neuropharmacology 22:907–914, 1983

Bradford HF, Norris PJ, Smith CC: Changes in transmitter release patterns in vitro induced by tremorgenic mycotoxins. J Environ Pathol Toxicol Oncol 10:17–30, 1990

Brown AW, Aldridge WN, Street BW, et al: Behavioral and neuropathological sequela of intoxication by trimethyltin compounds in the rat. Am J Pathol 97:59–82, 1979

Brown MA, Brix K: Review of health consequences from high-, intermediate- and low-level exposure to organophosphorus nerve agents. J Appl Toxicol 18:393–408, 1998

Bruyn GW, De Wolff FA: Plumbism, in Handbook of Clinical Neurology: Intoxications of the Nervous System. Edited by De Wolff FA. New York, Elsevier, 1994, pp 431–442

Bugiani O, Ghetti B: Aluminum encephalopathy: experimental vs human, in Aluminum and Renal Failure. Edited by De Broe ME, Coburn JW. Dordrecht, The Netherlands, Kluwer, 1990, pp 109–125

Campbell AW, Thrasher JD, Madison RA, et al: Neural autoantibodies and neurophysiologic abnormalities in patients exposed to molds in water-damaged buildings. Arch Environ Health 58:464–474, 2003

Campbell AW, Thrasher JD, Gray MR, et al: Mold and mycotoxins: effects on the neurological and immune systems in humans. Adv Appl Microbiol 55:375–406, 2004

Cavarati EM: Arsenic and arsine gas, in Medical Toxicology. Edited by Dart RC. Philadelphia, PA, Lippincott Williams & Wilkins, 2004, pp 1393–1401

Caravati EM, McCowan CL, Marshall SW: Plants, in Medical Toxicology. Edited by Dart RC. Philadelphia, PA, Lippincott Williams & Wilkins, 2004, pp 1671–1713

Cavanagh JB: Long term persistence of mercury in the brain. Br J Ind Med 45:649–651, 1988

Cavanagh JB, Holton JL, Nolan CC, et al: The effects of the tremorgenic mycotoxin penitrem A on the rat cerebellum. Vet Pathol 35:53–63, 1998

Chandra SV, Seth PK, Mankeshwar JK: Manganese poisoning: clinical and biochemical observations. Environ Res 7:374–380, 1974

Chandrasekaran A, Ponnambalam G, Kaur C: Domoic acid-induced neurotoxicity in the hippocampus of adult rats. Neurotox Res 6:105–117, 2004

Chen JW, Luo YL, Hwang MJ, et al: Territrem B, a tremorgenic mycotoxin that inhibits acetylcholinesterase with a noncovalent yet irreversible binding mechanism. J Biol Chem 274:34916–34923, 1999

Cherington M: Botulism: ten year experience. Arch Neurol 30:432–437, 1974

Cherington M: Botulism. Semin Neurol 10:27–31, 1990

Cook DG, Fahn S, Brait KA: Chronic manganese intoxication. Arch Neurol 30:59–64, 1974

Costa LG, Sulaiman R: Inhibition of protein synthesis by trimethyltin. Toxicol Appl Pharmacol 86:189–196, 1986

Crago BR, Gray MR, Nelson LA, et al: Psychological, neuropsychological, and electrocortical effects of mixed mold exposure. Arch Environ Health 58:452–463, 2003

Crystal HA, Schaumburg HH, Grober E, et al: Cognitive impairment and sensory loss associated with chronic low level ethylene oxide exposure. Neurology 29:978–983, 1988

Curley A, Gerrettson L: Acute chlordane poisoning. Arch Environ Health 18:211–215, 1969

Curtis L, Lieberman A, Stark M, et al: Adverse health effects of indoor molds. Journal of Nutritional and Environmental Medicine 14:1–14, 2004

Daniel S, Limson JL, Dairam A, et al: Through metal binding, curcumin protects against lead- and cadmium-induced lipid peroxidation in rat brain homogenates and against lead-induced tissue damage in rat brain. J Inorg Biochem 98:266–275, 2004

Dart RC: Introduction to plants, in Medical Toxicology. Edited by Dart RC. Philadelphia, PA, Lippincott Williams & Wilkins, 2004a, pp 1665–1671

Dart RC (ed): Medical Toxicology. Philadelphia, PA, Lippincott Williams & Wilkins, 2004b

Dart RC, Hurlbut KM, Boyer-Hassen L: Lead, in Medical Toxicology. Edited by Dart RC. Philadelphia, PA, Lippincott Williams & Wilkins, 2004, pp 1423–1431

Dart RC, Sullivan JB: Mercury, in Medical Toxicology. Edited by Dart RC. Philadelphia, PA, Lippincott Williams & Wilkins, 2004, pp 1437–1448

Davidovics Z, Cicco-Bloom E: Moderate lead exposure elicits neurotrophic effects in cerebral cortical precursor cells in culture. J Neurosci Res 80:817–825, 2005

De Wolff FA, Van der Voet GB: Biological monitoring of aluminum in renal patients. Clin Chim Acta 160:183–188, 1986

Desai K, Sullards MC, Allegood J, et al: Fumonisins and fumonisin analogs as inhibitors of ceramide synthase and inducers of apoptosis. Biochim Biophys Acta 1585:188–192, 2002

Didricksen N: Neurocognitive deficits in individuals exposed to toxigenic molds. Presented at 21st Annual Symposium on Man and His Environment in Health and Disease, Dallas, TX, June 19, 2003

Doctor SV, Costa LG, Kendall DA, et al: Trimethyltin inhibits the uptake of neurotransmitters into mouse forebrain synaptosomes. Toxicol Appl Pharmacol 25:213–221, 1982

Dunbar EM: Botulism. J Infect 20:1–3, 1990

Dunn MA, Sidell FR: Progress in medical defense against nerve agents. JAMA 262:649–652, 1989

Dyer RS, Walsh TJ, Wonderlin WF, et al: The trimethyltin syndrome in rats. Neurobehav Toxicol Teratol 4:127–133, 1982

Elhassani SB: The many faces of methylmercury poisoning. J Toxicol Clin Toxicol 19:875–906, 1983

Ellenhorn MJ: Ellenhorn's Medical Toxicology: Diagnosis and Treatment of Human Poisoning. Baltimore, MD, Williams & Wilkins, 1997

Erdman AR: Pesticides, in Medical Toxicology. Edited by Dart RC. Philadelphia, PA, Lippincott Williams & Wilkins, 2004, pp 1475–1496

Erikson KM, Aschner M: Increased manganese uptake by primary astrocyte cultures with altered iron status is mediated primarily by divalent metal transporter. Neurotoxicology 27:125–130, 2006

Erin N, Billingsley ML: Domoic acid enhances Bcl-2-calcineurin-inositol-1,4,5-trisphosphate receptor interactions and delayed neuronal death in rat brain slices. Brain Res 1014:45–52, 2004

Farnsworth NR: Hallucinogenic plants. Science 162:1086–1092, 1986

Feldman RG: Manganese, in Handbook of Clinical Neurology: Intoxications of the Nervous System. Edited by De Wolff FA. New York, Elsevier, 1994, pp 303–322

Flannigan SA, Tucker SB, Key MM: Prophylaxis of synthetic pyrethroid exposure. J Soc Occup Med 34:24–26, 1984

Food and Agriculture Organization/World Health Organization: 2,4,5-T Data Sheet on Pesticides. WHO/FAO Bulletin. Geneva, Switzerland, World Health Organization, 1975

Fortemps E, Amand G, Bomboir A, et al: Trimethyltin poisoning: report of two cases. Int Arch Occup Health 41:1–6, 1978

Garner CD, Nachtman JP: Manganese catalyzed auto-oxidation of dopamine to 6-hydroxydopamine in vitro. Chem Biol Interact 69:345–351, 1989

Garruto RM: Pacific paradigms of environmentally induced neurological disorders: clinical, epidemiological and molecular perspectives. Neurotoxicology 12:347–378, 1991

Ginsberg MD: Carbon monoxide intoxication: clinical features, neuropathology and mechanisms of injury. Clin Toxicol 23:281–288, 1985

Godwin HA: The biological chemistry of lead. Curr Opin Chem Biol 5:223–227, 2001

Goetz CG: Neurotoxins in Clinical Practice. Jamaica, NY, Spectrum, 1985

Gordon W, Johanning E, Haddad L: Cognitive Impairment Associated With Exposure to Toxigenic Fungi in Bioaerosols, Fungi and Mycotoxins: Health Effects Assessments, Prevention and Control. Albany, NY, Eastern New York Occupational and Health Center, 1999, pp 94–105

Graham DG: Catecholamine toxicity: a proposal for the molecular pathogenesis of manganese neurotoxicity and Parkinson's disease. Neurotoxicology 5:83–96, 1984

Gray MR, Thrasher JD, Crago R, et al: Mixed mold mycotoxicosis: immunological changes in humans following exposure in water-damaged buildings. Arch Environ Health 58:410–420, 2003

Gross JA: Ethylene oxide toxicity. Neurology 29:978–983, 1979

Habermann E: Tetanus, in Handbook of Clinical Neurology. Edited by Vinker PJ, Bruyn GW. Amsterdam, The Netherlands, Elsevier/North-Holland, 1978, pp 491–547

Hall AH, Robertson WO: Arsenic and other heavy metals, in Clinical Management of Poisoning and Drug Overdose. Edited by Haddad LM, Winchester JF. Philadelphia, PA, WB Saunders, 1990, pp 1024–1028

Harris WR: Equilibrium model for speciation of aluminum in serum. Clin Chem 38:1809–1882, 1992

Hartman DE: Neuropsychological Toxicology: Identification and Assessment of Human Neurotoxic Syndromes. New York, Pergamon, 1988

He F, Wang X, Zhow X, et al: Clinical observations on two patients of acute deltamethrin poisoning (abstract), in Proceedings of the 21st International Congress on Occupational Health, Dublin, Ireland, September 9–14, 1984, p 354

Holstege CP, Kirk M, Sidell FR: Chemical warfare: nerve agent poisoning. Crit Care Clin 13:923–942, 1997

Horowitz AL, Kaplan R, Sarpel G: Carbon monoxide toxicity: MRI imaging in the brain. Radiology 62:787–788, 1987

Hunter D, Benford R, Russell D: Poisoning by methylmercury compounds. Q J Med 9:193–213, 1940

Inoue N: [Neurological effects of chemical and biological weapons] (Japanese). Rinsho Shinkeigaku 43:880–882, 2003

Jeffery B, Barlow T, Moizer K, et al: Amnesic shellfish poison. Food Chem Toxicol 42:545–557, 2004

Jokanovic M, Stukalov PV, Kosanovic M: Organophosphate induced delayed polyneuropathy. Curr Drug Targets CNS Neurol Disord 1:593–602, 2002

Josephs KA, Ahlskog JE, Klos KJ, et al: Neurologic manifestations in welders with pallidal MRI T1 hyperintensity. Neurology 64:2033–2039, 2005

Kanchanapongkul J: Puffer fish poisoning: clinical features and management experience in 25 cases. J Med Assoc Thai 84:385–389, 2001

Kannan K, Yun SH, Evans TJ: Chlorinated, brominated, and perfluorinated contaminants in livers of polar bears from Alaska. Environ Sci Technol 39:9057–9063, 2005

Kawada T, Katsumata M, Suzuki H, et al: Insomnia as a sequela of sarin toxicity several years after exposure in Tokyo subway trains. Percept Mot Skills 100:1121–1126, 2005

Kerr DNS, Ward MK, Ellis W, et al: Aluminum intoxication in renal disease, in Aluminum in Biology and Medicine. Edited by Chadwick PJ, Whelan J. Chichester, England, Wiley, 1992, pp 123–141

Kerr HD, Saryan LA: Arsenic content of homeopathic medicines. Clin Toxicol 24:451–459, 1986

Keyes D: Chemical warfare agents, in Medical Toxicology. Edited by Dart RC. Philadelphia, PA, Lippincott Williams & Wilkins, 2004, pp 1777–1794

Kilburn KH: Indoor mold exposure associated with neurobehavioral and pulmonary impairment: a preliminary report. Arch Environ Health 58:390–398, 2003a

Kilburn KH: Summary of the 5th International Conference on Bioaerosols, Fungi, Bacteria, Mycotoxins, and Human Health. Arch Environ Health 58:538–542, 2003b

Kim SS, Kwack SJ, Lee RD, et al: Assessment of estrogenic and androgenic activities of tetramethrin in vitro and in vivo assays. J Toxicol Environ Health A 68:2277–2289, 2005

Kitazawa M, Anantharam V, Yang Y, et al: Activation of protein kinase C delta by proteolytic cleavage contributes to manganese-induced apoptosis in dopaminergic cells: protective role of Bcl-2. Biochem Pharmacol 69:133–146, 2005

Klaassen CD: Heavy metals and heavy-metal antagonists, in Goodman and Gilman's The Pharmacological Basis of Therapeutics, 9th Edition. Edited by Hardman JG, Limbird L, Goodman-Gilman A. New York, McGraw-Hill Professional, 2001a, pp 1851–1877

Klaassen CD: Nonmetallic environmental toxicants, air pollutants, solvents, vapors, and pesticides, in Goodman and Gilman's The Pharmacological Basis of Therapeutics, 9th Edition. Edited by Hardman JG, Limbird L, Goodman-Gilman A. New York, McGraw-Hill Professional, 2001b, pp 1877–1900

Korcheva V, Wong J, Corless C, et al: Administration of ricin induces a severe inflammatory response via nonredundant stimulation of ERK, JNK, and P38 MAPK and provides a mouse model of hemolytic uremic syndrome. Am J Pathol 166:323–339, 2005

Kreppel H, Reichl FX, Szinicz L, et al: Efficacy of various dithiol compounds in acute As_2O_3 poisoning in mice. Arch Toxicol 64:387–392, 1990

Kuzuhara S, Kanazawa S, Nakanishi T, et al: Ethylene oxide polyneuropathy. Neurology 33:377–380, 1983

Lallement G, Clarencon D, Brochier G, et al: Efficacy of atropine/pralidoxime/diazepam or atropine/HI-6/prodiazepam in primates intoxicated by soman. Pharmacol Biochem Behav 56:325–332, 1997

Lallement G, Clarencon D, Masqueliez C, et al: Nerve agent poisoning in primates: antilethal, anti-epileptic and neuroprotective effects of GK-11. Arch Toxicol 72:84–92, 1998

Lallement G, Demoncheaux JP, Foquin A, et al: Subchronic administration of pyridostigmine or huperzine to primates: compared efficacy against soman toxicity. Drug Chem Toxicol 25:309–320, 2002

Landrigan PJ: Occupational and community exposures to toxic metals: lead, cadmium, mercury and arsenic. West J Med 137:531–539, 1982

Lauwerys RR, Buchet JP, Roels H: The determination of trace levels of arsenic in human biological materials. Arch Toxicol 41:239–247, 1979

Le Quesne PM, Maxwell IC, Butterworth STG: Transient facial sensory symptoms following exposure to synthetic pyrethroids: a clinical and electrophysiological assessment. Neurotoxicology 2:1–11, 1980

Lerman Y, Hirshberg A, Shteger Z: Organophosphate and carbamate pesticide poisoning: the usefulness of a computerized clinical information system. Am J Ind Med 6:17–26, 1984

Lieberman A: Explosion of mold cases in homes, workplaces, and occupational medicine practices. Presented at 21st Annual Symposium on Man and his Environment in Health and Disease, Dallas, TX, June 19, 2003

Liu Y, Imai H, Sadamatsu M, et al: Cytokines participate in neuronal death induced by trimethyltin in the rat hippocampus via type II glucocorticoid receptors. Neurosci Res 51:319–327, 2005

Longland CL, Dyer JL, Michelangeli F: The mycotoxin paxilline inhibits the cerebellar inositol 1,4, 5-trisphosphate receptor. Eur J Pharmacol 408:219–225, 2000

Louria DB: Trace metal poisoning, in Cecil Textbook of Medicine. Edited by Wyngaarden JB, Smith LHJ. Philadelphia, PA, WB Saunders, 1988, pp 2385–2393

Lukiw WJ, McLachlan DRC: Aluminum neurotoxicity, in Handbook of Neurotoxicology: Effects and Mechanisms. Edited by Chang LW, Dyer RS. New York, Marcel Dekker, 1993, pp 105–142

Magee PN, Stoner HB, Barnes JM: The experimental production of oedema in the central nervous system of rats by triethyltin compounds. J Pathol Bacteriol 73:107–124, 1957

Major RH: Classic Descriptions of Disease. Springfield, IL, Charles C Thomas, 1945

Marasas WF, Riley RT, Hendricks KA, et al: Fumonisins disrupt sphingolipid metabolism, folate transport, and neural tube development in embryo culture and in vivo: a potential risk factor for human neural tube defects among populations consuming fumonisin-contaminated maize. J Nutr 134:711–716, 2004

Marks JD: Medical aspects of biologic toxins. Anesthesiol Clin North America 22:vii, 509–532, 2004

Mena I: Manganese, in Metals in the Environment. Edited by Waldron H. New York, Academic Press, 1980, pp 199–220

Metter JE, Bleecker ML: Quantitative neurological examination, in Occupational Neurology and Clinical Neurotoxicology. Edited by Bleecker ML, Hansen J. Baltimore, MD, Williams & Wilkins, 1994, pp 207–233

Min SK: A brain syndrome associated with delayed neuropsychiatric sequelae following acute carbon monoxide intoxication. Acta Psychiatr Scand 73:80–86, 1986

Mitchell-Heggs CAW, Conway M, Cassar J: Herbal medicine as a cause of combined lead and arsenic poisoning. Hum Exp Toxicol 9:195–196, 1990

Morgan JP, Penovich P: Jamaica ginger paralysis. Arch Neurol 35:530–532, 1978

Murphy VA, Adhwani KC, Smith QR, et al: Saturable transport of manganese (II) across the rat blood brain barrier. J Neurochem 57:948–954, 1991

Nagashima Y, Hamada Y, Ushio H, et al: Subcellular distribution of tetrodotoxin in puffer fish liver. Toxicon 37:1833–1837, 1999

Nakamura M, Yasumoto T: Tetrodotoxin derivatives in puffer fish. Toxicon 23:271–276, 1985

Naude TW, O'Brien OM, Rundberget T, et al: Tremorgenic neuromycotoxicosis in 2 dogs ascribed to the ingestion of penitrem A and possibly roquefortine in rice contaminated with Penicillium crustosum. J S Afr Vet Assoc 73:211–215, 2002

Nelson BK: Snake envenomation: incidence, clinical presentation and management. Med Toxicol Adverse Drug Exp 4:17–31, 1989

Ngim CH, Foo SC, Boey KW, et al: Chronic neurobehavioral effects of elemental mercury in dentists. Br J Psychiatry 167:95–98, 1995

Nishiyama M, Kuga T: Pharmacological effects of the tremorgenic mycotoxin fumitremorgin A. Jpn J Pharmacol 40:481–489, 1986

Normandin L, Hazell AS: Manganese neurotoxicity: an update of pathophysiologic mechanisms. Metab Brain Dis 17:375–387, 2002

Norris PJ, Smith CC, De BJ, et al: Actions of tremorgenic fungal toxins on neurotransmitter release. J Neurochem 34:33–42, 1980

Parenti M, Rusconi L, Cappabianca V, et al: Role of dopamine in manganese neurotoxicity. Brain Res 473:236–240, 1988

Perez-Mendes P, Cinini SM, Medeiros MA, et al: Behavioral and histopathological analysis of domoic acid administration in marmosets. Epilepsia 46 (suppl 5):148–151, 2005

Perl DP, Brody AR: Alzheimer's disease: x-ray spectrometric evidence of aluminum accumulation in neurofibrillary tangle bearing neurons. Science 208:297–299, 1980

Perl TM, Bedard L, Kosatsky T, et al: An outbreak of toxic encephalopathy caused by eating mussels contaminated with domoic acid. N Engl J Med 322:1775–1780, 1990

Peterson DW, Bradford HF, Mantle PG: Actions of a tremorgenic mycotoxin on amino acid transmitter release in vivo. Biochem Pharmacol 31:2807–2810, 1982

Petsas T, Fezoulidis I, Ziogas D: Gehirn Verkalkung bei chronischer Bleivergiftung [Cerebral calcification in chronic lead poisoning]. Rofo 157:192–193, 1992

Prockop LD: Neuroimaging in neurotoxicology, in Neurotoxicology: Approaches and Methods. Edited by Chang LW, Slikker W. New York, Academic Press, 1995, pp 753–763

Proudfoot AT: Poisoning due to pyrethrins. Toxicol Rev 24:107–113, 2005

Rea WJ, Didriksen N, Simon TR, et al: Effects of toxic exposure to molds and mycotoxins in building-related illnesses. Arch Environ Health 58:399–405, 2003

Roberts L: EPA moves to reassess the risk of dioxin. Science 252:911, 1991a

Roberts L: More pieces in the dioxin puzzle. Science 254:377, 1991b

Roels H, Lauwerys R, Genet P, et al: Relationship between external and internal parameters of exposure to manganese in workers from a manganese oxide and salt producing plant. Am J Ind Med 11:297–305, 1987

Ross WD, Emmett EA, Steiner J, et al: Neurotoxic effects of occupational exposure to organotins. Am J Psychiatry 138:1092–1095, 1981

Rouzaud M, Lutier J: Oedeme subaigu cerebromeninge du a une intoxication d'actualite. Presse Med 62:1075–1079, 1954

Russell FE: Snake Venom Poisoning. Great Neck, NY, Scholiom International, 1983

Ryan DW, Cherington M: Human type A botulism. JAMA 216:513–514, 1971

Saddik B, Williamson A, Nuwayhid I, et al: The effects of solvent exposure on memory and motor dexterity in working children. Public Health Rep 120:657–663, 2005

Scallet AC, Schmued LC, Johannessen JN: Neurohistochemical biomarkers of the marine neurotoxicant, domoic acid. Neurotoxicol Teratol 27:745–752, 2005

Schonwald S: Aluminum, in Medical Toxicology. Edited by Dart RC. Philadelphia, PA, Lippincott Williams & Wilkins, 2004a, pp 1387–1390

Schonwald S: Mushrooms, in Medical Toxicology. Edited by Dart RC. Philadelphia, PA, Lippincott Williams & Wilkins, 2004b, pp 1719–1735

Segura-Aguilar J, Lind C: On the mechanism of the Mn^{3+}-induced neurotoxicity of dopamine: prevention of quinone-derived oxygen toxicity by DT diaphorase and superoxide dismutase. Chem Biol Interact 72:309–324, 1989

Selwyn MJ: Triorganotin compounds as ionophores and inhibitors of ion translocating ATPases, in Organotin Compounds: New Chemistry and Applications. Edited by Zuckerman J. Washington, DC, American Chemical Society, 1976, pp 204–226

Shukla GS, Singhal RL: The present status of biological effects of toxic metals in the environment: lead, cadmium and manganese. Can J Physiol Pharmacol 62:1015–1031, 1984

Sidell FR: Soman and sarin: clinical manifestations and treatment of accidental poisoning by organophosphates. Clin Toxicol 7:1–17, 1974

Sidell FR: Clinical considerations in nerve agent intoxication, in Chemical Warfare Agents. Edited by Somani SM. New York, Academic Press, 1992, p 163

Silva VS, Duarte AI, Rego AC, et al: Effect of chronic exposure to aluminum on isoform expression and activity of rat (Na+/K+)ATPase. Toxicol Sci 88:485–494, 2005

Simon TR, Rea WJ: Use of functional brain imaging in the evaluation of exposure to mycotoxins and toxins encountered in Desert Storm/Desert Shield. Arch Environ Health 58:406–409, 2003

Smallwood P, Murray GB: Neuropsychiatric aspects of carbon monoxide poisoning: a review and single case report suggesting a role for amphetamines. Ann Clin Psychiatry 11:21–27, 1999

Spengos K, Schwartz A, Hennerici M: Multifocal cerebral demyelination after magic mushroom abuse. J Neurol 247:224–225, 2000

Steenland K: Chronic neurological effects of organophosphate pesticides. BMJ 312:1312–1313, 1996

Stommel EW, Watters MR: Marine neurotoxins: ingestible toxins. Curr Treat Options Neurol 6:105–114, 2004

Stranger J, Kerridge G: Multiple fractures of the dorsal part of the spine following chlordane poisoning. Med J Aust 1:267–268, 1968

Sudakin DL: Mycotoxins and toxigenic fungi, in Medical Toxicology. Edited by Dart RC. Philadelphia, PA, Lippincott Williams & Wilkins, 2004, pp 1714–1719

Taylor JR, Selhorst JB, Houff SA, et al: Chlordecone intoxication in man: clinical observations. Neurology 28:626–630, 1978

Teitelbaum JS, Zatorre RJ, Carpenter S, et al: Neurological sequela of domoic acid intoxication due to the ingestion of contaminated mussels. N Engl J Med 322:1781–1787, 1990

Toscano CD, Guilarte TR: Lead neurotoxicity: from exposure to molecular effects. Brain Res Brain Res Rev 49:529–554, 2005

Traverso HP, Kamil S, Rahim H, et al: A reassessment of risk factors for neonatal tetanus. Bull World Health Organ 69:573–579, 1991

Tryphonas L, Truelove J, Nera E, et al: Acute neurotoxicity of domoic acid in the rat. Toxicol Pathol 18:1–9, 1990

U.S. Central Intelligence Agency: Iraq's Weapons of Mass Destruction Programs. Washington, DC, U.S. Central Intelligence Agency, 2002

U.S. Department of State: Saddam's Chemical Weapons Campaign: Halabja, March 16, 1988. Washington, DC, Bureau of Public Affairs, U.S. Department of State, 2003

Usuki F, Yasutake A, Umehara F, et al: In vivo protection of a water-soluble derivative of vitamin E, Trolox, against methylmercury-intoxication in the rat. Neurosci Lett 304:199–203, 2001

Van der Voet GB: Intestinal absorption of aluminum, in Aluminum in Biology and Medicine (Ciba Foundation Symposium No 169). Edited by Chadwick DJ, Whelan J. Chichester, England, Wiley, 1992a, pp 109–122

Van der Voet GB: Intestinal absorption of aluminum: relation to neurotoxicity, in The Vulnerable Brain and Environmental Risks: Toxins in Food. Edited by Isaacson RL, Jensen KF. New York, Plenum, 1992b, pp 35–47

Van Poorten JF, Stienstra R, Dworacek B, et al: Physostigmine reversal of psilocybin intoxication (letter). Anesthesiology 56:313, 1982

Weinstein L: Current concepts: tetanus. N Engl J Med 289:1293–1296, 1973

White J: Elapid snakes, in Medical Toxicology. Edited by Dart RC. Philadelphia, PA, Lippincott Williams & Wilkins, 2004a, pp 1566–1578

White J: An overview of the venomous snakes of the world, in Medical Toxicology. Edited by Dart RC. Philadelphia, PA, Lippincott Williams & Wilkins, 2004b, pp 1543–1559

White J: Viperid snakes, in Medical Toxicology. Edited by Dart RC. Philadelphia, PA, Lippincott Williams & Wilkins, 2004c, pp 1579–1591

Wide C: Mercury hazards arising from the repair of sphygmomanometers. BMJ 293:1409–1410, 1986

Wilhelm JM, Jager DE, Ohnesorge FK: Aluminum toxicokinetics. Pharmacol Toxicol 66:4–9, 1990

Winship KA: Toxicity of inorganic arsenic salts. Adverse Drug React Acute Poisoning Rev 3:129–160, 1984

Wolters E, Huang CC, Clark C, et al: Positron emission tomography in manganese intoxication. Ann Neurol 26:647–651, 1989

Worek F, Widmann R, Knopff O, et al: Reactivating potency of obidoxime, pralidoxime, HI 6 and HLo 7 in human erythrocyte acetylcholinesterase inhibited by highly toxic organophosphorus compounds. Arch Toxicol 72:237–243, 1998

World Health Organization: Expanded Program on Immunization. Geneva, World Health Organization, 1988

Wu DJ, Li FQ: Domoic acid and human health. Wei Sheng Yan Jiu 34:378–381, 2005

Wu Z, Yang Y, Xie L, et al: Toxicity and distribution of tetrodotoxin-producing bacteria in puffer fish *Fugu rubripes* collected from the Bohai Sea of China. Toxicon 46:471–476, 2005

Wynter JE: The prevention of manganese poisoning. Indust Med Surg 31:308–310, 1962

Yang CC, Liao SC, Deng J: Tetrodotoxin poisoning in Taiwan: an analysis of poison center data. Vet Hum Toxicol 38:282–286, 1996

Yang SJ, Huh JW, Lee JE, et al: Inactivation of human glutamate dehydrogenase by aluminum. Cell Mol Life Sci 11:2538–2546, 2003

23

NEUROPSYCHIATRIC ASPECTS OF ETHANOL AND OTHER CHEMICAL DEPENDENCIES

Eric J. Nestler, M.D., Ph.D.
David W. Self, Ph.D.

Drug addiction continues to exact enormous human and financial costs on society, at a time when available treatments remain inadequately effective for most people. Given that advances in treating other medical disorders have resulted directly from research of the molecular and cellular pathophysiology of the disease process, an improved understanding of the basic neurobiology of addiction should likewise translate into more efficacious treatments.

Our knowledge of the basic neurobiology of drug addiction is leading psychiatric neuroscience in establishing the biological basis of a complex and clinically important behavioral abnormality. This is because many features of drug addiction in people can be reproduced in laboratory animals, in which findings are directly referable back to the clinical situation. Earlier work on drug reinforcement mechanisms, and more recently developed animal models that target the addiction process and drug craving, have made it possible to identify regions of the brain that play important roles in distinct behavioral features of addiction. These neural substrates are now the focus of extensive research on the molecular and cellular alterations that underlie these behavioral changes.

In this chapter we provide an overview of recent progress made in our understanding of the neurobiological basis of drug addiction. After providing brief definitions of commonly used terminology, we summarize the anatomical and neurochemical substrates that mediate the reinforcing effects of short-term drug exposure. We then describe how repeated drug exposure can induce gradually developing, progressive alterations in molecular and cellular signaling pathways, and how these neuroadaptive changes may ultimately contribute to addictive behavior.

DEFINITION OF TERMS

From a pharmacological perspective, drug addiction can be defined by processes such as tolerance, sensitization, dependence, and withdrawal. *Tolerance* refers to a pro-

---

This work was supported by grants from the National Institute on Drug Abuse.

gressive weakening of a given drug effect after repeated exposure, which may contribute to an escalation of drug intake as the addiction process proceeds. *Sensitization,* or *reverse tolerance,* refers to the opposite circumstance, whereby repeated administration of the same drug dose elicits an even stronger effect; sensitization to certain "incentive motivational" effects of drugs is believed to contribute to high relapse rates seen in addicted individuals. Thus, both tolerance and sensitization to different aspects of drug action can occur simultaneously. *Dependence* is defined as the need for continued drug exposure to avoid a withdrawal syndrome, which is characterized by physical or motivational disturbances when the drug is withdrawn. Presumably, the processes of tolerance, sensitization, dependence, and withdrawal are each caused by molecular and cellular adaptations in specific brain regions in response to repeated drug exposure. It is important to emphasize that these phenomena are not associated uniquely with drugs of abuse, as many clinically used medications that are not addicting (e.g., clonidine, propranolol, most antidepressants) can also produce similar phenomena. Rather, the manifestation of tolerance, sensitization, dependence, and withdrawal specifically in brain regions that regulate motivation is believed to underlie addiction-related changes in behavior.

Drugs of abuse are unique in terms of their reinforcing properties. A drug is defined as a reinforcer if the probability of a drug-seeking response is increased and maintained by pairing drug exposure with the response. Initially, most abused drugs function as positive reinforcers, presumably because they produce a positive affective state (e.g., euphoria). Such rapid and powerful associations between a drug reinforcer and a drug-seeking response probably reflect the drug's ability to usurp preexisting brain reinforcement mechanisms, which normally mediate the reinforcing effects of natural rewards such as food, sex, and social interaction.

Long-term exposure to reinforcing drugs can lead to drug addiction, which is characterized by an escalation in both the frequency and the amount of drug use and by intense drug craving during withdrawal despite grave adverse consequences. In the context of long-term drug use, a drug may serve not only as a positive reinforcer, but also as a negative reinforcer by alleviating the negative consequences of drug withdrawal. The persistence of drug craving and drug seeking (relapse) despite prolonged periods of abstinence suggests that long-lasting adaptations have occurred in the neural substrates that mediate acute drug reinforcement.

Addictive disorders are often defined clinically as a state of "psychological dependence," for example, in DSM-IV-TR (American Psychiatric Association 2000).

However, it is important to emphasize that in more precise pharmacological terms, we do not yet know the relative contributions of neurobiological changes that underlie tolerance, sensitization, or dependence/withdrawal to the compulsive drug-seeking behavior that is the clinical hallmark of an addictive disorder. It is possible that drug craving and relapse involve dependence-related dysphoria associated with drug withdrawal. Such factors are likely to be important during the relatively early phases of abstinence. However, a major question remains regarding the types of adaptations that underlie particularly long-lived aspects of addiction, for example, the increased risk of relapse that many addicts show even after years of abstinence. As stated above, such persistent drug craving may involve adaptations that underlie sensitization to the incentive motivational properties of drugs, drug-associated (conditioned) stimuli, and stressful events. In other words, sensitization to these various stimuli would increase their ability to "reinstate"—or "prime"—drug seeking despite prolonged abstinence. Identification of long-lasting adaptations that underlie these persisting behavioral changes is paramount to the ultimate development of truly effective treatments.

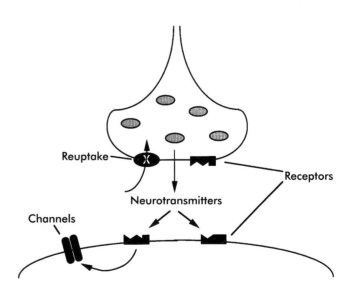

FIGURE 23–1.   A classic working model of synaptic transmission. In classic terms, synaptic transmission was conceived as the release of neurotransmitter from a nerve terminal, the binding of the neurotransmitter to specific receptor sites on target neurons, and the resulting alterations in the conductances of specific ion channels. The action of the neurotransmitter is then terminated by its reuptake into the nerve terminal or by enzymatic degradation (not shown).

TABLE 23–1. Examples of acute pharmacological actions of drugs of abuse

Drug	Action
Amphetamine	Stimulates monoamine release
Cannabinoids	Agonist at CB_1 cannabinoid receptors[a]
Cocaine	Inhibits monoamine reuptake transporters
Ethanol	Facilitates $GABA_A$ receptor function and inhibits NMDA glutamate receptor function[b]
Hallucinogens	Partial agonist at $5\text{-}HT_{2A}$ serotonin receptors
Nicotine	Agonist at nicotinic acetylcholine receptors
Opiates	Agonist at μ, δ, and κ opioid receptors[c]
Phencyclidine (PCP)	Antagonist at NMDA glutamate receptors

Note. $GABA_A = \gamma$-aminobutyric acid type A; NMDA = N-methyl-D-aspartate; $5\text{-}HT_2 = 5$-hydroxytryptamine (serotonin) type 2.
[a]The endogenous ligand(s) for this receptor has not yet been definitively identified; one candidate is anandamide.
[b]The mechanism by which ethanol produces these effects has not been established. In addition, ethanol affects many other neurotransmitter systems in brain.
[c]Activity at μ and δ receptors is thought to mediate the reinforcing actions of opiates.

THE SYNAPSE AS THE IMMEDIATE TARGET OF DRUGS OF ABUSE

The initial actions of drugs of abuse on the brain can be understood at the level of synaptic transmission. Figure 23–1 depicts a classic view of a synapse, in which a presynaptic nerve terminal, in response to a nerve impulse along its axon, releases a neurotransmitter that acts on a postsynaptic receptor to elicit changes in neuronal excitability of the postsynaptic neuron. The activity of the neurotransmitter is then turned off by its reuptake into the nerve terminal, or by enzymatic degradation (for review, see Nestler et al. 2001).

All drugs of abuse initially affect the brain by influencing the amount of a neurotransmitter present at the synapse or by interacting with specific neurotransmitter receptors. Table 23–1 lists examples of such acute pharmacological actions of some commonly used drugs of abuse. The fact that drugs of abuse initially influence different neurotransmitter and receptor systems in the brain explains the very different actions produced by these drugs acutely. For example, the presence of high levels of opioid receptors in the brain stem and spinal cord explains why opiates can exert such profound effects on respiration, level of consciousness, and nociception. In contrast, the importance of noradrenergic mechanisms in the regulation of cardiac function explains why cocaine can exert potent cardiotoxic effects.

In contrast to the many disparate acute actions of drugs of abuse, the drugs do appear to exert some common behavioral effects: as discussed above, they are all positively reinforcing after short-term exposure and cause a similar behavioral syndrome (addiction) after long-term exposure. This suggests that there are certain regions of the brain where the distinct acute pharmacological actions of these drugs converge at the level of a common reinforcement substrate. That is, in certain regions of the brain, which are discussed below, activation of opioid receptors (by opiates), inhibition of monoamine reuptake (by cocaine), or facilitation of GABAergic and inhibition of N-methyl-D-aspartate (NMDA) glutamatergic neurotransmission (by ethanol) would appear to elicit some common neurobiological response(s) that mediates their reinforcing properties.

MOLECULAR AND CELLULAR ADAPTATIONS AS THE LONG-TERM CONSEQUENCES OF DRUGS OF ABUSE

The acute pharmacological actions of a drug of abuse per se do not explain the long-term effects of repeated drug exposure. To understand such long-term effects, it is necessary to move beyond the classic view of a synapse, such as that shown in Figure 23–1. We now know that neurotransmitter-receptor activation does more to influence a target neuron than simply regulate its ion channels and immediate electrical properties: virtually every process in a neuron can be affected by neurotransmitter-receptor activation (Hyman et al. 2006; Nestler et al. 2001) (Figure

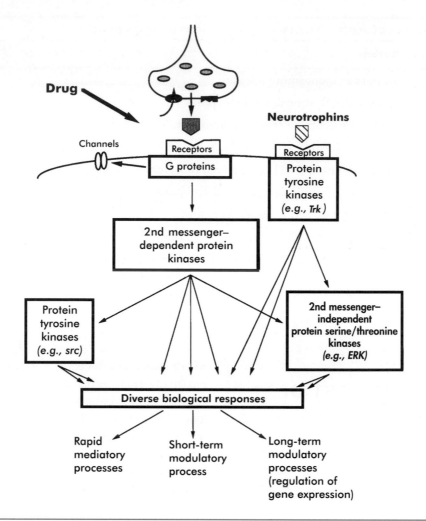

FIGURE 23–2.   A working model of synaptic transmission. Studies in basic neuroscience have provided a much more complex view of synaptic transmission than that shown in Figure 23–1. These studies focused on the involvement of intracellular messenger systems involving coupling factors (termed G proteins), second messengers (e.g., cyclic adenosine monophosphate [cAMP], calcium, nitric oxide, and the metabolites of phosphatidylinositol), and protein phosphorylation (involving the phosphorylation of phosphoproteins by protein kinases and their dephosphorylation by protein phosphatases) in mediating multiple actions of neurotransmitters on their target neurons. Second messenger–dependent protein kinases (e.g., those activated by cAMP or calcium) are classified as protein serine/threonine kinases, because they phosphorylate substrate proteins on serine or threonine residues. Each second messenger–dependent protein kinase phosphorylates a specific array of substrate proteins (which can be considered third messengers) and thereby leads to multiple biological responses of the neurotransmitter. Brain also contains many important intracellular regulatory pathways in addition to those regulated directly by G proteins and second messengers. This includes numerous protein serine/threonine kinases (e.g., the extracellular signal–regulated kinases [ERKs] or mitogen-activated protein [MAP] kinases), as well as numerous protein tyrosine kinases (which phosphorylate substrate proteins on tyrosine residues), some of which reside in the receptors for neurotrophins and most other growth factors (e.g., the trk proteins), and others that are not associated with growth factor receptors (e.g., src kinase). Each of these various protein kinases is highly regulated by extracellular stimuli. The second messenger–dependent protein kinases are regulated by receptor–G protein–second messenger pathways as mentioned above. The receptor-associated protein tyrosine kinases are activated on growth factor binding to the receptor. The second messenger–independent protein serine/threonine kinases and the protein tyrosine kinases that are not receptor associated seem to be regulated indirectly via the second messenger–dependent and growth factor–dependent pathways as depicted in the figure. The brain also contains numerous types of protein serine/threonine and protein tyrosine phosphatases, not shown in the figure, which are also subject to regulation by extracellular and intracellular stimuli. Thus, the binding of neurotransmitter to its receptor extracellularly results in numerous short-term and long-term biological responses through the complex regulation of multiple intracellular regulatory pathways and the phosphorylation or dephosphorylation of numerous substrate proteins.

23–2). Such effects are mediated by modulating the functional activity of proteins that are already present in the neuron or by regulating the actual amount of the proteins. Most neurotransmitters and receptors produce these diverse effects through biochemical cascades of intracellular messengers, which involve G proteins (guanosine triphosphate–binding membrane proteins that couple extracellular receptors to intracellular effector proteins), and the subsequent regulation of second messengers (such as cyclic adenosine monophosphate [cAMP], calcium, phosphatidylinositol, or nitric oxide) and protein phosphorylation (see Nestler et al. 2001). Protein phosphorylation is a process whereby phosphate groups are added to proteins by protein kinases or are removed from proteins by protein phosphatases. The addition or removal of phosphate groups dramatically alters protein function and leads to the myriad biological responses in question.

Neurotransmitter receptors function presynaptically to regulate the synthesis and storage of neurotransmitter via phosphorylation of synthetic enzymes and transporter proteins. In addition, altered phosphorylation of synaptic vesicle–associated proteins can modulate the release of neurotransmitters from presynaptic nerve terminals. Postsynaptically, altered phosphorylation of receptors and ion channels can modify the ability of neurotransmitters to regulate the physiological responses to the same or different neurotransmitter stimuli. Neurotransmitter-mediated phosphorylation of cytoskeletal proteins can produce structural and morphological changes in target neurons. Finally, altered phosphorylation of nuclear or ribosomal proteins can alter gene transcription and protein synthesis and hence the total amounts of these various types of proteins in the target neurons. Given the gradual development of drug addiction in most people and the persistence of drug craving for long periods after cessation of drug exposure, it is likely that repeated drug exposure causes altered patterns of gene expression and protein synthesis that underlie some of these long-term actions of drugs of abuse on the nervous system (Chao and Nestler 2004; Hyman et al. 2006; Nestler 1992).

Neurotransmitter regulation of G proteins and second messenger–dependent protein phosphorylation is a small part of a neuron's intracellular regulatory machinery (see Figure 23–2) (Nestler et al. 2001). Neurons also express high levels of protein tyrosine kinases (e.g., Trk proteins) that mediate the actions of neurotrophins and other growth factors. Growth factors play an important role in neuronal development, but more recently they have been shown to exert powerful effects on fully differentiated adult neurons. This implies that the traditional distinction between neurotransmitters and growth factors is becoming increasingly arbitrary. In addition,

neurons contain high levels of protein kinases that are not regulated directly by extracellular signals but are influenced by those signals indirectly via "crosstalk" among various intracellular pathways. Thus, each neurotransmitter-receptor system can interact with others via secondary, tertiary, etc., effects on various intracellular signaling pathways, all of which will contribute to the myriad effects of the original neurotransmitter stimulus.

This means that despite the initial actions of a drug of abuse on the activity of a neurotransmitter or receptor system, the many actions of drugs of abuse on brain function are achieved ultimately through the complex network of intracellular messenger pathways that mediate physiological responses to neurotransmitter-receptor interactions. Moreover, repeated exposure to drugs of abuse would be expected to produce molecular and cellular adaptations as a result of repeated perturbation of these intracellular pathways. These adaptations may be responsible for tolerance, sensitization, dependence, withdrawal, and, ultimately, the addiction process.

We begin our discussion of specific molecular and cellular adaptations that result from long-term drug exposure by considering the locus coeruleus, where adaptations in the cAMP pathway have been implicated in the molecular, cellular, and behavioral changes associated with physical signs of opiate dependence and withdrawal. Because similar molecular adaptations to long-term drug exposure are seen in brain regions associated with drug reinforcement and craving, the locus coeruleus has served as a model system to guide investigations into the molecular mechanisms underlying motivational dependence. These studies suggest that both physical and motivational changes associated with drug addiction are caused by some similar molecular adaptations, but in distinct neural substrates that regulate these behaviors (Nestler 2001).

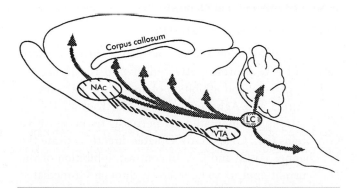

FIGURE 23–3. Locations of the locus coeruleus (LC), ventral tegmental area (VTA), and nucleus accumbens (NAc) in rat brain.

MOLECULAR MECHANISMS OF OPIATE DEPENDENCE IN THE LOCUS COERULEUS

The locus coeruleus is located on the floor of the fourth ventricle in the anterior pons (Figure 23–3). It contains the major noradrenergic nucleus in the brain with widespread projections to both the brain and spinal cord. This diffuse innervation allows the locus coeruleus to regulate the animal's general state of arousal, attention, and autonomic tone. An important role for the locus coeruleus in opiate physical dependence and withdrawal has been established at both the behavioral and electrophysiological levels: overactivation of locus coeruleus neurons is both necessary and sufficient for producing many behavioral signs of opiate withdrawal (see Aghajanian 1978; Koob et al. 1992; Maldonado and Koob 1993; Nestler 1992; Nestler and Aghajanian 1997; Rasmussen et al. 1990). Indeed, it was this knowledge of the role of the locus coeruleus in physical dependence to opiates that led to the introduction of clonidine—an α_2-adrenergic agonist that produces effects similar to those of morphine on neurons of the locus coeruleus (Aghajanian 1978)—as the first nonopiate treatment for opiate withdrawal in humans (Gold et al. 1978). Overactivation of locus coeruleus neurons during withdrawal arises from both extrinsic and intrinsic sources. The extrinsic source involves a hyperactive, excitatory glutamatergic input to the locus coeruleus from the nucleus paragigantocellularis (PGi) (Akaoka and Aston-Jones 1991; Rasmussen and Aghajanian 1989). This increased excitatory drive must arise in molecular adaptations within these afferent neurons or in their afferents, but the nature of these underlying mechanisms is still unknown. The intrinsic source involves intracellular adaptations in opioid receptor–coupled signal transduction pathways in locus coeruleus neurons.

MECHANISMS INTRINSIC TO THE LOCUS COERULEUS

Acutely, opiates inhibit locus coeruleus neurons via activation of a G protein–activated inward-rectifying K^+ (GIRK) channel and inhibition of an inward Na^+ current (e.g., Alreja and Aghajanian 1993; North et al. 1987). Both actions are mediated via pertussis toxin–sensitive G proteins (i.e., Gi and Go). Opiates directly activate the K^+ channel via Gi and Go. In contrast, inhibition of the Na^+ current appears to be indirect, through Gi-mediated inhibition of cAMP formation and reduced activation of cAMP-dependent protein kinase (protein kinase A). The identity of the channel that mediates this Na^+ current remains unknown. Biochemical studies confirm that opiates acutely inhibit adenylyl cyclase activity and cAMP-dependent protein phosphorylation in the locus coeruleus (Figure 23–4, top) (Nestler 1992).

With long-term exposure, locus coeruleus neurons develop tolerance to these acute inhibitory actions, as neuronal activity recovers toward preexposure levels (Aghajanian 1978; Williams et al. 2001). Administration of an opioid receptor antagonist causes a rebound increase in neuronal firing rates above preexposure levels both in vivo and in isolated slice preparations (Aghajanian 1978; Aston-Jones et al. 1997; Kogan et al. 1992; Rasmussen et al. 1990). These electrophysiological correlates of tolerance, dependence, and withdrawal are mediated in part via upregulation of the cAMP pathway as a compensatory, or homeostatic, adaptation to long-term exposure to opiates. Long-term opiate exposure increases locus coeruleus levels of Gi and Go, adenylyl cyclase types I and VIII, catalytic and regulatory subunits of protein kinase A, and several phosphoprotein substrates for the kinase (see Lane-Ladd et al. 1997; Nestler 1992; Nestler and Aghajanian 1997). One of these substrates, tyrosine hydroxylase, is the rate-limiting enzyme in the biosynthesis of norepinephrine (and other catecholamines), which suggests that norepinephrine synthesis is increased after long-term opiate administration.

The mechanisms by which long-term opiate exposure upregulates the cAMP pathway are complex (Nestler 2004). Some of the adaptations, including induction of adenylyl cyclase VIII and tyrosine hydroxylase, occur via increased gene expression that involves the transcription factor cAMP response element binding protein (CREB) (Boundy et al. 1998b; Chao et al. 2002; Lane-Ladd et al. 1997). CREB is activated when it is phosphorylated by protein kinase A or other protein kinases, and it is itself upregulated in the locus coeruleus after long-term morphine administration (see Nestler and Aghajanian 1997). A role for CREB-regulated genes in opiate physical dependence is consistent with the observation that mice lacking CREB show reduced opiate withdrawal symptoms (Maldonado et al. 1996). Other aspects of the upregulated cAMP pathway—for example, induction of protein kinase A subunits—appear to occur at a posttranscriptional level, apparently independent of gene transcription (Boundy et al. 1998a).

The upregulated cAMP pathway is thought to contribute to the reduced ability of opiates to inhibit the activity of locus coeruleus neurons and thus accounts, at least in part, for opiate tolerance. In addition, these compensatory adaptations contribute to the intrinsic hyperexcitability of locus coeruleus neurons seen during withdrawal (Aston-Jones et al. 1997; Kogan et al. 1992; Nestler and Aghajanian 1997) (Figure 23–4, bottom). This scheme is similar to

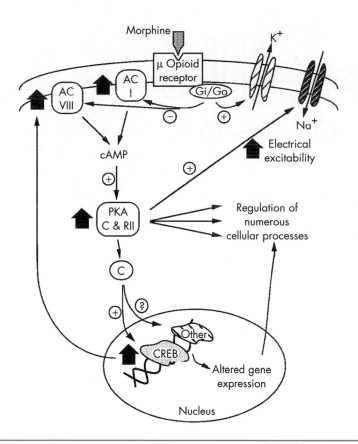

FIGURE 23–4. Schematic illustration of opiate actions in the locus coeruleus (LC). Opiates acutely inhibit LC neurons by increasing the conductance of an inwardly rectifying K^+ channel (*light crosshatch*) via coupling with subtypes of Gi and Go and by decreasing an Na^+-dependent inward current (*dark crosshatch*) via coupling with Gi and Go and the consequent inhibition of adenylyl cyclase. Reduced levels of cyclic adenosine monophosphate (cAMP) decrease protein kinase A (PKA) activity and the phosphorylation of the responsible channel or pump. Inhibition of the cAMP pathway also decreases phosphorylation of numerous other proteins and thereby affects many additional processes in the neuron. For example, it reduces the phosphorylation state of cAMP response element binding protein (CREB), which may initiate some of the longer-term changes in locus coeruleus function. *Upward bold arrows* summarize effects of long-term morphine use in the locus coeruleus. Long-term morphine use increases levels of types I and VIII adenylyl cyclase (AC), PKA catalytic (C) and regulatory type II (RII) subunits, and several phosphoproteins, including CREB. These changes contribute to the altered phenotype of the drug-addicted state. For example, the intrinsic excitability of LC neurons is increased via enhanced activity of the cAMP pathway and Na^+-dependent inward current, which contributes to the tolerance, dependence, and withdrawal exhibited by these neurons. Upregulation of type VIII adenylyl cyclase is mediated via CREB, whereas upregulation of type I adenylyl cyclase and of the PKA subunits appears to occur via CREB-independent mechanisms not yet identified.

Source. Reprinted from Nester EJ, Aghajanian GK: "Molecular and Cellular Basis of Addiction." *Science* 278:58–63, 1997. Used with permission.

one proposed earlier based on studies of neuroblastoma x glioma cells (Sharma et al. 1975). Although other mechanisms of opiate dependence in the locus coeruleus and elsewhere likely exist, manifestations of opiate dependence can be attributed directly to molecular and cellular adaptations in the cAMP pathway in specific neurons (Nestler and Aghajanian 1997). Related work suggests that similar types of adaptations underlie the long-term actions of opiates in other regions of the central nervous system (see, for example, Bonci and Williams 1997; Jolas et al. 2000; Terwilliger et al. 1991; Tjon et al. 1994; Unterwald et al. 1993).

Alterations in the ability of opioid receptors to couple to G proteins also could contribute to opiate tolerance (Figure 23–5). For example, an upregulated cAMP system could enhance the degree of opioid receptor desensitization through phosphorylation of the receptor. By promoting desensitization, the upregulated cAMP system in the tolerant state could lead to a reduced ability of opiates to acutely activate G proteins, the K^+ channel, and the Na^+ current. Chronic opiate-induced alterations in β-adrenergic receptor kinases (βARKs)—more generally referred to as G protein–coupled receptor kinases (GRKs)—or other

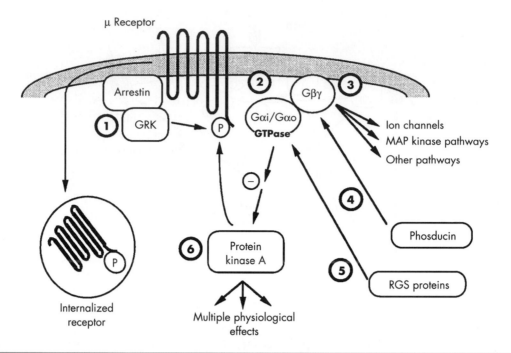

FIGURE 23–5.   Schematic illustration of possible mechanisms of drug-induced changes in opioid receptor sensitivity. Drug-induced adaptations in the efficacy of receptor-Gi/Go coupling could contribute to aspects of drug tolerance or sensitization. One possible mechanism is adaptations in processes that mediate acute desensitization of receptor function, such as receptor phosphorylation by G protein–coupled receptor kinases (GRKs) *(1)*. Other possible mechanisms include alterations in levels of G protein α *(2)* or βγ *(3)* subunits or of other proteins [for example, phosducin *(4)*; regulators of G protein signaling (RGS) proteins *(5)*, activators of G protein signaling (AGS) proteins (not depicted)] that modulate G protein function. Phosphorylation of the receptor by protein kinase A could not mediate acute receptor desensitization (since receptor activation leads to inhibition of the kinase); however, upregulation of the kinase *(6)* after long-term drug administration (see Figure 23–2) could phosphorylate and regulate receptor function during withdrawal states. Also shown in the figure is agonist-induced receptor internalization, which may be mediated via receptor phosphorylation. MAP=mitogen-activated protein.

Source.   Reprinted from Nestler EJ, Aghajanian GK: "Molecular and Cellular Basis of Addiction." *Science* 278:58–63, 1997. Used with permission.

protein components of this system (e.g., the arrestins) could also be involved in tolerance. This possibility is based on the role of GRKs and arrestins in mediating ligand-induced desensitization of opioid and other G protein–coupled receptors, which occurs independently of second messengers such as cAMP (see Gainetdinov et al. 2004; Von Zastrow 2004). GRK-mediated desensitization is believed to occur via the following scheme: ligand binding to the receptor facilitates GRK phosphorylation of the receptor, which then triggers its binding to arrestin, thereby attenuating coupling of the receptor to its G protein. This process also probably stimulates receptor internalization via endocytosis. Still another potential mechanism of opioid receptor desensitization involves drug-induced adaptations in G proteins themselves or in proteins that modulate the function of G proteins, such as the recently discovered family of regulators of G protein signaling (RGS) proteins (Gold et al. 2003). Each of these mechanisms has been shown to op-

erate in vitro, but the extent to which each contributes to opiate tolerance and dependence at the electrophysiological and behavioral levels is not yet known.

ROLE OF THE MESOLIMBIC DOPAMINE SYSTEM IN DRUG REINFORCEMENT

A substantial body of literature has established the mesolimbic dopamine system as a major neural substrate for the reinforcing effects of opiates, psychostimulants, ethanol, nicotine, and cannabinoids in animals (see Dworkin and Smith 1993; Ikemoto and Wise 2004; Koob et al. 1998; Kuhar et al. 1991; Olds 1982). This system consists of dopaminergic neurons in the ventral tegmental area (VTA) of the midbrain and their target neurons in forebrain regions such as the nucleus accumbens (NAc) and other ventral striatal regions (see Figure 23–3). For example, rats will self-administer dopamine, amphetamine (which releases dopamine), and cocaine and nomifensine (which elevate dopamine levels by blocking reuptake) directly into the NAc or olfactory tubercle, suggesting that dopamine receptors in the NAc mediate reinforcing stimuli. Opiates are self-administered directly into the dopamine cell body region of the VTA, where they activate dopamine neurons via disinhibitory mechanisms (see Johnson and North 1992) and thereby stimulate dopamine release in the NAc. Other drugs of abuse, such as ethanol, nicotine, and cannabinoids, also cause increased dopamine release in the NAc (Chen et al. 1990; Di Chiara and Imperato 1988), possibly through similar disinhibition of VTA dopamine neurons (Tanda et al. 1997). These findings have led some investigators to suggest that dopamine release in the NAc is a final common mechanism in the acute reinforcing effects of opiates, psychostimulants, and other abused drugs.

However, there is strong evidence that opiates such as heroin and morphine can produce reinforcement independently of the dopamine system, by acting directly on opioid receptors in the NAc and other brain regions (for review, see Bardo 1998). Dopamine antagonists and lesions of mesolimbic dopamine neurons, for example, fail to affect intravenous heroin self-administration. Animals also will self-administer opiates directly into the NAc, where opioid receptors on NAc neurons in essence bypass dopamine inputs. These data indicate that opiates can utilize both dopaminergic and nondopaminergic mechanisms in the NAc to produce reinforcement of drug self-administration. Importantly, lesions of NAc neurons attenuate both cocaine and heroin self-administration, suggesting that the NAc is a critical neural substrate for both psychostimulant and opiate reinforcement.

NEUROBIOLOGICAL MECHANISMS OF RELAPSE

Whereas drug self-administration is thought to provide a measure of the acute reinforcing properties of a drug, it is quite different from drug craving and drug seeking, which are the core behavioral abnormalities that define a state of addiction. Drug craving and drug seeking are cognitive states that are measured by subjective reports in humans and cannot be directly measured in laboratory animals. However, relapse is an operational event that can be measured directly when a laboratory animal reinitiates lever-press responding after abstaining from drug self-administration. To measure relapse in an experimental setting, investigators first introduce extinction conditions to animals with drug self-administration experience, thereby

attenuating reinforcement of further lever-press responding. As animals learn that the drug is no longer available, their efforts to self-administer the drug quickly diminish. After a given period of abstinence, the animals are presented with specific stimuli that induce responding at the lever that previously delivered drug injections. This reinitiation of responding is interpreted as relapse to drug-seeking behavior. The level of drug-seeking behavior is measured by the amount of effort (lever-pressing) exerted by the animals to self-administer the drug. Because these efforts are no longer reinforced by drug infusions, this behavior is also referred to as nonreinforced responding. In essence, this behavioral paradigm separates the incentive motivational component of drug reinforcement (drug seeking) from the consummatory component (drug taking) and is believed to measure changes in the motivational state of the animal in the absence of drug reinforcement.

Only three types of stimuli have been shown to induce relapse to drug-seeking behavior in animals. These stimuli consist of low doses of the drug that was previously self-administered, drug-associated (conditioned) cues, and stressful situations (for a review, see Self and Nestler 1998; Shaham et al. 2003). Because all three of these stimuli also trigger drug craving in human drug abusers, relapse to drug-seeking behavior in animals may represent a valid model of drug craving. Moreover, given that measures of drug craving can be confounded by the subjective nature of self-reports in humans (Tiffany et al. 1993), animal models of relapse may offer a more direct and objective measure of relapse to drug seeking than human reports of drug craving.

DRUG-INDUCED RELAPSE TO DRUG-SEEKING BEHAVIOR

A powerful trigger of relapse in animal models is a low "priming" injection with the drug that was self-administered by the animal on previous occasions (see Self and Nestler 1998; Shaham et al. 2003). This priming effect has been demonstrated for both opiates and psychostimulants. Interestingly, opiates such as morphine can trigger relapse to cocaine-seeking behavior and vice versa. Such "cross-priming" may reflect activation of a common neural substrate, perhaps the common ability of these drugs to activate the mesolimbic dopamine system.

Indeed, considerable evidence suggests that relapse triggered by priming injections of opiates and psychostimulants is mediated by the mesolimbic dopamine system. For example, microinfusion of amphetamine directly into the NAc, where it causes local dopamine release, effectively induces relapse to heroin-seeking behavior (Stewart and Vezina 1988). Conversely, microinfusion of morphine into the VTA, which indirectly activates dopamine neurons and consequently increases dopamine release in the NAc, induces relapse to heroin- and cocaine-seeking behavior (Stewart et al. 1984). In contrast, microinfusion of morphine into other brain regions rich in opioid receptors is ineffective at inducing relapse to drug-seeking behavior. Dopaminergic involvement in drug-induced relapse is further supported by the fact that several directly acting dopaminergic agonists are powerful inducers of relapse to both cocaine- and heroin-seeking behavior (De Wit and Stewart 1981; Self et al. 1996; Wise et al. 1990), whereas dopamine antagonists can block the priming effects of heroin, amphetamine, and cocaine (Ettenberg 1990; Shaham and Stewart 1996; Weissenborn et al. 1996). Taken together, these studies suggest that dopamine release in the NAc is both necessary and sufficient for inducing relapse to opiate- and psychostimulant-seeking behavior that is elicited by priming injections of the drugs (Figure 23–6).

Human neuroimaging studies corroborate a role for the NAc in cocaine-induced cocaine craving and also indicate a role for the left amygdala and right parahippocampal gyrus (Breiter et al. 1997). Functional inactivation studies in animals suggest that information flow from the prefrontal cortex through the NAc and descending to the ventral pallidum is necessary for cocaine-induced, cocaine-seeking behavior (McFarland and Kalivas 2001). Thus, motivational output ultimately could be determined by dopaminergic modulation of excitatory drive of NAc neurons that project to the ventral pallidum.

CUE-INDUCED RELAPSE TO DRUG-SEEKING BEHAVIOR

Cue-induced relapse to drug-seeking behavior involves the process of classical conditioning, whereby environmental stimuli, through repeated and specific association with drug exposure, acquire the ability to trigger relapse when presented in the absence of the drug (e.g., Ehrman et al. 1992; O'Brien et al. 1992; Robinson and Berridge 2003). The fact that these drug-associated cues can trigger appetitive or approach behavior has led investigators to hypothesize that these conditioned stimuli also activate the mesolimbic dopamine system (Ikemoto and Wise 2004; Robinson and Berridge 2003; Stewart et al. 1984), a possibility supported by several studies (Di Ciano et al. 1998; Ito et al. 2004; Phillips et al. 2003). In addition, others have found that presentation of cues associated with food rewards also activates dopamine neurons in the VTA, suggesting that cue-induced dopamine release is a neural signal for reward availability (Mirenowicz and Schultz 1996).

The amygdala is a critical substrate for cue-induced relapse to drug-seeking behavior. For example, lesions of

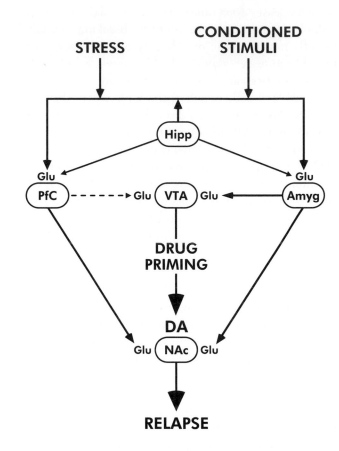

FIGURE 23–6.   Schematic representation of the primary pathways through which stress, drugs of abuse, and drug-associated conditioned stimuli are hypothesized to trigger drug craving and relapse to drug seeking. Stress and conditioned stimuli can activate excitatory glutamatergic projections (Glu) to the ventral tegmental area (VTA) from the amygdala (Amyg) and perhaps other regions, and indirectly (*dotted line*) from the prefrontal cortex (PfC) and hippocampus (Hipp), whereas priming injections of drugs directly stimulate dopamine (DA) release in the nucleus accumbens (NAc). In this sense, dopamine release in the NAc may be a final common trigger of drug craving by all three stimuli. At the level of NAc neurons, dopamine from the VTA modulates direct excitatory signals from the PfC, Amyg, and Hipp, where complex spatiotemporal integration of relapse-related information occurs. Studies showing involvement of these brain regions in relapse to drug seeking suggest that long-term changes in gene expression in these regions would alter the functionality of this circuitry and thus could produce profound changes in reactivity to stimuli that would trigger drug craving and relapse to drug seeking.

Source.   Adapted from Self DW, Nestler EJ: "Relapse to Drug Seeking: Neural and Molecular Mechanisms." *Drug and Alcohol Dependence* 51:49–60, copyright 1998, with permission from Elsevier.

the amygdala attenuate the ability of drug-associated cues to induce relapse (Meil and See 1997). Cue-induced relapse is attenuated even when the lesions are produced after learned associations between cues and drugs have already formed, which suggests that conditioned cues utilize the amygdala to access and activate appetitive motivational systems. In this regard, projections from the amygdala are known to activate VTA dopamine neurons through both monosynaptic and polysynaptic pathways, presumably leading to increased dopaminergic transmission in the NAc. Figure 23–6 illustrates this pathway whereby drug-associated cues can activate the mesolimbic dopamine system via known excitatory (glutamatergic) inputs from the amygdala. Also illustrated is an amygdalar projection to the prefrontal cortex, which could form an indirect pathway whereby drug-associated cues activate VTA dopamine neurons.

STRESS-INDUCED RELAPSE TO DRUG-SEEKING BEHAVIOR

Psychological stress can also trigger drug craving in humans and relapse to drug seeking in animals. In animals, stress-induced relapse is triggered after a brief period of mild intermittent footshock. Presentation of this stress effectively induces relapse to both cocaine- and heroin-seeking behavior (Ahmed and Koob 1997; Erb et al. 1996; Shaham and Stewart 1995). Interestingly, stress-induced relapse to heroin-seeking behavior is equally effective whether animals are physically dependent on heroin or not (Shaham et al. 1996). Similar to drug- and cue-induced relapse, stress-induced relapse also may involve activation of the mesolimbic dopamine system. This idea is supported by the finding that stress-induced dopamine release in the NAc correlates temporally with relapse to heroin-seeking behavior (Shaham and Stewart 1995). Moreover, stress-induced relapse is partially attenuated by pretreatment with dopamine antagonists (Shaham and Stewart 1996). A primary neural pathway through which stress can stimulate dopamine release in the NAc may involve stress-induced activation of the prefrontal cortex (Karreman and Moghaddam 1996; Moghaddam and Jackson 2004; Taber et al. 1995) and, indirectly, activation of VTA dopamine neurons through excitatory projections from other brain regions (see Figure 23–6).

Another pathway by which stress can activate the mesolimbic dopamine system involves the ability of stress to stimulate release of the neuropeptide corticotropin-releasing factor (CRF). Infusion of CRF into the cerebral ventricles mimics the effects of stress in inducing relapse to heroin-seeking behavior, and similar infusions of a CRF antagonist reduce stress-induced relapse (Shaham et al. 1997). Because CRF can activate central dopamine systems (e.g., via the hypothalamic-pituitary-adrenal axis and corticosterone secretion [Overton et al. 1996; Piazza et al. 1996]), CRF-induced relapse may also involve activation of the mesolimbic dopamine system. Indeed, systemic injections of corticosterone can induce relapse to cocaine-seeking behavior in animals, and psychosocial stress causes dopamine release in the NAc (Deroche et al. 1997; Pruessner et al. 2004). However, because stress can trigger relapse in adrenalectomized animals (Shaham et al. 1997) and stress-induced relapse is associated with relatively small increases in dopamine release in the NAc (Shaham et al. 1996), stress-induced relapse likely involves corticosterone- and dopamine-independent mechanisms as well.

Clearly, the effects of stress, cues, and drugs themselves on the mesolimbic dopamine system resemble druglike, or proponent, processes. In contrast, drug opposite or withdrawal-like processes fail to induce relapse to drug-seeking behavior in animal models. For example, the precipitation of opiate withdrawal with naltrexone fails to induce relapse in animals with heroin self-administration experience, even when the animals are markedly physically dependent on the opiate (Shaham et al. 1996). Similarly, blockade of dopamine receptors with dopamine antagonists fails to induce heroin- or cocaine-seeking behavior (Shaham and Stewart 1996; Weissenborn et al. 1996), despite their ability to produce aversive consequences. Although these data contrast sharply with human studies in which drug craving is associated with negative emotionality during opiate and ethanol withdrawal, they agree with reports of druglike, and even mood-elevating, symptoms of craving in cocaine-addicted individuals (Childress et al. 1988; Robbins et al. 1997).

Even though naltrexone-precipitated withdrawal fails to trigger relapse to heroin-seeking behavior in animals, spontaneous withdrawal from heroin has been associated with relapse in the same models (Shaham et al. 1996). It is possible that CRF plays a role in such withdrawal-induced relapse, because central CRF pathways are activated during withdrawal from virtually any drug of abuse (Heinrichs and Koob 2004). Withdrawal-related relapse may be relevant to factors involved in maintaining daily drug use in active drug abusers. In this sense, dependence and withdrawal may play a more prominent role in drug craving during periods of active drug use, whereas druglike processes (e.g., sensitization) may be more important in triggering drug craving and relapse after prolonged periods of abstinence, when withdrawal symptoms are no longer apparent. In addition, the alleviation of withdrawal by drug use (negative reinforcement) may facilitate drug reinforcement, leading indirectly to enhanced craving elicited by conditioned stimuli even after withdrawal symptoms subside (Hutcheson et al. 2001).

Although it has not been clearly resolved, cue- and stress-induced reinstatement of drug-seeking behavior also may involve dopamine-independent neural substrates (reviewed in Self 1998). Thus, the basolateral and central nuclei of the amygdala, as well as the prefrontal cortex and hippocampus, send direct excitatory projections to the NAc. Excitatory inputs from these regions converge with VTA dopamine inputs at the level of NAc neurons, where excitatory transmission in the NAc has been implicated in relapse to cocaine-seeking behavior (Di Ciano and Everitt 2004; Kalivas and McFarland 2003; McFarland et al. 2004). Together, these brain regions all form a complex circuit with primary sites of convergence in both the VTA and the NAc of the mesolimbic dopamine system, as depicted in Figure 23–6. Given the central role of the NAc in the output of these circuits, regulation of NAc neuronal activity, whether by dopamine or glutamate, may be a critical event in triggering drug craving.

MECHANISMS OF DOPAMINE-INDUCED RELAPSE

The studies described in the preceding sections suggest that relapse to drug seeking can be triggered by activation of dopamine receptors on NAc neurons. Dopamine receptors are divided into two general classes that are distinguishable by their structural properties and opposite modulation of adenylyl cyclase. The D_1-like receptors (D_1 and D_5) are positively coupled to adenylyl cyclase activity, whereas the D_2-like receptors (D_2, D_3, and D_4) either are negatively coupled or have no detectable effect on the enzyme. The two receptor classes also exert opposite effects on phosphatidylinositol turnover. Neurons intrinsic to the NAc express both D_1-like and D_2-like dopamine receptors, but in somewhat different neuronal populations (Curran and Watson 1995; Meador-Woodruff et al. 1991). In most cases, these receptors produce similar, even synergistic, responses at the physiological and behavioral levels (Hu and White 1994; Waddington and Daly 1993).

In contrast to these cooperative actions, activation of D_2-like, but not of D_1-like, dopamine receptors induces a profound and prolonged relapse to cocaine-seeking behavior in rats (De Vries et al. 1999; Self et al. 1996). These findings suggest that D_2-like receptors are primarily involved in inducing drug-seeking behavior by priming stimuli that release dopamine in the NAc. Although selective activation of D_1-like receptors fails to markedly induce cocaine-seeking behavior, D_1 receptors may have a permissive role in the priming effects mediated by D_2 receptors, as both D_1 and D_2 receptor antagonists can block the priming effects of cocaine and heroin (Shaham and Stewart 1996; Weissenborn et al. 1996). Thus, trans-

mission of D_2-mediated priming signals may require some minimal level of D_1 receptor activation. Interestingly, however, D_1-like receptor activation completely abolishes the ability of cocaine to induce relapse (Self et al. 1996). The opposing influence of D_1-like and D_2-like dopamine receptor activation on relapse to cocaine-seeking behavior is intriguing, because both D_1 and D_2 receptor agonists have reinforcing properties, have similar abilities to mimic the subjective effects of cocaine, and stimulate locomotor activity. One possible explanation for these findings is that D_2-like receptors mediate the incentive to seek further drug reinforcement, whereas D_1-like receptors could mediate some aspect of drug reward related to gratification, drive reduction, or satiety.

Opposite modulation of drug-seeking behavior by D_1 and D_2 dopamine receptors could involve their opposite effects on cAMP formation. In this regard, microinfusion of a selective inhibitor of protein kinase A into the NAc triggers relapse to cocaine-seeking behavior and potentiates cocaine-induced relapse to cocaine-seeking behavior in rats (Self et al. 1998). The effect of the protein kinase inhibitor resembles the effect of D_2 receptor stimulation, suggesting that dopamine triggers relapse by stimulating D_2 receptors that function via inhibition of protein kinase A activity. In any event, these findings suggest that protein kinase A activity in certain NAc neurons could play a pivotal role in regulating incentive motivation during drug craving and relapse.

ADAPTATIONS IN THE MESOLIMBIC DOPAMINE SYSTEM AFTER LONG-TERM DRUG EXPOSURE

Although symptoms of physical withdrawal from opiates and other drugs typically persist for short periods of time after cessation of long-term drug exposure, drug addicts report intense drug craving long after these physical symptoms have subsided. This suggests that different brain regions mediate physical and motivational symptoms of drug dependence, a view supported by direct experimental evidence (e.g., Koob et al. 1992). The motivational symptoms, which include an escalation of drug intake (tolerance), increased drug craving (sensitization), and withdrawal-induced dysphoria (dependence), could result from drug-induced adaptations in the normal functioning of reinforcement-related brain regions, such as the VTA and NAc. Recent studies have found that long-term drug exposure produces adaptations at the molecular and cellular levels in VTA dopamine neurons, and in their target neurons in the NAc, that may underlie motivational aspects of tolerance, sensitization, and dependence associated with drug addiction (e.g., see Hyman et al. 2006; Kalivas et al. 2005; Nestler 2001; Self 2004; Self and Nestler 1998; White and Kalivas 1998; M.E. Wolf 1998). The results from these studies provide the basis for specific hypotheses that now guide future investigations to test, more directly, the role of specific adaptations in mediating drug craving in addicted subjects.

The ability of various drugs of abuse to produce similar types of changes in drug-taking and drug-seeking behavior after repeated administration raises the possibility that these drugs also produce similar types of molecular and cellular adaptations in specific brain regions. Support for this possibility comes from behavioral data, in which long-term exposure to stimulants, opiates, or ethanol can cross-sensitize the animal to the effects of the other drugs (e.g., see Kelley 2004; Stewart 2003; Vezina 2004). As demonstrated below, there is also now considerable biochemical evidence that different drugs of abuse can produce similar molecular adaptations in the VTA–NAc pathway after long-term administration. These adaptations may be part of a common general mechanism of drug addiction and craving (Figure 23–7) (Nestler 2005).

REGULATION OF DOPAMINE IN THE VENTRAL TEGMENTAL AREA– NUCLEUS ACCUMBENS PATHWAY

A widely held view is that repeated exposure to a drug of abuse may produce some of its behavioral effects (e.g., drug craving or locomotor sensitization) by facilitating drug-induced dopamine release in the NAc. This possibility is best established for stimulants and opiates, which can result in augmented synaptic levels of dopamine as measured by in vivo microdialysis, under some experimental conditions. However, the large body of literature on this subject is inconsistent and confusing overall, given that these drugs have been reported to both increase and decrease synaptic levels of dopamine depending on the drug-treatment regimen employed and the time of withdrawal studied (for references, see Kalivas 2004; Robinson and Berridge 2003; Self and Nestler 1995; Spanagel and Weiss 1999; White and Kalivas 1998; M.E. Wolf 1998). Although altered regulation of dopamine release in the NAc or other brain regions is one likely mechanism underlying aspects of long-term drug exposure, its precise role remains uncertain.

It also has been difficult to identify the precise molecular targets of drugs of abuse that mediate the altered synaptic levels of dopamine observed. Long-term exposure to cocaine upregulates dopamine reuptake transporter proteins specifically in the mesolimbic dopamine system during late phases of withdrawal from the drug (Pilotte 1997). By increasing dopamine reuptake at the synapse, this molecular change would be expected to reduce synaptic levels of dopamine in the VTA–NAc pathway. Long-term exposure to opiates, cocaine, amphetamine, or ethanol has been shown to increase levels of tyrosine hydroxylase in the VTA but to reduce the total amount and phosphorylation state (and hence the enzymatic activity) of the enzyme in the NAc during early phases of withdrawal (Nestler 1992; Ortiz et al. 1995; Schmidt et al. 2001). Decreases in tyrosine hydroxylase activity in the NAc and increases in presynaptic dopamine reuptake could contribute to the reductions in basal extracellular dopamine levels and anhedonia seen during withdrawal (see Koob et al. 2004).

REGULATION OF OPIOID AND DOPAMINE RECEPTORS IN THE VENTRAL TEGMENTAL AREA AND NUCLEUS ACCUMBENS

It also has been proposed that altered levels of various opioid, dopamine, or other neurotransmitter receptors in the mesolimbic dopamine system could mediate some of the long-term effects of drugs of abuse on this neural pathway. The literature on this subject, although vast, is unsatisfying. In general it has been difficult to establish altered levels of opioid receptors in the VTA and NAc or any other brain regions in response to long-term opiate treatment, although μ and κ receptors are reported to be upregulated by long-term cocaine treatment (Unterwald et al. 1994). There have also been numerous reports of stimulant regulation of dopamine receptors in specific brain regions. Although conflicting data exist, most studies have found reductions in D_1 and D_2 receptors in the NAc in early withdrawal from self-administration or bingelike administration of cocaine. An in vivo positron emission tomographic study in rats found reductions in D_1 receptor binding that were mainly attributable to a reduced receptor affinity (Tsukada et al. 1996). In contrast, long-term self-administration or bingelike administration of cocaine is associated with a reduction in D_1 and D_2 receptor numbers in the NAc and with a reduction in maximal D_1-stimulated adenylyl cyclase activity (De Montis et al. 1998; Maggos et al. 1998; Moore et al. 1998), consistent with receptor downregulation. These findings in laboratory animals are consistent with observations in human cocaine and methamphetamine addicts, in whom decreases in D_2 receptor binding have been documented by brain imaging (Volkow et al. 1999).

The various changes seen at the receptor level cannot, however, explain consistent effects of stimulants on

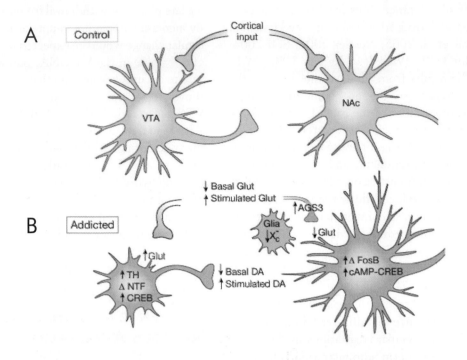

FIGURE 23–7.   Schematic summary of some common, chronic actions of drugs of abuse on the ventral tegmental area (VTA)–nucleus accumbens (NAc) circuit. *Panel A* (Control) shows a VTA neuron innervating an NAc neuron, and glutamatergic inputs to the VTA and NAc neurons, under normal conditions. *Panel B* (Addicted) illustrates several adaptations that occur after chronic drug administration. In the VTA, drug exposure induces tyrosine hydroxylase (TH) and increases α-amino-3-hydroxy-5-methyl-4-isoxalone propionic acid (AMPA) glutamatergic responses (Glut), possibly via induction of GluR1 (an AMPA glutamate receptor subunit) and altered trafficking of AMPA receptors. There is also evidence that VTA dopamine neurons decrease in size, an effect demonstrated thus far with chronic opiates only, but presumed for other drugs of abuse due to common associated biochemical adaptations (e.g., reduced levels of neurofilament proteins). Induction of cyclic adenosine monophosphate (cAMP) response element binding protein (CREB) activity and alterations in neurotrophic factor (NTF) signaling may partly mediate these various effects. In the NAc, all drugs of abuse induce the transcription factor ΔFosB, which may then mediate some of the shared aspects of addiction via regulation of numerous target genes. Several, but not all, drugs of abuse also induce CREB activity in this region, which may be mediated via upregulation of the cAMP pathway. Several additional changes have been found for stimulant exposure; it is not yet known whether they generalize to other drugs. Stimulants decrease AMPA glutamatergic responses in NAc neurons, possibly mediated via induction of GluR2 or repression of several postsynaptic density proteins (e.g., PSD95, Homer-1). These changes in postsynaptic glutamate responses are associated with complex changes in glutamatergic innervation of the NAc, including reduced glutamatergic transmission at baseline and in response to normal rewards, but enhanced transmission in response to cocaine and associated cues, effects mediated in part via upregulation of AGS3 (activator of G protein signaling) in cortical neurons and downregulation of the cystine-glutamate transporter (system X$_c^-$) in glia. Stimulants and nicotine also induce dendritic outgrowth of NAc neurons, although opiates are reported to produce the opposite action. The net effect of this complex dysregulation in glutamate function and synaptic structure is not yet known.

Source.   Reprinted from Nestler EJ: "Is There a Common Molecular Pathway for Addiction?" *Nature Neuroscience* 8:1445–1449, 2005. Used with permission.

dopamine receptor function, which have been well documented in recent years. Electrophysiological studies have shown that long-term exposure to cocaine or other stimulants causes transient subsensitivity of D$_2$-like autoreceptors in the VTA as well as longer-lasting supersensitivity to the effects of D$_1$-like receptor activation in the NAc at later withdrawal times (see White and Kalivas 1998; M.E. Wolf 1998). These changes in dopamine receptor function in both the VTA and the NAc are not accom-

panied by corresponding changes in dopamine receptor levels, which suggests that they are mediated via adaptations in postreceptor, intracellular signaling pathways.

ROLE OF GLUTAMATERGIC SYSTEMS IN LONG-TERM DRUG ACTION

Adaptations in glutamatergic systems have gained significant attention because of their prominent interactions with central dopamine function and their reported role in locomotor sensitization (see Kalivas 2004; White and Kalivas 1998; M.E. Wolf 1998). Specifically, glutamate receptor antagonists can block the development of locomotor sensitization to stimulants and opiates as well as the electrophysiological perturbations in mesolimbic dopamine function that accompany repeated stimulant exposure. Repeated stimulant exposure has been shown to increase the electrophysiological responsiveness of VTA dopamine neurons to glutamate and to decrease the responsiveness of NAc neurons to glutamate (White et al. 1995). These observations are consistent with the ability of drug exposure to induce a long-term potentiation-like effect in the VTA, and a long-term depression-like effect in the NAc, with respect to synaptic responses to glutamate (Thomas and Malenka 2003).

Supersensitivity of VTA dopamine neurons to glutamate could be mediated via upregulation of specific glutamate receptor subunits in this region, specifically GluR1 (an α-amino-3-hydroxy-5-methyl-4-isoxalone propionic acid [AMPA] glutamate receptor subunit), which has been seen after long-term administration of cocaine, opiates, or ethanol (Carlezon and Nestler 2002). Thus, mimicking drug-induced increases in GluR1 in the VTA, by use of viral-mediated gene transfer, causes sensitized responses to drugs of abuse. Altered levels of glutamate receptor subunits in the NAc are more variable, with different changes observed in early and late withdrawal (Churchill et al. 1999; Kelz et al. 1999; Lu and Wolf 1999). Changes in postsynaptic glutamate responses in the NAc could also be mediated by altered AMPA receptor trafficking or by adaptations in the neurons' postsynaptic densities, including reduced levels of PSD95 (postsynaptic density-95) and Homer or increased levels of F-actin, all of which help anchor AMPA receptors at the synapse (Kalivas et al. 2005; Yao et al. 2004).

In addition, chronic administration of stimulants is reported to alter glutamatergic innervation of the NAc by decreasing levels of the cystine-glutamate transporter in glial cells in this brain region (Kalivas 2004). This transporter normally promotes release of glutamate from prefrontal cortical glutamatergic nerve terminals. These findings highlight the complexity of drug-induced adaptations in glutamate function in the brain's reward circuitry (see Figure 23–7) and would suggest a profound dysfunction in cortical control over the NAc, which could in turn relate to the impulsive and compulsive features of drug addiction (Kalivas et al. 2005). A critical question remains as to whether dysfunctional cortical-NAc glutamatergic transmission in addiction involves a decrease in basal function, an increase in stimulated function, or both, and how these changes contribute to a loss of control over drug use.

REGULATION OF G PROTEINS AND cAMP PATHWAY IN THE VENTRAL TEGMENTAL AREA AND NUCLEUS ACCUMBENS

Repeated cocaine treatment produces transient decreases in the level of inhibitory G protein subunits, Gi and Go, that couple to D_2 autoreceptors in the VTA (Nestler 1992; Striplin and Kalivas 1992). The level of these G proteins in the VTA is negatively correlated with the initial level of locomotor activation produced by cocaine (Striplin and Kalivas 1992). In addition, pertussis toxin injected directly into the VTA, which functionally inactivates these G proteins, increases the locomotor activating effects of cocaine and thereby mimics locomotor sensitization. Together, these findings support the possibility that reduced levels of Gi and Go could account for the D_2 receptor subsensitivity observed electrophysiologically after long-term cocaine exposure and may play a role in some of the long-term effects of cocaine on mesolimbic dopamine function.

Repeated cocaine treatment also decreases levels of Gi and Go in the NAc (Nestler 1992; Striplin and Kalivas 1993) and increases levels of adenylyl cyclase and of cAMP-dependent protein kinase in this brain region (Terwilliger et al. 1991). Together, these changes would be expected to result in a concerted upregulation in the functional activity of the cAMP pathway. Because D_1 receptors are generally thought to produce their effects via activation of the cAMP pathway, these molecular adaptations could account for D_1 receptor supersensitivity observed during later withdrawal times. Long-term exposure to morphine, cocaine, heroin, or ethanol—but not to several drugs without reinforcing properties—produces similar changes in G proteins and the cAMP pathway (Ortiz et al. 1995; Self et al. 1995; Terwilliger et al. 1991). Although the long-term effects of morphine and ethanol on the electrophysiological state of NAc neurons have not yet been investigated, the biochemical findings suggest that an upregulated cAMP pathway may be part of a common mechanism of altered NAc function associated with the drug-treated state (see Figure 23–7). A critical question regarding these neuroadaptations is whether they contribute to changes in drug self-administration habits and to drug craving and relapse during abstinence.

We tested the former possibility by artificially upregulating the cAMP pathway in the NAc of animals during drug self-administration tests (Self et al. 1994, 1998). In these studies, escalation of drug self-administration is produced by inactivation of inhibitory G proteins with pertussis toxin or by sustained protein kinase A activity after microinfusion of a membrane-permeable cAMP analog into the NAc. Artificially mimicking the drug-induced neuroadaptations by sustained downregulation of inhibitory G proteins or by sustained increases in protein kinase A activity produces increases in drug self-administration. This effect is usually interpreted as a reduction in drug reward, with animals compensating by increasing their drug intake. These findings suggest that neuroadaptations in the NAc–cAMP pathway caused by repeated drug use may represent an intracellular mechanism of tolerance to the rewarding effects of drugs, which leads to escalating drug intake during drug self-administration. One possible mechanism for such tolerance may involve protein kinase A–mediated phosphorylation, desensitization, and downregulation of D_1 receptors (see Sibley et al. 1998). On the other hand, activation of the cAMP pathway in the NAc was shown to produce an enhancement of conditioned reinforcement produced by cues associated with food reward (Kelley and Holahan 1997) and to facilitate the ability of D_2 receptors to trigger cocaine seeking (Self 2004). This suggests that upregulation of the cAMP pathway in the NAc may potentiate the incentive motivational effects of reward-associated cues, and possibly their ability to elicit craving. Although further work is needed, these studies suggest that upregulation of cAMP–protein kinase A signaling in the NAc can produce both tolerance and sensitization-like effects associated with addiction.

EVIDENCE FOR STRUCTURAL CHANGES IN THE VENTRAL TEGMENTAL AREA–NUCLEUS ACCUMBENS PATHWAY

Although changes in levels of signal transduction proteins could mediate some of the long-term actions of drugs of abuse, they are unlikely to be responsible for the extremely long-lived adaptations that characterize an addicted state. One hypothesis is that adaptations in signaling pathways may cause longer-lasting structural changes in neurons (Bolaños and Nestler 2004). Several examples of such changes have been documented in recent years.

Long-term administration of morphine, for example, has been shown to decrease the size of VTA dopamine neurons as well as the caliber of their proximal processes (Sklair-Tavron et al. 1996). This is depicted in Figure 23–7. Morphine also causes a reduction in axoplasmic transport from the VTA to the NAc (see Nestler 1992). These findings may be related to the observation that long-term morphine use decreases levels of neurofilament proteins in this brain region, an effect also seen after long-term cocaine or ethanol exposure (Beitner-Johnson et al. 1992; Nestler 1992; Ortiz et al. 1995). The observed decrease in axonal transport rates could decrease the amount of tyrosine hydroxylase transported from dopamine cell bodies in the VTA to nerve terminals in the NAc. At a constant rate of tyrosine hydroxylase synthesis, this would tend to lead to the buildup of tyrosine hydroxylase observed in the VTA (as described in the earlier section on dopamine regulation in the VTA–Nac pathway) and to decreased levels of enzyme in the NAc. Such decreased levels of tyrosine hydroxylase, along with its reduced phosphorylation, have been reported (Nestler 1992; Schmidt et al. 2001; Self et al. 1995). Decreases in tyrosine hydroxylase in the NAc could explain the short-term reductions (also described earlier) in levels of basal and stimulated dopamine release during early phases of drug withdrawal.

Long-term morphine, cocaine, or ethanol treatment also increases levels of glial fibrillary acidic protein, specifically in the VTA (Beitner-Johnson et al. 1993; Ortiz et al. 1995). Drug-induced decreases in neurofilament proteins and increases in glial filament proteins in the VTA are reminiscent of neural insult or injury (see Figure 23–7). Such findings raise the possibility that perturbations in neurotrophic factor signaling are involved in long-term drug action. Indeed, direct infusion of any of several neurotrophic factors into the VTA has been shown to oppose the ability of long-term drug exposure to produce some of its characteristic biochemical and morphological changes in the VTA (Berhow et al. 1995; Messer et al. 2000; Sklair-Tavron et al. 1996). Such infusions of neurotrophic factors also potently modify behavioral responses to drug exposure (Bolaños and Nestler 2004; Horger et al. 1999; Lu et al. 2004; Pierce and Bari 2001). Of particular interest are the abnormal biochemical and behavioral responses to drugs of abuse in mice lacking brain-derived neurotrophic factor or glial cell line–derived neurotrophic factor and the alterations in certain neurotrophic factor signaling proteins after long-term drug exposure (Bolaños et al. 2003; He et al. 2005; Horger et al. 1999; Messer et al. 2000; D.H. Wolf et al. 1999). Together, these results indicate not only that exogenous neurotrophic factors can modify responses to drugs of abuse, but also that endogenous neurotrophic factor pathways are involved in mediating some of the long-term effects of drug exposure on the brain.

Drugs of abuse also cause structural changes in the medium spiny neurons of the NAc. Long-term administration of cocaine, amphetamine, or nicotine increases the dendritic arborizations of these neurons as well as the density of their terminal dendritic spines (Robinson and Kolb 1997). Similar changes have been found for pyramidal neurons in the prefrontal cortex. In contrast, long-term morphine administration causes the opposite changes in dendritic structure in the NAc (Robinson and Kolb 2004). Because alterations in dendritic spines are implicated in controlling the efficacy of synaptic transmission in other regions of brain, the observed drug-induced changes in the NAc represent an attractive mechanism by which long-

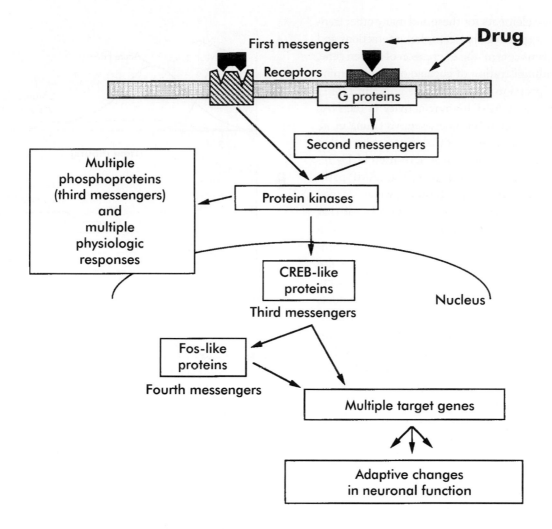

FIGURE 23–8.   Schematic illustration of the hypothetical role played by gene expression in drug addiction. According to this scheme, an initial extracellular effect of a drug of abuse would trigger changes in multiple intracellular messenger pathways in target neurons. Changes in the intracellular messengers would result in numerous physiologic responses to the drug (as shown in Figure 23–2), including alterations in gene expression. The latter types of alterations would occur through the regulation of many classes of nuclear, DNA-binding proteins termed transcription factors, such as cyclic adenosine monophosphate (cAMP) response element binding protein (CREB) and Fos. CREB exemplifies a transcription factor that is regulated by extracellular agents primarily through changes in its degree of phosphorylation. Fos exemplifies a transcription factor that is expressed at very low levels under basal conditions and is regulated by extracellular agents primarily through induction of its expression (in some cases via CREB). Both types of transcription factors would then result in altered levels of expression of specific target proteins that underlie the adaptive changes in brain function associated with addiction.

term drug exposure might produce very long-lived changes in NAc function and, hence, motivational processes.

MOLECULAR MECHANISMS UNDERLYING DRUG-INDUCED ADAPTATIONS IN THE NUCLEUS ACCUMBENS

The precise mechanisms by which long-term drug treatment alters levels of specific proteins in the VTA–NAc path-

way are still unknown, but there are now many studies that show that gene expression can be regulated by drug exposure (see Chao and Nestler 2004; Nestler 1992). Such studies have focused on the role played by two families of transcription factors (shown in Figure 23–8): CREB and CREB-like proteins and the products of certain immediate early genes (IEGs), such as the Fos and Jun family proteins (see Nestler 2001). Fos and Jun proteins form heterodimeric complexes that bind to specific DNA sequences referred to as activator protein 1 (AP-1) sites to regulate transcription of a target gene. Most genes likely contain numerous response elements for these and many other transcription factors, suggesting that complex interactions and multiple mechanisms control the expression of a given gene.

Short-term administration of cocaine or amphetamine increases the expression of several Fos and Jun family members and increases AP-1 binding activity in the NAc and dorsal striatum (for references, see McClung et al. 2004). One possible mechanism of cocaine action is that the drug induces c-Fos via dopamine activation of D_1 receptors and the subsequent activation of the cAMP pathway. These drugs also induce Egr1 (also known as Zif268) in these brain regions. Egr1 is a transcription factor that binds to a distinct response element but is regulated as an IEG product in a fashion similar to Fos- and Jun-like proteins (O'Donovan et al. 1999). Other drugs of abuse also induce these various IEGs in the NAc and dorsal striatum.

The ability to induce c-Fos and the other IEG products in the NAc is attenuated on repeated cocaine treatment, whereas the increased AP-1 binding activity persists for weeks after drug treatment ceases (Daunais and McGinty 1994; Hope et al. 1994). We now know that this persistent AP-1 binding activity is caused by the long-lived expression of biochemically modified isoforms of ΔFosB, a member of the Fos family of transcription factors. ΔFosB persists in the brain for a long time due to its extraordinary stability mediated in part by its phosphorylation by casein kinase II. Thus, it could represent a type of sustained molecular switch that contributes to prolonged aspects of cocaine addiction (Figure 23–9). Similar induction of ΔFosB is seen after long-term (but not after short-term) administration of opiates, nicotine, alcohol, cannabinoids, and phencyclidine (see McClung et al. 2004). Studies of transgenic mice in which ΔFosB, or an antagonist of ΔFosB, can be induced in adult animals selectively within the NAc and dorsal striatum demonstrate that ΔFosB expression increases an animal's sensitivity to the rewarding and locomotor-activating effects of cocaine and may increase the motivation to pursue cocaine reward as well (Colby et al. 2003; Kelz et al. 1999; Peakman et al. 2003). ΔFosB causes this behavioral phenotype via the regulation of numerous target genes, which are just now beginning to be identified and characterized (McClung and Nestler 2003). Interestingly, some of these target genes have been related to the decreased glutamate sensitivity and increased dendritic spine densities of NAc neurons observed after chronic drug exposure (see McClung et al. 2004).

Because long-term cocaine and morphine treatments upregulate the cAMP pathway in the NAc, the CREB family of transcription factors is also likely influenced by these drugs. Indeed, long-term drug treatments regulate CREB phosphorylation and functional activity in this brain region (see Cole et al. 1995; Shaw-Lutchman et al.

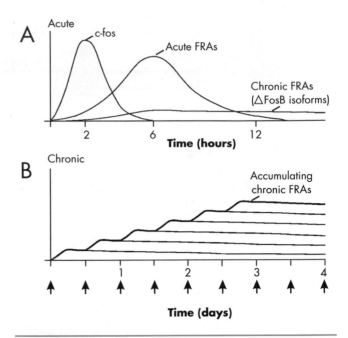

FIGURE 23–9.   Scheme for the gradual accumulation of ΔFosB (also called chronic Fos-related antigens [FRAs]) versus the rapid and transient induction of acute FRAs in the brain. *Panel A.* Several waves of FRAs are induced in neurons by many acute stimuli. c-Fos is induced rapidly and degrades within several hours of the acute stimulus, whereas other "acute FRAs" (e.g., FosB, FRA-1, and FRA-2) are induced somewhat later and persist somewhat longer than c-Fos. The chronic FRAs are phosphorylated isoforms of ΔFosB; they, too, are induced (although at low levels) after a single acute stimulus but persist in the brain for long periods (with a half-life longer than 1 week). In a complex with Jun-like proteins, these waves of FRAs form activator protein 1 (AP-1)–binding complexes with shifting composition over time. *Panel B.* With repeated (e.g., twice daily) stimulation, each acute stimulus induces a low level of ΔFosB. This is indicated by the lower set of overlapping lines, which indicates ΔFosB induced by each acute stimulus. The result is a gradual increase in the total levels of ΔFosB with repeated stimuli during a course of long-term treatment. This is indicated by the increasing stepped line in the graph. The increasing levels of ΔFosB with repeated stimulation would result in the gradual induction of significant levels of a long-lasting AP-1 complex, which could underlie persisting forms of neural plasticity in the brain.

Source.   Adapted from Hope BT, Nye HE, Kelz MB, et al: "Induction of a Long-Lasting AP1 Complex Composed of Altered Fos-like Proteins in Brain by Chronic Cocaine and Other Chronic Treatments. *Neuron* 13:1235–1244, copyright 1994, with permission from Elsevier.

2003). By use of viral-mediated gene transfer, it has been shown that increases in CREB levels in the NAc decrease an animal's sensitivity to the rewarding effects of cocaine and of morphine, whereas inactivation of CREB has the opposite effect (Barrot et al. 2002; Carlezon et al. 1998).

The effects of CREB are mediated in part by the opioid peptide dynorphin, which is increased by CREB and decreased on inactivation of CREB. Dynorphin acts on κ opioid receptors within the NAc and VTA to produce aversive effects by reducing dopamine release from presynaptic terminals. Thus, activation of CREB, and the resulting induction of dynorphin, in response to long-term drug exposure would appear to represent a mechanism of tolerance to drug reward as well as dysphoria during drug withdrawal (dependence) (Carlezon et al. 2005).

Current research is focused on identifying additional target genes for CREB and for ΔFosB and on identifying additional transcriptional control mechanisms that mediate the long-term actions of drugs of abuse on the mesolimbic dopamine system (McClung and Nestler 2003).

CONCLUSION

The availability of animal models that accurately reproduce important features of drug addiction in humans has made it possible to identify specific regions in the brain that play an important role in addictive disorders. Whereas the locus coeruleus plays an important role in physical dependence on opiates, it is the mesolimbic dopamine system as well as regions of the prefrontal cortex and amygdala that appear to be integrally involved in drug-seeking behavior, the essential clinical feature of drug addiction. Basic neurobiological investigations are now providing an increasingly complete understanding of the adaptations at the molecular and cellular levels that occur in these various brain regions and are responsible for behavioral features of drug addiction. Work to date has focused on adaptations in intracellular messenger pathways, particularly G proteins and the cAMP pathway, although many other types of adaptations will also prove to be involved. As the pathophysiological mechanisms underlying drug addiction become increasingly understood, it will be possible to develop more efficacious pharmacotherapies for the treatment of addictive disorders. Parallel studies, not covered in this chapter, of different inbred animal strains and of individual differences among large outbred populations promise to yield information concerning the specific proteins that underlie inherent differences in an individual's responsiveness to drugs of abuse. This work will lead eventually to the identification of specific genes and environmental factors that control individual variations in the susceptibility to drug addiction. Ultimately, this work could lead to the development of specific interventions that prevent drug addiction in particularly vulnerable individuals.

Highlights for the Clinician

Definition of terms	
Addiction	Compulsive drug use despite adverse consequences; loss of control over drug use
Craving	Incentive drive to seek and take drug
Dependence	Altered physiological state that causes a withdrawal syndrome when drug taking ceases
Reinforcement	Action of a stimulus that increases a behavioral response
Reward	Positive emotional response to a stimulus
Sensitization	Increased drug effect at constant dose
Tolerance	Reduced drug effect at constant dose

Acute actions of drugs of abuse	
Alcohol	GABA$_A$ receptor agonist; NMDA glutamate receptor antagonist; other actions
Amphetamine	Dopamine release potentiator
Cocaine	Dopamine reuptake transporter inhibitor
Marijuana	CB$_1$ cannabinoid receptor agonist
Nicotine	Nicotinic acetylcholine receptor agonist
Opiates	μ Opioid receptor agonists
Phencyclidine (PCP)	NMDA glutamate receptor antagonist

(continued)

Highlights for the Clinician *(continued)*

Role of locus coeruleus

✦ The major noradrenergic nucleus in the brain—one mediator of opiate physical dependence and withdrawal.

Features of mesolimbic dopamine reward circuit

✦ Site of cAMP pathway upregulation induced by chronic opiate administration (includes induction of adenylyl cyclase, protein kinase A, and transcription factor CREB). This upregulation represents one mechanism of opiate tolerance and physical dependence-withdrawal.

✦ Consists of dopamine neurons in VTA and their targets in NAc and several other limbic structures such as amygdala and frontal cortex.

✦ Mediates positive reinforcing and rewarding effects of all drugs of abuse as well as natural rewards (e.g., food, sex, social interaction).

✦ Drug-induced adaptations in mesolimbic dopamine system (includes common adaptations to many different drugs) mediate changes in reward mechanisms that in part underlie addiction—including tolerance, dependence-withdrawal, sensitization, and relapse.

Examples of drug-induced adaptations:

- Regulation of dopamine and opioid systems (mechanisms of tolerance and sensitization)

- Regulation of glutamate systems (influences drug-related memories)

- Upregulation of the cAMP pathway and transcription factor CREB (mechanisms of drug tolerance, dependence, and withdrawal)

- Structural changes in VTA neurons (influence drug tolerance)

- Structural changes in NAc neurons (influence drug sensitization)

- Role of transcription factor ΔFosB (influences drug sensitization)

Note.   cAMP = cyclic adenosine monophosphate; CREB = cAMP response element binding protein; GABA$_A$ = γ-aminobutyric acid type A; NAc = nucleus accumbens; NMDA = N-methyl-D-aspartate; VTA = ventral tegmental area.

RECOMMENDED READINGS

Goldstein A: Addiction: From Biology to Drug Policy, 2nd Edition. New York, Oxford University Press, 2001

Hyman SE, Malenka RC: Addiction and the brain: the neurobiology of compulsion and its persistence. Nature Rev Neurosci 2:695–703, 2001

Kalivas PW, Volkow N, Seamans J: Unmanageable motivation in addiction: a pathology in prefrontal-accumbens glutamate transmission. Neuron 45:647–650, 2005

Koob GF, Sanna PP, Bloom FE: Neuroscience of addiction. Neuron 21:467–476, 1998

Nestler EJ: Molecular basis of neural plasticity underlying addiction. Nature Rev Neurosci 2:119–128, 2001

Nestler EJ, Malenka RC: The addicted brain. Sci Am 290:78–85, 2004

Robinson TE, Kolb B: Structural plasticity associated with exposure to drugs of abuse. Neuropharmacology 47 (suppl 1):33–46, 2004

REFERENCES

Aghajanian GK: Tolerance of locus coeruleus neurons to morphine and suppression of withdrawal response by clonidine. Nature 276:186–188, 1978

Ahmed SH, Koob GF: Cocaine- but not food-seeking behavior is reinstated by stress after prolonged extinction. Psychopharmacology (Berl) 132:289–295, 1997

Akaoka A, Aston-Jones G: Opiate withdrawal-induced hyperactivity of locus coeruleus neurons is substantially mediated by augmented excitatory amino acid input. J Neurosci 11:3830–3839, 1991

Alreja M, Aghajanian GK: Opiates suppress a resting sodium-dependent inward current in addition to activating an outward potassium current in locus coeruleus neurons. J Neurosci 13:3525–3532, 1993

American Psychiatric Association: Diagnostic and Statistical Manual of Mental Disorders, 4th Edition, Text Revision. Washington, DC, American Psychiatric Association, 2000

Aston-Jones G, Hirata H, Akaoka H: Local opiate withdrawal in locus coeruleus in vivo. Brain Res 765:331–336, 1997

Bardo MT: Neuropharmacological mechanisms of drug reward: beyond dopamine in the nucleus accumbens. Crit Rev Neurobiol 12:37–67, 1998

Barrot M, Olivier JDA, Perrotti LI: CREB activity in the nucleus accumbens shell controls gating of behavioral responses to emotional stimuli. Proc Natl Acad Sci U S A 99:11435–11440, 2002

Beitner-Johnson D, Guitart X, Nestler EJ: Neurofilament proteins and the mesolimbic dopamine system: common regulation by chronic morphine and chronic cocaine in the rat ventral tegmental area. J Neurosci 12:2165–2176, 1992

Beitner-Johnson D, Guitart X, Nestler EJ: Glial fibrillary acidic protein and the mesolimbic dopamine system: regulation by chronic morphine and Lewis-Fischer strain differences in the rat ventral tegmental area. J Neurochem 61:1766–1773, 1993

Berhow MT, Russell DS, Terwilliger RZ, et al: Influence of neurotrophic factors on morphine- and cocaine-induced biochemical changes in the mesolimbic dopamine system. Neuroscience 68:969–979, 1995

Bolaños CA, Nestler EJ: Neurotrophic mechanisms in drug addiction. Neuromolecular Med 5:69–83, 2004

Bolaños CA, Perrotti LI, Edwards S, et al: Viral-mediated expression of phospholipase Cγ in distinct regions of the ventral tegmental area differentially modulates mood-related behaviors. J Neurosci 23:7569–7576, 2003

Bonci A, Williams JT: Increased probability of GABA release during withdrawal from morphine. J Neurosci 17:796–803, 1997

Boundy VA, Chen JS, Nestler EJ: Regulation of cAMP-dependent protein kinase subunit expression in CATH.a and SH-SY5Y cells. J Pharmacol Exp Ther 286:1058–1065, 1998a

Boundy VA, Gold SJ, Messer CJ, et al: Regulation of tyrosine hydroxylase promoter activity by chronic morphine in TH9.0-LacZ transgenic mice. J Neurosci 18:9989–9995, 1998b

Breiter HC, Gollub RL, Weisskoff RM, et al: Acute effects of cocaine on human brain activity and emotion. Neuron 19:591–611, 1997

Carlezon WA Jr, Nestler EJ: Elevated levels of GluR1 in the midbrain: a trigger for sensitization to drugs of abuse? Trends Neurosci 25:610–615, 2002

Carlezon WA Jr, Thome J, Olson VG, et al: Regulation of cocaine reward by CREB. Science 282:2272–2275, 1998

Carlezon WA Jr, Duman RS, Nestler EJ: The many faces of CREB. Trends Neurosci 28:436–445, 2005

Chao J, Nestler EJ: Molecular neurobiology of drug addiction. Annu Rev Med 55:113–132, 2004

Chao JR, Ni YG, Bolaños CA, Chen JS, et al: Characterization of the mouse adenylyl cyclase type VIII gene promoter: regulation by cAMP and CREB. Eur J Neurosci 16:1284–1294, 2002

Chen J, Paredes W, Li J, et al: Delta 9-tetrahydrocannabinol produces naloxone blockable enhancement of presynaptic dopamine efflux in nucleus accumbens of conscious, freely moving rats as measured by intracerebral microdialysis. Psychopharmacology (Berl) 102:156–162, 1990

Childress AR, McLellan AT, O'Brien CP: Extinguishing conditioned responses in drug dependent persons, in Learning Factors in Drug Dependence: NIDA Research Monograph. Edited by Ray B. Washington, DC, U.S. Government Printing Office, 1988, pp 137–144

Churchill L, Swanson CJ, Urbina M, et al: Repeated cocaine alters glutamate receptor subunit levels in the nucleus accumbens and ventral tegmental area of rats that develop behavioral sensitization. J Neurochem 72:2397–2403, 1999

Colby CR, Whisler K, Steffen C, et al: FosB enhances incentive for cocaine. J Neurosci 23:2488–2493, 2003

Cole RL, Konradi C, Douglass J, et al: Neuronal adaptation to amphetamine and dopamine: molecular mechanisms of prodynorphin gene regulation in rat striatum. Neuron 14:813–823, 1995

Curran EJ, Watson SJ: Dopamine receptor mRNA expression patterns by opioid peptide cells in the nucleus accumbens of the rat: a double in situ hybridization study. J Comp Neurol 361:57–76, 1995

Daunais JB, McGinty JF: Acute and chronic cocaine administration differentially alters striatal opioid and nuclear transcription factor mRNAs. Synapse 18:35–46, 1994

De Montis MG, Co C, Dworking SI, et al: Modifications of dopamine D1 receptor complex in rats self-administering cocaine. Eur J Pharmacol 362:9–15, 1998

Deroche V, Marinelli M, Le Moal M, et al: Glucocorticoids and behavioral effects of psychostimulants, II: cocaine intravenous self-administration and reinstatement depend on glucocorticoid levels. J Pharmacol Exp Ther 281:1401–1407, 1997

De Vries TJ, Schoffelmeer ANM, Binnekade R, et al: Dopaminergic mechanisms mediating the incentive to seek cocaine and heroin following long-term withdrawal of IV drug self-administration. Psychopharmacology (Berl) 143:254–260, 1999

De Wit H, Stewart J: Reinstatement of cocaine-reinforced responding in the rat. Psychopharmacology (Berl) 75:134–143, 1981

Di Chiara G, Imperato A: Drugs abused by humans preferentially increase synaptic dopamine concentrations in the mesolimbic system of freely moving rats. Proc Natl Acad Sci U S A 85:5274–5278, 1988

Di Ciano P, Everitt BJ: Direct interactions between the basolateral amygdala and nucleus accumbens core underlie cocaine-seeking behavior by rats. J Neurosci 24:7167–7173, 2004

Di Ciano P, Blaha CD, Phillips AG: Conditioned changes in dopamine oxidation currents in the nucleus accumbens of rats by stimuli paired with self-administration or yoked-administration of d-amphetamine. Eur J Neurosci 10:1121–1127, 1998

Dworkin SI, Smith JE: Opiates/opioids and reinforcement, in Biological Basis of Substance Abuse. Edited by Korenman SG, Barchas JD. New York, Oxford University Press, 1993, pp 327–338

Ehrman RN, Robbins SJ, Childress AR, et al: Conditioned responses to cocaine-related stimuli in cocaine abuse patients. Psychopharmacology (Berl) 107:523–529, 1992

Erb S, Shaham Y, Stewart J: Stress reinstates cocaine-seeking behavior after prolonged extinction and a drug-free period. Psychopharmacology (Berl) 128:408–412, 1996

Ettenberg A: Haloperidol prevents the reinstatement of amphetamine-rewarded runway responding in rats. Pharmacol Biochem Behav 36:635–638, 1990

Gainetdinov RR, Premont RT, Bohn LM, et al: Desensitization of G protein-coupled receptors and neuronal functions. Annu Rev Neurosci 27:107–144, 2004

Gold MS, Redmond DE, Kleber HD: Clonidine in opiate withdrawal. Lancet 11:599–602, 1978

Gold SJ, Han MH, Herman AE, et al: Regulation of RGS proteins in the locus coeruleus by chronic morphine. Eur J Neurosci 17:971–980, 2003

He DY, McGough NN, Ravindranathan A, et al: Glial cell line-derived neurotrophic factor mediates the desirable actions of the anti-addiction drug ibogaine against alcohol consumption. J Neurosci 25:619–628, 2005

Heinrichs SC, Koob GF: Corticotropin-releasing factor in brain: a role in activation, arousal, and affect regulation. J Ther Exp Pharmacol 311:427–440, 2004

Hope BT, Nye HE, Kelz MB, et al: Induction of a long-lasting AP1 complex composed of altered Fos-like proteins in brain by chronic cocaine and other chronic treatments. Neuron 13:1235–1244, 1994

Horger BA, Iyasere CA, Berhow MT, et al: Enhancement of locomotor activity and conditioned reward to cocaine by brain-derived neurotrophic factor. J Neurosci 19:4110–4122, 1999

Hu XT, White FJ: Loss of D_1/D_2 dopamine receptor synergisms following repeated administration of D_1 or D_2 receptor selective antagonists: electrophysiological and behavioral studies. Synapse 17:43–61, 1994

Hutcheson DM, Everitt BJ, Robbins TW, et al: The role of withdrawal in heroin addiction: enhances reward or promotes avoidance? Nat Neurosci 4:943–947, 2001

Hyman SE, Malenka RC, Nestler EJ: Neural mechanisms of addiction: the role of reward-related learning and memory. Annu Rev Neurosci 29:565–598, 2006

Ikemoto S, Wise RA: Mapping of chemical trigger zones for reward. Neuropharmacology 47 (suppl 1):190–201, 2004

Ito R, Dalley JW, Howes SR, et al: Dissociation in conditioned dopamine release in the nucleus accumbens core and shell in response to cocaine cues and during cocaine-seeking behavior in rats. J Neurosci 20:7489–7495, 2004

Johnson SW, North RA: Opioids excite dopamine neurons by hyperpolarization of local interneurons. J Neurosci 12:483–488, 1992

Jolas T, Nestler EJ, Aghajanian GK: Chronic morphine increases GABA tone on serotonergic neurons of the dorsal raphe nucleus: association with an upregulation of the cyclic AMP pathway. Neuroscience 95:433–443, 2000

Kalivas PW: Glutamate systems in cocaine addiction. Curr Opin Pharmacol 4:23–29, 2004

Kalivas PW, McFarland K: Brain circuitry and the reinstatement of cocaine-seeking behavior. Psychopharmacology 168:44–56, 2003

Kalivas PW, Volkow N, Seamans J: Unmanageable motivation in addiction: a pathology in prefrontal-accumbens glutamate transmission. Neuron 45:647–650, 2005

Karreman M, Moghaddam B: The prefrontal cortex regulates the basal release of dopamine in the limbic striatum: an effect mediated by ventral tegmental area. J Neurochem 66:589–598, 1996

Kelley AE: Memory and addiction: shared neural circuitry and molecular mechanisms. Neuron 44:161–179, 2004

Kelley AE, Holahan MR: Enhanced reward-related responding following cholera toxin infusion into the nucleus accumbens. Synapse 26:46–54, 1997

Kelz MB, Chen JS, Carlezon WA, et al: Expression of the transcription factor deltaFosB in the brain controls sensitivity to cocaine. Nature 401:272–276, 1999

Kogan JH, Nestler EJ, Aghajanian GK: Elevated basal firing rates and enhanced responses to 8-Br-cAMP in locus coeruleus neurons in brain slices from opiate-dependent rats. Eur J Pharmacol 211:47–53, 1992

Koob GF, Maldonado R, Stinus L: Neural substrates of opiate withdrawal. Trends Neurosci 15:186–191, 1992

Koob GF, Sanna PP, Bloom FE: Neuroscience of addiction. Neuron 21:467–476, 1998

Koob GF, Ahmed SH, Boutrel B, et al: Neurobiological mechanisms in the transition from drug use to drug dependence. Neurosci Biobehav Rev 27:739–749, 2004

Kuhar MJ, Ritz MC, Boja JW: The dopamine hypothesis of the reinforcing properties of cocaine. Trends Neurosci 14:299–302, 1991

Lane-Ladd SB, Pineda J, Boundy V, et al: CREB in the locus coeruleus: biochemical, physiological, and behavioral evidence for a role in opiate dependence. J Neurosci 17:7890–7901, 1997

Lu W, Wolf ME: Repeated amphetamine administration alters AMPA receptor subunit expression in rat nucleus accumbens and medial prefrontal cortex. Synapse 32:119–131, 1999

Lu L, Dempsey J, Liu SY, et al: A single infusion of brain-derived neurotrophic factor into the ventral tegmental area induces long-lasting potentiation of cocaine seeking after withdrawal. J Neurosci 24:1604–1611, 2004

Maggos CE, Tsukada H, Kakiuchi T, et al: Sustained withdrawal allows normalization of in vivo [^{11}C]N-methylspiperone dopamine D2 receptor binding after chronic binge cocaine: a positron emission tomography study in rats. Neuropsychopharmacology 19:146–153, 1998

Maldonado R, Koob GF: Destruction of the locus coeruleus decreases physical signs of opiate withdrawal. Brain Res 605:128–138, 1993

Maldonado R, Blendy JA, Tzavara E, et al: Reduction of morphine abstinence in mice with a mutation in the gene encoding CREB. Science 273:657–659, 1996

McClung CA, Nestler EJ: Regulation of gene expression and cocaine reward by CREB and FosB. Nat Neurosci 11:1208–1215, 2003

McClung CA, Ulery PG, Perrotti LI, et al: FosB: A molecular switch for long-term adaptation. Brain Res Mol Brain Res 132:146–154, 2004

McFarland K, Kalivas PW: The circuitry mediating cocaine-induced reinstatement of drug-seeking behavior. J Neurosci 21:8655–8663, 2001

McFarland K, Davidge SB, Lapish CC, et al: Limbic and motor circuitry underlying footshock-induced reinstatement of cocaine-seeking behavior. J Neurosci 24:1551–1560, 2004

Meador-Woodruff JH, Mansour A, Healy DJ, et al: Comparison of the distribution of D1 and D2 dopamine receptor mRNAs in rat brain. Neuropsychopharmacology 5:231–242, 1991

Meil WM, See RE: Lesions of the basolateral amygdala abolish the ability of drug associated cues to reinstate responding during withdrawal from self-administered cocaine. Behav Brain Res 87:139–148, 1997

Messer CJ, Eisch AJ, Carlezon WA Jr, et al: Role of GDNF in biochemical and behavioral adaptations to drugs of abuse. Neuron 26:247–257, 2000

Mirenowicz J, Schultz W: Preferential activation of midbrain dopamine neurons by appetitive rather than aversive stimuli. Nature 379:449–451, 1996

Moghaddam B, Jackson M: Effect of stress on prefrontal cortex function. Neurotox Res 6:73–78, 2004

Moore RJ, Vinsant SL, Nader MA, et al: Effect of cocaine self-administration on striatal dopamine D1 receptors in rhesus monkeys. Synapse 28:1–9, 1998

Nestler EJ: Molecular mechanisms of drug addiction. J Neurosci 12:2439–2450, 1992

Nestler EJ: Molecular basis of long-term plasticity underlying addiction. Nat Rev Neurosci 2:119–128, 2001

Nestler EJ: Historical review: molecular and cellular mechanisms of opiate and cocaine addiction. Trends Pharmacol Sci 25:210–218, 2004

Nestler EJ: Is there a common molecular pathway for addiction? Nat Neurosci 8:1445–1449, 2005

Nestler EJ, Aghajanian GK: Molecular and cellular basis of addiction. Science 278:58–63, 1997

Nestler EJ, Hyman SE, Malenka RC: Molecular Neuropharmacology: A Foundation for Clinical Neuroscience. New York, McGraw-Hill, 2001

North RA, Williams JT, Suprenant A, et al: Mu and delta receptors belong to a family of receptors that are coupled to potassium channels. Proc Natl Acad Sci U S A 84:5487–5491, 1987

O'Brien C, Childress A, McLellan A, et al: A learning model of addiction, in Addictive States. Edited by O'Brien CP, Jaffe JH. New York, Raven, 1992, pp 157–177

O'Donovan KJ, Tourtellotte WG, Millbrandt J, et al: The EGR family of transcription-regulatory factors: progress at the interface of molecular and systems neuroscience. Trends Neurosci 22:167–173, 1999

Olds ME: Reinforcing effects of morphine in the nucleus accumbens. Brain Res 237:429–440, 1982

Ortiz J, Fitzgerald LW, Charlton M, et al: Biochemical actions of chronic ethanol exposure in the mesolimbic dopamine system. Synapse 21:289–298, 1995

Overton PG, Tong ZY, Brain PF, et al: Preferential occupation of mineralocorticoid receptors by corticosterone enhances glutamate-induced burst firing in rat midbrain dopaminergic neurons. Brain Res 737:146–154, 1996

Peakman MC, Colby C, Perrotti LI, et al: Inducible, brain region specific expression of a dominant negative mutant of c-Jun in transgenic mice decreases sensitivity to cocaine. Brain Res 970:73–86, 2003

Phillips PE, Stuber GD, Heien ML, et al: Subsecond dopamine release promotes cocaine seeking. Nature 422:614–618, 2003

Piazza PV, Rouge-Pont F, Deroche V, et al: Glucocorticoids have state-dependent stimulant effects on the mesencephalic dopamine transmission. Proc Natl Acad Sci USA 93:8716–8720, 1996

Pierce RC, Bari AA: The role of neurotrophic factors in psychostimulant-induced behavioral and neuronal plasticity. Rev Neurosci 12:95–110, 2001

Pilotte NS: Neurochemistry of cocaine withdrawal. Curr Opin Neurol 10:534–538, 1997

Pruessner JC, Champagne F, Meaney MJ, et al: Dopamine release in response to a psychological stress in humans and its relationship to early life maternal care: a positron emission tomography study using [^{11}C] raclopride. J Neurosci 24:2825–2831, 2004

Rasmussen K, Aghajanian GK: Withdrawal-induced activation of locus coeruleus neurons in opiate-dependent rats: attenuation by lesions of the nucleus paragigantocellularis. Brain Res 505:346–350, 1989

Rasmussen K, Beitner-Johnson D, Krystal JH, et al: Opiate withdrawal and the rat locus coeruleus: behavioral, electrophysiological, and biochemical correlates. J Neurosci 10:2308–2317, 1990

Robbins SJ, Ehrman RN, Childress AR, et al: Relationships among physiological and self-report responses produced by cocaine-related cues. Addict Behav 22:157–167, 1997

Robinson TE, Berridge KC: Addiction. Annu Rev Psychol 54:25–53, 2003

Robinson TE, Kolb B: Persistent structural modifications in nucleus accumbens and prefrontal neurons produced by previous experience with amphetamine. J Neurosci 17:8491–8497, 1997

Robinson TE, Kolb B: Structural plasticity associated with exposure to drugs of abuse. Neuropharmacology 47 (suppl 1):33–46, 2004

Schmidt EF, Sutton MA, Schad CA, et al: Extinction training regulates tyrosine hydroxylase during withdrawal from cocaine self-administration (rapid communication). J Neurosci 21 (RC137):1–5, 2001

Self DW: Neural substrates of drug craving and relapse in drug addiction. Ann Med 30:379–389, 1998

Self DW: Regulation of drug-taking and -seeking behaviors by neuroadaptations in the mesolimbic dopamine system. Neuropharmacology 47:242–255, 2004

Self DW, Nestler EJ: Molecular mechanisms of drug reinforcement and addiction. Annu Rev Neurosci 18:463–495, 1995

Self DW, Nestler EJ: Relapse to drug seeking: neural and molecular mechanisms. Drug Alcohol Depend 51:49–60, 1998

Self DW, Terwilliger RZ, Nestler EJ, et al: Inactivation of Gi and Go proteins in nucleus accumbens reduces both cocaine and heroin reinforcement. J Neurosci 14:6239–6247, 1994

Self DW, McClenahan AW, Beitner-Johnson D, et al: Biochemical adaptations in the mesolimbic dopamine system in response to heroin self-administration. Synapse 21:312–318, 1995

Self DW, Barnhart WJ, Lehman DA, et al: Opposite modulation of cocaine-seeking behavior by D1-like and D2-like dopamine receptor agonists. Science 271:1586–1589, 1996

Self DW, Genova LM, Hope BT, et al: Involvement of cAMP-dependent protein kinase in the nucleus accumbens in cocaine self-administration and relapse of cocaine-seeking behavior. J Neurosci 18:1848–1859, 1998

Shaham Y, Stewart J: Stress reinstates heroin-seeking in drug-free animals: an effect mimicking heroin, not withdrawal. Psychopharmacology (Berl) 119:334–341, 1995

Shaham Y, Stewart J: Effects of opioid and dopamine receptor antagonists on relapse induced by stress and re-exposure to heroin in rats. Psychopharmacology (Berl) 125:385–391, 1996

Shaham Y, Rajabi H, Stewart J: Relapse to heroin-seeking in rats under opioid maintenance: the effects of stress, heroin priming, and withdrawal. J Neurosci 16:1957–1963, 1996

Shaham Y, Funk D, Erb S, et al: Corticotropin-releasing factor in stress-induced relapse to heroin-seeking in rats. J Neurosci 17:2605–2614, 1997

Shaham Y, Shalev U, Lu L, et al: The reinstatement model of drug relapse: history, methodology and major findings. Psychopharmacology 168:3–20, 2003

Sharma SK, Klee WA, Nirenberg M: Dual regulation of adenylate cyclase accounts for narcotic dependence and tolerance. Proc Natl Acad Sci U S A 72:3092–3096, 1975

Shaw-Lutchman SZ, Impey S, Storm D, et al: Regulation of CRE-mediated transcription in mouse brain by amphetamine. Synapse 48:10–17, 2003

Sibley DR, Ventura AL, Jiang D, et al: Regulation of the D1 receptor through cAMP-mediated pathways. Adv Pharmacol 42:447–450, 1998

Sklair-Tavron L, Shi W-X, Lane SB, et al: Chronic morphine induces visible changes in the morphology of mesolimbic dopamine neurons. Proc Natl Acad Sci U S A 93:11202–11207, 1996

Spanagel R, Weiss F: The dopamine hypothesis of reward: past and current status. Trends Neurosci 22:521–527, 1999

Stewart J: Stress and relapse to drug seeking: studies in laboratory animals shed light on mechanisms and sources of long-term vulnerability. Am J Addict 12:1–17, 2003

Stewart J, Vezina P: A comparison of the effects of intra-accumbens injections of amphetamine and morphine on reinstatement of heroin intravenous self-administration behavior. Brain Res 457:287–294, 1988

Stewart J, De Wit H, Eikelboom R: Role of unconditioned and conditioned drug effects in the self-administration of opiates and stimulants. Psychol Rev 91:251–268, 1984

Striplin CD, Kalivas PW: Correlation between behavioral sensitization to cocaine and G protein ADP-ribosylation in the ventral tegmental area. Brain Res 579:181–186, 1992

Striplin CD, Kalivas PW: Robustness of G protein changes in cocaine sensitization shown with immunoblotting. Synapse 14:10–15, 1993

Taber MT, Das S, Fibiger HC: Cortical regulation of subcortical dopamine release: mediation via the ventral tegmental area. J Neurochem 65:1407–1410, 1995

Tanda G, Pontieri FE, Di Chiara G: Cannabinoid and heroin activation of mesolimbic dopamine transmission by a common mu1 opioid receptor mechanism. Science 276:2048–2050, 1997

Terwilliger RZ, Beitner-Johnson D, Sevarino KA, et al: A general roll for adaptations in G-proteins and the cyclic AMP system in mediating the chronic actions of morphine and cocaine on neuronal function. Brain Res 548:100–110, 1991

Thomas MJ, Malenka RC: Synaptic plasticity in the mesolimbic dopamine system. Philos Trans R Soc Lond B Biol Sci 358:815–819, 2003

Tiffany ST, Singleton E, Haertzen CA, et al: The development of a cocaine craving questionnaire. Drug Alcohol Depend 34:19–28, 1993

Tjon GH, De Vries TJ, Ronken E, et al: Repeated and chronic morphine administration causes differential long-lasting changes in dopaminergic neurotransmission in rat striatum without changing its delta- and kappa-opioid receptor regulation. Eur J Pharmacol 252:205–212, 1994

Tsukada H, Kreuter J, Maggos CE, et al: Effects of binge pattern cocaine administration on dopamine D1 and D2 receptors in the rat brain: an in vivo study using positron emission tomography. J Neurosci 16:7670–7677, 1996

Unterwald EM, Cox BM, Creek MJ, et al: Chronic repeated cocaine administration alters basal and opioid-regulated adenylyl cyclase activity. Synapse 15:33–38, 1993

Unterwald EM, Rubenfeld JM, Kreek MJ: Repeated cocaine administration up-regulates kappa and mu, but not delta, opioids. Neuroreport 5:1613–1616, 1994

Vezina P: Sensitization of midbrain dopamine neuron reactivity and the self-administration of psychomotor stimulant drugs. Neurosci Biobehav Rev 27:827–839, 2004

Volkow ND, Fowler JS, Wang GJ: Imaging studies on the role of dopamine in cocaine reinforcement and addiction in humans. J Psychopharmacol 13:337–345, 1999

Von Zastrow M: Opioid receptor regulation. Neuromolecular Med 5:51–58, 2004

Waddington JL, Daly SA: Regulation of unconditioned motor behaviour by D1:D2 interaction, in D-1:D-2 Dopamine Receptor Interactions. Edited by Waddington JL. London, Academic Press, 1993, pp 203–233

Weissenborn R, Deroche V, Koob G, et al: Effects of dopamine agonists and antagonists on cocaine-induced operant responding for a cocaine-associated stimulus. Psychopharmacology (Berl) 126:311–322, 1996

White FJ, Kalivas PW: Neuroadaptations involved in amphetamine and cocaine addiction. Drug Alcohol Depend 51:141–153, 1998

White FJ, Hu X-T, Zhang X-F, et al: Repeated administration of cocaine or amphetamine alters neuronal responses to glutamate in the mesoaccumbens dopamine system. J Pharmacol Exp Ther 273:445–454, 1995

Williams JT, Christie MJ, Manzoni O: Cellular and synaptic adaptations mediating opioid dependence. Physiol Rev 81:299–343, 2001

Wise RA, Murray A, Bozarth MA: Bromocriptine self-administration and bromocriptine-reinstatement of cocaine-trained and heroin-trained lever pressing in rats. Psychopharmacology (Berl) 100:355–360, 1990

Wolf DH, Numan S, Nestler EJ, et al: Regulation of phospholipase Cgamma in the mesolimbic dopamine system by chronic morphine administration. J Neurochem 73:1520–1528, 1999

Wolf ME: The role of excitatory amino acids in behavioral sensitization to psychomotor stimulants. Prog Neurobiol 54:679–720, 1998

Yao WD, Gainetdinvo RR, Arbuckle MI, et al: Identification of PSD-95 as a regulator of dopamine-mediated synaptic and behavioral plasticity. Neuron 41:625–638, 2004

24

NEUROPSYCHIATRIC ASPECTS OF DEMENTIAS ASSOCIATED WITH MOTOR DYSFUNCTION

Alan J. Lerner, M.D.

David Riley, M.D.

The degenerative dementias associated with motor system dysfunction are diverse disorders that present a particular challenge to the clinician. Depending on where the primary pathology occurs in the motor system (basal ganglia, cerebellum, or motor neuron), symptoms can include abnormal movements, incoordination, or weakness in addition to the neuropsychiatric features. In this chapter, we review Huntington's disease (HD), Parkinson's disease (PD), progressive supranuclear palsy (PSP), and other conditions in which movement or motor disorders are cardinal clinical features (Table 24–1). In contrast, in primary degenerative dementias such as Alzheimer's disease (AD) and frontotemporal dementia (FTD), motor signs are relatively incidental and usually become prominent only in later stages of the disease.

As degenerative disorders, the dementias included in this chapter are characterized by gradual loss of function caused by progressive loss of neurons in specific regions of the brain associated with pathological hallmarks that are characteristic of the individual diseases. The specific etiologies of these diseases are often unknown, and clinical features frequently overlap among different conditions, making a clear nosology difficult.

As the genetic basis of these conditions is being elucidated (Table 24–2), a firmer basis has developed for de-ciphering the variability in clinical and neuropsychiatric symptoms. Despite these impressive, concerted advances in knowledge, specific biological interventions are limited in effectiveness.

The combination of motor, cognitive, and behavioral abnormalities is particularly stressful for patients, family members, and professional caregivers because of the multifaceted impairment in quality of life. It also poses difficult challenges for clinicians. Although medications are available to treat the motor symptoms for some of these conditions, these drugs frequently aggravate the cognitive and behavioral dysfunction. In addition, the motor impairments themselves create special difficulties in neuropsychiatric and neuropsychological testing of the cognitive and psychiatric dysfunction.

The classification of the dementias included in this chapter and their nosological relations to those considered in Apostolova and Cummings, Chapter 25 in this volume, are controversial. Ideally, classification depends on proper understanding of essential clinical and biological features. However, our understanding of the relations between brain changes and behavioral alterations in these disorders is limited. Many attempts have been made to define subtypes of dementia; for example, age at onset has been used

TABLE 24–1.   Degenerative dementias associated with motor system impairment

Extrapyramidal diseases

  Huntington's disease

  Parkinson's disease

  Dementia with Lewy body disease

  Progressive supranuclear palsy

  Cortical–basal ganglionic degeneration

  Multiple system atrophy

  Thalamic dementias

  Wilson's disease

  Pantothenate kinase–associated neurodegeneration

  Calcification of the basal ganglia (Fahr's disease)

  Frontotemporal dementia

Cerebellar diseases

  Olivopontocerebellar atrophy

  Friedreich's ataxia

  Spinocerebellar degenerations

Motor neuron diseases

  Motor neuron disease with dementia

  Amyotrophic lateral sclerosis/parkinsonism
  dementia complex

Other

  Normal-pressure hydrocephalus

  Creutzfeldt-Jakob disease

to characterize different forms of AD, HD, and PD. Another approach to develop a classification of dementia based on biology is the development of the concept of cortical and subcortical dementia (Albert et al. 1974; McHugh and Folstein 1975). AD and Pick's disease (now subsumed under FTD [see section "Frontotemporal Dementia" later in this chapter]) are thought to represent cortical dementias in which the predominant pathology is neocortical and the clinical symptoms—such as aphasia, apraxia, and agnosia—supposedly reflect cortical pathology. Subcortical dementias are conceptualized as showing prominent deficits in processing speed, memory dysfunction, and affective changes. However, it is apparent that all dementias cannot be easily classified into these two large categories. For example, the dementias of HD and PD are as clinically different from each other as they are from AD (Brown and Marsden 1988; Cummings 1990; Mayeux et al. 1983; Whitehouse 1986). Moreover, the pathological

basis for dementia in PD is now known to lie in the cerebral cortex (Apaydin et al. 2002), effectively rendering its designation as a "subcortical" dementia untenable.

HUNTINGTON'S DISEASE

HD is an autosomal dominantly transmitted, progressive neuropsychiatric disorder that can appear at any time in life. The peak period of onset is in the fourth and fifth decades. Because of their clinical prominence and central place in Huntington's (1872) description, dyskinesias, particularly chorea—defined as brief, random, nonstereotyped, purposeless movements—are usually considered the first sign of the disease. However, the clinical presentation is quite variable, and cognitive and psychiatric manifestations are often evident well before the movement disorder (S.E. Folstein 1989). Depression, irritability, and impulsive or erratic behavior are the most common psychiatric symptoms. Memory and concentration difficulties are early cognitive symptoms (S.E. Folstein 1989; Martin and Gusella 1986).

EPIDEMIOLOGY

Estimates of the prevalence of HD vary widely. S.E. Folstein (1989) concluded that the best estimate of point prevalence among Caucasians is 5–7 cases per 100,000. In general, the prevalence of HD in European populations is relatively uniform, although there are pockets of isolated populations in which the rates are much higher, as well as areas in Europe where the rates are much lower (e.g., Spain, Finland) (Harper 1992). Variability in rates may be artifacts of the instability of estimates based on small samples, but in the case of high prevalence, variability also may be the consequence of reproductive isolation.

HD is an autosomal dominant disorder with variable age at onset. Early onset is typically associated with paternal transmission and has a more rapid course (S.E. Folstein 1989; Martin and Gusella 1986). In adult-onset cases, death usually occurs after 16–20 years (S.E. Folstein 1989). The rate of decline may be slower in patients with onset after the fifth decade of life (Martin and Gusella 1986).

ETIOLOGY

George Huntington was fortunate to practice medicine in the same location as his father, giving him ample opportunity to observe the familial transmission of this disease (Huntington 1973). He correctly concluded that the familial transmission was hereditary and, although the concepts were not yet developed, appreciated that it was a dominant, fully penetrant, autosomal condition.

TABLE 24–2. Genes associated with degenerative disorders with motor involvement

Disease entity	Inheritance	Gene locus	Gene product
Huntington's disease	AD	4q16.3	Huntingtin
Parkinson's disease (PD)	AD	4q21	α-Synuclein
Early-onset PD	AR	1p36	PINK1; PARK6
PD type 8	AD	12q12	LRRK2; Dardarin
Atypical familial PD	AD	4q21	
Juvenile PD	AR	6q25.2–q27	PARK2
Dementia with Lewy bodies		5q35	Synuclein-β
Motor neuron disease with dementia	AD	15q21	
Friedreich's ataxia	AD	9q13	Frataxin
Frontotemporal dementia	AD	17q21.1	Tau
Wilson's disease	AR	13q14.1–q21.1	Adenosine triphosphatase
Pantothenate kinase–associated neurodegeneration	AR	20p13–p12.3	PANK2
Calcification of the basal ganglia (Fahr's disease)	AD	14q	
Spinocerebellar degenerations (multiple types; SCA-1 most common)	AD	6p23	Ataxin 1

Note. AD = autosomal dominant; AR = autosomal recessive; SCA = spinocerebellar atrophy.

In 1983, genetic linkage analysis, in a Venezuelan population with a very high prevalence of the disease, identified the HD gene locus at the distal end of the short arm of chromosome 4 (Gusella et al. 1983), and subsequently the gene itself was identified (Huntington's Disease Collaborative Research Group 1993). The mutant gene consists of a cytosine-adenine-guanine (CAG) trinucleotide repeat sequence that is longer than that of a normal gene. Normal alleles have a range of 9 to 30 CAG repeats, whereas the repeats in HD patients range from 40 to at least 121 (Albin and Tagle 1995; Huntington's Disease Collaborative Research Group 1993; Monckton and Caskey 1995). Patients with repeat lengths between 36 and 39 may or may not become symptomatic. The gene product of the HD gene is a protein called huntingtin. In unaffected individuals, it is a cytosolic protein, but in HD it is transported to the cell nucleus. The mechanism by which its abnormal transport and deposition in intraneuronal inclusions relate to molecular pathophysiology is currently unknown. Although age at onset is related to the number of gene repeats, environmental factors contribute as much as 38% of the variability in this important aspect of the disease (Wexler et al. 2004).

HD is one of many diseases characterized by trinucleotide repeats in the affected genes. These diseases include myotonic dystrophy, fragile X syndrome, spinobulbar muscular atrophy, and several of the spinocerebellar ataxias (SCAs 1, 2, 3, 7, and 17). The isolation of the gene has permitted some accounting for the apparent allelic heterogeneity of the disease, with family, race, and gender variation in age at onset (Farrer and Conneally 1985; S.E. Folstein et al. 1987). The CAG repeat length can be very unstable, particularly in males. Longer CAG repeats tend to be associated with earlier age at onset and male-to-male transmission, with the most repeats seen in patients with juvenile onset. However, the length of repeat does not have absolute correlation with motor symptomatology. Cases of what had been diagnosed as late-onset "senile chorea" have been recognized as late-onset HD, again with expanded gene repeats.

DIAGNOSIS AND CLINICAL FEATURES

Laboratory diagnosis of HD is straightforward; confirmation of the expanded trinucleotide repeat length is all that is required. The key step in diagnosis is to consider HD among the diagnostic possibilities. The classic clinical syndrome of HD consists of a combination of chorea and dementia in the setting of a positive family history consistent with autosomal dominant inheritance. Clinical diagnosis may become more problematic if patients present with other movement disorders, or psychiatric rather than cognitive dysfunction, and if the family history is incomplete or misleading (e.g., mistaken paternity). Cross-sectional assessment of patients may result in diagnostic inaccuracy because of this substantial variability in presentation early in the disease course and also because many conditions may present with chorea. In the 3%–9% of cases in which onset occurs before or during adolescence, the so-called Westphal variant, parkinsonism, myoclonus, or dystonia may be the predominant movements. Nearly half of HD patients initially present with emotional or cognitive symptoms. These symptoms are diverse and include depression, irritability, hallucinations, and apathy. Motor symptoms, if present, may be mild akinesia, restlessness, or involuntary movements that are easily attributable to another disorder. Other conditions such as PD, Sydenham's chorea, ataxias, cerebrovascular disease, systemic lupus erythematosus, schizophrenia, mood disorder, thyroid disease, acanthocytosis, drug-induced chorea, or alcoholism are other considerations in the differential diagnosis (see Table 24–1). However, when the patient has a positive family history consistent with autosomal dominant transmission, HD is a very likely explanation of these symptoms. Neuroimaging studies, especially positron emission tomography (PET) that shows glucose hypometabolism in the caudate nucleus, can be quite sensitive diagnostic aids (Furtado and Suchowersky 1995). Readily available direct genetic testing produces unequivocal diagnosis in uncertain cases.

The clinical and ethical issues involved in preclinical testing for HD—first considered when linkage studies became available (Brandt et al. 1989; Martin and Gusella 1986)—have become even more salient and critical because of the availability of HD gene analysis (Codori and Brandt 1994; Codori et al. 1994; Hayden et al. 1995; Hersch et al. 1994). These issues must be explored on an individual basis and may be aided by employing an experienced genetic counselor.

NEUROBIOLOGY

The most obvious gross pathology in HD occurs in the basal ganglia. The striatum is consistently affected, with degeneration beginning in the medial caudate nucleus and proceeding laterally to the putamen and occasionally to the globus pallidus. The actual mechanisms of cell destruction in the caudate nucleus are not known. Two models have been proposed. One focuses on abnormal posttranslation cleavage products that disturb cellular metabolism and function (Albin and Tagle 1995). A second model proposes an excitotoxic basis for HD involving the glutamate/N-methyl-D-aspartate (NDMA) receptor. This model rests heavily on the finding of abnormal 3-hydroxykynurenine levels in the brains of individuals with HD, which may indicate an excitotoxic basis for cell death. This model may be a valuable heuristic option for pharmacotherapeutic developments.

γ-Aminobutyric acid (GABA), the most abundant neurotransmitter of the spiny output neurons, and acetylcholine, the principal neurotransmitter of type I aspiny interneurons, are especially reduced (Martin and Gusella 1986). Other neurotransmitter changes in HD include increased concentrations of somatostatin (Albin and Tagle 1995; Pearson and Reynolds 1994). In the caudate nucleus, for example, somatostatin levels increase because of the selective survival of type II spiny interneurons. The alterations in absolute neurotransmitter concentrations and relative balance among different systems may account for some of the symptoms of HD (S.E. Folstein 1989).

Developing knowledge of basic neuroanatomy and neurochemistry has done much to elucidate the mechanisms of symptoms and symptom patterns in HD. Rich interconnections are found between the striatum and the prefrontal and parietal cortices (S.E. Folstein 1989; S.E. Folstein et al. 1990). Alexander et al. (1986) summarized evidence that there are five distinct parallel corticostriatal circuits subserving distinct neurobehavioral functions, including eye movements, motor behavior, emotion, and cognitive functions. Except for the motor circuit involving the putamen, the others are caudate nucleus–frontal circuits. Interestingly, lesions at any of the segments of the circuit produce similar functional consequences.

In addition, major sources of input to the basal ganglia (caudate nucleus and putamen) include limbic structures, the primary motor cortex, and motor association areas. These sources help to account for the co-occurrence of movement abnormalities and behavioral symptoms and for the often-noted influence of emotional states on the severity of motor symptoms.

There is substantial overlap in the neurotransmitter systems implicated in HD and those involved in extrapyramidal and psychiatric disorders. For example, caudate nucleus pathology and disruptions in caudate nucleus–prefrontal connections are associated with the mood disorders of HD (Mendez 1994).

The degree of atrophy of the caudate nucleus (Figure 24–1) correlates with cognitive dysfunction, including intelligence, memory, and visuospatial deficits (Bamford et al. 1989; Sax et al. 1983). Atrophy of the caudate nucleus is generally more consistently correlated than measures of frontal atrophy, with executive functions typically considered to be evidence of prefrontal cortical pathology (Bamford et al. 1989; Starkstein et al. 1988). Similar associations between functional impairments and caudate nucleus pathology have been reported with PET (Bamford et al. 1989). The deterioration in neuropsychological functions in HD appears to derive principally from disruptions in neural circuits caused by basal ganglia pathology (Bamford et al. 1989; M. Morris 1995).

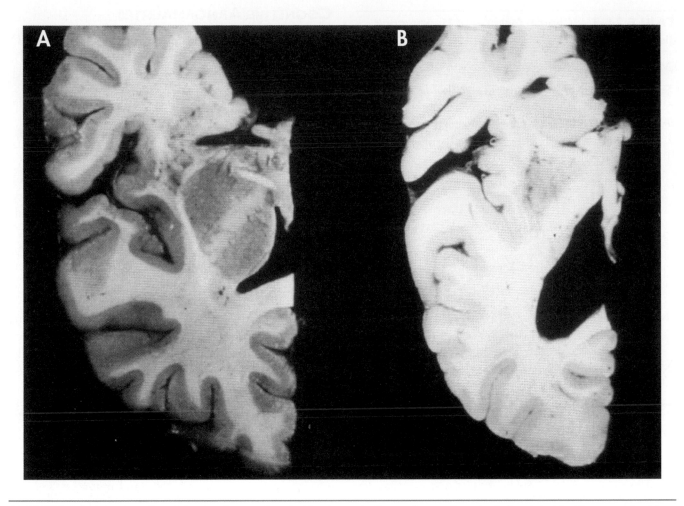

FIGURE 24–1. Atrophy of the caudate nucleus in Huntington's disease (coronal section). *Panel A.* Healthy control subject. *Panel B.* Patient with Huntington's disease. In this photograph, the frontal lobes are oriented inferiorly, the temporal lobes superiorly.

MOTOR ABNORMALITIES

HD was formerly known as Huntington's chorea, emphasizing the prominence of chorea, characterized by involuntary sudden, jerky movements of the limbs, face, or trunk, unpredictable in timing or distribution. Abnormalities of motor function in HD also include abnormal voluntary movements (Table 24–3). They can occur while the individual is at rest or in the course of planned movement (e.g., walking, reaching), although they are absent during sleep. Stress, such as that experienced during cognitive challenges (serial 7s, mental calculation), can increase chorea. Patients can generally suppress chorea for only short periods. Parkinsonism or dystonia, in the absence of chorea, is common in juvenile-onset (Westphal variant) cases.

Motor abnormalities change over the course of the disease. Early motor abnormalities include brief, irregular, jerky movements along with slower, writhing movements, which often occur in conjunction with the initia-

tion of action. Irregular flexion-extension of individual fingers ("piano playing") and ulnar deviation of the hands while walking are also common. Later, movements become almost constant, with severe grimacing, nodding, head bobbing, and a "dancing" gait. Chorea decreases and dystonia and an akinetic-rigid syndrome may supervene, especially in those with drug-induced parkinsonism (Feigin et al. 1995; Furtado and Suchowersky 1995).

Chorea may be misdiagnosed as nervousness, mannerisms, or intentional movements early in the course of the disease. Abnormalities in voluntary movements are helpful in the diagnosis because they are present in HD even in the absence of chorea. Patients have abnormalities in initiation and inhibition of eye movements (saccades, fixation, and smooth pursuit), coordination of limb movements, and articulation (Furtado and Suchowersky 1995; Leigh et al. 1983; Mendez 1994). Although they are nonspecific features of the illness, these abnormalities correlate more with intellectual impairment, memory disorder, and capacity for activities of daily living than does the chorea severity.

TABLE 24–3.   Clinical features of Huntington's disease

TABLE 24–3.   Clinical features of Huntington's disease

Motor symptoms

Chorea, consisting of nonrepetitive, nonperiodic, jerky movements of limbs, face, or trunk; exacerbated by stress; absent during sleep; may be consciously suppressed only for short periods

Parkinsonism

Dystonia

    Impaired initiation and inhibition of eye movements

    Incoordination of limb movements

    Articulation problems and dysphagia

    Myoclonus

    Gait and balance impairment

Neuropsychological symptoms

Declarative memory problems, with greater impairment in information retrieval than in recognition memory

Procedural memory deficits

Verbal fluency deficits

Impaired visuospatial skills

Problems with sustained concentration

Impaired executive functions (i.e., mental planning, organization of sequential actions, mental flexibility)

Language functions relatively preserved

Psychiatric features

Common symptoms

    Apathy

    Irritability

    Dysphoria

    Anxiety

Common syndromes

    Mood disorders (especially symptomatic major depression and bipolar disorder)

    Intermittent explosive disorder

    Schizophreniform disorder

    Atypical psychosis

COGNITIVE ABNORMALITIES

Cognitive deficits usually appear early in the course of HD and are progressive (M. Morris 1995) (see Table 24–3). When the deficits are severe, a brief mental status test is sufficient, such as the Mini-Mental State Examination (MMSE; M.F. Folstein et al. 1975). Very early in the disease, intelligence may be normal, and detailed neuropsychological testing is helpful. Although cognitive deficits can occur very early, it is questionable whether neuropsychological deficits appear before other clinical signs of the disease, but they can contribute to early disability (Diamond et al. 1992; Giordani et al. 1995; Jason et al. 1988; Mayeux et al. 1986a; Strauss and Brandt 1990).

Dementia of similar severity in different dementing illnesses is affected by different disabilities. Mendez (1994) found that for any given level of dementia, the pattern of failure is different in HD and AD. At mild levels of dementia (MMSE score of 20–24), HD patients are more impaired than AD patients are in the serial subtraction of 7 from 100, whereas AD patients are more likely to have errors in recalling the three items learned earlier in the examination. Naming and other language functions appear to be relatively preserved in HD, but not invariably, and may help differentiate HD from some forms of FTD (Butters et al. 1978; Cummings and Benson 1988).

The cognitive deficits of HD also include difficulties in sustained concentration and visuospatial skills. Visuospatial deficits are seen in tests measuring constructional ability. Patients with HD may have difficulty identifying or using their position in space relative to some fixed point (S.E. Folstein et al. 1990). This contrasts with AD, in which the deficit is mainly in the perception of extrapersonal space.

Executive dysfunction (problems with planning, organizing, and mental flexibility) is also affected early in HD. Examples of such tasks are those requiring keeping track of several things at once, discovering rules, or frequently changing mental sets (Bylsma et al. 1990; Starkstein et al. 1988; Wexler 1979).

Memory deficits are the best-characterized neuropsychological feature of the disease. Early studies (Brandt and Butters 1986) suggested that HD was characterized by major deficits in the encoding or storage of new information. However, deficits in retrieval of memories and the acquisition of procedural memory appear to be even more pronounced (S.E. Folstein et al. 1990).

Cognitive research on HD patients often contrasts them with AD and Korsakoff's disease patients. Unlike those groups, HD patients have better recognition memory for recent information and are able to make use of verbal mediators to improve performance. Moss et al.

(1986) found that recognition memory for designs, colors, or the positions of objects on a board was as impaired in HD patients as in those with AD or Korsakoff's disease. HD patients do not benefit from increased encoding opportunities and do not show a gradient of retrograde amnesia, such that more recent memories are more difficult to retrieve than more distant events.

Language, with the exception of verbal fluency and prosody, is relatively preserved in HD (Furtado and Suchowersky 1995; Mendez 1994; M. Morris 1995). Patients may answer questions with single words or short phrases, punctuated by pauses and silences. Patients have some deficit in the ability to understand prosodic elements of speech, which may contribute to the impairments in interpersonal relationships. Problems in writing often correlate with verbal difficulties.

PSYCHIATRIC ABNORMALITIES

Psychiatric symptoms are common in HD and are often the first signs of the disorder. "Insanity with a tendency to suicide" was one of the three cardinal features of the disease noted by Huntington (1973). Estimates of the proportion of patients who first present with psychiatric symptoms range from 24% to 79%, and the prevalence of psychiatric disorders in HD patients ranges from 35% to 73% (Cummings 1995; Mendez 1994).

Several studies have attempted to correlate genetic information with psychiatric symptoms. Shiwach and Norbury (1994) found no increase in schizophrenia, depression, psychiatric episodes, or behavior disorders in asymptomatic HD heterozygotes compared with their mutation-free siblings. HD family members did show more psychopathology than partner control subjects. The number of CAG repeats did not correlate with psychiatric symptoms or onset symptoms in two studies in which this variable was included (Claes et al. 1995; Zappacosta et al. 1996).

Although mood disorders have been emphasized in older studies (McHugh and Folstein 1975), a schizophreniform syndrome was once thought to be the most common psychiatric manifestation of HD. The early emphasis on schizophreniform syndromes probably related to ascertainment bias from reporting mental hospitals. Schizophrenic syndromes may be more common in more advanced cases of HD (S.E. Folstein 1989).

Studies that used explicit diagnostic criteria and standardized assessments suggested that intermittent explosive disorders and affective disorders are the most prevalent psychiatric conditions in HD (S.E. Folstein 1989; S.E. Folstein et al. 1990). Unipolar depression is common, but mania can also be seen in conjunction with HD. A markedly elevated risk of suicide is found in persons with HD, with the period of greatest risk in the 50s and 60s (Cummings 1995; Mendez 1994).

Personality changes—especially irritable, hostile, or angry mood—can be important harbingers of the onset of HD in at-risk individuals. Conduct disorder is not uncommon in the offspring of HD patients, even in those not carrying the genetic mutation. Although both of these disorders might be taken as results of limbic–basal ganglia–cortex disruptions, environmental factors associated with rearing by an affected parent may contribute to the personality disorders seen in the children of HD patients (Cummings 1995; Mendez 1994).

Irritability often precipitated by previously innocuous stimuli or events and anxiety are common in HD. Behavioral symptoms are more often reported in caregiver interviews and appear more frequently in early-onset patients. Approximately 30% of patients are reported to show altered sexual behavior, including sexual aggression, promiscuity, exhibitionism, voyeurism, and pedophilia (Cummings 1995; Mendez 1994). Whereas early HD may be accompanied by irritability, anxiety, aggression, and antisocial behavior, the middle stages often contain depression, psychosis, or mania. Later on in the disease, apathy and abulia are common psychiatric manifestations.

TREATMENT

No effective treatments are available for influencing the course of the disease. Several medical treatments may be used to palliate dementia, psychiatric disorders, and chorea. A combination of medical therapy and psychosocial intervention for patient and family can be beneficial in the management of the disease.

Early in the course of the disease, chorea can be treated with low-dose neuroleptic pharmacotherapy. The timing of this intervention is controversial. One approach is to withhold treatment until involuntary movements become disabling because of the dysphoria and feeling of cognitive dulling that neuroleptics can induce (S.E. Folstein 1989). Later in the disease course, combining a presynaptic (tetrabenazine or reserpine) and a postsynaptic dopamine blocker may be helpful. Treatment is not always effective, and use of dopamine blockade brings with it risk of tardive dyskinesia, worsening depression, and cognitive effects. Amantadine has been tried for chorea treatment with mixed results. An oral trial showed no benefit, but a small intravenous trial was promising (Lucetti et al. 2003; O'Suilleabhain and Dewey 2003). Because the impairment of voluntary movement persists, reducing chorea generally does not improve disability. Atypical neuroleptics may help to some degree but are less potent than haloperidol in suppressing involuntary movements. Their attractiveness in this setting is decreased risk of developing akathisia, parkinsonism, or tardive dyskinesia, albeit at a cost of reduced efficacy. For akinetic patients, antiparkinsonian drugs may be tried. No adequate controlled trials of the treatment of involuntary movements in HD have been done. Psychotic symptoms, especially hallucinations, are often responsive to neuroleptic therapy, and atypical neuroleptics are generally preferred.

Treatment of the emotional symptoms of HD can be more successful at times. Tricyclic antidepressants or lithium is often effective in the treatment of depressive symptoms. Improvement may be greater for the somatic-vegetative aspects of the syndrome than for the subjective elements of depression. The lessened responsiveness of helplessness-hopelessness to pharmacotherapy is understandable. Although rarely used, monoamine oxidase inhibitors and electroconvulsive therapy may be helpful (Ford 1986; Ranen et al. 1994).

Manic symptoms may respond to neuroleptics and carbamazepine more than to lithium (Mendez 1994). Irritability and aggressive outbursts respond to both environmental and pharmacological management. Irritability can be decreased by a reduction in environmental complexity and the institution of unchanging routines and also responds to neuroleptics. Successful treatment with β-adrenergic blockers has been reported in three patients who had aggressive outbursts but limited response to neuroleptics (Stewart et al. 1987). A paradoxical response in HD to pindolol has been reported (von Hafften and Jensen 1989).

Social support along with case management can be very important in the adaptation of the family to the diagnosis of HD and the management of the illness within the family (Shoulson 1982). Referral to the Huntington's Disease Society is helpful to provide educational materials and needed psychological support.

PARKINSON'S DISEASE

In 1817, James Parkinson described a new disorder he referred to as *the shaking palsy*, now referred to as *Parkinson's disease*. The cardinal neurological features include tremor, muscle rigidity, bradykinesia, and postural instability. When these features occur in another identified entity, the term *parkinsonism* or *secondary parkinsonism* is used. Neuropsychiatric symptoms, particularly dementia and depression, are frequently associated with PD or parkinsonism.

EPIDEMIOLOGY

PD affects perhaps 1 million individuals in North America and shows dramatic age-related increases in prevalence. The prevalence of PD is approximately 150 per

100,000, increasing after age 65 to nearly 1,100 per 100,000 (Kessler 1972). PD is found on every continent. Variations in prevalence have been reported, but ascertainment bias has not been excluded as the reason. No true clusters have been reported.

Dementia probably occurs in 20%–40% of patients with PD. Sample differences probably explain most of this variability, with early studies reporting the highest estimates (Ebmeier et al. 1990; Lieberman et al. 1979; Martilla and Rinne 1976; Rajput et al. 1984; Sutcliffe 1985). Mayeux (1990) found that the cumulative incidence of dementia in PD may be as high as 60% by age 88. In addition to age, family history of dementia, depression, and severe motor disability are risk factors for developing dementia in PD (Aarsland et al. 1996; Marder et al. 1990, 1995). The decline in mental status scores on the MMSE is similar to that observed in AD (Aarsland et al. 2004). In PD, depression occurs in up to 50% of patients.

ETIOLOGY

The role for genetic causes of PD has been growing since the 1997 discovery of an autosomal dominant mutation in the α-synuclein gene located on chromosome arm 4q21–q23 (Lucking et al. 2000). It was subsequently determined that α-synuclein is the major component of Lewy bodies, which are the pathological hallmark of PD and dementia with Lewy bodies (DLB), in all cases, whether familial or sporadic. This finding has led to a central role of α-synuclein in current concepts of the molecular pathogenesis of PD. However, α-synuclein mutations are rare causes of PD. Other genes, including *Parkin, LRRK2*, and the glucocerebrosidase gene, appear to account for far more cases of PD among the general population (Lucking et al. 2000).

A role for environmental factors cannot be excluded. Epidemiological studies have identified positive associations between the risk for PD and rural living and drinking well water, possibly mediated by pesticide exposure. However, no specific etiological agent has ever been identified. A negative association between the risk for PD and smoking has been established in numerous studies (Martilla et al. 1980). Parkinsonism has also been associated with use of a meperidine analog (Langston et al. 1983).

NEUROBIOLOGY

In several brain regions, the neuronal loss in PD is accompanied by the formation of Lewy bodies—hyaline inclusion bodies that were first described in the substantia innominata or nucleus basalis of Meynert. Lewy bodies also can be seen in the brain stem nuclei, particularly the substantia nigra and locus coeruleus (Jellinger 1986). In recent years, attention to Lewy bodies occurring in the neocortex has led to the recognition of DLB, which is described later in this chapter. Hurtig et al. (2000) found that cortical Lewy bodies were both sensitive and specific for dementia in PD in a prospectively studied cohort of patients with clinical PD. Braak and colleagues (2003) have provided evidence that the pathology of PD occurs sequentially, beginning in lower brain stem structures (an asymptomatic stage), followed by the substantia nigra (responsible for the onset of classic motor manifestations of PD), and ultimately into other cerebral structures, including the cortex. Although the concept of a rigid sequence of pathological evolution does not accord with the clinical variability of PD, the consistent distribution of PD lesions (Braak et al. 2003) provides a framework for understanding the numerous nonmotor manifestations of PD, including dementia.

The loss of dopaminergic cells in the substantia nigra relates most directly to the motor abnormalities—particularly the akinesia and rigidity—and can be compensated for by the administration of levodopa or dopamine agonists. Neuronal loss in the nucleus basalis of Meynert occurs to a small degree in all patients with idiopathic PD (Arendt et al. 1983; Tagliavini et al. 1984; Whitehouse et al. 1983). Some but not all dementia patients with PD develop senile plaques and neurofibrillary tangles (NFTs) identical to those found in AD (Boller et al. 1980; Chui et al. 1986; Hakim and Mathieson 1979). However, dementia in PD is most clearly associated with the finding of cortical Lewy body disease, consisting of neuronal degeneration and Lewy body formation in surviving neurons.

The pathological basis of depression in PD is unknown. Metabolic imaging shows bilateral decreases in regional cerebral blood flow in anteromedial frontal and cingulate cortex in depressed PD patients, overlapping with areas shown to be affected in primary depression (Ring et al. 1994). Mayeux et al. (1984, 1988) associated raphe pathology with depression by providing evidence of loss of serotonergic markers in cerebrospinal fluid (CSF). Also, alterations in noradrenaline and corticotropin-releasing factor may relate to psychiatric symptoms.

MOTOR SYMPTOMS

The most disabling motor features of PD are bradykinesia and rigidity (Table 24–4). The patient has difficulty initiating movements, and when movement is started, it is executed slowly. Poverty of associated movements (such as blinking or arm swing when walking) is characteristic. Lack of facial expression reflects akinesia of facial musculature. Rigidity can affect all muscle groups—proximal and distal, agonist and antagonist. Tremor is the presenting feature in most cases and is relatively slow (3–7 Hz),

TABLE 24–4.   Clinical features of Parkinson's disease

Motor symptoms

   Tremor

   Rigidity

   Akinesia

   Postural disturbances

Neuropsychological deficits

   Bradyphrenia

   Verbal and visual memory deficits

   Impaired visuospatial skills

   Executive dysfunction (e.g., sequencing, switching set)

   Language difficulties (e.g., naming)

Psychiatric features

   Possible premorbid personality characteristics

   Mood disorder

   Psychosis (usually medication-induced)

often occurs distally, and occurs most often at rest. It can be brought out with distraction and may be prominent in the upper limbs when walking. All of these motor manifestations typically occur asymmetrically in PD. Postural changes are a late development in PD and take two forms. One is a characteristic flexion at the neck, waist, elbows, and knees. The other, postural instability or disequilibrium, can lead to falls and serious injury. Early occurrence of postural instability should raise suspicion of a parkinsonian syndrome such as PSP, multiple system atrophy, or another akinetic-rigid syndrome. Treatment may improve tremor, rigidity, and akinesia but rarely has any effect on postural instability or dementia.

COGNITIVE IMPAIRMENTS

Many patients with PD show cognitive impairment; in some patients, the impairment may not be severe enough to warrant the label of dementia (see Table 24–4). Cognitive impairment may complicate PD at any time during its course, from preceding motor manifestations (Hedera et al. 1994) to occurring decades later.

A large body of literature exists describing visuospatial impairment, including spatial capacities, facial recognition, body schema, pursuit tracking, spatial attention, visual analysis, and judgments concerning position in space (Boller et al. 1984; Growdon and Corkin 1986; Levin 1990). Visuospatial function is composed of many separate abilities that are difficult to isolate and test separately (Brown and Marsden 1986). Visual analysis is impaired in PD (Levin et al. 1989; Pirozzolo et al. 1982; Villardita et al. 1982). Similarly, operating on objects in physical space (i.e., constructional praxis) is affected in PD, perhaps partly because of problems with spatial attention (Levin 1990). Abnormalities in memory involving verbal and nonverbal tasks with stimuli presented in different modalities occur.

The communication difficulties of PD are mostly a result of speech abnormalities, including hypophonia and dysarthria. However, language impairments can also occur and include reduced verbal fluency and naming difficulties (Matison et al. 1982). Abnormalities in syntax have been reported in PD (Cummings et al. 1988), although most studies have focused on semantics, comprehension, and naming (Bayles 1990).

Executive and attentional abnormalities also have been reported that are similar to deficits attributed to frontal lobe dysfunction (Freedman 1990). These deficits include sequencing voluntary motor activities, difficulties in maintaining and switching set, and abnormalities in selective attention. These abnormalities also may be seen in the setting of surgical treatments for PD, including pallidotomy and deep brain stimulation (see subsection "Surgical Treatment" later in this section).

The relations between the cognitive impairments in PD and the motor symptoms are complex. Poor performance on cognitive tests is not purely related to motor abnormalities. For example, visuospatial deficits continue to be detectable when tasks with limited roles for eye movements (e.g., tachistoscopy) are used. However, the presence of akinetic-rigid motor deficit makes comparisons with dementias such as AD or HD difficult to interpret.

PSYCHIATRIC ABNORMALITIES

Premorbid Personality

In the 1940s, patients who appeared to suppress anger and be quite perfectionistic ("masked personality") were claimed to be more at risk for developing PD (Booth 1948; Sands 1942). Later studies did not show such strong relations between premorbid personality and PD (Diller and Riklan 1956; Lishman 1978; Pollock and Hornabrook 1966). Nevertheless, the notion of a common premorbid personality in PD patients persists (Hubble and Koller 1995; Menza et al. 1993). Although they are difficult to undertake, new and better-designed studies with more modern personality inventories may help elucidate the relations between premorbid psychological characteristics and psychiatric sequelae of neurodegenerative disease.

Psychiatric Disturbances

Affective disorder is the most common psychiatric disturbance in PD, with estimated incidence from 20% to 90% (Mayeux et al. 1986b). Early in PD, some instances of depression are believed to be reactive. However, as in many chronic illnesses, the relation of disease severity to depression is nonlinear (Starkstein et al. 1989). Relatively few associations between depression and disease factors such as duration of disease, degree of disability, and response to medications have been established (Troster et al. 1995). A higher frequency of depression in early-onset cases being correlated with cognitive impairment and disease duration has been reported (Kostic et al. 1994). Menza and Mark (1994) found that depression did not correlate with novelty seeking, a personality trait related to dopaminergic systems. Harm avoidance, related to serotonergic systems, explained 31% of the variance in depression scores in PD. Schiffer and colleagues (1988) described a condition in which predominant anxiety occurs. Anxiety such as fear of falling (a real risk in advanced PD) is common. Sleep is frequently affected in PD, but this disturbance is frequently multifactorial, with medications, motor and nonmotor symptoms, and age playing as large a role as depression and anxiety (Menza and Rosen 1995). PD is frequently associated with development of restless legs syndrome, which responds to levodopa, dopamine agonists, or benzodiazepines.

Although depression is very common in PD, it often is not recognized, and when it is recognized, it is either untreated or undertreated. In a successive clinical sample, Weintraub et al. (2003) found that 33% met criteria for depression, but two-thirds of those had not received treatment, and a substantial proportion of those treated were receiving suboptimal doses, as indicated by ongoing depression. As in the secular trend, the use of selective serotonin reuptake inhibitors has increased in this population.

Psychosis

Psychosis of a schizophrenic nature has been reported in PD in the absence of medication effects (Mjones 1949). However, medications trigger the vast majority of episodes of psychosis in PD. The most important predisposing risk factor for psychosis is preexisting cognitive impairment. Age and visual impairment also contribute to risk. Celesia and Wanamaker (1972) observed psychotic episodes in 12% of their 153 patients. Most were caused by drugs and occurred in patients who were cognitively impaired. All of the antiparkinsonian medications have been implicated in the occurrence of hallucinations in PD. Of these, anticholinergic drugs, such as trihexyphenidyl, are the most notorious causes of delirium with psychotic features. Levodopa is the antiparkinsonian agent least likely to provoke hallucinations and delusions and is the preferred agent for management of PD symptoms and signs in psychotic patients.

Dementia

The occurrence of dementia in otherwise typical PD presents a diagnostic and therapeutic challenge. Because of the lack of distinctive biomarkers for the disorders under consideration, the diagnosis may change over time as the patient's full clinical picture develops. The clinician needs to consider each symptom both as part of the whole syndrome and in isolation for both diagnosis and therapy. Use of symptomatic therapy must be viewed in the context of what the patient, family, and clinician are attempting to accomplish. In a study of rivastigmine, moderate improvements occurred, but treated patients had higher rates of nausea, vomiting, and tremor (Emre et al. 2004).

TREATMENT

Great strides have been made in treating the motor dysfunction in PD. Six drugs, or classes of drugs, are currently available for this purpose, and surgery is being used increasingly. Medication classes include levodopa, which may be given with inhibitors of its breakdown such as monoamine oxidase–B (MAO-B) inhibitors and catechol-O-methyltransferase (COMT) inhibitors, dopamine agonists, amantadine, and anticholinergic agents. Levodopa and dopamine agonists are the two cornerstones of PD treatment. As PD progresses, treatment with levodopa is often complicated by dose-related fluctuations and dyskinesias, particularly in younger patients. Use of extended-release levodopa and MAO-B and COMT inhibitors can help with managing this symptom. Other agents that may help with motor fluctuations include selegiline and subcutaneous apomorphine (Bowron 2004). Besides the usual side effects of selegiline as an antiparkinsonian drug, an unusual side effect was transvestic fetishism, which resolved when selegiline was discontinued (Riley 2002).

Dopamine agonists are more often associated with cognitive side effects, postural hypotension, and peripheral edema. Besides psychosis, common to all antiparkinsonian therapy, dopamine agonists may cause sedation, including sleep attacks while driving, and compulsive behaviors related to gambling, sexual activity, and eating.

Treatment of the neuropsychiatric symptoms involves both behavioral and biological approaches. Behavioral treatment begins with a careful assessment of not only the medical aspects but also the functional effects of the illness on the patient's life and on the patient's family. Marriage therapy and family counseling may be appropriate in

some circumstances. Nursing and social work assessments can play an important role in providing a baseline for following the course of the illness. Frequent reassessments followed by modifications of care plans are necessary. Discussions with the individual and family members early in the disease when the patient can participate in decision making and prepare advance directives such as a living will are desirable. Early planning, both financial and legal, is helpful to minimize the difficulty of gaining access to and financing home care, day care, or institutional care.

A variety of interventions are available for the individual patient, including individual psychotherapy, particularly to deal with depression early in the illness. Particularly in the dementias associated with motor problems, physical and occupational therapy may be very helpful. A safety check at home—including the appropriate use of handrails, avoiding stairs if possible, and stowing away loose objects such as rugs and electrical cords—is the most important intervention to prevent falls.

Biological Treatment

The most important role for the physician in caring for patients with dementia is to use a preventive approach to avoid so-called excess disability, which is frequently a result of intercurrent illnesses, psychological stress, or iatrogenic disease, which is usually due to overuse of medication.

The most effective biological interventions are probably those for the treatment of mood disorders and psychosis. Treatment of depression in PD generally parallels that of non-PD depression. Virtually all antidepressants may aggravate tremor, with the notable exception of mirtazapine, which may improve tremor or dyskinesias (but which can be quite sedating). Despite their theoretical help in managing motor disability, antidepressants or other medications with significant anticholinergic potential can aggravate dementia or orthostatic hypotension.

Similarly, treatment of psychosis in PD is difficult because antipsychotics may worsen either motor symptoms or dementia, or both. A behavioral approach to identify drugs or other stressors contributing to psychosis is suggested (Saint-Cyr et al. 1993). Cholinesterase inhibitors may provide relief from psychosis in milder cases and spare patients from antipsychotic therapy. However, treatment with dopamine receptor blockers is often necessary. Fortunately, small doses of these agents are often sufficient to control PD-related hallucinosis. The atypical neuroleptics that produce little if any exacerbation of parkinsonism are quetiapine and clozapine (Motsinger et al. 2003; Parsa and Bastani 1998). Other atypical antipsychotics that were thought to cause few extrapyramidal side effects, such as risperidone, olanzapine, and aripiprazole, have been disappointments in this regard, and their use in PD must be monitored closely. Atypical antipsychotics have relatively high anticholinergic potential and can cause lethargy and conceivably affect cognition. Sleep disturbances are common with psychotic disorders, and the primary focus should be placed on sleep hygiene (i.e., increased daytime activity, a regular pattern of sleep preparation behavior, and avoidance of stimulants).

Treatment of dementia also follows the usual protocol for non-PD patients. Although cholinesterase inhibitors occasionally lead to worsening of parkinsonism, they are usually well tolerated and may produce measurable levels of cognitive enhancement that equals or surpasses their effectiveness in AD (Emre et al. 2004). The role of memantine in treating PD-related dementia is unclear, but no contraindication to its use is apparent.

Surgical Treatment

Patients whose PD motor manifestations become difficult to control consistently with medication, or who develop intolerable side effects, may be eligible for stereotactic surgery for their PD. The current surgical treatment of choice is deep brain stimulation (DBS) targeting the subthalamic nucleus, which has supplanted destructive lesioning such as internal pallidotomy. DBS surgery usually leads to more consistent, around-the-clock control of parkinsonian symptoms and allows for a reduction in antiparkinsonian medication. This reduction in medication can produce an amelioration of cognitive function. Rarely, electrode implantation results in deterioration in cognitive function that may be irreversible. Such a complication is much more likely to occur in elderly patients and those with preexisting dementia, making them riskier candidates for DBS surgery. Milder cognitive dysfunction is a more common outcome. A decrease in verbal fluency, particularly with left subthalamic nucleus stimulation, has been reported. Changes in personality and acute depression also have been reported (Hugdahl and Wester 2000; Kumar et al. 1999; Schmand et al. 2000; Starr et al. 1998). Some patients may experience improved cognitive scores secondary to surgery itself, such as improvements in cognitive flexibility (Witt et al. 2004). In most patients, surgery is well tolerated from a cognitive standpoint, and cognitive complications are typically transient.

DEMENTIA WITH LEWY BODIES

DLB is an increasingly recognized and studied form of dementia, accounting in some series for as many as 20% of cases. A complex relationship exists between DLB and AD. DLB occurs as the sole pathology but is often (approximately 50% of the time) mixed with AD pathology as the so-called Lewy body variant of AD.

CLINICAL DIAGNOSIS

Diagnostic criteria for DLB are based on the presence of two of three cardinal features: hallucinations, spontaneous parkinsonism, and daily fluctuations in cognition. The clinical criteria have been criticized as being of low sensitivity (Hohl et al. 2000). Verghese et al. (1999) concluded that the new criteria from the consortium on DLB have high negative predictive value and exclude patients without DLB. Litvan et al. (1998b) also examined sensitivity, specificity, and positive and negative predictive value of clinical criteria. They also determined that interrater reliability for diagnosis of DLB was not particularly good and varied across different visits as the disease evolved. An autopsy study that used the international consensus criteria (McKeith et al. 1996) and applied them strictly found that the 1996 criteria were both sensitive and specific, but false-negative DLB cases tended to lack hallucinations and spontaneous parkinsonism (McKeith et al. 2000).

In an attempt to improve the diagnostic sensitivity, a recent revision of the diagnostic criteria has been published (McKeith et al. 2006). Dementia is now obligatory for diagnosis of possible or probable DLB. In addition, the frequent occurrence of supportive features is now recognized, including rapid eye movement sleep behavior disorder, repeated falls and syncope, autonomic dysfunction, nonvisual hallucinations, delusions, depression, reduced occipital regional cerebral blood flow, abnormally low uptake of ^{123}I-metaiodobenzylguanidine (MIBG) on myocardial scintigraphy, and prominent slow-wave activity on electroencephalogram along with transient sharp waves in the temporal lobe (Table 24–5).

Compared with AD patients, DLB patients show no difference in age at onset, age at death, or duration of disease (Z. Walker et al. 2000). Rest tremor was more common in PD than in DLB, whereas myoclonus was more common in DLB. The frequency of rigidity, bradykinesia, dystonia, or gaze palsies did not differ (Louis et al. 1997). Litvan et al. (1998b) did not find postural imbalance helpful in differentiating DLB from PD. Response to levodopa is much more predictable in PD than in DLB.

One of the interesting clinical features of DLB is fluctuating consciousness. Ferman and colleagues (2004) identified four features of cognitive fluctuations in DLB: daytime drowsiness, sleep during the daytime of 2 hours or more, prolonged staring into space, and episodic disorganized speech. At least three of these features were present in 63% of their DLB patients but in only 12% of the AD patients (M.P. Walker et al. 2000).

TABLE 24–5. Clinical core characteristics of diffuse Lewy body disease

Dementia

Attentional impairment

Visuospatial difficulties

Fluctuations in cognitive functioning

Persistent, well-formed visual hallucinations

Parkinsonism

NEUROBIOLOGY

Genetic forms of DLB exist, including autosomal dominant forms. Ishikawa presented five cases with familial autosomal dominant DLB. These patients surprisingly responded well to levodopa therapy. As mentioned earlier, overlap occurs in clinical and pathological features of DLB, AD, and PD. DLB also overlaps with other degenerative syndromes, such as multiple system atrophy (Dickson et al. 1999), because both disorders are α-synucleinopathies. Autopsy studies have shown that DLB has similar numbers of neuritic plaques to AD but fewer NFTs (Samuel et al. 1997a). Attempts have been made to correlate pathological features with clinical findings. Samuel et al. (1997b) found that neocortical neuritic plaque burden and NFT counts in entorhinal cortex and loss of choline acetyltransferase were correlated with the severity of dementia. However, neocortical NFTs and synaptophysin were not correlated with dementia. The marked level of variability was reported in neuronal counts in entorhinal cortex in DLB—an area consistently and severely affected in AD. Sabbagh et al. (1999) also found that reductions in synaptophysin and choline acetyltransferase did not correlate with dementia severity in DLB as in AD.

Galvin et al. (1999) studied different forms of synuclein in PD and DLB. Antibodies to both α-synuclein and γ-synuclein detect aggregation of these products in dystrophic neurites. This supports a role for all three synucleins—α, β, and γ—in the pathology of both PD and DLB. Arima et al. (1999) studied the colocalization of α-synuclein with tau, which is associated with NFTs. Whereas NFTs or tau is rarely found in neurons in DLB, tau colocalizes with some Lewy bodies.

NEUROIMAGING

Standard structural imaging with computed tomography (CT) or magnetic resonance imaging (MRI) is not helpful in diagnosing DLB or in differential diagnosis. Frontal lobe atrophy may be prominent in DLB but is not sufficient to be clinically helpful. Attempts are being made to use other forms of neuroimaging to differentiate these conditions. Functional neuroimaging also has not proved to be specific in diagnosing DLB (Talbot et al. 1998)

TREATMENT

In addition to being monitored for responsiveness to levodopa, patients with DLB need to be watched carefully when neuroleptics are administered because they may develop complex and life-threatening neuroleptic malignant syndrome and related phenomena. In contrast, DLB patients may respond as well as or better to cholinesterase inhibitors than do AD patients (Fergusson and Howard 2000). No large controlled trials of memantine have been done yet to support a recommendation for its use in DLB.

PROGRESSIVE SUPRANUCLEAR PALSY

PSP (also known as Steele-Richardson-Olszewski syndrome) is a chronic, progressive disorder associated with eye movement abnormalities, parkinsonism, and dementia. It may have onset with deficient downward gaze, which causes trouble walking down stairs. The prevalence of PSP has been estimated at 1.4 per 100,000. Median age at onset of symptoms is approximately 63, with a median survival of 6–10 years (Golbe et al. 1988). Men are somewhat more likely to develop PSP. Postulated risk factors include history of hypertension, but no evidence shows that smoking cigarettes lowers PSP risk (Vanacore et al. 2000). Rare familial cases have been reported, and the disease may be more common, relative to PD, in Afro-Caribbeans and people from India (Chaudhuri et al. 2000).

DIAGNOSIS

The diagnosis of PSP is suggested by the presence of parkinsonism without tremor but with early disequilibrium and eye movement abnormalities. The earliest eye movement abnormalities include loss of vertical saccade velocity (Leigh and Riley 2000). This can be tested for by verbal request (e.g., "Look up, look down"). With disease progression, pursuit eye movements (e.g., following a moving object) are also impaired. When testing reflex eye movements with oculocephalic maneuvers (head turning), there is relative preservation of vertical eye movements. This has led to the designation of the eye movement abnormality in PSP as being supranuclear because the oculocephalic reflexes determine the integrity of the lower motor neuron pathways for up and down gaze. The lack of vertical eye movement abnormalities is the largest obstacle to correct antemortem diagnosis of PSP (Litvan et al. 1999). Ultimately, it is the constellation of clinical findings—that is, predominantly axial parkinsonism without tremor, unstable gait with postural instability, and vertical eye movement abnormality without "alien" limb movements (Table 24–6)—that best distinguishes PSP from PD, multiple system atrophy, cortical–basal ganglionic degeneration, and Pick's disease (Litvan et al. 1997).

Many patients with PSP have no noticeable dementia (Maher et al. 1985), and dementia is often not severe early in the course of PSP. It may be characterized by forgetfulness, slowing of thought processes, emotional or personality changes, and impaired ability to manipulate knowledge in the relative absence of aphasia, apraxia, or agnosia (Albert et al. 1974). PSP patients are particularly impaired on tests of frontal lobe function. PSP patients also may have deficits in visual scanning and search as well as verbal fluency, digit span, verbal memory, and logical memory.

Patients usually have extensor rigidity of the neck and face; bradykinetic, less rigid extremities; and a parkinsonian gait. Unlike PD or cortical–basal ganglionic degeneration, parkinsonism in PSP is almost always symmetrical in severity. Other signs include axial dystonia, bradyphrenia, perseveration, forced grasping, and utilization behaviors. Pseudobulbar palsy and pathological laughing and crying may be observed in the later stages. The gait disturbance is associated with postural instability and a tendency toward retropulsion. PSP may be misdiagnosed as PD, AD, hydrocephalus, or psychotic illness.

NEUROPSYCHIATRIC MANIFESTATIONS

PSP patients often have disturbances of sleep and depression and, occasionally, a schizophreniform psychosis (Aldrich et al. 1989). Also seen are memory loss, slowness of thought processes, changes in personality with apathy or depression, irritability, and forced inappropriate crying or laughing with outbursts of rage. PSP also may be associated with compulsive behaviors of the obsessive type (Destee et al. 1990).

TABLE 24–6.   Clinical characteristics of progressive supranuclear palsy

Gait instability with falls

Axial rigidity

Bradykinesia

Supranuclear gaze abnormalities

Dysarthria

Dementia

Apathy is particularly prominent in many cases and should be differentiated from concomitant depression. In a study that used the Neuropsychiatric Inventory, Levy et al. (1998) found that apathy correlated with lower cognitive function but not with depression subscale scores. Patients with PSP are particularly impaired in tasks requiring sequential movements, shifting of concepts, monitoring of the frequency of stimuli, or rapid retrieval of verbal information (Grafman et al. 1990). These symptoms, particularly the lack of motivation, are thought to be a reflection of frontal lobe impairment resulting from pathology in orbitofrontal-cortical circuits. Apraxia may be prominent in cases with prominent cerebral cortical involvement (Bergeron et al. 1997).

DIAGNOSTIC IMAGING

X-ray CT and MRI studies show early atrophy of midbrain structures with later atrophy of the pons and frontotemporal regions (Savoiardo et al. 1989). PET scanning has shown reduced spiperone binding in the basal ganglia. Fluorodeoxyglucose PET studies show marked frontal and temporal hypometabolism (Cambier et al. 1985; D'Antona et al. 1985; Maher et al. 1985). Fluorodopa uptake is also decreased in the striatum, which is reflective of decreased striatal dopamine formation and storage (Leenders et al. 1988). The loss of striatal dopamine receptors, as demonstrated by PET scanning, during life may explain the poor therapeutic efficacy of dopamine agonist therapy in PSP.

NEUROBIOLOGY

Neuropathological findings include neuronal loss associated with gliosis and NFTs, most marked in the substantia nigra, basal forebrain, subthalamic nucleus, pallidum, and superior colliculus. The tangles in PSP are straight filaments, not twisted as in AD (Takahashi et al. 1989). Extensive disruption occurs in fibrillar proteins in subcortical neurons, with antigenic similarities in neurofibrillary pathology between PSP and AD (Galloway 1988; Probst et al. 1988). Additional areas involved to a lesser extent include the locus coeruleus, striatum, and a variety of upper brain stem and midbrain structures (Agid et al. 1986). Standardized criteria for the neuropathological diagnosis of PSP have been proposed and should widen our understanding of the clinical spectrum of PSP (Litvan et al. 1996).

With the discovery that mutations in the tau gene on chromosome 17 are responsible for most clinical cases of PSP, similarities to other tauopathies such as FTD and cortical–basal ganglionic degeneration have emerged. In PSP, only the four-repeat-tau isoform aggregating into straight filaments is found. The relation of these neuronal pathologies to clinical phenotypes is unknown at present.

The neurochemistry of PSP is characterized by massive dopamine depletion in the striatum and reduced density of dopamine type 2 (D_2) receptors in the caudate nucleus and putamen (Pierot et al. 1988); widespread reduction in choline acetyltransferase levels in frontal cortex, basal forebrain, and basal ganglia (Whitehouse et al. 1988); diminished nicotinic receptors in the basal forebrain; diminished serotonin receptors in the temporal lobe (Maloteaux et al. 1988); and a variable reduction in GABAergic neurotransmitter systems in certain subcortical regions (Ruberg et al. 1985). Available evidence concerning cortical and subcortical as well as multiple neurotransmitter system abnormalities indicates that PSP is not a pure subcortical or dopaminergic dementia.

TREATMENT

No treatment has been found to be effective in relieving the motor or cognitive deficiencies in PSP. Levodopa treatment is generally not successful, correlating with the loss of postsynaptic striatal dopamine receptors. Indeed, it may worsen cognitive function, sometimes markedly. Poor responses with frequent dose-limiting side effects also occur with dopamine agonists. A report of effective treatment of violent behavior in a PSP patient with trazodone has been published and may be explained by the serotonergic effects of the drug (Schneider et al. 1989).

CORTICAL–BASAL GANGLIONIC DEGENERATION

Cortical–basal ganglionic degeneration presents with asymmetric basal ganglia (akinesia, rigidity, dystonia) and cerebral cortical (apraxia, cortical sensory loss, alien limb) manifestations (Riley et al. 1990) (Table 24–7). The alien limb is seen with parietal, medial frontal, and corpus callosum pathology. Dementia is a variable part of this syndrome but has been the presenting symptom in numerous case reports (Lang 2003). The neuropsychological profile is similar to that seen in PSP, with prominent executive dysfunction and explicit learning deficits without retention difficulties. However, asymmetric apraxias are frequent (Pillon et al. 1995). Depression is common, and other neuropsychiatric abnormalities include apathy or disinhibition, aberrant motor behaviors, and delusions (Litvan et al. 1998a). Oculomotor involvement similar to that in PSP may occur, particularly in advanced cases. Survival ranges from 2.5 to 12 years, with a median of about 8 years.

TABLE 24–7. Clinical characteristics of cortical–basal ganglionic degeneration

Akinesia and rigidity

Limb dystonia

Postural or action tremor

Focal reflex myoclonus

Apraxia

Cortical sensory loss

"Alien" limb phenomena

Dementia

Dysarthria

Highly asymmetric presentation

Classic cortical–basal ganglionic degeneration pathology shows abundant ballooned, achromatic neurons and focal cortical atrophy predominating in medial frontal and parietal lobes, plus degeneration of the substantia nigra. Astrocytic plaques are also seen in cortical–basal ganglionic degeneration cortex. The achromatic ballooned neurons are not found in increased numbers in other tauopathies. Cortical–basal ganglionic degeneration neuronal tau pathology shows wispy, fine-threaded tau inclusions, in comparison with the dense, compacted inclusions of PSP; the distribution of pathology falls mainly in basal ganglia and brain stem in PSP, whereas cortical–basal ganglionic degeneration shows widespread cerebral involvement as well (Dickson 1999). Differences in which tau isoforms accumulate in patients' brains may relate to different clinical phenotypes.

MRI may show asymmetric atrophy in the frontal and parietal lobes contralateral to the dominantly affected limbs (Soliveri et al. 1999). Cerebral blood flow studies show asymmetric decreased glucose utilization throughout the frontal cortex, superior parietal cortex, and caudate nucleus and thalamus contralateral to areas involved clinically and cognitive impairment (Hirono et al. 2000; Laureys et al. 1999; Yamauchi et al. 1998). Single-photon emission computed tomographic studies also show decreased blood flow in the basal ganglia and in widespread areas of frontal, temporal, and parietal cortex; however, PSP patients show only frontal hypoperfusion (Okuda et al. 2000). Dopamine binding is also reduced asymmetrically in cortical–basal ganglionic degeneration, as studied by both fluorodopa uptake and iodobenzamide single photon emission CT (Frisoni et al. 1995; Sawle et al. 1991). CSF tau levels are higher in patients with cortical–basal ganglionic degeneration than in patients with PSP or healthy control subjects, but the specificity of these findings is unclear.

Treatment of cortical–basal ganglionic degeneration is limited, with only a minority of patients responding to levodopa preparations given for parkinsonism. Myoclonus may respond to benzodiazepines, particularly clonazepam. No specific treatment for the dementia is available, but it may not be cholinergic in nature, suggesting that cholinesterase inhibitors are of limited value. Depression is common in cortical–basal ganglionic degeneration, but few data exist on response to antidepressants (Kampoliti et al. 1998; Litvan et al. 1998a).

FRONTOTEMPORAL DEMENTIA

The frontotemporal dementias constitute a heterogeneous group of conditions, often with prominent early behavioral disinhibitory symptoms. The clinical phenotypes that are now classified as FTD include Pick's disease, semantic aphasia, hereditary dysphasic dementia (J.C. Morris et al. 1984), and PSP and cortical–basal ganglionic degeneration. This familial syndrome may present with symptoms of Klüver-Bucy syndrome or social withdrawal, depression, and a schizophrenia-like picture in middle adulthood. Patients then develop parkinsonism and occasionally amyotrophy. Thus, not all of these patients have prominent motor disorders, often making diagnosis from primary psychiatric conditions difficult. Some patients with FTD have subclinical motor neuron disease apparent only at autopsy, suggesting that vigilance in this regard in patients complaining of weakness and showing muscle atrophy is warranted (Josephs et al. 2006).

The FTDs have been linked to mutations in the tau protein gene as described previously in the sections on PSP and cortical–basal ganglionic degeneration. Although consensus diagnostic criteria have been proposed, the incidence of these conditions has varied widely in different regions, possibly because of differences in case identification.

MULTIPLE SYSTEM ATROPHY

Multiple system atrophy is a disease concept that unifies three disorders previously thought to be disparate diseases but now commonly accepted as components of a clinical spectrum with a common pathological basis: striatonigral degeneration, Shy-Drager syndrome, and sporadic olivopontocerebellar atrophy. Consensus clinical diagnostic criteria for multiple system atrophy require that patients show evidence of autonomic dysfunction in the form of orthostatic hypotension or urinary incontinence in combination with either levodopa-unresponsive parkinsonism or cerebellar dysfunction (Gilman et al. 1998). In reality, many patients present with atypical parkinsonism or late-onset progressive ataxia without overt dysautonomia.

Cognitive dysfunction is so unusual in multiple system atrophy (Wenning et al. 2000) that dementia is considered an exclusionary criterion for diagnosis (Gilman et al. 1998). However, autopsy-proven cases of multiple system atrophy have been associated with clinically documented dementia (Schlossmacher et al. 2004). More often, formal neuropsychiatric studies report clinically unappreciated deficits in frontal lobe function (Robbins et al. 1992), verbal fluency, and verbal memory (Burk et al. 2006). Overall, multiple system atrophy is best thought of as the late-life parkinsonian disorder with the least tendency to produce cognitive impairment (Bak et al. 2005).

FRIEDREICH'S ATAXIA

Friedreich's ataxia presents with a slowly progressive ataxia, areflexia, pes cavus, and scoliosis. It is autosomal recessive, with mutations in the Frataxin gene on chromosome 9. Mental changes are present in about a quarter of cases but have not been well characterized. Some patients acquire a syndrome of "generalized intellectual deterioration." Others may show specific nonverbal intellectual impairments. In yet other cases, a variety of psychiatric disorders, including schizophrenia-like psychoses and depression, are the primary cognitive-behavioral abnormality. Changes in performance IQ, conceptual ability, and visual constructive tasks, as well as in tasks of three-dimensional spatial functions, have been found to be abnormal in Friedreich's ataxia. Personality abnormalities may be marked and are associated with juvenile delinquency and irritability. There may be excessive religiosity or mysticism.

OTHER SPINOCEREBELLAR ATAXIAS

The field of spinocerebellar ataxia has been revolutionized by the discovery of gene loci, which has finally allowed specificity of diagnosis for a large proportion of cases. Genetics studies have established that more than 25 separate disorders fall under the rubric of spinocerebellar ataxia. The molecular pathogenesis may involve excess polyglutamine repeats, channelopathies, or gene expression disorders but remains unknown in most cases.

Another complication is the appearance of cerebellar ataxia in other genetic syndromes (e.g., hereditary vitamin E deficiency, HD), acquired conditions (e.g., multiple sclerosis, ethanol abuse), and sporadic cases that cannot be further categorized. Among the best characterized are the autosomal dominant spinocerebellar ataxias. Abortive forms are common, and intrafamily variability is extremely common, with individuals sometimes showing little more than pes cavus or kyphoscoliosis. These disorders may present in childhood, early adulthood, or late adulthood and are usually slowly progressive. Associated findings of ataxic gait, intention tremor, decreased rapid alternating movements, past pointing, loss of the ability to check rebound, and dysarthria are common.

The ataxic disorders may not be accompanied by intellectual changes until late in the illness. In a study by Skre (1974), dementia was found in 36% of the patients with autosomal dominant spinocerebellar degeneration, 58% of the patients with autosomal recessive cerebellar disease, and 82% of the patients with autosomal recessive spinocerebellar degeneration. Memory and attentional deficits are found with apathy and psychomotor retardation and occasionally with depression or schizophrenia-like psychosis.

The recent literature contains syndrome-specific neuropsychiatric studies. Cognitive and behavior changes may be particularly prominent or presenting features of SCA-17, which can also have an HD-like phenotype (Bruni et al. 2004; Rolfs et al. 2003). SCA-1 can have prominent executive dysfunction, whereas mild verbal memory deficits can be seen in SCA-1, SCA-2, and SCA-3 (Burk et al. 2003) (SCA-3 is also known as Machado-Joseph disease). With disease progression, about one-third of patients with SCA-2 develop dementia (Geschwind 1999; Storey et al. 1999). SCA-12 is associated with cortical atrophy, and dementia can occur in later stages (O'Hearn et al. 2001). What is not yet clear from these studies is whether the similarities and overlaps in cognitive impairment are due to a common anatomical or pathophysiological basis, and many of the details regarding natural history remain to be elucidated (Kish et al. 1989).

Cerebellar ataxia itself is generally considered resistant to medications. Brief trials of many agents have been attempted, usually with minimal effect. Agents being investigated include buspirone, D-cycloserine, physostigmine, serotonergic agents, thyrotropin-releasing hormone, and acetazolamide (Ogawa 2004).

MOTOR NEURON DISEASE WITH DEMENTIA

Loss of strength with diminished muscle mass (amyotrophy) and dementia may be seen in motor neuron disease, also known as *amyotrophic lateral sclerosis* (ALS). Familial motor neuron disease may be isolated but has been reported within the setting of FTD, parkinsonism, and spinocerebellar degeneration (Rosenberg 1982).

Personality changes and hallucinations may occur in patients with ALS, and impairments in judgment, memory, abstract thinking, calculations, and anomia may occur

in individual patients. Whether patients without dementia but with sporadic ALS have a specific pattern of neuropsychological abnormalities remains to be elucidated (Gallassi et al. 1985; Montgomery and Erickson 1987).

The occurrence of dementia with ALS is the subject of a confusing classification, usually based on small clinical series. It has been called classic ALS with dementia (Wikstrom et al. 1982), dementia of motor neuron disease (Horoupian et al. 1984), progressive dementia with motor disease (Mitsuyama et al. 1985), and amyotrophy dementia complex (Morita et al. 1987). The disease may begin with personality changes or with motor system degeneration. Early personality changes may be seen in association with frontotemporal atrophy on CT, and the electroencephalogram result may be normal. Spongy changes are found in 90% of patients with gliosis. NFTs, Lewy bodies, and Pick bodies are not found. Extensive neuronal loss with gliosis is found in the substantia nigra in some cases (Horoupian et al. 1984). A loss of neurons occurs in layers 2 and 3 of the cortical mantle, particularly in the frontal and temporal regions. The syndrome of dementia with amyotrophy also may be found in Creutzfeldt-Jakob disease. In these latter cases, rapid decline is common, with an interval from onset to death of less than 1 year.

Western New Guinea, the Kii peninsula of Japan, and the island of Guam have a high incidence of ALS, often associated with parkinsonism and dementia. On Guam, 10% of adult deaths in the native Chomorro population result from ALS, and 7% are attributed to the Parkinson-dementia complex. In addition to bradykinesia and rigidity, mental slowing, apathy, and depression occur in the relative absence of aphasia, apraxia, or agnosia. Gross frontotemporal cortical atrophy is found at autopsy. NFTs are present in great abundance, with a relative absence of neuritic plaques in affected cortical regions, as well as in hippocampus, amygdala, and substantia nigra. Severe neuronal loss with depigmentation of the substantia nigra without Lewy body formation is seen. Pathological changes in the spinal cord include loss of anterior horn cells and neurofibrillary changes. Although various toxins have been implicated in its etiology, the exact cause of this symptom complex is unknown.

THALAMIC DEGENERATION

Thalamic degeneration may be found in isolation or rarely in association with multiple system atrophy. Abnormal movements of the limbs and trunk include tremor, choreoathetosis, and occasionally myoclonus. Alterations in sleep may be observed, such as in the prion-related disorder of fatal familial insomnia (Gambetti et al. 1995; Reder et al. 1995). Ataxia, paraparesis, blindness, spasticity, optic atrophy, nystagmus, and dysarthria also may be present. Aphasia, agnosia, and apraxia are usually absent. Depression may be prominent, and patients may be apathetic with personality changes and hypersomnolence. Memory and calculations are poor, and patients occasionally have incomprehensible spontaneous verbal output; judgment and calculations are impaired relatively early. Insight into the disease is limited. Severe gliosis and neuronal loss occur in the thalamus; gliosis and neuronal loss are also found in limbic projection nuclei.

Fatal familial insomnia is associated with a missense mutation at codon 178 and methionine homozygosity at codon 129 of the prion protein gene. In subjects who are heterozygotes at codon 129, expressing valine in the nonmutated allele, the disease has onset at a later age and slower progression. These latter individuals tend to have widespread cortical lesions along with ataxia and dysarthria. Fatal familial insomnia preferentially involves limbic thalamocortical circuits, correlating with the prominent sleep and autonomic disturbance, sympathetic hyperactivity, and flattening of circadian rhythms (Cortelli et al. 1999).

WILSON'S DISEASE

In Wilson's disease, also called hepatolenticular degeneration, the basal ganglia degenerate in association with abnormalities in liver function. It has autosomal recessive inheritance due to a mutation on chromosome 13 and is caused by a defect in copper metabolism, caused by a defective P-type adenosine triphosphatase (Cuthbert 1995; Petrukhin and Gilliam 1994). This leads to excessive copper deposition in the liver, corneas, and basal ganglia. Onset is usually in the second or third decade and is heralded by dystonia, parkinsonism, or cerebellar ataxia. Patients also may have dysarthria, dysphagia, hypophonia, or seizures. Chronic hepatitis or hemolytic anemia may be detected. Kayser-Fleischer rings are seen in nearly all patients with neurological Wilson's disease and consist of brown or green discolorations near the limbus of the cornea. Ventricular enlargement and cortical atrophy may be seen on computed tomographic scanning, and MRI detects abnormal signal in the lenticular nuclei, caudate nuclei, thalamus, dentate nuclei, and brain stem. The diagnosis may be established by slit-lamp examination of the cornea or laboratory studies reporting a serum ceruloplasmin level less than 20 mg/dL, a 24-hour copper excretion of more than 100 mg, or a liver biopsy showing increased hepatic copper concentration. Although the diagnosis may be relatively easy, Wilson's disease needs to be suspected in children and younger adults presenting with unknown hepatic or neuropsychiatric syndromes.

Affective and behavior changes may be the presenting symptoms of Wilson's disease and include schizophrenia-like changes, depression, or manic-depressive states. Sexual preoccupation and reduced sexual inhibitions are common. Aggressive and self-destructive or antisocial acts may be noted, and schizoid hysterical or sociopathic personality traits have been reported. Intellectual deterioration in Wilson's disease is relatively mild in the early symptomatic stages (Akil and Brewer 1995). Pathologically, patients have atrophy of the brain stem, dentate nucleus, and cerebellum with cavitary necrosis of the putamen.

Treatment of Wilson's disease consists of establishing and maintaining a negative copper balance. Induction is performed with either zinc or tetrathiomolybdate, and maintenance requires zinc or a copper-chelating agent such as trientine (trien) (Brewer 2005). D-Penicillamine has fallen out of favor because of multiple severe toxicities and the potential for severe worsening with initiation of therapy. Maintaining a copper-deficient diet also may be helpful. Patients with advanced disease may require liver transplantation. Neurological symptoms, including the dementia syndrome, improve with long-term therapy. Levodopa may be of some benefit in reversing neurological symptoms not improved by chelation or negative copper balance.

CALCIFICATION OF THE BASAL GANGLIA (FAHR'S DISEASE)

Calcification of the basal ganglia is a rare disorder that is sometimes inherited in an autosomal dominant fashion (Geschwind et al. 1999). Parkinsonism or dystonia may be combined with dementia and neuropsychiatric disturbances. Computed tomographic scans show extensive calcification of the basal ganglia and periventricular white matter. Patients may present in early adulthood with a schizophrenia-like psychosis or mood disorder or may present later in life with an extrapyramidal syndrome, dementia, and mood changes. Apathy, poor judgment, and memory are usually prominent, and language function is often spared. Cerebral blood flow to the calcified regions is markedly decreased and appears to correlate with the patient's condition (Uygur et al. 1995). Choreoathetosis, cerebellar ataxia, and dystonia also may be seen. Psychosis in calcification of the basal ganglia may respond to lithium.

Minor degrees of calcification in the basal ganglia or deep nuclei of the cerebellum are not uncommon and not pathological. However, dystrophic calcification occurs in pediatric acquired immune deficiency syndrome, Aicardi-Goutières syndrome, trisomy 21, Kearns-Sayre syndrome, and tumors or vascular lesions with dystrophic calcification. Pathological calcification of the basal ganglia has been associated with hypoparathyroidism, and there are case reports of association with astrocytomas. The pathogenesis of basal ganglia calcification is unknown (Baba et al. 2005).

PANTOTHENATE KINASE–ASSOCIATED NEURODEGENERATION

Pantothenate kinase–associated neurodegeneration was referred to in the past as Hallervorden-Spatz disease or as neurodegeneration with brain iron accumulation type 1 (NBIA-1; Arawaka et al. 1998). One reason that the newer name is preferred is the documentation of Hallervorden's association with euthanasia programs in Nazi Germany (Shevell 1992). NBIA-1 also has been supplanted because this term was thought to be too vague. Pantothenate kinase–associated neurodegeneration is a rare progressive autosomal recessive disease of childhood and adolescence characterized by stiffness of gait, distal wasting, dysarthria, and occasionally dementia. Brain iron accumulation also occurs in groups of nonspecific disorders encompassing the triad of pallidal iron deposition, axonal spheroids, and gliosis. This latter group has variable clinical findings and an age at onset from adolescence through middle age. Pantothenate kinase–associated neurodegeneration is part of the group of infantile neuraxonal dystrophies, of which it may be an allelic variant. Linkage to chromosome 20 has been documented (Gordon 2002).

Pathologically, olive or golden brown discoloration of the medial segment of the globus pallidus is seen. Some cases of pantothenate kinase–associated neurodegeneration show widespread α-synuclein–positive Lewy bodies and axonal swellings. Cases with and without lipid abnormalities, acanthocytosis, and pigmentary retinal degeneration have been reported (Arawaka et al. 1998; Halliday 1995; Newell et al. 1999). Neurochemical analysis in a single case of a 68-year-old man identified widespread dopamine deficiency in substantia nigra and striatum but relatively preserved limbic system dopamine concentrations (Jankovic et al. 1985).

CT shows mild atrophy with flattening of the caudate nucleus. MRI scans may show the so-called eye of the tiger sign, a result of bilateral hyperintensity of the rostral globus pallidus. There may be loss of T2-weighted signal in the substantia nigra pars reticularis, red nucleus, pulvinar, and globus pallidus resulting from iron accumulation (Lechner et al. 1999; Porter-Grenn et al. 1993; Tuite et al. 1996).

Granules of an iron-containing pigment similar to neuromelanin are found within and outside of neurons and hyperplastic astrocytes. Increased amounts of iron and other metals (zinc, copper, and calcium) are found in the affected tissue. Familial cases with autosomal recessive inheritance have been reported, and a gene localized to band 20p12.3–13 has been identified (Taylor et al. 1996).

Limited data on treatment of pantothenate kinase–associated neurodegeneration have been reported. Dystonia may respond to pallidotomy or thalamotomy, and dopa-responsive parkinsonism has been described (Justesen et al. 1999; Seibel et al. 1993; Tsukamoto et al. 1992; Tuite et al. 1996). No specific treatment for the dementia is available.

NORMAL-PRESSURE HYDROCEPHALUS

Normal-pressure hydrocephalus (NPH) is a syndrome composed of the triad of dementia, gait disturbance, and urinary incontinence. It may be associated with a history of meningitis, intracranial bleeding, or head injury (Friedland 1989). Idiopathic NPH cases are not uncommon among older patients presenting with hydrocephalus. A wide-based gait with slow steps and difficulty initiating locomotion are characteristic. Usually, no changes occur in motor strength or tone.

NPH is relatively easy to suspect, but difficult to diagnose. The diagnosis requires recognition of the symptoms and neuroimaging showing an enlarged ventricular system without corresponding cerebral atrophy. MRI scanning may show transependymal fluid flux. The difficulties in diagnosis arise in determining whether atrophy is congenital or merely age related, although enlargement of the temporal horns may be indicative of a true hydrocephalic picture. Conversely, it may be difficult to determine effectively that dementia in suspected NPH is not due to concomitant primary degenerative dementia. In series in which shunted patients also underwent brain biopsy, the prevalence of AD ranged from 31% to 50% (Savolainen et al. 1999).

The dementia of NPH presents primarily with attentional difficulties in the early stages. Anterograde memory deficits are usually absent in early NPH, although up to 50% of patients have some memory dysfunction (Fisher 1977). Language is typically spared early in the course, although late-stage patients may have an akinetic-mutism syndrome. "Frontal dysfunction," including apathy, lethargy, mental slowing, and perseveration, is extremely common in NPH. Occasional patients may present with psychosis as an initial symptom. The motor deficits of hydrocephalic patients may be similar to those seen in PD or other basal ganglia disorders. This may be because of the proximity of nigrostriatal pathways to the enlarged ventricles causing mass effect or ischemia (Curran and Lang 1994).

Dynamic testing begins with a high-volume lumbar puncture (up to 50 mL) and CSF pressure measurement and analysis, but this technique has low sensitivity. Transient improvement in gait, urinary incontinence, or neuropsychological functioning may help predict which individuals will respond to surgical treatment. Guidelines suggest that in equivocal cases or when the diagnosis is highly suspected, use of external lumbar drainage (up to 500 mL over several days) and CSF outflow resistance testing may confirm the diagnosis.

In carefully selected patients, CSF shunting may help up to 70% of patients (Bergsneider et al. 2005; Verrees and Selman 2004). The best cognitive results occur in patients whose cognitive disturbances are relatively mild and who have early onset of urinary incontinence and gait disturbance. Iddon and colleagues (1999) found that memory improved more than frontostriatal dysfunction after shunting. The presence of AD on concomitant brain biopsy does not preclude a successful outcome as measured by gait, restoration of urinary control, or psychometric study (Golomb et al. 2000). The use of programmable pressure valves reduces the complication rate of postshunting hematomas while ensuring optimal shunting in a given patient. Late shunt failure, as a result of mechanical failure or obstruction, may present as worsening clinical status (Williams et al. 1998).

Highlights for the Clinician

✦ **Accurate diagnosis** of dementias associated with motor dysfunction requires a full history, including family history of neurological and psychiatric disorders and medication exposures, and the physical examination is also key in differential diagnosis. Specific genetic testing may be available but often raises ethical questions.

✦ **The concept of cortical and subcortical dementias,** although heuristically useful, has serious anatomical, pathological, and neurochemical flaws.

✦ **Computed tomography and magnetic resonance neuroimaging** are useful primarily for excluding other sources of pathology in individuals with this class of disorders but are also important for diagnosis of normal-pressure hydrocephalus, Fahr's disease, neuropathological brain iron accumulation syndromes, and Wilson's disease. The role of functional imaging to differentiate disorders is limited at present.

✦ **The use of acetylcholinesterase inhibitors** is not universally indicated. Neurochemical evidence does not support the concept that all dementias are associated with degeneration of cholinergic markers. Evidence for use of memantine from well-controlled clinical trials is similarly lacking.

✦ **Huntington's disease** may present with motor, cognitive, or behavioral features, with onset most likely in the 40s and 50s. The age at onset is inversely related to the number of unstable trinucleotide repeats found on genetic testing.

✦ **Psychosis in Parkinson's disease** is often related to the use of dopaminergic agents and does not necessarily require neuroleptics for its treatment.

✦ **In individuals with a parkinsonian syndrome,** the symmetry of the rigidity is an important diagnostic feature: only Parkinson's disease and cortical–basal ganglionic degeneration show significant asymmetries. The rigidity in progressive supranuclear palsy is primarily in axial muscles.

✦ **Multiple system atrophy** is the least likely of the parkinsonian syndromes to be associated with dementia.

✦ **Dementia with Lewy bodies** may be underrecognized because of the low sensitivity of the diagnostic criteria.

✦ **Motor neuron disease** can be seen in isolation, in association with a frontal lobe syndrome, and in the context of a wider neurodegenerative disorder. A minority of such patients have a genetic disorder caused by mutations in the tau gene on chromosome 17.

✦ **Wilson's disease** may present with hepatic, psychiatric, or neurological symptoms, most commonly in adolescence or young adulthood. Recognition of its diagnostic possibility is the key to early diagnosis and treatment with good results through copper chelation therapy.

✦ **In normal-pressure hydrocephalus,** careful selection of patients for shunt placement can result in a high degree of success in symptom improvement. Dementia is the symptom least likely to improve, but the presence of concomitant Alzheimer's disease is not a complete contraindication to shunt placement.

RECOMMENDED READINGS

Huntington's Disease

Hague SM, Klaffke S, Bandmann O: Neurodegenerative disorders: Parkinson's disease and Huntington's disease. J Neurol Neurosurg Psychiatry 76:1058–1063, 2005

Landles C, Bates GP: Huntingtin and the molecular pathogenesis of Huntington's disease. Fourth in molecular medicine review series. EMBO Rep 5:958–963, 2004

Parkinson's Disease

Jankovic J: An update on the treatment of Parkinson's disease. Mt Sinai J Med 73:682–689, 2006

Savitt JM, Dawson VL, Dawson TM: Diagnosis and treatment of Parkinson disease: molecules to medicine. J Clin Invest 116:1744–1754, 2006

Dementia With Lewy Bodies

Lippa CF, Duda JE, Grossman M, et al: DLB and PDD boundary issues: diagnosis, treatment, molecular pathology, and biomarkers. Neurology 68:812–819, 2007

McKeith IG, Rowan E, Askew K, et al: Severe functional impairment in dementia with Lewy bodies than Alzheimer disease is related to extrapyramidal motor dysfunction. Am J Geriatr Psychiatry 14:582–588, 2006

Mosimann UP, Rowan EN, Partington CE, et al: Characteristics of visual hallucinations in Parkinson disease dementia and dementia with Lewy bodies. Am J Geriatr Psychiatry 14:153–160, 2006

Weisman D, McKeith I: Dementia with Lewy bodies. Semin Neurol 27:42–47, 2007

Progressive Supranuclear Palsy

Rampello L, Butta V, Raffaele R, et al: Progressive supranuclear palsy: a systematic review. Neurobiol Dis 20:179–186, 2005

Corticobasal Degeneration

Sha S, Hou C, Viskontas IV, et al: Are frontotemporal lobar degeneration, progressive supranuclear palsy and corticobasal degeneration distinct diseases? Nat Clin Pract Neurol 2:658–665, 2006

Frontotemporal Dementia

Boxer AL, Miller BL: Clinical features of frontotemporal dementia. Alzheimer Dis Assoc Disord 19 (suppl 1):S3–S6, 2005

Multiple System Atrophy

Bak TH, Rogers TT, Crawford LM, et al: Cognitive bedside assessment in atypical parkinsonian syndromes. J Neurol Neurosurg Psychiatry 76:420–422, 2005

Singer W, Opfer-Gehrking TL, McPhee BR, et al: Acetylcholinesterase inhibition: a novel approach in the treatment of neurogenic orthostatic hypotension. J Neurol Neurosurg Psychiatry 74:1294–1298, 2003

Freidreich's Ataxia and Spinocerebellar Ataxia

Geschwind DH: Focusing attention on cognitive impairment in spinocerebellar ataxia. Arch Neurol 56:20–22, 1999

Motor Neuron Disease With Dementia

Ringholz GM, Greene SR: The relationship between amyotrophic lateral sclerosis and frontotemporal dementia. Curr Neurol Neurosci Rep 6:387–392, 2006

Thalamic Degeneration

Montagna P, Gambetti P, Cortelli P, et al: Familial and sporadic fatal insomnia. Lancet Neurol 2:167–176. 2003

Wilson's Disease

Ala A, Walker AP, Ashkan K, et al: Wilson's disease. Lancet 369:397–408, 2007

Fahr's Disease

Geschwind DH, Loginov M, Stern JM: Identification of a locus on chromosome 14Q for idiopathic basal ganglia calcification (Fahr disease). Am J Hum Genet 65:764–772, 1999

Schmidt U, Mursch K, Halatsch ME: Symmetrical intracerebral and intracerebellar calcification ("Fahr's disease"). Funct Neurol 20:15, 2005

Pantothenate Kinase-Associated Neurodegeneration

Gregory A, Hayflick SJ: Neurodegeneration with brain iron accumulation. Folia Neuropathol 43:286–296, 2005

Nemeth AH: The genetics of primary dystonias and related disorders. Brain 125 (pt 4):695–721, 2002

Normal-Pressure Hydrocephalus

McGirt MJ, Woodworth G, Coon AL, et al: Diagnosis, treatment, and analysis of long-term outcomes in idiopathic normal-pressure hydrocephalus. Neurosurgery 57:699–705, 2005

Relkin N, Marmarou A, Klinge P, et al: Diagnosing idiopathic normal-pressure hydrocephalus. Neurosurgery 57 (3 suppl):S4–S16, 2005

REFERENCES

Aarsland D, Tandberg E, Larson JP, et al: Frequency of dementia in Parkinson's disease. Arch Neurol 53:538–542, 1996

Aarsland D, Andersen K, Larsen JP, et al: The rate of cognitive decline in Parkinson disease. Arch Neurol 61:1906–1911, 2004

Agid Y, Javoy-Agid F, Ruberg M, et al: Progressive supranuclear palsy: anatomoclinical and biochemical considerations, in Parkinson's Disease (Advances in Neurology Series, Vol 45). Edited by Yahr MD, Bergmann KJ. New York, Raven, 1986, pp 191–206

Akil M, Brewer GJ: Psychiatric and behavioral abnormalities in Wilson's disease, in Behavioral Neurology of Movement Disorders (Advances in Neurology Series, Vol 46). Edited by Weiner WS, Lang AE. New York, Raven, 1995, pp 171–178

Albert ML, Feldman RG, Willis AL: The "subcortical dementia" of progressive supranuclear palsy. J Neurol Neurosurg Psychiatry 37:121–130, 1974

Albin RL, Tagle DA: Genetics and molecular biology of Huntington's disease. Trends Neurosci 18:11–14, 1995

Aldrich MS, Foster NL, White RF, et al: Sleep abnormalities in progressive supranuclear palsy. Ann Neurol 25:577–581, 1989

Alexander GE, DeLong MR, Strick PL: Parallel organization of functionally segregated circuits linking basal ganglia and cortex. Annu Rev Neurosci 9:357–381, 1986

Apaydin H, Ahlskog JE, Parisi JE, et al: Parkinson disease neuropathology: later-developing dementia and loss of the levodopa response. Arch Neurol 59:102–112, 2002

Arawaka S, Saito Y, Murayama S, et al: Lewy body in neurodegeneration with brain iron accumulation type 1 is immunoreactive for alpha-synuclein. Neurology 51:887–889, 1998

Arendt T, Bigl V, Arendt A, et al: Loss of neurons in the nucleus basalis of Meynert in Alzheimer's disease, paralysis agitans, and Korsakoff's disease. Acta Neuropathol (Berl) 61:101–108, 1983

Arima K, Hirai S, Sunohara N, et al: Cellular co-localization of phosphorylated tau- and NACP/alpha-synuclein-epitopes in Lewy bodies in sporadic Parkinson's disease and in dementia with Lewy bodies. Brain Res 843:53–61, 1999

Baba Y, Broderick DF, Uitri RJ, et al: Heredofamilial brain calcinosis syndrome. Mayo Clin Proc 80:641–651, 2005

Bak TH, Rogers TT, Hearn VC, et al: Cognitive bedside assessment in atypical parkinsonian syndromes. J Neurol Neurosurg Psychiatry 76:420–422, 2005

Bamford K, Caine E, Kido D, et al: Clinical-pathologic correlation in Huntington's disease: a neuropsychological and computed tomography study. Neurology 39:796–801, 1989

Bayles KA: Language and Parkinson disease. Alzheimer Dis Assoc Disord 4:171–180, 1990

Bergeron C, Pollanen MS, Weyer L, et al: Cortical degeneration in progressive supranuclear palsy: a comparison with cortical-basal ganglionic degeneration. J Neuropathol Exp Neurol 56:726–734, 1997

Bergsneider M, Black PM, Klinge P, et al: Surgical management of idiopathic normal-pressure hydrocephalus. Neurosurgery 57 (3 suppl):S29–S39, 2005

Boller F, Mizutani R, Roessmann U, et al: Parkinson's disease, dementia, and Alzheimer's disease: clinicopathologic correlations. Ann Neurol 7:329–335, 1980

Boller F, Passafiume D, Keefe NC, et al: Visuospatial impairment in Parkinson's disease. Arch Neurol 41:485–490, 1984

Booth G: Psychodynamics in parkinsonism. Psychosom Med 10:1–14, 1948

Bowron A: Practical considerations in the use of apomorphine injectable. Neurology 62 (suppl 4):S32–S36, 2004

Braak H, Del Tredici K, Rub U, et al: Staging of brain pathology related to sporadic Parkinson's disease. Neurobiol Aging 24:197–211, 2003

Brandt J, Butters N: The neuropsychology of Huntington's disease. Trends Neurosci 9:118–120, 1986

Brandt J, Quaid SE, Folstein SE, et al: Presymptomatic diagnosis of delayed onset disease with linked DNA markers: the experience with Huntington's disease. JAMA 216:3108–3114, 1989

Brewer GJ: Neurologically presenting Wilson's disease: epidemiology, pathophysiology and treatment. CNS Drugs 19:185–192, 2005

Brown RE, Marsden CD: Visuospatial function in Parkinson's disease. Brain 109:987–1002, 1986

Brown RE, Marsden CD: "Subcortical dementia": the neuropsychological evidence. Neuroscience 25:363–387, 1988

Bruni AC, Takahashi-Fujigasaki J, Maltecca F, et al: Behavioral disorder, dementia, ataxia, and rigidity in a large family with TATA box-binding protein mutation. Arch Neurol 61:1314–1320, 2004

Burk K, Globas C, Bosch S, et al: Cognitive deficits in spinocerebellar ataxia type 1, 2, and 3. J Neurol 250:207–211, 2003

Burk K, Daum I, Rub U: Cognitive function in multiple system atrophy of the cerebellar type. Mov Disord 21:772–776, 2006

Butters N, Sax D, Montgomery K, et al: Comparison of the neuropsychological deficits associated with early and advanced Huntington's disease. Arch Neurol 35:585–589, 1978

Bylsma FW, Brandt J, Strauss ME: Aspects of procedural memory are differentially impaired in Huntington's disease. Arch Clin Neuropsychol 5:287–297, 1990

Cambier J, Masson M, Viader F, et al: Le syndrome frontal de la maladie de Steele-Richardson-Olszewski. Rev Neurol (Paris) 141:528–536, 1985

Celesia GG, Wanamaker WM: Psychiatric disturbances in Parkinson's disease. Dis Nerv Syst 33:577–583, 1972

Chaudhuri KR, Hu MT, Brooks DJ: Atypical parkinsonism in Afro-Caribbean and Indian origin immigrants to the UK. Mov Disord 15:18–23, 2000

Chui HC, Mortimer JA, Slager U, et al: Pathologic correlates of dementia in Parkinson's disease. Arch Neurol 43:991–995, 1986

Claes S, Van Zand K, Legius K, et al: Correlations between triplet repeat expansion and clinical features in Huntington's disease. Arch Neurol 52:749–753, 1995

Codori AM, Brandt J: Psychological costs and benefits of predictive testing for Huntington's disease. Am J Med Genet 54:174–184, 1994

Codori AM, Hanson R, Brandt J: Self-selection in predictive testing for Huntington's disease. Am J Med Genet 54:167–173, 1994

Cortelli P, Gambetti P, Montagna P, et al: Fatal familial insomnia: clinical features and molecular genetics. J Sleep Res 8 (suppl 1):23–29, 1999

Cummings JL (ed): Subcortical Dementia. New York, Oxford University Press, 1990

Cummings JL: Behavioral and psychiatric symptoms associated with Huntington's disease, in Behavioral Neurology of Movement Disorders (Advances in Neurology Series, Vol 65). Edited by Weiner WJ, Lang AE. New York, Raven, 1995, pp 179–186

Cummings JL, Benson DF: Psychological dysfunction accompanying subcortical dementias. Annu Rev Med 39:53–61, 1988

Cummings JL, Darkins A, Mendez M, et al: Alzheimer's disease and Parkinson's disease: comparison of speech and language alterations. Neurology 38:680–684, 1988

Curran T, Lang AE: Parkinsonian syndromes associated with hydrocephalus: case reports, a review of the literature, and pathophysiological hypotheses. Mov Disord 9:508–520, 1994

Cuthbert JA: Wilson's disease: a new gene and an animal model for an old disease. J Investig Med 43:323–326, 1995

D'Antona R, Baron JC, Samson Y, et al: Subcortical dementia: frontal cortex hypometabolism detected by positron tomography in patients with progressive supranuclear palsy. Brain 108:785–799, 1985

Destee A, Gray F, Parent M, et al: Obsessive-compulsive behavior and progressive supranuclear palsy. Rev Neurol 146:12–18, 1990

Diamond R, White RF, Myers RH, et al: Evidence of presymptomatic cognitive decline in Huntington's disease. J Clin Exp Neuropsychol 14:961–975, 1992

Dickson DW: Neuropathologic differentiation of progressive supranuclear palsy and corticobasal degeneration. J Neurol 246 (suppl 2):6–15, 1999

Dickson DW, Lin W, Liu WK, et al: Multiple system atrophy: a sporadic synucleinopathy. Brain Pathol 9:721–732, 1999

Diller L, Riklan M: Psychosocial factors in Parkinson's disease. J Am Geriatr Soc 4:1291–1300, 1956

Ebmeier KP, Calder SA, Craford JR, et al: Clinical features predicting dementia in idiopathic Parkinson's disease: a followup study. Neurology 40:1222–1224, 1990

Emre M, Aarsland D, Albanese A, et al: Rivastigmine for dementia associated with Parkinson's disease. N Engl J Med 351:2509–2518, 2004

Farrer LA, Conneally PM: A genetic model for age at onset in Huntington's disease. Am J Hum Genet 37:350–357, 1985

Feigin A, Kieburtz K, Bordwell K, et al: Functional decline in Huntington's disease. Mov Disord 10:211–214, 1995

Fergusson E, Howard R: Donepezil for the treatment of psychosis in dementia with Lewy bodies. Int J Geriatr Psychiatry 15:280–281, 2000

Ferman TJ, Smith GE, Boeve BF, et al: DLB fluctuations: specific features that reliably differentiate DLB from AD and normal aging. Neurology 62:181–187, 2004

Fisher CM: The clinical picture of normal pressure hydrocephalus. Clin Neurosurg 24:270–284, 1977

Folstein MF, Folstein SE, McHugh PR: Mini-Mental State: a practical method for grading the cognitive state of patients for the clinician. J Psychiatr Res 12:189–198, 1975

Folstein SE: Huntington's Disease: A Disorder of Families. Baltimore, MD, Johns Hopkins University Press, 1989

Folstein SE, Chase GA, Wahl WE, et al: Huntington's disease in Maryland: clinical aspects of racial variation. Am J Hum Genet 41:168–179, 1987

Folstein SE, Brandt J, Folstein MF: Huntington's disease, in Subcortical Dementia. Edited by Cummings JL. New York, Oxford University Press, 1990, pp 87–107

Ford MF: Treatment of depression in Huntington's disease with monoamine oxidase inhibitors. Br J Psychiatry 149:654–656, 1986

Freedman M: Parkinson's disease, in Subcortical Dementia. Edited by Cummings JL. New York, Oxford University Press, 1990, pp 108–122

Friedland RP: "Normal" pressure hydrocephalus and the saga of the treatable dementias. JAMA 262:2577–2581, 1989

Frisoni GB, Pizzolato G, Zanetti O, et al: Corticobasal degeneration: neuropsychological assessment and dopamine D_2 receptor SPECT analysis. Eur Neurol 35:50–54, 1995

Furtado S, Suchowersky O: Huntington's disease: recent advances in diagnosis and management. Can J Neurol Sci 22:5–12, 1995

Gallassi P, Montagna P, Ciardulli C, et al: Cognitive impairment in motor neuron disease. Acta Neurol Scand 71:480–484, 1985

Galloway PG: Antigenic characteristics of neurofibrillary tangles in progressive supranuclear palsy. Neurosci Lett 91:148–153, 1988

Galvin JE, Uryu K, Lee VM, et al: Axon pathology in Parkinson's disease and Lewy body dementia hippocampus contains alpha-, beta-, and gamma-synuclein. Proc Natl Acad Sci U S A 96:13450–13455, 1999

Gambetti P, Parchi P, Petersen RB, et al: Fatal familial insomnia and familial Creutzfeldt-Jakob disease: clinical, pathological and molecular features. Brain Pathol 5:43–51, 1995

Geschwind DH: Focusing attention on cognitive impairment in spinocerebellar ataxia. Arch Neurol 56:20–22, 1999

Geschwind DH, Loginov M, Stern JM: Identification of a locus on chromosome 14Q for idiopathic basal ganglia calcification (Fahr disease). Am J Hum Genet 65:764–772, 1999

Gilman S, Low PA, Quinn N, et al: Consensus statement on the diagnosis of multiple system atrophy. J Auton Nerv Syst 74:189–192, 1998

Giordani B, Berent S, Boivin MJ, et al: Longitudinal neuropsychological and genetic linkage analysis of persons at risk for Huntington's disease. Arch Neurol 52:59–64, 1995

Golbe LI, Davis PH, Schoenberg BS, et al: Prevalence and natural history of progressive supranuclear palsy. Neurology 38:1031–1034, 1988

Golomb J, Wisoff J, Miller DC, et al: Alzheimer's disease comorbidity in normal pressure hydrocephalus: prevalence and shunt response. J Neurol Neurosurg Psychiatry 68:778–781, 2000

Gordon N: Pantothenate kinase-associated neurodegeneration (Hallervorden-Spatz syndrome). Eur J Paediatr Neurol 6:243–247, 2002

Grafman J, Litvan I, Gomez C, et al: Frontal lobe function in progressive supranuclear palsy. Arch Neurol 47:553–558, 1990

Growdon JH, Corkin S: Cognitive impairments in Parkinson's disease, in Parkinson's Disease (Advances in Neurology Series, Vol 45). Edited by Yahr MD, Bergmann KJ. New York, Raven, 1986, pp 383–392

Gusella J, Wexler NS, Conneally PM, et al: A polymorphic DNA marker genetically linked to Huntington's disease. Nature 306:234–238, 1983

Hakim AM, Mathieson G: Dementia in Parkinson disease: a neuropathologic study. Neurology 29:1209–1214, 1979

Halliday W: The nosology of Hallervorden-Spatz disease. J Neurol Sci 134(suppl):84–91, 1995

Harper PS: The epidemiology of Huntington's disease. Hum Genet 89:365–376, 1992

Hayden MR, Bloch M, Wiggins S: Psychological effects of predictive testing for Huntington's disease, in Behavioral Neurology of Movement Disorders (Advances in Neurology Series, Vol 65). Edited by Weiner WS, Lang AE. New York, Raven, 1995, pp 201–210

Hedera P, Cohen ML, Lerner AJ, et al: Dementia preceding motor symptoms in Parkinson's disease: a case study. Neuropsychiatry Neuropsychol Behav Neurol 7:67–72, 1994

Hersch S, Jones R, Koroshetz W, et al: The neurogenetics genie: testing for the Huntington's disease mutation. Neurology 44:1369–1373, 1994

Hirono N, Ishii K, Sasaki M, et al: Features of regional cerebral glucose metabolism abnormality in corticobasal degeneration. Dement Geriatr Cogn Disord 11:139–146, 2000

Hohl U, Tiraboschi P, Hansen LA, et al: Diagnostic accuracy of dementia with Lewy bodies. Arch Neurol 57:347–351, 2000

Horoupian DL, Thal L, Katzman R, et al: Dementia and motor neuron disease: morphometric, biochemical, and Golgi studies. Ann Neurol 16:305–313, 1984

Hubble JP, Koller WC: The parkinsonian personality. Adv Neurol 65:43–48, 1995

Hugdahl K, Wester K: Neurocognitive correlates of stereotactic thalamotomy and thalamic stimulation in parkinsonian patients. Brain Cogn 42:231–252, 2000

Huntington G: On chorea, in Huntington's Chorea: 1872–1972 (Advances in Neurology Series, Vol 1). Edited by Barbeau A. New York, Raven, 1973, pp 33–35

Huntington's Disease Collaborative Research Group: A novel gene containing a trinucleotide repeat that is expanded and unstable on Huntington's disease chromosomes. Cell 72:971–983, 1993

Hurtig HI, Trojanowski JQ, Galvin J, et al: Alpha-synuclein cortical Lewy bodies correlate with dementia in Parkinson's disease. Neurology 54:1916–1921, 2000

Iddon JL, Pickard JD, Cross JJ, et al: Specific patterns of cognitive impairment in patients with idiopathic normal pressure hydrocephalus and Alzheimer's disease: a pilot study. J Neurol Neurosurg Psychiatry 67:723–732, 1999

Jankovic J, Kirkpatrick JB, Blomquist KA, et al: Late-onset Hallervorden-Spatz disease presenting as familial parkinsonism. Neurology 35:227–234, 1985

Jason GW, Pajurkova EM, Suchowersky O, et al: Presymptomatic neuropsychological impairment in Huntington's disease. Arch Neurol 45:769–773, 1988

Jellinger K: Overview of morphological changes in Parkinson's disease, in Parkinson's Disease (Advances in Neurology Series, Vol 45). Edited by Yahr MD, Bergmann KJ. New York, Raven, 1986, pp 1–18

Josephs KA, Parisi JE, Knopman DS, et al: Clinically undetected motor neuron disease in pathologically proven frontotemporal lobar degeneration with motor neuron disease. Arch Neurol 63:506–512, 2006

Justesen CR, Penn RD, Kroin JS, et al: Stereotactic pallidotomy in a child with Hallervorden-Spatz disease: case report. J Neurosurg 90:551–554, 1999

Kampoliti K, Goetz CG, Boeve BF, et al: Clinical presentation and pharmacological therapy in corticobasal degeneration. Arch Neurol 55:957–961, 1998

Kessler H: Epidemiological studies of Parkinson's disease, III: a community based study. Am J Epidemiol 96:242–254, 1972

Kish SJ, Robitaille Y, el-Awar M, et al: Non–Alzheimer-type pattern of brain choline acetyltransferase reduction in dominantly inherited olivopontocerebellar atrophy. Ann Neurol 26:362–367, 1989

Kostic VS, Filipovic SR, Lecic D, et al: Effect of age at onset on frequency of depression in Parkinson's disease. J Neurol Neurosurg Psychiatry 57:1265–1267, 1994

Kumar R, Lozano AM, Sime E, et al: Comparative effects of unilateral and bilateral subthalamic nucleus deep brain stimulation. Neurology 53:561–566, 1999

Lang AE: Corticobasal degeneration: selected developments. Mov Disord 18 (suppl 6):S51–S56, 2003

Langston JW, Ballard P, Tetrud JW, et al: Chronic parkinsonism in humans due to a product of meperidine-analog synthesis. Science 219:979–980, 1983

Laureys S, Salmon E, Garraux G, et al: Fluorodopa uptake and glucose metabolism in early stages of corticobasal degeneration. J Neurol 246:1151–1158, 1999

Lechner C, Meisenzahl EM, Uhlemann H, et al: [Hallervorden-Spatz syndrome: differential diagnosis of early onset dementia] (German). Nervenarzt 70:471–475, 1999

Leenders KL, Frackowiak RS, Lees AJ: Steele-Richardson-Olszewski syndrome: brain energy metabolism, blood flow and fluorodopa uptake measured by positron emission tomography. Brain 111:615–630, 1988

Leigh RJ, Riley DE: Eye movements in parkinsonism: it's saccadic speed that counts. Neurology 54:1018–1019, 2000

Leigh RJ, Newman SA, Folstein SE, et al: Abnormal ocular motor control in Huntington's disease. Neurology 33:1268–1275, 1983

Levin BE: Spatial cognition in Parkinson's disease. Alzheimer Dis Assoc Disord 4:161–170, 1990

Levin BE, Llabre MM, Weiner WJ: Cognitive impairments associated with early Parkinson's disease. Neurology 39:557–561, 1989

Levy ML, Cummings JL, Fairbanks LA, et al: Apathy is not depression. J Neuropsychiatry Clin Neurosci 10:314–319, 1998

Lieberman A, Dziatolowski M, Coopersmith M, et al: Dementia in Parkinson's disease. Ann Neurol 6:355–359, 1979

Lishman WA: Organic Psychiatry: The Psychological Consequences of Cerebral Disorder. Oxford, UK, Blackwell Scientific, 1978

Litvan I, Hauw JJ, Bartko JJ, et al: Validity and reliability of the preliminary NINDS neuropathologic criteria for progressive supranuclear palsy and related disorders. J Neuropathol Exp Neurol 55:97–105, 1996

Litvan I, Campbell G, Mangone CA, et al: Which clinical features differentiate progressive supranuclear palsy (Steele-Richardson-Olszewski syndrome) from related disorders? A clinicopathological study. Brain 120:65–74, 1997

Litvan I, Cummings JL, Mega M: Neuropsychiatric features of corticobasal degeneration. J Neurol Neurosurg Psychiatry 65:717–721, 1998a

Litvan I, MacIntyre A, Goetz CG, et al: Accuracy of the clinical diagnoses of Lewy body disease, Parkinson disease, and dementia with Lewy bodies: a clinicopathologic study. Arch Neurol 55:969–978, 1998b

Litvan I, Grimes DA, Lang AE, et al: Clinical features differentiating patients with postmortem confirmed progressive supranuclear palsy and corticobasal degeneration. J Neurol 246 (suppl 2):1–5, 1999

Louis ED, Klatka LA, Liu Y, et al: Comparison of extrapyramidal features in 31 pathologically confirmed cases of diffuse Lewy body disease and 34 pathologically confirmed cases of Parkinson's disease. Neurology 48:376–380, 1997

Lucetti C, Del Dotto P, Gambaccini G, et al: IV amantadine improves chorea in Huntington's disease: an acute randomized, controlled study. Neurology 60:1995–1997, 2003

Lucking CB, Durr A, Bonifati V, et al: Association between early onset Parkinson's disease and mutations in the Parkin gene. N Engl J Med 342:1560–1567, 2000

Maher ER, Smith EM, Lees AJ, et al: Cognitive deficits in the Steele-Richardson-Olszewski syndrome (progressive supranuclear palsy). J Neurol Neurosurg Psychiatry 48:1234–1239, 1985

Maloteaux JM, Vanisberg MA, Laterre C, et al: [^{3}H]GBR 12935 binding to dopamine uptake sites: subcellular localization and reduction in Parkinson's disease and progressive supranuclear palsy. Eur J Pharmacol 156:331–340, 1988

Marder K, Flood P, Cote, L, et al: A pilot study of risk factors for dementia in Parkinson's disease. Mov Disord 5:156–161, 1990

Marder K, Tang MX, Cote L, et al: The frequency and associated risk factors for dementia in patients with Parkinson's disease. Arch Neurol 52:695–701, 1995

Martilla RJ, Rinne UK: Dementia in Parkinson's disease. Acta Neurol Scand 54:431–441, 1976

Martilla RJ, Rinne UK: Smoking and Parkinson's disease. Acta Neurol Scand 62:322–325, 1980

Martin JB, Gusella JF: Huntington's disease: pathogenesis and management. N Engl J Med 20:1267–1276, 1986

Matison R, Mayeux R, Rosen J, et al: "Tip of the tongue" phenomenon in Parkinson's disease. Neurology 32:567–570, 1982

Mayeux R: Dementia in extrapyramidal disorders. Curr Opin Neurol Neurosurg 3:98–102, 1990

Mayeux R, Stern Y, Rosen J, et al: Is "subcortical dementia" a recognizable clinical entity? Ann Neurol 14:278–283, 1983

Mayeux R, Stern Y, Cote L, et al: Altered serotonin metabolism in depressed patients with Parkinson's disease. Neurology 34:642–646, 1984

Mayeux R, Stern Y, Herman A, et al: Correlates of early disability in Huntington's disease. Ann Neurol 20:727–731, 1986a

Mayeux R, Stern Y, Williams JBW, et al: Clinical and biochemical features of depression in Parkinson's disease. Am J Psychiatry 143:756–759, 1986b

Mayeux R, Stern Y, Sano M, et al: The relationship of serotonin to depression in Parkinson's disease. Mov Disord 3:236–244, 1988

McHugh PR, Folstein ME: Psychiatric syndromes in Huntington's disease: a clinical and phenomenologic study, in Psychiatric Aspects of Neurologic Disease. Edited by Benson DF, Blumer D. New York, Grune & Stratton, 1975, pp 267–285

McKeith IG, Galasko D, Kosaka K, et al: Consensus guidelines for the clinical and pathological diagnosis of dementia with Lewy bodies (DLB): report of the Consortium on DLB International Workshop. Neurology 47:1113–1124, 1996

McKeith IG, Ballard CG, Perry RH, et al: Prospective validation of consensus criteria for the diagnosis of dementia with Lewy bodies. Neurology 54:1050–1058, 2000

McKeith IG, Dickson DW, Lowe J, et al: Diagnosis and management of dementia with Lewy bodies: third report of the DLB Consortium. Neurology 65:1863–1872, 2006

Mendez MF: Huntington's disease: update and review of neuropsychiatric aspects. Int J Psychiatry Med 24:189–208, 1994

Menza MA, Mark MH: Parkinson's disease: the relationship to disability and personality. J Neuropsychiatry Clin Neurosci 6:165–169, 1994

Menza MA, Rosen RC: Sleep in Parkinson's disease: the role of depression and anxiety. Psychosomatics 36:262–266, 1995

Menza MA, Golbe LI, Cody RA, et al: Dopamine-related personality traits in Parkinson's disease. Neurology 43 (3 pt 1):505–508, 1993

Mitsuyama Y, Kogoh H, Ata K, et al: Progressive dementia with motor neuron disease: an additional case report and neuropathological review of 20 cases in Japan. Eur Arch Psychiatry Neurol Sci 235:1–8, 1985

Mjones H: Paralysis agitans, a clinical and genetic study. Acta Psychiatr Scand 54:1–195, 1949

Monckton DG, Caskey CT: Unstable triplet repeat diseases. Circulation 91:513–520, 1995

Montgomery GK, Erickson LM: Neuropsychological perspectives in amyotrophic lateral sclerosis. Neurol Clin 5:61–81, 1987

Morita K, Kaiya H, Ikeda T, et al: Presenile dementia combined with amyotrophy: a review of 34 Japanese cases. Arch Gerontol Geriatr 6:263–277, 1987

Morris JC, Cole M, Banker BQ, et al: Hereditary dysphasic dementia and the Pick-Alzheimer spectrum. Ann Neurol 16:455–466, 1984

Morris M: Dementia and cognitive changes in Huntington's disease, in Behavioral Neurology of Movement Disorders (Advances in Neurology Series, Vol 65). Edited by Weiner WS, Lang AE. New York, Raven, 1995, pp 187–200

Moss MB, Albert MS, Butters N, et al: Differential patterns of memory loss among patients with Alzheimer's disease, Huntington's disease, and alcoholic Korsakoff's syndrome. Arch Neurol 43:239–246, 1986

Motsinger CD, Perron GA, Lacy TJ: Use of atypical antipsychotic drugs in patients with dementia. Am Fam Physician 67:2335–2340, 2003

Newell KL, Boyer P, Gomez-Tortosa E, et al: Alpha-synuclein immunoreactivity is present in axonal swellings in neuroaxonal dystrophy and acute traumatic brain injury. J Neuropathol Exp Neurol 58:1263–1268, 1999

Ogawa M: Pharmacological treatments of cerebellar ataxia. Cerebellum 3:107–111, 2004

O'Hearn E, Holmes SE, Calvert PC, et al: SCA-12: tremor with cerebellar and cortical atrophy is associated with a CAG repeat expansion. Neurology 56:299–303, 2001

Okuda B, Tachibana H, Kawabata K, et al: Cerebral blood flow in corticobasal degeneration and progressive supranuclear palsy. Alzheimer Dis Assoc Disord 1491:46–52, 2000

O'Suilleabhain P, Dewey RB Jr: A randomized trial of amantadine in Huntington disease. Arch Neurol 60:996–998, 2003

Parsa MA, Bastani B: Quetiapine (Seroquel) in the treatment of psychosis in patients with Parkinson's disease. J Neuropsychiatry Clin Neurosci 10:216–219, 1998

Pearson SJ, Reynolds GP: Neocortical neurotransmitter markers in Huntington's disease. J Neural Transm Gen Sect 98:197–207, 1994

Petrukhin K, Gilliam TC: Genetic disorders of copper metabolism. Curr Opin Pediatr 6:698–701, 1994

Pierot L, Desnos C, Blin J, et al: D1 and D2-type dopamine receptors in patients with Parkinson's disease and progressive supranuclear palsy. J Neurol Sci 86:291–306, 1988

Pillon B, Blin J, Vidailhet M, et al: The neuropsychological pattern of corticobasal degeneration: comparison with progressive supranuclear palsy and Alzheimer's disease. Neurology 45:1477–1483, 1995

Pirozzolo FJ, Hansch EC, Mortimer JA, et al: Dementia in Parkinson disease: a neuropsychological analysis. Brain Cogn 1:71–83, 1982

Pollock M, Hornabrook RW: The prevalence, natural history and dementia of Parkinson's disease. Brain 89:429–448, 1966

Porter-Grenn L, Silbergleit R, Mehta BA: Hallervorden-Spatz disease with bilateral involvement of globus pallidus and substantia nigra: MR demonstration. J Comput Assist Tomogr 17:961–963, 1993

Probst A, Langui D, Lautenschlager C, et al: Progressive supranuclear palsy: extensive neuropil threads in addition to neurofibrillary tangles: very similar antigenicity of subcortical neuronal pathology in progressive supranuclear palsy and Alzheimer's disease. Acta Neuropathol 77:61–68, 1988

Rajput AH, Offord KP, Beard CM, et al: Epidemiology of parkinsonism: incidence, classification and mortality. Ann Neurol 16:278–282, 1984

Ranen NG, Peyser CE, Folstein SE: ECT as a treatment for depression in Huntington's disease. J Neuropsychiatry Clin Neurosci 6:154–159, 1994

Reder AT, Mednick AS, Brown P, et al: Clinical and genetic features of fatal familial insomnia. Neurology 45:1068–1075, 1995

Riley DE: Reversible transvestic fetishism in a man with Parkinson's disease treated with selegiline. Clin Neuropharmacol 25:234–237, 2002

Riley DE, Lang AE, Lewis A, et al: Cortical-basal ganglionic degeneration. Neurology 40:1203–1212, 1990

Ring HA, Bench CJ, Trimble MR, et al: Depression in Parkinson's disease: a positron emission study. Br J Psychiatry 165:333–339, 1994

Robbins TW, James M, Lange KW, et al: Cognitive performance in multiple system atrophy. Brain 115:271–291, 1992

Rolfs A, Koeppen AH, Bauer I, et al: Clinical features and neuropathology of autosomal dominant spinocerebellar ataxia (SCA17). Ann Neurol 54:367–375, 2003

Rosenberg RN: Amyotrophy in multisystem genetic diseases, in Human Motor Neuron Diseases. Edited by Rowland LP. New York, Raven, 1982, pp 149–157

Ruberg M, Javoy-Agid F, Hirsch E, et al: Dopaminergic and cholinergic lesions in progressive supranuclear palsy. Ann Neurol 18:523–529, 1985

Sabbagh MN, Corey-Bloom J, Tiraboschi P, et al: Neurochemical markers do not correlate with cognitive decline in the Lewy body variant of Alzheimer disease. Arch Neurol 45:1458–1461, 1999

Saint-Cyr JA, Taylor AE, Lang AE: Neuropsychological and psychiatric side effects in the treatment of Parkinson's disease. Neurology 43 (suppl 6):S47–S52, 1993

Samuel W, Alford M, Hofstetter CR, et al: Dementia with Lewy bodies versus pure Alzheimer disease: differences in cognition, neuropathology, cholinergic dysfunction, and synapse density. J Neuropathol Exp Neurol 56:499–508, 1997a

Samuel W, Crowder R, Hofstetter CR, et al: Neuritic plaques in the Lewy body variant of Alzheimer disease lack paired helical filaments. Neurosci Lett 223:73–76, 1997b

Sands IR: The type of personality susceptible to Parkinson disease. J Mt Sinai Hosp N Y 9:792–794, 1942

Savoiardo M, Strada L, Girotti F, et al: MR imaging in progressive supranuclear palsy and Shy-Drager syndrome. J Comput Assist Tomogr 13:555–560, 1989

Savolainen S, Paljarvi L, Vapalahti M: Prevalence of Alzheimer's disease in patients investigated for presumed normal pressure hydrocephalus: a clinical and neuropathological study. Acta Neurochir (Wien) 141:849–853, 1999

Sawle GV, Brooks DJ, Marsden CD, et al: Corticobasal degeneration: a unique pattern of regional cortical oxygen hypometabolism and striatal fluorodopa uptake demonstrated by positron emission tomography. Brain 114 (pt 1B):541–556, 1991

Sax DS, O'Donnell B, Butters N, et al: Computer tomographic, neurologic, and neuropsychological correlates of Huntington's disease. Int J Neurosci 18:21–36, 1983

Schiffer R, Kurlan R, Rubin AJ, et al: Evidence for atypical depression in Parkinson's disease. Am J Psychiatry 145:1020–1022, 1988

Schlossmacher MG, Hamann C, Cole AG, et al: Case records of the Massachusetts General Hospital: weekly clinicopathological exercises. Case 27-2004: a 79-year-old woman with disturbances in gait, cognition, and autonomic function. N Engl J Med 351:912–922, 2004

Schmand B, de Bie RM, Koning-Haanstra M, et al: Unilateral pallidotomy in PD: a controlled study of cognitive and behavioral effects. The Netherlands Pallidotomy Study (NEPAS) group. Neurology 54:1058–1064, 2000

Schneider LS, Gleason RP, Chui HC: Progressive supranuclear palsy with agitation: response to trazodone but not to thiothixene or carbamazepine. J Geriatr Psychiatry Neurol 2:109–112, 1989

Seibel MO, Date ES, Zeiner H, et al: Rehabilitation of patients with Hallervorden-Spatz syndrome. Arch Phys Med Rehabil 74:328–329, 1993

Shevell M: Racial hygiene, active euthanasia, and Julius Hallervorden. Neurology 42:2214–2219, 1992

Shiwach RS, Norbury CG: A controlled psychiatric study of individuals at risk for Huntington's disease. Br J Psychiatry 165:500–505, 1994

Shoulson I: Care of patients and families with Huntington's disease, in Movement Disorders. Edited by Marsden CD, Fahn S. London, Butterworths International Medical Reviews, 1982, pp 277–290

Skre H: Spino-cerebellar ataxia in western Norway. Clin Genet 6:265–288, 1974

Soliveri P, Monza D, Paridi D, et al: Cognitive and magnetic resonance imaging aspects of corticobasal degeneration and progressive supranuclear palsy. Neurology 53:502–507, 1999

Starkstein SE, Brandt J, Folstein S, et al: Neuropsychologic and neuropathologic correlates in Huntington's disease. J Neurol Neurosurg Psychiatry 51:1259–1263, 1988

Starkstein SE, Berthier ML, Bolduc PL, et al: Depression in patients with early versus late onset of Parkinson's disease. Neurology 39:1441–1445, 1989

Starr PA, Vitek JL, Bakay RAE: Ablative surgery and deep brain stimulation for Parkinson's disease. Neurosurgery 43:989–1015, 1998

Stewart JT, Mounts ML, Clark RL: Aggressive behavior in Huntington's disease: treatment with propranolol. J Clin Psychiatry 48:106–108, 1987

Storey E, Forrest SM, Shaw JH, et al: Spinocerebellar ataxia type 2: clinical features of a pedigree displaying prominent frontal-executive dysfunction. Arch Neurol 56:43–50, 1999

Strauss ME, Brandt J: Are there neuropsychologic manifestations of the gene for Huntington's disease in asymptomatic, at-risk individuals? Arch Neurol 47:905–908, 1990

Sutcliffe RLG: Parkinson's disease in the district of Northampton Health Authority, United Kingdom—a study of prevalence and disability. Acta Neurol Scand 72:363–379, 1985

Tagliavini F, Pilleri G, Bouras C, et al: The basal nucleus of Meynert in idiopathic Parkinson's disease. Acta Neurol Scand 69:20–28, 1984

Takahashi H, Oyanagi K, Takeda S, et al: Occurrence of 15-nm-wide straight tubules in neocortical neurons in progressive supranuclear palsy. Acta Neuropathol (Berl) 79:233–239, 1989

Talbot PR, Lloyd JJ, Snowden JS, et al: A clinical role for 99mTc-HMPAO SPECT in the investigation of dementia? J Neurol Neurosurg Psychiatry 64:306–313, 1998

Taylor ND, Litt M, Kramer P, et al: Homozygosity mapping of Hallervorden-Spatz syndrome to chromosome 20p12.3–p13. Nat Genet 16:479–481, 1996

Troster AI, Stalp LD, Paolo AM, et al: Neuropsychological impairment in Parkinson's disease with and without depression. Arch Neurol 52:1164–1169, 1995

Tsukamoto H, Inui K, Taniike M, et al: A case of Hallervorden-Spatz disease: progressive intractable dystonia controlled by bilateral thalamotomy. Brain Dev 14:269–272, 1992

Tuite PJ, Provias JP, Lang AE: Atypical dopa responsive parkinsonism in a patient with megalencephaly, midbrain Lewy body disease, and some pathological features of Hallervorden-Spatz disease. J Neurol Neurosurg Psychiatry 61:523–527, 1996

Uygur GA, Liu Y, Hellman RS, et al: Evaluation of regional cerebral blood flow in massive intracranial calcification. J Nucl Med 36:610–612, 1995

Vanacore N, Bonifati V, Fabbrini G, et al: Smoking habits in multiple system atrophy and progressive nuclear palsy. European Study Group on Atypical Parkinsonisms. Neurology 54:114–119, 2000

Verghese J, Crystal HA, Dickson DW, et al: Validity of clinical criteria for the diagnosis of dementia with Lewy bodies. Neurology 53:1974–1982, 1999

Verrees M, Selman WR: Management of normal pressure hydrocephalus. Am Fam Physician 70:1071–1078, 2004

Villardita C, Smirni P, Le Pira F, et al: Mental deterioration, visuoperceptive disabilities and constructional apraxia in Parkinson's disease. Acta Neurol Scand 66:112–120, 1982

von Hafften AH, Jensen CF: Paradoxical response to pindolol treatment for aggression in a patient with Huntington's disease. J Clin Psychiatry 50:230–231, 1989

Walker MP, Ayre GA, Cummings JL, et al: Quantifying fluctuation in dementia with Lewy bodies, Alzheimer's disease, and vascular dementia. Neurology 54:1616–1625, 2000

Walker Z, Allen RL, Shergill S, et al: Three years survival in patients with a clinical diagnosis of dementia with Lewy bodies. Int J Geriatr Psychiatry 15:267–273, 2000

Weintraub D, Moberg PJ, Duda JE, et al: Recognition and treatment of depression in Parkinson's disease. J Geriatr Psychiatry Neurol 16:178–183, 2003

Wenning G K, Ben-Shlomo Y, Hughes A, et al: What clinical features are most useful to distinguish definite multiple system atrophy from Parkinson's disease? J Neurol Neurosurg Psychiatry 68:434–440, 2000

Wexler NS: Perceptual, motor, cognitive, and emotional characteristics of persons at risk for Huntington's disease, in Huntington's Disease (Advances in Neurology Series, Vol 23). Edited by Chase TN, Wexler NS, Barbeau A. New York, Raven, 1979, pp 257–271

Wexler NS, Lorimer J, Porter J, et al: Venezuelan kindreds reveal that genetic and environmental factors modulate Huntington's disease age of onset. Proc Natl Acad Sci U S A 101:3498–3503, 2004

Whitehouse PJ: The concept of subcortical and cortical dementia: another look. Ann Neurol 19:1–6, 1986

Whitehouse PJ, Hedreen JC, White CL, et al: Basal forebrain neurons in the dementia of Parkinson's disease. Ann Neurol 13:243–248, 1983

Whitehouse PJ, Martino AM, Marcus KA, et al: Reductions in acetylcholine and nicotine binding in several degenerative diseases. Arch Neurol 45:722–724, 1988

Wikstrom J, Patenu A, Palo J, et al: Classic amyotrophic lateral sclerosis with dementia. Arch Neurol 39:681–683, 1982

Williams MA, Razumovsky AY, Hanley DF: Evaluation of shunt function in patients who are never better, or better than worse after shunt surgery for NPH. Acta Neurochir (Wien) 71:368–370, 1998

Witt K, Pulkowski U, Herzog J, et al: Deep brain stimulation of the subthalamic nucleus improves cognitive flexibility but impairs response inhibition in Parkinson disease. Arch Neurol 61:697–700, 2004

Yamauchi H, Fukuyama H, Nagahama Y, et al: Atrophy of the corpus callosum, cortical hypometabolism, and cognitive impairment in corticobasal degeneration. Arch Neurol 55:609–614, 1998

Zappacosta B, Monza D, Meoni C, et al: Psychiatric symptoms do not correlate with cognitive decline, motor symptoms, or CAG repeat length in Huntington's disease. Arch Neurol 53:493–497, 1996

25

NEUROPSYCHIATRIC ASPECTS OF ALZHEIMER'S DISEASE AND OTHER DEMENTING ILLNESSES

Liana G. Apostolova, M.D.

Jeffrey L. Cummings, M.D.

The dementias are a large group of neuropsychiatric disorders that preferentially affect the elderly. Their socioeconomic significance is steadily increasing as the number of elderly persons continues to rise. The most common dementia—Alzheimer's disease (AD)—accounts for 60%–70% of all dementias in older individuals. More than 90% of all patients with AD are 65 years or older. AD currently affects 4.5 million Americans, and the number will reach 13.2 million by the year 2050 in the United States alone (Hebert et al. 2003). The second most common dementia—dementia with Lewy bodies (DLB)—accounts for 15%–20% of the newly diagnosed cases, and vascular dementia (VaD) accounts for another 5%–10% (Corey-Bloom 2004; Grabowski et al. 2002). DLB and VaD also occur in seniors. Before age 65 years, frontotemporal dementia (FTD) is as common as AD; it accounts for 5%–9% of all newly diagnosed dementia cases (Grabowski et

al. 2002; Graff-Radford and Woodruff 2004). The dementias of the lenticulostriatal system are less common. They include Parkinson's disease dementia, progressive supranuclear palsy, Huntington's disease, corticobasal ganglionic degeneration, multiple system atrophy, Wilson's disease, neurodegeneration with brain iron accumulation, and Fahr's disease. The lenticulostriate dementias are discussed in Chapter 24 by Lerner and Riley. Of the prion disorders, Creutzfeldt-Jakob disease (CJD) and occasionally Gerstmann-Straussler Scheinker syndrome and fatal familial insomnia are associated with dementia. In this chapter, we focus on AD, DLB, FTD, VaD, and CJD.

DIAGNOSTIC CRITERIA

DSM-IV-TR (American Psychiatric Association 2000) defines *dementia* as an acquired cognitive syndrome of

This project was supported by a grant from the National Institute on Aging for the UCLA Alzheimer's Disease Research Center (P50 16570), the Kassel Parkinson's Disease Foundation, and the Sidell-Kagan Foundation. The authors would like to thank David Clark, M.D., and Ivan Klement, M.D., who contributed the frontotemporal dementia cortical thickness and pathology images.

TABLE 25–1. Diagnostic criteria for mild cognitive impairment

Cognitive complaint preferably corroborated by an informant

Impaired cognitive function—1.5 standard deviations below the age- and education-adjusted neuropsychological norms on one or more neuropsychological measures

Preserved general cognitive function

Intact activities of daily living

Not meeting DSM-IV-TR criteria for dementia

No evidence of concurrent general medical condition of sufficient severity to affect cognition

Source. Adapted from Petersen et al. 1999, 2001a.

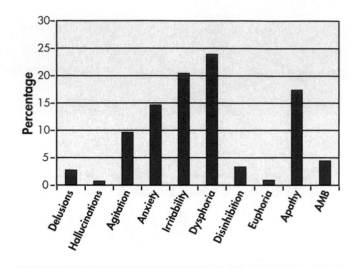

FIGURE 25–1. Frequency of neuropsychiatric symptoms in mild cognitive impairment. AMB=aberrant motor behavior.

Source. Data from Baquero et al. 2004; Geda et al. 2004; Hwang et al. 2004; Lyketsos et al. 2002.

sufficient severity to result in functional decline. Impairment of memory and at least one additional cognitive disturbance relative to prior level of functioning must be present. Functional decline can be manifested as impaired activities of daily living, vocational abilities, or social interactions. These criteria have been criticized for being too broad and nonspecific. Thus, expert groups have composed research criteria for each of the major dementia syndromes (Tables 25–1, 25–2, 25–4, 25–5, 25–6).

MILD COGNITIVE IMPAIRMENT

Mild cognitive impairment (Table 25–1) is an increasingly recognized intermediate stage between normal aging and dementia (Petersen et al. 1999, 2001a, 2001b), with an incidence of 10–26 per 10,000 elderly (Larrieu et al. 2002; Tervo et al. 2004) and annual conversion to dementia of 12%–15% (Petersen 2000; Petersen et al. 1999, 2001a; K. Ritchie and Touchon 2000). Mild cognitive impairment patients do not meet criteria for dementia because they do not show impairment in activities of daily living (American Psychiatric Association 2000). Following recognition of its etiological heterogeneity, mild cognitive impairment was subdivided into four major subtypes. The current research criteria define amnestic *mild cognitive impairment* as a cognitive state in which patients score 1.5 standard deviations (SD) below age- and education-adjusted normative values on various memory tests (Petersen et al. 1999, 2001a; Winblad et al. 2004). They may present with isolated memory impairment (e.g., single-domain amnestic mild cognitive impairment) or with associated impairment in one or more nonmemory domains such as executive, linguistic, or visuospatial abilities (e.g., multiple-domain amnestic

mild cognitive impairment). Likewise, nonamnestic mild cognitive impairment patients are subclassified under single-domain and multiple-domain subtype. They have preserved memory function but compromised nonmemory cognitive performances (Petersen et al. 1999, 2001a; Winblad et al. 2004).

Mild cognitive impairment outcomes are very heterogeneous. Although most patients develop dementia, some remain stable for many years, and some even improve (Wahlund et al. 2003). The pathological findings in mild cognitive impairment are most commonly consistent with impending AD, with neocortical senile plaques, neurofibrillary tangles, atrophy, and neuronal loss in layer II of the entorhinal cortex (Gomez-Isla et al. 1996; Haroutunian et al. 1998; Kordower et al. 2001; Price and Morris 1999; Troncoso et al. 1996). Nevertheless, the underlying pathogenesis is heterogeneous because mild cognitive impairment can evolve into various neurodegenerative disorders. Single-domain amnestic mild cognitive impairment can predate AD or rarely hippocampal sclerosis; multiple-domain amnestic and nonamnestic mild cognitive impairment can predate AD, VaD, DLB, or FTD; and single-domain nonamnestic mild cognitive impairment can evolve into FTD, VaD, DLB, Parkinson's disease dementia, progressive supranuclear palsy, or rarely AD (Petersen et al. 2001a; Winblad et al. 2004).

In addition to cognitive demise, mild cognitive impairment portends a host of behavior and personality changes. Administration of the Neuropsychiatric Inventory (NPI; Cummings et al. 1994) to caregivers of patients with mild cognitive impairment elicited one or more neuropsychiat-

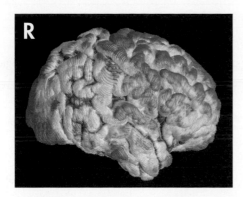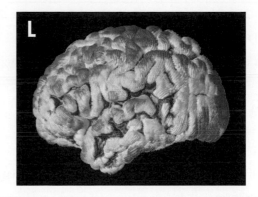

FIGURE 25–2. Gray matter atrophy in a patient with mild cognitive impairment showing involvement of the middle temporal gyrus and the temporo-parieto-occipital junction and mild involvement of the inferior dorsolateral prefrontal cortex and the superior parietal lobule. *Red*=most atrophic; *blue*=least atrophic; *yellow* and *green*=intermediate atrophy.

ric symptoms in 43%–59% of the patients with mild cognitive impairment (Feldman et al. 2004; Lyketsos et al. 2002). The most common symptoms are dysphoria (Baquero et al. 2004; Geda et al. 2004; Hwang et al. 2004; Lyketsos et al. 2002; Modrego and Ferrandez 2004), apathy, irritability (Baquero et al. 2004; Geda et al. 2004; Hwang et al. 2004; Lyketsos et al. 2002), and anxiety (Baquero et al. 2004; Geda et al. 2004; Hwang et al. 2004), whereas hallucinations, delusions (Baquero et al. 2004; Geda et al. 2004; Hwang et al. 2004; Lyketsos et al. 2002), euphoria, abnormal motor behavior, and disinhibition are relatively uncommon (Baquero et al. 2004; Geda et al. 2004; Lyketsos et al. 2002) (Figure 25–1). Neuropsychiatric symptoms correlate with more severe cognitive and functional impairment in mild cognitive impairment (Feldman et al. 2004; Ready et al. 2003). Depression conveys an increased likelihood for developing AD (Modrego and Ferrandez 2004). In mild cognitive impairment, depressive symptoms tend to persist and do not respond to medical therapy as readily as they do in elderly patients without cognitive impairment (Y.S. Li et al. 2001). The therapeutic challenge appears most pronounced for patients with mild cognitive impairment who go on to develop AD (Modrego and Ferrandez 2004).

Cortical and hippocampal atrophy is common in mild cognitive impairment. Figure 25–2 shows cortical atrophy in a patient with amnestic mild cognitive impairment.

Mild cognitive impairment is an important focus of the contemporary dementia-related research. As a strategic intermediate stage between normal aging and dementia, it is perceived as a critical therapeutic target. Two well-designed randomized clinical trials tested whether the acetylcholinesterase inhibitor donepezil is useful in mild cognitive impairment (Petersen et al. 2005; Salloway et al. 2004). The shorter 6-month trial assessed functional and cognitive improvement. The primary cognitive

and global functioning measures did not improve, but some of the secondary functional and cognitive outcomes showed a favorable response in treated patients relative to placebo (Salloway et al. 2004). The second trial followed up three groups of patients with mild cognitive impairment for 3 years after they were randomly assigned to donepezil, vitamin E, or placebo. The primary outcome was conversion to AD. In the first 18 months, donepezil-treated patients converted at a slower rate relative to both placebo and vitamin E. At the end of the 3-year period, the same proportion of patients from each group had progressed to AD. A more beneficial response was evident for those with an apolipoprotein epsilon 4 (*APOE*E4*) allele relative to those without (Petersen et al. 2005).

ALZHEIMER'S DISEASE

AD (Table 25–2) is the most common cause of cognitive decline among the elderly. It ranks third in health care cost after heart disease and cancer, approaching $100 billion annually (Schumock 1998). It frequently follows a prodromal stage of amnestic mild cognitive impairment during which amyloid pathology is already accumulating but has not reached the threshold for interfering with activities of daily living. As the disease progresses, the initially isolated memory deficits evolve into global cognitive decline with disturbance in language, visuospatial skills, and executive and social functioning. Early in the disease course, patients have deficient verbal and visual encoding, impaired delayed recall, concrete thinking, and mild anomia (Pasquier 1999). They may have trouble operating a vehicle and managing their finances. Patients may have deficient emotional processing manifested in difficulty with interpretation of facial expression and speech prosody (Cummings 2003a). As the disease progresses, patients develop transcortical sensory aphasia with relatively preserved syntax and phonological

TABLE 25–2. Diagnostic criteria for Alzheimer's disease (AD)

Probable AD

Dementia confirmed by clinical examination *and* mental status testing *and* formal neuropsychological testing

Deficits in two or more cognitive domains

Progressive cognitive decline

No disturbance of consciousness

Age at onset between 40 and 90 years

Absence of systemic medical, neurological, or psychiatric condition that could account for the cognitive decline

Supportive criteria

Progressive deterioration of language, motor skills, and/or perception

Impaired activities of daily living

Family history of dementia

Associated neuropsychiatric symptoms such as depression, insomnia, delusions, hallucinations, catastrophic reactions, sexual disorders, and weight loss

Features that make the diagnosis of AD questionable

Sudden onset

Focal neurological signs or symptoms

Seizures at onset of cognitive decline

Gait disturbance at onset of cognitive decline

Possible AD

Presence of a systemic medical, neurological, or psychiatric disease potentially capable of producing dementia but estimated an unlikely cause of the cognitive decline

Gradual decline in a single cognitive domain (e.g., aphasia)

Definite AD

Probable AD *and*

Histopathological evidence of AD

Source. Adapted from Corey-Bloom 2004; McKhann et al. 1984.

abilities (Pasquier 1999). Their judgment and ability to perform instrumental activities of daily living decline. Frequently, neurovegetative disturbances such as appetite loss and sleep-wake cycle disruption emerge (Cummings 2003a). As patients' conditions continue to deteriorate, they gradually lose the more basic activities of daily living such as dressing, eating, toileting, and finally communicating and ambulating. They typically succumb to the complications of immobilization (Beard et al. 1996; Hoyert and Rosenberg 1999; Kalia 2003; Kukull et al. 1994).

NEUROPSYCHIATRIC FEATURES OF ALZHEIMER'S DISEASE

Aside from cognitive decline, patients with AD experience a host of personality and behavior changes. Some

behaviors are more stage specific than are others (Figure 25–3). A graphic representation of the frequency of neuropsychiatric symptoms across the spectrum from normal aging to severe AD is presented in Figure 25–4.

Early in the disease course, AD patients have apathy, depressed mood, anxiety, and irritability (Lyketsos et al. 2000; Mega et al. 1996). Depressive symptoms—mild depression (dysphoria) or major depressive disorder—may predate the cognitive decline (Berger et al. 1999; Devanand et al. 1997) by as many as 10 years (Jost and Grossberg 1996; Speck et al. 1995). Lyketsos and Olin (2002) and Migliorelli et al. (1995) have estimated that dysphoria and major depression occur at approximately the same rate—that is, approximately half of the depressed AD patients would meet criteria for major depressive disorder, but the rest would not. Risk factors for

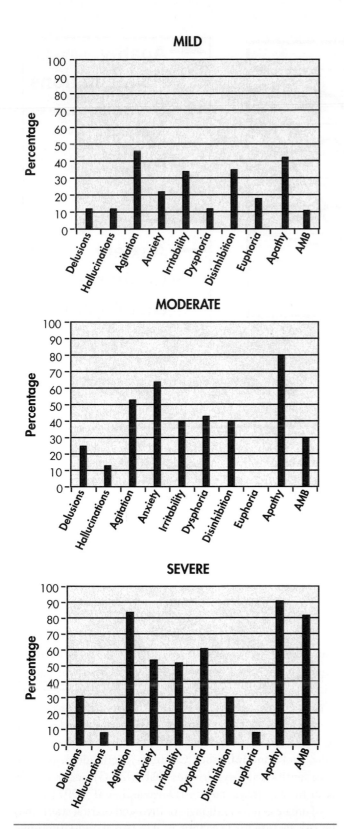

FIGURE 25–3. Frequency of neuropsychiatric symptoms in mild, moderate, and severe Alzheimer's disease. AMB=aberrant motor behavior.

Source. Data from Mega et al. 1996.

developing depression in AD are family or personal history of mood disorder, female gender, and younger age at onset of AD (Lyketsos and Olin 2002; Migliorelli et al. 1995). Depression in AD is associated with decreased quality of life, functional impairment, increased aggression, and increased institutionalization, as well as caregiver burden and caregiver depression (Cummings 2003b; Espiritu et al. 2001; Garre-Olmo et al. 2003; Lyketsos and Olin 2002). Depressed AD patients often have coexisting anxiety, agitation, disinhibition, and irritability (Frisoni et al. 1999; Garre-Olmo et al. 2003; Starkstein et al. 1997). Although depression has been linked to more precipitous cognitive decline by some (Heun et al. 2003), in most cases, improved mood has not been shown to correlate with improved cognition (Starkstein et al. 1997). In preliminary studies, depression in AD correlated with hypometabolism in bilateral superior frontal and left anterior cingulate gyri (Hirono et al. 1998). One positron emission tomography (PET) study reported hypometabolism of the parietal lobes (Sultzer et al. 1995). Pathologically, depression has been linked to monoaminergic dysfunction. AD patients with major depressive symptoms were found to have more profound degeneration of locus coeruleus and substantia nigra and associated reduction of norepinephrine and serotonin in the cortex (Forstl et al. 1992; Zubenko and Moossy 1988; Zubenko et al. 1990).

Apathy in AD is a complex syndrome consisting of loss of interest, motivation, volition, enjoyment, spontaneity, and emotional behavior. Apathy, the most common neuropsychiatric symptom in AD, affects 42% of the patients with mild, 80% with moderate, and 92% with advanced AD (see Figure 25–3) (Mega et al. 1996). It may occur up to 3 years prior to diagnosis (Jost and Grossberg 1996). Apathy and the associated executive dysfunction (Boyle et al. 2003; Kuzis et al. 1999; McPherson et al. 2002) result in inefficient social and environmental interaction, decreased engagement in day-to-day activities and personal care, and worse quality of life (Boyle et al. 2003; Freels et al. 1992). It increases caregiver burden and caregiver dissatisfaction and often leads to early institutionalization (Benoit and Robert 2003; Landes et al. 2001). Apathy most likely results from disruption of the anterior cingulate and dorsolateral prefrontal circuits (Cummings 1993; Damasio and Van Hoesen 1983; Landes et al. 2001; Mega and Cummings 1994). Lesions of the anterior cingulate or its disconnection from the supplementary motor area can cause the full spectrum of amotivational behavior, ranging from diminished initiative to akinetic mutism. AD patients with apathy have bilateral hypoperfusion of the anterior cingulate (Craig et al. 1996; Migneco et al. 2001); orbitofrontal, anterior temporal (Craig et al. 1996), dorsolateral prefrontal (Benoit

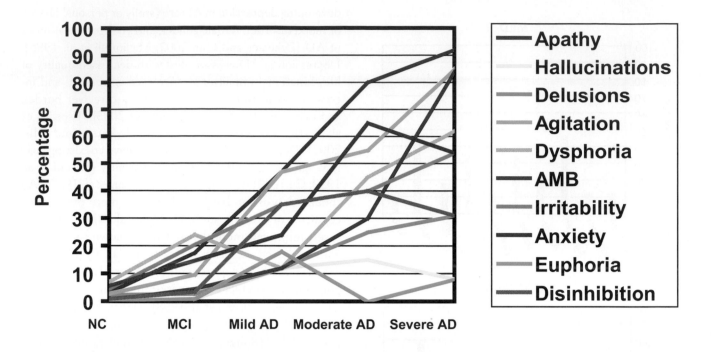

FIGURE 25–4. Frequency of neuropsychiatric symptoms from normal aging (NC) to severe Alzheimer's disease (AD). AMB=aberrant motor behavior; MCI=mild cognitive impairment.

Source.   Data from Baquero et al. 2004; Hwang et al. 2004; Lyketsos et al. 2000, 2002; Mega et al. 1996.

et al. 2002; Craig et al. 1996; Lopez et al. 2001b), and right temporoparietal (Ott et al. 1996) cortices; and basal ganglia (Lopez et al. 2001b). Neurofibrillary tangle (NFT) pathology in the left anterior cingulate gyrus has been linked to apathy in AD (Tekin et al. 2001).

Anxiety is another early feature of AD. It can present with apprehension and inner feelings of nervousness, with associated autonomic symptoms such as tachycardia, perspiration, dry mouth, and chest tightness. Relative to elderly persons without AD, in whom the prevalence of anxiety is 5.8% (Lyketsos et al. 2002), and to patients with mild cognitive impairment, in whom anxiety occurs in 11%–39% (Baquero et al. 2004; Geda et al. 2004; Hwang et al. 2004; Lyketsos et al. 2002), the frequency of anxiety in patients with AD averages to 48% (Mega et al. 1996).

Irritability increases from the cognitively normal elderly population, in which it is seen in 4.6% (Lyketsos et al. 2002), to mild cognitive impairment and to AD, in which it occurs in 29% and 42% of the patients, respectively.

As AD progresses, its behavioral profile expands. Some behaviors that are only rarely encountered in premorbid amnestic mild cognitive impairment or in the mild AD stages, such as disinhibition, aberrant motor behaviors, hallucinations, and delusions, ensue (Piccininni et al. 2005). In advanced AD, agitation, aggression, irritability, and violent behaviors may be prominent and prompt nursing home placement.

Disinhibition may manifest with impulsivity, tactlessness, loss of empathy, and violation of social boundaries. It results from dysfunction in the frontosubcortical circuits (Cummings 1993) and correlates with frontal and temporal hypoperfusion (Sultzer et al. 1995).

Aberrant motor behaviors include a variety of manifestations such as fidgetiness, pacing, and inability to stay still (Lyketsos et al. 2000; Mega et al. 1996; Petry et al. 1989). Its prevalence exponentially increases with disease progression.

Psychotic symptoms such as delusions and hallucinations are common features of AD and several other neurodegenerative disorders. They can result in patient distress, caregiver dissatisfaction, and early residential placement (Steele et al. 1990). The delusions are rarely as bizarre as in some primary psychiatric disorders such as schizophrenia. Common delusional themes are paranoia, theft, and infidelity. Content-specific delusions and misidentification syndromes (Table 25–3) occur mostly later in the disease course (Devanand et al. 1997).

Female gender and single or divorced marital status may be risk factors for psychosis in AD (Assal and Cummings 2002; Leroi et al. 2003). Hallucinations in AD are typically in the visual modality and tend to resolve (Marin et al. 1997). Both hallucinations and delusions correlate with poor insight (Migliorelli et al. 1995) and faster cognitive and functional decline (Rosen and Zubenko 1991). Func-

TABLE 25–3. Delusional misidentification syndromes

Syndrome	Content of delusion
Capgras' syndrome	That others (usually close relatives) have been replaced by impostors
Doppelganger/Heautoscopy	That one has a double
Fregoli's syndrome	That strangers have been replaced by familiar people
Intermetamorphosis	That two people have exchanged their appearance
Autoscopy	Perception of one's own body as a double
Foley's syndrome	That one's image in the mirror is that of another person
Reduplicative paramnesia	That a physical location (e.g., home) has been duplicated
Reduplication for time	That the chronological time is duplicated and one exists in two time points

tional imaging has indicated an association of psychotic symptoms in AD and right or left frontal (Kotrla et al. 1995; Lopez et al. 2001a; Mega et al. 2000; Sultzer et al. 1995), right or left parietal (Fukuhara et al. 2001; Lopez et al. 2001a; Mega et al. 2000), left medial temporal (Lopez et al. 2001a), bilateral temporal (Starkstein et al. 1994), and left anterior cingulate (Mega et al. 2000) abnormalities.

Other disturbing behaviors are wandering, occurring in as many as 43% of AD patients, and disturbed diurnal sleep pattern, occurring in 56% (Jost and Grossberg 1996).

PATHOLOGY OF ALZHEIMER'S DISEASE

AD is a neurodegenerative disorder that results from overproduction or accumulation of amyloid β (Aβ) and tau protein. Aβ is a segment of the amyloid precursor protein (APP) that is liberated by the joint action of two proteases—the β- and the γ-secretase. In healthy individuals, these two enzymes are responsible for only a small fraction of the APP cleavage, whereas the majority is accomplished by a third protease—the α-secretase, which splits the large APP molecule in the midst of the Aβ sequence and prevents the formation of the potentially toxic 39– to 43–amino acid Aβ protein (Mesulam 2000). Aβ polymerizes and produces first oligomeres and later polymers that clump together and form several types of amyloid inclusions. The diffuse and neuritic plaques deposit extracellularly (Figure 25–5). *Vascular amyloid* is the term for Aβ accumulation within the walls of cortical blood vessels (Duyckaerts and Dickson 2003). The first plaques appear in the temporo-occipital association regions (Duyckaerts and Dickson 2003; Mesulam 2000). Then they spread to the entorhinal and perirhinal, the parietal, and later the frontal association cortices (Braak and Braak 1997).

Tau is a structural protein of the microtubular transport system and plays a role in microtubule stabilization (Friedhoff et al. 1998; Ghetti et al. 2003; Giasson et al. 2003b;

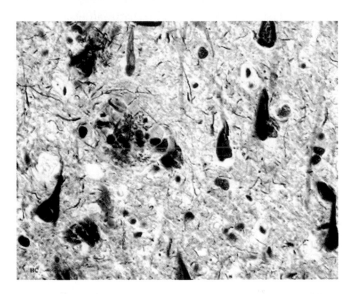

FIGURE 25–5. Amyloid plaques and neurofibrillary tangles stained with Bielschowsky's stain.

Source. Image courtesy of Ivan Klement.

Revesz and Holton 2003). Tau's affinity for microtubules is closely regulated by phosphorylation and dephosphorylation. AD tau is hyperphosphorylated with consequentially severely compromised function. Tau forms intracellular inclusions (NFTs) with highest density in the pyramidal cortical layer. Another site for tau accumulation is the dendritic tree of diseased neurons. Such accumulations are called neuropil threads when located in the neuropil and dystrophic neurites when located within neuritic plaques (Duyckaerts and Dickson 2003) (see Figure 25–5).

GENETICS OF ALZHEIMER'S DISEASE

Sporadic AD (e.g., late-onset AD) generally occurs after age 65. Its mode of inheritance is multifactorial with predisposition governed by the synergistic action of a constellation of genes that is further modified by epigenetic influences. The single most important risk factor for AD is age. Among 60- to 65-year-olds, its prevalence is 1%, but among those 85 years or older, it rises to 40% (von Strauss et al. 1999). Being female has been implicated in the likelihood of developing AD (Gao et al. 1998). The risk for and the age at onset of AD are modified by the apolipoprotein E (*APOE*) gene polymorphism on chromosome 19. The *APOE* gene has three major alleles—ε2, ε3, and ε4—and encodes a 299–amino acid glycoprotein functioning as a cholesterol transporter. *APOE*E4* promotes Aβ aggregation (Esler et al. 2002) and suppresses neural plasticity (Nathan et al. 2002; Teter et al. 1999). It also has been shown to accelerate disease onset in a dose-dependent fashion (Blacker et al. 1997; Corder et al. 1993; Hsiung et al. 2004; Khachaturian et al. 2004; Payami et al. 1997; Yoshizawa et al. 1994). The effect of *APOE*E4* is modified by race, being stronger in whites than in blacks (Evans et al. 2003), and inversely by advancing age (Blacker et al. 1997). Mental and physical exercise, a high education level, and a healthy diet rich in polyunsaturated as opposed to saturated fats offer protection from AD.

When AD presents before age 65 years (early-onset AD), instead of or in addition to the *APOE*E4* allele, consideration should be given to three autosomal dominant mutations—the APP gene mutation on chromosome 21, the presenilin-1 gene mutation on chromosome 14, and the presenilin-2 gene mutation on chromosome 1. Autosomal dominant early-onset AD is known for its atypical clinical features and shorter survival. Patients may have significant aphasia (Bertoli Avella et al. 2002; Binetti et al. 2003; Kennedy et al. 1995; Lampe et al. 1994; Lopera et al. 1997; Rippon et al. 2003), dysathria (Bird et al. 1989; Miklossy et al. 2003; P. Moretti et al. 2004; Nagano et al. 1992; Yasuda et al. 1999), early myoclonus, tonic-clonic or complex partial seizures (Bertoli Avella et al. 2002; Binetti et al. 2003; Bird et al. 1989; Campion et al. 1996; Fox et al. 1997; Kennedy et al. 1993, 1995; Lampe et al. 1994; Lopera et al. 1997; Miklossy et al. 2003; Newman et al. 1994; Rippon et al. 2003), spastic paraplegia or quadriplegia (Farlow et al. 1994; Miklossy et al. 2003; P. Moretti et al. 2004; Rippon et al. 2003; Verkkoniemi et al. 2001), dystonia (P. Moretti et al. 2004; Rippon et al. 2003), cerebellar ataxia (Miklossy et al. 2003), or marked cognitive fluctuations (Kennedy et al. 1993). Some of the atypical neuropsychiatric symptoms in early-onset AD's are emotional lability (Farlow et al. 1994; Nagano et al. 1992; Rippon et al. 2003), obsessive-compulsive behavior (Miklossy et al. 2003; Queralt et al. 2002; Rippon et al. 2003), an FTD type of presentation (Raux et al. 2000;

Tang-Wai et al. 2002), and hyperoral, hyperphagic, and hypersexual behavior resembling Klüver-Bucy syndrome (Tang-Wai et al. 2002).

NEUROIMAGING IN ALZHEIMER'S DISEASE

The American Academy of Neurology currently recommends a noncontrast structural image—either computed tomography (CT) or magnetic resonance imaging (MRI)—as part of the initial evaluation for cognitive impairment. MRI has several advantages—most notably, better resolution. The classical structural changes of AD are global cerebral atrophy with mesial temporal and parietal predilection. Hippocampal volume loss can be seen even premorbidly in the mild cognitive impairment stage (Jack et al. 2004). Gray matter atrophy can now be visualized easily with computational anatomy techniques (Apostolova et al. 2006; Apostolova et al., in press; Thompson et al. 2003, 2004). It is most pronounced in the association cortices, whereas primary cortices are relatively spared (Figure 25–6).

Functional neuroimaging techniques such as single-photon emission computed tomography (SPECT) and PET add another dimension to the dementia workup. They provide an estimate of neuronal function rather than cerebral structure and identify early hypoperfusion and hypometabolic changes in mesial temporal and parietal distribution and in the posterior cingulate (Figure 25–7). Later in the disease, global hypoperfusion or hypometabolism is the rule, with relative sparing of the basal ganglia and the primary sensorimotor and visual cortices (Silverman 2004).

THERAPY FOR ALZHEIMER'S DISEASE

The acetylcholinesterase inhibitors donepezil (Doody 2003), galantamine (Raskind 2003), and rivastigmine (Farlow 2003) were the first class of pharmaceuticals approved by the U.S. Food and Drug Administration for treatment of AD. Their effect is mediated by increased availability of acetylcholine in the synaptic cleft. Rivastigmine and galantamine have additional mechanisms of action. Rivastigmine blocks butyrylcholinesterase, and galantamine is an allosteric modulator of the nicotinic presynaptic receptors (Geerts et al. 2002). These three agents have modest cognitive, functional, and behavioral effects and a safe side-effect profile.

Memantine is approved for treatment of moderate to severe AD. Memantine is a weak *N*-methyl-D-aspartate receptor blocker and as such prevents the deleterious effects of continuous toxic low levels of glutamate while allowing the physiologically advantageous large glutamate

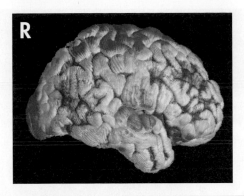
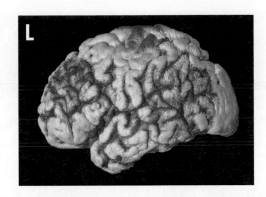

FIGURE 25–6. Gray matter atrophy in a patient with mild Alzheimer's disease showing involvement of the temporal, parietal, occipital, and frontal association cortices more severe on the left. Note the relative sparing of the primary sensory, motor, and visual cortices. *Red*=most atrophic; *blue*=least atrophic; *yellow* and *green*=intermediate atrophy.

surge to exert its required cognitive effect. More recently, memantine was shown to stimulate long-term potentiation and block tau hyperphosphorylation (L. Li et al. 2004; Voisin et al. 2004).

The symptomatic therapies described earlier have a modest effect. The need for disease-modifying therapy has long been recognized. In 1996, anti-Aβ monoclonal antibodies were developed. They were first shown to inhibit Aβ aggregation and later to promote dissolution of Aβ deposits and inhibit Aβ cytotoxicity in vitro (Solomon et al. 1996, 1997). These advances led to the development of an active Aβ vaccine that slowed down or abolished deposition of amyloid plaques in older and young APP transgenic mice, respectively (Schenk et al. 1999). Unfortunately, in the Phase II human vaccination trial, 6% of the patients developed meningoencephalitis (Orgogozo et al. 2003). Four of the patients were followed up until their death. In two patients, the autopsy showed greatly diminished amyloid plaque burden relative to what was expected for the stage of disease they were in, along with evidence of inflammatory response (Ferrer et al. 2004; Nicoll et al. 2003). In a post hoc analysis, cognitive improvement in a subgroup of patients who reacted to the vaccination with antibody synthesis relative to a group of patients who did not show antibody response was evident (Mattson 2004). Resources are currently invested in other methods targeting immune response against Aβ delivery such as the use of Aβ fragments or plasmid DNA encoding Aβ (Manea et al. 2004; Schiltz et al. 2004).

Passive immunization techniques also are under investigation. Passive immunization with mid-domain or amino-terminal Aβ antibodies results in decreased plaque burden in APP mice (Bard et al. 2000, 2003; Bussiere et al. 2004; Cribbs et al. 2003). Passive immunization may be safer because it is unlikely to illicit a T-cell autoimmune reaction, in addition to the short life of the anti-

bodies and the possibility of removing them via plasmapheresis.

Another focus for pharmaceutical development is Aβ production and aggregation. Several β- and γ-secretase inhibitors are currently being tested. Various peptide or nonpeptide inhibitors of Aβ polymerization are likewise being explored (Cohen and Kelly 2003; Wolfe 2002). Aβ aggregation needs copper and iron as cofactors. The antibiotic clioquinol chelates copper and showed activity in a Phase II clinical trial (C.W. Ritchie et al. 2004).

The presence of activated microglia in AD brains led to several anti-inflammatory clinical trials. Nevertheless, trials of prednisone (Aisen 2000; Aisen et al. 2000), diclofenac (Scharf et al. 1999), rofecoxib, and naproxen (Aisen et al. 2003) all had negative results (Weggen et al. 2003).

Of the antioxidants, standard therapy in AD is vitamin E (2,000 IU/dose). Its administration to AD patients in a large placebo-controlled trial resulted in functional benefit (Sano et al. 1997). Vitamin E failed to delay conversion of mild cognitive impairment to AD in a recent mild cognitive impairment trial (Petersen et al. 2005). Some have empirically recommended vitamin C on the basis of epidemiological evidence (Zandi et al. 2004). Two human trials of Ginkgo biloba reported conflicting results (Le Bars et al. 2000; van Dongen et al. 2003). Curcumin, a common neutraceutical ingredient of curry, seems to decrease Aβ deposition both in vitro and in transgenic mice (Lim et al. 2001; Ono et al. 2004). Curcumin therapeutic trials are currently under way. Other drugs under investigation are cholesterol-lowering agents. They also have been shown to reduce Aβ accumulation (Petanceska et al. 2002).

Several inhibitors of tau's hyperphosphorylation are being investigated (Iqbal et al. 2002). The most attractive agents appear to be lithium (Bhat et al. 2004), valproate (Loy and Tariot 2002), and memantine (L. Li et al. 2004).

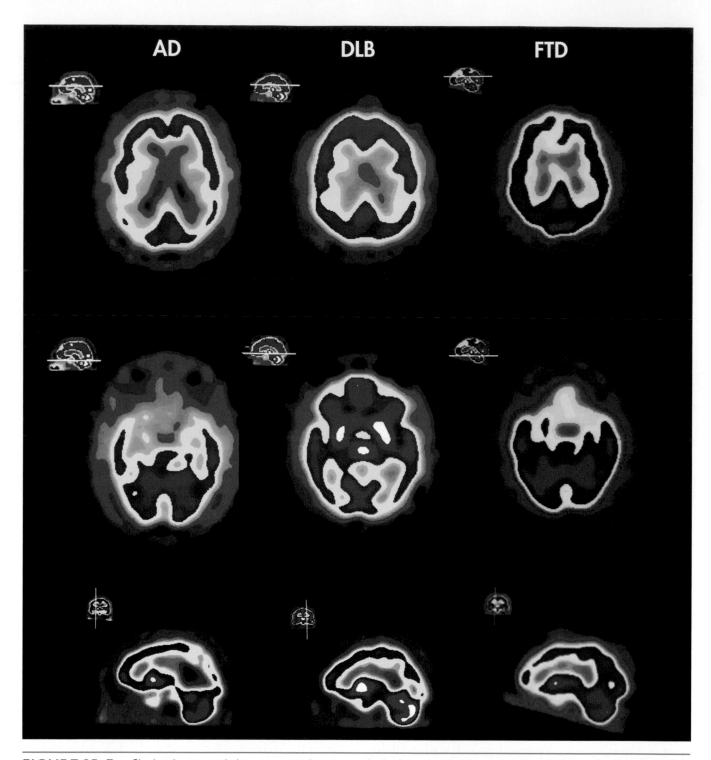

FIGURE 25–7.   Single-photon emission computed tomography in the primary dementias. In Alzheimer's disease (AD), there is bilateral mesial temporal and parietal hypoperfusion (left side). In dementia with Lewy bodies (DLB), bilateral parietal and occipital hypoperfusion is seen. Frontotemporal dementia (FTD) is characterized by frontotemporal hypoperfusion pattern.

MANAGEMENT OF NEUROPSYCHIATRIC DISTURBANCES IN ALZHEIMER'S DISEASE

In January 2005, the Expert Consensus Panel for Dementia published "Guidelines for Treatment of Behavioral Distur-

bances in Dementia" (Alexopoulos et al. 2005). For depression, the authors recommended antidepressant therapy with selective serotonin reuptake inhibitors (SSRIs) such as citalopram, sertraline, and escitalopram. If depressive symptoms persist, an acetylcholinesterase inhibitor, if not already prescribed, should be added. For depression with psychotic symptoms, the panel recommended risperidone, quetiapine, olanzapine, aripiprazole, or ziprasidone.

For long-term management of anxiety, the panel recommended SSRIs. Benzodiazepines or atypical antipsychotics are to be considered only for short-term management of severe anxiety until the SSRIs take effect.

For agitation and aggression, the experts emphasized the importance of environmental interventions such as structure, gentle reassurance, and redirection, as well as educational and emotional support for caregivers. When needed, the following medications are to be considered: atypical antipsychotics (risperidone, quetiapine, olanzapine, aripiprazole), SSRIs, or valproic acid.

For psychosis, the experts recommended risperidone and quetiapine as first-line therapy. The recommended second-line therapeutic agents were olanzapine and aripiprazole. High-potency antipsychotics were recommended only for short-term use.

For insomnia, the panel recommended trazodone or quetiapine as both short-term and long-term first-line agents. Other recommended agents were zolpidem, risperidone, mirtazapine, and olanzapine.

The expert guidelines described earlier preceded the U.S. Food and Drug Administration warning of the increased risk for stroke or death associated with the use of atypical antipsychotics in the elderly population with dementia. This warning is based on post hoc data analyses of randomized placebo-controlled trials of risperidone and olanzapine. The risk was highest for patients with risk factors for stroke such as hypertension, diabetes, and atrial fibrillation (Bullock 2005; Sink et al. 2005). Thus, prescribing physicians should consider carefully the risk-benefit ratio of antipsychotic therapy for treatment of behavioral and neuropsychiatric symptoms in dementia (Bullock 2005; Sink et al. 2005).

DEMENTIA WITH LEWY BODIES

DLB accounts for 15%–20% of all late-onset dementias and is the second most prevalent dementing disorder of the elderly (Corey-Bloom 2004; Grabowski et al. 2002). The most recent diagnostic criteria (McKeith et al. 1996) are listed in Table 25–4.

Cognitive decline in DLB is somewhat different than that observed in AD. Memory impairment is less severe in DLB, but attention and visuospatial and visuoperceptual functions can be severely affected early in the disease course. Cognitive fluctuations in AD are minor. In DLB, they are profound, and large variability in cognitive performance on attention and executive tasks has been de-

TABLE 25–4. Diagnostic criteria for dementia with Lewy bodies

Core features

Progressive cognitive decline interfering with activities of daily living (with prominent decline in attention, executive, or visuospatial performance)

Cognitive fluctuations

Recurrent visual hallucinations

Extrapyramidal symptoms (bradykinesia, rigidity, gait disturbance)

Supportive features

Repeated falls

Syncope

Transient loss of consciousness

Neuroleptic sensitivity

Delusions

Hallucinations in other modalities

Depression

Source. Adapted from McKeith et al. 1996.

scribed (Ballard et al. 2001a, 2001b). DLB patients often have fluctuating alertness and clear-cut episodes of delirium. Cognitive fluctuations could last a few minutes or persist for several days. Fluctuations are described in as many as 50%–75% of DLB patients (McKeith et al. 2004).

DLB is closely related to Parkinson's disease dementia, and both disorders are characterized by parkinsonism and dementia. It is arbitrarily accepted to diagnose Parkinson's disease dementia if motor symptoms precede cognitive decline by more than 12 months and to diagnose DLB if they occur within a year of each other. The extrapyramidal symptoms (EPS) observed in DLB are bradykinesia, rigidity, resting tremor, and gait disturbance. Relative to Parkinson's disease dementia, EPS are more symmetric (Del Ser et al. 2000). EPS coincide with DLB onset in 25%–50% of patients and develop later in the disease course in up to 100% of the patients (McKeith et al. 2003, 2004).

Several other supportive features help distinguish DLB from AD and VaD. Early falls and presyncopal or syncopal episodes are characteristic of DLB. DLB has prominent sleep disorders—most notably, rapid eye movement (REM) sleep behavior disorder. REM sleep behavior disorder can precede dementia onset by as long as a decade. It predates EPS and visual hallucinations in half and cognitive fluctuations in 80% of DLB patients (Ferman et al. 1999, 2002). Because REM sleep behavior disorder in a patient with dementia and parkinsonism

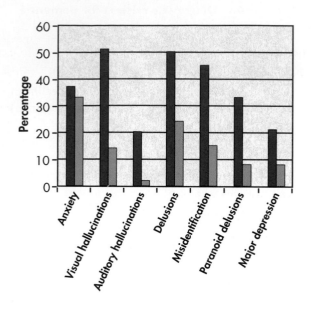

FIGURE 25–8. Prevalence of some neuropsychiatric features at disease onset in dementia with Lewy bodies (DLB; *blue*) and Alzheimer's disease (AD; *orange*).

Source. Data from Simard et al. 2000.

bears a positive predictive value of 92% for DLB (Boeve et al. 2001), some experts believe that it should be established as a supportive diagnostic criterion for DLB (Boeve et al. 2003b; Ferman et al. 2002; McKeith et al. 2003). It has been suggested that visual hallucinations are fragments of REM sleep intrusions into wakefulness (Arnulf et al. 2000).

A characteristic but ominous clinical symptom in DLB is the unusual sensitivity of DLB patients to neuroleptic medications. Adverse EPS have been reported in 81% of DLB patients compared with 19% of AD patients. The reactions included sedation, confusion, severe parkinsonism with extreme rigidity and immobility, and neuroleptic malignant syndrome. The mortality hazard ratio is 2.3 (McKeith et al. 1992). Thus, neuroleptic use is contraindicated in DLB.

NEUROPSYCHIATRIC FEATURES OF DEMENTIA WITH LEWY BODIES

Up to 98% of all DLB patients experience at least one psychiatric symptom during the course of their illness. Multiple simultaneous psychiatric symptoms are almost universal (Ballard et al. 1996). At disease onset, neuropsychiatric features are much more common in DLB than in AD (Simard et al. 2000) (Figure 25–8).

Hallucinations are exceedingly common in DLB. DLB patients may present with hallucinations prior to demen-

tia onset (Cercy and Bylsma 1997). As many as 65% of pathologically proven DLB cases but only 25% of AD cases are associated with visual hallucinations at disease onset. In mild dementia (Mini-Mental State Examination score of 20 or higher), 93% of the patients experiencing visual hallucinations had DLB pathology (Ballard et al. 1999). The content of visual hallucinations is similar in DLB, AD, and VaD and consists of complex, detailed, brightly colored three-dimensional images of people and animals. Less frequent are hallucinations of children, inanimate objects, insects, fire, and birds (Aarsland et al. 2001; Ballard et al. 1996, 1997a, 1997b, 1999). Most visual hallucinations are of normal size, complete, and animated, and half are associated with auditory hallucinations. Multiple visual hallucinations or visual hallucinations associated with auditory hallucinations are exceedingly rare in AD, but both are relatively common in DLB (Ballard et al. 1997a). Visual hallucinations remit in only 16% of DLB patients compared with 73% of AD and 70% of VaD patients (Ballard et al. 1996, 1997b). Visual hallucinations tend to worsen in the evening (Ballard et al. 1997a, McKeith et al. 1996), reflecting the effect of solitude, inactivity, and poor lighting. Patients are rarely disturbed by their visual hallucinations, although the occasional patient may feel fear, amusement, or anger (McKeith et al. 1992, 1996). The reported frequency of auditory hallucinations in DLB (19%–25%) is much greater than that observed in AD (4%–6%) (McKeith and O'Brien 1999; Simard et al. 2000); however, remission rates are similar (Ballard et al. 1996, 2001c). Olfactory hallucinations are reported in 7%–12% of DLB patients and tactile in up to 3% (Aarsland et al. 2001; Ballard et al. 1996; Simard et al. 2000).

Delusions are common in DLB; the prevalence is 49% compared with 31% in AD (Simard et al. 2000). The most common themes are delusional misidentification (see Table 25–3), followed by paranoid beliefs (theft, conspiracy, harassment, abandonment, infidelity) and phantom boarder (Aarsland et al. 2001; Hirono et al. 1999; Klatka et al. 1996; Simard et al. 2000; Weiner et al. 2002). Of the delusional misidentifications, mistaking television images for real occurs in 19%, followed by Capgras' syndrome in 10%, mistaking one's mirror image for another person in 9.5%, and reduplicative paramnesia in 2.4% (Ballard et al. 1996). Remission of DLB delusions is similar to that in AD and VaD (Ballard et al. 1997b, 2001c).

Depression is more common in DLB relative to AD (Ballard et al. 1999), although the symptomatology seems not to differ (Samuels et al. 2004). The depressed cognitively impaired patient has 16 times higher likelihood to have DLB pathology than to have AD pathology (Papka et al. 1998). Major depression per DSM-III-R (American Psychiatric Association 1987) criteria was observed in

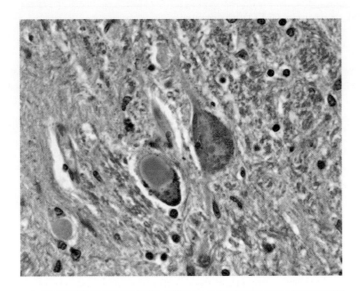

FIGURE 25–9. Lewy bodies stained with hematoxylin-eosin.

Source. Image courtesy of Ivan Klement.

33% of the patients with DLB (McKeith et al. 1992). Depression in DLB does not seem to correlate with cortical or subcortical Lewy body burden (Samuels et al. 2004).

Anxiety disorder meeting DSM-IV-TR criteria is rare in DLB, whereas feeling anxious is very common (Ballard et al. 1996). Up to 84% of DLB patients appear or feel anxious (Rockwell et al. 2000). Among three studies that used the NPI, two found anxiety was one of the most prominent neuropsychiatric features (Del Ser et al. 2000; Hirono et al. 1999; McKeith and Burn 2000).

Very few studies have assessed the full neuropsychiatric spectrum in DLB. Among the three NPI studies, apathy emerged as the most common psychiatric symptom. Agitation, aberrant motor behavior, and aggression were also significant in DLB, whereas euphoria and disinhibition rarely were reported (Del Ser et al. 2000; Hirono et al. 1999; McKeith and Burn 2000).

Neuropsychiatric remission occurs in 28% of DLB compared with 63% of AD and 33% of VaD patients largely because of persistent visual hallucinations.

PATHOLOGY OF DEMENTIA WITH LEWY BODIES

The major pathological finding in DLB is the Lewy body (Figure 25–9). Its major component—α-synuclein—is a natively unfolded 140–amino acid polypeptide. It localizes to the presynaptic terminals, where after binding to the cell membrane, it assumes a more structured conformation (Klucken et al. 2003; Spillantini 2003). α-Synuclein functions as a modulator of synaptic transmission and synaptic

vesicle transport. It also plays a role in neuronal plasticity (Giasson et al. 2003b; Jellinger 2003; Spillantini 2003).

Lewy bodies are frequently seen in the brain stem nuclei of patients with DLB, Parkinson's disease, and AD and occasionally in cognitively intact elderly. Cortical Lewy bodies, however, are seen in temporal, insular, and cingulate cortices in demented patients with DLB, Parkinson's disease dementia, and sometimes AD. Amygdalar Lewy bodies are common in DLB and AD (Jellinger 2003). Aβ pathology is frequently seen in DLB. When Aβ pathology is present, the patient is said to have the common form of DLB as opposed to pure DLB (Kosaka 1990). Aβ, tau, and α-synuclein pathology affect one another. α-Synuclein is a potent inducer of tau fibrillization. Both tau and α-synuclein mutually promote polymerization (Giasson et al. 2003a). Aβ has likewise been shown to promote Lewy body (Masliah et al. 2001) and NFT pathology in transgenic animals (Gotz et al. 2001; Lewis et al. 2001; Masliah et al. 2001).

NEUROIMAGING IN DEMENTIA WITH LEWY BODIES

DLB patients manifest brain atrophy in a similar pattern but with lesser severity compared with the atrophy observed in AD (Burton et al. 2002; Harvey et al. 1999; Hashimoto et al. 1998). When compared with nondemented elderly, hippocampal (Barber et al. 2000, 2001) and temporal lobe atrophy and ventricular enlargement are prominent (Barber et al. 1999, 2000). Involvement of the mesial temporal lobes, the frontal lobes, and the insular cortex is common (Burton et al. 2002).

Functional imaging has documented temporoparietal and occipital involvement in DLB. The latter helps differentiate DLB from AD (Colloby et al. 2002; Donnemiller et al. 1997; Imamura et al. 2001; Ishii et al. 1999; Lobotesis et al. 2001; Minoshima et al. 2001) (see Figure 25–7).

THERAPY FOR DEMENTIA WITH LEWY BODIES

DLB has significant cholinergic deficits surpassing those observed in AD. The two randomized placebo-controlled trials of the acetylcholinesterase inhibitor rivastigmine in DLB showed cognitive improvement specifically in vigilance, working memory, episodic memory, attention, and executive function (McKeith et al. 2000; Wesnes et al. 2002). The open-label studies of donepezil have been less consistent with respect to cognitive benefit (Simard and van Reekum 2004), whereas an open-label galantamine trial documented cognitive improvement (Edwards et al. 2004). Thus, acetylcholinesterase inhibitors are recommended in DLB (Swanberg and Cummings 2002).

TABLE 25–5. Diagnostic criteria for frontotemporal dementia (FTD) spectrum

Frontal variant FTD

Insidious onset and gradual progression

Early decline in interpersonal conduct

Early decline in personal conduct

Emotional blunting

Loss of insight

Decline in personal hygiene and grooming

Mental rigidity and inflexibility

Distractibility and impersistence

Hyperorality and dietary changes

Preparations and/or stereotyped behavior

Utilization behavior

Neuroimaging evidence of predominant frontal and temporal lobe involvement

Primary progressive aphasia

Insidious onset and gradual progression

Dysfluent speech output with at least one of the following: agrammatism, phonemic paraphasias, anomia

Supportive features: stuttering, apraxia of speech, impaired repetition, alexia, agraphia, early preservation of single-word comprehension, late mutism, early preservation of social skills, late behavior changes similar to frontal variant FTD

Neuroimaging evidence of predominant superior temporal, inferior frontal, and insular involvement

Semantic dementia

Insidious onset and gradual progression

Progressive fluent empty spontaneous speech

Loss of semantic word knowledge with impaired naming and single-word comprehension

Semantic paraphasias

Supportive features: pressured speech, idiosyncratic word substitution, surface dyslexia, and dysgraphia

Neuroimaging evidence of predominant anterior temporal lobe involvement

Source. Adapted from Neary et al. 1998.

Noncognitive symptoms in DLB also respond to anticholinergic treatment. Rivastigmine ameliorates neuropsychiatric symptoms (Maclean et al. 2001; McKeith et al. 2000) and improves mobility, functional dependence, and sleep (Maclean et al. 2001). The neuropsychiatric symptoms most responsive to acetylcholinesterase inhibitor therapy are hallucinations, paranoid delusions, daytime somnolence, apathy, aggression, and agitation (Simard and van Reekum 2004). Several open-label donepezil trials reported reduction of psychiatric symptoms (Simard and van Reekum 2004). Preliminary 12-week interim data from a 24-week multicenter, open-label galantamine trial in DLB reported improvement of delusions, hallucinations, apathy, and depression (Edwards et al. 2004).

Neuroleptic use is contraindicated in DLB because of the extreme risk of severe side effects such as neuroleptic malignant syndrome and death. Neuroleptic malignant syndrome is only rarely reported with atypical antipsychotics (McKeith et al. 1995). Extreme caution in instituting atypical antipsychotic therapy in DLB is advised. Treatment should begin with very low doses under close supervision for cognitive side effects or EPS (Swanberg and Cummings 2002). An open-label trial of melatonin for REM sleep behavior disorder that included seven DLB patients reported promising results (Boeve et al. 2003a).

FRONTOTEMPORAL DEMENTIA

FTD (Table 25–5) is a group of disorders that present with focal atrophy of the frontal and/or temporal lobes and evidence-specific behavioral and neuropsychological profiles. The age at onset varies between 35 and 75 years. Both sexes are equally affected. The three subtypes of FTD are frontal variant FTD (also known as Pick's disease), primary progressive aphasia, and semantic dementia. Onset around age 70 is typical for semantic dementia, whereas primary progressive aphasia and FTD tend to occur earlier.

FRONTAL VARIANT FRONTOTEMPORAL DEMENTIA

Frontal variant FTD is the most common subtype with a characteristic onset between age 45 and 60 years. It is characterized by insidious early behavioral disturbances such as changes of personal conduct and personality. Patients with frontal variant FTD characteristically show deficient social skills. They could be either socially inappropriate, overly familiar with random strangers, tactless and disinhibited, or aloof and seeking social isolation. Frontal variant FTD patients frequently disobey socially accepted norms and boundaries. They may become antisocial and even engage in criminal behavior. They become apathetic and self-centered and lack empathy and insight. These personality changes add enormous stress in their interpersonal relationships. Sometimes very unusual eating patterns may develop, such as carbohydrate cravings and the compulsive desire to eat the same food item (Bathgate et al. 2001).

Despite the paucity of cognitive complaints, neuropsychological testing shows deficits in verbal fluency and impaired frontal-executive functions such as abstract thinking, decision making, planning, sequencing, and set shifting. Diminished verbal free recall with benefit from semantic cueing is common, but visual memory is characteristically spared (Hodges and Miller 2001; Hou et al. 2003; Pasquier and Delacourte 1998).

PRIMARY PROGRESSIVE APHASIA

Primary progressive aphasia is an FTD variant characterized by early prominent language impairment. The patient's speech is dysfluent, effortful, and agrammatic. Language comprehension is preserved until late in the disease course with the exception of grammatically complex linguistic constructs. Anomia and phonemic paraphasic errors are pronounced. Despite the significant language involvement, these patients are frequently independent and continue to work until late in the disease course. Behavioral disturbances are mild in primary progressive aphasia.

In addition to the typical primary progressive aphasia presentation, two other variants of primary progressive aphasia recently have been defined: 1) progressive anarthria primary progressive aphasia variant and 2) logopenic progressive aphasia variant. In the former, the speech disorder is one of progressive difficulty with articulation; in the latter, the language output is anomic and dysfluent but nevertheless grammatically correct. Syntax, phonology, and semantic knowledge are relatively preserved, making the diagnoses of the classic primary progressive aphasia variant and semantic dementia unlikely (Gorno-Tempini et al. 2004).

SEMANTIC DEMENTIA

Semantic dementia presents with language impairment caused by semantic knowledge loss (e.g., concepts about word meaning, object use). The speech of patients with semantic dementia is fluent, well articulated, and grammatically correct but has simplified content and anomic substitutions with general words such as "thing" and "it." Semantic paraphasias of the supraordinate categories (e.g., "plant" for "flower") are frequent. The semantic knowledge dysfunction results in impaired receptive language function for both spoken and written language. Characteristically, patients with semantic dementia have surface dyslexia, in which they fail to correctly read or spell irregular words such as "yacht" or "pint" and instead use letter-by-letter reading or spelling (Gorno-Tempini et al. 2004). Frontal-type behaviors are frequently seen in semantic dementia (Bozeat et al. 2000; Hodges and Miller 2001). Semantic dementia patients have been reported to lack mental flexibility and to have significant depression (Bozeat et al. 2000).

NEUROPSYCHIATRIC FEATURES OF FRONTOTEMPORAL DEMENTIA

Figure 25–10 shows the frequency of neuropsychiatric symptoms in FTD assessed with the NPI. Relative to AD, FTD patients have significantly more apathy, euphoria, disinhibition, and abnormal motor behavior. The spectrum of neuropsychiatric symptoms in frontal variant FTD includes some specific behaviors such as obsessive-compulsive behavior, emotional lability, profound emotional coldness, loss of empathy, and dietary or eating changes. Obsessive-compulsive behavior is present in 24% of FTD patients at presentation and in 47% of FTD patients 2 years after diagnosis. It manifests as simple repetitive mannerisms such as lip smacking, hand clapping or rubbing, and counting or as complex compulsive acts such as hoarding, repeating a fixed route, having a strict routine, engaging in hyperorality, craving certain

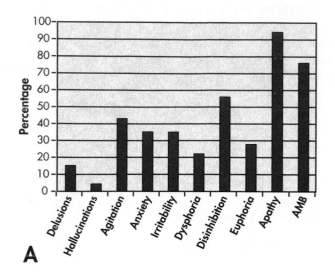

A

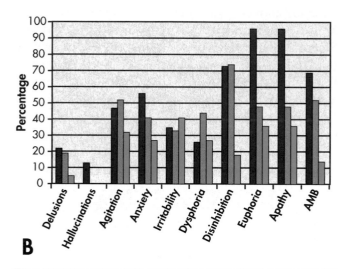

B

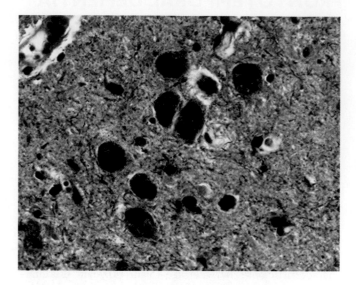

FIGURE 25–11.   Pick's bodies stained with Bielschow-sky's stain.

Source.   Image courtesy of Ivan Klement.

FIGURE 25–10.   *Panel A.* Frequency of neuropsychiatric symptoms in frontotemporal dementia (FTD). *Panel B.* Comparison of the frequency of neuropsychiatric symptoms in frontal variant FTD (fvFTD; *blue*), temporal variant FTD (tvFTD; *orange*), and Alzheimer's disease (AD; *green*). AMB=aberrant motor behavior.

Source.   Panel A data from Levy et al. 1996 and Mourik et al. 2004. Panel B data from Liu et al. 2004.

foods, eating the same food item every day, or performing complex ritualistic behaviors (Bathgate et al. 2001; Mendez and Perryman 2002).

PATHOLOGY OF FRONTOTEMPORAL DEMENTIA

FTD is generally considered a tauopathy. The tau gene is located on chromosome 17. Its product, the tau protein,

has four 31– to 32–amino acid repeats toward its carboxyl end. Tau exists in six isoforms—half are three-repeat (3R) and half are four-repeat (4R) tau. In healthy individuals, 3R and 4R tau are equally expressed. In most tauopathies, the ratio is changed. Patients with FTD sometimes have 3R and 4R tau disequilibrium.

Pick's disease (frontal variant FTD) is a 3R tau disorder. On gross inspection, the brain shows striking frontal, temporal, or combined frontotemporal atrophy. The microscopic imprint is the intraneuronal argyrophylic spherical tau inclusion called Pick's bodies (Figure 25–11). Other characteristic changes are striking neuronal loss and swollen neurons called Pick's cells (Bergeron et al. 2003; Lantos and Cairns 2001).

In most patients with hereditary FTD, tau inclusions in neurons and glia in addition to neuronal loss and vacuolation of the superficial cortical layers are seen (Ghetti et al. 2003; Lantos and Cairns 2001).

Tau-negative forms of FTD have been described. One is pathologically defined as dementia lacking distinctive histopathology, in which neuronal loss, gliosis, and microvacuolation are the sole pathological features. Nevertheless, when biochemical analyses were conducted, substantial reductions in the soluble brain tau content in both gray and white matter were found (Zhukareva et al. 2003).

The other form is the tau-negative ubiquitin-positive FTD that frequently presents with concomitant amyotrophic lateral sclerosis (ALS) (Lantos and Cairns 2001).

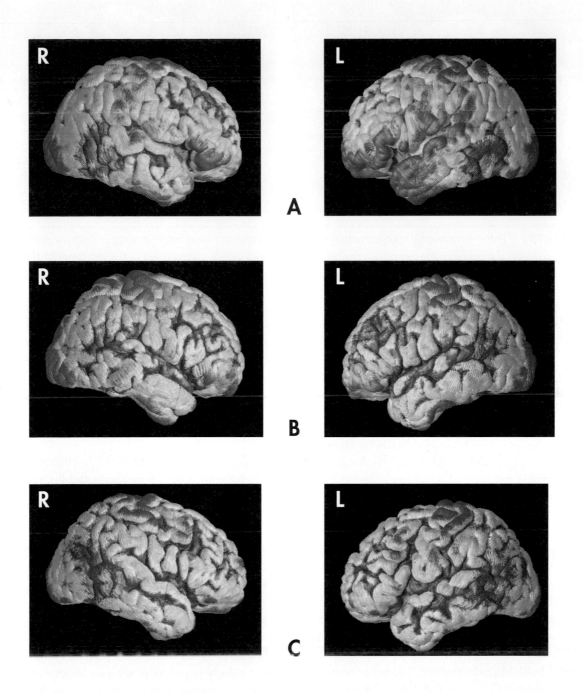

FIGURE 25–12.   Gray matter atrophy in frontotemporal dementia (FTD). In frontal variant FTD *(Row A)*, the frontal and temporal lobes are affected with right-sided predilection. In primary progressive aphasia *(Row B)*, left hemisphere involvement is more pronounced. The phonological centers—the left posterior inferior frontal gyrus and the left superior temporal gyrus—are characteristically affected. In semantic dementia *(Row C)*, the left hemisphere is more affected. The centers of semantic processing—the left anterior temporal lobe, the left middle temporal gyrus, and the left parietal cortex—are characteristically involved. *Red*=most atrophic; *blue*=least atrophic; *yellow* and *green*=intermediate atrophy.

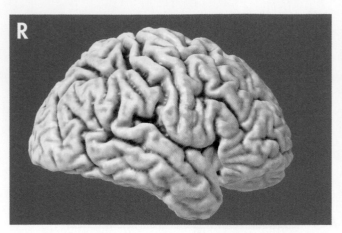
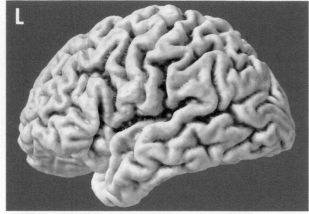

FIGURE 25–13.   Three-dimensional reconstruction of structural magnetic resonance imaging in primary progressive aphasia. Note the asymmetric atrophy of the perisylvian region on the left with severe involvement of the left superior temporal gyrus, a key area for phonological processing, and the left posterior inferior frontal gyrus (Broca's area), a key area for speech production.

GENETICS OF FRONTOTEMPORAL DEMENTIA

Approximately 40% of FTD patients have a family history suggestive of a similar disorder in a close relative. In 89% of the familial FTD cases, the inheritance pattern is autosomal dominant. The presentation in relatives is variable and includes personality and/or behavior changes, dementia, psychiatric illness, ALS, and parkinsonism (Chow et al. 1999).

Many causative mutations in the tau gene on chromosome 17 have been reported. In the central nervous system (CNS), 11 of the 16 exons of the tau gene are expressed. Mutations have been reported in exons 1, 9, 10, 11, 12, and 13. All mutations are autosomal dominant and have high penetrance, along with significant phenotypic variability (Ghetti et al. 2003; Hodges and Miller 2001).

In one family with FTD with dementia lacking distinctive histopathology, a linkage to chromosome 3 was found. Another with FTD-ALS had a mutation on chromosome 9, and a third had ubiquitin-positive, tau-negative inclusions on chromosome 17 (Lowe and Rossor 2003).

NEUROIMAGING IN FRONTOTEMPORAL DEMENTIA

The three subtypes of FTD have very distinct neuroimaging profiles. The behavioral variant of FTD has predominant frontal and to a lesser extent temporal atrophy, which is usually more significant on the right (Figure 25–12A). Primary progressive aphasia is associated with left inferior frontal, left insular, and left superior temporal involvement (Figures 25–12B and 25–13). Semantic

dementia is associated with atrophy of the left anterior temporal pole and gray matter loss in temporal, parietal, and frontal lobes (Figure 25–12C). Functional imaging shows frontotemporal changes (see Figure 25–7).

THERAPY FOR FRONTOTEMPORAL DEMENTIA

No effective therapy for FTD is currently available. SSRIs have been tested in open-label fashion. They provide symptomatic relief from compulsive behaviors, depression, disinhibition, and carbohydrate craving and reduce caregiver burden (R. Moretti et al. 2003a; Swartz et al. 1997). Selegiline, a monoamine oxidase–B inhibitor, may influence behavior and improve executive performance (R. Moretti et al. 2002).

VASCULAR DEMENTIA

VaD (Table 25–6) is the third leading cause of dementia in the elderly population, with an incidence of 6–12 per 1,000 in patients older than 70 years (Corey-Bloom 2004; Grabowski et al. 2002). It is caused by acquired ischemic or hemorrhagic brain damage; the most common etiologies are cerebrovascular and cardiovascular pathology. VaD is a heterogeneous dementia syndrome. It may be caused by small- or large-vessel arteriosclerotic disease, cardiac embolism, vasospasm, hypoperfusion, or hematological and rheological disturbances. Currently, the following VaD syndromes are recognized: multiinfarct dementia, single strategically placed infarct, lacunar state, and poststroke cognitive deterioration (Bowler 2002; Korczyn 2002). Rarer variants are Binswanger's

TABLE 25–6.   Diagnostic criteria for vascular dementia (VaD)

Probable VaD

Cognitive decline in two or more cognitive domains interfering with activities of daily living

Absence of delirium, aphasia, or sensorimotor impairment precluding administration of neuropsychological tests

Absence of another medical or psychiatric disorder that can cause cognitive decline

Focal neurological signs consistent with stroke

Neuroimaging evidence of extensive cerebrovascular disease

Onset of dementia within 3 months of a documented stroke

Abrupt onset, stepwise deterioration, and/or fluctuating course

Supporting features

Early gait disturbance

History of unsteadiness and frequent falls

Early urinary problems not explained by genitourinary condition

Pseudobulbar palsy

Neuropsychiatric manifestations such as mood changes, abulia, depression, and emotional incontinence

Psychomotor retardation or executive dysfunction

Possible VaD

Dementia otherwise meeting criteria for probable VaD but without neuroimaging confirmation of definite cerebrovascular disease

Dementia otherwise meeting criteria for probable VaD but without a clear temporal relation with a stroke event

Dementia otherwise meeting criteria for probable VaD but with subtle onset and gradual course of cognitive decline

Source.   Adapted from Roman et al. 1993.

disease, the genetic forms (such as cerebral autosomal dominant arteriopathy with subcortical infarcts and leukoencephalopathy, hypercoagulable states), and hypoxic-ischemic encephalopathy. Common risk factors for VaD are hypertension, hyperlipidemia, hyperhomocystinemia, diabetes mellitus, and smoking (Bowler 2002; Korczyn 2002). This discussion focuses primarily on the most common presentation—multi-infarct dementia.

Neuropsychological deficits in multi-infarct VaD are mostly suggestive of a subcortical dementia pattern, in which psychomotor slowing and executive dysfunction prevail. Relative to AD, VaD is associated with retrieval as opposed to encoding pattern of memory deficit. Decline in attention, processing speed, and set shifting are more readily observed (Schmidtke and Hull 2002). Language difficulties are common. Dysarthria may be present, along with shorter phrase length and simplified vocabulary and syntax. Confrontation naming is frequently impaired, albeit to a lesser extent when compared with AD. Visuospatial difficulties or problems with execution and planning may follow parietal involvement (McPherson and Cummings 1996).

The neurological examination is an important step in the evaluation of VaD patients because it frequently has abnormal results. Focal or generalized upper motor neuron signs (weakness, spasticity, hyperreflexia, extensor plantar reflex) and extrapyramidal findings (bradykinesia, rigidity, lower-body parkinsonism) are common. Gait abnormalities are frequently present, sometimes to the extent of gait apraxia. Dysarthria and/or aphasia and urinary incontinence also may be present (Chui 2001).

NEUROPSYCHIATRIC FEATURES OF VASCULAR DEMENTIA

Neuropsychiatric symptoms are common in VaD (Figure 25–14). Vascular depression is thought to occur from disruption of striato-pallido-thalamo-cortical pathways (Alexopoulos et al. 1997a, 1997b). Elderly depressed patients with new onset of depressive symptoms tend to have more white matter ischemic changes and more functional impairment than do elderly depressed patients with idiopathic depression. Functional impairment 3 months after stroke correlates highly with depressive

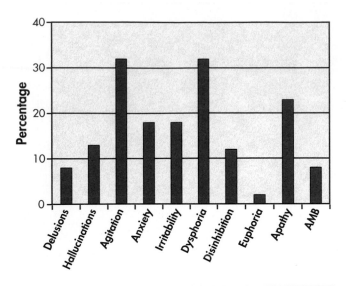

FIGURE 25–14.   Frequency of neuropsychiatric symptoms in vascular dementia. AMB=aberrant motor behavior.

Source.   Adapted from Lyketsos et al. 2000.

symptoms, whereas a year after the stroke, social isolation tends to associate better. In some studies, up to 94% of the patients with onset of depression after age 65 years have had silent strokes. Depression is highly prevalent among elderly with hypertension and coronary artery disease. Vascular depression leads to disturbance in attention, cognitive processing speed, and executive function (Alexopoulos et al. 1997b). Another study compared vascular depression with nonvascular depression and found that vascular depression tends to start later in life and is associated with significantly fewer psychotic features (Krishnan et al. 1997). Poststroke depression occurs more often after left hemispheric stroke, most frequently in the vascular territory of the middle cerebral artery, and with frontal lobe involvement. It shows a positive correlation with the size of the ischemic area (Joseph 1999; Paradiso and Robinson 1998; Shimoda and Robinson 1999). Relative to AD and mild cognitive impairment, VaD has the highest incidence of new-onset depression, and the mood changes are more refractory to therapy (Y.S. Li et al. 2001).

Psychosis is relatively common in VaD: 15.3% of patients are affected. Delusions are seen in 12.5% and hallucinations in 15.5%. Common delusional themes are delusions of theft, misidentification syndromes, phantom boarder, delusions of abandonment, and reduplicative paramnesia. Visual hallucinations were slightly more prevalent relative to auditory ones (Leroi et al. 2003).

A large epidemiological study of community-dwelling elderly with VaD used the NPI to assess the frequency

and severity of individual neuropsychiatric symptoms. Most common were depression and aggressive behaviors followed by apathy, irritability, and anxiety. Less frequent were delusions, hallucinations, disinhibition, and abnormal motor behaviors, and least common was euphoria (Lyketsos et al. 2000) (see Figure 25–14). Relative to AD, VaD has more severe depression, agitation, and apathy (Aharon-Peretz et al. 2000).

PATHOLOGY OF VASCULAR DEMENTIA

The pathological findings in VaD are heterogeneous. Multi-infarct dementia typically has underlying infarcts in the territory of the middle cerebral artery and the watershed regions. Microangiopathic changes and lacunar infarcts are commonly seen in the basal ganglia, periventricular white matter, or cortical and subcortical areas. They can lead to strategic infarct dementia syndrome in the case of thalamic, mesial temporal lobe, posterior cerebral artery territory, or basal forebrain strokes; to Binswanger's disease in the case of confluent lacunae and/or cystic infarcts in basal ganglia and periventicular white matter; or to multilacunar state in the case of basal ganglia and brain stem lacunar infarcts. Hypoperfusion VaD is characterized by multiple watershed cortical and subcortical microinfarcts and is most commonly a result of tight stenosis of the internal carotid or middle cerebral artery. Postischemic encephalopathy is characterized by cortical laminar necrosis and hippocampal and cerebellar ischemia and is most commonly due to cardiorespiratory collapse (Jellinger 2002).

NEUROIMAGING IN VASCULAR DEMENTIA

Chronic VaD lesions are best visualized on T2 and fluid attenuation inverse recovery (FLAIR) MRI sequences as hyperintense lesions (Figure 25–15). Acute infarcts are most easily appreciated on diffusion-weighted imaging as hyperintense lesions and on apparent diffusion coefficient maps as hypointense lesions. Functional imaging shows deficits in the areas corresponding with the stroke location.

THERAPY FOR VASCULAR DEMENTIA

The most important therapy in VaD is stroke prevention. Smoking cessation and tight control of hypertension, hyperlipidemia, and diabetes mellitus are imperative. Aspirin should be used for routine prophylaxis. Physical, occupational, and speech therapy may be beneficial for the functional recovery of many patients.

In VaD, cognitive, behavioral, and functional scales showed improvement in three acetylcholinesterase inhibitor trials (Black et al. 2003; Erkinjuntti et al. 2004;

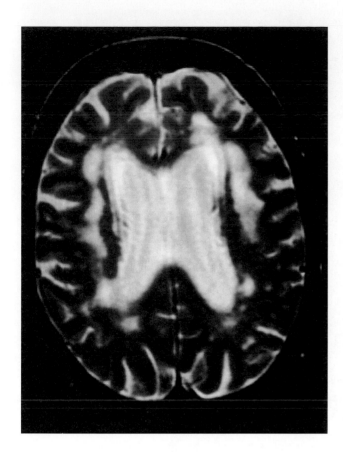

FIGURE 25–15. T2-weighted magnetic resonance imaging scan of a patient with vascular dementia showing confluent hyperintense white matter lesions of the periventricular white matter consistent with ischemic cerebral injury.

R. Moretti et al. 2003b; Passmore et al. 2005). Depression may respond to antidepressant therapy (Alexopoulos et al. 1997b; Starkstein and Robinson 1994). Pseudobulbar palsy may improve with antidepressant therapy or a fixed combination of dextromethorphan and quinidine. Atypical antipsychotics should be used only with greatest caution in this patient population because they have been shown to increase the risk for stroke and death in demented elderly patients with vascular risk factors (Bullock 2005; Sink et al. 2005).

CREUTZFELDT-JAKOB DISEASE

The prion disorders are a rare subgroup of the neurodegenerative diseases caused by infectious agents with proteinlike properties. Four prion disorders are known to affect humans—CJD, Gerstmann-Straussler-Scheinker syndrome, fatal familial insomnia, and kuru. CJD is the most common among them and is the one that character-

istically presents with rapid cognitive decline. Sporadic CJD is a disease that typically presents in the seventh decade of life (range 45–75 years) (Collinge and Palmer 1996). Familial CJD and new variant CJD (nvCJD) tend to present at a younger age.

The classic CJD presentation is that of rapidly progressing cognitive decline, with ataxia, multifocal myoclonic jerks, and startle myoclonus. Other features may include weakness, neuropathy, chorea, hallucinations, visual field cuts, language disturbance, and seizures. A third of the patients have prodromal fatigue, headache, insomnia, malaise, or depression. After myoclonus appears, electroencephalographic (EEG) recording typically shows periodic paroxysmal triphasic or sharp wave discharges against a slow background. EEG abnormalities are absent in as many as 30% of the patients. Cerebrospinal fluid (CSF) examination may show nonspecific abnormalities such as increased protein (Collinge and Palmer 1996). A sensitive but not highly specific CSF laboratory finding is the presence of protein 14–3–3 (Collinge and Palmer 1996; Mastrianni and Roos 2000). A promising diagnostic technique is tonsilar, olfactory mucosal, or muscle biopsy with immunostaining for the causative prion protein variant PrP^{sc}. Homozygosity for methionine at codon 129 of the prion gene is a predisposing factor for sporadic CJD (Collinge and Palmer 1996; Glatzel et al. 2005; Mastrianni and Roos 2000).

Iatrogenic CJD has been reported after inoculation of prion protein (PrP) via blood transfusions, inadequately sterilized surgical equipment or depth electrodes, dural grafts, corneal implants, and human pituitary–derived growth hormone. In these cases, ataxia may be the predominant presentation following severe cerebellar involvement. Genetic susceptibility may play a role (Collinge and Palmer 1996; Mastrianni and Roos 2000).

nvCJD was first reported in 1995 in the United Kingdom. It is thought to result from cow-to-human interspecies transmission of bovine spongiform encephalopathy via alimentary intake of beef or beef products. Early prominent neuropsychiatric disturbance with prominent anxiety, depression, and apathy with later progression to ataxia, dementia, chorea, or myoclonus is characteristic. Dysesthesias may be present. The inflicted are mostly children and adolescents (average age 26.3 years). The average survival is 14 months (Collinge and Palmer 1996; Ironside and Bell 1996).

Familial CJD accounts for about 15% of the CJD cases and is caused by point mutations, insertions, or deletions in the prion gene on chromosome 20. It tends to present a decade earlier than the sporadic variant and has a longer course (Collinge and Palmer 1996; Mastrianni and Roos 2000).

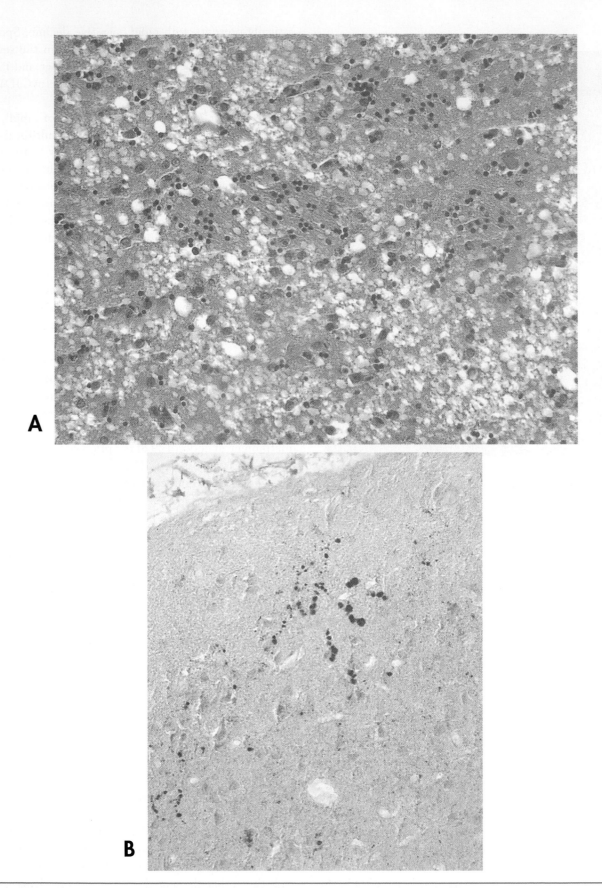

FIGURE 25–16.   *Panel A.* Spongiosis of the basal ganglia in Creutzfeldt-Jakob disease (CJD) stained with hematoxylin-eosin. *Panel B.* PrP^{Sc} immunostain in CJD.

NEUROPSYCHIATRIC FEATURES OF CREUTZFELDT-JAKOB DISEASE

Apathy, depression, sleep disorders, anorexia (Ajax and Rodnitzky 1998), and voracious appetite (personal observation) can occur. Hallucinations can occur in some (Mastrianni and Roos 2000). Prominent early neuropsychiatric changes are a classic feature in nvCJD (Collinge and Palmer 1996).

PATHOLOGY OF CREUTZFELDT-JAKOB DISEASE

PrP is a membrane-associated 253–amino acid protein in α-helical conformation. It is thought to play a role in signal transduction or as a serine protease or superoxide dismutase. PrP^{Sc} is a protease-resistant, β-pleated isoform of normal PrP. Disease progression is thought to occur by template-directed refolding when PrP^{Sc} serves as a template for normally folded PrP. Following the interaction, PrP is transformed into the infectious PrP^{Sc} isoform. Experimental interspecies transmission of prion in yeast cells was finally accomplished, which provided evidence for the primary role of the PrP in the infectious process (Tanaka et al. 2005).

The most striking microscopic abnormality in sporadic CJD is the pancortical vacuolation commonly referred to as *spongiosis* (Figure 25–16A). The vacuoles are axonal and dendritic swellings with accumulation of membranous material. Neuronal vacuolation may occasionally be present. Vacuoles can be seen in the cerebellum, white matter, basal ganglia, and brain stem. Reactive gliosis is present, but inflammatory cells are characteristically absent. The cortical areas most commonly showing spongiform changes are the occipital cortex, inferior temporal gyrus, and parietal cortex. Prion amyloid plaques are rarely seen in sporadic CJD and are only occasionally seen in familial CJD. They are more typical of nvCJD, iatrogenic CJD, kuru, and Gerstmann-Straussler-Scheinker syndrome (Ajax and Rodnitzky 1998; Ironside and Bell 1996).

Immunostaining of PrP^{Sc} (Figure 25–16B) is a sensitive technique allowing for definitive diagnosis of CJD and is extremely useful for questionable cases with very mild spongiform change. Immunostaining for PrP^{Sc} can be seen both in areas with spongiform change and in normal-appearing tissue (Ironside and Bell 1996).

NEUROIMAGING IN CREUTZFELDT-JAKOB DISEASE

MRI in CJD can show very specific abnormalities and aid the correct diagnosis. Increased T2 and FLAIR signal intensity in the basal ganglia (caudate, putamen) and in the pulvinar have been reported (Milton et al. 1991; Zeidler et al. 2000). Diffusion weighted images can show high signal in the basal ganglia and in the cortical ribbon most frequently in parieto-occipital distribution (Hirose et al. 1998; Matoba et al. 2001; Yee et al. 1999).

THERAPY FOR CREUTZFELDT-JAKOB DISEASE

No definite therapy for CJD is yet available. The antimalarial compound quinacrine cleared PrP^{Sc} in cell cultures. Despite lack of efficacy in a mouse prion model, two human trials are under way in the United States and the United Kingdom. Another potential agent, pentosan polyphosphate, was efficacious in animal models. Only anecdotal intraventricular application in humans has been conducted to date. Monoclonal anti-PrP antibodies have been very effective in cell cultures and mice, seemingly arresting prion infectivity. The antibodies, however, do not pass the blood-brain barrier and cannot be used for the CNS stage of the disorder. Their therapeutic potential lies only in secondary prevention after accidental inoculation. Another plausible therapeutic intervention is active immunization, but autoimmune sensitization and meningoencephalitis are potential complications (Mallucci and Collinge 2004).

CONCLUSION

The dementias are a prominent group of neurological disorders occurring mainly in the elderly. The full assessment of the patient with cognitive decline includes a thorough history of the current illness with particular attention to activities of daily living as well as social, family, and medication history. Alcohol and drug abuse and sexually transmitted diseases (e.g., syphilis, AIDS) need to be excluded in the appropriate patients. A detailed neuropsychiatric assessment of personality changes, mood disorders, and psychotic symptoms can help in the differential diagnosis. Such changes are sometimes present years before the onset of the cognitive decline. Genetic tests may be considered in young patients with a family history of dementia.

With advances in molecular biology and genetics, our understanding of the pathophysiology of dementia is steadily increasing. The pharmaceutical industry has many promising compounds in Phase I and II clinical trials. Candidate compounds are being identified to prevent or delay the onset or slow the decline in dementing illnesses.

Highlights for the Clinician

Approach	Notes	Comments
For all dementias:		
Inquire about behavioral changes	*Early in course:* Personality and mood changes, apathy, anxiety, irritability, appetite changes	✦ These features may precede cognitive decline.
	Later in course: Hallucinations, delusions, sundowning, disinhibition, agitation, aggression, aberrant motor behavior	✦ Family counseling and appropriate behavioral and pharmacological therapy help reduce patient and caregiver distress and delay nursing home placement.
Family education and counseling	A necessary intervention at each clinical visit	✦ Helps reduce caregiver distress and delay nursing home placement.
Treatment	Behavioral interventions	✦ Help reduce caregiver distress and delay nursing home placement.
	Medications	✦ Use cautiously and only when needed. ✦ Do not prescribe typical antipsychotics (high risk of parkinsonism and neuroleptic malignant syndrome). ✦ Treat with atypical antipsychotics only if psychosis is disturbing to patient and family. ✦ Consider acetylcholinesterase inhibitors as an alternative.
Always consider…	Dementia with Lewy bodies in patients with psychosis and parkinsonian features	

RECOMMENDED READINGS

Apostolova LG, Cummings JL: Neuropsychiatric features of dementia with Lewy bodies, in Dementia With Lewy Bodies and Parkinson's Disease. Edited by O'Brien J, McKeith I, Ames D, et al. Oxford, UK, Taylor and Francis, 2006, pp 73–94

Ballard C, Waite J, Birks J: Atypical antipsychotics for aggression and psychosis in Alzheimer's disease. Cochrane Database of Systematic Reviews. Wiley, 2006, pp 1–108

Craig D, Mirakhur A, Hart DJ, et al: A cross-sectional study of neuropsychiatric symptoms in 435 patients with Alzheimer's disease. Am J Geriatr Psychiatry 13:460–468, 2005

Lyketsos CG, Lopez O, Jones B, et al: Prevalence of neuropsychiatric symptoms in dementia and mild cognitive impairment: results from the cardiovascular health study. JAMA 288:1475–1483, 2002

McKeith IG, Dickson DW, Lowe J, et al: Diagnosis and management of dementia with Lewy bodies: third report of the DLB Consortium. Neurology 65:1863–1872, 2005

Sink KM, Holden KF, Yaffe K: Pharmacological treatment of neuropsychiatric symptoms of dementia: a review of the evidence. JAMA 293:596–608, 2005

REFERENCES

Aarsland D, Ballard C, Larsen JP, et al: A comparative study of psychiatric symptoms in dementia with Lewy bodies and Parkinson's disease with and without dementia. Int J Geriatr Psychiatry 16:528–536, 2001

Aharon-Peretz J, Kliot D, Tomer R: Behavioral differences between white matter lacunar dementia and Alzheimer's disease: a comparison on the neuropsychiatric inventory. Dement Geriatr Cogn Disord 11:294–298, 2000

Aisen PS: Anti-inflammatory therapy for Alzheimer's disease: implications of the prednisone trial. Acta Neurol Scand Suppl 176:85–89, 2000

Aisen PS, Davis KL, Berg JD, et al: A randomized controlled trial of prednisone in Alzheimer's disease. Alzheimer's Disease Cooperative Study. Neurology 54:588–593, 2000

Aisen PS, Schafer KA, Grundman M, et al: Effects of rofecoxib or naproxen vs placebo on Alzheimer disease progression: a randomized controlled trial. JAMA 289:2819–2826, 2003

Ajax T, Rodnitzky R: Creutzfeldt-Jacob disease. Home Healthcare Consultant 5:8–16, 1998

Alexopoulos GS, Meyers BS, Young RC, et al: Clinically defined vascular depression. Am J Psychiatry 154:562–565, 1997a

Alexopoulos GS, Meyers BS, Young RC, et al: "Vascular depression" hypothesis. Arch Gen Psychiatry 54:915–922, 1997b

Alexopoulos GS, Jeste D, Chung H, et al: The expert consensus guideline series. Treatment of dementia and its behavioral disturbances. Introduction: methods, commentary, and summary. Postgrad Med (special report):6–22, 2005

American Psychiatric Association: Diagnostic and Statistical Manual of Mental Disorders, 3rd Edition, Revised. Washington, DC, American Psychiatric Association, 1987

American Psychiatric Association: Diagnostic and Statistical Manual of Mental Disorders, 4th Edition, Text Revision. Washington, DC, American Psychiatric Association, 2000

Apostolova LG, Dinov ID, Dutton RA, et al: 3D comparison of hippocampal atrophy in amnestic mild cognitive impairment and Alzheimer's disease. Brain 129:2867–2873, 2006

Apostolova LG, Steiner CA, Akopyan GG, et al: 3D gray matter atrophy mapping in mild cognitive impairment and mild Alzheimer's disease. Arch Neurol (in press)

Arnulf I, Bonnet AM, Damier P, et al: Hallucinations, REM sleep, and Parkinson's disease: a medical hypothesis. Neurology 55:281–288, 2000

Assal F, Cummings JL: Neuropsychiatric symptoms in the dementias. Curr Opin Neurol 15:445–450, 2002

Ballard C, Lowery K, Harrison R, et al: Noncognitive symptoms in Lewy body dementia, in Dementia With Lewy Bodies. Edited by Perry R, McKeith I, Perry E. Cambridge, UK, Cambridge University Press, 1996, pp 67–84

Ballard C, McKeith I, Harrison R, et al: A detailed phenomenological comparison of complex visual hallucinations in dementia with Lewy bodies and Alzheimer's disease. Int Psychogeriatr 9:381–388, 1997a

Ballard C, O'Brien J, Coope B, et al: A prospective study of psychotic symptoms in dementia sufferers: psychosis in dementia. Int Psychogeriatr 9:57–64, 1997b

Ballard C, Holmes C, McKeith I, et al: Psychiatric morbidity in dementia with Lewy bodies: a prospective clinical and neuropathological comparative study with Alzheimer's disease. Am J Psychiatry 156:1039–1045, 1999

Ballard C, O'Brien J, Gray A, et al: Attention and fluctuating attention in patients with dementia with Lewy bodies and Alzheimer disease. Arch Neurol 58:977–982, 2001a

Ballard C, O'Brien J, Morris CM, et al: The progression of cognitive impairment in dementia with Lewy bodies, vascular dementia and Alzheimer's disease. Int J Geriatr Psychiatry 16:499–503, 2001b

Ballard CG, O'Brien JT, Swann AG, et al: The natural history of psychosis and depression in dementia with Lewy bodies and Alzheimer's disease: persistence and new cases over 1 year of follow-up. J Clin Psychiatry 62:46–49, 2001c

Baquero M, Blasco R, Campos-Garcia A, et al: [Descriptive study of behavioural disorders in mild cognitive impairment] (Spanish). Rev Neurol 38:323–326, 2004

Barber R, Gholkar A, Scheltens P, et al: Medial temporal lobe atrophy on MRI in dementia with Lewy bodies. Neurology 52:1153–1158, 1999

Barber R, Ballard C, McKeith IG, et al: MRI volumetric study of dementia with Lewy bodies: a comparison with AD and vascular dementia. Neurology 54:1304–1309, 2000

Barber R, McKeith IG, Ballard C, et al: A comparison of medial and lateral temporal lobe atrophy in dementia with Lewy bodies and Alzheimer's disease: magnetic resonance imaging volumetric study. Dement Geriatr Cogn Disord 12:198–205, 2001

Bard F, Cannon C, Barbour R, et al: Peripherally administered antibodies against amyloid beta-peptide enter the central nervous system and reduce pathology in a mouse model of Alzheimer disease. Nat Med 6:916–919, 2000

Bard F, Barbour R, Cannon C, et al: Epitope and isotype specificities of antibodies to beta-amyloid peptide for protection against Alzheimer's disease-like neuropathology. Proc Natl Acad Sci U S A 100:2023–2028, 2003

Bathgate D, Snowden JS, Varma A, et al: Behaviour in frontotemporal dementia, Alzheimer's disease and vascular dementia. Acta Neurol Scand 103:367–378, 2001

Beard CM, Kokmen E, Sigler C, et al: Cause of death in Alzheimer's disease. Ann Epidemiol 6:195–200, 1996

Benoit M, Robert P: [Depression and apathy in Alzheimer's disease] (French). Presse Med 32:S14–S18, 2003

Benoit M, Koulibaly PM, Migneco O, et al: Brain perfusion in Alzheimer's disease with and without apathy: a SPECT study with statistical parametric mapping analysis. Psychiatry Res 114:103–111, 2002

Berger AK, Fratiglioni L, Forsell Y, et al: The occurrence of depressive symptoms in the preclinical phase of AD: a population-based study. Neurology 53:1998–2002, 1999

Bergeron C, Morris HR, Rossor M: Pick's disease, in Neurodegeneration: The Molecular Pathology of Dementia and Movement Disorders. Edited by Dickson DW. Basel, Switzerland, ISN Neuropath Press, 2003, pp 124–131

Bertoli Avella AM, Marcheco Teruel B, Llibre Rodriguez JJ, et al: A novel presenilin 1 mutation (L174 M) in a large Cuban family with early onset Alzheimer disease. Neurogenetics 4:97–104, 2002

Bhat RV, Budd Haeberlein SL, Avila J: Glycogen synthase kinase 3: a drug target for CNS therapies. J Neurochem 89:1313–1317, 2004

Binetti G, Signorini S, Squitti R, et al: Atypical dementia associated with a novel presenilin-2 mutation. Ann Neurol 54:832–836, 2003

Bird TD, Sumi SM, Nemens EJ, et al: Phenotypic heterogeneity in familial Alzheimer's disease: a study of 24 kindreds. Ann Neurol 25:12–25, 1989

Black S, Roman GC, Geldmacher DS, et al: Efficacy and tolerability of donepezil in vascular dementia: positive results of a 24-week, multicenter, international, randomized, placebo-controlled clinical trial. Stroke 34:2323–2330, 2003

Blacker D, Haines JL, Rodes L, et al: ApoE-4 and age at onset of Alzheimer's disease: the NIMH genetics initiative. Neurology 48:139–147, 1997

Boeve BF, Silber MH, Ferman TJ, et al: Association of REM sleep behavior disorder and neurodegenerative disease may reflect an underlying synucleinopathy. Mov Disord 16:622–630, 2001

Boeve BF, Silber MH, Ferman TJ: Melatonin for treatment of REM sleep behavior disorder in neurologic disorders: results in 14 patients. Sleep Med 4:281–284, 2003a

Boeve BF, Silber MH, Parisi JE, et al: Synucleinopathy pathology and REM sleep behavior disorder plus dementia or parkinsonism. Neurology 61:40–45, 2003b

Bowler JV: The concept of vascular cognitive impairment. J Neurol Sci 203-204:11–15, 2002

Boyle PA, Malloy PF, Salloway S, et al: Executive dysfunction and apathy predict functional impairment in Alzheimer disease. Am J Geriatr Psychiatry 11:214–221, 2003

Bozeat S, Gregory CA, Ralph MA, et al: Which neuropsychiatric and behavioural features distinguish frontal and temporal variants of frontotemporal dementia from Alzheimer's disease? J Neurol Neurosurg Psychiatry 69:178–186, 2000

Braak H, Braak E: Frequency of stages of Alzheimer-related lesions in different age categories. Neurobiol Aging 18:351–357, 1997

Bullock R: Treatment of behavioural and psychiatric symptoms in dementia: implications of recent safety warnings. Curr Med Res Opin 21:1–10, 2005

Burton EJ, Karas G, Paling SM, et al: Patterns of cerebral atrophy in dementia with Lewy bodies using voxel-based morphometry. Neuroimage 17:618–630, 2002

Bussiere T, Bard F, Barbour R, et al: Morphological characterization of thioflavin-S-positive amyloid plaques in transgenic Alzheimer mice and effect of passive Abeta immunotherapy on their clearance. Am J Pathol 165:987–995, 2004

Campion D, Brice A, Dumanchin C, et al: A novel presenilin 1 mutation resulting in familial Alzheimer's disease with an onset age of 29 years. Neuroreport 7:1582–1584, 1996

Cercy SP, Bylsma FW: Lewy bodies and progressive dementia: a critical review and meta-analysis. J Int Neuropsychol Soc 3:179–194, 1997

Chow TW, Miller BL, Hayashi VN, et al: Inheritance of frontotemporal dementia. Arch Neurol 56:817–822, 1999

Chui H: Dementia attributable to subcortical ischemic vascular disease. Neurologist 7:208–219, 2001

Cohen FE, Kelly JW: Therapeutic approaches to protein-misfolding diseases. Nature 426:905–909, 2003

Collinge J, Palmer M: Human prion diseases, in Prion Diseases. Edited by Collinge J, Palmer M. New York, Oxford University Press, 1996, pp 18–56

Colloby SJ, Fenwick JD, Williams ED, et al: A comparison of (99m)Tc-HMPAO SPECT changes in dementia with Lewy bodies and Alzheimer's disease using statistical parametric mapping. Eur J Nucl Med Mol Imaging 29:615–622, 2002

Corder EH, Saunders AM, Strittmatter WJ, et al: Gene dose of apolipoprotein E type 4 allele and the risk of Alzheimer's disease in late onset families. Science 261:921–923, 1993

Corey-Bloom J: Alzheimer's disease. Continuum Lifelong Learning Neurol 10:29–57 2004

Craig AH, Cummings JL, Fairbanks L, et al: Cerebral blood flow correlates of apathy in Alzheimer disease. Arch Neurol 53:1116–1120, 1996

Cribbs DH, Ghochikyan A, Vasilevko V, et al: Adjuvant-dependent modulation of Th1 and Th2 responses to immunization with beta-amyloid. Int Immunol 15:505–514, 2003

Cummings JL: Frontal-subcortical circuits and human behavior. Arch Neurol 50:873–880, 1993

Cummings JL: Alzheimer's disease, in The Neuropsychiatry of Alzheimer's Disease and Related Dementias. Edited by Cummings JL. London, Martin Dunitz, 2003a, pp 57–116

Cummings JL: The impact of depressive symptoms on patients with Alzheimer disease (comment). Alzheimer Dis Assoc Disord 17:61–62, 2003b

Cummings JL, Mega M, Gray K, et al: The Neuropsychiatric Inventory: comprehensive assessment of psychopathology in dementia. Neurology 44:2308–2314, 1994

Damasio A, Van Hoesen G: Emotional disturbances associated with focal lesions of the limbic frontal lobe, in Neuropsychology of Human Emotion. Edited by Heilman K, Satz P. New York, Guilford, 1983, pp 85–108

Del Ser T, McKeith I, Anand R, et al: Dementia with Lewy bodies: findings from an international multicentre study. Int J Geriatr Psychiatry 15:1034–1045, 2000

Devanand DP, Jacobs DM, Tang MX, et al: The course of psychopathologic features in mild to moderate Alzheimer disease. Arch Gen Psychiatry 54:257–263, 1997

Donnemiller E, Heilmann J, Wenning GK, et al: Brain perfusion scintigraphy with 99mTc-HMPAO or 99mTc-ECD and 123I-beta-CIT single-photon emission tomography in dementia of the Alzheimer-type and diffuse Lewy body disease. Eur J Nucl Med 24:320–325, 1997

Doody RS: Update on Alzheimer drugs: donepezil. Neurologist 9:225–229, 2003

Duyckaerts C, Dickson DW: Neuropathology of Alzheimer's disease, in Neurodegeneration: The Molecular Pathology of Dementia and Movement Disorders. Edited by Dickson DW. Basel, Switzerland, ISN Neuropath Press, 2003, pp 47–65

Edwards KR, Hershey L, Wray L, et al: Efficacy and safety of galantamine in patients with dementia with Lewy bodies: a 12-week interim analysis. Dement Geriatr Cogn Disord 17 (suppl 1):40–48, 2004

Erkinjuntti T, Roman G, Gauthier S: Treatment of vascular dementia: evidence from clinical trials with cholinesterase inhibitors. J Neurol Sci 226:63–66, 2004

Esler WP, Marshall JR, Stimson ER, et al: Apolipoprotein E affects amyloid formation but not amyloid growth in vitro: mechanistic implications for apoE4 enhanced amyloid burden and risk for Alzheimer's disease. Amyloid 9:1–12, 2002

Espiritu DA, Rashid H, Mast BT, et al: Depression, cognitive impairment and function in Alzheimer's disease. Int J Geriatr Psychiatry 16:1098–1103, 2001

Evans DA, Bennett DA, Wilson RS, et al: Incidence of Alzheimer disease in a biracial urban community: relation to apolipoprotein E allele status. Arch Neurol 60:185–189, 2003

Farlow M: Update on rivastigmine. Neurologist 9:230–234, 2003

Farlow M, Murrell J, Ghetti B, et al: Clinical characteristics in a kindred with early onset Alzheimer's disease and their linkage to a G→T change at position 2149 of the amyloid precursor protein gene. Neurology 44:105–111, 1994

Feldman H, Scheltens P, Scarpini E, et al: Behavioral symptoms in mild cognitive impairment. Neurology 62:1199–1201, 2004

Ferman TJ, Boeve BF, Smith GE, et al: REM sleep behavior disorder and dementia: cognitive differences when compared with AD. Neurology 52:951–957, 1999

Ferman TJ, Boeve BF, Smith GE, et al: Dementia with Lewy bodies may present as dementia and REM sleep behavior disorder without parkinsonism or hallucinations. J Int Neuropsychol Soc 8:907–914, 2002

Ferrer I, Boada Rovira M, Sanchez Guerra ML, et al: Neuropathology and pathogenesis of encephalitis following amyloid-beta immunization in Alzheimer's disease. Brain Pathol 14:11–20, 2004

Forstl H, Burns A, Luthert P, et al: Clinical and neuropathological correlates of depression in Alzheimer's disease. Psychol Med 22:877–884, 1992

Fox NC, Kennedy AM, Harvey RJ, et al: Clinicopathological features of familial Alzheimer's disease associated with the M139V mutation in the presenilin 1 gene: pedigree but not mutation specific age at onset provides evidence for a further genetic factor. Brain 120 (pt 3):491–501, 1997

Freels S, Cohen D, Eisdorfer C, et al: Functional status and clinical findings in patients with Alzheimer's disease. J Gerontol 47:M177–M182, 1992

Friedhoff P, von Bergen M, Mandelkow EM, et al: A nucleated assembly mechanism of Alzheimer paired helical filaments. Proc Natl Acad Sci U S A 95:15712–15717, 1998

Frisoni GB, Rozzini L, Gozzetti A, et al: Behavioral syndromes in Alzheimer's disease: description and correlates. Dement Geriatr Cogn Disord 10:130–138, 1999

Fukuhara R, Ikeda M, Nebu A, et al: Alteration of rCBF in Alzheimer's disease patients with delusions of theft. Neuroreport 12:2473–2476, 2001

Gao S, Hendrie HC, Hall KS, et al: The relationships between age, sex, and the incidence of dementia and Alzheimer disease: a meta-analysis. Arch Gen Psychiatry 55:809–815, 1998

Garre-Olmo J, Lopez-Pousa S, Vilalta-Franch J, et al: Evolution of depressive symptoms in Alzheimer disease: one-year follow-up. Alzheimer Dis Assoc Disord 17:77–85, 2003

Geda YE, Smith GE, Knopman DS, et al: De novo genesis of neuropsychiatric symptoms in mild cognitive impairment (MCI). Int Psychogeriatr 16:51–60, 2004

Geerts H, Finkel L, Carr R, et al: Nicotinic receptor modulation: advantages for successful Alzheimer's disease therapy. J Neural Transm Suppl 62:203–216, 2002

Ghetti B, Hutton ML, Wszolek ZK: Frontotemporal dementia and parkinsonism linked to chromosome 17 associated with tau gene mutations, in Neurodegeneration: The Molecular Pathology of Dementia and Movement Disorders. Edited by Dickson DW. Basel, Switzerland, ISN Neuropath Press, 2003, pp 86–102

Giasson BI, Forman MS, Higuchi M, et al: Initiation and synergistic fibrillization of tau and alpha-synuclein. Science 300:636–640, 2003a

Giasson BI, Lee VM, Trojanowski JQ: Interactions of amyloidogenic proteins. Neuromolecular Med 4:49–58, 2003b

Glatzel M, Stoeck K, Seeger H, et al: Human prion diseases: molecular and clinical aspects. Arch Neurol 62:545–552, 2005

Gomez-Isla T, Price JL, McKeel DW Jr, et al: Profound loss of layer II entorhinal cortex neurons occurs in very mild Alzheimer's disease. J Neurosci 16:4491–4500, 1996

Gorno-Tempini ML, Dronkers NF, Rankin KP, et al: Cognition and anatomy in three variants of primary progressive aphasia. Ann Neurol 55:335–346, 2004

Gotz J, Chen F, van Dorpe J, et al: Formation of neurofibrillary tangles in P301l tau transgenic mice induced by Abeta 42 fibrils. Science 293:1491–1495, 2001

Grabowski TJ, Anderson SW, Cooper GE: Disorders of cognitive function. Continuum Lifetime Learning Neurol 8:177–226, 2002

Graff-Radford N, Woodruff B: Frontotemporal dementia. Continuum Lifetime Learning Neurol 10:58–80, 2004

Haroutunian V, Perl DP, Purohit DP, et al: Regional distribution of neuritic plaques in the nondemented elderly and subjects with very mild Alzheimer disease [see comment]. Arch Neurol 55:1185–1191, 1998

Harvey GT, Hughes J, McKeith IG, et al: Magnetic resonance imaging differences between dementia with Lewy bodies and Alzheimer's disease: a pilot study. Psychol Med 29:181–187, 1999

Hashimoto M, Kitagaki H, Imamura T, et al: Medial temporal and whole-brain atrophy in dementia with Lewy bodies: a volumetric MRI study. Neurology 51:357–362, 1998

Hebert LE, Scherr PA, Bienias JL, et al: Alzheimer disease in the US population: prevalence estimates using the 2000 census. Arch Neurol 60:1119–1122, 2003

Heun R, Kockler M, Ptok U: Lifetime symptoms of depression in Alzheimer's disease. Eur Psychiatry 18:63–69, 2003

Hirono N, Mori E, Ishii K, et al: Frontal lobe hypometabolism and depression in Alzheimer's disease. Neurology 50:380–383, 1998

Hirono N, Mori E, Tanimukai S, et al: Distinctive neurobehavioral features among neurodegenerative dementias. J Neuropsychiatry Clin Neurosci 11:498–503, 1999

Hirose Y, Mokuno K, Abe Y, et al: [A case of clinically diagnosed Creutzfeldt-Jakob disease with serial MRI diffusion weighted images] (Japanese). Rinsho Shinkeigaku 38:779–782, 1998

Hodges JR, Miller B: The neuropsychology of frontal variant frontotemporal dementia and semantic dementia: introduction to the special topic papers, part II. Neurocase 7:113–121, 2001

Hou C, Carlin D, Miller B: Non-Alzheimer's disease dementias: anatomic, clinical and molecular correlates. Can J Psychiatry 49:164–171, 2003

Hoyert DL, Rosenberg HM: Mortality from Alzheimer's disease: an update. Natl Vital Stat Rep 47:1–8, 1999

Hsiung GY, Sadovnick AD, Feldman H: Apolipoprotein E epsilon4 genotype as a risk factor for cognitive decline and dementia: data from the Canadian Study of Health and Aging. CMAJ 171:863–867, 2004

Hwang TJ, Masterman DL, Ortiz F, et al: Mild cognitive impairment is associated with characteristic neuropsychiatric symptoms. Alzheimer Dis Assoc Disord 18:17–21, 2004

Imamura T, Ishii K, Hirono N, et al: Occipital glucose metabolism in dementia with Lewy bodies with and without parkinsonism: a study using positron emission tomography. Dement Geriatr Cogn Disord 12:194–197, 2001

Iqbal K, Alonso Adel C, El-Akkad E, et al: Pharmacological targets to inhibit Alzheimer neurofibrillary degeneration. J Neural Transm Suppl (62):309–319, 2002

Ironside J, Bell J: Pathology of prion diseases, in Prion Diseases. Edited by Collinge J, Palmer M. Oxford University Press, 1996, pp 57–88

Ishii K, Yamaji S, Kitagaki H, et al: Regional cerebral blood flow difference between dementia with Lewy bodies and AD. Neurology 53:413–416, 1999

Jack CR Jr, Shiung MM, Gunter JL, et al: Comparison of different MRI brain atrophy rate measures with clinical disease progression in AD. Neurology 62:591–600, 2004

Jellinger KA: The pathology of ischemic-vascular dementia: an update. J Neurol Sci 203-204:153–157, 2002

Jellinger KA: Neuropathological spectrum of synucleinopathies. Mov Disord 18 (suppl 6):S2–S12, 2003

Joseph R: Frontal lobe psychopathology: mania, depression, confabulation, catatonia, perseveration, obsessive compulsions, and schizophrenia. Psychiatry 62:138–172, 1999

Jost BC, Grossberg GT: The evolution of psychiatric symptoms in Alzheimer's disease: a natural history study [see comment]. J Am Geriatr Soc 44:1078–1081, 1996

Kalia M: Dysphagia and aspiration pneumonia in patients with Alzheimer's disease. Metabolism 52:36–38, 2003

Kennedy AM, Newman S, McCaddon A, et al: Familial Alzheimer's disease: a pedigree with a mis-sense mutation in the amyloid precursor protein gene (amyloid precursor protein 717 valine→glycine). Brain 116 (pt 2):309–324, 1993

Kennedy AM, Newman SK, Frackowiak RS, et al: Chromosome 14 linked familial Alzheimer's disease: a clinico-pathological study of a single pedigree. Brain 118 (pt 1):185–205, 1995

Khachaturian AS, Corcoran CD, Mayer LS, et al: Apolipoprotein E epsilon4 count affects age at onset of Alzheimer disease, but not lifetime susceptibility: the Cache County Study. Arch Gen Psychiatry 61:518–524, 2004

Klatka LA, Louis ED, Schiffer RB: Psychiatric features in diffuse Lewy body disease: a clinicopathologic study using Alzheimer's disease and Parkinson's disease comparison groups. Neurology 47:1148–1152, 1996

Klucken J, McLean PJ, Gomez-Tortosa E, et al: Neuritic alterations and neural system dysfunction in Alzheimer's disease and dementia with Lewy bodies. Neurochem Res 28:1683–1691, 2003

Korczyn AD: The complex nosological concept of vascular dementia. J Neurol Sci 203-204:3–6, 2002

Kordower JH, Chu Y, Stebbins GT, et al: Loss and atrophy of layer II entorhinal cortex neurons in elderly people with mild cognitive impairment. Ann Neurol 49:202–213, 2001

Kosaka K: Diffuse Lewy body disease in Japan. J Neurol 237:197–204, 1990

Kotrla KJ, Chacko RC, Harper RG, et al: SPECT findings on psychosis in Alzheimer's disease. Am J Psychiatry 152:1470–1475, 1995

Krishnan KR, Hays JC, Blazer DG: MRI-defined vascular depression. Am J Psychiatry 154:497–501, 1997

Kukull WA, Brenner DE, Speck CE, et al: Causes of death associated with Alzheimer disease: variation by level of cognitive impairment before death. J Am Geriatr Soc 42:723–726, 1994

Kuzis G, Sabe L, Tiberti C, et al: Neuropsychological correlates of apathy and depression in patients with dementia. Neurology 52:1403–1407, 1999

Lampe TH, Bird TD, Nochlin D, et al: Phenotype of chromosome 14-linked familial Alzheimer's disease in a large kindred. Ann Neurol 36:368–378, 1994

Landes AM, Sperry SD, Strauss ME, et al: Apathy in Alzheimer's disease. J Am Geriatr Soc 49:1700–1707, 2001

Lantos PL, Cairns NJ: Neuropathology, in Early Onset Dementia. Edited by Hodges JR. New York, Oxford University Press, 2001, pp 227–262

Larrieu S, Letenneur L, Orgogozo JM, et al: Incidence and outcome of mild cognitive impairment in a population-based prospective cohort. Neurology 59:1594–1599, 2002

Le Bars PL, Kieser M, Itil KZ: A 26-week analysis of a double-blind, placebo-controlled trial of the ginkgo biloba extract EGb 761 in dementia. Dement Geriatr Cogn Disord 11:230–237, 2000

Leroi I, Voulgari A, Breitner JC, et al: The epidemiology of psychosis in dementia. Am J Geriatr Psychiatry 11:83–91, 2003

Levy ML, Miller BL, Cummings JL, et al: Alzheimer disease and frontotemporal dementias: behavioral distinctions. Arch Neurol 53:687–690, 1996

Lewis J, Dickson DW, Lin WL, et al: Enhanced neurofibrillary degeneration in transgenic mice expressing mutant tau and APP. Science 293:1487–1491, 2001

Li L, Sengupta A, Haque N, et al: Memantine inhibits and reverses the Alzheimer type abnormal hyperphosphorylation of tau and associated neurodegeneration. FEBS Lett 566:261–269, 2004

Li YS, Meyer JS, Thornby J: Longitudinal follow-up of depressive symptoms among normal versus cognitively impaired elderly. Int J Geriatr Psychiatry 16:718–727, 2001

Lim GP, Chu T, Yang F, et al: The curry spice curcumin reduces oxidative damage and amyloid pathology in an Alzheimer transgenic mouse. J Neurosci 21:8370–8377, 2001

Liu W, Miller BL, Kramer JH, et al: Behavioral disorders in the frontal and temporal variants of frontotemporal dementia. Neurology 62:742–748, 2004

Lobotesis K, Fenwick JD, Phipps A, et al: Occipital hypoperfusion on SPECT in dementia with Lewy bodies but not AD. Neurology 56:643–649, 2001

Lopera F, Ardilla A, Martinez A, et al: Clinical features of early onset Alzheimer disease in a large kindred with an E280A presenilin-1 mutation. JAMA 277:793–799, 1997

Lopez OL, Smith G, Becker JT, et al: The psychotic phenomenon in probable Alzheimer's disease: a positron emission tomography study. J Neuropsychiatry Clin Neurosci 13:50–55, 2001a

Lopez OL, Zivkovic S, Smith G, et al: Psychiatric symptoms associated with cortical-subcortical dysfunction in Alzheimer's disease. J Neuropsychiatry Clin Neurosci 13:56–60, 2001b

Lowe J, Rossor M: Frontotemporal lobar degeneration, in Neurodegeneration: The Molecular Pathology of Dementia and Movement Disorders. Edited by Dickson DW. Basel, Switzerland, ISN Neuropath Press, 2003, pp 342–348

Loy R, Tariot PN: Neuroprotective properties of valproate: potential benefit for AD and tauopathies. J Mol Neurosci 19:303–307, 2002

Lyketsos CG, Olin J: Depression in Alzheimer's disease: overview and treatment. Biol Psychiatry 52:243–252, 2002

Lyketsos CG, Steinberg M, Tschanz JT, et al: Mental and behavioral disturbances in dementia: findings from the Cache County Study on Memory in Aging. Am J Psychiatry 157:708–714, 2000

Lyketsos CG, Lopez O, Jones B, et al: Prevalence of neuropsychiatric symptoms in dementia and mild cognitive impairment: results from the cardiovascular health study. JAMA 288:1475–1483, 2002

Maclean LE, Collins CC, Byrne EJ: Dementia with Lewy bodies treated with rivastigmine: effects on cognition, neuropsychiatric symptoms, and sleep. Int Psychogeriatr 13:277–288, 2001

Mallucci G, Collinge J: Update on Creutzfeldt-Jakob disease. Curr Opin Neurol 17:641–647, 2004

Manea M, Mezo G, Hudecz F, et al: Polypeptide conjugates comprising a beta-amyloid plaque-specific epitope as new vaccine structures against Alzheimer's disease. Biopolymers 76:503–511, 2004

Marin DB, Green CR, Schmeidler J, et al: Noncognitive disturbances in Alzheimer's disease: frequency, longitudinal course, and relationship to cognitive symptoms. J Am Geriatr Soc 45:1331–1338, 1997

Masliah E, Rockenstein E, Veinbergs I, et al: Beta-amyloid peptides enhance alpha-synuclein accumulation and neuronal deficits in a transgenic mouse model linking Alzheimer's disease and Parkinson's disease. Proc Natl Acad Sci U S A 98:12245–12250, 2001

Mastrianni JA, Roos RP: The prion diseases. Semin Neurol 20:337–352, 2000

Matoba M, Tonami H, Miyaji H, et al: Creutzfeldt-Jakob disease: serial changes on diffusion-weighted MRI. J Comput Assist Tomogr 25:274–277, 2001

Mattson MP: Pathways towards and away from Alzheimer's disease. Nature 430:631–639, 2004

McKeith I, Burn D: Spectrum of Parkinson's disease, Parkinson's dementia and Lewy body dementia. Dementia 18:865–883, 2000

McKeith I, O'Brien J: Dementia with Lewy bodies. Aust N Z J Psychiatry 33:800–808, 1999

McKeith IG, Perry RH, Fairbairn AF, et al: Operational criteria for senile dementia of Lewy body type (SDLT). Psychol Med 22:911–922, 1992

McKeith IG, Ballard CG, Harrison RW: Neuroleptic sensitivity to risperidone in Lewy body dementia. Lancet 346:699, 1995

McKeith IG, Galasko D, Kosaka K, et al: Consensus guidelines for the clinical and pathologic diagnosis of dementia with Lewy bodies (DLB): report of the Consortium on DLB International Workshop. Neurology 47:1113–1124, 1996

McKeith I, Del Ser T, Spano P, et al: Efficacy of rivastigmine in dementia with Lewy bodies. a randomised, double-blind, placebo-controlled international study [see comment]. Lancet 356:2031–2036, 2000

McKeith IG, Burn DJ, Ballard CG, et al: Dementia with Lewy bodies. Semin Clin Neuropsychiatry 8:46–57, 2003

McKeith I, Mintzer J, Aarsland D, et al: Dementia with Lewy bodies. Lancet Neurol 3:19–28, 2004

McKhann G, Drachman D, Folstein M, et al: Clinical diagnosis of Alzheimer's disease: report of the NINCDS-ADRDA Work Group under the auspices of Department of Health and Human Services Task Force on Alzheimer's Disease. Neurology 34:939–944, 1984

McPherson SE, Cummings JL: Neuropsychological aspects of vascular dementia. Brain Cogn 31:269–282, 1996

McPherson S, Fairbanks L, Tiken S, et al: Apathy and executive function in Alzheimer's disease. J Int Neuropsychol Soc 8:373–381, 2002

Mega MS, Cummings JL: Frontal-subcortical circuits and neuropsychiatric disorders. J Neuropsychiatry Clin Neurosci 6:358–370, 1994

Mega MS, Cummings JL, Fiorello T, et al: The spectrum of behavioral changes in Alzheimer's disease. Neurology 46:130–135, 1996

Mega MS, Lee L, Dinov ID, et al: Cerebral correlates of psychotic symptoms in Alzheimer's disease. J Neurol Neurosurg Psychiatry 69:167–171, 2000

Mendez MF, Perryman KM: Neuropsychiatric features of frontotemporal dementia: evaluation of consensus criteria and review. J Neuropsychiatry Clin Neurosci 14:424–429, 2002

Mesulam MM: Aging, Alzheimer's disease and dementia, in Principles of Behavioral and Cognitive Neurology. Edited by Mesulam MM. Oxford, UK, Oxford University Press, 2000, pp 439–510

Migliorelli R, Teson A, Sabe L, et al: Prevalence and correlates of dysthymia and major depression among patients with Alzheimer's disease [see comment]. Am J Psychiatry 152:37–44, 1995

Migneco O, Benoit M, Koulibaly PM, et al: Perfusion brain SPECT and statistical parametric mapping analysis indicate that apathy is a cingulate syndrome: a study in Alzheimer's disease and nondemented patients. Neuroimage 13:896–902, 2001

Miklossy J, Taddei K, Suva D, et al: Two novel presenilin-1 mutations (Y256S and Q222H) are associated with early onset Alzheimer's disease. Neurobiol Aging 24:655–662, 2003

Milton WJ, Atlas SW, Lavi E, et al: Magnetic resonance imaging of Creutzfeldt-Jacob disease. Ann Neurol 29:438–440, 1991

Minoshima S, Foster NL, Sima AA, et al: Alzheimer's disease versus dementia with Lewy bodies: cerebral metabolic distinction with autopsy confirmation. Ann Neurol 50:358–365, 2001

Modrego PJ, Ferrandez J: Depression in patients with mild cognitive impairment increases the risk of developing dementia of Alzheimer type: a prospective cohort study. Arch Neurol 61:1290–1293, 2004

Moretti P, Lieberman AP, Wilde EA, et al: Novel insertional presenilin 1 mutation causing Alzheimer disease with spastic paraparesis. Neurology 62:1865–1868, 2004

Moretti R, Torre P, Antonello RM, et al: Effects of selegiline on fronto-temporal dementia: a neuropsychological evaluation. Int J Geriatr Psychiatry 17:391–392, 2002

Moretti R, Torre P, Antonello RM, et al: Frontotemporal dementia: paroxetine as a possible treatment of behavior symptoms: a randomized, controlled, open 14-month study. Eur Neurol 49:13–19, 2003a

Moretti R, Torre P, Antonello RM, et al: Rivastigmine in subcortical vascular dementia: a randomized, controlled, open 12-month study in 208 patients. Am J Alzheimers Dis Other Demen 18:265–272, 2003b

Mourik JC, Rosso SM, Niermeijer MF, et al: Frontotemporal dementia: behavioral symptoms and caregiver distress. Dement Geriatr Cogn Disord 18:299–306, 2004

Nagano K, Miki T, Yoshioka K, et al: [Two kindreds with familial Alzheimer's disease: analysis of the APP717 mutation and the mutated genes for the prion protein] (Japanese). Nippon Ronen Igakkai Zasshi 29:509–514, 1992

Nathan BP, Jiang Y, Wong GK, et al: Apolipoprotein E4 inhibits, and apolipoprotein E3 promotes neurite outgrowth in cultured adult mouse cortical neurons through the low-density lipoprotein receptor-related protein. Brain Res 928:96–105, 2002

Neary D, Snowden JS, Gustafson L, et al: Frontotemporal lobar degeneration: a consensus on clinical diagnostic criteria. Neurology 51:1546–1554, 1998

Newman SK, Warrington EK, Kennedy AM, et al: The earliest cognitive change in a person with familial Alzheimer's disease: presymptomatic neuropsychological features in a pedigree with familial Alzheimer's disease confirmed at necropsy. J Neurol Neurosurg Psychiatry 57:967–972, 1994

Nicoll JA, Wilkinson D, Holmes C, et al: Neuropathology of human Alzheimer disease after immunization with amyloid-beta peptide: a case report. Nat Med 9:448–452, 2003

Ono K, Hasegawa K, Naiki H, et al: Curcumin has potent anti-amyloidogenic effects for Alzheimer's beta amyloid fibrils in vitro. J Neurosci Res 75:742–750, 2004

Orgogozo JM, Gilman S, Dartigues JF, et al: Subacute meningoencephalitis in a subset of patients with AD after Abeta42 immunization. Neurology 61:46–54, 2003

Ott BR, Noto RB, Fogel BS: Apathy and loss of insight in Alzheimer's disease: a SPECT imaging study. J Neuropsychiatry Clin Neurosci 8:41–46, 1996

Papka M, Rubio A, Schiffer RB, et al: Lewy body disease: can we diagnose it? J Neuropsychiatry Clin Neurosci 10:405–412, 1998

Paradiso S, Robinson RG: Gender differences in poststroke depression. J Neuropsychiatry Clin Neurosci 10:41–47, 1998

Pasquier F: Early diagnosis of dementia: neuropsychology. J Neurol 246:6–15, 1999

Pasquier F, Delacourte A: Non-Alzheimer degenerative dementias. Curr Opin Neurol 11:417–427, 1998

Passmore AP, Bayer AJ, Steinhagen-Thiessen E: Cognitive, global, and functional benefits of donepezil in Alzheimer's disease and vascular dementia: results from large-scale clinical trials. J Neurol Sci 229-230:141–146, 2005

Payami H, Grimslid H, Oken B, et al: A prospective study of cognitive health in the elderly (Oregon Brain Aging Study): effects of family history and apolipoprotein E genotype. Am J Hum Genet 60:948–956, 1997

Petanceska SS, DeRosa S, Olm V, et al: Statin therapy for Alzheimer's disease: will it work? J Mol Neurosci 19:155–161, 2002

Petersen RC: Aging, mild cognitive impairment, and Alzheimer's disease. Neurol Clin 18:789–806, 2000

Petersen RC, Smith GE, Waring SC, et al: Mild cognitive impairment: clinical characterization and outcome [published erratum appears in Arch Neurol 56:760, 1999]. Arch Neurol 56:303–308, 1999

Petersen RC, Doody R, Kurz A, et al: Current concepts in mild cognitive impairment. Arch Neurol 58:1985–1992, 2001a

Petersen RC, Stevens JC, Ganguli M, et al: Practice parameter: early detection of dementia: mild cognitive impairment (an evidence-based review). Report of the Quality Standards Subcommittee of the American Academy of Neurology [see comment]. Neurology 56:1133–1142, 2001b

Petersen RC, Thomas RG, Grundman M, et al: Vitamin E and donepezil for the treatment of mild cognitive impairment. N Engl J Med 352:2379–2388, 2005

Petry S, Cummings JL, Hill MA, et al: Personality alterations in dementia of the Alzheimer type: a three-year follow-up study. J Geriatr Psychiatry Neurol 2:203–207, 1989

Piccininni M, Di Carlo A, Baldereschi M, et al: Behavioral and psychological symptoms in Alzheimer's disease: frequency and relationship with duration and severity of the disease. Dement Geriatr Cogn Disord 19:276–281, 2005

Price JL, Morris JC: Tangles and plaques in nondemented aging and "preclinical" Alzheimer's disease. Ann Neurol 45:358–368, 1999

Queralt R, Ezquerra M, Lleo A, et al: A novel mutation (V89L) in the presenilin 1 gene in a family with early onset Alzheimer's disease and marked behavioural disturbances. J Neurol Neurosurg Psychiatry 72:266–269, 2002

Raskind MA: Update on Alzheimer drugs: galantamine. Neurologist 9:225–229, 2003

Raux G, Gantier R, Thomas-Anterion C, et al: Dementia with prominent frontotemporal features associated with L113P presenilin 1 mutation. Neurology 55:1577–1578, 2000

Ready RE, Ott BR, Grace J, et al: Apathy and executive dysfunction in mild cognitive impairment and Alzheimer disease. Am J Geriatr Psychiatry 11:222–228, 2003

Revesz T, Holton JL: Anatamopathological spectrum of tauopathies. Mov Disord 18 (suppl 6):S13–S20, 2003

Rippon GA, Crook R, Baker M, et al: Presenilin 1 mutation in an African American family presenting with atypical Alzheimer dementia. Arch Neurol 60:884–888, 2003

Ritchie CW, Bush AI, Masters CL: Metal-protein attenuating compounds and Alzheimer's disease. Expert Opin Investig Drugs 13:1585–1592, 2004

Ritchie K, Touchon J: Mild cognitive impairment: conceptual basis and current nosological status [see comment]. Lancet 355:225–228, 2000

Rockwell E, Choure J, Galasko D, et al: Psychopathology at initial diagnosis in dementia with Lewy bodies versus Alzheimer disease: comparison of matched groups with autopsy-confirmed diagnoses. Int J Geriatr Psychiatry 15:819–823, 2000

Roman GC, Tatemichi TK, Erkinjuntti T, et al: Vascular dementia: diagnostic criteria for research studies. Report of the NINDS-AIREN International Workshop. Neurology 43:250–260, 1993

Rosen J, Zubenko GS: Emergence of psychosis and depression in the longitudinal evaluation of Alzheimer's disease. Biol Psychiatry 29:224–232, 1991

Salloway S, Ferris S, Kluger A, et al: Efficacy of donepezil in mild cognitive impairment: a randomized placebo-controlled trial. Neurology 63:651–657, 2004

Samuels SC, Brickman AM, Burd JA, et al: Depression in autopsy-confirmed dementia with Lewy bodies and Alzheimer's disease. Mt Sinai J Med 71:55–62, 2004

Sano M, Ernesto C, Thomas RG, et al: A controlled trial of selegiline, alpha-tocopherol, or both as treatment for Alzheimer's disease. The Alzheimer's Disease Cooperative Study. N Engl J Med 336:1216–1222, 1997

Scharf S, Mander A, Ugoni A, et al: A double-blind, placebo-controlled trial of diclofenac/misoprostol in Alzheimer's disease. Neurology 53:197–201, 1999

Schenk D, Barbour R, Dunn W, et al: Immunization with amyloid-beta attenuates Alzheimer-disease-like pathology in the PDAPP mouse. Nature 400:173–177, 1999

Schiltz JG, Salzer U, Mohajeri MH, et al: Antibodies from a DNA peptide vaccination decrease the brain amyloid burden in a mouse model of Alzheimer's disease. J Mol Med 82:706–714, 2004

Schmidtke K, Hull M: Neuropsychological differentiation of small vessel disease, Alzheimer's disease and mixed dementia. J Neurol Sci 203-204:17–22, 2002

Schumock GT: Economic considerations in the treatment and management of Alzheimer's disease. Am J Health Syst Pharm 55 (suppl 2):S17–S21, 1998

Shimoda K, Robinson RG: The relationship between poststroke depression and lesion location in long-term follow-up. Biol Psychiatry 45:187–192, 1999

Silverman DH: Brain 18F-FDG PET in the diagnosis of neurodegenerative dementias: comparison with perfusion SPECT and with clinical evaluations lacking nuclear imaging. J Nucl Med 45:594–607, 2004

Simard M, van Reekum R: The acetylcholinesterase inhibitors for treatment of cognitive and behavioral symptoms in dementia with Lewy bodies. J Neuropsychiatry Clin Neurosci 16:409–425, 2004

Simard M, van Reekum R, Cohen T: A review of the cognitive and behavioral symptoms in dementia with Lewy bodies. J Neuropsychiatry Clin Neurosci 12:425–450, 2000

Sink KM, Holden KF, Yaffe K: Pharmacological treatment of neuropsychiatric symptoms of dementia: a review of the evidence. JAMA 293:596–608, 2005

Solomon B, Koppel R, Hanan E, et al: Monoclonal antibodies inhibit in vitro fibrillar aggregation of the Alzheimer beta-amyloid peptide. Proc Natl Acad Sci U S A 93:452–455, 1996

Solomon B, Koppel R, Frankel D, et al: Disaggregation of Alzheimer beta-amyloid by site-directed mAb. Proc Natl Acad Sci U S A 94:4109–4112, 1997

Speck CE, Kukull WA, Brenner DE, et al: History of depression as a risk factor for Alzheimer's disease. Epidemiology 6:366–369, 1995

Spillantini MG: Introduction to synucleinopathies, in Neurodegeneration: The Molecular Pathology of Dementia and Movement Disorders. Edited by Dickson DW. Basel, Switzerland, ISN Neuropath Press, 2003, pp 156–158

Starkstein S, Robinson R: Neuropsychiatric aspects of stroke, in The American Psychiatric Press Textbook of Geriatric Neuropsychiatry. Edited by Coffey C, Cummings J. Washington, DC, American Psychiatric Press, 1994, pp 457–475

Starkstein SE, Vazquez S, Petracca G, et al: A SPECT study of delusions in Alzheimer's disease. Neurology 44:2055–2059, 1994

Starkstein SE, Chemerinski E, Sabe L, et al: Prospective longitudinal study of depression and anosognosia in Alzheimer's disease. Br J Psychiatry 171:47–52, 1997

Steele C, Rovner B, Chase GA, et al: Psychiatric symptoms and nursing home placement of patients with Alzheimer's disease. Am J Psychiatry 147:1049–1051, 1990

Sultzer DL, Mahler ME, Mandelkern MA, et al: The relationship between psychiatric symptoms and regional cortical metabolism in Alzheimer's disease. J Neuropsychiatry Clin Neurosci 7:476–484, 1995

Swanberg MM, Cummings JL: Benefit-risk considerations in the treatment of dementia with Lewy bodies. Drug Saf 25:511–523, 2002

Swartz JR, Miller BL, Lesser IM, et al: Frontotemporal dementia: treatment response to serotonin selective reuptake inhibitors. J Clin Psychiatry 58:212–216, 1997

Tanaka M, Chien P, Yonekura K, et al: Mechanism of cross-species prion transmission: an infectious conformation compatible with two highly divergent yeast prion proteins. Cell 121:49–62, 2005

Tang-Wai D, Lewis P, Boeve B, et al: Familial frontotemporal dementia associated with a novel presenilin-1 mutation. Dement Geriatr Cogn Disord 14:13–21, 2002

Tekin S, Mega MS, Masterman DM, et al: Orbitofrontal and anterior cingulate cortex neurofibrillary tangle burden is associated with agitation in Alzheimer disease. Ann Neurol 49:355–361, 2001

Tervo S, Kivipelto M, Hanninen T, et al: Incidence and risk factors for mild cognitive impairment: a population-based three-year follow-up study of cognitively healthy elderly subjects. Dement Geriatr Cogn Disord 17:196–203, 2004

Teter B, Xu PT, Gilbert JR, et al: Human apolipoprotein E isoform-specific differences in neuronal sprouting in organotypic hippocampal culture. J Neurochem 73:2613–2616, 1999

Thompson PM, Hayashi KM, de Zubicaray G, et al: Dynamics of gray matter loss in Alzheimer's disease. J Neurosci 23:994–1005, 2003

Thompson PM, Hayashi KM, de Zubicaray GI, et al: Mapping hippocampal and ventricular change in Alzheimer disease. Neuroimage 22:1754–1766, 2004

Troncoso JC, Martin LJ, Dal Forno G, et al: Neuropathology in controls and demented subjects from the Baltimore Longitudinal Study of Aging. Neurobiol Aging 17:365–371, 1996

van Dongen M, van Rossum E, Kessels A, et al: Ginkgo for elderly people with dementia and age-associated memory impairment: a randomized clinical trial. J Clin Epidemiol 56:367–376, 2003

Verkkoniemi A, Kalimo H, Paetau A, et al: Variant Alzheimer disease with spastic paraparesis: neuropathological phenotype. J Neuropathol Exp Neurol 60:483–492, 2001

Voisin T, Reynish E, Portet F, et al: What are the treatment options for patients with severe Alzheimer's disease? CNS Drugs 18:575–583, 2004

von Strauss E, Viitanen M, De Ronchi D, et al: Aging and the occurrence of dementia: findings from a population-based cohort with a large sample of nonagenarians. Arch Neurol 56:587–592, 1999

Wahlund LO, Pihlstrand E, Jonhagen ME: Mild cognitive impairment: experience from a memory clinic. Acta Neurol Scand Suppl 179:21–24, 2003

Weggen S, Eriksen JL, Sagi SA, et al: Evidence that nonsteroidal anti-inflammatory drugs decrease amyloid beta 42 production by direct modulation of gamma-secretase activity. J Biol Chem 278:31831–31837, 2003

Weiner MF, Doody RS, Sairam R, et al: Prevalence and incidence of major depressive disorder in Alzheimer's disease: findings from two databases. Dement Geriatr Cogn Disord 13:8–12, 2002

Wesnes K, McKeith I, Ferrara R, et al: Effects of rivastigmine on cognitive function in dementia with Lewy bodies: a randomized placebo-controlled international study using the cognitive drug research computerised assessment system. Dement Geriatr Cogn Disord 13:183–192, 2002

Winblad B, Palmer K, Kivipelto M, et al: Mild cognitive impairment: beyond controversies, towards a consensus. Report of the International Working Group on Mild Cognitive Impairment. J Intern Med 256:240–246, 2004

Wolfe MS: Therapeutic strategies for Alzheimer's disease. Nat Rev Drug Discov 1:859–866, 2002

Yasuda M, Maeda K, Hashimoto M, et al: A pedigree with a novel presenilin 1 mutation at a residue that is not conserved in presenilin 2. Arch Neurol 56:65–69, 1999

Yee AS, Simon JH, Anderson CA, et al: Diffusion-weighted MRI of right-hemisphere dysfunction in Creutzfeldt-Jakob disease. Neurology 52:1514–1515, 1999

Yoshizawa T, Yamakawa-Kobayashi K, Komatsuzaki Y, et al: Dose-dependent association of apolipoprotein E allele epsilon 4 with late-onset, sporadic Alzheimer's disease. Ann Neurol 36:656–659, 1994

Zandi PP, Anthony JC, Khachaturian AS, et al: Reduced risk of Alzheimer disease in users of antioxidant vitamin supplements: the Cache County Study. Arch Neurol 61:82–88, 2004

Zeidler M, Sellar RJ, Collie DA, et al: The pulvinar sign on magnetic resonance imaging in variant Creutzfeldt-Jakob disease. Lancet 355:1412–1418, 2000

Zhukareva V, Sundarraj S, Mann D, et al: Selective reduction of soluble tau proteins in sporadic and familial frontotemporal dementias: an international follow-up study. Acta Neuropathol (Berl) 105:469–476, 2003

Zubenko GS, Moossy J: Major depression in primary dementia: clinical and neuropathologic correlates. Arch Neurol 45:1182–1186, 1988

Zubenko GS, Moossy J, Kopp U: Neurochemical correlates of major depression in primary dementia. Arch Neurol 47:209–214, 1990

26

NEUROPSYCHIATRIC ASPECTS OF SCHIZOPHRENIA

Carol A. Tamminga, M.D.

Mujeeb U. Shad, M.D.

Subroto Ghose, M.D., Ph.D.

Despite centuries of curiosity and study focused on schizophrenia, its pathophysiology remains unknown. There are few medical illnesses for which the etiologies and mechanisms are so completely obscure. Although our eventual knowledge of this process is certain, the exact explanation has escaped current understanding. We know that schizophrenia is a psychiatric illness with well-established diagnostic criteria, clear signs and symptoms, and variably effective symptomatic treatments (Andreasen 1995; Carpenter and Buchanan 1994). However, not enough of the pieces of this puzzle have yet been manifested to arrange with any certainty the areas of sure knowledge into a complete disease picture. Having acknowledged this limitation, it is always a challenging exercise to lay out the current pieces of knowledge about schizophrenia, to examine all parts for level of certainty, and then to fit these ideas together into testable hypotheses of mechanism. Soon, relevant information will expand, both in quantity and in quality, because of the increased sensitivity of newer human research techniques—from rating precision to diagnostic specificity to functional imaging resolution—and because of the exponential increase in basic neuroscience knowledge, and now the completed human genome. In this chapter, we examine the pieces of knowledge we possess today that define the biology of schizophrenia and how we can view these pieces to rationally increase our understanding of the illness.

CLINICAL CHARACTERISTICS OF SCHIZOPHRENIA

Historically, schizophrenia-like conditions have been known for millennia. The Greeks clearly described the mental symptoms and personality deterioration of schizophrenia in the first and second centuries A.D. The Middle Ages brought a regression in any preexisting scientific approach to the illness and often completely misidentified the condition as willful or evil. Not until the eighteenth century did schizophrenia reappear as a disease construct; and it was not until the nineteenth century that psychotic disorders were viewed as entities, then called *insanity* or *madness*. Toward the end of the nineteenth century, moral treatment was practiced, whereby patients were treated with compassion and kindness in lieu of any other effective treatment. Broadly effective pharmacological treatments were not available until the mid-twentieth century; also, modern disease formulations were applied to the condition.

DIAGNOSIS

Throughout history, the identification of psychosis has always been straightforward because of its distinctive cognitive symptoms. Adequately distinguishing schizophrenia from other psychotic disorders was problematic but became clearer as etiologies and treatments of some of the other psychotic disorders were developed. For example, investigators discovered that niacin was an effective treatment for pellagra and that penicillin was effective for central nervous system (CNS) syphilis—both of which are diseases that can manifest themselves with psychotic conditions. Between the 1920s and the 1950s, the carving off of psychotic affective illness on the one hand, and schizotypal personality disorders on the other hand, created even clearer and more specific diagnostic criteria for schizophrenia (Carpenter and Buchanan 1995). DSM-IV-TR (American Psychiatric Association 2000) details clear diagnostic criteria accepted throughout North America and the worldwide scientific community; its criteria are based on extensive research, study, and review. The use of these criteria has led to the consistent and reliable diagnosis of schizophrenia. The DSM-IV-TR criteria and the tenth revision of the *International Statistical Classification of Diseases and Related Health Problems* (ICD-10; World Health Organization 1992) criteria are the world's two major diagnostic systems for schizophrenia; with the current editions, they have reconciled their major differences. Such structured diagnostic criteria have led to the examination and identification of schizophrenia around the world and to the observation that the incidence and the symptomatic expression are similar between countries and across cultures (Sartorius 1974).

Although the schizophrenia phenotype has been traditionally defined by chronic psychosis and functional deterioration, the boundary of the phenotype now is often viewed as broader than the schizophrenia diagnosis itself. Schizophrenia may well be the tip of an iceberg of schizophrenia-related diagnoses, augmented by the related personality disorders (Tsuang et al. 2000). Schizophrenia-related personality disorders evidence subtle symptoms and signs similar to schizophrenia, especially in some nonpsychotic first-degree relatives (Faraone et al. 2000). Moreover, antipsychotic treatment may improve functioning in persons with certain personality disorders (Tsuang et al. 1999).

SYMPTOMATOLOGY

In the International Pilot Study of Schizophrenia conducted by the World Health Organization (WHO; Sartorius 1974), symptoms were rated in schizophrenic persons in seven different countries. The symptoms were

TABLE 26–1.   Frequency of psychotic symptoms in schizophrenia

Symptom	Frequency (%)
Lack of insight	97
Hallucinations (auditory and verbal)	70–74
Ideas of reference	70
Suspiciousness	65
Flatness of affect	65
Paranoid state	64
Thought alienation	52
Thoughts spoken aloud	50

Source.   Reprinted from Sartorius N: "The International Pilot Study of Schizophrenia." *Schizophrenia Bulletin* (Winter):21–34, 1974. Used with permission.

noted to be similar around the world. The list of the most frequently reported symptoms (Table 26–1) is descriptive of the disease we see today.

Although the use of DSM-IV-TR clearly identifies a syndrome, investigators remain unsure that schizophrenia is a unitary illness with a single etiology and pathophysiology as opposed to a group of syndromes or a collection of interrelated conditions (Carpenter and Buchanan 1994). Therefore, various attempts have been made to delineate testable subtypes of the illness on the basis of clinical characteristics, which then can be evaluated for distinguishing brain characteristics (Carpenter et al. 1993). In several investigations of large populations of schizophrenic patients, the symptom presentations have been analyzed for the clustering of symptoms into symptomatic subgroups. These analyses have consistently identified three distinct symptom domains in schizophrenia: 1) psychosis domain—hallucinations, delusions, and paranoia; 2) cognitive deficit domain—thought disorder; and 3) negative symptom domain—anhedonia, social withdrawal, and thought poverty (Andreasen et al. 1995; Arndt et al. 1991; T.R. Barnes and Liddle 1990; Carpenter and Buchanan 1989; Kay and Sevy 1990; Lenzenweger et al. 1991; Liddle 1987).

Cognitive deficits are core symptoms of schizophrenia. Schizophrenic patients as a group perform poorly on most neuropsychological tests compared with healthy subjects. This poor performance is likely partly due to symptoms of schizophrenia (e.g., poor motivation or distraction from psychotic symptoms), and the negative effects of early onset of the illness and long-term institutionalization lead to the generalized deficits in these patients (Chapman and Chapman 1973). One approach to identify the specific neurocognitive deficits associated with schizophrenia is to examine the differential deficits associated with the illness (Chapman and Chapman 1973). A generalized neurocognitive impairment equally affects a person's performance on all tests, as long as these tests are approximately equal in difficulty. Measures that show selective impairment in testing when applied in schizophrenia are more likely to be associated with the pathophysiology of schizophrenia. Abnormalities in abstraction, problem solving, and other executive functions have been particularly noted in individuals with schizophrenia (Goldberg et al. 1987).

Specific neuropsychological deficits in schizophrenia are broad; they include memory, executive function, and motor performance (Braff et al. 1991; Gold et al. 1992; Goldberg et al. 1990; Gruzelier et al. 1988; R.C. Gur et al. 1991; Liddle and Morris 1991). No cognitive domains are entirely spared, and deficits in performance are highly intercorrelated within persons (Sullivan et al. 1994). Schizophrenic subjects in many of the studies show a pattern of deficits, ruling out a complete lack of motivation as a factor in performance. In schizophrenic persons, memory deficits occur (as shown, for example, in the recurring digit span test) that are consistent with temporohippocampal dysfunction (Gruzelier et al. 1988). Frontal cortical function is also abnormal (e.g., verbal fluency, spatial performance, pattern recognition), and long-term memory deficits have been documented (Gruzelier et al. 1988).

The study of identical twins discordant for schizophrenia has been a highly productive technique in providing a genetically matched control group, circumventing critical comparison confounds. In such a study, Goldberg and colleagues (1990) found that almost all schizophrenic twins performed more poorly than did their unaffected identical co-twins on all performance measures. Specifically, the schizophrenic twins performed significantly worse on assessments of intelligence, memory, attention, verbal fluency, and pattern recognition than did their identical twin control subjects. The performance of nonschizophrenic twins did not differ from that of unrelated healthy control subjects except for reduced performance in "logical memory" (Wechsler Adult Intelligence Scale [WAIS]) and on Trail Making Test A; in both of these cognitive areas, performance was still considerably different between the schizophrenic and the nonschizophrenic twins (Goldberg et al. 1990).

Similarly, persons with schizophrenia consistently perform poorly on tasks that require sustained attention or vigilance (Nuechterlein et al. 1992). Other studies document deficits in memory, including explicit memory and verbal memory (Gold et al. 1994; Saykin et al. 1991). Working memory, which permits task-relevant information to be kept active for brief periods, has received much attention in the schizophrenia literature. Individuals with schizophrenia

have difficulties maintaining working memory (Goldman-Rakic 1994; Park and Holzman 1992). Deficits in working memory may explain serious disorganization and functional deterioration observed in the schizophrenia spectrum. This is because the ability to hold information "online" is critical for organizing future thoughts and actions in the context of the recent past (Goldman-Rakic 1994).

The question of whether the cognitive deficits observed in schizophrenia are primary or secondary to the symptoms and related factors can be addressed more fully by studying nonpsychotic relatives of schizophrenic patients. Several studies have observed that the first-degree relatives of schizophrenic probands have many of the cognitive deficits observed in schizophrenia, even though these individuals do not experience overt psychosis (Asarnow et al. 1991; Balogh and Merritt 1985; Braff 1981; Cornblatt et al. 1989; Green et al. 1997; Park et al. 1995). These deficits include impairments in different dimensions of attention, language comprehension, verbal fluency, verbal memory, and spatial working memory. This pattern of findings has been documented by two of the most comprehensive studies of relatives of schizophrenic patients (T.D. Cannon et al. 1994; Faraone et al. 1995). These studies show that even after adjusting for IQ, measures of auditory attention, abstraction, and verbal memory differentiated relatives of patients with schizophrenia from the comparison groups. It is unclear whether the observed neurocognitive impairments in relatives were associated with schizophrenia-spectrum personality symptoms. Some studies show that relatives meeting criteria for definite or probable schizotypal personality disorder have the most pronounced impairment, although not all cognitively impaired relatives met the diagnostic criteria for the probable or definite schizotypal personality disorder (Condray et al. 1992, 1996). It is possible that a lower threshold for schizotypal diagnosis and/or inclusion of relatives with negative and paranoid symptoms would capture the remaining cognitively impaired subjects. Other investigators (Keefe et al. 1997, Pogue-Geile et al. 1991, Roxborough et al. 1993) used various instruments (Wisconsin Card Sorting Test, Trail Making Test, verbal fluency, Symbol Digit, and WAIS variables) to detect abnormalities among relatives of schizophrenic probands independent of schizotypal diagnosis.

Cohen and Serven-Schreiber (1992) suggested that these widespread disturbances in attention and language processing are caused by "a disturbance in the internal representation of contextual information," potentially arising from frontal cortical dysfunction and associated with dopamine deficiency. Cognitive psychologists have suggested that a defect in the connections between "cognitive modules" occurs in the illness rather than an abnormality within the individual module itself (Frith 1995). However, the concrete nature of that defect has been elusive. These data on neuropsychological function in schizophrenia are consistent with an overall brain disturbance in cognitive ability. To complicate these considerations further are the observations that the cognitive defects are not present in every person at all times and that the pattern of defects can change over time within an individual. This makes it difficult to propose permanent changes in connectivity in the illness and forces a concept of flexible or reversible functional changes.

When clinical symptoms (i.e., psychosis, cognitive deficits, and negative symptoms) are related to imaging findings, specific brain areas are found to be differentially involved in symptom manifestations in schizophrenia. Whether these regionally specific changes are a cause or an effect of the disorder is not known, but they do suggest the presence of distinct neuroanatomical substrates, possibly distinct cerebral systems, for the different symptom clusters. Although one cluster may predominate in some patients, the three clusters characteristically occur together, and one domain is not exclusive of another. It is not yet understood whether these symptom domains are meaningful as the multiple manifestations of a single disease pathophysiology or whether each is a partially independent disease construct of its own with distinct etiologies and partially independent pathophysiologies. One reason that this distinction is important lies in its therapeutic implications. Is there one treatment for schizophrenia? Or are there several treatments for symptom-specific domains of the illness? This question remains open, and its answer is being aggressively pursued in ongoing research.

COURSE

The diagnosis of schizophrenia usually implies a lifelong course of psychotic illness. Occasionally, the illness is of fast onset and episodic, with symptoms first occurring in late teenage and early adult years, and with satisfactory recovery between episodes. However, more often, other patterns of illness occur characterized by an insidious onset, a partial recovery, or a remarkable lack of recovery between episodes (Bleuler 1978; Ciompi and Müller 1976). In most schizophrenic patients, a profound deterioration in mental and social functioning occurs within the first few years of the illness. After the initial deteriorating years, the further course of illness settles at a low, but flat, plateau. Surprisingly, symptoms may improve in later life after age 50. Whereas schizophrenia was previously described as having an inevitably deteriorating long-term course, the Vermont longitudinal study of persons with severe mental illness found considerable heterogeneity in

outcome in later life among schizophrenic patients, including some frank late improvers; moreover, the Vermont study included chronically ill, poorly responsive patients who are most likely to have poor outcomes (Harding et al. 1987a, 1987b). Specifically, in this study of 269 patients (with a 97% follow-up rate), more than half of the individuals had no psychotic symptoms after 10 years of study (after approximately 15–20 years of illness), and most had a "good" level of functioning in their later life. These data are consistent with several other outcome studies conducted in Europe and the United States, which reported frequent good outcome in later years for individuals with schizophrenia (Bleuler 1978; Ciompi and Müller 1976; Huber et al. 1979; Tsuang et al. 1979). Whether elder years are merely less demanding periods for mental performance or whether the normal aging process is therapeutic in the illness is not known. That the disease course is generally flat in its middle years distinguishes schizophrenia from traditional neurodegenerative disorders in which the course is progressively downhill (such as Parkinson's disease or Alzheimer's dementia) and from traditional neurodevelopmental disorders (such as mental retardation) in which the course is steady and low from the beginning of life.

RISK FACTORS IN SCHIZOPHRENIA

Although the etiology of schizophrenia is not known, certain factors have been associated with a propensity toward the illness. Genetic predisposition is clear. Prenatal maternal illness and birth complications appear to be involved, at least as predisposing factors. In addition, winter birth of the proband is associated with a definite, although small, proportion of those with the diagnosis. Social adversity, migration, and cannabis use are risk factors during childhood and adolescence. Each risk factor alone confers a small risk, yet when they occur together, these risks may be multiplicative (Barr et al. 1990; Kendell and Kemp 1989; O'Callaghan et al. 1991). Moreover, these risk factors suggest the importance of early life events in the onset of an illness whose florid symptoms appear later in life.

GENETICS

The evidence is currently clear and consistent across many methodologically sound studies that schizophrenia aggregates in families. First-degree relatives of schizophrenic individuals have a lifetime risk of 3%–7% of manifesting schizophrenia compared with a 0.5%–1% lifetime risk for relatives of control subjects (Matthysse and Kidd

1976). Twin studies have been pivotal in identifying the familial factor as a genetic rather than an environmental risk (Gottesman and Shields 1982; Kety 1987). The monozygotic twin of a person with schizophrenia has a 31%–78% chance of contracting the illness, compared with a 0%–28% chance for a dizygotic twin. The heritability is estimated to be approximately 80% (Cardno and Gottesman 2000), with a complex mode of transmission (Gottesman and Shields 1967; McGue and Gottesman 1989). Two meta-analyses of schizophrenia linkage support the existence of susceptibility genes on chromosome arms 1q, 2q, 3p, 5q, 6p, 8p, 13q, 14p, 20q, and 22q (Badner and Gershon 2002; C.M. Lewis et al. 2003). These data support the idea that there may be several risk genes, each likely to be of small to moderate effect. Detailed studies of linked regions and other studies have identified several candidate genes (see reviews by Harrison and Weinberger 2005; Owen et al. 2005), and here we briefly review the genes for which strong evidence and biological plausibility exist.

Dystrobrevin Binding Protein-1 (*DTNBP1* or Dysbindin)

Dysbindin is one of the more promising candidate genes implicated in schizophrenia. The first study to implicate dysbindin determined that several single nucleotide polymorphisms (SNPs) and three-marker haplotypes spanning dysbindin were significantly associated with schizophrenia (Straub et al. 2002). The association between dysbindin and schizophrenia has since been shown in several other studies (Funke et al. 2004; Kirov et al. 2004; Numakawa et al. 2004; Schwab et al. 2003; Williams et al. 2004a) although not in all (Morris et al. 2003; Van Den Bogaert et al. 2003). The studies that implicate dysbindin differ in the risk alleles and haplotypes involved. Nonetheless, the evidence in favor of dysbindin as a susceptibility gene for schizophrenia is strong. The function of dysbindin in the human brain has not been determined. It is a 40- to 50-kDa protein that binds α- and β-dystrobrevins, components of the dystrophin glycoprotein complex. This complex is believed to play a role in stabilization of the postsynaptic membrane, cytoskeletal rearrangement (Adams et al. 2000; Grady et al. 2000), and signal transduction (Grady 1999). β-Dystrobrevin is expressed in neurons, where it is associated primarily with postsynaptic densities and may play a role in glutamatergic function (Talbot et al. 2004). A possible functional role of dysbindin in schizophrenia is supported by the finding of decreased mRNA and protein in human postmortem brain tissue from schizophrenic donors (Talbot et al. 2004; C.S. Weickert et al. 2004).

Neuregulin-1 (*NRG1*)

Stefansson et al. (2002) conducted an association analysis across 8p21–22 to determine a highly significant association between a seven-marker core haplotype in *NRG1* and schizophrenia. This was replicated in a second cohort (Stefansson et al. 2003). Other studies have provided further evidence of neuregulin as a susceptibility gene for schizophrenia (Corvin et al. 2004; Tang et al. 2004; Williams et al. 2003; Yang et al. 2003; Zhao et al. 2004), although, as in dysbindin studies, there are differences in risk alleles and SNPs implicated. Negative findings also have been reported (Iwata et al. 2004; Thiselton et al. 2004). Three studies (Stefansson et al. 2002, 2003; Williams et al. 2003) have implicated the specific core haplotype identified in the initial study. Taken together, these findings provide considerable evidence that neuregulin may be a risk gene for schizophrenia. Neuregulin is a large gene with 4 different isoforms that give rise to at least 15 different peptides (Harrison and Law 2006). Neuregulin peptides are involved in a host of physiological processes including neuronal migration, axon guidance, synaptogenesis, glial differentiation, myelination, neurotransmission, and synaptic plasticity.

D–Amino Acid Oxidase Activator and D–Amino Acid Oxidase

Association mapping in the linkage region on 13q22–34 found two genes—*G72* and *G30*—to be associated with schizophrenia in two populations (Chumakov et al. 2002). *G72* has been renamed D–amino acid oxidase activator (*DAOA*) after it was found to bind to and enhance activity of D–amino acid oxidase (DAO). DAO is involved in the metabolism of D-serine, a potent activator of *N*-methyl-D-aspartate (NMDA) glutamate receptor. Four SNPs in DAO itself were associated with schizophrenia. Thus, both DAO and *DAOA* were found to be associated with schizophrenia. Their potential to influence NMDA receptor function added credence to their importance as susceptibility genes of schizophrenia. Subsequent studies supported *DAOA* and DAO as important to the genetics of schizophrenia (Addington et al. 2004; Ma et al. 2006; Schumacher et al. 2004; Wang et al. 2004; Zou et al. 2005). Although these studies implicate the gene, differences regarding specific risk alleles or haplotypes are found across studies.

Regulator of G-Protein Signaling-4 (*RGS4*)

RGS4 is a gene that maps to 1q21–22, a region implicated in linkage studies. Decreased levels of this gene were found in human postmortem microarray studies in schizophrenia (Mirnics et al. 2001). Associations were found with four SNPs of various haplotypes in *RGS4* in three different populations of subjects (Chowdari et al. 2002). Later studies reported positive associations between *RGS4* and schizophrenia (Chen et al. 2004a; Fallin et al. 2005; Morris et al. 2004; Williams et al. 2004b; Zhang et al. 2005), but as for the other genes, the alleles and haplotypes implicated were inconsistent. Studies with no association between *RGS4* and schizophrenia also have been reported (Sobell et al. 2005). RGS proteins are a family of about 30 proteins that are guanosine triphosphatase–activating proteins serving to negatively regulate G protein–coupled receptors. *RGS4* is abundantly expressed in the brain and can regulate multiple G protein–coupled receptors, including dopaminergic and metabotropic glutamate receptors.

Catechol-O-Methyltransferase (*COMT*)

COMT maps to 22q11, the deletion of which produces velocardiofacial syndrome, a disease associated with a high incidence of psychosis. COMT is an enzyme involved in monoamine metabolism and a functional polymorphism at codon 108/158. A G-to-A substitution converts valine (Val) to methionine (Met), which influences COMT activity. Numerous association studies examining the COMT Val/Met polymorphism in schizophrenia have been inconsistent, and a recent meta-analysis reported no association (Glatt et al. 2003). A study examining a haplotype that included the Val158Met SNP reported a strong association to schizophrenia (Shifman et al. 2002), suggesting that the *COMT* gene may be a candidate gene but not because of the Val158Met SNP. Different haplotype associations at *COMT* also have been reported (Chen et al. 2004b; Sanders et al. 2005), with those carrying the Val158Met SNP showing stronger association. This polymorphism influences prefrontal cortical and hippocampal function (de Frias 2004; Egan et al. 2001; Goldberg et al. 2003; Joober et al. 2002; Malhotra et al. 2002) and the clinical response of schizophrenia to antipsychotic medication (Bertolino et al. 2004; T.W. Weickert et al. 2004).

Disrupted-in-Schizophrenia-1 and -2 (*DISC1* and *DISC2*)

A balanced translocation in chromosomes 1 and 11 (1;11) (q42.1;q14.3) linked to the major mental disorders—schizophrenia, depression, and mania—was found to disrupt two genes: *DISC1* and *DISC2* (St Clair et al. 1990). Linkage analysis indicated 1q42 as a possible locus for schizophrenia, and the strongest signal was found in a marker in the *DISC1* gene (Ekelund et al. 2001, 2004). Positive associations have been found in several later stud-

ies (Callicott et al. 2005; Hennah et al. 2003; Hodgkinson et al. 2004; Zhang et al. 2006). One negative study examined four SNPs in *DISC1* (Devon et al. 2001). The positive studies implicated *DISC1*, although the precise patterns of association differed. *DISC1* interacts with components of the cytoskeletal system such as NudE-like and the centromere proteins to impair neurite growth and development of the cerebral cortex (Kamiya et al. 2005).

Metabotropic Glutamate Receptor-3 (*GRM3*)

GRM3 was first implicated in a case–control study in which one of three SNPs (SNP1) in *GRM3* was significantly overrepresented in schizophrenia (Marti et al. 2002). In a subsequent study, a different SNP (SNP2) and a three-marker haplotype that included this SNP were found to be significantly associated with schizophrenia (Fujii et al. 2003). Egan et al. (2004) genotyped seven SNPs that included SNP1 and SNP2 implicated in the earlier studies. They found a positive association with a third SNP (SNP3) and trends for overtransmission of SNP1 and SNP2. A strong association was seen in haplotype analyses that included SNP1, SNP2, and SNP3. Functional effects of SNP3 on prefrontal- and hippocampal-dependent tasks were seen in both control and schizophrenic volunteers.

Understanding the effect of risk genes will undoubtedly be complex. Even though several risk genes have been implicated, the precise variations in the genes are inconsistent, and until specific mutations are identified, it will be difficult to determine the biological effect of each risk gene. Another level of complexity to factor in is the interaction between risk genes as well as the interaction between the risk genes and environmental factors.

ENVIRONMENTAL FACTORS

The role of environmental factors in the development of schizophrenia is evident from the fact that monozygotic twins have less than 100% concordance rates of schizophrenia. The neurodevelopmental hypothesis of schizophrenia suggests that a disruption of brain development underlies the later emergence of psychosis during adulthood. Brain development occurs well into the third decade of life, and environmental influences can have an effect at any time from the early prenatal to the late adolescent period.

Pre- and Perinatal Factors

Pre- and perinatal factors include in utero stress such as exposure to toxins, nutritional deficiencies and severe maternal duress, and obstetrical complications. Infections have been postulated to be responsible for the association between winter births and schizophrenia. Offspring of mothers who had influenza during the second trimester had a twofold risk of developing schizophrenia (Mednick 1988; O'Callaghan et al. 1991). Similarly, the risk of schizophrenia is increased in offspring exposed to famine during the prenatal period (Susser et al. 1996). Maternal experience of significant stress such as death of a spouse (Huttunen and Niskanen 1978) or living through catastrophes such as war (Van Os and Selten 1998) is associated with an increased risk of schizophrenia. Numerous studies have investigated obstetrical complications and schizophrenia. In a meta-analysis, factors associated with schizophrenia were found to be related to certain complications of pregnancy, abnormal fetal growth and development, and hypoxic delivery complications (M. Cannon et al. 2002).

Childhood and Adolescent Factors

Social stress has been postulated to be a factor in the development of schizophrenia. It is believed that there is a significant excess of life events prior to precipitation of the disease (Bebbington et al. 1993; Hirsch et al. 1996). Substantial evidence indicates that childhood physical, sexual, and emotional abuse are causal factors for schizophrenia (for review, see Read et al. 2005). A dose-response relation of abuse to severity of illness has been reported (Whitfield et al. 2005). Adverse socioeconomic position in childhood is also associated with the risk of developing psychosis (Wicks et al. 2005). Factors examined in this study included parental socioeconomic status, employment, housing situation, and welfare benefits. The greater the number of adverse social factors, the greater the risk of developing schizophrenia.

Evidence that migration is associated with schizophrenia has been accumulating over the years. Studies have reported that the African Caribbean population living in the United Kingdom have a sixfold higher increase in schizophrenia compared with the local white population (Hutchinson et al. 1996; Sugarman and Craufurd 1994). The increased risk was not seen in the adults who migrated but in the second generation who were raised in the United Kingdom. A recent meta-analysis supports the role of migration (Cantor-Graae and Selten 2005) in the development of schizophrenia. This association may be a reflection of social isolation in a vulnerable group.

Stimulant and cannabis use can induce psychosis. The association between cannabis use and psychosis is well established (Hall and Degenhardt 2000). In a study of 50,000 Swedish conscripts followed up for 15 years, Andreasson et al. (1987) reported that marijuana use during adolescence increased the risk for schizophrenia. This finding has now been replicated in several studies (Arseneault et al. 2002; Fergusson et al. 2003; Van Os et al. 2002; Weiser et al. 2002; Zammit et al. 2002), even after the ef-

fect of prodromal symptoms and other drug use was taken into account. Adolescent cannabis use is estimated to increase the risk for psychosis in adulthood by a factor of 2.9 (Semple et al. 2005). A recent study (Caspi et al. 2005) reported that cannabis use interacts with the genetic makeup of adolescents (described in the following section, "Gene–Environment Interactions"). It is important to put these risk factors in perspective. Although there is an association with the factors mentioned earlier, most individuals who experience these adversities do not develop schizophrenia.

GENE–ENVIRONMENT INTERACTIONS

Both genetic and environmental factors are clearly associated with schizophrenia. A currently accepted construct to understand schizophrenia entails a genetic vulnerability with environmental determinants of disease. Examples of this concept are seen in other psychiatric illnesses. The short (S) length polymorphism (*SLC6A4*) in the serotonin transporter-linked promoter region (5-HTTLPR) is linked to depression in individuals who are exposed to stressful life events (Caspi et al. 2003). In schizophrenia, evidence is starting to accumulate for a gene–environment interaction. For example, adolescent cannabis use in individuals with the *COMT* Val/Val genotype leads to almost a 10-fold increased risk for developing schizophrenia spectrum disorders in later life (Caspi et al. 2005). This dramatic increase was seen only in the *COMT* Val/Val group and only with adolescent, not adult, cannabis use. Another example is that high-risk adoptees raised in a dysfunctional adoptive family situation are more likely to develop schizophrenia or schizophrenia spectrum disorders (Tienari and Wynne 1994; Wahlberg et al. 1997). Complex interactions between genetic and environmental factors are likely to contribute to the etiology of schizophrenia.

Investigators argue that an important impediment in understanding the neurobiology of schizophrenia is disease heterogeneity. Gene–environment interactions may identify more homogeneous populations of schizophrenic persons. In fact, investigators have been attempting to define more homogeneous phenotypes of schizophrenia in persons with the illness and in family members ("endophenotypes") to test these genetically.

ENDOPHENOTYPES

The features most often used to develop phenotypes in the illness are neurocognitive characteristics, eye movements (Avila et al. 2002; Ross et al. 2002; Sweeney et al. 1998), prepulse inhibition (Braff and Geyer 1990; Swerdlow and Geyer 1998), evoked potentials (R. Freedman 2003), and in vivo brain imaging features (reviewed in Gottesman and

Gould 2003). These are spontaneous behaviors of the brain occurring in response to external cues that have a known neural anatomy and hence may be more direct reflections of neural pathology (Tregellas et al. 2004).

Smooth pursuit is the use of slow eye movement to track a small moving object. Normally, humans capture the image of the moving object onto the fovea, the most sensitive region of the retina, and approximately maintain the moving image on the fovea by generating smooth and slow predictive eye movements that match the velocity of the target (G. R. Barnes and Asselman 1991). To carry out this function, the ocular motor system processes the motion of the target image on the retina and then generates a combination of fast (i.e., saccadic) and slow (i.e., smooth pursuit) eye movements to capture the image quickly on the fovea (Lisberger et al. 1987). This is called the initiation phase of the smooth-pursuit eye movements and is subserved by a neuronal network of several brain regions, including mediotemporal cortex and brain stem ocular motor regions. Subsequently, the smooth-pursuit function becomes more complex during the so-called maintenance phase. The eye tracks the target mostly by predictive smooth-pursuit eye movements combined with some predictive saccades and occasional increases in smooth eye velocity or saccades to catch up with the target. Abnormalities in smooth-pursuit and saccadic eye movements have been extensively reported in schizophrenia (Holzman et al. 1984). The ability of some probands (60%–70%) with schizophrenia to follow a smooth pendulum movement with their eyes is deficient. Instead of describing smooth movements following a pendulum stimulus, some show jerky and irregular (delayed and catch-up movements) tracking patterns. Also, antisaccadic eye movements (those directed away from a stimulus) are abnormal in persons with the illness (Thaker et al. 1989, 2000). Studies that examined eye movements in individuals with schizophrenia spectrum personality with and without a known family history of schizophrenia noted smooth-pursuit deficits only in subjects who had a positive family history of schizophrenia (Thaker et al. 1996, 1998). A preliminary report found linkage of the smooth-pursuit eye movement abnormality to 6p21 in relatives of patients with schizophrenia (Arolt et al. 1996).

The influence of genetic variation on eye-tracking measures has been investigated. Thaker et al. (2004) reported that the predictive component is influenced by the COMT genotype in healthy subjects, explaining about 10% of the variance. Consistent with the effects of the Met/Met genotype on other prefrontal cortical functions, healthy subjects with this genotype performed better than those with the Val/Val genotype. Such an effect of COMT genotype was not observed in patients with schizophrenia.

If anything, there was an opposite, nonsignificant effect of the Met/Met genotype in subjects with schizophrenia: patients with schizophrenia who had the Met/Met genotype showed significantly poorer predictive pursuit than did healthy subjects who had the Met/Met genotype. This suggests a complex interaction between the COMT Val/Met genotype and other etiological factors (e.g., another gene) or prefrontal cortical dopaminergic activity.

Neurophysiological studies have identified abnormalities in information processing that often can be elicited in the absence of a behavioral response. Many studies have used signal averaging of electroencephalographic changes that are time-locked to sensory or cognitive events. Such event-related potentials have several time-bound segments that facilitate the examination of distinct aspects of information processing. In contrast to the neuropsychological and eye movement studies, P300 evoked potential response is a reliable positive change in potential occurring about 300 ms after a task-relevant stimulus or an unexpected stimulus. P300 has increased latency and decreased amplitude in persons with schizophrenia. Although these electroencephalographic measures may vary with changes in symptoms, the P300 amplitude is consistently small in schizophrenia even during relative remission of psychotic symptoms (Blackwood et al. 1991; Pfefferbaum et al. 1984). Other components of evoked potential are observed to be abnormal in schizophrenia. Mismatched negativity response that occurs earlier than P300 is observed to have smaller amplitude in schizophrenia, which suggests an abnormality in the early response to stimulus novelty (Javitt et al. 1995).

Measures of sensory gating are obtained by examining a process called prepulse inhibition. Prepulse inhibition is a normal phenomenon evident across all sensory modalities, in which a small initial ("pre") stimulus decreases the electrophysiological response to a second higher-intensity stimulus. In schizophrenia, many probands show abnormal prepulse inhibition, as do unaffected family members. The neural systems influencing both oculomotor movements and prepulse inhibition have been well described in animals and are believed to be highly conserved in humans (Swerdlow et al. 1994, 1999). P50 is an electrophysiological measure produced when two equal auditory stimuli are presented 500 ms apart and their evoked potential is measured. Healthy persons show a reduced response (in amplitude) to the second signal, whereas persons with schizophrenia (estimated at 80%) show less or no suppression. A linkage analysis showed evidence for linkage of the gating deficit in families of schizophrenic patients with markers of location in the 15q14 region (R. Freedman et al. 1997). This region has been shown to be the locus of the α_7 nicotinic cholinergic receptor subunit gene, although no molecular abnormality has yet been found in this region of linkage (R. Freedman et al. 1999).

Detection of endophenotypes will help identify candidate genes and allow rational selection of molecular targets for further investigation. Although genetic involvement in schizophrenia is certain, genetic makeup alone does not predict schizophrenia. Also, schizophrenia typically does not manifest until the second or third decade of life, implying an interaction between genotype and other factors prior to onset of the illness. It is possible that as the brain matures (e.g., during adolescence), neural networks in the brain are developing and becoming established, a time when molecular abnormalities may become apparent.

ANATOMICAL AND NEUROCHEMICAL FEATURES OF SCHIZOPHRENIA

IN VIVO BRAIN STRUCTURE USING MAGNETIC RESONANCE IMAGING

The application of magnetic resonance imaging (MRI) to the study of brain structure in schizophrenia, when adequate patient numbers and the sufficient image resolution of modern cameras have been used, has resulted in clear findings that have contributed greatly to our knowledge of the illness (R. E. Gur and Pearlson 1993). MRI studies have benefited from meticulous clinical technique and attention to the many possible sources of imaging artifacts. The first MRI studies detected a reduction in overall brain size, an increase in ventricular size, and variable cortical wasting in schizophrenia (Shelton and Weinberger 1987). The studies confirmed and extended older literature describing the examination of schizophrenic patients with computed axial tomography (CAT), which showed the ventricular enlargement with the cruder CAT technique (Johnstone et al. 1976). More recent MRI studies have frequently reported a volume decrease in the medial temporal cortical structures, hippocampus, amygdala, and parahippocampal gyrus with some consistency, especially in the studies with dense sampling (Barta et al. 1990; Bogerts et al. 1990; Breier et al. 1992; Kuperberg et al. 2003; Lawrie et al. 2002; Suddath et al. 1990). Newer analytic techniques allowing shape analysis of the hippocampus have identified striking regional shape differences in the hippocampus in schizophrenia (Csernansky et al. 1998). Not only has the volume of the superior temporal gyrus been reported to be reduced in schizophrenia, but the magnitude of the reduction has been correlated with the presence of hallucinations (Menon et al. 1995; Shenton et al. 1992) and with electrophysiological changes in the patients (McCarley et al. 1993). Other than volume reductions in these temporal

and limbic regions, reports of other structural changes assessed by MRI have been less consistent but not uninteresting. Some investigators have found increases in sulcal size, decreases in gray matter volume, and altered gyral patterns (Giuliani et al. 2005; Niznikiewicz et al. 2000; Pearlson and Marsh 1993). Even changes (increases) in white matter volume have been reported (Breier et al. 1992). Neocortical volume reduction may be present in only some symptomatic subgroups of schizophrenic subjects: for example, middle frontal cortex volume reduction in negative-symptom schizophrenia (Andreasen et al. 1992). The thalamus may have a reduced volume in schizophrenia, particularly the posterior portion (Andreasen et al. 1994; Csernansky et al. 2004); this is an observation that should direct future interest to this structure.

The extent to which overall volume of a brain structure reflects any internal pathology, especially if the pathology is subtle, is necessarily limited. Although positive MRI data can identify a brain area for further study, negative results do not rule out areas as pathological; moreover, MRI as a technique does not provide critical knowledge to differentiate functional relevance. Thus, it is important to follow up the identification of structural abnormalities with functional, pharmacological, or electrophysiological techniques.

MICROSCOPIC ANALYSIS OF POSTMORTEM CENTRAL NERVOUS SYSTEM TISSUE

The question of importance to be answered by the microscopic study of tissue from schizophrenic persons is whether a systematic neuropathological lesion can be identified, by type or location in the illness, that could provide a clue to pathophysiology. Here structure can more precisely indicate pathology than with in vivo imaging techniques because of the cellular resolution of this approach. It is widely accepted that no obvious, currently identifiable neuropathological lesion is present in schizophrenia as occurs in Parkinson's disease or Alzheimer's dementia. Certainly a more subtle pathology must be the expectation. Since the time when schizophrenia was called the "graveyard of neuropathology," a considerable resurgence of interest in the neuropathological characteristics of the schizophrenic brain has taken place, particularly within the last 10 years. Of universal caution in reviewing any schizophrenia neuropathological studies are careful attention to the possible confounds of tissue artifacts, long-term neuroleptic treatment, lifelong altered mental state, and relevant demographic factors.

A significant number of modern postmortem studies of pathology in tissue of schizophrenic persons have now been published (Bogerts 1993; Harrison 1999b). The technical range of measures performed on CNS tissue represents a great breadth of anatomical expertise. However, the application of these multiple techniques in the face of incomplete guiding hypotheses has left the postmortem literature of schizophrenia very broad and sometimes fragmented. The changes that have most consistently been found suggest a common localization for a neural defect in the illness (i.e., in limbic cortex) but not necessarily a common neuropathological feature. The primary limbic structures in brain (namely, hippocampus, cingulate cortex, anterior thalamus, and mammillary bodies) and their intimately associated cortical areas (entorhinal cortex) often have been found to have pathological abnormalities. These are abnormalities of cell size (Jeste and Lohr 1989), cell number (Falkai and Bogerts 1986), area (Suddath et al. 1989), neuronal organization (Scheibel and Kovelman 1981), and gross structure (Colter et al. 1987). Moreover, the entorhinal cortex has been observed to show abnormalities of cellular organization in layer 2 neurons (Arnold et al. 1991a). It is interesting to recall that both structural changes on MRI (Suddath et al. 1989) and (as is described shortly) functional changes in positron emission tomography (PET) (Tamminga et al. 1992) have targeted these same areas for interest in schizophrenia pathophysiology. The consistency of this localizing pathology, despite the variety of concrete findings, is striking across technically different studies. As increasingly sophisticated and diverse neuropathological techniques are applied to this analysis, important findings may emerge.

Even though they are consistently altered, limbic structures are not the only ones affected in the postmortem schizophrenic brain. The neocortex (especially frontal cortex) has been studied more recently, with varying reports of cell or tissue loss: one study reported volume reductions in gray matter (Pakkenberg 1987), two did not (Heckers et al. 1991; Rosenthal and Bigelow 1972), and one reported increased neuronal packing in frontal cortex (Goldman-Rakic 1995). The thalamus, because of its pivotal position in relation to afferent sensory information and as a station in the cortical-subcortical circuits, has been the occasional object of study with inconsistent but not negative results. Several studies reported cell loss and reduced tissue volume in the thalamus (Pakkenberg 1990; Treff and Hempel 1958), whereas another study reported none of these findings (Lesch and Bogerts 1984). Additional study in both frontal cortex and thalamus must be done before firm conclusions can be made. Moreover, it is possible that variability might be reduced (and the answer made clearer) by seeking neuropathological changes within symptom domains.

MARKERS OF BRAIN DEVELOPMENT

Findings from several kinds of postmortem investigations with CNS tissue of schizophrenic persons have suggested

abnormal cerebral development in the illness (Benes 1989; Benes et al. 1992; Goldman-Rakic et al. 1983; Weinberger 1987). Some studies have focused on the position in cortical layers (along an axis perpendicular to the brain surface) of particular neurons in schizophrenic brain, with an abnormally inferior position signaling abnormal development. During the second trimester of human fetal development as the cortex is forming, neurons migrate upward from the ventricular wall to their target cortical layer and form functional contacts. Regional studies of postmortem cortical tissue from schizophrenic individuals have generated several persuasive observations consistent with the idea that developmental mistakes in migratory pattern may be associated with schizophrenia. This evidence consists of cortical neurons appearing incorrectly in cortical layers lower (more inferior) than expected. Akbarian et al. (1993) reported a reduction in nicotinamide adenine dinucleotide phosphate (NADPH)–diaphorase staining neurons in the higher cortical layers of the schizophrenic dorsolateral prefrontal cortex and an increase ("trailing") in these neurons in underlying white matter layers. The researchers interpreted these findings as being consistent with an impairment of neuronal migration of these particular cells into upper layers of frontal cortex during their critical developmental period (second trimester) in schizophrenia. Earlier studies reported alterations in superficial cellular organization (e.g., in layer 2) in entorhinal cortex, with layer 2 cells "trailing" in the lower cortical layers, again consistent with a neuronal migratory failure in this area of cortex (Altshuler et al. 1987; Arnold et al. 1991a; Jakob and Beckmann 1986). Another study found cingulate and middle frontal cortices to have more neurons present in lower than in superficial layers, again consistent with a concept of migratory failure (Benes 1993).

Other kinds of developmental studies have focused on changes in structural and/or growth-related elements in the neurons themselves that would disturb normal development. The early observations of hippocampal neuronal disarray in schizophrenia are consistent with the more recently reported selective loss of two microtubule-associated proteins (MAP2 and MAP5) in schizophrenic postmortem hippocampal tissue (Arnold et al. 1991b). Another study found that the protein GAP-43 is increased in frontal and lingual gyral tissue of schizophrenic persons (Sower et al. 1995). GAP-43, a synaptic marker associated with the establishment and remodeling of synaptic connections, is normally enriched in associational cortex and hippocampus. This finding suggests the possibility of unusual synaptic remodeling in frontal and hippocampal cortices in schizophrenia and is consistent with altered neuronal activity in these areas, possibly secondary to failed or incomplete neuronal projection systems to or within these regions.

Akbarian and colleagues (1995) and Volk et al. (2000) reported decreased expression of glutamic acid decarboxylase (GAD) messenger ribonucleic acid (mRNA) in prefrontal cortex of schizophrenic persons without significant cell loss. It is thought that only one of the multiple types of γ-aminobutyric acid (GABA)–containing cortical neurons may be reduced in schizophrenia—the chandelier cell (D.A. Lewis 2000; D.A. Lewis et al. 2004). These alterations in GABA system activity may be the basis of the already observed frontal hypometabolism repeatedly reported in functional imaging studies of the illness. In the excitatory glutamatergic system, alteration in the composition of the NMDA-sensitive glutamate receptor in hippocampus has been reported (Gao et al. 2000), possibly reflecting disruption of limbic system function (Tamminga et al. 2000).

Although these postmortem findings are highly provocative and interesting, replication and extension studies are critical to confirm the initial results obtained and reported with low subject number and specialized technical procedures. Although it is necessary to report early on these findings to inform the field, further replication is certainly necessary. These kinds of postmortem results are compelling in schizophrenia because their presence is theoretically consistent with the cognitive changes of the illness.

NEURAL PLASTICITY

The brain remains a plastic organ throughout its life, even though neural plasticity is greatest in the developing brain. Developmental directives serve first to form the brain into its basic structure, with activity-dependent and activity-independent influences (Aoki and Siekevitz 1988); then, these same mechanisms and probably others remain operative in shaping the mature brain to conform to its task directives. These fascinating but incompletely understood processes influence the localization, extent, connectivity, and electrophysiological characteristics of specific cortical functions in the brain. Alterations in the spatial extent or the magnitude (over time) of sensory stimulation modify the somatosensory receptive field (in the groups of responsive neurons) in the cortex. That is, the functionally relevant neuronal field in the brain for a particular kind of sensory input depends on the characteristics of that input.

Extensive research suggests some generalizations about plasticity in the neocortex: 1) that the excitatory activity of neocortical neurons can change with use and is mediated by a dynamic cortical mechanism; 2) that the coincidence of inputs can strongly influence their shaping potency; and 3) that coincidence-based input selection may account, at least in part, for the creation and continuity of local representational organization in the cortex (Merzenich et al. 1988).

Neuronal functional integrity depends to a large degree on specific target-derived neurotrophic factors (Davies 1994; McAllister et al. 1999). Within the family of neurotrophic factors, brain-derived neurotrophic factor (BDNF) is the most predominantly expressed in postnatal brain, with the highest mRNA levels in hippocampus and neocortex (Ernfors et al. 1990; Hofer et al. 1990; Wetmore et al. 1990). Administration of BDNF (Cabelli et al. 1995) or molecules that neutralize its action (Cabelli et al. 1997) and experiments with transgenic mice (Hanover et al. 1999; Huang et al. 1999) show that BDNF changes the structural and functional development of the cortex. Infusion of BDNF can increase the branching and complexity of axons (Cohen-Cory and Fraser 1995) and dendrites (McAllister et al. 1995, 1997). Moreover, the morphoregulatory effects of BDNF are specific for particular neurons in specific layers, further indicating that neurotrophins have distinct functional roles in regulating neuronal form and connectivity in the CNS (McAllister et al. 1995). Alterations in the expression of BDNF and its receptor, TrkB, have been reported in human postmortem schizophrenic tissue (Durany et al. 2001; Hashimoto et al. 2005; Iritani et al. 2003; Takahashi et al. 2000; C.S. Weickert et al. 2003, 2005). Increased BDNF protein has been reported in the hippocampus in schizophrenia in some studies (Iritani et al. 2003; Takahashi et al. 2000), whereas others have reported decreased BDNF mRNA and protein expression in the hippocampus (Durany et al. 2001). Reduced BDNF is found in the prefrontal cortex (Hashimoto et al. 2005; C.S. Weickert et al. 2003). Expression of TrkB has been found to be decreased in the hippocampus and prefrontal cortex in schizophrenia (Hashimoto et al. 2005; Takahashi et al. 2000; C.S. Weickert et al. 2005). Although some studies are inconsistent with others, they suggest that the BDNF/TrkB system is altered in schizophrenia. This is an area of active research, and with the modern molecular neuroscience and neuroimaging tools available today, we can expect to gain greater understanding of the role of neurotrophins in schizophrenia in the near future.

BIOCHEMICAL STUDIES IN SCHIZOPHRENIA

The compelling impetus to study biochemical measures in schizophrenia derived from the early pharmacological observation that blockade of dopamine receptors in the brain reduces psychotic symptoms in schizophrenia (Carlsson and Lindquist 1963). The hypothesis derived from this observation—that dysfunction of the CNS dopaminergic system either in whole or in part accounts for psychosis in schizophrenia—has been explored in all body fluids and in various conditions of rest and stimulation over the last half-century (Davis et al. 1991; Elkashef et al. 1995) with little real support. The measurement of transmitters and metabolites in lumbar cerebrospinal fluid (CSF) as a reflection of neurotransmitter activity in the brain has not critically contributed to our understanding of schizophrenia pathophysiology, even though the CSF is in direct contact with brain tissue; moreover, its sampling and analysis are beset with potential confounds. Likewise, in the measurement of dopamine receptor density, studies have regularly reported increased dopamine type 2 (D_2)–family receptor density in caudate nucleus and putamen of schizophrenic individuals (Cross et al. 1981; Mackay et al. 1982; Reynolds and Mason 1995; Seeman et al. 1984). This latter change is almost always taken to be a consequence of long-term neuroleptic treatment and can be similarly shown in rats (Clow et al. 1980; Shirakawa and Tamminga 1994), monkeys (Lidow and Goldman-Rakic 1994), and neuroleptic-treated nonschizophrenic humans.

Interest in D_2-family receptor density in schizophrenia has been heightened by the report of increased D_4 density in the caudate nucleus and putamen of schizophrenic individuals (Seeman et al. 1993). However, because D_4 density is also known to increase with long-term neuroleptic treatment, further study of tissue from untreated schizophrenic individuals is needed to draw final conclusions. The work comparing individual D_2-family receptors (D_2, D_3, and D_4) in tissue from neuroleptic-free schizophrenic persons with caudate nucleus or putamen tissue from healthy control subjects showed no differences in density of the D_2-family subtypes in striatum (Lahti et al. 1995a; Reynolds and Mason 1995). More recent imaging studies, however, showed higher occupancy of D_2 receptors by dopamine in patients with schizophrenia (Abi-Dargham et al. 2000) and changes in dopamine release in acute illness phases (Laruelle et al. 1999), suggesting that a defect exists in the release of dopamine in the disease.

Other transmitter systems have more recently drawn interest as well, including serotonergic (Reynolds 1983; van Praag 1983), peptidergic (Nemeroff et al. 1983; Widerlöv et al. 1982), and most recently glutamatergic systems (reviewed in Tamminga 1998). Because of its ubiquitous and prominent location in the CNS, and because the antiglutamatergic drugs phencyclidine (PCP) and ketamine cause a schizophrenic-like reaction in humans, the glutamate system has become a focus of study. Several studies have examined ionotropic glutamate receptor subtypes (Meador-Woodruff and Healy 2000). Most studies have focused on the mesial temporal lobe, and many have reported abnormalities in α-amino-3-hydroxy-5-methylisoxazole-4-

propionic acid (AMPA), kainate (KA), and NMDA receptor expression at the mRNA, protein, and ligand-binding level. Studies in the prefrontal cortex have been inconsistent, although AMPA abnormalities probably exist (Dracheva et al. 2005; Scarr et al. 2005). Other brain regions, such as the thalamus, show abnormal ionotropic receptor expression (Ibrahim et al. 2000). The group II metabotropic glutamate (mGluR2 and 3) receptors are implicated in animal (Moghaddam and Adams 1998) and human (Krystal et al. 2005) studies of schizophrenia. An endogenous agonist of mGluR3, N-acetylaspartylglutamate (Coyle 1997; Neale et al. 2000), and its metabolic enzyme (Ghose et al. 2004; Tsai et al. 1995) are abnormally expressed in the schizophrenic brain. It is also interesting to note that mGluR3 may be a risk gene for schizophrenia (Egan et al. 2004).

Evidence of GABAergic involvement is found in reduced expression of presynaptic markers in subpopulations of interneurons in the frontal cortex and the hippocampal formation (Benes and Berretta 2001; D.A. Lewis et al. 2004). GABAergic neurons can be defined by the presence of one of three calcium-binding proteins—namely, parvalbumin, calretinin, and calbindin. The most characteristic morphological types of neurons that express parvalbumin are the large basket and chandelier cells (D.A. Lewis and Lund 1990). Decreased 67-kD glutamic acid decarboxylase (GAD 67) and GABA transporter subtype 1 (GAT1) are found in the parvalbumin-expressing prefrontal interneurons (D.A. Lewis et al. 2005).

Serotonin was hypothesized to be central to the pathophysiology of schizophrenia because of the psychotomimetic actions of serotonergic drugs, such as lysergic acid diethylamide (LSD) (D.X. Freedman 1975). More recently, the affinity of newer antipsychotic drugs for serotonergic receptors has raised further speculation over the role of this neurotransmitter system in the pathophysiology of the illness. Postmortem studies conducted to date have not found consistent changes in the serotonin chemistry or receptor expression (Harrison 1999a) in schizophrenia. Because serotonin has been shown to modify dopamine release in striatum (Kuroki et al. 2003; Marcus et al. 2000), the augmented antipsychotic action of the new drugs may be mediated through modulation of dopamine release into the synapse. Indeed, drugs without any dopamine receptor affinity, but with only serotonin type 2A ($5\text{-}HT_{2A}$) receptor antagonism, do behave as antipsychotic drugs in animal models and show antipsychotic activity in humans (de Paulis 2001). Because the serotonin system has diverse receptors and functions, it is not surprising that this aspect is not yet fully explored.

Clinically, it is well known that schizophrenic patients have a much higher incidence of cigarette smoking (Hughes et al. 1986). The upregulation in nicotinic receptors

(Benwell et al. 1988; Wonnacott 1990) seen in "normal" smokers is not seen in schizophrenia. On the contrary, decreased levels of nicotinic and muscarinic receptors are reported in the hippocampus, frontal cortex, thalamus, and striatum in schizophrenia (Hyde and Crook 2001). In addition, cholinergic neurotransmission is known to be integral to cognition and memory, functions disrupted in schizophrenia. These findings suggest cholinergic dysfunction in schizophrenia.

In summary, molecular abnormalities are found in several anatomical regions and in several neurotransmitter systems in the neuropathology of schizophrenia. Abnormalities in molecular targets should be examined in terms of pathways (not only neurotransmitter pathways) affecting circuit function. Additionally, identification of primary pathology from epiphenomena is essential. For example, neurotransmitter systems are dynamic, and disruption of one system would lead to compensatory mechanisms in other relevant pathways. A sound strategy to adopt once an abnormality is discovered is first to confirm the finding by replication in a second cohort and then to determine whether the molecular abnormality is part of the primary pathology. Converging data from in vivo human studies, postmortem human studies, and animal model studies would provide clues to the primary pathology.

FUNCTIONAL STUDIES IN SCHIZOPHRENIA WITH IN VIVO IMAGING TECHNIQUES

The advances made in neuroimaging technology now allow us to study neurochemical and physiological changes in the living human brain. Functional BOLD (blood oxygen level dependent) MRI indirectly measures changes in regional cerebral blood flow (rCBF), which reflects regional brain activity. Single-photon emission computed tomography (SPECT) and PET involve the use of a radioactive tracer to measure rCBF metabolic activity, with oxygen-15-labeled water ($H_2^{15}O$) or fluorine-18 fluorodeoxyglucose (FDG), or to quantify receptors using specific radioligands.

FUNCTIONAL IMAGING

rCBF studies were originally done with xenon-133 with individual cortical detectors. These studies originally identified frontal cortex blood flow abnormalities (Ingvar and Franzen 1971) and were later extended by Weinberger et al. (1986) to show abnormalities associated with impaired task performance. Schizophrenic subjects did not activate frontal cortex areas when performing a task known to involve frontal cortex activity (e.g., the Wisconsin Card

Sorting Test) in association with their inability to perform the task (reviewed in Holcomb et al. 1989). Subsequent imaging studies in schizophrenia produced inconsistent detection of frontal cortex hypometabolism, with some studies continuing to find it (Buchsbaum et al. 1984), others reporting no change in the measure (Tamminga et al. 1992), and still others finding frontal hypermetabolism (Cleghorn et al. 1989). A recent meta-analysis suggested that hypofrontality at rest is found in schizophrenia (Hill et al. 2004). However, two potential confounds must be considered. One confound is antipsychotic drug treatment, because neuroleptics are known to reduce neuronal activity in the frontal cortex. Second, deficit symptoms in schizophrenia are associated with reduced frontal cortex activation and could serve to confound observations. Studies have certainly confirmed frontal cortex alterations in schizophrenia with variable, complex, and still incompletely understood characteristics.

Our own studies with FDG PET were conducted in young, drug-free, floridly psychotic schizophrenic individuals (Tamminga et al. 1992). We detected metabolic differences in schizophrenia in limbic structures (anterior cingulate and hippocampal cortices), with both areas showing reduced metabolism (Figure 26–1). No other differences developed between the schizophrenic individuals and the healthy volunteers. However, within the schizophrenic group, primary negative-symptom patients showed the additional abnormalities of reduced metabolism in frontal and parietal cortices and thalamus compared with the non-negative-symptom group. Both of these findings (limbic changes overall in schizophrenia and frontal cortex reductions in negative symptoms) are consistent with considerable other literature in their regional localization (Andreasen et al. 1992; Tamminga et al. 1992. Reflecting the pathology found in postmortem tissue studies of schizophrenia, these results are consistent with limbic cortical dysfunction associated with the illness, particularly with its positive symptoms.

Because schizophrenic patients characteristically (although variably) perform many tasks more poorly than do nonschizophrenic persons, imaging assessment with a nongraded task will include a performance confound in its interpretation. The use of a variable error-rate task with all subjects fixed to the same performance level has been an innovation in this area, allowing comparisons without a prominent performance confound (Holcomb et al. 1996b, 2000). We have generated an rCBF comparison between schizophrenic patients and matched nonschizophrenic control subjects, conducted while both groups were performing a practiced auditory recognition task at a similar performance level (e.g., with task difficulty set to an 80% error level). The task involved discriminating between two audi-

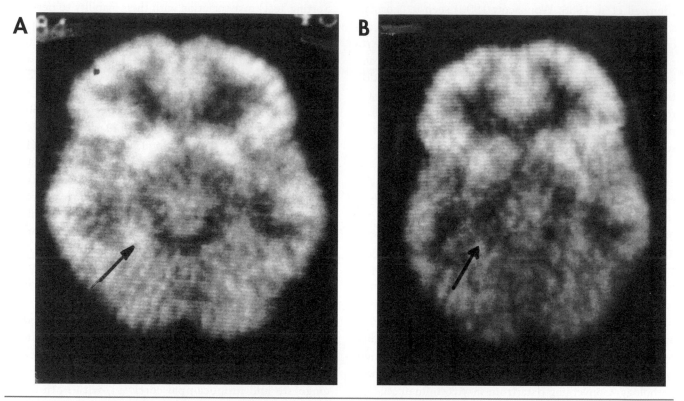

FIGURE 26–1.   Positron emission tomographic images with fluorodeoxyglucose. Both images are at the same axial level and show, among other areas, the medial temporal structures. *Panel A.* Image from a healthy control subject; the general area of parahippocampal gyrus/hippocampus is indicated by the arrow. *Panel B.* The schizophrenic individual has a remarkable reduction in glucose metabolism in the medial temporal structures (*arrow*). This reduction in parahippocampal gyrus metabolism is representative of differences in the entire schizophrenic group.

tory tones; the difference in tone frequency was varied to shape performance to 80% accuracy. Consistent with a priori predictions, the nonschizophrenic individuals activated a small area in the posterior superior temporal auditory cortex (right>left) and a spot in the left motor cortex in the control task. For the decision task, control subjects activated the anterior cingulate cortex, right insula, and right middle frontal cortex. The schizophrenic subjects had considerably more activation in extent and magnitude of response in the control task, showing activation not only in the superior temporal auditory cortex (left>right) but also in the left premotor cortex, left parietal cortex, right insula, and cingulate cortex. In the decision task (in which control subjects showed considerable activation in these regions), the schizophrenic subjects showed very little incremental increase in activation except for a mild flow increase in right frontal cortex (Figure 26–2). Overall, in comparing the "decision minus rest" subtraction between groups, the schizophrenic patients showed activation of approximately the same areas as did control subjects. Significantly more of this activation (which accompanied the decision task in nonschizophrenic subjects) was recruited for the relatively easy control (sensorimotor) task in the schizophrenic sub-

jects. Moreover, when the patients increased their performance in the decision task (indicated by reduced accuracy and slower response times), no additional flow changes were apparent. Patients were performing this task at an accuracy level similar to that of nonschizophrenic subjects.

Other scientists have used this method to understand the localization and type of functional defects in schizophrenia as well. Liddle and colleagues (1992) studied the correlation between well-delineated symptom clusters in schizophrenia (negative symptoms, hallucinations or delusions, and disorganization) and rCBF. Most interesting was the confirmation in this study, as well as elsewhere, that in vivo functional manifestations associated with schizophrenia are diverse. In overview, Liddle et al. reported that negative symptoms were negatively associated with rCBF in left frontal cortex and left parietal areas. Hallucinations and delusions were positively associated with flow in the left parahippocampal gyrus and the left ventral striatum. Disorganization was associated with flow in anterior cingulate cortex and mediodorsal thalamus. This study showed that brain areas are differently involved in symptom manifestations in schizophrenia, perhaps as either a cause or an effect of the disorder. Silbersweig et al. (1995)

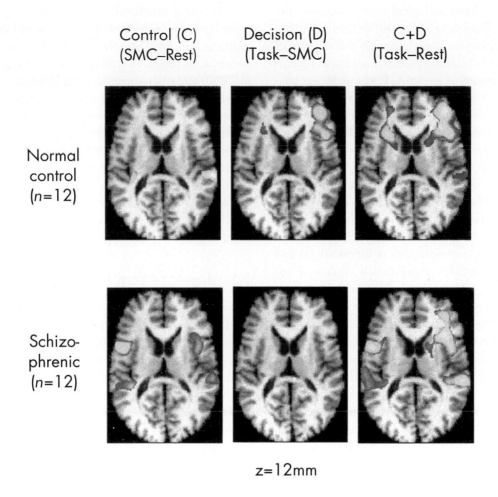

|Control (C) (SMC–Rest)|Decision (D) (Task–SMC)|C+D (Task–Rest)|

Normal control (n=12)

Schizo- phrenic (n=12)

z=12mm

FIGURE 26–2. Regional cerebral blood flow elevations seen at an axial level 12 mm above the anterior commissure–posterior commissure line in healthy control (*top row*) and schizophrenic (*bottom row*) subjects, each in a sensorimotor control (SMC) (*left column*) and a decision performance (*middle column*) condition. Control subjects merely activate the auditory cortex bilaterally (*upper left scan*) and the left motor cortex (data not shown) in the sensorimotor task, whereas the schizophrenic subjects activate those more and in more areas than do control subjects (*bottom left scan*). During the decision task, the control subjects activate middle and inferior frontal cortex (*upper middle scan*) and anterior cingulate gyrus (data not shown); however, the schizophrenic subjects do not recruit any additional areas or increase flow at all in their decision condition (*lower middle scan*). Overall, the schizophrenic subjects resemble the control subjects in the "task minus rest" analysis (*upper and lower right scans*), even though that activation occurred primarily in the control, not the decision, scan.

Source. Images contributed by Dr. Henry Holcomb and Dr. Adrienne Lahti.

scanned hallucinating schizophrenic persons to show involvement of specific brain regions with psychosis. This section is expanded on later in the chapter.

Other studies also have found evidence for limbic abnormalities in schizophrenia both at rest (Taylor et al. 1999) and with cognitive challenge (Artiges et al. 2000; Heckers et al. 1998; Spence et al. 1997). Heckers et al. (1998) found reduced hippocampal activation in schizophrenic subjects during a memory retrieval task of previously studied words. These findings complement other postmortem and structural imaging studies of abnormalities in medial temporal lobe structures of schizophrenic

individuals (Gao et al. 2000). Spence et al. (1997) studied schizophrenic subjects performing a complex motor task during an acute exacerbation of their illness and 4–6 weeks later, after their symptoms had improved. Although the subjects were acutely ill, they showed signs of prefrontal hypometabolism. When the schizophrenic volunteers' symptoms improved, the prefrontal regions were normal. However, when the schizophrenic patients were less symptomatic, rCBF in the anterior cingulate and bilateral parietal regions was still decreased. These limbic region abnormalities are probably the result of a dysfunctional network of regions and not a series of separate lesions.

Imaging during pharmacological manipulation of the NMDA-sensitive glutamate receptor system identifies specific brain regions that correlate with the severity of psychosis. PCP, an NMDA antagonist, produces a complex array of behaviors in humans. It can induce a psychotic state in nonschizophrenic persons (without delirium) that is characterized by many of the signs and symptoms often found in schizophrenia. Moreover, PCP (Luby et al. 1959) and ketamine (Lahti et al. 1995b) can both selectively exacerbate a patient's psychotic symptoms in schizophrenia, suggesting an action on (or near) the site of schizophrenia pathophysiology. Ketamine alters rCBF directly in the brain areas in which postmortem tissue and in vivo imaging studies indicate dysfunction in schizophrenic persons—specifically, in hippocampal and anterior cingulate cortices. Behaviorally, ketamine increases psychosis at subanesthetic doses in both neuroleptic-treated and neuroleptic-free schizophrenic patients to the same degree. Ketamine stimulates positive, not negative, symptoms in schizophrenia, and its action is not blocked by dopamine receptor antagonism (Lahti et al. 1995b). Symptoms that are stimulated by ketamine are that person's characteristic set of schizophrenic hallucinations, delusions, and/or thought disorder. This is unlike other psychotomimetics (e.g., amphetamine or muscimol), which stimulate psychotomimetic symptoms typical of the drug. This action of ketamine would be most parsimoniously explained by assuming that the drug stimulates a brain system that is already active in mediating (possibly even in originating) the psychosis.

We used $H_2^{15}O$ and PET to study the localization and time course of ketamine action in brain by measuring rCBF (Figure 26–3). Schizophrenic subjects who were taking a dose of ketamine active in exacerbating psychosis (0.3 mg/kg) showed increased rCBF in the anterior cingulate gyrus and decreased rCBF in hippocampus and lingual gyrus (Lahti et al. 1995a). The brain areas that showed a change had different time course patterns of rCBF over the 60 minutes after ketamine administration. This suggests that each area of brain has its own sensitivity to ketamine (which might be predicted on the basis of receptor localization and anatomical connections) and its own unique time course of response. Because other drugs have not been studied this way in humans, it is impossible to know whether this phenomenon is common, unusual, or unique. It does mean that ketamine at a behaviorally active (not anesthetic) dose produces rCBF actions in specific brain regions (more restricted than its receptor distribution would predict) and that the response of various cerebral regions appears independent. Questions of how this ketamine-induced psychosis stimulation might be related to schizophrenia still need to be answered.

Abnormal functional connections between brain regions have been suggested as the cause of abnormal rCBF patterns seen in schizophrenia (Frith et al. 1995; Weinberger et al. 1992). In studies of verbal fluency (Spence et al. 2000) and semantic processing (Jennings et al. 1998), a network analysis identified a functional disconnection between the anterior cingulate and prefrontal regions of schizophrenic subjects. Frontal lobe functional connectivity was abnormal in the schizophrenic subjects, even though they had significantly activated the regions and their behavior on the tasks was not impaired. These findings suggest that the abnormalities seen in the frontal lobes of schizophrenic persons may be a problem of integration across regions and not a specific regional abnormality.

NEURORECEPTOR IMAGING

Neuroreceptor SPECT and PET imaging allows the direct assessments of receptor density and indirect estimations of neurotransmitter release in the living brain. Human brain imaging ligand studies suggested abnormalities in D_1 receptor density in the frontal cortex of persons with schizophrenia (Karlsson et al. 2002), leading to speculation that an agonist at the D_1 receptor may be therapeutic in treating cognitive dysfunctions in schizophrenia (Goldman-Rakic et al. 2004). Imaging studies with D_2 receptor ligands reported increases in D_2 family receptors in neuroleptic-naive and neuroleptic-free schizophrenia (Wong et al. 1986), and a later report suggested the presence of increased D_2 receptor density in psychotic nonschizophrenic patients (Pearlson et al. 1995); however, subsequent studies that used various other D_2 ligands and replications with the initial ligand were unable to replicate this finding (Farde et al. 1990; Hietala et al. 1991; Martinot et al. 1990, 1991). All schizophrenic individuals do not have increased D_2 family receptors in the striatum, but an alteration in D_2 density may be characteristic of a subgroup of schizophrenic patients, perhaps those with a long duration of illness or other special clinical characteristics (Hietala et al. 1994).

The question remains whether D_2 family receptors are elevated in a subgroup of schizophrenic patients or reflect a confound of medication effect in the initial report. More recently, Laruelle et al. (1996) measured dopamine release into the synapse by using SPECT or PET imaging with low-affinity dopamine receptor ligands. They reported that persons with schizophrenia had an increased release of dopamine in the striatum during the acute phases of their illness in response to amphetamine challenge, compared with healthy control subjects (Abi-Dargham et al. 1998). A significant correlation was seen with dopamine release in the striatum and psychosis but not negative symptoms.

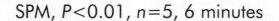

SPM, *P*<0.01, *n*=5, 6 minutes

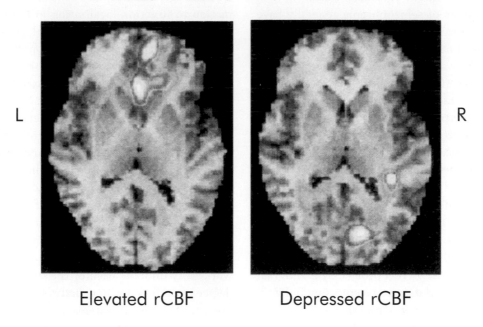

L   R

Elevated rCBF   Depressed rCBF

FIGURE 26–3. Regional cerebral blood flow (rCBF) localization of ketamine action in schizophrenic brain. rCBF increases occurred in anterior cingulate gyrus, extending to medial frontal areas (*left scan*); rCBF decreases are apparent in the hippocampus and lingual gyrus (*right scan*). The colored areas indicating significant flow change are plotted onto a magnetic resonance imaging template for ease of localization. SPM=statistical parametric mapping.

Source. Images contributed by Dr. Henry Holcomb and Dr. Adrienne Lahti.

Increased release seems not secondary to chronic antipsychotic treatment because augmented release also occurs in first-episode patients and some family members (Laruelle et al. 1999). This increase in dopaminergic tone in the striatum appears, at least in part, to be under glutamatergic regulation (Kegeles et al. 2000; Smith et al. 1998). Imaging glutamate receptors is of keen interest but is hampered by the difficulty in synthesis of such ligands, although efforts are under way (Waterhouse et al. 2004).

CLINICAL THERAPEUTICS IN SCHIZOPHRENIA

The clinical therapeutics of psychotic illness episodically but progressively advanced in the second half of the twentieth century. However, these advances have all been empirical, not theoretical, and rarely rational. Chlorpromazine was first tested in schizophrenic patients because of its known sedative properties as a preanesthetic agent (Delnay and Deniker 1952). Its selective antipsychotic activity was immediately noted and quickly established. This became the springboard for hypotheses of altered dopaminergic transmission in schizophrenia. In addition to this observation having generated decades of

research in therapeutics, it has been highly pivotal in promoting pharmacological approaches to the exploration of schizophrenia pathophysiology.

The conventional antipsychotics (butyrophenones, phenothiazines, and thioxanthenes) with potent antidopaminergic activity were used successfully to treat psychosis for 50 years, albeit with acute and chronic motor side effects. These drugs have vastly improved the lives of those afflicted with schizophrenia; however, these patients still endure considerable residual symptom burden and lifelong psychosocial impairments. In 1990, newer drugs were introduced with higher antiserotonergic potency accompanying the dopamine receptor blockade. These drugs were less likely to cause motor side effects and dysphoria but had their own serious side effects. The metabolic syndrome (weight gain, hyperlipidemia, diabetes, hypertension) is a side effect of concern with many of the new antipsychotics. Clozapine remains the only antipsychotic with demonstrably greater antipsychotic efficacy; the mechanism of its better effect is still not known. Recently, the concept of partial agonism at the D_2 receptors has added a novel and interesting perspective to the pharmacotherapy for schizophrenia (Carlsson et al. 2001). The efficacy of the first D_2 partial agonist— aripiprazole—has been established in preclinical trials, resulting in its approval by the U.S. Food and Drug Administration for the treatment of schizophrenia.

Existing treatments of schizophrenia generally have been unsuccessful in treating cognitive deficits in schizophrenia. There is controversy over whether second-generation antipsychotics improve cognition more than classic antipsychotics do (Green et al. 2002; Meltzer and McGurk 1999; Meltzer and Sumiyoshi 2003). The MATRICS (measurement and treatment research to improve cognition in schizophrenia) program was developed to identify potential molecular targets to treat cognitive deficits in schizophrenia (Geyer and Tamminga 2004). The molecular targets identified as having the greatest promise to improve cognition include the D_1 receptor (Goldman-Rakic et al. 2004), α_7 nicotinic receptor (Martin et al. 2004), muscarinic receptor (Friedman 2004), 5-HT_{1A} and 5-HT_{2A} receptors (Roth et al. 2004), noradrenergic receptors (Arnsten 2004), and the NMDA receptor (Coyle and Tsai 2004). The metabotropic glutamate receptors mGluR2, 3, and 5 modulate NMDA receptor function and also may provide a means to enhance cognition (Moghaddam 2004). Agonists of these receptors are being evaluated as new adjunctive drug treatments, and not as alternatives to current antipsychotics, in schizophrenia. Thus, they will be tested in volunteers whose positive symptoms are optimally treated and stable. For example, we are currently testing atomoxetine, a norepinephrine reuptake inhibitor that increases norepinephrine and dopamine levels in the frontal cortex, and M_1 muscarinic agonists (*N*-desmethyl clozapine, a derivative of clozapine with M_1 agonist properties).

Specific treatments are not available for primary negative symptoms. Antipsychotic drugs can diminish negative symptoms, an effect that may be secondary to the reduction of acute psychosis. Some studies suggest that the second-generation drugs are effective for secondary negative symptoms, but they have shown no efficacy for the deficit symptoms (Arango et al. 2004). In a longitudinal study, clozapine was found to be ineffective in treating deficit symptoms (Buchanan et al. 1998). Initial promise of glutamatergic agents such as D-cycloserine (Goff et al. 2004; Heresco-Levy et al. 2005) has not been replicated in the latest larger multicenter study (Carpenter et al. 2005).

INTEGRATIVE BASIC BRAIN MECHANISMS IMPORTANT TO UNDERSTANDING CEREBRAL FUNCTION

Advances in basic knowledge about the mammalian brain relevant to function have been not only fascinating but also pivotal to modern concepts of brain mechanisms. Decades ago, lesion studies contributed one kind of information to function localization in the CNS. Currently, more subtle, yet functionally critical, principles are emerging, which include evidence of complex neuronal pathways, strategies for connectivity between brain areas, neuronal plasticity, and cognitive strategies.

Because of its complexity, there remains much to learn about the principles of brain structure as they subserve function. Systems biology is an emerging concept of neuroscience (Kitano 2002) that is beginning to be applied to schizophrenia. Systems neuroscience, the study of the function of neural circuits, is concerned with the functional organization and processing of information in cellular networks, thereby linking molecular and cellular biology to behaviors such as cognitive, motivational, perceptual, and motor processes. In schizophrenia, specific neural networks may underlie each of the symptom domains. The degree of dysfunction in neural systems may vary, and predominantly affected systems may have a greater effect on the clinical presentation. The notion is that abnormal networks, not just an abnormal protein, are found in schizophrenia. This neural system–based approach provides a plausible and scientifically sound framework in which to conceptualize the pathophysiology of schizophrenia.

CORTICAL-SUBCORTICAL CIRCUITS

It is generally understood that local areas in brain perform delimited tasks; that is, they have a functional concentration. Clear examples of this are the role of the occipital cortex in visual perception and visually related memory; the superior temporal cortex in sound perception and auditory association functions; and the frontal cortex in integrative functions such as working memory, attention, and motor control. To coordinate these functions effectively, the brain must use a variety of communication systems to connect specialized areas with one another. One example of the way the brain has arranged such a system is the series of cortical-subcortical circuits described most recently by Alexander and DeLong (Alexander and Crutcher 1990; Alexander et al. 1986) and applied by them to a treatment approach in Parkinson's disease (DeLong 1990). These investigators have found evidence for multiple parallel segregated neural circuits that connect specific areas of the frontal cortex reciprocally with specific regions of the basal ganglia and thalamus. Additional investigators (M. Carlsson and Carlsson 1990; Graybiel 1990; Nauta 1989) have also speculated about such a system, usually with respect to motor functions and output because of their easy definition and quantitative convenience. Parallel, segregated neuronal tracts project from specific areas in the frontal cortex to homologous target areas of basal ganglia, organized somatotypically and by functional system (e.g., motor, oculomotor, limbic, prefrontal); within both the basal ganglia and the thalamus, the somatotopic organization is preserved. Within the basal ganglia (between striatum and substantia nigra pars reticulata), two legs of the pathway are connected in parallel, each having functionally opposite actions, presumably to subserve additional modulation. Efferents from the basal ganglia circuits project to their targets in thalamus. These thalamic areas project back to the originating frontal area, completing the feedback circuit. The neurochemical transmitters and firing characteristics of many of these pathways are known, thus providing possible sites and techniques for pharmacological intervention (M. Carlsson and Carlsson 1990; Graybiel 1990). Although our understanding of the contributions of basal ganglia and thalamus to cognitive activity is remarkably incomplete and not nearly as well studied as their involvement in motor function, these pathways must certainly set the tone for various cognitive activities just as they have more clearly been shown to do for motor functions. Concretely, one might imagine that the frontal cortex seeks to cue and to receive feedback from the basal ganglia and thalamus through these circuits, to set in motion other cerebral processing needed to accompany the cortically generated behavior, and also for sensitivity settings on planned behavior.

The potency of the influence of basal ganglia–thalamic feedback on frontal cortical activity is obvious in a neurological disorder such as Parkinson's disease, in which substantial motor feedback inhibition occurs (from the putamen) because of extreme deficiency there of nigral dopamine; this same feedback pathway may also function to mediate the antipsychotic action (and motor side effects) of neuroleptics in psychosis (Holcomb et al. 1996a). Alexander and DeLong (1986) have extrapolated from the importance of this feedback system in motor control that this same mechanism also should be operative in other frontal functions (memory, attention, and other aspects of cognition). They suggested that an area in the frontal cortex actually originates a voluntary cerebral (frontal) function but that the eventual expression of that function is powerfully modulated by the basal ganglia and thalamus through parallel segregated neuronal circuits.

Schizophrenia, by extrapolation, could hypothetically result from abnormal regulation of aspects of frontal cortical function. Findings from human imaging and postmortem studies in schizophrenia provide a basis for us to speculate on the neural circuits that may underlie symptom domains described earlier (Figure 26–4).

SYMPTOM CLUSTER CIRCUITS

Psychosis Neural Circuit

Earlier in this chapter, we discussed limbic abnormalities found in schizophrenia; these studies implicated the anterior cingulate cortex and the hippocampus in psychosis (Tamminga et al. 1992). Significant association between regional cerebral glucose metabolic rate in the limbic cortex (anterior cingulate cortex plus hippocampus) and the magnitude of positive symptoms was seen in medication-free schizophrenic volunteers. These studies allow us to speculate that the limbic cortex is associated with the positive symptoms of the illness, whereas the prefrontal cortex may support negative and cognitive symptoms. The anterior cingulate cortex and adjacent medial prefrontal cortex correlate with induction of positive symptoms with the NMDA antagonist ketamine (Lahti et al. 1995a). PET scanning in hallucinating schizophrenic persons is associated with activations in the medial prefrontal cortex, left superior temporal gyrus, right medial temporal gyrus, left hippocampus/parahippocampal region, thalamus, putamen, and cingulate (Copolov et al. 2003; Silbersweig et al. 1995). These studies provide clues to the anatomical structures that may be involved in a "psychosis neural circuit." Limbic regions, in particular, are frequently implicated in these in vivo studies. We postulate that a core pathology in the hippocampus affects other brain regions (e.g., the anterior cingulate cortex and medial prefrontal cortex) in the network. The proposed psychosis circuit consists of the anterior hippocampus, anterior cingulate, medial prefrontal cortex (Brodmann area 32), thalamus, ventral pallidum, striatum, and substantia nigra/ventral tegmental area (see Figure 26–4).

Negative Affect Neural Circuit

Brain activation patterns associated with negative symptoms show hypoactivation of the frontal lobe (Andreasen et al. 1992, 1994; Schroeder et al. 1994; Volkow et al. 1987; Wolkin et al. 1992). Decreased rCBF is seen in both the prefrontal and the parietal cortices of schizophrenic persons experiencing negative symptoms (Friston 1992; Liddle et al. 1992; Tamminga et al. 1992). The dorsolateral prefrontal cortex and parietal cortex have dense reciprocal interconnections, suggesting a close functional relation (Schwartz and Goldman-Rakic 1984). This may explain the observation that persons with deficit forms of schizophrenia have greater impairment in cognitive performance (Buchanan et al. 1994, 1997). Another study in patients with predominantly negative symptoms implicated the medial prefrontal, dorsolateral, and prefrontal cortices (Potkin et al. 2002). Lower activity also was noted in the thalamus (Tamminga et al. 1992), particularly the mediodorsal nucleus of the thalamus (Hazlett et al. 2004). The amygdala, a key component in the circuit of emotion, is implicated in emotional processing in schizophrenia (R..E. Gur et al. 2002). The neural system we propose for the negative symptom cluster includes the dorsolateral prefrontal cortex, parietal cortex, amygdala, anterior hippocampus, thalamus, ventral pallidum, striatum, and substantia nigra/ventral tegmental area.

Cognitive Deficit Neural Circuit

Abnormalities seen in the frontal lobes of schizophrenic patients may be the result of a problem of integration across regions and not a single regional abnormality (Jennings et al. 1998; Spence et al. 2000). Functional MRI studies that used cognitively demanding tasks, such as working memory tasks, produced diverse results. Research has shown that although rCBF increases in prefrontal regions with greater working memory demands, if working memory capacity is exceeded, the activation decreases (Callicott et al. 1999). In separate studies, disorganization was associated with flow in anterior cingulate and mediodorsal thalamus (Liddle et al. 1992), whereas apomorphine, a dopamine agonist that has antipsychotic properties, normalizes anterior cingulate blood flow of schizophrenic persons during verbal fluency task performance (Dolan et al. 1995). We propose that a neural system for cognitive deficits involves the dorsolateral prefrontal cortex, anterior hippocampus, anterior cingulate, thalamus, ventral pallidum, striatum, and substantia nigra/ventral tegmental area.

SYNTHESIS

CLINICAL OBSERVATIONS ABOUT SCHIZOPHRENIA IMPORTANT FOR FORMULATING PATHOPHYSIOLOGY

Several characteristics of schizophrenic illness are strikingly consistent across clinics, laboratories, and cultures, such that any theory of the illness must take them into account. These include but are not limited to the following: schizophrenic symptoms are clear and their clustering is common but not exclusive; symptoms fluctuate during the course of illness and may disappear entirely between episodes but then reappear; and the illness is most often lifelong, with the most flagrant symptoms and psychosocial deterioration appearing early in the illness, showing a plateau during middle years, and frequently ending with some degree of symptom resolution in later

years. The illness has a genetic component but is by no means fully genetically determined. Each candidate risk gene confers a small degree of risk, and it is likely that gene–environment interactions play a crucial etiological role in the disease. Although no traditional anatomical or biochemical change has come to be pathognomonic of the illness, it is in the limbic system (especially the hippocampus and entorhinal and cingulate cortices) that anatomical and functional changes, albeit of a varied pathological nature, are highly concentrated. Pharmacologically, only the antagonism of dopamine-mediated transmission with neuroleptics has been therapeutic. Other pharmacological approaches have so far resulted in negative outcomes. On the contrary, several pharmacological strategies are psychotomimetic, including drugs such as amphetamine, LSD, mescaline, muscimol, and PCP/ketamine. Of these, PCP/ketamine is the drug class that most faithfully mimics schizophrenia in nonschizophrenic persons and most potently and validly exacerbates schizophrenia symptoms in affected patients, even while inducing minimal primary drug symptoms. In addition, ketamine alters rCBF in cingulate cortex, hippocampus, and lingual gyrus; the first two areas were previously related to schizophrenia via other functional imaging techniques.

People with schizophrenia have pervasive, patterned, but interrelated cognitive dysfunction, suggesting a failure of an interactive connective function. Schizophrenic subjects, even when they are performing equivalently to healthy control subjects on a task, use similar brain areas but activate them prematurely and not in relation to difficulty, as is the case in nonschizophrenic individuals. The anterior cingulate cortex especially shows these differences. Moreover, whereas limbic areas might be broadly affected in all or most schizophrenic subjects, the frontal cortex and other neocortical areas seem to be associated with other discrete manifestations of illness, such as negative symptoms or deficit syndrome. Evidence of consistent, highly replicable biochemical change in the brain in schizophrenia has yet evaded the study of this illness. This does not mean that these parameters should not be studied, but it might suggest that only a composite biochemical change will give a clue (see, e.g., Issa et al. 1994a, 1994b) or that an entirely new (perhaps functional) approach is needed.

PITFALLS AND CONFOUNDS IN SCHIZOPHRENIA STUDIES

Schizophrenia is a difficult disease to study biologically for methodological and theoretical reasons. The brain is a highly protected organ whose tissue or integrated func-

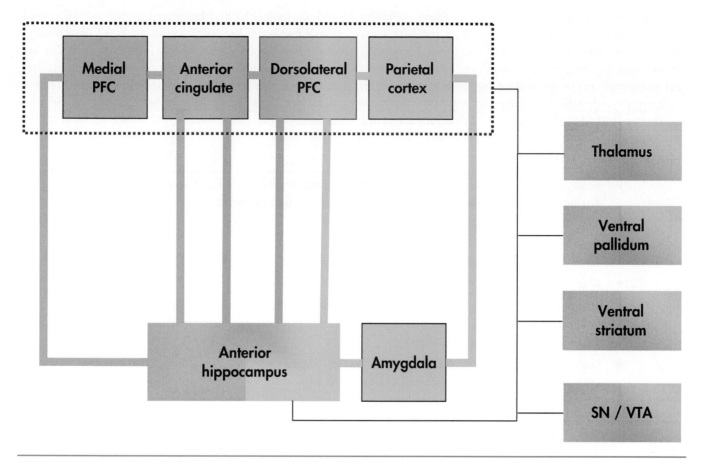

FIGURE 26–4. Hypothetical neural circuits underlying the three symptom domains of schizophrenia. In this model, a specific neural circuit underlies each of the symptom domains—the psychosis circuit (*orange*), cognitive deficit circuit (*blue*), and negative symptom circuit (*green*). The *dotted line* represents neocortex. Core deficits in the anterior hippocampus can influence functional integrity of each of these circuits. PFC=prefrontal cortex; SN/VTA=substantia nigra/ventral tegmental area.

tion cannot easily be sampled in vivo, even in illness. Schizophrenic individuals themselves often have compromised cognitive ability, and they may not be able to collaborate fully with a demanding research study. The long-term use of neuroleptic drugs is almost ubiquitous in schizophrenia and regularly confounds biological study. This long-term treatment alters much of the brain neurochemistry, as well as aspects of its structure, portions of its function, and probably more. Neuroleptic withdrawal for biological study is difficult because it frequently results in symptom reemergence. Symptom diversity is a hallmark of the illness, as is symptom fluctuation over time and within single individuals. Moreover, this diversity and fluctuation are most often masked by neuroleptic treatment in what we would have to assume is a complex manner.

Although they are difficult to manage for experimental designs, these issues can be worked with through careful clinical, pharmacological, genetic, and imaging assessment. Certainly these areas are always important parameters to assess in evaluating study results.

TOWARD A PATHOPHYSIOLOGY OF SCHIZOPHRENIA

Our understanding of the pathophysiology of schizophrenia is still obscure, and it is becoming evident that schizophrenia is not one disease but rather a syndrome. The identification of candidate risk genes, specific developmental environmental factors, and the effects of gene-environmental interactions speak to the heterogeneity we can expect to find in schizophrenia. A shift in conceptual framework from searching for a specific protein defect in schizophrenia to a search for defects in neural networks may represent a plausible biological approach to investigating the pathophysiology of schizophrenia. Identification of relevant neural systems and an understanding of the dynamics of the systems would provide a model to test function. As an initial formulation, we have proposed neural networks for each of the symptom domains. This formulation proposes that core pathology in the hippocampus influences the function of networks involving distinct cortical regions and subcortical structures.

Studies of schizophrenia are proceeding on many fronts. Investigators use information from patients, family members, birth records, and life histories, along with in vivo imaging, postmortem tissue, and phenomenological presentation, to formulate hypotheses. Research techniques with high sensitivity and resolution are now becoming available. Moreover, the techniques are broad and use molecular and functional probes as well as traditional measures. Productive leads are being used to target novel drug discovery, and new information in this area may inform our ideas of pathophysiology and etiology. Although the exact nature of schizophrenia is now unknown, it is not likely to remain unknown for much longer.

Highlights for the Clinician

- ✦ Schizophrenia is a disease composed of three symptom clusters, each of which may have a distinct molecular pathology and differ in its response to treatment:
    1. Deficits in cognition
    2. Psychosis
    3. Negative symptoms
- ✦ Cognitive deficits are arguably the core symptoms of schizophrenia.
- ✦ Current treatment strategies target the "psychosis" cluster. The "cognitive deficit" cluster is largely untreated. New adjunctive treatment strategies targeting cognitive dysfunction in schizophrenia are being evaluated.
- ✦ Gene–environment interactions are important etiological factors in schizophrenia. Minimizing environmental stressors in high-risk children and adolescents may reduce their risk of developing schizophrenia in adulthood.

RECOMMENDED READINGS

Harrison PJ, Weinberger DR: Schizophrenia genes, gene expression, and neuropathology: on the matter of their convergence. Mol Psychiatry 10:40–68, 2005

Maki P, Veijola J, Jones PB, et al: Predictors of schizophrenia: a review. Br Med Bull 73–74:1–15, 2005

REFERENCES

Abi-Dargham A, Gil R, Krystal J, et al: Increased striatal dopamine transmission in schizophrenia: confirmation in a second cohort. Am J Psychiatry 155:761–767, 1998

Abi-Dargham A, Rodenhiser J, Printz D, et al: Increased baseline occupancy of D_2 receptors by dopamine in schizophrenia. Proc Natl Acad Sci USA 97:8104–8109, 2000

Adams ME, Kramarcy N, Krall SP, et al: Absence of alpha-syntrophin leads to structurally aberrant neuromuscular synapses deficient in utrophin. J Cell Biol 150:1385–1398, 2000

Addington AM, Gornick M, Sporn AL, et al: Polymorphisms in the 13q33.2 gene G72/G30 are associated with childhood-onset schizophrenia and psychosis not otherwise specified. Biol Psychiatry 55:976–980, 2004

Akbarian S, Bunney WE, Potkin SG, et al: Altered distribution of nicotinamide-adenine dinucleotide phosphate-diaphorase cells in frontal lobe of schizophrenics implies disturbances of cortical development. Arch Gen Psychiatry 50:169–177, 1993

Akbarian S, Kim JJ, Potkin SG, et al: Gene expression for glutamic acid decarboxylase is reduced without loss of neurons in prefrontal cortex of schizophrenics. Arch Gen Psychiatry 52:258–266, 1995

Alexander GE, Crutcher MD: Functional architecture of basal ganglia circuits: neural substrates of parallel processing. Trends Neurosci 13:266–271, 1990

Alexander GE, DeLong MR, Strick PL: Parallel organization of functionally segregated circuits linking basal ganglia and cortex. Annu Rev Neurosci 9:357–381, 1986

Altshuler LL, Conrad A, Kovelman JA, et al: Hippocampal pyramidal cell orientation in schizophrenia. Arch Gen Psychiatry 44:1094–1098, 1987

American Psychiatric Association: Diagnostic and Statistical Manual of Mental Disorders, 4th Edition, Text Revision. Washington, DC, American Psychiatric Association, 2000

Andreasen NC: Symptoms, signs, and diagnosis of schizophrenia. Lancet 346:477–481, 1995

Andreasen NC, Rezai K, Alliger R, et al: Hypofrontality in neuroleptic-naive patients and in patients with chronic schizophrenia. Arch Gen Psychiatry 49:943–958, 1992

Andreasen NC, Arndt S, Swayze V II, et al: Thalamic abnormalities in schizophrenia visualized through magnetic resonance image averaging. Science 266:294–298, 1994

Andreasen NC, Arndt S, Alliger R, et al: Symptoms of schizophrenia: methods, meanings, and mechanisms. Arch Gen Psychiatry 52:341–351, 1995

Andreasson S, Allebeck P, Engstrom A, et al: Cannabis and schizophrenia: a longitudinal study of Swedish conscripts. Lancet 2:1483–1486, 1987

Aoki C, Siekevitz P: Plasticity in brain development. Sci Am 259(6):56–64, 1988

Arango C, Buchanan RW, Kirkpatrick B, et al: The deficit syndrome in schizophrenia: implications for the treatment of negative symptoms. Eur Psychiatry 19:21–26, 2004

Arndt S, Alliger RJ, Andreasen NC: The distinction of positive and negative symptoms: the failure of a two-dimensional model. Br J Psychiatry 158:317–322, 1991

Arnold SE, Hyman BT, Van Hoesen GW, et al: Some cytoarchitectural abnormalities of the entorhinal cortex in schizophrenia. Arch Gen Psychiatry 48:625–632, 1991a

Arnold SE, Lee VM-Y, Gur RE, et al: Abnormal expression of two microtubule-associated proteins (MAP2 and MAP5) in specific subfields of the hippocampal formation in schizophrenia. Proc Natl Acad Sci U S A 88:10850–10854, 1991b

Arnsten AFT: Adrenergic targets for the treatment of cognitive deficits in schizophrenia. Psychopharmacology (Berl) 174:25–31, 2004

Arolt V, Lencer R, Nolte A, et al: Eye tracking dysfunction is a putative phenotypic susceptibility marker of schizophrenia and maps to a locus on chromosome 6p in families with multiple occurrence of the disease. Am J Med Genet 67:564–579, 1996

Arseneault L, Cannon M, Poulton R, et al: Cannabis use in adolescence and risk for adult psychosis: longitudinal prospective study. BMJ 325:1212–1213, 2002

Artiges E, Salame P, Recasens C, et al: Working memory control in patients with schizophrenia: a PET study during a random number generation task. Am J Psychiatry 157:1517–1519, 2000

Asarnow RF, Granholm E, Sherman T: Span of apprehension in schizophrenia, in Handbook of Schizophrenia, Vol 5: Neuropsychology, Psychophysiology and Information Processing. Edited by Steinhauer SR, Gruzelier JH, Zubin J. Amsterdam, The Netherlands, Elsevier, 1991, pp 335–370

Avila MT, Hong E, Thaker GK: Current progress in schizophrenia research: eye movement abnormalities in schizophrenia: what is the nature of the deficit? J Nerv Ment Dis 190:179–180, 2002

Badner JA, Gershon ES: Meta-analysis of whole-genome linkage scans of bipolar disorder and schizophrenia. Mol Psychiatry 7:405–411, 2002

Balogh DW, Merritt RD: Susceptibility to type A backward pattern masking among hypothetically psychosis-prone college students. J Abnorm Psychol 94:377–383, 1985

Barnes GR, Asselman PT: The mechanism of prediction in human smooth pursuit eye movements. J Physiol (Lond) 439:439–461, 1991

Barnes TR, Liddle PF: Evidence for the validity of negative symptoms. Mod Probl Pharmacopsychiatry 24:43–72, 1990

Barr CE, Mednick SA, Munk-Jorgensen P: Exposure to influenza epidemics during gestation and adult schizophrenia: a 40-year study. Arch Gen Psychiatry 47:869–874, 1990

Barta PE, Pearlson GD, Powers RE, et al: Auditory hallucinations and smaller superior temporal gyral volume in schizophrenia. Am J Psychiatry 146:1457–1462, 1990

Bebbington P, Wilkins S, Jones P, et al: Life events and psychosis: initial results from the Camberwell Collaborative Psychosis Study. Br J Psychiatry 162:72–79, 1993

Benes FM: Myelination of cortical-hippocampal relays during late adolescence. Schizophr Bull 15:585–593, 1989

Benes FM: Neurobiological investigations in cingulate cortex of schizophrenic brain. Schizophr Bull 19:537–549, 1993

Benes FM, Berretta S: GABAergic interneurons: implications for understanding schizophrenia and bipolar disorder. Neuropsychopharmacology 25:1–27, 2001

Benes FM, Vincent SL, Alsterberg G, et al: Increased GABA$_A$-receptor binding in superficial layers of cingulate cortex in schizophrenics. J Neurosci 12:924–929, 1992

Benwell MEM, Balfour DJK, Anderson JM: Evidence that tobacco smoking increases the density of [3H]nicotine binding sites in human brain. J Neurochem 50:1243–1247, 1988

Bertolino A, Caforio G, Blasi G, et al: Interaction of COMT (Val(108/158)Met) genotype and olanzapine treatment on prefrontal cortical function in patients with schizophrenia. Am J Psychiatry 161:1798–1805, 2004

Blackwood DH, St Clair DM, Muir WJ, et al: Auditory P300 and eye tracking dysfunction in schizophrenic pedigrees. Arch Gen Psychiatry 48:899–909, 1991

Bleuler M: The Schizophrenic Disorders: Long-Term Patient and Family Studies. Translated by Clemens SM. New Haven, CT, Yale University Press, 1978

Bogerts B: Recent advances in the neuropathology of schizophrenia. Schizophr Bull 19:431–445, 1993

Bogerts B, Ashtari M, Degreef G, et al: Reduced temporal limbic structure volumes on magnetic resonance images in first episode schizophrenia. Psychiatry Res 35:1–13, 1990

Braff DL: Impaired speed of information processing in nonmedicated schizotypal patients. Schizophr Bull 7:499–508, 1981

Braff DL, Geyer MA: Sensorimotor gating and schizophrenia: human and animal model studies. Arch Gen Psychiatry 47:181–188, 1990

Braff DL, Heaton R, Kuck J, et al: The generalized pattern of neuropsychological deficits in outpatients with chronic schizophrenia with heterogeneous Wisconsin Card Sorting Test results. Arch Gen Psychiatry 48:891–898, 1991

Breier A, Buchanan RW, Elkashef A, et al: Brain morphology and schizophrenia: a magnetic resonance imaging study of limbic, prefrontal cortex, and caudate structures. Arch Gen Psychiatry 49:921–926, 1992

Buchanan RW, Strauss ME, Kirkpatrick B, et al: Neuropsychological impairments in deficit vs nondeficit forms of schizophrenia. Arch Gen Psychiatry 51:804–811, 1994

Buchanan RW, Strauss ME, Breier A, et al: Attentional impairments in deficit and nondeficit forms of schizophrenia. Am J Psychiatry 154:363–370, 1997

Buchanan RW, Breier A, Kirkpatrick B, et al: Positive and negative symptom response to clozapine in schizophrenic patients with and without the deficit syndrome. Am J Psychiatry 155:751–760, 1998

Buchsbaum MS, DeLisi LE, Holcomb HH, et al: Anteroposterior gradients in cerebral glucose use in schizophrenia and affective disorders. Arch Gen Psychiatry 41:1159–1166, 1984

Cabelli RJ, Hohn A, Shatz CJ: Inhibition of ocular dominance column formation by infusion of NT-4/5 or BDNF. Science 267:1662–1666, 1995

Cabelli RJ, Shelton DL, Segal RA, et al: Blockade of endogenous ligands of trkB inhibits formation of ocular dominance columns. Neuron 19:63–76, 1997

Callicott JH, Mattay VS, Bertolino A, et al: Physiological characteristics of capacity constraints in working memory as revealed by functional MRI. Cereb Cortex 9:20–26, 1999

Callicott JH, Straub RE, Pezawas L, et al: Variation in *DISC1* affects hippocampal structure and function and increases risk for schizophrenia. Proc Natl Acad Sci USA 102:8627–8632, 2005

Cannon M, Jones PB, Murray RM: Obstetric complications and schizophrenia: historical and meta-analytic review. Am J Psychiatry 159:1080–1092, 2002

Cannon TD, Mednick SA, Parnas J, et al: Developmental brain abnormalities in the offspring of schizophrenic mothers, II: structural brain characteristics of schizophrenia and schizotypal personality disorder. Arch Gen Psychiatry 51:955–962, 1994

Cantor-Graae E, Selten JP: Schizophrenia and migration: a meta-analysis and review. Am J Psychiatry 162:12–24, 2005

Cardno AG, Gottesman II: Twin studies of schizophrenia: from bow-and-arrow concordances to star wars Mx and functional genomics. Am J Med Genet 97:12–17, 2000

Carlsson A, Lindquist M: Effect of chlorpromazine and haloperidol on formation of 3-methoxytyramine and normetanephrine in mouse brain. Acta Pharmacol Toxicol 20:140–144, 1963

Carlsson A, Waters N, Holm-Waters S, et al: Interactions between monoamines, glutamate, and GABA in schizophrenia: new evidence. Annu Rev Pharmacol Toxicol 41:237–260, 2001

Carlsson M, Carlsson A: Interactions between glutamatergic and monoaminergic systems within the basal ganglia: implications for schizophrenia and Parkinson's disease. Trends Neurosci 13:272–276, 1990

Carpenter WT Jr, Buchanan RW: Domains of psychopathology relevant to the study of etiology and treatment in schizophrenia, in Schizophrenia: Scientific Progress. Edited by Schulz SC, Tamminga CA. New York, Oxford University Press, 1989, pp 13–22

Carpenter WT Jr, Buchanan RW: Schizophrenia. N Engl J Med 330:681–690, 1994

Carpenter WT Jr, Buchanan RW: Schizophrenia: introduction and overview, in Comprehensive Textbook of Psychiatry/VI. Edited by Kaplan HI, Sadock BJ. Baltimore, MD, Williams & Wilkins, 1995, pp 889–942

Carpenter WT Jr, Buchanan RW, Kirkpatrick B, et al: Strong inference, theory testing and the neuroanatomy of schizophrenia. Arch Gen Psychiatry 50:825–831, 1993

Carpenter WT, Buchanan RW, Javitt DC, et al: Testing two efficacy hypotheses for the treatment of negative symptoms. Abstract (115515) presented at the International Congress of Schizophrenia Research, Savannah, GA, 2005

Caspi A, Sugden K, Moffitt TE, et al: Influence of life stress on depression: moderation by a polymorphism in the 5-HTT gene. Science 301:386–389, 2003

Caspi A, Moffitt TE, Cannon M, et al: Moderation of the effect of adolescent-onset cannabis use on adult psychosis by a functional polymorphism in the catechol-O-methyltransferase gene: longitudinal evidence of a gene × environment interaction. Biol Psychiatry 57:1117–1127, 2005

Chapman LJ, Chapman JP: Problems in the measurement of cognitive deficit. Psychol Bull 79:380–385, 1973

Chen X, Dunham C, Kendler S, et al: Regulator of G-protein signaling 4 (*RGS4*) gene is associated with schizophrenia in Irish high density families. Am J Med Genet B Neuropsychiatr Genet 129:23–26, 2004a

Chen X, Wang X, O'Neill AF, et al: Variants in the catechol-O-methyltransferase (*COMT*) gene are associated with schizophrenia in Irish high-density families. Mol Psychiatry 9:962–967, 2004b

Chowdari KV, Mirnics K, Semwal P, et al: Association and linkage analyses of *RGS4* polymorphisms in schizophrenia. Hum Mol Genet 11:1373–1380, 2002

Chumakov I, Blumenfeld M, Guerassimenko O, et al: Genetic and physiological data implicating the new human gene *G72* and the gene for D-amino acid oxidase in schizophrenia. Proc Natl Acad Sci USA 99:13675–13680, 2002

Ciompi L, Müller C: Lebensweg und alter der schizophrenen: Eine katamnestische lonzeitstudies bis ins senium. Berlin, Springer-Verlag, 1976

Cleghorn JM, Kaplan RD, Nahmias C, et al: Inferior parietal region implicated in neurocognitive impairment in schizophrenia. Arch Gen Psychiatry 46:758–760, 1989

Clow A, Theodorou A, Jenner P, et al: Changes in cerebral dopamine function induced by a year's administration of trifluoperazine or thioridazine and their subsequent withdrawal. Adv Biochem Psychopharmacol 24:335–340, 1980

Cohen JD, Servan-Schreiber D: Context, cortex, and dopamine: a connectionist approach to behavior and biology in schizophrenia. Psychol Rev 99:45–77, 1992

Cohen-Cory S, Fraser SE: Effects of brain-derived neurotrophic factor on optic axon branching and remodelling in vivo. Nature 378:192–196, 1995

Colter N, Battal S, Crow TJ: White matter reduction in the parahippocampal gyrus of patients with schizophrenia. Arch Gen Psychiatry 44:1023–1026, 1987

Condray R, Steinhauer SR, Goldstein G: Language comprehension in schizophrenics and their brothers. Biol Psychiatry 32:790–802, 1992

Condray R, Steinhauer SR, van Kammen DP, et al: Working memory capacity predicts language comprehension in schizophrenic patients. Schizophr Res 20:1–13, 1996

Copolov DL, Seal ML, Maruff P, et al: Cortical activation associated with the experience of auditory hallucinations and perception of human speech in schizophrenia: a PET correlation study. Psychiatry Res 122:139–152, 2003

Cornblatt BA, Winters L, Erlenmeyer-Kimling L: Attentional markers of schizophrenia: evidence from the New York high-risk study, in Schizophrenia: Scientific Progress. Edited by Schulz S, Tamminga C. New York, Oxford University Press, 1989, pp 83–92

Corvin AP, Morris DW, McGhee K, et al: Confirmation and refinement of an "at-risk" haplotype for schizophrenia suggests the EST cluster, Hs.97362, as a potential susceptibility gene at the Neuregulin-1 locus. Mol Psychiatry 9:208–213, 2004

Coyle JT: The nagging question of the function of N-acetylaspartylglutamate. Neurobiol Dis 4:231–238, 1997

Coyle JT, Tsai G: The NMDA receptor glycine modulatory site: a therapeutic target for improving cognition and reducing negative symptoms in schizophrenia. Psychopharmacology (Berl) 174:32–38, 2004

Cross AJ, Crow TJ, Owen F: 3H-Flupenthixol binding in postmortem brains of schizophrenics: evidence for a selective increase in dopamine D2 receptors. Psychopharmacology 74:122–124, 1981

Csernansky JG, Joshi S, Wang L, et al: Hippocampal morphometry in schizophrenia by high dimensional brain mapping. Proc Natl Acad Sci U S A 95:11406–11411, 1998

Csernansky JG, Schindler MK, Splinter NR, et al: Abnormalities of thalamic volume and shape in schizophrenia. Am J Psychiatry 161:896–902, 2004

Davies AM: The role of neurotrophins in the developing nervous system. J Neurobiol 25:1334–1348, 1994

Davis KL, Kahn RS, Ko G, et al: Dopamine in schizophrenia: a review and reconceptualization. Am J Psychiatry 148:1474–1486, 1991

de Frias CM, Annerbrink K, Westberg L, et al: COMT gene polymorphism is associated with declarative memory in adulthood and old age. Behav Genet 34:533–539, 2004

Delay J, Deniker P, Harl JM: Traitements des états d'excitation et d'agitation par une méthode médicamenteuse derivée de l'hibernothérapie. Ann Med Psychol Paris 110:267–273, 1952

DeLong MR: Primate models of movement disorders of basal ganglia origin. Trends Neurosci 13:281–285, 1990

de Paulis T: M-100907 (Aventis). Curr Opin Investig Drugs 2:123–132, 2001

Devon RS, Anderson S, Teague PW, et al: Identification of polymorphisms within Disrupted in Schizophrenia 1 and Disrupted in Schizophrenia 2, and an investigation of their association with schizophrenia and bipolar affective disorder. Psychiatr Genet 11:71–78, 2001

Dolan RJ, Fletcher P, Frith CD, et al: Dopaminergic modulation of impaired cognitive activation in the anterior cingulate cortex in schizophrenia. Nature 378:180–182, 1995

Dracheva S, McGurk SR, Haroutunian V: mRNA expression of AMPA receptors and AMPA receptor binding proteins in the cerebral cortex of elderly schizophrenics. J Neurosci Res 79:868–878, 2005

Durany N, Michel T, Zochling R, et al: Brain-derived neurotrophic factor and neurotrophin 3 in schizophrenic psychoses. Schizophr Res 52:79–86, 2001

Egan MF, Goldberg TE, Kolachana BS, et al: Effect of COMT Val108/158 Met genotype on frontal lobe function and risk for schizophrenia. Proc Natl Acad Sci U S A 98:6917–6922, 2001

Egan MF, Straub RE, Goldberg TE, et al: Variation in GRM3 affects cognition, prefrontal glutamate, and risk for schizophrenia. Proc Natl Acad Sci U S A 101:12604–12609, 2004

Ekelund J, Hovatta I, Parker A, et al: Chromosome 1 loci in Finnish schizophrenia families. Hum Mol Genet 10:1611–1617, 2001

Ekelund J, Hennah W, Hiekkalinna T, et al: Replication of 1q42 linkage in Finnish schizophrenia pedigrees. Mol Psychiatry 9:1037–1041, 2004

Elkashef AM, Issa F, Wyatt RJ: The biochemical basis of schizophrenia, in Contemporary Issues in the Treatment of Schizophrenia. Edited by Shriqui CL, Nasrallah HA. Washington, DC, American Psychiatric Press, 1995, pp 3–41, 863

Ernfors P, Ibanez CF, Ebendal T, et al: Molecular cloning and neurotrophic activities of a protein with structural similarities to nerve growth factor: developmental and topographical expression in the brain. Proc Natl Acad Sci U S A 87:54–58, 1990

Falkai P, Bogerts B: Cell loss in the hippocampus of schizophrenics. Eur Arch Psychiatry Neurol Sci 236:154–161, 1986

Fallin MD, Lasseter VK, Avramopoulos D, et al: Bipolar I disorder and schizophrenia: a 440-single-nucleotide polymorphism screen of 64 candidate genes among Ashkenazi Jewish case-parent trios. Am J Hum Genet 77:918–936, 2005

Faraone SV, Seidman LJ, Kremen WS, et al: Neuropsychological functioning among the nonpsychotic relatives of schizophrenic patients: a diagnostic efficiency analysis. J Abnorm Psychol 104:286–304, 1995

Faraone SV, Seidman LJ, Kremen WS, et al: Neuropsychologic functioning among the nonpsychotic relatives of schizophrenic patients: the effect of genetic loading. Biol Psychiatry 48:120–126, 2000

Farde L, Wiesel FA, Stone-Elander S, et al: D_2 dopamine receptors in neuroleptic-naive schizophrenic patients: a positron emission tomography study with 11C raclopride. Arch Gen Psychiatry 47:213–219, 1990

Fergusson DM, Horwood LJ, Swain-Campbell NR: Cannabis dependence and psychotic symptoms in young people. Psychol Med 33:15–21, 2003

Freedman DX: LSD, psychotogenic procedures, and brain neurohumors. Psychopharmacol Bull 11:42–43, 1975

Freedman R: Electrophysiological phenotypes. Methods Mol Med 77:215–225, 2003

Freedman R, Coon H, Myles-Worsley M, et al: Linkage of a neurophysiological deficit in schizophrenia to a chromosome 15 locus. Proc Natl Acad Sci U S A 94:587–592, 1997

Freedman R, Adler LE, Leonard S: Alternative phenotypes for the complex genetics of schizophrenia. Biol Psychiatry 45:551–558, 1999

Friedman JI: Cholinergic targets for cognitive enhancement in schizophrenia: focus on cholinesterase inhibitors and muscarinic agonists. Psychopharmacology (Berl) 174:45–53, 2004

Friston KJ: The dorsolateral prefrontal cortex, schizophrenia and PET. J Neural Transm Suppl 37:79–93, 1992

Frith C: Functional imaging and cognitive abnormalities. Lancet 346:615–620, 1995

Frith CD, Friston KJ, Herold S, et al: Regional brain activity in chronic schizophrenic patients during the performance of a verbal fluency task. Br J Psychiatry 167:343–349, 1995

Fujii Y, Shibata H, Kikuta R, et al: Positive associations of polymorphisms in the metabotropic glutamate receptor type 3 gene (GRM3) with schizophrenia. Psychiatr Genet 13:71–76, 2003

Funke B, Finn CT, Plocik AM, et al: Association of the DTNBP1 locus with schizophrenia in a U.S. population. Am J Hum Genet 75:891–898, 2004

Gao X-M, Sakai K, Roberts RC, et al: Ionotropic glutamate receptors and expression of N-methyl-D-aspartate receptor subunits in subregions of human hippocampus: effects of schizophrenia. Am J Psychiatry 157:1141–1149, 2000

Geyer MA, Tamminga CA: Measurement and treatment research to improve cognition in schizophrenia: neuropharmacological aspects. Psychopharmacology (Berl) 174:1–2, 2004

Ghose S, Weickert CS, Colvin SM, et al: Glutamate carboxypeptidase II gene expression in the human frontal and temporal lobe in schizophrenia. Neuropsychopharmacology 29:117–125, 2004

Giuliani NR, Calhoun VD, Pearlson GD, et al: Voxel-based morphometry versus region of interest: a comparison of two methods for analyzing gray matter differences in schizophrenia. Schizophr Res 74:135–147, 2005

Glatt SJ, Faraone SV, Tsuang MT: Association between a functional catechol O-methyltransferase gene polymorphism and schizophrenia: meta-analysis of case-control and family based studies. Am J Psychiatry 160:469–476, 2003

Goff DC, Bottiglieri T, Arning E, et al: Folate, homocysteine, and negative symptoms in schizophrenia. Am J Psychiatry 161:1705–1708, 2004

Gold J, Goldberg T, Weinberger D: Prefrontal function and schizophrenic symptoms. Neuropsychiatry Neuropsychol Behav Neurol 5:253–261, 1992

Gold JM, Hermann BP, Randolph C, et al: Schizophrenia and temporal lobe epilepsy: a neuropsychological analysis. Arch Gen Psychiatry 51:265–272, 1994

Goldberg TE, Weinberger DR, Berman KF, et al: Further evidence for dementia of the prefrontal type in schizophrenia? A controlled study of teaching the Wisconsin Card Sorting Test. Arch Gen Psychiatry 44:1008–1014, 1987

Goldberg TE, Ragland D, Torrey EF, et al: Neuropsychological assessment of monozygotic twins discordant for schizophrenia. Arch Gen Psychiatry 47:1066–1072, 1990

Goldberg TE, Egan MF, Gscheidle T, et al: Executive subprocesses in working memory: relationship to catechol-O-methyltransferase Val158Met genotype and schizophrenia. Arch Gen Psychiatry 60:889–896, 2003

Goldman-Rakic PS: Working memory dysfunction in schizophrenia. J Neuropsychiatry Clin Neurosci 6:348–357, 1994

Goldman-Rakic PS: Psychopathology and neuropathology of prefrontal cortex in schizophrenia, in Schizophrenia: An Integrated View. Alfred Benzon Symposium 38. Edited by Fog R, Gerlach J, Hemmingsen R. Copenhagen, Denmark, Munksgaard, 1995, pp 126–138

Goldman-Rakic PS, Isseroff A, Schwartz ML, et al: The neurobiology of cognitive development, in Handbook of Child Psychology: Biology and Infancy Development. Edited by Mussen P. New York, Wiley, 1983, pp 281–344

Goldman-Rakic PS, Castner SA, Svensson TH, et al: Targeting the dopamine D1 receptor in schizophrenia: insights for cognitive dysfunction. Psychopharmacology 174:3–16, 2004

Gottesman II, Gould T: The endophenotype concept in psychiatry: etymology and strategic intentions. Am J Psychiatry 160:636–645, 2003

Gottesman II, Shields J: A polygenic theory of schizophrenia. Proc Natl Acad Sci U S A 58:199–205, 1967

Gottesman II, Shields J: Schizophrenia: The Epigenetic Puzzle. New York, Cambridge University Press, 1982

Grady RM, Grange RW, Lau KS, et al: Role for alpha-dystrobrevin in the pathogenesis of dystrophin-dependent muscular dystrophies. Nat Cell Biol 1:215–220, 1999

Grady RM, Zhou H, Cunningham JM, et al: Maturation and maintenance of the neuromuscular synapse: genetic evidence for roles of the dystrophin–glycoprotein complex. Neuron 25:279–293, 2000

Graybiel AM: Neurotransmitters and neuromodulators in the basal ganglia. Trends Neurosci 13:244–254, 1990

Green MF, Nuechterlein KH, Breitmeyer B: Backward masking performance in unaffected siblings of schizophrenic patients: evidence for a vulnerability indicator. Arch Gen Psychiatry 54:465–472, 1997

Gruzelier J, Seymour K, Wilson L: Impairments on neuropsychotic tests of temporohippocampal and frontohippocampal functions and word fluency in remitting schizophrenia and affective disorders. Arch Gen Psychiatry 45:623–629, 1988

Gur RC, Saykin AJ, Gur RE: Neuropsychological study of schizophrenia. Schizophr Res 1:153–162, 1991

Gur RE, Pearlson GD: Neuroimaging in schizophrenia research. Schizophr Bull 19:337–353, 1993

Gur RE, McGrath C, Chan RM, et al: An fMRI study of facial emotion processing in patients with schizophrenia. Am J Psychiatry 159:1992–1999, 2002

Hall W, Degenhardt L: Cannabis use and psychosis: a review of clinical and epidemiological evidence. Aust N Z J Psychiatry 34:26–34, 2000

Hanover JL, Huang ZJ, Tonegawa S, et al: Brain-derived neurotrophic factor overexpression induces precocious critical period in mouse visual cortex. J Neurosci 19:RC40, 1999

Harding CM, Brooks GW, Takamaru A, et al: The Vermont longitudinal study of persons with severe mental illness, I: methodology, study sample, and overall status 32 years later. Am J Psychiatry 144:718–726, 1987a

Harding CM, Brooks GW, Takamaru A, et al: The Vermont longitudinal study of persons with severe mental illness, II: long-term outcome of subjects who retrospectively met DSM-III criteria for schizophrenia. Am J Psychiatry 144:727–735, 1987b

Harrison PJ: Neurochemical alterations in schizophrenia affecting the putative receptor targets of atypical antipsychotics: focus on dopamine (D_1, D_3, D_4) and 5-HT$_{2a}$ receptors. Br J Psychiatry Suppl 38:12–22, 1999a

Harrison PJ: The neuropathology of schizophrenia: a critical review of the data and their interpretation. Brain 122:593–624, 1999b

Harrison PJ, Law AJ: Neuregulin 1 and schizophrenia: genetics, gene expression, and neurobiology. Biol Psychiatry 60:132–140, 2006

Harrison PJ, Weinberger DR: Schizophrenia genes, gene expression, and neuropathology: on the matter of their convergence. Mol Psychiatry 10:40–68, 2005

Hashimoto T, Bergen SE, Nguyen QL, et al: Relationship of brain-derived neurotrophic factor and its receptor TrkB to altered inhibitory prefrontal circuitry in schizophrenia. J Neurosci 25:372–383, 2005

Hazlett EA, Buchsbaum MS, Kemether E, et al: Abnormal glucose metabolism in the mediodorsal nucleus of the thalamus in schizophrenia. Am J Psychiatry 161:305–314, 2004

Heckers S, Heinsen H, Heinsen YC, et al: Cortex, white matter, and basal ganglia in schizophrenia: a volumetric postmortem study. Biol Psychiatry 29:556–566, 1991

Heckers S, Rauch SL, Goff D, et al: Impaired recruitment of the hippocampus during conscious recollection in schizophrenia. Nat Neurosci 1:318–323, 1998

Hennah W, Varilo T, Kestila M, et al: Haplotype transmission analysis provides evidence of association for DISC1 to schizophrenia and suggests sex-dependent effects. Hum Mol Genet 12:3151–3159, 2003

Heresco-Levy U, Javitt DC, Ebstein R, et al: D-Serine efficacy as add-on pharmacotherapy to risperidone and olanzapine for treatment-refractory schizophrenia. Biol Psychiatry 57:577–585, 2005

Hietala J, Syvälahti E, Vuorio K: Striatal dopamine D_2 receptor density in neuroleptic-naive schizophrenics studied with positron emission tomography, in Biological Psychiatry, Vol 2. Edited by Racagni G, Brunello N, Fukuda T. Amsterdam, The Netherlands, Excerpta Medica, 1991, pp 386–387

Hietala J, Syvälahti E, Vuorio K, et al: Striatal D_2 dopamine receptor characteristics in neuroleptic-naive schizophrenic patients studied with positron emission tomography. Arch Gen Psychiatry 51:116–123, 1994

Hill K, Mann L, Laws KR, et al: Hypofrontality in schizophrenia: a meta-analysis of functional imaging studies. Acta Psychiatr Scand 110:243–256, 2004

Hirsch S, Bowen J, Emami J, et al: A one year prospective study of the effect of life events and medication in the aetiology of schizophrenic relapse. Br J Psychiatry 168:49–56, 1996

Hodgkinson CA, Goldman D, Jaeger J, et al: Disrupted in schizophrenia 1 (DISC1): association with schizophrenia, schizoaffective disorder, and bipolar disorder. Am J Hum Genet 75:862–872, 2004

Hofer M, Pagliusi SR, Hohn A, et al: Regional distribution of brain-derived neurotrophic factor mRNA in the adult mouse brain. EMBO J 9:2459–2464, 1990

Holcomb HH, Links J, Smith C, et al: Positron emission tomography: measuring the metabolic and neurochemical characteristics of the living human nervous system, in Brain Imaging Applications in Psychiatry. Edited by Andreasen NC. Washington, DC, American Psychiatric Press, 1989, pp 235–370

Holcomb HH, Cascella NG, Thaker GK, et al: Functional sites of neuroleptic drug action in human brain: PET/FDG studies with and without haloperidol. Am J Psychiatry 153:41–49, 1996a

Holcomb HH, Gordon B, Loats HL, et al: Brain metabolism patterns are sensitive to attentional effort associated with a tone recognition task. Biol Psychiatry 39:1013–1022, 1996b

Holcomb HH, Lahti AC, Medoff DR, et al: Brain activation patterns in schizophrenic and comparison volunteers during a matched-performance auditory recognition task. Am J Psychiatry 157:1634–1645, 2000

Holzman PS, Solomon CM, Levin S, et al: Pursuit eye movement dysfunctions in schizophrenia: family evidence for specificity. Arch Gen Psychiatry 41:136–139, 1984

Huang ZJ, Kirkwood A, Pizzorusso T, et al: BDNF regulates the maturation of inhibition and the critical period of plasticity in mouse visual cortex. Cell 98:739–755, 1999

Huber G, Gross G, Schüttler R: Schizophrenie: Verlaufs und socialpsychiatrische langzeit unter suchungen an den 1945 bis 1959 in Bonn hospitalisierten schizophrenen Kranken: Monographien aus dem Gesamtgebiete der Psychiatrie, Bd 21. Berlin, Springer-Verlag, 1979

Hughes JR, Hatsukami DK, Mitchell JE, et al: Prevalence of smoking among psychiatric outpatients. Am J Psychiatry 143:993–997, 1986

Hutchinson G, Takei N, Fahy TA, et al: Morbid risk of schizophrenia in first-degree relatives of white and African-Caribbean patients with psychosis. Br J Psychiatry 169:776–780, 1996

Huttunen MO, Niskanen P: Prenatal loss of father and psychiatric disorders. Arch Gen Psychiatry 35:429–431, 1978

Hyde TM, Crook JM: Cholinergic systems and schizophrenia: primary pathology or epiphenomena? J Chem Neuroanat 22(1–2):53–63, 2001

Ibrahim HM, Hogg AJ Jr, Healy DJ, et al: Ionotropic glutamate receptor binding and subunit mRNA expression in thalamic nuclei in schizophrenia. Am J Psychiatry 157:1811–1823, 2000

Ingvar DH, Franzen G: Abnormalities of cerebral blood flow distribution in patients with chronic schizophrenia. Acta Psychiatr Scand 50:425–462, 1971

Iritani S, Niizato K, Nawa H, et al: Immunohistochemical study of brain-derived neurotrophic factor and its receptor, TrkB, in the hippocampal formation of schizophrenic brains. Prog Neuropsychopharmacol Biol Psychiatry 27:801–807, 2003

Issa F, Gerhardt GA, Bartko JJ, et al: A multidimensional approach to analysis of cerebrospinal fluid biogenic amines in schizophrenia, I: comparisons with healthy control subjects and neuroleptic-treated/unmedicated pairs analyses. Psychiatry Res 52:237–249, 1994a

Issa F, Kirch DG, Gerhardt GA, et al: A multidimensional approach to analysis of cerebrospinal fluid biogenic amines in schizophrenia, II: correlations with psychopathology. Psychiatry Res 52:251–258, 1994b

Iwata N, Suzuki T, Ikeda M, et al: No association with the neuregulin 1 haplotype to Japanese schizophrenia. Mol Psychiatry 9:126–127, 2004

Jakob H, Beckmann H: Prenatal development disturbances in the limbic allocortex in schizophrenics. J Neural Transm 65:303–326, 1986

Javitt DC, Doneshka P, Grochowski S, et al: Impaired mismatch negativity generation reflects widespread dysfunction of working memory in schizophrenia. Arch Gen Psychiatry 52:550–558, 1995

Jennings JM, McIntosh AR, Kapur S, et al: Functional network differences in schizophrenia: a rCBF study of semantic processing. Neuroreport 9:1697–1700, 1998

Jeste DV, Lohr JB: Hippocampal pathologic findings in schizophrenia. Arch Gen Psychiatry 46:1019–1026, 1989

Johnstone EC, Crow TJ, Frith CD, et al: Cerebral ventricular size and cognitive impairment in schizophrenia. Lancet 2:924–926, 1976

Joober R, Gauthier J, Lal S, et al: Catechol-O-methyltransferase Val-108/158-Met gene variants associated with performance on the Wisconsin Card Sorting Test. Arch Gen Psychiatry 59:662–663, 2002

Kamiya A, Kubo K, Tomoda T, et al: A schizophrenia-associated mutation of DISC1 perturbs cerebral cortex development. Nat Cell Biol 7:1067–1078, 2005

Karlsson P, Farde L, Halldin C, et al: PET study of D(1) dopamine receptor binding in neuroleptic-naive patients with schizophrenia. Am J Psychiatry 159:761–767, 2002

Kay SR, Sevy S: Pyramidical model of schizophrenia. Schizophr Bull 16:537–545, 1990

Keefe RS, Silverman JM, Mohs RC, et al: Eye tracking, attention, and schizotypal symptoms in nonpsychotic relatives of patients with schizophrenia. Arch Gen Psychiatry 54:169–176, 1997

Kegeles LS, Abi-Dargham A, Zea-Ponce Y, et al: Modulation of amphetamine-induced striatal dopamine release by ketamine in humans: implications for schizophrenia. Biol Psychiatry 48:627–640, 2000

Kendell RE, Kemp IW: Maternal influenza in the etiology of schizophrenia. Arch Gen Psychiatry 46:878–882, 1989

Kety SS: The significance of genetic factors in the etiology of schizophrenia: results from the national study of adoptees in Denmark. J Psychiatr Res 21:423–429, 1987

Kirov G, Ivanov D, Williams NM, et al: Strong evidence for association between the dystrobrevin binding protein 1 gene (DTNBP1) and schizophrenia in 488 parent-offspring trios from Bulgaria. Biol Psychiatry 55:971–975, 2004

Kitano H: Computational systems biology. Nature 420:206–210, 2002

Krystal JH, Abi-Saab W, Perry E, et al: Preliminary evidence of attenuation of the disruptive effects of the NMDA glutamate receptor antagonist, ketamine, on working memory by pretreatment with the group II metabotropic glutamate receptor agonist, LY354740, in healthy human subjects. Psychopharmacology (Berl) 179:303–309, 2005

Kuperberg GR, Broome MR, McGuire PK, et al: Regionally localized thinning of the cerebral cortex in schizophrenia. Arch Gen Psychiatry 60:878–888, 2003

Kuroki T, Meltzer HY, Ichikawa J: 5-HT 2A receptor stimulation by DOI, a 5-HT 2A/2C receptor agonist, potentiates amphetamine-induced dopamine release in rat medial prefrontal cortex and nucleus accumbens. Brain Res 972:216–221, 2003

Lahti AC, Holcomb HH, Medoff DR, et al: Ketamine activates psychosis and alters limbic blood flow in schizophrenia. Neuroreport 6:869–872, 1995a

Lahti AC, Koffel B, LaPorte D, et al: Subanesthetic doses of ketamine stimulate psychosis in schizophrenia. Neuropsychopharmacology 13:9–19, 1995b

Laruelle M, Abi-Dargham A, van Dyck CH, et al: Single photon emission computerized tomography imaging of amphetamine-induced dopamine release in drug-free schizophrenic subjects. Proc Natl Acad Sci U S A 93:9235–9240, 1996

Laruelle M, Abi-Dargham A, Gil R, et al: Increased dopamine transmission in schizophrenia: relationship to illness phases. Biol Psychiatry 46:56–72, 1999

Lawrie SM, Whalley HC, Abukmeil SS, et al: Temporal lobe volume changes in people at high risk of schizophrenia with psychotic symptoms. Br J Psychiatry 181:138–143, 2002

Lenzenweger MF, Dworkin RH, Wethington E: Examining the underlying structure of schizophrenic phenomenology: evidence for a three-process model. Schizophr Bull 17:515–524, 1991

Lesch A, Bogerts B: The diencephalon in schizophrenia: evidence for reduced thickness of the periventricular grey matter. Eur Arch Psychiatry Neurol Sci 234:212–219, 1984

Lewis CM, Levinson DF, Wise LH, et al: Genome scan meta-analysis of schizophrenia and bipolar disorder, part II: schizophrenia. Am J Hum Genet 73:34–48, 2003

Lewis DA: GABAergic local circuit neurons and prefrontal cortical dysfunction in schizophrenia. Brain Res 31:270–276, 2000

Lewis DA, Lund JS: Heterogeneity of chandelier neurons in monkey neocortex: corticotropin-releasing factor- and parvalbumin-immunoreactive populations. J Comp Neurol 293:599–615, 1990

Lewis DA, Volk DW, Hashimoto T: Selective alterations in prefrontal cortical GABA neurotransmission in schizophrenia: a novel target for the treatment of working memory dysfunction. Psychopharmacology (Berl) 174:143–150, 2004

Lewis DA, Hashimoto T, Volk DW: Cortical inhibitory neurons and schizophrenia. Nat Rev Neurosci 6:312–324, 2005

Liddle PF: The symptoms of chronic schizophrenia: a re-examination of the positive-negative dichotomy. Br J Psychiatry 151:145–151, 1987

Liddle PF, Morris DL: Schizophrenic syndromes and frontal lobe performance. Br J Psychiatry 158:340–345, 1991

Liddle PF, Friston KJ, Frith CD, et al: Patterns of cerebral blood flow in schizophrenia. Br J Psychiatry 160:179–186, 1992

Lidow MS, Goldman-Rakic PS: A common action of clozapine, haloperidol and remoxipride on D_1- and D_2-dopaminergic receptors in the primate cerebral cortex. Proc Natl Acad Sci U S A 91:4353–4356, 1994

Lisberger SG, Morris EJ, Tychsen L: Visual motion processing and sensory-motor integration for smooth pursuit eye movements. Annu Rev Neurosci 10:97–129, 1987

Luby ED, Cohen BD, Rosenbaum G, et al: Study of a new schizophrenomimetic drug; sernyl. Arch Neurol Psychiatr 81:363–369, 1959

Ma J, Qin W, Wang XY, et al: Further evidence for the association between G72/G30 genes and schizophrenia in two ethnically distinct populations. Mol Psychiatry 11:479–487, 2006

Mackay AVP, Iversen LL, Rossor M, et al: Increased brain dopamine and dopamine receptors in schizophrenia. Arch Gen Psychiatry 39:991–997, 1982

Malhotra AK, Kestler LJ, Mazzanti C, et al: A functional polymorphism in the COMT gene and performance on a test of prefrontal cognition. Am J Psychiatry 159:652–654, 2002

Marcus MM, Nomikos GG, Svensson TH: Effects of atypical antipsychotic drugs on dopamine output in the shell and core of the nucleus accumbens: role of 5-HT (2A) and alpha(1)-adrenoceptor antagonism. Eur Neuropsychopharmacol 10:245–253, 2000

Marti SB, Cichon S, Propping P, et al: Metabotropic glutamate receptor 3 (GRM3) gene variation is not associated with schizophrenia or bipolar affective disorder in the German population. Am J Med Genet 114:46–50, 2002

Martin LF, Kem WR, Freedman R: Alpha-7 nicotinic receptor agonists: potential new candidates for the treatment of schizophrenia. Psychopharmacology (Berl) 174:55–64, 2004

Martinot JL, Peron-Magnan P, Huret JD, et al: Striatal D_2 dopaminergic receptors assessed with positron emission tomography and [^{76}Br]bromospiperone in untreated schizophrenic patients. Am J Psychiatry 147:44–50, 1990

Martinot JL, Paillère-Martinot ML, Loch C, et al: The estimated density of D_2 striatal receptors in schizophrenia: a study with positron emission tomography and 76Br-bromolisuride. Br J Psychiatry 158:346–350, 1991

Matthysse SW, Kidd KK: Estimating the genetic contribution to schizophrenia. Am J Psychiatry 133:185–191, 1976

McAllister AK, Lo DC, Katz LC: Neurotrophins regulate dendritic growth in developing visual cortex. Neuron 15:791–803, 1995

McAllister AK, Katz LC, Lo DC: Opposing roles for endogenous BDNF and NT-3 in regulating cortical dendritic growth. Neuron 18:767–778, 1997

McAllister AK, Katz LC, Lo DC: Neurotrophins and synaptic plasticity. Annu Rev Neurosci 22:295–318, 1999

McCarley RW, Shenton ME, O'Donnell BF, et al: Auditory P300 abnormalities and left posterior superior temporal gyrus volume reduction in schizophrenia. Arch Gen Psychiatry 50:190–197, 1993

McGue M, Gottesman II: A single dominant gene still cannot account for the transmission of schizophrenia. Arch Gen Psychiatry 46:478–480, 1989

Meador-Woodruff JH, Healy DJ: Glutamate receptor expression in schizophrenic brain. Brain Res Brain Res Rev 31:288–294, 2000

Mednick SA, Machon RA, Huttunen MO, et al: Adult schizophrenia following prenatal exposure to an influenza epidemic. Arch Gen Psychiatry 45:189–192, 1988

Meltzer HY, McGurk SR: The effects of clozapine, risperidone, and olanzapine on cognitive function in schizophrenia. Schizophr Bull 25:233–255, 1999

Meltzer HY, Sumiyoshi T: Atypical antipsychotic drugs improve cognition in schizophrenia. Biol Psychiatry 53:265–267, 2003

Menon RR, Barta PE, Aylward EH, et al: Posterior superior temporal gyrus in schizophrenia: grey matter changes and clinical correlates. Schizophr Res 16:127–135, 1995

Merzenich MM, Recanzone G, Jenkins WM, et al: Cortical representational plasticity, in Neurobiology of Neocortex. Edited by Rakic P, Winger W. New York, Wiley, 1988, pp 41–67

Mirnics K, Middleton FA, Stanwood GD, et al: Disease-specific changes in regulator of G-protein signaling 4 (RGS4) expression in schizophrenia. Mol Psychiatry 6:293–301, 2001

Moghhadam BT: Targeting metabotropic glutamate receptors for treatment of the cognitive symptoms of schizophrenia. Psychopharmacology (Berl) 174:39–44, 2004

Moghaddam B, Adams BW: Reversal of phencyclidine effects by a group II metabotropic glutamate receptor agonist in rats. Science 281:1349–1352, 1998

Morris DW, McGhee KA, Schwaiger S, et al: No evidence for association of the dysbindin gene [DTNBP1] with schizophrenia in an Irish population-based study. Schizophr Res 60:167–172, 2003

Morris DW, Rodgers A, McGhee KA, et al: Confirming RGS4 as a susceptibility gene for schizophrenia. Am J Med Genet B Neuropsychiatr Genet 125:50–53, 2004

Nauta WJH: Reciprocal links of the corpus striatum with the cerebral cortex and limbic system: a common substrate for movement and thought? In Neurology and Psychiatry: A Meeting of Minds. Edited by Mueller J. Basel, Switzerland, Karger, 1989, pp 43–63

Neale JH, Bzdega T, Wroblewska B: N-Acetylaspartylglutamate: the most abundant peptide neurotransmitter in the mammalian central nervous system. J Neurochem 75:443–452, 2000

Nemeroff CB, Youngblood W, Manberg PJ, et al: Regional brain concentrations of neuropeptides in Huntington's chorea and schizophrenia. Science 221:972–975, 1983

Niznikiewicz M, Donnino R, McCarley RW, et al: Abnormal angular gyrus asymmetry in schizophrenia. Am J Psychiatry 157:428–437, 2000

Nuechterlein KH, Dawson ME, Gitlin M, et al: Developmental processes in schizophrenic disorders: longitudinal studies of vulnerability and stress. Schizophr Bull 18:387–425, 1992

Numakawa T, Yagasaki Y, Ishimoto T, et al: Evidence of novel neuronal functions of dysbindin, a susceptibility gene for schizophrenia. Hum Mol Genet 13:2699–2708, 2004

O'Callaghan E, Larkin C, Kinsella A, et al: Familial, obstetric, and other clinical correlates of minor physical anomalies in schizophrenia. Am J Psychiatry 148:479–483, 1991

Owen MJ, Craddock N, O'Donovan MC: Schizophrenia: genes at last? Trends Genet 21:518–525, 2005

Pakkenberg B: Postmortem study of chronic schizophrenic brains. Br J Psychiatry 151:744–752, 1987

Pakkenberg B: Pronounced reduction of total neuron number in mediodorsal thalamic nucleus and nucleus accumbens in schizophrenics. Arch Gen Psychiatry 47:1023–1028, 1990

Park S, Holzman PS: Schizophrenics show spatial working memory deficits. Arch Gen Psychiatry 49:975–982, 1992

Park S, Holzman PS, Goldman-Rakic PS: Spatial working memory deficits in the relatives of schizophrenic patients. Arch Gen Psychiatry 52:821–828, 1995

Pearlson GD, Marsh L: Magnetic resonance imaging in psychiatry, in American Psychiatric Press Review of Psychiatry, Vol 12. Edited by Oldham JM, Riba MB, Tasman A. Washington, DC, American Psychiatric Association, 1993, pp 347–381

Pearlson GD, Wong DF, Tune LE, et al: In vivo D_2 dopamine receptor density in psychotic and nonpsychotic patients with bipolar disorder. Arch Gen Psychiatry 52:471–477, 1995

Pfefferbaum A, Wenegrat BG, Ford JM, et al: Clinical application of the P3 component of event-related potentials, II: dementia, depression and schizophrenia. Electroencephalogr Clin Neurophysiol 59:104–124, 1984

Pogue-Geile MF, Garrett AH, Brunke JJ, et al: Neuropsychological impairments are increased in siblings of schizophrenic patients. Schizophr Res 4:390–395, 1991

Potkin SG, Alva G, Fleming K, et al: A PET study of the pathophysiology of negative symptoms in schizophrenia. Am J Psychiatry 159:227–237, 2002

Read J, Van Os J, Morrison AP, et al: Childhood trauma, psychosis and schizophrenia: a literature review with theoretical and clinical implications. Acta Psychiatr Scand 112:330–350, 2005

Reynolds GP: Increased concentrations and lateral asymmetry of amygdala dopamine in schizophrenia. Nature 305:527–529, 1983

Reynolds GP, Mason SL: Absence of detectable striatal dopamine D4 receptors in drug-treated schizophrenia. Eur J Pharmacol 281:R5–R6, 1995

Rosenthal R, Bigelow LB: Quantitative brain measurements in chronic schizophrenia. Br J Psychiatry 121:259–264, 1972

Ross RG, Olincy A, Mikulich SK, et al: Admixture analysis of smooth pursuit eye movements in probands with schizophrenia and their relatives suggests gain and leading saccades are potential endophenotypes. Psychophysiology 39:809–819, 2002

Roth BL, Hanizavareh SM, Blum AE: Serotonin receptors represent highly favorable molecular targets for cognitive enhancement in schizophrenia and other disorders. Psychopharmacology (Berl) 174:17–24, 2004

Roxborough H, Muir WJ, Blackwood DH, et al: Neuropsychological and P300 abnormalities in schizophrenics and their relatives. Psychol Med 23:305–314, 1993

Sanders AR, Rusu I, Duan J, et al: Haplotypic association spanning the 22q11.21 genes COMT and ARVCF with schizophrenia. Mol Psychiatry 10:353–365, 2005

Sartorius N: The International Pilot Study of Schizophrenia. Schizophr Bull (Winter):21–34, 1974

Saykin AJ, Gur RC, Gur RE, et al: Neuropsychological function in schizophrenia: selective impairment in memory and learning. Arch Gen Psychiatry 48:618–624, 1991

Scarr E, Beneyto M, Meador-Woodruff JH, et al: Cortical glutamatergic markers in schizophrenia. Neuropsychopharmacology 30:1521–1531, 2005

Scheibel AB, Kovelman JA: Disorientation of the hippocampal pyramidal cell and its processes in schizophrenia patients. Biol Psychiatry 16:101–102, 1981

Schroeder J, Buchsbaum MS, Siegel BV, et al: Patterns of cortical activity in schizophrenia. Psychol Med 24:947–955, 1994

Schumacher J, Jamra RA, Freudenberg J, et al: Examination of G72 and D-amino-acid oxidase as genetic risk factors for schizophrenia and bipolar affective disorder. Mol Psychiatry 9:203–207, 2004

Schwab SG, Knapp M, Mondabon S, et al: Support for association of schizophrenia with genetic variation in the 6p22.3 gene, dysbindin, in sib-pair families with linkage and in an additional sample of triad families. Am J Hum Genet 72:185–190, 2003

Schwartz ML, Goldman-Rakic PS: Callosal and intrahemispheric connectivity of the prefrontal association cortex in rhesus monkey: relation between intraparietal and principal sulcal cortex. J Comp Neurol 226:403–420, 1984

Seeman P, Ulpian C, Bergeron C, et al: Bimodal distribution of dopamine receptor densities in brains of schizophrenics. Science 225:728–731, 1984

Seeman P, Guan H-C, Van Tol HHM: Dopamine D_4 receptors are elevated in schizophrenia. Nature 365:441–445, 1993

Semple DM, McIntosh AM, Lawrie SM: Cannabis as a risk factor for psychosis: systematic review. J Psychopharmacol 19:187–194, 2005

Shelton RC, Weinberger DR: Brain morphology in schizophrenia, in Psychopharmacology: The Third Generation of Progress. Edited by Meltzer HY. New York, Raven, 1987, pp 773–781

Shenton ME, Kikinis R, Jolesz FA, et al: Abnormalities of the left temporal lobe and thought disorder in schizophrenia: a quantitative magnetic resonance imaging study. N Engl J Med 327:604–612, 1992

Shifman S, Bronstein M, Sternfeld M, et al: A highly significant association between a COMT haplotype and schizophrenia. Am J Hum Genet 71:1296–1302, 2002

Shirakawa O, Tamminga CA: Basal ganglia GABA$_A$ and dopamine D$_1$ binding site correlates of haloperidol-induced oral dyskinesias in rat. Exp Neurol 127:62–69, 1994

Silbersweig DA, Stern E, Frith C, et al: A functional neuroanatomy of hallucinations in schizophrenia. Nature 378:176–179, 1995

Smith GS, Schloesser R, Brodie JD, et al: Glutamate modulation of dopamine measured in vivo with positron emission tomography (PET) and 11C-raclopride in normal human subjects. Neuropsychopharmacology 18:18–25, 1998

Sobell JL, Richard C, Wirshing DA, et al: Failure to confirm association between RGS4 haplotypes and schizophrenia in Caucasians. Am J Med Genet B Neuropsychiatr Genet 139:23–27, 2005

Sower AC, Bird ED, Perrone-Bizzozero NI: Increased levels of GAP-43 protein in schizophrenic brain tissues demonstrated by a novel immunodetection method. Mol Chem Neuropathol 24:1–11, 1995

Spence SA, Brooks DJ, Hirsch SR, et al: A PET study of voluntary movement in schizophrenic patients experiencing passivity phenomena (delusions of alien control). Brain 120:1997–2011, 1997

Spence SA, Liddle PF, Stefan MD, et al: Functional anatomy of verbal fluency in people with schizophrenia and those at genetic risk: focal dysfunction and distributed disconnectivity reappraised. Br J Psychiatry 176:52–60, 2000

St Clair D, Blackwood D, Muir W, et al: Association within a family of a balanced autosomal translocation with major mental illness. Lancet 336:13–16, 1990

Stefansson H, Sigurdsson E, Steinthorsdottir V, et al: Neuregulin 1 and susceptibility to schizophrenia. Am J Hum Genet 71:877–892, 2002

Stefansson H, Sarginson J, Kong A, et al: Association of neuregulin 1 with schizophrenia confirmed in a Scottish population. Am J Hum Genet 72:83–87, 2003

Straub RE, Jiang Y, MacLean CJ, et al: Genetic variation in the 6p22.3 gene DTNBP1, the human ortholog of the mouse dysbindin gene, is associated with schizophrenia. Am J Hum Genet 71:337–348, 2002

Suddath RL, Casanova MF, Goldberg TE: Temporal lobe pathology in schizophrenia: a quantitative magnetic resonance imaging study. Am J Psychiatry 146:464–472, 1989

Suddath RL, Christison GW, Torrey EF, et al: Anatomical abnormalities in the brains of monozygotic twins discordant for schizophrenia. N Engl J Med 322:789–794, 1990

Sugarman PA, Craufurd D: Schizophrenia in the Afro-Caribbean community. Br J Psychiatry 164:474–480, 1994

Sullivan EV, Shear PK, Zipursky RB, et al: A deficit profile of executive, memory, and motor functions in schizophrenia. Biol Psychiatry 36:641–653, 1994

Susser E, Neugebauer R, Hoek HW, et al: Schizophrenia after prenatal famine: further evidence. Arch Gen Psychiatry 53:25–31, 1996

Sweeney JA, Luna B, Srinivasagam NM, et al: Eye tracking abnormalities in schizophrenia: evidence for dysfunction in the frontal eye fields. Biol Psychiatry 44:698–708, 1998

Swerdlow NR, Geyer MA: Using an animal model of deficient sensorimotor gating to study the pathophysiology and new treatments of schizophrenia. Schizophr Bull 24:285–301, 1998

Swerdlow NR, Braff DL, Taaid N, et al: Assessing the validity of an animal model of deficient sensorimotor gating in schizophrenic patients. Arch Gen Psychiatry 51:139–154, 1994

Swerdlow NR, Braff DL, Geyer MA: Cross-species studies of sensorimotor gating of the startle reflex. Ann N Y Acad Sci 877:202–216, 1999

Takahashi M, Shirakawa O, Toyooka K, et al: Abnormal expression of brain-derived neurotrophic factor and its receptor in the corticolimbic system of schizophrenic patients. Mol Psychiatry 5:293–330, 2000

Talbot K, Eidem WL, Tinsley CL, et al: Dysbindin-1 is reduced in intrinsic, glutamatergic terminals of the hippocampal formation in schizophrenia. J Clin Invest 113:1353–1363, 2004

Tamminga CA: Schizophrenia and glutamatergic transmission. Crit Rev Neurobiol 12:21–36, 1998

Tamminga CA, Thaker GK, Buchanan R, et al: Limbic system abnormalities identified in schizophrenia using positron emission tomography with fluorodeoxyglucose and neocortical alterations with deficit syndrome. Arch Gen Psychiatry 49:522–530, 1992

Tamminga CA, Vogel M, Gao X, et al: The limbic cortex in schizophrenia: focus on the anterior cingulate. Brain Res Brain Res Rev 31:364–370, 2000

Tang JX, Chen WY, He G, et al: Polymorphisms within 5' end of the neuregulin 1 gene are genetically associated with schizophrenia in the Chinese population. Mol Psychiatry 9:11–12, 2004

Taylor SF, Tandon R, Koeppe RA: Global cerebral blood flow increase reveals focal hypoperfusion in schizophrenia. Neuropsychopharmacology 21:368–371, 1999

Thaker GK, Nguyen JA, Tamminga CA: Increased saccadic distractibility in tardive dyskinesia: functional evidence for subcortical GABA dysfunction. Biol Psychiatry 25:49–59, 1989

Thaker GK, Cassady S, Adami H, et al: Eye movements in spectrum personality disorders: comparison of community subjects and relatives of schizophrenic patients. Am J Psychiatry 153:362–368, 1996

Thaker GK, Ross DE, Cassady SL, et al: Smooth pursuit eye movements to extraretinal motion signals: deficits in relatives of patients with schizophrenia. Arch Gen Psychiatry 55:830–836, 1998

Thaker GK, Ross DE, Cassady SL, et al: Saccadic eye movement abnormalities in relatives of patients with schizophrenia. Schizophr Res 45:235–244, 2000

Thaker GK, Wonodi I, Avila MT, et al: Catechol O-methyltransferase polymorphism and eye tracking in schizophrenia: a preliminary report. Am J Psychiatry 161:2320–2322, 2004

Thiselton DL, Webb BT, Neale BM, et al: No evidence for linkage or association of neuregulin-1 (NRG1) with disease in the Irish study of high-density schizophrenia families (ISHDSF). Mol Psychiatry 9:777–783, 2004

Tienari PJ, Wynne LC: Adoption studies of schizophrenia. Ann Med 26:233–237, 1994

Treff WM, Hempel KJ: Die Zelidichte bei Schizophrenen und klinisch Gesunden. J Hirnforsch 4:314–369, 1958

Tregellas JR, Tanabe JL, Miller DE, et al: Neurobiology of smooth pursuit eye movement deficits in schizophrenia: an fMRI study. Am J Psychiatry 161:315–321, 2004

Tsai G, Passani LA, Slusher BS, et al: Abnormal excitatory neurotransmitter metabolism in schizophrenic brains.Arch Gen Psychiatry 52:829–836, 1995

Tsuang MT, Woolson RD, Fleming JA: Long-term outcome of major psychoses, I: schizophrenia and affective disorders compared with psychiatrically symptom-free surgical conditions. Arch Gen Psychiatry 36:1295–1301, 1979

Tsuang MT, Stone WS, Seidman LJ, et al: Treatment of nonpsychotic relatives of patients with schizophrenia: four case studies. Biol Psychiatry 1:1412–1418, 1999

Tsuang MT, Stone WS, Faraone SV: Toward reformulating the diagnosis of schizophrenia. Am J Psychiatry 157:1041–1050, 2000

Van Den Bogaert A, Schumacher J, Schulze TG, et al: The DTNBP1 (dysbindin) gene contributes to schizophrenia, depending on family history of the disease. Am J Hum Genet 73:1438–1443, 2003

Van Os J, Selten JP: Prenatal exposure to maternal stress and subsequent schizophrenia: the May 1940 invasion of the Netherlands. Br J Psychiatry 172:324–326, 1998

Van Os J, Bak M, Hanssen M, et al: Cannabis use and psychosis: a longitudinal population-based study. Am J Epidemiol 156:319–327, 2002

van Praag HM: CSF 5-HIAA and suicide in non-depressed schizophrenics. Lancet 2:977–978, 1983

Volk DW, Austin MC, Pierri JN, et al: Decreased glutamic acid decarboxylase67 messenger RNA expression in a subset of prefrontal cortical gamma-aminobutyric acid neurons in subjects with schizophrenia. Arch Gen Psychiatry 57:237–245, 2000

Volkow ND, Wolf AP, Van Gelder P, et al: Phenomenological correlates of metabolic activity in 18 patients with chronic schizophrenia. Am J Psychiatry 144:151–158, 1987

Wahlberg KE, Wynne LC, Oja H, et al: Gene-environment interaction in vulnerability to schizophrenia: findings from the Finnish Adoptive Family Study of Schizophrenia. Am J Psychiatry 154:355–362, 1997

Wang X, He G, Gu N, et al: Association of G72/G30 with schizophrenia in the Chinese population. Biochem Biophys Res Commun 319:1281–1286, 2004

Waterhouse RN, Slifstein M, Dumont F, et al: In vivo evaluation of [^{11}C]N-(2-chloro-5-thiomethylphenyl)-N'-(3-methoxyphenyl)-N'-methylguanidine ([^{11}C]GMOM) as a potential PET radiotracer for the PCP/NMDA receptor. Nucl Med Biol 31:939–948, 2004

Weickert CS, Hyde TM, Lipska BK, et al: Reduced brain-derived neurotrophic factor in prefrontal cortex of patients with schizophrenia. Mol Psychiatry 8:592–610, 2003

Weickert CS, Straub RE, McClintock BW, et al: Human dysbindin (DTNBP1) gene expression in normal brain and in schizophrenic prefrontal cortex and midbrain. Arch Gen Psychiatry 61:544–555, 2004

Weickert CS, Ligons DL, Romanczyk T, et al: Reductions in neurotrophin receptor mRNAs in the prefrontal cortex of patients with schizophrenia. Mol Psychiatry 10:637–650, 2005

Weickert TW, Goldberg TE, Mishara A, et al: Catechol-O-methyltransferase val108/158met genotype predicts working memory response to antipsychotic medications. Biol Psychiatry 56:677–682, 2004

Weinberger DR: Implications of normal brain development for the pathogenesis of schizophrenia. Arch Gen Psychiatry 44:660–669, 1987

Weinberger DR, Berman KF, Zee RF: Physiologic dysfunction of dorso-lateral prefrontal cortex in schizophrenia, I: regional cerebral blood flow evidence. Arch Gen Psychiatry 43:114–124, 1986

Weinberger DR, Berman KF, Suddath R, et al: Evidence of dysfunction of a prefrontal-limbic network in schizophrenia: a magnetic resonance imaging and regional cerebral blood flow study of discordant monozygotic twins. Am J Psychiatry 149:890–897, 1992

Weiser M, Knobler HY, Noy S, et al: Clinical characteristics of adolescents later hospitalized for schizophrenia. Am J Med Genet 114:949–955, 2002

Wetmore C, Ernfors P, Persson H, et al: Localization of brain-derived neurotrophic factor mRNA to neurons in the brain by in situ hybridization. Exp Neurol 109:141–152, 1990

Whitfield CL, Dube SR, Felitti VJ, et al: Adverse childhood experiences and hallucinations. Child Abuse Negl 29:797–810, 2005

Wicks S, Hjern A, Gunnell D, et al: Social adversity in childhood and the risk of developing psychosis: a national cohort study. Am J Psychiatry 162:1652–1657, 2005

Widerlöv E, Lindstrom LH, Bissette G, et al: Subnormal CSF levels of neurotensin in a subgroup of schizophrenic patients: normalization after neuroleptic treatment. Am J Psychiatry 139:1122–1126, 1982

Williams NM, Preece A, Spurlock G, et al: Support for genetic variation in neuregulin 1 and susceptibility to schizophrenia. Mol Psychiatry 8:485–487, 2003

Williams NM, Preece A, Morris DW, et al: Identification in 2 independent samples of a novel schizophrenia risk haplotype of the dystrobrevin binding protein gene (*DTNBP1*). Arch Gen Psychiatry 61:336–344, 2004a

Williams NM, Preece A, Spurlock G, et al: Support for RGS4 as a susceptibility gene for schizophrenia. Biol Psychiatry 55:192–195, 2004b

Wolkin A, Sanfilipo M, Wolf AP, et al: Negative symptoms and hypofrontality in chronic schizophrenia. Arch Gen Psychiatry 49:959–965, 1992

Wong DF, Wagner HN Jr, Tune LE, et al: Positron emission tomography reveals elevated D_2 dopamine receptors in drug-naïve schizophrenics [published erratum appears in Science 235:623, 1987]. Science 234:1558–1563, 1986

Wonnacott S: The paradox of nicotinic acetylcholine receptor up-regulation by nicotine. Trends Pharmacol Sci 11:216–219, 1990

World Health Organization: International Statistical Classification of Diseases and Related Health Problems, 10th Revision. Geneva, Switzerland, World Health Organization, 1992

Yang JZ, Si TM, Ruan Y, et al: Association study of neuregulin 1 gene with schizophrenia. Mol Psychiatry 8:706–709, 2003

Zammit S, Allebeck P, Andreasson S, et al: Self reported cannabis use as a risk factor for schizophrenia in Swedish conscripts of 1969: historical cohort study. BMJ 325:1199, 2002

Zhang F, St Clair D, Liu X, et al: Association analysis of the RGS4 gene in Han Chinese and Scottish populations with schizophrenia. Genes Brain Behav 4:444–448, 2005

Zhang F, Sarginson J, Crombie C, et al: Genetic association between schizophrenia and the *DISC1* gene in the Scottish population. Am J Med Genet B Neuropsychiatr Genet 141:155–159, 2006

Zhao X, Shi Y, Tang J, et al: A case control and family based association study of the neuregulin1 gene and schizophrenia. J Med Genet 41:31–34, 2004

Zou F, Li C, Duan S, et al: A family-based study of the association between the *G72/G30* genes and schizophrenia in the Chinese population. Schizophr Res 73:257–261, 2005

27

NEUROPSYCHIATRIC ASPECTS OF MOOD DISORDERS

Paul E. Holtzheimer III, M.D.

Helen S. Mayberg, M.D.

Mood disorders are characterized by abnormalities of mood and affect regulation, cognitive changes, motor activity alterations, sleep abnormalities, appetite changes, and other disturbances of homeostatic and drive states (e.g., libido, motivation). Although the etiology of mood disorders in most patients is "idiopathic," neuropsychiatric disorders are commonly associated with disturbances of mood and affect, especially depressive syndromes. A growing database supports a similar neurobiological basis for mood disorders, regardless of etiology. However, rather than defining a single causative "lesion" or neurochemical abnormality, current models propose an integrated set of distinct, but interconnected, neural systems underlying the phenomenological features of mood disorders. Each of these systems may be more or less disturbed, resulting in variable symptomatic presentation and treatment response.

In this chapter, we review the neuropsychiatric aspects of mood disorders within this neural systems framework. We begin with a description of the clinical features of mood disorders that highlights the syndromal and multidimensional nature of these illnesses. We then discuss mood disorders commonly associated with neuropsychiatric conditions. The neurobiological bases for the various symptom clusters of mood disorders are then reviewed in detail, with an emphasis on specific domains associated with distinct neural systems. Finally, we present an integrated neural systems model for mood disorders.

CLINICAL FEATURES

TYPES OF MOOD DISORDERS

According to DSM-IV-TR (American Psychiatric Association 2000), mood disorders are typically characterized by the types of mood episodes that can occur over the course of the illness (Table 27–1). Thus, major depressive disorder (MDD) consists of one or more major depressive episodes (MDEs), whereas bipolar I disorder is defined by at least one manic episode and the possible occurrence of depressive, hypomanic, or mixed episodes over time; mixed episodes are mood episodes that include significant depressive and manic symptoms occurring simultaneously. Dysthymic disorder is not specifically characterized by distinct mood episodes but rather is defined as a chronic depressive syndrome consisting of symptoms that do not meet criteria for an MDE. Although distinct mood episodes are not used to characterize dysthymic disorder, other mood disorders (e.g., MDD) can be present as comorbid conditions. Each mood disorder and episode can be associated with several qualifiers (see Table 27–1).

This classification of mood disorders is useful for both clinical and research purposes. However, the simplicity of this schema belies the phenomenological complexity of mood disorders. Two patients with MDD, for example, may present with very different symptoms of an MDE.

TABLE 27–1. Current DSM-IV-TR nosology of mood disorders

Mood disorder	Mood episode required for diagnosis	Mood episodes that can occur	Other qualifiers
MDD	MDE	MDE only	Single versus recurrent Chronic With psychotic features With atypical features With melancholic features Severity of episode With postpartum onset With seasonal pattern
Bipolar I disorder	Manic episode	Manic episode, MDE, hypomanic episode, mixed	With psychotic features With rapid cycling With seasonal pattern Severity of episode
Bipolar II disorder	MDE and at least one hypomanic episode	MDE, hypomanic episode, ?mixed[a]	With rapid cycling With seasonal pattern Severity of episode
Dysthymia	None (see text)	None (see text)	None
Cyclothymia	Minor depressive episode and hypomanic episode	Hypomanic episode and minor depressive episodes only	None

Note.   MDD = major depressive disorder; MDE = major depressive episode.

[a]According to DSM-IV-TR, a mixed episode requires a patient to meet criteria for an MDE and a manic episode for at least 1 week; therefore, such a patient would be given an "official" diagnosis of bipolar I disorder. However, many investigators and clinicians support the concept of mixed episodes in bipolar II disorder as well; in other words, subjects can have mixed episodes but never have manic episodes.

One may have decreased sleep with early-morning awakening, severe psychomotor retardation, profound anhedonia, absence of mood reactivity, and a distinct quality of "depressed" mood that actually "feels" different from normal sadness (e.g., *melancholic* features). The other may present with sad mood and *atypical* features consisting of increased sleep, appetite, and mood reactivity. Both groups of symptoms meet the criteria for an MDD diagnosis, but the two illness presentations appear quite distinct. When mood disorders present in the context of neuropsychiatric conditions (such as Parkinson's disease), they can have even greater variability in presentation given the overlap between psychiatric and neurological symptoms. Because of this symptomatic variability, this section is organized by specific symptom clusters rather than specific mood disorder diagnoses. Within each symptom cluster, we describe the types of alterations seen with specific mood disorder diagnoses.

MOOD AND AFFECT

Disturbances of mood and affect are fundamental to a mood disorder diagnosis. Essentially every mood disorder requires a specific alteration of mood to justify the diagnosis (with the notable exception of MDD, which allows for no alteration of mood as long as anhedonia is present). Although the terms *mood* and *affect* are often used interchangeably, it is useful to make a semantic distinction between the two. Mood is used to refer to the subjective emotional state experienced by an individual (e.g., the subject *feels* happy, sad, anxious, numb). Affect is more objective and refers to the individual's emotional state as it appears to an outside observer (e.g., the subject *looks* happy, sad, anxious, numb). Importantly, affect also can be defined by the range of emotional states shown by a subject (e.g., during an interview), its stability and consistency over time, and how appropriate affect is, given the conversation, stated mood, and so forth.

Mood and affective states associated with specific mood episodes are often straightforward, and typically, mood and affect will correspond. Thus, the mood associated with depression is typically described as "sad," "blue," or simply "depressed," the associated affect is restricted in emotional range, and the patient looks sad. Conversely, patients with mania or hypomania usually describe an elevated mood and often appear excited and euphoric. Patients with a mixed episode often describe their mood as depressed or irritable but rarely elevated. However, affect in a mixed episode is often more labile than in depressed patients and may be inappropriate for the situation or stated mood.

Patients with neuropsychiatric disease often present with mood dissociated from affect. For example, a patient with Parkinson's disease may deny depressed mood or other symptoms of depression but present with severely restricted affect that looks depressed. Other neurological patients may deny feelings of depression or euphoria but present with prominent affective instability (e.g., inappropriate crying spells, laughing) called *pseudobulbar affect* (Husain 2005). These observed dissociations between mood and affect suggest that mood and affect are controlled by related but distinct neural systems.

INTEREST AND MOTIVATION

Mood episodes are commonly associated with disturbances of interest and motivation (i.e., perceived importance of and internal drive to engage with the external world). In fact, an MDE may be diagnosed in the absence of expressed depressed mood if significant anhedonia is present. In depressive states, interest and motivation are usually decreased—often dramatically so. Individuals with melancholic depression, for example, present with severe anhedonia such that they report no pleasure from even the most positive of stimuli. Conversely, patients with mania and hypomania typically have an exaggerated level of interest and increased responsiveness to positive stimuli; clinically, this may present as increased goal-directed activity (e.g., vigorous writing or cleaning) or engagement in pleasurable activity regardless of risks (e.g., promiscuity or substance abuse).

In the absence of a mood disorder, however, interest and motivation also may be disturbed. For example, apathy without associated depression is a common symptom associated with Parkinson's disease (Pluck and Brown 2002), Alzheimer's dementia (Landes et al. 2005; Starkstein et al. 2006), and some cases of traumatic brain injury (Kant et al. 1998). Furthermore, some neurological patients (often patients with traumatic brain injury, including stroke) show increased pleasure-seeking or disinhibition without having other symptoms associated with mania or hypomania (Dodd et al. 2005; Gorman and Cummings 1992; Starkstein et al. 2004).

It is important to recognize a distinction between anhedonia and apathy. *Anhedonia* is defined as a decreased ability to experience pleasure, whereas *apathy* is defined as primarily a decreased drive to engage in self-directed activity (Marin 1996; Snaith 1993).

SLEEP

Sleep is frequently abnormal in patients with mood disorders. Depressed patients often complain of decreased sleep characterized by difficulty falling asleep (early insomnia), frequent awakenings during the sleep cycle (middle insomnia), or early-morning awakening (late insomnia). Other patients describe hypersomnia (common in atypical depression). Manic and hypomanic patients typically report decreased *need* for sleep—that is, they feel capable of functioning "normally" on little or no sleep at all—in addition to an overall decreased amount of sleep. As with disturbances of affect, interest, and motivation, sleep abnormalities in the absence of a mood disorder are commonly found in neuropsychiatric patients, such as those with Parkinson's disease (Aarsland et al. 2005), Huntington's disease (Morton et al. 2005; Silvestri et al. 1995), and dementia (Grigg-Damberger 2004; Petit et al. 2004).

APPETITE

In patients with depression, appetite may be decreased, increased, or unchanged. The most common abnormality is a decrease in appetite with corresponding weight loss. However, some patients report increased appetite and weight gain during depressive episodes. In mania, appetite change is not a specific criterion for the disorder, although a decreased appetite (or decreased intake) is commonly observed. As with sleep abnormalities, appetite abnormalities are common in neuropsychiatric disease (Gillette-Guyonnet et al. 2000; Rosenberg et al. 1977; Trejo et al. 2005; Waxman et al. 1990).

PSYCHOMOTOR ACTIVITY

Motor and psychomotor deficits in depression involve a range of behaviors including changes in motility, mental activity, and speech (Sobin and Sackeim 1997). Depressed patients typically report a subjective sense of fatigue and a perceived and observed slowing of thought processes and physical activity. At the extreme, a depressed patient may present with catatonia. Conversely, mania is almost always associated with a dramatic increase in psychomotor speed (often reported as "racing" thoughts and associated with a corresponding increase in activity level [e.g., pressured speech and agitation]). These changes in psychomotor activity (including speech) tend to be state-related. Spontaneous motor activity is significantly lower when patients are depressed compared with the euthymic state (Dantchev and Widlocher 1998; Royant-Parola et al. 1986; Szabadi et al. 1976).

As with emotional state, psychomotor activity has a subjective and an objective component. Thus, a depressed patient may "feel" as if he or she has no energy but appear agitated and engage in increased physical activity; such a disconnect may be indicative of a mixed mood episode. Many neuropsychiatric illnesses are associated with a slowing of thought and motor activity without other symptoms of depression (e.g., Parkinson's disease). Agitation is also a common but nonspecific symptom in neuropsychiatric patients. Although agitation may be indicative of a manic episode, it also may arise as a response to pain or as a medication side effect (e.g., akathisia from antipsychotic medications).

EMOTIONAL BIAS

Patients with mood disorders commonly show mood-congruent emotional bias in cognitive processing (Murphy et al. 1999). For example, depressed subjects show better recall for negative words when presented with a word list varying in emotional tone (Bradley et al. 1997; Stip et al. 1994; Teasdale and Russell 1983) and are faster than nondepressed individuals at identifying negative adjectives as self-descriptive (Alloy et al. 1999). Depressed patients show worsening of performance in the context of negative feedback (Elliott et al. 1997b), and negative bias in emotional processing may predict treatment resistance (Levitan et al. 1998). In mania, subjects may have a strong positive emotional bias that presents as grandiosity and overfriendliness.

Neuroticism (as defined in the five-factor model of personality [McCrae and Costa 1987]) involves temperamental hypersensitivity to negative stimuli and the tendency to experience exaggerated negative mood states in situations of emotional instability or dissonance (Santor et al. 1997). High levels of neuroticism (especially when combined with low levels of extraversion) may indicate a predisposition to developing depression (Clark and Watson 1991; Fanous et al. 2002). Cloninger et al. (2006) used a different model of personality and suggested that personality traits involving negative bias (such as high "harm avoidance" and low "self-directedness") predict development of depression (Cloninger 1986; Cloninger et al. 2006). In the extreme, negative emotional bias in depression may present as excessive guilt and suicidal ideation.

COGNITION

The cognitive abnormalities typically seen in depressed patients include slowed thought processes and impaired attention and concentration. Depressed patients also have impaired executive functioning (planning, organization, short-term memory) (Austin et al. 2001). Manic patients also show impaired executive functioning (including disinhibition and impulsivity) and poor concentration and attention (Murphy and Sahakian 2001). Even in the absence of mood disorders, neurological patients commonly show cognitive impairment such that these symptoms may be nonspecific in neuropsychiatric conditions. However, in contrast to deficits associated with many structural neurological disorders, specific impairments in language, perception, and spatial abilities are not usually seen in patients with idiopathic mood disorders (except as a secondary consequence of poor attention, motivation, or organizational abilities). Cognitive deficits in mood disorders are typically of mild to moderate severity but can become quite severe in prolonged or intractable depression. Some patients, especially patients with late-life depression, may develop "pseudodementia" (Raskind 1998). Finally, cognitive disturbances may be exacerbated in neurological patients with a co-occurring mood disorder.

MOOD DISORDERS ASSOCIATED WITH NEUROPSYCHIATRIC CONDITIONS

DIFFICULTIES IN DIAGNOSIS

Correctly diagnosing a mood disorder in the neuropsychiatric patient can be difficult because symptoms of the neurological illness may mimic or mask the symptoms of mood disturbance. As discussed earlier, patients with neuropsychiatric disease may present with one or more symptoms without meeting other criteria for a mood disorder. For example, a patient with Parkinson's disease may present with flattened affect, apathy, and sleep disturbance, leading to a spurious diagnosis of MDD, even though other symptoms may not be present. On the other hand, the eventual development of a mood disorder in such a patient may be missed because the observable changes may be much more subtle (e.g., slight increase in apathy and withdrawal from others). Thus, when evaluating patients with neuropsychiatric disease, it is important to be vigilant for any and all symptoms of depression and to pay particular attention to symptoms less likely to be independently associated with the underlying neurological illness.

DEPRESSION

Depression is the most common mood disorder associated with neuropsychiatric illness. In patients with neurological illness, depression may result from the pathophysiology or treatment of the underlying neurological

TABLE 27–2. Common associations with depression in neuropsychiatric patients

Psychiatric (idiopathic)

Major depressive disorder

Bipolar disorder

Dysthymia

Cyclothymia

Neurological

Basal ganglia disease, especially:

Parkinson's disease

Huntington's disease

Wilson's disease

Cerebrovascular disease, especially:

Frontal cortical/subcortical stroke

Basal ganglia stroke

Multiple sclerosis

Infectious encephalitis

Neoplasm

Paraneoplastic syndrome

Traumatic brain injury

Dementia

Epilepsy

Pharmacological/iatrogenic

Corticosteroids

Thyroid ablation

α-Interferon

Deep brain stimulation (especially of subthalamic nucleus)

Substance intoxication or withdrawal

Other

Hypothyroidism

Cushing's syndrome

Vitamin deficiency (e.g., B_{12})

Autoimmune disease

disease, reaction to the psychosocial stress of having the underlying illness, recurrence of a premorbid depressive disorder, or a combination of all of these. Table 27–2 lists common associations of depression with various neuropsychiatric illnesses and treatments. In many patients, the etiology of depression may be multifactorial.

MANIA

Mania is seen less commonly than depression in neuropsychiatric patients. As with depression, mania may result from neuropathological changes associated with the underlying illness, medications used to treat the disorder, or progression or development of an underlying bipolar disorder. Table 27–3 lists known associations.

NEUROBIOLOGY OF MOOD DISORDERS

The neurobiology of mood disorders can be approached in two general ways: 1) defining the neurobiology of a mood disorder (or mood episode) as a distinct entity—a syndrome-specific approach, or 2) defining the neurobiology of specific phenomenological aspects of mood disorders (e.g., assessment of neuroanatomical correlates of sad mood)—a symptom-specific approach.

SYNDROME-SPECIFIC FINDINGS

Several studies have investigated the various neurophysiological and neuroanatomical correlates of specific mood disorders and mood episodes. Typically, these studies focused on patients with idiopathic mood disorders, although several included neurological patients with mood disorder syndromes. Broadly speaking, these studies suggested that mood disorders, regardless of etiology, share a similar neurobiology. However, these findings also showed that no single neurochemical or neuroanatomical abnormality fully explains the pathophysiology of mood disorders.

Neurochemical Findings

In depression, the main focus of neurochemical research has been driven by the "monoamine hypothesis" of depression (Schildkraut 1965). Of the monoamine neurotransmitter systems (serotonin, norepinephrine, and dopamine), serotonin has received the most attention, and strong evidence indicates that serotonergic dysfunction plays a major role in the pathophysiology of depression. Although the data are not unequivocal, patients with depression (compared with nondepressed subjects) show lower cerebrospinal fluid (CSF) levels of serotonin metabolites (Asberg et al. 1976; Mann et al. 1996), decreased serotonin transporter binding (Malison et al. 1998; Owens and Nemeroff 1994), and serotonin receptor abnormalities (D'Haenen et al. 1992; Drevets et al. 1999; Sargent et al. 2000). Medications (selective serotonin reuptake inhibitors [SSRIs]) that specifically target serotonin-mediated neurotransmission are effective in treating depression in up to 60% of patients

TABLE 27–3.   Common associations with mania in neuropsychiatric patients

Psychiatric (idiopathic)

Bipolar disorder

Cyclothymia

Neurological

Basal ganglia disease

Huntington's disease

Wilson's disease

Cerebrovascular disease

Frontal cortical/subcortical stroke

Basal ganglia stroke

Multiple sclerosis

Infectious encephalitis

Neoplasm

Paraneoplastic syndrome

HIV encephalopathy

Epilepsy

Pharmacological/iatrogenic

Dopaminergic agents

Corticosteroids

Substance intoxication or withdrawal

Surgical treatments, especially:

Pallidotomy

Deep brain stimulation

Antidepressant medications

Other

Cushing's syndrome

Vitamin deficiencies (e.g., B_{12} or niacin)

Hyperthyroidism

Systemic infections

Uremia

Electrolyte abnormality (e.g., hypocalcemia)

(Nelson 1999). Tryptophan depletion (Young et al. 1985), which results in an acute but transient decrease in available serotonin, can result in depressive relapse in patients previously responsive to SSRIs (Delgado et al. 1990; Neumeister et al. 2004). Gene–environment interaction studies suggest that subjects exposed to environmental stress are more likely to develop depression if they have at least one allele for a "low-efficiency" version of the serotonin transporter (Caspi et al. 2003; Kendler et al. 2005; Lenze et al. 2005).

Data supporting norepinephrine and dopamine dysfunction in the pathophysiology of depression are more limited but suggest a significant role for these neurotransmitters. Medications that increase noradrenergic neurotransmission are effective in treating depression (Arroll et al. 2005). In depressed patients taking noradrenergic antidepressants and euthymic patients with a history of depression, catecholamine depletion can result in depressive relapse (Berman et al. 1999; Charney 1998). CSF concentrations of homovanillic acid (the primary metabolite of dopamine) and urine levels of 3,4-dihydroxyphenylacetic acid (DOPAC; another dopamine metabolite) are decreased in depressed patients (Reddy et al. 1992; Roy et al. 1986, 1992). Various studies suggest that dopamine transporter activity may be reduced in patients with depression (Klimek et al. 2002; Meyer et al. 2001). Medications targeting the dopamine system, such as psychostimulants and pramipexole (and possibly bupropion), have shown antidepressant efficacy (Ferris and Beaman 1983; Goldberg et al. 2004; Meyer et al. 2002; Nierenberg et al. 1998; Zarate et al. 2004), particularly for depressive episodes in patients with bipolar disorder.

Neuroendocrine systems have been implicated in the pathophysiology of mood disorders. The hypothalamic-pituitary-adrenal (HPA) axis is clearly dysfunctional in at least some patients with depression (Arborelius et al. 1999; Nemeroff et al. 1991; Veith et al. 1993). The dexamethasone suppression test, previously tested as a specific marker of depressive illness, has abnormal results in subsets of depressed patients (Posener et al. 2000). Some reports of alterations in cortisol regulation associated with transient stress in patients with a history of early life trauma or abuse further suggest that HPA axis dysregulation may be an important marker of vulnerability to various types of mood disorders in later life (Heim et al. 2000); these data also suggest that HPA axis abnormalities may be causal for certain types of depression rather than the reverse. Corticotropin-releasing factor (CRF)—the hormone responsible for corticotropin release—has been shown to be an important modulator of monoaminergic activity and vice versa (Ruggiero et al. 1999; Zhang et al. 2004). More complex interactions of the HPA axis with other neuromodulatory systems are likely involved in the pathophysiology of mood disorders (e.g., interaction of gender, HPA axis function, and serotonin function [Barr et al. 2004] and interaction of HPA axis, serotonin, and γ-aminobutyric acid function [Tan et al. 2004]).

The hypothalamic-pituitary-thyroid axis has been linked with depression (Banki et al. 1988; Esposito et al. 1997; Kirkegaard et al. 1979; Musselman and Nemeroff

1996). Although clinical hypothyroidism is clearly associated with depressive symptoms, elevated levels of thyroid antibodies have been reported in patients with depression but without overt thyroid dysfunction (Nemeroff et al. 1985). A blunted response of thyrotropin to exogenous thyrotropin-releasing hormone (i.e., the thyroid stimulation test) has been described in depressed patients (Loosen 1985). Finally, thyroid hormone augmentation may be effective in treating antidepressant-resistant depression (Joffe and Sokolov 2000).

A role for other neuromodulatory systems in the pathophysiology of depression is likely. Glutamate and γ-aminobutyric acid dysfunction has been found in depressed patients and animal models of depression (Choudary et al. 2005; Kendell et al. 2005; Paul and Skolnick 2003; Zarate et al. 2003). The neurokinin system (known to be involved in nociception) also may play a role in the neurobiology of depression (Berrettini et al. 1985; Bondy et al. 2003; Rimon et al. 1984).

A growing database supports a role for inflammatory processes in mood disorders, especially depression (Raison et al. 2006). Certain immune mediators (such as corticosteroids and interferon-α) have been clearly associated with depressive and other mood disorder symptoms (Brown and Suppes 1998; Loftis and Hauser 2004). Also, depressed patients have higher levels of circulating inflammatory markers compared with nondepressed subjects (O'Brien et al. 2004). Inflammatory pathways may interact with stress-response systems (i.e., HPA axis) to mediate effects on mood and behavior (Raison et al. 2006).

An increasing number of studies have focused on dysregulation of second-messenger systems, gene transcription, various neurotrophic factors, and cell turnover in mood disorders (Manji et al. 2001; Taylor et al. 2005). Such pathways have been more extensively studied in bipolar disorder, for which medications (such as lithium) are known to have effects on these cell signaling systems (Einat and Manji 2006).

Genetics

The heritability of depression is 33%–50% (Fava and Kendler 2000; Kendler et al. 2006; Levinson 2006), and the heritability of bipolar disorder may be as high as 80%–90% (Kieseppa et al. 2004; McGuffin et al. 2003). Given the variability of mood disorders and the complex patterns of inheritance seen, these illnesses likely involve multiple genes and important genetic-environmental interactions.

As discussed earlier, monoaminergic neurotransmission has been strongly implicated in the pathophysiology of mood disorders. Consistent with this theory, several genes involved in monoamine function have been implicated in the vulnerability to depression and bipolar disorders

(Levinson 2006). One of the most consistent findings in genetic studies of mood disorders has been increased rates of depression in subjects with an "inefficient" form of the serotonin transporter (resulting from a functional single nucleotide polymorphism in the promoter region for the transporter gene) who are also exposed to stressful life events (Caspi et al. 2003; Kendler et al. 2005; Wilhelm et al. 2006). Serotonin transporter gene polymorphisms also have been implicated in bipolar disorder, although the data are contradictory (Levinson 2005; Mansour et al. 2005). Some data suggest that such polymorphisms may be associated with specific personality traits and symptoms of mood disorders, including neuroticism (Schinka et al. 2004) and suicidality (Levinson 2005).

Because monoamine dysfunction cannot fully explain the neurobiology of mood disorders, genes for other neuromodulators are another focus of investigation (Levinson 2006). For example, a functional polymorphism of the promoter region for the brain-derived neurotrophic factor gene may cause susceptibility to mood disorders, especially bipolar disorder (Green and Craddock 2003; Strauss et al. 2004).

Neuroanatomical Findings

The neuroanatomy of mood disorders has been of interest for decades. Early studies were limited to postmortem examinations given the absence or poor resolution of imaging techniques. Advances in structural and functional neuroimaging have allowed increasingly detailed investigation of brain anatomy and have greatly advanced our understanding of how parts of the brain are involved in the pathophysiology of depression.

The most common structural abnormalities associated with depression include decreased volumes of the prefrontal cortex, hippocampus, amygdala, and various basal ganglia structures, although data are inconsistent (Sheline 2003). Some, but not all, studies have also shown decreased volume of the subgenual medial frontal cortex in patients with depression when both magnetic resonance imaging (MRI) and postmortem anatomical measurements were used (Ballmaier et al. 2004; Botteron et al. 2002; Brambilla et al. 2002; Bremner et al. 2002; Drevets et al. 1997; Hastings et al. 2004; Hirayasu et al. 1999; Pizzagalli et al. 2004; Rajkowska 2000). Data suggest that structural differences in depressed patients may be at least partially determined by family history (Drevets et al. 1997; Hirayasu et al. 1999), gender (Botteron et al. 2002; Hastings et al. 2004), and age (Ballmaier et al. 2004). Also, variability in the structure of brain regions involved in mood regulation may be related to genetic factors, with polymorphisms of the promoter region for the serotonin transporter gene associated with

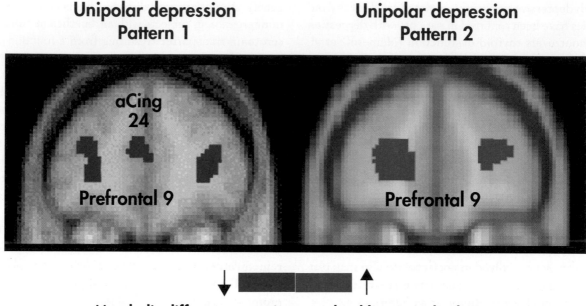

FIGURE 27–1.   Glucose metabolic positron emission tomography (PET) scan patterns in major depression. The most common pattern of resting brain activity measured with functional neuroimaging in depressed patients (vs. healthy control subjects) is prefrontal hypometabolism (*Pattern 1*). However, this is not universal; some studies identify increased prefrontal brain activity in comparably depressed patients (*Pattern 2*).

volume differences of the subgenual cingulate cortex and amygdala in healthy subjects (Pezawas et al. 2005).

The most common functional neuroanatomical abnormality associated with depression is resting state hypometabolism or decreased blood flow in the prefrontal cortex, including dorsolateral, ventrolateral, and orbitofrontal regions (Figure 27–1) (Baxter et al. 1989; Bench et al. 1992; Buchsbaum et al. 1986; Galynker et al. 1998; George et al. 1993; Goldapple et al. 2004; Gonul et al. 2004; Post et al. 1987; Videbech 2000), and activity of the prefrontal cortex has been inversely correlated with overall depression severity (Baxter et al. 1989; Drevets et al. 1992). However, hyperactivity of the prefrontal cortex also has been reported (Brody et al. 2001b; Drevets et al. 1992; Goldapple et al. 2004). Increased activity has been frequently described in various limbic-paralimbic subcortical regions (amygdala, anterior temporal, insula, basal ganglia, thalamus), but the data are less consistent than with the prefrontal findings (Buchsbaum et al. 1986; Drevets et al. 1992; Mayberg et al. 1994, 1997; Post et al. 1987). Hypoactivity in dorsal portions of the anterior cingulate cortex and hyperactivity in ventral regions have been frequently identified (Bauer et al. 2005; Bench et al. 1992; Ebert and Ebmeier 1996; Galynker et al. 1998; Gonul et al. 2004; Kennedy et al. 2001; Mayberg et al. 1994, 1997; Oda et al. 2003; Videbech et al.

2002), although not all studies have agreed (Drevets et al. 2002; Pizzagalli et al. 2004).

Taken together, these data suggest that depression (as a syndrome) is best characterized not by any single functional neuroanatomical abnormality but rather by a pattern of brain activity changes that includes decreased activity in dorsal regions and increased activity in ventral and limbic-paralimbic regions of a mood regulation network. Even in subjects who do not show this typical pattern, abnormal activity is seen in similar frontal cortical-subcortical brain regions.

Observations of patients undergoing surgery to alleviate treatment-refractory depression provide complementary evidence for such a neural systems conceptualization of the depression syndrome (Cosgrove and Rauch 2003; Malizia 1997; Mayberg et al. 2005). These studies suggest that surgical modulation of a putative mood regulation network (e.g., through tractotomy, vagus nerve stimulation, or deep brain stimulation) can alleviate depression, perhaps through "downstream" effects throughout this network (Mayberg 2003).

The neuroanatomy of bipolar disorder has been less well studied (for a review, see Strakowski et al. 2005). Generally, brain regions implicated in bipolar depression significantly overlap with those identified in unipolar depression (Sheline 2003). Neuroanatomical findings in mania are even more limited, likely because of the technical difficulties in studying manic patients. Interestingly, during mania, activity of prefrontal cortical regions may decrease (as often seen in depression), perhaps suggesting a valence-independent change in cortical activity during mood episodes (Strakowski et al. 2005).

These data indicate that mood disorders cannot be simply explained by a single-lesion model of regional brain dysfunction (just as no single neurotransmitter abnormality can explain all depressive syndromes). Rather, the functional neuroanatomy of mood disorders involves a diverse set of brain structures, including the prefrontal cortex, anterior cingulate cortex, subgenual cingulate cortex, medial temporal cortex, and parietal cortex, and various subcortical structures, including the ventral striatum, thalamus, hypothalamus, and brain stem. In addition, there is notable variability in neuroanatomical findings reported to date. Although some of this variability might be explained by inconsistencies in imaging technique and analysis (Videbech 2000; Videbech et al. 2002), this discordance likely results from underlying biological heterogeneity among patients with mood disorders.

Neurobiology of Mood Disorders in Neuropsychiatric Patients

Depression in patients with neurological disease is associated with many similar neurochemical findings as in patients with idiopathic major depression. All three monoamines are disrupted in Parkinson's disease, which is highly associated with depression (Chan-Palay and Asan 1989; D'Amato et al. 1987; Mayberg and Solomon 1995; Remy et al. 2005). Serotonergic dysfunction also has been linked to poststroke depression (Mayberg et al. 1988). Huntington's disease has been less clearly associated with monoaminergic abnormalities, but abnormalities of CRF and glutamate function have been suggested (Kurlan et al. 1988; Peyser and Folstein 1990; Slaughter et al. 2001).

The structural and functional neuroanatomy of depression associated with neurological disease also shares similarities with findings in idiopathic depression. Computed tomography and MRI studies in stroke patients with and without mood disorders have documented a high association of mood changes with infarctions of the frontal lobe and basal ganglia, particularly those occurring in close proximity to the frontal pole or involving the caudate nucleus (R.G. Robinson et al. 1984; Starkstein et al. 1987). Reports of patients with traumatic frontal lobe injury indicate a high correlation between affective disturbances and right hemisphere pathology (Grafman et al. 1986). Late-onset depression has been linked with MRI-defined white matter abnormalities likely related to otherwise subclinical

ischemic changes (Alexopoulos et al. 1997; Krishnan 2002). Secondary mania, although rare, is most consistently seen with right-sided basal frontal-temporal or subcortical damage (Starkstein et al. 1990). Studies of patients with head trauma, brain tumors, or ablative neurosurgery (Damasio and Van Hoesen 1983; Grafman et al. 1986; Stuss and Benson 1986) further suggest that dorsolateral lesions are associated with depression and depressive-like symptoms such as apathy and psychomotor slowing.

Several functional imaging studies of depressed patients with neurological disease have been conducted in which functional abnormalities would not be confounded by gross cortical lesions. These studies typically have included Parkinson's disease, Huntington's disease, and lacunar strokes of the basal ganglia—disorders with known or identifiable neurochemical, neurodegenerative, or focal changes in which the primary pathology spares frontal cortex (the region repeatedly implicated in idiopathic depression studies). These data have shown that depressed patients with Parkinson's disease have selective hypometabolism involving the caudate nucleus and prefrontal and orbitofrontal cortices (Jagust et al. 1992; Mayberg et al. 1990; Ring et al. 1994). Depressed patients with Huntington's disease show decreases in paralimbic orbitofrontal and inferior prefrontal cortices (as well as caudate abnormalities inherent to the disease) (Mayberg et al. 1992). Patients with depression following unilateral lacunar subcortical stroke also show cortical hypometabolism (Mayberg 1994), suggesting that subcortical lesions can affect function throughout a network of brain regions involved in mood regulation. These data suggest that the depressive syndrome, regardless of etiology, is associated with similar regional brain changes (Figure 27–2).

Together, imaging data for depressed patients with neurological disease help confirm that a cortical, subcortical, and limbic-paralimbic network of brain regions is involved in mood regulation. These data also support the notion that disturbance of the network at any critical node can result in behavioral effects and downstream activity changes consistent with idiopathic depression.

SYMPTOM-SPECIFIC FINDINGS

Another approach to the study of mood disorders has been to focus on the neurobiology of specific symptom clusters on the basis of the presumption that there will be greater homogeneity in the neural basis for a specific symptom than for the larger syndrome (in which symptom presentation may differ between subjects with the same disorder). In this section, we review the neurobiological bases for different symptoms and symptom clusters associated with mood disorders.

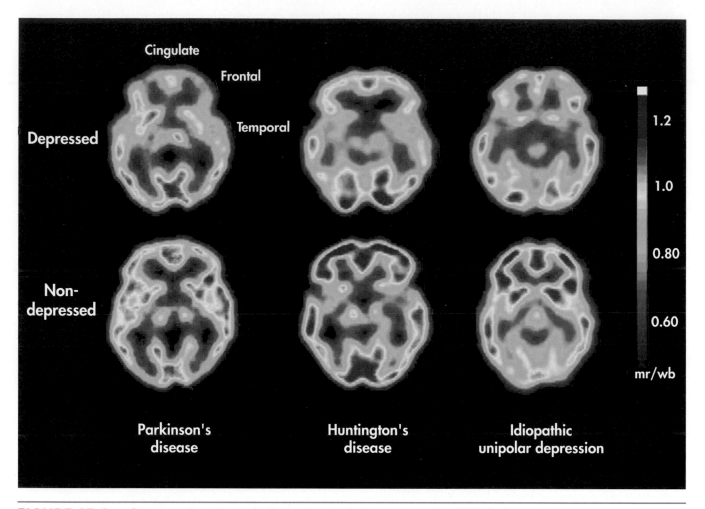

FIGURE 27–2.   Common glucose metabolic positron emission tomography (PET) findings in neurological and idiopathic depression. Decreased prefrontal, dorsal cingulate, and temporal cortical metabolism is a common finding across different depressive syndromes, including patients with Parkinson's disease, Huntington's disease, and idiopathic unipolar depression.

Mood and Affect

Neuroanatomical studies have played an important role in elucidating the neurobiology of emotions and emotional regulation. Broadly speaking, it has been shown that emotional processing occurs within neural networks that include predominantly ventral frontal brain structures (Phillips et al. 2003a, 2003b). In particular, sad mood has been correlated with increased activity in the ventral medial frontal cortex, with several studies implicating Brodmann area 25 of the subgenual cingulate cortex as a critical node in this network (Damasio et al. 2000; George et al. 1995; Kimbrell et al. 1999; Levesque et al. 2003b; Liotti et al. 2000; Talbot and Cooper 2006), and changes in this region have been associated with antidepressant treatments (George et al. 1999; Mayberg 2003; Mayberg et al. 2005; Nobler et al. 2001) (Figure 27–3).

Suppression of sadness in healthy subjects has been associated with activity of the dorsolateral prefrontal cortex (Levesque et al. 2003a), possibly suggesting a normal compensatory response in healthy subjects that may be abnormal in depressed patients (in whom abnormal dorsolateral prefrontal cortex activity is typically observed). Positive mood is associated with similar frontal, especially prefrontal, brain structures (Damasio et al. 2000; Gur et al. 2002; Habel et al. 2005; Killgore and Yurgelun-Todd 2004). Temporal lobe structures, especially the amygdala, also have been implicated in emotional processing (Phelps and LeDoux 2005). Furthermore, cortical-amygdala interactions may be involved in emotional reactivity, with variability between persons explained in part by genetic differences (Hariri et al. 2005; Pezawas et al. 2005). Some investigators have suggested that the brain has lateralized networks for emotional regulation, such that processing of positive emotions is more strongly associated with left-sided brain function and processing of negative emotions more strongly associated with right-sided neural systems (Davidson 1995).

Disturbance of affect (as distinct from mood) has been associated with dysfunction within the basal ganglia

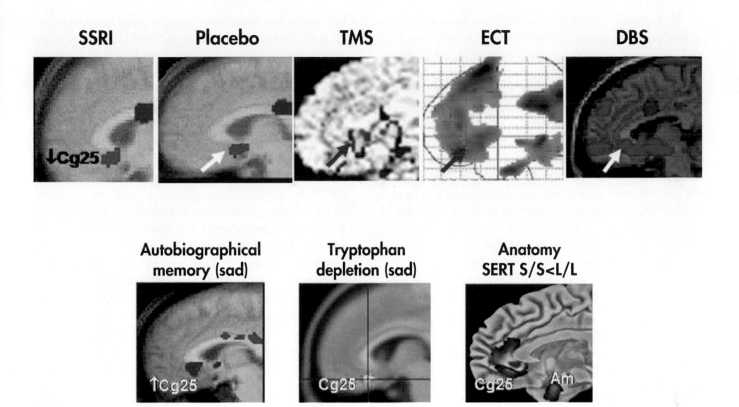

FIGURE 27–3. Imaging data supporting a role for Brodmann area 25 in depression. Decreased activity in the subgenual cingulate (Brodmann area 25; Cg25) is a consistent finding across numerous and diverse treatment studies (*top row*). Increased subgenual cingulate activity is associated with increased sadness, and functional connectivity of this region during processing of emotional stimuli may be mediated by genetics (*bottom row*). SSRI=selective serotonin reuptake inhibitor; TMS=transcranial magnetic stimulation; ECT=electroconvulsive therapy; DBS=deep brain stimulation; SERT=serotonin transporter.

Source. Adapted from George et al. 1999; Mayberg 2003; Mayberg et al. 2005; Nobler et al. 2001; Pezawas et al. 2005; Talbot and Cooper 2006.

and related structures. Patients with Parkinson's disease, for example, may have "depressive" affect in the absence of other depressive symptoms; furthermore, patients with Parkinson's disease may have greater difficulty demonstrating and recognizing facial expressions of emotion (Jacobs et al. 1995). Electrical stimulation of the subthalamic nucleus has been associated with pseudobulbar crying (Okun et al. 2004). Pseudobulbar affect in general (e.g., "pathological" crying or laughing) is associated with a few neurological diseases involving diverse brain structures (Okuda et al. 2005; Schiffer and Pope 2005; Zeilig et al. 1996). However, lesions almost always occur in motor neural systems (Schiffer and Pope 2005).

The neurochemical bases of mood and affect are not clear, although the involvement of monoaminergic systems has been suggested. Acute depletion of tryptophan (resulting in decreased available serotonin) can lead to a recurrence of "depressive symptoms" in vulnerable patients (Booij et al. 2002; Delgado et al. 1991), although it is not clear from the literature which depressive symptoms recur. Successful SSRI treatment is associated with decreased

activation of specific brain regions in response to sad stimuli in depressed patients (Fu et al. 2004). Dopamine function has been strongly associated with positive mood states (Burgdorf and Panksepp 2006; Drevets et al. 2001).

Interest and Motivation

Studies of interest and motivation strongly implicate function within ventral striatal and cortical systems, with the dopamine system likely involved. Ventral striatal dopaminergic pathways appear to play a critical role in motivation (Drevets et al. 2001; Goto and Grace 2005; Kalivas and Volkow 2005; Tremblay et al. 2005; Wise 2005). Interestingly, dopamine may be more important for motivation (seeking) behavior than for hedonic response or reward (Cagniard et al. 2005; S. Robinson et al. 2005). Orbitofrontal, anterior cingulate, and prefrontal cortices, as well as ventral basal ganglia (nucleus accumbens, ventral caudate, and ventral putamen), appear to be involved in the neurobiology of interest and hedonic response (Benoit et al. 2004; Cox et al. 2005; Roesch and Olson 2004; Tremblay et al. 2005; Volkow et al. 2005; Wallis and Miller 2003).

In depressed patients, anhedonia has been associated with decreased activity in ventral basal ganglia and ventral prefrontal cortical regions (Dunn et al. 2002; Keedwell et al. 2005), and altered reward processing has been identified with a dopaminergic probe (Tremblay et al. 2005). A study of hedonic response in schizophrenia patients (compared with healthy control subjects) found that patients failed to activate ventral cortical-subcortical regions (including insular cortex, nucleus accumbens, and parahippocampal gyrus) during an unpleasant experience but instead showed increased metabolism in frontal cortical regions (Crespo-Facorro et al. 2001). Studies of apathy (separate from depression and anhedonia) have implicated similar, but somewhat more dorsal, prefrontal and subcortical brain regions (van Reekum et al. 2005).

In summary, anhedonia and apathy appear to be mediated by overlapping brain regions that primarily include ventral cortical and subcortical areas. These regions largely overlap those involved in mood regulation described earlier. However, studies show that specific regions may be involved in decreased interest and motivation in the absence of the full depressive syndrome.

Sleep

Sleep physiology has been extensively studied in depressed patients. Sleep electroencephalogram (EEG) abnormalities in depression include prolonged sleep latency, decreased slow-wave sleep, and reduced rapid eye movement (REM) latency with disturbances in the relative time spent in both REM and non-REM sleep (Benca et al. 1992). Reduced REM latency is the best-studied and most reproducible sleep-related electroencephalography finding in depressed patients, and this abnormality is reversed by most antidepressants (Sharpley and Cowen 1995). Sleep deprivation, particularly if instituted in the second half of the night, has an effect similar to that of medication, although the rapid, dramatic improvement in depressive symptoms is short-lived (Wu and Bunney 1990). Imaging data have suggested that increased pretreatment activity in the ventral anterior cingulate cortex and ventromedial prefrontal cortex may predict antidepressant response to sleep deprivation (Wu et al. 1999, 2001). Changes in nocturnal body temperature and attenuation of the normal fluctuations in core body temperature during sleep further suggest a more generalized dysregulation of normal circadian rhythms in patients with depression (Benca 1994). To date, however, none of these markers has proven to be specific to depression, suggesting a neural system underlying sleep and circadian rhythms that is involved but not specific to mood disorder syndromes.

The physiology of sleep disturbances in patients with mania and bipolar depression is less well characterized.

Clinically, it has long been observed that sleep deprivation is a common precipitant of manic episodes, again suggesting an important biological link between sleep and affective symptoms. Patients with bipolar depression presenting with hypersomnia, however, do not show a consistent reduction in REM latency (Nofzinger et al. 1991). Marked changes in sleep continuity and other REM measures comparable to those seen in patients with MDD also have been described (Benca 1994).

Appetite

The neurobiology of appetite disturbance in patients with mood disorder and/or neuropsychiatric disease is not well understood. As described earlier, appetite and weight changes are common in these patients. Also, medications used to treat these conditions (e.g., anticonvulsants, lithium, neuroleptics) have clear effects on appetite, body weight, and metabolism. Brain regions involved in regulation of appetite and feeding include the hypothalamus and amygdala, and neuromodulatory systems involved include leptin (a peripheral hormone with central nervous system activity), melanocortin, neuropeptide Y, the HPA axis, and the monoamines (especially dopamine) (Kishi and Elmquist 2005). Leptin has been proposed as a potential target for novel antidepressant treatments (Lu et al. 2006).

Psychomotor Activity

Psychomotor abnormalities have largely been linked to monoaminergic neurotransmission and dorsal cortical and subcortical brain activity. Dopamine has been clearly implicated in the neurobiology of psychomotor activity. Patients with Parkinson's disease have decreased psychomotor activity (in the absence of depression) that clearly improves with dopaminergic therapies, and stimulant medications affecting dopaminergic function are associated with increased psychomotor activity. Mice bred to underexpress the gene for the dopamine transporter (leading to a hyperdopaminergic state) show hyperactivity in novel environments (but not in a home cage situation) (Zhuang et al. 2001). Decreased dopamine in the basal ganglia has been associated with psychomotor retardation in depressed patients (Martinot et al. 2001). Dorsolateral prefrontal cortex activity correlates with psychomotor activity in depressed patients, such that decreased blood flow or metabolism in the dorsal prefrontal cortex is associated with psychomotor retardation (Bench et al. 1993; Brody et al. 2001a; Videbech et al. 2002).

Emotional Bias

Emotional bias represents altered processing of emotional stimuli. Processing of positive and negative information (such as rewards and punishments) has been linked to the ventral prefrontal cortex, ventral striatum, midbrain, and hippocampus (Breiter and Rosen 1999; Elliott et al. 2000) and to dopamine function (Bressan and Crippa 2005; Vollm et al. 2004; Wise 2002). Depressed patients have shown abnormal activity in ventral cortical and subcortical brain regions associated with processing of feedback (Elliott et al. 1998) and negative emotional stimuli (Elliott et al. 2002; George et al. 1997). Depressed patients also may have heightened sensitivity to the rewarding effects of dextroamphetamine compared with healthy control subjects (suggesting a hypodopaminergic state); this sensitivity is associated with altered brain activity in ventral cortical and subcortical regions (Tremblay et al. 2005).

In this chapter, emotional bias is treated as a separate symptom. However, it may be better described as the cognitive processing of emotional stimuli. As such, it is not unreasonable to expect that emotional bias may reflect an interaction of neural systems involved in mood and cognition. For example, older patients with depression have shown slower performance on the emotional Stroop Test (compared with matched control subjects) as well as slower response for negative than for neutral or positive words (a pattern not seen in matched control subjects) (Dudley et al. 2002). Depressed patients show a different pattern of frontal-limbic brain activity during the standard and emotional Stroop Test compared with healthy control subjects (George et al. 1997), and interference on the emotional Stroop Test has been correlated with increased ventral anterior cingulate activity (Whalen et al. 1998) (as opposed to increased dorsal anterior cingulate activity with interference on a nonemotional Stroop Test; Bush et al. 1998).

Suicidal ideation might be viewed as an extreme of negative emotional bias. Postmortem brain studies of depressed people who committed suicide reported changes in a few additional serotonin markers, including regional transmitter and metabolite levels, transporter and postsynaptic receptor density, and second-messenger and transcription proteins (Arango et al. 1997, 2003; Mann et al. 2000).

Cognition

The neurobiology of cognition has been extensively investigated (Gazzaniga 2000). The cognitive processes disturbed in patients with mood disorders involve primarily dorsal frontal and subcortical brain regions. Working memory, planning, and organization are executive functions clearly linked with dorsolateral prefrontal cortical function and also known to be abnormal in depression (Rogers et al. 2004). Depressed patients have shown blunting of an expected left anterior cingulate increase during performance of a cognitive interference task (the Stroop Test) (George et al. 1997). These patients also have shown a

corresponding increase in function within the dorsolateral prefrontal cortex (a region not normally recruited during this task) (George et al. 1997), suggesting altered compensatory activity. During a planning task (the Tower of London), depressed patients show poor activation of the dorsal prefrontal cortex, anterior cingulate cortex, and dorsal caudate (Elliott et al. 1997a). Poor performance on the standard Stroop task in patients with late-life depression has been specifically associated with abnormalities in dorsal subcortical white matter (Alexopoulos et al. 2002).

Disinhibition (commonly seen in mania) has been associated with ventral cortical structures (Cummings 1995). Disinhibition in dementia, for example, is associated with tissue loss in the subgenual cingulate cortex (Rosen et al. 2005). Manic patients show poor activation in the orbitofrontal cortex during a response inhibition task (go/no-go) that reliably increases orbitofrontal activity in nonmanic control subjects (Altshuler et al. 2005).

A PUTATIVE NEURAL NETWORK MODEL OF MOOD DISORDERS

Similar neuropathological findings in mood disorders associated with diverse etiologies (e.g., idiopathic, Parkinson's disease, medication-induced) and specific neurobiological correlates for specific symptom clusters in mood disorders strongly suggest that mood disorder syndromes are best defined by dysfunction throughout several distinct, but interconnected, neural circuits. An extrapolation of this hypothesis implies that phenomenological differences among various patients with mood disorders might best be explained by differential dysfunction within these circuits.

Neural network models of mood regulation attempt to incorporate these findings into a coherent system and propose a set of testable hypotheses. One example of a neural network model for depression is presented here. This model has been confirmed in principle with the use of structural equation modeling of data from previous combined imaging-treatment studies (Seminowicz et al. 2004). Key features are as follows:

- Network dysfunction (i.e., mood disturbance) may be precipitated by dysfunction at any "critical node" within the network.
- Dysfunction at a critical node will have "upstream" and "downstream" effects that may result in further symptoms.
- Compensatory alterations within the network (in response to dysfunction) may lead to further alterations throughout the network, resulting in further symptomatic presentation.

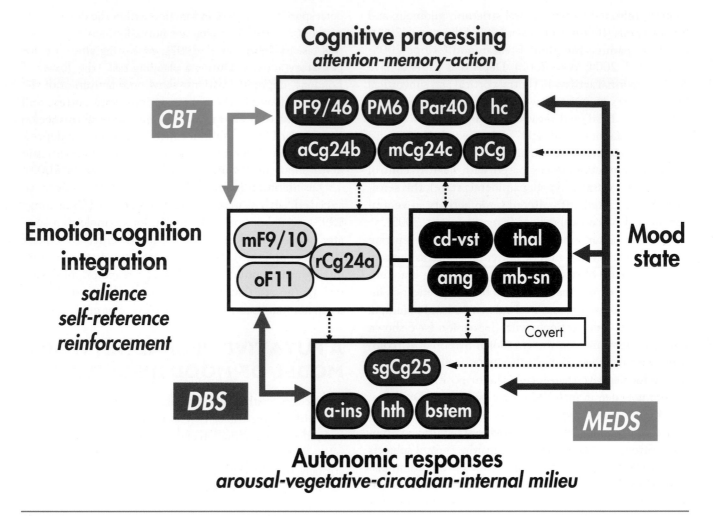

FIGURE 27–4.   A proposed model of mood regulation: Different sets of brain regions are involved in different aspects of mood experience and modulation. Numerous interconnections exist among these different regions, and the system is recognized to be dynamic and potentially modulated at any critical node. Different treatments for mood disorder syndromes may act primarily at different nodes within the system, with therapeutic downstream effects. Abbreviations: PF9/46 = dorsolateral prefrontal cortex; PM6 = premotor area; Par40 = dorsal parietal; hc = hippocampus; aCg24b = Brodmann area 24b/dorsal-perigenual anterior cingulate cortex; mCg24c = Brodmann area 24c/dorsal anterior cingulate cortex; pCg = posterior cingulate gyrus; mF9/10 = medial frontal cortex; rCg24a = Brodmann area 24a/perigenual-subgenual cingulate cortex; oF11 = orbitofrontal cortex; cd-vst = ventral caudate–ventral striatum; thal = thalamus; amg = amygdala; mb-sn = midbrain–subthalamic nuclei; sgCg25 = Brodmann area 25/subgenual cingulate cortex; a-ins = anterior insula, hth = hypothalamus, bstem = brain stem; CBT = cognitive-behavioral therapy; DBS = deep brain stimulation of Brodmann area 25; MEDS = antidepressant medications.

- Successful treatment of network dysfunction may occur through modulation of function at other critical nodes, presuming compensatory responses are intact.

Within this proposed model (Figure 27–4), distinct neural systems are associated with specific functions (and therefore associated with underlying symptom clusters). Cognitive, psychomotor, and sensorimotor processing are associated with dorsal prefrontal, dorsal anterior cingulate, parietal and posterior cingulate cortices, and hippocampus. Medial frontal, orbitofrontal, and perigen-

ual anterior cingulate cortices are associated with overt cognitive processing of emotional stimuli, including salience, reward value, and self-relevance. More covert or masked cognitive-emotional processing is associated with medial temporal and subcortical regions, including the amygdala, ventral basal ganglia, and midbrain structures and nuclei. Brain regions involved in homeostatic/drive processes (such as sleep and appetite) as well as body state representation (i.e., the physical aspects of emotional experience) include the subgenual anterior cingulate cortex, anterior insula, and hypothalamus. Brain stem nuclei are also included in these regions, although it is recognized that monoaminergic projections from these nuclei influence function throughout the entire network.

A key feature of this model is to recognize that these various brain regions, each involved in different aspects of mood and behavior, are relatively distinct but intricately connected to one another, typically in a bidirectional way. Emotional-behavioral states (e.g., depression) are then understood to be associated with alteration within several portions of this network, with symptomatic presentation corresponding to the direction and degree of dysfunction within each subregion. The source of dysfunction may vary (e.g., between idiopathic and neurologically related depression), but the neural systems involved are the same. It is further hypothesized that treatments with different primary mechanisms of action directly alter network activity at distinct nodes. Efficacy is then determined by how adequate the treatment site of action matches the source of dysfunction and/or the compensatory activity of the network. For example, certain "first-line" treatments, such as serotonergic antidepressant medications and cognitive-behavioral therapy (CBT), may have different primary sites of action within the network (frontal cortex for CBT and midbrain-subcortical regions for medications) but rely on intact connections between various regions of the circuit and the ability of these connected regions to respond appropriately (i.e., changes in midbrain-subcortical regions with medications must be able to result in downstream functional changes in frontal cortex and vice versa for CBT). Similarly, poor adaptive capacity within the network may underlie lack of response to common treatments and explain why progressively more aggressive treatments (such as electroconvulsive therapy and surgery) are needed to ameliorate symptoms.

Models such as this may further be used to develop testable hypotheses for novel treatments for mood disorders. For example, this model was used to develop deep brain stimulation of the subgenual cingulate cortex (Brodmann area 25), which has shown promising antidepressant effects in patients with treatment-resistant depression; these antidepressant effects were associated with systemwide changes in regional brain activity consistent with a combination of multiple treatments (Mayberg et al. 2005). The effects of other developing treatments (e.g., transcranial magnetic stimulation, vagus nerve stimulation, and deep brain stimulation of other targets such as the anterior internal capsule and nucleus accumbens) can be similarly tested within the context of this model.

CONCLUSION

Several distinct but interconnected neural systems regulate mood, affect, cognition, sleep, appetite, psychomotor activity, emotional regulation, and homeostatic/drive states. When these systems are disrupted, the resulting symptomatic presentation is broadly defined as a "mood disorder." Mood disorders may be associated with distinct neurological illnesses or other medical abnormalities (e.g., hypothyroidism), or they may be idiopathic. The etiologies of mood disorders may be diverse, but the neural dysfunction underlying the clinical manifestations is presumed to be the same. On this basis, models of brain systems involved in mood disorders can be developed and tested; we presented one possible model in this chapter.

Highlights for the Clinician

Symptoms of mood disorders in patients with neurological illness	
Less specific symptoms	**More specific symptoms**
✦ Affect disturbance	✦ Mood disturbance
✦ Apathy	✦ Anhedonia
✦ Agitation	✦ Excessive guilt
✦ Decreased psychomotor speed	✦ Suicidality
✦ Cognitive abnormalities	
✦ Sleep disturbance	
✦ Appetite disturbance	

RECOMMENDED READINGS

Drevets WC: Prefrontal cortical-amygdalar metabolism in major depression. Ann N Y Acad Sci 877:614–637, 1999

Mayberg HS: Modulating dysfunctional limbic-cortical circuits in depression: towards development of brain-based algorithms for diagnosis and optimised treatment. Br Med Bull 65:193–207, 2003

McDonald WM, Richard IH, DeLong MR: Prevalence, etiology, and treatment of depression in Parkinson's disease. Biol Psychiatry 54:363–375, 2003

REFERENCES

Aarsland D, Alves G, Larsen JP: Disorders of motivation, sexual conduct, and sleep in Parkinson's disease. Adv Neurol 96:56–64, 2005

Alexopoulos GS, Meyers BS, Young RC, et al: "Vascular depression" hypothesis. Arch Gen Psychiatry 54:915–922, 1997

Alexopoulos GS, Kiosses DN, Choi SJ, et al: Frontal white matter microstructure and treatment response of late-life depression: a preliminary study. Am J Psychiatry 159:1929–1932, 2002

Alloy LB, Abramson LY, Whitehouse WG, et al: Depressogenic cognitive styles: predictive validity, information processing and personality characteristics, and developmental origins. Behav Res Ther 37:503–531, 1999

Altshuler LL, Bookheimer SY, Townsend J, et al: Blunted activation in orbitofrontal cortex during mania: a functional magnetic resonance imaging study. Biol Psychiatry 58:763–769, 2005

American Psychiatric Association: Diagnostic and Statistical Manual of Mental Disorders, 4th Edition, Text Revision. Washington, DC, American Psychiatric Association, 2000

Arango V, Underwood MD, Mann JJ: Biologic alterations in the brainstem of suicides. Psychiatr Clin North Am 20:581–593, 1997

Arango V, Huang YY, Underwood MD, et al: Genetics of the serotonergic system in suicidal behavior. J Psychiatr Res 37:375–386, 2003

Arborelius L, Owens MJ, Plotsky PM, et al: The role of corticotropin-releasing factor in depression and anxiety disorders. J Endocrinol 160:1–12, 1999

Arroll B, Macgillivray S, Ogston S, et al: Efficacy and tolerability of tricyclic antidepressants and SSRIs compared with placebo for treatment of depression in primary care: a meta-analysis. Ann Fam Med 3:449–456, 2005

Asberg M, Thoren P, Traskman L, et al: "Serotonin depression"—a biochemical subgroup within the affective disorders? Science 191(4226):478–480, 1976

Austin MP, Mitchell P, Goodwin GM: Cognitive deficits in depression: possible implications for functional neuropathology. Br J Psychiatry 178:200–206, 2001

Ballmaier M, Toga AW, Blanton RE, et al: Anterior cingulate, gyrus rectus, and orbitofrontal abnormalities in elderly depressed patients: an MRI-based parcellation of the prefrontal cortex. Am J Psychiatry 161:99–108, 2004

Banki CM, Bissette G, Arato M, et al: Elevation of immunoreactive CSF TRH in depressed patients. Am J Psychiatry 145:1526–1531, 1988

Barr CS, Newman TK, Schwandt M, et al: Sexual dichotomy of an interaction between early adversity and the serotonin transporter gene promoter variant in rhesus macaques. Proc Natl Acad Sci U S A 101:12358–12363, 2004

Bauer M, London ED, Rasgon N, et al: Supraphysiological doses of levothyroxine alter regional cerebral metabolism and improve mood in bipolar depression. Mol Psychiatry 10:456–469, 2005

Baxter LR Jr, Schwartz JM, Phelps ME, et al: Reduction of prefrontal cortex glucose metabolism common to three types of depression. Arch Gen Psychiatry 46:243–250, 1989

Benca RM: Mood disorders, in Principles and Practice of Sleep Medicine. Edited by Kryger MH, Roth T, Dement WC. Philadelphia, PA, WB Saunders, 1994, pp 899–913

Benca RM, Obermeyer WH, Thisted RA, et al: Sleep and psychiatric disorders: a meta-analysis. Arch Gen Psychiatry 49:651–668; discussion 669–670, 1992

Bench CJ, Friston KJ, Brown RG, et al: The anatomy of melancholia: focal abnormalities of cerebral blood flow in major depression. Psychol Med 22:607–615, 1992

Bench CJ, Friston KJ, Brown RG, et al: Regional cerebral blood flow in depression measured by positron emission tomography: the relationship with clinical dimensions. Psychol Med 23:579–590, 1993

Benoit M, Clairet S, Koulibaly PM, et al: Brain perfusion correlates of the apathy inventory dimensions of Alzheimer's disease. Int J Geriatr Psychiatry 19:864–869, 2004

Berman RM, Narasimhan M, Miller HL, et al: Transient depressive relapse induced by catecholamine depletion: potential phenotypic vulnerability marker? Arch Gen Psychiatry 56:395–403, 1999

Berrettini WH, Rubinow DR, Nurnberger JI Jr, et al: CSF substance P immunoreactivity in affective disorders. Biol Psychiatry 20:965–970, 1985

Bondy B, Baghai TC, Minov C, et al: Substance P serum levels are increased in major depression: preliminary results. Biol Psychiatry 53:538–542, 2003

Booij L, Van der Does W, Benkelfat C, et al: Predictors of mood response to acute tryptophan depletion: a reanalysis. Neuropsychopharmacology 27:852–861, 2002

Botteron KN, Raichle ME, Drevets WC, et al: Volumetric reduction in left subgenual prefrontal cortex in early onset depression. Biol Psychiatry 51:342–344, 2002

Bradley BP, Mogg K, Lee SC: Attentional biases for negative information in induced and naturally occurring dysphoria. Behav Res Ther 35:911–927, 1997

Brambilla P, Nicoletti MA, Harenski K, et al: Anatomical MRI study of subgenual prefrontal cortex in bipolar and unipolar subjects. Neuropsychopharmacology 27:792–799, 2002

Breiter HC, Rosen BR: Functional magnetic resonance imaging of brain reward circuitry in the human. Ann N Y Acad Sci 877:523–547, 1999

Bremner JD, Vythilingam M, Vermetten E, et al: Reduced volume of orbitofrontal cortex in major depression. Biol Psychiatry 51:273–279, 2002

Bressan RA, Crippa JA: The role of dopamine in reward and pleasure behaviour—review of data from preclinical research. Acta Psychiatr Scand Suppl 427:14–21, 2005

Brody AL, Saxena S, Mandelkern MA, et al: Brain metabolic changes associated with symptom factor improvement in major depressive disorder. Biol Psychiatry 50:171–178, 2001a

Brody AL, Saxena S, Stoessel P, et al: Regional brain metabolic changes in patients with major depression treated with either paroxetine or interpersonal therapy: preliminary findings. Arch Gen Psychiatry 58:631–640, 2001b

Brown ES, Suppes T: Mood symptoms during corticosteroid therapy: a review. Harv Rev Psychiatry 5:239–246, 1998

Buchsbaum MS, Wu J, DeLisi LE, et al: Frontal cortex and basal ganglia metabolic rates assessed by positron emission tomography with [^{18}F]2-deoxyglucose in affective illness. J Affect Disord 10:137–152, 1986

Burgdorf J, Panksepp J: The neurobiology of positive emotions. Neurosci Biobehav Rev 30:173–187, 2006

Bush G, Whalen PJ, Rosen BR, et al: The counting Stroop: an interference task specialized for functional neuroimaging—validation study with functional MRI. Hum Brain Mapp 6:270–282, 1998

Cagniard B, Balsam PD, Brunner D, et al: Mice with chronically elevated dopamine exhibit enhanced motivation, but not learning, for a food reward. Neuropsychopharmacology 31:1362–1370, 2005

Caspi A, Sugden K, Moffitt TE, et al: Influence of life stress on depression: moderation by a polymorphism in the 5-HTT gene. Science 301(5631):386–389, 2003

Chan-Palay V, Asan E: Alterations in catecholamine neurons of the locus coeruleus in senile dementia of the Alzheimer type and in Parkinson's disease with and without dementia and depression. J Comp Neurol 287:373–392, 1989

Charney DS: Monoamine dysfunction and the pathophysiology and treatment of depression. J Clin Psychiatry 59 (suppl 14):11–14, 1998

Choudary PV, Molnar M, Evans SJ, et al: Altered cortical glutamatergic and GABAergic signal transmission with glial involvement in depression. Proc Natl Acad Sci U S A 102:15653–15658, 2005

Clark LA, Watson D: Tripartite model of anxiety and depression: psychometric evidence and taxonomic implications. J Abnorm Psychol 100:316–336, 1991

Cloninger CR: A unified biosocial theory of personality and its role in the development of anxiety states. Psychiatr Dev 4:167–226, 1986

Cloninger CR, Svrakic DM, Przybeck TR: Can personality assessment predict future depression? A twelve-month follow-up of 631 subjects. J Affect Disord 92:35–44, 2006

Cosgrove GR, Rauch SL: Stereotactic cingulotomy. Neurosurg Clin N Am 14:225–235, 2003

Cox SM, Andrade A, Johnsrude IS: Learning to like: a role for human orbitofrontal cortex in conditioned reward. J Neurosci 25:2733–2740, 2005

Crespo-Facorro B, Paradiso S, Andreasen NC, et al: Neural mechanisms of anhedonia in schizophrenia: a PET study of response to unpleasant and pleasant odors. JAMA 286:427–435, 2001

Cummings JL: Anatomic and behavioral aspects of frontal-subcortical circuits. Ann N Y Acad Sci 769:1–13, 1995

Damasio AR, Van Hoesen GW: Emotional disturbances associated with focal lesions of the limbic frontal lobe, in Neuropsychology of Human Emotion. Edited by Heilman KM, Satz P. New York, Guilford, 1983, pp 85–110

Damasio AR, Grabowski TJ, Bechara A, et al: Subcortical and cortical brain activity during the feeling of self-generated emotions. Nat Neurosci 3:1049–1056, 2000

D'Amato RJ, Zweig RM, Whitehouse PJ, et al: Aminergic systems in Alzheimer's disease and Parkinson's disease. Ann Neurol 22:229–236, 1987

Dantchev N, Widlocher DJ: The measurement of retardation in depression. J Clin Psychiatry 59 (suppl 14):19–25, 1998

Davidson R: Cerebral asymmetry, emotion, and affective style, in Brain Asymmetry. Edited by Davidson RJ, Hugdahl K. Cambridge, MA, MIT Press, 1995, pp 361–387

Delgado PL, Charney DS, Price LH, et al: Serotonin function and the mechanism of antidepressant action: reversal of antidepressant-induced remission by rapid depletion of plasma tryptophan. Arch Gen Psychiatry 47:411–418, 1990

Delgado PL, Price LH, Miller HL, et al: Rapid serotonin depletion as a provocative challenge test for patients with major depression: relevance to antidepressant action and the neurobiology of depression. Psychopharmacol Bull 27:321–330, 1991

D'Haenen H, Bossuyt A, Mertens J, et al: SPECT imaging of serotonin2 receptors in depression. Psychiatry Res 45:227–237, 1992

Dodd ML, Klos KJ, Bower JH, et al: Pathological gambling caused by drugs used to treat Parkinson disease. Arch Neurol 62:1377–1381, 2005

Drevets WC, Videen TO, Price JL, et al: A functional anatomical study of unipolar depression. J Neurosci 12:3628–3641, 1992

Drevets WC, Price JL, Simpson JR Jr, et al: Subgenual prefrontal cortex abnormalities in mood disorders. Nature 386(6627):824–827, 1997

Drevets WC, Frank E, Price JC, et al: PET imaging of serotonin 1A receptor binding in depression. Biol Psychiatry 46:1375–1387, 1999

Drevets WC, Gautier C, Price JC, et al: Amphetamine-induced dopamine release in human ventral striatum correlates with euphoria. Biol Psychiatry 49:81–96, 2001

Drevets WC, Bogers W, Raichle ME: Functional anatomical correlates of antidepressant drug treatment assessed using PET measures of regional glucose metabolism. Eur Neuropsychopharmacol 12:527–544, 2002

Dudley R, O'Brien J, Barnett N, et al: Distinguishing depression from dementia in later life: a pilot study employing the emotional Stroop task. Int J Geriatr Psychiatry 17:48–53, 2002

Dunn RT, Kimbrell TA, Ketter TA, et al: Principal components of the Beck Depression Inventory and regional cerebral metabolism in unipolar and bipolar depression. Biol Psychiatry 51:387–399, 2002

Ebert D, Ebmeier KP: The role of the cingulate gyrus in depression: from functional anatomy to neurochemistry. Biol Psychiatry 39:1044–1050, 1996

Einat H, Manji HK: Cellular plasticity cascades: genes-to-behavior pathways in animal models of bipolar disorder. Biol Psychiatry 59:1160–1171, 2006

Elliott R, Baker SC, Rogers RD, et al: Prefrontal dysfunction in depressed patients performing a complex planning task: a study using positron emission tomography. Psychol Med 27:931–942, 1997a

Elliott R, Sahakian BJ, Herrod JJ, et al: Abnormal response to negative feedback in unipolar depression: evidence for a diagnosis specific impairment. J Neurol Neurosurg Psychiatry 63:74–82, 1997b

Elliott R, Sahakian BJ, Michael A, et al: Abnormal neural response to feedback on planning and guessing tasks in patients with unipolar depression. Psychol Med 28:559–571, 1998

Elliott R, Friston KJ, Dolan RJ: Dissociable neural responses in human reward systems. J Neurosci 20:6159–6165, 2000

Elliott R, Rubinsztein JS, Sahakian BJ, et al: The neural basis of mood-congruent processing biases in depression. Arch Gen Psychiatry 59:597–604, 2002

Esposito S, Prange AJ Jr, Golden RN: The thyroid axis and mood disorders: overview and future prospects. Psychopharmacol Bull 33:205–217, 1997

Fanous A, Gardner CO, Prescott CA, et al: Neuroticism, major depression and gender: a population-based twin study. Psychol Med 32:719–728, 2002

Fava M, Kendler KS: Major depressive disorder. Neuron 28:335–341, 2000

Ferris RM, Beaman OJ: Bupropion: a new antidepressant drug, the mechanism of action of which is not associated with down-regulation of postsynaptic beta-adrenergic, serotonergic (5-HT$_2$), alpha 2-adrenergic, imipramine and dopaminergic receptors in brain. Neuropharmacology 22:1257–1267, 1983

Fu CH, Williams SC, Cleare AJ, et al: Attenuation of the neural response to sad faces in major depression by antidepressant treatment: a prospective, event-related functional magnetic resonance imaging study. Arch Gen Psychiatry 61:877–889, 2004

Galynker II, Cai J, Ongseng F, et al: Hypofrontality and negative symptoms in major depressive disorder. J Nucl Med 39:608–612, 1998

Gazzaniga MS (ed): The New Cognitive Neurosciences, 2nd Edition. Cambridge, MA, MIT Press, 2000

George MS, Ketter TA, Post RM: SPECT and PET imaging in mood disorders. J Clin Psychiatry 54(suppl):6–13, 1993

George MS, Ketter TA, Parekh PI, et al: Brain activity during transient sadness and happiness in healthy women. Am J Psychiatry 152:341–351, 1995

George MS, Ketter TA, Parekh PI, et al: Blunted left cingulate activation in mood disorder subjects during a response interference task (the Stroop). J Neuropsychiatry Clin Neurosci 9:55–63, 1997

George MS, Stallings LE, Speer AM, et al: Prefrontal rTMS reduces relative perfusion locally and trans-synaptically. Hum Psychopharmacol 14:161–170, 1999

Gillette-Guyonnet S, Nourhashemi F, Andrieu S, et al: Weight loss in Alzheimer disease. Am J Clin Nutr 71:637S–642S, 2000

Goldapple K, Segal Z, Garson C, et al: Modulation of cortical-limbic pathways in major depression: treatment-specific effects of cognitive behavior therapy. Arch Gen Psychiatry 61:34–41, 2004

Goldberg JF, Burdick KE, Endick CJ: Preliminary randomized, double-blind, placebo-controlled trial of pramipexole added to mood stabilizers for treatment-resistant bipolar depression. Am J Psychiatry 161:564–566, 2004

Gonul AS, Kula M, Bilgin AG, et al: The regional cerebral blood flow changes in major depressive disorder with and without psychotic features. Prog Neuropsychopharmacol Biol Psychiatry 28:1015–1021, 2004

Gorman DG, Cummings JL: Hypersexuality following septal injury. Arch Neurol 49:308–310, 1992

Goto Y, Grace AA: Dopaminergic modulation of limbic and cortical drive of nucleus accumbens in goal-directed behavior. Nat Neurosci 8:805–812, 2005

Grafman J, Vance SC, Weingartner H, et al: The effects of lateralized frontal lesions on mood regulation. Brain 109 (pt 6):1127–1148, 1986

Green E, Craddock N: Brain-derived neurotrophic factor as a potential risk locus for bipolar disorder: evidence, limitations, and implications. Curr Psychiatry Rep 5:469–476, 2003

Grigg-Damberger MM: Sleep in aging and neurodegenerative diseases. Suppl Clin Neurophysiol 57:508–520, 2004

Gur RC, Schroeder L, Turner T, et al: Brain activation during facial emotion processing. Neuroimage 16 (3 pt 1):651–662, 2002

Habel U, Klein M, Kellermann T, et al: Same or different? Neural correlates of happy and sad mood in healthy males. Neuroimage 26:206–214, 2005

Hariri AR, Drabant EM, Munoz KE, et al: A susceptibility gene for affective disorders and the response of the human amygdala. Arch Gen Psychiatry 62:146–152, 2005

Hastings RS, Parsey RV, Oquendo MA, et al: Volumetric analysis of the prefrontal cortex, amygdala, and hippocampus in major depression. Neuropsychopharmacology 29:952–959, 2004

Heim C, Newport DJ, Heit S, et al: Pituitary-adrenal and autonomic responses to stress in women after sexual and physical abuse in childhood. JAMA 284:592–597, 2000

Hirayasu Y, Shenton ME, Salisbury DF, et al: Subgenual cingulate cortex volume in first-episode psychosis. Am J Psychiatry 156:1091–1093, 1999

Husain MM: Emotional lability (pseudobulbar affect) in general psychiatry: an introduction. Am J Geriatr Pharmacother 3 (suppl 1):3, 2005

Jacobs DH, Shuren J, Bowers D, et al: Emotional facial imagery, perception, and expression in Parkinson's disease. Neurology 45:1696–1702, 1995

Jagust WJ, Reed BR, Martin EM, et al: Cognitive function and regional cerebral blood flow in Parkinson's disease. Brain 115 (pt 2):521–537, 1992

Joffe RT, Sokolov ST: Thyroid hormone treatment of primary unipolar depression: a review. Int J Neuropsychopharmacol 3:143–147, 2000

Kalivas PW, Volkow ND: The neural basis of addiction: a pathology of motivation and choice. Am J Psychiatry 162:1403–1413, 2005

Kant R, Duffy JD, Pivovarnik A: Prevalence of apathy following head injury. Brain Inj 12:87–92, 1998

Keedwell PA, Andrew C, Williams SC, et al: The neural correlates of anhedonia in major depressive disorder. Biol Psychiatry 58:843–853, 2005

Kendell SF, Krystal JH, Sanacora G: GABA and glutamate systems as therapeutic targets in depression and mood disorders. Expert Opin Ther Targets 9:153–168, 2005

Kendler KS, Kuhn JW, Vittum J, et al: The interaction of stressful life events and a serotonin transporter polymorphism in the prediction of episodes of major depression: a replication. Arch Gen Psychiatry 62:529–535, 2005

Kendler KS, Gatz M, Gardner CO, et al: A Swedish national twin study of lifetime major depression. Am J Psychiatry 163:109–114, 2006

Kennedy SH, Evans KR, Kruger S, et al: Changes in regional brain glucose metabolism measured with positron emission tomography after paroxetine treatment of major depression. Am J Psychiatry 158:899–905, 2001

Kieseppa T, Partonen T, Haukka J, et al: High concordance of bipolar I disorder in a nationwide sample of twins. Am J Psychiatry 161:1814–1821, 2004

Killgore WD, Yurgelun-Todd DA: Activation of the amygdala and anterior cingulate during nonconscious processing of sad versus happy faces. Neuroimage 21:1215–1223, 2004

Kimbrell TA, George MS, Parekh PI, et al: Regional brain activity during transient self-induced anxiety and anger in healthy adults. Biol Psychiatry 46:454–465, 1999

Kirkegaard C, Faber J, Hummer L, et al: Increased levels of TRH in cerebrospinal fluid from patients with endogenous depression. Psychoneuroendocrinology 4:227–235, 1979

Kishi T, Elmquist JK: Body weight is regulated by the brain: a link between feeding and emotion. Mol Psychiatry 10:132–146, 2005

Klimek V, Schenck JE, Han H, et al: Dopaminergic abnormalities in amygdaloid nuclei in major depression: a postmortem study. Biol Psychiatry 52:740–748, 2002

Krishnan KR: Biological risk factors in late life depression. Biol Psychiatry 52:185–192, 2002

Kurlan R, Caine E, Rubin A, et al: Cerebrospinal fluid correlates of depression in Huntington's disease. Arch Neurol 45:881–883, 1988

Landes AM, Sperry SD, Strauss ME: Prevalence of apathy, dysphoria, and depression in relation to dementia severity in Alzheimer's disease. J Neuropsychiatry Clin Neurosci 17:342–349, 2005

Lenze EJ, Munin MC, Ferrell RE, et al: Association of the serotonin transporter gene-linked polymorphic region (5-HTTLPR) genotype with depression in elderly persons after hip fracture. Am J Geriatr Psychiatry 13:428–432, 2005

Levesque J, Eugene F, Joanette Y, et al: Neural circuitry underlying voluntary suppression of sadness. Biol Psychiatry 53:502–510, 2003a

Levesque J, Joanette Y, Mensour B, et al: Neural correlates of sad feelings in healthy girls. Neuroscience 121:545–551, 2003b

Levinson DF: Meta-analysis in psychiatric genetics. Curr Psychiatry Rep 7:143–151, 2005

Levinson DF: The genetics of depression: a review. Biol Psychiatry 60:84–92, 2006

Levitan RD, Rector NA, Bagby RM: Negative attributional style in seasonal and nonseasonal depression. Am J Psychiatry 155:428–430, 1998

Liotti M, Mayberg HS, Brannan SK, et al: Differential limbic-cortical correlates of sadness and anxiety in healthy subjects: implications for affective disorders. Biol Psychiatry 48:30–42, 2000

Loftis JM, Hauser P: The phenomenology and treatment of interferon-induced depression. J Affect Disord 82:175–190, 2004

Loosen PT: The TRH-induced TSH response in psychiatric patients: a possible neuroendocrine marker. Psychoneuroendocrinology 10:237–260, 1985

Lu XY, Kim CS, Frazer A, et al: Leptin: a potential novel antidepressant. Proc Natl Acad Sci U S A 103:1593–1598, 2006

Malison RT, Price LH, Berman R, et al: Reduced brain serotonin transporter availability in major depression as measured by [^{123}I]-2 beta-carbomethoxy-3 beta-(4-iodophenyl)tropane and single photon emission computed tomography. Biol Psychiatry 44:1090–1098, 1998

Malizia AL: The frontal lobes and neurosurgery for psychiatric disorders. J Psychopharmacol 11:179–187, 1997

Manji HK, Drevets WC, Charney DS: The cellular neurobiology of depression. Nat Med 7:541–547, 2001

Mann JJ, Malone KM, Psych MR [sic], et al: Attempted suicide characteristics and cerebrospinal fluid amine metabolites in depressed inpatients. Neuropsychopharmacology 15:576–586, 1996

Mann JJ, Huang YY, Underwood MD, et al: A serotonin transporter gene promoter polymorphism (5-HTTLPR) and prefrontal cortical binding in major depression and suicide. Arch Gen Psychiatry 57:729–738, 2000

Mansour HA, Talkowski ME, Wood J, et al: Serotonin gene polymorphisms and bipolar I disorder: focus on the serotonin transporter. Ann Med 37:590–602, 2005

Marin RS: Apathy: concept, syndrome, neural mechanisms, and treatment. Semin Clin Neuropsychiatry 1:304–314, 1996

Martinot M, Bragulat V, Artiges E, et al: Decreased presynaptic dopamine function in the left caudate of depressed patients with affective flattening and psychomotor retardation. Am J Psychiatry 158:314–316, 2001

Mayberg HS: Frontal lobe dysfunction in secondary depression. J Neuropsychiatry Clin Neurosci 6:428–442, 1994

Mayberg HS: Modulating dysfunctional limbic-cortical circuits in depression: towards development of brain-based algorithms for diagnosis and optimised treatment. Br Med Bull 65:193–207, 2003

Mayberg HS, Solomon DH: Depression in Parkinson's disease: a biochemical and organic viewpoint. Adv Neurol 65:49–60, 1995

Mayberg HS, Robinson RG, Wong DF, et al: PET imaging of cortical S2 serotonin receptors after stroke: lateralized changes and relationship to depression. Am J Psychiatry 145:937–943, 1988

Mayberg HS, Starkstein SE, Sadzot B, et al: Selective hypometabolism in the inferior frontal lobe in depressed patients with Parkinson's disease. Ann Neurol 28:57–64, 1990

Mayberg HS, Starkstein SE, Peyser CE, et al: Paralimbic frontal lobe hypometabolism in depression associated with Huntington's disease. Neurology 42:1791–1797, 1992

Mayberg HS, Lewis PJ, Regenold W, et al: Paralimbic hypoperfusion in unipolar depression. J Nucl Med 35:929–934, 1994

Mayberg HS, Brannan SK, Mahurin RK, et al: Cingulate function in depression: a potential predictor of treatment response. Neuroreport 8:1057–1061, 1997

Mayberg HS, Lozano AM, Voon V, et al: Deep brain stimulation for treatment-resistant depression. Neuron 45:651–660, 2005

McCrae RR, Costa PT Jr: Validation of the five-factor model of personality across instruments and observers. J Pers Soc Psychol 52:81–90, 1987

McGuffin P, Rijsdijk F, Andrew M, et al: The heritability of bipolar affective disorder and the genetic relationship to unipolar depression. Arch Gen Psychiatry 60:497–502, 2003

Meyer JH, Kruger S, Wilson AA, et al: Lower dopamine transporter binding potential in striatum during depression. Neuroreport 12:4121–4125, 2001

Meyer JH, Goulding VS, Wilson AA, et al: Bupropion occupancy of the dopamine transporter is low during clinical treatment. Psychopharmacology (Berl) 163:102–105, 2002

Morton AJ, Wood NI, Hastings MH, et al: Disintegration of the sleep-wake cycle and circadian timing in Huntington's disease. J Neurosci 25:157–163, 2005

Murphy FC, Sahakian BJ: Neuropsychology of bipolar disorder. Br J Psychiatry Suppl 41:S120–S127, 2001

Murphy FC, Sahakian BJ, Rubinsztein JS, et al: Emotional bias and inhibitory control processes in mania and depression. Psychol Med 29:1307–1321, 1999

Musselman DL, Nemeroff CB: Depression and endocrine disorders: focus on the thyroid and adrenal system. Br J Psychiatry Suppl 30:S123–S128, 1996

Nelson JC: A review of the efficacy of serotonergic and noradrenergic reuptake inhibitors for treatment of major depression. Biol Psychiatry 46:1301–1308, 1999

Nemeroff CB, Simon JS, Haggerty JJ Jr, et al: Antithyroid antibodies in depressed patients. Am J Psychiatry 142:840–843, 1985

Nemeroff CB, Bissette G, Akil H, et al: Neuropeptide concentrations in the cerebrospinal fluid of depressed patients treated with electroconvulsive therapy: corticotrophin-releasing factor, beta-endorphin and somatostatin. Br J Psychiatry 158:59–63, 1991

Neumeister A, Nugent AC, Waldeck T, et al: Neural and behavioral responses to tryptophan depletion in unmedicated patients with remitted major depressive disorder and controls. Arch Gen Psychiatry 61:765–773, 2004

Nierenberg AA, Dougherty D, Rosenbaum JF: Dopaminergic agents and stimulants as antidepressant augmentation strategies. J Clin Psychiatry 59 (suppl 5):60–63; discussion 64, 1998

Nobler MS, Oquendo MA, Kegeles LS, et al: Decreased regional brain metabolism after ECT. Am J Psychiatry 158:305–308, 2001

Nofzinger EA, Thase ME, Reynolds CF 3rd, et al: Hypersomnia in bipolar depression: a comparison with narcolepsy using the multiple sleep latency test. Am J Psychiatry 148:1177–1181, 1991

O'Brien SM, Scott LV, Dinan TG: Cytokines: abnormalities in major depression and implications for pharmacological treatment. Hum Psychopharmacol 19:397–403, 2004

Oda K, Okubo Y, Ishida R, et al: Regional cerebral blood flow in depressed patients with white matter magnetic resonance hyperintensity. Biol Psychiatry 53:150–156, 2003

Okuda DT, Chyung AS, Chin CT, et al: Acute pathological laughter. Mov Disord 20:1389–1390, 2005

Okun MS, Raju DV, Walter BL, et al: Pseudobulbar crying induced by stimulation in the region of the subthalamic nucleus. J Neurol Neurosurg Psychiatry 75:921–923, 2004

Owens MJ, Nemeroff CB: Role of serotonin in the pathophysiology of depression: focus on the serotonin transporter. Clin Chem 40:288–295, 1994

Paul IA, Skolnick P: Glutamate and depression: clinical and preclinical studies. Ann N Y Acad Sci 1003:250–272, 2003

Petit D, Gagnon JF, Fantini ML, et al: Sleep and quantitative EEG in neurodegenerative disorders. J Psychosom Res 56:487–496, 2004

Peyser CE, Folstein SE: Huntington's disease as a model for mood disorders: clues from neuropathology and neurochemistry. Mol Chem Neuropathol 12:99–119, 1990

Pezawas L, Meyer-Lindenberg A, Drabant EM, et al: 5-HTTLPR polymorphism impacts human cingulate-amygdala interactions: a genetic susceptibility mechanism for depression. Nat Neurosci 8:828–834, 2005

Phelps EA, LeDoux JE: Contributions of the amygdala to emotion processing: from animal models to human behavior. Neuron 48:175–187, 2005

Phillips ML, Drevets WC, Rauch SL, et al: Neurobiology of emotion perception, I: the neural basis of normal emotion perception. Biol Psychiatry 54:504–514, 2003a

Phillips ML, Drevets WC, Rauch SL, et al: Neurobiology of emotion perception, II: implications for major psychiatric disorders. Biol Psychiatry 54:515–528, 2003b

Pizzagalli DA, Oakes TR, Fox AS, et al: Functional but not structural subgenual prefrontal cortex abnormalities in melancholia. Mol Psychiatry 9:393–405, 2004

Pluck GC, Brown RG: Apathy in Parkinson's disease. J Neurol Neurosurg Psychiatry 73:636–642, 2002

Posener JA, DeBattista C, Williams GH, et al: 24-Hour monitoring of cortisol and corticotropin secretion in psychotic and nonpsychotic major depression. Arch Gen Psychiatry 57:755–760, 2000

Post RM, DeLisi LE, Holcomb HH, et al: Glucose utilization in the temporal cortex of affectively ill patients: positron emission tomography. Biol Psychiatry 22:545–553, 1987

Raison CL, Capuron L, Miller AH: Cytokines sing the blues: inflammation and the pathogenesis of depression. Trends Immunol 27:24–31, 2006

Rajkowska G: Postmortem studies in mood disorders indicate altered numbers of neurons and glial cells. Biol Psychiatry 48:766–777, 2000

Raskind MA: The clinical interface of depression and dementia. J Clin Psychiatry 59 (suppl 10):9–12, 1998

Reddy PL, Khanna S, Subhash MN, et al: CSF amine metabolites in depression. Biol Psychiatry 31:112–118, 1992

Remy P, Doder M, Lees A, et al: Depression in Parkinson's disease: loss of dopamine and noradrenaline innervation in the limbic system. Brain 128 (pt 6):1314–1322, 2005

Rimon R, Le Greves P, Nyberg F, et al: Elevation of substance P-like peptides in the CSF of psychiatric patients. Biol Psychiatry 19:509–516, 1984

Ring HA, Bench CJ, Trimble MR, et al: Depression in Parkinson's disease: a positron emission study. Br J Psychiatry 165:333–339, 1994

Robinson RG, Kubos KL, Starr LB, et al: Mood disorders in stroke patients: importance of location of lesion. Brain 107 (pt 1):81–93, 1984

Robinson S, Sandstrom SM, Denenberg VH, et al: Distinguishing whether dopamine regulates liking, wanting, and/or learning about rewards. Behav Neurosci 119:5–15, 2005

Roesch MR, Olson CR: Neuronal activity related to reward value and motivation in primate frontal cortex. Science 304(5668):307–310, 2004

Rogers MA, Kasai K, Koji M, et al: Executive and prefrontal dysfunction in unipolar depression: a review of neuropsychological and imaging evidence. Neurosci Res 50:1–11, 2004

Rosen HJ, Allison SC, Schauer GF, et al: Neuroanatomical correlates of behavioural disorders in dementia. Brain 128 (pt 11):2612–2625, 2005

Rosenberg P, Herishanu Y, Beilin B: Increased appetite (bulimia) in Parkinson's disease. J Am Geriatr Soc 25:277–278, 1977

Roy A, Pickar D, Douillet P, et al: Urinary monoamines and monoamine metabolites in subtypes of unipolar depressive disorder and normal controls. Psychol Med 16:541–546, 1986

Roy A, Karoum F, Pollack S: Marked reduction in indexes of dopamine metabolism among patients with depression who attempt suicide. Arch Gen Psychiatry 49:447–450, 1992

Royant-Parola S, Borbely AA, Tobler I, et al: Monitoring of long-term motor activity in depressed patients. Br J Psychiatry 149:288–293, 1986

Ruggiero DA, Underwood MD, Rice PM, et al: Corticotropic-releasing hormone and serotonin interact in the human brainstem: behavioral implications. Neuroscience 91:1343–1354, 1999

Santor DA, Bagby RM, Joffe RT: Evaluating stability and change in personality and depression. J Pers Soc Psychol 73:1354–1362, 1997

Sargent PA, Kjaer KH, Bench CJ, et al: Brain serotonin1A receptor binding measured by positron emission tomography with [11C]WAY-100635: effects of depression and antidepressant treatment. Arch Gen Psychiatry 57:174–180, 2000

Schiffer R, Pope LE: Review of pseudobulbar affect including a novel and potential therapy. J Neuropsychiatry Clin Neurosci 17:447–454, 2005

Schildkraut JJ: The catecholamine hypothesis of affective disorders: a review of supporting evidence. Am J Psychiatry 122:509–522, 1965

Schinka JA, Busch RM, Robichaux-Keene N: A meta-analysis of the association between the serotonin transporter gene polymorphism (5-HTTLPR) and trait anxiety. Mol Psychiatry 9:197–202, 2004

Seminowicz DA, Mayberg HS, McIntosh AR, et al: Limbic-frontal circuitry in major depression: a path modeling metanalysis. Neuroimage 22:409–418, 2004

Sharpley AL, Cowen PJ: Effect of pharmacologic treatments on the sleep of depressed patients. Biol Psychiatry 37:85–98, 1995

Sheline YI: Neuroimaging studies of mood disorder effects on the brain. Biol Psychiatry 54:338–352, 2003

Silvestri R, Raffaele M, De Domenico P, et al: Sleep features in Tourette's syndrome, neuroacanthocytosis and Huntington's chorea. Neurophysiol Clin 25:66–77, 1995

Slaughter JR, Martens MP, Slaughter KA: Depression and Huntington's disease: prevalence, clinical manifestations, etiology, and treatment. CNS Spectr 6:306–326, 2001

Snaith P: Anhedonia: a neglected symptom of psychopathology. Psychol Med 23:957–966, 1993

Sobin C, Sackeim HA: Psychomotor symptoms of depression. Am J Psychiatry 154:4–17, 1997

Starkstein SE, Robinson RG, Price TR: Comparison of cortical and subcortical lesions in the production of poststroke mood disorders. Brain 110 (pt 4):1045–1059, 1987

Starkstein SE, Mayberg HS, Berthier ML, et al: Mania after brain injury: neuroradiological and metabolic findings. Ann Neurol 27:652–659, 1990

Starkstein SE, Garau ML, Cao A: Prevalence and clinical correlates of disinhibition in dementia. Cogn Behav Neurol 17:139–147, 2004

Starkstein SE, Jorge R, Mizrahi R, et al: A prospective longitudinal study of apathy in Alzheimer's disease. J Neurol Neurosurg Psychiatry 77:8–11, 2006

Stip E, Lecours AR, Chertkow H, et al: Influence of affective words on lexical decision task in major depression. J Psychiatry Neurosci 19:202–207, 1994

Strakowski SM, Delbello MP, Adler CM: The functional neuroanatomy of bipolar disorder: a review of neuroimaging findings. Mol Psychiatry 10:105–116, 2005

Strauss J, Barr CL, George CJ, et al: BDNF and COMT polymorphisms: relation to memory phenotypes in young adults with childhood-onset mood disorder. Neuromolecular Med 5:181–192, 2004

Stuss DT, Benson DF: The Frontal Lobes. New York, Raven, 1986

Szabadi E, Bradshaw CM, Besson JA: Elongation of pause-time in speech: a simple, objective measure of motor retardation in depression. Br J Psychiatry 129:592–597, 1976

Talbot PS, Cooper SJ: Anterior cingulate and subgenual prefrontal blood flow changes following tryptophan depletion in healthy males. Neuropsychopharmacology 31:1757–1767, 2006

Tan H, Zhong P, Yan Z: Corticotropin-releasing factor and acute stress prolongs serotonergic regulation of GABA transmission in prefrontal cortical pyramidal neurons. J Neurosci 24:5000–5008, 2004

Taylor C, Fricker AD, Devi LA, et al: Mechanisms of action of antidepressants: from neurotransmitter systems to signaling pathways. Cell Signal 17:549–557, 2005

Teasdale JD, Russell ML: Differential effects of induced mood on the recall of positive, negative and neutral words. Br J Clin Psychol 22 (pt 3):163–171, 1983

Trejo A, Boll MC, Alonso ME, et al: Use of oral nutritional supplements in patients with Huntington's disease. Nutrition 21:889–894, 2005

Tremblay LK, Naranjo CA, Graham SJ, et al: Functional neuroanatomical substrates of altered reward processing in major depressive disorder revealed by a dopaminergic probe. Arch Gen Psychiatry 62:1228–1236, 2005

van Reekum R, Stuss DT, Ostrander L: Apathy: why care? J Neuropsychiatry Clin Neurosci 17:7–19, 2005

Veith RC, Lewis N, Langohr JI, et al: Effect of desipramine on cerebrospinal fluid concentrations of corticotropin-releasing factor in human subjects. Psychiatry Res 46:1–8, 1993

Videbech P: PET measurements of brain glucose metabolism and blood flow in major depressive disorder: a critical review. Acta Psychiatr Scand 101:11–20, 2000

Videbech P, Ravnkilde B, Pedersen TH, et al: The Danish PET/depression project: clinical symptoms and cerebral blood flow: a regions-of-interest analysis. Acta Psychiatr Scand 106:35–44, 2002

Volkow ND, Wang GJ, Ma Y, et al: Activation of orbital and medial prefrontal cortex by methylphenidate in cocaine-addicted subjects but not in controls: relevance to addiction. J Neurosci 25:3932–3939, 2005

Vollm BA, de Araujo IE, Cowen PJ, et al: Methamphetamine activates reward circuitry in drug naive human subjects. Neuropsychopharmacology 29:1715–1722, 2004

Wallis JD, Miller EK: Neuronal activity in primate dorsolateral and orbital prefrontal cortex during performance of a reward preference task. Eur J Neurosci 18:2069–2081, 2003

Waxman MJ, Durfee D, Moore M, et al: Nutritional aspects and swallowing function of patients with Parkinson's disease. Nutr Clin Pract 5:196–199, 1990

Whalen PJ, Bush G, McNally RJ, et al: The emotional counting Stroop paradigm: a functional magnetic resonance imaging probe of the anterior cingulate affective division. Biol Psychiatry 44:1219–1228, 1998

Wilhelm K, Mitchell PB, Niven H, et al: Life events, first depression onset and the serotonin transporter gene. Br J Psychiatry 188:210–215, 2006

Wise RA: Brain reward circuitry: insights from unsensed incentives. Neuron 36:229–240, 2002

Wise RA: Forebrain substrates of reward and motivation. J Comp Neurol 493:115–121, 2005

Wu JC, Bunney WE: The biological basis of an antidepressant response to sleep deprivation and relapse: review and hypothesis. Am J Psychiatry 147:14–21, 1990

Wu J, Buchsbaum MS, Gillin JC, et al: Prediction of antidepressant effects of sleep deprivation by metabolic rates in the ventral anterior cingulate and medial prefrontal cortex. Am J Psychiatry 156:1149–1158, 1999

Wu JC, Buchsbaum M, Bunney WE Jr: Clinical neurochemical implications of sleep deprivation's effects on the anterior cingulate of depressed responders. Neuropsychopharmacology 25 (5 suppl):S74–S78, 2001

Young SN, Smith SE, Pihl RO, et al: Tryptophan depletion causes a rapid lowering of mood in normal males. Psychopharmacology (Berl) 87:173–177, 1985

Zarate CA Jr, Du J, Quiroz J, et al: Regulation of cellular plasticity cascades in the pathophysiology and treatment of mood disorders: role of the glutamatergic system. Ann N Y Acad Sci 1003:273–291, 2003

Zarate CA Jr, Payne JL, Singh J, et al: Pramipexole for bipolar II depression: a placebo-controlled proof of concept study. Biol Psychiatry 56:54–60, 2004

Zeilig G, Drubach DA, Katz-Zeilig M, et al: Pathological laughter and crying in patients with closed traumatic brain injury. Brain Inj 10:591–597, 1996

Zhang R, Tachibana T, Takagi T, et al: Serotonin modifies corticotropin-releasing factor-induced behaviors of chicks. Behav Brain Res 151:47–52, 2004

Zhuang X, Oosting RS, Jones SR, et al: Hyperactivity and impaired response habituation in hyperdopaminergic mice. Proc Natl Acad Sci U S A 98:1982–1987, 2001

28

NEUROPSYCHIATRIC ASPECTS OF ANXIETY DISORDERS

Dan J. Stein, M.D., Ph.D.
Scott L. Rauch, M.D.

Although anxiety has long held a central place in theories of psychopathology (Freud 1926/1959), it has only recently been appreciated that the anxiety disorders are among the most prevalent of the psychiatric disorders (Kessler et al. 1994, 2005) and that they account for perhaps a third of all costs of mental illness (Dupont et al. 1996). Furthermore, although it has long been recognized that specific neurological lesions may lead to anxiety symptoms (von Economo 1931), only in the past several years have advances in research allowed particular neuroanatomical hypotheses to be put forward about each of the different anxiety disorders. In this chapter, we review these developments in our understanding of the anxiety disorders from the perspective of neuropsychiatry. We begin by reviewing neurological disorders that may present with anxiety symptoms and then outline neuroanatomical models of each of the main anxiety disorders.

DSM-III (American Psychiatric Association 1980) provided significant impetus to research on the anxiety disorders by replacing the category of "anxiety neurosis" with several different conditions and by providing each with operational diagnostic criteria. DSM-IV-TR (American Psychiatric Association 2000) anxiety disorders include panic disorder with and without agoraphobia, social phobia (social anxiety disorder), posttraumatic stress disorder (PTSD), generalized anxiety disorder (GAD), obsessive-compulsive disorder (OCD), substance-induced anxiety disorder, and anxiety disorder due to a general medical condition. Although the inclusion of OCD in the category of anxiety disorders remains somewhat controversial (Montgomery 1993), for the purposes of this volume, we use the current DSM classification.

In each of the anxiety disorders, it is perhaps possible to discern a component comprising anxiety symptoms and a component comprising avoidance symptoms. In panic disorder, the anxiety symptoms are those of the panic attack—a discrete period of anxiety that develops rapidly, often spontaneously. The person also may develop agoraphobia symptoms, or avoidance of those stimuli that appear to promote panic attacks. In social phobia, panic attacks develop only in the context of social or performance situations in which the person fears embarrass-

Dr. Stein is supported by the Medical Research Council of South Africa.

ment or humiliation. As a result of these fears, the person may avoid these situations. In PTSD, in the aftermath of a traumatic event, the person has reexperiencing and hyperarousal symptoms, as well as a range of avoidance and numbing symptoms. In GAD, patients have anxiety about the future, and worry may serve as an avoidance behavior.

OCD is similarly characterized by both obsessions (intrusive thoughts or images that increase anxiety) and compulsions (repetitive behaviors or mental acts undertaken in response to obsessions or performed according to particular rules), which reduce anxiety. Several disorders have overlapping phenomenological and neurobiological features with OCD; these putative OCD spectrum disorders may include body dysmorphic disorder (characterized by intrusive thoughts of imagined ugliness), Tourette syndrome (in which OCD symptoms are often comorbid), and trichotillomania (characterized by repetitive hair pulling). Further brief notes on symptomatology are provided in the relevant sections below.

NEUROLOGICAL DISORDERS WITH ANXIETY SYMPTOMS

Neurological conditions that affect a range of different neuroanatomical structures may be associated with anxiety symptoms or disorders (Muller et al. 2005; Wise and Rundell 1999). Given that temporolimbic regions, striatum, and prefrontal cortex all likely play an important role in the pathogenesis of certain anxiety disorders, we begin by reviewing the association between lesions in these areas and subsequent anxiety symptoms before moving on to disorders with more widespread pathology. This literature not only is clinically relevant but also raises valuable questions for further research.

Various lesions of the temporolimbic regions have been associated with the subsequent development of panic disorder. Temporal lobe seizures (Bernik et al. 2002; Cavenar and Harris 1979), tumors (Kellner et al. 1996), arteriovenous malformation (Wall et al. 1985), lobectomy (Wall et al. 1986), and parahippocampal infarction (Maricle et al. 1991) all have been reported to present with panic attacks. The association seems particularly strong with right-sided lesions. (Conversely, removal of the amygdala results in both placidity toward previously feared objects [Klüver and Bucy 1939] and deficits in fear conditioning [Bechara et al. 1995].)

This literature, taken together with clinical observations that panic disorder may be accompanied by dissociation and depersonalization (Toni et al. 1996) and possibly by electroencephalographic abnormalities (Bystritsky et al. 1999) and temporal abnormalities (see "Panic Dis-

order" section below), as well as preliminary data that panic disorder can respond to anticonvulsants, raises the question of whether partially overlapping mechanisms may be at work in both temporal lobe seizure disorder and panic disorder (Weilburg et al. 1987). Certainly, it has been suggested that electroencephalogram (EEG) and anticonvulsant trials may be appropriate in patients with panic disorder refractory to conventional treatment (Kinrys and Wygant 2005; McNamara and Fogel 1990).

Lesions of the basal ganglia have been associated with obsessions and compulsions, a finding that has been crucial to the development of a "cortico-striatal-thalamic-cortical" (CSTC) hypothesis of OCD. An early "striatal topography" hypothesis was that caudate lesions in particular are associated with OCD, whereas putamen lesions result in tics (Rauch and Baxter 1998). On the other hand, there is also evidence that OCD is mediated by a range of CSTC circuits (Rosenberg and Keshavan 1998), and particular projection fields or cell types may be associated with specific kinds of symptoms.

The 1915–1926 pandemic of viral encephalitis lethargica provided early evidence of a specific neurological basis for OCD. The outbreak was followed by the presentation of numerous patients with a somnolent-like state and parkinsonian features. Various focal brain lesions, including involvement of the basal ganglia, were documented in these cases, and patients also were observed to have obsessive-compulsive symptoms and tics (Cheyette and Cummings 1995; von Economo 1931).

OCD symptoms also have been reported in a range of other basal ganglia lesions of various etiologies. Thus, OCD symptoms may be seen in Huntington's disease (Anderson et al. 2001), Parkinson's disease (Alegret et al. 2001), spasmodic torticollis (Wenzel et al. 1998), and basal ganglia lesions of a range of etiologies, including calcification, infarction, intoxication, and trauma (Cummings and Cunningham 1992). In this context, it is noteworthy that the basal ganglia may be particularly sensitive to prenatal and perinatal hypoxic-ischemic injury (in twins with Tourette syndrome, for example, an association exists between lower birth weight and increased severity of Tourette syndrome [Hyde and Weinberger 1995]).

Furthermore, early studies suggested a link between Sydenham's chorea and OCD symptoms (Grimshaw 1964), and a study by Swedo et al. (1989) reported that rheumatic fever patients with Sydenham's chorea had significantly more OCD symptoms than did those without chorea. This work has had exciting implications, insofar as it has formed the basis for an autoimmune theory of at least some cases of OCD. Swedo and colleagues have coined the term *PANDAS*, or pediatric autoimmune neuropsychiatric disorders associated with streptococcal infections, to describe patients who present with acute obsessive-compulsive or tic symptoms, hypothetically after developing antistriatal antibodies in response to infection (Swedo et al. 1998).

Some of the most promising research on the association between OCD and a movement disorder focused on the relation of OCD to Tourette syndrome. Gilles de la Tourette's (1885) initial description of the syndrome included a patient with tics, vocalizations, and perhaps obsessions. Increasing evidence suggests that a subgroup of patients with Tourette syndrome also has OCD (Sheppard et al. 1999). Conversely, a subgroup of OCD patients has tics (Goodman et al. 1990). Furthermore, family studies have found a high rate of OCD and/or tics in relatives of patients with Tourette syndrome and a high rate of Tourette syndrome and/or tics in relatives of OCD patients (Pato et al. 2001; Pauls et al. 1986).

Anxiety symptoms other than OCD may, however, also be seen in striatal disorders (Lauterbach et al. 1998). In Huntington's disease, for example, anxiety has been reported as a common prodromal symptom, with later development of several different anxiety disorders including OCD (Leroi and Michalon 1998; Tost et al. 2004). Anxiety symptoms and disorders are also common in Parkinson's disorder (Richard et al. 1996; Walsh and Bennett 2001) and may correlate inversely with left striatal dopamine transporter availability (Weintraub et al. 2005). Such findings arguably indicate that further attention should be paid to the role of the dopaminergic system in anxiety disorders (Stein et al. 2002), although other neurotransmitter systems also may be important in mediating anxiety symptoms in Parkinson's disorder (Menza et al. 1999, 2004).

Lesions of the frontal cortex may be associated with a range of perseverative symptoms. In the classic case of Phineas Gage, in addition to impairment in executive functions, the patient had perseverative symptoms and hoarding behaviors (Damasio 1994). Similarly, more recent cases of OCD after frontal lobe involvement have been documented. Ames et al. (1994) reviewed the literature on frontal lobe degeneration and subsequent obsessive-compulsive symptoms and noted descriptions of a range of repetitive behaviors from motor stereotypies to OCD.

Anxiety symptoms and disorders can, of course, be seen in a range of neurological disorders that affect multiple brain regions, including frontal cortex. In multiple sclerosis (MS), for example, anxiety symptoms may be found in up to 37% of subjects (Diaz-Olavarrieta et al. 1999), and anxiety disorders are also not uncommon (Riether 1999). Whether this anxiety reflects a psychological reaction or reflects the deposition of demyelinating plaques remains somewhat unclear, but treatment of symptoms should not be ignored (Riether 1999; Zorzon et al. 2001).

Similarly, anxiety symptoms have been noted to be common in Alzheimer's disease and in other dementias including vascular and frontotemporal dementias (Ballard et al. 2000; Porter et al. 2003). The relation between regional pathology and anxiety symptoms in these conditions deserves further attention. Additional work on the management of anxiety in dementia is also needed (Qazi et al. 2003).

Although the prevalence of depression after stroke has been well studied, less research has focused on anxiety after stroke. In one study, however, of 309 admissions to a stroke unit, DSM-III-R (American Psychiatric Association 1987) GAD was present in 26.9% of the patients (Castillo et al. 1993). The authors reported that anxiety plus depression was associated with left cortical lesions, whereas anxiety alone was associated with right hemisphere lesions. Also, worry was associated with anterior and GAD with right posterior lesions. Longitudinal studies have found that GAD can persist for several years after the stroke (Astrom 1996; Morrison et al. 2005). Again, anxiety plus depression may be associated with left hemisphere lesions and anxiety alone with right hemisphere lesions (Astrom 1996). Finally, it has been reported that agoraphobia was even more common than GAD after stroke (Burvill et al. 1995).

Anxiety disorders also have been reported in the aftermath of traumatic brain injury (Hiott and Labbate 2002). In one study, prevalence rates were 19% for PTSD, 15% for OCD, 14% for panic disorder, 10% for phobias, and 9% for GAD (Hibbard et al. 1998). Some evidence indicates relations between areas affected and risk for anxiety (Vasa et al. 2004). Of particular interest is the finding that PTSD can develop even when the patient has neurogenic amnesia for the traumatic event; this finding may suggest that implicit memories of trauma are sufficient for later PTSD to emerge, although subsequent appraisal processes also may be relevant (Joseph and Masterson 1999). In either event, PTSD in such patients may be unusual because reexperiencing symptoms are absent (Harvey et al. 2003; Warden et al. 1997).

NEUROANATOMY OF ANXIETY DISORDERS

In the following sections, we consider the neuropsychiatry of each of the major anxiety disorders. Each section begins by sketching a simplistic neuroanatomical model of the relevant anxiety disorder. This sketch is then used as a framework for attempting a more complex integration of animal data, clinical biological research (e.g., pharmacological probe studies), and brain imaging studies. Although much remains to be learned about the neurobiology of the anxiety disorders, there is a growing consolidation of different avenues of information, with increasingly specific models now existing for each of the major anxiety disorders.

GENERALIZED ANXIETY DISORDER

The term *generalized anxiety disorder* was first introduced in DSM-III, where it represented a refinement of the earlier concept of "anxiety neurosis." In DSM-III, GAD was viewed as a residual diagnosis, to be made in the absence of other disorders. More recent editions of DSM have, however, increasingly emphasized the cognitive symptoms of GAD and have also emphasized that GAD is an independent entity that may be found alone or comorbidly with other anxiety and mood conditions. GAD is the least common anxiety disorder in specialty anxiety clinics but the most common anxiety disorder in primary care practice (Kessler 2000).

Neuroanatomical models of GAD have not been well delineated to date. However, it may be speculated that GAD involves 1) a general "limbic circuit," including paralimbic cortex (e.g., anterior temporal cortex, posterior medial orbitofrontal cortex) and related subcortical structures (e.g., amygdala), which may be activated across a range of different anxiety disorders, and 2) perhaps some degree of prefrontal hyperactivity, which may represent an attempt across the anxiety disorders to suppress subcortically mediated anxiety or which may arguably reflect more specific GAD symptoms of excessive worrying and planning (Figure 28–1). In reviewing research relevant to this speculative model, we consider first neurochemical studies and then neuroanatomical findings.

Neurochemical Studies

Serotonergic mediation of GAD is supported by several findings. First, reduced cerebrospinal fluid levels of serotonin and reduced platelet paroxetine binding have been observed in this disorder (Iny et al. 1994). Second, administration of the pharmacological probe *m*-chlorophenylpiperazine (m-CPP), a serotonergic agonist, results in increased anxiety and hostility (Germine et al. 1992). Third, serotonergic compounds appear effective in the pharmacotherapy for GAD; buspirone, a serotonin type 1A (5-HT$_{1A}$) receptor partial agonist is effective in some studies, and growing evidence now shows the efficacy of the selective serotonin reuptake inhibitors (SSRIs) in this disorder (Baldwin and Polkinghorn 2005).

Animal work has long established the involvement of the locus coeruleus–norepinephrine–sympathetic nervous system in fear and arousal (Redmond 1986). In clinical studies of GAD, increased plasma norepinephrine

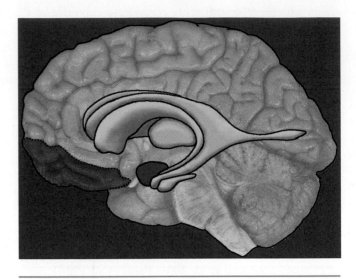

FIGURE 28–1.   Neuroanatomical model of generalized anxiety disorder. Note the increased activity in temporolimbic areas (Tiihonen et al. 1997b; Wu et al. 1991) as well as in prefrontal areas (Rauch et al. 1997; Wu et al. 1991).

Source.   Reprinted from Stein DJ: *False Alarm! How to Conquer the Anxiety Disorders.* Cape Town, South Africa, University of Stellenbosch, 2000. Used with permission.

and 3-methoxy-4-hydroxyphenylglycol (MHPG) and reduced platelet α_2-adrenergic peripheral receptor binding sites have been reported, although not all studies of static noradrenergic measures have produced consistent findings. Administration of more dynamic adrenergic probes has, however, indicated reduced adrenergic receptor sensitivity in GAD, perhaps an adaptation to high circulating catecholamines (Nutt 2001). The locus coeruleus system may well play a regulatory role in GAD, even if it is not the sole dysfunctional neurochemical system in the disorder. Indeed, dual serotonin and noradrenergic reuptake inhibitors have been shown effective in GAD. The locus coeruleus system projects to the amygdala and to other structures involved in anxiety responses, so that noradrenergic involvement is not inconsistent with the neuroanatomical model outlined earlier.

Involvement of the γ-aminobutyric acid (GABA)–benzodiazepine receptor complex in GAD is supported by several studies, including the responsiveness of this disorder to benzodiazepine treatment. Thus, anxious subjects (Weizman et al. 1987) and GAD patients (Rocca et al. 1991) have reduced benzodiazepine binding capacity, with normalization of findings after benzodiazepine treatment. GABA is the brain's predominant inhibitory neurotransmitter, and GABAergic pathways are widely distributed; nevertheless, the distribution of GABA and benzodiazepine receptors is particularly dense in limbic and paralimbic areas.

Neuroanatomical Studies

Neuroimaging research on GAD remains at a relatively preliminary stage. Nevertheless, findings are arguably consistent with involvement of limbic, paralimbic, and prefrontal regions. An early topographical EEG study indicated differences between patients with GAD and nonanxious control subjects in temporal and occipital regions (Buchsbaum et al. 1985). Later work by this group with positron emission tomography (PET) found that GAD patients had increased relative metabolic rates in right posterior temporal lobe, right precentral frontal gyrus, and left inferior area 17 in the occipital lobe but reduced absolute basal ganglia metabolic rates (Wu et al. 1991). Furthermore, benzodiazepine treatment resulted in decreases in absolute metabolic rates for limbic system and cortical surface (Wu et al. 1991). Studies that used magnetic resonance imaging and spectroscopy provided additional data on the involvement of these circuits in GAD (Mathew et al. 2004; Milham et al. 2005).

Preliminary imaging data on receptor binding in GAD are also available. In a study of female GAD patients, for example, left temporal pole benzodiazepine receptor binding was significantly reduced (Tiihonen et al. 1997b). This work suggested a role for temporolimbic regions and the GABA–benzodiazepine receptor complex in mediating GAD symptoms. At present, imaging studies do not suggest dysregulation of the serotonin transporter in GAD (Maron et al. 2004b). Nevertheless, serotonergic neurons branch widely throughout the brain, affecting each of the main regions postulated to mediate anxiety symptoms (Figure 28–2); and SSRI treatment may result in a normalization of neuronal activity in pooled anxiety disorder subjects (Carey et al. 2004) and in GAD patients (Hoehn-Saric et al. 2005).

OBSESSIVE-COMPULSIVE DISORDER

The characteristic obsessions and compulsions of OCD have a strikingly similar form and content across different patients and different contexts, an observation that perhaps immediately raises the question of a specific neuropsychiatric basis for this condition. In addition, OCD has a lifetime prevalence of 2%–3% in most countries in which data are available (Weissman et al. 1994), again supporting a biomedical model. Also remarkable is the finding that OCD is one of the most disabling of all medical conditions worldwide (Murray and Lopez 1996). Certainly the cost to the world economy of OCD is likely to run into the billions of dollars annually (Stein et al. 2000a).

Current neuroanatomical models of OCD emphasize the role of CSTC circuits (Figure 28–3). There is growing realization of the importance of various CSTC loops in a range of behavior disorders (Cummings 1993); ventral

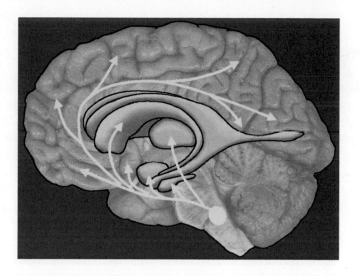

FIGURE 28–2. Serotonergic circuits project to key regions (prefrontal cortex, orbitofrontal cortex, anterior cingulate, amygdala, hippocampus, basal ganglia, thalamus) involved in the mediation of anxiety disorders.

Source. Reprinted from Stein DJ: *False Alarm! How to Conquer the Anxiety Disorders.* Cape Town, South Africa, University of Stellenbosch, 2000. Used with permission.

cognitive circuits, involving anterior and lateral orbitofrontal cortex, ventromedial caudate, and dorsomedial nuclei of the thalamus, appear to play a role in response inhibition, particularly in relation to certain kinds of cognitive-affective cues, and appear most relevant to OCD. This kind of model of OCD was first suggested by early findings of an association between neurological lesions of the striatum and OCD (see section "Neurological Disorders With Anxiety Symptoms" earlier in this chapter) and has been supported by a range of subsequent additional studies.

Similar CSTC circuits also have been hypothesized to be involved in various putative OCD spectrum disorders (such as Tourette syndrome). An early "striatal topography" model of OCD spectrum disorders suggested that whereas the ventral cognitive system mediated OCD symptoms, the sensorimotor cortex and putamen would instead be involved in Tourette syndrome and perhaps trichotillomania (Rauch and Baxter 1998). The data have not, however, fully supported such a model (Rosenberg and Keshavan 1998), and it is possible rather that particular striatal projection fields or cell types are involved in specific kinds of symptoms. We review findings relevant to the CSTC model in the following subsections on neurochemical and neuroanatomical studies in OCD.

Neurochemical Studies

Interest in the neurochemical substrate of OCD received significant impetus from the early finding that the disor-

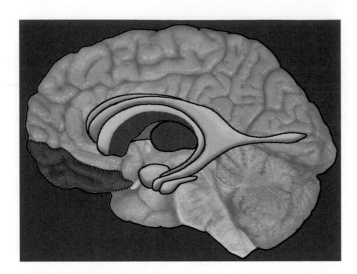

FIGURE 28–3. Neuroanatomical model of obsessive-compulsive disorder. Note the increased activity in the ventromedial cortico-striatal-thalamic-cortical circuit (Rauch and Baxter 1998).

Source. Reprinted from Stein DJ: *False Alarm! How to Conquer the Anxiety Disorders.* Cape Town, South Africa, University of Stellenbosch, 2000. Used with permission.

der responded to clomipramine, a serotonin reuptake inhibitor. Subsequent studies confirmed that clomipramine is more effective than desipramine, a noradrenergic reuptake inhibitor, in OCD (Zohar and Insel 1987). Furthermore, each of the SSRIs studied to date has been effective for the treatment of OCD (Vythilingum et al. 2000b). During effective treatment with a serotonin reuptake inhibitor, cerebrospinal fluid 5-hydroxyindoleacetic acid decreases (Thoren et al. 1980), and exacerbation of OCD symptoms by m-CPP is no longer seen after treatment with an SSRI (Zohar et al. 1988).

The serotonergic system innervates not only the basal ganglia but also the orbitofrontal cortex. Serotonergic abnormalities in OCD may be region specific; for example, in some studies, after administration of m-CPP, OCD symptoms are exacerbated (perhaps mediated by orbitofrontal cortex) but the neuroendocrine response is blunted (presumably mediated by hypothalamus) (Hollander et al. 1992). Of particular interest is animal work showing that downregulation of serotonin terminal autoreceptors in orbitofrontal cortex occurs only after a relatively long time and with relatively high doses of medication and does not occur after electroconvulsive therapy (El Mansari et al. 1995). This provides an elegant parallel with clinical findings that OCD pharmacotherapy differs from that used for depression.

Nevertheless, it is notable that many OCD patients do not respond to serotonin reuptake inhibitors, and not all patients show symptom exacerbation after m-CPP, suggesting that other neurochemical systems are also important. It is noteworthy that administration of dopamine agonists results in stereotypic behavior in animals and in tics in humans, and conversely, dopamine blockers are effective for the treatment of tics (Goodman et al. 1990). Furthermore, OCD patients with comorbid tics are less likely to respond to serotonin reuptake inhibitors but more likely to respond to augmentation of serotonin reuptake inhibitors with typical neuroleptics (McDougle et al. 1994).

Given the dopaminergic innervation of the striatum and the interaction between the serotonin and the dopaminergic systems (Kapur and Remington 1996), these findings are of course consistent with the CSTC model. Indeed, infusion of dopamine into the caudate results in stereotyped orofacial behaviors (grooming, gnawing) in animals (Fog and Pakkenberg 1971). Conversely, infusion of dopamine blockers into the same areas reduces amphetamine-induced stereotypy. Dopaminergic striatal circuits are presumably likely to be particularly important in OCD patients with tics and in patients with OCD spectrum disorders, such as Tourette syndrome, that are characterized by involuntary movements.

Other neurochemical systems, including glutamate and GABA, also play an important role in CSTC circuits (Carlsson 2001; Rosenberg and Keshavan 1998). In the future, manipulation of such systems may turn out to be useful for the pharmacotherapy of OCD.

Neuroanatomical Studies

A range of evidence indicates that corticostriatal circuits are important in mediating stereotypic behavior (Ridley 1994). Isolation of primates during development, for example, results in basal ganglia cytoarchitectural abnormalities and stereotypic behavior (Martin et al. 1991). MacLean (1973) noted that lesions of the striatum resulted in stereotypic behavior and suggested that this was a repository for fixed action patterns or inherited motor sequences (e.g., grooming, nest-building). Indeed, the animal literature on stereotypies and disorders of grooming parallels not only the phenomenology of OCD but also its psychopharmacology (Rapoport et al. 1992).

There is, however, a growing appreciation of the role of the striatum in cognition and learning. In particular, striatal function has increasingly been associated with the development, maintenance, and selection of motoric and cognitive procedural strategies. Different terms given to allude to this group of functions include *habit system* (Mishkin and Petri 1984), *response set* (Robbins and Brown 1990), and *procedural mobilization* (Saint-Cyr et al. 1995). Basal ganglia may play a particularly important role in the implicit learning of procedural strategies and their subsequent automatic execution. Certainly, neurological soft sign abnormalities and neuropsychological dysfunction in patients with OCD are consistent with dysfunction in CSTC circuits (Rauch et al. 1997, 2007; Stein et al. 1994).

Structural imaging studies are also consistent with a role for CSTC circuits in OCD. An early study found reduced caudate volume in OCD patients (Luxenberg et al. 1988), but not all subsequent research has replicated this finding. The finding that patients with PANDAS have increased basal ganglia volume (Giedd et al. 2000) may partly explain this inconsistency; in some OCD patients, basal ganglia volume initially may be increased, with subsequent reduction over time. Structural studies also have shown neuronal abnormalities or volume loss in orbitofrontal cortex, cingulate, amygdala, and thalamus in OCD (Valente et al. 2005). Also, putamen volume may be reduced in certain putative OCD spectrum disorders such as Tourette syndrome (Gerard and Peterson 2003) and trichotillomania (O'Sullivan et al. 1997).

Functional imaging studies, however, provide some of the most persuasive evidence of the role of CSTC circuits in OCD. OCD patients at rest, and especially when exposed to feared stimuli, show increased activity in the orbitofrontal cortex, anterior cingulate, and basal ganglia (Whiteside et al. 2004). A range of functional abnormalities also has been found in Tourette syndrome; one study, for example, found increased metabolism in the orbitofrontal cortex and putamen that correlated with complex behavioral and cognitive features (Braun et al. 1995). Interestingly, a single photon emission computed tomography (SPECT) study of patients with obsessive-compulsive symptoms found that regional cerebral blood flow (rCBF) differed depending on whether a family history of Tourette syndrome was present, with patterns similar to those seen in Tourette syndrome in patients from families affected with Tourette syndrome (Moriarty et al. 1997).

Functional imaging findings may have particular explanatory power when they also integrate cognitive neuroscience constructs and findings. Rauch and colleagues (1997), for example, have shown that during brain imaging of an implicit sequence learning task, control subjects without OCD showed striatal activation, but patients with OCD instead appeared to recruit medial temporal regions. These latter regions are typically involved in conscious cognitive-affective processing. Control subjects can process procedural strategies outside of awareness, but in OCD, these strategies intrude into consciousness. An additional set of studies has focused on the hypothesis that OCD is not a disorder of anxiety or fear but rather involves striatal disruption in the processing of disgust (Stein et al. 2001).

A further important set of findings that relate to the CSTC hypothesis of OCD emerges from work on neurosurgical treatments for OCD. Several different procedures have been used, but the general effect of these interventions is to interrupt CSTC circuits (Rauch et al. 2000). Some preliminary evidence suggests that right-sided neurosurgical lesions are most effective, a finding that raises interesting issues for future research on the laterality of OCD (Lippitz et al. 1999).

The "standard" neuroanatomical model of OCD may, however, be insufficiently complex to account for all cases. There is, for example, a literature on temporal lobe involvement in OCD. In some cases of OCD, temporal EEG abnormalities are seen (Jenike and Brotman 1984), and anticonvulsants may on occasion be useful (Khanna 1988). Similarly, in a study of OCD secondary to neurological abnormalities, SPECT scanning detected alterations not only in frontal areas but also in temporal regions (Hugo et al. 1999). A report described temporal lobe abnormalities in functional imaging of OCD patients with musical obsessions (Zungu-Dirwayi et al. 1999). Certainly, although OCD is in many ways a homogeneous entity, further research is necessary to delineate different neurobiological mechanisms, including divergent mediating neuronal circuitry, in symptom dimensions and subtypes of the disorder (Saxena and Rauch 2000).

Several studies have successfully integrated neurochemical and neuroimaging data. An early study reported that m-CPP exacerbation of OCD symptoms was associated with increased frontal rCBF (Hollander et al. 1995). A later SPECT study that used the $5-HT_{1D}$ probe sumatriptan also confirmed correlations between symptom changes and prefrontal rCBF, supporting a role for the terminal autoreceptor in OCD (Stein et al. 1999). In OCD, preliminary evidence now indicates alterations in components of the glutamatergic and serotonergic systems in frontostriatal circuitry (Adams et al. 2005; Rosenberg and Keshavan 1998) and disturbances in striatal dopamine transporter function (Talbot 2004; van der Wee et al. 2004). In Tourette syndrome, evidence also indicates alterations in striatal dopamine functioning (e.g., higher striatal binding to the dopamine transporter on imaging and in postmortem studies [Serra-Mestres et al. 2004]) and perhaps also disruptions in serotonin transporter function (Muller-Vahl et al. 2005). Finally, a seminal publication reported that patients with OCD treated with either serotonin reuptake inhibitors or behavior therapy had normalization of activity in CSTC circuits (Baxter et al. 1992); effective interventions appear to work via a final common pathway of specific brain structures.

Nevertheless, several important questions remain unresolved about the CSTC model of OCD. It is unclear, for example, how presumptive lesions to the CSTC occur. Despite the documentation of cases of PANDAS, the extent to which autoimmune processes contribute to OCD in general is not known. Also, there may be differential pathogenic mechanisms across different OCD spectrum disorders; for example, Tourette syndrome has been associated with autoantibodies against putamen but not caudate or globus pallidus (Singer et al. 1998). Finally, genetic variability may play some role; for example, some studies have found differences in polymorphisms in dopamine pathway candidate genes in OCD patients with and without tics (Pato et al. 2001).

Additionally, questions remain about the precise nature of CSTC dysfunction in OCD and its normalization by effective treatment. It is interesting, for example, that decreased orbitofrontal activity in OCD predicts positive response to pharmacotherapy, whereas higher orbitofrontal activity predicts positive response to behavior therapy (Brody et al. 1998). If the orbitofrontal cortex plays a role in extinguishing conditioned fear, then perhaps patients who already have increased activity are those for whom behavior therapy is possible. However, such hyperactivity may demand maximal serotonergic activation, and in patients who already have this, further SSRI-induced autoreceptor desensitization may be ineffective. Further work to consolidate fully a neuroanatomical model of both pharmacological and behavioral interventions in OCD is necessary.

PANIC DISORDER

Panic disorder is a highly prevalent disorder, with rates fairly similar across different social and cultural settings. It is now well recognized that panic disorder may be associated with significant morbidity (mood, anxiety, and substance use disorders) as well as with severe impairments in occupational and social functioning. Indeed, a growing pharmacoeconomic literature has emphasized the personal and financial costs of panic disorder; this is a serious disorder that has a substantial negative effect on quality of life.

Over the past decade or two, models of panic disorder have become increasingly sophisticated (Coplan et al. 1992; Gorman et al. 2000). Current neuroanatomical models of panic (Figure 28–4) emphasize 1) afferents from viscerosensory pathways to thalamus to the lateral nucleus of the amygdala, as well as from thalamus to cortical association areas to the lateral nucleus of the amygdala; 2) the extended amygdala, which is thought to play a central role in conditioned fear (Le Doux 1998) and anxiety (Davis and Whalen 2001); 3) the hippocampus, which is thought crucial for conditioning to the context of the fear (and so perhaps for phobic avoidance); and 4) efferent tracts from the amygdala to the hypothalamus and

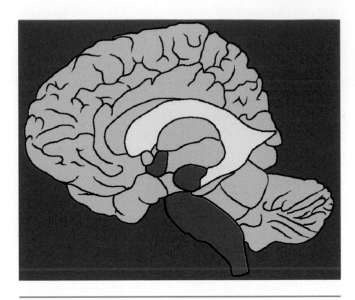

FIGURE 28–4. Neuroanatomical model of panic disorder. Note the activation of the amygdala, which has efferents to hypothalamus and brain stem sites (Gorman et al. 2000).

Source. Reprinted from Stein DJ: *False Alarm! How to Conquer the Anxiety Disorders.* Cape Town, South Africa, University of Stellenbosch, 2000. Used with permission.

brain stem structures, which mediate many of the symptoms of panic. Thus, efferents of the central nucleus of the amygdala include the lateral nucleus (autonomic arousal and sympathetic discharge) and paraventricular nucleus (increased adrenocorticoid release) of the hypothalamus and the locus coeruleus (increased norepinephrine release), parabrachial nucleus (increased respiratory rate), and periaqueductal gray (defensive behaviors and postural freezing) in the brain stem. This kind of general outline can be used as a starting framework for considering the range of data relevant to the neurobiology of panic disorder.

Neurochemical Studies

Early animal studies found that the locus coeruleus plays a key role in fear and anxiety (Redmond 1986), with both electrical and pharmacological stimulation resulting in fear responses. The locus coeruleus contains the highest concentration of noradrenergic-producing neurons in the brain. Viscerosensory input reaches the locus coeruleus via the nucleus tractus solitarius and the medullary nucleus paragigantocellularis, and the locus coeruleus sends efferents to a range of important structures, including the amygdala, hypothalamus, and brain stem periaqueductal gray (Coplan and Lydiard 1998).

Several clinical studies of panic disorder provide support for the role of the locus coeruleus; administration of yohimbine, for example, resulted in greater increases in MHPG in panic disorder patients than in control subjects without panic disorder. However, not all studies have replicated such findings, and studies of noradrenergic function in lactate-induced panic also have been inconsistent (Gorman et al. 2000), suggesting that additional neurochemical factors are important in the mediation of panic attacks.

Certainly, increasing evidence indicates that the serotonergic system plays a crucial role in panic disorder. A range of studies provides evidence for this; for example, several studies have found that m-CPP administration leads to an acute exacerbation of panic symptoms in panic disorder patients. Also, a good deal of evidence supports the efficacy of the SSRIs in panic disorder, with some indications that they may in fact be more effective than earlier classes of agents (Boyer 1995; Otto et al. 2001).

The serotonergic system interacts at several points with neuroanatomical structures thought important in panic disorder (Coplan and Lydiard 1998). First, serotonergic projections from the dorsal raphe nucleus generally inhibit the locus coeruleus, whereas projections from the locus coeruleus stimulate dorsal raphe nucleus serotonergic neurons and inhibit median raphe nucleus neurons. Furthermore, the dorsal raphe nucleus sends projections to prefrontal cortex, amygdala, hypothalamus, and periaqueductal gray among other structures. Thus, modulation of the serotonin system has the potential to influence the major regions of the panic disorder circuit, resulting in decreased noradrenergic activity, diminished release of corticotropin-releasing factor, and modification of defense and escape behaviors.

Indeed, clinical research confirms important interactions between the serotonin and the noradrenaline systems in panic disorder. In one study of fluoxetine treatment in panic disorder, degree of clinical global improvement correlated with the magnitude of plasma MHPG (a primary noradrenergic metabolite) decline, and significant elevations in plasma MHPG volatility during clonidine challenge in untreated panic disorder patients were normalized by SSRI treatment. The authors concluded that fluoxetine exerted a stabilizing influence on a dysregulated noradrenergic system (Coplan et al. 1997).

Peripheral benzodiazepine receptor binding is decreased in panic disorder (Marazziti et al. 1994), and benzodiazepines are effective in treating this condition (Gorman et al. 2000). In animal models, direct administration of a benzodiazepine agonist into the amygdala produces anxiolytic effects, which are weakened by pretreatment with a benzodiazepine receptor antagonist (Coplan and Lydiard 1998). GABA and benzodiazepine receptors are widely distributed in the brain, but the basolateral and lateral amygdala nucleus and the hippocampus, as well as frontal and occipital cortex, have high densities (see also the imaging studies in the following subsection).

A consideration of the various afferents to the locus coeruleus and amygdala is relevant to considering the extensive literature on panicogenic stimuli. It has been argued that respiratory panicogens (e.g., carbon dioxide, lactate), baroceptor stimulation (β agonists), and circulating peptides (cholecystokinin) promote panic via a limbic visceroreceptor pathway. In contrast, panic attacks that are conditioned by visuospatial, auditory, or cognitive cues may be mediated by pathways from cortical association areas to the amygdala (Coplan and Lydiard 1998). Ultimately, it may be possible to determine particular genetic loci that are involved in contextual fear conditioning, allowing for an integration of the neurochemical, genetic, and environmental data on panic disorder (Gorman et al. 2000).

Neuroanatomical Studies

Preliminary studies in nonanxious control subjects reported activation of amygdala and periamygdaloid cortical areas during conditioned fear acquisition and extinction (Gorman et al. 2000). Furthermore, in patients with panic disorder, increasing evidence suggests temporal or amygdalar-hippocampal abnormalities (Bisaga et al. 1998; Massana et al. 2003; Uchida et al. 2003; Vythilingam et al. 2000a), as well as frontal abnormalities (De Cristofaro et al. 1993; Nordahl et al. 1998; Wurthmann et al. 1998). Although hypocapnia-induced vasoconstriction has made the results of certain imaging studies in panic disorder difficult to interpret, it is noteworthy that imaging data may predict response to panicogens (Kent et al. 2005).

Advances in brain imaging methods have begun to allow the integration of neuroanatomical and neurochemical data. Thus, evidence indicates altered midbrain 5-HT$_{1A}$ receptor binding and serotonin transporter levels in panic disorder (Maron et al. 2004a; Neumeister et al. 2004). Several studies also have shown decreased benzodiazepine binding in temporal and frontal regions (Bremner et al. 2000; Kaschka et al. 1995; Marazziti et al. 1994). Preliminary data suggest that both pharmacotherapy and cognitive-behavioral therapy act to normalize the neurocircuitry thought to mediate panic disorder (Prasko et al. 2004).

POSTTRAUMATIC STRESS DISORDER

Posttraumatic stress disorders begin, by definition, in the aftermath of exposure to a trauma; in men, common traumas include combat exposure, and in women, the most common traumas include rape and sexual molestation (Kessler et al. 1995). Three sets of subsequent symptoms characterize PTSD: reexperiencing phenomena (such as visual flashbacks), avoidant and numbing symptoms, and hyperarousal. It should be emphasized

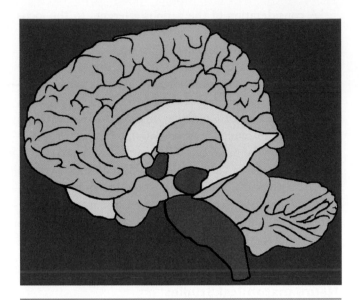

FIGURE 28–5. Neuroanatomical model of posttraumatic stress disorder. Note the increased activity in the amygdala and decreased activity in prefrontal areas (not anatomically to scale).

Source. Reprinted from Stein DJ: *False Alarm! How to Conquer the Anxiety Disorders.* Cape Town, South Africa, University of Stellenbosch, 2000. Used with permission.

that the prevalence of exposure to trauma is significantly higher than the prevalence of PTSD, indicating that most trauma does not lead to this disorder.

Indeed, an important development in the PTSD literature is a growing emphasis that this is not a "normal" reaction to an abnormal event (Yehuda and McFarlane 1995). Rather, PTSD is increasingly viewed as a serious disorder that is associated with significant morbidity and mediated by neurobiological and psychological dysfunctions.

Features of current neuroanatomical models of PTSD (Figure 28–5) include the following: 1) amygdalothalamic pathways are involved in the rapid, automatic (implicit) processing of incoming information; 2) hyperactivation of the amygdala, which sends afferents to other regions involved in the anxiety response (hypothalamus, brain stem nuclei), occurs; 3) the hippocampus is involved in (explicitly) remembering the context of traumatic memories; and 4) activity is decreased in certain frontal cortical areas, consistent with decreased verbalization during processing of trauma (e.g., deactivation of Broca's area), failure of fear extinction (e.g., failure to recruit medial and ventral prefrontal areas), and an inability to override automatic amygdala processing.

Neurochemical Studies

A range of neurochemical findings in PTSD are consistent with sensitization of various neurotransmitter systems (Charney 2004). In particular, there is evidence of hyperactive noradrenergic function and dopaminergic sensitization. Such sensitization is also consistent with the role of environmental traumas in PTSD; dopamine agonists and environmental traumas act as cross-sensitizers of each other. Evidence indicates that the amygdala and related limbic regions may play a particularly important role in the final common pathway of such hyperactivation.

Also, growing evidence suggests the importance of the serotonin system in mediating PTSD symptoms (Connor and Davidson 1998). Clinical studies of abnormal paroxetine binding and exacerbations of symptoms in response to administration of m-CPP are certainly consistent with a role for serotonin in PTSD (Southwick et al. 1997). Furthermore, the evidence for the efficacy of serotonin reuptake inhibitors in PTSD is increasing (Stein et al. 2000b), and some have argued that these agents may be more effective than other classes of medication (Dow and Kline 1997; Penava et al. 1996). These agents may act on amygdala circuits, helping to inhibit efferents to structures such as hypothalamus and brain stem nuclei, which mediate fear.

A third set of neurochemical findings in PTSD has focused on the hypothalamic-pituitary-adrenal (HPA) system. PTSD is characterized by decreased plasma levels of cortisol, as well as increased glucocorticoid receptor responsiveness, suggesting that negative feedback inhibition may play an important role in the pathogenesis of the disorder. Such findings differ from those found in other anxiety disorders and in depression (Yehuda 2002). Notably, cortisol-releasing factor receptors are also prominent in the amygdala, particularly in the central nucleus.

One important implication of the HPA findings is the possibility that dysfunction in this system results in neuronal damage, particularly to the hippocampus. Animal studies have documented hippocampal damage after exposure to either glucocorticoids or naturalistic psychosocial stressors (Sapolsky 2000). Parallel neurotoxicity in human PTSD could account for some of the cognitive impairments that are characteristic of this disorder.

Neuroanatomical Studies

A range of structural imaging studies are in fact consistent with the possibility of hippocampal dysfunction occurring in PTSD. A meta-analysis of magnetic resonance imaging studies, for example, emphasized the consistent finding of decreased hippocampal volume in PTSD secondary to adult or childhood trauma (Kitayama et al. 2005). In some studies, decreased volume has been associated with greater trauma exposure, increased symptom severity, or worse neuropsychological impairment. Nevertheless, evidence also shows that decreased hippocampal volume may precede the onset of PTSD and thus constitutes a risk factor for the development of this condition (Gilbertson et al. 2002). In addition, there are now increasing data suggesting decreased volume in medial and ventral prefrontal cortex (Rauch et al. 2006).

Functional imaging studies have provided additional information in support of a neuroanatomical model of PTSD. Several studies in control subjects without PTSD have provided evidence for subcortical processing of masked emotional stimuli by the amygdala. Furthermore, a range of studies found that PTSD patients exposed to audiotaped traumatic and neutral scripts had increases in neuronal activity in limbic and paralimbic areas (Taber et al. 2003). Also, areas of decreased activity may mediate symptoms; for example, decreased activity in Broca's area during exposure to trauma in PTSD is consistent with patients' inability to verbally process traumatic memories (Rauch et al. 1998). Subsequent studies have extended the work to address abnormalities during cognitive-affective processing of tasks in PTSD (Shin et al. 2004, 2005). The data support a view that there is deficient recruitment of medial and ventral prefrontal cortex in PTSD, consistent with dysfunction in fear extinction (Rauch et al. 2006).

Once again, modern techniques have allowed for the integration of neurochemical and neuroanatomical data. For example, PET has been used in combat veterans with PTSD and healthy control subjects after administration of yohimbine (Bremner et al. 1997); this noradrenergic agent resulted in a significant increase in anxiety in the patients with PTSD, and these subjects also had a decrease in activity in several areas, including prefrontal, temporal, parietal, and orbitofrontal cortex, a finding perhaps consistent with previous literature suggesting that rCBF decreases during intense anxiety states (Gur et al. 1987). The number of receptor binding studies in PTSD is also increasing (Bonne et al. 2005; Fujita et al. 2004). Finally, during treatment of PTSD with SSRIs, normalization of structure and activity in the limbic neurocircuitry occurs and is likely to mediate symptoms (Seedat et al. 2004; Vermetten et al. 2003).

SOCIAL PHOBIA (SOCIAL ANXIETY DISORDER)

Social phobia (social anxiety disorder) is characterized by a fear of social situations in which the individual may be exposed to the scrutiny of others. These fears may be divided into those that concern social interaction situations (such as dating and meetings) and performance fears (e.g., of talking, eating, or writing in public). These fears result in avoidance of social situations or endurance of these situations with considerable distress. Growing evidence indicates that social phobia is a chronic disorder, with sub-

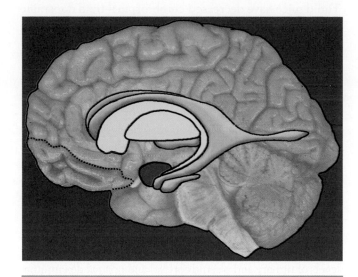

FIGURE 28–6. Neuroanatomical model of social phobia. Note the increased temporolimbic activity (van der Linden et al. 2000), decreased basal ganglia dopaminergic activity (Tiihonen et al. 1997a), and perhaps some increased prefrontal activity (Rauch et al. 1997; van der Linden et al. 2000).

Source. Reprinted from *Stein DJ: False Alarm! How to Conquer the Anxiety Disorders.* Cape Town, South Africa, University of Stellenbosch, 2000. Used with permission.

stantial comorbidity (particularly of mood and substance use disorders) and significant morbidity. Patients with social phobia are more likely to be unmarried, to have weaker social networks, to fail to complete high school and college, and to be unemployed (Ballenger et al. 1998).

Detailed neuroanatomical models of social phobia remain to be fully delineated. Nevertheless, it may be hypothesized again that temporolimbic circuitry is important in mediating the fear responses that characterize this disorder. Furthermore, serotonin and dopamine neurocircuitry, presumably involving prefrontal and basal ganglia regions, may also play a crucial role. We review some of the neurotransmitter and neuroimaging data that support such a model (Figure 28–6).

Neurochemical Studies

A range of evidence supports the role of serotonergic circuits in social phobia. A pharmacological probe study was performed with agents that affect the serotonergic (fenfluramine), dopaminergic (levodopa), and noradrenergic (clonidine) systems; the only positive finding was an augmented cortisol response to fenfluramine administration in patients with social phobia (Tancer et al. 1994). The authors concluded that patients with social phobia may have selective supersensitivity of serotonergic systems.

Also, a range of evidence indicates involvement of the dopaminergic system in social phobia (Stein et al. 2002).

Timid mice have decreased cerebrospinal fluid dopamine levels, and introverted depressed patients also may have decreased cerebrospinal fluid dopamine levels. Social status in monkeys may be reflected in differences in dopamine type 2 (D_2) striatal density. More persuasively, social phobia may develop in the context of Parkinson's disorder or after the administration of neuroleptics.

Evidence that the HPA axis may be dysfunctional in social phobia is inconsistent to date. Socially subordinate baboons have been reported to have elevated basal cortisol and to be less responsive to dexamethasone inhibition (Sapolsky et al. 1997). Also, children with a high frequency of wary behavior during peer play and behavioral inhibition had relatively high morning salivary cortisol levels (Schmidt et al. 1997). Patients with social phobia, however, have normal levels of urinary and plasma cortisol and normal dexamethasone suppression test results (Stein 1998), although some evidence shows an association between social phobia and hypothalamic growth hormone dysfunction (Uhde 1994).

Neuroanatomical Studies

Increasing evidence suggests that patients with social phobia have selective activation of the amygdala when exposed to potentially fear-relevant stimuli (Birbaumer et al. 1998; Nutt et al. 1998; Veit et al. 2002). Interestingly, subjects with behavioral inhibition, when studied as adults, also had heightened amygdala responses to novel fear-relevant stimuli (Schwartz et al. 2003). It is noteworthy that nonphobic control subjects with a particular variant in the serotonin transporter gene that is associated with anxiety traits, as well as subjects with social phobia, also have decreased volume or increased activity in amygdala or related circuitry (Furmark et al. 2004; Hariri et al. 2002; Pezawas et al. 2005). Treatment with an SSRI or with cognitive-behavioral therapy is able to normalize neuronal activity in such neurocircuitry (Furmark et al. 2002; Van der Linden et al. 2000).

Several molecular imaging studies provide additional data that are relevant to an integrated model of social phobia. Thus, evidence indicates that striatal dopamine reuptake site densities are markedly lower in patients with social phobia than in nonphobic control subjects (Tiihonen et al. 1997a). Other findings confirm abnormalities in components of the striatal dopaminergic system (Schneier et al. 2000), supporting the hypothesis that social phobia may be associated with a dysfunction of the striatal dopaminergic system. These types of data may point to a link between social phobia and dysfunctional processing of positive or rewarding information (Hare et al. 2005) and may ultimately suggest novel approaches to pharmacotherapy for this condition.

CONCLUSION

Several lessons emerge from a review of the neuropsychiatry of anxiety disorders. First, the anxiety disorders are common and disabling disorders not only in general clinical settings but also in patients with neurological illnesses such as Alzheimer's disease, stroke, and traumatic brain injury. Although the link between depression and neuropsychiatric disorders is increasingly recognized, the importance of anxiety disorders in this context has perhaps been relatively overlooked, paralleling their underdiagnosis and undertreatment in primary care settings. The anxiety disorders deserve to be carefully diagnosed, thoroughly assessed, and rigorously treated.

Second, both animal and clinical studies increasingly indicate that the amygdala and paralimbic structures play important roles in conditioned fear and in anxiety disorders. Amygdala lesions are classically associated with decreased fear responses, and conversely, limbic hyperactivation is characteristic of several different anxiety disorders. Paralimbic regions such as the anterior cingulate appear to play a key role at the interface of cognition and emotion. The apparent centrality of such systems to different anxiety disorders may account in part for their high comorbidity. Other limbic involvement may be specific to particular disorders (e.g., decreased hippocampal volume in PTSD or parahippocampal asymmetry in panic disorder).

Models of anxiety disorders increasingly integrate data from genetics, brain imaging, and treatment studies. Thus, particular genetic variants appear to be associated with increased activation of specific neuronal circuits during functional imaging, and effective pharmacotherapy and psychotherapy may act to normalize such circuitry. Serotonin reuptake inhibitors and CBT are increasingly viewed as first-line treatments for anxiety disorders. Innervation of amygdala and paralimbic structures by serotonergic neurons may be crucial in explaining their efficacy. Further advances in our understanding of the neurobiological bases of fear conditioning and extinction may lead to new therapeutic interventions (Ressler et al. 2004).

Finally, CTSC pathways are crucial in OCD, and data increasingly support a role for putative OCD spectrum disorders such as Tourette syndrome. It is particularly remarkable that CSTC pathways can be normalized by pharmacotherapy, by psychotherapy, and by neurosurgery. It can be argued that although OCD was once viewed as the key to a psychodynamic understanding of the mind, OCD and some OCD spectrum disorders such as Tourette syndrome are now the neuropsychiatric disorders par excellence. Certainly, such disorders provide a key paradigm and challenge for those who are interested in integrating "brain" and "mind" approaches to psychiatric disorders.

Highlights for the Clinician

♦ Anxiety symptoms and disorders are common in a range of neurological conditions.

♦ Although the literature on treatment is limited, in some cases standard antianxiety treatments may be useful.

♦ The neurocircuitry of the different anxiety disorders overlaps somewhat, but certain distinctive differences are seen, consistent with differences in symptomatology.

♦ The neurocircuitry of obsessive-compulsive disorder differs from that of other anxiety disorders, suggesting that this condition should be assessed and treated in a unique way.

♦ Genetic variations may account for some of the variance in functional neuroanatomy in studies of a particular disorder.

♦ Both effective pharmacotherapy and psychotherapy can normalize the functional neuroanatomy involved in mediating anxiety disorders.

RECOMMENDED READINGS

Furmark T, Tillfors M, Marteinsdottir I, et al: Common changes in cerebral blood flow in patients with social phobia treated with citalopram or cognitive-behavioral therapy. Arch Gen Psychiatry 59:425–433, 2002

Gorman JM, Kent JM, Sullivan GM, et al: Neuroanatomical hypothesis of panic disorder, revised. Am J Psychiatry 157:493–505, 2000

Kitayama N, Vaccarino V, Kutner M, et al: Magnetic resonance imaging (MRI) measurement of hippocampal volume in posttraumatic stress disorder: a meta-analysis. J Affect Disord 88:79–86, 2005

Talbot PS: The molecular neuroimaging of anxiety disorders. Curr Psychiatry Rep 6:274–279, 2004

Whiteside SP, Port JD, Abramowitz JS: A meta-analysis of functional neuroimaging in obsessive-compulsive disorder. Psychiatry Res 132:69–79, 2004

REFERENCES

Adams KH, Hansen ES, Pinborg LH, et al: Patients with obsessive-compulsive disorder have increased 5-HT2A receptor binding in the caudate nuclei. Int J Neuropsychopharmacol 8:391–401, 2005

Alegret M, Junque C, Valldeoriola F, et al: Obsessive-compulsive symptoms in Parkinson's disease. J Neurol Neurosurg Psychiatry 70:394–396, 2001

American Psychiatric Association: Diagnostic and Statistical Manual of Mental Disorders, 3rd Edition. Washington, DC, American Psychiatric Association, 1980

American Psychiatric Association: Diagnostic and Statistical Manual of Mental Disorders, 3rd Edition, Revised. Washington, DC, American Psychiatric Association, 1987

American Psychiatric Association: Diagnostic and Statistical Manual of Mental Disorders, 4th Edition, Text Revision. Washington, DC, American Psychiatric Association, 2000

Ames D, Cummings JL, Wirshing WC, et al: Repetitive and compulsive behavior in frontal lobe degenerations. J Neuropsychiatry Clin Neurosci 6:100–113, 1994

Anderson KE, Louis ED, Stern Y, et al: Cognitive correlates of obsessive and compulsive symptoms in Huntington's disease. Am J Psychiatry 158:799–801, 2001

Astrom M: Generalized anxiety disorder in stroke patients: a 3-year longitudinal study. Stroke 27:270–275, 1996

Baldwin DS, Polkinghorn C: Evidence-based pharmacotherapy of generalized anxiety disorder. Int Clin Psychopharmacol 8:293–302, 2005

Ballard C, Neill D, O'Brien J, et al: Anxiety, depression and psychosis in vascular dementia: prevalence and associations. J Affect Disord 59:97–106, 2000

Ballenger JC, Davidson JA, Lecrubier Y, et al: Consensus statement on social anxiety disorder from the International Consensus Group on Depression and Anxiety. J Clin Psychiatry 59 (suppl 17):54–60, 1998

Baxter LR, Schwartz JM, Bergman KS, et al: Caudate glucose metabolic rate changes with both drug and behavior therapy for OCD. Arch Gen Psychiatry 49:681–689, 1992

Bechara A, Tranel D, Damasio H, et al: Double dissociation of conditioning and declarative knowledge relative to the amygdala and hippocampus in humans. Science 269:1115–1118, 1995

Bernik MA, Corregiari FM, Braun IM: Panic attacks in the differential diagnosis and treatment of resistant epilepsy. Depress Anxiety 15:190–192, 2002

Birbaumer N, Grodd W, Diedrich O, et al: fMRI reveals amygdala activation to human faces in social phobics. Neuroreport 9:1223–1226, 1998

Bisaga A, Katz JL, Antonini A, et al: Cerebral glucose metabolism in women with panic disorder. Am J Psychiatry 155:1178–1183, 1998

Bonne O, Bain E, Neumeister A, et al: No change in serotonin type 1A receptor binding in patients with posttraumatic stress disorder. Am J Psychiatry 162:383–385, 2005

Boyer W: Serotonin uptake inhibitors are superior to imipramine and alprazolam in alleviating panic attacks: a meta-analysis. Int Clin Psychopharmacol 10:45–49, 1995

Braun AR, Randolph C, Stoetter B, et al: The functional neuroanatomy of Tourette's syndrome: an FDG-PET study, II: relationships between regional cerebral metabolism and associated behavioral and cognitive features of the illness. Neuropsychopharmacology 13:151–168, 1995

Bremner JD, Innis RB, Ng CK, et al: Positron emission tomography measurement of cerebral metabolic correlates of yohimbine administration in combat-related posttraumatic stress disorder. Arch Gen Psychiatry 54:246–254, 1997

Bremner JD, Innis RB, White T, et al: SPECT [I-123]iomazenil measurement of the benzodiazepine receptor in panic disorder. Biol Psychiatry 47:96–106, 2000

Brody AL, Saxena S, Schwartz JM, et al: FDG-PET predictors of response to behavioral therapy and pharmacotherapy in obsessive compulsive disorder. Psychiatry Res 84:1–6, 1998

Buchsbaum MS, Hazlett E, Sicotte N, et al: Topographic EEG changes with benzodiazepine administration in generalized anxiety disorder. Biol Psychiatry 20:832–842, 1985

Burvill PW, Johnson GA, Jamrozik KD, et al: Anxiety disorders after stroke: results from the Perth Community Stroke Study. Br J Psychiatry 166:328–332, 1995

Bystritsky A, Leuchter AF, Vapnik T: EEG abnormalities in non-medicated panic disorder. J Nerv Ment Dis 187:113–114, 1999

Carlsson ML: On the role of prefrontal cortex glutamate for the antithetical phenomenology of obsessive compulsive disorder and attention deficit hyperactivity disorder. Prog Neuropsychopharmacol Biol Psychiatry 25:5–26, 2001

Castillo CS, Starkstein SE, Fedoroff JP, et al: Generalized anxiety disorder after stroke. J Nerv Ment Dis 181:100–106, 1993

Cavenar JO, Harris MA: Temporal lobe seizures simulating anxiety attacks. US Navy Med 70:22–23, 1979

Charney DS: Psychobiological mechanisms of resilience and vulnerability: implications for successful adaptation to extreme stress. Am J Psychiatry 161:195–216, 2004

Cheyette SR, Cummings JL: Encephalitis lethargica: lessons for contemporary neuropsychiatry. J Neuropsychiatry Clin Neurosci 7:125–135, 1995

Connor KM, Davidson JRT: The role of serotonin in posttraumatic stress disorder: neurobiology and pharmacotherapy. CNS Spectr 3:43–51, 1998

Coplan JD, Lydiard RB: Brain circuits in panic disorder. Biol Psychiatry 44:1264–1276, 1998

Coplan JD, Gorman JM, Klein DF: Serotonin related functions in panic-anxiety: a critical overview. Neuropsychopharmacology 6:189–200, 1992

Coplan JD, Papp LA, Pine D, et al: Clinical improvement with fluoxetine therapy and noradrenergic function in patients with panic disorder. Arch Gen Psychiatry 54:643–648, 1997

Cummings JL: Frontal-subcortical circuits and human behavior. Arch Neurol 50:873–880, 1993

Cummings JL, Cunningham K: Obsessive-compulsive disorder in Huntington's disease. Biol Psychiatry 31:263–270, 1992

Damasio AR: Descartes' Error: Emotion, Reason, and the Human Brain. New York, HarperCollins, 1994

Davis M, Whalen PJ: The amygdala: vigilance and emotion. Mol Psychiatry 6:13–34, 2001

De Cristofaro MT, Sessarego A, Pupi A, et al: Brain perfusion abnormalities in drug-naive, lactate-sensitive panic patients: a SPECT study. Biol Psychiatry 33:505–512, 1993

Diaz-Olavarrieta C, Cummings JL, Velazquez J, et al: Neuropsychiatric manifestations of multiple sclerosis. J Neuropsychiatry Clin Neurosci 11:51–57, 1999

Dow B, Kline N: Antidepressant treatment of posttraumatic stress disorder and major depression in veterans. Ann Clin Psychiatry 9:1–5, 1997

Dupont RL, Rice DP, Miller LS, et al: Economic costs of anxiety disorders. Anxiety 2:167–172, 1996

El Mansari M, Bouchard C, Blier P: Alteration of serotonin release in the guinea pig orbito-frontal cortex by selective serotonin reuptake inhibitors. Neuropsychopharmacology 13:117–127, 1995

Fog R, Pakkenberg H: Behavioral effects of dopamine and p-hydroxyamphetamine injected into corpus striatum of rats. Exp Neurol 31:75–86, 1971

Freud S: Inhibitions, symptoms, and anxiety (1926), in The Standard Edition of the Complete Psychological Works of Sigmund Freud, Vol 20. Translated and edited by Strachey J. London, Hogarth Press, 1959, pp 75–175

Fujita M, Southwick SM, Denucci CC, et al: Central type benzodiazepine receptors in Gulf War veterans with posttraumatic stress disorder. Biol Psychiatry 56:95–100, 2004

Furmark T, Tillfors M, Marteinsdottir I, et al: Common changes in cerebral blood flow in patients with social phobia treated with citalopram or cognitive-behavioral therapy. Arch Gen Psychiatry 59:425–433, 2002

Furmark T, Tillfors M, Garpenstrand H, et al: Serotonin transporter polymorphism related to amygdala excitability and symptom severity in patients with social phobia. Neurosci Lett 362:189–192, 2004

Gerard E, Peterson BS: Developmental processes and brain imaging studies in Tourette syndrome. J Psychosom Res 55:13–22, 2003

Germine M, Goddard AW, Woods SW, et al: Anger and anxiety responses to m-chlorophenylpiperazine in generalized anxiety disorder. Biol Psychiatry 32:457–467, 1992

Giedd JN, Rapoport JL, Garvey MA, et al: MRI assessment of children with obsessive-compulsive disorder or tics associated with streptococcal infection. Am J Psychiatry 157:281–283, 2000

Gilbertson MW, Shenton ME, Ciszweski A, et al: Smaller hippocampal volume predicts pathological vulnerability to psychological trauma. Nat Neurosci 5:1242–1247, 2002

Goodman WK, McDougle CJ, Lawrence LP: Beyond the serotonin hypothesis: a role for dopamine in some forms of obsessive-compulsive disorder. J Clin Psychiatry 51 (suppl 8):36–43, 1990

Gorman JM, Kent JM, Sullivan GM, et al: Neuroanatomical hypothesis of panic disorder, revised. Am J Psychiatry 157:493–505, 2000

Grimshaw L: Obsessional disorder and neurological illness. J Neurol Neurosurg Psychiatry 27:229–231, 1964

Gur RC, Gur RE, Resnick ME, et al: The effect of anxiety on cortical cerebral blood flow and metabolism. J Cereb Blood Flow Metab 7:173–177, 1987

Hare TA, Tottenham N, Davidson MC, et al: Contributions of amygdala and striatal activity in emotion regulation. Biol Psychiatry 57:624–632, 2005

Hariri AR, Mattay VS, Tessitore A, et al: Serotonin transporter genetic variation and the response of the human amygdala. Science 297:400–403, 2002

Harvey AG, Brewin CR, Jones C, et al: Coexistence of posttraumatic stress disorder and traumatic brain injury: towards a resolution of the paradox. J Int Neuropsychol Soc 9:663–676, 2003

Hibbard MR, Uysal S, Kepler K, et al: Axis I psychopathology in individuals with traumatic brain injury. J Head Trauma Rehabil 13:24–39, 1998

Hiott DW, Labbate L: Anxiety disorders associated with traumatic brain injuries. Neurorehabilitation 17:345–355, 2002

Hoehn-Saric R, Schlund MW, Wong SH: Effects of citalopram on worry and brain activation in patients with generalized anxiety disorder. Psychiatry Res 131:11–21, 2005

Hollander E, DeCaria CM, Nitescu A, et al: Serotonergic function in obsessive-compulsive disorder: behavioral and neuroendocrine responses to oral m-chlorophenylpiperazine and fenfluramine in patients and healthy volunteers. Arch Gen Psychiatry 49:21–28, 1992

Hollander E, Prohovnik I, Stein DJ: Increased cerebral blood flow during m-CPP exacerbation of obsessive-compulsive disorder. J Neuropsychiatry Clin Neurosci 7:485–490, 1995

Hugo F, Van Heerden B, Zungu-Dirwayi N, et al: Functional brain imaging in obsessive-compulsive disorder secondary to neurological lesions. Depress Anxiety 10:129–136, 1999

Hyde TM, Weinberger DR: Tourette's syndrome: a model neuropsychiatric disorder. JAMA 273:498–501, 1995

Iny LJ, Pecknold J, Suranyi-Cadotte BE, et al: Studies of a neurochemical link between depression, anxiety, and stress from [3H] imipramine and [3H] paroxetine binding on human platelets. Biol Psychiatry 36:281–291, 1994

Jenike MA, Brotman AW: The EEG in obsessive-compulsive disorder. J Clin Psychiatry 45:122–124, 1984

Joseph S, Masterson J: Posttraumatic stress disorder and traumatic brain injury: are they mutually exclusive? J Trauma Stress 12:437–453, 1999

Kapur S, Remington G: Serotonin-dopamine interaction and its relevance to schizophrenia. Am J Psychiatry 153:466–476, 1996

Kaschka W, Feistel H, Ebert D: Reduced benzodiazepine receptor binding in panic disorders measured by iomazenil SPECT. J Psychiatr Res 29:427–434, 1995

Kellner M, Hirschmann M, Wiedemann K: Panic attacks caused by temporal tumors: an exemplary new case and a review. Depress Anxiety 4:243–245, 1996

Kent JM, Coplan JD, Mawlawi O, et al: Prediction of panic response to a respiratory stimulant by reduced orbitofrontal cerebral blood flow in panic disorder. Am J Psychiatry 162:1379–1381, 2005

Kessler RC: The epidemiology of pure and comorbid generalized anxiety disorder: a review and evaluation of recent research. Acta Psychiatr Scand Suppl 406:7–13, 2000

Kessler RC, McGonagle KC, Zhao S, et al: Lifetime and 12-month prevalence of DSM-III-R psychiatric disorders in the United States: results from the National Comorbidity Survey. Arch Gen Psychiatry 51:8–19, 1994

Kessler RC, Sonnega A, Bromet E, et al: Posttraumatic stress disorder in the National Comorbidity Survey. Arch Gen Psychiatry 52:1048–1060, 1995

Kessler RC, Chiu WT, Demler O, et al: Prevalence, severity, and comorbidity of 12-month DSM-IV disorders in the National Comorbidity Survey Replication. Arch Gen Psychiatry 62:617–627, 2005

Khanna S: Carbamazepine in obsessive-compulsive disorder. Clin Neuropharmacol 11:478–481, 1988

Kinrys G, Wygant LE: Anticonvulsants in anxiety disorders. Curr Psychiatry Rep 7:258–267, 2005

Kitayama N, Vaccarino V, Kutner M, et al: Magnetic resonance imaging (MRI) measurement of hippocampal volume in posttraumatic stress disorder: a meta-analysis. J Affect Disord 88:79–86, 2005

Klüver H, Bucy PC: Preliminary analysis of functions of the temporal lobes in monkeys. AMA Arch Neurol Psychiatry 42:979–1000, 1939

Lauterbach EC, Cummings JL, Duffy J, et al: Neuropsychiatric correlates and treatment of lenticulostriatal diseases: a review of the literature and overview of research opportunities in Huntington's, Wilson's, and Fahr's diseases—a report of the ANPA Committee on Research. American Neuropsychiatric Association. J Neuropsychiatry Clin Neurosci 10:249–266, 1998

Le Doux J: Fear and the brain: where have we been, and where are we going? Biol Psychiatry 44:1229–1238, 1998

Leroi I, Michalon M: Treatment of the psychiatric manifestations of Huntington's disease: a review of the literature. Can J Psychiatry 43:933–940, 1998

Lippitz BE, Mindus P, Meyerson BA, et al: Lesion topography after thermocapsulotomy or gamma knife capsulotomy for obsessive-compulsive disorder: relevance of the right hemisphere. Neurosurgery 44:452–458, 1999

Luxenberg JS, Swedo SE, Flament MF, et al: Neuroanatomical abnormalities in obsessive-compulsive disorder detected with quantitative x-ray computed tomography. Am J Psychiatry 145:1089–1093, 1988

MacLean PD: A Triune Concept of the Brain and Behavior. Toronto, ON, University of Toronto Press, 1973

Marazziti D, Rotondo A, Martini C, et al: Changes in peripheral benzodiazepine receptors in patients with panic disorder and obsessive-compulsive disorder. Neuropsychobiology 29:8–11, 1994

Maricle RA, Sennhauser S, Burry M: Panic disorder associated with right parahippocampal infarction. J Nerv Ment Dis 179:374–375, 1991

Maron E, Kuikka JT, Shlik J, et al: Reduced brain serotonin transporter binding in patients with panic disorder. Psychiatry Res 132:173–181, 2004a

Maron E, Kuikka JT, Ulst K, et al: SPECT imaging of serotonin transporter binding in patients with generalized anxiety disorder. Eur Arch Psychiatry Clin Neurosci 254:392–396, 2004b

Martin LJ, Spicer DM, Lewis MH, et al: Social deprivation of infant monkeys alters the chemoarchitecture of the brain, I: subcortical regions. J Neurosci 11:3344–3358, 1991

Massana G, Serra-Grabulosa JM, Salgado-Pineda P, et al: Amygdalar atrophy in panic disorder patients detected by volumetric magnetic resonance imaging. Neuroimage 19:80–90, 2003

Mathew SJ, Mao X, Coplan JD, et al: Dorsolateral prefrontal cortical pathology in generalized anxiety disorder: a proton magnetic resonance spectroscopic imaging study. Am J Psychiatry 161:1119–1121, 2004

McDougle CJ, Goodman WK, Leckman JF: Haloperidol addition in fluvoxamine-refractory obsessive-compulsive disorder: a double-blind placebo-controlled study in patients with and without tics. Arch Gen Psychiatry 51:302–308, 1994

McNamara ME, Fogel BS: Anticonvulsant-responsive panic attacks with temporal lobe EEG abnormalities. J Neuropsychiatry Clin Neurosci 2:193–196, 1990

Menza MA, Palermo B, DiPaola R, et al: Depression and anxiety in Parkinson's disease: possible effect of genetic variation in the serotonin transporter. J Geriatr Psychiatry Neurol 12:49–52, 1999

Menza M, Marin H, Kaufman K, et al: Citalopram treatment of depression in Parkinson's disease: the impact on anxiety, disability, and cognition. J Neuropsychiatry Clin Neurosci 16:315–319, 2004

Milham MP, Nugent AC, Drevets WC, et al: Selective reduction in amygdala volume in pediatric anxiety disorders: a voxel-based morphometry investigation. Biol Psychiatry 57:961–966, 2005

Mishkin M, Petri H: Memories and habits: some implications for the analysis of learning and retention, in Neuropsychology of Memory. Edited by Squire LR, Butters N. New York, Guilford, 1984, pp 287–296

Montgomery SA: Obsessive compulsive disorder is not an anxiety disorder. Int Clin Psychopharmacol 8 (suppl 1), 57–62, 1993

Moriarty J, Eapen V, Costa DC, et al: HMPAO SPECT does not distinguish obsessive-compulsive and tic syndromes in families multiply affected with Gilles de la Tourette's syndrome. Psychol Med 27:737–740, 1997

Morrison V, Pollard B, Johnston M, et al: Anxiety and depression 3 years following stroke: demographic, clinical, and psychological predictors. J Psychosom Res 59:209–213, 2005

Muller JE, Koen L, Stein DJ: Anxiety and medical disorders. Curr Psychiatry Rep 7:245–251, 2005

Muller-Vahl KR, Meyer GJ, Knapp WH, et al: Serotonin transporter binding in Tourette syndrome. Neurosci Lett 385:120–125, 2005

Murray CJL, Lopez AD: Global Burden of Disease: A Comprehensive Assessment of Mortality and Morbidity From Diseases, Injuries and Risk Factors in 1990 and Projected to 2020, Vol I: Harvard. Geneva, Switzerland, World Health Organization, 1996

Neumeister A, Bain E, Nugent AC, et al: Reduced serotonin type 1A receptor binding in panic disorder. J Neurosci 24:589–591, 2004

Nordahl TE, Stein MB, Benkelfat C, et al: Regional cerebral metabolic asymmetries replicated in an independent group of patients with panic disorders. Biol Psychiatry 44:998–1006, 1998

Nutt DJ: Neurobiological mechanisms in generalized anxiety disorder. J Clin Psychiatry 62 (suppl 11):22–27, 2001

Nutt DJ, Bell CJ, Malizia AL: Brain mechanisms of social anxiety disorder. J Clin Psychiatry 59 (suppl 17):4–11, 1998

O'Sullivan RL, Rauch SL, Breiter HC, et al: Reduced basal ganglia volumes in trichotillomania measured via morphometric magnetic resonance imaging. Biol Psychiatry 42:39–45, 1997

Otto MW, Tuby KS, Gould RA, et al: An effect-size analysis of the relative efficacy and tolerability of serotonin selective reuptake inhibitors for panic disorder. Am J Psychiatry 158:1989–1992, 2001

Pato MT, Schindler KM, Pato CN: The genetics of obsessive-compulsive disorder. Curr Psychiatry Rep 3:163–168, 2001

Pauls DL, Towbin KE, Leckman JF, et al: Gilles de la Tourette's syndrome and obsessive compulsive disorder: evidence supporting a genetic relationship. Arch Gen Psychiatry 43:1180–1182, 1986

Penava SJ, Otto MW, Pollack MH, et al: Current status of pharmacotherapy for PTSD: an effect size analysis of controlled studies. Depress Anxiety 4:240–242, 1996

Pezawas L, Meyer-Lindenberg A, Drabant EM, et al: 5-HTTLPR polymorphism impacts human cingulate-amygdala interactions: a genetic susceptibility mechanism for depression. Nat Neurosci 8:828–834, 2005

Porter VR, Buxton WG, Fairbanks LA, et al: Frequency and characteristics of anxiety among patients with Alzheimer's disease and related dementias. J Neuropsychiatry Clin Neurosci 15:180–186, 2003

Prasko J, Horacek J, Zalesky R, et al: The change of regional brain metabolism ([18]FDG PET) in panic disorder during the treatment with cognitive behavioral therapy or antidepressants. Neuro Endocrinol Lett 25:340–348, 2004

Qazi A, Shankar K, Orrell M: Managing anxiety in people with dementia: a case series. J Affect Disord 76:261–265, 2003

Rapoport JL, Ryland DH, Kriete M: Drug treatment of canine acral lick. Arch Gen Psychiatry 48:517–521, 1992

Rauch SL, Baxter LR: Neuroimaging in obsessive-compulsive and related disorders, in Obsessive-Compulsive Disorders: Practical Management, 3rd Edition. Edited by Jenike MA, Baer L, Minichiello WE. St. Louis, MO, Mosby, 1998, pp 289–316

Rauch SL, Savage CR, Alpert NM, et al: Probing striatal function in obsessive compulsive disorder: a PET study of implicit sequence learning. J Neuropsychiatry Clin Neurosci 9:568–573, 1997

Rauch SL, Shin LM, Whalen PJ, et al: Neuroimaging and the neuroanatomy of posttraumatic stress disorder. CNS Spectr 3:31–41, 1998

Rauch SL, Kim H, Makris N, et al: Volume reduction in the caudate nucleus following stereotactic placement of lesions in the anterior cingulate cortex in humans: a morphometric magnetic resonance imaging study. J Neurosurg 93:1019–1025, 2000

Rauch SL, Shin LM, Phelps EA: Neurocircuitry models of posttraumatic stress disorder and extinction: human neuroimaging research—past, present, and future. Biol Psychiatry 60:376–382, 2006

Rauch SL, Wedig MM, Wright CI, et al: Functional magnetic resonance imaging study of regional brain activation during implicit sequence learning in obsessive-compulsive disorder. Biol Psychiatry 61:330–336, 2007

Redmond DE Jr: The possible role of locus coeruleus noradrenergic activity in anxiety-panic. Clin Neuropharmacol 9 (suppl 4):40–42, 1986

Ressler KJ, Rothbaum BO, Tannenbaum L, et al: Cognitive enhancers as adjuncts to psychotherapy: use of D-cycloserine in phobic individuals to facilitate extinction of fear. Arch Gen Psychiatry 61:1136–1144, 2004

Richard IH, Schiffer RB, Kurlan R: Anxiety and Parkinson's disease. J Neuropsychiatry Clin Neurosci 8:383–392, 1996

Ridley RM: The psychology of perseverative and stereotyped behavior. Prog Neurobiol 44:221–231, 1994

Riether AM: Anxiety in patients with multiple sclerosis. Semin Clin Neuropsychiatry 4:103–113, 1999

Robbins TW, Brown VJ: The role of the striatum in the mental chronometry of action: a theoretical review. Rev Neurosci 2:181–213, 1990

Rocca P, Ferrero P, Gualerzi A, et al: Peripheral-type benzodiazepine receptors in anxiety disorders. Acta Psychiatr Scand 84:537–544, 1991

Rosenberg DR, Keshavan MS: Toward a neurodevelopmental model of obsessive-compulsive disorder. Biol Psychiatry 43:623–640, 1998

Saint-Cyr JA, Taylor AE, Nicholson K: Behavior and the basal ganglia, in Behavioral Neurology of Movement Disorders. Edited by Weinger EJ, Lang AE. New York, Raven, 1995, pp 1–28

Sapolsky RM: Glucocorticoids and hippocampal atrophy in neuropsychiatric disorders. Arch Gen Psychiatry 57:925–935, 2000

Sapolsky RM, Alberts SC, Altmann J: Hypercortisolism associated with social subordinance or social isolation among wild baboons. Arch Gen Psychiatry 54:1137–1143, 1997

Saxena S, Rauch SL: Functional neuroimaging and the neuroanatomy of obsessive-compulsive disorder. Psychiatr Clin North Am 23:563–586, 2000

Schmidt LA, Fox NA, Rubin KH, et al: Behavioral and neuroendocrine responses in shy children. Dev Psychobiol 30:127–140, 1997

Schneier FR, Liebowitz MR, Abi-Dargham A, et al: Low dopamine D(2) receptor binding potential in social phobia. Am J Psychiatry 157:457–459, 2000

Schwartz CE, Wright CI, Shin LM, et al: Inhibited and uninhibited infants "grown up": adult amygdalar response to novelty. Science 300(5627):1952–1953, 2003

Seedat S, Warwick J, van Heerden B, et al: Single photon emission computed tomography in posttraumatic stress disorder before and after treatment with a selective serotonin reuptake inhibitor. J Affect Disord 80:45–53, 2004

Serra-Mestres J, Ring HA, Costa DC, et al: Dopamine transporter binding in Gilles de la Tourette syndrome: a [^{123}I]FP-CIT/SPECT study. Acta Psychiatr Scand 109:140–146, 2004

Sheppard DM, Bradshaw JL, Purcell R, et al: Tourette's and comorbid syndromes: obsessive compulsive and attention deficit hyperactivity disorder: a common etiology? Clin Psychol Rev 19:531–552, 1999

Shin LM, Shin PS, Heckers S, et al: Hippocampal function in posttraumatic stress disorder. Hippocampus 14:292–300, 2004

Shin LM, Wright CI, Cannistraro PA, et al: A functional magnetic resonance imaging study of amygdala and medial prefrontal cortex responses to overtly presented fearful faces in posttraumatic stress disorder. Arch Gen Psychiatry 62:273–281, 2005

Singer HS, Guiliano JD, Hansen BH, et al: Antibodies against human putamen in children with Tourette syndrome. Neurology 50:1618–1624, 1998

Southwick SM, Krystal JH, Bremner JD, et al: Noradrenergic and serotonergic function in posttraumatic stress disorder. Arch Gen Psychiatry 54:749–758, 1997

Stein DJ, Hollander E, Cohen L: Neuropsychiatry of obsessive-compulsive disorder, in Current Insights in Obsessive-Compulsive Disorder. Edited by Hollander E, Zohar J, Marazziti D, et al. Chichester, England, Wiley, 1994, pp 167–182

Stein DJ, van Heerden B, Wessels CJ, et al: Single photon emission computed tomography of the brain with Tc-99m HMPAO during sumatriptan challenge in obsessive-compulsive disorder: investigating the functional role of the serotonin auto-receptor. Prog Neuropsychopharmacol Biol Psychiatry 23:1079–1099, 1999

Stein DJ, Allen A, Bobes J, et al: Quality of life in obsessive-compulsive disorder. CNS Spectr 5 (suppl 4):37–39, 2000a

Stein DJ, Zungu-Dirwayi N, van der Linden GJ, et al: Pharmacotherapy for posttraumatic stress disorder. Cochrane Database Syst Rev (4):CD002795, 2000b

Stein DJ, Liu Y, Shapira NA, et al: The psychobiology of obsessive-compulsive disorder: how important is the role of disgust? Curr Psychiatry Rep 3:281–287, 2001

Stein DJ, Westenberg HG, Liebowitz MR: Social anxiety disorder and generalized anxiety disorder: serotonergic and dopaminergic neurocircuitry. J Clin Psychiatry 63 (suppl 6):12–19, 2002

Swedo SE, Rapoport JL, Cheslow DL, et al: High prevalence of obsessive-compulsive symptoms in patients with Sydenham's chorea. Am J Psychiatry 146:246–249, 1989

Swedo SE, Leonard HL, Garvey M, et al: Pediatric autoimmune neuropsychiatric disorders associated with streptococcal infections: clinical description of the first 50 cases. Am J Psychiatry 155:264–271, 1998

Taber KH, Rauch SL, Lanius RA, et al: Functional magnetic resonance imaging: application to posttraumatic stress disorder. J Neuropsychiatry Clin Neurosci 15:125–129, 2003

Talbot PS: The molecular neuroimaging of anxiety disorders. Curr Psychiatry Rep 6:274–279, 2004

Tancer ME, Mailman RB, Stein MB, et al: Neuroendocrine responsivity to monoaminergic system probes in generalized social phobia. Anxiety 1:216–223, 1994

Thoren P, Asberg M, Bertilsson L: Clomipramine treatment of obsessive-compulsive disorder, II: biochemical aspects. Arch Gen Psychiatry 37:1289–1294, 1980

Tiihonen J, Kuikka J, Bergstrom K, et al: Dopamine reuptake site densities in patients with social phobia. Am J Psychiatry 154:239–242, 1997a

Tiihonen JF, Kuikka J, Rasanen P, et al: Cerebral benzodiazepine receptor binding and distribution in generalized anxiety disorder: a fractal analysis. Mol Psychiatry 2:463–471, 1997b

Toni C, Cassano GB, Perugi G, et al: Psychosensorial and related phenomena in panic disorder and in temporal lobe epilepsy. Compr Psychiatry 37:125–133, 1996

Tost H, Wendt CS, Schmitt A, et al: Huntington's disease: phenomenological diversity of a neuropsychiatric condition that challenges traditional concepts in neurology and psychiatry. Am J Psychiatry 161:28–34, 2004

Uchida RR, Del-Ben CM, Santos AC, et al: Decreased left temporal lobe volume of panic patients measured by magnetic resonance imaging. Braz J Med Biol Res 36:925–929, 2003

Uhde TW: Anxiety and growth disturbance: is there a connection? A review of biological studies in social phobia. J Clin Psychiatry 55(suppl):17–27, 1994

Valente AA Jr, Miguel EC, Castro CC, et al: Regional gray matter abnormalities in obsessive-compulsive disorder: a voxel-based morphometry study. Biol Psychiatry 58:479–487, 2005

van der Linden G, van Heerden B, Warwick J, et al: Functional brain imaging and pharmacotherapy in social phobia: single photon emission computed tomography before and after treatment with the selective serotonin reuptake inhibitor citalopram. Prog Neuropsychopharmacol Biol Psychiatry 24:419–438, 2000

van der Wee NJ, Stevens H, Hardeman JA, et al: Enhanced dopamine transporter density in psychotropic-naive patients with obsessive-compulsive disorder shown by [^{123}I]β-CIT SPECT. Am J Psychiatry 161:2201–2206, 2004

Vasa RA, Grados M, Slomine B, et al: Neuroimaging correlates of anxiety after pediatric traumatic brain injury. Biol Psychiatry 55:208–216, 2004

Veit R, Flor H, Erb M, et al: Brain circuits involved in emotional learning in antisocial behavior and social phobia in humans. Neurosci Lett 328:233–236, 2002

Vermetten E, Vythilingam M, Southwick SM, et al: Long-term treatment with paroxetine increases verbal declarative memory and hippocampal volume in posttraumatic stress disorder. Biol Psychiatry 54:693–702, 2003

von Economo C: Encephalitis Lethargica: Its Sequelae and Treatment. London, Oxford University Press, 1931

Vythilingam M, Anderson ER, Goddard A, et al: Temporal lobe volume in panic disorder: a quantitative magnetic resonance imaging study. Psychiatry Res 99:75–82, 2000a

Vythilingum B, Cartwright C, Hollander E: Pharmacotherapy of obsessive-compulsive disorder: experience with the selective serotonin reuptake inhibitors. Int Clin Psychopharmacol 15 (suppl 2):S7–S13, 2000b

Wall M, Tuchman M, Mielke D: Panic attacks and temporal lobe seizures associated with a right temporal lobe arteriovenous malformation: case report. J Clin Psychiatry 46:143–145, 1985

Wall M, Mielke D, Luther JS: Panic attacks and psychomotor seizures following right temple lobectomy (letter). J Clin Psychiatry 47:219, 1986

Walsh K, Bennett G: Parkinson's disease and anxiety. Postgrad Med J 77:89–93, 2001

Warden DL, Labbate LA, Salazar AM, et al: Posttraumatic stress disorder in patients with traumatic brain injury and amnesia for the event? J Neuropsychiatry Clin Neurosci 9:18–22, 1997

Weilburg JB, Bear DM, Sachs G: Three patients with concomitant panic attacks and seizure disorder: possible clues to the neurology of anxiety. Am J Psychiatry 144:1053–1056, 1987

Weintraub D, Newberg AB, Cary MS, et al: Striatal dopamine transporter imaging correlates with anxiety and depression symptoms in Parkinson's disease. J Nucl Med 46:227–232, 2005

Weissman MM, Bland RC, Canino GJ, et al: The cross national epidemiology of obsessive compulsive disorder. J Clin Psychiatry 55S:5–10, 1994

Weizman R, Tanne Z, Granek M, et al: Peripheral benzodiazepine binding sites on platelet membranes are increased during diazepam treatment of anxious patients. Eur J Pharmacol 138:289–292, 1987

Wenzel T, Schnider P, Wimmer A, et al: Psychiatric comorbidity in patients with spasmodic torticollis. J Psychosom Res 44:687–690, 1998

Whiteside SP, Port JD, Abramowitz JS: A meta-analysis of functional neuroimaging in obsessive-compulsive disorder. Psychiatry Res 132:69–79, 2004

Wise MG, Rundell JR: Anxiety and neurological disorders. Semin Clin Neuropsychiatry 4:98–102, 1999

Wu JC, Buchsbaum MS, Hershey TG, et al: PET in generalized anxiety disorder. Biol Psychiatry 29:1181–1199, 1991

Wurthmann C, Gregor J, Baumann B, et al: [Qualitative evaluation of brain structure in CT in panic disorders] [in German]. Nervenarzt 69:763–768, 1998

Yehuda R: Current status of cortisol findings in post-traumatic stress disorder. Psychiatr Clin North Am 25:341–368, 2002

Yehuda R, McFarlane AC: Conflict between current knowledge about posttraumatic stress disorder and its original conceptual basis. Am J Psychiatry 152:1705–1713, 1995

Zohar J, Insel TR: Drug treatment of obsessive-compulsive disorder. J Affect Disord 13:193–202, 1987

Zohar J, Insel TR, Zohar-Kadouch RC: Serotonergic responsivity in obsessive-compulsive disorder: effects of chronic clomipramine treatment. Arch Gen Psychiatry 45:167–172, 1988

Zorzon M, de Masi R, Nasuelli D, et al: Depression and anxiety in multiple sclerosis: a clinical and MRI study in 95 subjects. J Neurol 248:416–421, 2001

Zungu-Dirwayi N, Hugo F, van Heerden BB, et al: Are musical obsessions a temporal lobe phenomenon? J Neuropsychiatry Clin Neurosci 11:398–400, 1999

29

NEUROPSYCHIATRIC DISORDERS OF CHILDHOOD AND ADOLESCENCE

Martin H. Teicher, M.D., Ph.D.

Susan L. Andersen, Ph.D.

Carryl P. Navalta, Ph.D.

Akemi Tomoda, M.D., Ph.D.

Ann Polcari, Ph.D., R.N.

Dennis Kim, M.D.

In this chapter, we emphasize brain-based psychiatric disorders that invariably emerge during childhood and adolescence. Virtually all neuropsychiatric disorders can appear in pediatric patients; however, certain disorders such as attention-deficit/hyperactivity disorder (ADHD), mental retardation, autism, and Tourette syndrome (TS) must present before adulthood for diagnosis. These disorders are the focus of this chapter.

BRAIN DEVELOPMENT

The human brain is an enormously complex organ consisting, at the simplest level, of billions of neurons and trillions of synaptic interconnections. Genes provide the blueprint for our brain's architecture, which unfolds during the course of development. However, our genome, with only about 20,000 protein-coding genes, is insufficient to dictate the precise wiring schematic for our vast array of synaptic connections. Hence, the final form and function of our brain are sculpted by experience. Such an intrinsically complex process is inherently vulnerable to numerous errors, which set the stage for the emergence of childhood and adolescent neuropsychiatric disorders.

The brain develops through a series of overlapping stages, which are illustrated in Figure 29–1. The first stage is mitosis, in which neural progenitor cells multiply and divide in the neural tube in the area destined to become the ventricular surface. Eventually, during a specific delineated period of embryogenesis, the germinal cells undergo their final mitotic division to form immature nerve cells that can no longer reproduce. These neuroblasts are laid down inside out, with larger cells (e.g., pyramidal cells) generally appearing at an earlier stage than smaller cells (e.g., granule cells). During this period the brain produces two to three times the full adult complement of neurons. Neuronal mitosis is a critical process, and mitotic inhibi-

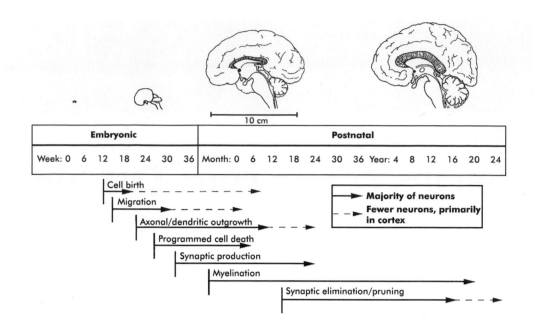

FIGURE 29–1.   Major overlapping stages of human brain development and approximate temporal sequence.

tors can exert devastating effects on brain development. Although neurogenesis ceases in most brain regions at birth, stem cells continue to generate neurons within the subventricular zone and hippocampal dentate gyrus throughout life (Kempermann and Gage 2000).

The second stage involves the migration of neurons to their final destination. This is a complex process in which immature neurons follow chemical, spatial, and mechanical gradients to reach their destination and establish connections with appropriate targets (Purves and Lichtman 1980). Glial cells also provide transient guide wires to facilitate migration (Rakic 1991). Once neurons reach their final destination at about the 16th fetal week, they branch in an attempt to establish appropriate connections (Sidman and Rakic 1973). Trophic factors, including brain-derived neurotrophic factor (BDNF), glial-derived neurotrophic factor (GDNF), and insulin-like growth factor (IGF-1), influence the migration or retraction of neurons during this process. In a striking turn of events, more than 50% of these neurons are eliminated before birth in a process known as *cell death* or *apoptosis* (Landmesser 1980). Cell survival depends on the level of activity the neuron receives and the presence of trophic factors that stabilize its growth (Cowan et al. 1984).

Synaptic development is also characterized by a distinct wave of overproduction. Synaptic density increases dramatically during the early postnatal period. Formation of synapses in the cerebellum peaks during the first 2–4 months, whereas synaptic density of the cortex continues to increase during childhood (Huttenlocher 1979). Changes in synaptic density are mirrored by changes in regional gray matter volume discernible on magnetic resonance imaging (MRI) (Giedd 2004). From birth to age 5, the brain triples in mass from 350 g to a near-adult weight of 1.2 kg. Part of this increase is a result of the marked arborization and enhanced connection of neurons. Much of the gain stems from the vigorous myelination of fiber tracts. Myelination markedly increases the speed of information exchange and is at least partially responsible for the emergence of our rich behavioral repertoire.

Myelination tends to progress in a posterior to anterior direction. Generally, projection fibers (connecting cortex with the lower parts of the brain and spinal cord) myelinate first, followed by commissural fibers, which connect the two hemispheres, and then association fibers, which interconnect cortical regions within the same hemisphere (Filley 2001). Diffusion tensor imaging shows that white matter integrity increases in the caudate nucleus and corpus callosum between ages 8–12 years and adulthood (Snook et al. 2005). Myelination of the frontal cortex continues between age 10 years and young adulthood (Suzuki et al. 2003). Left and right corticospinal pathways myelinate at the same rate, facilitating coordinated motor development. In contrast, frontotemporal pathways myelinate to a greater degree in the left hemisphere to support speech functions (Paus et al. 1999).

During the transition from childhood to adulthood, a dramatic elimination phase occurs in which synaptic contacts and neurotransmitter receptors overproduced during childhood are pruned back to final adult configuration.

Between ages 7 and 15 years, synaptic density in the frontal cortex decreases by approximately 40% (Huttenlocher 1979), along with gray matter volume (Giedd 2004). Similar changes occur in the density of dopamine (Seeman et al. 1987) (Figure 29–2), glutamate (Barks et al. 1988), and neurotensin (Mailleux et al. 1990) receptors. Overly extensive or insufficient pruning has been associated with autism (Courchesne et al. 2004) and some forms of mental retardation (Huttenlocher 1979), and has been hypothesized to play a key role in the emergence of schizophrenia (Feinberg 1982-1983; Keshavan et al. 1994). Teicher, Andersen, and colleagues (Andersen et al. 2000; Teicher et al. 1995) found that dopamine receptors prune very rapidly after the onset of puberty in the nigrostriatal system of rats, prune in early adulthood in the prefrontal cortex, but do not prune in the limbic connections to the nucleus accumbens. It is conceivable that pruning of striatal dopamine receptors is associated with the attenuation of hyperactivity and motor tics during adolescence (Andersen and Teicher 2000). Delayed pruning in the prefrontal cortex possibly unmasks an early lesion that may be associated with the emergence of schizophrenia.

Synaptic pruning drives an important developmental transition in which high synaptic density, facilitating acquisition of new knowledge and skills at considerable metabolic cost, is partially traded for a lower density system designed for rapid analysis and enhanced performance through use of established connections (Teicher et al. 1995). This maturational shift fits with more recent data on the relationship between intelligence and brain development. Researchers at the National Institutes of Health compared the patterns of brain growth in children with normal intelligence and children with superior intelligence (Shaw et al. 2006a). Level of intelligence was primarily associated with the developmental trajectory of frontal cortex. Children with superior intelligence had a particularly plastic cortex, which underwent an accelerated and prolonged phase of cortical thickening between 7 and 11 years of age, corresponding to the period of synaptic overproduction. An equally vigorous period of cortical thinning then ensued in early adolescence, in concert with the phase of synaptic pruning. It seems that the extent of overproduction and pruning and the timing of these processes are crucial determinants of adult outcome (Johnson 2003).

Overproduction and pruning shape the brain's response to cognitive tasks as measured by functional MRI (fMRI). Generally, younger children have a widespread and diffuse pattern of cortical activation that becomes more delineated and adultlike with maturation (Casey et al. 2000; Luna and Sweeney 2004). Pruning is regionally specific, and phylogenetically older regions, such as the striatum and motor cortex, prune earlier than higher

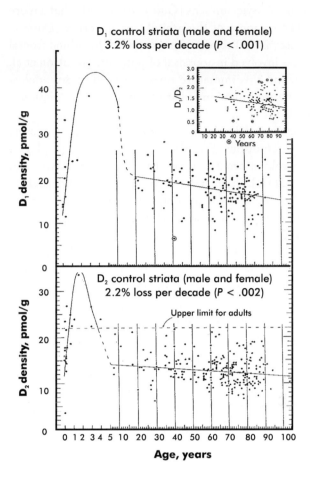

FIGURE 29–2. Overproduction and pruning of dopamine D_1 and D_2 receptors in human corpus striatum during childhood and adolescence.

Source. Reprinted from Seeman P, Bzowej N, Guan H, et al.: "Human Brain Receptors in Children and Aging Adults." *Synapse* 1:399–404, 1987. Used with permission.

level regions associated with cognition (Thompson et al. 2000). Synaptic pruning is probably responsible for the reduction in synaptic plasticity that occurs with maturation, attenuating our capacity to recover from injury. Synaptic pruning may also be responsible for the plateau in the growth of intellectual capacity (*mental age*) that occurs at about age 16 years (Walker 1994).

A crucial facet in brain development is the establishment and strengthening of connections between specific brain regions. Ernst et al. (2006) proposed a "triadic model" that endeavors to explain behavioral development in adolescence. According to their theory, risk taking and impulsivity associated with adolescence are attributable to 1) a strong reward system (nucleus accumbens), 2) a decreased harm-avoidance system (amygdala), and 3) "poor brakes" (prefrontal cortex). Functional imaging studies show that adolescents have an adultlike response of the nucleus accumbens (Galvan et al. 2005) but a more childlike response of the orbital frontal cortex (Durston and Casey 2006) to rewarding stimuli. The orbital frontal cortex is involved in appraisal of outcome (Knutson et al. 2001), and this immature response predisposes adolescents toward more immediate short-term over long-term gains (Ernst et al. 2006).

The amygdala plays an important role in processing negative emotions. Studies indicate that it also plays a similar role in processing positive emotions (Baxter and Murray 2002). In general, the response of the amygdala to affective stimuli, such as emotional faces, matures early in life and is important in associative learning (Killgore et al. 2001). Connections from the amygdala to the cortex develop gradually during the transition from adolescence to adulthood (Cunningham et al. 2002). These connections may foster the emergence of the "behavioral brake" of the prefrontal cortex, which helps to inhibit our engagement in activities with potential for harm (Amaral 2002).

Whereas many neurotransmitter systems follow the waxing and waning course of synaptogenesis, γ-aminobutyric acid (GABA)ergic transmission, like myelination, progressively increases in the cortex during adolescence (Lewis et al. 2004). Development of this major inhibitory transmitter presumably also facilitates emergence of enhanced cortical control over subcortical regions.

DEVELOPMENT OF LATERALIZATION AND HEMISPHERIC ASYMMETRY

The human brain is anatomically, neurochemically, and functionally asymmetric. Lateralization is largely established before age 5 years (Krashen 1973) and emerges through a multistage process that begins in utero (Chi et al. 1972; Molfese et al. 1975; Wada et al. 1975). Delayed myelination of the corpus callosum enables the two hemispheres to develop relatively independently. During the first few months, the right hemisphere develops more rapidly than the left, with more advanced dendritic outgrowth in Broca's area and motor cortex (Galaburda 1984; Simonds and Scheibel 1989). However, by age 5–6 months, dendritic growth in the left hemisphere surpasses that in the right and continues at a rapid pace for the next 2 years. Between ages 3 and 6 years, the right hemisphere accelerates in its development and helps provide the prosodic components of language that flower between ages 5 and 6 years. The left hemisphere, however, remains more differentiated. Early experience can exert a marked effect on lateralization in laboratory animals (Bulman-Fleming et al. 1992; Camp et al. 1984; Denenberg and Yutzey 1985). This effect may also be seen in humans and may be a factor in the genesis of psy-

chiatric disorders (Teicher 1994; Teicher et al. 1996a). Asymmetries do not appear to change significantly after childhood (Sowell et al. 2003).

The most frequently studied brain asymmetry is a planum temporale that is larger on the left than on the right (Galaburda et al. 1978; Geschwind and Levitsky 1968; Habib et al. 1995; Kulynych et al. 1994; Steinmetz et al. 1991; Wada et al. 1975). Conversely, gray matter density tends to be greater in the right posterior temporal regions than in the left (Watkins et al. 2001). These findings, which emerged through autopsy studies, have been confirmed with MRI (Blanton et al. 2001; Sowell et al. 2002).

SENSITIVE AND CRITICAL PERIODS

Brain development is sculpted by experience, but timing is crucial. There are specific stages when experience may exert a maximal effect on development (sensitive period) or when it must be present (critical period) for the formation of appropriate connections. The classic example is the development of ocular dominance columns, which can be disrupted by monocular deprivation before puberty but not after (Hubel and Wiesel 1998). Sensitive or critical periods have been delineated for neurotoxic effects on the fetus (Rice and Barone 2000), for capacity of androgens to masculinize the brain (Pardridge et al. 1982), and for development of speech, language (Doupe and Kuhl 1999; Eggermont and Ponton 2003; Sininger et al. 1999), and binocular vision (Goodyear et al. 2002). Sensitive and/or critical periods coincide with the increased expression of growth factors, which peak during periods of maximal synaptic plasticity (Berardi et al. 2000). Overexpression of BDNF can expand a critical period by provoking a precocious onset or by delaying its termination (Cabelli et al. 1995; Hanover et al. 1999). Expression of BDNF varies between brain regions and in response to stimuli (Majdan and Shatz 2006; Webster et al. 2006). Environmental enrichment can increase trophic factor production during sensitive periods (Meaney and Szyf 2005), and this increase may provide a means of altering brain development to compensate for deficiencies.

DISORDERS OF EXCESSIVE MOTOR ACTIVITY, MOVEMENT, IMPULSE, AND THOUGHT

One of the most prevalent clusters of childhood neuropsychiatric disorders includes ADHD, TS, and obsessive-compulsive disorder (OCD). These conditions often co-occur or run in families (Knell and Comings 1993; Pauls and Leckman 1986; Pauls et al. 1991). They likely occur as a consequence of different but interrelated defects in corticolimbic–basal ganglia circuits (Lou et al. 1990; Luxenberg et al. 1988; Peterson et al. 1993; Singer et al. 1993). TS and ADHD are discussed together to emphasize their commonality. OCD is discussed elsewhere in this book (see especially Chapter 28 by Stein and Rauch).

ATTENTION-DEFICIT/HYPERACTIVITY DISORDER

ADHD is one of the most common neuropsychiatric disorders of childhood, conservatively estimated to affect 3%–9% of school-age children (J.C. Anderson et al. 1987; Bird et al. 1988; Szatmari et al. 1989) and upwards of 18% as reported in systematic reviews (Rowland et al. 2002). ADHD is a serious disorder that is associated with a dramatically increased incidence of antisocial personality, drug abuse, delinquency, and criminality (Gittelman et al. 1985; Klein and Mannuzza 1991; Mannuzza et al. 1989, 1998; Satterfield et al. 1982; G. Weiss et al. 1985). Symptoms of ADHD often diminish with age, but about 65% of individuals with ADHD continue to experience significant symptoms in adulthood (Faraone et al. 2006).

ADHD was first identified as a medical disorder after the 1917 pandemic of von Economo's encephalitis. Affected adults who survived developed *encephalitis lethargica*, a severe form of Parkinson's disease, poignantly described in the film *Awakenings* (Sacks 1976). Affected children, in contrast, developed diametrically opposite symptoms of hyperactivity and impulsivity (Wender 1971). Subsequently, children presenting with problems of hyperactivity were given the diagnosis *minimal brain damage*, but, in the absence of direct evidence for brain damage, this term was changed to *minimal brain dysfunction*. DSM-III (American Psychiatric Association 1980) brought forth a new stage in our conceptualization of this condition when it renamed the syndrome *attention deficit disorder* and revised the name to *attention-deficit/hyperactivity disorder* in DSM-III-R (American Psychiatric Association 1987), a term retained in DSM-IV (American Psychiatric Association 1994). In contrast, the most comparable diagnosis in the International Classification of Diseases (ICD-10) (World Health Organization 1992) lexicon is *hyperkinetic disorder*, emphasizing the historical connection to hyperactivity.

Characteristic Features

ADHD is characterized by a triad of symptoms involving age-inappropriate problems with attention, impulse control, and hyperactivity (Barkley 1990; Tryon 1993). Currently, DSM-IV-TR (American Psychiatric Association 2000) divides the symptom triad into two factors: inattention and hyperactivity-impulsivity. To meet criteria for the disorder, children need to have, during the previous 6 months, at least six symptoms of inattention or six symptoms of hyperactivity-impulsivity. If they meet criteria for both inattention and hyperactivity-impulsivity, they receive a diagnosis of ADHD combined type, which is the most prevalent form. Otherwise, they are diagnosed with either ADHD predominantly inattentive type or ADHD predominantly hyperactive-impulsive type. In addition to the meeting of symptom criteria, accurate diagnosis requires that some of these symptoms emerge before age 7 years and be of sufficient severity to cause impairment. Symptoms must also be present in at least two different settings, must produce significant impairment in social or school endeavors, and must not be better accounted for by another mental disorder or occur exclusively during the course of a pervasive developmental disorder or psychotic disorder.

Although many sources state that ADHD is predominantly a disorder of males, substantial disparity exists in reported sex ratios (J.C. Anderson et al. 1987; Bird et al. 1988; Safer and Krager 1988). McGee et al. (1987) argued that sex differences were purely an artifact of the higher overall baseline rate of behavioral disturbance in boys. The Ontario Child Health Study (Szatmari et al. 1989) provides an interesting epidemiological perspective. According to parents' reports, boys had only a slightly greater prevalence of inattention, impulsivity, and hyperactivity. Even more striking was the observation that adolescent girls report that they had the same prevalence of symptoms as adolescent boys. This apparent equivalence was not an artifact of boys being unaware of their difficulties as they endorsed significantly more symptoms than their parents perceived. Only teachers found these symptoms to be significantly more prevalent in boys. In short, sex differences conceivably may be relatively minor. An increase in the diagnosing of ADHD in girls provides indirect support of this contention (Robison et al. 2002).

Although ADHD is defined by potentially measurable behavioral signs, it remains a controversial disorder, and its validity and prevalence have been disputed (Prior and Sanson 1986). Critics often point to the disparity in ADHD prevalence rates between the United States and England. This disparity is largely a result of differing diagnostic criteria, with ICD-10 criteria requiring all cases to have some symptoms of hyperactivity, impulsivity, and inattention. Further, the comorbid occurrence of ADHD and conduct disorder would be diagnosed as conduct disorder by ICD-10 and as ADHD with comorbid conduct disorder by DSM-IV (Popper and Steingard 1995). Converging evidence clearly supports the validity of ADHD as a psychiatric diagnosis with 1) specific and persistent disabling symptoms, 2) underlying biological basis, and 3) a characteristic response to treatment (Faraone 2005).

Studies using objective tests have documented the presence of hyperactivity (see Teicher 1995 for review) and have verified that this observation is not merely a subjective problem (Henker and Whalen 1989). Using a precise infrared motion analysis system to track body movement patterns during a computerized attention task, Teicher et al. (1996b) found that children with ADHD spent 66% less time immobile than normal, moved their head 3.4 times as far, and covered a 3.8 times greater area. Hyperactivity is most apparent when children with ADHD are required to sit still, and increased motor activity is also present while they are asleep (Porrino et al. 1983). However, they are no more active than normal when allowed to play (Porrino et al. 1983). Hence, their motor problem appears to stem from a diminished ability to inhibit activity to low levels (Teicher 1995). Deficient inhibition may also explain symptoms of inattention and impulsivity. Inattention usually manifests as failure to sustain interest in tasks that are boring or challenging and in distraction by irrelevant stimuli. These difficulties may arise from failure to inhibit initiation of competing actions. Impulsivity in ADHD largely manifests as impatience and social intrusion, which can be explained by a failure to inhibit immature behaviors through social learning. Conceptualizing ADHD as a primary defect in inhibitory capacity provides the foundation for specific pathophysiological models. This conceptualization is in accord with Robins (1992) and Korkman and Pesonen (1994), who found that impaired self-regulation and capacity to inhibit impulses, rather than inattention, were the factors that distinguished children with ADHD from children with learning disorders.

ADHD commonly occurs in conjunction with several other psychiatric disorders. Conduct disorder occurs in 40%–70% of subjects with ADHD. This disorder a serious behavioral problem in which afflicted children violate major societal rules and fail to respect individual rights. Conduct disorder appears to arise specifically in children who show signs of excessive aggressiveness (August et al. 1983). Learning disorders are also prevalent in children with ADHD (Semrud-Clikeman et al. 1992), as are mood disorders (Biederman et al. 2006; Spencer et al. 1999). Children abused early in life who develop symptoms of posttraumatic stress disorder (PTSD) also frequently meet criteria for ADHD (McLeer et al. 1994). Glod and Teicher (1996) found that 38% of hospitalized abused children with PTSD met criteria for ADHD and that on average these children were more active than normal children but were substantially less active than children with classic ADHD. It is, however, unclear whether abused children with PTSD actually have ADHD or a look-alike state (phenocopy). There is also a high incidence of ADHD among boys with TS (Comings and Comings 1987). Generalized resistance to thyroid hormone has also been associated with a high incidence of ADHD (P. Hauser et al. 1993), but this disorder is very rare and almost never found in children diagnosed with ADHD (R.E. Weiss et al. 1993). ADHD-like symptoms may also emerge as an indicator of genetic risk in children with a family history of schizophrenia (Marcus et al. 1985).

Clinical Course

Mothers often indicate that children with ADHD were extremely active in utero and that they started running and climbing as soon as they learned to walk. By the preschool years, symptoms of ADHD can be identified by teachers (Nolan et al. 2001), and these symptoms are associated with later learning problems, especially reading disabilities (Spira and Fischel 2005). However, diagnosing ADHD before age 4 or 5 years is a difficult task, and most cases remain undiagnosed until school age. Using older criteria, remission has been estimated to occur in 30% by adolescence and in 50%–70% by adulthood (Barkley 1990; Gittelman et al. 1985). Remission rates, however, depend on whether ADHD is assessed syndromically or symptomatically (Faraone et al. 2006). The most recent meta-analysis indicates that ADHD symptoms wane with age. Only 15% of children with ADHD will continue to meet full criteria for ADHD at age 25. However, about 65% will meet criteria for ADHD in partial remission and will show significant impairment (Faraone et al. 2006).

Adults with a childhood history of ADHD have increased rates of psychosocial impairment (including lower educational performance and attainment), social problems, and sexually transmitted diseases, as well as reduced employment success (Barkley et al. 2006). In persisting cases, the prevailing clinical dogma is that the hyperactivity abates but problems with inattention continue. Objective measures of activity in adults with ADHD indicate that many continue to have difficulty inhibiting activity to low levels (Teicher 1995).

Neuropsychological deficits are also common in ADHD. Working memory impairments specifically have been documented, especially problems in spatial storage and in the central executive control of spatial working memory (Martinussen et al. 2005). Children with ADHD also possess somewhat lower overall cognitive ability as measured by Full Scale intelligence scores of standardized tests (Frazier et al. 2004). Although executive functioning deficits in adults with ADHD appear to be less prominent than in children with ADHD (Schoechlin and Engel 2005), non-executive functions (e.g., response consistency, word reading, color naming) seem especially compromised (Boonstra et al. 2005).

Etiology and Pathophysiology

ADHD is perhaps best regarded as a syndrome in which the clinical phenotype may arise from multiple etiologies, probably through a number of different pathways. Worldwide, the leading cause of ADHD may be severe early malnutrition during the first year of life (Galler et al. 1983). In the United States, low birth weight, fetal alcohol exposure, and prenatal or postnatal lead exposure may be more common etiological factors. Genetic factors also play a major role. ADHD runs in families, particularly in the male relatives of ADHD children (Faraone and Biederman 1994). Girls with ADHD have a stronger family history than do boys, suggesting even greater genetic loading but lower penetrance. Twin studies indicate that heritability may be as high as 0.91 and that ADHD is inherited as a behavioral dimension rather than as a discrete disorder (Levy et al. 1997).

Efforts to identify a selective neurochemical imbalance in blood, urine, or cerebrospinal fluid (CSF) have been disappointing. Zametkin and Rapoport (1987) concluded that no reliable differences were found between control subjects without ADHD and boys with ADHD on measures of dopamine or norepinephrine metabolites. However, molecular studies focusing on the genes regulating response to dopamine and norepinephrine have provided some encouraging results. Cook et al. (1995) first suggested an association between polymorphisms of the dopamine transporter gene (*DAT1*) and ADHD. This association was later replicated in other studies (Comings et al. 1996; Daly et al. 1999; Gill et al. 1997; Waldman et al. 1998). This association makes sense because the dopamine transporter is the primary target of stimulant medications used to treat ADHD. However, three separate meta-analyses (Curran et al. 2001; Maher et al. 2002; Purper-Ouakil et al. 2005) and one recent comprehensive review (Bobb et al. 2005) emphasize that abnormalities in the dopamine transporter gene play only a modest role in enhancing susceptibility to the development of ADHD.

Other molecular genetic studies have disclosed a potential association between ADHD and a polymorphism of the dopamine D_4 receptor gene (e.g., LaHoste et al. 1996). The D_4 receptor is an interesting candidate gene in that it is preferentially located in prefrontal cortical regions (Durston et al. 2005; Sunahara et al. 1993) involved in executive control and regulation of attention. This gene has a 48-base-pair variable repeat in the third cytoplasmic loop that is associated with functional differences in re-

sponse to dopamine (Asghari et al. 1995). In particular, the 7-repeat allelic variant is less responsive to dopamine than other forms. LaHoste et al. (1996) found that 49% of the subjects with ADHD had at least one 7-repeat allele in comparison with only 21% of ethnically matched control subjects. Meta-analyses of case–control and family-based association studies reveal small but significant associations between ADHD and the presence of the 7-repeat allele (Faraone et al. 2001). Although this association has been frequently replicated, there have also been a significant number of negative studies (Bobb et al. 2005).

Comings et al. (2000) viewed ADHD as a complex disorder that emerges from the interaction of multiple genes. They examined the relationship between 20 genes for dopamine, serotonin, and noradrenergic metabolism and a quantitative score for ADHD in 336 unrelated subjects. Multivariate linear regression indicated that 3 dopamine genes, 3 serotonin genes, and 6 adrenergic genes contributed 2.3%, 3%, and 6.9%, respectively, to the variance. Altogether, polymorphisms in 12 genes explained 11.6% of the variance in symptom ratings. Although highly significant, it appears that a great deal remains to be learned regarding the role of genetic factors in the susceptibility to ADHD.

The findings of Comings et al. were somewhat surprising because they suggested that noradrenergic genes play a greater role than previously suspected, particularly in patients with both ADHD and learning disabilities (Comings et al. 2000). Recent studies have focused on the norepinephrine transporter and the α_{2A}-noradrenergic receptor as they serve as molecular targets for atomoxetine and clonidine. A significant association was reported between the G allele of the α_{2A} receptor promoter region and elevated inattentive and combined symptom scores (Roman et al. 2003), but a separate study failed to find an association when a diagnosis of ADHD was used as the benchmark (Xu et al. 2001). Studies of the norepinephrine transporter and ADHD have been discouraging to date (e.g., Barr et al. 2002; De Luca et al. 2004; McEvoy et al. 2002). Other genes under scrutiny include the serotonin transporter gene (Manor et al. 2001), dopamine D_5 receptor gene (Payton et al. 2001), and SNAP-25 (Mill et al. 2004, 2005). Future molecular genetic studies will likely investigate gene–environment interactions (Rutter 2006; Stevenson et al. 2005) in the context of developmental trajectories (Hay et al. 2004).

Imaging studies have helped to delineate a constellation of brain regions involved in ADHD. Abnormalities have been identified in the size or symmetry of the frontal cortex, caudate nucleus, corpus callosum, and cerebellar vermis (Tannock 1998). For example, Castellanos et al. (1996) reported a 4.7% smaller cerebral volume, a significant loss of normal right greater than left caudate asymmetry, smaller right globus pallidus, smaller anterior frontal region, and smaller cerebellum in children with ADHD. Regional morphometric differences may be apparent at some developmental stages but not others. For example, caudate volume appears to decrease with age in boys without ADHD, presumably as a consequence of pruning, but does not appear to change with age in boys with ADHD. Hence, Castellanos et al. (2003) found reduced caudate volumes in affected, but not unaffected, monozygotic twins discordant for ADHD. However, this difference in caudate volume faded by late adolescence (Castellanos et al. 2002).

Some studies reported that the anterior portion of the corpus callosum, which relays information between the left and right frontal cortex, is reduced in size in boys with ADHD (Giedd et al. 1994; Hynd et al. 1991). Other reports documented a decrease in size of the posterior corpus callosum (Hynd et al. 1991; Semrud-Clikeman et al. 1994). More recently, Hill et al. (2003) found that there was a reduction in total callosal area in a sample of boys and girls with ADHD. However, Castellanos et al. (1996), in the most comprehensive study with the largest sample size, failed to find a difference in any portion of the corpus callosum. Overmeyer et al. (2000) also found no corpus callosum differences between a subgroup of children with a refined subtype of ADHD and control subjects without ADHD who had siblings with ADHD.

In contrast, the most consistent morphometric difference between ADHD and control subjects has been a reduction in the size of the cerebellar vermis. This area is a midline gray and white matter region that connects left and right cerebellar hemispheres. Interestingly, it turns out to be the brain region that shows the greatest degree of growth during the postnatal period. Initial studies by Mostofsky et al. (1998) and Berquin et al. (1998) found significant reductions in the size of the posterior inferior lobe of the cerebellar vermis (lobules VIII–X). Follow-up studies (e.g., Castellanos et al. 2002; Durston et al. 2004) have further identified reduced cerebellar vermal volume as the most consistent anatomical finding in boys and girls with ADHD.

Functional imaging studies have also contributed in important ways to our understanding of the pathophysiology of ADHD. Initial studies documented resting state abnormalities in metabolism and regional blood flow in prefrontal cortex, caudate nucleus, and putamen (Ernst et al. 1994; Lou et al. 1990; Sieg et al. 1995; Zametkin et al. 1990). Teicher et al. (2000) developed a novel fMRI procedure called T2 relaxometry that provides a noninvasive indirect assessment of steady-state regional cerebral blood volume. Using this technique, we compared 11 boys with ADHD to 6 control subjects without ADHD. We found

significant elevations of T2 relaxation time (T_2RT) in the putamen, suggestive of diminished blood flow and neuronal activity. A robust relationship was found between T_2RT in the putamen and objective measures of hyperactivity (incapacity to sit still) and attention using infrared motion analysis. Additional correlates with hyperactivity and attention emerged in left dorsolateral prefrontal cortex (Teicher et al. 1996b) and cerebellar vermis (C.M. Anderson et al. 1999). Chronic treatment with methylphenidate altered T_2RT in each region, although the direction and magnitude of the effect were strongly dependent on the basal level of hyperactivity (Teicher et al. 2000). In those children with ADHD who were objectively hyperactive, methylphenidate reduced T_2RT (increased blood flow) in putamen and increased T_2RT in the cerebellar vermis. T_2RT changed in the opposite manner in ADHD children who had a more normal capacity to sit still. Similarly, methylphenidate markedly reduced seated activity in the objectively hyperactive children but either increased or exerted no effect on activity of nonhyperactive children with ADHD (Teicher et al. 2003b).

Functional imaging studies have also revealed corticostriatal defects during performance of cognitive tasks, particularly those that measure aspects of inhibitory control or working memory. Schweitzer et al. (2000) found that adults with ADHD had a more diffuse and predominantly occipital pattern of activation. Several groups have found a diminished degree of activation of dorsal anterior cingulate cortex (Bush et al. 1999; Durston et al. 2003; Tamm et al. 2004). Similarly, Rubia et al. (1999) found hypofunction of the right mesial and right inferior prefrontal cortex during motor inhibition tasks. Vaidya et al. (1998) found that ADHD children had greater blood oxygen level–dependent (BOLD) fMRI activation in frontal cortex on one attention task but reduced striatal activation on another, which increased with methylphenidate treatment. In a follow-up study, the caudate was again particularly hypoactive, which led the investigators to conclude that this diminished activity is a core abnormality in ADHD (Vaidya et al. 2005).

Imaging studies with single-photon emission computed tomography (SPECT) and positron emission tomography (PET) have detected regional neurochemical differences. A number of groups have focused on the dopamine transporter. A substantial increase in dopamine transporter density in striatum was first reported in adults with ADHD (Dougherty et al. 1999; K.H. Krause et al. 2000), and this increase was also observed in a small group of children (Cheon et al. 2003). A more recent study found only a slight difference in transporter density (Larisch et al. 2006), and two independent studies found no differences in striatal dopamine transporter density between control subjects and adolescents or adults with ADHD (Jucaite et al. 2005; van Dyck et al. 2002). ADHD subjects with a normal density of dopamine transporters may respond more poorly to methylphenidate than ADHD subjects with a high density of dopamine transporters (J. Krause et al. 2005).

Using 3,4-dihydroxyphenylalanine (DOPA) decarboxylase activity (a measure of dopamine innervation) with [^{18}F]DOPA PET, Ernst et al. (1998, 1999b) found evidence for prefrontal and midbrain (e.g., substantia nigra and ventral tegmental area) dopamine dysfunction in adults and children with ADHD, respectively. Similarly, Jucaite et al. (2005) found that there was a significant correlation between D_2 receptor density in right caudate nucleus and degree of objectively measured hyperactivity.

Magnetic resonance spectroscopy has also been used as a means of assessing neurochemical differences. Yeo et al. (2003) found that there were reduced levels of N-acetyl aspartate (suggestive of neuronal loss or dysfunction) in the dorsolateral prefrontal cortex of girls (but not boys) with ADHD. Sun et al. (2005) found that there were bilateral differences in the ratio of N-acetyl aspartate to creatine in the lenticular nucleus (putamen and globus pallidus) of schoolboys with the combined subtype of ADHD relative to control subjects and relative to boys with the predominantly inattentive subtype. Elevated frontal-striatal glutamatergic resonances were also observed in children with ADHD (Carrey et al. 2002, 2003; MacMaster et al. 2003), which could be diminished by treatment with methylphenidate (Carrey et al. 2003).

Altogether, these studies point to an array of morphometric and neurochemical abnormalities primarily in striatum (caudate/putamen), prefrontal cortex, and cerebellar vermis of individuals with ADHD. Together, these regions forms a circuit whose functionality may be impaired by a wide range of regional abnormalities that likely produce a similar array of syndromic manifestations.

Animal studies indicate that many forms of early brain injury produce hyperactivity. Of particular interest is the neonatal dopamine depletion model (B.A. Shaywitz et al. 1976a, 1976b), which is based on the von Economo's encephalitis paradox (i.e., that affected adults become parkinsonian, whereas affected children develop hyperactivity). Chemical ablation of dopamine nerve fibers produces a profound parkinsonian state in adult rats (Stricker 1976) but causes neonates to become hyperactive (B.A. Shaywitz et al. 1976b). These hyperactive rats perform poorly on a range of learning tasks, and stimulant drugs partially ameliorate these deficits (B.A. Shaywitz et al. 1976a). The hyperactivity often abates after puberty (B.A. Shaywitz et al. 1976b) unless the depletion is extremely profound (F.E. Miller et al.

1981). Curiously, the rats' hyperactivity is situationally specific (Teicher et al. 1981), and the degree and time course of the impairments are influenced by the rats' early experience (Pearson et al. 1980). Heffner et al. (1983) found that the critical feature of this model was depletion of dopamine within the frontal cortex. Early postnatal depletions of dopamine produced a concomitant increase in D_4 receptor binding in rats (Zhang et al. 2001). B.A. Shaywitz et al. (Raskin et al. 1983; B.A. Shaywitz et al. 1984) also found that relatively selective neonatal norepinephrine depletions produced impaired learning performance without hyperactivity. Thus, neonatal norepinephrine depletion may provide a model for the inattentive form of ADHD.

Pathophysiological Models of ADHD

A detailed pathophysiological model of ADHD needs to incorporate several factors. First, ADHD has a discrete time course. Symptoms emerge early in childhood (generally before age 7) and often abate or wane by adulthood. Second, many more boys than girls are diagnosed and treated for ADHD. However, ADHD symptoms are less likely to abate with age in girls. Third, pharmacological studies demonstrate that the most highly effective drugs for ADHD target either dopamine or norepinephrine. Fourth, imaging studies provide converging evidence for a disturbance in corticostriatal loops. Fifth, reverse asymmetries are found in brain structure and function in patients with ADHD. Malone et al. (1994) have argued that an imbalance exists between a left hemisphere (or anterior) attention system that provides focused sustained attention on a task (Jutai 1984) and a right (or posterior) attention system that regulates overall arousal and rapidly shifts attention to peripheral stimuli for processing novel information (Goldberg and Costa 1981; Heilman and Van Den Abell 1980). Finally, evidence suggests that the cerebellar vermis is affected in ADHD and may play a pivotal role in symptomatology.

We believe that the waxing and waning of symptoms with age, sex differences in prevalence, and greater persistence of ADHD symptoms in girls are all a consequence of the normal process of synaptic overproduction and pruning (Andersen and Teicher 2000). As illustrated in Figure 29–2, a marked overproduction of dopamine receptors in the striatum during childhood is pruned by adulthood. Furthermore, we have shown that this process occurs in male rats but is hardly apparent in female rats (Andersen et al. 1997). Sex differences in overproduction of dopamine receptors and other neural elements may account for the apparent shrinkage that occurs with age in the caudate nucleus of boys without ADHD but not girls (Castellanos et al. 1996). Our hypothesis is that at least one class of overexpressed receptors is a permissive factor in the clinical manifestation of ADHD. Overexpression in boys leads to greater clinical prevalence during the period of overproduction but may explain why fewer girls develop ADHD because this permissive factor is not expressed. Greater abatement of symptoms in boys occurs with pruning; however, girls with ADHD who remain symptomatic do so because the permissive factor is neither overproduced nor pruned in females. By adulthood, striatal D_2 density becomes equal (Teicher et al. 1995), and sex differences in prevalence largely disappear (Biederman et al. 1994). Further, the caudate nucleus apparently does not shrink with age in boys who meet diagnostic criteria for ADHD (Castellanos et al. 1996). We would hypothesize that this area shrinks in boys with ADHD who are no longer symptomatic. Andersen and Teicher (2000) also found that pruning of dopamine receptors in the prefrontal cortex occurs later in adulthood than pruning in the striatum. This process may help explain why symptoms of motor hyperactivity remit or diminish at an earlier age than attentional symptoms.

It is possible that the permissive factor may be a member of the dopamine D_2 receptor family (D_2, D_3, or D_4). D_2 family receptor density is a permissive factor in the expression of TS. Wolf et al. (1996) have shown that differences in Tourette's symptomatology between identical twins are completely explained by their differences in striatal D_2 receptor binding. However, this issue is an open question in ADHD because other neural elements are also overproduced and pruned in the striatum during the same period.

Figure 29–3 provides a schematic that integrates findings regarding drug response, hemispheric asymmetries in attention, and the role of corticostriatal circuits and the cerebellar vermis. As reviewed below, drugs that effectively treat ADHD act on catecholamine systems. Stimulant drugs bind to the dopamine transporter, attenuating dopamine reuptake and stimulating dopamine release (Breese et al. 1975; Gatley et al. 1996). This effect is attenuated and checked by the action of released dopamine on autoreceptors that control pulsatile release rates (Grace 1995; Seeman and Madras 1998). Stimulants also affect other monoamine systems and increase serotonin neurotransmission to variable degrees (Hernandez et al. 1987; Kuczenski et al. 1987). Methylphenidate appears to augment noradrenergic neurotransmission in humans, whereas dextroamphetamine decreases noradrenergic tone (Zametkin et al. 1985). This effect occurs because *p*-hydroxyamphetamine, the primary amphetamine metabolite, is taken up in the noradrenergic neuron and there converted into *p*-hydroxynorephedrine, a false neurotransmitter that displaces some of the active

transmitter (Lewander 1971a, 1971b; Rangno et al. 1973). Hence, treatment with methylphenidate increases levels of the norepinephrine metabolite 3-methoxy-4-hydroxyphenyl glycol (MHPG), whereas amphetamine causes MHPG levels to fall (Zametkin et al. 1985). ADHD symptoms are also attenuated by clonidine, which is an α_2-adrenoreceptor agonist (Hunt et al. 1985, 1986). Clonidine generally acts on noradrenergic autoreceptors within the locus coeruleus to attenuate noradrenergic neurotransmission. However, clonidine also acts as a partial agonist at postsynaptic α_2 receptors and can preserve or augment transmission through a component of the noradrenergic signal pathway, enhancing prefrontal cortex function (Arnsten et al. 1996). Selective norepinephrine reuptake inhibitors such as desipramine, nortriptyline, and atomoxetine have been shown to be effective in ADHD when administered in high doses (Popper 1997). Although these agents are highly selective in their action on the norepinephrine transporter, microdialysis studies show that they markedly increase levels of dopamine in the prefrontal cortex (Gresch et al. 1995). This increase occurs because dopamine axons in prefrontal cortex generally lack dopamine transporters, and a significant portion of dopamine released in prefrontal cortex is deactivated by uptake through noradrenergic transporters.

Dopamine and norepinephrine play pivotal roles in our two attentional systems. Dopamine is primarily involved in the left/anterior attention system that is predominantly a motor control system. This system modulates sustained focused attention within the foveal field of vision, facilitates visually guided motor behavior, and suppresses unnecessary movement in order to focus and attend (Malone et al. 1994). In contrast, norepinephrine is primarily involved in the right/posterior attention system that is primarily a sensory alerting system (Aston-Jones and Bloom 1981; Foote et al. 1980). This system modulates rapid phasic shifts in our attention, particularly to events in our peripheral field of vision. This system is a rapid one that can grab our attention and enhance arousal when salient or dangerous events are about to occur. The central amygdala, a key component of the fear and anxiety system (LaBar et al. 1998; LeDoux et al. 1988), connects to the locus coeruleus through corticotropin-releasing factor terminals that enhance noradrenergic activity (Van Bockstaele et al. 1998). Hence, the noradrenergically mediated right/posterior attentional system is coupled to fight-or-flight and startle responses.

The primary components of the left/anterior attention system are the corticostriatal pathways (prefrontal cortex, cingulate cortex, caudate, putamen, globus pallidus, and ventrolateral thalamus) along with dopamine projections

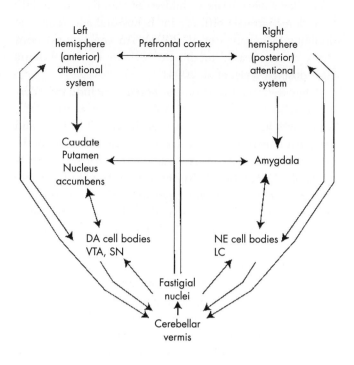

Left hemisphere (anterior) attentional system

Prefrontal cortex

Right hemisphere (posterior) attentional system

Caudate Putamen Nucleus accumbens

Amygdala

DA cell bodies VTA, SN

NE cell bodies LC

Fastigial nuclei

Cerebellar vermis

FIGURE 29–3. Simplified neural circuit diagram indicating the interconnections between brain regions and neurotransmitter systems involved in the regulation of activity and attention. Dysfunction in any component could induce symptoms of attention-deficit/hyperactivity disorder. DA = dopamine; LC = locus coeruleus; NE = norepinephrine; SN = substantia nigra; VTA = ventral tegmental area.

from the substantia nigra and ventral tegmental area. Major components of the right/posterior attention system are temporal and parietal cortex, locus coeruleus, amygdala, hippocampus, and thalamus. In general, patients with ADHD have a deficiency in the left/anterior attention system that leads to impaired focused attention, diminished capacity to suppress motor activity, and increased impulsivity (Malone et al. 1994). Some patients with ADHD may have (or also have) an overactive right/posterior system that can produce high distractibility and rapid intense shifts in attention and affect. It is also possible that some children with ADHD have an underactive right/posterior system, which can lead to left hemisphere-driven hyperfocus coupled with diminished awareness of the environment or external events. This situation may occur in some inattentive ADHD patients who are "spacey" and hypoactive. Recent quantitative electroencephalography (EEG) findings support the involvement of the temporal cortex and hippocampus in ADHD (Chabot et al. 2005), whereas MRI evidence of right parietal cortex thickness normalization in children with ADHD who had better outcomes may represent compensatory cortical change (Shaw et al. 2006b).

Stimulants, through their strong effects on the dopamine system, augment the left/anterior attention system and enhance focused attention and motor suppression. Clonidine, through its effects on norepinephrine, would likely suppress the right/posterior system and decrease distractibility and hyperarousal. Noradrenergic reuptake inhibitors should facilitate right/posterior function in situations in which norepinephrine is diminished. They may also bring an overactive noradrenergic system into better homeostasis, as they appear to do in panic disorder and PTSD (Goddard and Charney 1997). High doses of noradrenergic reuptake inhibitors also produce an indirect increase in prefrontal dopamine levels facilitating the left/anterior attention system.

Coordinated interplay and balance between these attentional systems is crucial for safety and success. The cerebellar vermis is in a key position to coordinate balance between these systems. First, the vermis receives multimodal sensory information (Brons et al. 1990; Donaldson and Hawthorne 1979; Huang and Liu 1990) and is intimately involved in the control of eye movements (Suzuki and Keller 1988). The vermis also receives vestibular (Denoth et al. 1979) and proprioceptive (Eccles et al. 1971) information to rapidly guide or adjust body position through its motor pathways. The vermis receives projections from prefrontal cortex (Schmahmann and Pandya 1995) along with noradrenergic and dopaminergic projections from the midbrain (Ariano et al. 1997a, 1997b; Dennett and Hubbard 1988; Melchitzky and Lewis 2000). The vermis outputs through the deep cerebellar fastigial nuclei. These nuclei exert robust effects on global cerebral blood flow and metabolism (Doba and Reis 1972; Goadsby and Lambert 1989). They also modulate the turnover of dopamine and norepinephrine (Dempsey and Richardson 1987). Hence, the vermis is ideally wired to affect cortical arousal and catecholamine neurotransmission in response to input from the prefrontal cortex and multimodal sensory systems. These observations underscore the tight association emerging between cerebellar vermis and prefrontal cortex in normal function and psychiatric disorders (Andreasen et al. 1996; Ciesielski et al. 1997; Sweeney et al. 1998).

We suspect that ADHD can arise in a number of ways from defects or imbalances in the activity and regulation of these attentional systems. The defect may be located specifically within an attentional system or may be vermal in origin, leading to an impaired capacity to balance and coordinate the systems. A variety of defects can produce similar syndromic manifestations and benefit from one or more drugs that enhance catecholamine neurotransmission. We suspect that, in the near future, use of objective behavioral measures, newer imaging technologies, and molecular studies will identify a number of specific etiologies that comprise the ADHD behavioral syndrome.

Treatment

Comprehensive treatment of ADHD includes both pharmacological and nonpharmacological interventions. Primary medication options include psychostimulants, antidepressants, and antihypertensives. Stimulants, the use of which continues to be clouded by unfounded concerns, remain the mainstay of treatment. In numerous studies, stimulants have been shown to attenuate hyperactivity, improve attention, and diminish impulsivity (Wilens and Biederman 1992). Methylphenidate, given in daily doses of 10–60 mg, and dextroamphetamine, in daily doses of 5–40 mg, are the major agents of choice. Unfortunately, both have a brief duration of action (as short as 3 hours). Effective treatment usually requires multiple daily doses, and children typically receive their first dose in the morning shortly before school and a second dose at lunchtime. Many children also benefit from a smaller dose after school. Older longer-acting preparations of methylphenidate and dextroamphetamine often failed to extend therapeutic duration (Brown et al. 1980; Pelham et al. 1987, 1990); however, newer long-acting formulations have succeeded in markedly extending duration of action. Adderall, a mixture of amphetamine and dextroamphetamine, has gained popularity as a single-dose preparation that provides a more gradual onset and longer duration. Pliszka et al. (2000) found that Adderall was at least as effective as regular methylphenidate, and 70% of their sample responded well to Adderall taken as a single dose. Average daily Adderall dose was 25 mg for preadolescents. Concerta was developed as a new delivery system for methylphenidate. Briefly, an osmotic minipump delivers methylphenidate in a manner that produces escalating blood levels throughout the day. The pump is surrounded by a shell of methylphenidate that provides an initial bolus. Studies suggest that once-daily Concerta is as effective as regular methylphenidate delivered in three equal doses throughout the day (Pelham et al. 2001). Metadate CD, Ritalin LA, and, most recently, Focalin XR are also among the second generation, once-daily methylphenidate preparations. Metadate CD and Ritalin LA are equivalent to twice-daily immediate-release methylphenidate with durations of action lasting 8–9 hours, and their effectiveness is relatively best earlier in the day when increased levels of methylphenidate are delivered (Liu et al. 2005). Immediate-release Focalin (D-methylphenidate) consists of the single dextro-isomer form of D,L-methylphenidate. Focalin XR uses an oral spheroidal drug absorption system to deliver 50% immediate medication and 50% delayed release approximately 4 hours after ingestion. Placebo-controlled clinical trials in children and adults with ADHD have demonstrated efficacy for behavioral and academic domains (McGough et al. 2005). An analog classroom study demonstrated medication effects up to 12 hours after dosing (Wigal et al. 2004).

New delivery forms on the horizon include transdermal methylphenidate (V.R. Anderson and Scott 2006), which was just recently approved by the U.S. Food and Drug Administration (FDA). Overall, transdermal methylphenidate appears to have significant efficacy in treatment of ADHD, but questions arise in terms of the rate of onset of benefits. We have recently reported that methylphenidate preparations that slowly rise to therapeutic dose appear to have less beneficial effects on objective measures of attention than preparations that provide a more rapid onset (Teicher et al. 2006a). Awaiting approval is NRP104/SPD489 (lisdexamfetamine dimesylate), a prodrug of amphetamine. This agent is cleaved and converted to amphetamine after oral absorption but is inactive if taken intravenously or intranasally. Hence, this agent may have limited abuse liability in adults and may not require FDA schedule 2 classification.

Methamphetamine, a much less frequently prescribed stimulant, is available in a sustained-release form (Desoxyn Gradumet) that seems to work reasonably well (Wender 1993). Pemoline is another effective stimulant with a longer duration of action and reduced potential for abuse. However, a relatively high (1%–3%) incidence of adverse hepatic effects has markedly restricted its use. High initial doses (37.5–112.5 mg) were found to produce rapid and sustained beneficial effects (Pelham et al. 1995). An average effective dose of pemoline for a child would be approximately 56 mg (Pelham et al. 1990). On the basis of advice from the FDA, pemoline is no longer available in the United States because of the overall risk of liver toxicity. Modafinil, a wakefulness-enhancing drug approved for treatment of narcolepsy, has been shown to be effective in randomized, double-blind, placebo-controlled trials (Biederman et al. 2005; Rugino and Samsock 2003). The mechanism of action of modafinil is uncertain. It appears to provide direct inhibition of dopamine reuptake, indirect inhibition of norepinephrine reuptake in the ventrolateral preoptic nucleus, and activation of the orexin/hyocretin brain peptide system.

Common side effects of stimulants include anorexia, stomachaches, insomnia, and mood changes (irritability, mood lability, dysphoria). Tics and stereotypic movements occur less commonly (discussion follows). Diminishing growth and stature from using stimulants are minimal. In the largest clinical trial to date (Multimodal Treatment Study of Children with ADHD [MTA]), mild growth suppression was observed at the 14-month and

24-month follow-ups (MTA Cooperative Group 2004). If stimulants attenuate final height, the consequence is less than an inch (Popper et al. 1995). Spencer et al. (1996) provide data that suggest that ADHD, as a disorder, is associated with delayed growth during early childhood, with compensatory growth by late adolescence. They found that stimulants played no role in the process.

Concern was raised by an FDA advisory committee in 2006 regarding the possible occurrence of sudden death in a small number of individuals treated with stimulants. The committee reviewed data from a 5-year period (1999–2003) and found that there were 12 deaths of children and adolescents on amphetamine-containing medications and 7 deaths on methylphenidate preparations. Overall, there were 0.36 deaths per 1 million amphetamine prescriptions written and 0.21 deaths per 1 million methylphenidate prescriptions written. However, the FDA has estimated that the basal rate of sudden death for children and adolescents ranges between 1.3 and 4.6 deaths per 100,000 person-years, suggesting that the incidence of sudden death on stimulants is well below the expected basal rate for spontaneous deaths (unrelated to treatment) reported in the literature.

Risk for stimulant abuse in the ADHD population appears small. Stimulants exert dysphoric, rather than euphoriant, effects on children (Rapoport et al. 1980), and compliance can be a significant problem. Individuals with ADHD do not generally like how the medication makes them feel, although many appreciate how the medication enhances performance and leads to greater acceptance by peers, teachers, or supervisors. Biederman et al. (1999), in an important study, found that stimulant treatment of ADHD in childhood actually diminished risk for substance abuse in adulthood. Subsequent studies by other researchers corroborated these initial findings and suggest that stimulant treatment of ADHD appears to reduce the risk for substance use disorders by 50% (Faraone and Wilens 2003). This outcome may be the result of a neuroprotective process affected by stimulant treatment (Andersen 2005; Andersen et al. 2002). Overall, psychostimulants are effective in the treatment of the core features of ADHD, particularly in children with very high levels of hyperactivity and inattention (Teicher et al. 2003b) and with significant fluctuations in attention and distractibility (Teicher et al. 2004b). Consistent and appropriate use can lead to enhanced self-esteem and improved quality of life. Even preschoolers with ADHD tolerate the medication well and can receive a significant benefit (Connor 2002; Short et al. 2004).

Although stimulants are the most proven efficacious treatments for ADHD, there has been widespread interest in nonstimulant alternatives. Atomoxetine (Strattera) is the first and only nonstimulant medication approved by the FDA for treating ADHD in children, adolescents, and adults. Atomoxetine selectively increases extracellular levels of norepinephrine and dopamine in the prefrontal cortex but does not affect dopamine in the striatum or nucleus accumbens (Bymaster et al. 2002). Hence, this agent should not have abuse liability in adults and should be less prone to induce or exacerbate tics. As described above under "Pathophysiological Models of ADHD," norepinephrine is intimately involved with the right/posterior attention system. Because noradrenergic activation affects attention and maintenance of arousal, this system has been implicated in the pathophysiology of ADHD (Biederman and Spencer 1999). Atomoxetine has been consistently demonstrated to be well tolerated and is free of the adverse cardiac conduction effects associated with tricyclic antidepressants. Atomoxetine has been shown to provide significant relief from the core symptoms of ADHD compared with placebo (Kelsey et al. 2004; M. Weiss et al. 2005). However, preliminary controlled trials suggest that stimulants generally outperform atomoxetine in direct therapeutic comparisons (Kemner et al. 2005; Wigal et al. 2005).

In terms of safety, atomoxetine provides marked therapeutic advantage over tricyclic antidepressants that selectively affect reuptake of norepinephrine, notably desipramine and nortriptyline. Several studies have demonstrated the effectiveness of these older agents in children with ADHD (Biederman and Spencer 2000). However, reports of sudden death in prepubertal children receiving desipramine have raised serious concerns about this agent and other tricyclic antidepressants (Abromowicz 1990; Geller et al. 1999; Popper 1997). The most common cardiac effects of tricyclic antidepressants in pediatric patients include sinus tachycardia, intraventricular conduction delay of the right bundle branch block type (QRS > 100 msec), and increased QTc intervals (Biederman et al. 1989; Leonard et al. 1995). For this reason, the maximum desipramine dosages should be 5 mg/kg/day, cardiac status and family cardiac history need to be carefully evaluated, and electrocardiogram and plasma levels need to be closely monitored. Although no direct causal relationship has been established between desipramine use and sudden death, cardiovascular toxicity remains a potential risk, and parents need to be informed of this possibility.

Studies also indicate that bupropion (Wellbutrin, 0.7 mg/kg/day), a second-generation antidepressant, can be effective in improving attention and reducing conduct problems (Barrickman et al. 1995). Venlafaxine (Effexor) exerts strong effects on both noradrenergic and serotonergic reuptake and should theoretically be beneficial for ADHD, with a more benign cardiac profile than that of tricyclic antidepressants. However, data are scant about its utility (Motavalli Mukaddes and Abali 2004; Olvera et al. 1996; Pleak and Gormly 1995; Wilens et al. 1995). Selective serotonin reuptake inhibitors (SSRIs), such as fluoxetine, were initially reported to be useful in an open trial (Barrickman et al. 1991). The general clinical consensus, however, is that SSRIs provide little effect on core symptoms of ADHD, can be helpful with comorbid mood and anxiety symptoms, but can also worsen ADHD symptoms (Popper 1997; Spencer et al. 2002). Although monoamine oxidase inhibitors are also effective in attenuating ADHD symptoms, dietary restrictions preclude their use in pediatric populations.

Evidence suggests that the α_2-adrenergic agonists clonidine and guanfacine are potentially effective treatments. Hunt and colleagues (Hunt 1987; Hunt et al. 1985, 1986) reported in a small sample that clonidine is comparable in efficacy to methylphenidate in reducing hyperactivity and impulsivity, although a meta-analysis of 11 studies found that the drug has an effect size less than that of stimulants (Connor et al. 1999). Oral doses are generally initiated at 0.025–0.05 mg and increased to a maximum of 3–10 µg/kg. Transdermal patches can provide more consistent drug effects and decreased propensity for allergic reactions. Common side effects include sedation, rash, and increased appetite and weight gain; less common reactions include headaches, rebound insomnia, cardiovascular effects, and mood lability. Rebound hypertension can occur upon abrupt cessation. In an open trial, guanfacine was reported to be efficacious in children with ADHD (Hunt et al. 1995) and those with comorbid TS (Chappell et al. 1995). Guanfacine may be especially effective in adults with ADHD (Taylor and Russo 2001) and produce less sedation and hypotension. Common initial doses are 0.25–0.5 mg, which can be titrated to up to 4 mg/day (Hunt et al. 1995).

Selection of a particular pharmacological agent depends on clinical presentation, comorbidity, duration of effect, and abuse potential by other family members. We find it useful to fully inform family members about potential risks and benefits of treatment and to have them decide which option they prefer. Effectiveness should be based on reports from the child, parents, and teachers. Standardized rating scales have been well validated and are often indispensable. We have also found that objective measures of activity and attention provide a very precise means for evaluation of therapeutic efficacy and dose titration (Teicher et al. 2003b, 2006a). Dosage adjustments are needed to optimize treatment and to compensate for growth and development. Some children and families tolerate reemergence of symptoms with medication discontinuation during weekends and summers. Most children require long-term treatment continuing into adolescence and possibly adulthood.

Despite the benefits of pharmacotherapy, additional treatment and support is often required. Environmental manipulation, such as reducing stimuli and distractions, may help modulate symptoms, and education tailored to the student's learning style may be necessary to improve academic performance. A variety of behavioral management programs have been created for parents (Barkley 1987; Robin and Foster 1989). Barkley et al. (1992) compared three different programs and found that they were all helpful, although clinically significant change was evident in only 5%–30% of subjects. The aforementioned MTA study evaluated the differential effects of a behavioral therapy strategy and a medication management strategy (MTA Cooperative Group 1999). Altogether, 579 children with ADHD combined type, ages 7–9.9 years, were assigned to 14 months of medication management (titration followed by monthly visits), intensive behavioral treatment (parent, school, and child components), the two combined, or standard community care. Children in the combined treatment and medication management groups showed significantly greater improvement than those given intensive behavioral treatment or community care. No significant differences were seen on any measure between combined treatment and medication management, although the combined and behavioral treatments had higher "consumer satisfaction" from both parents and teachers (P. S. Jensen 1999). Combined treatment may have advantages in more complex cases, such as when parents display negative or ineffective parenting practices (Hinshaw et al. 2000) or when children have comorbid anxiety or conduct disorders (P. S. Jensen et al. 2001). Unfortunately, children from all treatment groups remained significantly impaired in their peer relationships (Hoza et al. 2005). Medication management was superior to community treatment, in part because average methylphenidate dose was twice as high in the study, suggesting that subjects in the community did not receive an optimal dose. Methylphenidate was usually administered three times a day in the study versus twice daily in the community.

No studies support the effectiveness of psychotherapy alone, sugar toxicity or withdrawal, or restriction of salicylates or food dyes, although omitting food dyes may be helpful in a small minority. EEG biofeedback has been touted as an alternative to medications that can exert sustained beneficial effects (Lubar and Lubar 1984; Lubar et al. 1995; Nash 2000). A positive clinical response has been observed in approximately 75% of patients in case and controlled group studies of ADHD (Monastra et al. 2005). This treatment was shown to increase activation of the right anterior cingulate in an fMRI study (Levesque et al. 2006) and to enhance cortical activation on quantitative EEG (Monastra et al. 2005). Randomized, controlled studies are needed to determine its clinical efficacy.

TOURETTE SYNDROME AND OTHER TIC DISORDERS

TS is an intriguing neuropsychiatric disorder, presumably arising from deep within the basal ganglia, that illustrates the prominent associations between hyperactivity, impulsivity, tics, obsessions, and compulsions. Tics are stereotyped, brief, repetitive, purposeless, nonrhythmic motor and vocal responses. Although temporarily suppressible, tics are not under full voluntary control, and the individual often experiences increasing internal tension that is only relieved when the tic is released.

Clinically, tic disorders are divided into four categories: transient tic disorder, chronic tic disorder, TS, and tic disorder not otherwise specified. Transient tic disorder is diagnosed when an individual experiences either single or multiple motor and/or vocal tics many times a day on a near daily basis for at least 4 consecutive weeks but for no more than 12 months (American Psychiatric Association 2000). The tics must be distressing or cause significant impairment. Onset must occur before age 18 years, and tics may not be due to the direct effect of a drug or a more generalized neurological disorder such as Huntington's disease or postviral encephalitis. Transient tic disorder can be a single episode or can reoccur after a period of remission. Chronic tic disorder is diagnosed when an individual has motor tics or vocal tics (but not both) for more than a year with no more than a 3-month consecutive hiatus. Onset must be before 18 years, and the same exclusionary criteria apply as in transient tic disorder. TS is diagnosed when an individual meets criteria for a chronic tic disorder involving the presence of both motor and vocal tics. Tic disorder not otherwise specified is used for cases that fail to fall into one of these three primary categories.

Characteristic Features

Tics can be simple or complex. Simple motor tics include jerking movements, shrugging, and eye blinking. Simple vocal tics include grunting, sniffing, and throat clearing. More complex motor tics involve grimacing, banging, or temper tantrums, whereas complex vocal tics include echolalia and coprolalia. Tics wax and wane over time, and the primary muscle groups affected gradually change as well.

TS is a chronic condition in which both motor and vocal tics are observable. The tics are often presaged by premonitory sensory urges that build in tension until the tic is released (Leckman et al. 1993). Many patients feel more troubled by the pre-tic tension than by the tics themselves (Leckman et al. 1993), and some patients can successfully control their tics in public and unleash them when they are alone. Tics are markedly attenuated by sleep (Fish et al. 1991). TS waxes and wanes over time and can vary enormously in severity from mild and undiagnosed to disabling. Anxiety and stress can increase symptoms.

The modal age at onset is 6–7 years, but age at onset can range from 2 to 17 years (Leckman et al. 1995b). Tic symptoms are generally most severe during the period preceding puberty (average 10 ± 2.4 years of age) and gradually improve thereafter, except in the most severe cases (Leckman et al. 1998). For this reason, it is important to note that tic severity during childhood is not a predictor of tic severity at age 18 years (Leckman et al. 1998). In half of patients, symptoms start as a single tic involving eyes, face, or head and progress in a rostrocaudal manner. Before the first appearance of tics, 25%–50% of TS patients have a history of hyperactivity, inattention, and impulsivity consistent with ADHD (Comings and Comings 1987). Phonic and vocal tics generally emerge at about age 11 years, often starting with a single syllable and then progressing to longer exclamations. Coprolalia occurs in about 60% of patients and emerges in early adolescence.

Complex motor tics may be purposeless or camouflaged by a sequence of intentional actions and can be self-destructive or violent. In a pilot study, Budman et al. (1998) concluded that rage attacks are not related to tic severity but rather reflect an underlying pathophysiology with other comorbid conditions.

Obsessive-compulsive symptoms appear in 60% of cases (Leckman et al. 1995b), and OCD is observed in 7%–10%. Obsessive-compulsive symptoms usually emerge 5–10 years after the first appearance of simple tics (Bruun 1988). Tic-related OCD may differ from the classic OCD with an earlier age at onset; more prominent symptoms of ritualized touching, tapping, and rubbing; less satisfactory response to SSRIs; and an enhanced response to neuroleptic augmentation (Leckman et al. 1995b).

TS is not an uncommon condition of childhood and is believed to affect between one and six boys per thousand. The disorder is three- to fourfold more prevalent in boys than in girls. As TS often wanes after puberty, prevalence rates drop by about an order of magnitude (Leckman et al. 1995b).

Etiology and Pathophysiology

Tic disorders have a substantial genetic basis, but additional factors play a key role. A large study of affected sibpair families found that first-degree relatives had a tenfold increased risk (Tourette Syndrome Association International Consortium for Genetics 1999). Tics are present in about two-thirds of relatives of TS patients.

Monozygotic twins have about a 53% concordance rate versus an 8% concordance rate for dizygotic twins (Leckman et al. 1995b). In the past, mathematical models have suggested that TS and OCD may be transmitted by a single autosomal dominant gene with variable penetrance (Pauls and Leckman 1986), with sex differences explained by a substantially higher penetrance in males than females (Eapen et al. 1993). However, more recent etiological models of TS allow for multiple genes and gene-environment interactions (State et al. 2001). Currently, large-scale genetic studies are in progress in an attempt to identify genes associated with the development of TS (Black and Webb 2006). Smaller studies have suggested that the variable number of tandem repeat polymorphisms in the monoamine oxidase (MAO)-A gene may promote risk for TS, although there are discrepancies that remain to be worked out regarding whether increased risk results from a high- (Diaz-Anzaldua et al. 2004) or low-activity allele (Gade et al. 1998).

Although the TS gene is transmitted equally well by mothers and fathers, differences in clinical presentation can occur. Lichter et al. (1995) reported that maternal transmission was characterized by greater motor tic complexity and more frequent noninterfering rituals, whereas paternal transmission was associated with increased vocal tic frequency, earlier onset of vocal tics relative to motor tics, and more prominent ADHD behaviors. This mode of transmission is an example of genomic imprinting, in which certain genes may be differentially altered based on maternal or paternal lineage. Approximately 10% of individuals with TS have a nonfamilial version, which in all other ways is similar to the familial form.

Epigenetic factors play a role in the expression of TS. Examination of monozygotic twins discordant for TS indicates that the affected twin had a lower birth weight, suggesting involvement of perinatal factors. Other potential factors include exposure to high levels of gonadal androgens and stress hormones during early central nervous system (CNS) development or recurrent stress, anabolic steroids, cocaine, or other stimulants during postnatal development (Leckman et al. 1990). Emerging evidence suggests that Group A, β-hemolytic streptococcal infection can result in some forms of TS and OCD (Swedo 1994). (See section later in this chapter on PANDAS—pediatric autoimmune neuropsychiatric disorders associated with streptococcal infection.)

Although the definite pathophysiology of TS is not known, consensus has been reached that the basal ganglia and related thalamocortical circuitry are involved. Evidence derives from several sources, including the ameliorative effects of thalamic lesions and surgical disconnection of the prefrontal cortex (Leckman et al. 1991). MRI studies have revealed abnormalities in basal ganglia structures, corpus callosum morphology, and several cortical regions (Peterson et al. 1994, 2001, 2003). When monozygotic twins discordant for degree of TS severity were compared, Hyde et al. (1995) found that the more severely affected twin had a smaller right anterior caudate and smaller left lateral ventricle. Girls with TS alone had smaller lateral ventricles than did girls with TS and ADHD or control subjects (Zimmerman et al. 2000).

Functional imaging studies confirm the presence of altered striatal metabolism but also reveal more widespread involvement affecting frontal, cingulate, and insular cortex. George et al. (1992) found that TS subjects had significantly elevated right frontal cortex activity. Braun et al. (1993) found that regional glucose utilization was decreased in left hemispheric regions of the paralimbic and ventral prefrontal cortices (particularly orbitofrontal, inferior insular, and parahippocampal regions) and in subcortical regions including the nucleus accumbens and ventromedial caudate. Concomitant bilateral increases in regional glucose utilization in the supplementary motor, lateral premotor, and Rolandic cortices were also observed. In a more definitive study, Peterson et al. (1998) found that TS patients endeavoring to suppress their tics had increased neuronal activity in the right midfrontal cortex, bilateral superior and temporal gyrus, and right anterior cingulate and decreased neuronal activity in the ventral globus pallidus, putamen, midthalamus, right posterior cingulate, and left sensory motor cortex. When TS patients could freely express their tics, neuronal activity increased in the head of the caudate, primarily on the right side (Peterson et al. 1998). Neuroimaging findings significantly overlap among TS, ADHD, and OCD. OCD appears to involve metabolic changes in orbitofrontal cortex and caudate (Baxter 1992), whereas ADHD can involve prefrontal, cingulate, superior sensorimotor, and premotor cortex, along with the caudate, putamen, and cerebellar vermis (as discussed in the preceding section).

A variety of neurotransmitter abnormalities have been postulated to explain the pathophysiology of TS. However, the relationship between dopamine and TS is less than clear. For example, both presynaptic dopamine depletion and antipsychotic medication reduce tics, but in some cases dopamine agonists can also inhibit tic behavior (reviewed in Black et al. 2006). Actual measures of dopaminergic function have produced mixed results. CSF and tissue levels of the dopamine metabolite homovanillic acid (HVA) are reduced in TS (Leckman et al. 1995a). Reduced levels of HVA can arise from diminished dopamine turnover, which could result from postsynaptic supersensitivity. However, autopsy studies (Singer et al. 1991) and PET studies (Wong et al. 1997) have not found an elevation in dopamine D_2 receptor density in most subjects with TS that would be indicative of supersensitivity. Linkage studies have excluded dopamine D_1 and D_2 family receptors and the enzymes dopamine β-hydroxylase, tyrosinase, and tyrosine hydroxylase from being closely linked with TS (Barr et al. 1996, 1997; Brett et al. 1995b; Gelernter et al. 1995b; Ozbay et al. 2006). Thus, a mutation in a dopamine receptor gene or biosynthetic enzyme does not appear to be responsible for the genetic transmission of TS. Singer et al. (1991) found that TS patients at autopsy had a 37% greater density of dopamine transporter (reuptake) sites in caudate than did control subjects and 50% greater density in putamen. Malison et al. (1995) confirmed this finding with SPECT. Increased transporter density may explain the diminished HVA findings, as released dopamine recaptured by transport is predominantly converted into dihydroxyphenylacetic acid rather than HVA (Keller et al. 1973). TS patients also have greater accumulation of fluorodopa in the left caudate (a 25% increase) and right midbrain (53% increase) than do control subjects, suggesting an increase in DOPA decarboxylase enzyme activity (Ernst et al. 1999a). These findings are consistent with a greater degree of dopamine terminal innervation. Wolf et al. (1996) observed in monozygotic twins discordant for Tourette's severity that the more affected twin had a greater density of dopamine D_2 receptors in the caudate but not the putamen. Furthermore, within each twin pair a precise match was found between the degree of differences in D_2 binding in the head of the caudate and the degree of difference in severity. Thus, it appears that dopamine receptor density may be a modifying factor that helps explain the high degree of phenotypic variation in this disorder.

Noradrenergic theories about TS have also emerged based on the efficacy of clonidine, an α_2-agonist, which is believed to directly diminish firing rates of noradrenergic neurons and to indirectly modulate the activity of dopamine neurons (Leckman et al. 1995a). Adults with TS have elevated levels of CSF norepinephrine, a blunted growth hormone response to clonidine (Muller et al. 1994), and an abnormally high secretion of urinary norepinephrine in response to stress (Chappell et al. 1994). However, studies of the norepinephrine metabolite MHPG have been inconclusive (Leckman et al. 1995a).

Preliminary postmortem brain studies have shown that 5-hydroxytryptamine (5-HT) and its major metabolite 5-hydroxyindoleacetic acid (5-HIAA) may be globally decreased in the basal ganglia and other brain regions (G.M. Anderson et al. 1992). CSF studies have sometimes reported diminished levels of 5-HIAA (Leckman et al. 1995a, 1995b), and blood levels of 5-HT and tryptophan are also reduced (Comings 1990). Despite the well-known association between OCD and 5-HT, SSRIs have little efficacy against tics (Kurlan et al. 1993). Genetic studies exclude variation in the 5-HT$_{1A}$ and 5-HT$_7$ receptor genes and the tryptophan oxygenase gene from the etiology of TS (Brett et al. 1995a; Gelernter et al. 1995a).

Cholinergic interneurons play a critical role in modulating and balancing the effects of dopamine in the extrapyramidal system. Nicotine potentiates the therapeutic effects of neuroleptics (McConville et al. 1991), and muscarinic receptor binding is reduced in TS lymphocytes (Rabey et al. 1992). Clinical trials of choline, lecithin, and deanol have not been particularly efficacious (Leckman et al. 1995b). Treatment with a nicotine patch, which is believed to inactivate nicotinic receptors during chronic exposure, may potentiate the effects of neuroleptics in ameliorating TS symptoms (Sanberg et al. 1997; Silver et al. 2001).

Leckman et al. (1991) postulated that TS arises from a failure to habituate one or more components of the corticostriatal-thalamocortical circuit (see Figure 29–3). Oral facial tics may arise from insufficient habituation or excess excitation in circuits located within the ventromedian areas of the caudate and putamen that receive topographical projections from the orofacial regions of the primary motor and premotor cortex. It is also noteworthy that the amygdala projects to widespread areas of the nucleus accumbens and ventral portions of the caudate and putamen. Electrical stimulation of the amygdala produces motor and vocal responses resembling tics (Jadresic 1992). Based on the age at onset and proclivity for these conditions to attenuate or remit during puberty, we propose that they emerge during the period of synaptic overproduction and hyperinnervation that takes place during childhood (see Figure 29–2). Receptor overproduction may alter the balance between excitation and inhibition in circumscribed regions that control specific motor programs. Waning of symptoms after puberty may be related to the pruning of overproduced receptors and dopamine terminals.

Treatment

TS is a complicated and multifaceted condition in which there is enormous variability between patients. In some cases, ADHD is the major problem and tic symptoms may be relatively mild. For these individuals the risk of exacerbating tics with stimulant treatment may be a significant concern, but treatment can often be accomplished safely (Castellanos et al. 1997). Other patients are beset by tics that are disfiguring and result in social ostracism or unemployment. Still other patients have serious problems with premonitory sensory urges, obsessions, and compulsions, but in public have no discernible tics.

In general, neuroleptic drugs are effective in attenuating or suppressing tics in 60%–80% of patients (Singer 2005). Haloperidol (0.5–5 mg/day) and pimozide (1–3 mg/day) have been the drugs of choice. Both are high-potency dopamine D_2 receptor antagonists and are relatively nonsedating. Neuroleptic drugs will also attenuate symptoms of hyperactivity and impulsivity that emerge from comorbid ADHD. However, neuroleptics fail to facilitate attention and can cause substantial cognitive blunting. Pimozide may produce less cognitive blunting than haloperidol and can even have a beneficial cognitive effect in children with comorbid ADHD (Sallee et al. 1994). Pimozide is usually reserved for cases in which haloperidol has not proven entirely satisfactory, because pimozide can produce cardiac arrhythmias and requires more extensive monitoring. Atypical antipsychotic medications including risperidone, olanzapine, and ziprasidone, which may be associated with a lower incidence of extrapyramidal side effects than conventional neuroleptics, are commonly used in place of older neuroleptics (Black et al. 2006). Localized injections of botulinum toxin into the site of the most problematic tics has been highly effective. This treatment also attenuated premonitory sensations in 21 of 25 patients tested (Kwak et al. 2000). Muscle relaxants, benzodiazepines, presynaptic dopamine depleters, and dopamine agonists may be helpful in suppressing or inhibiting tics (Black et al. 2006).

The most serious side effect of neuroleptic treatment is the emergence of neuroleptic malignant syndrome, a potentially lethal state of muscle tension, hyperpyrexia, and autonomic nervous system lability. Reviews indicate that children are vulnerable to the emergence of neuroleptic malignant syndrome; however, there appear to be no reported cases in children treated with neuroleptics for TS (Steingard et al. 1992). An unusual but significant side effect of neuroleptic treatment is the development of phobic anxiety, which can result in school avoidance and social phobias (Linet 1985).

Clonidine is an often-prescribed alternative that may be useful in approximately 50% of cases (Leckman et al. 1982). It attenuates hyperactivity and impulsivity and may be valuable in children with comorbid ADHD and behavioral problems. Clonidine, however, is sedating and can blunt cognitive performance. In a double-blind placebo-controlled study, Singer et al. (1995) found that clonidine was less efficacious than desipramine for children with combined ADHD and TS. Efficacy of clonidine may increase over the course of 2–3 months, and dosage needs to be slowly titrated; blood pressure requires frequent monitoring, even after attaining stable dose. Guanfacine has been discussed as an alternative α_2-adrenoreceptor agonist. It produces less sedation and

hypotension, but it does not appear to be as efficacious as clonidine (Cummings et al. 2002).

Studies have produced a marked revision in our understanding of the use of stimulants to treat ADHD in children with TS. Initially, tics were viewed as a serious contraindication, as stimulants can worsen tics or bring tics forth in an otherwise asymptomatic individual (Denckla et al. 1976). However, studies by Sverd et al. (1989) and Gadow et al. (1992) have shown that children with stable TS can respond to stimulants without worsening of tics. In addition, any increase in tic behavior upon initiation of psychostimulant therapy is likely to be transient (Castellanos et al. 1997). As a general guideline, stimulants should not be used in a child in whom stimulants have previously brought forth or worsened tics. Stimulants can be cautiously administered to patients with stable TS. Patients should be carefully monitored for tic frequency or impairment, and in the absence of symptom exacerbation, treatment can continue and be adjusted for optimal efficacy. Evidence indicates that noradrenergic tricyclic antidepressants such as desipramine and nortriptyline are beneficial in patients with comorbid ADHD and chronic tic disorders (Spencer et al. 1993a, 1993b). More recent studies indicate that atomoxetine is also effective in these patients and is likely to be a safer choice (Allen et al. 2005).

TS with associated OCD can be relatively refractory to treatment with SSRIs and may require augmentation with a neuroleptic (McDougle et al. 1994). Although TS is clearly a brain-based disorder, it can be exacerbated by stress and anxiety and can be a severely stigmatizing illness with grievous psychosocial consequences. Habit reversal therapy can help control frequency of tics, and both this type of behavioral therapy and supportive psychotherapy can improve life quality in patients with TS (Deckersbach et al. 2006).

MENTAL RETARDATION

An enormous number of genetic, biochemical, and environmental factors can adversely affect brain development, leading to low general intelligence and limited adaptive capacity. Mental retardation is diagnosed when an individual presents, before 18 years of age, with an intelligence score of approximately 70 or below and concurrent deficits in adaptive functioning (American Psychiatric Association 2000). Mental retardation is a common syndrome, with an estimated prevalence of 1%–3% of the adult population. Clinically, mental retardation is divided by severity. The most prevalent form is mild mental retardation, in which intelligence scores range from 50 to 70. Nearly 90% of the mentally retarded population falls within this range. These individuals can learn many skills and generally achieve the equivalent of a sixth-grade education. They can live in the community, manage a job, and, with effort or assistance, handle financial matters, although they require support from families and communities to maintain this level of integration. Historically, mild mental retardation was thought to represent the lower end of the normal distribution of intelligence scores, and psychological factors were believed to play an important role. Studies continue to identify an increasing percentage of chromosomal abnormalities in patients who are mildly retarded (currently 4%–19%). Mild mental retardation is a heterogeneous set of disorders that sometimes arise from chromosomal abnormalities, environmental effects, or complex multifactorial polygenic inheritance (Thapar et al. 1994).

The next most prevalent cluster is moderate mental retardation, in which intelligence scores range from a low of 35–40 to a high of 50–55. Approximately 7% of the mentally retarded population falls within this range. These individuals can often learn to manage some aspects of daily living, such as making small change. They usually live in supervised residences and attain the equivalent of a second-grade education. They communicate at the level of a preschool or early grade school child.

About 3% of the mentally retarded population falls into the severe range, with intelligence scores ranging from 20–25 up to 35–40. These individuals typically learn few adaptive skills and live in highly structured and closely supervised settings. They have an increased prevalence of neurological complications such as seizures and spasticity, and often there is a discernible etiology, such as Down syndrome or fragile X syndrome.

Only about 1% of the mentally retarded population falls within the profound range, with IQ scores below 20–25. These individuals have a host of severe neurological and medical problems and typically die in their 20s. They need to live in highly structured and supervised settings and are completely dependent on others. Self-injurious behavior can occur in half of these patients.

Historically, it made sense to differentiate forms of mental retardation by severity because most cases arose from unknown etiologies. With the emergence of new molecular tools and the steady advance in behavioral phenotyping (State et al. 1997), this reliance on identification by severity alone is changing. In recent years there has been a marked increase in interest in specific genetic syndromes with mental retardation (Harris 2001; McElwee and Bernard 2002). There are known to be hundreds of genetic syndromes associated with mental retardation (Opitz 2000). Instead of attempting to distill the generic features of hundreds of different responsible disorders, it seems more reasonable to review some of the major known disorders that present with mental retardation. In addition, in this chapter we concentrate on the recent developments of research into X-chromosomal mental retardation and subtelomere deletions–related mental retardation.

DOWN SYNDROME

Down syndrome is the most common chromosomal abnormality that produces mental retardation. The incidence varies greatly with maternal age. In all newborns, the incidence is 1 per 1,000. However, if the mother is age 45 years or older, the incidence approaches 1 in 50. Down syndrome may be lethal, resulting in fetal death or still birth. Clinical presentation varies considerably. Characteristic features include microcephaly with large anterior fontanel, depressed nasal bridge, bilateral epicanthic folds, upward slanting (mongoloid) palpebral fissure, low set and misformed ears with hypoplastic tragus and narrow auditory meatus, and lingual protrusion with small mouth (Gold 1992). Other observable features include short stature, hands with a single transverse (simian) crease, brachyclinodactyly of the fifth finger, and wide separation between the large and second toe (Gold 1992). Neurologically, developmental delays and intellectual deficits are significant. Motor milestones are delayed as a result of generalized hypotonia, and expressive and receptive language is usually delayed and impaired. Hearing is also frequently affected as a result of middle ear disease or sensorineural hearing loss (Gold 1992). Seizures occur in less than 10% of cases but can emerge at any age. Quadriplegia can result at any time from cervical subluxation of the atlantoaxial process. Life expectancy is approximately 50 years, with about 40% developing Alzheimer's disease by this point (Holland et al. 1998). Factors that influence longevity include coexisting congenital heart disease and gastrointestinal anomalies (Gold 1992). Leukemia occurs with increased frequency, and neural changes characteristic of Alzheimer's disease begins to emerge in all who survive beyond the age of 30. Behaviorally, patients with Down syndrome tend to have more social skills and less psychopathology than patients with other forms of mental retardation (Harris 2001; State et al. 1997).

Etiology and Pathophysiology

Down syndrome is a prototypic chromosomal disorder involving extra replication of all or part of chromosome 21. The classic cause is nondisjunction during meiosis leading to trisomy 21, which is a noninherited genetic anomaly. The syndrome can also arise from inheritance of a translocation of part of chromosome 21 (most often to chromosomes 14 or 22) from asymptomatic mothers. It appears that extra replication of a 3,000-kilobase fragment of DNA in the 21q22 region is sufficient to produce many of the features of Down syndrome, including mental retardation (Park et al. 1987). Down syndrome arising from either nondisjunction or translocation can be diagnosed prenatally through chorionic villi sampling or amniocentesis. Although it is unclear how this extra genetic material leads to mental retardation, research has identified remarkable similarities between Down syndrome and Alzheimer's disease (Rumble et al. 1989). Patients with Down syndrome undergo progressive neuropathological changes leading to formation of neurofibrillary tangles and neuritic plaques at a relatively young adult age (Wisniewski et al. 1985). They also have other Alzheimer's-like neurochemical abnormalities, including a major loss of acetylcholine neurons in the nucleus basalis and of somatostatin neurons in the cerebral cortex, as well as reduced levels of norepinephrine and serotonin (Godridge et al. 1987). Chromosome 21 contains the precursor gene for β-amyloid, which is the protein that accumulates in neuritic plaques. Additional biochemical abnormalities include elevated levels of CuZn, superoxide dismutase, and protein $S100\beta$ (Huret et al. 1987; Lejeune 1990). Superoxide dismutase is an important housekeeping enzyme that prevents intracellular damage from free radicals; a mutation in the encoding gene is associated with the familial form of amyotrophic lateral sclerosis. Studies using model systems overexpressing this enzyme have found impaired monoamine neurotransmitter uptake and storage (Groner et al. 1994). The $S100\beta$ protein appears to target and activate astrocytes and specific neurons to stimulate neurite growth. Elevated levels of $S100\beta$ may lead to nonsensical growth of imperfect neurites, an early step in the formation of neuritic plaques (Sheng et al. 1994). As with Alzheimer's disease, apolipoprotein E4 is a risk factor associated with emergence of dementia in Down syndrome (Deb et al. 2000; Prasher and Haque 2000).

Pinter et al. (2001a, 2001b) used high-resolution MRI to compare patterns of brain volume in children and young adults with Down syndrome with a matched control group. They found that those with Down syndrome had smaller overall brain volumes and, after correction for overall gray and white matter volumes, had larger volumes of subcortical and parietal gray matter and temporal white matter (Pinter et al. 2001b). When corrected for overall brain volume, the Down syndrome group had significantly smaller hippocampal volumes (Pinter et al. 2001a).

FRAGILE X SYNDROME

Fragile X is the most common known inherited cause of mental retardation, with an estimated prevalence rate of 1 in 1,250 males and 1 in 2,000 females (Thapar et al. 1994). Fragile X accounts for approximately 7% of moderate and 4% of mild mental retardation in males and 2.5% of moderate and 3% of mild retardation in females (Thapar et al. 1994). The name derives from the observation that the X chromosome shows a "fragile" site, specifically a bent- or broken- appearing segment, when grown in the appropriate culture medium. The polymerase chain reaction provides a reliable and economic means for detecting this disorder (Thapar et al. 1994). The phenotypic presentation of this disorder is varied and more prominent in males. Infants present with relative macrocrania and facial edema, whereas older children and adults have a long face and a prominent chin. Large, floppy, seashell-shaped ears are characteristic at any age. Males entering adolescence have characteristic macroorchidism (enlarged testes) and a normal-size penis (Gold 1992). Affected individuals have an increased rate of psychiatric difficulties, with abnormal speech and language, impaired social relations, and ADHD (Hagerman and Hagerman 2004; Moore et al. 2004; Turk 1992). Many affected individuals show autistic features such as gaze avoidance, hand flapping, tactile defensiveness, and perseveration (Hagerman and Sobesky 1989; Harris 2001), although social withdrawal and reduced attachment to caregivers are not characteristic (State et al. 1997). Seventy percent of female carriers are not mentally retarded, but they have an increased prevalence of schizotypal features, depression, and below-average intelligence (Freund et al. 1992), and their level of symptomatology correlates with the degree of cytogenetically evident fragility (Chudley et al. 1983; Thapar et al. 1994). The American Academy of Neurology recommends screening for fragile X as a routine part of the evaluation of children with global developmental delays, even in the absence of dysmorphic features (Shevell et al. 2003).

Etiology and Pathophysiology

Fragile X has an unusual and important mode of inheritance that also appears in myotonic dystrophy and Huntington's chorea. In all of these disorders, the severity of the syndrome increases in successive generations. Other features of fragile X include the observation that phenotypically and cytogenetically normal males (normal transmitting males) can transmit the defect to apparently normal females who can then produce affected male offspring. These once puzzling clinical observations have been explained at the molecular level and stem from a process known as *anticipation*. The gene directly responsible for fragile X syndrome, *FMR1*, is located on the X chromosome at Xq27.3 (Verkerk et al. 1991). The 5′

untranslated region of the *FMR1* gene contains a polymorphic CGG trinucleotide repeat (6–60 repeats in normal subjects) that can be amplified to hundreds or thousands of repeats, producing the disorder (Verkerk et al. 1991). Fragile X usually results from expansion of the CGG repeats, leading to hypermethylation of the CpG island adjacent to *FMR1*, loss of transcription of the *FMR1* gene, and lack of FMR1 protein (Siomi et al. 1995). *FMR1* mRNA and protein are expressed in many tissues, but particularly high levels are found in brain and testes (Siomi et al. 1995). The role of FMR1 protein is incompletely understood but is known to serve as an RNA-binding protein (Siomi et al. 1995). Fragile X carriers, including normal transmitting males, have this elongated sequence of repeats, which increase in size, particularly when transmitted by females. If the permutation is transmitted by a normal transmitting male, the sequence is not elongated in the offspring (Thapar et al. 1994).

The past several years have seen remarkable growth in our understanding of the molecular processes underlying fragile X syndrome (Harikrishnan et al. 2005; Lim et al. 2005; O'Donnell and Warren 2002; Smith et al. 2004) and the potential role of *FMR1* in brain development (Jin and Warren 2000; Kogan et al. 2004; Zarnescu et al. 2005).

Eliez et al. (2001) reported MRI scans on 37 children and adolescents with fragile X. The subjects had increased caudate gray matter and volume of the lateral ventricle. Males with fragile X also had a slower rate of reduction in cortical gray matter with age than typically developing children.

X-Linked Mental Retardation

X-linked genetic defects are important causes of mental retardation and are probably responsible for 10%–12% of cases of mental retardation in males (Ropers et al. 2003). Considerable progress has been made in elucidating genetic factors associated with various forms of X-linked mental retardation (XLMR) (Kleefstra and Hamel 2005; Ropers and Hamel 2005; Suri 2005). The two main categories of XLMR are syndromic (S-XLMR), in which physical, neurological, and/or metabolic abnormalities exist in addition to mental retardation, and nonsyndromic (NS-XLMR), in which there are no consistent phenotypic manifestations other than mental retardation (Kerr et al. 1991).

Etiology and Pathophysiology

To date, the causative genes for 38 of the 136 known forms of S-XLMR have been identified (XLMR Genes Update Website 2005), and many of the remaining forms have been localized to specific portions of the X chromosome. Currently, 19 genes responsible for various forms of NS-XLMR have been identified (Renieri et al. 2005), although the majority remain unidentified and not yet localized. The lack of demonstrable phenotypic features other than mental retardation complicates the search for NS-XLMR genes.

The identification of XLMR-associated genes has provided insights into brain function. The genes affected in these conditions have roles in processes such as neuronal outgrowth, synaptic structure and function, synaptic plasticity, and learning and memory, and these genes might be determinants of intelligence.

Polymorphisms that predispose to mental retardation—but are not sufficient to cause symptoms on their own—might be present within the protein-coding regions of genes, in their regulatory regions, or in genes that encode small regulatory RNAs. Allelic variants of genes that are involved in XLMR might be candidates for such polymorphisms. Understanding the genetic causes of XLMR will be important in developing diagnostic, preventive, and therapeutic strategies for the treatment and management of this condition.

Subtelomere Deletion (Telomeric Defect)

Another recent advance in our understanding of mental retardation has been the recognition of subtelomeric rearrangements or deletions as a major etiological factor (de Vries et al. 2003). Mental retardation is the key consequence of subtelomeric defects, along with malformation syndromes. Some of the submicroscopic subtelomere deletions result in specific phenotypes, which may direct the clinician toward the diagnosis. In these patients, fluorescence in situ hybridization (FISH) analysis of a single and specific subtelomere may be sufficient to confirm the diagnosis. However, the majority of subjects with subtelomeric defects lack a characteristic phenotype. For these subjects, a general subtelomere screen is required to achieve a diagnosis. To date, about 2,500 individuals with mental retardation have been evaluated for subtelomere abnormalities, and these abnormalities have been found in about 5% of cases overall and in about 7% of cases with moderate to severe mental retardation. Some submicroscopic telomeric deletions are associated with a specific phenotype, such as 1p–, 4p–, 5p–, 9p–, 18p–, and 17p–. One of the more common submicroscopic telomeric deletions is 9q34.3. Patients with 9q– deletions have in common severe mental retardation, hypotonia, brachycephaly, flat face with hypertelorism, synophrys, anteverted nares, thickened lower lip, carp mouth with macroglossia, and conotruncal heart defects (Kleefstra et al. 2005). The minimum critical region responsible for this 9q– syndrome is approximately 1.2 Mb and encompasses at least 14 genes (Kleefstra et al. 2005).

Etiology and Pathophysiology

Telomeres are specialized protein-DNA constructs found at the ends of chromosomes, where they prevent degradation and end-to-end chromosomal fusion. Subtelomeres are gene-rich segments of DNA that are immediately adjacent to the telomeric caps and are characterized by both unique and repetitive stretches of DNA. Subtelomeres occupy the most distal region on the p and q ends of the chromosome that contain unique sequences of DNA. Research on subtelomeric syndromes is advancing at a rapid rate with availability of detection methods. As this work progresses, we will undoubtedly learn a great deal more about the roles of subtelomeric DNA in brain development.

PRADER-WILLI SYNDROME AND ANGELMAN'S SYNDROME

Prader-Willi syndrome and Angelman's syndrome are two distinct genetic forms of mental retardation that usually arise from de novo deletion of a tiny segment of chromosome 15. Prader-Willi syndrome is characterized by mental retardation or learning disability, infantile hypotonia and poor suck reflex, growth retardation, delayed sexual development, and childhood onset of pronounced obesity associated with hyperphagia, hypogenitalism, short stature, small hands and feet, almond-shaped eyes, strabismus, skin-picking, and low activity levels (State and Dykens 2000; Thapar et al. 1994). Food-related difficulties are the most striking and widely recognized sequelae of this syndrome. Without appropriate dietary and behavioral intervention, almost everyone with this syndrome will become dangerously obese. Although about 40% show mental retardation, most affected individuals are of normal or borderline IQ, but some may have associated behavior problems such as temper tantrums, stubbornness, foraging for food (Akefeldt and Gillberg 1999; Thapar et al. 1994), and OCD symptomatology (J.W. Kim et al. 2005; State et al. 1999), ADHD (Wigren and Hansen 2005), or a distinctive cognitive profile. Hypothalamic dysfunction may underlie the obesity that is typical of Prader-Willi syndrome (Kanumakala et al. 2005). The estimated incidence is approximately 1 in 25,000. Most cases are sporadic with a recurrence risk of less than 1 in 1,000 (Thapar et al. 1994).

Angelman's syndrome is characterized by severe mental retardation; stiff, jerky movements; ataxia; seizures; and unprovoked laughter. The estimated incidence is approximately 1 in 20,000, and most cases are sporadic (Thapar et al. 1994). Individuals with Angelman's syndrome also have severe learning disabilities, a happy disposition, subtly dysmorphic facial features, lack of speech, and sleep disorders (Clayton-Smith and Laan 2003; Watson et al. 2001).

Patients with paternal uniparental disomy of chromosome 15 or an imprinting defect are less severely affected (for review, see McElwee and Bernard 2002). They have a low incidence of severe seizures, hypopigmentation, and microencephaly and are more likely to have some speech. Some 70% are above the 80th percentile for weight. Patients with a mutation in *UBE3A* (E3 ubiquitin protein ligase gene) have features of both syndromes (Lossie et al. 2001).

Etiology and Pathophysiology

Prader-Willi and Angelman's syndromes illustrate an important genetic principle known as *genomic imprinting*. The majority of individuals with both disorders have remarkably similar deletions of a segment of chromosome 15, particularly surrounding 15q12 (Thapar et al. 1994). Most cases result from microdeletions in proximal chromosome 15q. The remainder result from maternal uniparental disomy of chromosome 15, from imprinting center defects, and rarely from balanced or unbalanced chromosome rearrangements involving chromosome 15. Structural rearrangements of chromosome 15 have been described in about 5% of the patients with a typical or an atypical Prader-Willi syndrome phenotype (Varela et al. 2004). The difference between Prader-Willi and Angelman's syndromes stems from the sex of the parent from whom the defective chromosome 15 is inherited. Prader-Willi syndrome emerges most frequently from 15q12 deletions of paternal origin. It can also occur in uniparental disomy where both chromosomes 15 are inherited from the mother (Nicholls et al. 1989), and this form is usually milder (Cassidy et al. 1997; Dykens et al. 1999; Roof et al. 2000). In contrast, Angelman's syndrome most often emerges from deletion in maternally derived chromosome 15 (15q11–13) or from uniparental disomy when both 15 chromosomes are inherited from the father (Knoll et al. 1991; Thapar et al. 1994). Angelman's syndrome can also emerge from point mutations or small deletions within the *UBE3A* gene, which lies within this region. *UBE3A* shows tissue-specific imprinting, with expression in the brain stemming exclusively from the maternal allele. The genetic mechanisms identified so far in Angelman's syndromes are found in 85%–90% of those with the clinical phenotype, and all interfere with *UBE3A* expression (Fang et al. 1999; Hitchins et al. 2004; Kishino et al. 1997; Malzac et al. 1998; Matsuura et al. 1997).

Neurochemical studies have found elevated levels of oxytocin (A. Martin et al. 1998), dopamine, and serotonin (Akefeldt et al. 1998) in the CSF of Prader-Willi patients. Administration of growth hormone has been reported to be helpful for somatic features of this disorder

(Lindgren and Ritzen 1999; Ritzen et al. 1999); however, this treatment may not improve the behavioral symptoms (Akefeldt and Gillberg 1999), and several cases of sudden unexpected death of subjects who received the growth hormone therapy have been reported (Nagai et al. 2005).

AUTISM AND PERVASIVE DEVELOPMENTAL DISORDERS

AUTISM

Autism was originally considered a rare childhood syndrome affecting only 4–5 children per 10,000 births (Fombonne 1996). This view has changed in recent years, and autism is now considered a fairly common disorder with prevalence rates ranging from 30–60 cases per 10,000 (Fombonne 2003; Rutter 2005b). However, a rigorous meta-analysis of epidemiological data from 37 studies suggested an overall prevalence of 7.1 per 10,000 (Williams et al. 2006). Boys are affected three- to four-fold more often than girls (Fombonne 1999; Wing and Gould 1979). Leo Kanner (1943) introduced the term *early infantile autism* to describe a group of 11 children. DSM-IV-TR (American Psychiatric Association 2000) distinguishes autistic disorder from other pervasive developmental disorders, including Rett's disorder, childhood disintegrative disorder, Asperger's disorder, and pervasive developmental disorder not otherwise specified. These disorders share a common set of severe disturbances in social recognition and interaction, impaired communication, and a restricted, stereotypic behavioral repertoire and range of interests.

Characteristic Features

Children with autism often seem indifferent to others. Their lack of interest may be manifested by minimal eye contact, delayed or absent facial signals, and impaired imitation of appropriate social behaviors. Autistic children have few (if any) friends; they may not engage in comfort seeking when distressed and often exhibit a preference for solitary play. Extreme cases find all physical contact aversive. Children with autism are frequently nonverbal when first diagnosed. If speech is present, it is often highly deviant and of limited communicative function. Abnormal speech patterns include echolalia, pronoun reversal, metaphorical language, poor grammatical structure, atonality, and arrhythmia. Autistic children also have deficient nonverbal communication skills.

Stereotypies are common in autism and can involve the flicking, twirling, or spinning of objects, or hand flapping, whirling, and posturing. Autistic children are often fascinated by spinning objects and other devices. Many autistic children resist change in their environment by ordering and arranging objects in precise ways to ensure sameness. Later in development, insistence on sameness can be observed in rigidified, ritualistic behavior patterns and routines. These symptoms may diminish with maturation in some individuals. Most, however, continue to display restricted and repetitive behaviors and are impaired by communication and social deficits (Seltzer et al. 2004).

Mental retardation is present in 75%–80% of children with autism and appears to be stable over time (Fombonne 1999; Freeman et al. 1985, 1991). Children with autism may be underresponsive or overresponsive to sensory stimuli (Ornitz 1974; Ornitz and Ritvo 1968)—an attribute that has spawned the popular but as yet unvalidated treatment known as *sensory integration therapy* (Dawson and Watling 2000; Smith et al. 2005). Many individuals with autism display a range of abnormal mood states that may include temper tantrums, aggression, self-injury, or unexplainable giggling. Toe walking and other forms of deviant motility are not uncommon.

Research suggests that the social problems of autistic children may stem, in part, from the inability to establish joint attention, such as pointing or showing objects (Baron-Cohen 1989), and this deficit may render them incapable of sharing mutual interests. Autistic children may also lack the ability to infer another person's state of mind—an inability that may be a core feature of the disorder (Leslie and Frith 1990; Perner et al. 1989) and is associated with other forms of executive dysfunction (Joseph and Tager-Flusberg 2004).

Newer approaches to screening have lowered the age of identification (Volkmar et al. 2005). Historically, an initial diagnosis was made when children were about 4 years old (Siegel et al. 1988). However, almost all parents recognize some type of abnormality by 24 months (De Giacomo and Fombonne 1998). In the first months of infancy, it is possible to discern a lack of social interest, including reduced levels of social engagement (Maestro et al. 1999, 2005). By 6–12 months it can become apparent that the child is failing to orient toward verbalization in general and to his or her own name in particular (Osterling et al. 2002; Werner et al. 2000). In a prospective study of high-risk infants, Zwaigenbaum et al. (2005) found that by 12 months, infants who were later diagnosed with autism were distinguishable from their nonaffected siblings and from low-risk infants. Major differences noted were atypical eye contact and imitation, prolonged latency to disengage visual attention, a characteristic pattern of early temperament, and delayed expressive and receptive language. Other behaviors that distinguish young children with autism include unusual gaze, finger mannerisms, atypical play, using people as tools, and limitations in response to speech, range of facial expression, use of conventional gesture, desire for shared enjoyment, offering of comfort, and attention to voice (Cox et al. 1999; Dahlgren and Gillberg 1989; Hoshino et al. 1982; Lord 1995; Wimpory et al. 2000).

Etiology and Pathophysiology

Autism appears to stem from both genetic and nongenetic factors that affect brain development (Ciaranello and Ciaranello 1995; Rutter 2005a). The concordance rate in monozygotic twins is 60%, but no concordance has been found between dizygotic twins (Bailey et al. 1995). Together with the prevalence of autism, these findings suggest that the heritability of the disorder is approximately 90%, which may be the highest of all multifactorial child psychiatric disorders (Rutter 2005a). Cognitive and social abnormalities (i.e., "broader autism phenotype") are nearly ubiquitous in monozygotic twins of affected probands. Dizygotic twins and siblings have a significant but much lower incidence of cognitive disturbance (August et al. 1981; Bailey et al. 1995). The prevalence rate of autism in siblings of children with the disorder is about 6%, which is a 60-fold increase over that found in the general population (Ritvo et al. 1985).

Although many etiological factors have been proposed, no single cause of autism has been elucidated. Minshew (1991) argued that less than 5% of individuals with autism have an identifiable etiology. Potential causal factors include tuberous sclerosis, cytomegalovirus, encephalitis, meningitis, congenital rubella, and fragile X. Immune abnormalities have also been proposed (Warren et al. 1995). Conservative sources estimate that fragile X may be present in 7% of males and 4% of females with autism (Bolton and Rutter 1990). Tuberous sclerosis is found in about 1%–3% of autism cases (Harrison and Bolton 1997). Recent speculations have targeted immunization, specifically the measles-mumps rubella (MMR) vaccine, and/or thimerosal, a mercury-based vaccine preservative, as causal factors. These hypotheses were carefully addressed by the Institute of Medicine of the National Academy of Science, which concluded that the body of epidemiological evidence favored rejection of a causal relationship between the MMR vaccine and autism, and thimerosal and autism, in their final report in 2004 (Institute of Medicine of the National Academies 2004). Removal of thimerosal from vaccines has not been associated with a reduction in new cases of autism (Fombonne et al. 2006).

Efforts are under way to identify candidate genes associated with autism. The combined twin and family prevalence data suggest that autism may emerge from the interaction of multiple (perhaps 3–15) susceptibility genes (Rutter 2005a; Wassink et al. 2004). In a review, Wassink et al. (2004) reported that at least 89 genes had been tested. Three genes may be viable candidates: neuroligin 3 and 4 (Jamain et al. 2003; Laumonnier et al. 2004), chromosome 15q11-q13 $GABA_A$ receptor subunits (Buxbaum et al. 2002; Nurmi et al. 2003), and the serotonin transporter (*SLC6A4*) (Conroy et al. 2004; Coutinho et al. 2004). Prior reports have documented deletions and duplications of the chromosome 15q11–q13 region (Cook 2001), especially when phenotypic information related to repetitive behavior and rigidity has been included (Shao et al. 2003). The serotonin transporter modulates levels of extracellular and synaptic serotonin, a neurotransmitter that has historically been associated with autism. However, supporting evidence for these candidate genes is lessened by internal inconsistencies and failures of replication (Wassink et al. 2004).

Neuroanatomical studies have suggested that autism arises from premature cessation of development in the cerebellum, cerebrum, and limbic system. Postmortem studies have identified regions of cellular loss unaccompanied by gliosis. These findings suggest that the lesion occurred in fetal life or was the result of misdirected development (Bauman 1991). Courchesne (1991) reported a 25% reduction in the size of cerebellar vermal lobes VI and VII in 14 of 18 subjects with autism. This reduction could result in faulty cortical projections. Differences in vermal size, however, correlated with low IQ rather than autism per se (Holttum et al. 1992; Levitt et al. 1999). Damage to the cerebellum may manifest as damage to the frontal lobes and affect attention, memory, and language (Riva and Giorgi 2000). Children with vermal lesions (as a consequence of CNS radiation or chemotherapy) can develop symptoms suggesting autism. Some theories propose that autism results from coordinated developmental anomalies affecting the posterior-superior vermis and frontal, temporal, and parietal lobes. Kemper and Bauman (1993) observed progressive developmental changes in neurons in the cerebellum, inferior olive, and diagonal band of Broca. In brains of young adults with autism, neurons in these regions were large and fetal in appearance. Brains of older adults with autism showed a marked decline in neuronal number, size, and extent of dendrites.

Reduced numbers of cerebellar Purkinje cells are the most consistent neuroanatomical findings in the autopsied autistic brain (Bauman and Kemper 2005). Kemper and Bauman (1993) theorized that deficient Purkinje cell production results in a failure to form appropriate corticocerebellar synaptic connections and that these circuits regress with age. This process may also explain the high density of small neurons observed in the hippocampus and amygdala (Bauman and Kemper 1985). Bailey et al.

(1998) found abnormal neuronal migration patterns in the brain stem and cerebellum, and reduced numbers of Purkinje cells in adult cases. A striking negative correlation was found between Purkinje cell number and cortical thickness. Carper and Courchesne (2000) also found a significant negative correlation between the size of vermal lobules VI–VII and volume of frontal gray matter in patients with autism, but not in control subjects. Numerous small and compact minicolumns have been reported in the frontal and temporal lobes of autistic brains (Casanova et al. 2002). Deficient development of corticocerebellar connections may have impaired the normal process of cortical development and attenuated pruning because this process depends on the establishment of strong appropriate connections. Lack of pruning is consistent with the elevated rates of glucose metabolism (Horwitz et al. 1988) and adenosine triphosphate utilization observed in the frontal and parietal lobes of patients with autism as well as the apparent brain enlargement in children, but not adults, with autism (Courchesne et al. 2003). Gyral malformations have also been found in the cortex and include pachygyria, polymicrogyria, heterotopia, and schizencephaly (Piven et al. 1990). Zoghbi (2003) has speculated that autism stems from the developmental dysregulation of mechanisms that pattern axonal outgrowth and/or dendritic arborizations and synaptic contacts between excitatory and inhibitory neurons in the cortex.

The deficits in cognitive functioning characteristic of autism have not been linked to specific anatomical defects. Individuals with autism perform normally on tasks that assess perception, attention, and classification of stimuli and appear to have intact sensory and basic memory functions. However, in children with autism, the slowed orientation to visual cues correlates with degree of cerebellar hypoplasia (Harris et al. 1999). Initial reaction time, orienting to sequential cues, and reorienting have all been observed to be slower in children with autism (Courchesne et al. 1994; Inui and Suzuki 1998; Townsend et al. 1999), consistent with disruption in the inferior olive—a brain structure associated with fast reaction time and temporal precision of coordinated muscle contractions (Welsh et al. 2005). Abnormalities have been observed in auditory P300 evoked potential responses that are probably indicative of deficient auditory processing (Novick et al. 1980). A reversal in hemispheric asymmetry has been proposed (Novick et al. 1980) and supported by MRI studies (Hashimoto et al. 1989). Glucose utilization is not as strongly correlated between the two hemispheres as it is in control subjects without autism (Horwitz et al. 1988). Thinning of the corpus callosum, especially the anterior subregions, has been found in 43% of subjects with autism (Egaas et al. 1995; Hardan et al.

2000) and is consonant with diminished hemispheric communication. This decrease in callosal size is more a consequence of diminished axon numbers than of decreased myelination (Belmonte et al. 1995).

Social deficits in autism have been examined with fMRI using facial perception tests. Patients with autism have attenuated responses in mesolimbic and temporal lobe cortical regions and in left cerebellum during facial processing (Critchley et al. 2000). Schultz et al. (2000) found that individuals with autism rely on feature-based strategies for facial recognition and have greater activation in the inferior temporal gyri. During facial processing, children with autism show less activity in the fusiform gyrus, increased activity in the precuneus and medial occipital gyrus, and nonmodulation of amygdala activity by task demands (Critchley et al. 2000; Hubl et al. 2003; Pierce et al. 2001; Schultz et al. 2000; Wang et al. 2004). These findings are consistent with structural MRI studies indicating fusiform enlargement (Waiter et al. 2004). Diminished amygdalar activity is consonant with emotion perception deficits observed in autism (Schultz 2005).

Neurochemically, the most noted observation has been a significant increase in whole-blood 5-HT levels in 30% of autistic individuals (Ritvo et al. 1970). High levels of 5-HT have also been found in most first-degree relatives (Piven et al. 1991). McBride et al. (1998) found that whole-blood 5-HT levels vary by race and pubertal status. They found, after correcting for race, a significant elevation in whole-blood 5-HT levels in about 25% of prepubertal but not postpubertal children with autism. Chugani et al. (1997, 1999) found decreased 5-HT synthesis and uptake in frontal cortex and thalamus, especially in boys. Using PET scans, this same group found asymmetries of 5-HT synthesis in frontal (90% of the children), temporal (47%), and parietal (30%) lobes, with the majority showing left-sided decreases (Chandana et al. 2005). Decreased left cortical 5-HT synthesis was associated with severe language impairment, whereas right-sided decreases in 5-HT synthesis tended to be associated with left or mixed handedness, suggesting some relationship to abnormal hemispheric specialization. These findings are consistent with the presence of smaller, more closely spaced minicolumns reported by Casanova et al. (2002) that would necessitate a compensatory shift in dominance to the right hemisphere. Mixed findings have emerged regarding a possible linkage of the 5-HT transporter gene and autism (Klauck et al. 1997; Maestrini et al. 1999). Elevated levels of endogenous opioids have also been noted in patients with autism. This observation emerged from the apparently high pain threshold of autistic individuals with self-abusive behaviors. Research suggests that levels of β-endorphin and endorphin fraction II may be elevated in the CSF (Ross et al. 1987).

Treatment

Pharmacotherapy for autism has had mixed results. However, many autistic children have appropriate target symptoms (e.g., hyperactivity, temper tantrums, irritability, stereotypies, self-injury, depression, and obsessive-compulsive behaviors) that warrant a therapeutic trial (Campbell et al. 1996). Although initial reports emerged that fenfluramine, an agent that stimulates 5-HT release, had promising effects (Ritvo et al. 1983, 1986), later studies were disappointing (Leventhal et al. 1993), and fenfluramine was withdrawn from the market by the manufacturer after it was found to be associated with heart valve abnormalities, primarily aortic regurgitation. Opiate antagonists such as naltrexone have been used to enhance cognitive processing (Bouvard et al. 1995) and reduce self-injury and hyperactivity (Campbell et al. 1993; Gillberg 1995), with equivocal results. Neuroleptics, particularly haloperidol, have been extensively evaluated in double-blind, placebo-controlled protocols (Campbell et al. 1996). Haloperidol reduces symptoms of anger, uncooperativeness, and hyperactivity and also exerts some effects on core features of autistic behavior and deviant speech (Campbell et al. 1996).

The newer atypical antipsychotics olanzapine and risperidone have shown some promise (Malone et al. 2001; McCracken et al. 2002), although weight gain, metabolic syndrome, and sedation can be problematic. Clomipramine has also been found to be effective in controlled studies in attenuating stereotypies, compulsions, ritualized behaviors, and aggression (Campbell et al. 1996). The few published reports indicate that SSRIs are modestly effective in decreasing hyperactivity, restlessness, agitation, obsessive thoughts, and preoccupations (McDougle et al. 1998; Posey et al. 1999). In a recent double-blind placebo-controlled crossover study of liquid fluoxetine, Hollander et al. (2005) found a significant decrease in the repetitive behaviors of a sample of children and adolescents with autism. Although anecdotal reports indicated that secretin, a gastrointestinal hormone, had therapeutic benefits, initial and subsequent controlled studies have been negative (Chez et al. 2000; Coplan et al. 2003; Molloy et al. 2002; Sandler et al. 1999). Further research needs to be conducted on SSRIs, lithium, and atypical antipsychotics (McDougle et al. 2000), especially research using randomized controlled trials and well-chosen and well-specified samples (Bodfish 2004).

Long-term interventions focus on community-based special educational programs and subsequent residential services for those who cannot be cared for at home. An initial study by Lovaas (1987) and a follow-up study (McEachin et al. 1993) suggest that as many as half of preschool-age children with autism can attain normal educational and intellectual function with extremely intensive early behavioral treatment. The interventions were designed to increase skills in the areas of attention, emotionality, language, toy play, peer interaction, and self-help while reducing tantrums, aggression, and self-stimulation (Lovaas and Smith 1989). Although Lovaas's findings are encouraging, the typical adult outcomes for children with autism are "poor" to "very poor" (Howlin et al. 2004), and long-term care continues to be the norm over the course of their lifetime (Nordin and Gillberg 1998).

RETT'S DISORDER

Rett's disorder is an X-linked dominant progressive degenerative disorder that is found exclusively in females, being lethal in males. Development often appears to be normal until about 18 months of age but is followed by the emergence of autistic symptoms, often leading to a diagnosis of autism. Development of distinctive hand stereotypies (i.e., twisting or wringing), deceleration in normal head growth leading to microcephaly, and progressive neurological deterioration help establish the correct diagnosis. Children develop gait ataxia between 1 and 4 years of age and may lose ambulation completely as they mature.

Monozygotic twins show complete concordance, whereas dizygotic twins are not concordant (Hagberg and Witt-Engerstrom 1987). Progressive clinical deterioration is mirrored by progressive cortical atrophy and neuronal loss (Zoghbi et al. 1985). There is a marked attenuation in levels of the noradrenergic metabolite MHPG and the dopamine metabolite HVA in the CSF (Zoghbi et al. 1985). Children with Rett's disorder show some of the motor problems observed in Parkinson's disease and suffer from reduced dopaminergic activity in the basal ganglia, substantia nigra, and cortex (Rett 1966; Wenk et al. 1991). Mutations in a gene called *MeCP2* is responsible for about one-third of cases (Amir et al. 1999).

Imaging and postmortem studies indicate that children with Rett's disorder have curtailed development, characterized by 1) reduced cerebral volume (Jellinger et al. 1988; Reiss et al. 1993), 2) cortical dysplasia with limited gliosis, 3) decreased cell size, 4) increased packing density (Bauman et al. 1995), 5) global reductions in gray and white matter volumes (Subramaniam et al. 1997), and 6) greater loss of gray matter versus white matter (Reiss et al. 1993), particularly in the prefrontal, posterior-frontal, and anterior-temporal regions (Subramaniam et al. 1997). Abnormalities in amino acid receptors have been demonstrated in basal ganglia (Blue et al. 1999a) and superior frontal gyrus (Blue et al. 1999b). *N*-methyl-D-aspartate (NMDA) receptor density in the superior frontal gyrus changes dramatically with age. Among patients with Rett's disorder, NMDA receptor density is higher in the brains of younger patients and lower in the brains of older patients compared with the brains of age-equivalent control subjects (Blue et al. 1999b). Dendritic arborization is reduced in many cortical regions (Armstrong et al. 1998).

PET scans demonstrate reduced frontal blood flow and reveal an immature blood flow and metabolism pattern comparable to that observed in early infancy (Nielsen et al. 1990). Magnetic resonance spectroscopy (MRS) imaging reveals a significant reduction of N-acetyl aspartate concentration and increased choline concentration in frontal, parietal, insular, and hippocampal regions. These findings are consistent with reduced neuronal arborization and gliosis in these regions (Horska et al. 2000).

ASPERGER'S DISORDER

Asperger's disorder is characterized by social dysfunction, pedantic speech, and idiosyncratic interests. Children with Asperger's disorder are distinguished from autistic children by better social function, normal intelligence, undelayed language development, and greater clumsiness. Although Asperger's disorder is, at present, nosologically distinct from autism, many argue that the disorder is merely a milder form of autism and should be categorized as such. For example, J.N. Miller and Ozonoff (2000) found no significant differences in motor, visuospatial, or executive functions between high-functioning patients with autism and subjects with Asperger's disorder, after controlling for the superior intellectual abilities of the group with Asperger's disorder.

SPECIFIC DISORDERS OF LEARNING

Learning disorders are specific deficits in the acquisition and performance of the academic skills of reading, writing, or arithmetic in the presence of normal intelligence and aptitude. These disorders often come to attention in grammar school when a child's academic performance falls substantially below expected levels. Learning disorders affect up to 10% of school-age children, although many cases go undiagnosed and frequently persist into adulthood (American Psychiatric Association 2000). Learning disorders appear to be a consequence of neurocortical impairments, yet their expression is affected by parental support, educational resources, and the individual's personality, initiative, and motivation. Clinically, it is important to distinguish learning disorders from a host of

other factors that can interfere with academic performance, such as mental retardation, sensory impairments, and psychiatric or neurological disorders that can affect attention, motivation, and behavior.

Intelligence tests, specific achievement tests, and a description of the child's classroom behavior are essential components of a learning disorder evaluation. Because learning disabilities often entitle children to special educational services, most states have codified legal guidelines for their diagnosis (Frankenberger and Fronzaglio 1991). Typically, the learning-disabled child demonstrates a significant discrepancy between nonverbal (performance) IQ and verbal IQ, with a history of delayed or impaired speech, language, or reading skills (American Academy of Child and Adolescent Psychiatry 1998; Tallal et al. 1991).

Overlooked or left untreated, learning disorders can lead to underachievement in a number of domains, along with diminished self-esteem, disinterest in school, truancy, misconduct, and substance abuse disorders (Benasich et al. 1993; Karacostas and Fisher 1993; Naylor et al. 1994; Rowe and Rowe 1992). Approximately 40% of children with learning disorders eventually drop out of school (Popper and Steingard 1995). Delinquent behaviors have been associated with learning disabilities; however, although reading disorders can worsen preexisting aggressive behavior, the current evidence is insufficient to presume that reading disability causes aggression (Cornwall and Bawden 1992).

CHARACTERISTIC FEATURES

At present, three identifiable learning disorders are recognized: reading disorder, mathematics disorder, and disorders of written expression. These disorders are often associated with each other, reading disorder being the most prevalent (American Psychiatric Association 2000). *Reading disorder*, often called *dyslexia*, is characterized by slow acquisition of reading skills despite normal intelligence, motivation, and emotional control. Prominent characteristics include letter and word reversals, word omissions and distortions, spelling errors, and substitution of words (American Psychiatric Association 2000). Left-right orientation, sound and phoneme discrimination, rapid visual and auditory sensory processing, and perceptual-motor skills are also impaired. Approximately 4% of school-age children in the United States are affected by reading disorder, and boys are affected three to four times more frequently than girls (C. Lewis et al. 1994). Some argue that this finding reflects referral bias, boys being more likely to receive evaluation as a consequence of their more disruptive classroom behaviors (American Psychiatric Association 2000). Reading ability can be improved with interventions. Problems with reading fluency and decoding of unfamiliar words do not generally remit on their own (S.E. Shaywitz and Shaywitz 2005). Affected adolescents and adults can continue to find reading effortful and slow, despite learning a fluent mini-vocabulary in their key areas of academic or career interest (S.E. Shaywitz and Shaywitz 2005).

Mathematics disorder is characterized by difficulty with counting, mathematical reasoning, calculations, and object conceptualization (American Psychiatric Association 2000). Impairment in spatial skills and in right-left, up-down, and east-west differentiation is frequently evident. Typically, children with mathematics disorder experience difficulty copying shapes, memorizing numbers, comprehending quantities, and sequencing tasks. About 1% of school-age children have mathematics disorder unaccompanied by any other specific learning disorder (American Psychiatric Association 2000). In contrast, 2% of children are affected by both mathematics and reading disorders (Lewis et al. 1994). Boys and girls appear to be equally affected (Lewis et al. 1994). A recent epidemiological study conducted in Greece found that 4.6% of a representative sample tested 2 standard deviations below the expected grade mean in mathematics, suggesting a higher prevalence rate than currently acknowledged (Koumoula et al. 2004).

Compared with reading and mathematics disorders, the *disorders of written expression* are not well characterized, and prevalence rates are unknown. Children have impairments in spelling, grammar, punctuation, sentence and paragraph formation, and organizational structure. These children will often have no difficulty verbalizing ideas and facts but are unable to write a paragraph about what they know. Characteristic features include slow ability to write or produce writing assignments, illegibility, letter reversals, word-finding and syntax errors, and punctuation and spelling problems (American Psychiatric Association 2000). It is important to distinguish disorders of written expression from developmental coordination disorder and ADHD, as children with the latter disorders may also present with illegible writing (American Psychiatric Association 2000).

ETIOLOGY AND PATHOPHYSIOLOGY

Learning disorders have both an environmental and a genetic basis. Environmental factors include prenatal ethanol exposure, perinatal complications, postnatal lead exposure, diminished parental and environmental stimulation, and head trauma (Ewing-Cobbs et al. 1998; Isaacs et al. 2001; Pennington and Smith 1983). A burgeoning literature suggests that some children with learning disorders have identifiable neurological abnormalities and that some

learning disorders follow simple genetic models (Galaburda et al. 2006; McGrath et al. 2006; Shalev 2004). Numerous studies have shown that learning disorders are highly heritable. Concordance for dyslexia may be as high as 91% in monozygotic twin pairs versus 31% for dizygotic twins (Pennington et al. 1983). Reading, mathematical, and spelling ability are all inherited traits, with heritability indices of 0.78 (Gillis et al. 1992), 0.51 (Gillis et al. 1992), and 0.53 (Stevenson et al. 1987), respectively.

Cardon et al. (1994, 1995) identified a quantitative trait locus on chromosome 6 (region 6p21.3–23) for reading disability in two carefully selected independent groups of sibling pairs. This region is found in the human leukocyte antigen encoding region, supporting the suspected association between autoimmune disorders and dyslexia (Geschwind and Behan 1982; Schachter and Galaburda 1986). The quantitative trait locus on chromosome 6p21.3–23 spans a 16.4-Mb (13.8 cM) interval from D6S109 to D6S291. Deffenbacher et al. (2004) refined this analysis to a 3.24 Mb region spanning D6S1597 to D6S1571 that was associated with severe scores and with maximal linkage converging at marker D6S1554 across phenotypes. More recently, Cope et al. (2005) found that *KIAA0319* was the specific gene most likely linked to dyslexia associated with chromosome 6p21.3–23 (specifically 6P22.2). The haplotype associated with dyslexia appears to lead to diminished production of *KIAA0319*, which plays a role in neuronal migration to the cerebral cortex (Paracchini et al. 2006).

Patterns of family inheritance have also helped to unravel the association between learning disorders and ADHD. Conservative estimates suggest that 8% of children with ADHD have a learning disorder, but actual estimates range from 0% to 92% (Semrud-Clikeman et al. 1992). Early studies showed that ADHD and learning disorders were transmitted independently (Faraone et al. 1993; Gilger et al. 1992) and suggested that comorbidity between ADHD and learning disorder may be a consequence of nonrandom mating (Faraone et al. 1993). However, a more recent study supported the independent transmission of ADHD and mathematical disabilities but found no evidence to support nonassortative mating in their sample of 464 probands (Monuteaux et al. 2005). Willcutt et al. (2000) found that there was a significant degree of heritability between reading disorder and ADHD symptoms of inattention but not between reading disorder and symptoms of hyperactivity/impulsivity. Approximately 95% of the phenotypic covariance between reading disorder and symptoms of inattention was attributable to common genetic influences versus only 21% of the phenotypic overlap between reading disorder and hyperactivity/impulsivity.

Evidence clearly suggests that there are heritable forms of learning disorders (Cardon et al. 1994, 1995; Pennington et al. 1983). However, critical questions about the nature of learning disorders color any discussion of etiology and pathophysiology. One major view is that learning disorders are relatively discrete neuropsychiatric syndromes affecting a specific set of higher cognitive functions without affecting general intelligence. Thus, learning disorders are identified by a clear discrepancy between aptitude and actual ability. Another view is that specific higher cognitive functions are not affected but that the neural circuits for lower-order cognitive functions are impaired, creating a block (S.E. Shaywitz and Shaywitz 2005). This view is supported by emerging data on dyslexia in which reading is affected by the lower-order function of decoding letters to their phonological sounds, which interferes with easy access to the intact higher cognitive function of comprehension (S.E. Shaywitz and Shaywitz 2005). This explains why an individual can have fluent speech and auditory word recognition but when reading cannot recognize unfamiliar words fluently. A contrasting view is that learning disorders are not discrete neurological syndromes and that they merely represent the tail end of a normal distribution of aptitudes and abilities (B.A. Shaywitz et al. 1995; S.E. Shaywitz et al. 1992). Evidence supporting the latter view derives mostly from the realm of psychological testing, in which an important study showed that reading ability scores were normally distributed, without an expected bimodal hump in the lower range that would have indicated a second population with lower mean value (S.E. Shaywitz et al. 1992; but see Rutter and Yule 1975).

Before the extensive use of MRI, scientists relied on autopsy findings to identify underlying anatomical differences in individuals with learning disorders. Autopsy findings in learning disorders include arteriovenous malformations, atypical gyral patterns in parietal lobes, thin corpus callosum in the region connecting the parietal lobes, and premature cessation of neuronal migration to the cortex, revealed by an excess number of neurons in white matter (Galaburda et al. 1985). Also, Galaburda (1993, 1994) observed anomalies in medial geniculate and lateral posterior thalamic nuclei. Perhaps the most interesting anomalies involve the cortex, particularly the left perisylvian region. These include neuronal ectopias in layer I, which are often nodular in appearance (brain warts) and associated with dysplasia of the underlying cortex. Micropolygyria has also been observed in some patients and in animals with autoimmune disorders that have deficient learning performance (Schrott et al. 1992).

Visual information from the retina is transmitted to the cerebral cortex by way of the lateral geniculate nucleus (LGN) in the thalamus. In primates, most of the retinal ganglion cells that project to the LGN belong to one of two classes, P and M, whose axons terminate in the parvocellular or magnocellular subdivisions of the LGN, respectively. These cell classes give rise to two channels that have been distinguished anatomically, physiologically, and behaviorally (DeYoe and Van Essen 1988). The magnocellular pathway has fast conduction velocities and large receptive fields, and it operates in a transient manner. In contrast, the parvocellular pathway is slow with much finer receptive fields (Mansilla et al. 1995). The visual cortex also can be subdivided into two pathways: one specialized for motion processing and the other for color and form information. Responses in the motion pathway depend primarily on magnocellular LGN, whereas visual responses in the color/form pathway depend on both P and M input (Ferrera et al. 1992). On the basis of electrophysiological studies and autopsy analysis of the LGN from five subjects, Livingstone et al. (1991) proposed that dyslexic subjects have a specific defect in the magnocellular pathway. They further suggested that dyslexic subjects perform poorly on auditory and somatosensory tests that require rapid discrimination and proposed an underlying defect in the fast subdivision of multiple cortical sensory systems. Evidence in support of this theory has been mixed. Studies using motion-based tests of the magnocellular pathway have been more supportive than tests using low-contrast stimuli (Demb et al. 1998a, 1998b; Greatrex and Drasdo 1995; Johannes et al. 1996; Kubova et al. 1996; Skottun 2000). J. Stein (2001) emphasized the importance of the magnocellular pathway in guiding visual attention and suggested that dyslexia in some individuals may result from impaired temporal processing in phonological, visual, and motor domains. Steinman et al. (1998) and Facoetti et al. (2000) also reiterated the association between magnocellular defects and impaired visuospatial attention in dyslexia.

Although researchers acknowledge that it is unlikely that a single deficit underlies dyslexia, competing theories focus on a specific factor such as a magnocellular, phonological, language, or cerebellar deficit. Ramus et al. (2003) conducted a study to ascertain the contribution of each type of deficit in a population of college students with dyslexia. Phonological deficits were found in all subjects, even in the absence of auditory, visual, and motor deficits. Additional auditory deficits were found along with phonological deficits in half of the subjects, and visual or cerebellar difficulties in less than a fourth of the subjects. A replication study with dyslexic children showed a similar pattern of prominent phonological deficits, concluding that sensory and motor deficits affect a subset of subjects with dyslexia but cannot independently explain a reading disability (White et al. 2006). Proponents of the role of sensory-motor deficits disagree, citing developmental maturational reasons for the findings (Tallal 2006).

Imaging studies reveal evidence for a diminished degree of anatomical and functional lateralization. For example, the planum temporale, which is normally asymmetrical with left-sided predominance, tends to be abnormally symmetrical in children with reading disorders. This symmetry suggests that individuals with reading disorders have an underdeveloped Broca's area relative to the homologous cortical area in the right hemisphere (Dalby et al. 1998; Haslam et al. 1981; Jernigan et al. 1991). Differences in the size of the perisylvian region may reflect a familial genetic factor (Plante 1991). Children with reading disorders have reduced activation of the left hemisphere (left temporoparietal cortex) under challenge conditions (Georgiewa et al. 1999; Lou et al. 1990; Rumsey et al. 1992; Simos et al. 2000) and may have reduced size of the left dorsolateral prefrontal cortex (Jernigan et al. 1991). Similarly, the cerebral blood flow pattern in the left angular gyrus of men with developmental dyslexia is not commensurate with blood flow in the extrastriate occipital and temporal lobes during single-word reading, suggesting a disconnection of the left angular gyrus in dyslexia (Horwitz et al. 1998).

Left hemisphere EEG activity is diminished relative to right-sided activity in children with reading disorders (Ackerman et al. 1998; Mattson et al. 1992), whereas right hemisphere activity is reduced in children with arithmetic disabilities (Mattson et al. 1992). Reduced lateralization of language centers is consistent with results from dichotic listening tasks (Morton 1994), which suggest either less efficient callosal transfer or right hemispheric processing of information. Curiously, corpus callosum area seems to be increased in some subjects with learning disorders and decreased in others. The corpus callosum is thicker in children with familial history of dysphasia/dyslexia, probably indicative of reduced cerebral dominance in this subgroup (Njiokiktjien 1994). In contrast, children who have suffered from perinatal adverse events that could impair cognitive skills have reduced corpus callosum area. Several mechanisms have been proposed to explain reductions in cerebral asymmetry, including reduced neuronal migration into the perisylvian region (Galaburda et al. 1985). At present these mechanisms require additional empirical support.

Left hemisphere specialization for language emerges over the course of maturation. An fMRI comparison of children and adults performing auditory/visual, phonological, semantic, and syntactic tasks demonstrated that adults have selective regional activation during each task, whereas children have overlapping activation during task performance

(Booth et al. 2001). Even considering this, fMRI studies comparing dyslexic children to age- and gender-matched control subjects consistently show a failure of the left hemisphere prefrontal brain systems to function properly (see review, S.E. Shaywitz and Shaywitz 2005). Dyslexic children fail to adequately engage specialized brain regions for language processing activated by normal reading children (left prefrontal cortex); instead they show more right than left inferior prefrontal activation (Backes et al. 2002). Similarly, brain activation during arithmetic calculation changes with age as functional specialization ensues. In a study of 8- to 19-year-old typical students, older adolescents demonstrated more activation in the left supramarginal gyrus and intraparietal sulcus as well as the left lateral occipital-temporal cortex—an area associated with visual word and symbol recognition (Rivera et al. 2005). The authors suggest that there is an early dependence on working memory and attention before specialization to the left posterior parietal cortex for math calculations (Rivera et al. 2005). Menon et al. (2000) reported that higher-order arithmetic processing in typical young adults activates the inferior and middle prefrontal gyri, as well as the angular and supramarginal gyri. Complex math also results in increased activation of the left and right caudate, left thalamus, and left- and right-middle (the corticothalamic) cerebellar circuits (Menon et al. 2000). Isaacs et al. (2001), in the first morphometric study of mathematics disorder, found gray matter volume reduced in the left intraparietal sulcus in neurologically healthy adolescents with mathematics disorder.

Studies of written expression in young adults identified an area in the left premotor cortex that was selectively activated when right-handed subjects observed or actually wrote single letters (Longcamp et al. 2003). A specific unilateral right ventral premotor region was activated by left-handed subjects during letter perception, demonstrating the existence of motor–perceptual interactions in letter reading (Longcamp et al. 2005). It is tempting to speculate that learning disorders affecting reading and spelling ability may stem from left hemisphere abnormalities, whereas disorders of arithmetic ability and social-emotional competence may arise from right hemisphere defects (Mattson et al. 1992; Semrud-Clikeman and Hynd 1990). Although this postulate may be true in many instances, it is not necessarily so. Sandson et al. (1994) described two patients with social-emotional processing disorder, a developmental syndrome usually ascribed to right hemisphere dysfunction. In these two patients, neurological examinations, EEG, and neuroimaging studies all revealed left hemisphere dysfunction. Both patients were left-handed and had findings suggestive of anomalous language dominance. Sandson et al. (1994) proposed that early injury to the left hemisphere can result in functional reorganization of the right hemisphere, sparing language and motor skills at the expense of functions that the right hemisphere normally subserves.

Nongenetic environmental factors clearly influence the appearance of learning disabilities. Fall conception significantly increases the risk of developing reading and arithmetic disabilities as well as mental retardation, presumably as a result of increased risk of viral infections during early stages of brain development (Liederman and Flannery 1994). Early exposure to environmental toxins can also manifest as learning disorders (Pihl and Parkes 1977). Prenatal and postnatal exposure to low-level lead is significantly associated with learning deficits in girls but not in boys (Leviton et al. 1993). Alcohol is another powerful factor that can produce learning disabilities in the presence of normal intelligence (Streissguth et al. 1990).

Geschwind and Galaburda (1985a, 1985b) proposed that increased fetal testosterone modifies neuronal, immune, and neural crest development. Testosterone can also inhibit neuronal migration by altering the ability of the CNS to identify trophic markers (Schachter et al. 1986). The Geschwind-Behan-Galaburda theory has been used to explain the relative superiority of males over females in spatial skills, the greater preponderance of learning disorders in males, the association between learning disorder and immune disorder, and the giftedness of left-handed individuals in other non–language-based skills (Geschwind and Behan 1982; Geschwind and Galaburda 1985a, 1985b). More recent studies have found that this influential theory is only partially supported by empirical evidence and is not consistent with current data on the development of the neural crest (Bryden et al. 1994).

TREATMENT

Mandated special education, provided in the least restrictive environment, is the current treatment for children with learning disorders. Special education is characterized by an individual educational plan and can include services provided as part of the usual classroom instruction, part-time removal from the classroom to designated "resource rooms," or work with an individual tutor. Specialized full-time classrooms, programs, or residential schools are usually reserved for those with lower IQ, severe learning disorders, or concomitant psychiatric or disruptive disorders.

Generally, alternative writing formats, skill building, and use of word processors can aid in the treatment of learning disorders, particularly disorders of written expression. Homework assignments for children with learning disabilities should emphasize simple, short tasks; careful monitoring and reinforcement by teachers; and parental involvement (Cooper and Nye 1994). Practical parent-based programs have become available (Jenson et al. 1994). In addition, efforts to increase the child's self-esteem are essential for successful treatment. One problem with special education programs is the low standard to which children are customarily held, which often causes them to progressively lose ground academically. Standards should be commensurate with a child's level of intelligence, not his or her deficits, recognizing that there are many ways to effectively educate children.

Efforts are under way to evaluate interventions to address dyslexia as a deficit in phonological ability. B.A. Shaywitz et al. (2004) provided evidence of the benefits of targeted intervention consisting of 50-minute daily tutorial of word-level instruction, blending letter sounds, oral reading, syllabic patterns, and timed reading to increase fluency. They evaluated groups of 6- to 9-year-old students and found that the group receiving phonological tutoring gained in reading accuracy and comprehension and demonstrated increased activation in left hemisphere regions, resembling that of normal readers. In contrast, the learning-disabled group that received community care was unchanged (B.A. Shaywitz et al. 2004).

Similarly, Tallal et al. (1996) found that intensive exposure to acoustically modified speech led to rapid gains in auditory comprehension in children with combined language-learning disorders. Tallal's group designed a computer program, now used in over 2,000 schools, that alters recorded speech by prolonging the duration of certain speech signals. Over time, comprehension can be maintained as the rapidity of these speech elements is gradually increased, resulting in enhanced capacity to understand normal speech (Tallal 2004).

No evidence supports the efficacy of medications to treat learning disorders. However, preliminary evidence suggests that response to stimulant treatment for ADHD may be diminished in children who have a co-occurring mathematics disorder, but not in children who have a reading disorder (Grizenko et al. 2006). This effect may be due to the higher level of executive dysfunction in children with mathematics disorder (Grizenko et al. 2006).

No direct evidence supports the efficacy of dietary or vitamin supplementation to treat learning disorders. However, a study to treat developmental coordination disorder in children with co-occurring learning and behavioral problems reported significant improvement in reading, spelling, and behavior, but not in the primary motor measures, during a 3-month placebo-controlled crossover study of supplemental fatty acids (Richardson and Montgomery 2005). Sensory integration therapy has little empirical support as a beneficial intervention for learning disorders (Hoehn and Baumeister 1994; Humphries et al. 1992; Kaplan et al. 1993).

SEIZURE DISORDERS

Epilepsy is a recurrent paroxysmal disorder involving excessive neural firing. It is a relatively common disorder with an incidence of 0.5%. Onset most often occurs before adulthood. It is estimated to affect 0.15% of preschoolers and 0.5% of school-age children. Seizures are more prevalent in boys than in girls, and the incidence is higher in nonwhites (W.A. Hauser 2003). Seizure disorders can present at birth and can be associated with chromosomal or structural abnormalities or in utero infections. Epilepsy can develop as a consequence of meningitis, encephalitis, head trauma, exposure to environmental toxins such as lead, inborn errors of metabolism, arteriovenous malformations, abnormalities in brain development—in short, from virtually any form of cerebral pathology that increases the excitability of brain tissue. Differential diagnosis is crucial. Many children suspected of having epilepsy have pseudoseizures or other paroxysmal nonepileptiform events (Andriola and Ettinger 1999; Rothner 1992). These events include mitral valve prolapse, cardiac arrhythmias, sleep disorders (pavor nocturnus, cataplexy, somnambulism), migraine headaches, movement disorders (e.g., TS, paroxysmal choreoathetosis), episodic dyscontrol, and panic disorder.

Seizure etiologies can be divided into genetic and acquired brain lesions. The latter may be focal, multifocal, or diffuse. Specific epilepsy syndromes with predominantly genetic basis (e.g., Lennox-Gastaut syndrome) can emerge in infancy or childhood (Blume 2004). A genetic etiology may be present in about 40% of cases. Newly identified genes and functional studies have reshaped our understanding of the pathophysiology of epilepsy (Gutierrez-Delicado and Serratosa 2004; Mulley et al. 2003). Genes associated with idiopathic generalized epilepsies are typically members of the ion channel family. Mutations in non–ion channel genes are responsible for autosomal dominant lateral temporal lobe epilepsy, at least one form of idiopathic focal epilepsy, cortical malformations, and syndromes that combine X-linked mental retardation and epilepsy (Hedera et al. 2004; Michelucci et al. 2003; Mulley et al. 2003; Stromme et al. 2002b). Most genetic epilepsies have a complex mode of inheritance, and genes identified so far account only for a minority of familial and sporadic cases.

Neuroimaging plays an important role in the investigation and treatment of patients with epilepsy. Diagnosis of the underlying substrate in a given patient with epilepsy determines prognosis with higher accuracy than EEG. MRI is the most sensitive technique for the diagnosis of hippocampal sclerosis, tumors, and malformations of cortical development (Kuzniecky 2005). Other imaging techniques such as PET, SPECT, and electromagnetic source imaging with magnetoencephalography are often reserved for patients with intractable epilepsy when surgery is contemplated (Bast et al. 2004). New developments such as MRS, receptor PET, and magnetic source imaging combined with electrocorticography are emerging clinical tools that give promise of improvements in diagnosis (Asano et al. 2004; Hudgins et al. 2005).

CLASSIFICATION AND FEATURES

Epilepsies are broadly classified by the location of the seizure focus. Primarily, generalized seizures involve the simultaneous emergence of seizure activity in both hemispheres, presumably from a subcortical focus. Partial seizures, in contrast, begin with discharge arising in a focal cortical area, though seizure activity can then spread (Dreifuss 1989). The major forms of generalized seizures are tonic-clonic seizures, absence seizures, myoclonic seizures, and infantile spasms. The major forms of partial seizures are simple seizures, complex partial seizures, and partial seizures secondarily generalized.

Generalized Seizures

Epilepsies with generalized tonic-clonic seizures, absence epilepsies, and myoclonic epilepsies often belong to the family of idiopathic generalized epilepsies (W.A. Hauser 1994). In more recent studies, mutations in the chloride channel gene CLCN2 have been associated with the most common forms of idiopathic generalized epilepsies (Gutierrez-Delicado et al. 2004; Niemeyer et al. 2004).

Tonic-clonic seizures are also known as *grand mal seizures*. Both hemispheres are simultaneously involved at the outset, producing immediate loss of consciousness, tonic extension, muscular stiffness, and inhibition of respiration. During the clonic phase of the attack, symmetrical jerking of all extremities occurs and is usually accompanied by oral and fecal incontinence (Rothner 1992). Typically tonic-clonic seizures last 2–5 minutes and are followed by somnolence and confusion. Severe headaches and muscle aches are also common in the postictal period.

There is convincing evidence that generalized tonic-clonic seizures are more likely to impair cognitive functions than are simple or complex partial seizures. Only the occurrence of status epilepticus increases the risk of cognitive impairments beyond that of generalized tonic-clonic seizures (Rausch 2002). There is still ongoing controversy as to whether these seizures originate in the cortex or in the thalamus. However, there is considerable evidence that frontal lobe structures play a major role in generating epileptic activity in generalized epilepsies (Pavone and Niedermeyer 2000). Imaging studies have revealed reduced basal rates of prefrontal glucose metabolism and reduced concentrations of N-acetyl aspartate (Savic et al. 2000; Swartz et al. 1996) indicative of neuronal loss or injury. Neuropsychological tests demonstrate impairment of prefrontal functions such as working memory and mental flexibility (Devinsky et al. 1997; Swartz et al. 1996).

Absence seizures are also known as *petit mal seizures*. They are characterized by abrupt onset of impaired consciousness that generally lasts for 10–20 seconds. During this period, children typically stare straight ahead and may flutter their eyelids, but there is usually an absence of movement. Posture is maintained and incontinence does not occur. Immediately after the seizure, consciousness is regained without postictal confusion. However, petit mal seizures can occur up to 20–30 times per day, taking a serious toll on attention, and can be brought on by stress and exercise. EEG reveals a highly characteristic 3 Hz spike-and-wave pattern (Rothner 1992). In some children, absence seizures remit during adolescence; in others, they are replaced by tonic-clonic seizures.

Infantile spasms, also known as *West syndrome*, are relatively uncommon, accounting for about 2% of childhood cases of epilepsy but about 25% of epilepsy cases with onset in the first year of life. This condition is one of the catastrophic epileptic syndromes in infancy characterized by a triad of symptoms involving infantile spasms, an interictal EEG pattern termed *hypsarrhythmia*, and mental retardation, although the diagnosis can be made even if one of these elements is missing. The disorder typically emerges between 3 months and 1 year of age. The spasms involve a brief jackknife-like flexion or extension of arms and legs. The spasms occur in clusters, particularly around sleep-wake transitions. They are associated with characteristic hypsarrhythmic EEG, a chaotic mixture of irregular high-voltage spike-and-wave discharge, multifocal sharp waves, and burst suppression. Most children with infantile spasms demonstrate moderate to profound mental retardation and will suffer from lifelong intractable seizures and impaired cognitive and psychosocial functioning (Pellock 1998; Riikonen 2004, Rothner 1992). The serine–threonine kinase 9 gene (*STK9*) has been associated with some cases of X-linked infantile spasms (Kalscheuer et al. 2003), whereas mutations in the aristaless-related homeobox gene (*ARX*) have been tied to other cases of X-linked and sporadic infantile spasms (Stromme et al. 2002a).

Myoclonic seizures, including atonic, akinetic, and tonic forms, usually emerge during the first 10 years of life and affect 0.1% of children. The combination of mental retardation, myoclonic seizures, and other seizure types is called *Lennox-Gastaut syndrome*. The myoclonic seizures are brief but frequent, and they are largely refractory to treatment. Ketogenic diet and corpus callostomy can be of benefit to some children (Pellock 1998; Rothner 1992).

Juvenile myoclonic epilepsy often emerges in adolescence and is a more benign and treatment-responsive condition. The seizures most frequently occur in the morning and take the form of myoclonic jerks or tonic-clonic convulsions. The EEG reveals characteristic generalized polyspikes. Children who develop this disorder are often healthy and free of neurological disturbance until the onset of the seizures. This condition persists throughout life but usually responds well to treatment with sodium valproate (Pellock 1998; Rothner 1992). Recently, *autosomal dominant juvenile myoclonic epilepsy* has been shown to be a channelopathy associated with a mutation in the $GABA_A$ receptor α_1 subunit (Cossette et al. 2002).

Partial Seizures

Simple partial seizures may be motor or sensory. A simple partial motor seizure consists of recurrent clonic movements of one part of the body without loss of consciousness. Sometimes motor activity can spread ipsilaterally (jacksonian march) or even spread to the contralateral hemisphere, resulting in a secondarily generalized tonic-clonic seizure. *Partial sensory seizures* consist of paresthesias or pain referred to a single part of the body. They also can spread. In general, partial seizures last 1–2 minutes and are not associated with loss of consciousness unless they generalize to the contralateral hemisphere (Rothner 1992).

Rolandic epilepsy is a benign, inherited focal epileptic disorder of childhood that is the most common form of focal seizure seen in children less than 15 years old (Rothner 1992). These seizures are characterized by emergence of sharp waves in the central temporal region and may or may not be accompanied by either seizure or neurological deficits. Children often report an aura around the mouth preceding the seizure, which is followed by the jerking of the mouth and face before spreading to the rest of the body. Children retain consciousness and do not have postictal confusion. The seizure lasts between 30 seconds and 3 minutes and usually occurs during sleep. Prognosis for spontaneous remission is excellent, and treatment is rarely required (Rothner 1992).

Complex partial seizures, also known as *psychomotor* or *temporal lobe seizures*, are the most frequent form of focal epilepsy and are distinguished from other partial seizures by alterations in consciousness. Auras such as unpleasant odors, tastes, or sensations frequently precede the seizure. The seizure may be characterized by staring, altered consciousness, and eye blinking with maintenance of balance. Approximately 80% of patients with complex partial seizures engage in simple, repetitive, and purposeless automatism, which can include swallowing, kissing, lip smacking, fumbling, scratching, or rubbing movements. Rarely, special sensory phenomena can occur that can include visual distortions or hallucinations, auditory hallucinations, dreamlike or dissociative states, and abnormal body sensations (Kaufman 2001). Déjà vu is widely recognized to be associated with temporal lobe epilepsy (Wild 2005). The seizures last about 2 minutes and are often followed by confusion, drowsiness, and amnesia for the events. The EEG often shows sharp waves or spikes from the temporal region (Rothner 1992). Partial complex seizure attacks occur far less frequently than absence spells.

Histopathological studies have revealed that the majority of patients with temporal lobe epilepsy (70%) have hippocampal sclerosis (Jokeit and Ebner 2002). Mesial temporal lobe epilepsy (MTLE) is rarely controlled to a sufficient degree by antiepileptic drugs. There is controversy as to whether chronic refractory temporal lobe epilepsies are associated with the risk of cognitive deterioration, although dementia is a very rare phenomenon in patients with MTLE. Bonilha et al. (2004) reported that patients with MTLE exhibit a reduction in gray matter concentration in regions outside the temporal lobe, specifically in areas that are connected to the hippocampus and parahippocampal region, suggesting an anatomical route for atrophy.

A rare familial epilepsy with onset in adolescence or early adulthood, *autosomal dominant lateral temporal lobe epilepsy*, has been associated with a mutation in the leucine-rich, glioma-inactivated 1 gene (*LGI1*) (also known as epitempin) (Pisano et al. 2005).

Frontal lobe epilepsy is the second most frequent localized form of epilepsy. Initial manifestation of frontal lobe seizures depends on the location of the epileptogenic zone. Focal clonic motor seizures result from epileptic activity within the primary motor cortex. Tonic seizures originate in the supplementary motor area and complex partial seizures in orbital frontal, medial frontal, frontal polar, and dorsal lateral regions. The complexity and diversity of frontal lobe functions are reflected in the variability of symptoms found in frontal lobe seizures and by the variability of related neuropsychological deficits. Neuropsychological studies have compared patients with frontal lobe and temporal lobe epilepsy to control subjects to measure nonspecific effects of focal epilepsy on cognition. Frontal lobe epilepsy is often associated with reduced attention span and psychomotor speed, whereas temporal lobe epilepsy is more often associated with impaired episodic memory (Exner et al. 2002; Helmstaedter et al. 1996).

Pseudoseizures

Pseudoseizures are also known as *dissociative convulsions* (ICD-10) or *nonepileptic seizures*. These are unintentional paroxysmal episodes of altered sensation, movement, perception, or emotion that clinically resemble epileptic seizures but are not accompanied by epileptiform neurophysiological changes (Krumholz 1999). Patients may suffer considerable disability, but early diagnosis and psychotherapeutic intervention can lead to improvement, reduce undue hospital attendance, and avoid unnecessary anticonvulsant treatment (R. Martin et al. 1998). In spite of characteristic differences in semiology, course, and response to treatment, the distinction between epileptic seizures and pseudoseizures can be extremely difficult and may ultimately depend on capturing a typical attack during prolonged video-EEG monitoring (Krumholz 1999). Interestingly, pseudoseizures and epilepsy often coexist (Lesser 1996), with incidence rates of 3–5 per 100,000 (Sigurdardottir and Olafsson 1998). As many as 20% of patients treated for intractable epilepsy may have pseudoseizures (Krumholz 1999). Research into risk factors for pseudoseizures has shown comorbidity with depression and personality disorder (A.M. Kanner et al. 1999; Wyllie et al. 1999). Early reports suggested that about 30% of individuals with pseudoseizures report a history of physical or sexual abuse (Alper et al. 1993; Betts and Boden 1992). They also have an increased history of brain injury (Pakalnis and Paolicchi 2000) and asthma (de Wet et al. 2003), suggesting that these conditions may be significant risk factors.

PSYCHIATRIC CONSEQUENCES OF EPILEPSY

Bear and Fedio (1977) proposed that patients with temporal lobe epilepsy had distinctive personality aberrations. Many were hyposexual, humorless, circumstantial, overly metaphysical, hyperreligious, hypergraphic, and interpersonally viscous. It was also proposed that right-sided foci predisposed a patient to anger, sadness, and elation, whereas left-sided foci led to ruminative and intellectual tendencies. More recent studies, however, have cast doubt on these theories (Kaufman 2001; Rodin and Schmaltz 1984).

An association exists between childhood epilepsy and behavioral, academic, and cognitive problems (Dunn and Austin 1999; Metz-Lutz et al. 1999). Indeed, cognitive impairment is the most common comorbid condition found in children with epilepsy (Aldenkamp 2001a, 2001b). Children with epilepsy often have academic difficulties and perform more poorly in school than would be expected based on their IQ scores (Dunn and Austin 1999; Williams 2003). Specific cognitive deficits associated with underachievement include impairments of language, memory, executive function, and attention (Fastenau et al. 2004). Problems with attention may be particularly important. Williams et al. (2001) found that after controlling for intelligence, impaired attention was a more significant predictor of academic problems than memory, self-esteem, or socioeconomic factors. Children with epilepsy also have a disproportionately high incidence of behavioral problems and comorbid psychiatric disorders.

Deficits in global mental functions such as consciousness, arousal, and activation, or in specific cognitive functions such as attention, memory, and language, may be more debilitating than the seizures themselves. These deficits may arise from underlying neurological dysfunction, seizure factors, and/or adverse CNS effects of antiepileptic drugs (Aldenkamp et al. 2005).

Several studies have reported symptoms of inattention, hyperactivity, or impulsivity consistent with a diagnosis of ADHD. Austin et al. (2001) found higher rates of attentional and behavioral problems 6 months before seizure onset in a sample of children with new-onset epilepsy than in their closest-aged healthy sibling. Children with partial seizures have more behavior problems than children with generalized seizures. Dunn et al. (2003) found evidence of ADHD in 37.7% of children with epilepsy present for at least 6 months. About two-thirds had the predominantly inattentive subtype. There was no statistically significant difference in rate of ADHD by seizure type or focus of epileptiform activity. Hesdorffer et al. (2004) looked for a past history of ADHD in a population-based study of children with new-onset epilepsy. They found that ADHD, predominantly inattentive type, was associated with new-onset seizures. Thome-Souza et al. (2004) used a structured psychiatric history to assess behavioral problems and classified seizures as partial or generalized. They found that 29.1% of the 78 children and adolescents studied met criteria for ADHD. The prevalence of ADHD was higher in the patients with partial seizures (62.5%) than in patients with generalized seizures (37.5%). Overall, these studies suggest that about a third of children with epilepsy will meet criteria for comorbid ADHD.

Early evidence suggested that psychosis can emerge in patients with temporal lobe epilepsy. The seizure disorder most often emerged in childhood (5–10 years of age), whereas psychosis was generally delayed in onset until about age 30 years. Left-handed patients with left-sided seizure foci were believed to be the most susceptible to psychosis (Perez and Trimble 1980). Interestingly, we have found that childhood abuse is associated with an increased incidence of left hemisphere EEG abnormalities (Ito et al. 1993) and indices of decreased left cortical differentiation (Ito et al. 1998). Davies (1978-1979) previously reported that childhood incest was associated with a high incidence of abnormal EEGs and seizure disorder in 36% of survivors. The stress of childhood trauma can affect aspects of brain development (as discussed in the later section "Neuropsy-

chiatric Consequences of Childhood Abuse"), thereby increasing the risk for emergence of seizures. Moreover, this type of trauma can be associated with development of serious psychopathology, including dissociation and perception of internal voices that can be mistaken for psychosis.

There appears to be a significant association between epilepsy and criminality. Incarcerated men have a fourfold increased incidence of epilepsy compared with the general population (Kaufman 2001). It is likely that both epilepsy and criminality result from common causes such as brain trauma and stressors associated with low socioeconomic status. As suggested above, a common association may exist among childhood abuse, EEG abnormalities, and criminal behavior. In a study of 14 juvenile murderers condemned to death, 12 had a history of brutal physical abuse and 5 had been sodomized by relatives (D.O. Lewis et al. 1988). EEG abnormalities and seizure disorders were common in this group (D.O. Lewis et al. 1988). Sexual trauma has often been identified in the life histories of sex offenders (Seghorn et al. 1987). Thus, early abuse can lead to a vicious cycle of intergenerational transmission and perpetuation associated with neuropsychiatric sequelae.

Affective disorders are more common in children with epilepsy than in healthy control subjects (Gilliam 2005). Thome-Souza et al. (2004) reported that depression occurred in 36.4% of children and adolescents with epilepsy. Whereas ADHD was particularly prevalent in prepubertal children, depression predominated in adolescents. Williams et al. (2003) reported the occurrence of mild to moderate symptoms of anxiety in 23% of children and adolescents with epilepsy and related presence of symptoms to comorbid learning or behavioral difficulties, ethnicity, and polytherapy. Children and adolescents with epilepsy should be periodically assessed for mood disorders to facilitate timely treatment.

Finally, there is a marked but substantially underappreciated association between epilepsy, suicidality, and self-destructive behavior. One of the earliest pioneering studies on the physiological determinants of suicide reported a strong positive association between paroxysmal EEG disturbances and suicidal ideation, suicide attempts, and assaultive-destructive behavior (Struve et al. 1972). It has also been reported that the risk of completed suicide is four to five times greater in individuals with epilepsy than among patients without epilepsy and that this risk may be 25-fold greater in patients with temporal lobe epilepsy (Barraclough 1987; Matthews and Barabas 1981). As many as one-third of all patients with epilepsy have attempted suicide at some point in their lives (Delay et al. 1957; I. Jensen and Larsen 1979). This risk is far greater for patients with epilepsy than patients with other medical disorders producing comparable degrees of handicap or disability (Mendez et al. 1986).

Mendez et al. (1989) provided data suggesting that this risk can be related to interictal psychopathological changes, particularly the high prevalence of borderline personality disorder. Brent et al. (1987) examined 15 children with epilepsy treated with phenobarbital and 24 children with epilepsy treated with carbamazepine. The groups were similar across a wide range of demographic, seizure-related, familial, and environmental factors. Patients treated with phenobarbital had a much higher prevalence of major depression (40% versus 4%, $P=0.02$) and a much greater prevalence of suicidal ideation (47% versus 4%, $P=0.005$). It is unclear whether phenobarbital produced these psychiatric disturbances or failed to alleviate them. However, the implications for treatment are clear.

TREATMENT

Antiepileptic drugs modify the balance between neuronal excitation and inhibition via their influence on cerebral transmitter systems and/or ion channel activities. Tonic-clonic seizures are often responsive to valproic acid, phenytoin, carbamazepine, phenobarbital, or topiramate. Valproic acid and ethosuximide are useful for the treatment of generalized absence seizures. Infantile spasms and myoclonic seizures of childhood are often treatment refractory. Potentially useful medications include adrenocorticotropic hormone, valproic acid, benzodiazepines, and vigabatrin (Gupta and Appleton 2005; Riikonen 2004). Lennox-Gastaut syndrome may be treated with valproate, lamotrigine, topiramate, or felbamate. There is usually no single antiepileptic medication that will control seizures in this disorder. Juvenile myoclonic epilepsy often responds favorably to valproic acid. Uncomplicated partial seizures are treated with carbamazepine, phenytoin, or phenobarbital. Partial complex seizures are also treated with carbamazepine, phenytoin, or phenobarbital. Many cases of partial complex seizure fail to fully respond to monotherapy and may require combination treatment. Gabapentin, lamotrigine, tiagabine, levetiracetam, zonisamide, and pregabalin are indicated for adjunctive therapy of partial seizures. The use of adjunctive therapy is a new approach to seizure management. The old rule was to pursue monopharmacy even to extreme doses to avoid polypharmacy, in the belief that multiple anticonvulsants would produce supra-additive toxicity. Controlled trials indicate that these newer adjunctive agents can potentiate anticonvulsant efficacy with little increase in side effects. Neurosurgery to remove an underlying lesion may be the treatment of choice for focal seizures, depending on the region affected (Wyllie et al. 1989).

Duration of medication treatment needs to be individualized. After a child has been free of seizures for 2–5 years, it may be possible to discontinue seizure medications. Discontinuation is less likely to succeed if the child has had a persistently abnormal EEG, known structural lesion, mental retardation, focal complex partial seizures, or multiple seizure types. Medications should be withdrawn slowly, generally one medication at a time (Rothner 1992).

Phenobarbital, and its associated congener primidone, acts on the $GABA_A$ receptor complex to increase the action of the inhibitory neurotransmitter GABA on chloride channels. It also appears to inhibit the release of glutamate (an excitatory neurotransmitter) from nerve endings. These agents are associated with hyperactivity, fussiness, lethargy, disturbed sleep, irritability, depression, and cognitive disturbance in children (Rothner 1992) and should not be used as drugs of first choice in the pediatric population.

Phenytoin was introduced in 1938 by Merritt and Putnamm and has been used ever since. It appears to act on voltage- and frequency-dependent sodium channels (Schwarz and Grigat 1989). It binds to the fast inactivated state of the channel, reducing high-frequency neuronal firing. Phenytoin may also have mild effects on the excitatory glutamate system and on the inhibitory GABA system, and chronic administration can lead to gingival hyperplasia and hirsutism. Phenytoin is a less frequent cause of behavioral problems than phenobarbital, but it can impair attention and coordination and can produce dizziness, ataxia, and diplopia. Phenytoin may provoke schizophrenia-like psychoses at high serum levels (McDanal and Bolman 1975; Schmitz 1999). In a study on 45 patients with drug related psychoses, 25 (56%) were attributed to treatment with phenytoin (Kanemoto et al. 2001).

Carbamazepine is structurally similar to tricyclic antidepressants but lacks prominent effects on monoamine reuptake. The main anticonvulsant mechanism of action is similar to that of phenytoin but with less "slowing" effect on the recovery state of the sodium channel. Common side effects include diplopia, dizziness, drowsiness, and transient leukopenia. Carbamazepine can also impair neuropsychological performance but is usually less problematic than phenobarbital or phenytoin (Rothner 1992). Rarely, aplastic anemia and hepatotoxicity can occur.

Valproic acid is one of the most effective drugs against generalized absence seizures. Proposed mechanisms of action include effects on sodium and T-type calcium channels and enhancement of GABA neurotransmission. Valproic acid is often the most tolerated anticonvulsant for children and adolescents. Common side effects include gastrointestinal distress and thinning of the hair. Rare cases of fetal hepatotoxicity have occurred, though these cases are almost entirely limited to infants and young children, and most instances occurred in conjunction with other drugs known to induce hepatic microsomal enzymes, which can foster buildup of a toxic valproate metabolite.

Pancreatitis is another rare complication. Occasionally drowsiness may arise, which can be related to elevated ammonia levels. Valproic acid is associated in a few instances with acute or chronic encephalopathies. These encephalopathies are related to dose, and perhaps to polytherapy, and are reversible with dose reduction (Schmitz 1999).

Isojarvi et al. (1993) reported the possibility that valproic acid was associated with polycystic ovaries, elevated levels of testosterone, and menstrual disturbances. Eighty percent of young women in their sample who started treatment with valproic acid prior to age 18 years had these findings. This issue remains controversial (Genton et al. 2001), but women should be cautioned about the risk for weight gain and be told to promptly report menstrual disturbances or signs of hirsutism. Switching treatment from valproic acid to lamotrigine fostered recovery in a small series of cases (Isojarvi and Tapanainen 2000).

Absence seizures are also treated with ethosuximide, which modifies the properties of voltage-dependent calcium channels, reducing T-type currents and thereby preventing synchronized firing. Although ethosuximide is useful in the treatment of absence seizures, it has no effect against possible coexisting major motor seizures. Major side effects include nausea, vomiting, and anorexia. Cognitive and behavioral side effects are uncommon. Psychosis has been reported to occur in about 2% of children treated with ethosuximide, typically following cessation of seizure.

Vigabatrin is an irreversible inhibitor of GABA transaminase, the enzyme responsible for the catabolism of GABA in the brain. It is used for treatment of infantile spasms unresponsive to other treatments (Gupta et al. 2005; Riikonen 2004). Vigabatrin has been associated with both psychosis and depression. Its use is limited because it can produce concentric visual field defects (Besag 2004).

Felbamate is used only in those patients who have not responded to more conventional treatment and whose seizures are so severe as to warrant treatment with a drug associated with markedly increased risk of aplastic anemia and hepatic failure. In children, the main indication is multiple seizures of the Lennox-Gastaut syndrome type (Schmidt and Bourgeois 2000). Felbamate may lead to increased alertness, sleep disturbance, and behavioral problems related to agitation (McConnell et al. 1996). The psychotropic effects of felbamate may be particularly problematic for anxious children, whereas sedated children may benefit from its stimulating properties (Ketter et al. 1996, 1997).

Gabapentin is a cyclic GABA analogue, originally designed as a GABA agonist (Macdonald and Kelly 1995). Initial research postulated that gabapentin exerted a selective effect on GABA neurotransmission; however, more recent studies indicate that it acts via selective inhibition of voltage-gated calcium channels containing the $\alpha_2\delta_1$ subunit.

The most common side effects of gabapentin include somnolence, ataxia, fatigue, and nausea. Gabapentin appears to be relatively free of adverse cognitive effects (Leach et al. 1997; R. Martin et al. 1999; Meador et al. 1999). However, a number of studies suggest that gabapentin may induce behavioral problems such as aggression in children with learning disabilities and adults with mental handicaps (Lee et al. 1996; Tallian et al. 1996; Wolf et al. 1995). Adverse behavioral effects may be minimized by gradual dose titration.

Lamotrigine is a phenyltriazine that acts by blocking voltage-dependent sodium channels producing voltage- and frequency-dependent inhibition. It also appears to inhibit presynaptic release of excitatory neurotransmitters. Lamotrigine is sometimes associated with the development of a rash that can presage serious dermatological consequences. Common side effects include dizziness, ataxia, diplopia, blurred vision, and nausea. Lamotrigine has gained a reputation for having positive psychotropic properties, improving both mood and cognitive functions. Severe psychiatric complications seem to be uncommon with lamotrigine, and psychosis and depression occurred only in very few cases in the trials (Fitton and Goa 1995). Insomnia, which may be associated with irritability, anxiety, or even hypomania, is the only significant psychiatric side effect, occurring in 6% of patients treated in monotherapy, compared with 2% in patients treated with carbamazepine and 3% in patients treated with phenytoin (Brodie et al. 1995). Children with learning difficulties and adults with mental handicaps may develop behavioral problems such as aggression (Beran and Gibson 1998; Ettinger et al. 1998). Lamotrigine is associated with fewer neuropsychological side effects than carbamazepine (Meador et al. 2001).

Tiagabine potentiates GABA neurotransmission by antagonizing presynaptic reuptake of GABA. Common side effects include dizziness, headache, sleepiness, inability to concentrate, and tremor. Tiagabine appears to be associated with a low incidence of depression or psychosis (Besag 2004); however, its use has been tied to the paradoxical provocation of de novo nonconvulsive status epilepticus because of a relatively narrow therapeutic index (Schapel and Chadwick 1996). Therefore, EEG assessment may be necessary to evaluate behavioral problems, particularly those associated with mutism, qualitative change in consciousness, or symptoms of autism or myoclonus.

Topiramate is a sulfamate-substituted monosaccharide. At pharmacologically relevant concentrations it blocks voltage-dependent sodium channels, augments the activity of the GABA at some subtypes of the $GABA_A$ receptor, antagonizes the 2-(aminomethyl)phenylacetic acid (AMPA)/kainate glutamate receptor subtype, and inhibits carbonic anhydrase. Common side effects in children include weight decrease, upper respiratory tract infection, paresthesia, anorexia, diarrhea, and mood problems. Topiramate may precipitate both psychosis and depression, but these are less likely to occur if currently recommended lower starting doses, escalation rates, and target doses are used. A significant proportion of topiramate-associated psychoses may occur as an alternative syndrome in patients who become seizure free (Mula et al. 2003a). An unusual idiosyncratic side effect of topiramate is amnestic or motor aphasia, and in controlled trials 17%–28% of patients developed symptoms classified as "abnormal thinking" (Mula et al. 2003b).

Levetiracetam does not affect voltage-gated sodium or T-type calcium channels and does not appear to directly facilitate GABA neurotransmission. However, it may antagonize the activity of negative modulators of GABA and glycine. Electrophysiologically, levetiracetam appears to prevent hypersynchronization of epileptiform burst firing and propagation of seizure activity. Common side effects include cough, dizziness, dry or sore throat, hoarseness, loss of energy or strength, muscle pain or weakness, runny nose, unusual drowsiness, tender swollen glands in the neck, difficulty swallowing, and changes in voice. Levetiracetam is not associated with a high risk for psychotic or depressive reactions. Significant affective episodes were reported in 2% and psychoses in 0.7% of patients treated in preclinical trials. Levetiracetam may exacerbate behavioral problems in children (Lagae et al. 2005) and may markedly increase their risk for aggression, including suicidal behavior.

Zonisamide is a sulfonamide that blocks sodium channels and reduces voltage-dependent, T-type calcium currents. Zonisamide facilitates dopaminergic and serotonergic neurotransmission and has weak inhibitory effects on carbonic anhydrase. Common side effects include sleepiness or fatigue, dizziness, loss of appetite, upset stomach, headache, agitation or irritability, poor coordination or tremor, speech problems, poor concentration, itching, and vision problems. Zonisamide may exert positive psychiatric benefits in some patients (Besag 2004). However, there are also indications of significant psychiatric adverse events, including depression and psychoses. In a Japanese series of patients with psychotic episodes, half of drug-related episodes were triggered by zonisamide (Besag 2001, 2004; Hirai et al. 2002; Hirose et al. 2003; Kimura 1994; Matsuura 1999).

Pregabalin was designed as a more potent successor to gabapentin and also exerts a selective inhibitory effect on voltage-gated calcium channels containing the $\alpha_2\delta_1$ subunit (Sills 2006). The most common side effects are dizziness, sleepiness, dry mouth, swelling of hands and feet, blurry vision, weight gain, and trouble concentrating. There is no evidence for significant psychiatric adverse events from controlled trials with pregabalin. However, clinical experience with this recently introduced drug is still limited.

TRAUMA, INFECTIONS, AND STRESS

The developing brain is highly susceptible to adverse environmental factors. In the final section, we summarize recent research on the neuropsychiatric consequences of traumatic brain injury, streptococcal infection, and physical, sexual, and emotional abuse during childhood. These are all too common occurrences that can produce severe neuropsychiatric sequelae.

TRAUMATIC BRAIN INJURY

The leading cause of disability in children between birth and age 19 years is injury. Data from the National Pediatric Trauma Registry indicate that more than 25% of children injured and admitted for hospital care receive a diagnosis of head injury. Traumatic brain injury is classified as penetrating or closed. After discharge from the hospital, a significant number of children continue to present with potentially detrimental psychiatric sequelae (Russo and Navalta 1995). Outcome is most strongly related to the severity of brain injury, although posttraumatic amnesia, length of coma, presence of brain stem injury, seizures, and increased intracranial pressure also affect prognosis (Beers 1992). Intelligence, fine motor skills, sensorimotor function, problem-solving ability, memory, adaptive function, attention, and language processing can all be affected (for a review, see Michaud et al. 1993a). In addition, the presence of posttraumatic behavioral disorders compounds these problems (Michaud et al. 1993b). Aggression, poor anger control, hyperactivity, and deficient social skills are typical behavioral symptoms (Asarnow et al. 1991). The emergence of these symptoms depends on the severity (Brown et al. 1981) and location of the injury (Sollee and Kindlon 1987). The symptoms are exacerbated by premorbid factors, including substance abuse, psychiatric disability, and dysfunctional family relations (Rivara et al. 1993).

The remarkable capacity of the developing brain to adapt to certain congenital anomalies and injuries has led many to believe that children will invariably show greater recovery than adults to traumatic brain injury (Rosner 1974). Others have hypothesized that children can be more vulnerable than adults. The relationship between age of injury and extent of disability is complex. Before puberty, a high density of synaptic connections allows for considerable adaptive plasticity, which is most evident in the capacity to develop language after severe left hemisphere injury. However, there are also sensitive and critical periods for establishment of connections and synaptic relations, and if these opportunities are lost, enduring consequences can result.

Max and colleagues (1997b, 1998a, 1998b, 1998c, 1999, 2000, 2004, 2006) have published extensively on the psychiatric consequences of brain trauma. A retrospective analysis revealed that 5.6% of 1,333 consecutive patients presenting to a child psychiatry outpatient clinic had a definite history of traumatic brain injury (Max and Dunisch 1997). In a large prospective study, 50 subjects were evaluated upon hospitalization for traumatic brain injury and reassessed upon follow-up at 3, 6, 12, and 24 months (Max et al. 1997a, 1997b, 1997c). The most consistently significant factors associated with the development of subsequent psychiatric disorders were increased severity of injury, family psychiatric history, and family dysfunction. Posttraumatic psychiatric disorders included organic personality syndrome, major depression, ADHD, oppositional defiant disorder, PTSD, simple phobia, separation anxiety disorder, OCD, adjustment disorder, mania, hypomania, and marijuana dependence. Some psychiatric sequelae were clinically apparent by 3 months after injury.

Secondary ADHD is a common sequela of traumatic brain injury that can affect 15%–20% of children (Max et al. 2005c) and may relate directly to damage to the orbital frontal gyrus (Max et al. 2005b) or severity of injury (Max et al. 2004), though preinjury adaptive function and psychosocial adversity may be important determinants of outcome 2 years post-trauma (Max et al. 2005c). Max et al. (1998a, 1998b) found that development of oppositional symptomatology in the first year after injury was strongly associated with psychosocial factors, whereas its persistence in the second year was more significantly related to severity of brain injury (Max et al. 1998a). Sixty-eight percent of the subjects experienced at least one PTSD symptom in the first 3 months, decreasing to 12% of the subjects at 2 years. Only 4% of the subjects met criteria for PTSD at any point in the study (Max et al. 1998b). Personality change occurred in 22% of participants in a prospective study in the first 6 months after injury. Severity of injury predicted personality change. Lesions of the dorsal prefrontal cortex, specifically the superior frontal gyrus, were associated with personality change after controlling for severity of injury or presence of other lesions (Max et al. 2005a). Personality disorder persisted in 12% after 2 years and was specifically related to injury to frontal lobe white matter (Max et al. 2006). Overall, severe traumatic brain injury is significantly associated with a greater incidence of psychiatric disorders (63%) compared with mild injury (21%) and orthopedic injury (4%) (Max et al. 1998d). Psychosocial intervention and family support may contribute to more effective treatment of brain-injured patients throughout the first 2 years after injury (Kinsella et al. 1999), although their therapeutic efficacy remains to be established.

PEDIATRIC AUTOIMMUNE NEUROPSYCHIATRIC DISORDERS

Pediatric autoimmune neuropsychiatric disorders, or PANDAS, represents a recently described clinical syndrome involving the emergence of OCD or tic disorders in the context of group A β-hemolytic streptococcal (GABHS) infection (reviewed in Snider and Swedo 2004). Swedo et al. (1998) provided the first characterization of 50 cases of PANDAS and proposed that patients with PANDAS could be identified by the following five criteria: 1) presence of OCD and/or a tic disorder, 2) age at onset before puberty, 3) episodic course of symptom severity, 4) association with GABHS infection, and 5) association with neurological abnormalities. PANDAS is thought to be the result of the development of an autoimmune reaction precipitated by GABHS infection resulting in antineuronal antibodies that target neurons in the basal ganglia (Pavone et al. 2004; Singer et al. 2004). This in turn gives rise to OCD, tic disorders including TS (Church et al. 2003; Muller et al. 2001), and possibly Sydenham's chorea—a similar neuropsychiatric syndrome that develops in association with rheumatic fever (Murphy et al. 2000). Initial reports indicated that antineuronal antibodies directed against neurons in the putamen could be isolated from sera of TS patients (Singer et al. 1998). Stereotypies and episodic utterances, analogous to involuntary movements seen in TS, were induced in rats by intrastriatal microinfusion of sera or gamma immunoglobulins from patients with TS (Hallett et al. 2000). However, a recent study found no differences between patients with PANDAS, patients with TS, and healthy control subjects in titers of antineuronal antibodies directed against putamen, caudate, or prefrontal cortex (Snider et al. 2005). It has been hypothesized that the episodic worsening of symptoms characteristic of PANDAS may result from additional occurrences of GABHS infection (S.W. Kim et al. 2004). Plasma exchange therapy and intravenous immunoglobulin treatment have produced mixed results in reducing the neuropsychiatric symptoms associated with PANDAS (Hoekstra et al. 2004; Perlmutter et al. 1999). Treatment with antibiotic prophylaxis using azithromycin and penicillin has also been studied, with some promising results (Garvey et al. 1999; Snider et al. 2005). It should be noted that only a modest subset of cases of OCD and TS are the result of PANDAS (Singer et al. 1999).

NEUROPSYCHIATRIC CONSEQUENCES OF CHILDHOOD ABUSE

Physical, sexual, or emotional traumatization during childhood can contribute to the development of a spectrum of psychiatric disorders (Teicher et al. 2006b). Early traumatization can be a risk factor in dissociative identity disorder (Wilbur 1984), refractory psychosis (Beck and van der Kolk 1987), borderline personality disorder (Herman et al. 1989; Stone 1981), somatoform disorder (Krystal 1978), depression (Fergusson et al. 1996), bipolar disorder (Post et al. 2001), and panic disorder (Faravelli et al. 1985). Childhood physical abuse can also sensitize patients to the development of PTSD (Bremner et al. 1993). Animal studies clearly suggest that early deprivation or stress can result in neurobiological abnormalities (Hofer 1975; Hubel 1978; McEwen 2000). However, little evidence for this has been shown in humans (van der Kolk and Greenberg 1987). Teicher and colleagues hypothesized that early traumatic experience in the form of childhood abuse could affect the development of the cerebral cortex and limbic system (for reviews, see Teicher 1989, 1994, 2002; Teicher et al. 2003a).

This hypothesis was studied in a variety of ways, one of which was to review EEG recordings from 115 consecutive admissions to the child and adolescent program at McLean Hospital (Ito et al. 1993). Psychiatrically ill children with abuse histories had a greater incidence of clinically significant EEG abnormalities (i.e., spike waves, sharp waves, paroxysmal slowing) than psychiatrically ill children without abuse. Hospitalized children with a documented history of severe physical and/or sexual abuse had a 72% incidence of abnormal EEG readings. This very high rate mirrored the rate reported by Davies (1978–1979) (72% abnormal EEGs, 36% clinical seizures) for individuals who were involved as the younger member of an incestuous relationship. However, Davies (1978–1979) proposed that this neurological abnormality made the individuals easier to victimize and that it was not a consequence of abuse but a predisposing risk factor.

Preclinical studies, however, suggest that exposure to early stress can indeed induce EEG abnormalities. Heath (1972) provided a powerful demonstration of this possibility by implanting depth electrodes in monkeys raised in isolation by Harry F. Harlow, M.D. Heath found that these monkeys had spike waves in their hippocampus and fastigial nuclei (which project from the cerebellar vermis to a variety of brain structures including the hippocampus). There are a variety of mechanisms that could produce this outcome. We have hypothesized that it may come about as a consequence of early stress-induced alterations in the structure and function of GABA$_A$ receptors (Teicher 2002), which has been observed in rats that were subjected to low levels of maternal care (Caldji et al. 2003). GABA is a major inhibitory neurotransmitter, and functional alterations in the structure of GABA$_A$ receptors would likely result in significant electrophysiological abnormalities, as has

been reported in patients with autosomal dominant juvenile myoclonic epilepsy (Cossette et al. 2002).

Ito et al. (1993) also found that abused and nonabused patients differed only in the prevalence of left hemisphere EEG abnormalities. Neuropsychological testing confirmed that left hemisphere deficits were 6.7-fold more prevalent than right hemisphere deficits in the abused group, whereas this ratio was 3-fold less in nonabused patients. EEG coherence (a measure of cortical interconnectivity that displays a prominent developmental sequence that parallels cortical maturation) was used in a follow-up study as a means of assessing cortical development (Ito et al. 1998; Teicher et al. 1997b). Abused children had higher overall levels of left hemisphere coherence and a reversed hemispheric asymmetry. These findings strongly suggest that abused adolescent patients had a deficient degree of left cortical differentiation and development.

Evidence for left hemisphere disturbance has also emerged in a number of imaging studies. Bremner et al. (1997) compared MRI scans of 17 adults with physical or sexual abuse and PTSD with scans of 17 matched subjects with no abuse history or PTSD. The left hippocampus was 12% smaller in the abused group than that in the nonabused adults. Stein et al. (1997) measured hippocampal volume in 21 women with childhood sexual abuse. Fifteen patients had current PTSD, and 15 had dissociative disorder. There was a significant reduction in left hippocampal size, which also correlated inversely with dissociative symptoms. Driessen et al. (2000) studied 21 adult women with borderline personality disorder and a history of childhood abuse and compared them with healthy control subjects. They found that patients with borderline personality disorder had nearly a 16% reduction in both left and right hippocampal volume. Vythilingam et al. (2002) found that depressed women with a history of childhood abuse had an 18% smaller left hippocampus than nonabused depressed subjects and a 15% smaller left hippocampus than healthy subjects. Right hippocampal volume was similar across the three groups. More recently, we have found that repeated episodes of childhood sexual abuse were associated with marked reduction in gray matter volume of left primary and secondary visual cortex and that prolonged and intense history of parental verbal abuse was associated with gray matter volume reduction in left hemisphere auditory cortex (Navalta et al., in press).

Because childhood abuse appeared to be associated with altered left hemisphere development and diminished right/left hippocampal development, we examined the corpus callosum as the major fiber tract connecting the hemispheres. MRI scans were obtained from 51 child psychiatric patients. We found that there was a substantial reduction in the midsaggital area of the corpus callosum in psychiatrically ill children with a history of abuse or neglect and that males were more affected than females (Teicher et al. 1997a). In a more comprehensive study, De Bellis et al. (1999) found that the most significant difference in brain morphology between abused children with PTSD and healthy control subjects was a reduction in the midsagittal area of the corpus callosum and that males were again more affected than females. More recently, we reported that there was a substantial reduction in corpus callosum area in psychiatrically ill children with a history of abuse or neglect relative to healthy control subjects, that males were more affected by neglect than any other adverse experience, and that girls were more affected by exposure to sexual abuse (Teicher et al. 2004a). The likelihood that abnormal development of the corpus callosum was a consequence of adverse early experience is supported by a study by Sanchez et al. (1998), who found that there was a substantial reduction in midsagittal area of the corpus callosum of male rhesus monkeys that were raised in the more isolated confines of the laboratory environment than in the richer and more attentive seminatural environment afforded by a colony.

Other studies suggest that developmental stage is a crucial factor in determining both the outcome and manifestation of abuse. As noted previously, four studies demonstrated an association between history of childhood abuse and reduced hippocampal volume in adults with a variety of psychiatric disorders. In contrast, at least three studies have failed to find an association between childhood abuse and hippocampal volume in children and adolescents with PTSD (Carrion et al. 2001; De Bellis et al. 1999, 2002). Myriad hypotheses can be put forth to explain why exposure to childhood abuse appears to be associated with reduced hippocampal volume in adulthood but normal hippocampal volume in childhood. We hypothesized that early abuse might exert an effect on brain development that only emerges at a much later stage of brain maturation. To test this hypothesis, we conducted a preclinical investigation of the time course of effect of early stress on hippocampal development (Andersen and Teicher 2004). Briefly, developing rats were subject to early stress and were sacrificed during different stages of development. We found that there was no significant difference in hippocampal synaptic density prior to or during puberty but that a robust difference emerged by early adulthood and persisted thereafter (Andersen and Teicher 2004). We further confirmed that a reduction in hippocampal volume could be observed in young women with a history of childhood sexual abuse by the time they were 18–22 years of age.

We have also begun to examine the effects of early abuse from a sensitive period perspective. Repeated episodes of childhood sexual abuse were associated, in the same group of subjects, with reduced hippocampal volume if the abuse was reported to occur between 3–5 years of age, but with reduced corpus callosal area if the abuse occurred between 9–10 years of age, and with reduced frontal cortex gray matter volume if it occurred during adolescence (Teicher 2005). This finding suggests that there may be distinctly different neuropsychological and neuropsychiatric sequelae of early abuse, depending in part on the age or developmental stage when the insult occurred.

The impact of adverse childhood experience is also strongly influenced by genetic factors. Caspi et al. (2002) found that polymorphisms in the gene associated with expression of MAO-A (which catabolizes monoaminergic neurotransmitters) played a pivotal role in determining whether childhood abuse led to the emergence of aggressive and antisocial behaviors. They also found that polymorphisms in the serotonin transporter played an important role in the association between early stress or loss and the development of depression (Caspi et al. 2003).

These studies provide evidence that early experience is a powerful chisel that shapes the developing brain in enduring ways that can lead to the emergence of neuropsychiatric disorders (Teicher 2002). The impact, however, depends on genetic susceptibility, timing of the exposure, age of the subject, and occurrence of subsequent events that may augment or attenuate the consequences of early stress.

Highlights for the Clinician

Synaptic pruning and brain development

✦ Axons, dendrites, synapses, and receptors in many brain regions are overproduced during childhood and scaled back ("pruned") during the transition from puberty to adulthood.

✦ In synaptic pruning, high synaptic density, facilitating *acquisition of new knowledge and skills*, may be partially traded for a lower-density system designed for *rapid analysis and enhanced performance* through utilization of established connections (Teicher et al. 1995). This process may represent an important developmental stage.

✦ Overproduction and pruning of dopamine receptors (more extensive in males than in females) may account for the *waxing and waning of symptom severity* in ADHD and Tourette syndrome.

Highlights for the Clinician *(continued)*

Sensitive and critical periods for brain development

✦ Brain development is sculpted by experience, but timing is crucial.

✦ Specific stages exist in which experience may maximally affect development (*sensitive period*) or must be present (*critical period*) for the formation of appropriate connections.

✦ *Environmental enrichment* during sensitive periods may provide a means of altering brain development to compensate for deficiencies.

Attention-deficit/hyperactivity disorder (ADHD)

✦ ADHD is characterized by age-inappropriate problems with attention, impulse control, and hyperactivity.

✦ ADHD commonly occurs in conjunction with conduct disorder, learning disorders, and mood disorders (Biederman et al. 2006; Spencer et al. 1999).

✦ ADHD is highly heritable, but no single gene has been found to have more than a modest influence.

✦ The major brain regions affected by ADHD include prefrontal and orbital cortex, striatum (caudate and putamen), and cerebellar vermis.

✦ Primary medication treatment options for ADHD include psychostimulants and atomoxetine.

✦ Stimulants are still the mainstay of treatment but can be combined with behavioral treatment when parenting issues arise or when co-occurring disorders are present.

Tics and Tourette syndrome (TS)

✦ Tics are stereotyped, brief, repetitive, purposeless, nonrhythmic motor and vocal responses.

✦ Tics can be simple or complex, and they can be chronic or transient.

✦ Simple motor tics include jerking movements, shrugging, and eye blinking. Simple vocal tics include grunting, sniffing, and throat clearing.

✦ More complex motor tics involve grimacing, banging, or temper tantrums.

✦ Tourette syndrome is diagnosed when both chronic motor and vocal tics are present.

✦ The modal age at onset of TS is 6–7 years. Tic symptoms are generally most severe during the period preceding puberty and gradually improve thereafter, except in the most severe cases.

✦ Although TS is clearly a brain-based disorder, the condition can be exacerbated by stress and anxiety and can be a severely stigmatizing illness.

✦ The basal ganglia and related thalamocortical circuitry have been implicated in the underlying pathophysiology of TS.

✦ Primary medication treatment options for tics include typical and atypical neuroleptics.

✦ Habit reversal therapy can help control the frequency of tics, and both this type of behavior therapy and supportive psychotherapy can improve quality of life (Deckersbach et al. 2006).

Mental retardation

✦ Mental retardation is diagnosed when an individual <18 years of age presents with an intelligence score of ≤70 and concurrent deficits in adaptive functioning (American Psychiatric Association 2000).

✦ Individuals with only mild deficits make up the vast majority of all cases (90%).

✦ Hundreds of genetic syndromes are known to be associated with mental retardation (Opitz 2000). The major ones are Down syndrome, fragile X syndrome, various forms of X-linked mental retardation, subtelomeric defects, Prader-Willi syndrome, and Angelman's syndrome.

Highlights for the Clinician (*continued*)

◆ Available treatments include special education for children and adolescents, residential services for adults, and newer atypical antipsychotics (such as risperidone) for severe behavior problems.

Autism and pervasive developmental disorders

◆ Autism is characterized by severe disturbances in social recognition and interaction, impaired communication, and a restricted, stereotypic behavioral repertoire and range of interests.

◆ Other pervasive developmental disorders share these characteristics, including Rett's disorder, childhood disintegrative disorder, Asperger's disorder, and pervasive developmental disorder not otherwise specified

◆ Stereotypies, which can involve the flicking, twirling, or spinning of objects, or hand flapping, whirling, and posturing, may diminish with maturation.

◆ Restricted and repetitive behaviors, as well as impaired communication and social deficits, continue into adulthood (Seltzer et al. 2004).

◆ Premature cessation of development in the cerebellum, cerebrum, and limbic system may be the neuroanatomical process by which autism results.

◆ Pharmacotherapy for autism has had mixed results, but appearance of target symptoms such as hyperactivity, irritability, depression, and obsessive-compulsive behaviors may warrant a therapeutic trial (Campbell et al. 1996).

◆ Primary medication treatment options include neuroleptics, atypical antipsychotics, and antidepressants.

◆ Nonpharmacological treatments include extremely intensive behavioral treatment initiated during preschool, designed to increase skills in the areas of attention, emotionality, language, toy play, peer interaction, and self-help while reducing tantrums, aggression, and self-stimulation (Lovaas and Smith 1989).

◆ Long-term interventions focus on community-based special educational programs and subsequent residential services for those who cannot be cared for at home.

Learning disorders

◆ Learning disorders are specific deficits in the acquisition and performance of the academic skills of reading, writing, or arithmetic skills in the presence of normal intelligence and aptitude.

◆ Heritability across learning disorders is quite high (e.g., 91% concordance rate for monozygotic twins with a reading disorder).

◆ Imaging studies reveal evidence for diminished anatomical and functional lateralization in reading disorders.

◆ Mandated special education, provided in the least restrictive environment, is the current treatment for children with learning disorders.

◆ Empirically based interventions that target certain aspects of speech (e.g., phonology) have shown promise in remediating reading and language deficits.

◆ No evidence supports the efficacy of medications, diet alterations, or vitamin supplementation to treat learning disorders.

Seizure disorders

◆ Seizures are classified according to whether the initial locus of activity is bilateral and subcortical (generalized seizures) or unilateral and cortical (partial seizures).

◆ The primary types of generalized seizures are tonic-clonic, absence, myoclonic, and infantile spasms.

Highlights for the Clinician *(continued)*

- ✦ The major types of partial seizures are simple seizures, complex partial seizures, and partial seizures secondarily generalized.

- ✦ Seizure etiologies can be divided into genetic and acquired brain lesions. The latter may be focal, multifocal, or diffuse.

- ✦ Specific epilepsy syndromes with a predominantly genetic basis (e.g., Lennox-Gastaut syndrome) can emerge in infancy or childhood (Blume 2004).

- ✦ An association exists between childhood epilepsy and behavioral, academic, and cognitive problems (Dunn and Austin 1999; Metz-Lutz et al. 1999), although such problems may or may not actually occur.

- ✦ Emotional disorders (i.e., depression and anxiety) as well as suicidality can be co-occurring conditions with epilepsy.

- ✦ Anticonvulsants can modify the balance between neuronal excitation and inhibition via their influence on cerebral transmitter systems and/or ion channel activities.

- ✦ Newer adjunctive agents can potentiate anticonvulsant efficacy with little increase in side effects.

Traumatic brain injury

- ✦ The leading cause of disability in children between birth and 19 years of age is injury.

- ✦ Traumatic brain injury affects intelligence, fine motor skills, sensorimotor function, problem-solving ability, memory, adaptive function, attention, and language processing (Michaud et al. 1993).

- ✦ By 3 months after injury, some psychiatric sequelae become apparent.

- ✦ Posttraumatic psychiatric disorders include organic personality syndrome, mood disorders, anxiety disorders, disruptive behavior disorders, adjustment disorders, and substance use disorders.

- ✦ Psychosocial intervention and family support can be helpful during the first 2 years after injury (Kinsella et al. 1999).

Pediatric autoimmune neuropsychiatric disorders (PANDAS)

- ✦ In this recently described clinical syndrome, obsessive-compulsive disorder or tic disorders emerge in the context of group A β-hemolytic streptococcal infection (Snider and Swedo 2004).

- ✦ Plasma exchange therapy and intravenous immunoglobulin treatment have produced mixed results.

- ✦ Antibiotic prophylaxis using azithromycin and penicillin have produced some promising results (Snider et al. 2005).

Trauma, brain development, and psychiatric disorders

- ✦ Physical, sexual, or emotional traumatization during childhood can contribute to the development of a spectrum of psychiatric disorders (Teicher et al. 2006).

- ✦ Such disorders include dissociative identity disorder, psychosis, borderline personality disorder, depression, bipolar disorder, and posttraumatic stress disorder.

- ✦ Converging evidence from imaging, electrophysiological, neuropsychological, and preclinical studies indicates that early traumatic stress detrimentally affects the development of the cerebral cortex, corpus callosum, and limbic system.

- ✦ These effects may depend, in part, on the age or developmental stage when the insult occurred as well as genetic factors.

RECOMMENDED READINGS

American Psychiatric Association: Diagnostic and Statistical Manual of Mental Disorders, 4th Edition, Text Revision. Washington, DC, American Psychiatric Association, 2000

Biederman J, Monuteaux MC, Mick E, et al: Psychopathology in females with attention-deficit/hyperactivity disorder: a controlled, five-year prospective study. Biol Psychiatry 60:1098–1105, 2006

Blume WT: Lennox-Gastaut syndrome: potential mechanisms of cognitive regression. Ment Retard Dev Disabil Res Rev 10:150–153, 2004

Campbell M, Schopler E, Cueva JE, et al: Treatment of autistic disorder. J Am Acad Child Adolesc Psychiatry 35:134–143, 1996

Deckersbach T, Rauch S, Buhlmann U, et al: Habit reversal versus supportive psychotherapy in Tourette's disorder: a randomized controlled trial and predictors of treatment response. Behav Res Ther 44:1079–1090, 2006

Dunn DW, Austin JK: Behavioral issues in pediatric epilepsy. Neurology 53 (5 suppl 2):S96–S100, 1999

Kinsella G, Ong B, Murtagh D, et al: The role of the family for behavioral outcome in children and adolescents following traumatic brain injury. J Consult Clin Psychol 67:116–123, 1999

Lovaas OI, Smith T: A comprehensive behavioral theory of autistic children: paradigm for research and treatment. J Behav Ther Exp Psychiatry 20:17–29, 1989

Metz-Lutz MN, Kleitz C, de Saint Martin A, et al: Cognitive development in benign focal epilepsies of childhood. Dev Neurosci 21:182–190, 1999

Michaud LJ, Duhaime AC, Batshaw ML: Traumatic brain injury in children. Pediatr Clin North Am 40:553–565, 1993

Opitz JM: Vision and insight in the search for gene mutations causing nonsyndromal mental deficiency. Neurology 55:328–330, 2000

Seltzer MM, Shattuck P, Abbeduto L, et al: Trajectory of development in adolescents and adults with autism. Ment Retard Dev Disabil Res Rev 10:234–247, 2004

Snider LA, Swedo SE: PANDAS: current status and directions for research. Mol Psychiatry 9:900–907, 2004

Spencer T, Biederman J, Wilens T: Attention-deficit/hyperactivity disorder and comorbidity. Pediatr Clin North Am 46:915–927, 1999

Teicher MH, Andersen SL, Hostetter JC Jr: Evidence for dopamine receptor pruning between adolescence and adulthood in striatum but not nucleus accumbens. Brain Res Dev Brain Res 89:167–172, 1995

Teicher MH, Samson JA, Polcari A, et al: Sticks, stones, and hurtful words: relative effects of various forms of childhood maltreatment. Am J Psychiatry 163:993–1000, 2006

REFERENCES

Abromowicz ME: Sudden death in children treated with a tricyclic antidepressant. Med Lett Drugs Ther 32:53, 1990

Ackerman PT, McPherson WB, Oglesby DM, et al: EEG power spectra of adolescent poor readers. J Learn Disabil 31:83–90, 1998

Akefeldt A, Gillberg C: Behavior and personality characteristics of children and young adults with Prader-Willi syndrome: a controlled study. J Am Acad Child Adolesc Psychiatry 38:761–769, 1999

Akefeldt A, Ekman R, Gillberg C, et al: Cerebrospinal fluid monoamines in Prader-Willi syndrome. Biol Psychiatry 44:1321–1328, 1998

Aldenkamp AP: Cognitive and behavioural assessment in clinical trials: when should they be done? Epilepsy Res 45:155–161, 2001a

Aldenkamp AP: Effects of antiepileptic drugs on cognition. Epilepsia 42 (suppl 1):46–49, discussion 50–51, 2001b

Aldenkamp AP, Weber B, Overweg-Plandsoen WC: Educational underachievement in children with epilepsy: a model to predict the effects of epilepsy on educational achievement. J Child Neurol 20:175–180, 2005

Allen AJ, Kurlan RM, Gilbert DL, et al: Atomoxetine treatment in children and adolescents with ADHD and comorbid tic disorders. Neurology 65:1941–1949, 2005

Alper K, Devinsky O, Perrine K, et al: Nonepileptic seizures and childhood sexual and physical abuse. Neurology 43:1950–1953, 1993

Amaral DG: The primate amygdala and the neurobiology of social behavior: implications for understanding social anxiety. Biol Psychiatry 51:11–17, 2002

American Academy of Child and Adolescent Psychiatry: Summary of the practice parameters for the assessment and treatment of children and adolescents with language and learning disorders. J Am Acad Child Adolesc Psychiatry 37:1117–1119, 1998

American Psychiatric Association: Diagnostic and Statistical Manual for Mental Disorders, 3rd Edition. Washington, DC, American Psychiatric Association, 1980

American Psychiatric Association: Diagnostic and Statistical Manual of Mental Disorders, 3rd Edition, Revised. Washington, DC, American Psychiatric Association, 1987

American Psychiatric Association: Diagnostic and Statistical Manual of Mental Disorders, 4th Edition. Washington, DC, American Psychiatric Association, 1994

American Psychiatric Association: Diagnostic and Statistical Manual of Mental Disorders, 4th Edition, Text Revision. Washington, DC, American Psychiatric Association, 2000

Amir RE, Van den Veyver IB, Wan M, et al: Rett syndrome is caused by mutations in X-linked MECP2, encoding methyl-CpG-binding protein 2. Nat Genet 23:185–188, 1999

Andersen SL: Stimulants and the developing brain. Trends Pharmacol Sci 26:237–243, 2005

Andersen SL, Teicher MH: Sex differences in dopamine receptors and their relevance to ADHD. Neurosci Biobehav Rev 24:137–141, 2000

Andersen SL, Teicher MH: Delayed effects of early stress on hippocampal development. Neuropsychopharmacology 29:1988–1993, 2004

Andersen SL, Rutstein M, Benzo JM, et al: Sex differences in dopamine receptor overproduction and elimination. Neuroreport 8:1495–1498, 1997

Andersen SL, Thompson AT, Rutstein M, et al: Dopamine receptor pruning in prefrontal cortex during the periadolescent period in rats. Synapse 37:167–169, 2000

Andersen SL, Arvanitogiannis A, Pliakas AM, et al: Altered responsiveness to cocaine in rats exposed to methylphenidate during development. Nat Neurosci 5:13–14, 2002

Anderson CM, Polcari AM, McGreenery CE, et al: Cerebellar vermis blood flow: associations with psychiatric symptoms in child abuse and ADHD. Abstr Soc Neurosci 25:1637, 1999

Anderson GM, Pollak ES, Chatterjee D, et al: Postmortem analysis of subcortical monoamines and amino acids in Tourette syndrome. Adv Neurol 58:123–133, 1992

Anderson JC, Williams S, McGee R: DSM-III disorders in preadolescent children: prevalence in a large sample from the general population. Arch Gen Psychiatry 44:69–76, 1987

Anderson VR, Scott LJ: Methylphenidate transdermal system in attention-deficit hyperactivity disorder in children. Drugs 66:1117–1126, 2006

Andreasen NC, O'Leary DS, Cizadlo T, et al: Schizophrenia and cognitive dysmetria: a positron-emission tomography study of dysfunctional prefrontal-thalamic-cerebellar circuitry. Proc Natl Acad Sci U S A 93:9985–9990, 1996

Andriola MR, Ettinger AB: Pseudoseizures and other nonepileptic paroxysmal disorders in children and adolescents. Neurology 53(suppl):S89–S95, 1999

Ariano MA, Wang J, Noblett KL, et al: Cellular distribution of the rat D_{1B} receptor in central nervous system using anti-receptor antisera. Brain Res 746:141–150, 1997a

Ariano MA, Wang J, Noblett KL, et al: Cellular distribution of the rat D_4 dopamine receptor protein in the CNS using anti-receptor antisera. Brain Res 752:26–34, 1997b

Armstrong DD, Dunn K, Antalffy B: Decreased dendritic branching in frontal, motor and limbic cortex in Rett syndrome compared with trisomy 21. J Neuropathol Exp Neurol 57:1013–1017, 1998

Arnsten AF, Steere JC, Hunt RD: The contribution of alpha 2-noradrenergic mechanisms of prefrontal cortical cognitive function: potential significance for attention-deficit hyperactivity disorder. Arch Gen Psychiatry 53:448–455, 1996

Asano E, Benedek K, Shah A, et al: Is intraoperative electrocorticography reliable in children with intractable neocortical epilepsy? Epilepsia 45:1091–1099, 2004

Asarnow RF, Satz P, Light R, et al: Behavior problems and adaptive functioning in children with mild and severe closed head injury. J Pediatr Psychol 16:543–555, 1991

Asghari V, Sanyal S, Buchwaldt S, et al: Modulation of intracellular cyclic AMP levels by different human dopamine D_4 receptor variants. J Neurochem 65:1157–1165, 1995

Aston-Jones G, Bloom FE: Norepinephrine-containing locus coeruleus neurons in behaving rats exhibit pronounced responses to non-noxious environmental stimuli. J Neurosci 1:887–900, 1981

August GJ, Stewart MA, Tsai L: The incidence of cognitive disabilities in the siblings of autistic children. Br J Psychiatry 138:416–422, 1981

August GJ, Stewart MA, Holmes CS: A four-year follow-up of hyperactive boys with and without conduct disorder. Br J Psychiatry 143:192–198, 1983

Austin JK, Harezlak J, Dunn DW, et al: Behavior problems in children before first recognized seizures. Pediatrics 107:115–122, 2001

Backes W, Vuurman E, Wennekes R, et al: Atypical brain activation of reading processes in children with developmental dyslexia. J Child Neurol 17:867–871, 2002

Bailey A, Le Couteur A, Gottesman I, et al: Autism as a strongly genetic disorder: evidence from a British twin study. Psychol Med 25:63–77, 1995

Bailey A, Luthert P, Dean A, et al: A clinicopathological study of autism. Brain 121 (pt 5):889–905, 1998

Barkley RA: Defiant children: a clinician's manual for parent training. New York, Guilford, 1987

Barkley RA: A critique of current diagnostic criteria for attention deficit hyperactivity disorder: clinical and research implications. J Dev Behav Pediatr 11:343–352, 1990

Barkley RA, Guevremont DC, Anastopoulos AD, et al: A comparison of three family therapy programs for treating family conflicts in adolescents with attention-deficit hyperactivity disorder. J Consult Clin Psychol 60:450–462, 1992

Barkley RA, Fischer M, Smallish L, et al: Young adult outcome of hyperactive children: adaptive functioning in major life activities. J Am Acad Child Adolesc Psychiatry 45:192–202, 2006

Barks JD, Silverstein FS, Sims K, et al: Glutamate recognition sites in human fetal brain. Neurosci Lett 84:131–136, 1988

Baron-Cohen S: The autistic child's theory of mind: a case of specific developmental delay. J Child Psychol Psychiatry 30:285–297, 1989

Barr CL, Wigg KG, Zovko E, et al: No evidence for a major gene effect of the dopamine D_4 receptor gene in the susceptibility to Gilles de la Tourette syndrome in five Canadian families. Am J Med Genet 67:301–305, 1996

Barr CL, Wigg KG, Zovko E, et al: Linkage study of the dopamine D_5 receptor gene and Gilles de la Tourette syndrome. Am J Med Genet 74:58–61, 1997

Barr CL, Kroft J, Feng Y, et al: The norepinephrine transporter gene and attention-deficit hyperactivity disorder. Am J Med Genet 114:255–259, 2002

Barraclough BM: The suicide rate of epilepsy. Acta Psychiatr Scand 76:339–345, 1987

Barrickman L, Noyes R, Kuperman S, et al: Treatment of ADHD with fluoxetine: a preliminary trial. J Am Acad Child Adolesc Psychiatry 30:762–767, 1991

Barrickman LL, Perry PJ, Allen AJ, et al: Bupropion versus methylphenidate in the treatment of attention-deficit hyperactivity disorder. J Am Acad Child Adolesc Psychiatry 34:649–657, 1995

Bast T, Oezkan O, Rona S, et al: EEG and MEG source analysis of single and averaged interictal spikes reveals intrinsic epileptogenicity in focal cortical dysplasia. Epilepsia 45:621–631, 2004

Bauman ML: Microscopic neuroanatomic abnormalities in autism. Pediatrics 87:791–796, 1991

Bauman ML, Kemper TL: Histoanatomic observations of the brain in early infantile autism. Neurology 35:866–874, 1985

Bauman ML, Kemper TL: Neuroanatomic observations of the brain in autism: a review and future directions. Int J Dev Neurosci 23:183–187, 2005

Bauman ML, Kemper TL, Arin DM: Pervasive neuroanatomic abnormalities of the brain in three cases of Rett's syndrome. Neurology 45:1581–1586, 1995

Baxter LR Jr: Neuroimaging studies of obsessive compulsive disorder. Psychiatr Clin North Am 15:871–884, 1992

Baxter MG, Murray EA: The amygdala and reward. Nat Rev Neurosci 3:563–573, 2002

Bear DM, Fedio P: Quantitative analysis of interictal behavior in temporal lobe epilepsy. Arch Neurol 34:454–467, 1977

Beck JC, van der Kolk B: Reports of childhood incest and current behavior of chronically hospitalized psychotic women. Am J Psychiatry 144:1474–1476, 1987

Beers SR: Cognitive effects of mild head injury in children and adolescents. Neuropsychol Rev 3:281–320, 1992

Belmonte M, Egaas B, Townsend J, et al: NMR intensity of corpus callosum differs with age but not with diagnosis of autism. Neuroreport 6:1253–1256, 1995

Benasich AA, Curtiss S, Tallal P: Language, learning, and behavioral disturbances in childhood: a longitudinal perspective. J Am Acad Child Adolesc Psychiatry 32:585–594, 1993

Beran RG, Gibson RJ: Aggressive behaviour in intellectually challenged patients with epilepsy treated with lamotrigine. Epilepsia 39:280–282, 1998

Berardi N, Pizzorusso T, Maffei L: Critical periods during sensory development. Curr Opin Neurobiol 10:138–145, 2000

Berquin PC, Giedd JN, Jacobsen LK, et al: Cerebellum in attention-deficit hyperactivity disorder: a morphometric MRI study. Neurology 50:1087–1093, 1998

Besag FM: Behavioural effects of the new anticonvulsants. Drug Saf 24:513–536, 2001

Besag FM: Behavioural effects of the newer antiepileptic drugs: an update. Expert Opin Drug Saf 3:1–8, 2004

Betts T, Boden S: Diagnosis, management and prognosis of a group of 128 patients with non-epileptic attack disorder, part II: previous childhood sexual abuse in the aetiology of these disorders. Seizure 1:27–32, 1992

Biederman J, Spencer T: Attention-deficit/hyperactivity disorder (ADHD) as a noradrenergic disorder. Biol Psychiatry 46:1234–1242, 1999

Biederman J, Spencer T: Non-stimulant treatments for ADHD. Eur Child Adolesc Psychiatry 9 (suppl 1):I51–I59, 2000

Biederman J, Baldessarini RJ, Wright V, et al: A double-blind placebo controlled study of desipramine in the treatment of ADD, I: efficacy. J Am Acad Child Adolesc Psychiatry 28:777–784, 1989

Biederman J, Faraone SV, Spencer J: Gender differences in a sample of adults with attention deficit hyperactivity disorder. Psychiatry Res 53:13–29, 1994

Biederman J, Wilens T, Mick E, et al: Pharmacotherapy of attention-deficit/hyperactivity disorder reduces risk for substance use disorder. Pediatrics 104:E20, 1999

Biederman J, Swanson JM, Wigal SB, et al: Efficacy and safety of modafinil film-coated tablets in children and adolescents with attention-deficit/hyperactivity disorder: results of a randomized, double-blind, placebo-controlled, flexible-dose study. Pediatrics 116:E777–E784, 2005

Biederman J, Monuteaux MC, Mick E, et al: Psychopathology in females with attention-deficit/hyperactivity disorder: a controlled, five-year prospective study. Biol Psychiatry 60:1098–1105, 2006

Bird HR, Canino G, Rubio-Stipec M: Estimates of the prevalence of childhood maladjustment in a community survey in Puerto Rico. Arch Gen Psychiatry 45:1120–1126, 1988

Black KJ, Webb H: Tourette syndrome and other tic disorders. eMedicine Journal, 2006. Available at: http://www.emedicine.com/neuro/topic664.htm. Accessed November 9, 2006

Blanton RE, Levitt JG, Thompson PM, et al: Mapping cortical asymmetry and complexity patterns in normal children. Psychiatry Res 107:29–43, 2001

Blue ME, Naidu S, Johnston MV: Altered development of glutamate and GABA receptors in the basal ganglia of girls with Rett syndrome. Exp Neurol 156:345–352, 1999a

Blue ME, Naidu S, Johnston MV: Development of amino acid receptors in frontal cortex from girls with Rett syndrome. Ann Neurol 45:541–545, 1999b

Blume WT: Lennox-Gastaut syndrome: potential mechanisms of cognitive regression. Ment Retard Dev Disabil Res Rev 10:150–153, 2004

Bobb AJ, Castellanos FX, Addington AM, et al: Molecular genetic studies of ADHD: 1991 to 2004. Am J Med Genet B Neuropsychiatr Genet 132:109–125, 2005

Bodfish JW: Treating the core features of autism: are we there yet? Ment Retard Dev Disabil Res Rev 10:318–326, 2004

Bolton P, Rutter M: Genetic influences in autism. Int Rev Psychiatry 2:67–80, 1990

Bonilha L, Rorden C, Castellano G, et al: Voxel-based morphometry reveals gray matter network atrophy in refractory medial temporal lobe epilepsy. Arch Neurol 61:1379–1384, 2004

Boonstra AM, Oosterlaan J, Sergeant JA, et al: Executive functioning in adult ADHD: a meta-analytic review. Psychol Med 35:1097–1108, 2005

Booth JR, Burman DD, Van Santen FW, et al: The development of specialized brain systems in reading and oral-language. Child Neuropsychol 7:119–141, 2001

Bouvard MP, Leboyer M, Launay JM, et al: Low-dose naltrexone effects on plasma chemistries and clinical symptoms in autism: a double-blind, placebo-controlled study. Psychiatry Res 58:191–201, 1995

Braun AR, Stoetter B, Randolph C, et al: The functional neuroanatomy of Tourette's syndrome: an FDG-PET study, I: regional changes in cerebral glucose metabolism differentiating patients and controls. Neuropsychopharmacology 9:277–291, 1993

Breese GR, Cooper BR, Hollister AS: Involvement of brain monoamines in the stimulant and paradoxical inhibitory effects of methylphenidate. Psychopharmacologia 44:5–10, 1975

Bremner JD, Southwick SM, Johnson DR, et al: Childhood physical abuse and combat-related posttraumatic stress disorder in Vietnam veterans. Am J Psychiatry 150:235–239, 1993

Bremner JD, Randall P, Vermetten E, et al: Magnetic resonance imaging-based measurement of hippocampal volume in posttraumatic stress disorder related to childhood physical and sexual abuse: a preliminary report. Biol Psychiatry 41:23–32, 1997

Brent DA, Crumrine PK, Varma RR, et al: Phenobarbital treatment and major depressive disorder in children with epilepsy. Pediatrics 80:909–917, 1987

Brett PM, Curtis D, Robertson MM, et al: Exclusion of the 5-HT1A serotonin neuroreceptor and tryptophan oxygenase genes in a large British kindred multiply affected with Tourette's syndrome, chronic motor tics, and obsessive-compulsive behavior. Am J Psychiatry 152:437–440, 1995a

Brett PM, Curtis D, Robertson MM, et al: The genetic susceptibility to Gilles de la Tourette syndrome in a large multiple affected British kindred: linkage analysis excludes a role for the genes coding for dopamine D_1, D_2, D_3, D_4, D_5 receptors, dopamine beta hydroxylase, tyrosinase, and tyrosine hydroxylase. Biol Psychiatry 37:533–540, 1995b

Brodie MJ, Richens A, Yuen AW: Double-blind comparison of lamotrigine and carbamazepine in newly diagnosed epilepsy: UK Lamotrigine/Carbamazepine Monotherapy Trial Group. Lancet 345:476–479, 1995

Brons J, Robertson LT, Tong G: Somatosensory climbing fiber responses in the caudal posterior vermis of the cat cerebellum. Brain Res 519:243–248, 1990

Brown GL, Ebert MH, Mikkelsen EJ, et al: Behavior and motor activity response in hyperactive children and plasma amphetamine levels following a sustained release preparation. J Am Acad Child Psychiatry 19:225–239, 1980

Brown GL, Chadwick O, Shaffer D, et al: A prospective study of children with head injuries, III: psychiatric sequelae. Psychol Med 11:63–78, 1981

Bruun RD: Subtle and underrecognized side effects of neuroleptic treatment in children with Tourette's disorder. Am J Psychiatry 145:621–624, 1988

Bryden MP, McManus IC, Bulman-Fleming MB: Evaluating the empirical support for the Geschwind-Behan-Galaburda model of cerebral lateralization. Brain Cogn 26:103–167, 1994

Budman CL, Bruun RD, Park KS, et al: Rage attacks in children and adolescents with Tourette's disorder: a pilot study. J Clin Psychiatry 59:576–580, 1998

Bulman-Fleming B, Wainwright PE, Collins RL: The effects of early experience on callosal development and functional lateralization in pigmented BALB/c mice. Behav Brain Res 50:31–42, 1992

Bush G, Frazier JA, Rauch SL, et al: Anterior cingulate cortex dysfunction in attention-deficit/hyperactivity disorder revealed by fMRI and the Counting Stroop. Biol Psychiatry 45:1542–1552, 1999

Buxbaum JD, Silverman JM, Smith CJ, et al: Association between a GABRB3 polymorphism and autism. Mol Psychiatry 7:311–316, 2002

Bymaster FP, Katner JS, Nelson DL, et al: Atomoxetine increases extracellular levels of norepinephrine and dopamine in prefrontal cortex of rat: a potential mechanism for efficacy in attention deficit/hyperactivity disorder. Neuropsychopharmacology 27:699–711, 2002

Cabelli RJ, Hohn A, Shatz CJ: Inhibition of ocular dominance column formation by infusion of NT-4/5 or BDNF. Science 267:1662–1666, 1995

Caldji C, Diorio J, Meaney MJ: Variations in maternal care alter GABA(A) receptor subunit expression in brain regions associated with fear. Neuropsychopharmacology 28:1950–1959, 2003

Camp DM, Robinson TE, Becker JB: Sex differences in the effects of early experience on the development of behavioral and brain asymmetries in rats. Physiol Behav 33:433–439, 1984

Campbell M, Anderson LT, Small AM, et al: Naltrexone in autistic children: behavioral symptoms and attentional learning. J Am Acad Child Adolesc Psychiatry 32:1283–1291, 1993

Campbell M, Schopler E, Cueva JE, et al: Treatment of autistic disorder. J Am Acad Child Adolesc Psychiatry 35:134–143, 1996

Cardon LR, Smith SD, Fulker DW, et al: Quantitative trait locus for reading disability on chromosome 6. Science 266:276–279, 1994

Cardon LR, Smith SD, Fulker DW, et al: Quantitative trait locus for reading disability [correction]. Science 268:1553, 1995

Carper RA, Courchesne E: Inverse correlation between frontal lobe and cerebellum sizes in children with autism. Brain 123 (pt 4):836–844, 2000

Carrey N, MacMaster FP, Sparkes SJ, et al: Glutamatergic changes with treatment in attention deficit hyperactivity disorder: a preliminary case series. J Child Adolesc Psychopharmacol 12:331–336, 2002

Carrey N, MacMaster FP, Fogel J, et al: Metabolite changes resulting from treatment in children with ADHD: a ^{1}H-MRS study. Clin Neuropharmacol 26:218–221, 2003

Carrion VG, Weems CF, Eliez S, et al: Attenuation of frontal asymmetry in pediatric posttraumatic stress disorder. Biol Psychiatry 50:943–951, 2001

Casanova MF, Buxhoeveden DP, Switala AE, et al: Minicolumnar pathology in autism. Neurology 58:428–432, 2002

Casey BJ, Giedd JN, Thomas KM: Structural and functional brain development and its relation to cognitive development. Biol Psychol 54:241–257, 2000

Caspi A, McClay J, Moffitt TE, et al: Role of genotype in the cycle of violence in maltreated children. Science 297:851–854, 2002

Caspi A, Sugden K, Moffitt TE, et al: Influence of life stress on depression: moderation by a polymorphism in the 5-HTT gene. Science 301:386–389, 2003

Cassidy SB, Forsythe M, Heeger S, et al: Comparison of phenotype between patients with Prader-Willi syndrome due to deletion 15q and uniparental disomy 15. Am J Med Genet 68:433–440, 1997

Castellanos FX, Giedd JN, Marsh WL, et al: Quantitative brain magnetic resonance imaging in attention-deficit hyperactivity disorder. Arch Gen Psychiatry 53:607–616, 1996

Castellanos FX, Giedd JN, Elia J, et al: Controlled stimulant treatment of ADHD and comorbid Tourette's syndrome: effects of stimulant and dose. J Am Acad Child Adolesc Psychiatry 36:589–596, 1997

Castellanos FX, Lee PP, Sharp W, et al: Developmental trajectories of brain volume abnormalities in children and adolescents with attention-deficit/hyperactivity disorder. JAMA 288:1740–1748, 2002

Castellanos FX, Sharp WS, Gottesman RF, et al: Anatomic brain abnormalities in monozygotic twins discordant for attention deficit hyperactivity disorder. Am J Psychiatry 160:1693–1696, 2003

Chabot RJ, di Michele F, Prichep L: The role of quantitative electroencephalography in child and adolescent psychiatric disorders. Child Adolesc Psychiatr Clin N Am 14:21–53, 2005

Chandana SR, Behen ME, Juhasz C, et al: Significance of abnormalities in developmental trajectory and asymmetry of cortical serotonin synthesis in autism. Int J Dev Neurosci 23:171–182, 2005

Chappell P, Riddle M, Anderson G, et al: Enhanced stress responsivity of Tourette syndrome patients undergoing lumbar puncture. Biol Psychiatry 36:35–43, 1994

Chappell PB, Riddle MA, Scahill L, et al: Guanfacine treatment of comorbid attention-deficit hyperactivity disorder and Tourette's syndrome: preliminary clinical experience. J Am Acad Child Adolesc Psychiatry 34:1140–1146, 1995

Cheon KA, Ryu YH, Kim YK, et al: Dopamine transporter density in the basal ganglia assessed with [^{123}I]IPT SPET in children with attention deficit hyperactivity disorder. Eur J Nucl Med Mol Imaging 30:306–311, 2003

Chez MG, Buchanan CP, Bagan BT, et al: Secretin and autism: a two-part clinical investigation. J Autism Dev Disord 30:87–94, 2000

Chi J, Dooling E, Giles F: Left-right asymmetries of the temporal speech areas of the human fetus. Arch Neurol 34:346–348, 1972

Chudley AE, Knoll J, Gerrard JW, et al: Fragile (X) X-linked mental retardation, I: relationship between age and intelligence and the frequency of expression of fragile (X)(q28). Am J Med Genet 14:699–712, 1983

Chugani DC, Muzik O, Rothermel R, et al: Altered serotonin synthesis in the dentatothalamocortical pathway in autistic boys. Ann Neurol 42:666–669, 1997

Chugani DC, Muzik O, Behen M, et al: Developmental changes in brain serotonin synthesis capacity in autistic and nonautistic children. Ann Neurol 45:287–295, 1999

Church AJ, Dale RC, Lees AJ, et al: Tourette's syndrome: a cross sectional study to examine the PANDAS hypothesis. J Neurol Neurosurg Psychiatry 74:602–607, 2003

Ciaranello AL, Ciaranello RD: The neurobiology of infantile autism. Annu Rev Neurosci 18:101–128, 1995

Ciesielski KT, Harris RJ, Hart BL, et al: Cerebellar hypoplasia and frontal lobe cognitive deficits in disorders of early childhood. Neuropsychologia 35:643–655, 1997

Clayton-Smith J, Laan L: Angelman syndrome: a review of the clinical and genetic aspects. J Med Genet 40:87–95, 2003

Comings DE: Blood serotonin and tryptophan in Tourette syndrome. Am J Med Genet 36:418–430, 1990

Comings DE, Comings BG: A controlled study of Tourette syndrome, I: attention-deficit disorder, learning disorders, and school problems. Am J Hum Genet 41:701–741, 1987

Comings DE, Wu S, Chiu C, et al: Polygenic inheritance of Tourette syndrome, stuttering, attention deficit hyperactivity, conduct, and oppositional defiant disorder: the additive and subtractive effect of the three dopaminergic genes: *DRD2, D beta H*, and *DAT1*. Am J Med Genet 67:264–288, 1996

Comings DE, Gade-Andavolu R, Gonzalez N, et al: Comparison of the role of dopamine, serotonin, and noradrenaline genes in ADHD, ODD and conduct disorder: multivariate regression analysis of 20 genes. Clin Genet 57:178–196, 2000

Connor DF: Preschool attention deficit hyperactivity disorder: a review of prevalence, diagnosis, neurobiology, and stimulant treatment. J Dev Behav Pediatr 23(suppl):S1–S9, 2002

Connor DF, Fletcher KE, Swanson JM: A meta-analysis of clonidine for symptoms of attention-deficit hyperactivity disorder. J Am Acad Child Adolesc Psychiatry 38:1551–1559, 1999

Conroy J, Meally E, Kearney G, et al: Serotonin transporter gene and autism: a haplotype analysis in an Irish autistic population. Mol Psychiatry 9:587–593, 2004

Cook EH Jr: Genetics of autism. Child Adolesc Psychiatr Clin N Am 10:333–350, 2001

Cook EH Jr, Stein MA, Krasowski MD, et al: Association of attention-deficit disorder and the dopamine transporter gene. Am J Hum Genet 56:993–998, 1995

Cooper H, Nye B: Homework for students with learning disabilities: the implications of research for policy and practice. J Learn Disabil 27:470–479, 1994

Cope N, Harold D, Hill G, et al: Strong evidence that KIAA0319 on chromosome 6p is a susceptibility gene for developmental dyslexia. Am J Hum Genet 76:581–591, 2005

Coplan J, Souders MC, Mulberg AE, et al: Children with autistic spectrum disorders, II: parents are unable to distinguish secretin from placebo under double-blind conditions. Arch Dis Child 88:737–739, 2003

Cornwall A, Bawden HN: Reading disabilities and aggression: a critical review. J Learn Disabil 25:281–288, 1992

Cossette P, Liu L, Brisebois K, et al: Mutation of GABRA1 in an autosomal dominant form of juvenile myoclonic epilepsy. Nat Genet 31:184–189, 2002

Courchesne E: Neuroanatomic imaging in autism. Pediatrics 87:781–790, 1991

Courchesne E, Townsend J, Akshoomoff NA, et al: Impairment in shifting attention in autistic and cerebellar patients. Behav Neurosci 108:848–865, 1994

Courchesne E, Carper R, Akshoomoff N: Evidence of brain overgrowth in the first year of life in autism. JAMA 290:337–344, 2003

Courchesne E, Redcay E, Kennedy DP: The autistic brain: birth through adulthood. Curr Opin Neurol 17:489–496, 2004

Coutinho AM, Oliveira G, Morgadinho T, et al: Variants of the serotonin transporter gene (SLC6A4) significantly contribute to hyperserotonemia in autism. Mol Psychiatry 9:264–271, 2004

Cowan WM, Fawcett JW, O'Leary DD, et al: Regressive events in neurogenesis. Science 225:1258–1265, 1984

Cox A, Klein K, Charman T, et al: Autism spectrum disorders at 20 and 42 months of age: stability of clinical and ADI-R diagnosis. J Child Psychol Psychiatry 40:719–732, 1999

Critchley HD, Daly EM, Bullmore ET, et al: The functional neuroanatomy of social behaviour: changes in cerebral blood flow when people with autistic disorder process facial expressions. Brain 123 (pt 11):2203–2212, 2000

Cummings DD, Singer HS, Krieger M, et al: Neuropsychiatric effects of guanfacine in children with mild Tourette syndrome: a pilot study. Clin Neuropharmacol 25:325–332, 2002

Cunningham MG, Bhattacharyya S, Benes FM: Amygdalocortical sprouting continues into early adulthood: implications for the development of normal and abnormal function during adolescence. J Comp Neurol 453:116–130, 2002

Curran S, Mill J, Tahir E, et al: Association study of a dopamine transporter polymorphism and attention deficit hyperactivity disorder in UK and Turkish samples. Mol Psychiatry 6:425–428, 2001

Dahlgren SO, Gillberg C: Symptoms in the first two years of life: a preliminary population study of infantile autism. Eur Arch Psychiatry Neurol Sci 238:169–174, 1989

Dalby MA, Elbro C, Stodkilde-Jorgensen H: Temporal lobe asymmetry and dyslexia: an in vivo study using MRI. Brain Lang 62:51–69, 1998

Daly G, Hawi Z, Fitzgerald M, et al: Mapping susceptibility loci in attention deficit hyperactivity disorder: preferential transmission of parental alleles at DAT1, DBH and DRD5 to affected children. Mol Psychiatry 4:192–196, 1999

Davies RK: Incest: some neuropsychiatric findings. Int J Psychiatry Med 9:117–121, 1978-1979

Dawson G, Watling R: Interventions to facilitate auditory, visual, and motor integration in autism: a review of the evidence. J Autism Dev Disord 30:415–421, 2000

De Bellis MD, Keshavan MS, Clark DB, et al: Developmental traumatology, part II: brain development. Biol Psychiatry 45:1271–1284, 1999

De Bellis MD, Keshavan MS, Shifflett H, et al: Brain structures in pediatric maltreatment-related posttraumatic stress disorder: a sociodemographically matched study. Biol Psychiatry 52:1066–1078, 2002

De Giacomo A, Fombonne E: Parental recognition of developmental abnormalities in autism. Eur Child Adolesc Psychiatry 7:131–136, 1998

De Luca V, Muglia P, Jain U, et al: No evidence of linkage or association between the norepinephrine transporter (NET) gene MnlI polymorphism and adult ADHD. Am J Med Genet B Neuropsychiatr Genet 124:38–40, 2004

de Vries BB, Winter R, Schinzel A, et al: Telomeres: a diagnosis at the end of the chromosomes. J Med Genet 40:385–398, 2003

de Wet CJ, Mellers JD, Gardner WN, et al: Pseudoseizures and asthma. J Neurol Neurosurg Psychiatry 74:639–641, 2003

Deb S, Braganza J, Norton N, et al: APOE epsilon 4 influences the manifestation of Alzheimer's disease in adults with Down's syndrome. Br J Psychiatry 176:468–472, 2000

Deckersbach T, Rauch S, Buhlmann U, et al: Habit reversal versus supportive psychotherapy in Tourette's disorder: a randomized controlled trial and predictors of treatment response. Behav Res Ther 44:1079–1090, 2006

Deffenbacher KE, Kenyon JB, Hoover DM, et al: Refinement of the 6p21.3 quantitative trait locus influencing dyslexia: linkage and association analyses. Hum Genet 115:128–138, 2004

Delay J, Deniker P, Barande R: Le suicide des epileptiques. Encephale 46:401–436, 1957

Demb JB, Boynton GM, Best M, et al: Psychophysical evidence for a magnocellular pathway deficit in dyslexia. Vision Res 38:1555–1559, 1998ba

Demb JB, Boynton GM, Heeger DJ: Functional magnetic resonance imaging of early visual pathways in dyslexia. J Neurosci 18:6939–6951, 1998b

Dempsey CW, Richardson DE: Paleocerebellar stimulation induces in vivo release of endogenously synthesized [^{3}H]dopamine and [^{3}H]norepinephrine from rat caudal dorsomedial nucleus accumbens. Neuroscience 21:565–571, 1987

Denckla MB, Bemporad JR, MacKay MC: Tics following methylphenidate administration: a report of 20 cases. JAMA 235:1349–1351, 1976

Denenberg VH, Yutzey DA: Hemispheric laterality, behavioral asymmetry, and the effects of early experience in rats, in Cerebral Lateralization in Nonhuman Species. Edited by Glick SD. Orlando, FL, Academic Press, 1985, pp 109–133

Dennett ER, Hubbard JI: Noradrenaline excites neurons in the guinea pig cerebellar vermis in vitro. Brain Res Bull 21:245–249, 1988

Denoth F, Magherini PC, Pompeiano O, et al: Responses of Purkinje cells of the cerebellar vermis to neck and macular vestibular inputs. Pflugers Arch 381:87–98, 1979

Devinsky O, Gershengorn J, Brown E, et al: Frontal functions in juvenile myoclonic epilepsy. Neuropsychiatry Neuropsychol Behav Neurol 10:243–246, 1997

DeYoe EA, Van Essen DC: Concurrent processing streams in monkey visual cortex. Trends Neurosci 11:219–226, 1988

Diaz-Anzaldua A, Joober R, Riviere JB, et al: Tourette syndrome and dopaminergic genes: a family based association study in the French Canadian founder population. Mol Psychiatry 9:272–277, 2004

Doba N, Reis DJ: Changes in regional blood flow and cardiodynamics evoked by electrical stimulation of the fastigial nucleus in the cat and their similarity to orthostatic reflexes. J Physiol 227:729–747, 1972

Donaldson IM, Hawthorne ME: Coding of visual information by units in the cat cerebellar vermis. Exp Brain Res 34:27–48, 1979

Dougherty DD, Bonab AA, Spencer TJ, et al: Dopamine transporter density in patients with attention deficit hyperactivity disorder. Lancet 354:2132–2133, 1999

Doupe AJ, Kuhl PK: Birdsong and human speech: common themes and mechanisms. Annu Rev Neurosci 22:567–631, 1999

Dreifuss FE: Classification of epileptic seizures and the epilepsies. Pediatr Clin North Am 36:265–279, 1989

Driessen M, Herrmann J, Stahl K, et al: Magnetic resonance imaging volumes of the hippocampus and the amygdala in women with borderline personality disorder and early traumatization. Arch Gen Psychiatry 57:1115–1122, 2000

Dunn DW, Austin JK: Behavioral issues in pediatric epilepsy. Neurology 53 (5 suppl 2):S96–S100, 1999

Dunn DW, Austin JK, Harezlak J, et al: ADHD and epilepsy in childhood. Dev Med Child Neurol 45:50–54, 2003

Durston S, Casey BJ: What have we learned about cognitive development from neuroimaging? Neuropsychologia 44:2149–2157, 2006

Durston S, Tottenham NT, Thomas KM, et al: Differential patterns of striatal activation in young children with and without ADHD. Biol Psychiatry 53:871–878, 2003

Durston S, Hulshoff Pol HE, Schnack HG, et al: Magnetic resonance imaging of boys with attention-deficit/hyperactivity disorder and their unaffected siblings. J Am Acad Child Adolesc Psychiatry 43:332–340, 2004

Durston S, Fossella JA, Casey BJ, et al: Differential effects of DRD4 and DAT1 genotype on fronto-striatal gray matter volumes in a sample of subjects with attention deficit hyperactivity disorder, their unaffected siblings, and controls. Mol Psychiatry 10:678–685, 2005

Dykens EM, Cassidy SB, King BH: Maladaptive behavior differences in Prader-Willi syndrome due to paternal deletion versus maternal uniparental disomy. Am J Ment Retard 104:67–77, 1999

Eapen V, Pauls DL, Robertson MM: Evidence for autosomal dominant transmission in Tourette's syndrome: United Kingdom cohort study. Br J Psychiatry 162:593–596, 1993

Eccles JC, Sabah NH, Schmidt RF, et al: Significance of dual input to cat cerebellum via mossy and climbing fibres. J Physiol 218:90P–91P, 1971

Egaas B, Courchesne E, Saitoh O: Reduced size of corpus callosum in autism. Arch Neurol 52:794–801, 1995

Eggermont JJ, Ponton CW: Auditory-evoked potential studies of cortical maturation in normal hearing and implanted children: correlations with changes in structure and speech perception. Acta Otolaryngol 123:249–252, 2003

Eliez S, Blasey CM, Freund LS, et al: Brain anatomy, gender and IQ in children and adolescents with fragile X syndrome. Brain 124:1610–1618, 2001

Ernst M, Liebenauer L, Fitzgerald G, et al: Reduced brain metabolism in hyperactive girls. J Am Acad Child Adolesc Psychiatry 33:858–868, 1994

Ernst M, Zametkin AJ, Matochik JA, et al: DOPA decarboxylase activity in attention deficit hyperactivity disorder adults: a [fluorine-18]fluorodopa positron emission tomographic study. J Neurosci 18:5901–5907, 1998

Ernst M, Zametkin AJ, Jons PH, et al: High presynaptic dopaminergic activity in children with Tourette's disorder. J Am Acad Child Adolesc Psychiatry 38:86–94, 1999a

Ernst M, Zametkin AJ, Matochik JA, et al: High midbrain [^{18}F]DOPA accumulation in children with attention deficit hyperactivity disorder. Am J Psychiatry 156:1209–1215, 1999b

Ernst M, Pine DS, Hardin M: Triadic model of the neurobiology of motivated behavior in adolescence. Psychol Med 36:299–312, 2006

Ettinger AB, Weisbrot DM, Saracco J, et al: Positive and negative psychotropic effects of lamotrigine in patients with epilepsy and mental retardation. Epilepsia 39:874–877, 1998

Ewing-Cobbs L, Fletcher JM, Levin HS, et al: Academic achievement and academic placement following traumatic brain injury in children and adolescents: a two-year longitudinal study. J Clin Exp Neuropsychol 20:769–781, 1998

Exner C, Boucsein K, Lange C, et al: Neuropsychological performance in frontal lobe epilepsy. Seizure 11:20–32, 2002

Facoetti A, Paganoni P, Lorusso ML: The spatial distribution of visual attention in developmental dyslexia. Exp Brain Res 132:531–538, 2000

Fang P, Lev-Lehman E, Tsai TF, et al: The spectrum of mutations in UBE3A causing Angelman syndrome. Hum Mol Genet 8:129–135, 1999

Faraone SV: The scientific foundation for understanding attention-deficit/hyperactivity disorder as a valid psychiatric disorder. Eur Child Adolesc Psychiatry 14:1–10, 2005

Faraone SV, Biederman J: Is attention deficit hyperactivity disorder familial? Harv Rev Psychiatry 1:271–287, 1994

Faraone SV, Wilens T: Does stimulant treatment lead to substance use disorders? J Clin Psychiatry 64 (suppl 11):9–13, 2003

Faraone SV, Biederman J, Lehman BK, et al: Evidence for the independent familial transmission of attention deficit hyperactivity disorder and learning disabilities: results from a family genetic study. Am J Psychiatry 150:891–895, 1993

Faraone SV, Doyle AE, Mick E, et al: Meta-analysis of the association between the 7-repeat allele of the dopamine D(4) receptor gene and attention deficit hyperactivity disorder. Am J Psychiatry 158:1052–1057, 2001

Faraone SV, Biederman J, Mick E: The age-dependent decline of attention deficit hyperactivity disorder: a meta-analysis of follow-up studies. Psychol Med 36:159–165, 2006

Faravelli C, Webb T, Ambonetti A: Prevalence of traumatic early life events in 31 agoraphobic patients with panic attacks. Am J Psychiatry 142:1493–1494, 1985

Fastenau PS, Shen J, Dunn DW, et al: Neuropsychological predictors of academic underachievement in pediatric epilepsy: moderating roles of demographic, seizure, and psychosocial variables. Epilepsia 45:1261–1272, 2004

Feinberg I: Schizophrenia: caused by a fault in programmed synaptic elimination during adolescence? J Psychiatr Res 17:319–334, 1982-1983

Fergusson DM, Horwood LJ, Lynskey MT: Childhood sexual abuse and psychiatric disorder in young adulthood, II: psychiatric outcomes of childhood sexual abuse. J Am Acad Child Adolesc Psychiatry 35:1365–1374, 1996

Ferrera VP, Nealey TA, Maunsell JH: Mixed parvocellular and magnocellular geniculate signals in visual area V4. Nature 358:756–761, 1992

Filley CM: The Behavioral Neurology of White Matter. New York, Oxford University Press, 2001

Fish DR, Sawyers D, Allen PJ, et al: The effect of sleep on the dyskinetic movements of Parkinson's disease, Gilles de la Tourette syndrome, Huntington's disease, and torsion dystonia. Arch Neurol 48:210–214, 1991

Fitton A, Goa KL: Lamotrigine: an update of its pharmacology and therapeutic use in epilepsy. Drugs 50:691–713, 1995

Fombonne E: Is the prevalence of autism increasing? J Autism Dev Disord 26:673–676, 1996

Fombonne E: The epidemiology of autism: a review. Psychol Med 29:769–786, 1999

Fombonne E: Epidemiological surveys of autism and other pervasive developmental disorders: an update. J Autism Dev Disord 33:365–382, 2003

Fombonne E, Zakarian R, Bennett A, et al: Pervasive developmental disorders in Montreal, Quebec, Canada: prevalence and links with immunizations. Pediatrics 118:E139–E150, 2006

Foote SL, Aston-Jones G, Bloom FE: Impulse activity of locus coeruleus neurons in awake rats and monkeys is a function of sensory stimulation and arousal. Proc Natl Acad Sci U S A 77:3033–3037, 1980

Frankenberger W, Fronzaglio K: A review of states' criteria and procedures for identifying children with learning disabilities. J Learn Disabil 24:495–500, 1991

Frazier TW, Demaree HA, Youngstrom EA: Meta-analysis of intellectual and neuropsychological test performance in attention-deficit/hyperactivity disorder. Neuropsychology 18:543–555, 2004

Freeman BJ, Ritvo ER, Needleman R, et al: The stability of cognitive and linguistic parameters in autism: a five-year prospective study. J Am Acad Child Psychiatry 24:459–464, 1985

Freeman BJ, Rahbar B, Ritvo ER, et al: The stability of cognitive and behavioral parameters in autism: a twelve-year prospective study. J Am Acad Child Adolesc Psychiatry 30:479–482, 1991

Freund LS, Reiss AL, Hagerman R, et al: Chromosome fragility and psychopathology in obligate female carriers of the fragile X chromosome. Arch Gen Psychiatry 49:54–60, 1992

Gade R, Muhleman D, Blake H, et al: Correlation of length of VNTR alleles at the X-linked MAOA gene and phenotypic effect in Tourette syndrome and drug abuse. Mol Psychiatry 3:50–60, 1998

Gadow KD, Nolan EE, Sverd J: Methylphenidate in hyperactive boys with comorbid tic disorder, II: short-term behavioral effects in school settings. J Am Acad Child Adolesc Psychiatry 31:462–471, 1992

Galaburda AM: Anatomical asymmetries in the human brain, in Biological Foundations of Cerebral Dominance. Edited by Geschwind N, Galaburda AM. Cambridge, MA, Harvard University Press, 1984, pp 11–25

Galaburda AM: Neuroanatomic basis of developmental dyslexia. Neurol Clin 11:161–173, 1993

Galaburda AM: Developmental dyslexia and animal studies: at the interface between cognition and neurology. Cognition 50:133–149, 1994

Galaburda AM, LeMay M, Kemper TL, et al: Right-left asymmetries in the brain. Science 199:852–856, 1978

Galaburda AM, Sherman GF, Rosen GD, et al: Developmental dyslexia: four consecutive patients with cortical anomalies. Ann Neurol 18:222–233, 1985

Galaburda AM, LoTurco J, Ramus F, et al: From genes to behavior in developmental dyslexia. Nat Neurosci 9:1213–1217, 2006

Galler JR, Ramsey F, Solimano G, et al: The influence of early malnutrition on subsequent behavioral development, II: classroom behavior. J Am Acad Child Psychiatry 22:16–22, 1983

Galvan A, Hare TA, Davidson M, et al: The role of ventral frontostriatal circuitry in reward-based learning in humans. J Neurosci 25:8650–8656, 2005

Garvey MA, Perlmutter SJ, Allen AJ, et al: A pilot study of penicillin prophylaxis for neuropsychiatric exacerbations triggered by streptococcal infections. Biol Psychiatry 45:1564–1571, 1999

Gatley SJ, Pan D, Chen R, et al: Affinities of methylphenidate derivatives for dopamine, norepinephrine and serotonin transporters. Life Sci 58:231–239, 1996

Gelernter J, Rao PA, Pauls DL, et al: Assignment of the 5HT7 receptor gene (*HTR7*) to chromosome 10q and exclusion of genetic linkage with Tourette syndrome. Genomics 26:207–209, 1995a

Gelernter J, Vandenbergh D, Kruger SD, et al: The dopamine transporter protein gene (*SLC6A3*): primary linkage mapping and linkage studies in Tourette syndrome. Genomics 30:459–463, 1995b

Geller B, Reising D, Leonard HL, et al: Critical review of tricyclic antidepressant use in children and adolescents. J Am Acad Child Adolesc Psychiatry 38:513–516, 1999

Genton P, Bauer J, Duncan S, et al: On the association between valproate and polycystic ovary syndrome. Epilepsia 42:295–304, 2001

George MS, Trimble MR, Costa DC, et al: Elevated frontal cerebral blood flow in Gilles de la Tourette syndrome: a 99Tcm-HMPAO SPECT study. Psychiatry Res 45:143–151, 1992

Georgiewa P, Rzanny R, Hopf JM, et al: fMRI during word processing in dyslexic and normal reading children. Neuroreport 10:3459–3465, 1999

Geschwind N, Behan P: Left-handedness: association with immune disease, migraine, and developmental learning disorder. Proc Natl Acad Sci U S A 79:5097–5100, 1982

Geschwind N, Galaburda AM: Cerebral lateralization: biological mechanisms, associations, and pathology, I: a hypothesis and a program for research. Arch Neurol 42:428–459, 1985a

Geschwind N, Galaburda AM: Cerebral lateralization: biological mechanisms, associations, and pathology, II: a hypothesis and a program for research. Arch Neurol 42:521–552, 1985b

Geschwind N, Levitsky W: Human brain: left-right asymmetries in temporal speech region. Science 161:186–187, 1968

Giedd JN: Structural magnetic resonance imaging of the adolescent brain. Ann N Y Acad Sci 1021:77–85, 2004

Giedd JN, Castellanos FX, Casey BJ, et al: Quantitative morphology of the corpus callosum in attention deficit hyperactivity disorder. Am J Psychiatry 151:665–669, 1994

Gilger JW, Pennington BF, DeFries JC: A twin study of the etiology of comorbidity: attention-deficit hyperactivity disorder and dyslexia. J Am Acad Child Adolesc Psychiatry 31:343–348, 1992

Gill M, Daly G, Heron S, et al: Confirmation of association between attention deficit hyperactivity disorder and a dopamine transporter polymorphism. Mol Psychiatry 2:311–313, 1997

Gillberg C: Endogenous opioids and opiate antagonists in autism: brief review of empirical findings and implications for clinicians. Dev Med Child Neurol 37:239–245, 1995

Gilliam FG: Diagnosis and treatment of mood disorders in persons with epilepsy. Curr Opin Neurol 18:129–133, 2005

Gillis JJ, DeFries JC, Fulker DW: Confirmatory factor analysis of reading and mathematics performance: a twin study. Acta Genet Med Gemellol (Roma) 41:287–300, 1992

Gittelman R, Mannuzza S, Shenker R, et al: Hyperactive boys almost grown up, I: psychiatric status. Arch Gen Psychiatry 42:937–947, 1985

Glod CA, Teicher MH: Relationship between early abuse, post-traumatic stress disorder, and activity levels in prepubertal children. J Am Acad Child Adolesc Psychiatry 35:1384–1393, 1996

Goadsby PJ, Lambert GA: Electrical stimulation of the fastigial nucleus increases total cerebral blood flow in the monkey. Neurosci Lett 107:141–144, 1989

Goddard AW, Charney DS: Toward an integrated neurobiology of panic disorder. J Clin Psychiatry 58 (suppl 2):4–12, 1997

Godridge H, Reynolds GP, Czudek C, et al: Alzheimer-like neurotransmitter deficits in adult Down's syndrome brain tissue. J Neurol Neurosurg Psychiatry 50:775–778, 1987

Gold AP: Evaluation and diagnosis by inspection, in Child and Adolescent Neurology for Psychiatrists. Edited by Kaufman DM, Solomon GE, Pfeffer CR. Baltimore, MD, Williams & Wilkins, 1992, pp 1–12

Goldberg E, Costa LD: Hemisphere differences in the acquisition and use of descriptive systems. Brain Lang 14:144–173, 1981

Goodyear BG, Nicolle DA, Menon RS: High resolution fMRI of ocular dominance columns within the visual cortex of human amblyopes. Strabismus 10:129–136, 2002

Grace AA: The tonic/phasic model of dopamine system regulation: its relevance for understanding how stimulant abuse can alter basal ganglia function. Drug Alcohol Depend 37:111–129, 1995

Greatrex JC, Drasdo N: The magnocellular deficit hypothesis in dyslexia: a review of reported evidence. Ophthalmic Physiol Opt 15:501–506, 1995

Gresch PJ, Sved AF, Zigmond MJ, et al: Local influence of endogenous norepinephrine on extracellular dopamine in rat medial prefrontal cortex. J Neurochem 65:111–116, 1995

Grizenko N, Kovacina B, Amor LB, et al: Relationship between response to methylphenidate treatment in children with ADHD and psychopathology in their families. J Am Acad Child Adolesc Psychiatry 45:47–53, 2006

Groner Y, Elroy-Stein O, Avraham KB, et al: Cell damage by excess CuZnSOD and Down's syndrome. Biomed Pharmacother 48:231–240, 1994

Gupta R, Appleton R: Corticosteroids in the management of the paediatric epilepsies. Arch Dis Child 90:379–384, 2005

Gutierrez-Delicado E, Serratosa JM: Genetics of the epilepsies. Curr Opin Neurol 17:147–153, 2004

Habib M, Robichon F, Levrier O, et al: Diverging asymmetries of temporo-parietal cortical areas: a reappraisal of Geschwind/Galaburda theory. Brain Lang 48:238–258, 1995

Hagberg B, Witt-Engerstrom I: Rett syndrome: epidemiology and nosology—Progress in Knowledge 1986—a conference communication. Brain Dev 9:451–457, 1987

Hagerman PJ, Hagerman RJ: The fragile-X premutation: a maturing perspective. Am J Hum Genet 74:805–816, 2004

Hagerman RJ, Sobesky WE: Psychopathology in fragile X syndrome. Am J Orthopsychiatry 59:142–152, 1989

Hallett JJ, Harling-Berg CJ, Knopf PM, et al: Anti-striatal antibodies in Tourette syndrome cause neuronal dysfunction. J Neuroimmunol 111:195–202, 2000

Hanover JL, Huang ZJ, Tonegawa S, et al: Brain-derived neurotrophic factor overexpression induces precocious critical period in mouse visual cortex. J Neurosci 19:RC40, 1999

Hardan AY, Minshew NJ, Keshavan MS: Corpus callosum size in autism. Neurology 55:1033–1036, 2000

Harikrishnan KN, Chow MZ, Baker EK, et al: Brahma links the SWI/SNF chromatin-remodeling complex with *MeCP2*-dependent transcriptional silencing. Nat Genet 37:254–264, 2005

Harris JC: Advances in genetic medicine applied to mental retardation syndromes. Curr Opin Psychiatry 14:427–430, 2001

Harris NS, Courchesne E, Townsend J, et al: Neuroanatomic contributions to slowed orienting of attention in children with autism. Brain Res Cogn Brain Res 8:61–71, 1999

Harrison JE, Bolton PF: Annotation: tuberous sclerosis. J Child Psychol Psychiatry 38:603–614, 1997

Hashimoto T, Tayama M, Mori K, et al: Magnetic resonance imaging in autism: preliminary report. Neuropediatrics 20:142–146, 1989

Haslam RH, Dalby JT, Johns RD, et al: Cerebral asymmetry in developmental dyslexia. Arch Neurol 38:679–682, 1981

Hauser P, Zametkin AJ, Martinez P, et al: Attention deficit-hyperactivity disorder in people with generalized resistance to thyroid hormone. N Engl J Med 328:997–1001, 1993

Hauser WA: The prevalence and incidence of convulsive disorders in children. Epilepsia 35 (suppl 2):S1–S6, 1994

Hauser WA: Epilepsy epidemiology, in Encyclopedia of the Neurological Sciences. Edited by Aminoff MJ, Daroff RB. San Diego, CA, Academic Press, 2003, pp 201–202

Hay D, Bennett K, McStephen M, et al: Attention deficit-hyperactivity disorder in twins: a developmental genetic analysis. Aust J Psychol 56:99–107, 2004

Heath RG: Electroencephalographic studies in isolation-raised monkeys with behavioral impairment. Dis Nerv Syst 33:157–163, 1972

Hedera P, Abou-Khalil B, Crunk AE, et al: Autosomal dominant lateral temporal epilepsy: two families with novel mutations in the LGI1 gene. Epilepsia 45:218–222, 2004

Heffner TG, Heller A, Miller FE, et al: Locomotor hyperactivity in neonatal rats following electrolytic lesions of mesocortical dopamine neurons. Brain Res 285:29–37, 1983

Heilman KM, Van Den Abell T: Right hemisphere dominance for attention: the mechanism underlying hemispheric asymmetries of inattention (neglect). Neurology 30:327–330, 1980

Helmstaedter C, Kemper B, Elger CE: Neuropsychological aspects of frontal lobe epilepsy. Neuropsychologia 34:399–406, 1996

Henker B, Whalen CK: Hyperactivity and attention deficits. Am Psychol 44:216–223, 1989

Herman JL, Perry JC, van der Kolk BA: Childhood trauma in borderline personality disorder. Am J Psychiatry 146:490–495, 1989

Hernandez L, Lee F, Hoebel BG: Simultaneous microdialysis and amphetamine infusion in the nucleus accumbens and striatum of freely moving rats: increase in extracellular dopamine and serotonin. Brain Res Bull 19:623–628, 1987

Hesdorffer DC, Ludvigsson P, Olafsson E, et al: ADHD as a risk factor for incident unprovoked seizures and epilepsy in children. Arch Gen Psychiatry 61:731–736, 2004

Hill DE, Yeo RA, Campbell RA, et al: Magnetic resonance imaging correlates of attention-deficit/hyperactivity disorder in children. Neuropsychology 17:496–506, 2003

Hinshaw SP, Owens EB, Wells KC, et al: Family processes and treatment outcome in the MTA: negative/ineffective parenting practices in relation to multimodal treatment. J Abnorm Child Psychol 28:555–568, 2000

Hirai K, Kimiya S, Tabata K, et al: Selective mutism and obsessive compulsive disorders associated with zonisamide. Seizure 11:468–470, 2002

Hirose M, Yokoyama H, Haginoya K, et al: [A five-year-old girl with epilepsy showing forced normalization due to zonisamide] (Japanese). No To Hattatsu 35:259–263, 2003

Hitchins MP, Rickard S, Dhalla F, et al: Investigation of *UBE3A* and *MECP2* in Angelman syndrome (AS) and patients with features of AS. Am J Med Genet A 125:167–172, 2004

Hoehn TP, Baumeister AA: A critique of the application of sensory integration therapy to children with learning disabilities. J Learn Disabil 27:338–350, 1994

Hoekstra PJ, Minderaa RB, Kallenberg CG: Lack of effect of intravenous immunoglobulins on tics: a double-blind placebo-controlled study. J Clin Psychiatry 65:537–542, 2004

Hofer MA: Studies on how early maternal deprivation produces behavioral change in young rats. Psychosom Med 37:245–264, 1975

Holland AJ, Hon J, Huppert FA, et al: Population-based study of the prevalence and presentation of dementia in adults with Down's syndrome. Br J Psychiatry 172:493–498, 1998

Hollander E, Phillips A, Chaplin W, et al: A placebo controlled crossover trial of liquid fluoxetine on repetitive behaviors in childhood and adolescent autism. Neuropsychopharmacology 30:582–589, 2005

Holttum JR, Minshew NJ, Sanders RS, et al: Magnetic resonance imaging of the posterior fossa in autism. Biol Psychiatry 32:1091–1101, 1992

Horska A, Naidu S, Herskovits EH, et al: Quantitative ^{1}H MR spectroscopic imaging in early Rett syndrome. Neurology 54:715–722, 2000

Horwitz B, Rumsey JM, Grady CL, et al: The cerebral metabolic landscape in autism: intercorrelations of regional glucose utilization. Arch Neurol 45:749–755, 1988

Horwitz B, Rumsey JM, Donohue BC: Functional connectivity of the angular gyrus in normal reading and dyslexia. Proc Natl Acad Sci U S A 95:8939–8944, 1998

Hoshino Y, Kumashiro H, Yashima Y, et al: Early symptoms of autistic children and its diagnostic significance. Folia Psychiatr Neurol Jpn 36:367–374, 1982

Howlin P, Goode S, Hutton J, et al: Adult outcome for children with autism. J Child Psychol Psychiatry 45:212–229, 2004

Hoza B, Gerdes AC, Mrug S, et al: Peer-assessed outcomes in the multimodal treatment study of children with attention deficit hyperactivity disorder. J Clin Child Adolesc Psychol 34:74–86, 2005

Huang C, Liu G: Organization of the auditory area in the posterior cerebellar vermis of the cat. Exp Brain Res 81:377–383, 1990

Hubel DH: Effects of deprivation on the visual cortex of cat and monkey. Harvey Lect 72:1–51, 1978

Hubel DH, Wiesel TN: Early exploration of the visual cortex. Neuron 20:401–412, 1998

Hubl DH, Bolte S, Feineis-Matthews S, et al: Functional imbalance of visual pathways indicates alternative face processing strategies in autism. Neurology 61:1232–1237, 2003

Hudgins RJ, Flamini JR, Palasis S, et al: Surgical treatment of epilepsy in children caused by focal cortical dysplasia. Pediatr Neurosurg 41:70–76, 2005

Humphries T, Wright M, Snider L, et al: A comparison of the effectiveness of sensory integrative therapy and perceptual-motor training in treating children with learning disabilities. J Dev Behav Pediatr 13:31–40, 1992

Hunt RD: Treatment effects of oral and transdermal clonidine in relation to methylphenidate: an open pilot study in ADD-H. Psychopharmacol Bull 23:111–114, 1987

Hunt RD, Minderaa RB, Cohen DJ: Clonidine benefits children with attention deficit disorder and hyperactivity: report of a double-blind placebo-crossover therapeutic trial. J Am Acad Child Psychiatry 24:617–629, 1985

Hunt RD, Minderaa RB, Cohen DJ: The therapeutic effect of clonidine in attention deficit disorder with hyperactivity: a comparison with placebo and methylphenidate. Psychopharmacol Bull 22:229–236, 1986

Hunt RD, Arnsten AF, Asbell MD: An open trial of guanfacine in the treatment of attention-deficit hyperactivity disorder. J Am Acad Child Adolesc Psychiatry 34:50–54, 1995

Huret JL, Delabar JM, Marlhens F, et al: Down syndrome with duplication of a region of chromosome 21 containing the CuZn superoxide dismutase gene without detectable karyotypic abnormality. Hum Genet 75:251–257, 1987

Huttenlocher PR: Synaptic density in human frontal cortex: developmental changes and effects of aging. Brain Res 163:195–205, 1979

Hyde TM, Stacey ME, Coppola R, et al: Cerebral morphometric abnormalities in Tourette's syndrome: a quantitative MRI study of monozygotic twins. Neurology 45:1176–1182, 1995

Hynd GW, Semrud-Clikeman M, Lorys AR, et al: Corpus callosum morphology in attention deficit-hyperactivity disorder: morphometric analysis of MRI. J Learn Disabil 24:141–146, 1991

Institute of Medicine of the National Academies: Immunization Safety Review: Vaccines and Autism. May 17, 2004. Available at: http://www.iom.edu/CMS/3793/4705/20155.aspx. Accessed November 22, 2006.

Inui N, Suzuki K: Practice and serial reaction time of adolescents with autism. Percept Mot Skills 86:403–410, 1998

Isaacs EB, Edmonds CJ, Lucas A, et al: Calculation difficulties in children of very low birthweight: a neural correlate. Brain 124:1701–1707, 2001

Isojarvi JI, Tapanainen JS: Valproate, hyperandrogenism, and polycystic ovaries: a report of 3 cases. Arch Neurol 57:1064–1068, 2000

Isojarvi JI, Laatikainen TJ, Pakarinen AJ, et al: Polycystic ovaries and hyperandrogenism in women taking valproate for epilepsy. N Engl J Med 329:1383–1388, 1993

Ito Y, Teicher MH, Glod CA, et al: Increased prevalence of electrophysiological abnormalities in children with psychological, physical, and sexual abuse. J Neuropsychiatry Clin Neurosci 5:401–408, 1993

Ito Y, Teicher MH, Glod CA, et al: Preliminary evidence for aberrant cortical development in abused children: a quantitative EEG study. J Neuropsychiatry Clin Neurosci 10:298–307, 1998

Jadresic D: The role of the amygdaloid complex in Gilles de la Tourette's syndrome. Br J Psychiatry 161:532–534, 1992

Jamain S, Quach H, Betancur C, et al: Mutations of the X-linked genes encoding neuroligins NLGN3 and NLGN4 are associated with autism. Nat Genet 34:27–29, 2003

Jellinger K, Armstrong D, Zoghbi HY, et al: Neuropathology of Rett syndrome. Acta Neuropathol (Berl) 76:142–158, 1988

Jensen I, Larsen JK: Mental aspects of temporal lobe epilepsy: follow-up of 74 patients after resection of a temporal lobe. J Neurol Neurosurg Psychiatry 42:256–265, 1979

Jensen PS: Fact versus fancy concerning the multimodal treatment study for attention-deficit hyperactivity disorder. Can J Psychiatry 44:975–980, 1999

Jensen PS, Hinshaw SP, Kraemer HC, et al: ADHD comorbidity findings from the MTA study: comparing comorbid subgroups. J Am Acad Child Adolesc Psychiatry 40:147–158, 2001

Jenson WR, Sheridan SM, Olympia D, et al: Homework and students with learning disabilities and behavior disorders: a practical, parent-based approach. J Learn Disabil 27:538–548, 1994

Jernigan TL, Hesselink JR, Sowell E, et al: Cerebral structure on magnetic resonance imaging in language- and learning-impaired children. Arch Neurol 48:539–545, 1991

Jin P, Warren ST: Understanding the molecular basis of fragile X syndrome. Hum Mol Genet 9:901–908, 2000

Johannes S, Kussmaul CL, Munte TF, et al: Developmental dyslexia: passive visual stimulation provides no evidence for a magnocellular processing defect. Neuropsychologia 34:1123–1127, 1996

Johnson MH: Development of human brain functions. Biol Psychiatry 54:1312–1316, 2003

Jokeit H, Ebner A: Effects of chronic epilepsy on intellectual functions. Prog Brain Res 135:455–463, 2002

Joseph RM, Tager-Flusberg H: The relationship of theory of mind and executive functions to symptom type and severity in children with autism. Dev Psychopathol 16:137–155, 2004

Jucaite A, Fernell E, Halldin C, et al: Reduced midbrain dopamine transporter binding in male adolescents with attention-deficit/hyperactivity disorder: association between striatal dopamine markers and motor hyperactivity. Biol Psychiatry 57:229–238, 2005

Jutai JW: Cerebral asymmetry and the psychophysiology of attention. Int J Psychophysiol 1:219–225, 1984

Kalscheuer VM, Tao J, Donnelly A, et al: Disruption of the serine/threonine kinase 9 gene causes severe X-linked infantile spasms and mental retardation. Am J Hum Genet 72:1401–1411, 2003

Kanemoto K, Tsuji T, Kawasaki J: Reexamination of interictal psychoses based on DSM-IV psychosis classification and international epilepsy classification. Epilepsia 42:98–103, 2001

Kanner AM, Parra J, Frey M, et al: Psychiatric and neurologic predictors of psychogenic pseudoseizure outcome. Neurology 53:933–938, 1999

Kanner L: Autistic disturbances of affective contact. Nervous Child 2:217–250, 1943

Kanumakala S, Greaves R, Pedreira CC, et al: Fasting ghrelin levels are not elevated in children with hypothalamic obesity. J Clin Endocrinol Metab 90:2691–2695, 2005

Kaplan BJ, Polatajko HJ, Wilson BN, et al: Reexamination of sensory integration treatment: a combination of two efficacy studies. J Learn Disabil 26:342–347, 1993

Karacostas DD, Fisher GL: Chemical dependency in students with and without learning disabilities. J Learn Disabil 26:491–495, 1993

Kaufman DM: Clinical Neurology for Psychiatrists, 5th Edition. St. Louis, MO, WB Saunders, 2001

Keller HH, Bartholini G, Pletscher A: Spontaneous and drug-induced changes of cerebral dopamine turnover during postnatal development of rats. Brain Res 64:371–378, 1973

Kelsey DK, Sumner CR, Casat CD, et al: Once-daily atomoxetine treatment for children with attention-deficit/hyperactivity disorder, including an assessment of evening and morning behavior: a double-blind, placebo-controlled trial. Pediatrics 114:E1–E8, 2004

Kemner JE, Starr HL, Ciccone PE, et al: Outcomes of OROS methylphenidate compared with atomoxetine in children with ADHD: a multicenter, randomized prospective study. Adv Ther 22:498–512, 2005

Kemper TL, Bauman ML: The contribution of neuropathologic studies to the understanding of autism. Neurol Clin 11:175–187, 1993

Kempermann G, Gage FH: Neurogenesis in the adult hippocampus. Novartis Found Symp 231:220–235; discussion 235–241, 302–306, 2000

Kerr B, Turner G, Mulley J, et al: Non-specific X linked mental retardation. J Med Genet 28:378–382, 1991

Keshavan M, Anderson S, Pettegrew JW: Is schizophrenia due to excessive synaptic pruning in the prefrontal cortex? The Feinberg hypothesis revisited. J Psychiatr Res 28:239–265, 1994

Ketter TA, Malow BA, Flamini R, et al: Felbamate monotherapy has stimulant-like effects in patients with epilepsy. Epilepsy Res 23:129–137, 1996

Ketter TA, Malow BA, Post RM, et al: Psychiatric effects of felbamate. J Neuropsychiatry Clin Neurosci 9:118–119, 1997

Killgore WD, Oki M, Yurgelun-Todd DA: Sex-specific developmental changes in amygdala responses to affective faces. Neuroreport 12:427–433, 2001

Kim JW, Yoo HJ, Cho SC, et al: Behavioral characteristics of Prader-Willi syndrome in Korea: comparison with children with mental retardation and normal controls. J Child Neurol 20:134–138, 2005

Kim SW, Grant JE, Kim SI, et al: A possible association of recurrent streptococcal infections and acute onset of obsessive-compulsive disorder. J Neuropsychiatry Clin Neurosci 16:252–260, 2004

Kimura S: Zonisamide-induced behavior disorder in two children. Epilepsia 35:403–405, 1994

Kinsella G, Ong B, Murtagh D, et al: The role of the family for behavioral outcome in children and adolescents following traumatic brain injury. J Consult Clin Psychol 67:116–123, 1999

Kishino T, Lalande M, Wagstaff J: UBE3A/E6-AP mutations cause Angelman syndrome. Nat Genet 15:70–73, 1997

Klauck SM, Poustka F, Benner A, et al: Serotonin transporter (5-HTT) gene variants associated with autism? Hum Mol Genet 6:2233–2238, 1997

Kleefstra T, Hamel BC: X-linked mental retardation: further lumping, splitting and emerging phenotypes. Clin Genet 67:451–467, 2005

Kleefstra T, Smidt M, Banning MJ, et al: Disruption of the gene Euchromatin Histone Methyl Transferase1 (Eu-HMTase1) is associated with the 9q34 subtelomeric deletion syndrome. J Med Genet 42:299–306, 2005

Klein RG, Mannuzza S: Long-term outcome of hyperactive children: a review. J Am Acad Child Adolesc Psychiatry 30:383–387, 1991

Knell ER, Comings DE: Tourette's syndrome and attention-deficit hyperactivity disorder: evidence for a genetic relationship. J Clin Psychiatry 54:331–337, 1993

Knoll JH, Glatt KA, Nicholls RD, et al: Chromosome 15 uniparental disomy is not frequent in Angelman syndrome. Am J Hum Genet 48:16–21, 1991

Knutson B, Fong GW, Adams CM, et al: Dissociation of reward anticipation and outcome with event-related fMRI. Neuroreport 12:3683–3687, 2001

Kogan CS, Boutet I, Cornish K, et al: Differential impact of the FMR1 gene on visual processing in fragile X syndrome. Brain 127:591–601, 2004

Korkman M, Pesonen AE: A comparison of neuropsychological test profiles of children with attention deficit-hyperactivity disorder and/or learning disorder. J Learn Disabil 27:383–392, 1994

Koumoula A, Tsironi V, Stamouli V, et al: An epidemiological study of number processing and mental calculation in Greek schoolchildren. J Learn Disabil 37:377–388, 2004

Krashen S: Lateralization, language learning, and the critical period: some new evidence. Language Learning 23:63–74, 1973

Krause J, la Fougere C, Krause KH, et al: Influence of striatal dopamine transporter availability on the response to methylphenidate in adult patients with ADHD. Eur Arch Psychiatry Clin Neurosci 255:428–431, 2005

Krause KH, Dresel SH, Krause J, et al: Increased striatal dopamine transporter in adult patients with attention deficit hyperactivity disorder: effects of methylphenidate as measured by single photon emission computed tomography. Neurosci Lett 285:107–110, 2000

Krumholz A: Nonepileptic seizures: diagnosis and management. Neurology 53(suppl):S76–S83, 1999

Krystal H: Trauma and affects. Psychoanal Study Child 33:81–116, 1978

Kubova Z, Kuba M, Peregrin J, et al: Visual evoked potential evidence for magnocellular system deficit in dyslexia. Physiol Res 45:87–89, 1996

Kuczenski R, Segal DS, Leith NJ, et al: Effects of amphetamine, methylphenidate, and apomorphine on regional brain serotonin and 5-hydroxyindole acetic acid. Psychopharmacology (Berl) 93:329–335, 1987

Kulynych JJ, Vladar K, Jones DW, et al: Gender differences in the normal lateralization of the supratemporal cortex: MRI surface-rendering morphometry of Heschl's gyrus and the planum temporale. Cereb Cortex 4:107–118, 1994

Kurlan R, Como PG, Deeley C, et al: A pilot controlled study of fluoxetine for obsessive-compulsive symptoms in children with Tourette's syndrome. Clin Neuropharmacol 16:167–172, 1993

Kuzniecky RI: Neuroimaging of epilepsy: therapeutic implications. NeuroRx 2:384–393, 2005

Kwak CH, Hanna PA, Jankovic J: Botulinum toxin in the treatment of tics. Arch Neurol 57:1190–1193, 2000

LaBar KS, Gatenby JC, Gore JC, et al: Human amygdala activation during conditioned fear acquisition and extinction: a mixed-trial fMRI study. Neuron 20:937–945, 1998

Lagae L, Buyse G, Ceulemans B: Clinical experience with levetiracetam in childhood epilepsy: an add-on and monotherapy trial. Seizure 14:66–71, 2005

LaHoste GJ, Swanson JM, Wigal SB, et al: Dopamine D_4 receptor gene polymorphism is associated with attention deficit hyperactivity disorder. Mol Psychiatry 1:121–124, 1996

Landmesser LT: The generation of neuromuscular specificity. Annu Rev Neurosci 3:279–302, 1980

Larisch R, Sitte W, Antke C, et al: Striatal dopamine transporter density in drug naive patients with attention-deficit/hyperactivity disorder. Nucl Med Commun 27:267–270, 2006

Laumonnier F, Bonnet-Brilhault F, Gomot M, et al: X-linked mental retardation and autism are associated with a mutation in the NLGN4 gene, a member of the neuroligin family. Am J Hum Genet 74:552–557, 2004

Leach JP, Girvan J, Paul A, et al: Gabapentin and cognition: a double blind, dose ranging, placebo controlled study in refractory epilepsy. J Neurol Neurosurg Psychiatry 62:372–376, 1997

Leckman JF, Cohen DJ, Detlor J, et al: Clonidine in the treatment of Tourette syndrome: a review of data. Adv Neurol 35:391–401, 1982

Leckman JF, Dolnansky ES, Hardin MT, et al: Perinatal factors in the expression of Tourette's syndrome: an exploratory study. J Am Acad Child Adolesc Psychiatry 29:220–226, 1990

Leckman JF, Knorr AM, Rasmusson AM, et al: Basal ganglia research and Tourette's syndromes. Trends Neurosci 14:94, 1991

Leckman JF, Walker DE, Cohen DJ: Premonitory urges in Tourette's syndrome. Am J Psychiatry 150:98–102, 1993

Leckman JF, Goodman WK, Anderson GM, et al: Cerebrospinal fluid biogenic amines in obsessive compulsive disorder, Tourette's syndrome, and healthy controls. Neuropsychopharmacology 12:73–86, 1995a

Leckman JF, Pauls D, Cohen D: Tic disorders, in Psychopharmacology: The Fourth Generation of Progress. Edited by Bloom F, Kupfer D. New York, Raven, 1995b, pp 1665–1674

Leckman JF, Zhang H, Vitale A, et al: Course of tic severity in Tourette syndrome: the first two decades. Pediatrics 102:14–19, 1998

LeDoux JE, Iwata J, Cicchetti P, et al: Different projections of the central amygdaloid nucleus mediate autonomic and behavioral correlates of conditioned fear. J Neurosci 8:2517–2529, 1988

Lee DO, Steingard RJ, Cesena M, et al: Behavioral side effects of gabapentin in children. Epilepsia 37:87–90, 1996

Lejeune J: Pathogenesis of mental deficiency in trisomy 21. Am J Med Genet Suppl 7:20–30, 1990

Leonard HL, Meyer MC, Swedo SE, et al: Electrocardiographic changes during desipramine and clomipramine treatment in children and adolescents. J Am Acad Child Adolesc Psychiatry 34:1460–1468, 1995

Leslie AM, Frith U: Prospects for a cognitive neuropsychology of autism: Hobson's choice. Psychol Rev 97:122–131, 1990

Lesser RP: Psychogenic seizures. Neurology 46:1499–1507, 1996

Leventhal BL, Cook EH Jr, Morford M, et al: Clinical and neurochemical effects of fenfluramine in children with autism. J Neuropsychiatry Clin Neurosci 5:307–315, 1993

Levesque J, Beauregard M, Mensour B: Effect of neurofeedback training on the neural substrates of selective attention in children with attention-deficit/hyperactivity disorder: a functional magnetic resonance imaging study. Neurosci Lett 394:216–221, 2006

Leviton A, Bellinger D, Allred EN, et al: Pre- and postnatal low-level lead exposure and children's dysfunction in school. Environ Res 60:30–43, 1993

Levitt JG, Blanton R, Capetillo-Cunliffe L, et al: Cerebellar vermis lobules VIII–X in autism. Prog Neuropsychopharmacol Biol Psychiatry 23:625–633, 1999

Levy F, Hay DA, McStephen M, et al: Attention-deficit hyperactivity disorder: a category or a continuum? Genetic analysis of a large-scale twin study. J Am Acad Child Adolesc Psychiatry 36:737–744, 1997

Lewander T: Displacement of brain and heart noradrenaline by p-hydroxynorephedrine after administration of p-hydroxyamphetamine. Acta Pharmacol Toxicol (Copenh) 29:20–32, 1971a

Lewander T: On the presence of p-hydroxynorephedrine in the rat brain and heart in relation to changes in catecholamine levels after administration of amphetamine. Acta Pharmacol Toxicol (Copenh) 29:3–48, 1971b

Lewis C, Hitch GJ, Walker P: The prevalence of specific arithmetic difficulties and specific reading difficulties in 9- to 10-year-old boys and girls. J Child Psychol Psychiatry 35:283–292, 1994

Lewis DA, Cruz D, Eggan S, et al: Postnatal development of prefrontal inhibitory circuits and the pathophysiology of cognitive dysfunction in schizophrenia. Ann N Y Acad Sci 1021:64–76, 2004

Lewis DO, Pincus JH, Bard B, et al: Neuropsychiatric, psychoeducational, and family characteristics of 14 juveniles condemned to death in the United States. Am J Psychiatry 145:584–589, 1988

Lichter DG, Jackson LA, Schachter M: Clinical evidence of genomic imprinting in Tourette's syndrome. Neurology 45:924–928, 1995

Liederman J, Flannery KA: Fall conception increases the risk of neurodevelopmental disorder in offspring. J Clin Exp Neuropsychol 16:754–768, 1994

Lim JH, Booker AB, Fallon JR: Regulating fragile X gene transcription in the brain and beyond. J Cell Physiol 205:170–175, 2005

Lindgren AC, Ritzen EM: Five years of growth hormone treatment in children with Prader-Willi syndrome: Swedish National Growth Hormone Advisory Group. Acta Paediatr Suppl 88:109–111, 1999

Linet LS: Tourette syndrome, pimozide, and school phobia: the neuroleptic separation anxiety syndrome. Am J Psychiatry 142:613–615, 1985

Liu F, Muniz R, Minami H, et al: Review and comparison of the long acting methylphenidate preparations. Psychiatr Q 76:259–269, 2005

Livingstone MS, Rosen GD, Drislane FW, et al: Physiological and anatomical evidence for a magnocellular defect in developmental dyslexia. Proc Natl Acad Sci U S A 88:7943–7947, 1991

Longcamp M, Anton JL, Roth M, et al: Visual presentation of single letters activates a premotor area involved in writing. Neuroimage 19:1492–1500, 2003

Longcamp M, Anton JL, Roth M, et al: Premotor activations in response to visually presented single letters depend on the hand used to write: a study on left-handers. Neuropsychologia 43:1801–1809, 2005

Lord C: Follow-up of two-year-olds referred for possible autism. J Child Psychol Psychiatry 36:1365–1382, 1995

Lossie AC, Whitney MM, Amidon D, et al: Distinct phenotypes distinguish the molecular classes of Angelman syndrome. J Med Genet 38:834–845, 2001

Lou HC, Henriksen L, Bruhn P: Focal cerebral dysfunction in developmental learning disabilities. Lancet 335:8–11, 1990

Lovaas OI: Behavioral treatment and normal educational and intellectual functioning in young autistic children. J Consult Clin Psychol 55:3–9, 1987

Lovaas OI, Smith T: A comprehensive behavioral theory of autistic children: paradigm for research and treatment. J Behav Ther Exp Psychiatry 20:17–29, 1989

Lubar JO, Lubar JF: Electroencephalographic biofeedback of SMR and beta for treatment of attention deficit disorders in a clinical setting. Biofeedback Self Regul 9:1–23, 1984

Lubar JF, Swartwood MO, Swartwood JN, et al: Evaluation of the effectiveness of EEG neurofeedback training for ADHD in a clinical setting as measured by changes in T.O.V.A. scores, behavioral ratings, and WISC-R performance. Biofeedback Self Regul 20:83–99, 1995

Luna B, Sweeney JA: The emergence of collaborative brain function: fMRI studies of the development of response inhibition. Ann N Y Acad Sci 1021:296–309, 2004

Luxenberg JS, Swedo SE, Flament MF, et al: Neuroanatomical abnormalities in obsessive-compulsive disorder detected with quantitative x-ray computed tomography. Am J Psychiatry 145:1089–1093, 1988

Macdonald RL, Kelly KM: Antiepileptic drug mechanisms of action. Epilepsia 36 (suppl 2):S2–S12, 1995

MacMaster FP, Carrey N, Sparkes S, et al: Proton spectroscopy in medication-free pediatric attention-deficit/hyperactivity disorder. Biol Psychiatry 53:184–187, 2003

Maestrini E, Lai C, Marlow A, et al: Serotonin transporter (5-HTT) and gamma-aminobutyric acid receptor subunit beta3 (GABRB3) gene polymorphisms are not associated with autism in the IMGSA families: The International Molecular Genetic Study of Autism Consortium. Am J Med Genet 88:492–496, 1999

Maestro S, Casella C, Milone A, et al: Study of the onset of autism through home movies. Psychopathology 32:292–300, 1999

Maestro S, Muratori F, Cesari A, et al: Course of autism signs in the first year of life. Psychopathology 38:26–31, 2005

Maher BS, Marazita ML, Ferrell RE, et al: Dopamine system genes and attention deficit hyperactivity disorder: a meta-analysis. Psychiatr Genet 12:207–215, 2002

Mailleux P, Pelaprat D, Vanderhaeghen JJ: Transient neurotensin high-affinity binding sites in the human inferior olive during development. Brain Res 508:345–348, 1990

Majdan M, Shatz CJ: Effects of visual experience on activity-dependent gene regulation in cortex. Nat Neurosci 9:650–659, 2006

Malison RT, McDougle CJ, van Dyck CH, et al: [^{123}I]beta-CIT SPECT imaging of striatal dopamine transporter binding in Tourette's disorder. Am J Psychiatry 152:1359–1361, 1995

Malone MA, Kershner JR, Swanson JM: Hemispheric processing and methylphenidate effects in attention-deficit hyperactivity disorder. J Child Neurol 9:181–189, 1994

Malone RP, Cater J, Sheikh RM, et al: Olanzapine versus haloperidol in children with autistic disorder: an open pilot study. J Am Acad Child Adolesc Psychiatry 40:887–894, 2001

Malzac P, Webber H, Moncla A, et al: Mutation analysis of UBE3A in Angelman syndrome patients. Am J Hum Genet 62:1353–1360, 1998

Mannuzza S, Klein RG, Konig PH, et al: Hyperactive boys almost grown up, IV: criminality and its relationship to psychiatric status. Arch Gen Psychiatry 46:1073–1079, 1989

Mannuzza S, Klein RG, Bessler A, et al: Adult psychiatric status of hyperactive boys grown up. Am J Psychiatry 155:493–498, 1998

Manor I, Eisenberg J, Tyano S, et al: Family based association study of the serotonin transporter promoter region polymorphism (*5-HTTLPR*) in attention deficit hyperactivity disorder. Am J Med Genet 105:91–95, 2001

Mansilla AO, Barajas HM, Arguero RS, et al: Receptors, photoreception and brain perception: new insights. Arch Med Res 26:1–15, 1995

Marcus J, Hans SL, Lewow E, et al: Neurological findings in high-risk children: childhood assessment and 5-year follow-up. Schizophr Bull 11:85–100, 1985

Martin A, State M, Anderson GM, et al: Cerebrospinal fluid levels of oxytocin in Prader-Willi syndrome: a preliminary report. Biol Psychiatry 44:1349–1352, 1998

Martin R, Gilliam F, Kilgore M, et al: Improved health care resource utilization following video-EEG-confirmed diagnosis of nonepileptic psychogenic seizures. Seizure 7:385–390, 1998

Martin R, Kuzniecky R, Ho S, et al: Cognitive effects of topiramate, gabapentin, and lamotrigine in healthy young adults. Neurology 52:321–327, 1999

Martinussen R, Hayden J, Hogg-Johnson S, et al: A meta-analysis of working memory impairments in children with attention-deficit/hyperactivity disorder. J Am Acad Child Adolesc Psychiatry 44:377–384, 2005

Matsuura M: Epileptic psychoses and anticonvulsant drug treatment. J Neurol Neurosurg Psychiatry 67:231–233, 1999

Matsuura T, Sutcliffe JS, Fang P, et al: De novo truncating mutations in E6-AP ubiquitin-protein ligase gene (*UBE3A*) in Angelman syndrome. Nat Genet 15:74–77, 1997

Matthews WS, Barabas G: Suicide and epilepsy: a review of the literature. Psychosomatics 22:515–524, 1981

Mattson AJ, Sheer DE, Fletcher JM: Electrophysiological evidence of lateralized disturbances in children with learning disabilities. J Clin Exp Neuropsychol 14:707–716, 1992

Max JE, Dunisch DL: Traumatic brain injury in a child psychiatry outpatient clinic: a controlled study. J Am Acad Child Adolesc Psychiatry 36:404–411, 1997

Max JE, Lindgren SD, Robin DA, et al: Traumatic brain injury in children and adolescents: psychiatric disorders in the second three months. J Nerv Ment Dis 185:394–401, 1997a

Max JE, Robin DA, Lindgren SD, et al: Traumatic brain injury in children and adolescents: psychiatric disorders at two years. J Am Acad Child Adolesc Psychiatry 36:1278–1285, 1997b

Max JE, Smith WL Jr, Sato Y, et al: Traumatic brain injury in children and adolescents: psychiatric disorders in the first three months. J Am Acad Child Adolesc Psychiatry 36:94–102, 1997c

Max JE, Castillo CS, Bokura H, et al: Oppositional defiant disorder symptomatology after traumatic brain injury: a prospective study. J Nerv Ment Dis 186:325–332, 1998a

Max JE, Castillo CS, Robin DA, et al: Posttraumatic stress symptomatology after childhood traumatic brain injury. J Nerv Ment Dis 186:589–596, 1998b

Max JE, Lindgren SD, Knutson C, et al: Child and adolescent traumatic brain injury: correlates of disruptive behaviour disorders. Brain Inj 12:41–52, 1998c

Max JE, Lindgren SD, Knutson C, et al: Child and adolescent traumatic brain injury: correlates of injury severity. Brain Inj 12:31–40, 1998d

Max JE, Roberts MA, Koele SL, et al: Cognitive outcome in children and adolescents following severe traumatic brain injury: influence of psychosocial, psychiatric, and injury-related variables. J Int Neuropsychol Soc 5:58–68, 1999

Max JE, Koele SL, Castillo CC, et al: Personality change disorder in children and adolescents following traumatic brain injury. J Int Neuropsychol Soc 6:279–289, 2000

Max JE, Lansing AE, Koele SL, et al: Attention deficit hyperactivity disorder in children and adolescents following traumatic brain injury. Dev Neuropsychol 25:159–177, 2004

Max JE, Levin HS, Landis J, et al: Predictors of personality change due to traumatic brain injury in children and adolescents in the first six months after injury. J Am Acad Child Adolesc Psychiatry 44:434–442, 2005a

Max JE, Schachar RJ, Levin HS, et al: Predictors of attention-deficit/hyperactivity disorder within 6 months after pediatric traumatic brain injury. J Am Acad Child Adolesc Psychiatry 44:1032–1040, 2005b

Max JE, Schachar RJ, Levin HS, et al: Predictors of secondary attention-deficit/hyperactivity disorder in children and adolescents 6 to 24 months after traumatic brain injury. J Am Acad Child Adolesc Psychiatry 44:1041–1049, 2005c

Max JE, Levin HS, Schachar RJ, et al: Predictors of personality change due to traumatic brain injury in children and adolescents six to twenty-four months after injury. J Neuropsychiatry Clin Neurosci 18:21–32, 2006

McBride PA, Anderson GM, Hertzig ME, et al: Effects of diagnosis, race, and puberty on platelet serotonin levels in autism and mental retardation. J Am Acad Child Adolesc Psychiatry 37:767–776, 1998

McConnell H, Snyder PJ, Duffy JD, et al: Neuropsychiatric side effects related to treatment with felbamate. J Neuropsychiatry Clin Neurosci 8:341–346, 1996

McConville BJ, Fogelson MH, Norman AB, et al: Nicotine potentiation of haloperidol in reducing tic frequency in Tourette's disorder. Am J Psychiatry 148:793–794, 1991

McCracken JT, McGough J, Shah B, et al: Risperidone in children with autism and serious behavioral problems. N Engl J Med 347:314–321, 2002

McDanal CE Jr, Bolman WM: Delayed idiosyncratic psychosis with diphenylhydantoin. JAMA 231:1063, 1975

McDougle CJ, Goodman WK, Price LH: Dopamine antagonists in tic-related and psychotic spectrum obsessive compulsive disorder. J Clin Psychiatry 55 (suppl):24–31, 1994

McDougle CJ, Brodkin ES, Naylor ST, et al: Sertraline in adults with pervasive developmental disorders: a prospective open-label investigation. J Clin Psychopharmacol 18:62–66, 1998

McDougle CJ, Scahill L, McCracken JT, et al: Research Units on Pediatric Psychopharmacology (RUPP) Autism Network: background and rationale for an initial controlled study of risperidone. Child Adolesc Psychiatr Clin N Am 9:201–224, 2000

McEachin JJ, Smith T, Lovaas OI: Long-term outcome for children with autism who received early intensive behavioral treatment. Am J Ment Retard 97:359–391, 1993

McElwee C, Bernard S: Genetic syndromes and mental retardation. Curr Opin Psychiatry 15:469–475, 2002

McEvoy B, Hawi Z, Fitzgerald M, et al: No evidence of linkage or association between the norepinephrine transporter (*NET*) gene polymorphisms and ADHD in the Irish population. Am J Med Genet 114:665–666, 2002

McEwen BS: Effects of adverse experiences for brain structure and function. Biol Psychiatry 48:721–731, 2000

McGee R, Williams S, Silva PA: A comparison of girls and boys with teacher-identified problems of attention. J Am Acad Child Adolesc Psychiatry 26:711–717, 1987

McGough JJ, Pataki CS, Suddath R: Dexmethylphenidate extended-release capsules for attention deficit hyperactivity disorder. Expert Rev Neurother 5:437–441, 2005

McGrath LM, Smith SD, Pennington BF: Breakthroughs in the search for dyslexia candidate genes. Trends Mol Med 12:333–341, 2006

McLeer SV, Callaghan M, Henry D, et al: Psychiatric disorders in sexually abused children. J Am Acad Child Adolesc Psychiatry 33:313–319, 1994

Meador KJ, Loring DW, Ray PG, et al: Differential cognitive effects of carbamazepine and gabapentin. Epilepsia 40:1279–1285, 1999

Meador KJ, Loring DW, Ray PG, et al: Differential cognitive and behavioral effects of carbamazepine and lamotrigine. Neurology 56:1177–1182, 2001

Meaney MJ, Szyf M: Environmental programming of stress responses through DNA methylation: life at the interface between a dynamic environment and a fixed genome. Dialogues Clin Neurosci 7:103–123, 2005

Melchitzky DS, Lewis DA: Tyrosine hydroxylase- and dopamine transporter-immunoreactive axons in the primate cerebellum: evidence for a lobular- and laminar-specific dopamine innervation. Neuropsychopharmacology 22:466–472, 2000

Mendez MF, Cummings JL, Benson DF: Depression in epilepsy: significance and phenomenology. Arch Neurol 43:766–770, 1986

Mendez MF, Lanska DJ, Manon-Espaillat R, et al: Causative factors for suicide attempts by overdose in epileptics. Arch Neurol 46:1065–1068, 1989

Menon V, Rivera SM, White CD, et al: Dissociating prefrontal and parietal cortex activation during arithmetic processing. Neuroimage 12:357–365, 2000

Metz-Lutz MN, Kleitz C, de Saint Martin A, et al: Cognitive development in benign focal epilepsies of childhood. Dev Neurosci 21:182–190, 1999

Michaud LJ, Duhaime AC, Batshaw ML: Traumatic brain injury in children. Pediatr Clin North Am 40:553–565, 1993a

Michaud LJ, Rivara FP, Jaffe KM, et al: Traumatic brain injury as a risk factor for behavioral disorders in children. Arch Phys Med Rehabil 74:368–375, 1993b

Michelucci R, Poza JJ, Sofia V, et al: Autosomal dominant lateral temporal epilepsy: clinical spectrum, new epitempin mutations, and genetic heterogeneity in seven European families. Epilepsia 44:1289–1297, 2003

Mill J, Richards S, Knight J, et al: Haplotype analysis of SNAP-25 suggests a role in the aetiology of ADHD. Mol Psychiatry 9:801–810, 2004

Mill J, Xu X, Ronald A, et al: Quantitative trait locus analysis of candidate gene alleles associated with attention deficit hyperactivity disorder (ADHD) in five genes: *DRD4, DAT1, DRD5, SNAP-25,* and *5HT1B.* Am J Med Genet B Neuropsychiatr Genet 133:68–73, 2005

Miller FE, Heffner TG, Kotake C, et al: Magnitude and duration of hyperactivity following neonatal 6-hydroxydopamine is related to the extent of brain dopamine depletion. Brain Res 229:123–132, 1981

Miller JN, Ozonoff S: The external validity of Asperger disorder: lack of evidence from the domain of neuropsychology. J Abnorm Psychol 109:227–238, 2000

Minshew NJ: Indices of neural function in autism: clinical and biologic implications. Pediatrics 87:774–780, 1991

Molfese DL, Freeman RB Jr, Palermo DS: The ontogeny of brain lateralization for speech and nonspeech stimuli. Brain Lang 2:356–368, 1975

Molloy CA, Manning-Courtney P, Swayne S, et al: Lack of benefit of intravenous synthetic human secretin in the treatment of autism. J Autism Dev Disord 32:545–551, 2002

Monastra VJ, Lynn S, Linden M, et al: Electroencephalographic biofeedback in the treatment of attention-deficit/hyperactivity disorder. Appl Psychophysiol Biofeedback 30:95–114, 2005

Monuteaux MC, Faraone SV, Herzig K, et al: ADHD and dyscalculia: evidence for independent familial transmission. J Learn Disabil 38:86–93, 2005

Moore CJ, Daly EM, Schmitz N, et al: A neuropsychological investigation of male premutation carriers of fragile X syndrome. Neuropsychologia 42:1934–1947, 2004

Morton LL: Interhemispheric balance patterns detected by selective phonemic dichotic laterality measures in four clinical subtypes of reading-disabled children. J Clin Exp Neuropsychol 16:556–567, 1994

Mostofsky SH, Reiss AL, Lockhart P, et al: Evaluation of cerebellar size in attention-deficit hyperactivity disorder. J Child Neurol 13:434–439, 1998

Motavalli Mukaddes N, Abali O: Venlafaxine in children and adolescents with attention deficit hyperactivity disorder. Psychiatry Clin Neurosci 58:92–95, 2004

MTA Cooperative Group: A 14-month randomized clinical trial of treatment strategies for attention-deficit/hyperactivity disorder. The MTA Cooperative Group Multimodal Treatment Study of Children with ADHD. Arch Gen Psychiatry 56:1073–1086, 1999

MTA Cooperative Group: National Institute of Mental Health Multimodal Treatment Study of ADHD follow-up: changes in effectiveness and growth after the end of treatment. Pediatrics 113:762–769, 2004

Mula M, Trimble MR, Lhatoo SD, et al: Topiramate and psychiatric adverse events in patients with epilepsy. Epilepsia 44:659–663, 2003a

Mula M, Trimble MR, Thompson P, et al: Topiramate and word-finding difficulties in patients with epilepsy. Neurology 60:1104–1107, 2003b

Muller N, Putz A, Klages U, et al: Blunted growth hormone response to clonidine in Gilles de la Tourette syndrome. Psychoneuroendocrinology 19:335–341, 1994

Muller N, Kroll B, Schwarz MJ, et al: Increased titers of antibodies against streptococcal M12 and M19 proteins in patients with Tourette's syndrome. Psychiatry Res 101:187–193, 2001

Mulley JC, Scheffer IE, Petrou S, et al: Channelopathies as a genetic cause of epilepsy. Curr Opin Neurol 16:171–176, 2003

Murphy TK, Goodman WK, Ayoub EM, et al: On defining Sydenham's chorea: where do we draw the line? Biol Psychiatry 47:851–857, 2000

Nagai T, Obata K, Tonoki H, et al: Cause of sudden, unexpected death of Prader-Willi syndrome patients with or without growth hormone treatment. Am J Med Genet A 136:45–48, 2005

Nash JK: Treatment of attention deficit hyperactivity disorder with neurotherapy. Clin Electroencephalogr 31:30–37, 2000

Navalta CP, Tomoda A, Teicher MH: Trajectories of neurobehavioral development: the clinical neuroscience of child abuse, in Stress, Trauma, and Children's Memory Development: Neurobiological, Cognitive, and Clinical Perspectives. Edited by Howe ML, Goodman GS, Cicchetti D. Oxford, UK, Oxford University Press (in press)

Naylor MW, Staskowski M, Kenney MC, et al: Language disorders and learning disabilities in school-refusing adolescents. J Am Acad Child Adolesc Psychiatry 33:1331–1337, 1994

Nicholls RD, Knoll JH, Butler MG, et al: Genetic imprinting suggested by maternal heterodisomy in nondeletion Prader-Willi syndrome. Nature 342:281–285, 1989

Nielsen JB, Friberg L, Lou H, et al: Immature pattern of brain activity in Rett syndrome. Arch Neurol 47:982–986, 1990

Niemeyer MI, Yusef YR, Cornejo I, et al: Functional evaluation of human ClC-2 chloride channel mutations associated with idiopathic generalized epilepsies. Physiol Genomics 19:74–83, 2004

Njiokiktjien C: Dyslexia: a neuroscientific puzzle. Acta Paedopsychiatr 56:157–167, 1994

Nolan EE, Gadow KD, Sprafkin J: Teacher reports of DSM-IV ADHD, ODD, and CD symptoms in schoolchildren. J Am Acad Child Adolesc Psychiatry 40:241–249, 2001

Nordin V, Gillberg C: The long-term course of autistic disorders: update on follow-up studies. Acta Psychiatr Scand 97:99–108, 1998

Novick B, Vaughan HG Jr, Kurtzberg D, et al: An electrophysiologic indication of auditory processing defects in autism. Psychiatry Res 3:107–114, 1980

Nurmi EL, Amin T, Olson LM, et al: Dense linkage disequilibrium mapping in the 15q11-q13 maternal expression domain yields evidence for association in autism. Mol Psychiatry 8:624–634, 2003

O'Donnell WT, Warren ST: A decade of molecular studies of fragile X syndrome. Annu Rev Neurosci 25:315–338, 2002

Olvera RL, Pliszka SR, Luh J, et al: An open trial of venlafaxine in the treatment of attention-deficit/hyperactivity disorder in children and adolescents. J Child Adolesc Psychopharmacol 6:241–250, 1996

Opitz JM: Vision and insight in the search for gene mutations causing nonsyndromal mental deficiency. Neurology 55:328–330, 2000

Ornitz EM: The modulation of sensory input and motor output in autistic children. J Autism Child Schizophr 4:197–215, 1974

Ornitz EM, Ritvo ER: Perceptual inconstancy in early infantile autism: the syndrome of early infant autism and its variants including certain cases of childhood schizophrenia. Arch Gen Psychiatry 18:76–98, 1968

Osterling JA, Dawson G, Munson JA: Early recognition of 1-year-old infants with autism spectrum disorder versus mental retardation. Dev Psychopathol 14:239–251, 2002

Overmeyer S, Simmons A, Santosh J, et al: Corpus callosum may be similar in children with ADHD and siblings of children with ADHD. Dev Med Child Neurol 42:8–13, 2000

Ozbay F, Wigg KG, Turanli ET, et al: Analysis of the dopamine beta hydroxylase gene in Gilles de la Tourette syndrome. Am J Med Genet B Neuropsychiatr Genet 141:673–677, 2006

Pakalnis A, Paolicchi J: Psychogenic seizures after head injury in children. J Child Neurol 15:78–80, 2000

Paracchini S, Thomas A, Castro S, et al: The chromosome 6p22 haplotype associated with dyslexia reduces the expression of KIAA0319, a novel gene involved in neuronal migration. Hum Mol Genet 15:1659–1666, 2006

Pardridge WM, Gorski RA, Lippe BM, et al: Androgens and sexual behavior. Ann Intern Med 96:488–501, 1982

Park JP, Wurster-Hill DH, Andrews PA, et al: Free proximal trisomy 21 without the Down syndrome. Clin Genet 32:342–348, 1987

Pauls DL, Leckman JF: The inheritance of Gilles de la Tourette's syndrome and associated behaviors: evidence for autosomal dominant transmission. N Engl J Med 315:993–997, 1986

Pauls DL, Raymond CL, Stevenson JM, et al: A family study of Gilles de la Tourette syndrome. Am J Hum Genet 48:154–163, 1991

Paus T, Zijdenbos A, Worsley K, et al: Structural maturation of neural pathways in children and adolescents: in vivo study. Science 283:1908–1911, 1999

Pavone A, Niedermeyer E: Absence seizures and the frontal lobe. Clin Electroencephalogr 31:153–156, 2000

Pavone P, Bianchini R, Parano E, et al: Anti-brain antibodies in PANDAS versus uncomplicated streptococcal infection. Pediatr Neurol 30:107–110, 2004

Payton A, Holmes J, Barrett JH, et al: Examining for association between candidate gene polymorphisms in the dopamine pathway and attention-deficit hyperactivity disorder: a family based study. Am J Med Genet 105:464–470, 2001

Pearson DE, Teicher MH, Shaywitz BA, et al: Environmental influences on body weight and behavior in developing rats after neonatal 6-hydroxydopamine. Science 209:715–717, 1980

Pelham WE Jr, Sturges J, Hoza J, et al: Sustained release and standard methylphenidate effects on cognitive and social behavior in children with attention deficit disorder. Pediatrics 80:491–501, 1987

Pelham WE Jr, Greenslade KE, Vodde-Hamilton M, et al: Relative efficacy of long-acting stimulants on children with attention deficit-hyperactivity disorder: a comparison of standard methylphenidate, sustained-release methylphenidate, sustained-release dextroamphetamine, and pemoline. Pediatrics 86:226–237, 1990

Pelham WE Jr, Swanson JM, Furman MB, et al: Pemoline effects on children with ADHD: a time-response by dose-response analysis on classroom measures. J Am Acad Child Adolesc Psychiatry 34:1504–1513, 1995

Pelham WE Jr, Gnagy EM, Burrows-Maclean L, et al: Once-a-day Concerta methylphenidate versus three-times-daily methylphenidate in laboratory and natural settings. Pediatrics 107:E105, 2001

Pellock JM: Treatment of seizures and epilepsy in children and adolescents. Neurology 51:S8–S14, 1998

Pennington BF, Smith SD: Genetic influences on learning disabilities and speech and language disorders. Child Dev 54:369–387, 1983

Perez MM, Trimble MR: Epileptic psychosis: diagnostic comparison with process schizophrenia. Br J Psychiatry 137:245–249, 1980

Perlmutter SJ, Leitman SF, Garvey MA, et al: Therapeutic plasma exchange and intravenous immunoglobulin for obsessive-compulsive disorder and tic disorders in childhood. Lancet 354:1153–1158, 1999

Perner J, Frith U, Leslie AM, et al: Exploration of the autistic child's theory of mind: knowledge, belief, and communication. Child Dev 60:688–700, 1989

Peterson B, Riddle MA, Cohen DJ, et al: Reduced basal ganglia volumes in Tourette's syndrome using three-dimensional reconstruction techniques from magnetic resonance images. Neurology 43:941–949, 1993

Peterson BS, Leckman JF, Duncan JS, et al: Corpus callosum morphology from magnetic resonance images in Tourette's syndrome. Psychiatry Res 55:85–99, 1994

Peterson BS, Skudlarski P, Anderson AW, et al: A functional magnetic resonance imaging study of tic suppression in Tourette syndrome. Arch Gen Psychiatry 55:326–333, 1998

Peterson BS, Staib L, Scahill L, et al: Regional brain and ventricular volumes in Tourette syndrome. Arch Gen Psychiatry 58:427–440, 2001

Peterson BS, Thomas P, Kane MJ, et al: Basal ganglia volumes in patients with Gilles de la Tourette syndrome. Arch Gen Psychiatry 60:415–424, 2003

Pierce K, Muller RA, Ambrose J, et al: Face processing occurs outside the fusiform "face area" in autism: evidence from functional MRI. Brain 124:2059–2073, 2001

Pihl RO, Parkes M: Hair element content in learning disabled children. Science 198:204–206, 1977

Pinter JD, Brown WE, Eliez S, et al: Amygdala and hippocampal volumes in children with Down syndrome: a high-resolution MRI study. Neurology 56:972–974, 2001a

Pinter JD, Eliez S, Schmitt JE, et al: Neuroanatomy of Down's syndrome: a high-resolution MRI study. Am J Psychiatry 158:1659–1665, 2001b

Pisano T, Marini C, Brovedani P, et al: Abnormal phonologic processing in familial lateral temporal lobe epilepsy due to a new LGI1 mutation. Epilepsia 46:118–123, 2005

Piven J, Berthier ML, Starkstein SE, et al: Magnetic resonance imaging evidence for a defect of cerebral cortical development in autism. Am J Psychiatry 147:734–739, 1990

Piven J, Tsai GC, Nehme E, et al: Platelet serotonin, a possible marker for familial autism. J Autism Dev Disord 21:51–59, 1991

Plante E: MRI findings in the parents and siblings of specifically language-impaired boys. Brain Lang 41:67–80, 1991

Pleak RR, Gormly LJ: Effects of venlafaxine treatment for ADHD in a child. Am J Psychiatry 152:1099, 1995

Pliszka SR, Browne RG, Olvera RL, et al: A double-blind, placebo-controlled study of Adderall and methylphenidate in the treatment of attention-deficit/hyperactivity disorder. J Am Acad Child Adolesc Psychiatry 39:619–626, 2000

Popper CW: Antidepressants in the treatment of attention-deficit/hyperactivity disorder. J Clin Psychiatry 58 (suppl 14):14–31, 1997

Popper CW, Steingard RJ: Disorders usually first diagnosed in infancy, childhood, or adolescence, in The American Psychiatric Press Textbook of Psychiatry, Second Edition. Edited by Hales RE, Yudofsky SC, Talbott JA. Washington, DC, American Psychiatric Press, 1995, pp 729–832

Porrino LJ, Rapoport JL, Behar D, et al: A naturalistic assessment of the motor activity of hyperactive boys, I: comparison with normal controls. Arch Gen Psychiatry 40:681–687, 1983

Posey DI, Litwiller M, Koburn A, et al: Paroxetine in autism. J Am Acad Child Adolesc Psychiatry 38:111–112, 1999

Post RM, Leverich GS, Xing G, et al: Developmental vulnerabilities to the onset and course of bipolar disorder. Dev Psychopathol 13:581–598, 2001

Prasher VP, Haque MS: Apolipoprotein E, Alzheimer's disease, and Down's syndrome. Br J Psychiatry 177:469–470, 2000

Prior M, Sanson A: Attention deficit disorder with hyperactivity: a critique. J Child Psychol Psychiatry 27:307–319, 1986

Purper-Ouakil D, Wohl M, Mouren MC, et al: Meta-analysis of family based association studies between the dopamine transporter gene and attention deficit hyperactivity disorder. Psychiatr Genet 15:53–59, 2005

Purves D, Lichtman JW: Elimination of synapses in the developing nervous system. Science 210:153–157, 1980

Rabey JM, Lewis A, Graff E, et al: Decreased (3H) quinuclidinyl benzilate binding to lymphocytes in Gilles de la Tourette syndrome. Biol Psychiatry 31:889–895, 1992

Rakic P: Development of the primate cerebral cortex, in Child and Adolescent Psychiatry. Edited by Lewis M. Baltimore, MD, Williams & Wilkins, 1991, pp 11–28

Ramus F, Rosen S, Dakin SC, et al: Theories of developmental dyslexia: insights from a multiple case study of dyslexic adults. Brain 126:841–865, 2003

Rangno RE, Kaufmann JS, Cavanaugh JH, et al: Effects of a false neurotransmitter, p-hydroxynorephedrine, on the function of adrenergic neurons in hypertensive patients. J Clin Invest 52:952–960, 1973

Rapoport JL, Buchsbaum MS, Weingartner H, et al: Dextroamphetamine: its cognitive and behavioral effects in normal and hyperactive boys and normal men. Arch Gen Psychiatry 37:933–943, 1980

Raskin LA, Shaywitz BA, Anderson GM, et al: Differential effects of selective dopamine, norepinephrine or catecholamine depletion on activity and learning in the developing rat. Pharmacol Biochem Behav 19:743–749, 1983

Rausch R: Epilepsy surgery within the temporal lobe and its short-term and long-term effects on memory. Curr Opin Neurol 15:185–189, 2002

Reiss AL, Faruque F, Naidu S, et al: Neuroanatomy of Rett syndrome: a volumetric imaging study. Ann Neurol 34:227–234, 1993

Renieri A, Pescucci C, Longo I, et al: Non-syndromic X-linked mental retardation: from a molecular to a clinical point of view. J Cell Physiol 204:8–20, 2005

Rett A: Uber Ein Zerebral-Atrophisches Syndrom Bei Hyperammonamie. Vienna, Austria, Bruder Hollinek, 1966

Rice D, Barone S Jr: Critical periods of vulnerability for the developing nervous system: evidence from humans and animal models. Environ Health Perspect 108 (suppl 3):511–533, 2000

Richardson AJ, Montgomery P: The Oxford-Durham study: a randomized, controlled trial of dietary supplementation with fatty acids in children with developmental coordination disorder. Pediatrics 115:1360–1366, 2005

Riikonen R: Infantile spasms: therapy and outcome. J Child Neurol 19:401–404, 2004

Ritvo ER, Yuwiler A, Geller E, et al: Increased blood serotonin and platelets in early infantile autism. Arch Gen Psychiatry 23:566–572, 1970

Ritvo ER, Freeman BJ, Geller E, et al: Effects of fenfluramine on 14 outpatients with the syndrome of autism. J Am Acad Child Psychiatry 22:549–558, 1983

Ritvo ER, Freeman BJ, Mason-Brothers A, et al: Concordance for the syndrome of autism in 40 pairs of afflicted twins. Am J Psychiatry 142:74–77, 1985

Ritvo ER, Freeman BJ, Yuwiler A, et al: Fenfluramine treatment of autism: UCLA collaborative study of 81 patients at nine medical centers. Psychopharmacol Bull 22:133–140, 1986

Ritzen EM, Lindgren AC, Hagenas L, et al: Growth hormone treatment of patients with Prader-Willi syndrome: Swedish Growth Hormone Advisory Group. J Pediatr Endocrinol Metab 12 (suppl 1):345–349, 1999

Riva D, Giorgi C: The cerebellum contributes to higher functions during development: evidence from a series of children surgically treated for posterior fossa tumours. Brain 123 (pt 5):1051–1061, 2000

Rivara JB, Jaffe KM, Fay GC, et al: Family functioning and injury severity as predictors of child functioning one year following traumatic brain injury. Arch Phys Med Rehabil 74:1047–1055, 1993

Rivera SM, Reiss AL, Eckert MA, et al: Developmental changes in mental arithmetic: evidence for increased functional specialization in the left inferior parietal cortex. Cereb Cortex 15:1779–1790, 2005

Robin AL, Foster SL: Negotiating Parent-Adolescent Conflict: A Behavioral-Family Systems Approach. New York, Guilford, 1989

Robins PM: A comparison of behavioral and attentional functioning in children diagnosed as hyperactive or learning-disabled. J Abnorm Child Psychol 20:65–82, 1992

Robison LM, Skaer TL, Sclar DA, et al: Is attention deficit hyperactivity disorder increasing among girls in the US? Trends in diagnosis and the prescribing of stimulants. CNS Drugs 16:129–137, 2002

Rodin E, Schmaltz S: The Bear-Fedio Personality Inventory and temporal lobe epilepsy. Neurology 34:591–596, 1984

Roman T, Schmitz M, Polanczyk GV, et al: Is the alpha-2A adrenergic receptor gene (ADRA2A) associated with attention-deficit/hyperactivity disorder? Am J Med Genet B Neuropsychiatr Genet 120:116–120, 2003

Roof E, Stone W, MacLean W, et al: Intellectual characteristics of Prader-Willi syndrome: comparison of genetic subtypes. J Intellect Disabil Res 44 (pt 1):25–30, 2000

Ropers HH, Hamel BC: X-linked mental retardation. Nat Rev Genet 6:46–57, 2005

Ropers HH, Hoeltzenbein M, Kalscheuer V, et al: Nonsyndromic X-linked mental retardation: where are the missing mutations? Trends Genet 19:316–320, 2003

Rosner BS: Recovery of function and localization of function in historical perspective, in Plasticity and Recovery of Function in the Central Nervous System. Edited by Stein DG, Rosen JJ, Butters N. New York, Academic Press, 1974, pp 1–29

Ross DL, Klykylo WM, Hitzemann R: Reduction of elevated CSF beta-endorphin by fenfluramine in infantile autism. Pediatr Neurol 3:83–86, 1987

Rothner AD: Epilepsy, in Child and Adolescent Neurology for Psychiatrists. Edited by Kaufman DM, Solomon GE, Pfeffer CR. Baltimore, MD, Williams & Wilkins, 1992, pp 96–113

Rowe KJ, Rowe KS: The relationship between inattentiveness in the classroom and reading achievement (Part B): an explanatory study. J Am Acad Child Adolesc Psychiatry 31:357–368, 1992

Rowland AS, Lesesne CA, Abramowitz AJ: The epidemiology of attention-deficit/hyperactivity disorder (ADHD): a public health view. Ment Retard Dev Disabil Res Rev 8:162–170, 2002

Rubia K, Overmeyer S, Taylor E, et al: Hypofrontality in attention deficit hyperactivity disorder during higher-order motor control: a study with functional MRI. Am J Psychiatry 156:891–896, 1999

Rugino TA, Samsock TC: Modafinil in children with attention-deficit hyperactivity disorder. Pediatr Neurol 29:136–142, 2003

Rumble B, Retallack R, Hilbich C, et al: Amyloid A4 protein and its precursor in Down's syndrome and Alzheimer's disease. N Engl J Med 320:1446–1452, 1989

Rumsey JM, Andreason P, Zametkin AJ, et al: Failure to activate the left temporoparietal cortex in dyslexia: an oxygen 15 positron emission tomographic study. Arch Neurol 49:527–534, 1992

Russo DC, Navalta CP: Some new dimensions of behavioral analysis and therapy, in Behavioral Approaches for Children and Adolescents: Challenges for the Next Century. Edited by Van Bilsen HPJG, Kendall PC, Slavenberg JH. New York, Plenum, 1995, pp 19–39

Rutter M: Aetiology of autism: findings and questions. J Intellect Disabil Res 49:231–238, 2005a

Rutter M: Incidence of autism spectrum disorders: changes over time and their meaning. Acta Paediatr 94:2–15, 2005b

Rutter M: Genes and Behavior. Malden, MA, Blackwell, 2006

Rutter M, Yule W: The concept of specific reading retardation. J Child Psychol Psychiatry 16:181–197, 1975

Sacks O: Awakenings. Cambridge, MA, Da Capo Press, 1976

Safer DJ, Krager JM: A survey of medication treatment for hyperactive/inattentive students. JAMA 260:2256–2258, 1988

Sallee FR, Sethuraman G, Rock CM: Effects of pimozide on cognition in children with Tourette syndrome: interaction with comorbid attention deficit hyperactivity disorder. Acta Psychiatr Scand 90:4–9, 1994

Sanberg PR, Silver AA, Shytle RD, et al: Nicotine for the treatment of Tourette's syndrome. Pharmacol Ther 74:21–25, 1997

Sanchez MM, Hearn EF, Do D, et al: Differential rearing affects corpus callosum size and cognitive function of rhesus monkeys. Brain Res 812:38–49, 1998

Sandler AD, Sutton KA, DeWeese J, et al: Lack of benefit of a single dose of synthetic human secretin in the treatment of autism and pervasive developmental disorder. N Engl J Med 341:1801–1806, 1999

Sandson TA, Manoach DS, Price BH, et al: Right hemisphere learning disability associated with left hemisphere dysfunction: anomalous dominance and development. J Neurol Neurosurg Psychiatry 57:1129–1132, 1994

Satterfield JH, Hoppe CM, Schell AM: A prospective study of delinquency in 110 adolescent boys with attention deficit disorder and 88 normal adolescent boys. Am J Psychiatry 139:795–798, 1982

Savic I, Lekvall A, Greitz D, et al: MR spectroscopy shows reduced frontal lobe concentrations of N-acetyl aspartate in patients with juvenile myoclonic epilepsy. Epilepsia 41:290–296, 2000

Schachter SC, Galaburda AM: Development and biological associations of cerebral dominance: review and possible mechanisms. J Am Acad Child Psychiatry 25:741–750, 1986

Schapel G, Chadwick D: Tiagabine and non-convulsive status epilepticus. Seizure 5:153–156, 1996

Schmahmann JD, Pandya DN: Prefrontal cortex projections to the basilar pons in rhesus monkey: implications for the cerebellar contribution to higher function. Neurosci Lett 199:175–178, 1995

Schmidt D, Bourgeois B: A risk-benefit assessment of therapies for Lennox-Gastaut syndrome. Drug Saf 22:467–477, 2000

Schmitz B: Psychiatric syndromes related to antiepileptic drugs. Epilepsia 40 (suppl 10):S65–S70, 1999

Schoechlin C, Engel RR: Neuropsychological performance in adult attention-deficit hyperactivity disorder: meta-analysis of empirical data. Arch Clin Neuropsychol 20:727–744, 2005

Schrott LM, Denenberg VH, Sherman GF, et al: Environmental enrichment, neocortical ectopias, and behavior in the autoimmune NZB mouse. Brain Res Dev Brain Res 67:85–93, 1992

Schultz RT: Developmental deficits in social perception in autism: the role of the amygdala and fusiform face area. Int J Dev Neurosci 23:125–141, 2005

Schultz RT, Gauthier I, Klin A, et al: Abnormal ventral temporal cortical activity during face discrimination among individuals with autism and Asperger syndrome. Arch Gen Psychiatry 57:331–340, 2000

Schwarz JR, Grigat G: Phenytoin and carbamazepine: potential- and frequency-dependent block of Na currents in mammalian myelinated nerve fibers. Epilepsia 30:286–294, 1989

Schweitzer JB, Anderson C, Ernst M: ADHD: neuroimaging and behavioral/cognitive probes, in Functional Neuroimaging in Child Psychiatry. Edited by Ernst M, Rumsey JM. Cambridge, England, Cambridge University Press, 2000, 278–297

Seeman P, Madras BK: Anti-hyperactivity medication: methylphenidate and amphetamine. Mol Psychiatry 3:386–396, 1998

Seeman P, Bzowej NH, Guan HC, et al: Human brain dopamine receptors in children and aging adults. Synapse 1:399–404, 1987

Seghorn TK, Prentky RA, Boucher RJ: Childhood sexual abuse in the lives of sexually aggressive offenders. J Am Acad Child Adolesc Psychiatry 26:262–267, 1987

Seltzer MM, Shattuck P, Abbeduto L, et al: Trajectory of development in adolescents and adults with autism. Ment Retard Dev Disabil Res Rev 10:234–247, 2004

Semrud-Clikeman M, Hynd GW: Right hemispheric dysfunction in nonverbal learning disabilities: social, academic, and adaptive functioning in adults and children. Psychol Bull 107:196–209, 1990

Semrud-Clikeman M, Biederman J, Sprich-Buckminster S, et al: Comorbidity between ADDH and learning disability: a review and report in a clinically referred sample. J Am Acad Child Adolesc Psychiatry 31:439–448, 1992

Semrud-Clikeman M, Filipek PA, Biederman J, et al: Attention-deficit hyperactivity disorder: magnetic resonance imaging morphometric analysis of the corpus callosum. J Am Acad Child Adolesc Psychiatry 33:875–881, 1994

Shalev RS: Developmental dyscalculia. J Child Neurol 19:765–771, 2004

Shao Y, Cuccaro ML, Hauser ER, et al: Fine mapping of autistic disorder to chromosome 15q11-q13 by use of phenotypic subtypes. Am J Hum Genet 72:539–548, 2003

Shaw P, Greenstein D, Lerch J, et al: Intellectual ability and cortical development in children and adolescents. Nature 440:676–679, 2006a

Shaw P, Lerch J, Greenstein D, et al: Longitudinal mapping of cortical thickness and clinical outcome in children and adolescents with attention-deficit/hyperactivity disorder. Arch Gen Psychiatry 63:540–549, 2006b

Shaywitz BA, Klopper JH, Yager RD, et al: Paradoxical response to amphetamine in developing rats treated with 6-hydroxydopamine. Nature 261:153–155, 1976a

Shaywitz BA, Yager RD, Klopper JH: Selective brain dopamine depletion in developing rats: an experimental model of minimal brain dysfunction. Science 191:305–308, 1976b

Shaywitz BA, Teicher MII, Cohen DJ, et al: Dopaminergic but not noradrenergic mediation of hyperactivity and performance deficits in the developing rat pup. Psychopharmacology 82:73–77, 1984

Shaywitz BA, Fletcher JM, Shaywitz SE: Defining and classifying learning disabilities and attention-deficit/hyperactivity disorder. J Child Neurol 10 (suppl 1):S50–S57, 1995

Shaywitz BA, Shaywitz SE, Blachman B, et al: Development of left occipitotemporal systems for skilled reading in children after a phonologically based intervention. Biol Psychiatry 55:926–933, 2004

Shaywitz SE, Shaywitz BA: Dyslexia (specific reading disability). Biol Psychiatry 57:1301–1309, 2005

Shaywitz SE, Escobar MD, Shaywitz BA, et al: Evidence that dyslexia may represent the lower tail of a normal distribution of reading ability. N Engl J Med 326:145–150, 1992

Sheng JG, Mrak RE, Griffin WS: S100 beta protein expression in Alzheimer disease: potential role in the pathogenesis of neuritic plaques. J Neurosci Res 39:398–404, 1994

Shevell M, Ashwal S, Donley D, et al: Practice parameter: evaluation of the child with global developmental delay: report of the Quality Standards Subcommittee of the American Academy of Neurology and the Practice Committee of the Child Neurology Society. Neurology 60:367–380, 2003

Short EJ, Manos MJ, Findling RL, et al: A prospective study of stimulant response in preschool children: insights from ROC analyses. J Am Acad Child Adolesc Psychiatry 43:251–259, 2004

Sidman RL, Rakic P: Neuronal migration, with special reference to developing human brain: a review. Brain Res 62:1–35, 1973

Sieg KG, Gaffney GR, Preston DF, et al: SPECT brain imaging abnormalities in attention deficit hyperactivity disorder. Clin Nucl Med 20:55–60, 1995

Siegel B, Pliner C, Eschler J, et al: How children with autism are diagnosed: difficulties in identification of children with multiple developmental delays. J Dev Behav Pediatr 9:199–204, 1988

Sigurdardottir KR, Olafsson E: Incidence of psychogenic seizures in adults: a population-based study in Iceland. Epilepsia 39:749–752, 1998

Sills GJ: The mechanisms of action of gabapentin and pregabalin. Curr Opin Pharmacol 6:108–113, 2006

Silver AA, Shytle RD, Philipp MK, et al: Transdermal nicotine and haloperidol in Tourette's disorder: a double-blind placebo-controlled study. J Clin Psychiatry 62:707–714, 2001

Simonds RJ, Scheibel AB: The postnatal development of the motor speech area: a preliminary study. Brain Lang 37:42–58, 1989

Simos PG, Breier JI, Fletcher JM, et al: Brain activation profiles in dyslexic children during non-word reading: a magnetic source imaging study. Neurosci Lett 290:61–65, 2000

Singer HS: Tourette's syndrome: from behaviour to biology. Lancet Neurol 4:149–159, 2005

Singer HS, Hahn IH, Moran TH: Abnormal dopamine uptake sites in postmortem striatum from patients with Tourette's syndrome. Ann Neurol 30:558–562, 1991

Singer HS, Reiss AL, Brown JE, et al: Volumetric MRI changes in basal ganglia of children with Tourette's syndrome. Neurology 43:950–956, 1993

Singer HS, Brown J, Quaskey S, et al: The treatment of attention-deficit hyperactivity disorder in Tourette's syndrome: a double-blind placebo-controlled study with clonidine and desipramine. Pediatrics 95:74–81, 1995

Singer HS, Giuliano JD, Hansen BH, et al: Antibodies against human putamen in children with Tourette syndrome. Neurology 50:1618–1624, 1998

Singer HS, Giuliano JD, Hansen BH, et al: Antibodies against a neuron-like (HTB-10 neuroblastoma) cell in children with Tourette syndrome. Biol Psychiatry 46:775–780, 1999

Singer HS, Loiselle CR, Lee O, et al: Anti-basal ganglia antibodies in PANDAS. Mov Disord 19:406–415, 2004

Sininger YS, Doyle KJ, Moore JK: The case for early identification of hearing loss in children: auditory system development, experimental auditory deprivation, and development of speech perception and hearing. Pediatr Clin North Am 46:1–14, 1999

Siomi MC, Siomi H, Sauer WH, et al: FXR1, an autosomal homolog of the fragile X mental retardation gene. EMBO J 14:2401–2408, 1995

Skottun BC: The magnocellular deficit theory of dyslexia: the evidence from contrast sensitivity. Vision Res 40:111–127, 2000

Smith KT, Coffee B, Reines D: Occupancy and synergistic activation of the FMR1 promoter by Nrf-1 and Sp1 in vivo. Hum Mol Genet 13:1611–1621, 2004

Smith T, Mruzek DW, Mozingo D: Sensory integrative therapy, in Controversial Therapies for Developmental Disabilities: Fad, Fashion and Science in Professional Practice. Edited by Jacobson JW, Foxx RM, Mulick JA. Mahwah, NJ, Lawrence Erlbaum, 2005, pp 331–350

Snider LA, Swedo SE: PANDAS: current status and directions for research. Mol Psychiatry 9:900–907, 2004

Snider LA, Lougee L, Slattery M, et al: Antibiotic prophylaxis with azithromycin or penicillin for childhood-onset neuropsychiatric disorders. Biol Psychiatry 57:788–792, 2005

Snook L, Paulson LA, Roy D, et al: Diffusion tensor imaging of neurodevelopment in children and young adults. Neuroimage 26:1164–1173, 2005

Sollee ND, Kindlon DJ: Lateralized brain injury and behavior problems in children. J Abnorm Child Psychol 15:479–491, 1987

Sowell ER, Thompson PM, Rex D, et al: Mapping sulcal pattern asymmetry and local cortical surface gray matter distribution in vivo: maturation in perisylvian cortices. Cereb Cortex 12:17–26, 2002

Sowell ER, Thompson PM, Welcome SE, et al: Cortical abnormalities in children and adolescents with attention-deficit hyperactivity disorder. Lancet 362:1699–1707, 2003

Spencer T, Biederman J, Kerman K, et al: Desipramine treatment of children with attention-deficit hyperactivity disorder and tic disorder or Tourette's syndrome. J Am Acad Child Adolesc Psychiatry 32:354–360, 1993a

Spencer T, Biederman J, Wilens T, et al: Nortriptyline treatment of children with attention-deficit hyperactivity disorder and tic disorder or Tourette's syndrome. J Am Acad Child Adolesc Psychiatry 32:205–210, 1993b

Spencer TJ, Biederman J, Harding M, et al: Growth deficits in ADHD children revisited: evidence for disorder-associated growth delays? J Am Acad Child Adolesc Psychiatry 35:1460–1469, 1996

Spencer T, Biederman J, Wilens T: Attention-deficit/hyperactivity disorder and comorbidity. Pediatr Clin North Am 46:915–927, 1999

Spencer TJ, Biederman J, Wilens TE, et al: Novel treatments for attention-deficit/hyperactivity disorder in children. J Clin Psychiatry 63 (suppl 12):16–22, 2002

Spira EG, Fischel JE: The impact of preschool inattention, hyperactivity, and impulsivity on social and academic development: a review. J Child Psychol Psychiatry 46:755–773, 2005

State MW, Dykens EM: Genetics of childhood disorders, XV: Prader-Willi syndrome: genes, brain, and behavior. J Am Acad Child Adolesc Psychiatry 39:797–800, 2000

State MW, King BH, Dykens E: Mental retardation: a review of the past 10 years, part II. J Am Acad Child Adolesc Psychiatry 36:1664–1671, 1997

State MW, Dykens EM, Rosner B, et al: Obsessive-compulsive symptoms in Prader-Willi and "Prader-Willi-Like" patients. J Am Acad Child Adolesc Psychiatry 38:329–334, 1999

State MW, Pauls DL, Leckman JF: Tourette's syndrome and related disorders. Child Adolesc Psychiatr Clin N Am 10:317–331, 2001

Stein J: The magnocellular theory of developmental dyslexia. Dyslexia 7:12–36, 2001

Stein MB: Hippocampal volume in women victimized by childhood sexual abuse. Psychol Med 27:951–999, 1997

Steingard R, Khan A, Gonzalez A, et al: Neuroleptic malignant syndrome: review of experience with children and adolescents. J Child Adolesc Psychopharmacol 2:183–198, 1992

Steinman SB, Steinman BA, Garzia RP: Vision and attention, II: is visual attention a mechanism through which a deficient magnocellular pathway might cause reading disability? Optom Vis Sci 75:674–681, 1998

Steinmetz H, Volkmann J, Jancke L, et al: Anatomical left-right asymmetry of language-related temporal cortex is different in left- and right-handers. Ann Neurol 29:315–319, 1991

Stevenson J, Graham P, Fredman G, et al: A twin study of genetic influences on reading and spelling ability and disability. J Child Psychol Psychiatry 28:229–247, 1987

Stevenson J, Asherson P, Hay D, et al: Characterizing the ADHD phenotype for genetic studies. Dev Sci 8:115–121, 2005

Stone MH: Borderline syndromes: a consideration of subtypes and an overview, directions for research. Psychiatr Clin North Am 4:3–13, 1981

Streissguth AP, Barr HM, Sampson PD: Moderate prenatal alcohol exposure: effects on child IQ and learning problems at age 7 1/2 years. Alcohol Clin Exp Res 14:662–669, 1990

Stricker EM: Recovery of function following brain damage: implications for motivated ingestive behaviors, in Appetite and Food Intake: Report of the Dahlem Workshop. Edited by Silverstone T. Oxford, England, Abakon Verlagsgesellschaft, 1976

Stromme P, Mangelsdorf ME, Scheffer IE, et al: Infantile spasms, dystonia, and other X-linked phenotypes caused by mutations in Aristaless related homeobox gene, ARX. Brain Dev 24:266–268, 2002a

Stromme P, Mangelsdorf ME, Shaw MA, et al: Mutations in the human ortholog of Aristaless cause X-linked mental retardation and epilepsy. Nat Genet 30:441–445, 2002b

Struve FA, Klein DF, Saraf KR: Electroencephalographic correlates of suicide ideation and attempts. Arch Gen Psychiatry 27:363–365, 1972

Subramaniam B, Naidu S, Reiss AL: Neuroanatomy in Rett syndrome: cerebral cortex and posterior fossa. Neurology 48:399–407, 1997

Sun L, Jin Z, Zang YF, et al: Differences between attention-deficit disorder with and without hyperactivity: a ^{1}H-magnetic resonance spectroscopy study. Brain Dev 27:340–344, 2005

Sunahara RK, Seeman P, Van Tol HH, et al: Dopamine receptors and antipsychotic drug response. Br J Psychiatry Suppl 31–38, 1993

Suri M: The phenotypic spectrum of ARX mutations. Dev Med Child Neurol 47:133–137, 2005

Suzuki DA, Keller EL: The role of the posterior vermis of monkey cerebellum in smooth-pursuit eye movement control, II: target velocity-related Purkinje cell activity. J Neurophysiol 59:19–40, 1988

Suzuki Y, Matsuzawa H, Kwee IL, et al: Absolute eigenvalue diffusion tensor analysis for human brain maturation. NMR Biomed 16:257–260, 2003

Sverd J, Gadow KD, Paolicelli LM: Methylphenidate treatment of attention-deficit hyperactivity disorder in boys with Tourette's syndrome. J Am Acad Child Adolesc Psychiatry 28:574–582, 1989

Swartz BE, Simpkins F, Halgren E, et al: Visual working memory in primary generalized epilepsy: an ^{18}FDG-PET study. Neurology 47:1203–1212, 1996

Swedo SE: Sydenham's chorea: a model for childhood autoimmune neuropsychiatric disorders. JAMA 272:1788–1791, 1994

Swedo SE, Leonard HL, Garvey M, et al: Pediatric autoimmune neuropsychiatric disorders associated with streptococcal infections: clinical description of the first 50 cases. Am J Psychiatry 155:264–271, 1998

Sweeney JA, Strojwas MH, Mann JJ, et al: Prefrontal and cerebellar abnormalities in major depression: evidence from oculomotor studies. Biol Psychiatry 43:584–594, 1998

Szatmari P, Offord DR, Boyle MH: Ontario Child Health Study: prevalence of attention deficit disorder with hyperactivity. J Child Psychol Psychiatry 30:219–230, 1989

Tallal P: Improving language and literacy is a matter of time. Nat Rev Neurosci 5:721–728, 2004

Tallal P: What happens when "dyslexic" subjects do not meet the criteria for dyslexia and sensorimotor tasks are too difficult even for the controls? Dev Sci 9:262–269, 2006

Tallal P, Townsend J, Curtiss S, et al: Phenotypic profiles of language-impaired children based on genetic/family history. Brain Lang 41:81–95, 1991

Tallal P, Miller SL, Bedi G, et al: Language comprehension in language-learning impaired children improved with acoustically modified speech. Science 271:81–84, 1996

Tallian KB, Nahata MC, Lo W, et al: Gabapentin associated with aggressive behavior in pediatric patients with seizures. Epilepsia 37:501–502, 1996

Tamm L, Menon V, Ringel J, et al: Event-related fMRI evidence of frontotemporal involvement in aberrant response inhibition and task switching in attention-deficit/hyperactivity disorder. J Am Acad Child Adolesc Psychiatry 43:1430–1440, 2004

Tannock R: Attention deficit hyperactivity disorder: advances in cognitive, neurobiological, and genetic research. J Child Psychol Psychiatry 39:65–99, 1998

Taylor FB, Russo J: Comparing guanfacine and dextroamphetamine for the treatment of adult attention-deficit/hyperactivity disorder. J Clin Psychopharmacol 21:223–228, 2001

Teicher MH: Psychological factors in neurological development, in Neurobiological Development. Edited by Evrard P, Minkowski A. New York, Raven, 1989, pp 243–258

Teicher MH: Early abuse, limbic system dysfunction, and borderline personality disorder, in Biological and Neurobehavioral Studies of Borderline Personality Disorder. Edited by Silk K. Washington, DC, American Psychiatric Press, 1994, pp 177–207

Teicher MH: Actigraphy and motion analysis: new tools for psychiatry. Harv Rev Psychiatry 3:18–35, 1995

Teicher MH: Scars that won't heal: the neurobiology of child abuse. Sci Am 286:68–75, 2002

Teicher MH: Childhood abuse and regional brain development: evidence for sensitive periods. Paper presented at the annual meeting of the American Academy of Child and Adolescent Psychiatry, Toronto, ON, October, 2005, p 78

Teicher MH, Shaywitz BA, Kootz HL, et al: Differential effects of maternal and sibling presence of hyperactivity of 6-hydroxydopamine-treated developing rats. J Comp Physiol Psychol 95:134–145, 1981

Teicher MH, Andersen SL, Hostetter JC Jr: Evidence for dopamine receptor pruning between adolescence and adulthood in striatum but not nucleus accumbens. Brain Res Dev Brain Res 89:167–172, 1995

Teicher MH, Ito Y, Glod CA, et al: Neurophysiological mechanisms of stress response in children, in Severe Stress and Mental Disturbance in Children. Edited by Pfeffer C. Washington, DC, American Psychiatric Press, 1996a, pp 59–84

Teicher MH, Ito Y, Glod CA, et al: Objective measurement of hyperactivity and attentional problems in ADHD. J Am Acad Child Adolesc Psychiatry 35:334–342, 1996b

Teicher MH, Ito Y, Glod CA, et al: Preliminary evidence for abnormal cortical development in physically and sexually abused children using EEG coherence and MRI, in Psychobiology of Posttraumatic Stress Disorder. Edited by Yehuda R, McFarlane AC. New York, New York Academy of Science, 1997, pp 160–175

Teicher MH, Anderson CM, Polcari A, et al: Functional deficits in basal ganglia of children with attention-deficit/hyperactivity disorder shown with functional magnetic resonance imaging relaxometry. Nat Med 6:470–473, 2000

Teicher MH, Andersen SL, Polcari A, et al: The neurobiological consequences of early stress and childhood maltreatment. Neurosci Biobehav Rev 27:33–44, 2003a

Teicher MH, Polcari A, Anderson CM, et al: Rate dependency revisited: understanding the effects of methylphenidate in children with attention deficit hyperactivity disorder. J Child Adolesc Psychopharmacol 13:41–52, 2003b

Teicher MH, Dumont NL, Ito Y, et al: Childhood neglect is associated with reduced corpus callosum area. Biol Psychiatry 56:80–85, 2004a

Teicher MH, Lowen SB, Polcari A, et al: Novel strategy for the analysis of CPT data provides new insight into the effects of methylphenidate on attentional states in children with ADHD. J Child Adolesc Psychopharmacol 14:219–232, 2004b

Teicher MH, Polcari A, Foley M, et al: Methylphenidate blood levels and therapeutic response in children with ADHD, I: effects of different dosing regimens. J Child Adolesc Psychopharmacol 16:416–431, 2006a

Teicher MH, Samson JA, Polcari A, et al: Sticks, stones, and hurtful words: relative effects of various forms of childhood maltreatment. Am J Psychiatry 163:993–1000, 2006b

Thapar A, Gottesman II, Owen MJ, et al: The genetics of mental retardation. Br J Psychiatry 164:747–758, 1994

Thome-Souza S, Kuczynski E, Assumpcao F Jr, et al: Which factors may play a pivotal role on determining the type of psychiatric disorder in children and adolescents with epilepsy? Epilepsy Behav 5:988–994, 2004

Thompson PM, Giedd JN, Woods RP, et al: Growth patterns in the developing brain detected by using continuum mechanical tensor maps. Nature 404:190–193, 2000

Tourette Syndrome Association International Consortium for Genetics: A complete genome screen in sib pairs affected by Gilles de la Tourette syndrome. Am J Hum Genet 65:1428–1436, 1999

Townsend J, Courchesne E, Covington J, et al: Spatial attention deficits in patients with acquired or developmental cerebellar abnormality. J Neurosci 19:5632–5643, 1999

Tryon WW: The role of motor excess and instrumented activity measurement in attention deficit hyperactivity disorder. Behav Mod 17:371–406, 1993

Turk J: The fragile-X syndrome: on the way to a behavioural phenotype. Br J Psychiatry 160:24–35, 1992

Vaidya CJ, Austin G, Kirkorian G, et al: Selective effects of methylphenidate in attention deficit hyperactivity disorder: a functional magnetic resonance study. Proc Natl Acad Sci U S A 95:14494–14499, 1998

Vaidya CJ, Bunge SA, Dudukovic NM, et al: Altered neural substrates of cognitive control in childhood ADHD: evidence from functional magnetic resonance imaging. Am J Psychiatry 162:1605–1613, 2005

Van Bockstaele EJ, Colago EE, Valentino RJ: Amygdaloid corticotropin-releasing factor targets locus coeruleus dendrites: substrate for the co-ordination of emotional and cognitive limbs of the stress response. J Neuroendocrinol 10:743–757, 1998

van der Kolk B, Greenberg MS: The psychobiology of the trauma response: hyperarousal, constriction, and addiction to traumatic reexposure, in Psychological Trauma. Edited by van der Kolk B. Washington, DC, American Psychiatric Press, 1987, pp 63–87

van Dyck CH, Quinlan DM, Cretella LM, et al: Unaltered dopamine transporter availability in adult attention deficit hyperactivity disorder. Am J Psychiatry 159:309–312, 2002

Varela MC, Lopes GM, Koiffmann CP: Prader-Willi syndrome with an unusually large 15q deletion due to an unbalanced translocation t(4;15). Ann Genet 47:267–273, 2004

Verkerk AJ, Pieretti M, Sutcliffe JS, et al: Identification of a gene (FMR-1) containing a CGG repeat coincident with a breakpoint cluster region exhibiting length variation in fragile X syndrome. Cell 65:905–914, 1991

Volkmar F, Chawarska K, Klin A: Autism in infancy and early childhood. Annu Rev Psychol 56:315–336, 2005

Vythilingam M, Heim C, Newport J, et al: Childhood trauma associated with smaller hippocampal volume in women with major depression. Am J Psychiatry 159:2072–2080, 2002

Wada JA, Clarke R, Hamm A: Cerebral hemispheric asymmetry in humans: cortical speech zones in 100 adults and 100 infant brains. Arch Neurol 32:239–246, 1975

Waiter GD, Williams JH, Murray AD, et al: A voxel-based investigation of brain structure in male adolescents with autistic spectrum disorder. Neuroimage 22:619–625, 2004

Waldman ID, Rowe DC, Abramowitz A, et al: Association and linkage of the dopamine transporter gene and attention-deficit hyperactivity disorder in children: heterogeneity owing to diagnostic subtype and severity. Am J Hum Genet 63:1767–1776, 1998

Walker EF: Developmentally moderated expressions of the neuropathology underlying schizophrenia. Schizophr Bull 20:453–480, 1994

Wang AT, Dapretto M, Hariri AR, et al: Neural correlates of facial affect processing in children and adolescents with autism spectrum disorder. J Am Acad Child Adolesc Psychiatry 43:481–490, 2004

Warren RP, Yonk J, Burger RW, et al: DR-positive T cells in autism: association with decreased plasma levels of the complement C4B protein. Neuropsychobiology 31:53–57, 1995

Wassink TH, Brzustowicz LM, Bartlett CW, et al: The search for autism disease genes. Ment Retard Dev Disabil Res Rev 10:272–283, 2004

Watkins KE, Paus T, Lerch JP, et al: Structural asymmetries in the human brain: a voxel-based statistical analysis of 142 MRI scans. Cereb Cortex 11:868–877, 2001

Watson P, Black G, Ramsden S, et al: Angelman syndrome phenotype associated with mutations in MECP2, a gene encoding a methyl CpG binding protein. J Med Genet 38:224–228, 2001

Webster MJ, Herman MM, Kleinman JE, et al: BDNF and trkB mRNA expression in the hippocampus and temporal cortex during the human lifespan. Gene Expr Patterns 6:941–951, 2006

Weiss G, Hechtman L, Milroy T, et al: Psychiatric status of hyperactives as adults: a controlled prospective 15-year follow-up of 63 hyperactive children. J Am Acad Child Psychiatry 24:211–220, 1985

Weiss M, Tannock R, Kratochvil C, et al: A randomized, placebo-controlled study of once-daily atomoxetine in the school setting in children with ADHD. J Am Acad Child Adolesc Psychiatry 44:647–655, 2005

Weiss RE, Stein MA, Trommer B, et al: Attention-deficit hyperactivity disorder and thyroid function. J Pediatr 123:539–545, 1993

Welsh JP, Ahn ES, Placantonakis DG: Is autism due to brain desynchronization? Int J Dev Neurosci 23:253–263, 2005

Wender PH: Minimal Brain Dysfunction in Children. New York, Wiley, 1971

Wender PH: Methamphetamine in child psychiatry. J Child Adolesc Psychopharmacol 3:iv–vi, 1993

Wenk GL, Naidu S, Casanova MF, et al: Altered neurochemical markers in Rett's syndrome. Neurology 41:1753–1756, 1991

Werner E, Dawson G, Osterling J, et al: Brief report. Recognition of autism spectrum disorder before one year of age: a retrospective study based on home videotapes. J Autism Dev Disord 30:157–162, 2000

White S, Milne E, Rosen S, et al: The role of sensorimotor impairments in dyslexia: a multiple case study of dyslexic children. Dev Sci 9:237–259, 2006

Wigal S, Swanson JM, Feifel D, et al: A double-blind, placebo-controlled trial of dexmethylphenidate hydrochloride and *d,l-threo*-methylphenidate hydrochloride in children with attention-deficit/hyperactivity disorder. J Am Acad Child Adolesc Psychiatry 43:1406–1414, 2004

Wigal SB, McGough JJ, McCracken JT, et al: A laboratory school comparison of mixed amphetamine salts extended release (Adderall XR) and atomoxetine (Strattera) in school-aged children with attention deficit/hyperactivity disorder. J Atten Disord 9:275–289, 2005

Wigren M, Hansen S: ADHD symptoms and insistence on sameness in Prader-Willi syndrome. J Intellect Disabil Res 49:449–456, 2005

Wilbur CB: Multiple personality and child abuse: an overview. Psychiatr Clin North Am 7:3–7, 1984

Wild E: Deja vu in neurology. J Neurol 252:1–7, 2005

Wilens TE, Biederman J: The stimulants. Psychiatr Clin North Am 15:191–222, 1992

Wilens TE, Biederman J, Spencer TJ: Venlafaxine for adult ADHD. Am J Psychiatry 152:1099–1100, 1995

Willcutt EG, Pennington BF, DeFries JC: Twin study of the etiology of comorbidity between reading disability and attention-deficit/hyperactivity disorder. Am J Med Genet 96:293–301, 2000

Williams J: Learning and behavior in children with epilepsy. Epilepsy Behav 4:107–111, 2003

Williams J, Phillips T, Griebel ML, et al: Factors Associated With Academic Achievement in Children with Controlled Epilepsy. Epilepsy Behav 2:217–223, 2001

Williams J, Steel C, Sharp GB, et al: Anxiety in children with epilepsy. Epilepsy Behav 4:729–732, 2003

Williams JG, Higgins JP, Brayne CE: Systematic review of prevalence studies of autism spectrum disorders. Arch Dis Child 91:8–15, 2006

Wimpory DC, Hobson RP, Williams JM, et al: Are infants with autism socially engaged? A study of recent retrospective parental reports. J Autism Dev Disord 30:525–536, 2000

Wing L, Gould J: Severe impairments of social interaction and associated abnormalities in children: epidemiology and classification. J Autism Dev Disord 9:11–29, 1979

Wisniewski KE, Wisniewski HM, Wen GY: Occurrence of neuropathological changes and dementia of Alzheimer's disease in Down's syndrome. Ann Neurol 17:278–282, 1985

Wolf S, Shinnar S, Kang H, et al: Gabapentin toxicity in children manifesting as behavioral changes. Epilepsia 36:1203–1205, 1995

Wolf S, Jones D, Knable M, et al: Tourette syndrome: prediction of phenotypic variation in monozygotic twins by caudate nucleus D_2 receptor binding. Science 273:1225–1227, 1996

Wong DF, Singer HS, Brandt J, et al: D_2-like dopamine receptor density in Tourette syndrome measured by PET. J Nucl Med 38:1243–1247, 1997

World Health Organization: The ICD-10 Classification of Mental and Behavioural Disorders: Clinical Descriptions and Diagnostic Guidelines. Geneva, World Health Organization, 1992

Wyllie E, Rothner AD, Luders H: Partial seizures in children: clinical features, medical treatment, and surgical considerations. Pediatr Clin North Am 36:343–364, 1989

Wyllie E, Glazer JP, Benbadis S, et al: Psychiatric features of children and adolescents with pseudoseizures. Arch Pediatr Adolesc Med 153:244–248, 1999

XLMR Genes Update Website, 2005. Available at: http://xlmr.interfree.it/home.htm. Accessed November 21, 2006.

Xu C, Schachar R, Tannock R, et al: Linkage study of the alpha2A adrenergic receptor in attention-deficit hyperactivity disorder families. Am J Med Genet 105:159–162, 2001

Yeo RA, Hill DE, Campbell RA, et al: Proton magnetic resonance spectroscopy investigation of the right frontal lobe in children with attention-deficit/hyperactivity disorder. J Am Acad Child Adolesc Psychiatry 42:303–310, 2003

Zametkin AJ, Rapoport JL: Neurobiology of attention deficit disorder with hyperactivity: where have we come in 50 years? J Am Acad Child Adolesc Psychiatry 26:676–686, 1987

Zametkin AJ, Karoum F, Linnoila M, et al: Stimulants, urinary catecholamines, and indoleamines in hyperactivity: a comparison of methylphenidate and dextroamphetamine. Arch Gen Psychiatry 42:251–255, 1985

Zametkin AJ, Nordahl TE, Gross M, et al: Cerebral glucose metabolism in adults with hyperactivity of childhood onset. N Engl J Med 323:1361–1366, 1990

Zarnescu DC, Jin P, Betschinger J, et al: Fragile X protein functions with lgl and the par complex in flies and mice. Dev Cell 8:43–52, 2005

Zhang K, Tarazi FI, Baldessarini RJ: Role of dopamine D(4) receptors in motor hyperactivity induced by neonatal 6-hydroxydopamine lesions in rats. Neuropsychopharmacology 25:624–632, 2001

Zimmerman AM, Abrams MT, Giuliano JD, et al: Subcortical volumes in girls with Tourette syndrome: support for a gender effect. Neurology 54:2224–2229, 2000

Zoghbi HY: Postnatal neurodevelopmental disorders: meeting at the synapse? Science 302:826–830, 2003

Zoghbi HY, Percy AK, Glaze DG, et al: Reduction of biogenic amine levels in the Rett syndrome. N Engl J Med 313:921–924, 1985

Zwaigenbaum L, Bryson S, Rogers T, et al: Behavioral manifestations of autism in the first year of life. Int J Dev Neurosci 23:143–152, 2005

Part V

Neuropsychiatric Treatments

30

INTRACELLULAR AND INTERCELLULAR PRINCIPLES OF PHARMACOTHERAPY FOR NEUROPSYCHIATRIC DISORDERS

W. Dale Horst, Ph.D.

Michael J. Burke, M.D., Ph.D.

The technical advances for identifying the genes responsible for specific protein components of the neurotransmission process are revolutionizing psychopharmacology. These molecular biological methods are changing the manner in which new drugs are being discovered, providing more specific knowledge of the biological nature of mental illness, and redefining basic concepts of psychopharmacological therapy and even the lexicon of psychopharmacology.

For example, psychotherapeutic drugs traditionally have been referred to by the disorders that they treat, such as *antidepressants*, *anxiolytics*, and *antipsychotics*. This nomenclature is understandable in the case of drugs such as the tricyclic antidepressants, which have multiple sites of actions and complex pharmacodynamics, but it is inadequate in terms of newer, more specific therapeutic agents. Thus, it has become more common to speak of *benzodiazepine receptor agonists*, *antagonists*, *inverse agonists*, or *selective serotonin reuptake inhibitors* (SSRIs), terms that not only define the site of action but also characterize the type of activity of the agent.

New advances always bring new questions and new problems. The ability to develop agents with ever-increasing specificity may give rise to the question of whether this is a desirable goal. Is it reasonable to assume that disorders such as major depression and schizophrenia are the result of one specific lesion in the neurotransmission process? Are several concurrent lesions necessary to express the disorder, or can any one of several different lesions be responsible for similar symptoms and the same diagnosis?

The answers to such basic questions not only will influence the development of new therapeutic agents but also will have a major effect on how physicians diagnose disorders in their patients and how they arrive at an effective course of therapy. In this chapter, we summarize our understanding of the basic elements of neurotransmission and how this knowledge is influencing drug development and treatment strategies.

HISTORICAL PERSPECTIVES

For centuries, humankind has been taking drugs and concoctions to relieve the symptoms of abnormal behavior. As far back as the third century B.C., cathartic herbs were used to cure melancholy (Burton 1927a). Even though these treatments could not have been effective, the traditions surrounding their use lasted for centuries. Not until early in the twentieth century were attempts made to scientifically evaluate the effectiveness of drugs in mental illness (Wright 1926).

Modern psychopharmacology began rather dramatically in the 1950s when a series of serendipitous observations revealed the therapeutic properties of several psychotherapeutic agents. These new agents not only proved useful in therapy but also served as important research tools for the discovery of new frontiers of neurochemistry and neurophysiology. This process encouraged the development of theories based on the organic nature of brain function and mental dysfunction (Wooley 1962). The development of these frontiers has, in turn, led to the development of better drugs for the treatment of mental illnesses.

The therapeutic effect of chlorpromazine in psychotic patients was documented in 1952. Chlorpromazine was under development as a drug to reduce fluid loss in surgery. At about the same time, the tranquilizing properties of a *Rauwolfia* extract, reserpine, were being observed in psychotic patients (for a review of these developments, see Cole 1959). Iproniazid, a drug used in the treatment of tuberculosis, was observed to have antidepressant effects in 1952 and became available to practicing physicians in 1957. In 1954, meprobamate was identified as a specific anxiolytic and was used in the treatment of neuroses (Caldwell 1978).

The discovery of drugs that appeared to be effective in alleviating the symptoms of specific mental illnesses such as depression, psychosis, and neurosis led to an intensive search for additional drugs of this type. Because chlorpromazine was a tricyclic compound, many drugs with this basic structure were tested for antipsychotic activity. This research eventually led to the discovery of the antidepressant class of tricyclics, for many years the drugs of choice in treating depression. Similarly, the search for new chemical structures with antipsychotic activity led to the discovery of the benzodiazepines as specific anxiolytics (Sternbach and Horst 1982).

The rapid and dramatic developments in psychopharmacology during the 1950s had an equally dramatic influence on psychiatry and how the human brain was viewed by society ("Pills for the Mind" 1955). Over the years, our ability to treat mental illness with drugs promoted the chemical nature of the brain and deemphasized Freudian concepts (Wallis and Willwerth 1992). This change in view was further enhanced by our knowledge of mind-altering drugs such as lysergic acid diethylamide (LSD). Although LSD did not achieve therapeutic status, its influences on mental functions were well known (Rosenfeld 1966) by the lay public and by psychopharmacologists.

The development of modern neuropsychopharmacology not only provided tools with which neurophysiologists and neurochemists could learn more about brain function, but more importantly, this era stimulated great interest in the neurosciences. As a result, the increase in basic knowledge of brain function has enhanced the discovery of newer, better therapeutic agents for the treatment of mental illness.

NEUROBIOLOGY

During the past several decades, tremendous strides have been made in understanding the basic mechanisms of brain function. Progress has been aided by advances in neuropsychopharmacology and the availability of technologies such as receptor-binding techniques, patch clamp techniques, and, more recently, molecular genetic procedures. The advances in understanding the basic process of brain function permit a better understanding of the brain in dysfunction, which assists in the development of specifically targeted therapeutic agents.

The brain consists of approximately 100 million neurons, which account for one-half of the brain's volume, the other half being made up of glial cells. Glial cells guide the synaptic formation of neurons during brain development (Bacci et al. 1999), influence the extracellular environment of the neurons (Bullock et al. 2005), synthesize neurotransmitter precursors (D.L. Martin 1992), and respond to, or in some cases cause, brain damage (Aschner et al. 1999; McGeer and McGeer 1998; Raivich et al. 1999). In turn, neurons are known to produce factors influencing the development and function of glia (Melcangi et al. 1999; Vardimon et al. 1999).

GLIA

For many years, glia were thought to have a somewhat limited or passive role in brain function, but more recent revelations indicate that glia have receptors, uptake mechanisms, and enzymes for several neurotransmitters, suggesting that the functions of these cells are closely integrated with neuronal functions (Inagaki and Wada 1994; D.L. Martin 1992; Otero and Merrill 1994; Ransom and Sontheimer 1992; Theis et al. 2005) (Table 30–1).

An important example of this type of interaction is shown in Figure 30–1. Glutamate and γ-aminobutyric acid (GABA) are ubiquitous neurotransmitters in the brain, serving as primary excitatory and inhibitory neurotransmitters. Glial cells (astrocytes) play a prominent role in recycling and conserving both glutamate and GABA by recapturing them from the synapse, converting them to glutamine, and then returning glutamine to the presynaptic neurons for conversion back to the appropriate neurotransmitter (Shank et al. 1989). In addition to the conservation of neurotransmitter, glia protect neurons by limiting synaptic levels of glutamate (Bacci et al. 1999; Vardimon et al. 1999). Prominent among glutamate's several cellular influences is the opening of specific calcium channels that allow the influx of calcium ions into neurons. The overstimulation of neurons via this mechanism has been associated with neurotoxicity and neuronal death. Thus, it is of considerable importance that extraneuronal concentrations of glutamate be controlled and that mechanisms exist to limit the synaptic activity of this neurotransmitter. Glial cells have been shown to possess membrane transporters or uptake sites for glutamate; it also has been found that

glutamate uptake into glial cells is the primary route for clearing synaptic glutamate. Once inside the glial cell, the glutamate is metabolized to glutamine, a neuronally inactive substance. The conversion of glutamate to glutamine occurs primarily in glial cells via the enzyme glutamine synthetase. Thus, glial cells play a critical role in limiting synaptic concentrations of glutamate and conserving the neurotransmitter for reuse. An important element in the above functions is the maintenance of appropriate levels of glutamine synthetase activity in glial cells. Significant factors in the regulation of glutamine synthetase activity are glucocorticoid stimulation of gene expression and the absolute requirement for the astrocyte and neuron to be in juxtaposition. The critical neuronal factor required for gene expression of glutamine synthetase has not been identified (Vardimon et al. 1999).

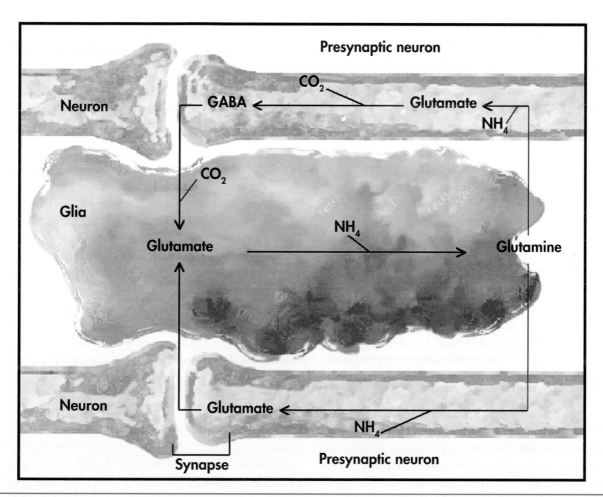

FIGURE 30–1. The role of glia (astrocytes) in accumulating, metabolizing, and conserving synaptic γ-aminobutyric acid (GABA) and glutamate. Specific membrane transporters move GABA and glutamate into glia cells, where GABA is carboxylated (combined with CO_2) to form glutamate; glutamate is in turn aminated (combined with NH_4) to create glutamine. Glutamine is then transported out of the glia and is available to GABAergic and glutamatergic presynaptic neurons for conversion to their respective neurotransmitters. Through these mechanisms, glia play an important role in maintaining synaptic concentrations below neurotoxic levels and salvage two ubiquitous and important neurotransmitters.

TABLE 30–1.   Membrane elements of mammalian glia

Receptors[a]	Response mode
Noradrenergic (α and β)	G protein
Adenosine	G protein
Acetylcholine (muscarinic)	G protein
Neuropeptides (substance P)	G protein
Glutamate (quisqualate, kainate)	Ion gating
γ-Aminobutyric acid (GABA$_A$)	Ion gating

Ion channels (voltage sensitive)
Potassium (inwardly rectifying, outwardly rectifying, and transient A-type)
Sodium—tetrodotoxin sensitive ("neuronal") and tetrodotoxin resistant ("glial")
Calcium (L- and T-type)
Chloride

Transporters (uptake sites)
GABA
Glutamate
Glycine
Alanine

[a]Although nearly all neuronal-type neuroreceptors have been shown to occur on glial membranes, only those that have been shown to produce a response have been included here.

Source.   Adapted from Bordey and Sontheimer 2000; Krantz, Chaudhry, Edwards 1999; Marcaggi and Attwell 2004; Ransom and Sontheimer 1992; Sontheimer 1994.

Further evidence of the role astrocytes play in limiting synaptic levels of glutamate is indicated by the influence that neuronal factors play in the regulation of glutamate transporter expression in glial membranes (Schlag et al. 1998; Swanson et al. 1997). A soluble, diffusible substance secreted by neurons has been shown to increase the expression of glutamate transporter molecules in astrocytes. Thus, it would appear that the level of neuronal activity plays a role in regulating the rate at which glutamate is transported into the glia for inactivation as described earlier. Although the substance has not been identified, the previously mentioned effects can be mimicked by cyclic adenosine monophosphate (cAMP) analogues (Schlag et al. 1998; Swanson et al. 1997).

Two types of neurotransmitter-activated calcium channels have been seen in astrocytes (Gebremedhin et al. 2003). In addition, a significant amount of communication between neurons and glia is now known to occur via direct interaction of neurotransmitters such as glutamate and GABA with membrane surface receptors on astrocytes adjacent to neuronal synapses (Lin and Bergles 2004; Schipke and Kettenmann 2004). Evidence also shows neuronal synaptic junctions formed with some types of progenitor cells (Lin and Bergles 2004). The local effects of these interactions of neurotransmitters with glia are likely to influence brain activity over long distances through the establishment of glial calcium waves (Schipke and Kettenmann 2004).

Investigations have reported a metabolic coupling between glia and neurons (Bacci et al. 1999; Poitry-Yamate et al. 1995; Tsacopoulos and Magistretti 1996). Considerable energy is consumed in the various processes of synaptic transmission. The preferred energy source for brain function is glucose. Astrocytes are capable of transporting glucose across the cell membrane via an active, carrier-assisted mechanism. Because astrocytes are well known to be in intimate contact with the brain's vascular system, it is assumed that glucose is transported directly into the glia from the circulation. Inside the glia, glycolysis transforms the glucose to lactose and in the process provides energy for the transport of neurotransmitters and ions across the glial membrane. Lactose is then transferred out of the glia and accumulated by neurons, where it is the preferred substrate for oxidative metabolism. This energy transfer process is stimulated by the uptake of neurotransmitters such as glutamate and GABA. Neurotransmitter uptake by glia is accompanied by the influx of sodium ions. The accumulation of sodium ions stimulates a sodium/potassium adenosine triphosphatase (Na$^+$/K$^+$-ATPase) pump, which consumes adenosine triphosphate (ATP) and exchanges intracellular sodium ions for extracellular potassium ions. The activity of the ATPase stimulates the metabolism of glucose, resulting in increased lactose production. Thus, the production of metabolic precursor keeps pace with the overall synaptic activity.

Astroglia are known to play a pivotal role in the regulation of brain physiology and neuronal activity via the nitric oxide (NO) pathway (for a review of glial involvement in the synthesis of NO, see Wiesinger 2001). Thus, they accumulate and store L-arginine, the precursor of NO, and, at least under some circumstances, can accumulate the metabolic precursors of L-arginine and synthesize L-arginine. The L-arginine stored in the astroglia is then available for NO synthesis and modification of neuronal activity, neuronal energy metabolism, and regulation of local blood flow through NO action on epithelial cells lining the microvasculature. More details on the actions of NO on brain function are found in a later section.

In some cases, astrocytes have been shown to possess functional ion channels controlled by neurotransmitter receptors. In this way, glia have been associated with long-distance signal transmission in the brain via gap junctions across glial membranes (Cornell-Bell and Finkbeiner 1991; Cornell-Bell et al. 1990; Sohl et al. 2005). The observation that glial gap junctions are in part controlled by components of second-messenger systems (Enkvist and McCarthy 1992) supports the active role of glial cells in brain function. Glial dysfunction has been suggested to play a role in epilepsy and the degenerative diseases, Parkinson's and Huntington's (Ransom and Sontheimer 1992; Schousboe et al. 2004). Although several psychopharmacological agents interact with glial elements, as well as those same elements found on neurons, the contributions of these glial interactions to the agents' overall pharmacodynamics remain the subject of intensive investigation.

One exciting potential therapeutic lead is represented by research with glial cell line–derived neurotrophic factor (GDNF). GDNF was isolated from a culture of glial cells and found to stimulate the growth of embryonic dopamine neurons (Bohn 1999). Since this observation on dopaminergic neurons, GDNF has been found to elicit a trophic response on several other brain neuron types, including motor neurons and noradrenergic, cholinergic, and serotonergic neurons (Bohn 1999). In addition, other neurotrophic factors have been identified with activity similar to that of GDNF (Saarma and Sariola 1999); these factors include neurturin, persephin, and artemin. GDNF, a chain of 134 peptides synthesized from a larger propeptide, exerts its biological activity through a series of complex receptor interactions, requiring cofactors, and a tyrosine kinase receptor (Grondin and Gash 1998; Saarma and Sariola 1999). Although the exact role of GDNF in brain development and maintenance is not known, it has been shown to be active in a variety of animal models for Parkinson's disease (Bohn 1999; Grondin and Gash 1998; Lapchak 1998).

Although GDNF showed great promise in preclinical studies, initial clinical trials with GDNF have been disappointing. First, the physiology of GDNF is more complex than previously appreciated (Sariola and Saarma 2003); biological activity requires specific receptor sites and cofactors. Second, important considerations for the therapeutic use of GDNF must include the site of action and a suitable delivery system. Early studies in which GDNF was administered into the lateral ventricles resulted in no therapeutic effect while producing significant side effects. However, a subsequent trial in which GDNF was infused directly into the putamen did provide effective treatment with no significant side effects (Gill et al. 2003). Thus, the therapeutic use of GDNF for Parkinson's and other neurodegenerative brain disorders will await improvements in GDNF delivery (Kirik et al. 2004).

NEURONS

The basic function of neurons is to convey electrical signals in a highly organized and integrated way, each neuron receiving input from many other neurons and in turn providing input to many other neurons. This function is the product of complex chemical processes transmitting signals across neuronal synapses—a symphony of intraneuronal and interneuronal events, layers of feedback, and control mechanisms ensuring the correct or appropriate response. Although chemical transmission is a complex, multistepped system, it provides for maximum flexibility and unidirectional flow of neuronal signals.

Resting neurons maintain an electrical polarization between the inside and the outside of the cellular membrane. This polarization is negative on the inside and positive on the outside of the neuron. Key elements in maintaining the polarized state include the presence of large (nondiffusible) intracellular, negatively charged proteins and specific ion pumps, located in the neuronal membrane, that use cellular energy to pump ions against concentration gradients. Changes in the state of transmembranal polarization are effected by a system of specific ion channels activated by neurotransmitter substances or by the degree of transmembrane (voltage-sensitive) depolarization. Ions move through the channels because of concentration (from high to low concentrations) or electrogenic (opposite charges attract) gradients. Activation of neurotransmitter-controlled ion channels reduces the level of polarization to a critical level at which voltage-sensitive channels open and permit the rapid influx of cations (e.g., Na^+). This influx completely depolarizes the neuron and even reverses the polarization for a brief period. Membrane ion channels adjacent to the area of depolarization open, thus extending the depolarization along the neuron and causing the formation of an action potential. In this way, electrical signals are carried from one end of the neuron to the other. Repolarization occurs by the opening of voltage-sensitive K^+ channels. Because K^+ concentrations are high inside the neuron and low outside, K^+ carries positive charges to the outside of the membrane, making the inside more negative. The restoration of conditions in the resting state is completed by the exchange of intracellular Na^+ ions for extracellular K^+ ions. The ion exchange is accomplished by an energy-dependent pump. (Excellent reviews of the electrical nature of neurons may be found in Levitan and Kaczmarek 2002.)

Synapse

The *synapse* is defined as the juncture of two neurons. The neuron from which the signal is coming is known as the *presynaptic neuron*, whereas the receiving neuron is called the *postsynaptic neuron*. Signals are passed across the synapse by either of two mechanisms. The first is by direct connection of the presynaptic and postsynaptic neurons via gap junctions (similar to the connection of astrocytes described earlier). The physiological significance of this type of connection is that transmission is rapid, can occur in two directions, and can synchronize the activity of many neurons. Electrogenic coupling of neurons occurs in only a few populations of neurons located primarily in the brain stem (Baker and Llinas 1971; Korn et al. 1973; Llinas et al. 1974). Cortical precursor cells are also known to communicate via gap junctions (LoTurco and Kriegstein 1991), although this function is lost as the cells develop into mature functioning neurons. Other neurons in the suprachiasmatic nucleus are also known to transmit signals via gap junctions, which are at least partially influenced by the neurotransmitter GABA (Shinohara et al. 2000). These gap junctions can be unique in that they are electrogenic in nature but are influenced by a neurotransmitter. Thus, they may have the advantages of both modes of interneuronal communication.

Chemical Transmission

By far, the dominant means of neuron-to-neuron communication or transmission is through specific chemicals or neurotransmitters. To operate effectively, chemical transmission requires the presence of several elements (Table 30–2). These elements consist of specific proteins in the form of enzymes, storage-binding proteins, uptake and membrane transport structures, receptors, and response systems (ion channels and second-messenger systems). Each element represents an opportunity for malfunction (disease state) or a point for modulation of transmission through pharmacological intervention. In fact, the manipulation of these elements serves as the basis of modern psychopharmacology. The functional relation of the elements of neurotransmission is illustrated in Figures 30–2 and 30–3.

TABLE 30–2.   Elements required for chemical transmission

Presynaptic

Enzymes for neurotransmitter synthesis

Mechanism for neurotransmitter storage

Mechanism for appropriate neurotransmitter release

Neurotransmitter receptors for feedback modification of neurotransmitter release

Synaptic

Mechanism for terminating neurotransmitter action

Postsynaptic

Neurotransmitter receptors to initiate response

Coupler proteins

Mechanism for response (ion channels/second-messenger systems)

Neurotransmitter synthesis.   The final enzymatic steps in synthesizing a neurotransmitter generally occur in or near the storage site. This ensures maximum efficiency in the neurotransmitter molecules getting to the storage sites. Neuropeptides are a notable exception to this rule because their synthesis involves gene activation followed by DNA transcription and RNA translation to form large polypeptides. The polypeptides are then broken down into the component neuropeptides. This all occurs within the neuronal soma, so that the neuropeptides must be transported along the axon to the nerve terminal for storage. In several cases, neurotransmitter-synthesizing enzymes are shared by more than one neurotransmitter system. For example, the neurotransmitters norepinephrine and dopamine share the enzymes tyrosine hydroxylase and L-3,4-dihydroxyphenylalanine decarboxylase, whereas several peptides share common peptidases. Although many drugs inhibit specific neurotransmitter-synthesizing enzymes, these drugs have not proven useful as therapeutic agents, either because the neurotransmitters they influence are ubiquitous and important to many life processes or because the enzymes influence multiple neurotransmitters and thus produce broad, nonspecific effects.

Neurotransmitter storage and release.   Many neurotransmitters are stored in organelles known as *synaptic vesicles* (Thiel 1995). These structures, constructed in the soma and transported along the axons with their full complement of neurotransmitter, concentrate near the nerve terminal. The vesicular membranes contain many specific protein structures involved in the multiple functions of the storage vesicles (Kelly 1999; Krantz et al. 1999; Rahami-

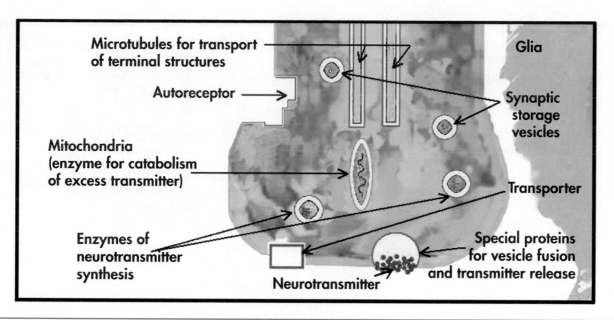

FIGURE 30–2. Typical presynaptic neuron with key structures relevant to neurotransmission. Microtubules transport storage vesicles, enzymes, and a variety of proteins from the neuronal soma, where they are synthesized, to the nerve ending, where they are required for carrying out their physiological functions. Storage vesicles maintain stores of neurotransmitter molecules for eventual release into the synaptic cleft. Mitochondria contain enzymes vital to providing energy to the neuron; in many cases (such as the biogenic amines) they contain enzymes, such as monoamine oxidase, which help to regulate neurotransmitter levels in the nerve ending. Calcium and a variety of special fusion proteins fuse the storage vesicle membranes with the neuronal membrane to release the neurotransmitter into the synaptic cleft. Transporter pumps are proteins incorporated into the neuronal membrane that transport the neurotransmitter from the synapse into the neuron, where it can be reincorporated into the storage vesicle. Autoreceptors respond to neurotransmitter released from the nerve ending to provide feedback regulation of presynaptic depolarization.

moff et al. 1999). Vesicular functions include neurotransmitter synthesis, neurotransmitter transport across the vesicular membrane, neurotransmitter binding inside the vesicle, docking proteins for attaching to the neuronal plasma membrane, calcium-binding proteins for membrane fusion and neurotransmitter release, and special coating proteins for vesicular endocytosis and recycling processes.

Calcium ions are an essential element for the release of neurotransmitters. A major mechanism for calcium entry results from the activation of voltage-gated ion channels located in the plasma membrane (Rahamimoff et al. 1999; Zhang and Ramaswami 1999). The activation of the voltage-gated ion channels depends on many factors such as the activity of numerous other membrane ion channels (Rahamimoff et al. 1999) and a variety of presynaptic ligand-gated ion channels (MacDermott et al. 1999) as well as autoreceptors (MacDermott et al. 1999). Given the absolute requirement for Ca^{2+} in the neurotransmitter release process, it is perhaps not surprising that the proteins that compose the voltage-gated calcium channel are intimately bound to specific proteins associated with storage vesicle docking and fusion pro-

cesses (Catterall 1999). This would ensure that neurotransmitter release is occurring in a microenvironment containing an appropriate concentration of calcium.

Proteins involved in the storage and release mechanisms of neurotransmitters are well conserved in many different neurotransmitter systems so that drugs that interfere with storage and release tend to have broad, nonspecific effects. Reserpine is a well-known example of such a drug. Reserpine destroys the ability of presynaptic storage vesicles to transport and store all biogenic amines, including norepinephrine, dopamine, serotonin, and histamine (Krantz et al. 1999). Because this effect is not reversible, recovery from the effects of reserpine requires the synthesis and transport of new storage vesicles to the nerve terminals, a process that requires several days. For these reasons, reserpine has had a short-lived and limited use in psychiatry.

The pharmacology surrounding the control of neurotransmitter release via heterosynaptic, ligand-gated mechanisms presents some clinically significant examples. Neurotransmitters for the presynaptic, ligand-gated channels include GABA, glutamate, acetylcholine, serotonin, and ATP (MacDermott et al. 1999).

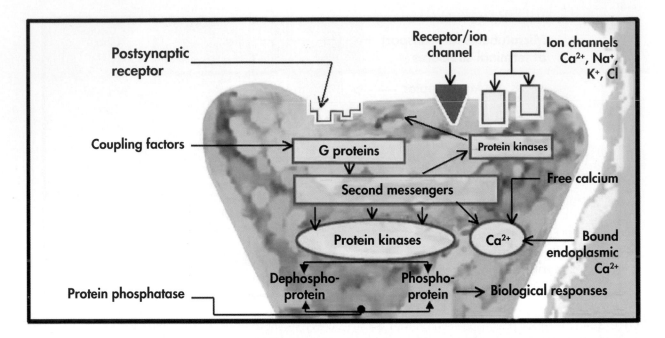

FIGURE 30–3.   Typical postsynaptic neuron with key structures relevant to neurotransmission. Neurotransmitter substances bind to postsynaptic receptors that may be one of two major types, G protein or ion channel coupled. Other ion channels are regulated by intraneuronal ions such as calcium or potassium, as well as by transmembrane voltages. G proteins couple receptors with second-messenger systems that in turn regulate a variety of protein kinases that are responsible for initiating biological responses. Second messengers also directly regulate intraneuronal calcium levels. The various elements in the illustration are shown in their functional sequence, not in their anatomical domains. Postsynaptic receptors, G proteins, and second messengers are in fact neuronal membrane–associated elements.

Presynaptic GABA receptors are of the GABA$_A$ type and thus relevant to the inhibitory actions of the benzodiazepines (Tallman et al. 1999). The presynaptic GABA$_A$ receptors are channels for chloride ions, and their activation hyperpolarizes the presynaptic neuron, resulting in inhibition of presynaptic release of neurotransmitters. Presynaptic cholinergic receptors are of the nicotinic type and, when activated, tend to depolarize the neuron by admitting sodium and calcium ions. The activation of these presynaptic receptors by nicotine is the source of tobacco's central pharmacological and addictive properties (Grady et al. 1992; MacDermott et al. 1999; Watkins et al. 1999; Wonnacott 1997; Yeomans and Baptista 1997). Presynaptic serotonin receptors such as the 5-hydroxytryptamine type 3 (5-HT$_3$), when activated, admit calcium into the neuron, thus promoting depolarization and neurotransmitter release (Ronde and Nichols 1998). As with all other serotonergic receptors, the activity of the 5-HT$_3$ receptors is enhanced by drugs that block the reuptake of serotonin (MacDermott et al. 1999).

In addition, ethanol has been shown to influence several of these presynaptic receptors such as GABA$_A$; glutamate; and nicotinic, cholinergic, and 5-HT$_3$ serotonergic types (Lovinger 1997; Narahashi et al. 1999). The relevance of ethanol's influence on these structures to its pharmacological actions is the subject of continued investigations.

Neurotransmitter inactivation.   Once liberated into the synapse, neurotransmitters are available to transmit their signals until they are removed or inactivated in some manner. Thus, neurotransmitter inactivation is an important element in controlling synaptic transmission. Rapid inactivation would attenuate transmission, whereas slow inactivation would accentuate signal transmission. Three major routes for neurotransmitter inactivation are known. First, neurotransmitters may be removed by washout or turnover of the extraneuronal fluid. This occurs at a relatively slow rate in the brain and would appear to be inadequate for rapid control of neurotransmitter activity.

A second mode of neurotransmitter inactivation is by enzymatic degradation of the neurotransmitter. A notable example of this mode is with acetylcholine, a major excitatory neurotransmitter in the brain, in which the time span in the synapse is vital for proper function. Acetylcholine is rapidly metabolized in the synapse by acetylcholinesterase, a process that splits the neurotransmitter into two parts: acetate and choline. These two components are then transported back into the presynaptic neuron where another enzyme, choline acetyltransferase, rejoins them to form acetylcholine. Thus, these two enzymes and the transport of the precursors across the membrane form an effective and efficient means of rapidly terminating the synaptic activity of the neurotransmitter while protecting the availability of the precursors required for neurotransmitter synthesis.

A third mechanism for neurotransmitter inactivation is a variation of the second. In this case, rather than transporting the individual components of the neurotransmitter, the intact neurotransmitter is transported across the presynaptic neuronal membrane and into the cytoplasm, where it is eventually accumulated by storage vesicles and available for release once again. This transport, or reuptake, is accomplished by special transmembrane proteins that serve as carriers. Because the concentrations of neurotransmitter are generally greater in the presynaptic terminal than in the synaptic fluid, cellular energy in the form of ATP is expended in the reuptake process. Many major neurotransmitters are primarily inactivated by this reuptake process. These include the biogenic amines norepinephrine, dopamine, and serotonin and the amino acids GABA, glycine, and glutamate. The transporter proteins for most neurotransmitters have similar properties (Krantz et al. 1999; Nelson 1998) such as a requirement for sodium and chloride ions. The transporters characteristically have 12 transmembrane sections, with a large extracellular loop between the third and fourth sections. This third loop contains a site or sites for glycosylation (Blakely et al. 1997; Gegelashvili and Schousboe 1997; Krantz et al. 1999; Nelson 1998). Inhibition of glycosylation at these sites appears to diminish the function or efficiency of the transporter but does not influence substrate affinity (Melikian et al. 1996).

A second set of transporters, similar to, but genetically distinct from, those found in the neuronal membrane, is located within the membranes of the neurotransmitter storage vesicles. These transporters move the neurotransmitters from the neuronal cytoplasm to the interior of the vesicles, where they are ready for release once again (Krantz et al. 1999).

The serotonin transporter has been the subject of intensive investigation because it is the site of action for the SSRIs, the drugs of choice in the treatment of major depression. A transporter protein structure approximating the serotonin transporter is shown in Figure 30–4. In common with other neurotransmitter transporters, the serotonergic transporter has 12 transmembrane sections with both the amino and the carboxyl terminals within the neuron (Blakely et al. 1997; Nelson 1998). The serotonin transporter molecule includes intraneuronal sites for phosphorylation that are critical for the regulation of

transporter activity (Blakely et al. 1997, 1998). These sites appear to be primarily phosphorylated by kinase C and dephosphorylated via the action of phosphatase 2A (Blakely et al. 1998). Phosphorylation inactivates the transporter molecules and therefore slows the clearing of serotonin from the synaptic cleft. This phosphorylation process is likely to serve as a kind of feedback control because kinase C activity is regulated via neurotransmitter interaction with neuroreceptors (see subsection "Second Messengers" and Figure 30–7 later in this chapter).

Recognition, or binding, sites for serotonin to the transporter are located at extraneuronal loops of the molecule. A precondition for substrate binding is the binding of one each of sodium and chloride ions to the transporter (Krantz et al. 1999; Nelson 1998). Presumably, the binding of these ions places the tertiary configuration of the transporter in the best position for substrate binding. The exact location of the site of attachment of inhibitory drugs, such as many of the antidepressant compounds, is not known for all drugs but is most likely to occur at a variety of external sites. The tricyclic antidepressants are known to bind to the central loops (Blakely et al. 1991; Nelson 1998) in the transport domain for serotonin.

The transporters for several types of neurotransmitters, including those for the amino acids GABA and glutamate, the catecholamines dopamine and norepinephrine, and the biogenic amine serotonin, have long been known to have a requirement for the presence of sodium and chloride ions in order to function. In general, binding of these monovalent ions appears to be required for the neurotransmitter to bind to the transporter. Studies have suggested that transporters for the neurotransmitters may actually serve a significant role as ion channels and thus play a part in neuronal function and regulation of neuronal activity (Galli et al. 1997; Krantz et al. 1999; Lester et al. 1996; Nelson 1998). Although the ion requirements can vary, depending on which transporter is involved, the basic mechanisms appear to be similar for the entire family of transporters.

As an example, the serotonin transporter appears to function with neutral stoichiometry. Thus, $Na^+/Cl^-/$ serotonin are transported into the neuron while K^+ is transported out, resulting in no net transfer of charge (Galli et al. 1997; Krantz et al. 1999); however, it has been found that significant charge transfer does occur through the serotonin transporter (Galli et al. 1997). The exact nature of this transfer is not known, but clearly the transporter is acting as an ion channel.

This raises interesting questions as to the primary function of transporters. It has always been assumed that their primary role is to remove neurotransmitters from the synapse and to do so in such a way as to conserve neu-

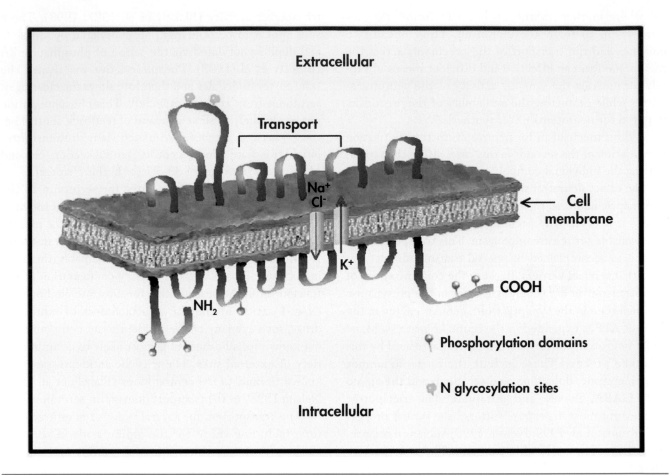

FIGURE 30–4.   A typical neurotransmitter transporter protein. Although neurotransmitter transporters exhibit specificity for the neurotransmitter transported, they have many structural features in common. Each has 12 transmembrane sections, a large extraneuronal loop between the third and fourth transmembrane sections, intraneuronal sites for phosphorylation, and a requirement for ion binding. The figure approximates a serotonin transporter.

rotransmitters for reuse. This information presents the possibility that the transporters' primary role is as an ion channel with the transport of neurotransmitters as a channel-regulating mechanism in addition to providing for the conservation of neurotransmitters (Galli et al. 1997; Krantz et al. 1999; Lester et al. 1996).

This novel perspective of the neurotransporters may provide a solution to an old puzzle concerning the mechanism of action of antidepressants. It is well known that antidepressants require a few weeks of treatment before the onset of clinical response, and yet their blockade of neurotransmitter reuptake is immediate. Because reuptake blockers appear to block the ion channel activity of the transporters as well as their transport function (Galli et al. 1997; Lester et al. 1996), the reuptake inhibitor antidepressants' significant pharmacological action may relate more to the presynaptic, intraneuronal, ionic milieu than to increased synaptic neurotransmitter concentrations.

Whether transporter or ion channel, these structures are important for proper brain function. Approximately

4% of the human population has been found to have a genetic defect that reduces the transcription process for the serotonin gene, resulting in individuals with reduced transporter function (Lesch et al. 1996). Such individuals have been found to have relatively high anxiety–related traits (Lesch et al. 1996). In addition, this defect has been suggested as having a possible link to neurodevelopment and neurodegenerative disorders (Lesch and Mossner 1998).

In the case of the biogenic amines, although reuptake is the major means of limiting their synaptic activity, significant contributions to inactivation are made via the enzymes catechol-O-methyltransferase (Guldberg and Marsden 1975; Mannisto et al. 1992) and monoamine oxidase (Singer and Ramsay 1995). Inactivation by these enzymes does not result in any known reusable or physiologically active products. The reuptake sites for the biogenic amines show some specificity for each amine, but the sites for each amine appear to be identical on all neurons and in all brain regions containing that amine. Thus, it is possible to design a drug that will specifically block the reuptake of a particular biogenic amine, but that drug will influence reuptake to the same extent at all neurons containing that amine. As is discussed later, this specificity is an important factor in therapeutic drug design.

Unlike the biogenic amines, the amino acid neurotransmitters are taken up by both presynaptic neurons and adjacent glial cells (Gadea and Lopez-Colome 2001a, 2001b, 2001c) (see Figure 30–1). Also, unlike the biogenic amines, amino acid transporters occur in multiple variations for each of the neurotransmitters. Thus, five variations of the glutamate transporter (Gadea and Lopez-Colome 2001a) have been identified, whereas four are known for GABA (Gadea and Lopez-Colome 2001b) and three for glycine (Gadea and Lopez-Colome 2001c). As more is learned about the physiological role of these various transporter subtypes, they may prove to be useful sites for specific modification by drugs.

The pharmacological manipulation of reuptake or transport sites has been an area of intensive activity in developing drugs for the treatment of major depression. The discovery of the ability of tricyclic antidepressants such as imipramine and amitriptyline to be potent reuptake blockers of norepinephrine and serotonin led to the early hypothesis that depression resulted from an insufficiency of these biogenic amines and that this insufficiency was corrected by reducing the rate at which these neurotransmitters were removed from the synapse. This hypothesis was supported by other pharmacological and biological observations. More recent clinical success with a new class of antidepressants, the SSRIs, underscores the importance of amine reuptake as an appropriate mechanism of action for antidepressant activity, although it is now apparent that reuptake inhibition alone may not be directly responsible for the antidepressant activity. Rather, reuptake inhibition initiates changes or adjustments in receptors, ion fluxes, and intracellular messenger systems, which alter neurotransmission in key pathways (Galli et al. 1997; Kilts 1994; Paul et al. 1994).

Receptors.   Neuroreceptors are specific, membrane-bound proteins that bind neurotransmitter molecules and translate that molecular attachment into a physiological response. The amino acid sequence of each receptor type imparts a specificity for the particular neurotransmitter that will bind to it. Of particular importance in defining a receptor is that a physiological response results when the receptor is activated. Many proteins are capable of binding neurotransmitter substances but are not capable of eliciting a response. Such binding proteins are better referred to as *acceptors*.

Neuroreceptors can be placed into four broad categories, depending on the mode of action of their physiologi-

cal response. The most prevalent of these are those receptors that connect to a second-messenger system through one of a family of proteins referred to as G proteins. This receptor type is characterized by having seven transmembrane sections of the protein with extracellular and intracellular loops that serve as neurotransmitter binding sites and as sites for receptor regulation (Figure 30–5).

A second class of receptors consists of those receptors that form membrane ion channels or ionophores. Stimulation of receptors in this class opens ion channels specific for sodium, potassium, calcium, and chloride ions. The receptor/ion channel consists of five individual proteins, each with four transmembrane sections. The receptors are made up of a combination of protein subtypes; each subtype can exist in several variations. Thus, receptor/ion channels for a specific neurotransmitter can exist in several variations.

The third receptor class consists of receptors that attach to allosteric sites on other neuroreceptors regulating receptor ligand affinities. Examples of receptors that act at allosteric sites include the benzodiazepine and associated receptors that modify GABA receptor activity, as well as the glycine B receptor, associated with the N-methyl-D-aspartate (NMDA) subtype of glutamate receptor. The presence of glycine on the glycine B receptor is one of the requirements for glutamate activation of the NMDA receptor.

The fourth receptor class is made up of intraneuronal receptors best characterized by steroid transcription factor binding and the synthesis of various components of synaptic transmission, such as enzymes, receptors, and second-messenger systems (Joels and de Kloet 1994). As might be expected, the effects mediated by these receptors have a slow onset and last over an extended time.

Neuroreceptors generally show specificity for neurotransmitters and usually are identified by the neurotransmitter that binds to them and to which they elicit a response. The existence of subtypes of receptors for specific neurotransmitters has been known for several decades. For example, acetylcholine receptors were traditionally thought of as being either nicotinic or muscarinic, according to their pharmacological response. It is now known that they not only have different pharmacological characteristics but also are entirely different in their functions and modes of responses. The nicotinic acetylcholine receptor is a five-protein sodium ion channel that is opened in the presence of acetylcholine, whereas the muscarinic receptor is a single-protein unit coupled to a second-messenger system (inositol phosphate) by a G protein.

Historically, receptor subtypes have been identified by pharmacological studies in which specific drugs are used to stimulate or block receptor activity. Such techniques are limited in that they do not differentiate between receptor subtypes as either two different proteins

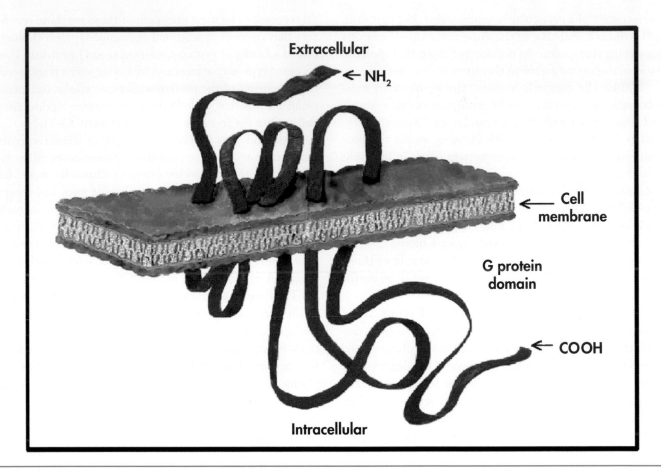

FIGURE 30–5.   A typical G protein–coupled neurotransmitter receptor. The receptors of this type have seven transmembrane sections, with the carboxyl terminal on the inside of the neuron. The figure approximates a serotonin type 1A receptor. Receptors of this type vary with regard to their amino acid composition and the lengths of the extracellular and intracellular segments.

or one protein in different membrane configurations. Pharmacological techniques are also limited in the number of subtypes that can be identified, particularly as the pharmacological differences become more subtle or if specific pharmacological agents are not available.

In recent years, biomolecular techniques have been used to identify and characterize many new receptor subtypes. Specific genes have been identified that express neuroreceptor subtypes for many of the neurotransmitters. Through these techniques, populations of "pure" receptor types have been produced, which may then be used for identifying specific ligands for the receptors. Specific ligands are in turn useful for determining the location and density of specific receptors. Methods also exist by which transcription paths are altered to prevent the expression of specific receptors (Lucas and Hen 1995), thus providing animal models that are lacking specific receptors. Such studies provide important clues as to the physiological function of specific receptors (Furth et al. 1994; Lai et al. 1994; Saudou et al. 1994; Silvia et al. 1994; Stan-

difer et al. 1994; Tecott et al. 1995; Thomas and Capecchi 1990; Wahlestedt et al. 1993; Zhou et al. 1994).

As can be seen in Table 30–3, receptors for various neurotransmitters come in many subtypes. For example, 14 subtypes have been identified for serotonin, with the possibility of more to be discovered (Hoyer et al. 2002). Nearly all receptors for the various neurotransmitters come in several subtypes. This fact is important from a pharmacological perspective because it means that it is possible to identify compounds for a specific receptor subtype, thus limiting the pharmacological effects.

Neuroreceptors are important sites for pharmacological intervention in psychiatric disorders. For example, all antipsychotic medications are known to have antagonist activity at dopamine receptors. Antidepressant drugs are well known to influence receptors either directly as antagonists or indirectly by up- or downregulation of receptor populations (Kilts 1994). Many antidepressants, the tricyclic antidepressants in particular, are known to interact with receptors of several neurotransmitter systems.

TABLE 30–3. Some major types of neurotransmitters

Neurotransmitter	Mode of response	Messenger system	Receptor subtypes	
Amines				
Acetylcholine	Ionophore	$Na^+/K^+/Ca^{2+}$ channels	Nicotinic	Multiple subunit variations
	G protein	cAMP IP_3	Muscarinic	5
Norepinephrine	Ionophore and G protein	Ca^{2+} channels and cAMP	α	6
	G protein	cAMP	β	3
Dopamine	G protein	cAMP		5
Serotonin	G protein	cAMP	5-HT_{1A-F} 5-HT_{2A-C} 5-HT_{4-7}	13
	Ionophore	Cation channel	5-HT_3	1
Amino acids				
Glutamate (ionotropic)	Ionophore	Na^+/K^+	Kainate, quisqualate	2
Glutamate	Ionophore	Ca^{2+}	NMDA	1
Glutamate (metabotropic)	G protein	cAMP, IP_3	$mGlu_{1-7}$	7
Glycine	Ionophore	Cl^-		Multiple subunit variations
	Allosteric site on glutamate receptor	Required for glutamate (NMDA) receptor activation		
GABA	Ionophore	Cl^-	$GABA_A$	1
	G protein	cAMP	$GABA_B$	1
Benzodiazepine	Allosteric site	Occupation of this site increases efficacy of GABA receptor		
Purines				
Adenosine	G protein		A_1 A_{2a-b} A_3	4
ATP/ADP/XDP	Ionophore			4
	G protein			
Peptides				
Opioid (enkephalins/ endorphins)	G protein	cAMP	μ, σ, κ	3
Angiotensin	G protein	cGMP	AT_1 and AT_2	2
Cholecystokinin	G protein		CCK_A and CCK_B	2
Vasopressin/oxytocin	G protein		V_{1A}, V_{1B}, V_2; OT	3; 1
Somatostatin	G protein		SST_{1-5}	5
Neurotensin	G protein			1
Steroids				
Corticosterone/ cortisol	Gene transcription	Modification of neurotransmission elements	Mr_s Gr_s	2

Note. A = adenosine; ADP = adenosine diphosphate; AT = angiotensin; ATP = adenosine triphosphate; cAMP = cyclic adenosine monophosphate; CCK = cholecystokinin; cGMP = cyclic guanosine monophosphate; GABA = γ-aminobutyric acid; Gr = glucocorticoid; IP_3 = inositol-1,4,5-triphosphate; 5-HT = 5-hydroxytryptamine; mGlu = metabotropic glutamate; Mr = mineralocorticoid; NMDA = N-methyl-D-aspartate; OT = oxytocin; SST = somatostatin; V = vasopressin; XDP = xanthine diphosphate.

Anxiolytic agents, the benzodiazepines and buspirone, exert their pharmacological actions through interaction with benzodiazepine and serotonin type 1A (5-HT$_{1A}$) receptors, respectively.

Drugs can interact with receptors in one of several ways. They can bind to the receptor and cause a physiological response similar to that of a natural neurotransmitter; such a drug would be referred to as an *agonist*. Other drugs can also bind to the receptor and not elicit a physiological response, but instead prevent agonists from binding to the receptor; this would describe *antagonist* activity. A third type of ligand-receptor interaction is referred to as *inverse agonism*. An inverse agonist is a drug that binds to a receptor but produces an effect opposite that of agonist activity. This type of action has been described in studies of the benzodiazepine receptor (Stephens et al. 1986); a single receptor mediates agonist, antagonist, and inverse agonist activities. Pharmaceutical agents appear to produce mixtures of these basic reactions; for example, mixed antagonist and agonist actions may produce partial or limited agonist activities but when in the presence of full agonists may behave as antagonists.

Another distinctive interaction between psychotropic drugs and receptors is well known to occur with long-term antidepressant treatment. Multiple but not single doses of many antidepressant compounds are known to downregulate β-adrenergic receptors (Wolfe et al. 1978) and NMDA receptors in brain tissue (Paul et al. 1994); that is, they reduce the actual number of receptor sites. Because many of these drugs do not interact with these receptor populations directly, the induced changes may be the result of some second-messenger system activity, although the precise mechanisms for these effects are not known. Because the slow onset of the receptor adaptations is similar to the timing of the onset of the clinical antidepressant effect (Oswald et al. 1972), it has been suggested that one or the other of these changes may be related to the antidepressant effect itself (Caldecott-Hazard et al. 1991; Paul et al. 1994).

G proteins. Serving as linking proteins between extracellular receptors and intracellular effector mechanisms (second messengers), the G proteins (regulatory guanosine triphosphate [GTP]-binding proteins) constitute a large family of related structures vital to the transmission of interneuronal signals. G proteins are actually heterotrimeric structures composed of one each of three protein subunits termed α, β, and γ (Rens-Domiao and Hamm 1995). To date, 18 specific α subunits, 5 β subunits, and 7 γ subunits have been identified. The various subunits are not all interchangeable, and some combinations of the subunits are not compatible.

The α subunits play a key role in the transduction process. The α unit binds the guanine nucleotide and has intrinsic GTPase activity. The α subunit also interacts with the neuroreceptor to initiate the transduction process. Frequently, the α subunit interacts with the effector proteins, although this function has been attributed to the β or γ subunit in some instances (Clapham and Neer 1993; Haga and Haga 1992; Pitcher et al. 1992). Although the α subunit disengages from the other two subunits at certain stages of transduction, the β and γ subunits remain bound to each other at all times.

The sequence of events of the G protein transduction cycle are illustrated in Figure 30–6. The binding of an agonist to a neuroreceptor causes the release of guanine diphosphate (GDP) from the α subunit with the subsequent binding of GTP. The binding of GTP releases the α subunit from the β/γ subunit complex and at the same time binds the α subunit to the effector protein. After the interaction with the effector, the α subunit converts GTP to GDP (intrinsically) and recombines with the β and γ subunits to begin the cycle over again.

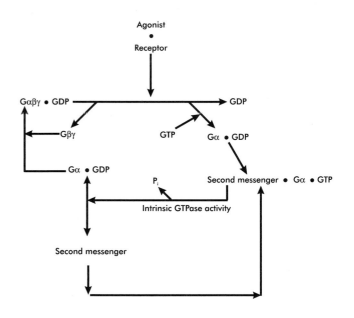

FIGURE 30–6. Regulatory cycle of G protein signal coupling. G protein exists as a triprotein with α, β, and γ subunits. Binding of an agonist to a receptor induces the release of the α subunit from the β/γ subunits and guanine diphosphate (GDP) from the α subunit. Guanosine triphosphate (GTP) binds to the α subunit; this complex then binds to a second messenger (adenylate cyclase or phospholipase C). The intrinsic GTPase converts GTP to GDP, which results in the uncoupling of the α subunit from the second messenger. The second messenger is then available for recoupling to an α/GTP complex. The α/GDP complex then binds to a β/γ subunit complex, and the cycle is ready to begin again.

All of the neuroreceptors that are known at this time to stimulate G protein regulatory units are of the seven-transmembrane helical type. G proteins are known to interact with a variety of effectors, which include adenyl cyclase, phosphodiesterase (phosphatidylinositol turnover), calcium and potassium channels, and receptor-coupled kinases. Through these effectors, G proteins are involved in both excitatory and inhibitory roles. Through the stimulation of receptor-coupled kinases and the phosphorylation of specific intracellular domains of the receptor proteins, G proteins provide feedback control of receptor sensitivity (Hausdorff et al. 1990).

Relatively little is known about drug influences on G protein functions. Lithium inhibits G protein function in the adrenergic stimulation of adenylate cyclase (Belmaker et al. 1990); however, the role of this effect in the therapeutics of lithium is not known. G proteins are only recently being considered as sites for drug actions (see section "Novel Targets for Pharmacotherapy" later in this chapter). No psychiatric disorders have been identified that result from defects in the G protein regulatory systems. As more is learned about this vital link in neuronal transmission, opportunities for pharmacological manipulation may become increasingly evident.

Second messengers. As stated earlier, many types of neuroreceptors are connected via a family of G proteins to one of two classes of second-messenger systems, the cAMP/protein phosphorylation system or the inositol triphosphate/diacylglycerol system. Each of these two systems is regulated by the action of G proteins, and the effectors for each system include protein kinases, which catalyze the transfer of the terminal phosphate group of ATP to a wide variety of substrate proteins (Table 30–4). In addition to activating protein kinases, the inositol triphosphate pathway is directly involved in the regulation of intraneuronal calcium concentrations. Unlike the localized effects of changes in ions, second-messenger actions are known to spread over long distances in neurons, thus influencing many types of neuronal functions (Kasai and Petersen 1994).

Neuroreceptors, through specific G proteins, either stimulate or inhibit the enzyme adenylate cyclase, which catalyzes the formation of cAMP (Gilman 1989) (Figure 30–7). cAMP binds to protein kinases, which activate specific effector proteins through the process of phosphorylation (see Figure 30–7 and Table 30–4). A key element in this pathway is the intraneuronal concentration of cAMP. The rate of synthesis of cAMP is the ratio of stimulatory to inhibitory receptor input, whereas the rate of metabolic degradation of cAMP is determined by the activity of the enzyme phosphodiesterase. Multiple ge-

TABLE 30–4. Classes of proteins that are targets for phosphorylation by protein kinases

G proteins
Microtubule-associated proteins or neurofilaments
Synaptic vesicle proteins
Neurotransmitter-synthesizing enzymes
Neurotransmitter receptors
Ion channel proteins
Neurotransmitter transporters

netic forms of adenylate cyclase (D.M. Cooper et al. 1995) and phosphodiesterase (McKnight 1991) have been identified. More than 300 specific forms of protein kinase are known (Walsh and Van Patten 1994), and they result in diverse activities.

In the case of the inositol/diacylglycerol system, extraneuronal signals are transmitted via a neurotransmitter receptor through a G protein to a phosphodiesterase, phospholipase C, which in turn hydrolyzes phosphatidylinositol 4,5-biphosphate (PIP_2), an intermembrane-bound phospholipid (Figure 30–8). The products of this hydrolyzation are inositol 1,4,5-triphosphate (IP_3) and diacylglycerol, both of which serve second-messenger roles (Hokin and Dixon 1993). IP_3 diffuses to the endoplasmic reticulum and stimulates a specific IP_3 receptor to release sequestered Ca^{2+}. The IP_3 receptor is now known to exist in multiple subtypes (Danoff and Ross 1994; Marshall and Taylor 1993). The activity of IP_3 receptors is regulated by several allosteric sites for Ca^{2+}, adenine nucleotides, and protein kinases. IP_3 is inactivated by the removal of phosphate through a series of phosphatase enzymes, and the inositol moiety is recycled back to phosphatidylinositol.

The diacylglycerol formed by the action of phospholipase C activates a widely distributed kinase, kinase C. Kinase C phosphorylates several proteins associated with a variety of neuronal membranes, such as those of synaptic vesicles, microtubules, receptor proteins (Nalepa 1994; Premont et al. 1995), and transporters (Blakely et al. 1998). The action of diacylglycerol is quite short, and it is rapidly recycled into phosphatidylinositol or metabolized to enter prostaglandin synthetic pathways.

The activity level of a protein that is activated by phosphorylation is determined by the relative rates of phosphorylation versus dephosphorylation. Calcineurin has been identified as a major factor in the dephosphorylation of a wide variety of proteins with key roles in synaptic transmission (Yakel 1997). These processes include ion channels (receptor and voltage gated), neurorecep-

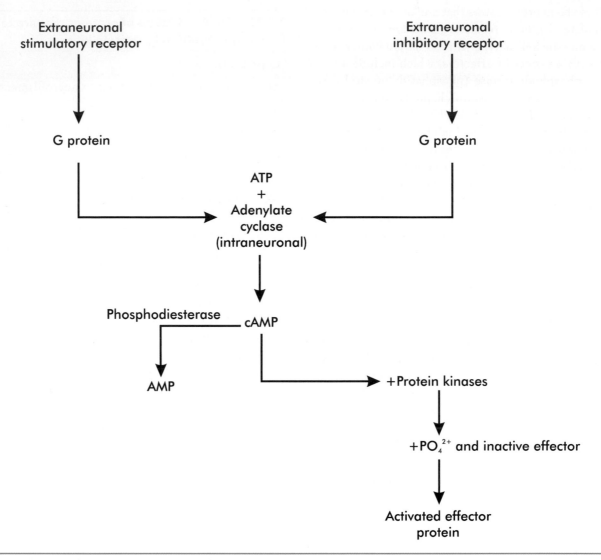

FIGURE 30–7.   Regulation and actions of the second messenger adenylate cyclase. Adenylate cyclase is either stimulated or inhibited in its production of cyclic adenosine monophosphate (cAMP) by specific receptors and G proteins. cAMP stimulates a variety of protein kinases, which in turn phosphorylate (combine with PO_4^{2+}) an effector that activates it and produces biological responses. cAMP is inactivated by the enzyme phosphodiesterase, which converts cAMP to AMP.
ATP=adenosine triphosphate.

tors, and neurotransmitter release. Calcineurin is approximately 50% bound to the neuronal membrane and thus influences many membrane-bound processes.

Calcineurin is composed of two subunits, designated A and B. The A subunit binds Ca^{2+} and calmodulin; Ca^{2+} binding is required for the binding of calmodulin. The B unit also binds Ca^{2+}, and full phosphatase activity is not realized unless all of these components are in place (Yakel 1997).

Calcineurin has been shown to regulate receptor-gated ion channels such as those gated by glutamate (NMDA), GABA, serotonin (5-HT$_3$), and acetylcholine (nicotinic type). Calcineurin appears to have a major influence on voltage-gated Ca^{2+} channels. Calcineurin is

also implicated in the processes of synaptic release of neurotransmitters and the recycling of the synaptic structures themselves. NO synthetase is a substrate for calcineurin; the dephosphorylation of NO synthetase increases its activity and enhances the production of NO. This latter process may be involved in certain neurotoxicity mechanisms. Finally, calcineurin regulates gene transcription and synaptic plasticity in learning and memory-related processes through influences on cAMP response element–binding protein (CREB) (Yakel 1997).

Although no psychotherapeutic agents are known to influence calcineurin, immunosuppressant drugs such as cyclosporine A and FK506 are potent inhibitors of calcineurin (Yakel 1997). The clinical significance of these

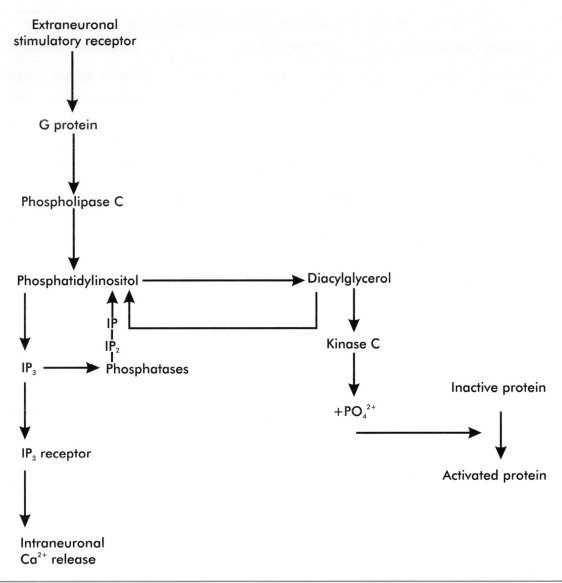

FIGURE 30–8.   Intraneuronal actions of phospholipase C activity. Phospholipase C is activated via a receptor-stimulated G protein. Phospholipase C splits phosphatidylinositol into inositol triphosphate (IP$_3$) and diacylglycerol moieties. The diacylglycerol stimulates kinase C, which activates effector proteins through phosphorylation. The inositol triphosphate binds to a receptor on the endoplasmic reticulum. Stimulation of this receptor releases bound calcium into the cytoplasm. Inositol triphosphate is inactivated by a series of phosphatases. Inositol is reincorporated into phosphatidylinositol. The antimanic drug lithium is a potent inhibitor of phosphatase and blocks the reincorporation of inositol into phosphatidylinositol.

immunosuppressant drugs with respect to their inhibition of calcineurin is not known; however, these drugs caused neurotoxicity and sympathetic hypertension in in vivo animal studies (Hughes 1990; Lyson et al. 1993; Yakel 1997).

Traditionally, the components of second-messenger systems have not been the primary targets of psychopharmacological agents. This is because second messengers are few in number and therefore not specific or selective compared with neurotransmitter receptors or reuptake sites. For example, a drug that influences the intracellular

levels of cAMP would be expected to have the same influence in many types of synapses simultaneously or, for that matter, in many kinds of tissues because second messengers exist in many types of cells outside the nervous system (Nishizuka 1995). Now that subtypes of elements such as phospholipase, phosphodiesterase, adenylate cyclase, and IP$_3$ receptors are known, the identification of more selective agents may be possible.

At this time, there is only one known psychotherapeutic agent that likely has its mechanism of action in a second-messenger system. Lithium, as an agent for treat-

TABLE 30–5.   Characteristics of the subtypes of nitric oxide synthase (NOS)

Subtype	Primary cellular location	Ca^{++} dependent	Role of NO production
NOS$_1$	Neuronal	Yes	Modification of synaptic activity
NOS$_2$	Glial	No	Inflammatory reactions
NOS$_3$	Endothelial	Yes	Local vascular responses
			Smooth muscle relaxant

Source.   Adapted from Calabrese et al. 2004; Galea and Feinstein 1999; Heales et al. 1999; Krukoff 1999.

ing mania, is well known to block inositol monophosphatase, a critical enzyme in the synthesis of phosphatidylinositol and the subsequent production of IP$_3$ (Hokin and Dixon 1993; Parthasarathy et al. 1994). This is a suggested mechanism of lithium's antimanic action because the influences on IP$_3$ occur at therapeutic doses (Baraban et al. 1989; Belmaker et al. 1990). Other pharmacological observations support this hypothesis (Brunello and Tascedda 2003). It is becoming more evident that a great deal of interaction takes place among the various components of the second-messenger systems and that some drug effects may be accounted for in this way. For example, the antidepressants affect cAMP levels through their influences on adrenergic receptors; however, they also influence the inositol/diacylglycerol system by modifying the action of kinase C (Nalepa 1994). Thus, antidepressant effects may be produced through more than one neurotransmitter system.

The ultimate influence that an agonist exerts on a neuronal system depends on a complex series of interactions between the agonist and the receptor, the receptor and the G protein, and the G protein and the second-messenger system (Kenakin 1995a, 1995b). Although it has not yet been documented, different agonists may influence receptors in ways that alter the interaction of the receptors with a variety of G proteins. Receptors may activate more than one kind of G protein, thus providing qualitatively differing biological responses. It also has been reported that the relative concentrations of receptors to G proteins may be an important determinant in the qualitative response to agonist activity. High concentrations of receptors relative to G proteins result in interactions with multiple types of G proteins providing multiple effects. The role that these factors play in disease states or drug mechanisms of action is not known at this time, but certainly psychotropic agents such as antidepressants and antipsychotics are well known for their influences on receptor populations, and some of their pharmacological actions may result from changes in the interaction of these crucial elements in neurotransmission.

Other Modulators of Neuronal Function

Nitric oxide.   Although synaptic transmission, via specific neurotransmitters, has long been considered the mainstay of brain function and served as the focus of pharmacological interventions, in recent years other substances have been shown to play key roles in brain activity. The establishment of NO as a neuromodulatory substance in the brain has opened new avenues of research in brain function and dysfunction.

Unlike other neurotransmitters, NO is not stored and released by specific presynaptic nerve endings and does not interact with specific receptors. NO is a gas and is synthesized on demand and diffuses rapidly through aqueous and lipid beds; thus, its influence is not synaptic in nature. Furthermore, it is capable of interacting with any molecule existing in an appropriate electrogenic state (Dawson and Snyder 1994).

NO is synthesized by one of three isoenzymes referred to as nitric oxide synthase (NOS); some characteristics of these isoenzymes can be found in Table 30–5. Once formed, NO reacts with the heme group of soluble guanyl cyclase, which then catalyzes the formation of cyclic guanosine monophosphate (cGMP) from GTP. cGMP then elicits several biological effects through interaction with specific protein kinases, phosphorolases, and ion channels. The biochemistry of NO synthesis and activity is summarized in Figure 30–9. Often, the Ca^{++} for the stimulation of NOS$_1$ and NOS$_2$ activities comes from the activation of glutamatergic NMDA-type receptors or possibly from intracellular sources through the action of inositol triphosphate.

NO derived from NOS$_2$ is primarily induced by a variety of cellular stresses such as cytokines and other substances associated with inflammation and is often associated with neurotoxicity. In these circumstances, NO interacts with superoxide anion radicals to form peroxynitrite (Pfeiffer and Mayer 2001), a strong oxidant that is widely believed to be associated with neurotoxicity and many neurodegenerative diseases (Heales et al. 1999; Liu et al. 2002).

The influences of NO on brain function are numerous and widespread. NO has been implicated in neuronal processes for long-term depression and potentiation, synaptic

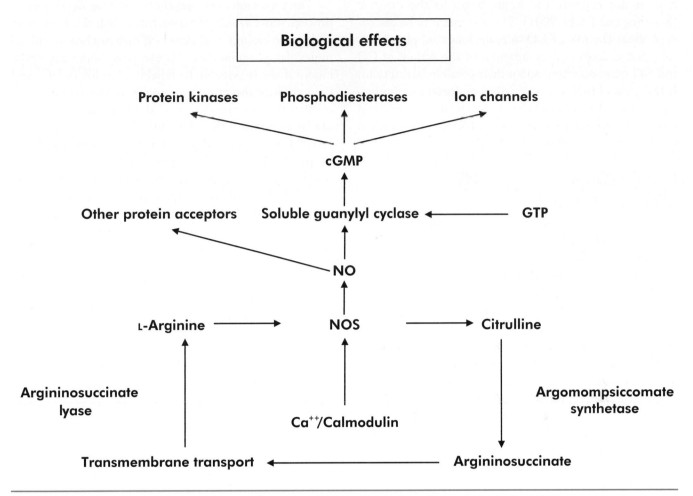

FIGURE 30–9. Biochemical events related to the synthesis and biological effects of nitric oxide (NO) occur in both neurons and glial cells. Intracellular calcium to activate nitric oxide synthase (NOS$_1$ and NOS$_3$) is derived from the activation of membrane receptors such as glutamate N-methyl-D-aspartate (NMDA) receptors or intracellular receptors such as inositol triphosphate receptors. cGMP=cyclic guanosine monophosphate; GTP=guanosine triphosphate.

Source. Adapted from Kiss and Vizi 2001; Seminara et al. 2001; Wiesinger 2001.

plasticity in the developing brain, and regulation of gap junction activity (Garthwaite 2001). NO has been found to alter the activity of the monoamines, norepinephrine, dopamine, serotonin (Kiss and Vizi 2001), glutamate, and GABA (Ferraro and Sardo 2004; Sequeira et al. 2001). Because of its nonsynaptic nature, NO's influence on overall brain function has been difficult to describe (Kiss 2000).

In addition to direct influences on synaptic brain activity, NO plays an important role in regulating blood flow to local areas of the brain. NO is a powerful smooth muscle relaxant and therefore dilates small arterioles and capillaries. Through this effect, NO provides increased blood supplies to active areas of the brain and thus ensures adequate supplies of oxygen and glucose to support glial and neuronal functions (Tsai et al. 1999). NO released from glial cells appears to play an important role in regulating blood flow (Schipke and Kettenmann 2004).

Carbon monoxide. During the past two decades, evidence has been accumulated suggesting that carbon monoxide (CO) is a neuroactive substance with some similarities to NO (Dawson and Snyder 1994; Hawkins et al. 1994; Morse et al. 2002). CO is synthesized in neuronal tissue via the enzyme heme oxygenase 2 (HO2) (Baranano and Snyder 2001). The action of HO2 produces biliverden (quickly reduced to bilirubin) in addition to CO. Bilirubin has been shown to be an effective antioxidant and thus can protect against neurotoxicity when synthesized locally through this reaction. Like NO, CO binds to and activates soluble guanyl cyclase to promote the conversion of GTP to cGMP. Although CO binds to soluble guanyl cyclase with equal affinity compared with NO, the two gases produce different reactions (Koesling and Friebe 2001). CO is a much weaker stimulator of soluble guanyl cyclase, presumably because it does not rupture the heme bond to the enzyme (Koesling and Friebe 2001). There is much to be discovered about the role of CO in brain function, physiologically and in disease. A comparison of the actions of CO and NO raises questions about their possible interactions: Is the ratio of their concentrations important in producing a particular effect? What is the influence on brain functions resulting from exogenous NO and CO, such as would occur with tobacco smoking?

PSYCHOTROPIC DRUG DEVELOPMENT

In the last century, efforts to refine psychiatric diagnoses and uncover the biological bases of psychiatric disorders have typically followed advances in neuroscience in general and neuropharmacology in particular. Historically, identification of the sites of action of clinically effective psychotropic drugs led to hypotheses of disease pathophysiology, many of which have now been held for decades with only slight modification. A case in point is the *dopamine hyperactivity* hypothesis of psychosis, supported by the discovery of the dopamine antagonist properties of chlorpromazine (Snyder et al. 1974). This hypothesis provided the framework for subsequent research and development of other dopamine antagonist drugs over the last 50 years.

In the latter half of the twentieth century, the psychotropic drug development process was based on the use of animal tests that modeled the responses to the index drug, which often had been discovered serendipitously (e.g., chlorpromazine, amitriptyline). Because the animal models were selected on the basis of drug response rather than disease pathophysiology, the new drugs tended to have pharmacological profiles similar to those drugs used to establish the research models. Hence successive generations of psychotropic drugs were developed, with some improvements relating to side-effect profiles and pharmacokinetic features, but there were no major advances.

ADVANCES IN MOLECULAR PHARMACOLOGY

Twenty years ago, it would have been difficult to imagine that an alternative strategy to animal models of psychiatric disorders could be used in behavioral pharmacology to rationally develop psychotropic drugs. Even more difficult to imagine at that time is a debate of the wisdom of choosing to develop one new drug over another on the basis of its relative potency for specific biological targets in the central nervous system (CNS). Only in recent times have new approaches become a possibility, and now rational or targeted drug development includes psychopharmacology.

The transition in the psychotropic drug development process was a result of powerful technical advances in molecular biology and genetics, which revolutionized molecular pharmacology. These new laboratory techniques make it possible to reliably identify, isolate, and then produce the protein components of synaptic transmission. In this process, once identified, a new protein can be cloned and then functionally assessed for effects on cell metabolism and protein synthesis. For new receptor proteins, specific ligands are synthesized and radiolabeled to examine their location, density, and function in the CNS. The role of receptor proteins can be further elucidated with modified gene expression in vivo (e.g., gene-specific suppression, splice variants, functional "knockout" of a specific receptor). Together these techniques are helping us understand how heretofore undiscovered components of neurotransmission may be at fault in psychiatric disorders and then provide a means to correct the function of the errant component.

NEURORECEPTOR PHARMACOLOGY

The benefits of the technical advances in molecular biology are nowhere more apparent in psychiatry than in the area of receptor pharmacology. In little over a decade, numerous new receptors have been identified and cloned (see Table 30–3). These receptors are characterized with respect to second-messenger systems, cellular locations, and regional distribution in the CNS. At last count, 14 serotonin receptor subtypes have been successfully cloned and are being studied with selective ligands and knockout mice (Hoyer et al. 2002; Sanders-Bush and Canton 1995). This is a dramatic advance considering that less than 20 years ago, only 2 serotonin receptor subtypes were known to exist. During this same period, 5 dopamine receptor subtypes and 5 muscarinic acetylcholine receptor subtypes have been isolated, and at least 12 protein subunits have been described that associate in various combinations to form numerous pentameric nicotinic acetylcholine receptor subtypes (Hogg et al. 2003; Holmes et al. 2004). As quickly as new receptor subtypes are identified, agonist and antagonists, and more recently gene-knockout animals, have been developed to explore their clinical significance. The result has been a cascade of new research, some of which has already led to the development of successful therapeutics (e.g., the 5-HT$_{1A}$ agonist buspirone, the 5-HT$_{1D}$ agonist sumatriptan, the 5-HT$_3$ antagonist ondansetron).

As new neuroreceptor subtypes are identified, several phenomena now occur in a relatively efficient manner: exploration of receptor action on cellular function in vitro and in vivo, evaluation of established therapeutic agents for binding affinity at the newly identified sites, generation of new theories of disease pathophysiology, and subsequent clinical evaluation of selective receptor ligands. This dynamic process has been recently illustrated in the area of antipsychotic drug development.

Antipsychotic Pharmacodynamics

For several decades, it has been recognized that all effective antipsychotic drugs inhibit dopamine receptors in the brain (Spano et al. 1978). It was widely believed that two types of dopamine receptors existed and that antipsychotic activity was related to inhibition of one of these, the dopamine type 2 (D_2) receptor (Stoof and Kebabian 1984). With the successful identification of at least five functional dopamine receptors came the consideration that perhaps a subtype other than the D_2 might be a more effective target for antipsychotic drugs (Meador-Woodruff 1994).

After its identification in brain tissue, the dopamine D_4 receptor subtype attracted particular attention as a target for antipsychotic drug therapy for a few reasons. This particular dopamine receptor was identified to be present in relatively high concentrations in the mesocortical areas of the brain but in relatively low concentrations in nigrostriatal regions (Todd and O'Malley 1993). Because blockade of dopamine receptors in the nigrostriatal regions is thought to be responsible for the unwanted movement disorders associated with antipsychotic drugs, the distribution of D_4 receptors suggested a means of selectively blocking dopamine transmission with respect to brain regions. With the recognition that clozapine had relatively high affinity for D_4 receptors, the theory was proposed that this biological activity might be responsible for the unique clinical features of clozapine (e.g., minimal extrapyramidal effects, efficacy in treating negative signs and symptoms of schizophrenia) (Seeman and Van Tol 1993; Van Tol et al. 1991).

The D_4 hypothesis provided the basis for broad investigation, including receptor binding studies, assay of D_4 messenger RNA (mRNA) in the brains of patients with schizophrenia, production of a D_4 receptor knockout mouse line, and clinical trials of a D_4 antagonist (Kramer et al. 1997; Mulcrone and Kerwin 1996; Rubinstein et al. 1997; Seeman et al. 1995). The D_4 antagonist did not show efficacy for treating acute psychosis, and taken together, the basic science studies did not identify an abnormality in this receptor associated with schizophrenia. Although the enthusiasm about a primary role of the D_4 receptor subtype in the pathophysiology of schizophrenia or as a preferred target of antipsychotic therapy has been dampened, the "D_4 Schizophrenia Story" is still an achievement (Kerwin and Owen 1999). It illustrates our current capabilities and the efficiency of the process from rational hypothesis to molecular research to clinical

analysis. Findings from the previous investigation now inform current studies of D_4 receptors and their role in cognition, attention, and behavioral inhibition (Holmes et al. 2004; Wong and Van Tol 2003).

Recent data continue to support the consensus that the D_2 binding affinity of antipsychotic drugs predicts their clinical efficacy (Holmes et al. 2004; Kapur et al. 2000). However, as new, nondopamine neuroreceptors are identified, it has been recognized that many antipsychotic drugs bind with relatively high affinity to these sites. Thus, nondopamine receptors are being considered as sites of action for antipsychotic drugs, which may mitigate some of the adverse effects or enhance the efficacy of D_2 receptors (L. F. Martin et al. 2004; Millan 2005; Richelson 1999).

Atypical antipsychotic drugs.   The so-called atypical antipsychotic drugs are characterized clinically by a relative decrease in extrapyramidal symptoms (EPS) and increased efficacy in treating negative symptoms of schizophrenia. Pharmacologically, this class of drugs is characterized by a higher binding affinity for 5-HT_{2A} receptors over dopamine D_2 receptors (Bymaster et al. 1996; Seeman and Van Tol 1993) (Table 30–6). With the clinical success of the atypical agents, the combination of 5-HT_{2A} and D_2 receptor binding properties has become a prototype for identifying compounds to develop as antipsychotic agents (Remington and Kapur 1999; Richelson 1999). How these two mechanisms interact to mediate the clinically desirable effects of atypical antipsychotics remains unclear. Studies in rats suggest that 5-HT_{2A} antagonism increases serotonin and dopamine levels in the rat brain (Devaud et al. 1992). Based on this observation, it has been advanced that 5-HT_{2A} antagonism could have effects on the negative symptoms of schizophrenia by increasing prefrontal dopamine transmission and mitigate the EPS of D_2 blockade through an increased dopamine synaptic tone (Hoyer et al. 2002; Richelson 1999).

Another area of investigation into the serotonergic pharmacodynamics of antipsychotic drugs follows the observation that some atypical antipsychotic agents bind with relatively high affinity and act as antagonists to the 5-HT_6 and 5-HT_7 receptor subtypes (Glatt et al. 1995; Hoyer et al. 2002; Roth et al. 1994) (see Table 30–6). These findings have drawn attention to the possible psychoactive properties of perhaps the relatively least studied serotonin receptor subtypes, 5-HT_6 and 5-HT_7. Although clinical trials with selective 5-HT_6 and 5-HT_7 ligands are lacking, mounting evidence indicates that these receptors play a prominent role in the regulation and maintenance of multiple neuronal systems and contribute to psychotropic drug efficacy. In the rat, 5-HT_6 receptors appear to modulate central cholinergic activity

TABLE 30–6.   Receptor binding affinity for selected antipsychotic drugs

Drug	D_2	D_4	$5\text{-}HT_{2A}$	$5\text{-}HT_6$	$5\text{-}HT_7$	$5\text{-}HT_{2A}/D_2$
Clozapine	125	21	12	4	63	0.1
Olanzapine	11	27	4	2.5	104	0.4
Risperidone	3	7	0.6	425	1.4	0.2
Haloperidol	1	5	78	>5,000	263	78

Note.   The affinity constants (Ki values in nanomolar) were determined in vitro using both rat and human brain tissue. A lower numerical value of Ki indicates greater receptor binding affinity. D_2, D_4 = dopamine receptor subtypes; $5\text{-}HT_{2A}$, $5\text{-}HT_6$, $5\text{-}HT_7$ = serotonin receptor subtypes; $5\text{-}HT_{2A}/D_2$ = ratio of binding affinities for the serotonin and dopamine receptor subtypes.

Source.   Data adapted from Bymaster et al. 1996; Roth et al. 1994; Seeman and Van Tol 1993.

(Hoyer et al. 2002). This observation has led to speculation that the beneficial effects of clozapine on cognitive dysfunction in schizophrenia may be mediated by the high-affinity binding to $5\text{-}HT_6$ receptors and stimulated further investigation of this receptor subtype as a putative target for the treatment of cognitive disorders.

First postulated to be a serotonin autoreceptor, $5\text{-}HT_7$ heteroreceptors recently have been identified on astrocytes throughout the CNS, on GABAergic interneurons in the dorsal raphe nucleus, and on glutamatergic cortico-raphe neurons (Harsing et al. 2004; Hirst et al. 1997; Roberts et al. 2004). In these various sites, the $5\text{-}HT_7$ heteroreceptors appear to modulate serotonin tone in several ways, including regulation of neuronal release of GABA and glutamate. The high-affinity binding of atypical antipsychotic agents to the $5\text{-}HT_7$ receptor provide a provocative alternative hypothesis for the "atypicality" of these drugs (i.e., decreased negative symptoms and EPS resulting from a $5\text{-}HT_7$-mediated increase in basal serotonergic tone). Taken together, these findings suggest an intimidating system complexity, yet they are a source of considerable enthusiasm. Unraveling the interactions of $5\text{-}HT_6$ and $5\text{-}HT_7$ receptors will advance our understanding of the pathophysiology of psychosis and other neuropsychiatric disorders and in so doing will determine whether these serotonin receptor subtypes are incidental or pivotal targets for psychotropic drug development (Hoyer et al. 2002; Leopoldo 2004).

MERITS OF PSYCHOTROPIC DRUG SELECTIVITY

The first successful drugs for treating depression and psychosis were characterized by having complicated pharmacodynamic profiles with multiple biological activities at clinically relevant doses. Over time, it was realized that for drugs such as imipramine and chlorpromazine, certain biological actions (e.g., α-adrenergic receptor blockade) con-

tributed little to the therapeutic effect of the drugs but were responsible for a variety of adverse effects. At best, these adverse effects were a nuisance for the patient and compromised treatment compliance; at worst, they narrowed the therapeutic index with resultant safety concerns.

The further disadvantage of a drug with multiple mechanisms of action is that the ratio of potency of the various components is fixed, which limits the ability to adjust treatment with dosing (e.g., poor tolerability of one mechanism prevents advancing the drug dose to increase another action). In this sense, when treating a condition for which multiple drug actions are necessary, it would be preferable to have an armamentarium of highly selective agents that would permit each action in a therapeutic regimen to be adjusted independently. Hence the concept of selectivity arose as a desirable feature for psychotropic agents. The concept became a reality with the advent of the SSRIs.

The SSRIs represented the first generation of psychotropic drugs to be rationally designed to target a selected site in the CNS with minimal biological effects at other sites. The selected target for SSRIs is the presynaptic transmembrane protein that transports serotonin from the synapse back into the cell, hence "reuptake." The logic held true, and this class of antidepressants went on to become the current cornerstone of antidepressant pharmacotherapy. A key feature in the success of the SSRIs has been that by virtue of their selectivity, drug tolerability and safety were greatly improved over their antidepressant predecessors. In the wake of the SSRIs, other selective agents targeting the traditional biogenic monoamines have been developed, marketed, and widely adopted in clinical use. These include the so-called dual-action selective serotonin-norepinephrine reuptake inhibitors (SNRIs) (e.g., venlafaxine), the selective norepinephrine and dopamine reuptake inhibitors (NDRIs) (e.g., bupropion), and the selective norepinephrine reuptake inhibitors (NRIs) (e.g., atomoxetine).

As we depart down the path of synthesizing highly selective ligands for newly identified sites in the CNS, one wonders if the time has come when a psychotropic drug may be made selective to the point that its utility can no longer be detected by conventional clinical investigation. Particularly for psychiatric disorders, which are syndromal in nature and lack distinct biological markers, one is likely to have a heterogeneous clinical population. In such a population, with the potential for diverse pathophysiology, the effects of a drug with a highly specific mechanism of action may improve too few subjects to be detected reliably. Hence agents that are particularly beneficial for some but not all patients could fail to be identified. Continued achievement in drug development for psychiatric disorders necessitates that efforts in molecular pharmacology proceed hand in hand with efforts to identify genotypes or physiological measures that characterize subpopulations of patients with similar pathophysiology.

Despite the clinical benefits of drug selectivity, within the context of the current capabilities in molecular pharmacology, how selective can a new drug be and still be practical to develop and useful in therapy? Is a highly selective, single-mechanism drug an end in and of itself? Are psychiatric disorders such as depression and schizophrenia likely to be the result of a single malfunctioning component in the chain of events of neurotransmission and hence treatable by selecting a singular target? The ancient advice of Burton (1927b) may still apply:

> Mixed diseases must have mixed remedies, and such simples are commonly mixed as have reference to the part affected, some to qualify, the rest to comfort, some one part, some another.

Several examples of post-SSRI-era psychotropic agents are nonselective, with multiple biological activities. Many of these agents have proven clinically useful (e.g., mirtazapine, a 5-HT_{2A}, 5-HT_{2C}, and 5-HT_3 antagonist). In some cases, these agents have even become prototypes for developing new therapies (e.g., clozapine, a 5-HT_{2A}, 5-HT_6, 5-HT_7, D_1, D_2, and D_4 antagonist). If the focus in drug development had been selectivity at all cost, these agents, and the provocative research directions they have provided, may not have been identified. Drug selectivity, albeit a feature of importance, only represents a refinement that enhances clinical effectiveness. Although the SSRIs revolutionized antidepressant pharmacotherapy, they did so with the same basic mechanism of action as the earliest antidepressants. For major advances in drug development, the novelty of the pharmacological profile is of principal importance. Efforts are under way to explore strategies for incorporating novel mechanisms into SSRIs to enhance efficacy (Pacher and Kecskemeti 2004).

NOVEL TARGETS FOR PHARMACOTHERAPY

Development of new drugs with novel mechanisms of action to treat psychiatric disorders has been constrained by our limited understanding of disease pathophysiology and the mechanisms that mediate the therapeutic effects of established treatments. Newer psychotropic drugs provide many therapeutic advantages, but they essentially recapitulate the mechanisms of action of their earliest predecessors. Antidepressant therapy is a case in point. Although the antidepressant drug armamentarium has expanded at an unprecedented rate over the last 15 years, the new agents retain a traditional focus on biogenic monoamine neurotransmitters and extracellular neuronal membranes (Coyle and Duman 2003).

Clearly, the expanded antidepressant armamentarium has advanced the clinical treatment of depression. The skillful clinician can now select from among these agents with regard to the specific neurotransmitter target(s) (e.g., serotonin, norepinephrine, dopamine) and mechanism of action (e.g., transport protein inhibitor, autoreceptor and heteroreceptor antagonist, enzyme inhibitor) (Pacher and Kecskemeti 2004; Stahl and Grady 2003). However, despite this increase in antidepressant options and a rationale for treatment selection, drug therapy remains ineffective in many patients, is often associated with distressing adverse effects, and may take a prolonged period to be effective. The same drawbacks exist for other psychotropic drug therapies (e.g., antipsychotics, mood stabilizers, anxiolytics). Hence the search for improved psychotropic drugs must continue. With our new skill in studying and manipulating the components of neurotransmission, researchers are enthusiastic that novel molecular targets will be identified for drug therapy. Developing psychotropic agents with completely novel mechanisms of action is of considerable interest, not only among clinicians (Pacher and Kecskemeti 2004; Stahl 1998a, 1998b; Stahl and Grady 2003; Triggle 1999) and the pharmaceutical industry (Hoyer et al. 2002; Nutt 1998, Wahlestedt 1998) but also in the financial world (Langreth 1998, 1999).

In psychotropic drug development, numerous possibilities are open to explore in the search for novel mechanisms of action. In large part, research efforts have been focused on the "first messenger" in neurotransmission—namely, the neurotransmitter and its membrane-binding site. This remains an exciting and potentially profitable level of exploration. New receptors are being identified at an unprecedented rate, and each represents a possible therapeutic target. At the same time, nonclassical neurotransmitters and the elements of intracellular signaling pathways are being investigated as possible targets for psychotropic pharmacotherapies.

Substance P and Neuropeptides

Substance P is the most abundant of several neurokinins and perhaps one of the best known neuropeptides in the CNS (J.R. Cooper et al. 2003; Herpfer and Lieb 2005; Pacher and Kecskemeti 2004). Three neurokinin receptors have been identified and isolated (i.e., NK-1, NK-2, NK-3). Substance P binds preferentially to the NK-1 receptor but also has agonist properties at the NK-2 and NK-3 receptors. Numerous indications suggest that substance P may be a reasonable target for novel antidepressant therapy. These preclinical findings have been summarized recently and include the following observations (Adell 2004; Herpfer and Lieb 2005; Kramer et al. 1998):

- Substance P and its binding sites are expressed in regions of the brain involved in stress and emotional response (e.g., amygdala, hippocampus, hypothalamus).
- Substance P content in these brain regions changes in response to stressful stimuli.
- Central administration of substance P produces aversion and anxiogenic behavioral responses in rodents.
- Traditional antidepressant drugs induce a decrease in substance P in rat brain.

These observations led to the development of NK-1 antagonists and a series of preliminary clinical trials. In some of the trials, the NK-1 antagonists appeared to be well tolerated and to produce significant reductions in both depression and anxiety rating scale scores, but in other studies, the results were disappointing (Herpfer and Lieb 2005; Kramer et al. 1998). Taken together, the equivocal results of the clinical trials have not dampened enthusiasm for further investigation of neurokinins as antidepressant targets. More recent data suggest that selective antagonists for all three neurokinin receptors have antidepressant properties, and it has been speculated that blockade of more than one neurokinin receptor subtype may have additive effects (Dableh et al. 2005). Development of substances that block more than one neurokinin receptor and clinical trials of selective NK-2 receptor antagonists are under way (Herpfer and Lieb 2005).

Glutamate Transmission and NMDA Receptors

As the understanding of glutamate transmission has progressed and with an appreciation of glutamate as a primary excitatory neurotransmitter in the CNS, efforts are ongoing to explore the role of glutamate in a wide range of neuropsychiatric disorders, including psychosis, anxiety, dementia, depression, stroke, and epilepsy (Goff et al. 1999; Javitt 2004; Posey et al. 2004; Tsai et al. 1999). Neurotransmission involving the NMDA subtype of the glutamate receptor has received particular attention (Millan 2002, 2005). Because direct NMDA recognition site agonists appear to be excitotoxic, modulatory sites of glutamatergic transmission are being investigated as potential therapeutic targets. These modulatory mechanisms include allosteric binding sites on NMDA receptors for glycine and D-serine; glycine transporter proteins expressed on neurons and glia, which tightly control synaptic glycine concentration; and metabotropic receptors that regulate glutamate release (Javitt 2004; Kew and Kemp 2005).

Glutamate in schizophrenia.   Several lines of evidence suggest that at least some of the symptoms of schizophrenia may result from a lack of activity at the NMDA type of glutamate receptors in corticolimbic brain areas (Coyle and Tsai 2004; Coyle et al. 2003; Kanai and Hediger 2003). In addition, several lines of evidence suggest that NMDA receptors are very much involved in the regulation of dopamine activity in the brain (Javitt 2004; Sur and Kinney 2004). Subsequently, the NMDA receptor, along with its modulatory site, the glycine B receptor, has been the target of recent clinical evaluations in subjects with schizophrenia (Millan 2002). The presence of glycine on its recognition site is a requirement for operation of the NMDA receptor. Because the NMDA receptor is a Ca^{++} ion channel when activated, and excessive intracellular calcium is associated with neurotoxicity, direct stimulation of the NMDA receptor may yield undesirable effects. A less severe way of stimulating NMDA influences may be through the use of agonists at the glycine B site (Coyle and Tsai 2004). Three glycine B agonists have been evaluated for their influence on the symptoms of schizophrenia: glycine, D-serine, and D-cycloserine (see Millan 2005 for a review of these studies). The full agonists, glycine and D-serine, resulted in some improvement in positive and cognitive symptoms, with the greatest improvement in negative symptoms. However, large doses are required to obtain significant concentrations in the brain: 40–60 g/day of glycine and 2 g/day of D-serine. D-Cycloserine is a partial agonist at the glycine receptor and therefore may act as an agonist or antagonist depending on the concentration of glycine available to the receptor site. D-Cycloserine also has been shown to improve symptoms of schizophrenia in some studies (Coyle and Tsai 2004) but not in others (van Berckel et al. 1999).

Another pharmacological approach to increasing glycine activity is to block the reuptake of synaptic glycine (Javitt 2004; Sur and Kinney 2004). *N*-methylglycine (sarcosine), a naturally occurring inhibitor of the glycine transporter, has been reported to improve multiple symptoms of schizophrenia (Tsai et al. 2004). Specific, high-affinity blockers of glycine reuptake have been identified and shown to modulate dopamine activity in preclinical investigations (Javitt et al. 2005).

Although the results of limited clinical studies with agents acting at the NMDA and glycine B sites are consistent with the suggestion that alterations in NMDA function are relevant to treating symptoms of schizophrenia and that agents working at these sites may prove useful, additional drug development is required to provide practical therapeutic agents for clinical use.

Intracellular Messenger Systems

There is intense interest in looking for therapeutic targets distal to the neurotransmitter membrane receptor along the intracellular signal transduction pathways (Coyle and Duman 2003; Pacher and Kecskemeti 2004; Paul 1999). The family of G proteins and the second-messenger systems that act to regulate gene expression are considered attractive potential targets for antidepressant drugs. Data already show that long-term administration of a wide variety of established antidepressant drugs regulates G protein α subunit expression (Lesch and Manji 1992). This finding suggests that G protein alteration may be an integral part of the neuroadaptive mechanisms that underlie therapeutic response (Rasenick et al. 1996). Additionally, considerable evidence suggests that antidepressant drug therapies affect second-messenger systems such as the cAMP pathway and in this way modulate gene expression in the CNS to bring about their therapeutic effects (G. Chen et al. 1999; Nibuya et al. 1996).

With the advances in molecular biology and genetics, the intracellular messenger systems in neurotransmission can now be investigated for novel therapeutic targets. At this level of signal transduction, protein kinase–mediated phosphoproteins regulate gene expression. This area of research is particularly provocative, focusing attention away from the acute biochemical response to pharmacological interventions to the long-term neuroadaptive mechanisms that more likely mediate therapeutic response. As these neuroadaptive mechanisms are elucidated, the possibilities for novel therapies increase dramatically, from drugs that alter the protein phosphorylation cascade to agents that directly modify encoding of specific genes.

Several research teams have already identified changes in neuronal gene expression and protein synthesis that occur in response to diverse antidepressant therapies and are commensurate with the 2- to 3-week lag time to onset of therapeutic effect. Tricyclic antidepressants, SSRIs, and even electroconvulsive therapy, but not selected nonantidepressant drugs, have been found to increase transcription of CREB and the mitochondrial protein cytochrome b in brain tissue (Huang et al. 1997;

Nibuya et al. 1996). Tricyclic antidepressants and the SSRI paroxetine have been found to increase glucocorticoid receptor gene expression in rodent and human tissue (Barden 1999; Okugawa et al. 1999; Vedder et al. 1999). The significance of these particular proteins to antidepressant efficacy remains obscure. However, the antidepressant-mediated upregulation and expression of CREB are particularly provocative in light of the recognition that CREB regulates expression of multiple genes, including the gene for brain-derived neurotrophic factor (BDNF) (B. Chen et al. 2001; Thome et al. 2000). Both CREB and BDNF have been shown to increase synaptic integrity and neuronal growth; in animal models of depression, they have antidepressant properties (e.g., reversal of learned helplessness) (A.C. Chen et al. 2001; Shirayama et al. 2002). In the search for new psychotropic drugs, intracellular cascade elements that activate transcription factors such as CREB or stimulate translation of proteins such as BDNF represent novel therapeutic targets for further investigation (Coyle and Duman 2003).

CONCLUSION

Considering the relative lack of effective treatments for mental illness during the first half of the twentieth century, the discovery of effective drugs in the 1950s was a milestone. The availability of these agents not only provided relief of symptoms to millions of patients but also opened the door to our understanding of basic brain physiology and chemistry. Increased knowledge of brain diseases and of psychopharmacology has led to the reality of rational drug design and targeted drug discovery. As knowledge increases, the targets become smaller and the drug effects more specific.

The ability to target drug action has totally changed the preclinical processes of drug development. The process is faster and more efficient and depends more on logic and knowledge than on luck. The clinical elements of drug development in psychiatry, on the contrary, have not kept pace. Clinical trials still require large-scale multisite studies of patients with vaguely defined psychiatric syndromes that may consist of multiple disorders as defined by pathophysiology. The approach is one of sheer numbers to determine drug efficacy. Many useful drugs may actually be determined to be ineffective through this methodology because they may improve symptoms in only a small subset of the study population.

The clinical phase of drug development therefore should be upgraded coincident with the advances being made in preclinical development. Such an upgrade would include a return to open-label studies, in either late Phase I or early Phase II. These studies would represent advanced behavioral pharmacology studies to better characterize the drugs and effects seen at particular doses. Such studies would include both behavioral observations and surrogate markers to measure clinical response when possible. When possible and appropriate, studies would be done both in psychiatrically healthy volunteers and in patients with the target illness. The goals of such studies would be to define 1) the dose response and time curves, 2) the measures that would be most suited for the larger studies needed to document efficacy, and 3) the types of patients that should be enrolled in those later pivotal studies.

The discipline of neuropharmacology is poised to identify novel therapeutic targets for psychiatric disorders. At this time, the possible sites for pharmacological intervention in the neurotransmission process seem endless. As research efforts progress, many of the novel sites of action that are explored likely will not become preferred targets for psychotropic pharmacotherapy. However, the ultimate achievement is that each attempt to develop a novel psychotropic agent brings us closer to understanding the complex process of neurotransmission and the pathophysiology of neuropsychiatric disorders.

Highlights for the Clinician

Historical perspective

- ✦ Development of modern psychopharmacology in the 1950s was via serendipity.

- ✦ Psychopharmacology has contributed to understanding the organic nature of brain functions.

Neurobiology

- ✦ Glia make up approximately one half of the brain's volume and contribute significantly to brain functions through chemical interactions with neurons.

- ✦ The predominant means of synaptic communication between neurons is via chemical transmission.

- ✦ Five essential processes involved in chemical transmission include (presynaptic) synthesis, storage, release, (postsynaptic) inactivation, and receptors; these processes provide many targets for drug-induced modifications of neuronal activity.

- ✦ G proteins serve as important molecular mediators between neuroreceptors and intraneuronal second-messenger systems.

- ✦ Phosphorylation of proteins provides an important means of regulating neuronal activity through increasing and decreasing protein activity.

- ✦ The gases nitric oxide and carbon monoxide are important neuromodulatory agents and may be involved in psychiatric disorders and neurodegenerative events.

Psychotropic drug development

- ✦ Advances in molecular pharmacology have streamlined the search for new and novel psychotherapeutic agents by providing specific molecular targets.

- ✦ Examples of the new technologies can be seen in the identification and characterization of neurotransmitter receptors, allowing for the development of specific, limited-action drugs for these sites.

- ✦ As technology permits the development of more selective therapeutic agents, a better understanding of how specific proteins are involved in brain dysfunction is required to make optimum therapeutic use of novel therapeutics.

- ✦ Novel sites under investigation for drug intervention in psychotherapeutics include neuropeptides and glutamate receptors.

- ✦ Intracellular processes that regulate gene expression also represent new areas for the development of novel psychotherapeutic agents.

RECOMMENDED READING

Charney DS, Nestler EJ: Neurobiology of Mental Illness, 2nd Edition. New York, Oxford University Press, 2004

REFERENCES

Adell A: Antidepressant properties of substance P antagonists: relationship to monoaminergic mechanisms? [published erratum appears in Curr Drug Targets CNS Neurol Disord 3:269, 2004] Curr Drug Targets CNS Neurol Disord 3:113–121, 2004

Aschner M, Allen JW, Kimelberg HK, et al: Glial cells in neurotoxicity development. Annu Rev Pharmacol Toxicol 39:151–173, 1999

Bacci A, Verderio C, Pravettoni E, et al: The role of glial cells in synaptic function. Philos Trans R Soc Lond B Biol Sci 354:403–409, 1999

Baker R, Llinas R: Electronic coupling between neurons in the rat mesencephalic nucleus. J Physiol 212:45–63, 1971

Baraban JM, Worley PF, Snyder SH: Second messenger systems and psychoactive drug action: focus on the phosphoinositide system and lithium. Am J Psychiatry 146:1251–1259, 1989

Baranano DE, Snyder SH: Neural roles for heme oxygenase: contrasts to nitric oxide synthase. Proc Natl Acad Sci U S A 98:10996–11002, 2001

Barden N: Regulation of corticosteroid receptor gene expression in depression and antidepressant action. J Psychiatry Neurosci 24:25–39, 1999

Belmaker RH, Livine A, Agam G, et al: Role of inositol-1-phosphatase inhibition in the mechanism of action of lithium. Pharmacol Toxicol 66 (suppl 3):76–83, 1990

Blakely RD, Berson HE, Fremeau RTJ, et al: Cloning and expression of a functional serotonin transporter from rat brain. Nature 354:66–70, 1991

Blakely RD, Ramamoorthy S, Qian Y, et al: Regulation of antidepressant-sensitive serotonin transporters, in Neurotransmitter Transporters: Structure, Function, and Regulation. Edited by Reith MEA. Totowa, NJ, Humana Press, 1997, pp 29–72

Blakely RD, Ramamoorthy S, Schroeter S, et al: Regulated phosphorylation and trafficking of antidepressant-sensitive serotonin transporter proteins. Biol Psychiatry 44:169–178, 1998

Bohn MC: A commentary on glial cell line-derived neurotrophic factor (GDNF): from a glial secreted molecule to gene therapy. Biochem Pharmacol 57:135–142, 1999

Bordey A, Sontheimer H: Ion channel expression by astrocytes in situ: comparison of different CNS regions. Glia 30:27–38, 2000

Brunello N, Tascedda F: Cellular mechanisms and second messengers: relevance to the psychopharmacology of bipolar disorders. Int J Neuropsychopharmacol 6:181–189, 2003

Bullock TH, Bennett MV, Johnston D, et al: Neuroscience: the neuron doctrine, redux. Science 310:791–793, 2005

Burton R: The Anatomy of Melancholy. Edited by Dell F, Jordan-Smith P. New York, Farrar & Rinehart, 1927a, pp 574–582

Bymaster FP, Hemrick-Luecke SK, Perry KW, et al: Neurochemical evidence for antagonism by olanzapine of dopamine, serotonin, alpha 1-adrenergic and muscarinic receptors in vivo in rats. Psychopharmacology (Berl) 124:87–94, 1996

Calabrese V, Boyd-Kimball D, Scapagnini G, et al: Nitric oxide and cellular stress response in brain aging and neurodegenerative disorders: the role of vitagenes. In Vivo 18:245–267, 2004

Caldecott-Hazard S, Morgan DG, DeLeon-Jones F, et al: Clinical and biochemical aspects of depressive disorders, II: transmitter/receptor theories. Synapse 9:251–301, 1991

Caldwell AE: History of psychopharmacology, in Principles of Psychopharmacology, 2nd Edition. Edited by Clark WG, Delgiudice J. New York, Academic Press, 1978, pp 9–40

Catterall WA: Interactions of presynaptic Ca^{2+} channels and snare proteins in neurotransmitter release, in Molecular and Functional Diversity of Ion Channels and Receptors. Edited by Rudy B, Seeburg P. New York, New York Academy of Sciences, 1999, pp 144–159

Chen AC, Shirayama Y, Shin KH, et al: Expression of the cAMP response element binding protein (CREB) in hippocampus produces an antidepressant effect. Biol Psychiatry 49:753–762, 2001

Chen B, Dowlatshahi D, MacQueen GM, et al: Increased hippocampal BDNF immunoreactivity in subjects treated with antidepressant medication. Biol Psychiatry 50:260–265, 2001

Chen G, Hasanat K, Bebchuk J, et al: Regulation of signal transduction pathways and gene expression by mood stabilizers and antidepressants. Psychosom Med 61:599–617, 1999

Clapham DE, Neer EJ: New roles for G-protein beta gamma-dimers in transmembrane signaling. Nature 365:403–406, 1993

Cole JO: Psychopharmacology: problems in evolution, in National Research Council Information. Edited by Cole JO, Gerard RW. Washington, DC, National Academy of Sciences, 1959, pp 92–107

Cooper DM, Mons N, Karpen JW: Adenylyl cyclases and the interaction between calcium and cAMP signaling. Nature 374:421–424, 1995

Cooper JR, Bloom FE, Roth RH: The Biochemical Basis of Neuropharmacology, 8th Edition. New York, Oxford University Press, 2003, pp 423–426

Cornell-Bell AH, Finkbeiner SM: Ca^{2+} waves in astrocytes. Cell Calcium 12:185–204, 1991

Cornell-Bell AH, Finkbeiner SM, Cooper MS, et al: Glutamate induced calcium waves in cultured astrocytes: long-range glial signaling. Science 247:470–473, 1990

Coyle JT, Duman RS: Finding the intracellular signaling pathways affected by mood disorder treatments. Neuron 38:157–160, 2003

Coyle JT, Tsai G: The NMDA receptor glycine modulatory site: a therapeutic target for improving cognition and reducing negative symptoms in schizophrenia. Psychopharmacology (Berl) 174:32–38, 2004

Coyle JT, Tsai G, Goff D: Converging evidence of NMDA receptor hypofunction in the pathophysiology of schizophrenia. Ann N Y Acad Sci 1003:318–327, 2003

Dableh LJ, Yashpal K, Rochford J, et al: Antidepressant-like effects of neurokinin receptor antagonists in the forced swim test in the rat. Eur J Pharmacol 507:99–105, 2005

Danoff SK, Ross CA: The inositol trisphosphate receptor gene family: implications for normal and abnormal brain function. Prog Neuropsychopharmacol Biol Psychiatry 18:1–16, 1994

Dawson TM, Snyder SH: Gases as biological messengers: nitric oxide and carbon monoxide in the brain. J Neurosci 14:5147–5159, 1994

Devaud LL, Hollingsworth EB, Cooper BR: Alterations in extracellular and tissue levels of biogenic amines in rat brain induced by the serotonin(2) receptor antagonist, ritanserin. J Neurochem 59:1459–1466, 1992

Enkvist MOK, McCarthy KD: Activation of protein kinase C blocks astroglial gap junction communication and inhibits the spread of calcium waves. J Neurochem 59:519–526, 1992

Ferraro G, Sardo P: Nitric oxide and brain hyperexcitability. In Vivo 18:357–366, 2004

Furth PA, St. Onge L, Boger H, et al: Temporal control of gene expression in transgenic mice by a tetracycline-responsive promoter. Proc Natl Acad Sci U S A 91:9302–9306, 1994

Gadea A, Lopez-Colome AM: Glial transporters for glutamate, glycine and GABA, I: glutamate transporters. J Neurosci Res 63:453–460, 2001a

Gadea A, Lopez-Colome AM: Glial transporters for glutamate, glycine and GABA, II: GABA transporters. J Neurosci Res 63:461–468, 2001b

Gadea A, Lopez-Colome AM: Glial transporters for glutamate, glycine and GABA, III: glycine transporters. J Neurosci Res 64:218–222, 2001c

Galea E, Feinstein DL: Regulation of the expression of the inflammatory nitric oxide synthase (NOS2) by cyclic AMP. FASEB J 13:2125–2137, 1999

Galli A, Petersen CI, deBlaquiere M, et al: Drosophila serotonin transporters have voltage-dependent uptake coupled to a serotonin-gated ion channel. J Neurosci 17:3401–3411, 1997

Garthwaite J: The physiological roles of nitric oxide in the central nervous system, in Nitric Oxide. Edited by Mayer B. Berlin, Springer-Verlag, 2001, pp 259–275

Gebremedhin D, Yamaura K, Zhang C, et al: Metabotropic glutamate receptor activation enhances the activities of two types of Ca2+-activated k+ channels in rat hippocampal astrocytes. J Neurosci 23:1678–1687, 2003

Gegelashvili G, Schousboe A: High affinity glutamate transporters: regulation of expression and activity. Mol Pharmacol 52:6–15, 1997

Gill SS, Patel NK, Hotton GR, et al: Direct brain infusion of glial cell line-derived neurotrophic factor in Parkinson disease. Nat Med 9:589–595, 2003

Gilman AG: G proteins and regulation of adenylyl cyclase. JAMA 262:1819–1825, 1989

Glatt CE, Snowman AM, Sibley DR, et al: Clozapine: selective labeling of sites resembling 5HT$_6$ serotonin receptors may reflect psychoactive profile. Mol Med 1:398–406, 1995

Goff DC, Tsai G, Levitt J, et al: A placebo-controlled trial of D-cycloserine added to conventional neuroleptics in patients with schizophrenia. Arch Gen Psychiatry 56:21–27, 1999

Grady S, Marks MJ, Wonnacott S, et al: Characterization of nicotinic receptor-mediated [^{3}H] dopamine release from synaptosomes prepared from mouse striatum. J Neurochem 59:848–856, 1992

Grondin R, Gash DM: Glial cell line-derived neurotrophic factor (GDNF): a drug candidate for the treatment of Parkinson's disease. J Neurol 245:35–42, 1998

Guldberg HC, Marsden CA: Catechol-O-methyl transferase: pharmacological aspects and physiological role. Pharmacol Rev 27:135–206, 1975

Haga K, Haga T: Activation by G protein beta gamma subunits of agonist- or light-dependent phosphorylation of muscarinic acetylcholine receptors and rhodopsin. J Biol Chem 267:2222–2227, 1992

Harsing LGJ, Prauda I, Barkoczy J, et al: A 5-HT$_7$ heteroreceptor-mediated inhibition of [^{3}H]serotonin release in raphe nuclei slices of the rat: evidence for a serotonergic-glutamatergic interaction. Neurochem Res 29:1487–1497, 2004

Hausdorff WP, Caron MG, Lefkowitz RJ: Turning off the signal: desensitization of β-adrenergic receptor function. FASEB J 4:2881–2889, 1990

Hawkins RD, Zhuo M, Arancio O: Nitric oxide and carbon monoxide as possible retrograde messengers in hippocampal long-term potentiation. J Neurobiol 25:652–665, 1994

Heales SJ, Bolanos JP, Stewart VC, et al: Nitric oxide, mitochondria and neurological disease. Biochem Biophys Acta 1410:215–228, 1999

Herpfer I, Lieb K: Substance P receptor antagonists in psychiatry: rationale for development and therapeutic potential. CNS Drugs 19:275–293, 2005

Hirst WD, Price GW, Rattray M, et al: Identification of 5-hydroxytryptamine receptors positively coupled to adenylyl cyclase in rat cultured astrocytes. Br J Pharmacol 120:509–515, 1997

Hogg RC, Raggenbass M, Bertrand D: Nicotinic acetylcholine receptors: from structure to brain function. Rev Physiol Biochem Pharmacol 147:1–46, 2003

Hokin LE, Dixon JF: The phosphoinositide signalling system, I: historical background, II: effects of lithium on the accumulation of second messenger inositol 1,4,5-trisphosphate in brain cortex slices. Prog Brain Res 98:309–315, 1993

Holmes A, Lachowicz JE, Sibley DR: Phenotypic analysis of dopamine receptor knockout mice: recent insights into the functional specificity of dopamine receptor subtypes. Neuropharmacology 47:1117–1134, 2004

Hoyer D, Hannon JP, Martin GR: Molecular, pharmacological and functional diversity of 5-HT receptors. Pharmacol Biochem Behav 71:533–554, 2002

Huang N, Strakhova M, Layer R, et al: Chronic antidepressant treatments increase cytochrome β mRNA levels in mouse cerebral cortex. J Mol Neurosci 9:167–176, 1997

Hughes RL: Cyclosporine-related central nervous system toxicity in cardiac transplantation (letter). N Engl J Med 323:420–421, 1990

Inagaki N, Wada H: Histamine and prostanoid receptors on glial cells. Glia 11:102–109, 1994

Javitt DC: Glutamate as a therapeutic target in psychiatric disorders. Mol Psychiatry 9:984–997, 2004

Javitt DC, Hashim A, Sershen H: Modulation of striatal dopamine release by glycine transport inhibitors. Neuropsychopharmacology 30:649–656, 2005

Joels M, de Kloet ER: Mineralcorticoid and glucocorticoid receptors in the brain: implications for ion permeability and transmitter systems. Prog Neurobiol 43:1–36, 1994

Kanai Y, Hediger MA: The glutamate and neutral amino acid transporter family: physiological and pharmacological implications. Eur J Pharmacol 479:237–247, 2003

Kapur S, Zipursky R, Jones C, et al: Relationship between dopamine D_2 occupancy, clinical response, and side effects: a double blind PET study of first-episode schizophrenia. Am J Psychiatry 157:514–520, 2000

Kasai H, Petersen OH: Spatial dynamics of second messengers: IP3 and cAMP as long-range and associative messengers. Trends Neurosci 17:95–101, 1994

Kelly RB: An introduction to the nerve terminal, in Neurotransmitter Release. Edited by Bellen HJ. Oxford, UK, Oxford University Press, 1999, pp 1–33

Kenakin T: Agonist-receptor efficacy, I: mechanisms of efficacy and receptor promiscuity. Trends Pharmacol Sci 16:188–192, 1995a

Kenakin T: Agonist-receptor efficacy, II: agonist trafficking of receptor signals. Trends Pharmacol Sci 16:232–238, 1995b

Kerwin R, Owen M: Genetics of novel therapeutic targets in schizophrenia. Br J Psychiatry 174:1–4, 1999

Kew JN, Kemp JA: Ionotropic and metabotropic glutamate receptor structure and pharmacology. Psychopharmacology (Berl) 179:4–29, 2005

Kilts CD: Recent pharmacologic advances in antidepressant therapy. Am J Med 97 (suppl 6A):3S–12S, 1994

Kirik D, Georgievska B, Bjorklund A: Localized striatal delivery of GDNF as a treatment for Parkinson disease. Nat Neurosci 7:105–110, 2004

Kiss JP: Role of nitric oxide in the regulation of monoaminergic neurotransmission. Brain Res Bull 52:459–466, 2000

Kiss JP, Vizi ES: Nitric oxide: a novel link between synaptic and nonsynaptic transmission. Trends Neurosci 24:211–215, 2001

Koesling D, Friebe A: Enzymology of soluble guanylyl cyclase, in Nitric Oxide. Edited by Mayer B. Berlin, Springer-Verlag, 2001, pp 93–109

Korn H, Sotelo C, Crepel F: Electronic coupling between neurons in rat lateral vestibular nucleus. Exp Brain Res 16:255–275, 1973

Kramer MS, Last B, Getson A, et al: The effects of a selective D_4 dopamine receptor antagonist (L-745,870) in acutely psychotic inpatients with schizophrenia. Arch Gen Psychiatry 54:567–572, 1997

Kramer MS, Cutler N, Feighner J, et al: Distinct mechanism for antidepressant activity by blockade of central substance P receptors (comments). Science 281:1640–1645, 1998

Krantz DE, Chaudhry FA, Edwards RH: Neurotransmitter transporters, in Neurotransmitter Release. Edited by Bellen HJ. Oxford, UK, Oxford University Press, 1999, pp 145–207

Krukoff TL: Central actions of nitric oxide in regulation of autonomic functions. Brain Res Brain Res Rev 30:52–65, 1999

Lai J, Bilsky EJ, Rothman RB, et al: Treatment with antisense oligodeoxynucleotide to the opioid delta receptor selectively inhibits delta 2-agonist antinociception. Neuroreport 5:1049–1052, 1994

Langreth R: Merck reports positive test results for new type of antidepressant drug. Wall Street Journal, September 11, 1998, p B7

Langreth R: Merck and Co. hits a stumbling block in testing experimental antidepressant. Wall Street Journal, January 25, 1999, p B6

Lapchak PA: A preclinical development strategy designed to optimize the use of glial cell line-derived neurotrophic factor in the treatment of Parkinson's disease. Mov Disord 13:49–54, 1998

Leopoldo M: Serotonin(7) receptors (5-HT(7)Rs) and their ligands. Curr Med Chem 11:629–661, 2004

Lesch K, Manji H: Signal-transducing G proteins and antidepressant drugs: evidence for modulation of alpha subunit gene expression in rat brain. Biol Psychiatry 32:549–579, 1992

Lesch KP, Mossner R: Genetically driven variation in serotonin uptake: is there a link to affective spectrum, neurodevelopmental, and neurodegenerative disorders? Biol Psychiatry 44:179–192, 1998

Lesch KP, Bengel D, Heils A, et al: Association of anxiety-related traits with a polymorphism in the serotonin transporter gene regulatory region. Science 274:1527–1531, 1996

Lester HA, Cao Y, Mager S: Listening to neurotransmitter transporters. Neuron 17:807–810, 1996

Levitan IB, Kaczmarek LK: The Neuron: Cell and Molecular Biology, 3rd Edition. New York, Oxford University Press, 2002

Lin SC, Bergles DE: Synaptic signaling between neurons and glia. Glia 47:290–298, 2004

Liu B, Gao HM, Wang JY, et al: Role of nitric oxide in inflammation-mediated neurodegeneration. Ann N Y Acad Sci 962:318–331, 2002

Llinas R, Baker R, Sotelo C: Electronic coupling between neurons in the cat inferior olive. J Neurophysiol 37:560–571, 1974

LoTurco JJ, Kriegstein AR: Clusters of coupled neuroblasts in embryonic neocortex. Science 252:563–566, 1991

Lovinger DM: Alcohols and neurotransmitter gated ion channels: past, present and future. Naunyn Schmiedebergs Arch Pharmacol 356:267–282, 1997

Lucas JJ, Hen R: New players in the 5-HT receptor field: genes and knockouts. Trends Pharmacol Sci 16:246–252, 1995

Lyson T, Ermel LD, Belshaw PJ, et al: Cyclosporine- and FK506-induced sympathetic activation correlates with calcineurin-mediated inhibition of T-cell signaling. Circ Res 73:596–602, 1993

MacDermott AB, Role LW, Siegelbaum SA: Presynaptic ionotropic receptors and the control of transmitter release. Annu Rev Neurosci 22:443–485, 1999

Mannisto PT, Ulmanen I, Lundstrom K, et al: Characteristics of catechol-O-methyltransferase (COMT) and properties of selective COMT inhibitors. Prog Drug Res 39:291–350, 1992

Marcaggi P, Attwell D: Role of glial amino acid transporters in synaptic transmission and brain energetics. Glia 47:217–225, 2004

Marshall IC, Taylor CW: Regulation of inositol 1,4,5-trisphosphate receptors. J Exp Biol 184:161–182, 1993

Martin DL: Synthesis and release of neuroactive substances by glial cells. Glia 5:81–94, 1992

Martin LF, Kem WR, Freedman R: Alpha-7 nicotinic receptor agonists: potential new candidates for the treatment of schizophrenia. Psychopharmacology (Berl) 174:54–64, 2004

McGeer PL, McGeer EG: Glial cell reactions in neurodegenerative diseases: pathophysiology and therapeutic interventions. Alzheimer Dis Assoc Disord 12 (suppl 2):S1–S6, 1998

McKnight GS: Cyclic AMP second messenger systems. Curr Opin Cell Biol 3:213–217, 1991

Meador-Woodruff JH: Update on dopamine receptors. Ann Clin Psychiatry 6:79–90, 1994

Melcangi RC, Magnaghi V, Martini L: Steroid metabolism and effects in central and peripheral glial cells. J Neurobiol 40:471–483, 1999

Melikian HE, Ramamoorthy S, Tate CG, et al: Inability to N-glycosylate the human norepinephrine transporter reduces protein stability, surface trafficking, and transport activity but not ligand recognition. Mol Pharmacol 50:266–276, 1996

Millan MJ: N-methyl-D-aspartate receptor-coupled glycineB receptors in the pathogenesis and treatment of schizophrenia: a critical review. Curr Drug Targets CNS Neurol Disord 1:191–213, 2002

Millan MJ: N-Methyl-D-aspartate receptors as a target for improved antipsychotic agents: novel insights and clinical perspectives. Psychopharmacology (Berl) 179:30–53, 2005

Morse D, Sethi J, Choi AM: Carbon monoxide-dependent signaling. Crit Care Med 30:S12–S17, 2002

Mulcrone J, Kerwin RW: No difference in the expression of the D4 gene in post-mortem frontal cortex from controls and schizophrenics. Neurosci Lett 219:163–166, 1996

Nalepa I: The effect of psychotropic drugs on the interaction of protein kinase C with second messenger systems in the rat cerebral cortex. Pol J Pharmacol 46:1–14, 1994

Narahashi T, Aistrup GL, Marszalec W, et al: Neuronal nicotinic acetylcholine receptors: a new target site of ethanol. Neurochem Int 35:131–141, 1999

Nelson N: The family of Na$^+$/Cl$^-$ neurotransmitter transporters. J Neurochem 71:1785–1803, 1998

Nibuya M, Nestler E, Duman R: Chronic antidepressant administration increases the expression of cAMP response element binding protein (CREB) in rat hippocampus. J Neurosci 316:2365–2372, 1996

Nishizuka Y: Protein kinase C and lipid signaling for sustained cellular responses. FASEB J 9:484–496, 1995

Nutt D: Substance-P antagonists: a new treatment for depression? Lancet 352:1644–1646, 1998

Okugawa G, Omori K, Suzukawa J, et al: Long-term treatment with antidepressants increases glucocorticoid receptor binding and gene expression in cultured rat hippocampal neurons. J Neuroendocrinol 11:887–895, 1999

Oswald I, Brezinova V, Dunleavy DLF: On the slowness of action of tricyclic antidepressant drugs. Br J Psychiatry 120:673–677, 1972

Otero GC, Merrill JE: Cytokine receptors on glial cells. Glia 11:117–128, 1994

Pacher P, Kecskemeti V: Trends in the development of new antidepressants: is there a light at the end of the tunnel? Curr Med Chem 11:925–943, 2004

Parthasarathy L, Vadnal RE, Parthasarathy R, et al: Biochemical and molecular properties of lithium-sensitive *myo*-inositol monophosphatase. Life Sci 54:1127–1142, 1994

Paul IA, Nowak G, Layer RT, et al: Adaptation of the N-methyl-D-aspartate receptor complex following chronic antidepressant treatments. J Pharmacol Exp Ther 269:95–102, 1994

Paul S: CNS drug discovery in the 21st century: from genomics to combinatorial chemistry and back. Br J Psychiatry 174:23–25, 1999

Pfeiffer S, Mayer B: The biological chemistry of nitric oxide and peroxynitrite, in Nitric Oxide: Basic Research and Clinical Applications. Edited by Gryglewski RJ, Minuz P. Amsterdam, The Netherlands, IOS Press, 2001, pp 35–43

Pills for the mind: new era in psychiatry. Time 65(10):63–69, March 7, 1955

Pitcher JA, Inglese J, Higgins JB, et al: Role of by subunits of G proteins in targeting the β-adrenergic receptor kinase to membrane-bound receptors. Science 257:1264–1267, 1992

Poitry-Yamate CL, Poitry S, Tsacopoulos M: Lactate released by Muller glial cells is metabolized by photoreceptors from mammalian retina. J Neurosci 15:5179–5191, 1995

Posey DJ, Kem DL, Swiezy NB, et al: A pilot study of D-cycloserine in subjects with autistic disorder. Am J Psychiatry 161:2115–2117, 2004

Premont RT, Inglese J, Lefkowitz RJ: Protein kinases that phosphorylate activated G protein-coupled receptors. FASEB J 9:175–182, 1995

Rahamimoff R, Butkevich A, Duridanova D, et al: Multitude of ion channels in the regulation of transmitter release. Philos Trans R Soc Lond B Biol Sci 354:281–288, 1999

Raivich G, Jones LL, Werner A, et al: Molecular signals for glial activation: pro- and anti-inflammatory cytokines in the injured brain. Acta Neurochir Suppl (Wien) 73:21–30, 1999

Ransom BR, Sontheimer H: The neurophysiology of glial cells. J Clin Neurophysiol 9:224–251, 1992

Rasenick M, Chaney K, Chen J: G protein-mediated signal transduction as a target of antidepressant and antibipolar drug action: evidence from model systems. J Clin Psychiatry 57:49–55, 1996

Remington G, Kapur S: D2 and 5-HT-2 receptor effects of antipsychotics: bridging basic and clinical findings using PET. J Clin Psychiatry 60:15–19, 1999

Rens-Domiao S, Hamm HE: Structural and functional relationships of heterotrimeric G-proteins. FASEB J 9:1059–1066, 1995

Richelson E: Receptor pharmacology of neuroleptics: relation to clinical effects. J Clin Psychiatry 60:5–14, 1999

Roberts C, Thomas DR, Bate ST, et al: GABAergic modulation of 5-HT$_7$ receptor-mediated effects on 5-HT efflux in the guinea-pig dorsal raphe nucleus. Neuropharmacology 46:935–941, 2004

Ronde P, Nichols RA: High calcium permeability of serotonin 5-HT$_3$ receptors on presynaptic nerve terminals from rat striatum. J Neurochem 70:1094–1103, 1998

Rosenfeld A: The vital facts about the drug and its effects. Life 60:30–31, 1966

Roth BL, Craigo SC, Choudhary MS, et al: Binding of typical and atypical antipsychotic agents to 5-hydroxytryptamine-6 and 5-hydroxytryptamine-7 receptors. J Pharmacol Exp Ther 268:1403–1410, 1994

Rubinstein M, Phillips TJ, Bunzow JR, et al: Mice lacking dopamine D$_4$ receptors are supersensitive to ethanol, cocaine, and methamphetamine. Cell 90:991–1001, 1997

Saarma M, Sariola H: Other neurotrophic factors: glial cell line-derived neurotrophic factor (GDNF). Microsc Res Tech 45:292–302, 1999

Sanders-Bush E, Canton H: Serotonin receptors: signal transduction pathways, in Psychopharmacology: The Fourth Generation of Progress. Edited by Bloom FE, Kupfer DJ. New York, Raven, 1995, pp 431–441

Sariola H, Saarma M: Novel functions and signalling pathways for GDNF. J Cell Sci 116:3855–3862, 2003

Saudou F, Amara DA, Dierich A, et al: Enhanced aggressive behavior in mice lacking 5-HT$_{1B}$ receptor. Science 265:1875–1878, 1994

Schipke CG, Kettenmann H: Astrocyte responses to neuronal activity. Glia 47:226–232, 2004

Schlag BD, Vondrasek JR, Munir M, et al: Regulation of the glial Na$^+$-dependent glutamate transporters by cyclic AMP analogs and neurons. Mol Pharmacol 53:355–369, 1998

Schousboe A, Sarup A, Larsson OM, et al: GABA transporters as drug targets for modulation of GABAergic activity. Biochem Pharmacol 68:1557–1563, 2004

Seeman P, Van-Tol HH: Dopamine receptor pharmacology. Curr Opin Neurol Neurosurg 6:602–608, 1993

Seeman P, Guan HC, Van Tol HH: Schizophrenia: elevation of dopamine D$_4$-like sites, using [^{3}H]nemonapride and [^{125}I]epidepride. Eur J Pharmacol 286:R3–R5, 1995

Seminara AR, Krumenacker JS, Murad F: Signal transduction with nitric oxide, guanylyl cyclase and cyclic guanosine monophosphate, in Nitric Oxide: Basic Research and Clinical Applications. Edited by Gryglewski RJ, Minuz P. Amsterdam, IOS Press, 2001, pp 5–22

Sequeira SM, Carvalho AP, Carvalho CAM, et al: Mechanisms of regulation of neurotransmitter release by nitric oxide, in Nitric Oxide: Basic Research and Clinical Applications. Edited by Gryglewski RJ, Minuz P. Amsterdam, The Netherlands, IOS Press, 2001, pp 212–215

Shank RP, William JB, Charles WA: Glutamine and 2-oxoglutarate as metabolic precursors of the transmitter pools of glutamate and GABA: correlation of regional uptake by rat brain synaptosomes. Neurochem Res 16:29–34, 1989

Shinohara K, Hiruma H, Funabashi T, et al: GABAergic modulation of gap junction communication in slice cultures of the rat suprachiasmatic nucleus. Neuroscience 96:591–596, 2000

Shirayama Y, Chen AC, Nakagawa S, et al: Brain-derived neurotrophic factor produces antidepressant effects in behavioral models of depression. J Neurosci 22:3251–3261, 2002

Silvia CP, King GR, Lee TH, et al: Intranigral administration of D$_2$ dopamine receptor antisense oligodeoxynucleotides establishes a role for nigrostriatal D$_2$ autoreceptors in the motor actions of cocaine. Mol Pharmacol 46:51–57, 1994

Singer TP, Ramsay RR: Monoamine oxidases: old friends hold many surprises. FASEB J 9:605–610, 1995

Snyder SH, Banerjee SP, Yamamura HI, et al: Drugs, neurotransmitters, and schizophrenia. Science 184:1243–1253, 1974

Sohl G, Maxeiner S, Willecke K: Expression and functions of neuronal gap junctions. Nat Rev Neurosci 6:191–200, 2005

Sontheimer H: Voltage-dependent ion channels in glial cells. Glia 11:156–172, 1994

Spano PF, Govoni S, Trabucchi M: Studies on the pharmacological properties of dopamine receptors in various areas of the central nervous system. Adv Biochem Psychopharmacol 19:155–165, 1978

Stahl SM: Basic psychopharmacology of antidepressants, part 1: antidepressants have seven distinct mechanisms of action. J Clin Psychiatry 59:5–14, 1998a

Stahl SM: Selecting an antidepressant by using mechanism of action to enhance efficacy and avoid side effects. J Clin Psychiatry 59:23–29, 1998b

Stahl SM, Grady MM: Differences in mechanism of action between current and future antidepressants. J Clin Psychiatry 64:13–17, 2003

Standifer KM, Chien CC, Wahlestedt C, et al: Selective loss of delta opioid analgesia and binding by antisense oligodeoxynucleotides to a delta opioid receptor. Neuron 12:805–810, 1994

Stephens DN, Kehr W, Duka T: Anxiolytic and anxiogenic beta-carbolines: tools for the study of anxiety mechanisms, in GABAergic Transmission and Anxiety. Edited by Biggio G, Costa E. New York, Raven, 1986, pp 91–106

Sternbach LH, Horst WD: Psychopharmacological agents, in Kirk-Othmer Encyclopedia of Chemical Technology, 3rd Edition. Edited by Grayson M, Eckroth D. New York, Wiley, 1982, pp 342–379

Stoof JC, Kebabian JW: Two dopamine receptors: biochemistry, physiology and pharmacology. Life Sci 35:2281–2296, 1984

Sur C, Kinney GG: The therapeutic potential of glycine transporter-1 inhibitors. Expert Opin Investig Drugs 13:515–521, 2004

Swanson RA, Liu J, Miller JW, et al: Neuronal regulation of glutamate transporter subtype expression in astrocytes. J Neurosci 17:932–940, 1997

Tallman JF, Cassela JV, White G, et al: GABA$_A$ receptors: diversity and its implications for CNS disease. Neuroscientist 5:351–361, 1999

Tecott LH, Sun LM, Akana SF, et al: Eating disorder and epilepsy in mice lacking 5-HT2c serotonin receptors. Nature 374:542–546, 1995

Theis M, Sohl G, Eiberger J, et al: Emerging complexities in identity and function of glial connexins. Trends Neurosci 28:188–195, 2005

Thiel G: Recent breakthroughs in neurotransmitter release: paradigm for regulated exocytosis? News in Physiological Science 10:42–46, 1995

Thomas KR, Capecchi MR: Targeted disruption of the murine int-1 proto-oncogene resulting in severe abnormalities in midbrain and cerebellar development. Nature 346:847–850, 1990

Thome J, Sakai N, Shin K, et al: cAMP response element-mediated gene transcription is upregulated by chronic antidepressant treatment. J Neurosci 20:4030–4036, 2000

Todd RD, O'Malley KL: Family ties: dopamine D$_2$-like receptors. Neurotransmissions 9:1–4, 1993

Triggle DJ: The pharmacology of ion channels: with particular reference to voltage-gated Ca2$^+$ channels. Eur J Pharmacol 375:311–325, 1999

Tsacopoulos M, Magistretti PJ: Metabolic coupling between glia and neurons. J Neurosci 16:877–885, 1996

Tsai G, Lane HY, Yang P, et al: Glycine transporter I inhibitor, N-methylglycine (sarcosine), added to antipsychotics for the treatment of schizophrenia. Biol Psychiatry 55:452–456, 2004

Tsai GE, Falk WE, Gunther J, et al: Improved cognition in Alzheimer's disease with short-term D-cycloserine treatment. Am J Psychiatry 156:467–469, 1999

van Berckel BN, Evenblij CN, van Loon BJ, et al: D-Cycloserine increases positive symptoms in chronic schizophrenic patients when administered in addition to antipsychotics: a double-blind, parallel, placebo-controlled study. Neuropsychopharmacology 21:203–210, 1999

Van Tol HH, Bunzow JR, Guan HC, et al: Cloning of the gene for a human dopamine D$_4$ receptor with high affinity for the antipsychotic clozapine. Nature 350:610–614, 1991

Vardimon L, Ben-Dror I, Avisar N, et al: Glucocorticoid control of glial gene expression. J Neurobiol 40:513–527, 1999

Vedder H, Bening-Abu-Shach U, Lanquillon S, et al: Regulation of glucocorticoid receptor mRNA in human blood cells by amitriptyline and dexamethasone. J Psychiatr Res 33:303–308, 1999

Wahlestedt C: Reward for persistence in substance P research [comment]. Science 281:1624–1625, 1998

Wahlestedt C, Pich EM, Koob GF, et al: Modulation of anxiety and neuropeptide Y-Y1 receptors by antisense oligodeoxynucleotides. Science 259:528–531, 1993

Wallis C, Willwerth J: Schizophrenia: a new drug brings patients back to life. Time 140:52–58, 1992

Walsh DA, Van Patten SM: Multiple pathway signal transduction by the cAMP-dependent protein kinase. FASEB J 8:1227–1236, 1994

Watkins SS, Epping-Jordan MP, Koob GF, et al: Blockade of nicotine self-administration with nicotinic antagonists in rats. Pharmacol Biochem Behav 62:743–751, 1999

Wiesinger H: Arginine metabolism and the synthesis of nitric oxide in the nervous system. Prog Neurobiol 64:365–391, 2001

Wolfe BB, Harden TK, Sporn JR, et al: Presynaptic modulation of *beta* adrenergic receptors in rat cerebral cortex after treatment with antidepressants. J Pharmacol Exp Ther 207:446–457, 1978

Wong AH, Van Tol HH: The dopamine D$_4$ receptors and mechanisms of antipsychotic atypicality. Prog Neuropsychopharmacol Biol Psychiatry 27:1091–1099, 2003

Wonnacott S: Presynaptic nicotinic ACh receptors. Trends Neurosci 20:92–98, 1997

Wooley DW: The Biochemical Bases of Psychoses: Serotonin Hypothesis About Mental Diseases. New York, Wiley, 1962

Wright WW: Results obtained by the intensive use of bromides in functional psychoses. Am J Psychiatry 82:365–389, 1926

Yakel JL: Calcineurin regulation of synaptic function: from ion channels to transmitter release and gene transcription. Trends Pharmacol Sci 18:124–134, 1997

Yeomans J, Baptista M: Both nicotinic and muscarinic receptors in ventral tegmental area contribute to brain-stimulation reward. Pharmacol Biochem Behav 57:915–921, 1997

Zhang B, Ramaswami M: Synaptic vesicle endocytosis and recycling, in Neurotransmitter Release. Edited by Bellen HJ. Oxford, UK, Oxford University Press, 1999, pp 389–431

Zhou LW, Zhang SP, Qin ZH, et al: In vivo administration of an oligodeoxynucleotide antisense to the D$_2$ dopamine receptor messenger RNA inhibits D$_2$ dopamine receptor-mediated behavior and the expression of D$_2$ dopamine receptors in mouse striatum. J Pharmacol Exp Ther 268:1015–1023, 1994

31

PSYCHOPHARMACOLOGICAL TREATMENTS FOR PATIENTS WITH NEUROPSYCHIATRIC DISORDERS

Paul E. Holtzheimer III, M.D.

Mark Snowden, M.D., M.P.H.

Peter P. Roy-Byrne, M.D.

Modern neuropsychiatry is concerned with the understanding and treatment of cognitive, emotional, and behavioral syndromes in patients with known neurological illness or central nervous system (CNS) dysfunction. Although some syndromes in patients with neurological disease (e.g., depression following stroke) are clinically similar to those seen in patients experiencing the syndrome de novo, treatment response may be quite different. Furthermore, the neuropsychiatric sequelae of several neurological disorders frequently seem an amalgam of several syndromes and often do not fit neatly into DSM-IV-TR syndromal definitions (American Psychiatric Association 2000). Does the combative, irritable, agitated, brain-injured patient have dysphoric mania, agitated depression, or posttraumatic stress disorder (PTSD)? Does the apathetic, withdrawn poststroke patient really have major depression? Although DSM-IV-TR may be a useful starting point, departing from it is a frequent necessity.

Despite dissimilarities in the pathophysiology, clinical presentation, and treatment response of neuropsychiatric and "idiopathic" psychiatric syndromes, the treatment of neuropsychiatric illness has largely been modeled on known treatments of idiopathic psychiatric disorders (e.g., depression, mania, psychosis). Unfortunately, the lack of a strong evidence base for treatments of neuropsychiatric disorders (e.g., the paucity of double-blind, placebo-controlled treatment studies or even large case series) makes treatment more art than science. In addition to identifying efficacious treatments, attention to altered side-effect sensitivity and pertinent interactions with commonly used neurological drugs is an especially important aspect of the treatment of neuropsychiatric patients.

For this reason, this chapter does not duplicate material commonly found in textbooks of psychopharmacology and psychiatric treatment. The neuropsychiatrist specifically needs information on the psychopharmacological treatment of neuropsychiatric syndromes rather than drug treatment of psychiatric illness in general. The reader is referred to other standard textbooks for this latter information (Schatzberg and Nemeroff 1998). The chapter is not organized by medication but rather by syndrome so that the interested physician and trainee can more easily locate information relevant to a specific patient with a specific array of cognitive, emotional, and behavioral abnormalities. Side effects, drug interactions, and pharmacokinetic considerations are included to the extent they pertain to the neuropsychiatric context.

We begin with an overview of how to approach the neuropsychiatric patient for pharmacological treatment. The chapter then focuses on five major syndromes commonly seen in neuropsychiatric patients: 1) depression, including apathy and "deficit" states; 2) psychosis, including a variety of disturbances of perception and thought; 3) states of agitation, including anxiety and mania; 4) aggression, impulsivity, and behavioral dyscontrol; and 5) cognitive disturbance, including amnesia and dementia. These syndromes are seen more often in combination than in isolation, and the presence of one often increases the chance of another (e.g., cognitive impairment increases risk for depression in both Parkinson's disease [Tandberg et al. 1997] and Alzheimer's disease [Payne et al. 1998]). Throughout the chapter, a common organization is used. Each syndrome is defined in enough detail to indicate how it borders on and overlaps with the others. The most common etiologies and possible neuroanatomical-neurochemical substrates of these syndromes are reviewed. Following this, data on treatment are reviewed, emphasizing the quality of the data. Issues of dosage, treatment duration, and response course are considered. Finally, side effects, pharmacokinetic considerations, and drug interactions are highlighted. Considerations related to the particular neuropsychiatric condition involved (e.g., Parkinson's disease versus Huntington's disease) are discussed when appropriate.

APPROACH TO THE NEUROPSYCHIATRIC PATIENT

The psychiatrist who is asked to assess a neuropsychiatric patient for pharmacological treatment first must become familiar with the nature and course of the underlying neurological illness. This includes an understanding of the disorder's neuroanatomy and neurochemistry because apparently distinct neurological and psychiatric symptoms often arise from similar mechanisms intrinsic to the neurological disorder (e.g., psychosis in CNS neoplasms). Conversely, similar symptoms can be caused by distinct neurological and psychiatric disorders as well as by the side effects and interactions of neurological and psychotropic medications (e.g., both Parkinson's bradykinesia and phenytoin-induced lethargy may be mistaken for signs of depression). Furthermore, many psychiatric medications can worsen

the neurological illness (e.g., neuroleptics administered for Parkinson's psychosis; antidepressants administered for multiple sclerosis mood lability), whereas neurological medications can precipitate psychiatric syndromes (e.g., psychosis and anxiety related to dopamine agonists in Parkinson's disease; steroid-induced mania in CNS lupus). Therefore, treatment must first consider the primary neurological disorder and its medications.

Other medical conditions and treatments, recent surgeries, and health habits also should be considered. Pallidotomy and deep brain stimulation for Parkinson's disease can produce cognitive or other psychiatric effects (Bejjani et al. 1999; Stefurak et al. 2003). Herbal medicines can produce neuropsychiatric symptoms and interact with medications (LaFrance et al. 2000). History of alcohol and drug use must be explored because substance abuse, intoxication, and withdrawal can lead to a vast array of psychiatric symptoms that might otherwise be inappropriately attributed to neurological illness (e.g., depression, anxiety, psychosis, impulsivity, and cognitive impairment) (Rosse et al. 1997).

Establishing rapport with the patient before delving into details of the history and treatment options can greatly enhance the patient's willingness to discuss symptoms and concerns, as well as increase the likelihood of adherence to recommendations. Many patients have no prior experience with the mental health system and may feel surprised and even threatened that a psychiatrist has been consulted. The fear of further loss of control in a situation that already feels out of control may be quite profound. Awareness of and empathy for these reactions are necessary. It can also be helpful to explain carefully that the patient's psychological and behavioral symptoms are frequently encountered as part of the symptom complex of the underlying neurological disorder and that they can be treated. Presenting the pharmacological intervention as a way to assist recovery during a period of intense stress and adaptation will help the patient feel more hopeful and maintain an internal locus of control. Realistic expectations, including the possibility of incomplete remission of symptoms, must be conveyed from the outset so that the patient and his or her family do not become more distressed if some symptoms persist. All of the psychiatric symptoms may not be alleviated, but treatment may significantly benefit the rehabilitation process; a focus on improving overall function should be emphasized throughout the treatment process.

The neuropsychiatrist must be aware of the strong effect of not only the patient's and family's urgent wish to have the patient's psychiatric symptoms treated but also the clinician's intense desire to help. The frequent urge to "do something...anything" must be resisted. Some symptoms may be long-standing and unlikely to resolve quickly, whereas others may result from an adjustment disorder that may dissipate without pharmacological treatment. Treatments themselves may be associated with significant side effects and risks. A rash decision to treat can cause more problems than it solves.

Patients with neuropsychiatric illnesses often do not fit into "classic" diagnostic categories as defined by DSM-IV-TR. Thus, when assessing a neurological patient for psychopathology, the clinician must be able to look beyond DSM-IV-TR criteria when appropriate. A careful, detailed focus on identifying problematic symptoms may establish clear symptom clusters (e.g., anhedonia, apathy, poor energy) that may respond to pharmacological intervention, even when specific diagnostic criteria for a particular disorder (e.g., major depression) are not fully met.

The next step in evaluating a neurological patient's appropriateness for psychotropic medication involves obtaining a careful history of premorbid psychiatric problems, personality traits, and coping styles. Multiple informants will minimize informational bias (Strauss et al. 1997). Optimal treatment must take into account whether the psychiatric symptoms preexisted the neurological disorder or arose as a neurologically or psychologically mediated result of the neurological disease. Because CNS insults, particularly in the frontal lobe, can amplify underlying character traits (Prigatano 1992), it may not be possible to eradicate completely behaviors that at first appear to be a direct result of the neurological insult. In addition, certain premorbid traits, such as IQ, may have important implications for course of illness (Palsson et al. 1999).

During the patient interview, the clinician must remember that the neurological disorder may dampen (or heighten) the patient's emotional expressivity, especially in older patients. Thus, the clinician must rely equally on the patient's subjective and somatic complaints and the reports of friends, family members, and caregivers to accurately identify and characterize emotional and behavior problems requiring intervention. Importantly, patients and their caregivers may differ in their view of which symptoms are most troubling; for example, a patient often reports cognitive difficulties as more disabling, whereas family members may view the patient's emotional or behavior changes as more problematic (Hendryx 1989). Careful prospective documentation of symptoms will help in tracking what are often slow improvements that seem subjectively inconsequential to the patient and caregiver but lead to noticeable improvements in overall functioning. Although it may be impractical to document all symptoms completely, specific target symptoms and functional goals should be measured in as much detail as

possible. A simple procedure is to have caregivers, significant others, and patients use simple, anchored 0–10 scales to rate the severity of symptoms, distress, and functional impairment over time. Similar documentation of symptoms that may worsen with treatment (such as rigidity in a patient with Parkinson's disease being treated for psychosis) will allow optimal management. Figure 31–1 depicts one simple example of such a scale, which allows the clinician to fill in items tailored to the particular patient's symptoms and problems.

A basic tenet of treating psychiatric symptoms in patients with neurological disorders is to limit polypharmacy—that is, treat as many signs and symptoms with as few medications as possible. Patients with CNS pathology are more susceptible to CNS medication side effects (e.g., sedative, anticholinergic, extrapyramidal, and epileptogenic effects). Therefore, a patient with a severe head injury having complex partial seizures and agitation, mood lability, and impulsivity should be considered for treatment with an anticonvulsant such as carbamazepine or valproate rather than a combination of an anticonvulsant (such as phenytoin) and lithium. A single appropriate anticonvulsant may treat both the seizures and the behavioral disturbance and limit the potential side effects associated with two separate medications. Treatment of symptoms secondary to the primary neurological disorder, such as pain and sleep disturbance, may decrease psychiatric symptoms sufficiently to allow avoidance of further psychopharmacotherapy. For example, analgesia has been shown to alleviate agitation, irritability, and anger in both patients and caregivers (Perry et al. 1991). Similarly, appropriate treatment of psychiatric symptoms early in presentation (e.g., early treatment of depression with a serotonin reuptake inhibitor) can prevent exacerbation of the underlying neurological disorder. For example, emotional distress has been shown to worsen, and even precipitate, exacerbations of multiple sclerosis (Grant et al. 1989). Potential "neuroprotective" effects of psychotropic medications should be considered in patients who have had a stroke or head injury (Alexopoulos et al. 1997), as should the rare possibility that the effects of medications could worsen the underlying illness.

Detailed knowledge of the patient's stage in rehabilitation as well as the patient's current social, occupational, and interpersonal status is required to tailor the pharmacological regimen to specific practical needs and limitations. For example, starting a potentially sedating medication at a time when a rigorous physical therapy regimen is being initiated or during a long-awaited reentry into the workplace would be ill-advised. Social and interpersonal status can affect access to treatment (Ferrando et al. 1999), ability of caregivers to participate in treatment

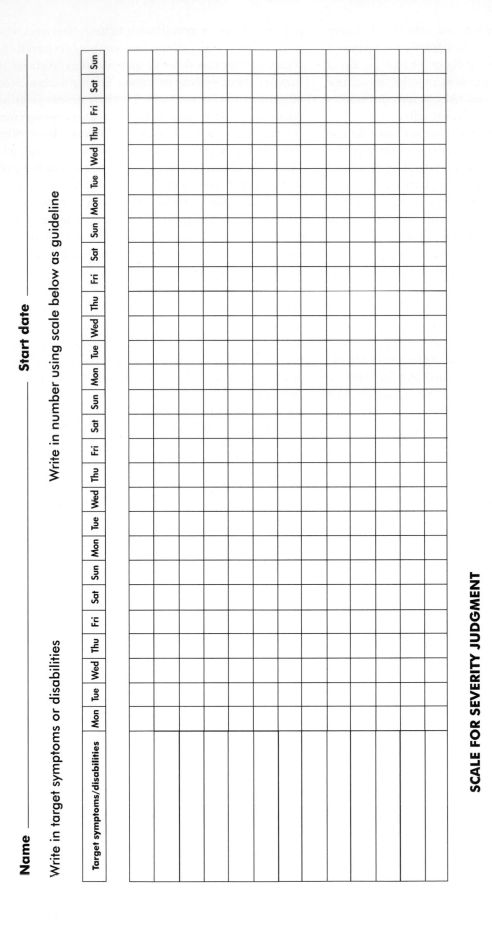

FIGURE 31–1.   Rating scale for the assessment of medication efficacy.

(Donaldson et al. 1998), vulnerability of patients to domestic violence (Diaz-Olavarrieta et al. 1999), and psychiatric outcome (Max et al. 1998).

Before psychotropic medications are administered, an appropriate medical workup should be done. Because of the patient's susceptibility to medication side effects, the clinician should start at a lower dose of medication and titrate more slowly, although the patient may ultimately require the same dose of medication as the non-neurological patient does (i.e., "Start low and go slow…but go!"). Side effects should be well documented, and standardized measures should be used whenever possible. Because neurological patients may have cognitive deficits, the anticipated benefit of the medication, the dosing regimen, and any potential side effects must be thoroughly explained to the patient and caregiver as well as all other physicians caring for the patient. For example, a patient who is receiving meperidine for pain from his neurologist and is also receiving a selective serotonin reuptake inhibitor (SSRI) for depressive symptoms from his psychiatrist may be at risk for developing a life-threatening serotonin syndrome. Also, a patient who has experienced a stroke may be susceptible to low blood pressure and should be prescribed drugs with anticholinergic and alpha-blocking properties only with great caution.

Once medication has been initiated, all available tools to subjectively monitor pharmacokinetics and pharmacological efficacy must be considered. Objective rating scales for symptoms and side effects (as discussed earlier in this section) should be considered. Additionally, monitoring medication blood levels and physiological response (such as vital signs), as well as other laboratory monitoring when appropriate (such as electroencephalography in a patient with seizure disorder or delirium), can be helpful. Medication blood levels do not always correlate with medication efficacy but can still give information about compliance, drug metabolism, and potential toxicity. It should be remembered that some neuropsychiatric patients with impaired cognition or communication ability may not be able to convey information adequately about efficacy and side effects, requiring more objective monitoring.

DEPRESSION, APATHY, AND "DEFICIT" STATES

Major depression and dysthymia are among the most common psychiatric disorders. Although decades of clinical observation and research have clearly delineated various subtypes of idiopathic major depression (e.g., retarded versus agitated, melancholic versus atypical), few consis-

tent clinical or biological differences between these subtypes have emerged (Goodwin and Jamison 1990). Even the clinical maxim of avoiding the use of "activating" antidepressants in anxious depressed individuals has not been supported (Tollefson et al. 1994). In contrast, subtype distinction may be more important in the assessment and treatment of neuropsychiatric disorders. In these patients, agitated states may overlap significantly with behavioral dyscontrol, delirium, and occasionally psychosis, whereas retarded depression may overlap with apathetic and other deficit-like states, including states in which cognitive slowing and amotivation occur in the absence of a clear mood disturbance (Levy et al. 1998). It is reasonable then that these subtypes may suggest different pathophysiologies and treatments.

COMMON ETIOLOGIES

Depression and apathy are extremely common following stroke or traumatic brain injury (TBI); with Parkinson's disease or Huntington's disease; with multiple sclerosis or epilepsy; in association with diencephalic, frontal, and temporal lobe tumors; and during the course of Alzheimer's and multi-infarct dementias. Depression, when it occurs in patients with human immunodeficiency virus (HIV) infection—although not more prevalent than in matched control subjects (Williams et al. 1991)—is often associated with marked apathy and subtle deficits in neurocognitive function (Castellon et al. 1998) that can progress in later stages to dementia. Most studies, except those in HIV infection, have reported a prevalence of depression greater than that in comparably disabling physical illness not involving the CNS and have failed to find a consistent association of severity of depression with progression of neurological illness or subsequent disability. This outcome argues that depression is not simply a reaction to neurological illness or subsequent disability but, when it occurs, is a core feature of these illnesses, with partially overlapping pathophysiology (Lyketsos et al. 1998). Nonetheless, psychological reactions to either the causative event (e.g., a posttraumatic stress reaction—see Bryant et al. 2000) or the subsequent neurological disability (e.g., an adjustment disorder or grief reaction), as well as discomfort related to the underlying illness (e.g., pain, insomnia), may contribute significantly to the overall clinical presentation and must be considered and addressed separately (and before initiating psychotropic medications). The possibility that currently prescribed medications might be contributing to depression also needs to be carefully considered. These include anticonvulsants, sedative-hypnotics, α- and β-adrenergic blockers, corticosteroids, antiretrovirals, alpha interferon, metoclopramide, histamine type 2 receptor (H_2) blockers, calcium channel blockers, and angiotensin-converting enzyme inhibitors. Patients with histories of depression may be more likely to develop depression side effects from some drugs (e.g., depression following interferon treatment of multiple sclerosis [D.C. Mohr et al. 1999]). Withdrawal from some agents, including anticonvulsants, benzodiazepines, and stimulants, also may be associated with depression.

ANATOMY AND NEUROCHEMISTRY

The range of neuroanatomical and neurochemical substrates that have been associated with depressive and apathetic states in neurologically ill patients is extremely wide. The most common pathophysiological substrates include disruption of frontal lobe cortical-subcortical circuits and perturbation of ascending monoaminergic pathways. This is supported by the greater incidence of depression with left frontal strokes (Morris et al. 1996) and left frontal and basal ganglia TBI, the predominance of depression or apathy compared with other psychiatric disturbances in basal ganglia disease (Lauterbach et al. 1997), greater frontostriatal involvement detected on postmortem examination in depressed Alzheimer's disease patients (Zubenko and Moossy 1988), and consistent data from neuroimaging studies of depression associated with several neuropsychiatric conditions (Mayberg 1994). Patients with temporal lobe epilepsy and depression also show similar left frontal hypometabolism on positron emission tomography (PET) scan (Bromfield et al. 1992), and more than 50% of those with depression have no further depressive episodes after temporal lobe surgery (Altshuler et al. 1999). Multiple sclerosis patients with depression show disturbed blood flow only in limbic cortex (Sabatini et al. 1996), consistent with notions that dysregulation of paralimbic areas such as the cingulate cortex can disconnect intact frontal cortical and subcortical areas, producing depression in the absence of frontostriatal damage (Mayberg 2003). Patients who develop depression in later years show increased abnormalities in white matter likely related to vascular damage; this further supports the notion that depression in some patients may be a "disconnection syndrome" in which frontal and subcortical regions involved in mood regulation cannot communicate efficiently because of white matter disruption (Alexopoulos 2002; Taylor et al. 2003).

A convergence of data from human postmortem pathological (C.P. Chen et al. 1996; Zubenko and Moossy 1988), cerebrospinal fluid (CSF) (Mayeux et al. 1988), genetic (Mossner et al. 2001), imaging (Mayberg et al. 1988), and neuroendocrine (Kostic et al. 1996) studies

support a role for serotonin (5-hydroxytryptamine; 5-HT) in the depression of Parkinson's disease, stroke, and Alzheimer's dementias. Frontal lobe damage from TBI is also selectively associated with reduced brain serotonin function (van Woerkom et al. 1977), and even depressed patients with mild TBI have altered serotonin function on neuroendocrine testing compared with nondepressed mild TBI patients (Mobayed and Dinan 1990). Depressed Alzheimer's disease patients have greater locus coeruleus neuronal loss than do those without depression (Forstl et al. 1992), implicating central noradrenergic activity. Finally, dopaminergic pathways are likely involved in the pathophysiology of depression (Dailly et al. 2004), especially in disorders such as Parkinson's disease (Remy et al. 2005).

These abnormalities are particularly relevant in the pathophysiology of depressive syndromes in neuropsychiatry because most currently available antidepressants affect these transmitter systems. However, it should be emphasized that monoamine neurotransmitter hypotheses of depression are giving way to considerably more sophisticated models emphasizing alterations in multiple receptor subtypes and associated signal transduction mechanisms, as well as changes in other transmitter (e.g., glutamate, γ-aminobutyric acid [GABA]) and neuropeptide systems (Duman 1998; Hindmarch 2002). These more complex models of depression may give rise to novel therapeutic approaches.

TREATMENT

In contrast to the plethora of double-blind, placebo-controlled trials of various antidepressants in major depression, relatively few such studies have been done in depressed patients with neurological illness. Several open studies have suggested efficacy for typical antidepressant medications in depressive syndromes in neuropsychiatric patients, including those with TBI (Fann et al. 2000; Muller et al. 1999; Newburn et al. 1999; Turner-Stokes et al. 2002), epilepsy (Kuhn et al. 2003; Specchio et al. 2004), multiple sclerosis (Benedetti et al. 2004), Parkinson's disease (McDonald et al. 2003), Alzheimer's dementia (Lyketsos and Olin 2002), and stroke (Kimura et al. 2003; Niedermaier et al. 2004; Spalletta and Caltagirone 2003). Placebo-controlled studies have examined the efficacy of nortriptyline (Lipsey et al. 1984; Robinson et al. 2000), trazodone (Reding et al. 1986), citalopram (G. Andersen et al. 1994), and fluoxetine (Fruehwald et al. 2003; Robinson et al. 2000; Wiart et al. 2000) in depressed stroke patients; of imipramine (Strang 1965), nortriptyline (J. Andersen et al. 1980), desipramine (Laitinen 1969), citalopram (Wermuth et al. 1998), and sertraline (Leentjens et al. 2003) in depressed Parkinson's disease patients; of desipramine in depressed multiple sclerosis patients (Schiffer and Wineman 1990); of imipramine (Reifler et al. 1989), clomipramine (Petracca et al. 1996), moclobemide (Roth et al. 1996), maprotiline (Fuchs et al. 1993), citalopram (Nyth et al. 1992), fluoxetine (Petracca et al. 2001), and sertraline (Lyketsos et al. 2003; Magai et al. 2000) in depressed Alzheimer's disease patients; of desipramine in depressed TBI patients (Wroblewski et al. 1996); and of fluoxetine in depressed patients with Huntington's disease (Como et al. 1997). Although studies have documented efficacy for SSRIs (Elliott et al. 1998; Zisook et al. 1998) and imipramine (Elliott et al. 1998) in depressed patients with HIV disease, most patients in these studies were not in the late stages of HIV illness and potentially had major depression unrelated to CNS viral involvement. Several studies of the monoamine oxidase–B (MAO-B) inhibitor selegiline in Parkinson's disease patients measured effects on depression as a secondary phenomenon (Klaassen et al. 1995).

Most of the placebo-controlled studies cited earlier reported a greater efficacy of the active drug compared with placebo in the course of trial durations between 4 and 8 weeks. Type of illness (e.g., Huntington's disease [Como et al. 1997]) and stage of illness (e.g., advanced Alzheimer's disease [Magai et al. 2000]) may have affected response in negative studies; also, several studies may not have been powered adequately to show a statistically significant difference between the groups. The group of Parkinson's disease studies generally report response rates somewhat lower (i.e., 60%) than in non–medically ill depressed patients. Many studies have purposely used lower doses (e.g., trazodone 200 mg [Reding et al. 1986]), as would be used in elderly patients, and earlier studies using normal doses of tricyclics sometimes showed a high frequency of side effects (e.g., 18% rate of delirium in stroke patients [Lipsey et al. 1984]) and an inability to reach therapeutic blood levels (Schiffer and Wineman 1990).

Although many of the studies listed earlier showed efficacy for SSRIs in treating depression in neuropsychiatric patients, a provocative 12-week placebo-controlled study showed that nortriptyline was superior to fluoxetine in depressed stroke patients (Robinson et al. 2000). A comparison of amitriptyline and fluoxetine in depressed patients with Alzheimer's disease showed equal efficacy (Taragano et al. 1997), although this study did not include a placebo control group. A study of nondepressed stroke patients with hemiplegia showed that fluoxetine was superior to both maprotiline and placebo in facilitating rehabilitation therapy, supporting a distinct functional effect in the absence of depression (Dam et al. 1996). SSRIs also have been shown to improve "emo-

tional incontinence" in neuropsychiatric patients (Iannaccone and Ferini-Strambi 1996; Muller et al. 1999; Nahas et al. 1998; Tan and Dorevitch 1996).

SSRIs also may have a more favorable side-effect profile compared with tricyclic antidepressants (TCAs) in neuropsychiatric patients. Sedation, postural hypotension, modest hypertension, and seizure threshold–lowering effects are common with TCAs and may be more pronounced in medically ill, especially neuropsychiatric, patients. In one study of 68 brain-injured patients taking TCAs, 20% developed seizures (Wroblewski et al. 1990). In HIV disease patients, imipramine was much less tolerable than paroxetine (Elliott et al. 1998), and in multiple sclerosis patients, TCAs produced twice the side-effect rate of SSRIs (Scott et al. 1996). Among isolated reports noting CNS side effects with SSRIs, extrapyramidal side effects (EPS) were most common (Leo 1996), although large case series suggested that these effects are not typical for more obviously vulnerable patients with either Parkinson's disease (Caley and Friedman 1992) or multiple sclerosis (Flax et al. 1991), and one study in Parkinson's disease patients suggested that SSRIs may actually improve bradykinesia (Rampello et al. 2002).

Given their side-effect burden, potential for adverse events, and potential for serious interaction with multiple other medications, there would seem to be little reason to use nonselective monoamine oxidase inhibitors (MAOIs) in treating depressed neuropsychiatric patients. Selegiline, a selective MAO-B inhibitor, would seem to be a good choice for Parkinson's disease patients because it has primary effects on the underlying illness. However, the lower doses used to treat Parkinson's disease symptoms generally have not been effective in studies of primary major depression, which usually requires higher doses that also inhibit MAO-A. Finally, bupropion was found to be effective in fewer than half of Parkinson's disease patients in one study (Goetz et al. 1984); also, bupropion can lower the seizure threshold, which may limit its usefulness in many neuropsychiatric patients. Few reports have examined the use of other antidepressants in neuropsychiatric patients.

Although strategies using dopaminergic agents have been particularly recommended for states of apathy often seen in Parkinson's disease patients, sometimes without accompanying depression (Chatterjee and Fahn 2002), Parkinson's disease patients do not experience euphoria in response to methylphenidate, possibly reflecting degeneration of dopaminergic neurons with decreased dopamine availability (Cantello et al. 1989). However, more direct-acting agonists such as bromocriptine and amantadine have been found to be effective in these groups of patients (Jouvent et al. 1983) as well as in individual patients with TBI-associated apathy (Van Reekum et al. 1995). Pramipexole, a dopamine agonist, may be effective in treating depression in Parkinson's disease patients (Moller et al. 2005; Rektorova et al. 2003). Stimulants such as methylphenidate have shown efficacy in treating apathy related to Alzheimer's dementia and vascular dementia (Galynker et al. 1997) and stroke patients (Grade et al. 1998; Watanabe et al. 1995), can work within 2 days (Masand et al. 1991), and promote improved participation in rehabilitation and enhanced functioning (Crisostomo et al. 1988). One retrospective case series documented efficacy in depressed stroke patients comparable to that of nortriptyline, with a more rapid onset of effect and a similar side-effect profile (Lazarus et al. 1994). A tendency for stimulants to reduce seizure frequency (Wroblewski et al. 1992) or to enhance neuronal recovery (Feeney et al. 1982) in brain injury patients may be other advantages. Methylphenidate also has been effective in improving impairments in psychomotor speech and arousal in three apathetic patients with brain tumors (Weitzner et al. 1995). A documented effect of pemoline compared with placebo on fatigue in 50% of multiple sclerosis patients is noteworthy (Weinshenker et al. 1992), although the drug was not very well tolerated because of anorexia, irritability, and insomnia. Patients with HIV-related apathetic depression have done particularly well with methylphenidate in case reports (White et al. 1992). However, other reports have claimed that even though dopaminergic agents improve affect and cognitive function, they may be less effective on core symptoms of apathy such as lack of initiative (Salloway 1994), and they could provoke psychosis in Parkinson's disease and other vulnerable patients.

A growing database suggests that various brain stimulation techniques may have efficacy in treating depression, although they have not been extensively studied in neuropsychiatric patients. Electroconvulsive therapy (ECT) is an effective treatment for depression in Parkinson's disease patients that can also transiently improve core motor symptoms (Factor et al. 1995; Fall et al. 1995; Fregni et al. 2005; Kellner et al. 1994; Moellentine et al. 1998; Pridmore and Pollard 1996). Five of six patients with Huntington's disease also improved with ECT, although one patient developed delirium and another developed a worsening of the movement disorder (Ranen et al. 1994). ECT has been used to treat depression in a patient with frontal craniotomy and residual meningioma (Starkstein and Migliorelli 1993). Reports of a high rate of ECT-induced delirium in Parkinson's disease patients, alone (Oh et al. 1992) and in comparison with stroke patients (Figiel 1992), have been interpreted as being due to denervation supersensitivity of dopamine

receptors, and reduction of dopaminergic drugs before ECT has been advised (Rudorfer et al. 1992). In general, patients with more severe depression often accompanied by psychosis may be the best candidates for ECT.

Repetitive transcranial magnetic stimulation (rTMS) has shown efficacy in treating depression in depressed patients without neurological disease (Burt et al. 2002; Holtzheimer et al. 2001; Kozel and George 2002), and some data suggest efficacy in depressed patients with Parkinson's disease (Dragasevic et al. 2002; Fregni et al. 2004) and poststroke depression (Jorge et al. 2004). Vagus nerve stimulation has led to mood improvements in patients with epilepsy (Elger et al. 2000) and was recently approved by the U.S. Food and Drug Administration (FDA) for the treatment of treatment-resistant depression (George et al. 2005; Rush et al. 2005). Deep brain stimulation of the subthalamic nucleus and internal globus pallidus has shown efficacy in treating the motor symptoms associated with Parkinson's disease (The Deep Brain Stimulation for Parkinson's Disease Study Group 2001), essential tremor (Schuurman et al. 2000), and dystonia (Lozano and Abosch 2004) but also has been associated with negative mood changes (Bejjani et al. 1999; Berney et al. 2002). However, a study of high-frequency deep brain stimulation of the white matter adjacent to the subgenual cingulate region in nonneuropsychiatric patients showed potential antidepressant efficacy (Mayberg et al. 2005).

In summary, SSRIs are generally considered the treatment of choice in neuropsychiatric patients with depression; in no condition are SSRIs contraindicated as a first-line treatment for depressive syndromes. The question of whether tricyclics are superior to SSRIs in some neuropsychiatric patients (such as those with poststroke depression) requires further study and must include a careful analysis of relative tolerability and potential for adverse events. SSRIs with relatively shorter half-lives (paroxetine, fluvoxamine) or absence of inhibition of select microsomal enzyme systems (citalopram, sertraline, paroxetine, fluvoxamine) may be advantageous in some cases. Because of the potentially activating properties of the SSRIs, they should be started at about half the usual starting dose and titrated up to standard antidepressant doses in the first 1–3 weeks. Venlafaxine at lower doses is less likely to cause hypertension but also acts more like a pure SSRI, with noradrenergic properties requiring higher (225 mg or greater) doses. Mirtazapine's effect of increased appetite could be advantageous in HIV (Elliott and Roy-Byrne 2000) or Alzheimer's (Raji and Brady 2001) patients with wasting, although sedative side effects may limit its use in some patients. More apathetic states could be treated with dopaminergic strategies, including bupropion, bromocriptine, amantadine, and stimulants. TCAs, if used, should probably be limited to desipramine (lowest anticholinergic effects) and nortriptyline (lowest hypotensive effects, low anticholinergic effects, and good blood level data for interpretation). Nonselective MAOIs should probably be avoided in neuropsychiatric patients. Table 31–1 lists characteristic antidepressants recommended in this section, dose ranges, side effects, and relevant drug interactions.

In patients who do not respond or cannot tolerate pharmacological treatments, ECT is a very reasonable treatment option. Other brain stimulation techniques (rTMS, vagus nerve stimulation, deep brain stimulation) have shown promising results in treating depression but require much further study before their usefulness in treating depressed neuropsychiatric patients can be determined.

PSYCHOSIS

Psychotic states (hallucinations, delusions, and formal thought disorder) principally occur in schizophrenia and less commonly in mania and depression. Psychosis occurs less frequently overall in neurological patients than does depression, agitation, or cognitive impairment and often may be associated with and a result of cognitive impairment, as in paranoid delusions in Alzheimer's disease patients. When it occurs, psychosis can have a serious effect on patient care, causing noncompliance with needed medical interventions, behavior that may lead to self-harm or injury, and caregiver withdrawal from the patient. In these circumstances, rapid and definitive treatment of psychosis is warranted whether it occurs in isolation or, more commonly, in combination with states of agitation, cognitive impairment, depression, or mania.

COMMON ETIOLOGIES

Unlike depression and agitation, psychosis is relatively uncommon in stroke and multiple sclerosis and is less common in TBI and early and middle-phase Parkinson's disease. It is more commonly seen in association with complex partial epilepsy, Huntington's disease and late-stage Parkinson's disease, HIV infection, limbic encephalitis (e.g., herpes simplex), multi-infarct (i.e., subcortical) and Alzheimer's dementias, and tumors involving the temporal lobe and diencephalon (Feinstein and Ron 1998). In these latter conditions, most of which involve characteristic temporal lobe subcortical-limbic anatomical regions, the rate of occurrence is also greater than in the general population (Bredkjaer et al. 1998). Psychosis in HIV infection is often associated with greater neurocognitive impairment (i.e., dementia) but is also associated with prior substance abuse, suggesting that extra-

neurological factors often may be relevant (Sewell et al. 1994a). In contrast to HIV infection, in Alzheimer's dementia, psychosis is associated with more severe dementia and rapid disease progression. Psychosis in Parkinson's disease is often a complication of antiparkinsonian treatment and ranges from benign hallucinations in a clear sensorium to delusions with or without delirium. More advanced disease and cognitive impairment seem to increase the risk (Aarsland et al. 1999). Psychosis is an uncommon initial presentation of these conditions but must be particularly considered as a disguised presentation of HIV infection, mass lesions, limbic encephalitis, Huntington's disease, and temporal lobe epilepsy. Metachromatic leukodystrophy often presents with psychosis as the first symptom (Hyde et al. 1992). Psychosis in epilepsy can occur in three forms: a more common chronic interictal psychosis, a much rarer alternating psychosis that remits with seizure activity (forced normalization) (Sachdev 1998), and, even more rarely, peri-ictal or postictal psychotic behavior. A host of toxic-metabolic etiologies can cause psychosis, mostly in combination with a delirious picture. Antiparkinsonian drugs, primarily dopamine analogues and other dopamine receptor agonists, are a common cause of psychosis in Parkinson's disease patients. Corticosteroids used to treat many neuropsychiatric illnesses can cause psychosis. Digitalis, propranolol, anticonvulsants, H_2 blockers, and nonsteroidal anti-inflammatory drugs (NSAIDs), usually in high doses, have rarely been associated with psychotic symptoms. Thus, when evaluating the psychotic neuropsychiatric patient, careful assessment of the patient's metabolic status, medications, and history of exposure to various toxins and chemicals is crucial.

ANATOMY AND NEUROCHEMISTRY

Anatomical and neurochemical correlates of psychotic symptoms in schizophrenia and of the overall illness have been better delineated than those of almost any other behavioral syndrome. Some studies have suggested that schizophrenia is a neurodevelopmental illness that begins with in utero defects in the medial temporal lobe and midline periventricular (i.e., brain stem) structures (Pantelis et al. 2003; Shapiro 1993). The former results in disturbed development, both cytoarchitecturally and neurochemically, of multiple components of a neural limbic loop (one of several parallel cortico-striato-thalamo-cortical circuits) including ventral striatum and cingulate, entorhinal, and temporal cortices, whereas the latter may give rise to subfrontal and striatal circuit disturbances thought to underlie the negative (cognitive and affective) schizophrenic symptoms. "Neural connectivity" is disturbed in both prefrontal

TABLE 31–1.   Antidepressants

Drug	Starting daily dose (mg)	Target daily dose (mg)	Neuropsychiatric side effects	Neuropsychiatric drug interactions	Comments
Tricyclic antidepressants (TCAs)					
Nortriptyline	10	30–100	Dizziness, fatigue, drowsiness, tremor, nervousness, confusion, insomnia, headache, seizures, anticholinergic effects Other: orthostatic hypotension, ECG alterations, cardiac conduction delay, tachycardia, sexual dysfunction, weight gain	Increased blood levels with SSRIs, neuroleptics, methylphenidate, VPA, opioids Decreased blood levels with CBZ, phenytoin, barbiturates Increased blood levels of neuroleptics, CBZ, opioids Decreased blood levels of levodopa Additive anticholinergic effects with neuroleptics, antiparkinsonian agents, antihistamines	Low, but present, anticholinergic and hypotensive potential Blood level monitoring available Antiarrhythmic properties Analgesic effects, even at low doses, for neuropathic pain
Desipramine	25	75–200			
Amitriptyline	10	50–150			
Imipramine	10	50–200			
Clomipramine	25	75–200			
Doxepin	10	50–200			
Protriptyline	2.5	10–30			

TABLE 31–1. Antidepressants (continued)

Drug	Starting daily dose (mg)	Target daily dose (mg)	Neuropsychiatric side effects	Neuropsychiatric drug interactions	Comments
SSRIs and serotonin-norepinephrine reuptake inhibitors (SNRIs)					
Fluoxetine	5	10–80	Drowsiness (especially with paroxetine, fluvoxamine), nervousness or agitation (especially with fluoxetine), fatigue (especially with paroxetine), insomnia, tremor, dizziness, headache, confusion, paresthesia Other: nausea, diarrhea, sexual dysfunction, weight loss, hyponatremia, blood pressure changes (especially with venlafaxine)	Increased sedation with hypnotics, chloral hydrate, antihistamines Lethargy, impaired consciousness with metoprolol, propranolol Excitation and hallucinations with narcotics EPS with neuroleptics Neurotoxicity with lithium Serotonergic effects with lithium, buspirone, sumatriptan Serotonin syndrome with other serotonergic drugs (e.g., TCAs, MAOIs, atypical neuroleptics, opioids) Contraindicated with MAOIs (hypertensive crisis) Increased blood levels with valproate Decreased blood levels with CBZ Increased blood levels of TCAs, neuroleptics, BZDs, CBZ, valproate, phenytoin, propranolol (especially with fluoxetine, paroxetine)	Fluoxetine: may require up to 8 weeks to reach steady state; most inhibition of hepatic cytochrome P450 2D6 enzymes; also inhibits 2C and 3A4; potential use in cataplexy; antimyoclonic adjunct with oxitriptan Sertraline: increased blood level with food; most likely to cause diarrhea; least inhibition of cytochrome P450 2D6 but does inhibit 2C and 3A4 Paroxetine: more sedating, less stimulating, and shorter half-life than fluoxetine, sertraline; withdrawal syndrome more likely/severe; inhibition of cytochrome P450 2D6 but not 2C and 3A4; can inhibit trazodone metabolism Fluvoxamine: use twice-daily administration; most sedating and shortest half-life of SSRIs; withdrawal syndrome most likely; least bound to plasma proteins and no inhibition of hepatic cytochrome P450 2D6 enzymes; does inhibit 1A2, 2C, and 3A4 enzymes; less ejaculatory delay compared with fluoxetine, sertraline, paroxetine Citalopram: Minimal to no cytochrome inhibition; most purely serotonergic in vitro Venlafaxine: hypertensive exacerbation likely dose related; extended-release formulation much better tolerated than immediate release Duloxetine: cytochrome inhibition similar to fluoxetine; less hypertensive exacerbation than venlafaxine
Sertraline	25	50–200			
Paroxetine	10	20–50			
Fluvoxamine	25	50–300			
Citalopram	10	20–60			
Escitalopram	5–10	10–20			
Venlafaxine	37.5	150–300			
Duloxetine	20–30	60			

TABLE 31–1. Antidepressants (continued)

Drug	Starting daily dose (mg)	Target daily dose (mg)	Neuropsychiatric side effects	Neuropsychiatric drug interactions	Comments
Other antidepressants					
Bupropion	75–150	200–450	Nervousness, tremor, dizziness, insomnia, headache, confusion, paresthesia, drowsiness, seizures	Contraindicated with MAOIs Decreased blood level with CBZ	Risk of seizures, especially with dosages >450 mg/day, >150 mg/dose Contraindicated in seizure disorders, bulimia, anorexia nervosa Fewer drug interactions than SSRIs
Mirtazapine	15	30–60	Sedation (less with higher doses); weight gain, agranulocytosis (very rare)	Contraindicated with MAOIs	No in vitro cytochrome enzyme inhibition May be more effective at higher doses (>60 mg/day) but few controlled data
Psychostimulants					
Methylphenidate	5–30	10–90	Nervousness, insomnia, dizziness, headache, dyskinesia, drowsiness, confusion, delusions, rebound depression, hallucinations, Tourette's, tics Other: anorexia, palpitations, blood pressure and pulse changes, cardiac arrhythmia, weight loss	Hypertension with MAOIs Increased blood levels of TCAs, phenytoin, phenobarbital, primidone Antagonistic effect by neuroleptics, phenobarbital	Contraindicated in marked anxiety, tension, agitation Fast onset of action Give early in day, divided doses (methylphenidate three times daily, dextroamphetamine twice daily) Dependence rare in medically ill May precipitate or worsen Tourette's or dyskinesia
Dextroamphetamine	2.5–20	5–60			

Note. BZDs=benzodiazepines; CBZ=carbamazepine; ECG=electrocardiogram; EPS=extrapyramidal side effects; MAOIs=monoamine oxidase inhibitors; SSRIs=selective serotonin reuptake inhibitors; TCAs=tricyclic antidepressants; VPA=valproic acid.

and temporal areas (Benes 1999; Kegeles et al. 1998; Selemon and Goldman-Rakic 1999), and some abnormalities are lateralized for both neuroanatomical (Levitan et al. 1999) and neurochemical (Laakso et al. 2000) findings. Metabolic changes in superior temporal gyrus (Suzuki et al. 1993), cingulate (Cleghorn et al. 1990), and striatum (Cleghorn et al. 1992) have been associated specifically with hallucinations. Frontal lobe dysfunction also plays a role in nonschizophrenic psychotic symptoms (Simpson et al. 1999) and, in schizophrenia, may play a role in "releasing" subcortical dopamine activity (Bertolino et al. 1999).

All three major monoamine neurotransmitters play a role in the limbic loop (Joyce 1993). Dopamine type 2 (D_2) receptors in ventral striatum, temporal cortex, perirhinal cortex, and hippocampus, along with ventral striatal glutamate and $5\text{-}HT_2$ receptors in ventral striatum and temporal cortex, are well positioned to modulate activity in the loop.

Anatomical and neurochemical findings in psychosis in neurological patients are surprisingly consistent with these abnormalities. Epileptic patients with psychosis more often have lesions that originated prenatally or perinatally and that affect medial temporal lobe neurons on the left (Roberts et al. 1990; Sachdev 1998), have reductions in left medial temporal lobe blood flow on single photon emission computed tomography (SPECT) (Marshall et al. 1993), have higher magnetic resonance imaging (MRI) T1 values in the left temporal lobe (Conlon et al. 1990), and have increased striatal dopamine metabolism (Reith et al. 1994). Patients with metachromatic leukodystrophy and psychosis have demyelinating lesions of subfrontal white matter disconnecting frontotemporal and frontal striatal circuits (Hyde et al. 1992). The rare occurrence of psychosis in multiple sclerosis is associated with MRI lesions in temporoparietal areas (Feinstein et al. 1992). In contrast, psychosis in Alzheimer's disease is associated with less specific findings, including abnormalities in the parietal lobe (Kotrla et al. 1995; Mentis et al. 1995), occipital lobe (Hirono et al. 1998), basal ganglia (Caligiuri and Peavy 2000), temporoparietal areas (Lopez et al. 1991), and frontotemporal regions (Lopez et al. 2001) and with reduced levels of serotonin in multiple areas (Zubenko et al. 1991). In Parkinson's disease, intraventricular infusions of dopamine produce psychosis (Kulkarni et al. 1992), as do dopaminergic medications used to treat the illness (Poewe 2003). Despite loss of nigrostriatal dopamine neurons in Parkinson's disease, supersensitive dopamine receptors in other areas (e.g., the limbic loop) may be responsible for the psychotic effects. "Release" of subcortical dopamine in frontotemporal dementia may occur secondary to cortical damage (Nitrini and Rosenberg 1998), a potential mechanism of action in idiopathic schizophrenia (Bertolino et al. 1999).

TREATMENT

Neuroleptic (antipsychotic) medications remain the mainstay in the pharmacological treatment of psychosis. Little evidence shows that other agents sometimes used as effective adjuncts to neuroleptics (e.g., anticonvulsants, benzodiazepines) have primary antipsychotic effects of their own. Although typical neuroleptics (e.g., haloperidol, perphenazine, chlorpromazine) have proven efficacy in the treatment of psychosis related to multiple causes, the side-effect profiles of these medications, including the risk of severe adverse reactions (such as tardive dyskinesia and neuroleptic malignant syndrome), can limit their usefulness. Alternatively, the atypical neuroleptics (clozapine, risperidone, olanzapine, quetiapine, ziprasidone, and aripiprazole) have been shown to be as effective as typical neuroleptics in the treatment of psychosis and are generally associated with different, somewhat more tolerable side effects. (However, note that the association of these medications with alterations in metabolism of glucose and cholesterol may present difficulties for the long-term use of these medications in certain susceptible patients; also, these medications have been associated with tardive dyskinesia and neuroleptic malignant syndrome, although at much lower rates than with the typical neuroleptics.) These advantages are even more prominent in neuropsychiatric patients, who are more prone to neurological side effects. For example, patients with HIV psychosis have a several-fold higher rate of side effects, even at daily doses as low as 100–250 mg in chlorpromazine equivalents (Sewell et al. 1994b), when compared with medically ill control subjects (Ramachandran et al. 1997).

Typical neuroleptics have been most often studied in the mixed psychosis and agitation of dementia patients. Although an early placebo-controlled study showing superiority of both haloperidol (mean dose = 4.6 mg) and loxapine (mean dose = 22 mg) reported that only one-third of the patients showed significant improvement (Petrie et al. 1982), a more recent study (Devanand et al. 1998) showed a response rate of 55%–60% with 2–3 mg of haloperidol, superior to a 30% response rate with 0.5 mg and consistent with the high correlation obtained between blood levels of haloperidol and change on the psychosis factor of the Brief Psychiatric Rating Scale (BPRS) in an earlier study (Devanand et al. 1992). In contrast, correlations between blood level and hostility/agitation were much lower. Unfortunately, studies still suggest that patients with dementia are overtreated with neuroleptics, with 20 of 22 nursing home patients able to discontinue these drugs successfully in one study (Bridges-Parlet et al. 1997).

Despite a long history of use of typical neuroleptics in epilepsy-related psychosis, the treatment of psychosis in epilepsy has not been subjected to controlled study, and even uncontrolled reports are scarce. The often-cited phenomenon of forced normalization (i.e., worsening psychosis with better seizure control) is actually quite rare. However, if psychosis can be documented to worsen with better seizure control, a slight increase in seizure frequency in someone with nondangerous complex partial seizures could improve psychosis. The more common syndrome of chronic interictal psychosis should be treated with neuroleptics, with careful attention to effects on seizure frequency. In one report (Onuma et al. 1991), 11 of 21 patients (52%) showed aggravation of symptoms with decrease or discontinuation of neuroleptics. This suggests that patients should be carefully monitored to determine whether ongoing neuroleptics are truly required.

Much of the literature on atypical antipsychotics in neuropsychiatric patients has focused on Parkinson's disease patients because of their unique sensitivity to EPS and frequency of psychotic side effects from antiparkinsonian medications. The only medication with confirmed antipsychotic benefit without worsening Parkinson's disease in double-blind, placebo-controlled trials is clozapine at a dosage less than 50 mg/day (Pollak et al. 2004; The Parkinson Study Group 1999). The only other placebo-controlled data suggest no benefit (and worsening of parkinsonian symptoms) with olanzapine (Breier et al. 2002). Several chart reviews and open or active medication comparison studies suggest that quetiapine may be useful in treating psychosis in Parkinson's disease patients (Fernandez et al. 1999, 2002, 2003; Juncos et al. 2004; Morgante et al. 2002, 2004; Parsa and Bastani 1998; Reddy et al. 2002; Targum and Abbott 2000; Wijnen et al. 2003); however, no placebo-controlled data are available to support this conclusion. Open data suggest that risperidone may have antipsychotic efficacy in Parkinson's disease patients (E. Mohr et al. 2000), although risperidone may worsen parkinsonian symptoms more than clozapine does (Ellis et al. 2000). One open study did not suggest any benefit for aripiprazole in Parkinson's disease psychosis (Fernandez et al. 2004). A case report (Connemann and Schonfeldt-Lecuona 2004) and two small open studies (Gomez-Esteban et al. 2005; Oechsner and Korchounov 2005) suggest a potential benefit for ziprasidone.

Thus, the data to date suggest clozapine as the most efficacious atypical antipsychotic for psychosis in Parkinson's disease. However, several side effects and potential adverse reactions limit the use of clozapine. Clozapine is associated with significant weight gain, abnormalities in glucose and cholesterol metabolism, and autonomic reactions (increased salivation, increased heart rate, constipation, hypotension). There is an approximately 1% risk of agranulocytosis with clozapine, and close monitoring of

white blood cell counts is required. Clozapine also significantly lowers the seizure threshold and produces electroencephalographic abnormalities in most non–neurologically ill patients at some time during treatment (Malow et al. 1994; Welch et al. 1994). In schizophrenic patients, seizures are dose dependent (Haller and Binder 1990), and both slow titration and lower ceiling doses (below 600 mg) may reduce the likelihood of seizures. In the neuropsychiatric population, doses far lower than these may be likely to provoke seizures. Both seizures and myoclonus due to clozapine may respond to valproate (Meltzer and Ranjan 1994). Reports in neuropsychiatric groups suggest that preexisting electroencephalographic abnormalities predict liability to develop delirium with clozapine (Duffy and Kant 1996).

Beyond clozapine, quetiapine and risperidone have the next strongest database in Parkinson's disease psychosis. Quetiapine and risperidone have both been associated with weight gain and metabolic abnormalities but to a lesser degree than clozapine has; also, the risk of agranulocytosis appears to be much lower with these medications. Risperidone may worsen parkinsonism to a greater degree than clozapine does (and possibly quetiapine), but this risk is most likely still lower than with the typical neuroleptics.

There is growing evidence for the efficacy of atypical antipsychotics in dementia-related psychoses, with risperidone and olanzapine supported by the strongest database (Sink et al. 2005). Reports in severe Lewy body dementia suggest the potential for marked confusion with clozapine (Burke et al. 1998) and intolerance in three of eight patients taking olanzapine (Walker et al. 1999); however, other reports with risperidone and clozapine suggest good tolerability (Allen et al. 1995; Chacko et al. 1993). Atypical antipsychotics may increase the risk of stroke in patients with dementia (Sink et al. 2005), and the U.S. FDA recently required a black box warning on all atypical antipsychotic medications indicating that they may be associated with increased mortality when used to treat agitation in patients with dementia.

Results are mixed in other neuropsychiatric patient groups. Singh et al. (1997) reported substantial efficacy without EPS for risperidone in 20 of 21 psychotic HIV patients, and Lera and Zirulnik (1999) reported good efficacy for clozapine in psychotic HIV patients who experienced EPS with typical neuroleptics. Other reports have shown EPS with risperidone and akathisia with olanzapine (Meyer et al. 1998). For Huntington's disease, atypical antipsychotics can benefit the movement disorder as well as the psychiatric complications, although the database is limited (Bonelli et al. 2004). Some data suggest that atypical antipsychotics may be beneficial in Huntington's disease only when doses equivalent to 6 mg of risperidone are used (Dallocchio et al. 1999; Parsa et al. 1997), and Huntington's disease patients may have difficulty tolerating these doses. With clozapine, marked disability was seen in most patients at doses of 150 mg—lower than needed for maximal benefit (van Vugt et al. 1997). Atypical antipsychotics are considered first-line agents for the treatment of psychosis in patients with TBI (McAllister and Ferrell 2002). Risperidone has been effective in 5 of 6 patients with TBI without EPS (Duffy and Kant 1996). In other reports, risperidone was superior to conventional neuroleptics in improving TBI psychosis, sleep and daytime alertness (Schreiber et al. 1998), and psychosis following ischemic brain damage (Zimnitzky et al. 1996). Finally, risperidone has been effective for psychosis associated with neurosarcoidosis (Popli 1997). Doses between 3 and 6 mg were used in these studies.

Few novel treatments for psychosis are available. One report noted good antipsychotic efficacy without worsening of motor symptoms in 15 of 16 Parkinson's disease patients given the 5-HT$_3$ antagonist antiemetic ondansetron at dosages of 12–24 mg/day (Zoldan et al. 1995). This drug has not been found to be effective in schizophrenia (Newcomer et al. 1992), suggesting some divergence of mechanism in Parkinson's disease psychosis and schizophrenia. In contrast, glutamatergic medications offer a potential avenue for antipsychotic effects in Parkinson's disease patients based on pathophysiological theories of schizophrenia, the psychotomimetic potential of N-methyl-D-aspartate (NMDA) antagonists (Knable and Rickler 1995), their possible benefit in treating the overall syndrome of Parkinson's disease (Lange and Riederer 1994), and the potential utility of D-cycloserine, an NMDA receptor–complex agonist at the glycine site, in the treatment of schizophrenia (Goff et al. 1999). ECT may improve treatment-resistant psychosis, especially if the psychosis presents acutely and/or within the context of a mood disorder.

In summary, neuroleptic medications should be considered first-line agents for the treatment of psychosis across the full range of neuropsychiatric conditions. Clozapine is least likely to have motor side effects, although seizure threshold–lowering effects are more problematic in neurologically compromised patients. It may be preferred in unusually EPS-sensitive patients with Parkinson's disease, Huntington's disease, and other conditions with basal ganglia involvement, although other side effects may limit the ability to reach therapeutic doses in certain disorders (such as Huntington's disease). In most neurological disorders, patients will show exaggerated sensitivity to motor side effects, making atypical antipsychotics the treatment of choice. Table 31–2 lists characteristic antipsychotics recommended in this section, dose ranges, side effects, and relevant drug interactions.

AGITATED STATES, INCLUDING ANXIETY AND MANIA

Syndromes of agitation span the entire spectrum of psychiatric illness, occurring in mood disorders, anxiety disorders, psychosis, dementia, and impulse-control disorders. In the absence of frank psychosis, dementia, or delirium, the differential diagnosis of prominent agitation remains extremely difficult because states of agitated depression, mixed bipolar mood states/dysphoric mania, and severe panic or anxiety overlap substantially in phenomenology.

COMMON ETIOLOGIES

Stroke is commonly associated with generalized anxiety at a rate comparable to depression; it is more rarely associated with mania (Robinson 1997). In contrast, there is a much greater incidence of mania in TBI than in the general population (Jorge et al. 1993). Patients with multiple sclerosis are more likely to have mania compared with both general and psychiatric inpatient populations (Joffe et al. 1987; Pine et al. 1995; Schiffer et al. 1986). Temporal lobe epilepsy is among the most common causes of secondary mania seen in the general medical setting (Barczak et al. 1988; Chakrabarti et al. 1999; Gillig et al. 1988; Guillem et al. 2000; Pascualy et al. 1997). In stroke, patients with both anxiety and depression are more likely to have cortical lesions (and to have a poorer prognosis [Shimoda and Robinson 1998]), whereas patients with depression alone are more likely to have subcortical lesions (Starkstein et al. 1990). The same exclusively cortical pattern has been found for pure mania versus mixed bipolar states (Starkstein et al. 1991). Similarly, the high incidence of agitation in Alzheimer's dementia (its most common behavioral disturbance [Devanand 1997]), but not in multi-infarct dementias, highlights the importance of cortical damage and subcortical preservation. However, the high rate of anxiety disorders and symptoms in patients with Parkinson's disease, occurrence of mania with brain stem lesions (Drake et al. 1990), elevated rates of mania in the HIV-infected population (Lyketsos et al. 1997), and findings that poststroke bipolar disorder is strongly associated with right hemisphere lesions that involve subcortical and midline structures (Berthier et al. 1996) suggest that subcortical involvement alone is capable of producing states of agitation, although more likely with manic appearance.

Most studies show that these conditions occur for the most part at rates greater than in the general population, are not necessarily associated with a greater rate of familial psychiatric illness, and have characteristic lesion location (discussed in more detail below), suggesting that

TABLE 31–2.   Antipsychotics/neuroleptics

Drug	Starting daily dose (mg)	Target daily dose (mg)	Neuropsychiatric side effects	Neuropsychiatric drug interactions	Comments
Typical neuroleptics					
Haloperidol	1–5	2–20	Parkinsonism, dystonia, akathisia, perioral (rabbit) tremor, anticholinergic effects, sedation, confusion, impaired psychomotor performance, TD, NMS, orthostatic hypotension, ejaculatory inhibition, priapism, dysphagia, urinary incontinence, temperature dysregulation, sudden death (possibly due to cardiac arrhythmia) Other: slowed cardiac repolarization, photosensitivity, hyperthermia, hyperprolactinemia, weight gain	Additive CNS depressant effects with other CNS depressants Additive anticholinergic effects with other anticholinergic drugs Increased EPS with SSRIs, lithium, buspirone Neurotoxicity with lithium Increased blood level of TCAs, valproate, phenytoin, β-adrenergic blockers Decreased blood level with lithium, CBZ, phenytoin, phenobarbital, antiparkinsonian agents Increased blood level with TCAs, SSRIs, MAOIs, alprazolam, buspirone, β-adrenergic blockers	Haloperidol: most EPS potential, especially with low calcium, akathisia with low iron; intravenous route provides rapid onset of action with potentially lower risk of EPS; available in decanoate form; useful in Huntington's, Tourette's Perphenazine: available in decanoate form
Perphenazine	4–16	8–40			
Atypical antipsychotics					
Risperidone	0.25–1	2–6	Sedation, insomnia, agitation, EPS, headache, anxiety, dizziness, aggressive reaction, NMS Other: anticholinergic side effects, weight gain, possible glucose control and cholesterol abnormalities	May antagonize effects of levodopa and dopamine agonists Increased blood level with clozapine, inhibitor of cytochrome P450 2D6 Decreased blood level with CBZ	Maximum efficacy for most patients at 4–6 mg/day Less EPS potential than haloperidol but more than other atypical agents Typically use two divided daily doses

TABLE 31–2. Antipsychotics/neuroleptics (continued)

Drug	Starting daily dose (mg)	Target daily dose (mg)	Neuropsychiatric side effects	Neuropsychiatric drug interactions	Comments
Clozapine	15–50	200–600	Drowsiness, dizziness, headache, tremor, syncope, insomnia, restlessness, hypokinesia/akinesia, agitation, seizures, rigidity, akathisia, confusion, fatigue, hyperkinesia, weakness, lethargy, ataxia, slurred speech, depression, abnormal movements, anxiety, EPS, NMS, obsessive-compulsive symptoms Other: salivation, weight gain, glucose intolerance, hypercholesterolemia agranulocytosis	Additive CNS depressant effects with other CNS depressants Occasional collapse (hypotension, respiratory depression, loss of consciousness) with BZDs Increased risk of bone marrow suppression with CBZ, possibly lithium Increased risk of NMS with other antipsychotics, lithium, CBZ Decreased blood level with CBZ, phenytoin Serotonin syndrome with other serotonergic drugs	Initially monitor WBC count weekly; may increase interval if stable for several months; lower risk of EPS, TD, NMS, and higher risk of lowering seizure threshold than do typical neuroleptics May improve motor function in Tourette's, Huntington's, drug-induced persistent dyskinesia, spasmodic torticollis, essential tremor
Olanzapine	5	10–20	Somnolence, headache, dizziness, NMS Other: dry mouth, weight gain, glucose control abnormalities, hypercholesterolemia, nausea, constipation, elevated transaminase	Additive CNS depressant effects with other CNS depressants Increased blood level with fluoxetine, duloxetine Decreased blood level with smoking and CBZ	Once-daily dosing
Quetiapine	12.5–25	300–450	Sedation, EPS, dizziness, agitation Other: moderate weight gain, postural hypotension, dry mouth, elevated transaminase, glucose control abnormalities, lipid abnormalities	Additive CNS depressant effects with other CNS depressants	Very sedating; often used in low doses for treating insomnia
Ziprasidone	20–40	120–160	Agitation, akathisia, insomnia, NMS Other: QT prolongation possible, may affect lipid and glucose metabolism	Serotonin syndrome with other serotonergic drugs Increased cardiac rhythm effects with other medications that affect conduction	Use divided daily doses Appears to cause little weight gain and few effects on glucose and lipid metabolism
Aripiprazole	5–15	20–30	Agitation, akathisia, insomnia, NMS	Decreased blood level with barbiturates, CBZ	Appears to cause little weight gain and few effects on glucose and lipid metabolism Long half-life

Note. BZDs = benzodiazepines; CBZ = carbamazepine; CNS = central nervous system; EPS = extrapyramidal side effects; MAOIs = monoamine oxidase inhibitors; NMS = neuroleptic malignant syndrome; SSRIs = selective serotonin reuptake inhibitors; TCAs = tricyclic antidepressants; TD = tardive dyskinesia; WBC = white blood cell.

these symptoms are not merely a reaction to illness. Treatment of the underlying illness sometimes ameliorates symptoms (e.g., reduced mania in zidovudine [AZT]-treated HIV illness [Mijch et al. 1999]). However, other conditions (besides the underlying illness) should be considered in the differential diagnosis of these agitated states. Agitation plays a prominent role in the phenomenology of PTSD, which may result following the trauma leading to TBI. A broad spectrum of drugs, including corticosteroids, thyroid hormone, psychostimulants, appetite suppressants, cocaine, caffeine, other dopaminergic agents (levodopa, bromocriptine), felbamate, dextromethorphan, alpha interferon, and angiotensin-converting enzyme inhibitors, have all been associated with agitation, anxiety, and mania. Withdrawal states from alcohol, sedative-hypnotics, and opiate drugs also can produce significant agitation. Finally, withdrawal from SSRIs may produce agitation, along with dizziness, malaise, headache, and nausea.

ANATOMY AND NEUROCHEMISTRY

As with depression, a variety of neuroanatomical and neurochemical substrates have been associated with agitated states. Converging data implicate the right anterior inferior temporal lobe and its connections to orbital frontal and related limbic circuits (including cingulate, amygdala, hippocampus, and parahippocampus) in the pathophysiology of both anxious and manic states. Lesion studies involving poststroke mania (Robinson and Starkstein 1989), poststroke anxiety (Castillo et al. 1993), and TBI mania (Jorge et al. 1993) implicated right anterior temporal and limbic structures. Other neuroimaging findings include lower perfusion in right temporal basal cortex in primary mania with SPECT (Migliorelli et al. 1993), medial temporal lobe hypoplasia in bipolar patients (Strakowski et al. 2002), decreased right caudate volume compared with healthy older control subjects (Beyer et al. 2004), right temporal lobe abnormalities in panic disorder patients with MRI (Ontiveros et al. 1989) and electroencephalography (Weilburg et al. 1995), and decreased right posterotemporal and right medial frontal cortex blood flow during induced anxiety in healthy control subjects with PET (Kimbrell et al. 1999). Mania has been shown to improve with right prefrontal rTMS (Grisaru et al. 1998; Michael and Erfurth 2004; Saba et al. 2004). Neurochemical perturbations associated with agitated states are less clear. Despite the potential efficacy of neuroleptics in the treatment of agitated states, one study found no association between agitation and postmortem indices of dopaminergic function (Bierer et al. 1993). Although consistent evidence indicates serotonergic defi-

ciencies in Alzheimer's disease patients (Raskind and Peskind 1994), these deficiencies have been inconsistently related to agitation (Mintzer et al. 1998). One study has implicated increased central noradrenergic function in agitated states (Elrod et al. 1997).

TREATMENT

An important step in treating agitated states in neuropsychiatric patients is identifying and addressing medical and pharmacological factors that may be causing or contributing to symptoms. Patients with neurological injury are likely to be quite susceptible to medical conditions (e.g., infection, electrolyte imbalance, or metabolic abnormalities) and medications (e.g., corticosteroids, thyroid hormone replacements, antiemetics, or anticholinergics) that can cause anxiety, mania, or agitation in the absence of delirium or psychosis. Although specific pharmacological management of the agitated state still may be required, it is equally if not more important to treat associated medical conditions and stop offending medications if possible.

Numerous medications have been used in the treatment of agitated states in neuropsychiatric patients, although few double-blind, placebo-controlled studies are available. Across multiple neuropsychiatric syndromes associated with agitation, anticonvulsants (particularly carbamazepine and valproate) have shown consistent efficacy and reasonable tolerability. Anticonvulsants have been recommended for secondary mania–associated "neurological" factors, including substance abuse (Pope et al. 1988). Scattered reports have suggested efficacy for carbamazepine in mentally retarded manic patients (Glue 1989), in patients with HIV-related mania resistant to lithium (Halman et al. 1993), in TBI patients with agitation (Azouvi et al. 1999), and in patients with Alzheimer's-related agitation resistant to neuroleptics (Olin et al. 2001). A placebo-controlled trial in 51 agitated patients with dementia showed a 77% response rate for carbamazepine compared with a 21% response for placebo (Tariot et al. 1998a).

Valproate has shown efficacy in mentally retarded manic patients (Sovner 1989) and in agitated patients with brain injury (Horne and Lindley 1995). Valproate has shown potential efficacy in agitated patients with dementia (Kunik et al. 1998; Porsteinsson et al. 1997); however, a large randomized, placebo-controlled trial showed no efficacy (Tariot et al. 2005). Blood levels have varied widely (14–107 µg/mL), although studies showed some responders at levels lower than 50 µg/mL. One placebo-controlled trial with open follow-up showed good efficacy and reasonable tolerability for valproate in agitated demented patients (Porsteinsson et al. 2001, 2003). It is of interest that one survey noted that valproate is preferred by clinicians to carbamazepine (The Expert Consensus Panel for Agitation in Dementia 1998); this is perhaps related to more clinical experience with valproate (given its widespread use in bipolar disorder).

Because of the potential for bone marrow suppression with carbamazepine and for hepatotoxicity and thrombocytopenia with valproate, complete blood cell count and liver function tests should be monitored. Carbamazepine and valproate blood levels do not necessarily correlate with clinical response but should be used to monitor compliance and drug metabolism.

A very preliminary database suggests a possible role for gabapentin in the treatment of agitation in neuropsychiatric patients. Given its relatively mild side-effect profile and few drug-drug interactions, gabapentin would be an attractive treatment option if efficacy could be documented. Several case reports and case series have shown that gabapentin has potential efficacy for agitation in patients with dementia (Goldenberg et al. 1998; Miller 2001; Regan and Gordon 1997; Roane et al. 2000), stroke (Low and Brandes 1999), and mental retardation (Bozikas et al. 2001). However, other reports have shown gabapentin to be minimally effective in agitated dementia patients (Herrmann et al. 2000) or associated with increases in anxiety and restlessness in TBI patients (Childers and Holland 1997). No placebo-controlled data are available. Several other anticonvulsants are available (including oxcarbazapine, topiramate, tiagabine, zonisamide, levetiracetam) but have not been well studied in neuropsychiatric patients. Lamotrigine has a growing database showing efficacy in treating patients with bipolar disorder (Bowden et al. 2003; Calabrese et al. 1999) but limited data supporting its use in other neuropsychiatric patients.

Lithium, a first-line agent in the management of mania and bipolar disorder in younger patients, has been used successfully in manic patients with neurological illness but may have significantly more side effects in this population (Himmelhoch et al. 1980; Kemperman et al. 1989; Roose et al. 1979; Smith and Helms 1982). These side effects can include tremor, gastrointestinal complaints, increased thirst, cardiac abnormalities, muscle weakness, and fatigue. Neurological side effects of lithium may be greater in patients with underlying neurological disease. Finally, the narrow therapeutic window may make it difficult to use lithium appropriately in patients who have poor medication compliance (because of memory problems and confusion), who have decreased renal clearance, and who are taking concomitant medications that may result in clinically significant interactions (such as thiazide diuretics). Two reports have shown that lithium, even at low levels, was less effective and produced severe side effects in bipolar patients after head trauma

(Hornstein and Seliger 1989) and stroke (Moskowitz and Altshuler 1991). Lithium also has been shown to be inadequate without clozapine augmentation in Parkinson's disease (Kim et al. 1994) and to be less effective in patients with mental retardation (Glue 1989). Except for a possibly unique effect on steroid-induced mania and agitation (Falk et al. 1979), lithium would appear not to be considered a first-line choice for many neuropsychiatric patients. Its proconvulsant effect (Moore 1981; Parmelee and O'Shanick 1988; Sacristan et al. 1991) and ability to cause or aggravate EPS (Lecamwasam et al. 1994) are other shortcomings. In dementia, most reports show that it has minimal effect (Holton and George 1985; Kunik et al. 1994), although it may be useful in certain HIV-related manic syndromes (Halman et al. 1993).

Benzodiazepines are potent inhibitors of both primary mania and anxiety. However, in agitated states secondary to neurological illness, these agents can cause confusion, cognitive impairment, psychomotor slowing, and disinhibition presenting as a paradoxical reaction; also, their short- and long-term efficacy have not been established. Studies in patients with dementia have shown that the beneficial effects of oxazepam over placebo are lost at 8 weeks as a result of tolerance (Sanders 1965) and that benzodiazepines are generally inferior to typical neuroleptics in the treatment of behavioral disturbances (Coccaro et al. 1990; Herz et al. 1992; Kirven and Montero 1973). A double-blind study in hospitalized patients with acquired immunodeficiency syndrome (AIDS) and delirium showed that lorazepam was markedly inferior to both haloperidol and chlorpromazine and was associated with such severe, treatment-limiting adverse effects that this arm of the study was prematurely terminated (Breitbart et al. 1996). A drug discontinuation study showed that dementia patients tapered from long-term use of benzodiazepines had improved memory without worsening of anxiety (Salzman 2000). Despite these findings, the judicious use of benzodiazepines could be considered in extremely difficult cases that do not respond to other interventions. Low doses and careful titration are necessary to minimize side effects, and agents with short half-lives and without active metabolites should be used preferentially.

Typical neuroleptics have been used frequently to treat nonspecific agitation with reasonably good effect in some studies (Breitbart et al. 1996; Salzman 1987). However, EPS, sedation, and hypotension limit these medications, and several placebo-controlled studies have shown these drugs to be only marginally more effective in the absence of more classic psychotic symptoms (Lonergan et al. 2002; Raskind 1993). Additionally, neurological patients appear to be at increased risk for developing tardive dyskinesia and akathisia (Lonergan et al. 2002), and animal studies have implicated typical neuroleptics in being deleterious to cortical recovery (Feeney et al. 1982). In general, the typical neuroleptics have largely been replaced by the atypical antipsychotics in clinical practice (Alexopoulos et al. 2004; Kasckow et al. 2004). Risperidone was effective at a low dose in two placebo-controlled studies (Brodaty et al. 2003; Katz et al. 1999), although the data are not consistent (De Deyn et al. 1999). Other studies have shown efficacy for olanzapine (Meehan et al. 2001; Street et al. 2000), although, again, the data are not consistent (De Deyn et al. 2004). A greater rate of EPS has been associated with risperidone, even at low doses, in dementia patients (Herrmann et al. 1998). Prior studies have shown an increased risk of stroke with atypical antipsychotics (Sink et al. 2005), but this may be related to factors not associated with the medications themselves (Herrmann and Lanctot 2005). However, atypical antipsychotics may be associated with increased mortality when used in agitated patients with dementia (Schneider et al. 2005). In 15 placebo-controlled trials enrolling a total of 5,106 patients, mortality rose from 2.6% in subjects taking placebo to 4.5% in drug-treated subjects, for an increased mortality risk between 1.6 and 1.7 in the drug-treated subjects. Because atypical antipsychotics across different classes were studied, the FDA warning applies to all the atypical antipsychotics, including those not systematically studied. The published warning suggests a similar risk for older, traditional antipsychotics and that an official warning for those medications may be forthcoming. It should be recognized that not treating agitation is also associated with significant risks, including danger to the patient and caregivers and loss of living situation. Thus, the documented risks must be weighed alongside the efficacy data cited earlier even in the absence of an official FDA indication for use in agitated dementia patients.

Typical antidepressant medications also have shown mixed efficacy in treating agitation in neuropsychiatric patients. Citalopram was effective for anxiety, fear, and panic in 65 Alzheimer's dementia patients but not in 24 patients with vascular dementia (Nyth and Gottfries 1990); fluoxetine was no more effective than placebo or haloperidol in reducing agitation in Alzheimer's patients in another small study (Auchus and Bissey-Black 1997). Although SSRIs are known to cause agitation as a side effect in primary depression, they work equally well in patients with agitated and retarded primary depression (Tollefson et al. 1994). Other reports have noted the utility of TCAs in brain injury–related agitation (Mysiw et al. 1988), in states of pathological emotional lability in stroke (Robinson et al. 1993), and in multiple sclerosis (Schiffer et al. 1985). Fluoxetine also has reportedly

been effective for emotional lability in stroke, multiple sclerosis, brain injury, amyotrophic lateral sclerosis, and encephalitis (Iannaccone and Ferini-Strambi 1996; Sloan et al. 1992; W.C. Tsai et al. 1998). Sertraline also may be effective (Burns et al. 1999; Peterson et al. 1996), although the data are somewhat mixed (Lanctot et al. 2002). Although some studies have suggested trazodone may be helpful in treating agitation in patients with dementia (Lawlor et al. 1994; Sultzer et al. 1997), an analysis of double-blind, placebo-controlled data found that the data were insufficient to support the use of trazodone for agitation (Martinon-Torres et al. 2004).

Other agents may be beneficial in treating agitation in neurological patients, although further study is clearly necessary. β-Adrenergic blockers have shown efficacy for treating agitation and aggression in patients with TBI (Fleminger et al. 2003). Evidence is also emerging that cholinergic medications, discussed in detail in the "Cognitive Disturbance" section later in this chapter, may have antiagitation effects (Lanctot and Herrmann 2000; Mega et al. 1999; Rosler et al. 1998). The nonbenzodiazepine anxiolytic buspirone has shown some efficacy in agitated states associated with dementia (Colenda 1988; Cooper 2003) and TBI (Levine 1988), especially when no severe motor or cognitive deficits were present (Gualtieri 1991). In Huntington's disease, one study reported improvement in both agitation and choreoathetoid movements with buspirone 120 mg/day (Hamner et al. 1996). In developmentally delayed patients, 16 of 22 had a good response to 15–45 mg/day (Buitelaar et al. 1998). Although one study showed that low-dose buspirone was superior to haloperidol in agitated dementia, the effects were extremely modest (Cantillon et al. 1996). Despite these promising studies, no placebo-controlled data are available.

In summary, several pharmacological agents have some data supporting efficacy in the treatment of agitation and anxiety in neuropsychiatric patients. More well-designed clinical trials are needed to better guide treatment selection. The anticonvulsants carbamazepine and valproate have a reasonably strong database supporting their use in treating agitation and anxiety across a range of neuropsychiatric conditions and generally would be considered first-line agents; however, the side effects and risks associated with these medications are not inconsequential. In the presence of prominent anxiety or dysphoria (suggesting perhaps an underlying depressive syndrome), antidepressant medications, particularly the SSRIs, should be considered first- or second-line treatments. Benzodiazepines should be reserved for severe or treatment-resistant cases; when used, agents with shorter half-lives and no active metabolites should be chosen, and doses should be started very low and titrated carefully. In the absence of clear mania, lithium does not appear to be supported as a first- or even second-line agent at this time. Neuroleptics, which have long been a mainstay in the treatment of agitated neuropsychiatric patients, are coming under closer scrutiny given recent concerns about increased mortality risk when used in agitated patients with dementia. However, these agents, especially the atypical antipsychotics, have shown efficacy in treating agitation across a range of conditions. Before using these agents, a careful risk-benefit analysis should be performed, and informed consent should be carefully documented. Tables 31–3 and 31–4 list characteristic mood stabilizers and anxiolytics recommended in this section, with dose ranges, side effects, and relevant drug interactions.

AGGRESSION, IMPULSIVITY, AND BEHAVIORAL DYSCONTROL

Behavioral dyscontrol is a common complication in neuropsychiatric patients and includes aggressive acts, paraphilias, compulsions, rituals, self-mutilation, and other socially inappropriate behaviors. Such symptoms can be associated with psychosis, agitated or manic states, depression, or cognitive impairment. They may also be part of acute delirium or chronic severe brain dysfunction. Less often, behavioral dyscontrol (e.g., aggression, hypersexuality) may result from more specific neurological lesions (Mendez et al. 2000). The severity of symptoms can range from mild irritability to marked physical violence. As more severely compromised neurological patients survive as a result of improved medical care, the neuropsychiatrist will increasingly confront this problem. Because behavioral dyscontrol may consist of a complex admixture of symptoms, thorough exploration of potential neurological and psychiatric etiologies is required. It is important to document the behavioral dysfunction and its potential response to treatment with observer ratings. The Overt Aggression Scale (Yudofsky et al. 1986) is one reliable and valid method. The Aberrant Behavior Checklist, which measures irritability, social withdrawal, stereotyping, hyperactivity, and excessive speech, is another (Aman et al. 1985). Although behavioral management remains a core treatment of impulsivity and aggression (Wong et al. 1988), psychopharmacological interventions have become increasingly important.

COMMON ETIOLOGIES

Behavioral dyscontrol has been associated with a broad range of neurological disorders. It has been most frequently observed in disorders involving diffuse and global neurological dysfunction such as TBI, mental retardation, delirium, and dementia. However, more focal disease of the prefrontal cortical and basal ganglia regions (frontal strokes, Huntington's disease, and Parkinson's disease) and temporal lobes (epilepsy, Klüver-Bucy syndrome, and frontotemporal dementia) can also lead to aggression, impulsivity, hypersexuality, and other forms of behavioral dyscontrol.

The psychodynamic significance of a chronically debilitating neurological illness can play a role in further exacerbating any premorbid maladaptive characterological traits and coping strategies. Furthermore, an inability to carry out adaptive planning, problem solving, and other executive functions, caused by CNS damage, can lead to frustration, anxiety, and nonproductive, impulsive acts when a patient is confronted with external stressors. Hence it may be useful to understand dyscontrol as a maladaptive attempt by an individual with a limited behavioral repertoire to deal with a stressful environment or event (Halliday and Mackrell 1998).

Many neurological medications can cause or exacerbate behavior problems by agitating or activating the patient. Such medications include levodopa, corticosteroids, amantadine, bromocriptine, interferon, selegiline, and antiviral agents (such as AZT). Sedative-hypnotics (such as barbiturates and benzodiazepines), analgesics (opiates and other narcotics), anabolic steroids, antidepressants, stimulants, antipsychotics, and anticholinergic drugs also have been associated with aggression. Stimulants, dopaminergic agents, and testosterone-containing medications may increase sexual drive. Alcohol and drugs of abuse, such as cocaine, amphetamines, barbiturates, and phencyclidine, can cause or exacerbate behavioral dyscontrol and adversely interact with medications.

ANATOMY AND NEUROCHEMISTRY

Damage to the frontal and basotemporal lobes has been shown to be associated with impulsivity, aggression, and violence, although data in neuropsychiatric patients are limited (Fornazzari et al. 1992; Starkstein et al. 1994; Tonkonogy 1991). A lateral orbitofrontal circuit involving orbitofrontal cortex, striatum, subthalamic nucleus, substantia nigra, and thalamus is thought to regulate empathic and socially appropriate behavior (Mega and Cummings 1994). Damage may lead to irritability, tactlessness, impulsivity, environmental dependency, and mood lability. On the contrary, obsessive-compulsive spectrum disorders, which involve increased behavioral control and concern for social behavioral appropriateness, have been shown to be associated with increased metabolic activity in the orbitofrontal cortex and caudate nucleus (Baxter et al. 1987; Braun et al. 1995). Damage

TABLE 31–3.   Mood stabilizers

Drug	Starting daily dose (mg)	Target daily dose (mg)	Neuropsychiatric side effects	Neuropsychiatric drug interactions	Comments
Lithium	300–900	600–2,400	Lethargy, fatigue, muscle weakness, tremor, headache, confusion, dulled senses, ataxia, dysarthria, aphasia, muscle hyperirritability, hyperactive deep tendon reflexes, hypertonia, choreoathetoid movements, cogwheel rigidity, dizziness, drowsiness, disturbed accommodation, dystonia, seizures, EPS Other: nausea, diarrhea, polyuria, nephrogenic diabetes insipidus, hypothyroidism, hyperparathyroidism, T-wave depression, acne, leukocytosis	EPS and NMS with neuroleptics Neurotoxicity with SSRIs, neuroleptics, CBZ, valproate, phenytoin, calcium channel blockers Increased blood level with SSRIs, NSAIDs, dehydration Increased or decreased blood levels with diuretics Increased or decreased blood level of neuroleptics	Lowers seizure threshold Predominantly renally excreted Once-daily dosing more tolerable with less renal toxicity Blood levels correlate with therapeutic response and toxicity Used in Huntington's, cluster headaches, torticollis, Tourette's, SIADH, leukopenia
Carbamazepine	200–600	400–2,000	Dizziness, drowsiness, incoordination, confusion, headache, fatigue, blurred vision, hallucinations, diplopia, oculomotor disturbance, nystagmus, speech disturbance, abnormal involuntary movement, peripheral neuritis, paresthesia, depression, agitation, talkativeness, tinnitus, hyperacusis Other: nausea, bone marrow suppression, hepatotoxicity, SIADH	Additive CNS depressant effects with other CNS depressants Contraindicated with MAOIs Neurotoxicity with lithium, neuroleptics Bone marrow suppression with clozapine Increased blood level with SSRIs, verapamil Decreased blood level with TCAs, haloperidol, valproate, phenytoin, phenobarbital Decreased blood levels of TCAs, BZDs, neuroleptics, valproate, phenytoin, phenobarbital, methadone, propranolol	Induces own hepatic metabolism (2–5 weeks) Monitor CBC, LFTs, electrolytes Blood level of approximately 4–12 µg/mL Useful in trigeminal neuralgia, neuropathic pain, sedative-hypnotic withdrawal

TABLE 31–3. Mood stabilizers (*continued*)

Drug	Starting daily dose (mg)	Target daily dose (mg)	Neuropsychiatric side effects	Neuropsychiatric drug interactions	Comments
Valproate	250–750	500–3,300	Sedation, tremor, paresthesia, headache, lethargy, dizziness, diplopia, confusion, incoordination, ataxia, dysarthria, psychosis, nystagmus, asterixis, "spots before eyes" Other: nausea, hair loss, thrombocytopenia, impaired platelet aggregation, elevated liver transaminases, hepatotoxicity, pancreatitis	Additive CNS depressant effects with other CNS depressants Increased blood level with chlorpromazine Decreased blood level with SSRIs, CBZ, phenytoin, phenobarbital Increased blood level of TCAs, chlorpromazine, CBZ, phenytoin, phenobarbital, primidone, BZDs	Monitor CBC with platelets, LFTs Blood level of approximately 50–150 μg/mL Useful in neuropathic pain

Note. BZDs = benzodiazepines; CBC = complete blood count; CBZ = carbamazepine; CNS = central nervous system; EPS = extrapyramidal side effects; LFTs = liver function tests; MAOIs = monoamine oxidase inhibitors; NMS = neuroleptic malignant syndrome; NSAIDs = nonsteroidal anti-inflammatory drugs; SIADH = syndrome of inappropriate antidiuretic hormone; SSRIs = selective serotonin reuptake inhibitors; TCAs = tricyclic antidepressants.

TABLE 31–4.   Anxiolytics and sedative-hypnotics

Drug	Starting daily dose (mg)	Target daily dose (mg)	Neuropsychiatric side effects	Neuropsychiatric drug interactions	Comments
Benzodiazepines					
Alprazolam	0.25–0.50	0.75–6.00	Drowsiness, incoordination, confusion, dysarthria, fatigue, agitation, dizziness, akathisia, anterograde amnesia (especially alprazolam, lorazepam) Other: sexual dysfunction	Augments respiratory depression with opioids	May develop tolerance to psychotropic and anticonvulsant effects
Lorazepam	0.5–1.0	1.5–12.0		Neurotoxicity and sexual dysfunction with lithium	Do not induce own metabolism
Clonazepam	0.25–0.50	1–5		Additive CNS depressant effects with other CNS depressants	Addictive potential
				Increased blood level with SSRIs, phenytoin	May cause withdrawal syndrome
				Decreased blood level with CBZ	May cause EEG changes
				Decreased blood level of levodopa, phenytoin	May worsen delirium and dementia
					May be useful in treating akathisia
					Clonazepam may accumulate in bloodstream
					May have utility in pain syndromes, movement disorders
Others					
Buspirone	10–15	15–60	Nervousness, headache, confusion, weakness, numbness, drowsiness, tremor, paresthesia, incoordination	EPS with neuroleptics Hypertension with MAOIs Increased ALT with trazodone Increased blood level of BZDs, haloperidol	Has antidepressant effects as adjunct to SSRI but may produce dysphoria at higher doses Slow onset of action Nonaddictive Usually does not impair psychomotor performance
Diphenhydramine	25–50	25–200	Drowsiness, fatigue, dizziness, confusion, anticholinergic effects, incoordination, tremor, nervousness, insomnia, euphoria, paresthesia	Additive CNS depressant effects with other CNS depressants Increased anticholinergic effects with MAOIs, TCAs	Minimal effects on EEG Anticholinergic effects may decrease EPS but may exacerbate delirium May help with insomnia; tolerance may develop Unpredictable anxiolytic properties

TABLE 31–4. Anxiolytics and sedative-hypnotics (continued)

Drug	Starting daily dose (mg)	Target daily dose (mg)	Neuropsychiatric side effects	Neuropsychiatric drug interactions	Comments
Clonidine	0.05–0.20	0.15–0.80	Nervousness, agitation, depression, headache, insomnia, vivid dreams or nightmares, behavior changes, restlessness, anxiety, hallucinations, delirium, sedation, weakness, fatigue	Additive CNS depressant effects with other CNS depressants Impaired blood pressure control with neuroleptics Decreased blood level with TCAs	Useful in opiate withdrawal, Tourette's, and possibly mania, anxiety, akathisia, ADHD, aggression Available in transdermal form

Note. ADHD = attention-deficit/hyperactivity disorder; ALT = alanine aminotransferase; BZDs = benzodiazepines; CNS = central nervous system; EEG = electroencephalogram; EPS = extrapyramidal side effects; MAOIs = monoamine oxidase inhibitors; SSRIs = selective serotonin reuptake inhibitors; TCAs = tricyclic antidepressants.

to the dorsolateral prefrontal cortex, causing executive cognitive dysfunction, also may lead to aggressive behavior by impairing the patient's problem-solving ability, resulting in frustration over his or her inability to rely on previously familiar coping strategies. More subtle dysfunction in this area may be associated with reduction in autonomic activity that could impede the fear conditioning needed to have a "conscience" and inhibit antisocial behavior (Raine et al. 2000). Damage to basotemporal lobe and related areas (amygdala, septum, hippocampus) that project to orbitofrontal cortex also may disrupt behavioral programs and result in disinhibition (Starkstein and Robinson 1997). The beneficial effect of stereotactic amygdalotomy for intractable aggression is instructive in this regard (Lee et al. 1998). More diffuse white matter injury, such as in multiple sclerosis, HIV encephalopathy, and diffuse axonal injury from TBI, also can produce behavioral dyscontrol, possibly by damaging the connections between brain regions within these networks.

Animal and human studies show that norepinephrine enhances aggressive behavior (Brown et al. 1979; Higley et al. 1992), consistent with findings of MAO dysfunction in violent kindreds (Brunner et al. 1993) and aggression in MAO "knockout" mice (Cases et al. 1995). Low serotonin levels in the prefrontal regions have been associated with impulsivity, aggression, and completed suicide (Linnoila and Virkkunen 1992; Owen et al. 1986). Preservation of neurons in substantia nigra pars compacta is associated with aggression in Alzheimer's disease patients (possibly by providing normal dopamine input to degenerated supersensitive target neurons) (Victoroff et al. 1996). Aggression in Alzheimer's disease is also associated with genetic variation in genes for D_1 and D_3 receptors (Sweet et al. 1998). GABA may play an indirect modulatory role; increasing GABA levels in animals has been shown to reduce aggressive behavior, whereas acetylcholine has been reported to increase aggressive behaviors (J.J. Mann 1995). The endogenous opioid system also has been implicated in the development of self-injurious, stereotypic, and deviant social behavior, but treatment studies with opioid antagonists have yielded equivocal results (discussion follows), calling this hypothesis into question. Finally, aggression has been associated with elevated levels of arginine vasopressin in CSF (Coccaro et al. 1998) in personality disorder patients and with elevated levels of testosterone in elderly men with dementia (Orengo et al. 2002).

TREATMENT

As with other behavioral syndromes in neuropsychiatric patients, limited data support treatment choices for behavioral dyscontrol. Treatment often targets the clinical syndromes associated with the maladaptive behavior. Thus, the irritable, depressed patient should first be given an antidepressant; the agitated, paranoid patient should receive a trial of a neuroleptic; and the agitated, angry patient may benefit from an anticonvulsant. However, common side effects of medications used to treat anger and aggression can themselves exacerbate the symptoms (e.g., akathisia from neuroleptics; benzodiazepine-induced disinhibition; overactivation from antidepressants), and anticholinergic agents can aggravate cognitive deficits, lower seizure threshold, and promote delirium, particularly when combined with other delirium-promoting agents.

β-Adrenergic receptor blockers have been studied in a wide range of neuropsychiatric disorders and shown to be efficacious in both open (Alpert et al. 1990; Connor et al. 1997; Greendyke and Kanter 1986; Greendyke et al. 1986; Ratey et al. 1992b) and double-blind, placebo-controlled trials (Allan et al. 1996; Ratey et al. 1992b); however, not all data are consistent (Allan et al. 1996; Silver et al. 1999). β-Blockers are effective in reducing anger and aggression in patients with acute TBI (Fleminger et al. 2003). Other patients with more clear-cut brain damage, as in developmental disability (Connor et al. 1997), may also do better with β-blockers. Response may take up to 8 weeks, and both central and peripheral effects may contribute to therapeutic action (Ruedrich 1996). Pindolol is less likely to cause bradycardia, and nadolol and long-acting propranolol allow once-daily dosing, which may be necessary in the noncompliant or cognitively impaired patient. Secondary depression resulting from β-blockers appears to be a rare occurrence, but these medications are contraindicated in patients with asthma, chronic obstructive pulmonary disease, type 1 diabetes, congestive heart failure, persistent angina, significant peripheral vascular disease, and hyperthyroidism (Yudofsky et al. 1987). Yudofsky et al. (1987) proposed titrating the dose of propranolol as high as 12 mg/kg or up to 800 mg and maintaining maximum tolerable dosages for up to 8 weeks to achieve the desired clinical response, although dosages in the range of 160–320 mg/day have been effective.

Parenteral benzodiazepines are often used to manage both acute aggression and behavioral dyscontrol and can be as effective as neuroleptics (Dorevitch et al. 1999). However, they can also produce disinhibition, which worsens agitation and arousal (Yudofsky et al. 1987). Benzodiazepines with rapid onset of action and relatively short half-lives that can be given intramuscularly or intravenously, such as lorazepam, are most useful in the acute situation. Diazepam and chlordiazepoxide are less reliably and rapidly absorbed intramuscularly (Garza-Trevino et al. 1989). Although longer-acting benzodiazepines, such as clonazepam (Freinhar and Alvarez 1986), can be useful in patients with more chronic agitation and aggression, particularly when symptoms of anxiety coexist, their use in treating or preventing more chronic aggression is not supported (Salzman 1988). Impairment of cognitive function by benzodiazepines could potentially aggravate aggression by increasing confusion.

Buspirone can reduce anxiety-associated agitation and has a benign side-effect profile. It has been reported to be effective in treating aggression in patients with head injury (Gualtieri 1991), developmental disability (Verhoeven and Tuinier 1996), dementia (Colenda 1988; Tiller et al. 1988), and Huntington's disease (Byrne et al. 1994). Although the effect of buspirone on anxiety can reduce agitation, its effect on aggression is probably independent of anxiolysis. The usual dose is between 30 and 60 mg (Verhoeven and Tuinier 1996), but lower doses (5–15 mg) have been useful in some reports (Ratey et al. 1991, 1992a).

Serotonergic antidepressants also have been effective in the treatment of aggression and behavioral dyscontrol. Open trials support efficacy for fluoxetine in depressed (Fava et al. 1991), brain-injured (Sobin et al. 1989), and mentally retarded (Cook et al. 1992; Markowitz 1992) patients; sertraline in mentally retarded (Hellings et al. 1996), Huntington's disease (Ranen et al. 1996), developmentally disabled (J.J. Campbell and Duffy 1995), and intermittent explosive disorder (Feder 1999) patients; paroxetine in mentally retarded patients (although the effect wore off after 1 month) (Davanzo et al. 1998) and in patients with dementia (J.R. Swartz et al. 1997); and citalopram in patients with dementia (Pollock et al. 1997). Standard dose ranges were typically used. Two controlled studies showed effects superior to those of placebo for fluoxetine in patients with personality disorder (Coccaro and Kavoussi 1997) and for fluvoxamine in adult autistic patients (McDougle et al. 1996). Two case reports showed fluoxetine to be effective in treating obsessive-compulsive disorder in HIV-infected persons (McDaniel and Johnson 1995). Trazodone may be effective in reducing aggression secondary to organic mental disorders and dementia (Greenwald et al. 1986; Mashiko et al. 1996; Pinner and Rich 1988; D.M. Simpson and Foster 1986; Zubieta and Alessi 1992). Concomitant use of tryptophan in some of these reports confounds interpretation of efficacy, however.

Although anticonvulsants are particularly effective in treating mood lability, impulsivity, and aggression in patients with known seizure disorders, lack of electroencephalographic abnormalities does not preclude potential benefit from anticonvulsants (Mattes 1990). Carbamazepine has been effective in managing aggression and irritability in a variety of patients with CNS impairment, including dementia, developmental disorders, schizo-

phrenia, seizures, and TBI (Chatham-Showalter 1996; Evans and Gualtieri 1985; Luchins 1984; Mattes 1990; McAllister 1985; Yatham and McHale 1988). However, a placebo-controlled trial in children with conduct disorder showed no benefit (Cueva et al. 1996). Valproate has been found to be effective for aggression in patients with mental retardation (Ruedrich et al. 1999), TBI (Wroblewski et al. 1997), dementia (Haas et al. 1997), and personality disorder (Kavoussi and Coccaro 1998) and may be better tolerated than carbamazepine; however, placebo-controlled data are generally lacking (Lindenmayer and Kotsaftis 2000). Blood levels below 50 µg/mL have been effective in some reports (Mazure et al. 1992) but not others (Sival et al. 2002). A review of 17 reports showed a 77% response rate with normal blood level range (Lindenmayer and Kotsaftis 2000). Phenytoin has been effective for impulsive aggression in inmates (Barratt 1993; Barratt et al. 1991; Stanford et al. 2005). Limited data are available for other anticonvulsants.

Lithium was effective in treating aggressive behavior and affective instability in brain-injured patients (Glenn et al. 1989) and in a double-blind, placebo-controlled trial with 42 adult mentally retarded patients (M. Craft et al. 1987). Open trials in aggressive children with mental retardation and patients chronically hospitalized for severe aggression also support its use (Bellus et al. 1996; M. Campbell et al. 1995). Although higher plasma levels are more likely to result in clinical improvement, the potential for lower serum levels of lithium to cause neurotoxicity in neuropsychiatric patients may limit its use.

Neuroleptics are effective in treating aggression in neuropsychiatric patients (Rao et al. 1985). They should be reserved, however, for patients who have psychotic symptoms or who require rapid behavioral control. Although typical neuroleptics may decrease arousal and agitation in the acute setting, the extrapyramidal and anticholinergic properties of these medications can further increase agitation, particularly when combined with other drugs with anticholinergic properties (Tune et al. 1992). Akathisia can be confused with worsening aggression, thus prompting a detrimental increase in neuroleptic dose. Neuroleptics can also, in some cases, impair executive cognitive functioning (Medalia et al. 1988). In the chronically aggressive psychotic patient, clozapine at doses of 300–500 mg may be the most effective antipsychotic (Cohen and Underwood 1994; Michals et al. 1993). Risperidone is certainly better tolerated, but placebo-controlled evidence is conflicting: two studies (Czobor et al. 2002; De Deyn et al. 1999) showed superior effects to haloperidol in schizophrenia and dementia, whereas another study (Beck et al. 1997) found no difference in a small but select group of forensic schizophrenic subjects. Open studies showed good effects in autistic (Horrigan and Barnhill 1997) and mentally retarded (Cohen et al. 1998) patients. Overall, risperidone, olanzapine, and quetiapine have data to support their use in patients with dementia, although side effects can still limit their use (DeVane and Mintzer 2003; Kindermann et al. 2002; Lawlor 2004; Tariot et al. 2004b); also, the potentially increased mortality of patients with dementia taking atypical antipsychotics raises serious questions about the use of these agents. Various atypical antipsychotics have also shown efficacy in treating aggression in patients with developmental disability, including autism, and mental retardation (Barnard et al. 2002; Buitelaar et al. 2001; Janowsky et al. 2003; Maneeton et al. 2001; McCracken et al. 2002; Posey and McDougle 2000; Zarcone et al. 2001, 2004); again, side effects and potential long-term risks should be considered when deciding whether to use these medications.

Other medications, such as amantadine, a dopamine agonist, and clonidine, an α-adrenergic agonist, have been used to treat aggression. Gualtieri et al. (1989) used amantadine successfully in dosages of 50–400 mg/day in agitated patients recovering from coma. Clonidine at 0.6 mg/day reduced violent outbursts in an autistic adult (Koshes and Rock 1994), but its depressogenic and hypotensive risks may be problematic in the neurological patient. Clearly, more study is needed before use of these agents can be generally recommended.

In summary, truly evidence-based treatment of aggression and behavioral dyscontrol in neuropsychiatric populations is difficult because of the lack of consistent placebo-controlled data. Although clear ethical issues are involved in carrying out placebo-controlled studies in aggressive neuropsychiatric patients, developing concerns over increased risks with currently available pharmacotherapies highlight the importance of generating a database of studies that confirm or refute the efficacy and the safety of various psychopharmacological agents.

COGNITIVE DISTURBANCE

Unlike depression, anxiety, mania, and psychosis, all of which can occur as "primary" disorders independent of gross neurological disease, cognitive disturbance is almost always a result of etiologically identifiable brain dysfunction and has previously served largely to define disorders known as organic brain syndromes. Moreover, cognitive impairment is often associated with other mood and behavioral features (e.g., agitation and depression predict greater cognitive disturbance in Alzheimer's disease and Parkinson's disease, respectively [S.T. Chen et al. 1998; Kuzis et al. 1997]), as well as with functional status and

survival time (e.g., in HIV illness [Wilkie et al. 1998]). However, difficulties with concentration, memory, and more complicated executive cognitive functions occur not just as primary components of neurological disease and CNS dysfunction but also as epiphenomena in the course of major mood disturbance (i.e., pseudodementia) and as a core feature of schizophrenia (Lancon et al. 2000) and chronic bipolar disorder (Ferrier and Thompson 2002), as a measurable but more subtle aspect of PTSD and obsessive-compulsive disorder, and secondary to many medications used to treat neurological and other medical illnesses. Most important, even minor improvements in cognition can produce substantial health care cost savings (Ernst and Hay 1997). Although the increasing sophistication of modern neuropsychological testing has allowed extensive batteries to dissect cognitive dysfunction into multiple, partially overlapping components, thereby serving to better define the deficits of individual patients, these multiple components have, for the most part, not yet been related to distinct neuropathological or neurochemical processes, nor have they been used in aggregate to evaluate the effects of novel treatments that seek to retard or arrest cognitive dysfunction in the dementias or promote and enhance cognitive function in healthy subjects.

COMMON ETIOLOGIES

The list of neuropsychiatric conditions characterized by cognitive disturbance includes virtually every neuropsychiatric disorder; the most important causes include the primary dementias (Alzheimer's and vascular), later-occurring dementias associated with subcortical degenerative diseases (Parkinson's disease and Huntington's disease), TBI, stroke, chronic alcoholism (Korsakoff's syndrome), a host of rarer degenerative dementias, and CNS infectious disease, the most commonly seen now being HIV infection with its late-occurring subcortical dementia. The neuropathological processes associated with these conditions are thought to be irreversible, although there is hope that speed of neurodegeneration can be retarded. For example, AZT has been shown to have an effect in slowing cognitive deterioration in HIV-dementia patients (Portegies et al. 1989), and cholinergic medications are thought to act similarly in patients with Alzheimer's dementia. The advent of an NMDA antagonist (memantine) in the treatment of dementia (Molinuevo et al. 2005) suggests that other avenues for neuroprotection may be possible.

Other etiologies of cognitive impairment might be thought of as potentially reversible processes depending on whether their severity and duration are sufficient to produce more permanent neurological damage. These include CNS inflammatory disease (e.g., lupus); exposure to heavy metals, organophosphates, and organic solvents; endocrinopathies; and other toxic or infectious processes. Additional CNS inflammatory processes may contribute to the cognitive impairment seen in both HIV infection (Glass et al. 1993; Tyor et al. 1992) and Alzheimer's dementia (Aisen and Davis 1994) and provide another target for treatment intervention. Finally, the list of medications able to impair cognitive functions is widespread and includes commonly used neurological medications (anticonvulsants, barbiturates, steroids, β-blockers), cardiac medications (digoxin, procainamide, calcium channel blockers), chemotherapeutic agents (especially biological response modifiers such as interleukin-2), and H_2 blockers.

ANATOMY AND NEUROCHEMISTRY

The range of disorders associated with cognitive impairment produces neuropathological deficits covering the entire spectrum of cortical and subcortical areas. Thus, it is difficult to implicate damage to one structure or set of structures. The important role of the hippocampus and adjacent inferior temporal neocortical and limbic areas in mediating memory is well known (Squire and Zola-Morgan 1991), and these areas are commonly affected in Alzheimer's dementia, dementias of other etiology, and TBI. The frontal lobe and related striatal circuits play a key role in organizational and retrieval strategies as well as working memory (Petrides et al. 1993; B.E. Swartz et al. 1996). These areas are obviously affected in Huntington's disease, Parkinson's disease, and HIV-related and Korsakoff's dementia and have been implicated in the executive dysfunction of multiple sclerosis (Foong et al. 1999) and the cognitive impairment of neurosyphilis (Russouw et al. 1997). However, imaging studies clearly show that abnormal activation patterns in patients with memory disturbance extend far beyond morphological deficits detected by computed tomography or MRI scanning (Heiss et al. 1992). For example, subcortical stroke produces cortical hypometabolism that correlates with degree of cognitive impairment (Kwan et al. 1999).

Many biochemical processes influence memory and cognition, among them acetylcholine, the monoamine neurotransmitters, intracellular signaling enzymes, cyclic nucleotides and other second and third messengers, and hormones such as vasopressin and oxytocin. Alzheimer's disease patients have loss of cerebral choline acetyltransferase—the biosynthetic enzyme for acetylcholine that correlates with decreasing cognitive function (Baskin et al. 1999)—once the disease has progressed beyond the early phases. In contrast, changes in the locus coeruleus of these patients (D.M. Mann et al. 1984) and decreases in serotonin (Zubenko et al. 1990) seem more related to depression

than to dementia severity. However, in stroke patients, cognitive function was positively correlated with right frontal cortical serotonin receptor binding in one PET scan study (Morris et al. 1993), suggesting differing neurochemical substrates for cognitive impairments of different etiology. Korsakoff's disease patients have lowered levels of CSF 3-methoxy-4-hydroxyphenylglycol (MHPG), homovanillic acid (HVA), and, in some patients, 5-hydroxyindoleacetic acid (5-HIAA) (Halliday et al. 1993), along with a small change in cholinergic neurons (McEntee and Mair 1990). Alzheimer's disease patients have increased levels of plasma MHPG that directly correlate with increasing cognitive impairment (Lawlor et al. 1995). In Parkinson's disease patients, a loss of cortical cholinergic markers also occurs (Perry et al. 1991), and Parkinson's disease patients with dementia, compared with those without dementia, have a greater loss of midbrain dopaminergic neurons (Rinne et al. 1989a, 1989b). Disturbances of calcium homeostasis are thought to play some role in Alzheimer's and vascular (Fischhof 1993) as well as HIV (Lipton 1991) dementias. High levels of corticosteroids are thought to be capable of damaging hippocampal neurons and may contribute to the cognitive impairment in both Korsakoff's (Emsley et al. 1994) and Alzheimer's (Sunderland et al. 1989) dementias. Glutamate and NMDA receptors and subsequent calcium-dependent biochemical processes may play a key role in linking physiology to structural change (both the cellular damage that results from ischemic injury and TBI and the laying down of longer-term memory traces via long-term potentiation). Neuropeptide systems are also differentially affected by neurodegeneration, with decreases in corticotropin-releasing hormone, β-endorphin, and somatostatin being prominent in Alzheimer's and vascular dementias (Heilig et al. 1995), and corticotropin-releasing hormone decreases occurring in the earliest stage of Alzheimer's dementia when cholinergic markers are still preserved (Davis et al. 1999). Finally, genotyping may inform clinical practice in the future. The apolipoprotein E4 allele has been associated with greater cognitive impairment in Alzheimer's disease patients (Rasmusson et al. 1996) and with greater sensitivity to drug-induced cognitive impairment in elderly patients (Pomara et al. 1998, 2005), and the number of trinucleotide repeats in Huntington's disease is related to cognitive decline in early stages of the disease (Jason et al. 1997).

TREATMENT

Most treatment studies continue to focus on Alzheimer's dementia, the most prevalent cause of cognitive impairment in the U.S. population. During the past 5 years, a growing number of studies have documented the palliative efficacy of reversible cholinesterase inhibitors in these patients. Available FDA-approved medications include donepezil, rivastigmine, and galantamine, and all have better tolerability than and an absence of liver transaminase toxicity seen with tacrine hydrochloride (Greenberg et al. 2000; S.L. Rogers et al. 1998, 2000). The available cholinesterase inhibitors typically have shown similar efficacy and tolerability (Farlow et al. 2000; McKeith et al. 2000; Rosler et al. 1999; Wilcock 2000; Wilkinson and Murray 2001). Depending on the specific study and medication examined, 25%–50% of drug-treated subjects had a four-point change in Alzheimer's Disease Assessment Scale cognition scores (ADAS-cog), an amount comparable to about 6 months' deterioration in untreated patients (Cummings 2004). The effect may delay the need for nursing home placement (Knopman et al. 1996), although it does not appear to halt the long-term trajectory of the illness. Evidence also suggests beneficial psychotropic effects in patients with problematic depression, psychosis, agitation, and disinhibition, although other patients without obvious behavior problems may experience behavioral worsening (Mega et al. 1999). It also may have efficacy in vascular dementia (Erkinjuntti et al. 2002; Mendez et al. 1999; Wilkinson et al. 2003) and for psychotropic-induced memory loss in patients without dementia (Jacobsen and Comas-Diaz 1999). The long-term benefits of treatment have been questioned because a prospective 3-year cost-effectiveness study from the United Kingdom found cognitive improvement but no advantages in delays in institutionalization, progression of disability, costs of care, or caregiver psychopathology (Courtney et al. 2004).

The NMDA receptor antagonist memantine reduces glutamatergic CNS toxicity and has been approved for use in treatment of moderate to severe Alzheimer's disease. Compared with placebo control subjects, patients taking memantine had improved activities of daily living scores as well as global improvement as measured with the Clinician's Interview-Based Impression of Change Plus Caregiver Input (Reisberg et al. 2003). The improvement was modest and of the magnitude seen in cholinesterase inhibitor trials. When memantine was added to donepezil, limited data suggest significantly better outcomes in activities of daily living function and Clinician's Interview-Based Impression of Change Plus Caregiver Input scores compared with the group receiving donepezil and placebo (Tariot et al. 2004a). In the absence of a memantine plus placebo group, it is unclear if the benefit is truly additive or if switching patients from donepezil to memantine at the point of moderate severity would have resulted in the same degree of disease slowing.

Although use of muscarinic agonists has not been practical because of requirements for either frequent in-

travenous (arecoline) or intracerebroventricular (bethanechol) administration and because of high rates of nausea and other side effects, studies have documented the efficacy of arecoline (Raffaele et al. 1991) and bethanechol (Penn et al. 1988), suggesting that newer muscarinic agonists, now under development, may prove to be more practically effective (Fisher et al. 2003). Nicotine agonists also may prove useful in both Alzheimer's and Parkinson's (Newhouse et al. 1997) dementias. Although galantamine has nicotinic effects in addition to its cholinesterase inhibition (Maelicke et al. 2001), no advantage over other marketed inhibitors has been identified.

Selegiline, an MAO-B inhibitor commonly used in Parkinson's disease, was initially shown at an open daily dose of 20 mg to improve cognitive performance of 14 Alzheimer's dementia patients (Schneider et al. 1991). Subsequently, double-blind studies of selegiline at low 10-mg doses likely to act principally by increasing CNS dopamine showed superiority to placebo (Finali et al. 1991), to phosphatidylserine (Monteverde et al. 1990), and to oxiracetam (Falsaperla et al. 1990) on a variety of cognitive tests. However, as summarized in a negative crossover study (Tariot et al. 1998b), positive effects of this drug on agitation and depression in some patients make it difficult to separate mood-state dependent effects on cognition from a primary cognitive effect. One other study showed no effect (Freedman et al. 1998), and still another showed a modest effect on delaying functional impairment (Sano et al. 1997). Because the former study was one of the few longer-term evaluations, the utility of the agent requires further study.

Several naturalistic case–control studies have shown that anti-inflammatory drugs may help Alzheimer's dementia patients. In one study, patients taking daily NSAIDs or aspirin had shorter duration of illness and better cognitive performance (Rich et al. 1995). In another study, the onset of Alzheimer's dementia in monozygotic twin pairs was inversely proportional to prior use of steroids or corticotropin (Breitner et al. 1994). Finally, a third naturalistic study (Prince et al. 1998) showed that NSAID use was associated with less cognitive decline, particularly in younger subjects. One placebo-controlled study of 44 patients actually supported an effect for indomethacin (J. Rogers et al. 1993), and NSAIDs are associated with histopathological evidence of slowed progression of Alzheimer's dementia (Alafuzoff et al. 2000). However, another study failed to show an effect for diclofenac/misoprostol (Scharf et al. 1999), and a study of prednisone also had negative findings (Aisen et al. 2000), although the dose was quite low, and adverse effects on hippocampal cells could have counteracted anti-inflammatory effects. Although no reports have examined effects of therapy aimed at the cytokine-related inflammatory pathways in HIV disease patients, this strategy also holds some promise.

Before the approval of the acetylcholinesterase inhibitors and memantine, the only approved cognitive drugs were ergoloid mesylates (Hydergine). Their cognitive benefits have always been said to be modest at best and hard to distinguish from nonspecific activating properties. A review (Schneider and Olin 1994) confirmed this, showing effect sizes of 0.56 for clinical ratings but only 0.27 for neuropsychological measures. Furthermore, patients with vascular dementia did better than Alzheimer's dementia patients. A previous study in 80 Alzheimer's dementia patients that failed to show an effect (Thompson et al. 1990) may have been compromised by its 3 mg/day dosage because there is a strong dose-response relation with this drug, and some investigators believe that higher doses (e.g., 8 mg) might be better (Schneider and Olin 1994). One study showed increases in glucose metabolism on PET scan in both cortical and basal ganglia areas with the drug (Nagasawa et al. 1990).

Two studies support very modest effects of antioxidants. Le Bars et al. (1997) showed that Ginkgo biloba was superior to placebo by 1.4 ADAS-cog points in a mixed Alzheimer's and vascular dementia group. These results are inferior to those seen with tacrine or donepezil, and the predominance of mild cases makes the generalizability of results unclear. A meta-analysis of studies with this agent (Oken et al. 1998) showed that few reports were well designed with clearly described patient groups, although these few also showed similar modest effects. An increase in bleeding risk, especially for patients taking anticoagulants, warrants caution, however. A second study (Sano et al. 1997) showed that 2,000 IU of α-tocopherol slowed functional decline in Alzheimer's disease patients, with a delay of about a half-year over a 2-year period. However, no cognitive improvements were noted, despite these functional benefits.

Initial studies showing that fewer Alzheimer's and vascular dementia patients take replacement estrogen than do matched control subjects (Mortel and Meyer 1995) and that those who do have better cognitive function than those who do not (Henderson et al. 1994) have been replicated in several other uncontrolled naturalistic designs showing that estrogen use is associated with reduced incidence of Alzheimer's disease (Slooter et al. 1999). These associations were convergent with preclinical studies showing genomic and receptor-mediated effects of estrogen on learning, memory, and neuronal growth and connections (Shaywitz and Shaywitz 2000). Unfortunately, well-designed treatment studies (Henderson et al. 2000; Mulnard et al. 2000) failed to show a beneficial effect of estrogen supplements for mildly to moderately impaired elderly women with Alzheimer's disease, although beneficial effects in postmenopausal women without dementia (Kampen and Sherwin 1994) suggest that preventive effects might be possible.

Based on the possibility that calcium blockade will slow mechanisms of neuronal death that depend on increased free intracellular calcium in Alzheimer's disease, studies of 90 mg/day of nimodipine in these patients have shown some promise. Ban et al. (1990) showed 12 weeks of nimodipine to be more effective than placebo on the Mini-Mental State Examination and the Wechsler Memory Scale; improvement continued between 60 and 90 days. Tollefson (1990) showed that the same dose improved recall on the Buschke test, although 180 mg proved worse than placebo. However, one naturalistic study showed that elderly patients taking calcium channel blockers are more likely to develop dementia (Maxwell et al. 1999). Unique calcium channel effects of nimodipine could explain some of these differences.

A variety of other agents have been either tested briefly or reported on. Stimulants (methylphenidate or dextroamphetamine) have been found in one open trial (Angrist et al. 1992) to improve scores on several neuropsychological tests in HIV disease patients and have been found in a placebo-controlled crossover trial to improve cognition in cognitively impaired HIV disease patients (van Dyck et al. 1997). Methylphenidate and dextroamphetamine can be useful in patients with distractibility, impaired attention, impulsivity, and irritability (Mooney and Haas 1993), symptoms also seen in attention-deficit/hyperactivity disorder. These stimulants are generally well tolerated in the neurological patient (Kaufmann et al. 1984), do not appear to lower the seizure threshold at therapeutic doses (Wroblewski et al. 1992), and may even enhance cortical recovery (Feeney et al. 1982). However, they should be used with caution because of their potential to aggravate irritability and delusional thought content. Opiate antagonists helped improve TBI-associated memory impairment in one case series (Tennant and Wild 1987). The serotonergic antidepressant fluvoxamine has improved memory impairment in Korsakoff's dementia in two studies (Martin et al. 1989, 1995). Clonidine variably improved memory in Korsakoff's dementia, and this was correlated with increased cingulate gyrus and thalamic blood flow (Moffoot et al. 1994). Both clonidine and another α_2 agonist, guanfacine, improve various aspects of cognition in healthy humans (Jakala et al. 1999a, 1999b, 1999c).

Phosphatidylserine, a lipid membrane processor, improved several cognitive measures in Alzheimer's dementia patients (Crook et al. 1992). Citicoline, a metabolic intermediate that enhances the formation of neural

TABLE 31–5.   Cognitive agents

Drug	Starting daily dose (mg)	Target daily dose (mg)	Neuropsychiatric side effects	Neuropsychiatric drug interactions	Comments
Acetylcholinesterase inhibitors					
Donepezil	5	10	Headache, fatigue, dizziness, insomnia	Effects antagonized by anticholinergic drugs	Donepezil has once-daily dosing
Rivastigmine	3	12			Rivastigmine and galantamine have twice-daily dosing; once-daily formulation for galantamine also available
Galantamine	8	24	Other: nausea, diarrhea, weight loss, muscle cramps, joint pain		
NMDA antagonist					
Memantine	5	20	Fatigue, headache, dizziness, psychosis, confusion. Other: nausea, diarrhea, pain, increased blood pressure	Carbonic anhydrase inhibitors (such as acetazolamide) may increase blood levels. Possible interactions with other NMDA antagonists (such as amantadine) are unknown	Twice-daily dosing

Note.   NMDA = *N*-methyl-D-aspartate.

membranes and promotes acetylcholine biosynthesis, improved verbal memory in older individuals with "inefficient" memories who did not have dementia (Spiers et al. 1996). Milacemide, a prodrug for glycine (Dysken et al. 1992), did not work in Alzheimer's dementia patients despite the plausibility of NMDA-glutamate theories of cognition (Ingram et al. 1994) and increased word retrieval in young and old subjects without dementia taking it (Schwartz et al. 1991). However, cycloserine improved cognition relative to placebo in 17 Alzheimer's disease patients, suggesting that NMDA strategies need to be pursued further (G.E. Tsai et al. 1999). Finally, preliminary studies show a beneficial effect for both insulin and somatostatin acutely administered to Alzheimer's disease patients (S. Craft et al. 1999), whereas peptide T may be associated with improved performance in more cognitively impaired HIV disease patients with relatively preserved immunological status (Heseltine et al. 1998).

In conclusion, only a few approved treatments for cognitive impairment, principally in Alzheimer's dementia, are available. Donepezil, rivastigmine, and galantamine are generally well tolerated, with modest efficacy at slowing cognitive decline. Memantine may have benefit in patients with moderate to severe dementia and as a combination therapy. It is actively being studied as a potential neuroprotective agent. Other agents have been investigated, but data are too limited to provide strong recommendations. Table 31–5 lists characteristic cognitive agents recommended in this section, dose ranges, side effects, and relevant drug interactions.

Highlights for the Clinician

Overall approach

+ Establish rapport early.

+ Be aware of patient and family discomfort with discussing psychiatric issues.

+ Be aware of the multiple etiological possibilities.

+ Consider presenting the diagnosis in terms of symptom clusters rather than formal DSM-IV-TR diagnoses.

Highlights for the Clinician *(continued)*

✦ Obtain all collateral information possible.

✦ Limit polypharmacy.

✦ Aim for adequate doses and duration of medication trials.

Depression and similar states

✦ These are the most common syndromes associated with neurological disease.

✦ SSRIs are generally considered to be the first-line treatment choice given apparent efficacy and reasonable tolerability.

✦ TCAs can be efficacious but may be difficult for patients to tolerate.

✦ Atypical antidepressants (bupropion, mirtazapine) also may be efficacious.

✦ ECT is effective for patients with treatment-resistant depression.

✦ Other brain stimulation techniques (TMS, VNS, DBS) may be useful, but data are sparse.

Psychosis

✦ Typical antipsychotic medications are efficacious but can have significant adverse effects in neurological patients.

✦ Atypical antipsychotics should be considered the first-line treatment choice.

✦ Clozapine has the strongest database but is generally considered second- or third-line because of side effects.

Anxiety, mania, and agitated states

✦ Anxiety and agitation are common in neurological patients; mania is much less common.

✦ Etiology is often comorbid conditions (e.g., urinary tract infection) or medications.

✦ First-line treatment choice depends on symptom presentation and etiology:

• For agitated or manic patients, consider anticonvulsants and/or atypical antipsychotics.

• For anxious patients, consider SSRIs.

✦ Benzodiazepines can be effective but can have significant adverse effects in neurological patients.

✦ Atypical antipsychotics have been associated with increased mortality in agitated patients with dementia.

Aggression, impulsivity, and behavioral dyscontrol

✦ These states are common in neurological patients and should be carefully distinguished from anxiety, agitation, or mania.

✦ First-line treatment choice will depend heavily on associated neurological illness, comorbidities, and acuity.

✦ For acute agitation, parenteral atypical antipsychotics are a first-line choice; parenteral benzodiazepines can be used with caution.

✦ For prolonged states, consider SSRIs, anticonvulsants, and possibly atypical antipsychotics.

Cognitive disturbance

✦ Acetylcholinesterase inhibitors are first-line agents for most patients with dementia.

✦ Memantine may be effective alone or in combination with acetylcholinesterase inhibitors, especially in patients with moderate to severe dementia.

Note. DBS = deep brain stimulation; ECT = electroconvulsive therapy; SSRIs = selective serotonin reuptake inhibitors; TCAs = tricyclic antidepressants; TMS = transcranial magnetic stimulation; VNS = vagus nerve stimulation.

RECOMMENDED READINGS

Charney D, Nestler E (eds): Neurobiology of Mental Illness, 2nd Edition. New York, Oxford University Press, 2005

Davis KL, Charney D, Coyle JT, et al (eds): Neuropsychopharmacology: The Fifth Generation of Progress. American College of Neuropsychopharmacology. Philadelphia, PA, Lippincott Williams & Wilkins, 2002

Nestler EJ, Hyman SE, Malenka RC (eds): Molecular Basis of Neuropharmacology: A Foundation for Clinical Neuroscience. New York, McGraw-Hill, 2001

REFERENCES

Aarsland D, Larsen JP, Cummins JL, et al: Prevalence and clinical correlates of psychotic symptoms in Parkinson disease: a community-based study. Arch Neurol 56:595–601, 1999

Aisen PS, Davis KL: Inflammatory mechanisms in Alzheimer's disease: implications for therapy. Am J Psychiatry 151:1105–1113, 1994

Aisen PS, Davis KL, Berg JD, et al: A randomized controlled trial of prednisone in Alzheimer's disease. Alzheimer's Disease Cooperative Study. Neurology 54:588–593, 2000

Alafuzoff I, Overmyer M, Helisalmi S, et al: Lower counts of astroglia and activated microglia in patients with Alzheimer's disease with regular use of non-steroidal anti-inflammatory drugs. J Alzheimers Dis 2:37–46, 2000

Alexopoulos GS: Frontostriatal and limbic dysfunction in late-life depression. Am J Geriatr Psychiatry 10:687–695, 2002

Alexopoulos GS, Meyers BS, Young RC, et al: "Vascular depression" hypothesis. Arch Gen Psychiatry 54:915–922, 1997

Alexopoulos GS, Streim J, Carpenter D, et al: Using antipsychotic agents in older patients. J Clin Psychiatry 65 (suppl 2):5–99, 2004

Allan ER, Alpert M, Sison CE, et al: Adjunctive nadolol in the treatment of acutely aggressive schizophrenic patients. J Clin Psychiatry 57:455–459, 1996

Allen RL, Walker Z, D'Ath PJ, et al: Risperidone for psychotic and behavioural symptoms in Lewy body dementia. Lancet 346:185, 1995

Alpert M, Allan ER, Citrome L, et al: A double-blind, placebo-controlled study of adjunctive nadolol in the management of violent psychiatric patients. Psychopharmacol Bull 26:367–371, 1990

Altshuler L, Rausch R, Delrahim S, et al: Temporal lobe epilepsy, temporal lobectomy, and major depression. J Neuropsychiatry Clin Neurosci 11:436–443, 1999

Aman MG, Singh NN, Stewart AW, et al: The Aberrant Behavior Checklist: a behavior rating scale for the assessment of treatment effects. Am J Ment Defic 89:485–491, 1985

American Psychiatric Association: Diagnostic and Statistical Manual of Mental Disorders, 4th Edition, Text Revision. Washington, DC, American Psychiatric Association, 2000

Andersen G, Vestergaard K, Lauritzen L: Effective treatment of poststroke depression with the selective serotonin reuptake inhibitor citalopram. Stroke 25:1099–1104, 1994

Andersen J, Aabro E, Gulmann N, et al: Anti-depressive treatment in Parkinson's disease: a controlled trial of the effect of nortriptyline in patients with Parkinson's disease treated with L-dopa. Acta Neurol Scand 62:210–219, 1980

Angrist B, d'Hollosy M, Sanfilipo M, et al: Central nervous system stimulants as symptomatic treatments for AIDS-related neuropsychiatric impairment. J Clin Psychopharmacol 12:268–272, 1992

Auchus AP, Bissey-Black C: Pilot study of haloperidol, fluoxetine, and placebo for agitation in Alzheimer's disease. J Neuropsychiatry Clin Neurosci 9:591–593, 1997

Azouvi P, Jokic C, Attal N, et al: Carbamazepine in agitation and aggressive behaviour following severe closed-head injury: results of an open trial. Brain Inj 13:797–804, 1999

Ban TA, Morey L, Aguglia E, et al: Nimodipine in the treatment of old age dementias. Prog Neuropsychopharmacol Biol Psychiatry 14:525–551, 1990

Barczak P, Edmunds E, Betts T: Hypomania following complex partial seizures: a report of three cases. Br J Psychiatry 152:137–139, 1988

Barnard L, Young AH, Pearson J, et al: A systematic review of the use of atypical antipsychotics in autism. J Psychopharmacol 16:93–101, 2002

Barratt ES: The use of anticonvulsants in aggression and violence. Psychopharmacol Bull 29:75–81, 1993

Barratt ES, Kent TA, Bryant SG, et al: A controlled trial of phenytoin in impulsive aggression. J Clin Psychopharmacol 11:388–389, 1991

Baskin DS, Browning JL, Pirozzolo FJ, et al: Brain choline acetyltransferase and mental function in Alzheimer disease. Arch Neurol 56:1121–1123, 1999

Baxter LR Jr, Phelps ME, Mazziotta JC, et al: Local cerebral glucose metabolic rates in obsessive-compulsive disorder: a comparison with rates in unipolar depression and in normal controls. Arch Gen Psychiatry 44:211–218, 1987

Beck NC, Greenfield SR, Gotham H, et al: Risperidone in the management of violent, treatment-resistant schizophrenics hospitalized in a maximum security forensic facility. J Am Acad Psychiatry Law 25:461–468, 1997

Bejjani BP, Damier P, Arnulf I, et al: Transient acute depression induced by high-frequency deep-brain stimulation. N Engl J Med 340:1476–1480, 1999

Bellus SB, Stewart D, Vergo JG, et al: The use of lithium in the treatment of aggressive behaviours with two brain-injured individuals in a state psychiatric hospital. Brain Inj 10:849–860, 1996

Benedetti F, Campori E, Colombo C, et al: Fluvoxamine treatment of major depression associated with multiple sclerosis. J Neuropsychiatry Clin Neurosci 16:364–366, 2004

Benes FM: Evidence for altered trisynaptic circuitry in schizophrenic hippocampus. Biol Psychiatry 46:589–599, 1999

Berney A, Vingerhoets F, Perrin A, et al: Effect on mood of subthalamic DBS for Parkinson's disease: a consecutive series of 24 patients. Neurology 59:1427–1429, 2002

Berthier ML, Kulisevsky J, Gironell A, et al: Poststroke bipolar affective disorder: clinical subtypes, concurrent movement disorders, and anatomical correlates. J Neuropsychiatry Clin Neurosci 8:160–167, 1996

Bertolino A, Knable MB, Saunders RC, et al: The relationship between dorsolateral prefrontal N-acetylaspartate measures and striatal dopamine activity in schizophrenia. Biol Psychiatry 45:660–667, 1999

Beyer JL, Kuchibhatla M, Payne M, et al: Caudate volume measurement in older adults with bipolar disorder. Int J Geriatr Psychiatry 19:109–114, 2004

Bierer LM, Knott PJ, Schmeidler JM, et al: Post-mortem examination of dopaminergic parameters in Alzheimer's disease: relationship to noncognitive symptoms. Psychiatry Res 49:211–217, 1993

Bonelli RM, Wenning GK, Kapfhammer HP: Huntington's disease: present treatments and future therapeutic modalities. Int Clin Psychopharmacol 19:51–62, 2004

Bowden CL, Calabrese JR, Sachs G, et al: A placebo-controlled 18-month trial of lamotrigine and lithium maintenance treatment in recently manic or hypomanic patients with bipolar I disorder. Arch Gen Psychiatry 60:392–400, 2003

Bozikas V, Bascialla F, Yulis P, et al: Gabapentin for behavioral dyscontrol with mental retardation. Am J Psychiatry 158:965–966, 2001

Braun AR, Randolph C, Stoetter B, et al: The functional neuroanatomy of Tourette's syndrome: an FDG-PET Study, II: relationships between regional cerebral metabolism and associated behavioral and cognitive features of the illness. Neuropsychopharmacology 13:151–168, 1995

Bredkjaer SR, Mortensen PB, Parnas J: Epilepsy and non-organic non-affective psychosis: national epidemiologic study. Br J Psychiatry 172:235–238, 1998

Breier A, Sutton VK, Feldman PD, et al: Olanzapine in the treatment of dopamimetic-induced psychosis in patients with Parkinson's disease. Biol Psychiatry 52:438–445, 2002

Breitbart W, Marotta R, Platt MM, et al: A double-blind trial of haloperidol, chlorpromazine, and lorazepam in the treatment of delirium in hospitalized AIDS patients. Am J Psychiatry 153:231–237, 1996

Breitner JC, Gau BA, Welsh KA, et al: Inverse association of anti-inflammatory treatments and Alzheimer's disease: initial results of a co-twin control study. Neurology 44:227–232, 1994

Bridges-Parlet S, Knopman D, Steffes S: Withdrawal of neuroleptic medications from institutionalized dementia patients: results of a double-blind, baseline-treatment-controlled pilot study. J Geriatr Psychiatry Neurol 10:119–126, 1997

Brodaty H, Ames D, Snowdon J, et al: A randomized placebo-controlled trial of risperidone for the treatment of aggression, agitation, and psychosis of dementia. J Clin Psychiatry 64:134–143, 2003

Bromfield EB, Altshuler L, Leiderman DB, et al: Cerebral metabolism and depression in patients with complex partial seizures. Arch Neurol 49:617–623, 1992

Brown GL, Goodwin FK, Ballenger JC, et al: Aggression in humans correlates with cerebrospinal fluid amine metabolites. Psychiatry Res 1:131–139, 1979

Brunner HG, Nelen M, Breakefield XO, et al: Abnormal behavior associated with a point mutation in the structural gene for monoamine oxidase A. Science 262:578–580, 1993

Bryant RA, Marosszeky JE, Crooks J, et al: Posttraumatic stress disorder after severe traumatic brain injury. Am J Psychiatry 157:629–631, 2000

Buitelaar JK, van der Gaag RJ, van der Hoeven J: Buspirone in the management of anxiety and irritability in children with pervasive developmental disorders: results of an open-label study. J Clin Psychiatry 59:56–59, 1998

Buitelaar JK, van der Gaag RJ, Cohen-Kettenis P, et al: A randomized controlled trial of risperidone in the treatment of aggression in hospitalized adolescents with subaverage cognitive abilities. J Clin Psychiatry 62:239–248, 2001

Burke WJ, Pfeiffer RF, McComb RD: Neuroleptic sensitivity to clozapine in dementia with Lewy bodies. J Neuropsychiatry Clin Neurosci 10:227–229, 1998

Burns A, Russell E, Stratton-Powell H, et al: Sertraline in stroke-associated lability of mood. Int J Geriatr Psychiatry 14:681–685, 1999

Burt T, Lisanby SH, Sackeim HA: Neuropsychiatric applications of transcranial magnetic stimulation: a meta-analysis. Int J Neuropsychopharmacol 5:73–103, 2002

Byrne A, Martin W, Hnatko G: Beneficial effects of buspirone therapy in Huntington's disease (letter). Am J Psychiatry 151:1097, 1994

Calabrese JR, Bowden CL, Sachs GS, et al: A double-blind placebo-controlled study of lamotrigine monotherapy in outpatients with bipolar I depression. Lamictal 602 Study Group. J Clin Psychiatry 60:79–88, 1999

Caley CF, Friedman JH: Does fluoxetine exacerbate Parkinson's disease? J Clin Psychiatry 53:278–282, 1992

Caligiuri MP, Peavy G: An instrumental study of the relationship between extrapyramidal signs and psychosis in Alzheimer's disease. J Neuropsychiatry Clin Neurosci 12:34–39, 2000

Campbell JJ 3rd, Duffy JD: Sertraline treatment of aggression in a developmentally disabled patient (letter). J Clin Psychiatry 56:123–124, 1995

Campbell M, Kafantaris V, Cueva JE: An update on the use of lithium carbonate in aggressive children and adolescents with conduct disorder. Psychopharmacol Bull 31:93–102, 1995

Cantello R, Aguggia M, Gilli M, et al: Major depression in Parkinson's disease and the mood response to intravenous methylphenidate: possible role of the "hedonic" dopamine synapse. J Neurol Neurosurg Psychiatry 52:724–731, 1989

Cantillon M, Brunswick R, Molina D, et al: A double-blind trial for agitation in a nursing home population with Alzheimer's disease. Am J Geriatr Psychiatry 4:263–267, 1996

Cases O, Seif I, Grimsby J, et al: Aggressive behavior and altered amounts of brain serotonin and norepinephrine in mice lacking MAOA. Science 268:1763–1766, 1995

Castellon SA, Hinkin CH, Wood S, et al: Apathy, depression, and cognitive performance in HIV-1 infection. J Neuropsychiatry Clin Neurosci 10:320–329, 1998

Castillo CS, Starkstein SE, Fedoroff JP, et al: Generalized anxiety disorder after stroke. J Nerv Ment Dis 181:100–106, 1993

Chacko RC, Hurley RA, Jankovic J: Clozapine use in diffuse Lewy body disease. J Neuropsychiatry Clin Neurosci 5:206–208, 1993

Chakrabarti S, Aga VM, Singh R: Postictal mania following primary generalized seizures. Neurol India 47:332–333, 1999

Chatham-Showalter PE: Carbamazepine for combativeness in acute traumatic brain injury. J Neuropsychiatry Clin Neurosci 8:96–99, 1996

Chatterjee A, Fahn S: Methylphenidate treats apathy in Parkinson's disease. J Neuropsychiatry Clin Neurosci 14:461–462, 2002

Chen CP, Alder JT, Bowen DM, et al: Presynaptic serotonergic markers in community-acquired cases of Alzheimer's disease: correlations with depression and neuroleptic medication. J Neurochem 66:1592–1598, 1996

Chen ST, Sultzer DL, Hinkin CH, et al: Executive dysfunction in Alzheimer's disease: association with neuropsychiatric symptoms and functional impairment. J Neuropsychiatry Clin Neurosci 10:426–432, 1998

Childers MK, Holland D: Psychomotor agitation following gabapentin use in brain injury. Brain Inj 11:537–540, 1997

Cleghorn JM, Garnett ES, Nahmias C, et al: Regional brain metabolism during auditory hallucinations in chronic schizophrenia. Br J Psychiatry 157:562–570, 1990

Cleghorn JM, Franco S, Szechtman B, et al: Toward a brain map of auditory hallucinations. Am J Psychiatry 149:1062–1069, 1992

Coccaro EF, Kavoussi RJ: Fluoxetine and impulsive aggressive behavior in personality-disordered subjects. Arch Gen Psychiatry 54:1081–1088, 1997

Coccaro EF, Kramer E, Zemishlany Z, et al: Pharmacologic treatment of noncognitive behavioral disturbances in elderly demented patients. Am J Psychiatry 147:1640–1645, 1990

Coccaro EF, Kavoussi RJ, Hauger RL, et al: Cerebrospinal fluid vasopressin levels: correlates with aggression and serotonin function in personality-disordered subjects. Arch Gen Psychiatry 55:708–714, 1998

Cohen SA, Underwood MT: The use of clozapine in a mentally retarded and aggressive population. J Clin Psychiatry 55:440–444, 1994

Cohen SA, Ihrig K, Lott RS, et al: Risperidone for aggression and self-injurious behavior in adults with mental retardation. J Autism Dev Disord 28:229–233, 1998

Colenda CC 3rd: Buspirone in treatment of agitated demented patient (letter). Lancet 1:1169, 1988

Como PG, Rubin AJ, O'Brien CF, et al: A controlled trial of fluoxetine in nondepressed patients with Huntington's disease. Mov Disord 12:397–401, 1997

Conlon P, Trimble MR, Rogers D: A study of epileptic psychosis using magnetic resonance imaging. Br J Psychiatry 156:231–235, 1990

Connemann BJ, Schonfeldt-Lecuona C: Ziprasidone in Parkinson's disease psychosis (letter). Can J Psychiatry 49:73, 2004

Connor DF, Ozbayrak KR, Benjamin S, et al: A pilot study of nadolol for overt aggression in developmentally delayed individuals. J Am Acad Child Adolesc Psychiatry 36:826–834, 1997

Cook EH Jr, Rowlett R, Jaselskis C, et al: Fluoxetine treatment of children and adults with autistic disorder and mental retardation. J Am Acad Child Adolesc Psychiatry 31:739–745, 1992

Cooper JP: Buspirone for anxiety and agitation in dementia (letter). J Psychiatry Neurosci 28:469, 2003

Courtney C, Farrell D, Gray R, et al: Long-term donepezil treatment in 565 patients with Alzheimer's disease (AD2000): randomised double-blind trial. Lancet 363 (9427):2105–2115, 2004

Craft M, Ismail IA, Krishnamurti D, et al: Lithium in the treatment of aggression in mentally handicapped patients: a double-blind trial. Br J Psychiatry 150:685–689, 1987

Craft S, Asthana S, Newcomer JW, et al: Enhancement of memory in Alzheimer disease with insulin and somatostatin, but not glucose. Arch Gen Psychiatry 56:1135–1140, 1999

Crisostomo EA, Duncan PW, Propst M, et al: Evidence that amphetamine with physical therapy promotes recovery of motor function in stroke patients. Ann Neurol 23:94–97, 1988

Crook T, Petrie W, Wells C, et al: Effects of phosphatidylserine in Alzheimer's disease. Psychopharmacol Bull 28:61–66, 1992

Cueva JE, Overall JE, Small AM, et al: Carbamazepine in aggressive children with conduct disorder: a double-blind and placebo-controlled study. J Am Acad Child Adolesc Psychiatry 35:480–490, 1996

Cummings JL: Alzheimer's disease. N Engl J Med 351:56–67, 2004

Czobor P, Volavka J, Sheitman B, et al: Antipsychotic-induced weight gain and therapeutic response: a differential association. J Clin Psychopharmacol 22:244–251, 2002

Dailly E, Chenu F, Renard CE, et al: Dopamine, depression and antidepressants. Fundam Clin Pharmacol 18:601–607, 2004

Dallocchio C, Buffa C, Tinelli C, et al: Effectiveness of risperidone in Huntington chorea patients. J Clin Psychopharmacol 19:101–103, 1999

Dam M, Tonin P, De Boni A, et al: Effects of fluoxetine and maprotiline on functional recovery in poststroke hemiplegic patients undergoing rehabilitation therapy. Stroke 27:1211–1214, 1996

Davanzo PA, Belin TR, Widawski MH, et al: Paroxetine treatment of aggression and self-injury in persons with mental retardation. Am J Ment Retard 102:427–437, 1998

Davis KL, Mohs RC, Marin DB, et al: Neuropeptide abnormalities in patients with early Alzheimer disease. Arch Gen Psychiatry 56:981–987, 1999

De Deyn PP, Rabheru K, Rasmussen A, et al: A randomized trial of risperidone, placebo, and haloperidol for behavioral symptoms of dementia. Neurology 53:946–955, 1999

De Deyn PP, Carrasco MM, Deberdt W, et al: Olanzapine versus placebo in the treatment of psychosis with or without associated behavioral disturbances in patients with Alzheimer's disease. Int J Geriatr Psychiatry 19:115–126, 2004

Devanand DP: Behavioral complications and their treatment in Alzheimer's disease. Geriatrics 52 (suppl 2):S37–S39, 1997

Devanand DP, Cooper T, Sackeim HA, et al: Low dose oral haloperidol and blood levels in Alzheimer's disease: a preliminary study. Psychopharmacol Bull 28:169–173, 1992

Devanand DP, Marder K, Michaels KS, et al: A randomized, placebo-controlled dose-comparison trial of haloperidol for psychosis and disruptive behaviors in Alzheimer's disease. Am J Psychiatry 155:1512–1520, 1998

DeVane CL, Mintzer J: Risperidone in the management of psychiatric and neurodegenerative disease in the elderly: an update. Psychopharmacol Bull 37:116–132, 2003

Diaz-Olavarrieta C, Campbell J, Garcia de la Cadena C, et al: Domestic violence against patients with chronic neurologic disorders. Arch Neurol 56:681–685, 1999

Donaldson C, Tarrier N, Burns A: Determinants of carer stress in Alzheimer's disease. Int J Geriatr Psychiatry 13:248–256, 1998

Dorevitch A, Katz N, Zemishlany Z, et al: Intramuscular flunitrazepam versus intramuscular haloperidol in the emergency treatment of aggressive psychotic behavior. Am J Psychiatry 156:142–144, 1999

Dragasevic N, Potrebic A, Damjanovic A, et al: Therapeutic efficacy of bilateral prefrontal slow repetitive transcranial magnetic stimulation in depressed patients with Parkinson's disease: an open study. Mov Disord 17:528–532, 2002

Drake ME Jr, Pakalnis A, Phillips B: Secondary mania after ventral pontine infarction. J Neuropsychiatry Clin Neurosci 2:322–325, 1990

Duffy JD, Kant R: Clinical utility of clozapine in 16 patients with neurological disease. J Neuropsychiatry Clin Neurosci 8:92–96, 1996

Duman RS: Novel therapeutic approaches beyond the serotonin receptor. Biol Psychiatry 44:324–335, 1998

Dysken MW, Mendels J, LeWitt P, et al: Milacemide: a placebo-controlled study in senile dementia of the Alzheimer type. J Am Geriatr Soc 40:503–506, 1992

Elger G, Hoppe C, Falkai P, et al: Vagus nerve stimulation is associated with mood improvements in epilepsy patients. Epilepsy Res 42:203–210, 2000

Elliott AJ, Roy-Byrne PP: Mirtazapine for depression in patients with human immunodeficiency virus. J Clin Psychopharmacol 20:265–267, 2000

Elliott AJ, Uldall KK, Bergam K, et al: Randomized, placebo-controlled trial of paroxetine versus imipramine in depressed HIV-positive outpatients. Am J Psychiatry 155:367–372, 1998

Ellis T, Cudkowicz ME, Sexton PM, et al: Clozapine and risperidone treatment of psychosis in Parkinson's disease. J Neuropsychiatry Clin Neurosci 12:364–369, 2000

Elrod R, Peskind ER, DiGiacomo L, et al: Effects of Alzheimer's disease severity on cerebrospinal fluid norepinephrine concentration. Am J Psychiatry 154:25–30, 1997

Emsley RA, Roberts MC, Aalbers C, et al: Endocrine function in alcoholic Korsakoff's syndrome. Alcohol Alcohol 29:187–191, 1994

Erkinjuntti T, Kurz A, Gauthier S, et al: Efficacy of galantamine in probable vascular dementia and Alzheimer's disease combined with cerebrovascular disease: a randomised trial. Lancet 359:1283–1290, 2002

Ernst RL, Hay JW: Economic research on Alzheimer disease: a review of the literature. Alzheimer Dis Assoc Disord 11 (suppl 6):135–145, 1997

Evans RW, Gualtieri CT: Carbamazepine: a neuropsychological and psychiatric profile. Clin Neuropharmacol 8:221–241, 1985

Factor SA, Molho ES, Brown DL: Combined clozapine and electroconvulsive therapy for the treatment of drug-induced psychosis in Parkinson's disease. J Neuropsychiatry Clin Neurosci 7:304–307, 1995

Falk WE, Mahnke MW, Poskanzer DC: Lithium prophylaxis of corticotropin-induced psychosis. JAMA 241:1011–1012, 1979

Fall PA, Ekman R, Granerus AK, et al: ECT in Parkinson's disease: changes in motor symptoms, monoamine metabolites and neuropeptides. J Neural Transm Park Dis Dement Sect 10(2–3):129–140, 1995

Falsaperla A, Monici Preti PA, Oliani C: Selegiline versus oxiracetam in patients with Alzheimer-type dementia. Clin Ther 12:376–384, 1990

Fann JR, Uomoto JM, Katon WJ: Sertraline in the treatment of major depression following mild traumatic brain injury. J Neuropsychiatry Clin Neurosci 12:226–232, 2000

Farlow M, Anand R, Messina J Jr, et al: A 52-week study of the efficacy of rivastigmine in patients with mild to moderately severe Alzheimer's disease. Eur Neurol 44:236–241, 2000

Fava M, Rosenbaum JF, McCarthy M, et al: Anger attacks in depressed outpatients and their response to fluoxetine. Psychopharmacol Bull 27:275–279, 1991

Feder R: Treatment of intermittent explosive disorder with sertraline in 3 patients. J Clin Psychiatry 60:195–196, 1999

Feeney DM, Gonzalez A, Law WA: Amphetamine, haloperidol, and experience interact to affect rate of recovery after motor cortex injury. Science 217:855–857, 1982

Feinstein A, Ron M: A longitudinal study of psychosis due to a general medical (neurological) condition: establishing predictive and construct validity. J Neuropsychiatry Clin Neurosci 10:448–452, 1998

Feinstein A, du Boulay G, Ron MA: Psychotic illness in multiple sclerosis: a clinical and magnetic resonance imaging study. Br J Psychiatry 161:680–685, 1992

Fernandez HH, Friedman JH, Jacques C, et al: Quetiapine for the treatment of drug-induced psychosis in Parkinson's disease. Mov Disord 14:484–487, 1999

Fernandez HH, Trieschmann ME, Burke MA, et al: Quetiapine for psychosis in Parkinson's disease versus dementia with Lewy bodies. J Clin Psychiatry 63:513–515, 2002

Fernandez HH, Trieschmann ME, Burke MA, et al: Long-term outcome of quetiapine use for psychosis among parkinsonian patients. Mov Disord 18:510–514, 2003

Fernandez HH, Trieschmann ME, Friedman JH: Aripiprazole for drug-induced psychosis in Parkinson disease: preliminary experience. Clin Neuropharmacol 27:4–5, 2004

Ferrando SJ, Rabkin JG, de Moore GM, et al: Antidepressant treatment of depression in HIV-seropositive women. J Clin Psychiatry 60:741–746, 1999

Ferrier IN, Thompson JM: Cognitive impairment in bipolar affective disorder: implications for the bipolar diathesis. Br J Psychiatry 180:293–295, 2002

Figiel GS: ECT and delirium in Parkinson's disease (letter; author reply appears in Am J Psychiatry 149:1759–1760, 1992). Am J Psychiatry 149:1759, 1992

Finali G, Piccirilli M, Oliani C, et al: L-deprenyl therapy improves verbal memory in amnesic Alzheimer patients. Clin Neuropharmacol 14:523–536, 1991

Fischhof PK: Divergent neuroprotective effects of nimodipine in PDD and MID provide indirect evidence of disturbances in Ca2+ homeostasis in dementia. Methods Find Exp Clin Pharmacol 15:549–555, 1993

Fisher A, Pittel Z, Haring R, et al: M1 muscarinic agonists can modulate some of the hallmarks in Alzheimer's disease: implications in future therapy. J Mol Neurosci 20:349–356, 2003

Flax JW, Gray J, Herbert J: Effect of fluoxetine on patients with multiple sclerosis (letter). Am J Psychiatry 148:1603, 1991

Fleminger S, Greenwood RJ, Oliver DL: Pharmacological management for agitation and aggression in people with acquired brain injury. Cochrane Database Syst Rev (1): CD003299, 2003

Foong J, Rozewicz L, Davie CA, et al: Correlates of executive function in multiple sclerosis: the use of magnetic resonance spectroscopy as an index of focal pathology. J Neuropsychiatry Clin Neurosci 11:45–50, 1999

Fornazzari L, Farcnik K, Smith I, et al: Violent visual hallucinations and aggression in frontal lobe dysfunction: clinical manifestations of deep orbitofrontal foci. J Neuropsychiatry Clin Neurosci 4:42–44, 1992

Forstl H, Burns A, Luthert P, et al: Clinical and neuropathological correlates of depression in Alzheimer's disease. Psychol Med 22:877–884, 1992

Freedman M, Rewilak D, Xerri T, et al: L-Deprenyl in Alzheimer's disease: cognitive and behavioral effects. Neurology 50:660–668, 1998

Fregni F, Santos CM, Myczkowski ML, et al: Repetitive transcranial magnetic stimulation is as effective as fluoxetine in the treatment of depression in patients with Parkinson's disease. J Neurol Neurosurg Psychiatry 75:1171–1174, 2004

Fregni F, Simon DK, Wu A, et al: Non-invasive brain stimulation for Parkinson's disease: a systematic review and meta-analysis of the literature. J Neurol Neurosurg Psychiatry 76:1614–1623, 2005

Freinhar JP, Alvarez WA: Clonazepam treatment of organic brain syndromes in three elderly patients. J Clin Psychiatry 47:525–526, 1986

Fruehwald S, Gatterbauer E, Rehak P, et al: Early fluoxetine treatment of post-stroke depression: a three-month double-blind placebo-controlled study with an open-label long-term follow up. J Neurol 250:347–351, 2003

Fuchs A, Hehnke U, Erhart C, et al: Video rating analysis of effect of maprotiline in patients with dementia and depression. Pharmacopsychiatry 26:37–41, 1993

Galynker I, Ieronimo C, Miner C, et al: Methylphenidate treatment of negative symptoms in patients with dementia. J Neuropsychiatry Clin Neurosci 9:231–239, 1997

Garza-Trevino ES, Hollister LE, Overall JE, et al: Efficacy of combinations of intramuscular antipsychotics and sedative-hypnotics for control of psychotic agitation. Am J Psychiatry 146:1598–1601, 1989

George MS, Rush AJ, Marangell LB, et al: A one-year comparison of vagus nerve stimulation with treatment as usual for treatment-resistant depression. Biol Psychiatry 58:364–373, 2005

Gillig P, Sackellares JC, Greenberg HS: Right hemisphere partial complex seizures: mania, hallucinations, and speech disturbances during ictal events. Epilepsia 29:26–29, 1988

Glass JD, Wesselingh SL, Selnes OA, et al: Clinical-neuropathologic correlation in HIV-associated dementia. Neurology 43:2230–2237, 1993

Glenn MB, Wroblewski B, Parziale J, et al: Lithium carbonate for aggressive behavior or affective instability in ten brain-injured patients. Am J Phys Med Rehabil 68:221–226, 1989

Glue P: Rapid cycling affective disorders in the mentally retarded. Biol Psychiatry 26:250–256, 1989

Goetz CG, Tanner CM, Klawans HL: Bupropion in Parkinson's disease. Neurology 34:1092–1094, 1984

Goff DC, Tsai G, Levitt J, et al: A placebo-controlled trial of D-cycloserine added to conventional neuroleptics in patients with schizophrenia. Arch Gen Psychiatry 56:21–27, 1999

Goldenberg G, Kahaner K, Basavaraju N, et al: Gabapentin for disruptive behaviour in an elderly demented patient. Drugs Aging 13:183–184, 1998

Gomez-Esteban JC, Zarranz JJ, Velasco F, et al: Use of ziprasidone in parkinsonian patients with psychosis. Clin Neuropharmacol 28:111–114, 2005

Goodwin FK, Jamison KR: Manic-Depressive Illness. New York, Oxford University Press, 1990

Grade C, Redford B, Chrostowski J, et al: Methylphenidate in early poststroke recovery: a double-blind, placebo-controlled study. Arch Phys Med Rehabil 79:1047–1050, 1998

Grant I, Brown GW, Harris T, et al: Severely threatening events and marked life difficulties preceding onset or exacerbation of multiple sclerosis. J Neurol Neurosurg Psychiatry 52:8–13, 1989

Greenberg SM, Tennis MK, Brown LB, et al: Donepezil therapy in clinical practice: a randomized crossover study. Arch Neurol 57:94–99, 2000

Greendyke RM, Kanter DR: Therapeutic effects of pindolol on behavioral disturbances associated with organic brain disease: a double-blind study. J Clin Psychiatry 47:423–426, 1986

Greendyke RM, Kanter DR, Schuster DB, et al: Propranolol treatment of assaultive patients with organic brain disease: a double-blind crossover, placebo-controlled study. J Nerv Ment Dis 174:290–294, 1986

Greenwald BS, Marin DB, Silverman SM: Serotoninergic treatment of screaming and banging in dementia. Lancet 2:1464–1465, 1986

Grisaru N, Chudakov B, Yaroslavsky Y, et al: Transcranial magnetic stimulation in mania: a controlled study. Am J Psychiatry 155:1608–1610, 1998

Gualtieri CT: Buspirone for the behavior problems of patients with organic brain disorders. J Clin Psychopharmacol 11:280–281, 1991

Gualtieri T, Chandler M, Coons TB, et al: Amantadine: a new clinical profile for traumatic brain injury. Clin Neuropharmacol 12:258–270, 1989

Guillem E, Plas J, Musa C, et al: Ictal mania: a case report. Can J Psychiatry 45:493–494, 2000

Haas S, Vincent K, Holt J, et al: Divalproex: a possible treatment alternative for demented, elderly aggressive patients. Ann Clin Psychiatry 9:145–147, 1997

Haller E, Binder RL: Clozapine and seizures. Am J Psychiatry 147:1069–1071, 1990

Halliday S, Mackrell K: Psychological interventions in self-injurious behaviour: working with people with a learning disability. Br J Psychiatry 172:395–400, 1998

Halliday G, Ellis J, Heard R, et al: Brainstem serotonergic neurons in chronic alcoholics with and without the memory impairment of Korsakoff's psychosis. J Neuropathol Exp Neurol 52:567–579, 1993

Halman MH, Worth JL, Sanders KM, et al: Anticonvulsant use in the treatment of manic syndromes in patients with HIV-1 infection. J Neuropsychiatry Clin Neurosci 5:430–434, 1993

Hamner M, Huber M, Gardner VT 3rd: Patient with progressive dementia and choreoathetoid movements treated with buspirone. J Clin Psychopharmacol 16:261–262, 1996

Heilig M, Sjogren M, Blennow K, et al: Cerebrospinal fluid neuropeptides in Alzheimer's disease and vascular dementia. Biol Psychiatry 38:210–216, 1995

Heiss WD, Pawlik G, Holthoff V, et al: PET correlates of normal and impaired memory functions. Cerebrovasc Brain Metab Rev 4:1–27, 1992

Hellings JA, Kelley LA, Gabrielli WF, et al: Sertraline response in adults with mental retardation and autistic disorder. J Clin Psychiatry 57:333–336, 1996

Henderson VW, Paganini-Hill A, Emanuel CK, et al: Estrogen replacement therapy in older women: comparisons between Alzheimer's disease cases and nondemented control subjects. Arch Neurol 51:896–900, 1994

Henderson VW, Paganini-Hill A, Miller BL, et al: Estrogen for Alzheimer's disease in women: randomized, double-blind, placebo-controlled trial. Neurology 54:295–301, 2000

Hendryx PM: Psychosocial changes perceived by closed-head-injured adults and their families. Arch Phys Med Rehabil 70:526–530, 1989

Herrmann N, Lanctot KL: Do atypical antipsychotics cause stroke? CNS Drugs 19:91–103, 2005

Herrmann N, Rivard MF, Flynn M, et al: Risperidone for the treatment of behavioral disturbances in dementia: a case series. J Neuropsychiatry Clin Neurosci 10:220–223, 1998

Herrmann N, Lanctot K, Myszak M: Effectiveness of gabapentin for the treatment of behavioral disorders in dementia. J Clin Psychopharmacol 20:90–93, 2000

Herz LR, Volicer L, Ross V, et al: Pharmacotherapy of agitation in dementia. Am J Psychiatry 149:1757–1758, 1992

Heseltine PN, Goodkin K, Atkinson JH, et al: Randomized double-blind placebo-controlled trial of peptide T for HIV-associated cognitive impairment. Arch Neurol 55:41–51, 1998

Higley JD, Mehlman PT, Taub DM, et al: Cerebrospinal fluid monoamine and adrenal correlates of aggression in free-ranging rhesus monkeys. Arch Gen Psychiatry 49:436–441, 1992

Himmelhoch JM, Neil JF, May SJ, et al: Age, dementia, dyskinesias, and lithium response. Am J Psychiatry 137:941–945, 1980

Hindmarch I: Beyond the monoamine hypothesis: mechanisms, molecules and methods. Eur Psychiatry 17 (suppl 3):294–299, 2002

Hirono N, Mori E, Ishii K, et al: Alteration of regional cerebral glucose utilization with delusions in Alzheimer's disease. J Neuropsychiatry Clin Neurosci 10:433–439, 1998

Holton A, George K: The use of lithium in severely demented patients with behavioural disturbance. Br J Psychiatry 146:99–100, 1985

Holtzheimer PE 3rd, Russo J, Avery DH: A meta-analysis of repetitive transcranial magnetic stimulation in the treatment of depression [published erratum appears in Psychopharmacol Bull 37:5, 2003]. Psychopharmacol Bull 35:149–169, 2001

Horne M, Lindley SE: Divalproex sodium in the treatment of aggressive behavior and dysphoria in patients with organic brain syndromes. J Clin Psychiatry 56:430–431, 1995

Hornstein A, Seliger G: Cognitive side effects of lithium in closed head injury. J Neuropsychiatry Clin Neurosci 1:446–447, 1989

Horrigan JP, Barnhill LJ: Risperidone and explosive aggressive autism. J Autism Dev Disord 27:313–323, 1997

Hyde TM, Ziegler JC, Weinberger DR: Psychiatric disturbances in metachromatic leukodystrophy: insights into the neurobiology of psychosis. Arch Neurol 49:401–406, 1992

Iannaccone S, Ferini-Strambi L: Pharmacologic treatment of emotional lability. Clin Neuropharmacol 19:532–535, 1996

Ingram DK, Spangler EL, Iijima S, et al: New pharmacological strategies for cognitive enhancement using a rat model of age-related memory impairment. Ann N Y Acad Sci 717:16–32, 1994

Jacobsen FM, Comas-Diaz L: Donepezil for psychotropic-induced memory loss. J Clin Psychiatry 60:698–704, 1999

Jakala P, Riekkinen M, Sirvio J, et al: Clonidine, but not guanfacine, impairs choice reaction time performance in young healthy volunteers. Neuropsychopharmacology 21:495–502, 1999a

Jakala P, Riekkinen M, Sirvio J, et al: Guanfacine, but not clonidine, improves planning and working memory performance in humans. Neuropsychopharmacology 20:460–470, 1999b

Jakala P, Sirvio J, Riekkinen M, et al: Guanfacine and clonidine, alpha 2-agonists, improve paired associates learning, but not delayed matching to sample, in humans. Neuropsychopharmacology 20:119–130, 1999c

Janowsky DS, Barnhill LJ, Davis JM: Olanzapine for self-injurious, aggressive, and disruptive behaviors in intellectually disabled adults: a retrospective, open-label, naturalistic trial. J Clin Psychiatry 64:1258–1265, 2003

Jason GW, Suchowersky O, Pajurkova EM, et al: Cognitive manifestations of Huntington disease in relation to genetic structure and clinical onset. Arch Neurol 54:1081–1088, 1997

Joffe RT, Lippert GP, Gray TA, et al: Mood disorder and multiple sclerosis. Arch Neurol 44:376–378, 1987

Jorge RE, Robinson RG, Starkstein SE, et al: Secondary mania following traumatic brain injury. Am J Psychiatry 150:916–921, 1993

Jorge RE, Robinson RG, Tateno A, et al: Repetitive transcranial magnetic stimulation as treatment of poststroke depression: a preliminary study. Biol Psychiatry 55:398–405, 2004

Jouvent R, Abensour P, Bonnet AM, et al: Antiparkinsonian and antidepressant effects of high doses of bromocriptine: an independent comparison. J Affect Disord 5:141–145, 1983

Joyce JN: The dopamine hypothesis of schizophrenia: limbic interactions with serotonin and norepinephrine. Psychopharmacology (Berl) 112 (1 suppl):S16–S34, 1993

Juncos JL, Roberts VJ, Evatt ML, et al: Quetiapine improves psychotic symptoms and cognition in Parkinson's disease. Mov Disord 19:29–35, 2004

Kampen DL, Sherwin BB: Estrogen use and verbal memory in healthy postmenopausal women. Obstet Gynecol 83:979–983, 1994

Kasckow JW, Mulchahey JJ, Mohamed S: The use of novel antipsychotics in the older patient with neurodegenerative disorders in the long-term care setting. J Am Med Dir Assoc 5:242–248, 2004

Katz IR, Jeste DV, Mintzer JE, et al: Comparison of risperidone and placebo for psychosis and behavioral disturbances associated with dementia: a randomized, double-blind trial. Risperidone Study Group. J Clin Psychiatry 60:107–115, 1999

Kaufmann MW, Cassem NH, Murray GB, et al: Use of psychostimulants in medically ill patients with neurological disease and major depression. Can J Psychiatry 29:46–49, 1984

Kavoussi RJ, Coccaro EF: Divalproex sodium for impulsive aggressive behavior in patients with personality disorder. J Clin Psychiatry 59:676–680, 1998

Kegeles LS, Humaran TJ, Mann JJ: In vivo neurochemistry of the brain in schizophrenia as revealed by magnetic resonance spectroscopy. Biol Psychiatry 44:382–398, 1998

Kellner CH, Beale MD, Pritchett JT, et al: Electroconvulsive therapy and Parkinson's disease: the case for further study. Psychopharmacol Bull 30:495–500, 1994

Kemperman CJ, Gerdes JH, De Rooij J, et al: Reversible lithium neurotoxicity at normal serum level may refer to intracranial pathology. J Neurol Neurosurg Psychiatry 52:679–680, 1989

Kim E, Zwil AS, McAllister TW, et al: Treatment of organic bipolar mood disorders in Parkinson's disease. J Neuropsychiatry Clin Neurosci 6:181–184, 1994

Kimbrell TA, George MS, Parekh PI, et al: Regional brain activity during transient self-induced anxiety and anger in healthy adults. Biol Psychiatry 46:454–465, 1999

Kimura M, Tateno A, Robinson RG: Treatment of poststroke generalized anxiety disorder comorbid with poststroke depression: merged analysis of nortriptyline trials. Am J Geriatr Psychiatry 11:320–327, 2003

Kindermann SS, Dolder CR, Bailey A, et al: Pharmacological treatment of psychosis and agitation in elderly patients with dementia: four decades of experience. Drugs Aging 19:257–276, 2002

Kirven LE, Montero EF: Comparison of thioridazine and diazepam in the control of nonpsychotic symptoms associated with senility: double-blind study. J Am Geriatr Soc 21:546–551, 1973

Klaassen T, Verhey FR, Sneijders GH, et al: Treatment of depression in Parkinson's disease: a meta-analysis. J Neuropsychiatry Clin Neurosci 7:281–286, 1995

Knable MB, Rickler K: Psychosis associated with felbamate treatment. J Clin Psychopharmacol 15:292–293, 1995

Knopman D, Schneider L, Davis K, et al: Long-term tacrine (Cognex) treatment: effects on nursing home placement and mortality. Tacrine Study Group. Neurology 47:166–177, 1996

Koshes RJ, Rock NL: Use of clonidine for behavioral control in an adult patient with autism. Am J Psychiatry 151:1714, 1994

Kostic VS, Lecic D, Doder M, et al: Prolactin and cortisol responses to fenfluramine in Parkinson's disease. Biol Psychiatry 40:769–775, 1996

Kotrla KJ, Chacko RC, Harper RG, et al: SPECT findings on psychosis in Alzheimer's disease. Am J Psychiatry 152:1470–1475, 1995

Kozel FA, George MS: Meta-analysis of left prefrontal repetitive transcranial magnetic stimulation (rTMS) to treat depression. J Psychiatr Pract 8:270–275, 2002

Kuhn KU, Quednow BB, Thiel M, et al: Antidepressive treatment in patients with temporal lobe epilepsy and major depression: a prospective study with three different antidepressants. Epilepsy Behav 4:674–679, 2003

Kulkarni J, Horne M, Butler E, et al: Psychotic symptoms resulting from intraventricular infusion of dopamine in Parkinson's disease. Biol Psychiatry 31:1225–1227, 1992

Kunik ME, Yudofsky SC, Silver JM, et al: Pharmacologic approach to management of agitation associated with dementia. J Clin Psychiatry 55(suppl):13–17, 1994

Kunik ME, Puryear L, Orengo CA, et al: The efficacy and tolerability of divalproex sodium in elderly demented patients with behavioral disturbances. Int J Geriatr Psychiatry 13:29–34, 1998

Kuzis G, Sabe L, Tiberti C, et al: Cognitive functions in major depression and Parkinson disease. Arch Neurol 54:982–986, 1997

Kwan LT, Reed BR, Eberling JL, et al: Effects of subcortical cerebral infarction on cortical glucose metabolism and cognitive function. Arch Neurol 56:809–814, 1999

Laakso A, Vilkman H, Alakare B, et al: Striatal dopamine transporter binding in neuroleptic-naive patients with schizophrenia studied with positron emission tomography. Am J Psychiatry 157:269–271, 2000

LaFrance WC Jr, Lauterbach EC, Coffey CE, et al: The use of herbal alternative medicines in neuropsychiatry: a report of the ANPA Committee on Research. J Neuropsychiatry Clin Neurosci 12:177–192, 2000

Laitinen L: Desipramine in treatment of Parkinson's disease: a placebo-controlled study. Acta Neurol Scand 45:109–113, 1969

Lancon C, Auquier P, Nayt G, et al: Stability of the five-factor structure of the Positive and Negative Syndrome Scale (PANSS). Schizophr Res 42:231–239, 2000

Lanctot KL, Herrmann N: Donepezil for behavioural disorders associated with Lewy bodies: a case series. Int J Geriatr Psychiatry 15:338–345, 2000

Lanctot KL, Herrmann N, van Reekum R, et al: Gender, aggression and serotonergic function are associated with response to sertraline for behavioral disturbances in Alzheimer's disease. Int J Geriatr Psychiatry 17:531–541, 2002

Lange KW, Riederer P: Glutamatergic drugs in Parkinson's disease. Life Sci 55:2067–2075, 1994

Lauterbach EC, Jackson JG, Price ST, et al: Clinical, motor, and biological correlates of depressive disorders after focal subcortical lesions. J Neuropsychiatry Clin Neurosci 9:259–266, 1997

Lawlor BA: Behavioral and psychological symptoms in dementia: the role of atypical antipsychotics. J Clin Psychiatry 65 (suppl 11):5–10, 2004

Lawlor BA, Radcliffe J, Molchan SE, et al: A pilot placebo-controlled study of trazodone and buspirone in Alzheimer's disease. Int J Geriatr Psychiatry 9:55–59, 1994

Lawlor BA, Bierer LM, Ryan TM, et al: Plasma 3-methoxy-4-hydroxyphenylglycol (MHPG) and clinical symptoms in Alzheimer's disease. Biol Psychiatry 38:185–188, 1995

Lazarus LW, Moberg PJ, Langsley PR, et al: Methylphenidate and nortriptyline in the treatment of poststroke depression: a retrospective comparison. Arch Phys Med Rehabil 75:403–406, 1994

Le Bars PL, Katz MM, Berman N, et al: A placebo-controlled, double-blind, randomized trial of an extract of Ginkgo biloba for dementia. North American EGb Study Group. JAMA 278:1327–1332, 1997

Lecamwasam D, Synek B, Moyles K, et al: Chronic lithium neurotoxicity presenting as Parkinson's disease. Int Clin Psychopharmacol 9:127–129, 1994

Lee GP, Bechara A, Adolphs R, et al: Clinical and physiological effects of stereotaxic bilateral amygdalotomy for intractable aggression. J Neuropsychiatry Clin Neurosci 10:413–420, 1998

Leentjens AF, Vreeling FW, Luijckx GJ, et al: SSRIs in the treatment of depression in Parkinson's disease. Int J Geriatr Psychiatry 18:552–554, 2003

Leo RJ: Movement disorders associated with the serotonin selective reuptake inhibitors. J Clin Psychiatry 57:449–454, 1996

Lera G, Zirulnik J: Pilot study with clozapine in patients with HIV-associated psychosis and drug-induced parkinsonism. Mov Disord 14:128–131, 1999

Levine AM: Buspirone and agitation in head injury. Brain Inj 2:165–167, 1988

Levitan C, Ward PB, Catts SV: Superior temporal gyral volumes and laterality correlates of auditory hallucinations in schizophrenia. Biol Psychiatry 46:955–962, 1999

Levy ML, Cummings JL, Fairbanks LA, et al: Apathy is not depression. J Neuropsychiatry Clin Neurosci 10:314–319, 1998

Lindenmayer JP, Kotsaftis A: Use of sodium valproate in violent and aggressive behaviors: a critical review. J Clin Psychiatry 61:123–128, 2000

Linnoila VM, Virkkunen M: Aggression, suicidality, and serotonin. J Clin Psychiatry 53(suppl):46–51, 1992

Lipsey JR, Robinson RG, Pearlson GD, et al: Nortriptyline treatment of post-stroke depression: a double-blind study. Lancet 1:297–300, 1984

Lipton SA: Calcium channel antagonists and human immunodeficiency virus coat protein-mediated neuronal injury. Ann Neurol 30:110–114, 1991

Lonergan E, Luxenberg J, Colford J: Haloperidol for agitation in dementia. Cochrane Database Syst Rev (2):CD002852, 2002

Lopez OL, Becker JT, Brenner RP, et al: Alzheimer's disease with delusions and hallucinations: neuropsychological and electroencephalographic correlates. Neurology 41:906–912, 1991

Lopez OL, Smith G, Becker JT, et al: The psychotic phenomenon in probable Alzheimer's disease: a positron emission tomography study. J Neuropsychiatry Clin Neurosci 13:50–55, 2001

Low RA Jr, Brandes M: Gabapentin for the management of agitation. J Clin Psychopharmacol 19:482–483, 1999

Lozano AM, Abosch A: Pallidal stimulation for dystonia. Adv Neurol 94:301–308, 2004

Luchins DJ: Carbamazepine in violent non-epileptic schizophrenics. Psychopharmacol Bull 20:569–571, 1984

Lyketsos CG, Olin J: Depression in Alzheimer's disease: overview and treatment. Biol Psychiatry 52:243–252, 2002

Lyketsos CG, Schwartz J, Fishman M, et al: AIDS mania. J Neuropsychiatry Clin Neurosci 9:277–279, 1997

Lyketsos CG, Treisman GJ, Lipsey JR, et al: Does stroke cause depression? J Neuropsychiatry Clin Neurosci 10:103–107, 1998

Lyketsos CG, DelCampo L, Steinberg M, et al: Treating depression in Alzheimer disease: efficacy and safety of sertraline therapy, and the benefits of depression reduction: the DIADS. Arch Gen Psychiatry 60:737–746, 2003

Maelicke A, Samochocki M, Jostock R, et al: Allosteric sensitization of nicotinic receptors by galantamine, a new treatment strategy for Alzheimer's disease. Biol Psychiatry 49:279–288, 2001

Magai C, Kennedy G, Cohen CI, et al: A controlled clinical trial of sertraline in the treatment of depression in nursing home patients with late-stage Alzheimer's disease. Am J Geriatr Psychiatry 8:66–74, 2000

Malow BA, Reese KB, Sato S, et al: Spectrum of EEG abnormalities during clozapine treatment. Electroencephalogr Clin Neurophysiol 91:205–211, 1994

Maneeton N, Intaprasert S, Srisurapanont M: Risperidone for controlling aggressive behavior in a mentally retarded child: a case report. J Med Assoc Thai 84:893–896, 2001

Mann DM, Yates PO, Marcyniuk B: A comparison of changes in the nucleus basalis and locus coeruleus in Alzheimer's disease. J Neurol Neurosurg Psychiatry 47:201–203, 1984

Mann JJ: Violence and aggression, in Psychopharmacology: The Fourth Generation of Progress. Edited by Bloom FE, Kupfer DJ. New York, Raven, 1995, pp 1919–1928

Markowitz PI: Effect of fluoxetine on self-injurious behavior in the developmentally disabled: a preliminary study. J Clin Psychopharmacol 12:27–31, 1992

Marshall EJ, Syed GM, Fenwick PB, et al: A pilot study of schizophrenia-like psychosis in epilepsy using single-photon emission computerised tomography. Br J Psychiatry 163:32–36, 1993

Martin PR, Adinoff B, Eckardt MJ, et al: Effective pharmacotherapy of alcoholic amnestic disorder with fluvoxamine: preliminary findings. Arch Gen Psychiatry 46:617–621, 1989

Martin PR, Adinoff B, Lane E, et al: Fluvoxamine treatment of alcoholic amnestic disorder. Eur Neuropsychopharmacol 5:27–33, 1995

Martinon-Torres G, Fioravanti M, Grimley EJ: Trazodone for agitation in dementia. Cochrane Database Syst Rev (4): CD004990, 2004

Masand P, Murray GB, Pickett P: Psychostimulants in post-stroke depression. J Neuropsychiatry Clin Neurosci 3:23–27, 1991

Mashiko H, Yokoyama H, Matsumoto H, et al: Trazodone for aggression in an adolescent with hydrocephalus. Psychiatry Clin Neurosci 50:133–136, 1996

Mattes JA: Comparative effectiveness of carbamazepine and propranolol for rage outbursts. J Neuropsychiatry Clin Neurosci 2:159–164, 1990

Max JE, Robin DA, Lindgren SD, et al: Traumatic brain injury in children and adolescents: psychiatric disorders at one year. J Neuropsychiatry Clin Neurosci 10:290–297, 1998

Maxwell CJ, Hogan DB, Ebly EM: Calcium-channel blockers and cognitive function in elderly people: results from the Canadian Study of Health and Aging. CMAJ 161:501–506, 1999

Mayberg HS: Frontal lobe dysfunction in secondary depression. J Neuropsychiatry Clin Neurosci 6:428–442, 1994

Mayberg HS: Modulating dysfunctional limbic-cortical circuits in depression: towards development of brain-based algorithms for diagnosis and optimised treatment. Br Med Bull 65:193–207, 2003

Mayberg HS, Robinson RG, Wong DF, et al: PET imaging of cortical S2 serotonin receptors after stroke: lateralized changes and relationship to depression. Am J Psychiatry 145:937–943, 1988

Mayberg HS, Lozano AM, Voon V, et al: Deep brain stimulation for treatment-resistant depression. Neuron 45:651–660, 2005

Mayeux R, Stern Y, Sano M, et al: The relationship of serotonin to depression in Parkinson's disease. Mov Disord 3:237–244, 1988

Mazure CM, Druss BG, Cellar JS: Valproate treatment of older psychotic patients with organic mental syndromes and behavioral dyscontrol. J Am Geriatr Soc 40:914–916, 1992

McAllister TW: Carbamazepine in mixed frontal lobe and psychiatric disorders. J Clin Psychiatry 46:393–394, 1985

McAllister TW, Ferrell RB: Evaluation and treatment of psychosis after traumatic brain injury. NeuroRehabilitation 17:357–368, 2002

McCracken JT, McGough J, Shah B, et al: Risperidone in children with autism and serious behavioral problems. N Engl J Med 347:314–321, 2002

McDaniel JS, Johnson KM: Obsessive-compulsive disorder in HIV disease: response to fluoxetine. Psychosomatics 36:147–150, 1995

McDonald WM, Richard IH, DeLong MR: Prevalence, etiology, and treatment of depression in Parkinson's disease. Biol Psychiatry 54:363–375, 2003

McDougle CJ, Naylor ST, Cohen DJ, et al: A double-blind, placebo-controlled study of fluvoxamine in adults with autistic disorder. Arch Gen Psychiatry 53:1001–1008, 1996

McEntee WJ, Mair RG: The Korsakoff syndrome: a neurochemical perspective. Trends Neurosci 13:340–344, 1990

McKeith IG, Grace JB, Walker Z, et al: Rivastigmine in the treatment of dementia with Lewy bodies: preliminary findings from an open trial. Int J Geriatr Psychiatry 15:387–392, 2000

Medalia A, Gold J, Merriam A: The effects of neuroleptics on neuropsychological test results of schizophrenics. Arch Clin Neuropsychol 3:249–271, 1988

Meehan K, Zhang F, David S, et al: A double-blind, randomized comparison of the efficacy and safety of intramuscular injections of olanzapine, lorazepam, or placebo in treating acutely agitated patients diagnosed with bipolar mania. J Clin Psychopharmacol 21:389–397, 2001

Mega MS, Cummings JL: Frontal-subcortical circuits and neuropsychiatric disorders. J Neuropsychiatry Clin Neurosci 6:358–370, 1994

Mega MS, Masterman DM, O'Connor SM, et al: The spectrum of behavioral responses to cholinesterase inhibitor therapy in Alzheimer disease. Arch Neurol 56:1388–1393, 1999

Meltzer HY, Ranjan R: Valproic acid treatment of clozapine-induced myoclonus. Am J Psychiatry 151:1246–1247, 1994

Mendez MF, Younesi FL, Perryman KM: Use of donepezil for vascular dementia: preliminary clinical experience. J Neuropsychiatry Clin Neurosci 11:268–270, 1999

Mendez MF, Chow T, Ringman J, et al: Pedophilia and temporal lobe disturbances. J Neuropsychiatry Clin Neurosci 12:71–76, 2000

Mentis MJ, Weinstein EA, Horwitz B, et al: Abnormal brain glucose metabolism in the delusional misidentification syndromes: a positron emission tomography study in Alzheimer disease. Biol Psychiatry 38:438–449, 1995

Meyer JM, Marsh J, Simpson G: Differential sensitivities to risperidone and olanzapine in a human immunodeficiency virus patient. Biol Psychiatry 44:791–794, 1998

Michael N, Erfurth A: Treatment of bipolar mania with right prefrontal rapid transcranial magnetic stimulation. J Affect Disord 78:253–257, 2004

Michals ML, Crismon ML, Roberts S, et al: Clozapine response and adverse effects in nine brain-injured patients. J Clin Psychopharmacol 13:198–203, 1993

Migliorelli R, Starkstein SE, Teson A, et al: SPECT findings in patients with primary mania. J Neuropsychiatry Clin Neurosci 5:379–383, 1993

Mijch AM, Judd FK, Lyketsos CG, et al: Secondary mania in patients with HIV infection: are antiretrovirals protective? J Neuropsychiatry Clin Neurosci 11:475–480, 1999

Miller LJ: Gabapentin for treatment of behavioral and psychological symptoms of dementia. Ann Pharmacother 35:427–431, 2001

Mintzer J, Brawman-Mintzer O, Mirski DF, et al: Fenfluramine challenge test as a marker of serotonin activity in patients with Alzheimer's dementia and agitation. Biol Psychiatry 44:918–921, 1998

Mobayed M, Dinan TG: Buspirone/prolactin response in post head injury depression. J Affect Disord 19:237–241, 1990

Moellentine C, Rummans T, Ahlskog JE, et al: Effectiveness of ECT in patients with parkinsonism. J Neuropsychiatry Clin Neurosci 10:187–193, 1998

Moffoot A, O'Carroll RE, Murray C, et al: Clonidine infusion increases uptake of 99mTc-exametazime in anterior cingulate cortex in Korsakoff's psychosis. Psychol Med 24:53–61, 1994

Mohr DC, Likosky W, Dwyer P, et al: Course of depression during the initiation of interferon beta-1a treatment for multiple sclerosis. Arch Neurol 56:1263–1265, 1999

Mohr E, Mendis T, Hildebrand K, et al: Risperidone in the treatment of dopamine-induced psychosis in Parkinson's disease: an open pilot trial. Mov Disord 15:1230–1237, 2000

Molinuevo JL, Llado A, Rami L: Memantine: targeting glutamate excitotoxicity in Alzheimer's disease and other dementias. Am J Alzheimers Dis Other Demen 20:77–85, 2005

Moller JC, Oertel WH, Koster J, et al: Long-term efficacy and safety of pramipexole in advanced Parkinson's disease: results from a European multicenter trial. Mov Disord 20:602–610, 2005

Monteverde A, Gnemmi P, Rossi F, et al: Selegiline in the treatment of mild to moderate Alzheimer-type dementia. Clin Ther 12:315–322, 1990

Mooney GF, Haas LJ: Effect of methylphenidate on brain injury-related anger. Arch Phys Med Rehabil 74:153–160, 1993

Moore DP: A case of petit mal epilepsy aggravated by lithium. Am J Psychiatry 138:690–691, 1981

Morgante L, Epifanio A, Spina E, et al: Quetiapine versus clozapine: a preliminary report of comparative effects on dopaminergic psychosis in patients with Parkinson's disease. Neurol Sci 23 (suppl 2):S89–S90, 2002

Morgante L, Epifanio A, Spina E, et al: Quetiapine and clozapine in parkinsonian patients with dopaminergic psychosis. Clin Neuropharmacol 27:153–156, 2004

Morris PL, Mayberg HS, Bolla K, et al: A preliminary study of cortical S2 serotonin receptors and cognitive performance following stroke. J Neuropsychiatry Clin Neurosci 5:395–400, 1993

Morris PL, Robinson RG, Raphael B, et al: Lesion location and poststroke depression. J Neuropsychiatry Clin Neurosci 8:399–403, 1996

Mortel KF, Meyer JS: Lack of postmenopausal estrogen replacement therapy and the risk of dementia. J Neuropsychiatry Clin Neurosci 7:334–337, 1995

Moskowitz AS, Altshuler L: Increased sensitivity to lithium-induced neurotoxicity after stroke: a case report. J Clin Psychopharmacol 11:272–273, 1991

Mossner R, Henneberg A, Schmitt A, et al: Allelic variation of serotonin transporter expression is associated with depression in Parkinson's disease. Mol Psychiatry 6:350–352, 2001

Muller U, Murai T, Bauer-Wittmund T, et al: Paroxetine versus citalopram treatment of pathological crying after brain injury. Brain Inj 13:805–811, 1999

Mulnard RA, Cotman CW, Kawas C, et al: Estrogen replacement therapy for treatment of mild to moderate Alzheimer disease: a randomized controlled trial. Alzheimer's Disease Cooperative Study. JAMA 283:1007–1015, 2000

Mysiw WJ, Jackson RD, Corrigan JD: Amitriptyline for post-traumatic agitation. Am J Phys Med Rehabil 67:29–33, 1988

Nagasawa H, Kogure K, Kawashima K, et al: Effects of co-dergocrine mesylate (Hydergine) in multi-infarct dementia as evaluated by positron emission tomography. Tohoku J Exp Med 162:225–233, 1990

Nahas Z, Arlinghaus KA, Kotrla KJ, et al: Rapid response of emotional incontinence to selective serotonin reuptake inhibitors. J Neuropsychiatry Clin Neurosci 10:453–455, 1998

Newburn G, Edwards R, Thomas H, et al: Moclobemide in the treatment of major depressive disorder (DSM-3) following traumatic brain injury. Brain Inj 13:637–642, 1999

Newcomer JW, Faustman WO, Zipursky RB, et al: Zacopride in schizophrenia: a single-blind serotonin type 3 antagonist trial. Arch Gen Psychiatry 49:751–752, 1992

Newhouse PA, Potter A, Levin ED: Nicotinic system involvement in Alzheimer's and Parkinson's diseases: implications for therapeutics. Drugs Aging 11:206–228, 1997

Niedermaier N, Bohrer E, Schulte K, et al: Prevention and treatment of poststroke depression with mirtazapine in patients with acute stroke. J Clin Psychiatry 65:1619–1623, 2004

Nitrini R, Rosemberg S: Psychotic symptoms in dementia associated with motor neuron disease: a pathophysiological hypothesis. J Neuropsychiatry Clin Neurosci 10:456–458, 1998

Nyth AL, Gottfries CG: The clinical efficacy of citalopram in treatment of emotional disturbances in dementia disorders: a Nordic multicentre study. Br J Psychiatry 157:894–901, 1990

Nyth AL, Gottfries CG, Lyby K, et al: A controlled multicenter clinical study of citalopram and placebo in elderly depressed patients with and without concomitant dementia. Acta Psychiatr Scand 86:138–145, 1992

Oechsner M, Korchounov A: Parenteral ziprasidone: a new atypical neuroleptic for emergency treatment of psychosis in Parkinson's disease? Hum Psychopharmacol 20:203–205, 2005

Oh JJ, Rummans TA, O'Connor MK, et al: Cognitive impairment after ECT in patients with Parkinson's disease and psychiatric illness (letter). Am J Psychiatry 149:271, 1992

Oken BS, Storzbach DM, Kaye JA: The efficacy of Ginkgo biloba on cognitive function in Alzheimer disease. Arch Neurol 55:1409–1415, 1998

Olin JT, Fox LS, Pawluczyk S, et al: A pilot randomized trial of carbamazepine for behavioral symptoms in treatment-resistant outpatients with Alzheimer disease. Am J Geriatr Psychiatry 9:400–405, 2001

Ontiveros A, Fontaine R, Breton G, et al: Correlation of severity of panic disorder and neuroanatomical changes on magnetic resonance imaging. J Neuropsychiatry Clin Neurosci 1:404–408, 1989

Onuma T, Adachi N, Hisano T, et al: 10-Year follow-up study of epilepsy with psychosis. Jpn J Psychiatry Neurol 45:360–361, 1991

Orengo C, Kunik ME, Molinari V, et al: Do testosterone levels relate to aggression in elderly men with dementia? J Neuropsychiatry Clin Neurosci 14:161–166, 2002

Owen F, Chambers DR, Cooper SJ, et al: Serotonergic mechanisms in brains of suicide victims. Brain Res 362:185–188, 1986

Palsson S, Aevarsson O, Skoog I: Depression, cerebral atrophy, cognitive performance and incidence of dementia: population study of 85-year-olds. Br J Psychiatry 174:249–253, 1999

Pantelis C, Velakoulis D, McGorry PD, et al: Neuroanatomical abnormalities before and after onset of psychosis: a cross-sectional and longitudinal MRI comparison. Lancet 361:281–288, 2003

Parmelee DX, O'Shanick GJ: Carbamazepine-lithium toxicity in brain-damaged adolescents. Brain Inj 2:305–308, 1988

Parsa MA, Bastani B: Quetiapine (Seroquel) in the treatment of psychosis in patients with Parkinson's disease. J Neuropsychiatry Clin Neurosci 10:216–219, 1998

Parsa MA, Szigethy E, Voci JM, et al: Risperidone in treatment of choreoathetosis of Huntington's disease. J Clin Psychopharmacol 17:134–135, 1997

Pascualy M, Tsuang D, Shores M, et al: Frontal-complex partial status epilepticus misdiagnosed as bipolar affective disorder in a 75-year-old man. J Geriatr Psychiatry Neurol 10:158–160, 1997

Payne JL, Lyketsos CG, Steele C, et al: Relationship of cognitive and functional impairment to depressive features in Alzheimer's disease and other dementias. J Neuropsychiatry Clin Neurosci 10:440–447, 1998

Penn RD, Martin EM, Wilson RS, et al: Intraventricular bethanechol infusion for Alzheimer's disease: results of double-blind and escalating-dose trials. Neurology 38:219–222, 1988

Perry EK, McKeith I, Thompson P, et al: Topography, extent, and clinical relevance of neurochemical deficits in dementia of Lewy body type, Parkinson's disease, and Alzheimer's disease. Ann N Y Acad Sci 640:197–202, 1991

Peterson KA, Armstrong S, Moseley J: Pathologic crying responsive to treatment with sertraline (letter). J Clin Psychopharmacol 16:333, 1996

Petracca G, Teson A, Chemerinski E, et al: A double-blind placebo-controlled study of clomipramine in depressed patients with Alzheimer's disease. J Neuropsychiatry Clin Neurosci 8:270–275, 1996

Petracca GM, Chemerinski E, Starkstein SE: A double-blind, placebo-controlled study of fluoxetine in depressed patients with Alzheimer's disease. Int Psychogeriatr 13:233–240, 2001

Petrides M, Alivisatos B, Meyer E, et al: Functional activation of the human frontal cortex during the performance of verbal working memory tasks. Proc Natl Acad Sci U S A 90:878–882, 1993

Petrie WM, Ban TA, Berney S, et al: Loxapine in psychogeriatrics: a placebo- and standard-controlled clinical investigation. J Clin Psychopharmacol 2:122–126, 1982

Pine DS, Douglas CJ, Charles E, et al: Patients with multiple sclerosis presenting to psychiatric hospitals. J Clin Psychiatry 56:297–306; discussion 307–308, 1995

Pinner E, Rich CL: Effects of trazodone on aggressive behavior in seven patients with organic mental disorders. Am J Psychiatry 145:1295–1296, 1988

Poewe W: Psychosis in Parkinson's disease. Mov Disord 18 (suppl 6):S80–S87, 2003

Pollak P, Tison F, Rascol O, et al: Clozapine in drug induced psychosis in Parkinson's disease: a randomised, placebo controlled study with open follow up. J Neurol Neurosurg Psychiatry 75:689–695, 2004

Pollock BG, Mulsant BH, Sweet R, et al: An open pilot study of citalopram for behavioral disturbances of dementia: plasma levels and real-time observations. Am J Geriatr Psychiatry 5:70–78, 1997

Pomara N, Tun H, Deptula D, et al: ApoE-epsilon 4 allele and susceptibility to drug-induced memory impairment in the elderly. J Clin Psychopharmacol 18:179–181, 1998

Pomara N, Willoughby L, Wesnes K, et al: Apolipoprotein E epsilon4 allele and lorazepam effects on memory in high-functioning older adults. Arch Gen Psychiatry 62:209–216, 2005

Pope HG Jr, McElroy SL, Satlin A, et al: Head injury, bipolar disorder, and response to valproate. Compr Psychiatry 29:34–38, 1988

Popli AP: Risperidone for the treatment of psychosis associated with neurosarcoidosis. J Clin Psychopharmacol 17:132–133, 1997

Porsteinsson AP, Tariot PN, Erb R, et al: An open trial of valproate for agitation in geriatric neuropsychiatric disorders. Am J Geriatr Psychiatry 5:344–351, 1997

Porsteinsson AP, Tariot PN, Erb R, et al: Placebo-controlled study of divalproex sodium for agitation in dementia. Am J Geriatr Psychiatry 9:58–66, 2001

Porsteinsson AP, Tariot PN, Jakimovich LJ, et al: Valproate therapy for agitation in dementia: open-label extension of a double-blind trial. Am J Geriatr Psychiatry 11:434–440, 2003

Portegies P, de Gans J, Lange JM, et al: Declining incidence of AIDS dementia complex after introduction of zidovudine treatment. BMJ 299:819–821, 1989

Posey DJ, McDougle CJ: The pharmacotherapy of target symptoms associated with autistic disorder and other pervasive developmental disorders. Harv Rev Psychiatry 8:45–63, 2000

Pridmore S, Pollard C: Electroconvulsive therapy in Parkinson's disease: 30 month follow up (letter). J Neurol Neurosurg Psychiatry 60:693, 1996

Prigatano GP: Personality disturbances associated with traumatic brain injury. J Consult Clin Psychol 60:360–368, 1992

Prince M, Rabe-Hesketh S, Brennan P: Do antiarthritic drugs decrease the risk for cognitive decline? An analysis based on data from the MRC treatment trial of hypertension in older adults. Neurology 50:374–379, 1998

Raffaele KC, Berardi A, Asthana S, et al: Effects of long-term continuous infusion of the muscarinic cholinergic agonist arecoline on verbal memory in dementia of the Alzheimer type. Psychopharmacol Bull 27:315–319, 1991

Raine A, Lencz T, Bihrle S, et al: Reduced prefrontal gray matter volume and reduced autonomic activity in antisocial personality disorder. Arch Gen Psychiatry 57:119–127; discussion 128–129, 2000

Raji MA, Brady SR: Mirtazapine for treatment of depression and comorbidities in Alzheimer disease. Ann Pharmacother 35:1024–1027, 2001

Ramachandran G, Glickman L, Levenson J, et al: Incidence of extrapyramidal syndromes in AIDS patients and a comparison group of medically ill inpatients. J Neuropsychiatry Clin Neurosci 9:579–583, 1997

Rampello L, Chiechio S, Raffaele R, et al: The SSRI, citalopram, improves bradykinesia in patients with Parkinson's disease treated with L-dopa. Clin Neuropharmacol 25:21–24, 2002

Ranen NG, Peyser CE, Folstein SE: ECT as a treatment for depression in Huntington's disease. J Neuropsychiatry Clin Neurosci 6:154–159, 1994

Ranen NG, Lipsey JR, Treisman G, et al: Sertraline in the treatment of severe aggressiveness in Huntington's disease. J Neuropsychiatry Clin Neurosci 8:338–340, 1996

Rao N, Jellinek HM, Woolston DC: Agitation in closed head injury: haloperidol effects on rehabilitation outcome. Arch Phys Med Rehabil 66:30–34, 1985

Raskind MA: Geriatric psychopharmacology: management of late-life depression and the noncognitive behavioral disturbances of Alzheimer's disease. Psychiatr Clin North Am 16:815–827, 1993

Raskind MA, Peskind ER: Neurobiologic bases of noncognitive behavioral problems in Alzheimer disease. Alzheimer Dis Assoc Disord 8 (suppl 3):54–60, 1994

Rasmusson DX, Dal Forno G, Brandt J, et al: Apo-E genotype and verbal deficits in Alzheimer's disease. J Neuropsychiatry Clin Neurosci 8:335–337, 1996

Ratey J, Sovner R, Parks A, et al: Buspirone treatment of aggression and anxiety in mentally retarded patients: a multiple-baseline, placebo lead-in study. J Clin Psychiatry 52:159–162, 1991

Ratey JJ, Leveroni CL, Miller AC, et al: Low-dose buspirone to treat agitation and maladaptive behavior in brain-injured patients: two case reports. J Clin Psychopharmacol 12:362–364, 1992a

Ratey JJ, Sorgi P, O'Driscoll GA, et al: Nadolol to treat aggression and psychiatric symptomatology in chronic psychiatric inpatients: a double-blind, placebo-controlled study. J Clin Psychiatry 53:41–46, 1992b

Reddy S, Factor SA, Molho ES, et al: The effect of quetiapine on psychosis and motor function in parkinsonian patients with and without dementia. Mov Disord 17:676–681, 2002

Reding MJ, Orto LA, Winter SW, et al: Antidepressant therapy after stroke: a double-blind trial. Arch Neurol 43:763–765, 1986

Regan WM, Gordon SM: Gabapentin for behavioral agitation in Alzheimer's disease. J Clin Psychopharmacol 17:59–60, 1997

Reifler BV, Teri L, Raskind M, et al: Double-blind trial of imipramine in Alzheimer's disease patients with and without depression. Am J Psychiatry 146:45–49, 1989

Reisberg B, Doody R, Stoffler A, et al: Memantine in moderate-to-severe Alzheimer's disease. N Engl J Med 348:1333–1341, 2003

Reith J, Benkelfat C, Sherwin A, et al: Elevated dopa decarboxylase activity in living brain of patients with psychosis. Proc Natl Acad Sci U S A 91:11651–11654, 1994

Rektorova I, Rektor I, Bares M, et al: Pramipexole and pergolide in the treatment of depression in Parkinson's disease: a national multicentre prospective randomized study. Eur J Neurol 10:399–406, 2003

Remy P, Doder M, Lees A, et al: Depression in Parkinson's disease: loss of dopamine and noradrenaline innervation in the limbic system. Brain 128 (pt 6):1314–1322, 2005

Rich JB, Rasmusson DX, Folstein MF, et al: Nonsteroidal anti-inflammatory drugs in Alzheimer's disease. Neurology 45:51–55, 1995

Rinne JO, Rummukainen J, Paljarvi L, et al: Dementia in Parkinson's disease is related to neuronal loss in the medial substantia nigra. Ann Neurol 26:47–50, 1989a

Rinne JO, Rummukainen J, Paljarvi L, et al: Neuronal loss in the substantia nigra in patients with Alzheimer's disease and Parkinson's disease in relation to extrapyramidal symptoms and dementia. Prog Clin Biol Res 317:325–332, 1989b

Roane DM, Feinberg TE, Meckler L, et al: Treatment of dementia-associated agitation with gabapentin. J Neuropsychiatry Clin Neurosci 12:40–43, 2000

Roberts GW, Done DJ, Bruton C, et al: A "mock up" of schizophrenia: temporal lobe epilepsy and schizophrenia-like psychosis. Biol Psychiatry 28:127–143, 1990

Robinson RG: Neuropsychiatric consequences of stroke. Annu Rev Med 48:217–229, 1997

Robinson RG, Starkstein SE: Mood disorders following stroke: new findings and future directions. J Geriatr Psychiatry 22:1–15, 1989

Robinson RG, Parikh RM, Lipsey JR, et al: Pathological laughing and crying following stroke: validation of a measurement scale and a double-blind treatment study. Am J Psychiatry 150:286–293, 1993

Robinson RG, Schultz SK, Castillo C, et al: Nortriptyline versus fluoxetine in the treatment of depression and in short-term recovery after stroke: a placebo-controlled, double-blind study. Am J Psychiatry 157:351–359, 2000

Rogers J, Kirby LC, Hempelman SR, et al: Clinical trial of indomethacin in Alzheimer's disease. Neurology 43:1609–1611, 1993

Rogers SL, Farlow MR, Doody RS, et al: A 24-week, double-blind, placebo-controlled trial of donepezil in patients with Alzheimer's disease. Donepezil Study Group. Neurology 50:136–145, 1998

Rogers SL, Doody RS, Pratt RD, et al: Long-term efficacy and safety of donepezil in the treatment of Alzheimer's disease: final analysis of a US multicentre open-label study. Eur Neuropsychopharmacol 10:195–203, 2000

Roose SP, Bone S, Haidorfer C, et al: Lithium treatment in older patients. Am J Psychiatry 136:843–844, 1979

Rosler M, Retz W, Retz-Junginger P, et al: Effects of two-year treatment with the cholinesterase inhibitor rivastigmine on behavioural symptoms in Alzheimer's disease. Behav Neurol 11:211–216, 1998

Rosler M, Anand R, Cicin-Sain A, et al: Efficacy and safety of rivastigmine in patients with Alzheimer's disease: international randomised controlled trial. BMJ 318:633–638, 1999

Rosse RB, Riggs RL, Dietrich AM, et al: Frontal cortical atrophy and negative symptoms in patients with chronic alcohol dependence. J Neuropsychiatry Clin Neurosci 9:280–282, 1997

Roth M, Mountjoy CQ, Amrein R: Moclobemide in elderly patients with cognitive decline and depression: an international double-blind, placebo-controlled trial. Br J Psychiatry 168:149–157, 1996

Rudorfer MV, Manji HK, Potter WZ: ECT and delirium in Parkinson's disease. Am J Psychiatry 149:1758–1759; author reply 1759–1760, 1992

Ruedrich SL: Beta adrenergic blocking medications for treatment of rage outbursts in mentally retarded persons. Semin Clin Neuropsychiatry 1:115–121, 1996

Ruedrich S, Swales TP, Fossaceca C, et al: Effect of divalproex sodium on aggression and self-injurious behaviour in adults with intellectual disability: a retrospective review. J Intellect Disabil Res 43 (pt 2):105–111, 1999

Rush AJ, Marangell LB, Sackeim HA, et al: Vagus nerve stimulation for treatment-resistant depression: a randomized, controlled acute phase trial. Biol Psychiatry 58:347–354, 2005

Russouw HG, Roberts MC, Emsley RA, et al: Psychiatric manifestations and magnetic resonance imaging in HIV-negative neurosyphilis. Biol Psychiatry 41:467–473, 1997

Saba G, Rocamora JF, Kalalou K, et al: Repetitive transcranial magnetic stimulation as an add-on therapy in the treatment of mania: a case series of eight patients. Psychiatry Res 128:199–202, 2004

Sabatini U, Pozzilli C, Pantano P, et al: Involvement of the limbic system in multiple sclerosis patients with depressive disorders. Biol Psychiatry 39:970–975, 1996

Sachdev P: Schizophrenia-like psychosis and epilepsy: the status of the association. Am J Psychiatry 155:325–336, 1998

Sacristan JA, Iglesias C, Arellano F, et al: Absence seizures induced by lithium: possible interaction with fluoxetine. Am J Psychiatry 148:146–147, 1991

Salloway SP: Diagnosis and treatment of patients with "frontal lobe" syndromes. J Neuropsychiatry Clin Neurosci 6:388–398, 1994

Salzman C: Treatment of the elderly agitated patient. J Clin Psychiatry 48(suppl):19–22, 1987

Salzman C: Treatment of agitation, anxiety, and depression in dementia. Psychopharmacol Bull 24:39–42, 1988

Salzman C: Cognitive improvement after benzodiazepine discontinuation (letter). J Clin Psychopharmacol 20:99, 2000

Sanders JF: Evaluation of oxazepam and placebo in emotionally disturbed aged patients. Geriatrics 20:739–746, 1965

Sano M, Ernesto C, Thomas RG, et al: A controlled trial of selegiline, alpha-tocopherol, or both as treatment for Alzheimer's disease. The Alzheimer's Disease Cooperative Study. N Engl J Med 336:1216–1222, 1997

Scharf S, Mander A, Ugoni A, et al: A double-blind, placebo-controlled trial of diclofenac/misoprostol in Alzheimer's disease. Neurology 53:197–201, 1999

Schatzberg AF, Nemeroff CB (eds): The American Psychiatric Press Textbook of Psychopharmacology, 2nd Edition. Washington, DC, American Psychiatric Press, 1998

Schiffer RB, Wineman NM: Antidepressant pharmacotherapy of depression associated with multiple sclerosis. Am J Psychiatry 147:1493–1497, 1990

Schiffer RB, Herndon RM, Rudick RA: Treatment of pathologic laughing and weeping with amitriptyline. N Engl J Med 312:1480–1482, 1985

Schiffer RB, Wineman NM, Weitkamp LR: Association between bipolar affective disorder and multiple sclerosis. Am J Psychiatry 143:94–95, 1986

Schneider LS, Olin JT: Overview of clinical trials of hydergine in dementia. Arch Neurol 51:787–798, 1994

Schneider LS, Pollock VE, Zemansky MF, et al: A pilot study of low-dose L-deprenyl in Alzheimer's disease. J Geriatr Psychiatry Neurol 4:143–148, 1991

Schneider LS, Dagerman KS, Insel P: Risk of death with atypical antipsychotic drug treatment for dementia: meta-analysis of randomized placebo-controlled trials. JAMA 294:1934–1943, 2005

Schreiber S, Klag E, Gross Y, et al: Beneficial effect of risperidone on sleep disturbance and psychosis following traumatic brain injury. Int Clin Psychopharmacol 13:273–275, 1998

Schuurman PR, Bosch DA, Bossuyt PM, et al: A comparison of continuous thalamic stimulation and thalamotomy for suppression of severe tremor. N Engl J Med 342:461–468, 2000

Schwartz BL, Hashtroudi S, Herting RL, et al: Glycine prodrug facilitates memory retrieval in humans. Neurology 41:1341–1343, 1991

Scott TF, Allen D, Price TR, et al: Characterization of major depression symptoms in multiple sclerosis patients. J Neuropsychiatry Clin Neurosci 8:318–323, 1996

Selemon LD, Goldman-Rakic PS: The reduced neuropil hypothesis: a circuit based model of schizophrenia. Biol Psychiatry 45:17–25, 1999

Sewell DD, Jeste DV, Atkinson JH, et al: HIV-associated psychosis: a study of 20 cases. San Diego HIV Neurobehavioral Research Center Group. Am J Psychiatry 151:237–242, 1994a

Sewell DD, Jeste DV, McAdams LA, et al: Neuroleptic treatment of HIV-associated psychosis. HNRC group. Neuropsychopharmacology 10:223–229, 1994b

Shapiro RM: Regional neuropathology in schizophrenia: where are we? Where are we going? Schizophr Res 10:187–239, 1993

Shaywitz BA, Shaywitz SE: Estrogen and Alzheimer disease: plausible theory, negative clinical trial. JAMA 283:1055–1056, 2000

Shimoda K, Robinson RG: Effects of anxiety disorder on impairment and recovery from stroke. J Neuropsychiatry Clin Neurosci 10:34–40, 1998

Silver JM, Yudofsky SC, Slater JA, et al: Propranolol treatment of chronically hospitalized aggressive patients. J Neuropsychiatry Clin Neurosci 11:328–335, 1999

Simpson DM, Foster D: Improvement in organically disturbed behavior with trazodone treatment. J Clin Psychiatry 47:191–193, 1986

Simpson S, Baldwin RC, Jackson A, et al: The differentiation of DSM-III-R psychotic depression in later life from nonpsychotic depression: comparisons of brain changes measured by multispectral analysis of magnetic resonance brain images, neuropsychological findings, and clinical features. Biol Psychiatry 45:193–204, 1999

Singh AN, Golledge H, Catalan J: Treatment of HIV-related psychotic disorders with risperidone: a series of 21 cases. J Psychosom Res 42:489–493, 1997

Sink KM, Holden KF, Yaffe K: Pharmacological treatment of neuropsychiatric symptoms of dementia: a review of the evidence. JAMA 293:596–608, 2005

Sival RC, Haffmans PM, Jansen PA, et al: Sodium valproate in the treatment of aggressive behavior in patients with dementia—a randomized placebo controlled clinical trial. Int J Geriatr Psychiatry 17:579–585, 2002

Sloan RL, Brown KW, Pentland B: Fluoxetine as a treatment for emotional lability after brain injury. Brain Inj 6:315–319, 1992

Slooter AJ, Bronzova J, Witteman JC, et al: Estrogen use and early onset Alzheimer's disease: a population-based study. J Neurol Neurosurg Psychiatry 67:779–781, 1999

Smith RE, Helms PM: Adverse effects of lithium therapy in the acutely ill elderly patient. J Clin Psychiatry 43:94–99, 1982

Sobin P, Schneider L, McDermott H: Fluoxetine in the treatment of agitated dementia (letter). Am J Psychiatry 146:1636, 1989

Sovner R: The use of valproate in the treatment of mentally retarded persons with typical and atypical bipolar disorders. J Clin Psychiatry 50(suppl):40–43, 1989

Spalletta G, Caltagirone C: Sertraline treatment of post-stroke major depression: an open study in patients with moderate to severe symptoms. Funct Neurol 18:227–232, 2003

Specchio LM, Iudice A, Specchio N, et al: Citalopram as treatment of depression in patients with epilepsy. Clin Neuropharmacol 27:133–136, 2004

Spiers PA, Myers D, Hochanadel GS, et al: Citicoline improves verbal memory in aging. Arch Neurol 53:441–448, 1996

Squire LR, Zola-Morgan S: The medial temporal lobe memory system. Science 253:1380–1386, 1991

Stanford MS, Helfritz LE, Conklin SM, et al: A comparison of anticonvulsants in the treatment of impulsive aggression. Exp Clin Psychopharmacol 13:72–77, 2005

Starkstein SE, Migliorelli R: ECT in a patient with a frontal craniotomy and residual meningioma. J Neuropsychiatry Clin Neurosci 5:428–430, 1993

Starkstein SE, Robinson RG: Mechanism of disinhibition after brain lesions. J Nerv Ment Dis 185:108–114, 1997

Starkstein SE, Cohen BS, Fedoroff P, et al: Relationship between anxiety disorders and depressive disorders in patients with cerebrovascular injury. Arch Gen Psychiatry 47:246–251, 1990

Starkstein SE, Fedoroff P, Berthier ML, et al: Manic-depressive and pure manic states after brain lesions. Biol Psychiatry 29:149–158, 1991

Starkstein SE, Migliorelli R, Teson A, et al: Specificity of changes in cerebral blood flow in patients with frontal lobe dementia. J Neurol Neurosurg Psychiatry 57:790–796, 1994

Stefurak T, Mikulis D, Mayberg H, et al: Deep brain stimulation for Parkinson's disease dissociates mood and motor circuits: a functional MRI case study. Mov Disord 18:1508–1516, 2003

Strakowski SM, Adler CM, DelBello MP: Volumetric MRI studies of mood disorders: do they distinguish unipolar and bipolar disorder? Bipolar Disord 4:80–88, 2002

Strang RR: Imipramine in treatment of parkinsonism: a double-blind placebo study. BMJ 5452:33–34, 1965

Strauss ME, Lee MM, DiFilippo JM: Premorbid personality and behavioral symptoms in Alzheimer disease: some cautions. Arch Neurol 54:257–259, 1997

Street JS, Clark WS, Gannon KS, et al: Olanzapine treatment of psychotic and behavioral symptoms in patients with Alzheimer disease in nursing care facilities: a double-blind, randomized, placebo-controlled trial. The HGEU Study Group. Arch Gen Psychiatry 57:968–976, 2000

Sultzer DL, Gray KF, Gunay I, et al: A double-blind comparison of trazodone and haloperidol for treatment of agitation in patients with dementia. Am J Geriatr Psychiatry 5:60–69, 1997

Sunderland T, Merril CR, Harrington MG, et al: Reduced plasma dehydroepiandrosterone concentrations in Alzheimer's disease (letter). Lancet 2:570, 1989

Suzuki M, Yuasa S, Minabe Y, et al: Left superior temporal blood flow increases in schizophrenic and schizophreniform patients with auditory hallucination: a longitudinal case study using 123I-IMP SPECT. Eur Arch Psychiatry Clin Neurosci 242:257–261, 1993

Swartz BE, Halgren E, Simpkins F, et al: Primary or working memory in frontal lobe epilepsy: an 18FDG-PET study of dysfunctional zones. Neurology 46:737–747, 1996

Swartz JR, Miller BL, Lesser IM, et al: Frontotemporal dementia: treatment response to serotonin selective reuptake inhibitors. J Clin Psychiatry 58:212–216, 1997

Sweet RA, Nimgaonkar VL, Kamboh MI, et al: Dopamine receptor genetic variation, psychosis, and aggression in Alzheimer disease. Arch Neurol 55:1335–1340, 1998

Tan I, Dorevitch M: Emotional incontinence: a dramatic response to paroxetine (letter). Aust N Z J Med 26:844, 1996

Tandberg E, Larsen JP, Aarsland D, et al: Risk factors for depression in Parkinson disease. Arch Neurol 54:625–630, 1997

Taragano FE, Lyketsos CG, Mangone CA, et al: A double-blind, randomized, fixed-dose trial of fluoxetine vs. amitriptyline in the treatment of major depression complicating Alzheimer's disease. Psychosomatics 38:246–252, 1997

Targum SD, Abbott JL: Efficacy of quetiapine in Parkinson's patients with psychosis. J Clin Psychopharmacol 20:54–60, 2000

Tariot PN, Erb R, Podgorski CA, et al: Efficacy and tolerability of carbamazepine for agitation and aggression in dementia. Am J Psychiatry 155:54–61, 1998a

Tariot PN, Goldstein B, Podgorski CA, et al: Short-term administration of selegiline for mild-to-moderate dementia of the Alzheimer's type. Am J Geriatr Psychiatry 6:145–154, 1998b

Tariot PN, Farlow MR, Grossberg GT, et al: Memantine treatment in patients with moderate to severe Alzheimer disease already receiving donepezil: a randomized controlled trial. JAMA 291:317–324, 2004a

Tariot PN, Profenno LA, Ismail MS: Efficacy of atypical antipsychotics in elderly patients with dementia. J Clin Psychiatry 65 (suppl 11):11–15, 2004b

Tariot PN, Raman R, Jakimovich L, et al: Divalproex sodium in nursing home residents with possible or probable Alzheimer disease complicated by agitation: a randomized, controlled trial. Am J Geriatr Psychiatry 13:942–949, 2005

Taylor WD, MacFall JR, Steffens DC, et al: Localization of age-associated white matter hyperintensities in late-life depression. Prog Neuropsychopharmacol Biol Psychiatry 27:539–544, 2003

Tennant FS Jr, Wild J: Naltrexone treatment for postconcussional syndrome. Am J Psychiatry 144:813–814, 1987

The Deep Brain Stimulation for Parkinson's Disease Study Group: Deep-brain stimulation of the subthalamic nucleus or the pars interna of the globus pallidus in Parkinson's disease. N Engl J Med 345:956–963, 2001

The Expert Consensus Panel for Agitation in Dementia: Treatment of agitation in older persons with dementia. Postgrad Med Spec No:1–88, 1998

The Parkinson Study Group: Low-dose clozapine for the treatment of drug-induced psychosis in Parkinson's disease. N Engl J Med 340:757–763, 1999

Thompson TL 2nd, Filley CM, Mitchell WD, et al: Lack of efficacy of hydergine in patients with Alzheimer's disease. N Engl J Med 323:445–448, 1990

Tiller JW, Dakis JA, Shaw JM: Short-term buspirone treatment in disinhibition with dementia (letter). Lancet 2:510, 1988

Tollefson GD: Short-term effects of the calcium channel blocker nimodipine (Bay-e-9736) in the management of primary degenerative dementia. Biol Psychiatry 27:1133–1142, 1990

Tollefson GD, Greist JH, Jefferson JW, et al: Is baseline agitation a relative contraindication for a selective serotonin reuptake inhibitor: a comparative trial of fluoxetine versus imipramine. J Clin Psychopharmacol 14:385–391, 1994

Tonkonogy JM: Violence and temporal lobe lesion: head CT and MRI data. J Neuropsychiatry Clin Neurosci 3:189–196, 1991

Tsai GE, Yang P, Chung LC, et al: D-serine added to clozapine for the treatment of schizophrenia. Am J Psychiatry 156:1822–1825, 1999

Tsai WC, Lai JS, Wang TG: Treatment of emotionalism with fluoxetine during rehabilitation. Scand J Rehabil Med 30:145–149, 1998

Tune L, Carr S, Hoag E, et al: Anticholinergic effects of drugs commonly prescribed for the elderly: potential means for assessing risk of delirium. Am J Psychiatry 149:1393–1394, 1992

Turner-Stokes L, Hassan N, Pierce K, et al: Managing depression in brain injury rehabilitation: the use of an integrated care pathway and preliminary report of response to sertraline. Clin Rehabil 16:261–268, 2002

Tyor WR, Glass JD, Griffin JW, et al: Cytokine expression in the brain during the acquired immunodeficiency syndrome. Ann Neurol 31:349–360, 1992

van Dyck CH, McMahon TJ, Rosen MI, et al: Sustained-release methylphenidate for cognitive impairment in HIV-1-infected drug abusers: a pilot study. J Neuropsychiatry Clin Neurosci 9:29–36, 1997

Van Reekum R, Bayley M, Garner S, et al: N of 1 study: amantadine for the amotivational syndrome in a patient with traumatic brain injury. Brain Inj 9:49–53, 1995

van Vugt JP, Siesling S, Vergeer M, et al: Clozapine versus placebo in Huntington's disease: a double blind randomised comparative study. J Neurol Neurosurg Psychiatry 63:35–39, 1997

van Woerkom TC, Teelken AW, Minderhous JM: Difference in neurotransmitter metabolism in frontotemporal-lobe contusion and diffuse cerebral contusion. Lancet 1:812–813, 1977

Verhoeven WM, Tuinier S: The effect of buspirone on challenging behaviour in mentally retarded patients: an open prospective multiple-case study. J Intellect Disabil Res 40 (pt 6):502–508, 1996

Victoroff J, Zarow C, Mack WJ, et al: Physical aggression is associated with preservation of substantia nigra pars compacta in Alzheimer disease. Arch Neurol 53:428–434, 1996

Walker Z, Grace J, Overshot R, et al: Olanzapine in dementia with Lewy bodies: a clinical study. Int J Geriatr Psychiatry 14:459–466, 1999

Watanabe MD, Martin EM, DeLeon OA, et al: Successful methylphenidate treatment of apathy after subcortical infarcts. J Neuropsychiatry Clin Neurosci 7:502–504, 1995

Weilburg JB, Schachter S, Worth J, et al: EEG abnormalities in patients with atypical panic attacks. J Clin Psychiatry 56:358–362, 1995

Weinshenker BG, Penman M, Bass B, et al: A double-blind, randomized, crossover trial of pemoline in fatigue associated with multiple sclerosis. Neurology 42:1468–1471, 1992

Weitzner MA, Meyers CA, Valentine AD: Methylphenidate in the treatment of neurobehavioral slowing associated with cancer and cancer treatment. J Neuropsychiatry Clin Neurosci 7:347–350, 1995

Welch J, Manschreck T, Redmond D: Clozapine-induced seizures and EEG changes. J Neuropsychiatry Clin Neurosci 6:250–256, 1994

Wermuth L, Sorensen PS, Timm B, et al: Depression in idiopathic Parkinson's disease treated with citalopram: a placebo controlled trial. Nord J Psychiatry 52:163–169, 1998

White JC, Christensen JF, Singer CM: Methylphenidate as a treatment for depression in acquired immunodeficiency syndrome: an n-of-1 trial. J Clin Psychiatry 53:153–156, 1992

Wiart L, Petit H, Joseph PA, et al: Fluoxetine in early poststroke depression: a double-blind placebo-controlled study. Stroke 31:1829–1832, 2000

Wijnen HH, van der Heijden FM, van Schendel FM, et al: Quetiapine in the elderly with parkinsonism and psychosis. Eur Psychiatry 18:372–373, 2003

Wilcock GK: Treatment for Alzheimer's disease. Int J Geriatr Psychiatry 15:562–565, 2000

Wilkie FL, Goodkin K, Eisdorfer C, et al: Mild cognitive impairment and risk of mortality in HIV-1 infection. J Neuropsychiatry Clin Neurosci 10:125–132, 1998

Wilkinson D, Murray J: Galantamine: a randomized, double-blind, dose comparison in patients with Alzheimer's disease. Int J Geriatr Psychiatry 16:852–857, 2001

Wilkinson D, Doody R, Helme R, et al: Donepezil in vascular dementia: a randomized, placebo-controlled study. Neurology 61:479–486, 2003

Williams JB, Rabkin JG, Remien RH, et al: Multidisciplinary baseline assessment of homosexual men with and without human immunodeficiency virus infection, II: standardized clinical assessment of current and lifetime psychopathology. Arch Gen Psychiatry 48:124–130, 1991

Wong SE, Woolsey JE, Innocent AJ, et al: Behavioral treatment of violent psychiatric patients. Psychiatr Clin North Am 11:569–580, 1988

Wroblewski BA, McColgan K, Smith K, et al: The incidence of seizures during tricyclic antidepressant drug treatment in a brain-injured population. J Clin Psychopharmacol 10:124–128, 1990

Wroblewski BA, Leary JM, Phelan AM, et al: Methylphenidate and seizure frequency in brain injured patients with seizure disorders. J Clin Psychiatry 53:86–89, 1992

Wroblewski BA, Joseph AB, Cornblatt RR: Antidepressant pharmacotherapy and the treatment of depression in patients with severe traumatic brain injury: a controlled, prospective study. J Clin Psychiatry 57:582–587, 1996

Wroblewski BA, Joseph AB, Kupfer J, et al: Effectiveness of valproic acid on destructive and aggressive behaviours in patients with acquired brain injury. Brain Inj 11:37–47, 1997

Yatham LN, McHale PA: Carbamazepine in the treatment of aggression: a case report and a review of the literature. Acta Psychiatr Scand 78:188–190, 1988

Yudofsky SC, Silver JM, Jackson W, et al: The Overt Aggression Scale for the objective rating of verbal and physical aggression. Am J Psychiatry 143:35–39, 1986

Yudofsky SC, Silver JM, Schneider SE: Pharmacologic treatment of aggression. Psychiatr Ann 17:397–407, 1987

Zarcone JR, Hellings JA, Crandall K, et al: Effects of risperidone on aberrant behavior of persons with developmental disabilities, I: a double-blind crossover study using multiple measures. Am J Ment Retard 106:525–538, 2001

Zarcone JR, Lindauer SE, Morse PS, et al: Effects of risperidone on destructive behavior of persons with developmental disabilities, III: functional analysis. Am J Ment Retard 109:310–321, 2004

Zimnitzky BM, DeMaso DR, Steingard RJ: Use of risperidone in psychotic disorder following ischemic brain damage. J Child Adolesc Psychopharmacol 6:75–78, 1996

Zisook S, Peterkin J, Goggin KJ, et al: Treatment of major depression in HIV-seropositive men. HIV Neurobehavioral Research Center Group. J Clin Psychiatry 59:217–224, 1998

Zoldan J, Friedberg G, Livneh M, et al: Psychosis in advanced Parkinson's disease: treatment with ondansetron, a 5-HT$_3$ receptor antagonist. Neurology 45:1305–1308, 1995

Zubenko GS, Moossy J: Major depression in primary dementia: clinical and neuropathologic correlates. Arch Neurol 45:1182–1186, 1988

Zubenko GS, Moossy J, Kopp U: Neurochemical correlates of major depression in primary dementia. Arch Neurol 47:209–214, 1990

Zubenko GS, Moossy J, Martinez AJ, et al: Neuropathologic and neurochemical correlates of psychosis in primary dementia. Arch Neurol 48:619–624, 1991

Zubieta JK, Alessi NE: Acute and chronic administration of trazodone in the treatment of disruptive behavior disorders in children. J Clin Psychopharmacol 12:346–351, 1992

32

PSYCHOTHERAPY FOR PATIENTS WITH NEUROPSYCHIATRIC DISORDERS

David V. Forrest, M.D.

Preston McLean (1959, p. 1765), writing about the philosophy of psychiatry and anticipating similar remarks by Kendler (2005), pointed out that there are many pseudoconflicts in psychiatry and that "there is no genuine opposition between science and common sense." No longer in dualistic conflict, the neurological and psychiatric domains are increasingly viewed as a mutually interacting continuum, and neurologists and psychiatrists agree that ideally they should be addressed together in an empathic manner. Pressures on physicians from medical payment organizations currently not only marginalize and limit empathic care but also tend to deprive patients of their foremost asset in responding to the challenge of illness: the sense of control of their own care. Although this decreases morale in all illnesses, neuropsychiatric patients are especially threatened by losses of control because, as this chapter shows, their conditions so typically and devastatingly impair control.

As crucial as empathy is, or an awareness of the intersubjective relatedness of the minds of physician and patient, neuropsychiatry must be expertly informed by the knowledge of the natural and pathological processes of the brain. Just as contact with patients with gross neurological impairment helps us assess neurological abnormalities in

psychiatric patients, so, too, can familiarity with the needs of more impaired psychiatric patients—especially those with schizophrenia, organic mental disorders, and substance use disorders—help us frame a psychotherapeutic approach that is tailored to the cognitive and affective needs of patients with neurological disorders.

Many of the same mechanisms overlap in neurological and psychiatric conditions. Deep brain stimulation has been used to treat epilepsy, essential tremor, Tourette syndrome, dystonia, Parkinson's disease, obsessive-compulsive disorder, chronic pain, and depression—all disorders also exquisitely sensitive to emotional conditions and susceptible to psychotherapeutic interventions. Kanner (2004) noted that depression is a risk factor for, has similar structural and functional changes to, and negatively affects the course of neurological disorders such as Alzheimer's disease, epilepsy, Parkinson's disease, and stroke. Woods and Short (1985) found that 50% of 270 newly admitted patients with major psychiatric disorders had neurological abnormalities, and Schiffer (1983) established psychiatric diagnoses in 41.9% of 241 neurology patients. Thus, in formulating an approach to neuropsychiatry, empathic medical psychotherapy techniques must be adapted to the specific neurological features of the patient.

PSYCHODYNAMIC ASPECTS OF THE MENTAL EXAMINATION

Structured examinations and formal neuropsychological testing do not bring out the information necessary to formulate a comprehensive treatment plan and only hint at the difficulties that will be encountered as the psychiatrist adjusts the treatment to an individual's treatment course. At some point, the checklist is set aside, and a shift is made to a psychodynamically oriented interview with ample open-ended questions that will enable the psychiatrist to appreciate each patient's unique personality and affective qualities. Such an interview should provide an understanding of the hereditary, constitutional, developmental, experiential, and interpersonal contributions to the formation of personality structure and the major traumata and conflicts the patient has encountered along the way. The effect of the illness is assessed similarly and placed in the context of the person's longitudinal history. The psychiatrist goes beyond assessing the elements of function, as in physical medicine, and is interested in the operational aspects of how the patient will fare while at home and at work, as in rehabilitation medicine.

The administration of any structured mental examination marks a shift away from a psychotherapeutic relatedness to the patient toward an evaluative mode that always has a distancing effect and sometimes is experienced as threatening by the patient. The analogy to the physical examination is not complete because the patient's very ability to make sense of the proceedings is being questioned. This is a time for warmth and reassurance on the part of the examiner, which pay the scientific dividend of eliciting the patient's best performance. The patient may experience emotions as strong as self-loathing and humiliation, depending on the deficits involved and the degree of investment in the integrity of those functions.

The examining psychiatrist must ensure that a methodical approach is not mistaken by the patient for scorn and must avoid a smug supplying of the correct answers, which could be taken for an air of superiority. Seemingly "playing to the crowd" at the patient's expense, whether before assembled family or in front of residents and medical students, is to be scrupulously avoided. Sympathetic recognition of all deficits should be directed first to the patient. Even complex concepts such as the operationally crucial faculty of constructional ability can be evaluated empathetically. For example, the psychiatrist may ask, "Has it been difficult lately to plan your day or to grasp the overall picture in complicated situations? Have you noticed difficulty in getting things together to do something?"

CONTACT IN NEUROPSYCHIATRIC PATIENTS

On entering the patient's room, the psychiatrist should be aware that impairments in the patient's hierarchy of capacities are likely to impede any beneficial encounter between patient and physician in specific ways that require adaptations and compensations in psychotherapeutic technique. In general, each capacity listed in Table 32–1 is dependent on the integrity of those that precede it.

DEFENSES: THE NEUROPSYCHODYNAMIC CONTINUUM

The psychiatrist who is well trained in psychodynamic psychotherapy brings to the study of defense mechanisms in neuropsychiatry a relevant but incomplete description. Defenses are psychodynamic mechanisms used by a person interacting with the surprises and dangers of the world and with drives and emotions from within. Traditionally, defenses have been classified on a dimension from the most mature to the most immature (Forrest 1980). The most mature defenses (such as sublimation, suppression, and laughter) are viewed as the healthiest ones. Less mature defenses (such as reaction formation, rationalization, displacement, and isolation) are thought to be characteristic of a neurotic level of function. The most immature defenses (such as denial, splitting, merging, projection, and projective identification) are considered the most unhealthy, typifying psychotic functioning. Although psychodynamic theory originally recognized a somatic contribution to the mental defenses, it did not specify which mental defenses are associated with organic impairment or how the defenses are related to organic processes.

In approaching defenses in neuropsychiatry, parallels may be sought between the mental mechanisms of defense and defensive brain (or cortical) reactions. At the very least, patient and family can be helped to see which defensive reactions are exacerbations of characterological armor (under varying degrees of voluntary control and amenable to interpretation) and which are more primitive, automatic defenses of an injured brain that may be compensated for by tolerant understanding and environmental manipulation. Between these two extremes lie defensive formations that are rooted in both psyche and brain. Finally, one must not assume that a learning process is absent in cortical defenses, so that improvement occurs only with spontaneous recovery, or that the mental defenses always have a plasticity that is completely reeducable by psychotherapy.

Comparisons on the basis of operational principles may be made among cortical defenses, mental defenses, and a bridging area of what might be termed *neuropsychic*

TABLE 32–2. Neuropsychiatric defense continuum *(continued)*

Continuum	Mental defenses	Neuromental defenses	Cortical reactions
Impaired world view	"My relationship to the world has changed."	"The world is bigger, harder to deal with, more confusing," or (in schizophrenia) more aesthetically awesome	"The world has been changed, reduplicated, substituted" in patients with brain injury
Impaired view of others	Transference reactions: "It's I who have changed, my perceptions differ because I'm injured"; degrees of insight; interpersonal shallowness and manipulativeness	Misidentification: "People have changed, are different, are to blame, have been replaced by impostors"; splitting and projective identification; "underlying defect" in borderline syndrome of failure of delineation	Prosopagnosia: state-dependent change in cognition of people or their relation to self
Sex object shift	Avoidance of parental object to preserve ties to family	Failure to integrate affects and sexuality	Failure to differentiate sexual object (Klüver-Bucy syndrome of bilateral hippocampal damage) or own gender
Impaired ego boundary	Creativity and regression in the service of the ego	Disturbing nightmares, other vulnerability to internal and external processes, and schizophrenia	Diminished stimulus barrier
Impairment of conation or will	Identification with the aggressor, and introjection and incorporation in health, neurosis, and depression	Made cognition, made volition, and command hallucinations in schizophrenia	Echolalia, echopraxia, and involuntary reflex activity in brain injury
Impaired movement or spatial play	Disorientation, agoraphobia, diminished sense of mastery and mobility and of bodily feedback and control, and lowered confidence in actions	Vestibular defensiveness, fear of moving, fear of falling or of whirling (twirling a soft sign in children), incoordination, and clumsiness	Vertigo, motor or proprioceptive impairment, incoordination, poor eye tracking, ataxia, and tremor

whereas in schizophrenia, cognitive and linguistic elements—often exaggerated and fanciful—are recruited to compensate for poor command of affects, and the result often frustrates interpersonal sense. The abnormally small thalamus visualized by Andreasen et al. (1994) through magnetic resonance imaging (MRI) averaging is in keeping with the basic schizophrenic difficulty with attaching affective valuations to (and thereby organizing) thoughts, sensations, and perceptions (Forrest 1983a, 1983d).

BASIC APPROACHES TO NEUROPSYCHIATRIC PATIENTS

The neuropsychiatrist must be crucially attuned to nuances of a patient's affect. One's own perception of affect can be

calibrated against the highly reliable means of affect scoring of short videotaped interview segments by professional audiences (Forrest 2003) or any peer group. The six general affect categories—joy, fear, anger, shame, guilt, and sadness—can each be rated on a scale of 0 to 4+, like any other medical measurement. At the beginning of an interview, the patient's more specific manifest affect (e.g., under anger, boredom, irritation, annoyance) can be read and reflected back as the single most powerful means of establishing rapport. Patients may show several emotions in one interview. For example, a middle-aged man who has had a small stroke may feel joyous relief at his progressing recovery, fear of extension or recurrence, anger at discomfort of hospital procedures, shame at his altered appearance, guilt that illness has interrupted his breadwinning and hopes for raises, and sad-

TABLE 32–3.   Modalities of psychotherapy in neuropsychiatry

Helpful aspects of the psychoanalytic approach for neuropsychiatry

1. Respect for the patient's autonomy and self-determination

2. Theoretical concept of defense organization

3. Most sufficient map of mental, cognitive, and emotional function

4. Model based on conflict among mental structures

5. Emphasis on shared meaning, attunement, affirmative empathy, intersubjective awareness, and emotions in general (Anshin 1995)

Inappropriate aspects of the psychoanalytic approach for neuropsychiatry

1. Too passive a receptiveness rather than making affective contact

2. Too much reliance on free association and dreams

3. Search for remote causes and relationships

4. Attribution of treatment events to abstract forces and entities in talking to patients

5. Overemphasis on transference versus reality issues

6. Intentional lack of frames and structures

7. Interpersonal relationships considered as inner object relations

8. Avoidance of direct answers or being a "blank screen" rather than being a beacon to security

9. Use of the couch, which is powerful, disorienting, and emotionally abandoning (Forrest 2004b)

Other modalities of psychotherapy in neuropsychiatry

1. Behaviorist approaches to the patient's learning system as a black box may be helpful in structuring relearning, but they are "brainless" in their theoretic avoidance of capacities, defenses, conflicts, recruitment of affect to aid cognition, and other neuromental dynamics that are helpful in explanation.

2. Interpersonal and family approaches are surprisingly helpful communication systems despite the clear nidus of difficulty in a neuropathologically "designated patient" because of the effect on relatives and their involvement in the care of the patient's disabilities. Often lacking the hereditary and imitative influences found in neurotic, characterological, and major psychiatric disorders, the families of patients with acquired neuropsychiatric disorders may themselves be less disordered and more of a help in the treatment.

3. Cognitive approaches help in an educative way to spell out the "baby steps" that need to be accomplished to achieve complex goals, but to work better, they require attention to intersubjective emotions, conflicts, and goals.

ness at the loss of his sense of youthful invulnerability and bodily integrity. A common error in treating impaired brain function is not adjusting one's own projection of emotional tone to the patient's needs (Forrest 1983b). For example, patients with hyperemotionalism (as in pseudobulbar cases) may require neuropsychiatrists to throttle down their own emotions. But the challenge for most neuropsychiatrists is to *increase* the benevolent emotion they project toward certain patients who for various reasons are receiving signals poorly (as in apathetic patients). Psychotherapy in neuropsychiatry should be eclectic, adapting elements that are helpful from various modalities (Table 32–3).

The varieties of personality characteristics and defenses (obsessive, histrionic, paranoid, depressive, hypo-

manic, phobic, counterphobic, sociopathic, schizoid, narcissistic) that are used in prescribing medications psychodynamically (Forrest 2004a, 2004c) are also discernible in neuropsychiatric patients and can guide therapy.

Finally, Vaillant (2003) and Bromley (2005) have tried to describe positive mental health as strengths, the obverse of psychopathology, preferring the concept of resilience to concepts of superiority, positivism, maturity, sociability, and subjective well-being. I agree that resilience is less controversial but is relative to the burdens suffered and have called for new categories of "offenses," or capabilities for taking on challenges such as neuropsychiatric illness (Forrest 2005a), in addition to defenses.

TRAUMATIC BRAIN INJURY

Traumatic brain injury results principally from vehicular accidents, falls, acts of violence, and sports injuries and is more than twice as likely to occur in men as in women. The highest incidence is among persons ages 15–24 years and 75 years or older, with a less striking peak in children age 5 years or younger (National Institutes of Health Consensus Development Panel 1999). Thus, these patients may not be very mature, resilient, or resourceful.

Childs (1985) stated that the most difficult sequelae of head injury to treat are the psychosocial disabilities; impaired cognition is next in degree of difficulty, and impaired physical abilities are the least difficult. Also, perhaps contrary to common assumption, the patient's family suffers most severely from the disruption of emotions and object relations, next most from the intellectual impairments, and least from the physical impairments. For these reasons, psychotherapy can play a crucial role in individual and family recovery after head injury.

The emotional climate is worsened by the typical emergence of bad temper in the patient 3 or more months after the injury. The family's optimism that full recovery will occur, based on successes in physical rehabilitation, turns to disappointment when the patient's impulse control worsens. The doctors often bear the transferred brunt of family anger. Interventions should aim at legitimizing family disappointment and avoiding comments that abet the splitting. Unconscious or unacknowledged family anger at the patient for being injured contributes to the patient's internalized anger within the family system and must be addressed to head off severe self-loathing or suicidal trends as the protection of denial wears off.

Regression in the patient's mental processes may parallel neurological regression, and both mental and neuromental defenses parallel pathological brain reactions. Often, borderline or other organic personality disorders result that comprise an array roughly paralleling functional personality syndromes (Childs 1985). It is important to interview family and friends to determine the premorbid personality of the patient in calculating effects of injury, which may be easier to change.

Psychotherapeutic interventions optimally begin soon after the patient is hospitalized, and management of the emotional climate is crucial to recovery. Childs (1985) recommended placing a priority on the reestablishment of object constancy in cognitively impaired patients by staff members who are carefully selected for their lack of personal tension or anger and work one-on-one all day with each patient. This familiar and consistent other person enacts an early stage in cognitive retraining of a regressively lost relational skill. This is accomplished with a

TABLE 32–4. Measures to assist recovery of patients with brain injury

1. Relate interventions to family grieving stage (denial, anger, grief resolution).

2. Structure daily events to assist patient in internalizing routine and reestablishing circadian rhythms.

3. Establish positive rewards to reinforce responsible behavior; individualize rewards to what patient likes.

4. Approach disabilities with expectancy they will be overcome cheerfully, never as excuse for misbehavior.

5. Individualize treatment goals to patient's specific problems; for example, reward withdrawn frontal patients for conversation and reward aggressive patients for not reacting.

6. Break maladaptive habits by vigilance and restraint because motivation to become involved in positive change follows elimination of irresponsible behavior.

7. Orient family extensively to structure needed before discharge to home so that gains are maintained.

Source. Adapted from Berry 1984.

soothing voice and touch, with the limitation of talk to familiar subjects and to the patient only, and with the restriction of stimulation to a single channel. Later, active exercises include practice in following directions requiring progressively more sequential steps (Luria 1973), problem solving, and movement from the concrete to the abstract, retracing developmental steps and hoping for generalization of learning. Martelli et al. (1999) reported that posttraumatic headache, estimated to persist for 6 months in up to 44% of patients, exerts a significant negative effect on postconcussive adaptation and therefore should be managed. Other measures the psychiatrist should consider are summarized in Table 32–4.

Prigatano et al. (2003) suggested an approach to psychotherapy for traumatic brain injury organized under the mnemonic ICAR, which refers to providing *information* to restore hope and help the patient grasp the deficits, setting up *contingency* incentives to promote cooperative behavior; improving self-*awareness* and self-monitoring of behavior and recovering skills, and establishing a *relationship* in which the therapist can provide experiences that stimulate emotion but permit the patient self-mastery and constructive dealing with the emotion. The authors consider developing the therapeutic relationship to be a combination of art and science, requiring a knowledge of brain-behavior disturbances, an appreciation of psychodynamics and learning theory, and the ability to consider existential issues.

LANGUAGE AND OTHER PSYCHOTHERAPEUTIC CORRELATES

Verbal impairment to some degree is found in all patients with closed head injuries who have been referred to a rehabilitation medicine center. Sarno (1980) found that 32% of the patients with brain injury had classic aphasia, 38% had motor dysarthria, and 30% had no discernible aphasic deficit in spontaneous speech but clear evidence of verbal deficit on testing. Dysarthric patients, without exception, showed subclinical linguistic effects. Because psychotherapy depends on the use of language with an emotional dimension, the psychiatrist should be alert to subtle evidence of dysarthria, identify any linguistic problems, and consciously adapt the psychotherapeutic technique to the deficit in the particular patient.

The task of psychotherapy for the patient with brain damage is to assess his or her capability for each step in the cognitive sequence of defenses against threat, to help break down difficult steps into subroutines, and to assist in bridging gaps with the psychiatrist's own analytic functions. Hamburg (1985) outlined a sequence of cognitive defenses, which includes 11 elements:

1. Regulate the timing and dosage of the threat.
2. Deal with stresses one at a time.
3. Seek information from multiple sources.
4. Formulate expectations.
5. Delineate manageable goals.
6. Rehearse coping strategies, and practice in safe situations.
7. Test coping strategies in situations of moderate risk.
8. Appraise feedback from those situations.
9. Try more than one approach, keeping several options open.
10. Commit to one approach.
11. Develop buffers against disappointment, and develop contingency plans.

The psychiatrist should consider how the person stressed with brain damage is deprived of each and all of these optimal mental and psychosocial mechanisms of mastery. The stress arises from within and cannot be eliminated by avoidance or flight. The organic disease cannot be viewed at a distance from the self because it is in the very organ of self-perception. On the contrary, the cognitively distorted perceptions of a paralyzed limb involve

highly metaphoric removals from the self and illustrate the difficulty one has in grasping an illness of one's own brain. The virtual impossibility of clearly grasping the disease of the perceiving organ itself renders the regulation of the timing, dosage, and sequence of multiple threats as formidable problems for psychotherapy. Formulation of expectations and delineation of goals are frequently impossible when the requisite cognitive skills are absent. "Safe" and "moderate-risk" situations are lacking for the patient haunted by a global sense of impairment that intrudes into every pleasurable aspect of life. Finally, the choice of multiple options, the use of feedback from situations, and the possibility of contingency plans are all techniques that may be quite unreachable for the patient with brain damage.

In one study by Andersson et al. (1999), the two-thirds of the traumatic brain injury patients classified as more apathetic had a poorer response to the rehabilitation process. Associated factors during the therapy were decreased autonomic reactivity in cardiovascular and electrodermal monitoring, less perceived emotional discomfort, and reduced self-awareness and insight, with disengagement and lack of concern about their situation. An implication is that psychotherapy should be aimed at improving self-awareness in apathetic patients.

Mateer (1999) recommended that frontal lobe disorders of executive function impairing initiation, sequencing of impulse control, attention, prospective memory, and self-awareness, leading to disorganized and maladaptive behaviors, can be approached through environmental manipulations, training in compensatory strategies, and techniques to improve underlying skills, including attention and prospective memory. The goal is movement from dependent external to independent internal self-regulation of behavior. Environmental manipulations, behavioral strategies, and external cueing are used early and with those who have little initiative and response to internal cues; later, and with patients who have more self-direction and awareness, cognitive training, compensatory devices such as memory books, and self-instructional and metacognitive strategies are more appropriate. Metacognitive strategies regulate behavior by replacing lost implicit and unconscious inner speech controls with explicit and conscious control through self-talk, covert internalized self-monitoring, and behavioral schemas for specified situations. Practice on attentional tasks is supplemented with proactive practice in identifying potentially difficult situations. Prospective memory, or remembering to remember (e.g., to take medications or call in), is more correlated with functional independence than is cued recall and is trained by practice carrying out actions with more and more intervening distractions and tasks. Problem-solving training involves brainstorming alternatives, comparing information from multiple sources (e.g., several clothing catalogues), and drawing inferences (e.g., perusing short detective stories for clues). Although growth in self-awareness of deficits may initiate emotional problems, improved awareness of internal and external emotional cues that signal or trigger emotions may lead to better self-management. Matteer and Bogod (2003) emphasized strategies for promoting maintenance and generalization of what is learned. Other behavioral and emotional residua noted by Delmonico et al. (1998) include substance abuse, depression, anxiety, chronic suicidal or homicidal ideation, poor impulse control, and degrees of frustration and anger. These are all approachable in group psychotherapy.

Grosswasser and Stern (1998) proposed a psychodynamic model of the neurobehavioral manifestations, which are viewed as a default means of emotional expression by the patients and therefore not entirely abnormal in the patients' interpersonal contexts. Anderson and Silver (1998), citing Yudofsky et al. (1990), noted the characteristic inappropriate features of aggression in patients with brain injury. Aggression is reactive, triggered by trivial stimuli; nonreflective and unpremeditated; nonpurposeful, serving no long-term goals; explosive, not gradual, in buildup; periodic, occurring in brief outbursts punctuating long periods of calm; and ego-dystonic, followed by embarrassment and regret rather than blaming others or justifying it. All these features can and should be approached by the behavioral techniques in addition to pharmacotherapy. Corrigan and Bach (2005) spell out aggression replacement strategies (e.g., assertiveness replacement strategies for patients who become angry when their needs are not met) and decelerative techniques, such as social extinction (for the socially responsive), contingent observation of self-controlled peer models, suggested time-outs, overcorrection requiring effort (e.g., throw a tray at lunch and have to clean several other tables as well), and as a last resort to prevent harm, contingent restraint and seclusion (within statutes, never as punishment, and not when it reinforces the aggressive or sexual behavior).

Flashman et al. (1998) suggested an approach to a lack of awareness that begins with ascertaining whether the patient has a lack of knowledge of the deficit, an inappropriate response to it, or an inability to appreciate its consequences on daily living. The therapeutic relationship is primary to helping the patient approach the likely combination of neurological and psychological denial along the neuromental spectrum. Treatment judiciously validates the self view and world view without fostering unrealistic expectations or forcing complete awareness all at once. Some deficits such as anosognosia with hemiplegia usually resolve in weeks, but other deficits, especially in social behavior and anger management, may persist and may

include resistance to the need for help. Relying on an established relationship, explorations identify the discrepancies between the patients' own views of their strengths and abilities and the feedback from others. Education and supportive therapy for significant others, and modeling for them a process of gentle teaching, play a vital role in appreciating the issues regarding awareness in their loved one. Awareness alone does not ensure application to real-life situations. A common cueing system uses simple, affectively neutral, nonthreatening cues the patient finds easy to detect to alert the patient to target behaviors that are occurring. Group therapy and other feedback also may be helpful. Bellus et al. (1998) pointed out that despite early success with the cognitive symptoms of schizophrenia, little effort at cognitive remediation is directed to long-term psychiatric patients, including those who have brain injury; however, in the brain injury rehabilitation community, there is strong support for cognitive remediation despite mixed results in the literature. A single case study reported improved verbal and nonverbal cognitive functioning on IQ testing over 20 years. Treatment included "low-tech" small group interventions within intensive behavioral rehabilitation programs.

SEXUAL DISTURBANCES AFTER BRAIN INJURY

Sexual disturbances may follow brain injury, especially damage to the limbic system. According to Weinstein (1974), "Changes in sexual behavior observed in brain-damaged patients are often abnormal by reason of the [inappropriate] circumstances in which they occur, rather than their intrinsic nature" (p. 16) or by their being different from the person's habitual conduct. It is often helpful to make it clear to the family that the patient with a brain injury has not become oversexed and that the patient is just enacting a normal sexuality in the wrong context because of a more general disorder of judgment.

Sexual behavior in individuals with brain damage usually is marked by a loss of specificity as to objects or forms of excitation rather than a new focus. Although specific behavior such as fetishism has been linked to temporal lobe seizure activity (as well as hyper- and hyposexuality), intermediary personality factors and learning are more likely the cause than postulated so-called sexual centers, as has been suggested for heterosexual pursuit.

Verbal seductiveness frequently occurs in a situation of stress, such as when a patient is asked about his or her illness or is being tested, and thus may have a defensive, avoidant quality. Another stress-related phenomenon is ludic play, which appears as punning or joking about illness, caricaturing disabilities, or imitating or mimicking the examiner's behavior. Often patients classify their disabilities in sexual terms, or sex enters into the content of their confabulations and delusions in the acute state, which Weinstein (1974) declared are useful signs that sexual behavior will be acted out later in a real-life situation. Some patients seek relatedness through physical contact that may "put off" visitors or staff, all the more so when the dementia is secondary to a contagious disease.

A study of the psychosexual consequences of brain injury by Kreutzer and Zasler (1989) showed that most patients reported a lessening of sexual drive, erectile function, and frequency of intercourse; reduced self-esteem and self-perceived sex appeal; and no relation between the level of affect and sexual behavior. Despite the changes, the quality of the patients' marital relationships appeared preserved.

OTHER THERAPEUTIC EMOTIONAL ISSUES

To some, patients with traumatic brain injury may seem remote from the usual psychodynamic practice, which lacks patients with dementia pugilistica or of the status in which being knocked out is a regular occurrence. However, automobile accidents are common; sports as diverse as football, soccer, and competitive diving include head trauma (from the water alone in the high dive, apart from hitting the board); and many elderly and alcoholic patients have had falls with blows to the head. Concussion, or "immediate and transient loss of consciousness accompanied by a brief period of amnesia after a blow to the head," is common, affecting 50 people per 100,000 population per year in the United States (Ropper and Gorson 2007). Thus, traumatic components may enter into many psychiatric disorders. Pollack (1994) provided a comprehensive approach to the psychotherapeutic processes and goals in more significant traumatic brain injury. Particularly valuable, and often ignored, are the affective and countertransferential aspects of work with these patients, to which therapist overidentification, overoptimism, impatience, inflexibility, and unfamiliarity with the neuropsychiatry of traumatic brain injury may contribute, as Pollack (2005) has pointed out.

Chief among the affects encountered is sadness arising in loneliness from the social isolation that results. A loss of morale afflicts both patient and family and requires the psychiatrist to instill hope without making insubstantial predictions of a successful outcome, especially in the face of the usual uncertainty of the recovery process. Pollack (2005) noted that incomprehension of the changes the brain injury has wrought in relationships and impairments in self-monitoring lead to appraising others' intentions erroneously, and sometimes negatively, so that paranoia results. Inappropriate or exaggerated guilt and shame about

responsibility for the trauma may occur and should not be countered too early in the therapeutic relationship.

Countertransference is complicated by the limits of the patient's self-awareness and self-monitoring. Frequent problems are the wishful underestimation of the severity of the disabilities, the premature returning of the patient to challenging situations with resulting catastrophic reactions, and a lack of patience with the patient's problems with memory, comprehension, or executive inflexibility. Lack of recovery, inactivity, and behavior problems may be misinterpreted as a lack of motivation or sabotage.

Frustration and anger may lead to a wish to abandon the patient, who reacts with hurt feelings and even hate. Sometimes the patients are stimulus-seeking adolescent males who view seeking even necessary help as compromising their proud independence.

Maintaining good boundaries in the treatment process can moderate the intensity of the countertransference.

FAMILY APPROACH TO TRAUMATIC BRAIN INJURY

In a very real psychiatric sense, the locus of traumatic brain injury is not within a single cranium but in a family. As Solomon and Scherzer (1991), suggesting a more "ecological" approach, have reported:

> [T]here is a severe increase in the level of stress within the family....Wives and mothers of the TBI [traumatic brain-injured] victim experience increases in anxiety, social dysfunction and perceived burden as a function of the severity of the injury, and these symptoms persist at least 1–2 years post-trauma.... The cognitive and affective changes rather than the physical deficits are the most troublesome for the family.... Whereas the family plays out their own dynamics in the hospital room, the hospital staff is often guilty of both condescension and wrongly attributing pathology to the family in order to explain conflicts with the hospital staff. The consequences of such conflict include the alienation of the family, who often represent the last resource of the patient, and the loss of potential allies in the rehabilitation process....We have interviewed over 100 families... these interviews reveal that the father is least likely to be able to tolerate the stress. He may abandon the family either physically or psychologically....When the father leaves, the mother is left with full parental responsibility for looking after the traumatically brain-injured member and feels overwhelmed....When the offspring is discharged from the hospital, it is usually the mother who takes on the role of case manager. (p. 255)

The mother as caregiver must deal with the patient's depressed, apathetic, or abusive emotions and obscene language. The male patient may be sexually harassing, the female lewd and aggressive. The mother is confused by the strange behavior, but with partial recovery, the patient, still not ready to be independent, no longer listens to her. The effects on the mothers parallel those on the wives of brain-injured patients, who have a deterioration in social and marital adjustment during the first year. Children find that they have to compete for attention, cannot express anger, and are often assigned responsibilities that are not age appropriate.

Ideally, the family should be integrated into the treatment process from the beginning. Solomon and Scherzer (1991) proposed detailed guidelines for the therapist, who should be highly directive, informed, and informing; an advocate for brain-injured patients; a guardian against exploitation; and a model for both patient and family while showing the family members that they are also models for the patient. The therapist should monitor comprehension, assist generalization of learning from one situation to another, and help the family to avoid being manipulated and to be free to protect themselves and to refuse to tolerate unacceptable behavior. Braga et al. (2005) found that the families of 5- to 12-year-old brain-injured children can efficiently acquire the skills to make physical and cognitive interventions in the children's everyday routines at home, with results at 1 year significantly superior to those from clinician-delivered interventions. Wade et al. (2005) had the parents complete self-guided exercises via supplied high-speed Internet access on problem solving, communication, and antecedent (precipitating) behavior management and found improvement in parental burden, stress, and depression, as well as the brain-injured child's antisocial behavior. Weekly videoconferences were accomplished with Web cameras that were also supplied.

STROKE

According to a study of stroke survivors by Kotila et al. (1984), clear improvement can be expected after stroke from the acute stage to 3 months, continuing to a lesser degree to 12 months. At 12 months, 78% of the patients who had survived strokes were living at home, and 58% were independent in activities of daily living. Of those patients who were gainfully employed before having a stroke, 55% had returned to work after 12 months. The authors emphasized that emotional reactions as well as neurological deficits influence outcome and should be considered in assessing prognosis.

A stroke is unwelcome at any age, but Goodstein (1983) noted that for older patients, a stroke activates preexisting fears of losing control or sanity, dying, and becoming disfigured or impaired physically or sexually. The elderly also are more insecure about sudden recurrences, long stays away from home, and running out of retirement funds.

The useful British term *emotionalism* has been defined by House et al. (1989, p. 991) as "an increase in frequency of crying or laughing, where the crying or laughing comes with little or no warning, and emotional expression is outside normal control, so that the subject cries or laughs in social situations where he or she would not previously have done so." It affects 20%–25% of stroke survivors in the first 6 months. Also referred to as *emotional lability* or *pseudobulbar affect*, it is not limited to bilateral brain damage and not predicted by unilateral lesion location. Calvert et al. (1998) compared emotionalism with posttraumatic stress disorder; in both, the patient experiences irritability and recurring, uncontrollable, emotionally charged mental events. Calvert et al. noted that emotionalism is not a meaningless accompaniment of brain injury; patients consider the precipitating thoughts and memories meaningful, and just as in posttraumatic stress disorder, the patient relives meaningful experiences. Ideas of reference were present in about a third of the stroke patients with emotionalism as compared with a tenth of those without, and this may be a product of embarrassment and social unease. Although antidepressive agents may aid these pathological affects, psychotherapeutic attention should be directed to the patient's subjective experience of meaningful content.

Lorig et al. (1999) reported that a self-management program for chronic diseases, including stroke, improved self-reported health; decreased distress, fatigue, disability, and social role activities limitations; and led to fewer hospitalizations and hospital days. No differences were found in pain or psychological well-being. Suhr and Anderson (1998) treated medication-resistant hallucinations in a 52-year-old patient with a right middle cerebral artery stroke with cognitive restructuring that included education of the patient and his family and training in compensatory strategies for the effect of symptoms on daily activities. Similarly, Goldenberg and Hagman (1998) trained patients with aphasia and right-sided hemiplegia after left hemisphere stroke, whose apraxia prevented activities of daily living, and found that no generalization occurred from trained to nontrained activities and that success was preserved at 6 months only in those who had practiced the specific activities in their daily routines at home.

Friefeld et al. (2004) found that stroke in childhood is more devastating to quality of life than are other chronic diseases such as diabetes and cancer. The severity of neurological outcome did not correlate with emotional quality-of-life ratings by children and parents. Girls were more anxious, discontented, and negative about their strokes than were boys. Deficits affecting schoolwork may become more apparent with time, lead to frustration, and require support and special education.

POSTDISCHARGE PLANNING

Several studies have underscored the importance of social support in the patient's adjustment to physical deficits from a stroke. Evans and Northwood (1983) related the wide variation in individual differences in adjustment to expressed interpersonal needs for social support. Labi et al. (1980) studied long-term survivors of stroke and found that a significant proportion manifested social disability, despite complete physical restoration. The parameters of social function in the study were socialization inside and outside the home, hobbies, and interests; much of the subjects' disability could not be accounted for by age, physical impairment, or specific neurological deficits. The distribution of documented functional disabilities suggested that in addition to organic deficits, psychosocial factors were major determinants.

The psychiatrist should be aware, as T. Wilson and Smith (1983) determined, that poststroke patients often will attempt to drive. However, these patients may have special difficulty handling all aspects of driving. Many of these difficulties are predictable from the clinical examination, and the patient should be warned. In addition to these deficits, problems with diminished vision, personality change, the prominence of denial and projection as mental defenses, and alcoholism are likely to increase the risks of driving for these patients. I have noted, in an era of availability of oversize vehicles, that feelings of vulnerability from subconsciously perceived mental deficits sometimes lead a patient with multi-infarct dementia and depression with gait difficulties to purchase a larger vehicle for self-protection, when switching to a slower-moving, three-wheeled motorized cart would be more appropriate to the patient's skills.

DEFENSES AND OBJECT RELATIONS IN HEMIPLEGIA

A discussion by Critchley (1979) of patients' reactions to hemiplegia contains observations of a variety of defensive maneuvers that epitomize the "neurologizing" of the dynamic defenses of psychiatry. In the loss of the sensation and control of parts of the body, remarkable changes occur in relation to those parts that Critchley calls "personification of the paralyzed limbs" (p. 117). This develops after an initial period of anosognosia and may be an overcompensation. The patient becomes a detached onlooker and the limb a foreign body outside the self. A patient may refer to the paralyzed limb as if it were an object such as a pet, a plaything, or a person of another sex, often with attributed personality traits. Splitting and lateralization into good and bad sides of the body, which ordinarily require a psychotic personality to

be manifested in the absence of neurological disease, become accessible and readily used defenses against the changed representation of the impaired body part, in brain and mind. Patients may insult or scream abuse at the limb. Beneath the level of denotative meaning and concrete representation that neurology comprehends, metaphors appear that speak to psychiatrists in fuller connotations about the state of the personality in relation to the diseased limb.

APPROACH TO PATIENTS WHO ARE UNSTABLE ON THEIR FEET

The fearful (usually elderly) patient who feels unstable on his or her feet is a common neuropsychiatric problem. An educational therapeutic approach is often helpful and may serve as a model of that approach within the context of an ongoing therapeutic relationship. The patient is taught that there are at least six components of balance, any and all of which, once improved, will contribute to them all. This immediately begins to dispel the sense of helplessness and maps a multipronged offensive effort that the patient can marshal.

Treatment of gait can target 1) muscular conditioning, 2) footing and dorsal-column feedback from legs, 3) vestibular and circulatory dizziness, 4) visual input to balance, 5) basal ganglia function, and 6) phobic and other neuromental content. The neuromental dimension is often the most important. The patient may express the feeling of a lack of support in symbolic somatic language of unsteadiness and a fear of falling. Often, the patient has become isolated through the deaths of relatives and friends, and therapy must deal with a resistance to affiliate that usually expresses the sentiment that the loved ones cannot be replaced. This sentiment must be given its due because it is a form of loving memorial. But progress is rapid once the patient sees associating with others as compatible with loving memories. Even the acquisition of a pet that stays in the home can improve the sense of security. Physical immobility diminishes the patient's sense of participation in life. While not working on the gait in the ways described earlier, patients are encouraged to correspond with distant friends, authors whose books and articles they have enjoyed, and new contacts through clubs and interests that encourage correspondence via letter and e-mail.

SPINAL CORD INJURY

A quarter of a million Americans live permanently paralyzed from spinal cord injuries, and 10,000 new cases occur each year (most often in young persons), with devastating effects on career and emotional costs for the patients and their families (National Advisory Neurological Disorders and Stroke Council 1990). These patients, insofar as they are brain intact, may have emotional reactions that are similar to those mourning the death of a loved one or other situations of severe loss (Bracken and Shepard 1980). Consequently, premorbid personality and the influence of significant others play a central role in coping with injury. These devastating injuries attract the greatest sympathy when they are sustained by famous figures in sports or entertainment, and the leadership of those who have adapted well to the most severe limitations, as in high cervical lesions, can provide role models for patient identification. An overly sympathetic "kindness mode" or "kid glove treatment" based on countertransference reactions to the devastating disability can be less helpful to patients with spinal cord injuries and may contribute to denial when they are also substance abusers (Perez and Pilsecker 1994).

Manifest depression is not an inevitable psychological sequel to spinal cord injury. Howell et al. (1981) found diagnosable depression in only 5 of 22 patients with spinal cord injuries of less than 6 months' duration. Bodenhamer et al. (1983) found that patients with spinal cord injuries reported less depression and more anxiety and optimism than their caregivers predicted. Bodenhamer et al. (1983) also pointed out that traditional stage theories of what is said to be a mourninglike adjustment must be individualized.

One of the most sophisticated accounts of the experiential dimension of spinal cord injury has been contributed by the noted anthropologist Robert Murphy (1987), who some 18 years before his death developed a spinal cord tumor that eventually separated him from the sense of his body. The *social* estrangement that resulted, which he compared to turning into a bug in Kafka's *Metamorphosis* (p. 108), despite his continued abilities to work, is discussed sensitively and professionally. He felt that he was "undergoing a savage parody of life itself" (Murphy 1987, p. 221) and that "the most important aspect of human behavior is that it derives its organization and content in the interaction of our biological drives with culture" (p. 225). He found that

> the four most far-reaching changes in consciousness of the disabled are: lowered self-esteem; the invasion of thought by physical deficits; a strong undercurrent of anger; and the acquisition of a new, total, and undesirable identity. I can only liken the situation to a curious kind of "invasion of the body snatchers," in which the alien intruder and the old occupant coexist in mutual hostility in the same body. (Murphy 1987, p. 108)

In correspondence (R.F. Murphy, personal communication, May 1987), Murphy responded to my inquiry about his dreams, reporting that they were only about his condition and often denied its reality. They began with

his walking and then remembering that he was paralyzed and also could not drive a car, so he could not get home. There was no resolution of the dilemma, and eventually the dreams began only with his being able to pull himself up to use a walker and take a few steps, also long impossible. His book has helped others in the same situation; reading this first-person account in a professional voice also can help the treating psychiatrist develop empathic understanding of the patient with spinal cord injury.

The best predictor of future self-care by these patients is past self-care behavior, augmented by knowledge of personality tendencies. Green et al. (1984), studying persons who had had spinal cord injuries at least 4 years previously, administered the Tennessee Self-Concept Scale (Fitts 1965) and found, in comparison with scale norms, that the respondents had significantly *higher* personal self, moral-ethical self, and social self scores, although they had significantly lower physical self scores. The higher-than-normal self-concept scores were related to perceived independence, provision of one's own transportation, assistance needed, and living arrangements. These findings suggest the possibility of *enhanced* self-concepts through mastery of handicaps and that the psychiatrist often need not settle for limitations in the patient's mental health.

Craig et al. (1999) found that persons who initially perceived life as externally controlled and who received structured cognitive-behavioral therapy in specialized groups during the rehabilitation phase were more likely than control subjects to feel in control of themselves 2 years postinjury and had fewer readmissions, used fewer drugs, and reported higher levels of adjustment. An external locus of control was associated with depressive mood 2 years after admission. Not everyone with spinal cord injury needs cognitive-behavioral therapy during their hospitalized phase, but those who reported high levels of depressive mood benefited greatly.

The psychotherapeutic approach to the chronic pain that is a persistent problem for 50% of the patients with spinal cord injuries also emphasizes the development of patient self-management, as reviewed by Umlauf (1992). The patient's responsibility is to himself or herself, not the physician. Coping abilities already shown with the injury are reinforced and applied to the problem of pain, which is never minimized or generalized in conversations with the patient. For this reason, a period of stability in postinjury adaptation should be established before beginning the intervention of a self-management program, which can otherwise seem intimidating and disheartening. Increased physical activity and decreased sedentary or prone time are often combined with increased supervised aerobic and strength exercise, with the involvement of the personal care attendant in therapy. The goals of pain management include increasing positive affects, improving sleep despite care demands such as a midnight turning schedule for skin care, learning to self-monitor emotions and situations that promote pain, and improvement in self-appraisal in coping with severe pain episodes. A useful question suggested by Umlauf (1992) is, "If we took away your pain, what activities would you be able to do that you are not able to do now?" (p. 114). Thus, an attempt is made to separate the patient's perspective on achievement from his or her pain problems. Clear distinctions are taught between the levels of nocioception (a reflex nerve arc), pain perception (e.g., "a hot poker shoved up my spine"), suffering (including dysphoric emotions, anger, insomnia), and pain behavior (rubbing, verbalizing, grimacing) to instruct that the intervention is aimed at the latter two levels. Muscle relaxation techniques and self-hypnosis depend on and are attuned to patient ability. Peer support groups and role models are helpful here. Stress reduction focuses on situations that contribute to both pain and spasticity, and cognitive interventions emphasize rational thinking, attention distraction, and pain reinterpretation (e.g., "It's not killing me").

The social level demands analysis of pain as a communication. The patient can learn that when he or she is silent because of pain, others may interpret this as negativity. Integration of pain management strategies into workplace adaptation is much needed in view of the low percentage of patients with spinal cord injuries who return to work. Social skills training and videotapes may be useful. Demographically, these patients are young men who are activity oriented rather than passive and introspective and may resist group or individual therapy that is not action oriented and peer involving. Appropriate use of pain medications; dealing with anger at the situation, oneself, and one's doctors; developing purposes for the rest of one's life; and avoiding compensation neuroses are major therapy themes.

In a longitudinal study, Rosenstiel and Roth (1981) found that their best-adjusted patients with spinal cord injuries predominantly used the defenses of rationalization and denial, in keeping with the notion that the psychiatrist ought to respect the so-called more primitive defenses, if they work. Other traits that favored adjustment were avoidance of catastrophizing and of worrying what their lives would be like, thinking about goals to be achieved after leaving the rehabilitation center, and use of internal forms of mental rehearsal in anticipation of going home. DeJong et al. (1984) found that the best predictors of independent living outcome were marital status, education, transportation barriers, economic disincentives, and severity of disability. Table 32–5 summarizes management issues for patients who have spinal cord injuries.

SEXUAL THERAPY FOR PATIENTS WITH SPINAL CORD INJURIES

Sexual therapy for the patient with a spinal cord injury, like sexual counseling for other patients, requires that the psychiatrist be comfortable and specially trained in such work. Schuler (1982) culled the techniques from five programs. The myth that patients with spinal cord injuries are asexual should be dispelled, and these patients should be helped to derive satisfaction from their sexual relations. The psychiatrist should emphasize resolving the high rate of marital discord. This includes not provoking guilt in the spouse with homilies about mutual responsibility, but instead giving close attention to the spouse's role in the vital area of sexuality. Ovulation still occurs in women with spinal cord injuries, and testicular atrophy is avoided in many men who receive excellent care. Pregnancy is possible with artificial insemination. Attitudes toward sexuality may be changed with the exploration of neglected erogenous zones in each partner, and sexuality should be redefined as any activity that is mutually stimulating.

A person with spinal cord injury can be taught to prepare a new partner by explaining the physical condition and improving communication. New techniques that use mechanical devices for stimulation and the expanded use of fantasy may be introduced. The psychiatrist should be sensitive to a patient's embarrassment and should be willing to spend sufficient time to discuss the topics. A psychosexual history may be used to obtain information that initially may be controversial (e.g., prosthetic devices, oral sex, and masturbation). Disabled male patients and their spouses must be helped to avoid rigid sex-role stereotypes of male domination and female passivity.

THE FAMILY MODEL IN SPINAL CORD INJURY

Whereas family attitudes about the injured person's entitlements are pervasive, all members of the family are affected differently according to their roles. Children must be specially prepared for their first confrontation with their parent's disability (Romano 1976), especially in dealing with fantasies of divine punishment. Children and other family members who construe human relationships in overly corporeal terms may also fear that with paralysis, the disabled parent has lost all effectiveness as an authority to admire or control them. Questions about the meaning of suffering almost always arise in persons with strong religious beliefs; often persons whose religiousness is less than mature have fantasies that they or their entire families are being punished for their intrinsic "badness." Steinglass et al. (1982) considered the suddenness of the effect

TABLE 32–5. Management issues for patients with spinal cord injury

1. Recognize that injured patients are not generally greater risk takers.

2. Expect mourning reactions to loss of use of body.

3. Evaluate premorbid personality to understand coping techniques.

4. Consider anxiety and optimism as well as depression.

5. Individualize traditional stage theories of mourning.

6. Avoid giving priority to medication over psychotherapy.

7. Gauge self-care ability based on past self-care.

8. Expect enhanced self-concepts with experience of mastery.

9. Avoid learned helplessness with early rehabilitation.

10. Treat interfering affective reactions before discharge.

11. Respect "primitive" rationalization and denial if they work.

12. Help avoid catastrophizing and worrying.

13. Encourage mental rehearsal for goals after discharge.

14. Consider spouse and socioeconomic and educational levels in plans.

of spinal cord injury on families and how an overemphasis on short-term stability of family life may lead patients to sacrifice family needs for growth and development. Family involvement with the rehabilitation process decreases feelings of anxiety, helplessness, and isolation.

EPILEPSY

Twenty million Americans will have at least one seizure during their lives, and 2 million will have spontaneously recurrent seizures. Although seizures generally can be controlled and patients remain relatively well adjusted, in one study of patients with epilepsy, Roberts and Guberman (1989) found that 33% had been treated for a mental disorder.

In formulating psychotherapy, the neuropsychiatrist may consider the functional context in which epilepsy occurs (Sands 1982). Differing age-related needs and tasks may be delayed or arrested at each stage of life by seizures, which usually have a regressive, exhibitionistic, and

shame-producing effect. In preschool-age children, it is important to consider what the effect on the affective climate of the family is and whether the family reaction manifests enlightenment or neurotic enmeshment. In the school-age child, the psychiatrist should consider the effects of peer acceptance or scapegoating on the patient's compliance with medication regimens. In the adolescent, issues related to epilepsy and driving, dating, sexuality, employability, and substance abuse should be explored. It is also important to determine whether seizure occurrence is linked to menstruation and, if so, what the teenage girl's ideas about this relationship may be. The visibility of medication side effects may be mortifying for an adolescent. For a young adult, the psychiatrist should help the patient consider the degree of autonomy as opposed to inhibition of independence. Travel becomes relevant for such a patient, as do issues regarding the pursuit of a career and the acceptance of seizures by employers, prospective mates, or the patient's own family. In the older adult, the psychiatrist needs to help the patient accept any necessary limitations on living alone or to face issues such as forced retirement or placement in a nursing home.

Kanner and Balabanov (2002) have cautioned that a seemingly reactive depression that persists after several months should not be considered a normal reaction to the stresses of having epilepsy, which often would be self-limited. A bidirectional augmenting relationship is seen between epilepsy and depressive disorders, which may be comorbid. Epileptic patients have less flexibility in mental processing and coping. Furthermore, Kanner and Palac (2000) have found that epilepsy patients considered depressive by neurologists may have appetite, sleep, and concentration difficulties, but they more prominently had intermittent anhedonia, irritability, poor frustration tolerance, mood lability, anxiety, and fatigue, with symptom-free days, short of a definitive DSM diagnosis. Even in these cases, antidepressive medication may be indicated and can be synergistic with psychotherapy.

MANAGEMENT OF INTERICTAL BEHAVIOR AND PERSONALITY CHANGES

From Blumer (1982), we may adapt hints for the management of the behavior and personality changes that he associated with the interictal states of temporal lobe epilepsy (complex partial seizure state) and that may occur in other seizure states:

- Viscosity, or stickiness, to a subject in conversation (or to the interviewer) by a laborious, detailed, and emphatic conversation and delay at the door on the way out may be worked with if the psychiatrist is neither rejecting nor overly passive. Self-critical patients with left temporal foci accept this issue better than do patients with right temporal foci, who tend to deny it.

- Deepened emotionality is associated with conflict around a hyperreligious overpreoccupation with righteousness and a Dostoevskian concern with crime and punishment. In these patients, cheerful hypermoralism alternates with briefer episodes of explosive verbalized anger and threatened violence, followed by remorse or denial. A patient may benefit from the psychiatrist's explaining how others learn to avoid the patient because of this deepened emotionality. These patients also may be coached to drop the proselytizing mode and remove themselves physically from entanglements.
- Hyposexuality is seldom complained of but further isolates patients with temporal lobe epilepsy, especially males. Although the hyposexuality may be drug responsive, the psychiatrist should address the isolation and the needs of the spouse and encourage closeness.
- Mood swings, especially those that build up over several days to a seizure, may be difficult for relatives, who try to avoid outbursts.
- Schizophrenia-like psychosis may occur after many years in the presence of a personality more like that of the patient with temporal lobe epilepsy than that of the schizoid patient. The psychiatrist should adapt the treatment approach to specific features, as with patients who are schizophrenic. Psychosis may diminish when anticonvulsants are discontinued for a few days.
- Memory disorders, which are related in severity to seizure severity and bitemporality, occur retrograde and anterograde during postictal confusion. Having the patient write memos at the first sign of an aura may help. Psychomotor automatisms also are a postictal phenomenon to be identified and explained.

ALZHEIMER'S DISEASE

Cummings and Jeste (1999) stated that demographic projections to the year 2010 indicate a 25% increase in Alzheimer's disease and other dementias and call for advocacy and education of those involved in managed care organizations.

The neuropsychiatrist should approach the effect of Alzheimer's disease on the patient and his or her family in a way that is comprehensive yet sensitive to the stage of the disease. The following suggestions are adapted and amplified from Aronson (1984), Jenicke (1985), and Rabins et al. (1982).

Because attention and memory are impaired in patients with Alzheimer's disease, a dyadic psychothera-

peutic learning process is usually impossible. In speaking with the patient and the family together, however, the psychiatrist should convey by affects directed toward the patient that the patient is valued by the psychiatrist. This provides for attitudinal modeling by the family and helps prevent retaliatory behavior by the patient against the family. It may be difficult for physicians and other professionals to have genuine feelings of appreciation of the Alzheimer's patient because professionals are selected and trained to value intellect and memory in themselves over personality, sensation, or pleasure.

The single overriding principle for treatment of the family of the Alzheimer's patient is the maintenance of family homeostasis and equilibrium despite the great changes in roles that result. Both patient and family benefit most if the family life can preserve its function as a holding environment for all its members and a social entity in which the members can feel loved and be loving.

Sleep is the first consideration in home care. The family cannot care for the patient and will resent the patient more if family members have sleep deficits caused by the patient's reversed sleep cycle. A strict diurnal schedule is prescribed, as with any insomnia, with sufficient daily activity and exercise so that the characteristically physically vigorous patient does not have an unusual amount of leftover energy during the night.

Quality-of-life considerations for the family should be immediately addressed by the psychiatrist. Discussions should counter the family's irrational feelings of guilt, family shame, punitive self-denial, and personal responsibility for the disease, all of which may lead to resentment and the potential for abuse of the patient. The physician must *prescribe* family fun with and without the patient. Small et al. (1997) reported that psychotherapeutic intervention with family members is often indicated because nearly half of all caregivers become depressed. Teri et al. (1997), in a controlled study of two nine-session behavioral treatments for depression in dementia—one emphasizing patient-pleasant events and one emphasizing caregiver problem solving—showed that both yielded significant patient and caregiver improvement in depressive symptoms lasting to 6-month follow-up, as compared with control subjects receiving typical care or assigned to a wait list. In the pleasant-events therapy (lacking behavioral strategies), after an introductory session, four sessions were devoted to identifying, planning, and increasing pleasant events for the patient; following this, caregiver problems and pleasant-event planning for themselves were addressed. In the problem-solving therapy, the focus was on patients' depressive behaviors of specific concern to caregivers. It is significant that the caregivers, many of whom were significantly depressed, also had improved depression scores, even though they were not seeking treatment for themselves and treatment was not targeted to them but rather trained them to aid the patient.

Financial planning based on clinical reality should be addressed as soon as possible after diagnosis. Early consultation with a social worker to access available care resources and legal advice about the shifting of financial responsibility can help avoid bankrupting the family. The psychiatrist should neither shun relevant financial concerns nor take sides in financial disputes. Aspects of the patient's clinical condition may enter into court proceedings, and the psychiatrist should keep clinical notes grounded in specific observations, quotes, and evaluations.

Care of the patient, a new dependent, requires help from the whole family, but children and other immature family members may find it especially taxing and may be less than helpful because of their own unanswered needs for support and their inability to tolerate a situation that does not conform with ideal expectations. The psychiatrist should assist the family in avoiding situations that are stressful to the patient's diminished processing ability. Just as a person with cardiac failure should not be physically overtaxed, a person with brain failure should not be pressed to evaluate multiple inputs or to negotiate complex interpersonal situations, to compensate for changes in plans or schedules that were attuned to bodily cycles, or to weather a physical illness without special help.

The family can prevent the patient from making errors and straying by eliminating dangerous choices, an elder version of childproofing. Weapons, dangerous tools, or substances that could be erroneously ingested by the patient must be locked away, and outside door locks that cannot be opened at night should be installed. Keys to the car can be made unavailable, knobs can be removed from stoves, and matches should be hidden. The patient should not be left alone with minors who would be vulnerable to molestation. Secondary systems of memory enhancement, such as posted signs, arrows, daily schedules, and identifying labels on objects or clothes, may be used. Simple syntax should be used in all conversations so that the patient's memory and attention are not taxed.

Monacelli et al. (2003) have shown that when Alzheimer's patients become lost even in familiar surroundings, this reflects an impairment in spatial disorientation that is distinct from their memory impairment. This impairment may identify Alzheimer-prone older adults and should be addressed separately in evaluation and remediation, especially as it affects ambulation and vehicular navigation.

Frank fear in the patient should be investigated as a possible index of victimization by the family. The psychiatrist should use knowledge of the 15 predictable functional assessment stages in the progression of both normal aging and Alzheimer's disease, as described by Reisberg (1985), to weigh the presence of other, treatable factors. For example, incontinence should only occur late in Alzheimer's disease; if the patient experiences this problem sooner, there may be a treatable infection. Loss of the ability to dress properly never precedes loss of the ability to choose clothing properly and could mean the patient is misbehaving. However, skills that the patient had yesterday may be gone today, and the family should be helped to accept the deterioration. As the sad saying goes, first it's forgetting names, then forgetting to zip up, then forgetting to zip down.

Katz (1998), noting that depression with reversible cognitive impairment may be a prodrome for dementia, concluded that research supports the reliability of assessment of typical depressive symptoms, even in patients with mild to moderate cognitive impairment, by self-rating with the Geriatric Depression Scale, which remains valid in patients with a Mini-Mental State Examination (Folstein et al. 1975) score of 15 or more. Potential difficulties with assessment include families' tendencies to report greater depression in patients than clinicians do and the ambiguity of apathy and related symptoms that can result from both depression and Alzheimer's disease. R.S. Wilson et al. (2003), evaluating older Catholic clergy members, found that those in the 90th percentile of the stable personality trait of proneness to experience psychological distress had twice the risk of developing Alzheimer's disease as did those in the 10th percentile. Distress proneness was particularly related to decline in episodic memory and was independent of pathological markers such as plaques and tangles. The authors commented that depression, a common form of mental distress, is also associated with Alzheimer's risk and decline in episodic memory and may be a remediable contribution to the disorder or its progression.

Chen et al. (1991) found that in the early stages of Alzheimer's disease, extrapyramidal signs and psychosis were more likely to develop than myoclonus but that as the disease progressed, the risk of developing myoclonus equaled that of the other two signs. They concluded that all three signs are developmental features marking the progression of the disease rather than disease subtypes. Although it may reflect their negative stereotyping of psychiatric illness, families frequently prefer to view psychosis as secondary to the progression of Alzheimer's disease rather than as a primary disease. When the symptoms or brain imagery suggest elements of vascular dementia, the family may prefer to emphasize that their loved one is having "a series of little strokes," even though the impeded ambulation in patients with subcortical multi-infarct dementia is among the most trying of symptoms for caregivers. Although the psychiatrist stands for medical reality, clinical tact dictates forbearance in not hammering insistently at diagnostic classification. Relatives may see themselves as future patients. Mayeux et al. (1991) found a 50% chance of dementia by age 91 years in the first-degree relatives of patients with Alzheimer's disease but almost the same percentage in the relatives of patients with other dementias and cognitive disorders in Parkinson's disease, a sixfold higher incidence than in the relatives of healthy elderly subjects.

It is an emotional reality that the family of an Alzheimer's patient may "pre-mourn" the loss of the patient's personality before his or her death and may thereby devalue what is left of the person. Often the patient is protected by the disease from awareness of this emotional abandonment, but at times when sensibility lingers, the caring physician remains the last real representative of "other people." Table 32–6 summarizes management issues for patients with Alzheimer's disease.

OTHER SUGGESTIONS FOR PSYCHOTHERAPY WITH MEMORY-IMPAIRED PATIENTS

Clinicians should facilitate trust by establishing a therapeutic relationship with the memory-impaired patient, as much as possible, that has a higher priority than that with relatives and caregivers. Hushed-voice discussions with family should be particularly avoided. The memory impaired are *not* hard of hearing and may piece together overheard fragments into planning that excludes their interests and wishes. The psychiatrist should avoid causing iatrogenic paranoia. His or her respect for the patient serves as a model for imitation by family and caregivers.

More than most patients, memory-impaired patients track affects. They pay particular attention not so much to what is said but to the expressiveness with which it is said. Memory of affective experiences with the psychiatrist persists when cognitive recall of what was said does not. The psychiatrist must tune his or her own affect projections up or down as dictated by the patient's condition.

It is helpful to get the patient on a platform of familiarity to optimize mnemonic function. An example is asking the patient to say something in a language learned as a youth. One patient, remembering early French studies, enjoyed recalling and repronouncing the historical name *Vercingetorix*.

Sessions should be scheduled at the same time of day to capitalize on continuity of state-dependent memory based on circadian rhythms. Registration can be facilitated by not overloading the patient with too much information or gratuitous elaboration. The patient's attention

can be maintained by projection of affect and sympathetic interest. Distractions, especially ambient noise but also clutter and unessential comments, should be eliminated.

The patient should not be expected to converse while walking into the consulting room; the psychiatrist should wait to talk until the patient is settled in a chair and should not speak while the patient is speaking or engaged in an action, such as signing a Medicare form. The psychiatrist must be tolerant of perseveration at session's end; it is usually a sign that the therapeutic relationship is beneficial.

The patient should always be allowed to complete a thought, even if it is repetitive, stereotyped, or perseverative. For the patient, it may have the power of repeating reassuring prayers or imprecations to ward off chaos. An example is one patient who would recite the names of his former caregivers in reverse whenever the current one was brought up. Another patient described the frail memory structures that would reemerge as she spoke animatedly about a topic as "a house of cards" that would collapse when she would be interrupted by a person intent on another mission, however trivial, such as arranging a pillow behind her.

Repeating and, if possible, restating in a briefer and more pithy way what patients say helps them remember and feel welcome.

Patients should be taught to use notes to keep track and helped to construct hierarchies. A labeled photograph album of familiar persons can be shared with the psychiatrist.

Interpretations, communications, or instructions should be broken down into simpler steps in sequence. Statements should be to the point and not overly drawn out or complex in syntax. I use the term *sound bites* in instructing families and spouses not to string together chained associations. If ideas require multiple sentences, topic sentences and summaries should be used.

The patient's ability to abstract and generalize should be reevaluated periodically. If the patient generalizes poorly, he or she should be allowed to approach and master each situation as separate and distinct.

Patients should be affectively rewarded with varying facial expressions and tones to praise achievements of insight. The psychiatrist should express therapeutic reactions and interventions without delay to underscore emphases and facilitate recall. For example, one gentleman with preserved fastidiousness about hanging up his clothing and preserving the creases saved his family cleaning and pressing expenses and effort.

An incessant or haranguing style that might overtire the patient should be avoided. Chronic brain failure, like heart failure, requires rests. Things that were automatic before require effort at every step.

Burns et al. (2005) attempted six sessions of psychodynamic interpersonal therapy with early Alzheimer's patients

TABLE 32–6. Management issues for patients with Alzheimer's disease

1. Convey valuation of patient for attitudinal modeling.
2. Maintain equilibrium of family when roles must shift.
3. Prescribe sleep and exercise schedule so patient sleeps at night.
4. Discuss family guilt and shame about affected member.
5. Prescribe family fun with and without patient.
6. Refer to social worker to access care resources.
7. Suggest legal help with financial responsibility.
8. Avoid taking sides in family financial disputes.
9. Encourage log of incapacities in advanced-disease patient.
10. Note effect of newly dependent patient on dependent family members.
11. Attend to age-specific needs of children and teenagers.
12. Encourage substitute role models for children.
13. Discuss wounded pride about loss of ideal family image.
14. Assist family in avoiding situations that tax brain failure.
15. Coach family in avoiding changes in plans and schedules.
16. Give added help at times of stress, such as during physical illness.
17. Capitalize on poor memory to distract patient from stress.
18. Lock up weapons, poisons, money, and car keys.
19. Remove matches, lighters, and stove knobs.
20. Do not leave patient alone with minors vulnerable to molestation.
21. Set timers for comforting radio and television programs in patient's room.
22. Post signs, labels, and arrows as memory reinforcers.
23. Avoid household clutter and distracting background sounds.
24. Speak in short clauses and simple syntax to patient.
25. Investigate frank fear in patient for possible abuse.
26. Check emerging problems against known stages to see if avoidable.
27. Help patient find appropriate substitute activities with friends.
28. Attend closely to mental health needs of spouse.
29. Note overconcern about care, concealing feeling of family that patient would be "better off dead."
30. Note that patient gait impediments are among the most frustrating for caregivers.
31. Recognize that family may premourn physical death of patient.

and did not find improvement; thus, they argued that no evidence supports brief psychotherapy for these patients, although the technique was accepted and helped individually.

The more general premise that life is worth living may be more tenuously held by aging patients who are losing their memory and feel like they are losing their personality with it. A useful interpretation is that the patient's presence, which everyone but the patient is aware of, is more important to his or her family and friends than is his or her memory. The family may be enlisted to reinforce this. In one case of vascular dementia, the patient's daughter, unprompted, told her memory-impaired mother that her dignity in the face of her impairment had been a model for her and her siblings and reminded her how much her grandson had looked forward to introducing his fiancée to her. Prior to this, the mother had reported lying in bed each night praying that God would take her away and said, "To live without a memory is to live without a consciousness of yourself." Now she said, "You all have to stay close to me and preserve what's left of me to matter to you all."

Matteson et al. (1997) helpfully approached treating the regressive aspects of Alzheimer's disease and related disorders within a Piagetian framework. Patients with normal forgetfulness maintain formal operations (age 12 and older), those with borderline or mild disease use concrete operations (ages 7–12) and benefit by set routines; those with moderate disease use preoperational thinking (ages 2–7) and benefit by instructions one at a time and aid with bathing and dressing; and those with moderately severe and late-stage disease use sensorimotor cognition (ages 0–2) and benefit by assistance in daily and basic activities, such as hygiene, toileting, and eating.

CARE FOR THE CAREGIVER

Maintenance of the caregiver, sometimes just referred to as the carer, is of prime importance. Mittleman et al. (2004) found in a study of 406 spouse caregivers of patients with Alzheimer's disease that fewer depressive symptoms emerged in those caregivers who received enhanced counseling and support treatments. Caregivers were taught to improve caregiving skills and to mobilize the support of family networks and were given counseling as needed over the entire disease course.

The defense mechanism I have termed *heterostasis*, the reliance on another to maintain one's cognitive and emotional integrity, commonly appears in the memory-impaired person reliant on a spouse or other caregiver. The patient's separation anxiety, although more understandable, is also more imprisoning for the caregiver, who may need to run errands and write checks as well as have time to herself or himself. Some suggestions for the caregiver include ways of taking leave of the patient.

When leaving, the caregiver should break cleanly and move out smartly. The analogous situation is the mother of a kindergartner, but one for whom every day seems like the first day. The child fusses until the mother is gone and then begins to relate to whomever he or she is left with. The presence of the spouse may be extended in various ways:

- *The visual souvenir.* A smiling portrait of the spouse is produced and placed prominently, with the time of return noted.
- *The auditory fetish.* The sound of the caregiver's voice is reassuring. For example, a spouse who had experience reading for the blind was encouraged to produce a reassuring script recalling pleasant times together that could be played in her absence on a tape recorder.

- *The video surrogate.* With the help of other family members, a videotaped interview with the spouse, on whom the patient relies for heterostasis, is prepared. This runs from 2 to 6 hours and allows the spouse sufficient time away. The camera is kept largely on the full face. With poor enough memory, it remains fresh.
- *The cellular telephone umbilical link.* Cellular telephones are ideal for the caregiver to take with him or her when the memory-impaired patient is able to answer the telephone or be directed to it. Finding the ringing telephone usually is no problem. After suddenly or surreptitiously leaving, the caregiver immediately dials the home number from the hallway. When the patient answers the telephone, he or she is told the caregiver is completing an errand and will be home soon. The timing of the next call is based on experience with the latency of the patient's reaccumulating separation anxiety. The psychiatrist can help determine this by asking the patient to wait alone in the waiting room while consulting with the spouse. Usually, after a time the patient will knock on the door, if he or she still remembers the caregiver is behind it. Alternatively, the caregiver can be asked to leave and the patient's discomfort observed. Cellular telephones that transmit images may be still more effective.

In the happy situation of other patients who have an abundance of family or staff at hand to help, a great deal of heterostasis is adaptive, compensates greatly for the memory impairment, and may be praised as an accomplishment ("You have been very successful in using others for your memory"). But even here, tensions arise, and the patient may be ready for help with some more independent techniques, such as a memory book as described by Burke et al. (1994). As in all other matters, the patient can be helped to function as normally as possible by using a standard daily appointment reminder book with added sections on orientation, memory log, calendar, things to do, transportation, feelings log, names, and today's tasks. Reviewing of the memory book should be scheduled several times during the day and sometimes prompted by a wristwatch alarm. Practice sessions are essential, with shopping, outings, therapy assignments, and so forth. The physician adopts a coaching style, and the patient writes entries into the book.

TREATING THE WORKING MEMORY

Research by Goldman-Rakic (1992, 1994) and others has described a component of memory that is short term, accessed to be used or applied, and driven by attentional processes. It functions like random access memory (RAM) computer chips, which hold data temporarily for processing that have been stored in long-term components (the hard drive or CD-ROM in the computer analogy). Goldman-Rakic showed that the working memory, located in the prefrontal cortex, is connected to sensory memories and can be inactivated in specific segments, much like visual field cuts. Working memory lasts for 10 to 15 seconds of mental focus and has a span that includes the sentence before and after the one that is being spoken. It also differs in the right and left prefrontal cortices, similarly to differences in right and left cortices generally, in that the right side pictures the memory (of a face, for example) and the left side encodes information about it.

The working memory, especially the keeping of a train of thought, is hypothesized to be impaired in schizophrenia. Weinberger et al. (1986) have shown in positron emission tomography studies a diminished prefrontal cortical response to challenge by the Wisconsin Card Sorting Test (Heaton 1985), which constantly changes the rules of a classification task. But schizophrenia brings other problems, especially with attention itself, and other conditions with prefrontal damage (and damage to other areas of the brain where working memory may be distributed) can create problems with the working memory.

The spatiality of this memory (and in this, humans are like other mammals, such as rats) offers clues as to how to approach its impairment therapeutically. The patient can be encouraged to approach memory tasks spatially. Any of us who have moved our office and all of its books (especially in middle age) can appreciate how much of our functioning memory is pegged to the location of our printed sources. Visualizing a familiar room with objects positioned in familiar places may be helpful. Some computer programs have used this principle to become more user friendly. Anything that gets the patients to move, such as sports or dancing, is helpful, even if they do not recall the scores or the steps. Many patients recall essential contacts or resources in a maplike way, and this should be encouraged. Drawings, cartoons, and maps can be produced by the patient, sometimes with help, and kept for reference. Geography games are good, but work with maps should emphasize neighborhood and floor plans (e.g., the way to the psychiatrist's office) as well as countries and continents. In all of this, we count on some brain plasticity, which may lead to improvement with practice. Memory is only one component of general intelligence, and intellectual activity can help stave off its deterioration.

CONTRIBUTION OF THE SOMATIC MEMORY

The somatic, motoric, procedural, or action type of memory has been recognized as distinct from the explicit or declarative memory, and it may be preserved or im-

paired, with some independence and also some plasticity. Performing a neurological examination is valuable in evaluating the intactness or impairment of the motor and action systems, which I have classified functionally (Forrest 1994). People with motor impairment may have difficulty remembering or conceptualizing spatial relationships. This is one reason to prescribe exercise for patients with a variety of disorders from depression to Parkinson's disease. In aging and senile dementia of the Alzheimer's type, the declarative memory may be quite disturbed, with more preservation of the somatic procedural memory. If possible, the physician should try to link this with cortical spatiality by prescribing maintenance of physical mobility through exercise and sports and encouraging visual and pictorial activities such as the mapmaking and diagramming of familiar spaces mentioned earlier. Such exercises have more applicability and generalizability than do abstract cognitive remediation exercises. The rebuilding of habits capitalizes on the automatic activities being separately represented (and, rarely, vulnerable to loss in isolation—as of automatic speech such as prayer). Ordinarily, musical activities may be more easily recalled or performed. For example, Matteson et al. (1997) recommended the consistent use of certain songs to announce patient meetings.

APPROACH TO AGITATION IN PATIENTS WITH PROFOUND DEMENTIA

Cohen-Mansfield and Deutsch (1996) analyzed the catchall term *agitation* as meaningful communication and suggested therapeutic responses that are adapted to the patients' capabilities. Even though neurological impairment sets the stage, there is some indication that verbal agitation such as screams and abusive language, although usually undirected, occurs more on awakening, suggesting toilet needs, or preceding staff manipulation, perhaps to avoid painful handling. These behaviors also occurred when the patient was alone at night or fearful. Determining when a confused person is too cold or in pain requires careful attention. Individualized treatment included reinforcing desirable behavior and ignoring inappropriate behavior.

For physically aggressive persons, staff handling should be monitored. Physically nonaggressive behaviors often may be adaptive and can be accommodated in a protected manner (e.g., allowing the patient to pace in a sheltered garden or making meal and bath times flexible). Often, agitation signals nonphysical, existential needs, such as for human contact, meaningful activities, stimulation, and reassurance about fears and losses. Activities that are tailored to the patients' sense of identity, former work role, and preferences; to their sensory abilities (which may need to be augmented with eyeglasses or hearing aids); and to their current needs, such as for contact, stimulation, exercise, or a specific activity such as being helpful or useful can be provided to harness the patients' energy. Intact sensory modalities can be used. For example, visual capacity permits gazing at mirrors, windows, videotapes of family, and old movies. The patient can listen to audiotapes, telephone contacts, music, and religious services. Mobility permits social visits, rocking chairs, walks, and tasks. Intact touch can be occupied with massage, Jacuzzi, pillows or stuffed animals, exploration of materials, and pet care.

Patients can be helped to value the strengths and purposes of their minds at every stage. As the curve for raw memory retention falls, the curve for wisdom often rises, at least for a time. Capacities for loving and caring should be treasured. Later, the capability of mere sensual pleasure and comfort may be the best one can expect.

PARKINSON'S DISEASE

In describing the "shaking palsy" as a purely motor rather than mental degeneration, Parkinson (1817) referred to depression and terminal delirium, and it was once taught that the mind is not affected in patients with Parkinson's disease. Reflecting the more recent recognition of concomitant mental involvement, Mayeux and Stern (1983) described some of the specific mental processes that are impaired. Building on such observations, the psychiatrist may make a more educated psychotherapeutic approach to the patient with this syndrome.

TREATMENT CONSIDERATIONS IN EARLY PARKINSON'S DISEASE

Although the cognitive impairments of late Parkinson's disease may be underestimated under the surmise that it is purely a motor disorder, this is largely true at the onset of the disease when many years of good function are expected. Early cases should be exposed as little as possible to the most advanced cases in support groups or waiting areas. The patient's significant other should not be addressed as the *caregiver* because this conjures up for many people the specter of a complete dependent on their hands in the near future. The term *partner* is preferable, emphasizing that the couple are partners in living. As soon as possible after diagnosis, the couple should be urged to take a vacation, even a brief one, to stake out pleasure goals, which should be renewed on a continuing basis. Concealment of the diagnosis may be of the highest priority early in the disorder, depending on the patient's occupation, and demands for secrecy are realistic, not para-

noid. Whatever the pharmacological therapy, the couple can benefit from psychotherapy to counter stresses that amplify the tremor and bradykinesia. The couple should be encouraged to compensate for the parkinsonian facies by practice in remembering to animate the affect, enunciate clearly and loudly enough, and restore normal gestural fluency as much as possible. If aging ballerinas and actors can play young persons, Parkinson's patients can often imitate nonparkinsonian mannerisms. Just as inattention to or distraction from the affected parts can amplify symptoms, attention and volition can diminish them. The parkinsonian facies is a default position in the early stages, and interpersonal and videotaped feedback can teach the patient to be more facially expressive, to smile when encountering others, to move the eyes, and to avoid the fixed, astonished, expressionless mask that occurs in face-to-face listening. Figure 32–3 shows facial warm-up and facial affect exercises adapted from Côté et al. (undated) and Ekman and Friesen (2003).

Psychotherapeutic support of patient and partner is indicated. Waters (1999), following Golbe and Sage (1995), suggested a timetable for illness-related discussions:

- At diagnosis, the clinician should generalize about the disease and its treatability.
- At 1–2 months, the clinician should explain the typical prognosis (progression over two decades), tell of the promise of research, and recommend lay literature and *national* support societies.
- At 8 months, the clinician should educate about treatment complications if L-dopa has been started.
- At 2 years, the clinician should recommend a *local* support group and regular exercise if the patient is sedentary.

Although tremor, rigidity, and bradykinesia cannot be eliminated by nonpharmacological approaches, their functional effect can be modified by physical and occupational therapy. Waters (1999) illustrated helpful exercises and recommended walking a mile a day, swimming to aid symmetrical use of muscles, and doing favorite activities, such as ballroom dancing. Environmental measures include removing doorsills, scatter rugs, obstructing furniture, and difficult faucets or handles. Cathy Curtis, P.T. (personal communication, May 2000), recommended smooth, nonslippery flooring that does not have dazzling reflections. Montgomery et al. (1994), in a controlled study, found that even a supportive personalized educational program administered by mail to patients taking bromocriptine stabilized activities of daily living over 6 months compared with control subjects, who used more levodopa and whose disease progressed.

Warm-up exercises

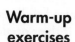

   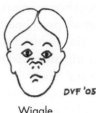 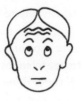

Raise brows Wrinkle forehead

Open mouth widely

Puff out cheeks

Whistle

Wiggle nose

DVF '05

Facial motion exercises

Joy, happiness | Fear | Anger | Sadness | Surprise | Disgust

 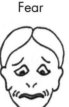 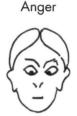 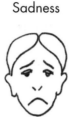 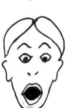 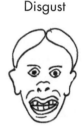

Raise mouth corners
Crinkle eyes

Raise inner brows
Widen and lower mouth
Open eyes wide

Lower inner brows
Tighten mouth

Lower corners, raise mid mouth
Raise inner brows

Raise brows
Lower lip and jaw

Nose upward
Mouth expanded
Lower brows

FIGURE 32–3. Facial warm-up and facial affect exercises.

In a controlled study of behavioral strategies in Parkinson's disease patients administered for 90 minutes twice a week over a 10-week period in which their medication was held constant, Müller et al. (1997) used an optoelectronic two-camera motion analysis system to show the improvement in postural control and the initiation of movement. As the authors noted, parkinsonian patients were able to improve their shuffling and small-stepped gait voluntarily as long as they concentrated. Difficulty initiating and maintaining stepping also can be influenced by external visual cues, such as a striped floor; auditory cues, such as a marching song; or internal cues, such as silently speaking a command to move oneself. Emotional or psychosocial stress also strongly influences gait posture and other motor performance. Behavioral interventions are aimed at standing straighter, balancing better, starting more quickly to walk, and stepping more rhythmically with normal arm swing. Special strategies taught include using external cues (visual, acoustic, or tactile) when walking or during motor freezing episodes and practice in getting up from a chair, turning in bed, and handwriting. Dividing complex movements into several simpler movements (chaining) is positively reinforced with the handwriting or longer-distance walking. When training the gait, videotaped feedback and rehearsals

are used, and progressive muscle relaxation is taught to control movements, especially when stressed. Social skills training helps to apply the new learning to problematic situations. Forward bending (a stooped posture) appeared to be very sensitive to behavior changes and may be clinically useful in quantifying disease progression. Similarly, Ellgring et al. (1993) found that stress management, relaxation training, cognitive restructuring, social skills training, modeling, and role-playing conferred techniques that could be effectively transferred into everyday life in most patients.

Dementia is estimated to affect 20% of the patients with Parkinson's disease (Waters 1999), more among older-than younger-onset disease, and usually is a subcortical dementia, with memory loss associated with poor concentration and initiative and slow responses (bradyphrenia) rather than with the aphasia, apraxia, and agnosia of cortical dementias such as Alzheimer's. Hallucinosis occurs in 30% of the L-dopa-treated patients, but the hallucinations are nonthreatening and can be managed without neuroleptics in most patients, some of whom even appear amused by them.

Because the degree of intellectual impairment tends to increase as the severity of motoric symptoms increases (Mayeux and Stern 1983), the psychiatrist should also assume that the patient will have greater impairment in the ability to make therapeutic contact if motor ability is more impaired. Furthermore, the psychiatrist should not conclude that all psychopathology is reactive to impairment or that the constriction of the patient's life is due solely to motoric limitations. Beatty et al. (1989) found the Mini-Mental State Examination useful in assessing the cognitive impairments of Parkinson's disease, and they also found that tests of frontal lobe function, such as the Wisconsin Card Sorting Test, did not indicate that the cognitive impairments experienced by these patients arose principally from typical frontal lobe dysfunction. Instead, such tests suggested that cerebral dysfunction extended beyond subcortical-frontal circuits.

Mayeux and Stern (1983) found that bradykinesia and rigidity, but not tremor, gait disturbance, or posture, predicted overall intellectual performance for a patient taking the Mini-Mental State Examination. The neuropsychiatrist should not hesitate to examine the patient neurologically to gauge potential areas of mental difficulty. Although this would appear to be a roundabout approach compared with doing a mental status examination, it is often less threatening and efficiently yields a preliminary clinical impression. The types of motor impairments tell us much about the patient's quality of thought, insight, and ability to relate to the therapist. Mayeux and Stern (1983) and Hallet (1979) noted that the activities that are impaired require directed attention to the task, sequencing of cognitive processes, and often additional motor interaction. In more psychiatric terms, these activities involve an inherent motoric or spatial mental action.

Other disturbances characteristic of patients with Parkinson's disease are impaired perceptual motor or visuospatial functions, especially the inability to perform sequential or predictive voluntary movements (Stern et al. 1984). This results in impaired internal spatial representation (from which may arise the initiation of independent thought and mental action) and articulatory difficulty without impaired language reception or production. In fact, Parkinson's disease is distinct from other neuropsychiatric disorders because of the paucity of language impairment, a significant boon to the psychiatrist trying to do psychotherapeutic work.

Memory in these patients is often slowed without being impaired. Trouble with word finding, which worsens with increased motoric symptoms in some parkinsonian patients, was considered a form of the "tip of the tongue" phenomenon similar to anomia in aphasic patients with frontal lobe lesions. Mayeux (1984) summarized a review of the literature on Parkinson's disease and Huntington's disease by stating that "nearly every patient with a movement disorder has some type of behavioral dysfunction, whether it is personality change or intellectual impair-

ment" (p. 537). The close linkage of motor and mental action may be turned to advantage by using some behavioral techniques.

For example, patients should be encouraged to keep fit by regular moderate exercise, especially if their occupations are sedentary. Fitness does not stop the progression of Parkinson's disease, but it does help patients cope with symptoms. Free-moving calisthenics and sports such as swimming are best, but safety, especially with patients who freeze motorically, must be considered.

It is important to employ sensory, rhythmic, and other cues and reminders to keep the bradykinetic patient moving. A patient can put taplike nails in the shoes to provide an auditory cue to keep the rhythm of walking constant and prevent festination. A small piece of raw carrot in the mouth may remind the patient to swallow and prevent drooling. Many techniques helpful to movement and mental state seem mechanical: wearing slippery rather than rubber soles to permit shuffling without falling, dispensing with canes and walkers when there is retropulsion, raising the back legs of chairs and toilet seats 2 inches to facilitate rising, and removing doorsills to prevent a patient from freezing in a doorway. An L-shaped extension at the tip of a cane can be stepped over so that the patient can keep moving. A simple device to quantify tremor (Forrest 1990) reassures patients of preserved control of intentional movements (Figure 32–4) and can be used to monitor other patients whose hands shake from a variety of causes, including familial tremor and medication, and who are sensitive about this, usually in social contexts where they may be mistaken for alcoholic persons.

Motor blocks are among the most disabling and therapeutically frustrating problems in the management of Parkinson's disease. Sudden transient freezing and related phenomena are associated with being in narrow spaces such as doorways in 25% of patients, with turning in 45% of patients, and with starting to walk in 86% of patients, according to a large database review by Giladi et al. (1992), and occur more often in patients whose symptoms began in the gait or trunk than in the upper body. Involving "the abnormal retrieval or execution of complex motor tasks" (Giladi et al. 1992, p. 333), whether from the disease itself or a side effect of L-dopa, motor blocks also are influenced by emotional factors and visual perceptual input. Hesitation at constricted points may be an atavistic feature resembling liminal cautiousness in animals, such as felines. The patients may be encouraged to focus on pattern continuities that may bring them past constricted points (see Figure 32–5), a feature that has been capitalized on in the experimental use of virtual-reality helmets that superimpose repetitive apparent perceptual stepping stones on the visual field.

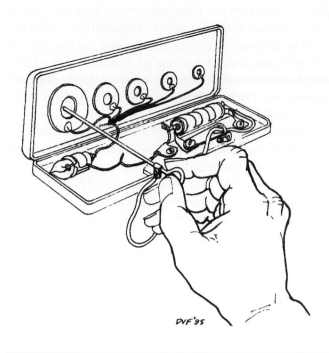

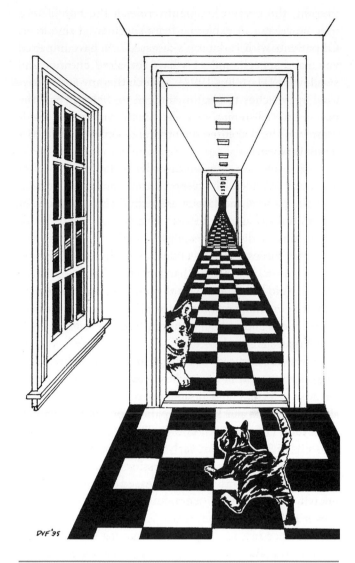

FIGURE 32–4. The tremometer is a simple device that closes a circuit and lights a bulb when the patient is unable to hold the probe in progressively smaller holes without touching the washers. The suggested sizes for the inside diameters of the washers are 9/16″, 3/8″, 5/16″, 1/4″, and 3/16″. Although the device quantitates tremor, it is most useful for reassuring patients that they are able to accomplish the task despite their shaky hands.

Source. Full instructions for the tremometer, suggestions for use, and clinical examples are presented in Forrest DV: "The Tremometer: A Convenient Device to Measure Postural Tremor From Lithium and Other Causes." *Journal of Neuropsychiatry and Clinical Neurosciences* 2:391–394, 1990.

NONMOTOR EXPERIENCES IN PARKINSONISM AND RELATED CONDITIONS

The somatosensory discomforts of parkinsonism, tardive conditions, and other movement disorders may be underestimated by the physician unfamiliar with them. Feelings of cold or burning; back, neck, and other pain; and peculiar dysphoric sensations are particularly troublesome at night, when external sensations are diminished and the rest tremor may be more noticeable, disturbing sleep. A thoracospinal (axial) vibration (internal tremor) often occurs as well. Position shifting is difficult, and stiffness and cramps are troublesome. Autonomic and myoclonic complications may be present in patients with multiple system atrophy and olivopontocerebellar atrophy, respectively, and impediments of information processing also result. Ford et al. (1994) described painful oral and genital sensations in 11 patients with tardive akathisia, tardive

FIGURE 32–5. Patients with parkinsonism may have difficulty with motor blocks, which often occur in narrowed spaces such as doorways. This behavior has an atavistic quality and resembles the liminal wariness of animals. Concentration on visual continuities may help to counter this problem.

dyskinesia, or tardive dystonia. Patients should be helped to learn to distract themselves from focusing on these internal symptoms. Pleasant music or reading at bedtime until sleepiness comes may be helpful, as in the psychotherapeutic approaches to insomnia generally.

Constipation is such a common feature that it has been called "the number one movement disorder" and requires paying constant attention to exercise, hydration, stool bulking, and balancing constipating anticholinergics against the need to reduce tremor. Patients often discontinue medications on their own and have difficulty distinguishing among the effects of polypharmacy (which is frequently used). When relief from medication is only partial, especially when striatonigral degeneration is present, the psychotherapeutic role of the psychiatrist may be greater in exploring fears and mental resources. Of patients with Parkinson's disease, 70% have impaired voice and speech, and 41% have impaired chewing and swallowing (Hartelius 1994). Speech therapy and behavioral approaches to swallowing can be helpful, but the psychiatrist's listening style also must be adapted considerately to the decreased quantity and forcefulness of the patients' speech.

Parkinson's disease is a disorder of knife-edge tolerances and balances. The response to L-dopa is so dramatic that the patient and family are exquisitely conscious of the central role of drug effects. Patient and family, building on this medication response, may try to convey the idea that the psychiatrist is dealing with a cumbersome apparatus—a thing rather than a person. The psychiatrist should avoid becoming so totally immersed in the intricacies of compelling medicomotor phenomena such as on-off reactions and sudden transient freezing that the emotional issues are neglected.

A previous strategy of being reluctant to make the diagnosis or treat it in the earliest stages may be changing because selegiline and rasagiline are now being used to slow the course and keep the patient employed (Parkinson Study Group 1993, 2004). The patient whose Parkinson's disease is in an early stage should be watched closely for symptoms of depression. The psychiatrist should seriously consider the increased risk of suicide, especially in males who overvalue physical mobility and power and are extremely anxious about their continued performance in competitive and exacting sports such as tennis and golf. Activities less aggravating for the patient with mild Parkinson's disease may be chosen. More confusion than meets the eye (because of the preservation of language) contributes to the consternation felt by these patients over adaptation to the new challenge of disability. Furthermore, early pharmacotherapy for the disorder often involves anticholinergic agents, which have an additional potential for confusion.

TREATMENT CONSIDERATIONS IN LATE PARKINSON'S DISEASE

Often, antiparkinsonian drugs lose their efficacy with time. This can result in severe disillusionment in patients and their families. Increasing the doses can aggravate side effects. Emotional sequelae of L-dopa treatment may include domineering behavior, increased libido, manic hyperactivity or depression, confused irrational behavior, activation of latent psychosis, vivid nightmares that may disturb sleep, and visual hallucinations. Psychiatrists may be called on to help with these effects. Paying attention to the requirements for a patient's orientation (e.g., nightlights and familiar schedules), decreasing the stimulus level to diminish irritability, encouraging the beleaguered spouse to set limits, informing the spouse that the libidinal changes seldom persist, and, most of all, ensuring compliance with the times of dosing all may be helpful.

Doonief et al. (1992), in a survey of 336 patients with Parkinson's disease from 1984 to 1989, found that depression had a prevalence of 47% and an incidence rate of 1.86% per year compared with an incidence rate of 0.17% for individuals older than 40 in the general population.

Starkstein et al. (1990) studied patients with Parkinson's disease and found that 40% had major or minor depression and that depression was associated with left hemisphere involvement in patients with unilateral symptoms. Thus, depression in the early stages of Parkinson's disease may be generally related to left hemisphere dysfunction, although some studies have not found a lateral bias. Another peak of depression late in the course of the disease correlated with impairment of activities of daily living and of cognitive function.

Evaluating depression in Parkinson's disease is confounded by the many motor and autonomic or vegetative features psychiatrists use to diagnose depression that are also caused by Parkinson's disease. The clinician must go beyond mammalian bodily signs and delve into the patient's uniquely human mental dynamics, as in the list of suggested questions shown in Table 32–7.

Suicide is comparatively rare in Parkinson's disease. The psychiatrist should explore the patient's image of the disease process. Parkinson's disease is common enough to be a vivid caricature in the minds of patients, who fear they will become an exaggeration of the motor tendencies of the aged that are assumed by stage actors and comics who portray shuffling old duffers. Fear of humiliation because of such an image may be allayed by emphasizing the medical manageability of the condition, its usual slow progression, and intense research efforts, including transplantation and brain stimulation, that are based on knowledge of the pathophysiology of the disease. Later symptoms of emotional flattening, apathy, and impoverishment of the ability to relate to loved ones can be especially painful for the spouse.

If the capability for empathic, loving relatedness is lost, as it frequently is late in a variety of organic and degenerative brain states such as Parkinson's disease, the patient may not be able to invest an inner representation of the spouse with emotion. The tragic result late in the course of the disease may be a lack of appreciation of the spouse's loving care. A patient in an advanced stage of the disease may not even miss the caregiving spouse on his or her death if the patient's practical needs are satisfied.

TABLE 32–7. Questions to evaluate depression in Parkinson's disease

1. Have you found it difficult to remember a time when you felt better?

2. Is it now difficult for you to imagine a time when you will again feel happy?

3. Have you been feeling angry at yourself lately?

4. Are you more critical of yourself than usual?

5. Do you feel you are guilty of something?

6. Do you feel your appearance is unattractive?

7. Do you feel ashamed and wish to avoid exposure?

8. Does time seem to move more slowly? More quickly?

9. Is it difficult to imagine the future?

10. Are you tormented by recollections?

11. Do you feel others find you uninteresting, boring, or dull?

12. Do you feel an inner anger you cannot let out?

13. Does it seem that everyone else is happier than you are?

14. Do you feel older?

15. Do you keep thinking about lost possibilities, opportunities, things, or relationships?

16. Do you feel you are headed for a life of poverty?

17. Are you denying yourself small pleasures you used to enjoy?

18. Are you overwearing the same clothing?

19. Have you stopped caring about bathing?

20. Do you have a heaviness in your chest?

21. Does everything you touch turn bad?

22. Do you feel your life is a failure?

23. Have you felt unbearably sad?

24. Have you wanted to cry but been unable to?

25. Do you feel stuck in a low mood?

26. Have you felt your life is not worth living?

27. Have you thought that your life would end by an accident?

28. Have you thought of ending your life?

29. Have you thought of a means to end your life?

30. Have you made plans to end your life?

31. Is there a change in your religious feelings?

32. Do you feel abandoned?

33. Have you lost hope?

This attitude, or lack of attitude, can alienate or demoralize the most important caregiver. Often the psychiatrist must sensitively weigh the couple's unequal relationship, including the need of the spouse to recognize the patient's discouraging lack of emotional mutuality. Lucien Côté, M.D., a neurologist with extensive experience in Parkinson's disease, noted (personal communication, February 2000) that in this primarily motoric disorder, the patients particularly fail to appreciate and come to take for granted the motor assistance that is given to them. Because they are so dependent on it, the caregiver's help becomes part of their physical self-concept, which is extraordinarily malleable in all of us, as Ramachandran (1998) elegantly demonstrated experimentally. An analogy would be the fighter pilot who begins to feel that his or her body is coextensive with the airplane and its control surfaces. Secker and Brown (2005) administered 12–14 cognitive-behavioral therapy sessions to "carers" of Parkinson's patients with sleep difficulty, depression, anxiety, loneliness, and other symptoms of mental strain and found significant improvement on the General Health Questionnaire.

Henchcliffe (2005) noted that dementia is common in Parkinson's disease, occurring in about 45%, contributing to both functional decline and reduced quality of life. It differs phenotypically from Alzheimer's disease in that relatively less memory impairment but more bradyphrenia and visuospatial deficits occur, and visual hallucinations are possible and are experienced as tolerable. Psychotherapeutic techniques described for Alzheimer's disease may be adapted accordingly, especially regarding a greater tolerance for spatial maneuvering.

Groves and Forrest (2005) pointed out that throughout the course of Parkinson's disease, opportunities abound for psychosocial interventions that can improve the lives of patients and caregivers, and they provide an expanded list of suggestions for early, middle, and late stages of the disease.

DOPAMINE AND PERSONALITY IN PARKINSON'S DISEASE

Personality is not only a learned and habitual phenomenon simply to be unlearned in the psychotherapeutic analysis of character defenses. Evidence is growing that neurotransmitters have specific influences on personality. Dopamine has been associated with novelty seeking (analogous to exploratory behavior in animals), serotonin with harm avoidance, and norepinephrine with reward dependence. Menza et al. (1990), viewing Parkinson's disease with its low dopamine levels as a natural experiment, showed by rating scales completed by patients and their families that patients with Parkinson's disease had significantly less novelty-seeking behavior, both currently and premorbidly, than did control subjects with rheumatological and orthopedic diseases, but no differences were seen in serotonin- and norepinephrine-mediated behaviors. The psychotherapeutic approach to the "reflective, rigid, stoic, slow-tempered, frugal, and orderly behaviors," as Menza et al. (1990, p. 286) characterized them, can include admiration of these traits as virtues. Dopamine agonists may alter some of these personality traits and even promote uncharacteristic impulsive gambling when a casino is accessible. One patient discovered that he could pursue coin collecting online and at auctions that ran all night, transforming sleepless fretting into a time of pleasure and of focusing on the perfection and durability of these objects. Table 32–8 summarizes management issues for patients with Parkinson's disease.

The patient with Parkinson's disease and bipolar disorder presents a special management problem because levodopa may trigger manic highs. A neuroleptic such as quetiapine should be added to the mood stabilizer while raising the levodopa-carbidopa doses gradually. In consultation with the patient and family members, the psychiatrist should establish a behavioral checklist of the order of past warning signs to recognize early an impending high. For example, the first warning sign in the case of a 56-year-old woman with mild tremor and prominent slowing was racing thoughts and voices instigating activities; second, she would compulsively clean and withdraw from others; and third, she would sleep poorly and spend wildly on clothes. Continuing relationships with her psychiatrist and neurologist anchored safe management of her medication for Parkinson's disease.

HUNTINGTON'S DISEASE

In a large kindred of Huntington's disease families from Venezuela, in whom the G8 DNA marker was localized to chromosome 4, all descendants were said to "inherit" the disease, but only those who were affected by it were said to "have" it (Gusella et al. 1983). Wexler (1985) pointed out that although this distorts genetic truth, it expresses the experience of being at risk as a distinct state of mind. Because this state is stressful and conflict ridden, the psychiatrist may be consulted on various issues. CAG repetitions within the Huntington gene usually account for only 44% of the variability in the age at onset, and a search is on for other genetic and environmental factors that may slow the time to onset so that it exceeds a typical life span (Phillips 2004). Among the variables being studied are diet, smoking, and alcohol use behavior.

Ambiguity about whether one will be affected, as

TABLE 32–8.   Management issues for patients with Parkinson's disease

1. Estimate problems of therapeutic contact by motor impairment.
2. Estimate cognitive impairment by bradykinesia and rigidity.
3. Use neurological examination readily because less threatening than cognitive examination.
4. Capitalize on language preservation without underestimating impairment of spatial planning.
5. Coordinate psychotherapy with occupational and physical therapy sessions.
6. Encourage exercise and fitness to help cope with symptoms.
7. Employ sensory, mechanical, and cognitive aids to movement.
8. Anticipate symbiotic relationship with pharmacotherapy process.
9. Avoid neglecting emotional issues amidst dosing schedule.
10. Observe early in course for depression and suicide risk.
11. Choose activities and sports appropriate to abilities.
12. Distinguish early neuropsychiatric depression from later reaction to impairment.
13. Explore patient's embarrassment about image of appearance.
14. Emphasize manageability and slow progression of illness.
15. Anticipate disillusionment as drugs lose efficacy in time.
16. Anticipate side effects of L-dopa treatment.
17. Aid orientation with night-lights and schedules.
18. Decrease stimulus level to decrease irritability.
19. Anticipate spouse's pain when confronted by affective flattening.
20. Praise reflective, stoic, frugal, and orderly premorbid personality.

with any late-onset autosomal dominant disease, may dominate the mental life of people at risk for Huntington's disease. Administration of the genetic test for persons at risk requires much sensitivity to the emotional dimensions of determining whether an individual has the gene, and the test should always be administered as part of a personal physician-patient relationship. Hayden and Bombard (2005) noted that the prevalence of catastrophic events—suicide, suicide attempt, and hospitalization—following predictive testing is only 0.97% over an 11-year follow-up and the incidence 0.44% per year. The direct mutation test is highly accurate and permits identifying patients without a family history. Testing can be done anonymously but may impede counseling and follow-up. Prenatal testing can be done by linkage analysis exclusion testing without revealing the parent's risk. Only a tiny percentage of those at risk have taken the test, for a variety of reasons, including cost and fears of discrimination, especially by insurers (Mechcatie 1990). The very success of identification of the gene may raise hopes that an effective therapy is imminent, reducing demand for testing. Leroi and Michalon (1998) recommended that minors usually not be tested, and a counseling program with preestablished guidelines should accompany testing of adults. Tibben (2002) reported more exhaustively the implications of the declining risk estimation with advancing age (past 30) for persons carrying the *HD* gene, the specific recommendations for counseling persons of differing risks from varying inheritances, the effects of testing and refusing to test (which may be seen as rejection rather than caution), the guidelines for minors and adolescents if testing is done and for prenatal testing, and the revolution in politics and insurance resulting from the advent of presymptomatic testing.

The overlap of the initial symptoms of Huntington's disease and everyday experience, such as incidences of clumsiness, irritability, nocturnal myoclonus, emotional instability, or infrequent lapses of memory or judgment, can lead to hypochondriacal worries. The psychiatrist may help the patient by taking over the responsibility of the symptom search, distinguishing between those symptoms that overlap with normality and the disease, or by teaching the patient to delegate this function to the neurologist.

MANAGEMENT OF AFFECTED PATIENTS

Van Vugt and Roos (1999) remarked that despite the discovery of the gene defect (an expanded trinucleotide repeat) and its product huntingtin, no curative therapy is available, and psychosocial support remains the hallmark in the care of patients and relatives confronted with genetically determined and inevitable functional decline. Management issues are summarized in Table 32–9.

Knowing that one has Huntington's disease and knowing which parent is affected often leads to an unreasonable conscious or unconscious blaming of the gene-donating parent. This can disrupt vital processes of internalization of character from that parent during development. Psychotherapy

---

TABLE 32–9. Management issues for patients with Huntington's disease

1. Interpret blaming of gene-donating parent.
2. Help patient internalize healthy heritage from affected parent.
3. Ventilate wishes for healthy parental model.
4. Work with envy and rage against unaffected siblings.
5. Discuss fantasies that disease is a punishment.
6. Recognize that ideas of blame and prevention are strategies for control.
7. Do not participate in denial of transmissibility.
8. Recognize that movement disorder adds disability to dementia.
9. Note that preservation of recognition may lead to depression.
10. Ensure that family has aid of physiatrists and nutritionists.
11. Improvise mechanical assistance to movement function.
12. Discuss family ambivalence about preserving life in downhill course.
13. Help family take pride in giving nutrition and learning Heimlich maneuver for choking.
14. Encourage caregivers to pace themselves and take recreation.

---

can help patients deal with their longings for a healthy parental model and control primitive, envious rage against unaffected siblings. Positive aspects of the affected parent as a model should be sought. Psychotherapy can help with fantasies that the disease is a punishment, that anyone is to blame, and that alternative behaviors could have prevented it, while recognizing that such thoughts are defenses against helplessness and lack of control. In some instances, knowledge of the risk of the disorder has been denied by persons at risk and even their professional caregivers, with the result of needless transmission of the gene to another generation.

Leroi and Michalon (1998) reviewed the sparse treatment literature, noting that the presence of major affective disorder in the patients (33%) is strongly correlated with that in their offspring and is associated with a positive diagnosis in the offspring. Small doses of nonsedating and nonanticholinergic antidepressants can spare remaining cognitive reserve and aid response to psychotherapy. Huntington's patients have more trouble with aggression than do Alzheimer's patients, and so do otherwise asymptomatic gene carriers (Anderson and Marshall 2005). Aggressiveness may constitute the main need for hospitalization of affected patients, but a careful search should be made to determine whether provocations such as pain, thirst, hunger, frustration at changing capabilities, and imposed changes in routine are present. Irritability and social withdrawal may respond to support and structuring, and situational apathy (withdrawal, poorer hygiene, decreased initiative and motivation) may respond to structured and stimulating settings.

The disease itself adds the further incapacitation of a movement disorder to a progressive, unremitting dementia affecting higher-level intellectual skills and judgment. Frequently, speech is impaired, and intelligibility of communication with loved ones may be better maintained through referral to speech therapy for help with the dysarthria; speech augmentation devices may become necessary. Patients with Huntington's disease remain oriented to their surroundings, are able to recognize family and caregivers, and are able to convey their likes and dislikes somewhat better than do patients with Alzheimer's disease and other dementias. In keeping with this, they have more depression and less psychosis. Choreic movements eventually may increase a patient's caloric needs to 6,000 calories per day, but the coordination required to eat and swallow the food is impaired.

Ambivalence on the part of family and staff may arise around the sad irony of the daily struggle to keep the patient adequately nourished, in view of the disease's progressive downhill course and the likelihood that the patient will one day die of choking. However, there is comfort for the family and staff in treating the patient properly, managing nutrition efficiently, and knowing the Heimlich maneuver. Care of patients with Huntington's disease is a great burden, and those who do it need to monitor and pace themselves to avoid undue discouragement while deriving the satisfaction of being compassionate and useful.

INFECTIONS AND AUTOIMMUNE DISORDERS OF THE CENTRAL NERVOUS SYSTEM

Fallon and Nields (1994), writing about the complications of Lyme disease, cautioned that previously in the history of many neuropsychiatrically significant infections—whether caused by other bacteria (neurosyphilis, tuberculosis), parasites (neurocysticercosis, toxoplasmosis), fungi (coccidiomycosis, cryptococcosis), or viruses (herpes simplex virus, human immunodeficiency virus [HIV])—as well as of autoimmune disorders of the central nervous system such as lupus and multiple sclerosis,

the associated psychiatric symptoms were thought to be functional or hysterical. Physiologically based cognitive and mood changes were erroneously attributed exclusively to emotional reactions to the illness.

This is not to say that these conditions have no functional dimension. Fallon et al. (1992) discussed the complex secondary reactions, on an emotional basis, to Lyme disease, with its peculiar constellation of a fluctuating course of bizarre symptoms, cognitive disability, chronic pain, and uncertainties of diagnosis and treatment.

However, the physiologically based symptoms of Lyme disease include some that are among those frequently chosen for histrionic conversion. Shadick et al. (1994) found that physiologically significant late symptoms include arthralgias ($P=0.0001$) and extremity numbness, tingling or burning, unusual fatigue, poor concentration and/or memory loss, emotional lability, and difficulty sleeping (all $P \leq 0.05$). Not significant were myalgias, seizures, and depression.

Clearly, the psychotherapeutic approach demands a high index of suspicion to credit a physiological basis. This is often a preferred strategy anyway in building a therapeutic alliance that will encourage the emergence of conflicts and secondary gain. Generally, the patient is reassured but not encouraged to act more ill. In the case of HIV infection, the appearance of the first noticeable neuropsychiatric symptoms may have a grave effect on the patient, so that it is good to consider other explanations for the symptoms. Substantial neurological involvement with the tick-borne Lyme spirochete indicates a more aggressive treatment with intravenous antibiotics to diminish, but not necessarily eliminate, late complications. Some patients with residual sequelae will require neuropsychiatrically informed psychotherapy.

MULTIPLE SCLEROSIS

The influential view of Cottrell and Wilson (1926) that 63% of multiple sclerosis patients were unusually euphoric has been supplanted by numerous studies, beginning with that of Braceland and Giffin (1950), which showed more depression among these patients.

Minden and Schiffer (1990), in reviewing affective disorders in patients with multiple sclerosis, stated that the euphoria is usually described as a mental serenity, a cheerful feeling of physical well-being found more frequently later in the course of the disease—an affect dissociated from the cognitive awareness of the disability. This is not a fluctuating, reversible affect but a persistent change of personality. Although a positive affect is unlikely to stir a clamor for psychotherapy, it is advisable to have a close look to address the patient's possible pain beneath the euphoria in view of the frequent depressive symptoms that do respond to psychotherapy. Minden and Schiffer (1990) noted a higher rate of bipolar disorder in multiple sclerosis patients. Minden (1992), plumbing more deeply into apparent euphoria in multiple sclerosis patients, did not view it as an unmitigated blessing, particularly when it is an outward affective display disconnected from subjectively experienced depressive feelings that become apparent on "patient and empathic inquiry" (p. 201). Emotional instability of a labile nature responds so well to antidepressants that psychotherapy alone should not be considered.

Ron and Logsdail (1989) found no evidence that psychiatric symptoms in isolation were the first manifestation of multiple sclerosis; in their study, elation was correlated with widespread MRI abnormalities, and flattening of affect, delusions, and thought disorder were correlated with temporoparietal pathology on MRI. Grant et al. (1989) found that 77% of new multiple sclerosis patients, compared with only 35% of control subjects, experienced marked life stress in the year before the onset of symptoms, perhaps explaining the timing of symptom exacerbation for some patients by a psychosomatic process of further destabilizing an already unstable neuroimmunological system.

Psychiatrists should help the patient focus on the lack of certainty in prognosis in a positive sense rather than on the myriad of possible symptoms. It is important to point out that the absence of sure knowledge reflects the general uncertainty of life, including variability of the disease over time. Many patients conceal their disease at work for long periods. About two-thirds of patients never lose their ability to walk (some with crutches), and life span is normal, according to the National Multiple Sclerosis Society. The psychiatrist should emphasize the presence of medical support and treatment rather than the lack of cure and should be aware that the mysterious nature of the disease encourages magical theories involving self-blame and interpretation of the illness as an ominous metaphor (Simons 1984).

The psychiatrist should not reinforce the sick role for these patients and instead can offer the concept that a patient with multiple sclerosis has a disease but is not ill in the traditional sense. Thus, encouraging the realistic, but temporary and selective, omission of activities that are onerous for the patient becomes important. However, family fun needs to be preserved as well. Psychiatrists should recognize differences in patients' expectations about self-reliance and involvement in their own care (compared with passivity toward medical authority) in this illness, which has a great capacity to stimulate dependence on physicians. Most patients with multiple sclerosis are unemployed (LaRocca et al. 1985), compounding the financial strain of medical expenses and prospects of nursing home care at an unacceptably early age. If direct questioning indicates that the patient with multiple sclerosis has sexual difficulties, the psychiatrist should distinguish between degrees of organic and psychogenic sexual dysfunction in males by nocturnal penile tumescence monitoring. Many people have erectile difficulties and anorgasmia unrelated to multiple sclerosis. A spouse's resistance to the labeling of a partner as "disabled" may indicate a lesser likelihood of marital breakdown than with immediate acceptance. Steck et al. (2005) found that psychotherapy was indicated in half of the children ages 6–18 of patients with multiple sclerosis.

In assessing the potential of multiple sclerosis for creating disappointment with the self, the psychiatrist needs to recognize that multiple sclerosis is a disease of young adults that occurs in the prime of their lives, when they may have the highest performance expectations of themselves. Because extensive frontal lobe involvement of multiple sclerosis greatly impairs analytic ability, planning and organizing, flexibility, and emotional lability and limits the value of psychotherapy, it is important not to reach beyond reasonable therapeutic goals or to attempt sweeping revision of defenses when neuropsychiatric assessment suggests such involvement of the frontal lobe. Psychiatrists should help these patients to manage fatigue and other limitations by assisting them in selecting and planning participation in activities rather than seeing the patients withdraw or regress as a result of frustration at attempting too much. It is imperative to focus on what the patient is able to do, not what he or she is unable to do. This means that the psychiatrist should advise the patient to avoid undue stress, which temporarily worsens symptoms, and should reassure the patient that these flare-ups do not permanently advance the disease.

In a discussion that could serve as a model approach to psychotherapy for a specific neuropsychiatric condition, with implications for any infectious or inflammatory condition with a remitting and recurrent course, Minden (1992) offered suggestions for treating multiple sclerosis that begin with the diagnostic difficulties and phenomenological variability and proceed from elemental principles of psychotherapy to issues of the therapeutic relationship, transference, and countertransference.

Of general interest for neuropsychiatry is Minden's advice to apply a spectrum of strategies, from insight-oriented to supportive, in a flexible way over time, as determined by the patient's needs in dealing with a fluctuating disorder and one that varies unpredictably in severity in individuals from little disability (20% of patients with multiple sclerosis have benign disease) and moderate disability (20%–30% have relapsing-remitting multiple sclerosis) to severe disability (50%–60% have chronic progressive multiple sclerosis). In summary, Minden (1992) offered "a simple principle: when external reality is overwhelming, it must be addressed before internal reality can be explored" (p. 207). Compounding the anxiety and dread of unpredictability, not only of the course but also of each acute episode, is the effect on the physician-patient relationship of the diagnostic difficulty: physicians are seen as evasive and insensitive and patients as demanding, annoying, or attention seeking. Fatigue (present in 90% of patients with multiple sclerosis and incapacitating for nearly 70%) and altered sensation and visual blurring are subjective symptoms that often fail to elicit sympathy from professionals and family.

Minden (1992) pointed out that when there are "few objective findings, unmistakable secondary gain, and perhaps hysterical personality traits or intense preoccupation with symptoms, it is not difficult to see why a person with MS [multiple sclerosis] may be thought to have conversion disorder, somatization disorder or hypochondriasis" (p. 200). Somatoform disorders or emotional elaboration may coexist with multiple sclerosis, especially in view of the reality of the frequent disruptions of the course of life originating in the body. Minden asks clinicians to consider whether bodily expression of emotions may be not only understandable but also healthy to some degree in patients with multiple sclerosis and, correspondingly, is concerned that physicians not discourage frank and frequent discussion of the symptoms that so trouble these patients.

The cognitive deficits of multiple sclerosis, as in other subcortical dementias, affect retrieval more than encoding and storage of information (Rao 1990, cited in Minden 1992) and are variable in degree but also in effect according to the demands of the patient's lifestyle for mental acuity. Although speech slurring is common, communication by language is less affected, and most difficulties with the larger aspects of mental planning require compensatory reevaluation and frank work with the patient.

Common themes that may be anticipated in psychotherapy for patients with multiple sclerosis arise at characteristic points in the illness course: when function deteriorates, when the patient must use crutches or a wheelchair, when employment ends, and when nursing home placement looms. Minden (1992) noted that the wheelchair is more threatening as a symbol of humiliating loss of control early in the disease than when it is helpful and needed. She found that wives fear abandonment by spouses more than husbands do (and twice as many women develop multiple sclerosis). Visible impairments such as the dragging of a foot or the use of a cane cause shame, and conflicts arise over unaccustomed wishes to be

cared for. Because patients attribute personal meanings to the illness, such as its being a punishment for something they were responsible for doing, Minden inferred that this may be easier to contemplate than their real powerlessness in the face of the disease. Defenses must be respected as positive attempts of the personality to cope and are not necessarily to be analyzed away unless they can be replaced with something better. For example, much as the psychiatrist may object on a scientific or moral basis to the implication that patients with multiple sclerosis have been bad persons, assumed guilt permits confession, expiation, and forgiveness by others or in structured religious resources. The occult origin of exacerbations may lead to a disease culture of paranoid blaming.

Minden (1992) suggested that the actual course of therapy should be tailored to the condition, beginning with reservations about loss of control in being sent to a psychiatrist. The therapeutic alliance is easier to build when the initial session resembles the familiar structure of medical consultations in which the physician actively questions the patient, replies directly to the patient's questions, and "asks about cognitive changes as easily as a neurologist asks about changes in walking" (Minden 1992, p. 204). The patient's defense of focusing on symptoms over feelings is not challenged, and there is no assumption that the patient will enter formal psychotherapy. Even if they do, patients should be encouraged to come and go in therapy according to the vicissitudes of the illness. Leaving may be more healthy than staying. Fixed rules about missed appointments are less appropriate with multiple sclerosis patients, in whom function is so medically context–dependent. Self-help groups such as those offered by the National Multiple Sclerosis Society should be encouraged, but fears of seeing others with advanced cases of the disease should be respected. Minden cited the work of Schiffer (1987), concluding that patients whose depression failed to improve and who were more concerned with losing their dependent gratifications had psychiatric problems that predated the multiple sclerosis and would be more effectively given psychiatric help.

Neuropsychological assessments can be useful in patients who are unaware of or are denying their deficits. Before tests are ordered for this purpose, however, the neuropsychological tester should be made aware of this intention so that the patient can be handled with tact and care.

Transference issues also were noted by Minden (1992) and include the perception of the psychiatrist as "a source of stability in an otherwise unpredictable life" (p. 210). As elsewhere, idealization may lead to devaluation and disappointment. Other patients may be suspicious and anxious. Transference is always noted but is not usually explored or analyzed. Countertransference problems include discomfort with chronic debilitation; embarrassment at unfamiliarity with the latest research; hesitation at necessary exploration in detail of daily dressing, bathing, and toilet function; feelings of defeat and hopelessness; impatience with scanning speech and dysarthria; guilt at being healthy and enjoying life when the patient is not; pain at watching intellectual impairment; and irritation at the patient's failure to follow therapeutic plans because of frontal lobe involvement. Valleroy and Kraft (1984) found that one-half to three-quarters of the persons with multiple sclerosis say that they have sexual impairment, which also requires special attention to transferential envy and countertransferential guilt, as in the case of other spinal cord disorders (see section "Spinal Cord Injury" earlier in this chapter).

Reflecting the murky waters of multiple sclerosis therapy, a meta-analysis by Mohr and Goodkin (1999) indicated that efficacy of psychotherapy versus antidepressants was not significantly different for depression in multiple sclerosis, that improving coping skills was better than increasing insight, and that all treatments were more effective than none. Jean et al. (1999) found that neuropsychological variables chosen for their sensitivity to multiple sclerosis did not predict coping styles or their effectiveness but that higher levels of distress were associated with emotion-focused coping strategies, indicating psychotherapeutic interventions aimed at improving ways of coping. Brassington and Marsh (1998) designated multiple sclerosis as a subcortical dementia and considered that cognitively heterogeneous patient groups may disguise more specific focal neuropsychological impairment; they called for more evaluation of psychological and rehabilitation interventions. Shnek et al. (1997) found that patients with multiple sclerosis have greater levels of depression and helplessness and lower levels of self-efficacy than do spinal cord injury patients, perhaps because of the unpredictable course and possibility of being affected in many different ways. Helplessness and lower self-efficacy predicted depression, but cognitive distortions had no independent effect. Mohr et al. (2005) administered 16 weeks of telephone therapy for depression in patients with multiple sclerosis and found cognitive-behavioral components outdid emotional support.

Minden (1992) also noted that what patients with multiple sclerosis want "is simply a compassionate, understanding person with whom to share their worries and sadness" (p. 211). Table 32–10 summarizes management issues for patients with multiple sclerosis.

Crayton et al. (2004), discussing multimodal management in an era of inconsistently effective disease-modifying agents, recommended the effectiveness of communication, education, exercise, and support. Cognitive deterioration may signify active disease, and associated fatigue, depression, and relationship issues may be treated by psychotherapy as well as pharmacotherapy, which may aggravate the typical sexual dysfunction. Birnbaum and Miller (2004) identified deficits in testing of the generation and application of working strategies in novel tasks in 76% of multiple sclerosis patients, which were not correlated with their depression or fatigue and could have implications for patients' coping with nonroutine tasks and the implementation of their cognitive rehabilitation.

PSYCHOGENIC MOVEMENT DISORDERS

Conventional psychiatric wisdom holds that psychoanalytic ideas are so pervasive in post-Freudian America that people rarely develop conversion hysteria as a symptomatic expression of conflict. But neurology clinics that deal with an active motor component, as in seizures and movement disorders, still resemble Charcot's Salpêtrière clinic (Forrest 2005b). Tremor and dystonia are most frequently imitated. Tremor is seldom mistaken and easily tested. The posturing of dystonia is another matter; before 1978, 44% of the real dystonia cases had been previously misdiagnosed as emotional in origin (Williams and Fahn 1988). Peculiarities of the disorder may mislead. A sensory trick, such as the patient touching his or her cheek, may correct cervical dystonia (Naumann et al. 2000); patients may be able to walk backward but not forward; and symptoms may vary with emotions. In an overcorrection, by 1975, for a time no case of proven psychogenic dystonia was acknowledged. According to Williams and Fahn (1988), about 3%–5% of the cases are now estimated to be psychogenic, more likely so if the dystonia begins in the foot and at rest rather than in action, is paroxysmal rather than continual, and is accompanied by other psychogenic features such as false weakness or sensory findings, self-inflicted injuries, or multiple somatizations. Jahanshahi (2005) reviewed the convoluted history of the psychiatric approach to dystonia and the evidence against psychogenesis of most dystonia. Williams et al. (2005) presented an expanded list of clues suggesting a nonneurological disorder and the primary and secondary gain factors with varying consciousness of intentionality.

GENERAL SUGGESTIONS FOR THE MANAGEMENT OF PSYCHOGENIC DYSTONIA

Williams and Fahn (1988) strongly suggested that patients with psychogenic dystonia be admitted to the hospital, not

TABLE 32–10. Management issues for patients with multiple sclerosis

1. Expect more depression than euphoria, especially early.
2. Look past euphoria for coexistent depressive symptoms.
3. Consider possible bipolar disease or steroid effects during psychotherapy.
4. Avoid relying on psychotherapy alone for treatment of emotional instability.
5. Avoid unnecessarily medicating euphoria.
6. Note likely presence of life stress before episode.
7. Suggest psychotherapy, especially after diagnosis.
8. Disclose diagnosis to significant others, not to all.
9. Assist those who are dating with disclosure after rapport with partner.
10. Help patient see uncertainty of prognosis in a positive sense of possibility.
11. Plan for the possibility of disability, as in choosing a new home, but hope for the best.
12. Anticipate magical theories of self-blame in view of mysterious nature of the disease's etiology and fluctuations.
13. Avoid reinforcing sick or disabled role.
14. Select activities to substitute for those posing difficulties.
15. Accept differences in patients' relying on selves versus doctors.
16. Inquire directly about sexual difficulties.
17. Approach sexual functioning discussion cautiously and involve spouse eventually.
18. Consider urologic treatment options for male patients.
19. Adapt therapeutic goals and discourse in impaired planning ability.
20. Help to manage fatigue by selection and planning.
21. Focus on capacities, not disabilities.
22. Advise avoidance of stresses that worsen symptoms.
23. Reassure that flare-ups do not permanently advance the disease.
24. Keep newly diagnosed patients from support groups for wheelchair-bound, blind, or incontinent patients.

Source.   Items 7–9 and 11 were adapted from Scheinberg 1983.

so much for the necessary diagnostic studies (such as a sleep study) as for support during the explanation that their symptoms are emotional in origin, and for effective behavior therapy employing rewards for progress. They have insisted that a neurologist be involved in the diagnosis. Placebo ruses may aid diagnosis but are not a lasting treatment, and the patient must be told immediately to avoid a sense of betrayal. The patient is told "firmly that he/she has dystonia and that it is caused by unconscious conflicts which cause real physical symptoms. Pent-up emotions need to be expressed, and when there has been some blockage of this process, they do so by producing these abnormal movements" (p. 453). Patronizing, condescending, or morally judgmental attitudes sabotage prospects for engagement.

Constricting reimbursement for care now makes hospitalization less often possible, yet an intervention is called for on an outpatient basis. The following are sug-

gestions from our experience at the Movement Disorder Clinic at the Neurological Institute of New York. Williams et al. (2005) noted the lack of controlled therapeutic trials but reported that we were pleasantly surprised by some good results from our outpatient approach.

STUDIES IN HYSTERIA REVISITED: MULTIDISCIPLINARY APPROACH TO CONVERSION DISORDER IN AN OUTPATIENT MOVEMENT DISORDER CLINIC

There are few such dramatic demonstrations of the dynamic unconscious as those patients whose conflicts are expressed in psychogenic movement disorders that are not conscious malingering. Yet a delving, uncovering approach may be especially unsuited to these patients' needs, at least initially, for several reasons. These cases also strain the diagnostic acumen of both psychiatrists and neurologists. It is possible to adopt a helpful psychotherapeutic stance that bridges the organic-functional dilemma before diagnostic certainty.

As in psychiatry generally, our cases are context dependent and our procedures are not rigid. But general guidelines are emerging from our experience. These apply to unconsciously or mostly unconsciously maintained symptoms rather than primarily malingering or compensation neuroses.

- *Use proximity, immediacy, and expectancy.* These three cardinal principles from military psychiatry denote the availability of psychiatric consultation at the site and at the time of the neurological consultation, together with a positively maintained expectancy of symptomatic improvement. The psychiatric function should appear to the patient to be naturally and seamlessly integrated into the consultation, rather than at a remove suggesting banishment.

- *Capitalize on the patient's wish to change.* The patient may be fed up with the inconvenience of the symptom and secretly disgusted with himself or herself. This may be more likely late in the chain of referral, when frustration has mounted.

- *Employ the cachet of the specialty clinic.* Prestige of place coupled with acceptance by the elite specialists, when these can be offered, provide a narcissistic booster.

- *Provide multidisciplinary attention.* Being presented before at least half a dozen clinic specialists fulfills a wish for attention and signals that a definitive opinion will be given. The presence of an overwhelming number of staff is sometimes also used in emergency department and military care stations to calm the obstreperous or violent patient. Here, the effect of group pressure applied with admiring and caring attentiveness has greater clout than an individual professional could muster.

- *Sort out the components of the patient's dilemma.* How can he or she extricate himself or herself from the limiting trap of the symptom formation, and what are the perpetuating rewards? Ideally, a psychodynamic formulation should be arrived at, but for numerous reasons, such as the press of time in a neurological clinic and the lower likelihood that the patient or relatives have insight or can provide in-depth information, a greater degree of inference may be needed.

- *Assess the patient's interpersonal world.* At the very least, the significant human connections should be inquired about to gauge the patient's main support system, particularly if the symptoms would be relinquished. Possible gain factors should be identified, with calculation as to how they might be diminished.

- *Limit disability rewards.* Psychogenic movement disorders on an unconscious conversion or factitious basis (as opposed to conscious malingering) confer genuine disability on the patient, but an attempt should be made to limit or wean from disability payments with positive expectancy and the reassurance that the muscles will learn to move more normally.

- *Read the patient's body language.* These physically, not mentally, oriented patients do not speak meaningfully in words about their conflicts. What could he or she be saying nonverbally? What do the movements say, considered as an expressive dance or pantomime? What is the emotion they express (joy, fear, anger, shame, guilt, sadness)? The term *alexithymia* describes having a lack of words for feelings, but these patients do not lack gestural language. Moreover, these patients are performers, albeit unconscious ones, putting on a show. They appreciate an audience, especially a large one of specialists intent on observing every last motion. Motoric alexithymia may result from poor intermodal connectivity in the brain and may be contrasted with the facility of synesthesia (Forrest 2005b).

- *Deconstruct the objective correlative.* The term comes from drama criticism (T. S. Eliot) and refers to the concrete bit of stage business that conveys the significant emotional action or vector of the moment. For example, Lear's helplessness is shown when he cannot undo a button. Some of the patient's gestural language is more pertinent than the rest.

- *Speak the patient's language.* If these patients wanted verbal psychotherapy, they would have asked for it. Just as they are not expressive in words, they do not comprehend very well the words that might be spoken by therapists about their conflicts. Instead, they may be acutely sensitive to facial expressions, tone of voice, and the speed with which a professional might whirl on his or her heel and leave the room. The patient's language is action and gesture, and the main brunt of the therapeutic intervention must be carried out nonverbally. The way in which the patient is touched, examined, and spoken to by the neurologist begins the treatment. Therapeutic actions include participation of nursing staff and social workers to assess situational factors. Specially prescribed maneuvers by physical therapy and rehabilitation medicine establish a graded timetable for progress. The psychiatrist assesses emotional expression and suggests medication for mood disorders.

- *Guard the patient's secret.* The patient's behavior conceals yet often betrays secrets that are strongly defended against. Early in the psychoanalytic movement, the simple goal was to make the unconscious conscious, but this did not do justice to the analysis of defenses that is usually necessary in psychodynamic treatment. Because of the limits of contact with these patients, usually the secret must be left unspoken and implicit, even if symptoms are relinquished. If the patient was sexually abused, for example, the patient still may repress or not have verbal access to the recollection. It may take months or years for a history of incest to emerge in the therapeutic process. Leading the witness can result in false memory syndrome. Aggressive "lancing of the boil" of the unconscious conflict is contraindicated. Setbacks have occurred when psychiatrists, flushed with joy about their patient's cooperative improvement and equating it with verbal comprehension, have said something overly interpretive or shown him or her something in writing about conversion symptoms that jarred the patient.

- *Medicate implicit mood disorders.* The patient may have entered this symptomatic detour from living well because of a depressive lack of confidence about succeeding in more usual ways. Antidepressant medication may help supply the mental energy to engage in psychotherapy and find the way back to the competitive real world. As an active placebo, it may provide a face-saving excuse to relinquish the symptom. Medication, like the physical examination, also reassures the patient of the physician's interest. Medication other than antidepressants may be helpful; for example, analgesics may ease the painful spasm from holding postures.

The following case illustrates psychogenic dystonia:

A 58-year-old Hispanic man, formerly a machinist, worked as a cook until 1 year ago, when he felt a pain in his right leg that developed into psychogenic dystonia, with a stiffly extended right leg while sitting or walking and back pain from the maintained posture. For 8 months, he had been walking with a cane. He had been given gabapentin, baclofen, and carisoprodol.

He did not want to see a psychiatrist but agreed to the psychiatrist's presence. The psychiatrist advised the neurologist in English, and the neurologist spoke to the patient in Spanish. On psychiatric examination, the patient had a forlorn affect, which he attributed to a divorce and his subsequent loneliness. The neurologist was encouraged to take an admiring stance and to tell the patient that he was a handsome man, looked young for his age, and should be attractive to women.

Further inquiry suggested by the symbolism of his symptom found that he had sexual dysfunction secondary to diabetes. The physical therapist suggested relaxation and strengthening exercises for his leg, and her demonstration was done in the presence of several of our female staff, who paid close attention. The neurol-

ogist, at the psychiatrist's suggestion, said that there was hope that his sexual dysfunction could be improved. A medicine with some of that effect, bupropion, would be begun. He also suggested that the patient obtain a job where he could work sitting down.

When the patient returned to the clinic in 6 weeks, he had been working part-time (3 hours a day) at a restaurant preparing food. He also noted that he had a little more sexual desire. He elaborated on the sensations he was feeling in his right leg. Not only did it stiffen up, but he saw the foot and leg get longer, and his right leg would swell and enlarge. These symptoms further pointed to the symbolic content of compensating for his acquired impotency by enacting an erect and tumescent leg. The patient was praised liberally by the assembled group for his progress in obtaining part-time work. The physical therapist gave him more exercises, and—with considerable attention and praise—convinced him to do modified deep knee bends. The group all paid attention to this and, in fact, actually applauded. The patient himself smiled in pride for the first time. He was told that we were impressed with his progress and that as his leg became less stiff and his back loosened up, we would consider further medication to aid his sexual recovery.

BRAIN TUMORS

The brain tumors most likely to produce behavioral difficulties in patients for which a psychiatrist might be consulted are those of the temporal lobe, and the tumors do so by becoming an irritative focus for temporal lobe epilepsy. Blumer and Benson (1975) noted the difficulties for psychotherapy that are caused by the viscous type of verbal expression in patients with temporal lobe epilepsy, including a deepening of emotional response that is not reversed by anticonvulsant therapy and the changes in sexuality and episodic aggressivity. These authors argued in favor of nondrug psychiatric management of temporal lobe emotional features.

Blumer and Benson (1975) stated that the "pseudodepressed" change in personality caused by lesions of the convexity of the frontal lobes warrants early and ongoing rehabilitative efforts and mobilization; that is, patients should not be allowed to sit around. Patients with the "pseudopsychopathic" alteration of personality, more attributed to lesions of the orbital surface, have misbehavior that tries the patience of family members, who may benefit from psychiatric support. In patients with recurrent or intractable central nervous system tumors, more diffuse signs of increased intracranial pressure sometimes supplant the specific personality changes already mentioned.

J. Jaffe (personal communication, August 1990) found that psychiatric consultation in several hundred patients with neurosurgical brain tumor and arteriovenous malfor-

TABLE 32–11.   Management issues for patients with brain tumors

1. Correlate observations of specific impairments with tumor location, as in the case of temporal lobe involvement.

2. Expect diffuse difficulties and trouble with novel situations.

3. Mobilize patients with frontal "pseudodepressed" changes.

4. Watch for communication of fears, sometimes nonverbally.

5. Provide warmth, understanding, and explanation as a consistent figure before and after surgery.

6. Explain puzzling anatomical symptoms, such as contralateral effects.

7. Discuss permissibility of exertion and sex in arteriovenous malformations.

8. Distinguish between growth and malignancy of tumor.

9. Explain that malignancy may differ in degree and is not black and white.

10. Invite reporting of psychotic symptoms on high-dose steroids.

11. Reassure about competency and arrange for wishes to be respected in terminal patients.

12. Reassure that death will come after a coma, and there will be little or controllable pain.

mation led to an appreciation of how much warm understanding and explanation by a consistent figure can minimize the distress before and after surgery. Certain communications are often useful. For example, the central nervous system anatomical basis of puzzling peripheral symptoms can be explained because patients are not as familiar with brain symptoms as they are with cardiac symptoms. In patients who face a terminal course, reassurance may be given to these patients about competency, with assistance in arranging for their wishes to be respected. The patient who fears a painful and frightening death can be told that death will likely come after lapsing into a coma and (with the exception of certain headache patients) will bring little, or controllable, pain. Table 32–11 summarizes management issues for patients with brain tumors.

Butler and Mulhern (2005) discussed neurocognitive costs of improving rates of cures of brain tumors in children and adolescents and suggested ways of reducing treatment-related late effects, including cognitive remediation and alterations in the classroom.

CONCLUSION

Neuropsychiatry has been thought to involve poor prognoses, but when the statistics are in the patient's favor, they may aid the psychiatrist's supportive role. For example, in a study by Thorngren et al. (1990) of stroke patients discharged from the hospital to independent living, 1 year later 90% were still in their own homes, 99% could walk independently, 92%–95% could climb a staircase, and 90% could manage their daily hygiene. Six percent had died, and 25% had been rehospitalized.

When the statistics are not so favorable, the psychiatrist's objective and relativistic viewpoint may be tested. Psychiatrists and other physicians often have such high demands for their own performance that they must guard against identifying too easily with suicidal impulses in impaired patients who might later be grateful for aggressive intervention against depression and suicide. Lessons that can be learned from this include the need for a relativistic viewpoint that can adopt the patients' differing standards for acceptable living. It is also imperative to recognize that emotional exhaustion and burnout sometimes may affect young professionals with high standards more than most people, who have more relaxed standards of performance and may be better able to contemplate enduring life with prolonged morbidity and a chronic downhill course. In general, patients with neurological deficits that affect their performance may be better able to accept them than are some of their physicians, and physicians need to help them make the most of living.

Highlights for the Clinician

+ **Contact:** The neuropsychiatric examination and psychotherapeutic interventions in patients with neuropsychiatric disorders require expert attention to a hierarchy of barriers to the establishment of empathic contact.

+ **Continuum:** Conceptualizing a mind-brain dichotomy is less useful than viewing patient responses on a continuum from cortical neurological reactions to psychodynamic defenses, with intermediate neuromental defenses that are formations in the mind that have a flavor of brain function rather than of an abstract psychology. Examples are the underappreciated misidentification syndromes, stereotypy, and perseverative repetitions.

+ **Traumatic change:** Traumatic brain injury epitomizes the special difficulty of neuropsychiatric disorders for the patient—that they are disorders of the organ of human self-control, adaptation, and mastery of challenges. The suddenness of the dramatic life changes brought about by the trauma adds to difficulty of grasp, loneliness, and projection of self-condemnation.

+ **Family needs:** In most neuropsychiatric disorders, the family, spouse, or caregiver should be integrated into the psychotherapeutic approach from the start. This is especially the case when the condition creates great dependency, such as spinal cord disorders and advanced motor and cognitive disorders. Caregivers need the support, and a family approach multiplies the efficacy of the clinician's interventions. The effect on children and adolescents of an impaired parent varies with their age and emotional stage.

+ **Unsteadiness:** Instability on the feet in the elderly, which may arise from difficulties at different levels of the neuraxis, should be addressed because of its effect on emotional insecurity.

+ **Epilepsy:** Epilepsy poses age-related needs and tasks, and interictal personality effects may be profound.

+ **Alzheimer's:** Care of the patient with Alzheimer's disease or other dementia includes thoughtful environmental precautions—an elder version of childproofing—as well as prompting signposts and other memory aids, including provisions for continuity of dependency on relationships. Encourage early help with financial planning. Capitalize on remaining spatial somatic, motoric, procedural, and action memory as explicit memory wanes. Patients may be premourned as if dead and emotionally abandoned, and frank fear in the patient may signal elder abuse.

+ **Early Parkinson's:** In early Parkinson's disease, the paucity of facial affect display is the chief obstacle to appearing unimpaired, and facial emotion exercises can be prescribed to help this, in addition to general exercises for mobility. The spouse should be referred to as a partner in living rather than as a caregiver at this stage, and, more than in most conditions, pleasure goals should be prescribed to counter the restrictions and anhedonia that accompany the disease. Do not neglect the nonmotor disorders of sensation, peristalsis, and sleep. Depression may be greater with left hemisphere involvement in unilateral patients (with more tremor and rigidity in the right extremities). Dopamine agonists may pose a risk of rash or compulsive gambling uncharacteristic of the personality.

+ **Late Parkinson's:** In late Parkinson's disease, depression correlates with impairment of cognition and activities of daily living. If the capacity for loving relatedness wanes late in the disorder, a lack of appreciation of the spouse's loving care may be especially difficult for the spouse.

+ **Huntington's:** Huntington's disease not only affects but also implicates the family, with the potential for blame dynamics, quandaries about premorbid testing, and shared mood disorder as well as motor inheritance. Speech therapy practically helps maintain contact, and Heimlich maneuver training for the family is a must.

Highlights for the Clinician (continued)

✦ **Multiple sclerosis:** In multiple sclerosis, do not reinforce the sick role, because the patient is not ill in the traditional sense. Omit onerous activities temporarily and selectively. Depression is more likely than, and may underlie, apparent euphoria. Help ambitious young patients to pace themselves. The occult origins of exacerbations may lead to a guilty, paranoid, or blaming culture of the disease.

✦ **Movement disorders:** Patients with psychogenic movement disorders tend to be alexithymic, lacking verbal but not gestural language, which they use like mime actors to portray their distress. Although hospital admission is preferable for explanation that they have dystonia or tremor of emotional origin, and for appropriate behavior therapy, this is often impossible because of constricted reimbursement. They do not receive verbal interpretation of their symptoms gladly and may be approached in an outpatient setting with the aid of a physical therapist and a strong ethos of expectancy of improvement. Often secret conflicts and traumata must remain secret for the time being.

✦ **Brain tumors:** Brain tumor patients benefit from much less disabling and pain-inducing techniques of treatment and can be supported with more optimism than in the past.

✦ **Prognosis and perspectives:** Neuropsychiatric prognoses are not necessarily grim. For example, 90% of stroke patients were still in their homes, and 99% could walk independently a year later. But when faced with a patient with a chronic downhill course, the young professional with high self-standards of performance must guard against countertransference feelings that reinforce temporary suicidal inclinations. Clinicians should recognize that the patients may be more able than they themselves are to contemplate their impaired lives with grace, equanimity, and gratitude.

RECOMMENDED READINGS

Anderson KE, Weiner WJ, Lang AE (eds): Advances in Neurology, Vol 96: Behavioral Neurology of Movement Disorders. Philadelphia, PA, Lippincott Williams & Wilkins, 2005

Schiffer RB, Rao SM, Fogel BS (eds): Neuropsychiatry, 2nd Edition. Philadelphia, PA, Lippincott Williams & Wilkins, 2003

Silver JM, McAllister TW, Yudofsky SC (eds): Textbook of Traumatic Brain Injury. Washington, DC, American Psychiatric Publishing, 2005

Yudofsky SC, Kim HF: Neuropsychiatric Assessment (Review of Psychiatry Series, Vol 23; Oldham JM and Riba MB, series eds). Washington, DC, American Psychiatric Publishing, 2004

REFERENCES

Anderson KE, Marshall FJ: Behavioral symptoms associated with Huntington's disease, in Advances in Neurology, Vol 96: Behavioral Neurology of Movement Disorders. Edited by Anderson KE, Weiner WJ, Lang AE. Philadelphia, PA, Lippincott Williams & Wilkins, 2005, pp 197–208

Anderson KE, Silver JM: Modulation of anger and aggression. Semin Clin Neuropsychiatry 3:232–241, 1998

Andersson S, Gundersen OM, Finset A: Emotional activation during therapeutic interaction in traumatic brain injury: effect of apathy, self-awareness and implications for rehabilitation. Brain Inj 13:393–404, 1999

Andreasen NC, Arndt S, Swayze V, et al: Thalamic abnormalities in schizophrenia visualized through magnetic resonance imaging. Science 266:294–298, 1994

Anshin RN: Intersubjectivity, creative uncertainty, and systems theory: an approach to the therapeutic use of empathy. J Am Acad Psychoanal 23:369–378, 1995

Aronson MK: Alzheimer's and Other Dementias. Carrier Letter No 102. Belle Meade, NJ, Carrier Foundation, November 1984

Beatty WW, Staton RD, Weir WS, et al: Cognitive disturbances in Parkinson's disease. J Geriatr Psychiatry Neurol 2:22–33, 1989

Bellus SB, Kost PP, Vergo JG, et al: Improvements in cognitive functioning following intensive behavioral rehabilitation. Brain Inj 12:139–145, 1998

Benson DF: Disorders of verbal expression, in Psychiatric Aspects of Neurological Disease. Edited by Benson DF, Blumer D. New York, Grune & Stratton, 1975, pp 121–135

Berry V: Partners/Families and Professionals Together: A Model of Posttraumatic Rehabilitation. Austin, TX, Ranch Treatment Center, 1984

Birnbaum S, Miller A: Cognitive strategies application of multiple sclerosis patients. Mult Scler 10:67–73, 2004

Blumer D: Specific psychiatric complications in certain forms of epilepsy and their treatment, in Epilepsy: A Handbook for the Mental Health Professional. Edited by Sands H. New York, Brunner/Mazel, 1982, pp 97–111

Blumer D, Benson DF: Personality changes with frontal and temporal lobe lesions, in Psychiatric Aspects of Neurologic Disease, Vol 1. Edited by Benson DF, Blumer D. New York, Grune & Stratton, 1975, pp 151–170

Bodenhamer E, Achterberg-Lawlis J, Kevorkian G, et al: Staff and patient perceptions of the psychosocial concerns of spinal cord injured persons. Am J Phys Med 62:182–193, 1983

Braceland FJ, Giffin ME: The mental changes associated with multiple sclerosis (an interim report). Res Publ Assoc Res Nerv Ment Dis 28:450–455, 1950

Bracken MB, Shepard MJ: Coping and adaptation following acute spinal cord injury: a theoretical analysis. Paraplegia 18:74–85, 1980

Braga LW, Da Paz AC, Ylvisaker M: Direct clinician-delivered versus indirect family supported rehabilitation of children with traumatic brain injury: a randomized controlled trial. Brain Inj 19:819–831, 2005

Brassington JC, Marsh NV: Neuropsychological aspects of multiple sclerosis. Neuropsychol Rev 8:42–77, 1998

Bromley E: Elements of Dynamics, V: resiliency and the narrative. J Am Acad Psychoanal Dyn Psychiatry 33:389–404, 2005

Burke JM, Danick JA, Bemis B, et al: A process approach to memory book training for neurological patients. Brain Inj 8:71–81, 1994

Burns A, Guthrie E, Marino-Francis F, et al: Brief psychotherapy in Alzheimer's disease: randomized controlled trial. Br J Psychiatry 187:143–147, 2005

Butler RW, Mulhern RK: Neurocognitive interventions for children and adolescents surviving cancer. J Pediatr Psychol 30:65–78, 2005

Calvert T, Knapp P, House A: Psychological associations with emotionalism after stroke. J Neurol Neurosurg Psychiatry 65:928–929, 1998

Chen JY, Stern Y, Sano M, et al: Cumulative risks of developing extrapyramidal signs, psychosis, or myoclonus in the course of Alzheimer's disease. Arch Neurol 48:1141–1143, 1991

Childs AH: Brain injury: "Now what shall we do?" Problems in treating brain injuries. Psychiatric Times, April 1985, pp 15–17

Cohen-Mansfield J, Deutsch LH: Agitation: subtypes and their mechanisms. Semin Clin Neuropsychiatry 1:325–339, 1996

Corrigan PW, Bach PA: Behavioral treatment, in Textbook of Traumatic Brain Injury. Edited by Silver JM, McAllister TM, Yudofsky SC. Washington, DC, American Psychiatric Publishing, 2005, pp 669–671

Côté L, Riedel G, Orr JDE: Exercises for the Parkinson Patient With Hints for Daily Living. New York, Parkinson's Disease Foundation, undated. Videotape version available from: http://www.pdf.org

Cottrell SS, Wilson SAK: The affective symptomatology of disseminated sclerosis. J Neurol Psychopathol 7:1, 1926

Craig A, Hancock K, Dickson H: Improving the long term adjustment of spinal cord injured persons. Spinal Cord 37:345–350, 1999

Crayton H, Heyman RA, Rossman HS: A multimodal approach to managing the symptoms of multiple sclerosis. Neurology 63 (suppl 5):S12–S18, 2004

Critchley M: The Divine Banquet of the Brain and Other Essays. New York, Raven, 1979

Cummings JL, Jeste DV: Alzheimer's disease and its management in the year 2010. Psychiatr Serv 50:1173–1177, 1999

DeJong G, Branch LG, Corcoran PJ: Independent living outcomes in spinal cord injury: multivariate analyses. Arch Phys Med Rehabil 65:66–73, 1984

Delmonico RL, Hanley-Peterson P, Englander J: Group psychotherapy for persons with traumatic brain injury: management of frustration and substance abuse. J Head Trauma Rehabil 13:10–22, 1998

Doonief G, Mirabello E, Bell K, et al: An estimate of the incidence of depression in idiopathic Parkinson's disease. Arch Neurol 49:305–307, 1992

Ekman P, Friesen WV: Unmasking the Face: A Guide to Recognizing Emotions From Facial Expressions. Cambridge, MA, Malor Books, 2003

Ellgring H, Seiler S, Perleth B, et al: Psychosocial aspects of Parkinson's disease. Neurology 43 (suppl 6):S41–S44, 1993

Evans RL, Northwood LK: Social support needs in adjustment to stroke. Arch Phys Med Rehabil 64:61–64, 1983

Fallon BA, Nields JA: Lyme disease: a neuropsychiatric illness. Am J Psychiatry 151:1571–1582, 1994

Fallon BA, Nields JA, Burrascano JJ, et al: The neuropsychiatric manifestations of Lyme borreliosis. Psychiatr Q 63:95–115, 1992

Fitts WH: Manual for Tennessee Self-Concept Scale. Nashville, TN, Counselor Recordings & Tests, 1965

Flashman LA, Amador A, McAllister TW: Lack of awareness of deficits in traumatic brain injury. Semin Clin Neuropsychiatry 3:201–210, 1998

Folstein MF, Folstein SE, McHugh PR: "Mini-Mental State": a practical method of grading the cognitive state of patients for the clinician. J Psychiatr Res 12:189–198, 1975

Ford B, Greene P, Fahn S: Oral and genital tardive pain syndromes. Neurology 44:2115–2119, 1994

Forrest DV: E. E. Cummings and the thoughts that lie too deep for tears: of defenses in poetry. Psychiatry 43:13–42, 1980

Forrest DV: Schizophrenic language: vantages from neurology, in Treating Schizophrenic Patients. Edited by Stone MH, Albert HD, Forrest DV, et al. New York, McGraw-Hill, 1983a, pp 325–335

Forrest DV: Therapeutic adaptations to the affective features of schizophrenia, in Treating Schizophrenic Patients. Edited by Stone MH, Albert HD, Forrest DV, et al. New York, McGraw-Hill, 1983b, pp 217–226

Forrest DV: Therapeutic adaptations to the cognitive features of schizophrenia, in Treating Schizophrenic Patients. Edited by Stone MH, Albert HD, Forrest DV, et al. New York, McGraw-Hill, 1983c, pp 165–182

Forrest DV: With two heads you can think twice: relations in the language of madness. J Am Acad Psychoanal 11:113–132, 1983d

Forrest DV: The tremometer: a convenient device to measure postural tremor from lithium and other causes. J Neuropsychiatry Clin Neurosci 2:391–394, 1990

Forrest DV: Mind, brain and machine: action and creation. J Am Acad Psychoanal 22:29–56, 1994

Forrest DV: Language and psychosis: seeking the poetry of malfunction in the spirit of Silvano Arieti. J Am Acad Psychoanal 27:563–574, 1999

Forrest DV: Freud's neuromental model: analytical structures and local habitations, in Whose Freud? The Place of Psychoanalysis in Contemporary Culture. Edited by Brooks P, Woloch A. New Haven, CT, Yale University Press, 2000, pp 255–266

Forrest DV: Elements of Dynamics, I: emotions and audiences. J Am Acad Psychoanal Dyn Psychiatry 31:705–720, 2003

Forrest DV: Elements of Dynamics, II: psychodynamic prescribing. J Am Acad Psychoanal Dyn Psychiatry 32:359–380, 2004a

Forrest DV: Elements of Dynamics, III: the face and the couch. J Am Acad Psychoanal Dyn Psychiatry 32:561–564, 2004b

Forrest DV: Elements of Dynamics, IV: afterword to "Neuronal Metaphors." J Am Acad Psychoanal Dyn Psychiatry 32:661–667, 2004c

Forrest DV: Elements of Dynamics, V: foreword to "Looking at Resilience." J Am Acad Psychoanal Dyn Psychiatry 33:385–387, 2005a

Forrest DV: Elements of Dynamics, VI: the dynamic unconscious and unconscious dynamics. J Am Acad Psychoanal Dyn Psychiatry 33:547–560, 2005b

Friefeld S, Yeboah O, Jones JE, et al: Health-related quality of life and its relationship to neurological outcome in child survivors of stroke. CNS Spectr 9:465–475, 2004

Giladi N, McMahon D, Przborski S, et al: Motor blocks in Parkinson's disease. Neurology 42:333–339, 1992

Golbe LI, Sage JI: Medical treatment of Parkinson's disease, in Treatment of Movement Disorders. Edited by Kurlan R. Philadelphia, PA, JB Lippincott, 1995, pp 1–56

Goldenberg G, Hagman S: Therapy of activities of daily living in patients with apraxia. Neuropsychological Rehabilitation 8:123–141, 1998

Goldman-Rakic PS: Working memory and the mind. Sci Am 267:110–117, 1992

Goldman-Rakic PS: Working memory dysfunction in schizophrenia. J Neuropsychiatry Clin Neurosci 6:348–357, 1994

Goldstein K: Aftereffects of Brain Injuries in War. New York, Grune & Stratton, 1942

Goodstein RK: Overview: cerebrovascular accident and the hospitalized elderly: a multidimensional clinical problem. Am J Psychiatry 140:141–147, 1983

Grant I, Brown GW, Harris T, et al: Severely threatening events and marked life difficulties preceding onset or exacerbation of multiple sclerosis. J Neurol Neurosurg Psychiatry 52:8–13, 1989

Green BC, Pratt CC, Grigsby TE: Self-concept among persons with long-term spinal cord injury. Arch Phys Med Rehabil 65:751–754, 1984

Grosswasser Z, Stern MJ: A psychodynamic model of behavior after acute central nervous system damage. J Head Trauma Rehabil 13:69–79, 1998

Groves MS, Forrest DV: Parkinson's disease as a model for psychosocial issues in chronic neurodegenerative disease, in Advances in Neurology, Vol 96: Behavioral Neurology of Movement Disorders. Edited by Anderson KE, Weiner WJ, Lang AE. Philadelphia, PA, Lippincott Williams & Wilkins, 2005, pp 65–83

Gusella JF, Wexler NS, Coneally PM, et al: A polymorphic DNA marker genetically linked to Huntington's disease. Nature 306:234–238, 1983

Hallet M: Physiology and pathophysiology of voluntary movement. Current Neurology 2:351–376, 1979

Hamburg D: Brain, behavior and health. VanGieson Award Address presented at the New York State Psychiatric Institute, New York, November 1985

Hartelius L: Speech and swallowing in Parkinson's disease. Folia Phoniatr Logop 46:9–17, 1994

Hayden MR, Bombard Y: Psychosocial effects of predictive testing for Huntington's disease, in Advances in Neurology, Vol 96: Behavioral Neurology of Movement Disorders. Edited by Anderson KE, Weiner WJ, Lang AE. Philadelphia, PA, Lippincott Williams & Wilkins, 2005, pp 226–239

Heaton R: Wisconsin Card Sorting Test. Odessa, TX, Psychological Assessment Resources, 1985

Henchcliffe C: Challenges in Parkinson's disease dementia treatment. Neurology Alert 23(6):45–46, 2005

House A, Dennis M, Molyneux A, et al: Emotionalism after stroke. BMJ 298:991–994, 1989

Howell T, Fullerton DT, Harvey RF, et al: Depression in spinal cord injured patients. Paraplegia 19:284–288, 1981

Jahanshahi M: Behavioral and psychiatric manifestations in dystonia, in Advances in Neurology, Vol 96: Behavioral Neurology of Movement Disorders. Edited by Anderson KE, Weiner WJ, Lang AE. Philadelphia, PA, Lippincott Williams & Wilkins, 2005, pp 291–319

Jean VM, Paul RH, Beatty WW: Psychological and neuropsychological predictors of coping patterns by patients with multiple sclerosis. J Clin Psychol 55:21–26, 1999

Jenicke MA: Alzheimer's Disease: Diagnosis, Treatment and Management. Philadelphia, PA, Clinical Perspectives on Aging, Wyeth Laboratories Division American Home Products Corporation, 1985

Kanner AM: Is major depression a neurologic disorder with psychiatric symptoms? Epilepsy Behav 5:636–644, 2004

Kanner AM, Balabanov A: Depression and epilepsy: how closely related are they? Neurology 58 (suppl 5):S27–S39, 2002

Kanner AM, Palac S: Depression in epilepsy: a common but often unrecognized comorbid malady. Epilepsy Behav 1:37–51, 2000

Katz IR: Diagnosis and treatment of depression in patients with Alzheimer's disease and other dementias. J Clin Psychiatry 59 (suppl 9):38–44, 1998

Kendler KS: Toward a philosophical structure for psychiatry. Am J Psychiatry 162:433–440, 2005

Kotila M, Waltimo O, Niemi ML, et al: The profile of recovery from stroke and factors influencing outcome. Stroke 15:1039–1044, 1984

Kreutzer JS, Zasler ND: Psychosexual consequences of traumatic brain injury: methodology and preliminary findings. Brain Inj 3:177–186, 1989

Labi MJ, Phillips TF, Greshman GE: Psychosocial disability in physically restored long-term stroke survivors. Arch Phys Med Rehabil 61:561–565, 1980

LaRocca N, Kalb R, Scheinberg L, et al: Factors associated with unemployment of patients with multiple sclerosis. J Chronic Dis 38:203–210, 1985

Leeman E, Leeman S: Neuronal metaphors: probing neurobiology for psychodynamic meaning. J Am Acad Psychoanal Dyn Psychiatry 32:645–659, 2004

Leroi I, Michalon M: Treatment of the psychiatric manifestations of Huntington's disease: a review of the literature. Can J Psychiatry 43:933–940, 1998

Lorig KR, Sobel DS, Stewart AL, et al: Evidence suggesting that a chronic disease self-management program can improve health status while reducing hospitalization. Med Care 37:5–14, 1999

Luria AR: The Working Brain: An Introduction to Neuropsychology. New York, Basic Books, 1973

Martelli MF, Grayson RL, Zasler ND: Posttraumatic headache: neuropsychological and psychological effects and treatment implications. J Head Trauma Rehabil 14:49–69, 1999

Mateer CA: Executive function disorders: rehabilitation challenges and strategies. Semin Clin Neuropsychiatry 4:50–59, 1999

Mateer CA, Bogod NM: Cognitive behavioral and selected pharmacologic interventions after acquired brain injury, in Neuropsychiatry, 2nd Edition. Edited by Schiffer RB, Rao SM, Fogel BS. Philadelphia, PA, Lippincott Williams & Wilkins, 2003, pp 165–186

Matteson MA, Linton AD, Cleary BL, et al: Management of problematic behavioral symptoms associated with dementia: a cognitive developmental approach. Aging (Milano) 9:342–355, 1997

Mayeux R: Behavior manifestations of movement disorders: Parkinson's and Huntington's disease. Neurol Clin 2:527–540, 1984

Mayeux R, Stern Y: Intellectual dysfunction and dementia in Parkinson disease, in The Dementias. Edited by Mayeux R, Rosen WG. New York, Raven, 1983, pp 211–227

Mayeux R, Sano M, Chen J, et al: Risk of dementia in first degree relatives of patients with Alzheimer's disease and related disorders. Arch Neurol 48:269–273, 1991

McLean PG: Psychiatry and philosophy, in The American Handbook of Psychiatry, Vol 2. Edited by Arieti S. New York, Basic Books, 1959, pp 1760–1776

Mechcatie E: Guidelines for Huntington's genetic testing, follow up. Clinical Psychiatry News 18:2, 22, 1990

Menza MA, Forman NE, Goldstein HS, et al: Parkinson's disease, personality and dopamine. J Neuropsychiatry Clin Neurosci 2:282–287, 1990

Minden SL: Psychotherapy for people with multiple sclerosis. J Neuropsychiatry Clin Neurosci 4:198–213, 1992

Minden SL, Schiffer RB: Affective disorders in multiple sclerosis: review and recommendations for clinical research. Arch Neurol 47:98–104, 1990

Mittleman MS, Roth DL, Coon DW, et al: Sustained benefit of supportive intervention for depressive symptoms in caregivers of patients with Alzheimer's disease. Am J Psychiatry 161:850–856, 2004

Mohr DC, Goodkin DE: Treatment of depression in multiple sclerosis: review and meta-analysis. Clinical Psychology— Science and Practice 6:1–9, 1999

Mohr DC, Hart SL, Julian L, et al: Telephone-administered psychotherapy for depression [in multiple sclerosis]. Arch Gen Psychiatry 62:1007–1014, 2005

Monacelli AM, Cushman LA, Kavcic V, et al: Spatial disorientation in Alzheimer's disease: the remembrance of things passed. Neurology 61:1491–1497, 2003

Montgomery EB Jr, Lieberman A, Sigh G, et al, on behalf of the PROPATH Advisory Board: Patient education and health promotion can be effective in Parkinson's disease: a randomized controlled trial. Am J Med 97:429–435, 1994

Müller V, Mohr B, Rosin R, et al: Short-term effects of behavioral treatment on movement initiation and postural control in Parkinson's disease: a controlled clinical study. Mov Disord 12:306–314, 1997

Murphy RF: The Body Silent. New York, Holt, 1987

National Institutes of Health Consensus Development Panel: Consensus conference: rehabilitation of persons with traumatic brain injury. NIH Consensus Development Panel on Rehabilitation of Persons With Traumatic Brain Injury. JAMA 282:974–983, 1999

Naumann M, Magyar-Lehmann S, Reiners K, et al: Sensory tricks in cervical dystonia: perceptual dysbalance of parietal cortex modulates frontal motor programming. Ann Neurol 47:322–328, 2000

Parkinson J: An Essay on the Shaking Palsy. London, England, Sherwood, Neely & Jones, 1817

Parkinson Study Group: Effects of tocopherol and deprenyl (selegiline) on the progression of disability in early Parkinson's disease. N Engl J Med 238:167–183, 1993

Parkinson Study Group: A controlled, randomised, delayed-start study of rasagiline in early Parkinson disease. Arch Neurol 61:561–566, 2004

Perez M, Pilsecker C: Group therapy with spinal cord injured substance abusers. Paraplegia 32:188–192, 1994

Phillips L: Genes and environment affect age of onset of Huntington disease. Neurology Today, May 2004, pp 21–22

Pollack IW: Individual psychotherapy, in Neuropsychiatry of Traumatic Brain Injury. Edited by Silver JM, Yudofsky SC, Hales RE. Washington, DC, American Psychiatric Press, 1994, pp 671–702

Pollack IW: Psychotherapy, in Textbook of Traumatic Brain Injury. Edited by Silver JM, McAllister TM, Yudofsky SC. Washington, DC, American Psychiatric Publishing, 2005, pp 641–654

Prigatano GP, Borgaro S, Caples H: Non-pharmacologic management of psychiatric disturbances after traumatic brain injury. Int Rev Psychiatry 15:371–379, 2003

Rabins PV, Mace NL, Lucas MJ: The impact of dementia on the family. JAMA 248:333–335, 1982

Ramachandran VS: Phantoms in the Brain: Exploring the Mysteries of the Human Mind. New York, William Morrow, 1998

Rao SM (ed): Neurobehavioral Aspects of Multiple Sclerosis. New York, Oxford University Press, 1990

Reisberg B: Alzheimer's disease update. Psychiatr Ann 15:319–322, 1985

Roberts JK, Guberman A: Religion and epilepsy. Psychiatr J Univ Ott 14:282–286, 1989

Romano MD: Preparing children for parental disability. Soc Work Health Care 1:309–315, 1976

Ron MA, Logsdail SJ: Psychiatric morbidity in multiple sclerosis: a clinical and MRI study. Psychol Med 19:887–895, 1989

Ropper AH, Gorson KC: Concussion. N Engl J Med 356:166–172, 2007

Rosenstiel AK, Roth S: Relationship between cognitive activity and adjustment in four spinal-cord-injured individuals: a longitudinal investigation. J Human Stress 7:35–43, 1981

Sands H: Psychodynamic management of epilepsy, in Epilepsy: A Handbook for the Mental Health Professional. Edited by Sands H. New York, Brunner/Mazel, 1982, pp 135–157

Sarno MT: The nature of verbal impairment after closed head injury. J Nerv Ment Dis 168:685–692, 1980

Scheinberg LC: Multiple Sclerosis: A Guide for Patients and Their Families. New York, Raven, 1983

Schiffer RB: Psychiatric aspects of clinical neurology. Am J Psychiatry 140:205–211, 1983

Schiffer RB: The spectrum of depression in multiple sclerosis: an approach for clinical management. Arch Neurol 44:596–599, 1987

Schuler M: Sexual counseling for the spinal cord injured: a review of 5 programs. J Sex Marital Ther 8:241–252, 1982

Secker DL, Brown RG: Cognitive behavior therapy (CBT) for carers of patients with Parkinson's disease: a preliminary randomized controlled trial. J Neurol Neurosurg Psychiatry 76:491–497, 2005

Shadick NA, Phillips CB, Logigian EL, et al: The long-term clinical outcomes of Lyme disease. Ann Intern Med 121:560–567, 1994

Shnek ZM, Foley FW, LaRocca NG, et al: Helplessness, self-efficacy, cognitive distortions, and depression in multiple sclerosis and spinal cord injury. Ann Behav Med 19:287–294, 1997

Signer SF: Capgras syndrome: the delusion of substitution. J Clin Psychiatry 481:47–50, 1987

Simons AF: Problems of providing support for people with MS and their families, in Multiple Sclerosis: Psychological and Social Aspects. Edited by Simons AF. London, England, Heinemann Medical Books, 1984, pp 1–20

Small GW, Rabins PV, Barry PP, et al: Diagnosis and treatment of Alzheimer disease and related disorders: consensus statement of the American Association of Geriatric Psychiatry, the Alzheimer's Association, and the American Geriatrics Society. JAMA 278:1363–1371, 1997

Solomon CR, Scherzer BP: Some guidelines for family therapists working with the traumatically brain injured and their families. Brain Inj 5:253–266, 1991

Starkstein SE, Preziosi TJ, Bolduc PL, et al: Depression in Parkinson's disease. J Nerv Ment Dis 178:27–31, 1990

Steck B, Amsler F, Schwald Dillar A, et al: Indication for psychotherapy in offspring of a parent affected by a chronic somatic disease (e.g., multiple sclerosis). Psychopathology 38:38–48, 2005

Steinglass P, Temple S, Lisman SA, et al: Coping with spinal cord injury: the family perspective. Gen Hosp Psychiatry 4:259–264, 1982

Stern Y, Mayeux R, Rosen J: Contribution of perceptual motor dysfunction to construction and tracing disturbances in Parkinson's disease. J Neurol Neurosurg Psychiatry 47:987–989, 1984

Suhr JA, Anderson SW: Behavioral management of chronic hallucinations and delusions following right middle cerebral artery stroke. Psychotherapy 35:464–471, 1998

Teri LA, Logsdon RG, Uomoto J, et al: Behavioral treatment of depression in dementia patients: a controlled clinical trial. J Gerontol B Psychol Sci Soc Sci 52:P159–P166, 1997

Thorngren M, Westling B, Norrving B: Outcome after stroke in patients discharged to independent living. Stroke 21:236–240, 1990

Tibben A: Genetic counseling and presymptomatic testing, in Huntington's Disease. Edited by Bates G, Harper PS, Jones L. London, England, Oxford University Press, 2002, pp 198–248

Umlauf RL: Psychological interventions for chronic pain following spinal cord injury. Clin J Pain 8:111–118, 1992

Vaillant GE: Mental health. Am J Psychiatry 160:1373–1384, 2003

Valleroy ML, Kraft GH: Sexual dysfunction in multiple sclerosis. Arch Phys Med Rehabil 65:125–128, 1984

van Vugt JPP, Roos RAC: Huntington's disease: options for controlling symptoms. CNS Drugs 11:105–123, 1999

Wade SL, Wolfe C, Brown TM, et al: Putting the pieces together: preliminary efficacy of a web-based family intervention for children with traumatic brain injury. J Pediatr Psychol 30:437–442, 2005

Waters CH: Diagnosis and Treatment of Parkinson's Disease. Caddo, OK, Professional Communications, 1999

Weinberger DR, Berman KF, Zec RF: Physiological dysfunction of dorsolateral prefrontal cortex in schizophrenia, I: regional cerebral blood flow (CBF) evidence. Arch Gen Psychiatry 43:114–125, 1986

Weinstein EA: Sexual disturbances after brain injury. Medical Aspects of Human Sexuality 8:10–31, 1974

Wexler NS: Genetic jeopardy and the new clairvoyance, in Progress in Medical Genetics, Vol 6. Edited by Beam A, Child B, Motulsky A. New York, Praeger, 1985, pp 277–304

Williams DT, Fahn S: Psychogenic dystonia, in Advances in Neurology, Vol 50: Dystonia 2. Edited by Fahn S, Marsden CD, Calne DB. New York, Raven, 1988, pp 431–455

Williams DT, Ford B, Fahn S: Treatment issues in psychogenic-neuropsychiatric movement disorders, in Advances in Neurology, Vol 96: Behavioral Neurology of Movement Disorders. Edited by Anderson KE, Weiner WJ, Lang AE. Philadelphia, PA, Lippincott Williams & Wilkins, 2005, pp 250–363

Wilson RS, Evans DA, Bienias JL, et al: Proneness to psychological distress is associated with risk of Alzheimer's disease. Neurology 61:1479–1485, 2003

Wilson T, Smith T: Driving after stroke. Int Rehabil Med 5:170–177, 1983

Woods BT, Short MP: Neurological dimensions of psychiatry. Biol Psychiatry 20:192–198, 1985

Yudofsky SC, Silver JM, Hales RE: Pharmacologic management of aggression in the elderly. J Clin Psychiatry 51(suppl):22–28; discussion 29–32, 1990

33

COGNITIVE REHABILITATION AND BEHAVIOR THERAPY FOR PATIENTS WITH NEUROPSYCHIATRIC DISORDERS

Michael D. Franzen, Ph.D.

Mark R. Lovell, Ph.D.

Increasing evidence indicates that the treatment of central nervous system (CNS) disorders is a viable and productive endeavor. Even traumatic brain injury, the effects of which were previously thought to be permanently devastating, has been found to be improved by a variety of treatments (Cicerone et al. 2000; NIH Consensus Statement 1998). Psychiatry plays a central role in the assessment and treatment of individuals with neurological impairment. There is an increasing need for a broad-based understanding of methods of promoting recovery from brain injury and disease. The role of the psychiatrist in the diagnosis and treatment of the sequelae of CNS dysfunction has become a crucial one and promises to become even more central with the continued development of sophisticated neuropharmacological treatments for both the cognitive and the psychosocial components of brain impairment (Gualtieri 1988).

In particular, the recent application of selective serotonin reuptake inhibitors with brain-injured patients appears to hold some promise. In addition to these exciting new developments, an understanding of nonpharmacological, behavioral methods of assessment and treatment can greatly enhance the patient's recovery from cognitive deficits and together with a pharmacological approach can improve the cognitive and behavioral effects of CNS dysfunction. In this chapter, we review the role of psychological treatments for the neuropsychological (cognitive) and behavioral consequences of CNS dysfunction.

In response to the increase in the number of patients requiring treatment for CNS dysfunction, there has been a proliferation of treatment agencies structured to provide rehabilitation services, as well as an accompanying increase in research efforts designed to assess the efficacy of these treatment programs. A particularly intense focus over the last few years has been the development of rehabilitation programs designed specifically to treat the neuropsychological and psychosocial sequelae of neuropsychiatric disorders. With evidence of the beneficial effects of rehabilitation have come modest increases in reimbursement, which in turn have fueled the increase in availability of services. Additionally, there has been an increasing awareness of the potential neuropsychological effects of disorders of other somatic systems that have some effect on CNS operations, such as cancer (Anderson-

Hanley et al. 2003) and hypertension (Muldoon et al. 2002), as well as potential neuropsychological side effects of the treatment for those disorders. Overall, identification of neuropsychological deficits has caused increased interest in developing treatments for the deficits. Before turning to a discussion of specific treatment modalities that may be useful with neuropsychiatric patients, we briefly review neuroanatomical influences on the recovery process.

NEUROANATOMICAL AND NEUROPHYSIOLOGICAL DETERMINANTS OF RECOVERY

Recovery from brain injury or disease can be conceptualized as involving a number of separate but interacting processes. Although a complete discussion of existing research concerning neuroanatomical and neurophysiological aspects of the recovery process is beyond the scope of this chapter, we provide here a brief review. (For a more complete review of current theories of recovery from brain injury, see Gouvier et al. 1986.)

After an acute brain injury, such as a stroke or head injury, some degree of improvement is likely because of a lessening of the temporary or treatable consequences of the injury. Factors such as degree of cerebral edema and extent of increased intracranial pressure are well known to temporarily affect brain function after a closed head injury or stroke (Lezak 1995). Extracellular changes after injury to the cell also have been shown to affect neural functioning. In addition, the regrowth of neural tissue to compensate for an injured area has been shown to occur to some minimal extent in animal studies on both anatomical (Kolata 1983) and physiological (Wall and Egger 1971) levels and may have some limited relevance for humans. With many acute brain injuries, functioning improves as these temporary effects subside. However, with degenerative illnesses, such as Alzheimer's disease and Huntington's disease, the condition actually worsens over time.

The differences in prognosis among various neurological disorders obviously affect the structure of the rehabilitation program. For example, the expectations and goals of a rehabilitation program that is structured to improve memory function in patients with head injury are likely to be much different from those of a program for patients with Alzheimer's disease. Similarly, the goals will vary as a function of the severity of memory impairment in patients with closed head injury. A program designed for patients with head injury and consequent moderate memory impairment is likely to focus on teaching alternative strategies for remembering new information. In contrast, a program designed for a patient with Alz-

heimer's disease would probably focus on improving the patient's functioning with regard to activities of daily living. Previously, the amount of time since the injury also was seen as a determining variable in the design of rehabilitation efforts, with treatment aimed at improving the skill or substituting other cognitive mechanisms used in the early stages of recovery and treatment aimed at compensatory behaviors in the late stages of recovery. However, some intriguing data suggest that at least for stroke, brain reorganization for motor skills may be possible even a decade past the time of the stroke (Liepert et al. 2000).

COGNITIVE REHABILITATION OF PATIENTS WITH NEUROPSYCHIATRIC DISORDERS

The terms *cognitive rehabilitation* and *cognitive retraining* have been variously used to describe treatments designed to maximize recovery of the individual's abilities in the areas of intellectual functioning, visual processing, language, attention, and memory. It is important to note that the techniques used to improve cognitive functioning after a neurological event represent an extremely heterogeneous group of procedures that vary widely in their focus according to the nature of the patient's cognitive difficulties, the specific skills and training of the staff members, and the medium through which information is presented (e.g., computer vs. individual therapy vs. group therapy). Ideally, a cognitive rehabilitation program should be tailored to each patient's particular needs and should be based on a thorough, individualized neuropsychological assessment of the patient's cognitive and behavioral deficits, as well as an estimation of how these deficits are likely to affect the patient in his or her daily life.

Because patients with different neurological or neuropsychiatric syndromes often have different cognitive deficits, the focus of the treatment is likely to vary greatly. For example, a treatment program designed primarily to treat patients with head injury is likely to focus on the amelioration of attentional and memory deficits, whereas a rehabilitation program designed for stroke patients is likely to focus on a more specific deficit, such as language disorders or other disorders that tend to occur after localized brain damage, and to have less emphasis on co-occurring attentional and memory deficits. For disorders with changing parameters such as the progressive neurological disorders, the stage of the illness and degree of impairment may also play a role in the development of a rehabilitation treatment plan. Sinforiani et al. (2004)

reported that a cognitive rehabilitation program was effective in reversing the cognitive deficits associated with the early stages of Parkinson's disease, but it may be unlikely that such a program would be effective in later stages.

Attention to psychiatric problems in patients with neurological impairment is an increasingly important component of rehabilitation efforts (e.g., Robinson 1997). The use of pharmacological agents in the treatment of affective and behavior changes following traumatic brain injury has been reported in case studies (Khouzam and Donnelly 1998; Mendez et al. 1999). Carbamazepine has been used in the treatment of behavioral agitation following severe traumatic brain injury (Azouvi et al. 1999).

The systematic research concerning the effectiveness of cognitive and behavioral treatment strategies in this group is increasing. However, this area is still a developing endeavor. Some work has been reported in the area of treating social skills deficits and anger control. Medd and Tate (2000) reported the effects of anger management training in individuals with traumatic brain injury. In addition to psychologically based methods, pharmacological methods have been used to treat the physical and emotional symptoms (Holzer 1998; McIntosh 1997; Wroblewski et al. 1997). Although amantadine was at first promising, it has not provided robust effects in improving cognitive and behavioral functioning in brain-injured subjects (Schneider et al. 1999). The treatment of frontal lobe injury with dopaminergic agents may beneficially affect other rehabilitation efforts (Kraus and Maki 1997). Furthermore, the use of psychostimulants in facilitating treatment effects has been reported for pediatric subjects with traumatic brain injury (Williams et al. 1998) as well as for adults (Glen 1998). Most of our information comes from experience with patients in rehabilitation settings. Following is a brief review of cognitive rehabilitation strategies designed to treat specific cognitive deficits that may be associated with neuropsychiatric disorders.

The results of psychological treatment methods for the cognitive deficits associated with traumatic brain injury generally show larger effects for skills as measured by standardized tests than as measured by ecologically relevant behaviors (Ho and Bennett 1997). This is a vexing problem because the ultimate goal of the treatment is to provide some socially relevant and valid effect. Future research is needed to investigate the variables that govern generalizability and ecological validity.

There has been some interest in the cognitive rehabilitation of individuals with schizophrenia. Although schizophrenia is not an acquired disorder of cognitive impairment, it does have similarities to other neuropsychiatric disorders that have received attention in the clinical neuropsychological literature. Flesher (1990) presented an intriguing discussion of an approach to using this type of intervention with schizophrenic patients; however, there have been limited reports of applications, an exception being Benedict et al. (1994), who reported on the use of information processing rehabilitation. In that study, computer vigilance training was used to treat the attentional deficits shown by a group of schizophrenic patients. Although it may be too early to critically evaluate the efficacy of this approach (Bellak and Mueser 1993), it certainly bears watching. In contrast, the use of behavioral methods for training in social skills in schizophrenic patients is well documented.

ATTENTIONAL PROCESSES

Disorders of attention are common sequelae of several neurological disorders, particularly traumatic brain injury. Recognition and treatment of attentional disorders are extremely important because an inability to focus and sustain attention may directly limit the patient's ability to actively participate in the rehabilitation program and may therefore affect progress in other areas of cognitive functioning. It must be stressed that attention is not a unitary process. A number of components of attention have been identified, including alertness and the ability to selectively attend to incoming information, as well as the capacity to focus and maintain attention or vigilance (Posner and Rafal 1987).

Rehabilitation programs designed to improve attention usually attempt to address all of these processes. One such program is the Orientation Remedial module developed by Ben-Yishay and associates (Ben-Yishay and Diller 1981) at New York University. The Orientation Remedial program consists of five separate tasks that are presented by microcomputer and vary in degree of difficulty; they involve training in the following areas:

1. Attending and reacting to environmental signals
2. Timing responses in relation to changing environmental cues
3. Being actively vigilant
4. Estimating time
5. Synchronizing of response with complex rhythms

Progress on these tasks is a prerequisite for further training on higher-level tasks. Because of the early position of attentional processes in the hierarchy of cognitive operations, many clinical researchers have targeted attention deficits using both behavioral and pharmacological methods. Modafinil has been found to improve performance on measures of attention, reaction time, and executive function in healthy subjects who have been sleep deprived (Walsh et al. 2004), but the generalizability of these findings to individuals with CNS injury has yet to be demonstrated.

MEMORY

Within the field of cognitive rehabilitation, much emphasis has been placed on the development of treatment approaches to improve memory. This is not surprising, given the importance of memory functions in everyday life and the pervasiveness of memory disorders in many different neurologically impaired populations. In reviewing the empirical literature, Franzen and Haut (1991) divided the strategies into three basic categories: 1) the use of spared skills in the form of mnemonic devices or alternative functional systems, 2) the use of direct retraining with repetitive practice and drills, and 3) the use of behavioral prosthetics or external devices or strategies to improve memory.

Use of Spared Skills

Because memory is not a unitary construct, impairment in one form of memory is often coupled with a spared skill in another form of memory. Mnemonic strategies are approaches to memory rehabilitation that are specifically designed to promote the encoding and remembering of a specific type of information, depending on the patient's particular memory impairment, by capitalizing on the spared skills. Currently, several different types of mnemonic strategies may be of use in neuropsychiatric settings. Visual imagery is one of the most well-known and commonly used mnemonic strategies (Glisky and Schacter 1986) and involves the use of visual images to assist in the learning and retention of verbal information. Probably the oldest and best-known visual imagery strategy is the method of loci, which involves the association of verbal information to be remembered with locations that are familiar to the patient (e.g., the room in a house or the location on a street). When recall of the information is required, the patient visualizes each room and the items that are to be remembered in each location (Moffat 1984). Initial research suggested that this method may be particularly useful for elderly patients (Robertson-Tchabo et al. 1976).

A related method of learning and remembering new information, generally referred to as *peg mnemonics*, requires the patient to learn a list of peg words and to associate these words with a given visual image, such as "one bun," "two shoe," and so on. After the learned association of the numbers with the visual image, sequential information can be remembered in order by association with the visual image (Gouvier et al. 1986). This strategy has been widely used by professional mnemonists and showed some early promise in patients with brain injuries (Patten 1972). More recent research, however, suggested that this approach may not be highly effective because patients with brain injuries are unable to generate visual images (Crovitz et al. 1979) and have difficulty maintaining this information over time.

Another type of visual imagery procedure that has been widely used in clinical settings and has been studied extensively is face-name association. As the name implies, this procedure has been used by patients with brain injuries to promote the remembering of people's names based on visual cues. The technique involves associating the components of the name with a distinctive visual image. For example, the name "Angela Harper" might be encoded by the patient by visualizing an angel playing a harp. Obviously, the ease with which this method can be used by patients with brain injuries depends on their ability to form internal visual images, as well as the ease with which the name can be transferred into a distinct visual image. Whereas it may be relatively easy to find visual associations for a name such as "Angela Harper," a name such as "Jane Johnson" may be much more difficult to encode in this manner.

Overall, visual imagery strategies may be useful for specific groups of patients (e.g., those with impairments in verbal memory who need to use nonverbal cues to assist them in recall) and in patients whose impairments are mild enough to allow them to recall the series of steps necessary to spontaneously use these strategies once they return to their natural environments. A series of single-subject experiments reported by Wilson (1987) indicated that the strategy of visual imagery to learn people's names may be differentially effective for different individuals, even when the etiology of memory impairment is similar.

In addition to the extensive use of visual imagery strategies for improving memory in patients with brain injuries, the use of verbally based mnemonic strategies also has become quite popular, particularly with patients who have difficulty using visual imagery. One such procedure, semantic elaboration, involves constructing a story out of new information to be remembered. This type of procedure may be particularly useful in patients who are unable to use imagery strategies because of a reduced ability to generate internal visual images.

Rhyming strategies involve remembering verbal information by incorporating the information into a rhyme. This procedure was originally demonstrated by Gardner (1977) with a globally amnesic patient who was able to recall pertinent personal information by the learning and subsequent singing of the following rhyme:

> Henry's my name/Memory's my game/
>   I'm in the V.A. in Jamaica Plain.
> My bed's on 7D/The year is '73/
>   Every day I make a little gain.

For patients who have difficulty learning and remembering written information, Glasgow et al. (1977) used a structured procedure called *PQRST*. This strategy involves application of the following five steps:

1. Preview the information.
2. Form Questions about the information.
3. Read the information.
4. State the questions.
5. Test for retention by answering the questions after the material has been read.

REPETITIVE PRACTICE

Cognitive rehabilitation strategies that emphasize repetitive practice of the information to be remembered have become extremely popular in rehabilitation settings despite little experimental evidence that these procedures produce lasting improvement in memory. Repetitive practice strategies rely heavily on the use of drills and appear to be based on a mental muscle conceptualization of memory (Harris and Sunderland 1981) in which it is assumed that memory can be improved merely by repeated exposure to the information to be learned. Although it is generally accepted that patients with brain injuries can learn specific pieces of information through repeated exposure, studies designed to show generalization of this training to new settings or tasks have not been encouraging. (For a review, see Schacter and Glisky 1986.)

In view of the lack of evidence that repetitive practice strategies are effective in producing improvement in memory in patients with brain damage, Glisky and Schacter (1986) suggested that attempts to remedy memory disorders should be focused on the acquisition of domain-specific knowledge that is likely to be relevant to the patient's ability to function in everyday life. This approach differs from the use of traditional cognitive remediation strategies in that 1) the goal of this treatment is not to improve memory functioning in general but rather to deal with specific problems associated with memory impairment, 2) the information acquired through this treatment has practical value to the individual, and 3) the information learned through training exercises is chosen on the basis of having some practical value in the patient's natural environment. Initial research has established that even patients with severe brain injuries are indeed capable of acquiring discrete pieces of information that are important to their ability to function on a daily basis (Glasgow et al. 1977; Wilson 1982). Similarly, Chiaravalloti et al. (2003) found that repetition was not helpful in remediating the memory deficits of individuals with multiple sclerosis (MS), who instead may benefit from other rehabilitation strategies in addition to the repetition.

EXTERNAL MEMORY AIDS

External aids to memory can take various forms, but generally they fall into the two categories of memory storage devices and memory-cuing strategies (Harris 1984). Probably the most basic memory storage devices are in the form of written lists and memory books. Lists and memory books are widely used by patients with brain injuries to record information that is vital to their daily function (e.g., the daily schedule of activities and chores to be performed) and that is then consulted at a given time. These strategies are not designed to provide a general improvement in the patient's ability to learn and retain new information but are used as memory support devices. A study reported by Schmitter-Edgecombe et al. (1995) supported the efficacy of memory notebook training to improve memory for everyday activities, although there was no difference in laboratory-based memory tasks, and the gains were not maintained as well at a 6-month follow-up evaluation.

With recent advances in the field of microelectronics, handheld electronic storage devices have become increasingly popular in rehabilitation settings. Although these devices allow for the storage of large amounts of information, their often complicated operation requirements may obviate their use in all but the mildest cases of brain injury or disease. Another problem inherent in the use of external storage devices is that the devices must be consulted at the appropriate time in order to be useful. This may be a difficult task for the patient with brain injury and often requires the use of cuing strategies that remind the patient to engage in a behavior at a given time.

The application of cuing involves the use of prompts designed to remind the patient to engage in a specific behavioral sequence at a given time. To be maximally effective, the cue should be given as close as possible to the time that the behavior is required, must be active (e.g., the use of an alarm clock) rather than passive, and should provide a reminder of the specific behavior that is desired (Harris 1984). One particularly useful cuing device currently in use is the alarm wristwatch. This device can be set to sound an alarm at a given time. Although this technique does not provide specific information about the desired response, it can provide a useful cue to prompt the patient to check a list or other storage device for further instructions. Thus, a patient with brain injury can be cued to engage in some behavior on a regular basis.

VISUAL-PERCEPTUAL DISORDERS

In addition to memory impairment, individuals with brain injuries may have difficulties with visual perception. Deficits in visual perception are most common in patients who have undergone right hemisphere cerebrovascular accidents (Gouvier et al. 1986). Given the importance of visual-perceptual processing to many occupational tasks and to the safe operation of an automobile (Sivak et al. 1985), the rehabilitation of deficits in this area could have important implications for the recovery of neuropsychiatric patients.

A deficit that is particularly common in stroke patients is hemispatial neglect syndrome. This deficit is characterized by an inability to recognize stimuli in the contralateral visual field. One strategy that has often been used to treat hemispatial neglect is visual scanning training. This procedure, which has been designed to promote scanning to the neglected hemifield, has been extensively used at the Rusk Institute of Rehabilitation of the New York Medical Center (Diller and Weinberg 1977), as well as by others (Gianutsos et al. 1983). The New York Medical Center program uses a light board with 20 colored lights and a target that can be moved around the board at different speeds. With this device, the patient can be systematically trained to attend to the neglected visual field. This procedure, with the addition of other tasks (e.g., a size estimation and body awareness task), was found to improve visual-perceptual functioning in a group of patients with brain injuries in comparison with a group of similar patients who received standard occupational therapy (Gordon et al. 1985). Other researchers have produced similar therapeutic gains in scanning and other aspects of visual-perceptual functioning through rehabilitation strategies. (For a more complete review of this area, see Gianutsos and Matheson 1987 and Gordon et al. 1985.)

PROBLEM SOLVING AND EXECUTIVE FUNCTIONS

Patients who have sustained brain injuries from closed head injuries often experience a breakdown in their ability to reason, to form concepts, to solve problems, to execute and terminate behavioral sequences, and to engage in other complex cognitive activities (F.C. Goldstein and Levin 1987). Similarly, executive dysfunction correlates with white matter changes seen in diffusion tensor magnetic resonance imaging of patients with vascular dementia (O'Sullivan et al. 2004). Deficits in these areas are among the most debilitating to the neuropsychiatric patient because they often underlie changes in the basic abilities to function interpersonally, socially, and vocationally. Executive function appears to have a relationship to other, simpler tasks. For example, performance on tests of executive function is correlated with lower-extremity coordination and walking speed in older healthy individuals (Ble et al. 2005). Because of increasing evidence that executive function affects lower-order tasks, more effort has been dedicated to the systematic development of

rehabilitation programs to ameliorate these disorders. These treatment programs can be difficult to plan and implement, partly due to the complex and multifaceted nature of intellectual and executive functions.

Intellectual and executive functioning cannot be conceptualized as unitary constructs but rather involve numerous processes that include motivation, abstract thinking, and concept formation, as well as the ability to plan, reason, and execute and terminate behaviors. Therefore, breakdowns in intellectual and executive functioning can occur for various reasons depending on the underlying core deficit(s) and can vary based on the area of the brain that is injured. For example, injury to the parieto-occipital area is likely to result in a problem-solving deficit secondary to difficulty with comprehension of logical-grammatical structure, whereas a frontal lobe injury may impede problem solving by disrupting the individual's ability to plan and to carry out the series of steps necessary to process the grammatical material (Luria and Tsvetkova 1990). The identification and possible treatment of executive dysfunction is important because of implications for the treatment of patients' other deficits, such as the impact of executive dysfunction on the capacity to consent to medical treatment in patients with Alzheimer's disease (Marson and Harrell 1999).

An apparent breakdown in the patient's ability to function intellectually also can occur secondary to deficits in other related areas of neuropsychological functioning, such as attention, memory, and language. The type of rehabilitation strategy best suited for such a patient depends on the underlying core deficit that needs to be addressed. The goal of rehabilitation for a patient with a left parieto-occipital lesion might be to help the patient develop the skill to correctly analyze the grammatical structure of the problem. Rehabilitation efforts for a patient with frontal lobe injury might emphasize impulse control and execution of the appropriate behavioral sequence to solve the problem.

Because of the multitude of factors that can result in difficulties in intellectual and executive functioning in patients with brain injuries, programs designed to rehabilitate these patients have necessarily involved attempts to address these deficits in a hierarchical manner, as originally proposed by Luria (1963). One such program was developed at New York University by Ben-Yishay and associates (Ben-Yishay and Diller 1983). They developed a two-tiered approach that defines five basic deficit areas—arousal and attention, memory, impairment in underlying skill structure, language and thought, and feeling tone—and two domains of higher-level problem solving. This model proposes that deficits in the higher-level skills are often produced by core deficits and that the patient's behavior is likely to depend on an interaction between the two domains (F.C. Goldstein and Levin 1987). Stablum et al. (2000) reported the effects of a treatment of executive dysfunction by training and practice in a dual-task procedure. They found improvements in executive function for both patients with closed head injury and patients with anterior communicating artery aneurysms (ACoA). This study is particularly noteworthy because the investigators provided data regarding maintenance of the gains at 3 months for the patients with closed head injury and at 12 months for ACoA patients.

SPEECH AND LANGUAGE

Disorders of speech and language are common sequelae of neurological damage, particularly when the dominant (usually left) hemisphere is injured. Because the ability to communicate is often central to the patient's personal, social, and vocational readjustment after brain injury or disease, rehabilitation efforts in this area are extremely important. In most rehabilitation settings, speech and language therapies have traditionally been the province of speech pathologists. Therapy has often involved a wide variety of treatments depending on the training, interest, and theoretic orientation of the therapist. The goal of therapy has variously been the improvement of comprehension (receptive language) and expression (expressive language), and it has been shown that patients who receive speech therapy after a stroke improve more than patients who do not (Basso et al. 1979).

In treating speech and language impairment, it is important to consider the reason for the observed speech deficit in designing the treatment; that is, it is not sufficient simply to identify the behavioral deficit and attempt to increase the rate of production (Franzen 1991). For example, Giles et al. (1988) increased appropriate verbalizations in a patient with head injury by providing cuing to keep verbalization short and to pause in planning his speech. Here the remediation attempted to affect the mediating behavior rather than to decrease unwanted behavior through extinction.

MOLAR BEHAVIORS

The final test of rehabilitation efforts is frequently the change in ecologically relevant molar behaviors—that is, in behaviors that would be used in the open environment. Examples of such molar behaviors include driving, completion of occupational work tasks, successful social interaction, and, at a simpler level, activities of daily living. The results of standardized testing may account for most of the variance reported for molar behaviors such as

driving skill (Galski et al. 1997). However, the improvement in these molar behaviors also may depend on treatment aimed directly at the production of the behaviors, even when the component cognitive skills have been optimized. Giles et al. (1997) used behavioral techniques to improve washing and dressing skills in a series of individuals with severe brain injury.

USE OF COMPUTERS IN COGNITIVE REHABILITATION

The use of microcomputers in cognitive rehabilitation, as in many other facets of everyday life, has increased dramatically over the last decade. The microcomputer has great potential for use in rehabilitation settings and may offer several advantages over more conventional, therapist-based treatments (Gourlay et al. 2000; Grimm and Bleiberg 1986). Microcomputers may have the advantage of being potentially self-instructional and self-paced, of requiring less direct staff time, and of accurately providing direct feedback to the patient about performance. Microcomputers also facilitate research by accurately and consistently recording the large amounts of potentially useful data that are generated during the rehabilitation process.

Notwithstanding these advantages, several cautions must be mentioned concerning the use of microcomputers in the rehabilitation process. First, it must be emphasized that the microcomputer is merely a tool (albeit a highly sophisticated one), and its usefulness is limited by the availability of software that meets the needs of the individual patient and the skill of the therapist in implementing the program(s). As noted by Harris (1984), the danger is that cognitive rehabilitation will become centered around the software that is available through a given treatment program rather than being based on the individual needs of the patient. Second, microcomputers are not capable of simulating human social interaction and should not be used in lieu of human therapeutic contact.

Despite these challenges, there is a significant potential advantage in the capacity to present precise stimuli and conditions and to readily measure and record the effects of the treatments (Rizzo and Buckwalter 1997), and the use of computer programs in cognitive rehabilitation is increasing in quantity and quality (Gontkovsky et al. 2002). There are reports of the effectiveness of computerized rehabilitation programs for patients with Parkinson's disease (Sinforiani et al. 2004), closed head injury (Grealy et al. 1999), and schizophrenia (da Costa and de Carvalho 2004). Bellucci et al. (2003) report that computerized cognitive rehabilitation has a positive effect on the negative symptoms of schizophrenic patients.

DISORDERS AND ASSOCIATED TREATMENTS

With the recognition that different disorders entail different cognitive deficits, programs have been developed to address these deficits. For example, Birnboim and Miller (2004) reported that patients with MS have specific deficits in working strategies and that interventions aimed at improving the capacity to develop and use these strategies may necessarily precede other cognitive rehabilitation interventions. In a review of studies using MS patients, Amato and Zipoli (2003) report limited evidence in support of existing programs that attempt to moderate the cognitive impairment associated with MS, but they also provide suggestions for future attempts and report optimism on the part of investigators involved in current research. Cuesta (2003) reviewed published studies involving the treatment of memory impairment following stroke and reported generally positive but moderate results. Particular interest has been focused on treatment of the dementias, especially Alzheimer's dementia (Clare et al. 2003). Some of these advances have involved novel pharmacological approaches, such as nicotinic substances, that can be combined with behavioral approaches (Newhouse et al. 1997). Another study involved the combination of cognitive rehabilitation methods with the use of cholinesterase inhibitors (Loewenstein et al. 2004). In this study, gains were reported at the end of 12 weeks of treatment and were maintained at a 3-month follow-up. Certain disorders may have their own specific considerations. For example, greater awareness of deficit is associated with greater improvement from cognitive rehabilitation in patients with Alzheimer's disease (Clare et al. 2002, 2004).

Patients with schizophrenia demonstrate significant cognitive impairment, and cognitive dysfunction is a prominent symptom of the disorder. This cognitive impairment can interfere with other treatment efforts, and cognitive rehabilitation has been reported to improve general aspects of other symptoms and problems exhibited by patients with schizophrenia (Lewis et al. 2003). A review of attempts to rehabilitate the attention deficits associated with schizophrenia indicates generally positive results (Suslow et al. 2001). The evidence is mixed regarding the extent to which brain perfusion changes as a result of cognitive rehabilitation in schizophrenia (Penades et al. 2000). However, a quantitative review of studies indicates that cognitive rehabilitation not only improves cognitive operations on the experimental tasks but also generalizes to improvement on tasks outside the experimental setting (Krabbendam and Aleman 2003).

BEHAVIORAL DYSFUNCTION AFTER BRAIN INJURY

Understanding of the full range of behavioral dysfunction in individuals with brain injury or disease is far from complete. Unfortunately, relatively few follow-up studies to date have systematically investigated the efficacy of neuropsychiatric treatment programs. In addition, as is the case with the literature on cognitive rehabilitation, much of what is known comes from studies conducted in rehabilitation settings rather than in hospitals specifically designed to treat patients with neuropsychiatric disorders. Most of the recent studies in this area have focused on patients with traumatic brain injuries.

Behavioral dysfunction associated with other neurological disorders, such as cerebrovascular accidents and progressive dementing disorders, also has received considerable attention but has not been the subject of a great deal of research to evaluate treatment procedures that are likely to be effective. Despite the relatively sparse amount of literature on treatment outcome in this area, the studies that have been reported have been useful in guiding the development of practical strategies for dealing with the behavioral-psychiatric consequences of brain injury. In particular, behaviorally based treatments have been heavily used. Behavioral dysfunction after brain injury can have a marked effect on the recovery process itself, as well as on the more general aspects of psychosocial adjustment. It is indeed ironic and unfortunate that the patients most needing cognitive rehabilitation services are often kept out of many treatment facilities because of their disruptive behavior. In fact, research studies (Levin et al. 1982; Lishman 1978; Weddell et al. 1980) have shown that behavioral dysfunction is often associated with reduced abilities to comply with rehabilitation programs, to return to work, to engage in recreational and leisure activities, and to sustain positive interpersonal relationships.

Levin and Grossman (1978) reported behavior problems that were present 1 month after traumatic brain injury and that occurred in areas such as emotional withdrawal, conceptual disorganization, motor slowing, unusual thought content, blunt affect, excitement, and disorientation. At 6 months after injury, those patients who had poor social and occupational recovery continued to manifest significant cognitive and behavioral disruption. Complaints of tangential thinking, fragmented speech, slowness of thought and action, depressed mood, increased anxiety, and marital and/or family conflict also were frequently noted (Levin et al. 1979). Other behavioral changes reported to have the potential to cause psychosocial disruption include increased irritability (Rosenthal 1983), social inappropriateness (Lewis et al. 1988), aggression (Mungas 1988), and expansiveness, helplessness, suspiciousness, and anxiety (Grant and Alves 1987). Rapoport et al. (2005) describe the deleterious effect of depressive reactions on cognitive functions in individuals who have experienced mild to moderate closed head injury. It appears that any cognitive rehabilitation program should also target the emotional reactions in order to optimize recovery.

Behavioral dysfunction is not limited to individuals with traumatic brain injuries. Patients with lesions in specific brain regions secondary to other pathological conditions also can have characteristic patterns of dysfunctional behavior. For example, frontal lobe dysfunction secondary to stroke, tumor, or other disease processes is often associated with a cluster of symptoms, including social disinhibition, reduced attention, distractibility, impaired judgment, affective lability, and more pervasive mood disorder (Bond 1984; Stuss and Benson 1984). In contrast, Prigatano (1987) noted that individuals with temporal lobe dysfunction can show heightened interpersonal sensitivity, which can evolve into frank paranoid ideation.

In addition to differences between patients with different types of brain injury or disease, the variability in the severity and extent of behavioral disruption after injury within each patient group is remarkable. Eames and Wood (1985), for example, vividly described the variability in severity of impairment in a group of patients who received treatment on a special unit for patients with behavior disorders and head injuries. Verbal and physical aggression, inappropriate social and sexual behavior, self-injury, irritability, and markedly altered levels of drive and motivation represent the kinds of behaviors shown by their patients. The magnitude of their dysfunction precluded many of the patients from participating in traditional rehabilitation programs. They could not be managed at home, in extended-care facilities, or even in general inpatient psychiatric settings. Perhaps not too surprisingly, individuals with mild head injuries are less prone to debilitating behavioral changes but still can experience physical, cognitive, and affective changes of sufficient magnitude to affect their ability to return to preaccident activities (Dikmen et al. 1986; Levin et al. 1987).

It seems clear that adjustment (and failure to adjust) after brain injury appears to be related to a multitude of neurological and nonneurological factors, each of which requires consideration in the choice of an appropriate course of intervention for any observed behavioral dysfunction. In addition to the extent and severity of the neurological injury itself, some of the other factors that can contribute to the presence and type of behavioral dysfunction include the amount of time elapsed since the injury, premorbid psychiatric and psychosocial adjust-

ment, financial resources, social supports, and personal awareness of (and reaction to) acquired deficits (Eames 1988; G. Goldstein and Ruthven 1983; Gross and Schutz 1986; Meier et al. 1987).

Given the large number of factors that influence recovery from brain injury, a multidimensional approach to the behavioral treatment of patients with brain injury is likely to result in an optimal recovery. This approach should take into consideration the patient's premorbid level of functioning (in terms of both psychological adjustment and neuropsychological functioning), as well as his or her current psychological and neuropsychological resources. Individuals with more severe cognitive impairments are more likely to profit from highly structured behavioral programs. Those whose neuropsychological functioning is more intact, in contrast, may profit from interventions with a more active cognitive component that requires them to use abstract thought as well as self-evaluative and self-corrective processes. Not surprisingly, therapeutic approaches that fall under the general heading of behavior therapy represent an approach that is gaining increasing interest as a component of the overall treatment plan for patients with neuropsychiatric impairment. Ackerman (2004) presents a case study of treatment for a patient with mild traumatic brain injury and posttraumatic stress disorder in which the treatment required coordinated application of cognitive rehabilitation techniques, biofeedback, and psychotherapy. Although there were no experimental controls such as could be applied using single-subject design methods, this report does illustrate the need for a multidimensional approach to the treatment of patients with cognitive deficits.

BEHAVIOR THERAPY FOR PATIENTS WITH BRAIN IMPAIRMENT

The domain of behavior therapy has expanded considerably in the past 20 years. Although it is not the primary purpose of this chapter to review the history of behaviorally based therapies, it is useful to keep in mind that behavioral assessment and treatment have extended far beyond their early roots in classical and operant conditioning and have been adapted for use with numerous special populations, most recently including persons with brain injuries. (For more comprehensive and critical presentations of the recent status and direction of behavior therapies, see Haynes 1984, Hersen and Bellack 1985, and Kazdin 1979; for excellent compendia describing both assessment and treatment approaches in clinically useful terms, see Bellack and Hersen 1985a and Hersen and Bellack 1988.)

Despite a broadening scope that has included the treatment of patients with neurological impairment, behavioral approaches remain committed to the original principles derived from experimental and social psychology. They also emphasize the empirical and objective implementation and evaluation of treatment (Bellack and Hersen 1985b).

The general assumptions about the nature of behavior disorders that form the basis of behavioral approaches include the following (Haynes 1984):

- Disordered behavior can be expressed through overt actions, thoughts, verbalizations, and physiological reactions.
- These reactions do not necessarily vary in the same way for different individuals or for different behavior disorders.
- Changing one specific behavior may result in changes in other related behaviors.
- Environmental conditions play an important role in the initiation, maintenance, and alteration of behavior.

These assumptions have led to approaches emphasizing the objective evaluation of observable aspects of the individual and his or her interaction with the environment. The range of observable events is limited only by the clinician's ability to establish a reliable, valid quantification of the target behavior or environmental condition. As previously noted, this could range from a specific physiological reaction, such as heart rate, to a self-report of the number of obsessive thoughts occurring during a 24-hour period.

Intervention focuses on the active interaction between the individual and the environment. The goal of treatment is to alter those aspects of the environment that have become associated with the initiation or maintenance of maladaptive behaviors or to alter the patient's response to those aspects of the environment in some way.

The application of a behavioral intervention with a neuropsychiatric patient requires careful consideration of both the neuropsychological and the environmental aspects of the presenting problem. Although this may seem obvious, the attempted synthesis of these two separate disciplines is still in the early stages of development. Few clinicians have the training, time, or energy to become and remain equally competent in both neuropsychology and behavioral psychology. There is, however, a growing effort to explore areas of commonality between these two specialties. Professional interest groups among behavioral psychologists are attempting to define more precisely the domain of behavioral neuropsychology (Horton and Barrett 1988).

At present, the accumulated body of evidence remains limited regarding the specific types of behavioral interventions that are most effective in treating the various dysfunc-

tional behaviors observed in individuals with different kinds of brain injuries. Despite this limitation, there is optimism, based on the current literature, that behavior therapy can be effective for patients with brain injuries (Horton and Miller 1985). Indeed, an increasing number of books, primarily on the rehabilitation of patients with brain injuries, describe the potential applications of behavioral approaches for persons with neurological impairment (Edelstein and Couture 1984; G. Goldstein and Ruthven 1983; Seron 1987; Wood 1984). Such sources provide an excellent introduction to the basic models, methods, and limitations of behavioral treatments of patients with brain injuries.

Behavioral approaches can be broadly classified into at least three general models (Calhoun and Turner 1981): 1) a traditional behavioral approach, 2) a social learning approach, and 3) a cognitive-behavioral approach. The degree to which the client or patient is required to participate actively in the identification and alteration of the environmental conditions assumed to be supporting the maladaptive behavior varies across these models.

TRADITIONAL BEHAVIORAL APPROACH

The traditional behavioral approach emphasizes the effects of environmental events that occur after (consequences), as well as before (antecedents), a particular behavior of interest. We address these two aspects of environmental influence separately.

Interventions Aimed at the Consequences of Behavior

A consequence that increases the probability of a specific behavior occurring again under similar circumstances is termed a *reinforcer*. Consequences can either increase or decrease the likelihood of a particular behavior occurring again.

A behavior followed by an environmental consequence that increases the likelihood that the behavior will occur again is called a *positive reinforcer*. A behavior followed by the removal of a negative or aversive environmental condition is called a *negative reinforcer*. A behavior followed by an aversive environmental event is termed a *punishment*. The effect of punishment is to reduce the probability that the behavior will occur under similar conditions. There has often been confusion concerning the difference between negative reinforcers and punishments. It is useful to remember that reinforcers (positive or negative) always increase the likelihood of the behavior occurring again, whereas punishments decrease the likelihood of a behavior occurring again. When the reliable relation between a specific behavior and an environmental consequence is removed, the behavioral effect is to reduce the target behavior to a near-zero level of occurrence. This process is called *extinction*. Self-management skills (relaxation training, biofeedback) have been used in the treatment of ataxia (Guercio et al. 1997).

Interventions Aimed at the Antecedents of Behavior

Behavior is controlled or affected not only by the consequences that follow it but also by events that precede it. These events are called *antecedents*. For example, an aggressive patient may have outbursts only in the presence of the nursing staff and never in the presence of the physician. In this case, a failure to search for potential antecedents (e.g., female sex or physical size) that may be eliciting the behavior may leave half of the behavioral assessment undone and may result in difficulty decreasing the aggressive behavior. This type of approach may be particularly useful in patients for whom the behavior is disruptive enough that approaches aimed at manipulation of consequences hold some danger for staff and family (e.g., in the case of a patient with explosive or violent outbursts). In this situation, treatment is structured to decrease the likelihood of an outburst by restructuring the events that lead to the violent behavior. Some patients are able to learn to anticipate these antecedents themselves, whereas for others, it becomes the task of the treatment staff to identify and modify the antecedents that lead to unwanted behavior. For example, if the stress of verbal communication leads to aggressive behavior in an aphasic patient, the patient may be initially trained to use an alternative form of communication, such as writing or sign language (Franzen and Lovell 1987).

Other Behavioral Approaches

Yet another class of approaches involves the use of differential reinforcement of other behaviors. In this approach, the problem behavior is not consequated—that is, the effect of the problem behavior is not addressed. Instead, another behavior that is inconsistent with the problem target behavior is reinforced. As the other behavior increases in frequency, the problem behavior decreases. Hegel and Ferguson (2000) reported the successful use of this approach in reducing aggressive behavior in a subject with brain injury. Differential reinforcement of low rates of responding also may be used to reduce undesired behaviors (Alderman and Knight 1997). Finally, noncontingent reinforcement in the form of increased attention to a subject resulted in a decrease in aggression toward others and a decrease in self-injurious behaviors (Persel et al. 1997).

SOCIAL LEARNING APPROACH

With the social learning approach, cognitive processes that mediate between environmental conditions and behavioral responses are included in explanations of the learning process. Social learning approaches take advantage of learning through modeling—by systematically arranging opportunities for patients to observe socially adaptive examples of social interaction. Emphasis is also placed on practicing the components of social skills in role-playing situations, where the patient can receive corrective feedback. Intervention that focuses on social skills training is one example of a treatment that is often useful for patients with brain injuries who have lost the ability to effectively monitor their behavior and to respond appropriately in a given situation.

Socially skilled behavior is generally divided into three components: 1) social perception, 2) social problem solving, and 3) social expression. Training can occur at any one of these levels. For the patient who has lost the ability to interact appropriately with conversational skills, this behavior may be modeled by staff members. (For a comprehensive review, see Bandura 1977.)

COGNITIVE-BEHAVIORAL APPROACH

The term *cognitive-behavioral approach* refers to a heterogeneous group of procedures that emphasizes the individual's cognitive mediation (self-messages) in explaining behavioral responses within environmental contexts. The thoughts, beliefs, and predictions about one's own actions and their potential environmental consequences are emphasized. Treatment focuses on changing maladaptive beliefs and increasing an individual's self-control within the current social environment by changing maladaptive thoughts or beliefs. This approach is particularly useful with patients who have relatively intact language and self-evaluative abilities.

Cognitive-behavioral treatments originally were designed to treat affective disorders and symptoms. However, the use of the approach has widened to include anxiety, personality disorders, and skills deficits. For example, Suzman et al. (1997) used cognitive-behavioral methods to improve the problem-solving skills of children with cognitive deficits following traumatic brain injury.

ASSESSMENT OF TREATMENT EFFECTS

In addition to providing a set of methodologies to affect the disordered behavior produced by cognitive deficits, the literature on behavior therapy has provided a conceptual scheme for evaluating the effects of intervention. One of the most influential products of the tradition of behavior therapy has been the development of single-subject designs to evaluate the effect of interventions. Although originally conceived as a method of evaluating the effect of

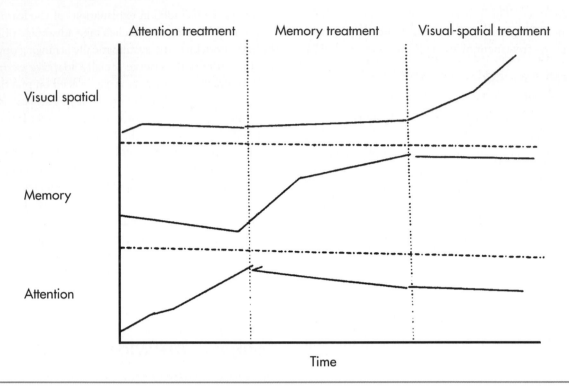

FIGURE 33–1.   Multiple-baseline design for the treatment of a patient with brain injury and deficits in attention, memory, and visual-spatial processing. Attention, memory, and visual-spatial skills are each treated in sequence; improvement is seen in one area before beginning the next phase of treatment, and performance in untreated skill areas is used as a comparison for the treated areas. The vertical axis represents level of performance in each skill area (visual spatial, memory, and attention). The passage of time is represented on the horizontal axis. The dotted vertical lines are those times at which treatment was switched from the previous focus to the current focus, such as from attention training to memory training.

environmental interventions, the single-subject design has been successfully applied in the evaluation of pharmacological interventions as well. Because each patient is an individual and treatment of cognitive dysfunction is still a relatively nascent endeavor, interventions often need to be specifically tailored to the individual patient. Interventions often must be applied before the period of spontaneous recovery has ended, and a method to distinguish the effects of intervention from the effects of recovery of acute physiological disturbance is needed. The multiple-baseline design is a single-subject design that addresses these issues (Franzen and Iverson 1990).

The design of multiple baselines across behaviors involves the evaluation of more than one behavior taking place at the same time. However, only one of the behaviors is targeted for intervention at a time. In this way, the non-targeted behaviors are used as control comparisons for the targeted behaviors. For example, behavior A is targeted for intervention first, and monitors on behaviors B and C are used as control comparisons. After completion of the treatment phase for behavior A, an intervention is implemented for behavior B, and monitors on behaviors A and C are used as control comparisons.

Figure 33–1 presents an example of a multiple baseline design in the treatment of an individual with brain injury and deficits in memory, attention, and visual-spatial processing. The attention skills receive treatment in the first phase, with a concomitant improvement in skill level. At the second phase, memory skills are treated, with a concomitant improvement. Finally, visual-spatial skills are treated at the third phase, and improvement is seen there. At each phase, performance in the other untreated skill areas is used as a control comparison for the treated skill areas.

In an application of the multiple-baseline design to the treatment of a patient with brain injury, Franzen and Harris (1993) reported a case in which a patient had deficits in attention-based memory and in abstraction and planning as the result of a closed head injury. This patient was first seen 23 days after the closed head injury occurred. He was seen for a series of weekly appointments. At these appointments, the emotional adjustment was discussed and support was provided. Additionally, the patient received psychotherapy in the form of anger control training and social reinforcement for increasing his daily level of activity and self-initiated social interactions, two areas identified as problems during the evaluation. Finally, cognitive retraining exercises were implemented and taught to the patient and his family so that home practice could take place on a daily basis. The family was instructed in the methods used to record the scores from the exercises, which were then entered into a daily log.

The cognitive retraining was conducted according to a design in which multiple baselines across behaviors were used. Cognitive retraining treatment was first aimed at improving attention and memory with a set of four exercises implemented both during outpatient appointments and at home. An assessment conducted on both of the targeted treatment areas of memory and abstraction and planning skills indicated improvement in the memory realm but not in the abstraction and planning realm. During the second phase, treatment was aimed at improving abstraction and planning skills with a set of exercises that were again implemented during outpatient appointments and at home. Evaluations during this phase indicated improvement in abstraction and planning skills but no further improvement in memory skills. A complete neuropsychological battery of tests was administered at the first contact and again after the termination of treatment. Additionally, short tests of relevant neuropsychological function were administered before the initiation of treatment, at each phase change, and at the termination of treatment. The results of the standardized neuropsychological tests were consistent with the behavioral monitoring conducted on the skill exercises, namely, improvement in attention and memory as a result of the treatment in the first phase and improvement in abstraction and planning skills as a result of the treatment in the second phase.

CASE EXAMPLES OF BEHAVIORAL INTERVENTION

In this section, we present two case examples of how behavioral interventions can be applied within the context of the comprehensive care provided in an acute neuropsychiatric inpatient setting. Although the focus of the cases is on behavioral treatment, patients are monitored by an interdisciplinary treatment team representing neuropsychiatry, neuropsychology, psychiatric nursing, occupational therapy, recreational therapy, speech-language pathology, and physical therapy. The emphasis here is on the application of behavioral procedures, not on the attribution of outcome. The cases selected represent typical behavior complaints within this type of setting. In this chapter, we have discussed the application of behavioral technology to the remediation of cognitive deficits. A more common use of behavioral methods is in the treatment of problematic behavior that might otherwise interfere with the rehabilitation process.

CASE EXAMPLE 1: INAPPROPRIATE SEXUAL AND AGGRESSIVE LANGUAGE AND BEHAVIOR

Mr. A, a 27-year-old single man, had received a closed head injury as the result of a suicide attempt at age 19. He had been significantly involved with drug abuse and had attempted suicide while intoxicated after discharge from a substance treatment center to which he had been sent by his parents. Before his suicide attempt, he had been involved in a motorcycle accident while intoxicated, and the accident had left him unable to ambulate without the use of a wheelchair. The suicide attempt involved taking an overdose of sleeping pills with alcohol and firing a pistol into his right temple. He was discovered by his mother after the shot was fired. He had a significant and noticeable cranial depression as the result of his injury.

Mr. A had received inpatient acute rehabilitation services and had been placed in various personal-care facilities. Each time, he was discharged because of disruptive behavior, including sexually inappropriate language, touching of staff and female residents, and aggressive language, with occasional escalation to aggressive behavior. Although at first he expressed relief at being sent to a rehabilitation hospital, where "at least the staff know what they're doing," he soon became involved in conflicts with the staff and began showing the inappropriate behavior that had been the cause of his referral to the rehabilitation hospital. He made sexual comments directed at female staff and would attempt to fondle them. He would place his wheelchair in the hallway such that it was difficult for people to walk past him without his grabbing them. On his third night at the hospital, he was found behind the closed door of a confused female patient's room. Mr. A was found with his hands beneath her bedclothes, although he was fully clothed and still in his wheelchair. Mr. A also was seen lighting his cigarettes in his bedroom instead of in the smoking area outside of the hospital. There were circumscribed times for smoking, but Mr. A insisted on smoking throughout the day. He would use threats of physical violence or legal action against any staff who would attempt to control his behavior. In fact, he had obtained the services of a pro bono lawyer to file suit against a previous placement because of what he termed "abuse by the staff." The suit was dismissed by a judge, but the reputation he acquired from this behavior made it difficult to find another personal-care facility to house him afterward.

The neuropsychological evaluation indicated an average IQ, with a value of 107 for the Full-Scale IQ. His Wechsler Memory Scale—Revised (WMS-R; Wechsler 1987) General Memory Index was 96, and his Delayed Recall Index was somewhat lower, at 87. His performance on the Halstead Category Test (Reitan and Wolfson 1985) indicated only mild problems with abstract problem solving. Verbal generativity and naming were intact. Motor speed was slowed, especially on the right side. Visual-perceptual performance was adequate. There were no signs of significant cognitive impairment otherwise. Performance on the Trail Making Test (Reitan and Wolfson 1985) and on the Stroop Color-Word Test (Golden 1978) was adequate. There were no signs of an organic basis for impulsivity or perseveration.

Although his free behavior might be construed as being a manifestation of impulsivity, Mr. A did not show signs of that problem on standardized tests. He also showed reasonable problem-solving and planning skills, both on standardized tests and on the basis of his history (e.g., hiring the lawyer to press suit against the personal-care facility). However, the fact that he engaged the attorney while still a resident in the facility in question indicated a tendency to let his negative feelings override his better judgment. His memory test performance indicated that he should be able to remember a contingency system if it were described to him in simple terms and on multiple occasions.

On the basis of the evaluation, a behavior management program was designed in which Mr. A received full information about the contingencies and the reasons for implementing them, namely, to help him control his behavior and to learn more appropriate and, ultimately, more effective ways of pursuing his wants. The underlying principles involved were to minimize punishment because he used aggression to escape punishing situations and to increase social reinforcement and social control over his behavior so that the treatment gains could be maintained in a nonhospital setting.

A functional analysis of the aggressive behavior indicated that Mr. A used aggressive language when it appeared that limits would be placed on his behaviors. For example, if a staff member attempted to enforce the rules regarding smoking or keeping perishable food in his room, Mr. A would threaten to physically attack the staff member or would engage in verbal vituperation and vulgarity. Especially because of his history, the staff members would typically back down and leave Mr. A to his own desires. This appeared to be a pattern at several care facilities, especially after the unsuccessful lawsuit.

A functional analysis of the sexual behavior indicated that Mr. A initiated sexual behavior against individuals who could not retaliate. For example, he would fondle confused patients, or female staff members would be constrained in their responses to him. He did not approach the nonprofessional staff, who would presumably be more inclined to provide a negative consequence to his behavior.

Mr. A was able to escape or avoid undesirable circumstances (e.g., frustration of his desire to smoke or to engage in desired behaviors contrary to hospital policy or schedule) by engaging in aggressive behavior. The contingency management program included informing Mr. A that aggressive behavior would not result in being allowed to have his way. Instead, Mr. A would be reminded of the rules regarding the issue in question. If he continued to threaten aggression, he would be escorted to his room. If he threatened to sue the hospital, he would be advised to discuss all such matters with the hospital counsel, who had been briefed on the situation. Mr. A also was informed of the usual grievance procedure already implemented in the hospital and was introduced to the patient representative.

Mr. A was hypothesized to be seeking sexual contact with individuals who could not refuse him because of his concerns about rejection. Therefore, the contingency management system used to treat this problem behavior included a verbal indication that such behavior would not be tolerated. If Mr. A initiated fondling or sexual language with a patient, his access to that patient would be severely limited. If he initiated it with a staff member, that staff member would immediately leave the room and be replaced by a male staff member. Additionally, Mr. A received individual counseling regarding sexuality in disabled individuals. He was given the opportunity to attend social mixers with the local paraplegic and head injury survivor groups, where he could meet young people with similar concerns.

The result of the treatment intervention was a dramatic reduction in aggressive behavior in a short time. The inappropriate sexual behavior decreased, although the inappropriate sexual verbalizations remained. An interview with Mr. A's mother indicated that vulgar and, at times, explicit sexual talk was a premorbid behavior pattern for Mr. A. It was not thought that treatment would be effective in totally changing that aspect.

CASE EXAMPLE 2: DEPRESSION WITH FAILURE TO USE AMBULATORY ASSISTANCE

Ms. B, a 68-year-old right-handed woman with a high school education, had a history of diabetes and moderate hypertension, both of which were of recent onset. She lived alone and one evening had a stroke that left her with ambulatory difficulties, significant memory deficits, and depression. She was receiving inpatient rehabilitation, including physical therapy, memory retraining, and psychotherapy. She tended to try to ambulate without her walker, which was a concern to the staff because of the potential for falls and injury.

The neuropsychological evaluation indicated generally intact language skills. Her motor functions were slow in comparison with age-appropriate norms, and her left side showed relatively more slowing. Motor strength was attenuated on the left side, and balance and gait problems were noted. Attention was moderately impaired; she had the ability to repeat up to six digits, but only inconsistently. She showed difficulty on tasks requiring concentration and mental manipulation of information. Her Visual Memory Index on the WMS-R was 82, Verbal Memory Index was 91, and Delayed Memory Index was 71. Her performance on abstract problem-solving tasks was adequate but somewhat lower than average.

Ms. B often would attempt to walk without the use of her walker. She would attempt to rise from a chair or from her bed without calling for assistance or using the walker to steady herself. In physical therapy sessions, she willingly used the walker or the assistance of the physical therapist. Individual psychotherapy with Ms. B centered on the themes of change and aging. She had been relatively healthy until approximately 4 years earlier and had been living independently until the time of her stroke. She had been driving and had been a resource for her children by baby-sitting and running errands for them. The conceptualization of her failure to use the walker involved her memory deficits, whereby she would forget that the use of a walker was necessary. A secondary reason involved her difficulty in accepting the changes in her situation.

The individual psychotherapist addressed the issues of accepting her current situation. Ms. B was helped to focus on her abilities rather than on her disabilities. The importance of realistically evaluating her needs was emphasized. Other staff members were instructed to remind Ms. B of her strengths whenever she became focused on her difficulties. Staff members, including housekeeping and transportation workers, were encouraged not to minimize her difficulties while not focusing extensively on them.

As intervention for her memory difficulties, Ms. B was given overlearning procedures involving getting out of bed and rising from a chair. Each day, Ms. B would practice (with supervision and feedback) getting out of bed and reaching for her walker for 30 minutes. In the afternoon, she would receive 15 minutes of practice in rising from a chair and reaching for her walker. It was believed that overlearning with dense practice would help make the use of the walker second nature. Ms. B was taught to repeat the phrase "Before I stand, I need my walker" multiple times and to use that phrase each time she wanted to stand. Each staff member also repeated that phrase each time they helped Ms. B get out of bed or up from a chair.

A small can was attached to the frame of her walker. Staff members were given tokens and instructed to randomly provide social reinforcement and to place a token in the can when they saw Ms. B using the walker. Twenty tokens could be exchanged for an extra time period in the crafts room. This procedure was chosen to develop a positive valence toward the use of the walker as well as to increase use of the walker. Staff members also randomly quizzed Ms. B on the pro-

cedures needed to arise from bed and arise from a chair. The dependent measures used were the number of times that Ms. B needed to be reminded to use the walker, the number of tokens collected in the can attached to the walker, and the number of correct answers to the quiz questions.

Ms. B showed appropriate changes in behavior in response to the contingencies. The staff felt that the treatment was successful when, on awakening and not finding her walker, Ms. B called for a nurse rather than attempting to stand on her own.

CONCLUSION

Neuropsychological and behavioral dysfunction associated with brain injury can be varied and complex. Effective intervention requires an integrated interdisciplinary approach that focuses on the individual patient and his or her specific needs. There may be an interactive effect in that improvement in cognitive operations may result in improvement in emotional and behavioral adaptation. Behaviorally based formulations can provide a valuable framework from which to understand the interaction between an individual with compromised physical, neuropsychological, and emotional functioning, as well as the psychosocial environment in which he or she is trying to adjust.

Much work remains to define the most effective cognitive and behaviorally based treatments for various neuropsychiatric disorders. There is increasing evidence that computerized approaches may be helpful. A combined behavioral and pharmacological approach may be more effective than either strategy alone. The evidence to date suggests that cognitive rehabilitation is indeed an area worthy of continued pursuit.

Highlights for the Clinician

- ✦ The neuroanatomical and neurophysiological determinants of recovery vary by etiology; therefore, treatment in different disorders will vary.

- ✦ Rehabilitation efforts have been developed to address deficits in attention, memory, visual-perceptual skills, executive functions, and speech and language.

- ✦ Behavioral dysfunction is a frequent effect of acquired brain impairment and can complicate treatment of cognitive deficits as well as be a target for intervention in itself.

- ✦ Pharmacological and behavioral interventions optimally are integrated to increase the success of rehabilitative efforts.

- ✦ The assessment of treatment effects can be documented by using single-subject experimental designs.

RECOMMENDED READINGS

Halligan PW, Wade DT (eds): The Effectiveness of Rehabilitation for Cognitive Deficits. New York, Oxford University Press, 2005

High WM Jr, Sander AM, Struchen MA, et al (eds): Rehabilitation for Traumatic Brain Injury. New York, Oxford University Press, 2005

Klein R, McNamara P, Albert ML): Neuropharmacologic approaches to cognitive rehabilitation. Behav Neurol 17:1–3, 2006

León-Carrión J, von Wild KRH, Zitnay GA (eds): Brain Injury Treatment: Theories and Practices. New York, Taylor & Francis, 2006

Loewenstein D, Acevedo A: Training of cognitive and functionally relevant skills in Mild Alzheimer's disease: an integrated approach, in Geriatric Neuropsychology: Assessment and Intervention. Edited by Attix DK, Welsh-Bohmer KA. New York, Guilford, 2006, pp 261–274

Murrey GJ: Alternate Therapies in the Treatment of Brain Injury and Neurobehavioral Disorders: A Practical Guide. New York, Haworth Press, 2006

REFERENCES

Ackerman RJ: Applied psychophysiology, clinical biofeedback, and rehabilitation neuropsychology: a case study—mild traumatic brain injury and post-traumatic stress disorder. Phys Med Rehabil Clin N Am 15:919–931, 2004

Alderman N, Knight C: The effectiveness of DRL in the management of severe behaviour disorders following brain injury. Brain Inj 11:79–101, 1997

Amato MP, Zipoli V: Clinical management of cognitive impairment in multiple sclerosis: a review of current evidence. Int MS J 1072–1083, 2003

Anderson-Hanley C, Sherman ML, Riggs R, et al: Neuropsycholgoical effects of treatments for adults with cancer: a meta-analysis and review of the literature. J Int Neuropsychol Soc 9:967–982, 2003

Azouvi P, Jokic C, Attal N, et al: Carbamazepine in agitation and aggressive behaviour following severe closed-head injury. Brain Inj 13:797–804, 1999

Bandura A: Social Learning Theory. Englewood Cliffs, NJ, Prentice-Hall, 1977

Basso A, Capotani E, Vignolo L: Influence of rehabilitation on language skills in aphasic patients. Arch Neurol 36:190–196, 1979

Bellack AS, Hersen M: Dictionary of Behavior Therapy Techniques. New York, Pergamon, 1985a

Bellack AS, Hersen M: General considerations, in Handbook of Clinical Behavior Therapy With Adults. Edited by Hersen M, Bellack AS. New York, Plenum, 1985b, pp 3–19

Bellack AS, Mueser KT: Psychosocial treatment for schizophrenia. Schizophr Bull 19:317–336, 1993

Bellucci DM, Glaberman K, Haslam N: Computer assisted cognitive rehabilitation reduces negative symptoms in the severely mentally ill. Schizophr Res 59:225–232, 2003

Ben-Yishay Y, Diller L: Rehabilitation of cognitive and perceptual deficits in people with traumatic brain damage. Int J Rehabil Res 4:208–210, 1981

Ben-Yishay Y, Diller L: Cognitive deficits, in Rehabilitation of the Head-Injured Adult. Edited by Griffith EA, Bond M, Miller J. Philadelphia, PA, FA Davis, 1983, pp 167–183

Benedict RH, Harris AE, Markow T, et al: Effects of attention training on information processing in schizophrenia. Schizophr Bull 20:537–546, 1994

Birnboim S, Miller A: Cognitive strategies application of multiple sclerosis patients. Mult Scler 10:67–73, 2004

Ble A, Volpato S, Zuliani G, et al: Executive function correlates with walking speed in older person: the InCHIANTI study. J Am Geriatr Soc 3:410–415, 2005

Bond M: The psychiatry of closed head injury, in Closed Head Injury: Psychosocial, Social and Family Consequences. Edited by Brooks PN. Oxford, England, Oxford University Press, 1984, pp 148–178

Calhoun KS, Turner SM: Historical perspectives and current issues in behavior therapy, in Handbook of Clinical Behavior Therapy. Edited by Turner SM, Calhoun KS, Adams HE. New York, Wiley, 1981, pp 1–11

Chiaravalloti ND, Demaree H, Gaudino EA, et al: Can the repetition effect maximize learning multiple sclerosis? Clin Rehabil 17:58–68, 2003

Cicerone KD, Dahlberg C, Kalmar K, et al: Evidence-based cognitive rehabilitation: recommendations for clinical practice. Arch Phys Med Rehabil 81:1596–1615, 2000

Clare L, Wilson BA, Carter G, et al: Relearning face-name associations in early Alzheimer's disease. Neuropsychology 16:538–547, 2002

Clare L, Carter G, Hodges JR: Cognitive rehabilitation as a component of early intervention in Alzheimer's disease: a single case study. Aging Ment Health 7:15–21, 2003

Clare L, Wilson BA, Carter G, et al: Awareness in early stage Alzheimer's disease: relation to outcome of cognitive rehabilitation. J Clin Exp Neuropsychol 26:215–226, 2004

Crovitz H, Harvey M, Horn R: Problems in the acquisition of imagery mnemonics: three brain damaged cases. Cortex 15:225–234, 1979

Cuesta GM: Cognitive rehabilitation of memory following stroke. Adv Neurol 92:415–421, 2003

da Costa RM, de Carvalho LA: The acceptance of virtual realist devices for cognitive rehabilitation: a report of positive results with schizophrenia. Comput Methods Programs Biomed 73:173–182, 2004

Dikmen S, McLean A, Temkin N: Neuropsychological and psychosocial consequences of minor head injury. J Neurol Neurosurg Psychiatry 49:1227–1232, 1986

Diller L, Weinberg J: Hemi-inattention in rehabilitation: the evolution of a rational remediation program. Adv Neurol 18:63–82, 1977

Eames P: Behavior disorders after severe head injury: their nature, causes and strategies for management. J Head Trauma Rehabil 3:1–6, 1988

Eames P, Wood R: Rehabilitation after severe brain injury: a follow-up study of a behavior modification approach. J Neurol Neurosurg Psychiatry 48:613–619, 1985

Edelstein BA, Couture ET: Behavioral Assessment and Rehabilitation of the Traumatically Brain-Damaged. New York, Plenum, 1984

Flesher S: Cognitive habilitation in schizophrenia: a theoretical review and model of treatment. Neuropsychol Rev 1:223–246, 1990

Franzen MD: Behavioral assessment and treatment of brain-impaired individuals, in Progress in Behavior Modification. Edited by Hersen M, Eisler RM. Newbury Park, CA, Sage, 1991, pp 56–85

Franzen MD, Harris CV: Neuropsychological rehabilitation: application of a modified multiple baseline design. Brain Inj 7:525–534, 1993

Franzen MD, Haut MW: The psychological treatment of memory impairment: a review of empirical studies. Neuropsychol Rev 2:29–63, 1991

Franzen MD, Iverson GL: Applications of single subject design to cognitive rehabilitation, in Neuropsychology Across the Lifespan. Edited by Horton AM. New York, Springer, 1990, pp 155–174

Franzen MD, Lovell MR: Behavioral treatments of aggressive sequelae of brain injury. Psychiatr Ann 17:389–396, 1987

Galski T, Ehle HT, Williams JB: Off-road driving evaluations for persons with cerebral injury: a factor analytic study of pre-driver and simulator testing. Am J Occup Ther 51:352–359, 1997

Gardner H: The Shattered Mind: The Person After Brain Damage. London, Routledge & Kegan Paul, 1977

Gianutsos R, Matheson P: The rehabilitation of visual perceptual disorders attributable to brain injury, in Neuropsychological Rehabilitation. Edited by Meier MJ, Benton AL, Diller L. New York, Guilford, 1987, pp 202–241

Gianutsos R, Glosser D, Elbaum J, et al: Visual imperception in brain injured adults: multifaceted measures. Arch Phys Med Rehabil 64:456–461, 1983

Giles GM, Pussey I, Burgess P: The behavioral treatment of verbal interaction skills following severe head injury: a single case study. Brain Inj 2:75–79, 1988

Giles GM, Ridley JE, Dill A, et al: A consecutive series of adults with brain injury treated with a washing and dressing retraining program. Am J Occup Ther 51:256–266, 1997

Glasgow RE, Zeiss RA, Barrera M, et al: Case studies on remediating memory deficits in brain damaged individuals. J Clin Psychol 33:1049–1054, 1977

Glen MB: Methylphenidate for cognitive and behavioral dysfunction after traumatic brain injury. J Head Trauma Rehabil 13:87–90, 1998

Glisky EL, Schacter DL: Remediation of organic memory disorders: current status and future prospects. J Head Trauma Rehabil 4:54–63, 1986

Golden CJ: The Stroop Color-Word Test: Clinical and Experimental Manual. Chicago, IL, Stoelting, 1978

Goldstein FC, Levin HS: Disorders of reasoning and problem solving ability, in Neuropsychological Rehabilitation. Edited by Meier MJ, Benton AL, Diller L. New York, Guilford, 1987, pp 327–354

Goldstein G, Ruthven L: Rehabilitation of the Brain-Damaged Adult. New York, Plenum, 1983

Gontkovsky ST, McDonald NB, Clark PG, et al: Current directions in computer-assisted cognitive rehabilitation. NeuroRehabilitation 17:195–199, 2002

Gordon W, Hibbard M, Egelko S, et al: Perceptual remediation in patients with right brain damage: a comprehensive program. Arch Phys Med Rehabil 66:353–359, 1985

Gourlay D, Lun KC, Liya G: Telemedicinal virtual reality for cognitive rehabilitation. Stud Health Technol Inform 77:1181–1186, 2000

Gouvier WD, Webster JS, Blanton PD: Cognitive retraining with brain damaged patients, in The Neuropsychology Handbook: Behavioral and Clinical Perspectives. Edited by Wedding D, Horton AM, Webster J. New York, Springer, 1986, pp 278–324

Grant I, Alves W: Psychiatric and psychosocial disturbances in head injury, in Neurobehavioral Recovery From Head Injury. Edited by Levin HS, Grafman J, Eisenberg HM. New York, Oxford University Press, 1987, pp 222–246

Grealy MA, Johnson DA, Rushton SK: Improving cognitive function after brain injury: the use of exercise and virtual reality. Arch Phys Med Rehabil 80:661–667, 1999

Grimm BH, Bleiberg J: Psychological rehabilitation in traumatic brain injury, in Handbook of Clinical Neuropsychology, Vol 2. Edited by Filskov SB, Boll TJ. New York, Wiley, 1986, pp 495–560

Gross Y, Schutz LF: Intervention models in neuropsychology, in Clinical Neuropsychology of Intervention. Edited by Uzzell BP, Gross Y. Boston, MA, Martinus Highoff, 1986, pp 179–204

Gualtieri CT: Pharmacotherapy and the neurobehavioral sequelae of traumatic brain injury. Brain Inj 2:101–109, 1988

Guercio J, Chittum R, McMorrow M: Self-management in the treatment of ataxia: a case study in reducing ataxic tremor through relaxation and biofeedback. Brain Inj 11:353–362, 1997

Harris JE: Methods of improving memory, in Clinical Management of Memory Problems. Edited by Wilson BA, Moffat N. Rockville, MD, Aspen, 1984, pp 46–62

Harris JE, Sunderland A: A brief survey of the management of memory disorders in rehabilitation units in Britain. Int Rehabil Med 3:206–209, 1981

Haynes SN: Behavioral assessment of adults, in Handbook of Psychological Assessment. Edited by Goldstein G, Hersen M. New York, Pergamon, 1984, pp 369–401

Hegel MT, Ferguson RJ: Differential reinforcement of other behavior (DRO) to reduce aggressive behavior following traumatic brain injury. Behav Modif 24:94–101, 2000

Hersen M, Bellack AS: Handbook of Clinical Behavior Therapy With Adults. New York, Plenum, 1985

Hersen M, Bellack AS: Dictionary of Behavioral Assessment Techniques. New York, Pergamon, 1988

Ho MR, Bennett TL: Efficacy of neuropsychological rehabilitation of mild-moderate traumatic brain injury. Arch Clin Neuropsychol 12:1–11, 1997

Holzer JC: Buspirone and brain injury (letter). J Neuropsychiatry Clin Neurosci 10:113, 1998

Horton AM, Barrett D: Neuropsychological assessment and behavior therapy: new directions in head trauma rehabilitation. J Head Trauma Rehabil 3:57–64, 1988

Horton AM, Miller WA: Neuropsychology and behavior therapy, in Progress in Behavior Modifications. Edited by Hersen M, Eisler R, Miller PM. New York, Academic Press, 1985, pp 1–55

Kazdin AE: Fictions, factions, and functions of behavior therapy. Behav Ther 10:629–654, 1979

Khouzam HR, Donnelly NJ: Remission of traumatic brain injury-induced compulsions during venlafaxine treatment. Gen Hosp Psychiatry 20:62–63, 1998

Kolata G: Brain-grafting work shows promise (letter). Science 221:1277, 1983

Krabbendam L, Aleman A: Cognitive remediation in schizophrenia: a quantitative review of controlled studies. Psychopharmacology 169:376–382, 2003

Kraus MF, Maki M: Effect of amantadine hydrochloride on symptoms of frontal lobe dysfunction in brain injury: case studies and review. J Neuropsychiatry Clin Neurosci 9:222–230, 1997

Levin HS, Grossman RG: Behavioral sequelae of closed head injury: a quantitative study. Arch Neurol 35:720–727, 1978

Levin HS, Grossman RG, Ross JE, et al: Long-term neuropsychological outcome of closed head injury. J Neurosurg 50:412–422, 1979

Levin HS, Benton AL, Grossman RG: Neurobehavioral Consequences of Closed Head Injury. New York, Oxford University Press, 1982

Levin HS, Mattis S, Ruff R, et al: Neurobehavioral outcome following minor head injury: a three center study. J Neurosurg 66:234–243, 1987

Lewis FD, Nelson J, Nelson C, et al: Effects of three feedback contingencies on the socially inappropriate talk of a brain-injured adult. Behav Ther 19:203–211, 1988

Lewis L, Unkefer EP, O'Neal SK, et al: Cognitive rehabilitation with patients having severe psychiatric disabilities. Psychiatr Rehabil J 26:325–331, 2003

Lezak MD: Neuropsychological Assessment, 3rd Edition. New York, Oxford University Press, 1995

Liepert J, Bauder H, Miltner WHR, et al: Treatment-induced cortical reorganization after stroke in humans. Stroke 31:1210–1216, 2000

Lishman WA: Organic Psychiatry. St. Louis, MO, Blackwell Scientific, 1978

Loewenstein DA, Acevedo AS, Czaja SJ, et al: Cognitive rehabilitation of mildly impaired Alzheimer's disease patients on cholinesterase inhibitors. Am J Geriatr Psychiatry 12:395–402, 2004

Luria AR: Restoration of Function After Brain Injury. New York, Macmillan, 1963

Luria AR, Tsvetkova LS: The Neuropsychological Analysis of Problem Solving. Orlando, FL, Paul Deutsch, 1990

Marson D, Harrell L: Executive dysfunction and loss of capacity to consent to medical treatment in patients with Alzheimer's disease. Semin Clin Neuropsychiatry 4:41–49, 1999

McIntosh GC: Medical management of noncognitive sequelae of minor traumatic brain injury. Appl Neuropsychol 4:62–68, 1997

Medd J, Tate RL: Evaluation of anger management therapy programme following acquired brain injury: a preliminary study. Neuropsychol Rehabil 10:185–201, 2000

Meier MJ, Strauman S, Thompson WG: Individual differences in neuropsychological recovery: an overview, in Neuropsychological Rehabilitation. Edited by Meier MJ, Benton AL, Diller L. New York, Guilford, 1987, pp 71–110

Mendez MF, Nakawatase TV, Brown CV: Involuntary laughter and inappropriate hilarity. J Neuropsychiatry Clin Neurosci 11:253–258, 1999

Moffat N: Strategies of memory therapy, in Clinical Management of Memory Problems. Edited by Wilson BA, Moffat N. Rockville, MD, Aspen, 1984, pp 63–88

Muldoon MF, Waldstein SR, Ryan CM, et al: Effects of six anti-hypertensive medications on cognitive performance. J Hypertens 20:1643–1652, 2002

Mungas D: Psychometric correlates of episodic violent behavior: a multidimensional neuropsychological approach. Br J Psychiatry 152:180–187, 1988

Newhouse PA, Potter A, Levin ED: Nicotinic system involvement in Alzheimer's and Parkinson's diseases: implications for therapeutics. Drugs Aging 11:206–228, 1997

NIH Consensus Statement: Rehabilitation of Persons With Traumatic Brain Injury, Vol 16, No 1, October 26–28, 1998. Available at: http://consensus.nih.gov/1998/1998TraumaticBrainInjury109html.htm. Accessed January 6, 2007.

O'Sullivan M, Morris RG, Huckstep B, et al: Diffusion tensor MRI correlates with executive dysfunction in patients with ischaemic leukoariaosis. J Neurol Neurosurg Psychiatry 75:441–447, 2004

Patten BM: The ancient art of memory. Arch Neurol 26:25–31, 1972

Persel CS, Persel CH, Ashley MJ, et al: The use of noncontingent reinforcement and contingent restrain to reduce physical aggression and self-injurious behaviour in a traumatically brain injured adult. Brain Inj 11:751–760, 1997

Penades R, Boget T, Lomena F, et al: Brain perfusion and neuropsychological changes in schizophrenic patients after cognitive rehabilitation. Psychiatry Res 98:127–132, 2000

Posner HI, Rafal RD: Cognitive theories of attention and the rehabilitation of attentional deficits, in Neuropsychological Rehabilitation. Edited by Meier MJ, Benton AL, Diller L. New York, Guilford, 1987, pp 182–201

Prigatano GP: Personality and psychosocial consequences after brain injury, in Neuropsychological Rehabilitation. Edited by Meier MJ, Benton AL, Diller L. New York, Guilford, 1987, pp 355–378

Rapoport MJ, McCullagh S, Shami P, et al: Cognitive impairment associated with major depression following mild and moderate traumatic brain injury. J Neuropsychiatry Clin Neurosci 17:61–65, 2005

Reitan RM, Wolfson D: The Halstead-Reitan Neuropsychological Test Battery: Theory and Clinical Interpretation. Tucson, AZ, Neuropsychology Press, 1985

Rizzo AA, Buckwalter JG: Virtual reality and cognitive assessment and rehabilitation: the state of the art. Stud Health Technol Inform 44:123–145, 1997

Robertson-Tchabo EA, Hausman CP, Arenberg D: A classical mnemonic for older learners: a trip that works. Educational Gerontologist 1:215–216, 1976

Robinson RG: Neuropsychiatric consequences of stroke. Annu Rev Med 48:217–229, 1997

Rosenthal M: Behavioral sequelae, in Rehabilitation of the Head Injured Adult. Edited by Rosenthal M, Griffith ER, Bond MR, et al. Philadelphia, PA, FA Davis, 1983, pp 297–308

Schacter DL, Glisky EL: Memory rehabilitation: restoration, alleviation, and the acquisition of domain specific knowledge, in Clinical Neuropsychology of Intervention. Edited by Uzzell B, Gross Y. Boston, MA, Martinus Nijhof, 1986, pp 257–287

Schmitter-Edgecombe M, Fahy JF, Whelan JP, et al: Memory remediation after severe closed head injury: notebook training versus supportive therapy. J Consult Clin Psychol 63:484–489, 1995

Schneider WN, Drew-Cates J, Wong TM, et al: Cognitive and behavioural efficacy of amantadine in acute traumatic brain injury: an initial double-blind placebo-controlled study. Brain Inj 13:863–872, 1999

Seron X: Operant procedures and neuropsychological rehabilitation, in Neuropsychological Rehabilitation. Edited by Meier MJ, Benton AL, Diller L. New York, Guilford, 1987, pp 132–161

Sinforiani E, Banchieri L, Zuchella C, et al: Cognitive rehabilitation in Parkinson's disease. Arch Gerontol Geriatr Suppl 9:387–391, 2004

Sivak M, Hill C, Henson D, et al: Improved driving performance following perceptual training of persons with brain damage. Arch Phys Med Rehabil 65:163–167, 1985

Stablum F, Umilta C, Mogentale C, et al: Rehabilitation of executive deficits in closed head injury and anterior communicating artery aneurysm patients. Psychol Res 63:265–278, 2000

Stuss DT, Benson DF: Neuropsychological studies of the frontal lobes. Psychol Bull 95:3–28, 1984

Suslow T, Schonauer K, Arolt V: Attention training in the cognitive rehabilitation of schizophrenic patients: a review of efficacy studies. Acta Psychiatr Scand 103:15–23, 2001

Suzman KB, Morris RD, Morris MK, et al: Cognitive remediation of problem solving deficits in children with acquired brain injury. J Behav Ther Exp Psychiatry 28:203–212, 1997

Wall P, Egger M: Mechanisms of plasticity of new connection following brain damage in adult mammalian nervous systems, in Recovery of Function: Theoretical Considerations for Brain Injury Rehabilitation. Edited by Bach-y-Rita P. Baltimore, MD, University Park Press, 1971, pp 117–129

Walsh JK, Randazzo AC, Stone KL, et al: Modafinil improves alertness, vigilance, and executive function during simulated night shifts. Sleep 27:434–439, 2004

Wechsler D: Wechsler Memory Scale—Revised. San Antonio, TX, Psychological Corporation, 1987

Weddell R, Oddy M, Jenkins D: Social adjustment after rehabilitation: a two year follow up of patients with severe head injury. Psychol Med 10:257–263, 1980

Williams SE, Ris DM, Ayyangar R, et al: Recovery in pediatric brain injury: is psychostimulant medication beneficial? J Head Trauma Rehabil 13:73–81, 1998

Wilson B: Success and failure in memory training following a cerebral vascular accident. Cortex 18:581–594, 1982

Wilson B: Identification and remediation of everyday problems in memory-impaired patients, in Neuropsychology of Alcoholism: Implications for Diagnosis and Treatment. Edited by Parsons GA, Butters N, Nathan PE. New York, Guilford, 1987, pp 322–338

Wood RL: Behavior disorders following severe brain injury: their presentation and psychological management, in Closed Head Injury: Psychological, Social and Family Consequences. Edited by Brooks N. New York, Oxford University Press, 1984, pp 195–219

Wroblewski BA, Joseph AB, Kupfer J, et al: Effectiveness of valproic acid on destructive and aggressive behaviours in patients with acquired brain injury. Brain Inj 11:37–47, 1997

INDEX

*Page numbers in **boldface** type refer to tables or figures.*